THIRD EDITION

Pharmacotherapeutics for Nurse Practitioner Prescribers

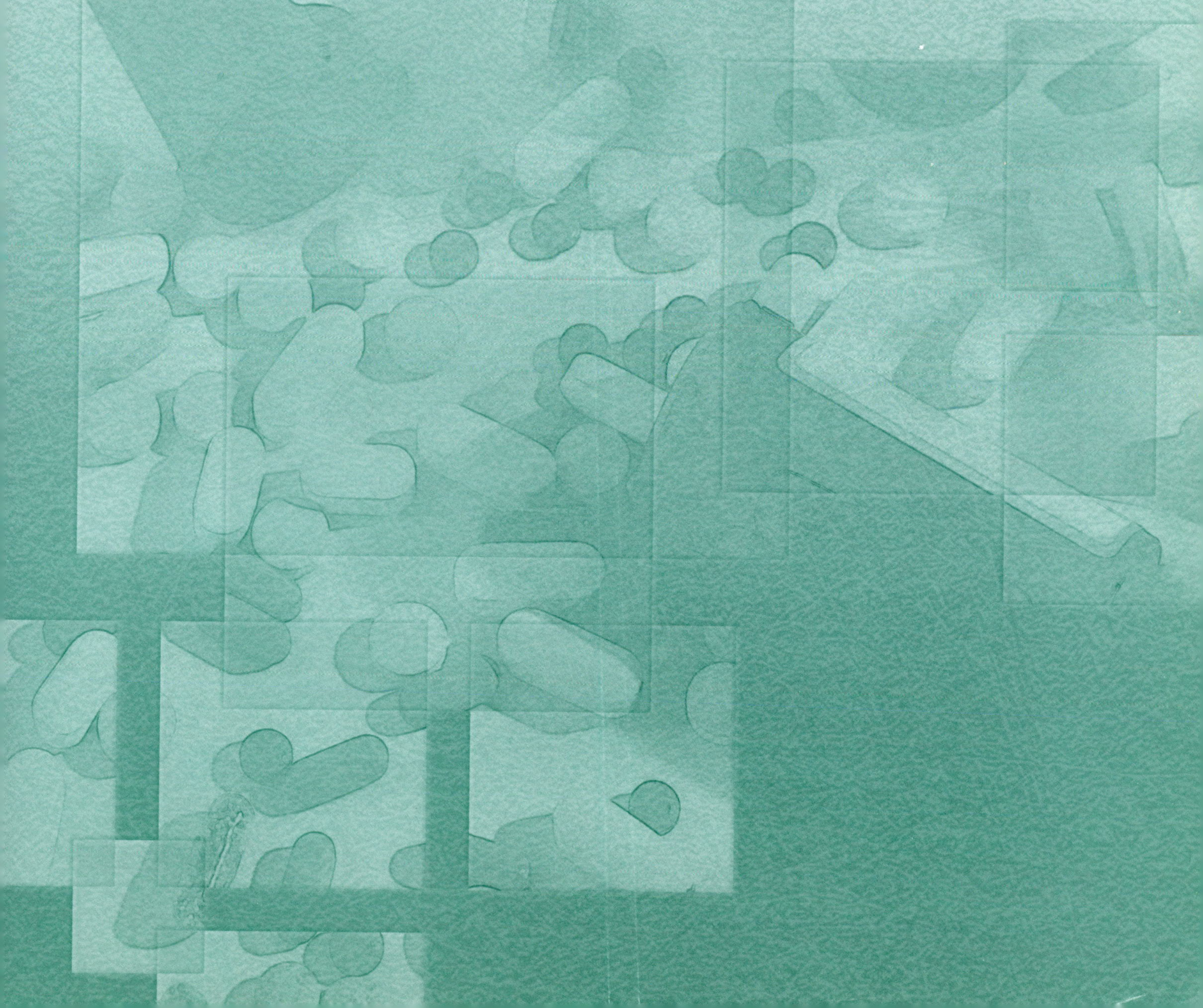

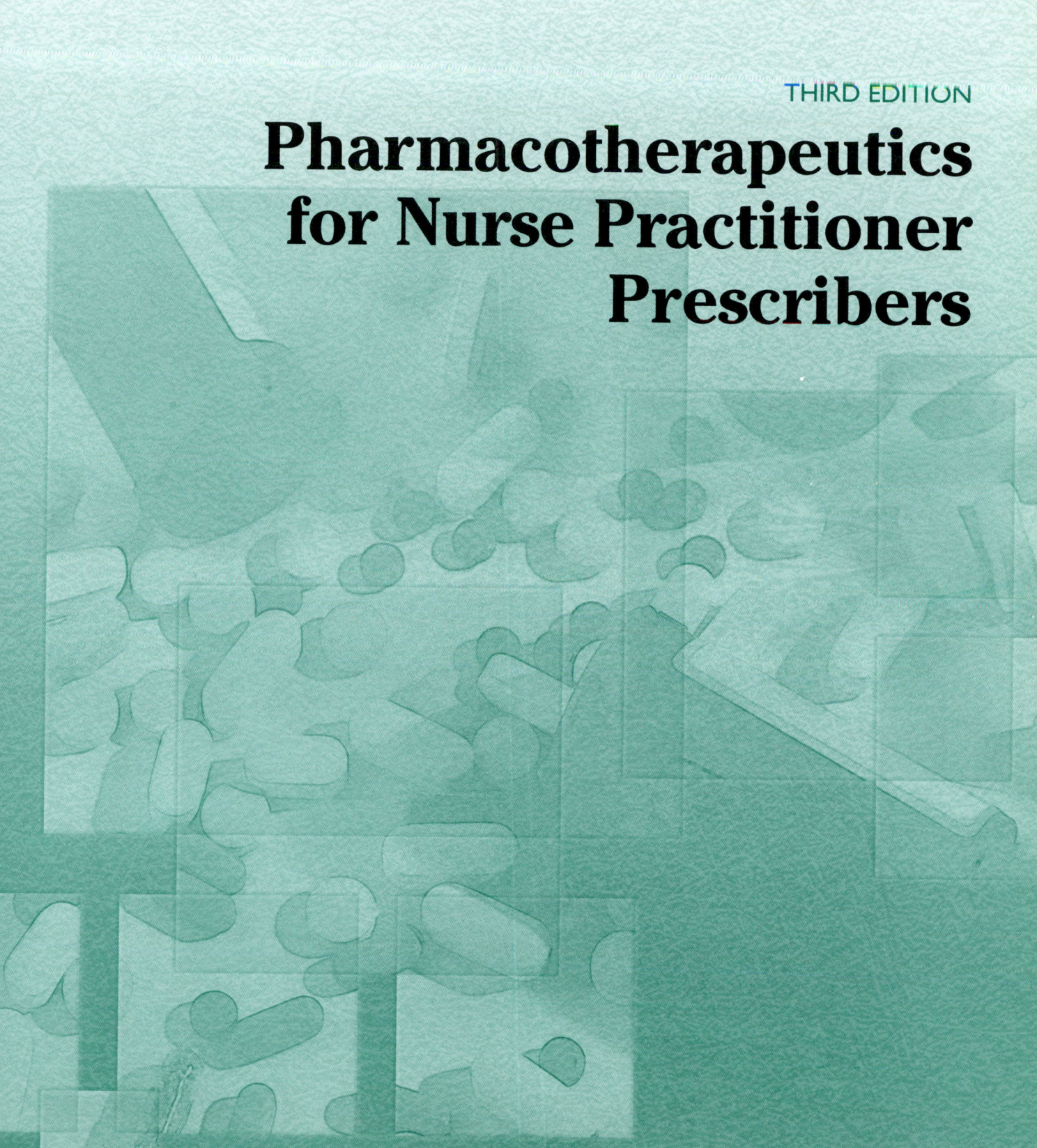

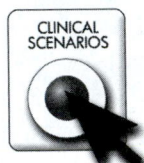

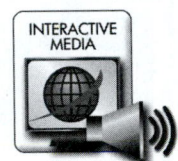

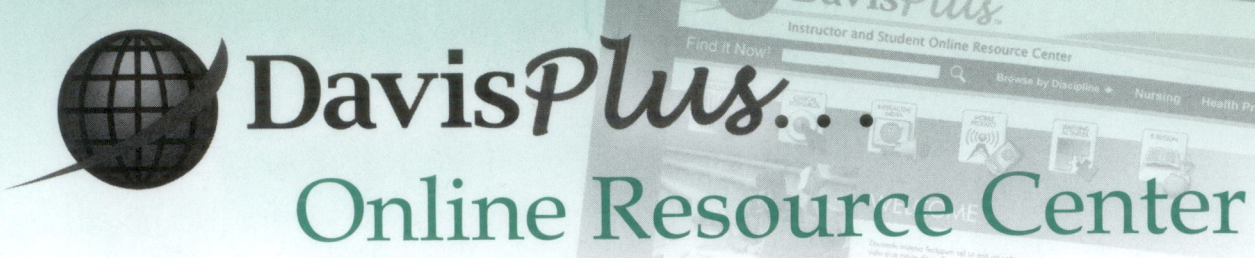

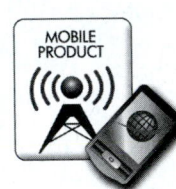

THIRD EDITION

Pharmacotherapeutics for Nurse Practitioner Prescribers

Teri Moser Woo, RN, PhD, CPNP
Associate Professor of Nursing
University of Portland
School of Nursing
Portland, Oregon
and
Pediatric Nurse Practitioner
Kaiser Permanente Northwest Region

Anita Lee Wynne, PhD, FNP-retired
Professor Emeritus of Nursing
School of Nursing
University of Portland
Portland, Oregon

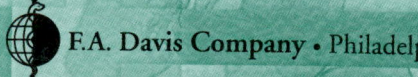

F.A. Davis Company • Philadelphia

F. A. Davis Company
1915 Arch Street
Philadelphia, PA 19103
www.fadavis.com

Printed in the United States of America

Last digit indicates print number: 10 9 8 7 6 5 4 3 2 1

Publisher: Joanne Patzek DaCunha, RN, MSN
Director of Content Development: Darlene D. Pedersen
Project Editor: Jamie M. Elfrank
Design & Illustration Coordinator: Carolyn O'Brien

Library of Congress Cataloging-in-Publication Data

Woo, Teri Moser, 1962–
Pharmacotherapeutics for nurse practitioner prescribers / Teri Moser Woo, Anita Lee Wynne. — 3rd ed.
p. ; cm.
Rev. ed. of: Pharmacotherapeutics for nurse practitioner prescribers / Anita Lee Wynne, Teri Moser Woo, Ali J. Olyaei.
Includes bibliographical references and index.
ISBN-13: 978-0-8036-2235-7
ISBN-10: 0-8036-2235-X
1. Pharmacology. 2. Therapeutics. 3. Nurse practitioners. I. Wynne, Anita Lee, 1941– II. Wynne, Anita Lee, 1941– Pharmacotherapeutics for nurse practitioner prescribers. III. Title.
[DNLM: 1. Pharmacological Phenomena—Nurses' Instruction. 2. Drug Prescriptions—Nurses' Instruction. 3. Drug Therapy—nursing. 4. Nurse Practitioners. QV 38]
RM300.W96 2011
615'.1—dc22
2011006059

I would like to dedicate this book to my family.
My husband, John, and my three sons, Michael,
Patrick, and Nicholas, have been wonderfully
supportive as I have completed this project.

TMW

To my loving husband and my family without
whose patience and support this book never would
have been completed; and to my children and
grandchildren, who daily make my life complete.
In loving memory of my mother, who died in 2006,
and my father, who consistently taught me to shoot
for the stars and who died in 2010.

ALW

PREFACE

The increasing volume of pharmacology-related information presents a challenge to acquire and maintain current knowledge in the area of pharmacotherapeutics. The number of new drugs coming on the market each year, the changes in "the best" drugs to use for any given disease state based on the latest research, the influence on patient and practitioner alike of advertising and promotion, and the increasing incursion of managed care and restricted formularies into practice decisions about drug selection are phenomenal. This book is designed to provide nurse practitioner students and the nurse practitioner in the primary care setting with a thorough, current, and usable pharmacology text and reference to address these challenges.

The design of this book assumes knowledge of basic pharmacology from one's undergraduate education in nursing. Although a brief review of basic pharmacology is presented in **Chapter 2**, the focus of the book is on advanced pharmacology and the role of the advanced practice nurse in pharmacotherapeutics. The authors of the text are practicing nurse practitioners or selected specialists in a field. The book is by nurse practitioners, for nurse practitioners and other health-care providers who prescribe drugs

ORGANIZATION

This book is organized around four distinct content areas: The Foundation, Pharmacotherapeutics With Single Drugs, Pharmacotherapeutics With Multiple Drugs, and Special Drug Treatment Considerations.

The Foundation

The 13 chapters in **Unit I** provide the foundation of advanced pharmacology and the link between this knowledge and professional practice. **Chapter 1** discusses the role of the nurse practitioner in both the United States of America and Canada as prescriber and the knowledge needed to actualize this role. Current issues about the evolving role and education of these providers are also presented in this edition including discussion of the Doctorate of Nursing Practice.

Discussion of the roles of other advanced practice nurses and physicians assistants in prescribing has also been added. Factors involved in clinical judgment related to prescribing are a central focus, and collaboration with other health-care providers is also presented.

The pharmacology knowledge required for rational drug selection requires more depth than that given in undergraduate pharmacology, where the focus is on safe administration of drugs prescribed by someone else. Advanced pharmacology information on receptor reserve and regulation, bioavailability and bioequivalence, metabolism of drugs including a focus on the cytochrome P450 microsomal enzyme system, half-life, and steady state are provided in **Chapters 3** and **8**. Information central to the prescribing role includes an in-depth discussion of volume of distribution and therapeutic drug monitoring. Volume of distribution is important in prescribing drugs with very large or very small volumes of distribution and for selecting drugs for patients with cardiac or renal failure, during pregnancy, or when a patient is underweight or obese. Knowing what tests to order and when to order them to assess plasma drug levels by bioassay and to monitor for adverse drug reactions is necessary to make choices about when or if dosage alterations are required or drugs need to be stopped. These are also covered in **Unit I**.

Legal and professional aspects of the prescriber role are presented in **Chapter 4**. Issues surrounding the legal authority of a nurse practitioner to prescribe a drug, the conditions under which the prescription may be written, and how to write the prescription are presented. Risk management issues are also discussed, including informed consent, dealing with multiple providers, and substance abuse and drug-seeking behaviors.

Nurse practitioners have a history of high levels of patient satisfaction with the care provided. This is related, in part, to their holistic approach to each patient. Several chapters are devoted to information that reflects this approach. Cost, knowledge deficits, dealing with complex treatment regimens, and negotiating a shared responsibility for drug management are discussed in **Chapter 6**. Many patients choose to use complementary therapies such as herbal remedies. **Chapter 10** discusses herbal therapy and other complementary therapies and provides a list of resources in this area.

A relatively new area in pharmacotherapeutics is ethnopharmacology. As more research is occurring in this area, treatment guidelines are beginning to include which drugs are best for different racial groups. Cultural and ethnic considerations in prescribing drugs are the subject of **Chapter 7**. Pharmacogenomics involves the influence of both race/ethnicity and individual genetic makeup on drug metabolism. **Chapter 8** provides a greatly expanded discussion of the role of pharmacogenomics in prescribing.

Consideration of drug and food interactions has long been a part of nursing knowledge, but the interrelationship between nutrition and drug therapy beyond these interactions has been largely missed. **Chapter 9** provides a discussion of this interrelationship including nutritional supplementation and nutrition as therapy. The third edition also includes discussion of nutraceuticals, in which foods are prescribed for their health benefits.

In an age of increasing use of technology, the nurse practitioner must be able to acquire information about drugs and to deliver care to patients using this technology. The push for use of electronic health records (EHRs) has made **Chapter 11** critical information with its discussion of computers and other data and communication devices and the Internet as sources of information and for care delivery This chapter has been restructured in the third edition to focus on the use of information technology directly related to patient encounters. Especially helpful is a large table that presents up-to-date sites for drug information from government, commercial, organizational, and other sources. Where it is possible to determine, each site has a discussion of its content, reliability, frequency of update, link to other sites, charges or fees, and who is the "owner or operator" of the site. If the site is supported by advertising, this is also mentioned. The future use of information technology in obtaining drug-related information and the delivery of health-care services is also included.

Cost issues are increasingly central to prescribing decisions. **Chapter 12** provides an expanded discussion of pharmacoeconomics. Written by a nurse practitioner in the third edition, the focus is more directly on the prescriber's role.

Over-the-counter drugs may be prescribed by the practitioner or chosen by patients on their own. These drugs are often erroneously perceived to be less powerful and having fewer adverse reactions than prescription drugs. Understanding their role in pharmacotherapeutics is the focus of **Chapter 13**.

Pharmacotherapeutics With Single Drugs

The next two units are organized around specific drugs and the diseases they are used to treat. The chapters in **Unit II** are organized to provide easy access to information based on specific drug classes. Many practitioners have a personal formulary of drugs they use for disease processes that they commonly see. When presented with a patient requiring drug therapy, they know the class of drug from which they will make a rational drug choice. The information they seek is about drugs within that class that would be most appropriate for this patient.

Pharmacokinetics, pharmacodynamics, and pharmacotherapeutics for each drug class are discussed. Tables with easy-to-access information on pharmacokinetic properties of each drug, drug interactions, clinical use and dosing, and available dosing forms are presented. There is a major focus on rational drug selection and on monitoring parameters. Patient education specific to each drug class is provided—designed around administration of the drug, adverse drug reactions to monitor for and what to do if they occur, and lifestyle modifications that complement the drug therapy.

To provide the most up-to-date, accurate, and relevant information possible, contributors to this unit are practicing clinicians and the newest published guidelines are consistently used. Clinical pearls drawn from the daily practice world of these contributors are incorporated throughout the text. Drugs currently in development that may influence drug choices in the near future are also included in the On-the-Horizon feature.

Pharmacotherapeutics With Multiple Drugs

Unit III chapters provide access to drug information from the viewpoint of the disease processes they are commonly used to treat. Patients often have complex health and illness issues and treatment needs. Nurse practitioner students find these especially perplexing, and these patients may have disease processes that extend beyond those a given nurse practitioner commonly sees. The knowledge the student or practitioner needs to select the appropriate drug to treat a given disease may be limited. **Unit III** facilitates acquisition of this knowledge by providing access to information from a disease process format. The diseases in this unit are those commonly seen in primary care and for which multidrug therapy from more than one drug class may be recommended.

Pharmacotherapeutics is discussed in relation to the pathophysiology of the disease and the goals of treatment. Each chapter explores how patient variables, economic considerations, concurrent diseases, and drug characteristics influence rational drug selection. Outcome evaluation is presented with guidelines for consultation and referral. Where relevant the newest published professional guidelines are incorporated. Each patient is unique and no set of guidelines or treatment algorithm applies to each patient. However, these tools, drawn from the clinical knowledge and experience of experts in a given specialty, are helpful in rational drug selection, especially for the student and novice practitioner. Clinically based case studies provide a framework for application of pharmacotherapeutic knowledge and are provided in an online supplement to this edition.

Special Drug Treatment Considerations

Unit IV focuses on special populations. Age-related variables are explored in **Chapter 50**, Pediatric Patients, and **Chapter 51**, Geriatric Patients. Gender variables are considered in **Chapter 48**, Women as Patients, and **Chapter 49**, Men as Patients. **Chapter 49** is a new addition to the book. Information on safe prescription of drugs for lactating patients is often difficult to find, and tables with the most current information on the effect of drugs on the nursing infant are found in **Chapter 50**.

The prevalence of chronic illness is increasing as acute illnesses that formerly accounted for most of the morbidity and mortality in developed countries have been eradicated or come under control. **Chapter 52** discusses the modification of pharmacotherapeutics in patient populations with chronic illness or in long-term care facilities.

The final chapter in the book deals with one of the most common yet often perplexing issues with which prescribers deal: pain. **Chapter 53** focuses on management of both acute and chronic pain across the age continuum. The third edition includes the most current information on newer drugs used to treat chronic pain and new pain assessment tools for patients with dementia. Expanded discussion of the legal aspects of prescribing related to drug dependent patients includes Material Risk Assessment and Pain Management Contract documents.

FEATURES

Throughout the text, care has been taken to provide the reader with a consistent and logical presentation of material. Visual appeal is provided through the generous use of tables, illustrations, and flowcharts. Other features are unique to the specific units:

Unit I Chapters

In-depth pharmacology base for advanced pharmacotherapeutics
Herbal and complimentary therapies
Ethnopharmacology and pharmacogenomics
Nutrition and nutraceuticals as therapy
Pharmacoeconomics
Information technolo gy including EHR and how it is used in a busy practice

Unit II Chapters

Tables for ease of access to information
- Pharmacokinetics tables
- Drug Interactions tables
- Dosage Schedule tables
- Available Drug Dosage Forms tables

Rational drug selection and monitoring parameters
- Patient Education
- Clinical Pearls
- On-the-Horizon feature

Unit III Chapters

Integration of pathophysiology and pharmacotherapeutics
Integration of professional treatment guidelines
Drugs Commonly Used tables
Patient Education displays

Unit IV Chapters

Variables related to special populations
- Pediatrics
- Geriatrics
- Women
- Men
- Chronically ill and long-term care
- Pain management

SUMMARY

Every effort has been made to make this text as comprehensive, accurate, and user friendly as possible. The generous use of tables for ease of access to information, the focus on rational drug selection, the inclusion of often hard to find monitoring parameters, and the integration of patient education throughout the text are examples of this user-friendly approach. The authors hope that you will find this a valuable resource both as a student and in your practice.

TMW
ALW

ACKNOWLEDGMENTS

I would like to acknowledge my mentors who have supported me throughout my nursing career. Included in this list are Dr. Sheila Kodadek, who has been my mentor and friend throughout my nursing career, and the late Dr. Terry Misener. I would also like to acknowledge the faculty at University of Portland who have offered me support, encouragement, and advice as I completed these chapters while teaching full-time.

TMW

The authors would also like to acknowledge our previous co-authors, Michael Millard, RPh and Ali J. Olyaei, PharmD. They contributed to the development and refinement of multiple foundational chapters in the first two editions of the text and their work is acknowledged here.

TMW
ALW

ABOUT THE AUTHORS

TERI MOSER WOO, RN, PHD, CPNP, CNL

Teri has been a pediatric health-care provider for 25 years. She received her BSN from Oregon Health Sciences University (OHSU) in 1985. Teri earned a MSN in Childrearing Family Nursing in 1989 and a Post-Masters Pediatric Nurse Practitioner Certificate in 1993 from OHSU. In 2008 she earned a PhD in Nursing from University of Colorado Denver College of Nursing. Teri was president of the Oregon Pediatric Nurse Practitioner Association from 1998–2000 and is currently president-elect of OPNPA. She is an Associate Professor at University of Portland School of Nursing, teaching undergraduate and graduate courses in pharmacology and is the Director of the Clinical Nurse Leader masters program. Teri continues to practice as a PNP for Kaiser Permanente in both Ambulatory Care and Urgent Care.

ANITA LEE WYNNE, PHD, FNP (RETIRED)

Anita Lee received her Bachelor of Science in nursing from San Diego State University, a Master of Science in Nursing with a focus in Adult Health from the University of Colorado Health Science Center, and a Master of Public Health and PhD with a focus in Health Behavior from the University of Oklahoma College of Health. She received her Family Nurse Practitioner preparation at Gonzaga University in the Post Master's Certificate Option program. Her 25 years of teaching experience include baccalaureate and master's degree programs in Oklahoma and Oregon, and her favorite teaching areas are pathophysiology, pharmacotherapeutics, and health assessment. She has retired from teaching and clinical practice.

CONTRIBUTORS

Kathleen Bell, MS, RN, CNM
Instructor
University of Portland
School of Nursing
Portland, Oregon

Gina Dobbs, MSN, CRNP
Nurse Practitioner and Sub-Investigator
1917 HIV/AIDS Outpatient/Research Clinic
University of Alabama Birmingham
Birmingham, Alabama

Danita Lee Ewing, RN, PHD
Assistant Professor of Nursing
Oregon Health and Sciences University
Portland, Oregon

Teral Gerlt, MS, RN, WHCNP-E
Instructor
Oregon Health & Science University School of Nursing
Portland, Oregon

Kathryn A. Hanavan, RN, MSN, ANP-C, BC-ADM
Adult Nurse Practitioner
Harold Schnitzer Diabetes Health Center
Oregon Health & Science University
Portland, Oregon

Tracy Klein, PhD, FNP, FAANP
Advanced Practice Consultant
Oregon State Board of Nursing
Family Practice Nurse Practitioner
SW Family Physicians
Tigard, Oregon

Taynin Kopanos, FNP, DNP
Family Nurse Practitioner
Denver, Colorado

Victoria LaPorte, RN, MS, ANP
Family Nurse Practitioner
Pain Relief Specialists Northwest
Milwaukie, Oregon

Sharon Maxey, DNP(c), FNP
Kaiser Permanente
Portland, Oregon

Fugio McPherson, RN, FNP
Family Nurse Practitioner, Acupuncturist
Internal Medicine Clinic
Madigan Army Medical Center
Fort Lewis, Washington

James L. Raper, DSN, CRNP, JD, FAANP, FAAN
Director & NP, HIV/AIDS Outpatient, Research and Dental Clinic
Associate Professor of Medicine & Nursing
University of Alabama at Birmingham
Birmingham, Alabama

Marylou Robinson, PhD, FNP-C
Assistant Professor of Nursing
University of Colorado Denver College of Nursing
Denver, Colorado

Margaret Scharf, DNP, PMHNP, FNP
Psychiatric Mental Health Nurse Practitioner
Assistant Professor
Chair, Biobehavioral Faculty
Coordinator PMHNP/DNP program
Oregon Health & Science University School of Nursing
Portland, Oregon

Casey R. Shillam, RN, PhD
John A. Hartford Foundation
Building Academic Geriatric Nursing Capacity Scholar
Post-Doctoral Fellow
Betty Irene Moore School of Nursing
University of California Davis
School of Nursing
Sacramento, California

Diane Vines, PhD, RN, RTRT
Associate Professor
University of Portland School of Nursing
Rapid Trauma Resolution Therapist
Private Practice
Portland, Oregon

Jacqueline Webb, MS, FNP
Instructor
University of Portland School of Nursing
Family Nurse Practitioner
PACS Clinic
Portland, Oregon

REVIEWERS

Samuel Marfo Addae, PharmD
Clinical Pharmacist
Heart of the Rockies Regional Medical Center
Salida, Colorado

Carol E. Agana, MSNc, RNP, APN
Instructor
University of Arkansas
Fayetteville, Arkansas

Gwendolyn H. Blatnak, PharmD
Clinical Content Specialist
Greenwood Village, Colorado

Douglas E. Boggs, PharmD, MS, BCPP
Faculty Research Associate
Maryland Psychiatric Research Center
University of Maryland School of Medicine
Baltimore, Maryland

Benjamin Brooks, PharmD
Clinical Pharmacist
Medical Center of Aurora
Aurora, Colorado

Jennifer Christensen, PharmD
University of Colorado
Commerce City, Colorado

Paul Cernak, PharmD
Medical Science Liaison
Elan Pharmaceuticals
Adjunct Faculty
Millersville University
Millersville, Pennsylvania
Weidner University
Chester, Pennsylvania

Charlotte Covington, MSN, APRN, FNP-BC
Associate Professor
Vanderbilt School of Nursing
Nashville, Tennessee

Mary Kate Friess, RN, BSN, MSN, FNP-BC
Family Nurse Practitioner
Assistant Professor of Nursing
Marian University
Fond du Lac, Wisconsin

Joan P. Frizzell, PhD, CRNP, ANP-BC
Associate Professor
La Salle University
Philadelphia, Pennsylvania

Rebecca J. Gyrka, PharmD, PhD
Associate Professor
Director of Therapeutics
Loma Linda University
School of Pharmacy
Loma Linda, California

Emily Hajjar, PharmD, BCPS, CGP
Assistant Professor
Jefferson School of Pharmacy
Philadelphia, Pennsylvania

Brenda Hoskins, DNP, ARNP, GNP-BC, FAANP
Associate Clinical Professor
University of Iowa School of Nursing
Iowa City, Iowa

Timothy R. Hudd, BS, PharmD, RPh, AE-C
Assistant Professor of Pharmacy Practice
Massachusetts College of Pharmacy and Health Sciences
Boston, Massachusetts

Donald Lamprecht, PharmD, BCPS
Clinical Pharmacy Specialist
Kaiser Permanente Colorado
University of Colorado-Denver
School of Pharmacy
Aurora, Colorado

Adrienne Mackzum, PharmD, MS, BCPS
Clinical Pharmacist
Craig Hospital
Englewood, Colorado

Joel C. Marrs, PharmD, BCPS (AQ Cardiology), CLS
Assistant Professor
Department of Pharmacy
University of Colorado
School of Pharmacy
Aurora, Colorado

Lori Martin-Plank, PhD, MSN, FNP-BC, GNP-BC
Clinical Assistant Professor, Track Coordinator
FNP Program
Temple University College of Health Professions
Philadelphia, Pennsylvania

Carla G. May, BS Pharmacy
Program Director
Vance Granville Community College
Henderson, North Carolina

Nelda New, PhD, APRN
Graduate Nursing Program Director
University of Central Arkansas
Conway, Arkansas

Monika Nuffer, PharmD
Academic and Experiential Program Coordinator, NTPD & Instructor
Department of Clinical Pharmacy
University of Colorado, School of Pharmacy
Aurora, Colorado

Jim Pace, DSN, ANP-BC
Professor of Nursing
Vanderbilt University School of Nursing
Nashville, Tennessee

Debra Ann Quadrani, PharmD, MHCA
Pharmacist
Veteran's Administration
Denver, Colorado

Dr. Dana Clawson Roe, DNS, WHNP-BC
Associate Professor of Nursing
Coordinator of Women's Health Nurse Practitioner Program
Northwestern State University College of Nursing
Shreveport, Louisiana

Connie Roppolo, MSN, APRN, FNP-BC
Assistant Professor of Nursing in Graduate Studies
Northwestern University
Shreveport, Louisiana

Marilyn D. Saulsbury, PhD, RPh
Associate Professor of Pharmacology
Hampton University – Department of Pharmaceutical Sciences
Hampton, Virginia

Timothy Schardt, PharmD, BCPS
Inpatient Pharmacist
Denver Health Medical Center
Denver, Colorado

Gwen Smith, PharmD
Clinical Content Specialist
Greenwood Village, Colorado

Michelle D. Thomas, PharmD
Clinical Pharmacist
University of Maryland
Springfield Hospital Center
Sykesville, Maryland

Paul R. Yaft, PharmD, CACP, BCPS
Clinical Pharmacy Specialist
Kaiser Permanente
Aurora, Colorado

CONTENTS

UNIT I

The Foundation

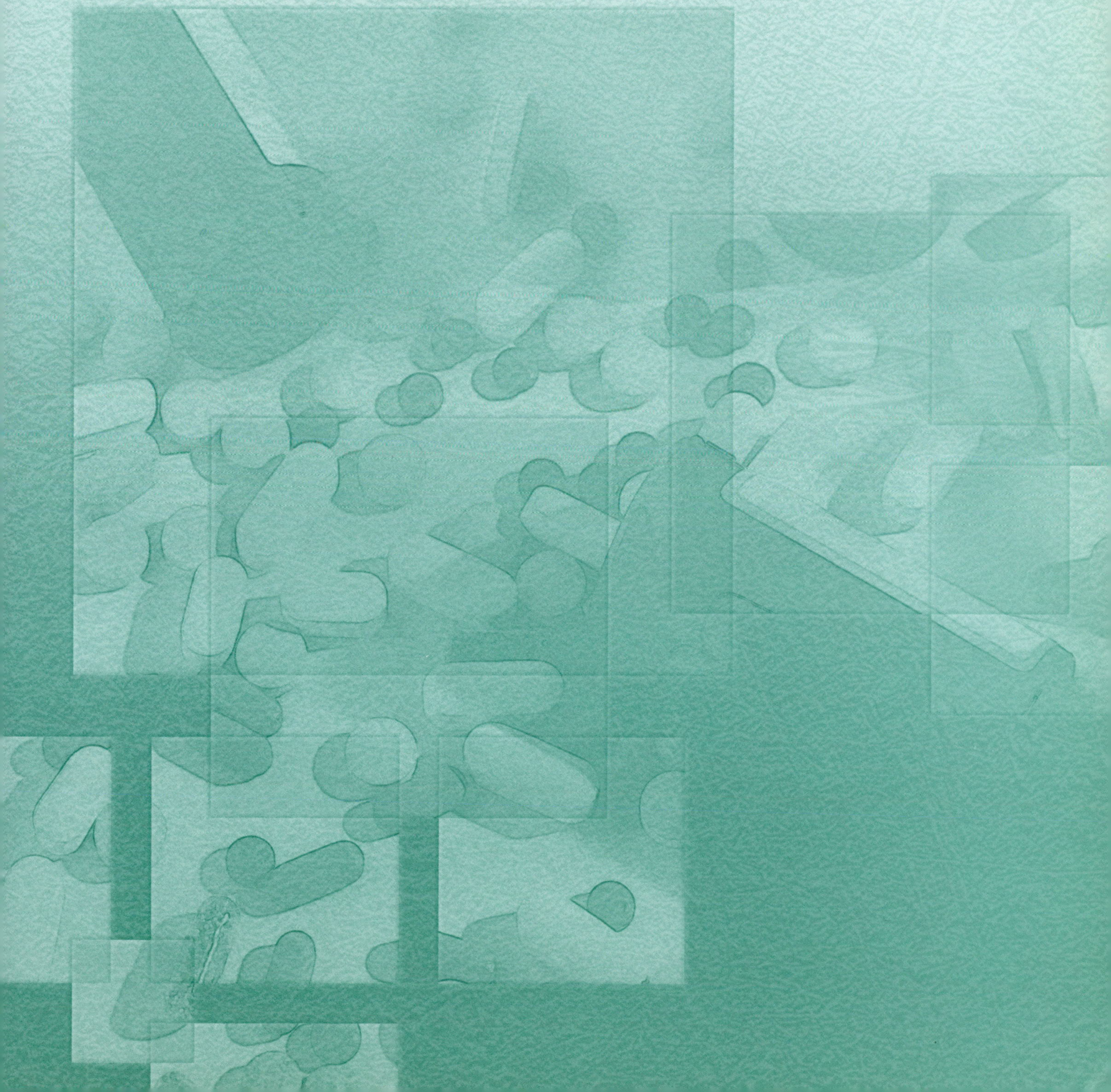

CHAPTER 1

THE ROLE OF THE NURSE PRACTITIONER AS PRESCRIBER

Anita Lee Wynne • Teri Moser Woo

Chapter Outline

Nurses have been administering medications prescribed by another provider for many years. The knowledge base to safely perform this activity has been an integral part of basic nursing programs. With the advent of the advanced practice nurse (APN), especially the nurse practitioner (NP), the role of the nurse in relation to medications evolved to include prescribing the medications as well as administering them. The prescriber role requires additional knowledge beyond that taught in undergraduate nursing programs. More than that, it requires the willingness and ability to assume a different kind of responsibility for this activity.

Other health-care providers, most notably physician assistants (PAs), have also been added to the list of prescribers in primary care. Although they are not nurses, their role is also included in this chapter.

ROLES OF REGISTERED NURSES AND ADVANCED PRACTICE NURSES WHO ARE NOT NURSE PRACTITIONERS

Registered Nurses

Experienced registered nurses (RNs) often find themselves in the position of discussing what might be the "best" drug a patient should receive with a physician or other provider. The RN is an advocate for the patient and his or her input is sought and highly valued. Collaboration of this nature increases the nurse's self-esteem and results in improved patient care as the disciplines of medicine and nursing work together. The responsibility for the final decision, however, remains with the physician or other provider in this case.

Advanced Practice Nurses

APNs have a higher level of responsibility than the RN related to pharmacotherapeutics. The nature of this responsibility depends on whether the nurse can prescribe drugs. States vary in their laws related to prescriptive authority for non-NP APNs. Often, APNs who are not NPs do not have prescriptive authority. Because they have in-depth knowledge of the drugs used in their specialty area, their collaboration with the health-care provider who is prescribing is at a different level from that of the registered nurse. They may assist in determining the pharmacotherapeutic protocols for their patients and select drugs within those protocols to be administered to their patients. These roles related to pharmacotherapeutics represent an intermediate level of responsibility between the RN, who administers drugs chosen by another provider, and the NP, who prescribes a drug without the need for a protocol. APNs also often collaborate with other providers in designing and implementing research protocols to test the efficacy of a new drug. They also have a central role in educating nurses and other providers in the appropriate use of these new drugs.

ROLES AND RESPONSIBILITIES OF NURSE PRACTITIONERS

NPs exist in a range of types of practice that include certified registered nurse anesthetists, certified nurse midwives, and others whose title includes the words *nurse practitioner*. NPs often differ from other nurses and other primary care providers in their prescriptive authority. The role of the NP as prescriber places the responsibility for the final decision of which drug to use and how to use it in the hands of the NP. The degree of autonomy in this role and the breadth of drugs that can be prescribed vary from state to state, based on the nurse practice act of that state. Every year the January issue of the journal *The Nurse Practitioner* and an issue of *The American Journal for Nurse Practitioners* present a summary of each state's practice acts as they relate to titling, roles, and prescriptive authority. As of January 2009 (Pearson, 2009; Phillips, 2009), the following were true of NP regulation of practice and prescribing authority:

- All states have title protection for NPs.
- In all but five states, the control of practice and licensure is within the sole authority of the Board of Nursing. These five states have joint control in the Board of Nursing and the Board of Medicine.
- Scope of practice is determined by the individual NP's license.
- In 24 states, NPs are totally autonomous in their practice In 20, they are required to have some physician collaboration, and in three, there is physician supervision. In the remaining states, requirements include practicing by protocol, using a collaborative practice agreement, and having some degree of physician supervision, which may be by electronic means.
- Fourteen states and the District of Columbia have total autonomy in prescriptive authority. The remaining states require some degree of physician involvement. Although a few states have been able to increase NP autonomy in this area, it is important to maintain a constant vigil on the legislative and regulatory issues related to prescriptive authority and autonomy as they are under regular assault (American Medical Association, 2009; Partin, 2008; Pearson, 2009).
- Two states exclude controlled substances from the prescriptive authority of NPs, but all other states permit it, most with Schedules II to V.

ADVANCED KNOWLEDGE

Knowledge about the pharmacokinetics and pharmacodynamics of drugs, how to administer them safely, and what to teach the patient are learned in undergraduate nursing courses and refined in practice. This knowledge is critical to the decision the NP is about to make, but additional knowledge and responsibility are required to assume the prescriber role. The advanced practice role of the NP, although clearly an example of expanded nursing role functions and not "junior doctoring," is, nonetheless, a blending of the disciplines of medicine and nursing. Medical, pharmacological, and nursing knowledge intertwine in the NP role. It now becomes the role and responsibility of the NP to determine the diagnosis for which the drug will be prescribed and to prescribe the appropriate drug.

The NP role requires advanced knowledge about pathophysiology and medical diagnoses and their relationship to choosing an appropriate drug. Determining the medical diagnosis is not within the scope of this book, but rational drug selection requires knowledge of the disease processes (medical diagnoses) for which a drug may be prescribed and the mechanism of action of a specific drug and how it affects this disease process. Rational drug selection is discussed throughout the book.

The NP role also requires advanced pharmacology knowledge beyond that taught in undergraduate education. Knowledge required for rational drug selection includes bioequivalence and cost for deciding whether to use a generic form of a given drug; the enzyme systems used to metabolize a drug for deciding about potential drug interactions; and the pharmacokinetics of a drug for determining the loading, maintenance, and tapering doses. The terms may sound familiar, but the underlying depth of information and the role of this information in determining the best drug to prescribe are beyond basic knowledge. Volume of distribution, for example, receives little discussion in undergraduate nursing pharmacology texts, but it is often critical in determining dosage for drugs with very large or small volumes of distribution and in selecting drugs for patients with cardiac or renal failure, pregnant patients, or patients who are underweight or obese. Assessment of plasma drug levels by bioassay may be familiar, but the use of this knowledge to determine whether a drug should be prescribed or the prescription altered will be new. The RN may know a given drug's effect on renal functioning, but the prescribing NP needs to know what tests to order and when to order them to appropriately monitor that functioning, as well as when or if to alter the dosage or stop the drug. Diagnostic tests and their role in drug monitoring will be new. Additional knowledge is also needed about prescriptive authority. Does the chosen drug fit within the legal authority of an NP to prescribe in this state? What are the conditions under which the prescription may be written, and how does one correctly write it? What constraints may be in place because of the patient's health insurer or lack of health insurance?

BENEFITS OF A NURSE PRACTITIONER AS PRESCRIBER

Although the focus of this book is on pharmacotherapeutic intervention, other treatment options are also part of the NP armamentarium to treat a given disorder and often interact with the pharmacotherapeutic intervention to provide the desired outcome. Common therapies that may be chosen as treatment options or that are integral to drug therapy are integrated throughout the drug-specific and disease-specific chapters. Some of them have traditionally been part of what all nurses teach, and they remain central to the role of the NP: for example, lifestyle management issues for a cardiac patient, relaxation techniques for a patient experiencing stress, and appropriate exercise for a patient with low back pain or arthritis. Herbal therapies have been part of the health practices of people throughout history, but only recently have health-care providers acknowledged them and considered them in planning treatment. If the NP chooses to use herbal therapy or the patient is using this therapy from another provider, the NP must have reliable information sources about this therapy. This book includes a chapter on herbal therapy and the uses of complementary therapies as well as the use of herbal interventions integrated throughout the rest of the book. Nutrition is also a common issue in nursing, but often the nurse's knowledge of nutrition related to pharmacology is limited to food–drug interactions or the low-sodium diet for a patient with hypertension. Knowledge regarding how foods and nutrition affect drug prescribing is integrated throughout the book; how foods are used as therapy is included in Chapter 9, Nutraceuticals.

Choosing among pharmacological and other treatment options also involves advanced knowledge. The right choice depends on accurate information about the patient and his or her situation and about the effects of the alternative treatment options on health outcomes. Choices also depend on the patient's culture, preferences for different health outcomes, attitudes toward taking risks, and willingness to endure morbidity now for some possible future benefit. Characteristic of NPs and their practice are consideration of the whole patient, the joint setting of therapeutic goals, and the inclusion of the patient in each decision about care. This holistic approach remains a central element in NP practice and is often cited by patients and other providers as a hallmark and distinguishing feature of NP practice. Adherence to a drug treatment regimen has traditionally been poor or less than optimal. Statistics cited often place patient adherence (taking the drugs as prescribed) at less than 50 percent. Research shows that adherence is better for prescriptions given by NPs, and the proposed reasons for the difference are these very issues of consideration of the whole patient and inclusion of the patient in decision making. Another factor in improved adherence is patient education; NPs spend more time than other providers in teaching their patients about their disease process and the relationship of the treatment regimen to it. Each of these important aspects of drug choice and utilization is covered in the book.

ROLES AND RESPONSIBILITIES OF PHYSICIAN ASSISTANTS

PAs have title protection in all states. As of May 2008, all states have some form of legal definition of prescriptive authority. The laws vary, but the following are generally true:

- Five states require drugs be limited to a specific formulary that is often practice specific. This is down from ten states in 2004. Some states also require that the prescription of any drugs be limited by protocol devised by the supervising physician.
- Fifteen states permit prescription of only Schedules III to V and five states do not permit prescription of any scheduled drugs.
- All states have some form of practice oversight or supervision by a physician. These requirements vary from on-site supervision to oversight in some form of communication. Some states require that charts and/or prescriptions be reviewed and cosigned on a regular basis.
- Control of practice and licensing is usually by the State Medical Board of Examiners or its equivalent. PAs may have one to five members on that board, but in only a few states do they have controlling numbers and in one state, PA presence is only required

on task forces and committees of the Medical Board. Some states have specific Boards for PAs, but once again there is a strong medical presence on these Boards. However, the PAs have controlling numbers in a few states; in Tennessee, total control of PA practice is by the Tennessee Physician Assistant Committee. This increase in control of their practice is an important goal of the PA community.

As with NPs, PAs often have their own U.S. Drug Enforcement Agency (DEA) number and have in-depth knowledge of drugs within their specialty area. Unlike NPs, this specialty area is defined by the scope of practice of their supervising physician in most states, but this includes family practice physicians who have a very wide scope of practice (American Academy of Physician Assistants, 2008).

CLINICAL JUDGMENT IN PRESCRIBING

Prescribing a drug results from clinical judgment based on a thorough assessment of the patient and the patient's environment, the determination of medical and nursing diagnoses, a review of potential alternative therapies, and specific knowledge about the drug chosen and the disease process it is designed to treat. In general, the best therapy is the least invasive, least expensive, and least likely to cause adverse reactions. Frequently, the choice is to have nonpharmacological and pharmacological therapies working together. When the choice of treatment options is a drug, several questions arise.

Is There a Clear Indication for Drug Therapy?

In the age of managed care and increased awareness of the limitations of drugs, this has become an important question. For example, in treating otitis media, the use of antibiotics is controversial. A high percentage of otitis media infections resolve on their own, so how do we know that the antibiotic was the cause of the cure? Antibiotic resistance of organisms is on the rise. Is overtreatment with antibiotics a contributing factor? Before drug therapy is chosen, the indication for using a drug should be carefully considered.

What Drugs Are Effective in Treating This Disorder?

Several drugs are often effective; which is the best one for this unique patient? Even if only the most effective class of drug is considered, few classes of drugs have only one drug in them. How does one determine "best"; what are the criteria? Are there nationally recognized guidelines that can be used as criteria? The Agency for Health Care Quality (AHCQ), the National Institutes of Health (NIH), and many specialty organizations publish disease-specific treatment guidelines that include both pharmacological and nonpharmacological therapies.

What Is the Goal of Therapy With This Drug?

What is the best drug to achieve treatment goals? A variety of goals are possible in the choice of any therapy. The goal may be cure of the disease and short term in nature. If cure is the goal, troublesome adverse effects may be better tolerated, and cost may be less of an issue. If the goal is long-term treatment for a chronic condition, adverse effects and costs take on a different level of importance, and how well the drug fits into the lifestyle of the patient can be a critical issue.

Under What Conditions Is It Determined That a Drug Is Not Meeting the Goal and a Different Therapy or Drug Should Be Tried?

At the onset of therapy, monitoring times are established to see how well the drug is meeting the goal. Monitoring parameters are often published for the drug, but they may need to be adjusted, based on the age or concurrent disease processes of the patient. Part of this decision making may include questions about when to consult or refer the patient.

Are There Unnecessary Duplications With Other Drugs the Patient Is Already Taking?

Sometimes drugs from different classes are given together to achieve a desired effect, and this is a therapeutic choice. It may also be that the provider is not aware of the overlap, especially if the patient is seeing several different providers. For example, a patient who is on a **diuretic** to treat hypertension may have potassium supplementation. Another provider may decide to use an **angiotensin-converting enzyme (ACE) inhibitor** to treat heart failure. An **ACE inhibitor** can also be used to treat hypertension. Rather than a treatment regimen with three drugs, it may be possible to use a combination of an **ACE inhibitor** with a **diuretic** in one tablet and, because **ACE inhibitors** cause potassium retention, no supplemental potassium would be needed. Any time a regimen can be simplified, adherence is more likely.

Would an Over-the-Counter Drug Be Just as Useful as a Prescription Drug?

Increasing numbers of drugs are being moved from prescription-only to over-the-counter (OTC) status. Often, this results in a significant reduction in cost for the patient. It also can create problems, however, unless the provider takes a good drug history because many patients do not consider these as "drugs" once they are not prescribed.

What About Cost?

Who will pay for this drug? Can the patient afford it? What patient advocacy issue does this raise? Will these issues affect adherence to the treatment regimen? Cost is an issue for several reasons. Many insurance policies do not cover the cost of drugs so the patient must pay "out of pocket." The newer the drug, the more likely the cost is to be high, based on the drug manufacturer's need to reclaim research and development costs while the corporation still holds the patent on that drug. Newest is not always best, and consideration of cost is a major factor in choosing between newer drugs and ones that have been around long enough to be available in generic form. Multiple national retail pharmacies have developed $4.00 prescription formularies. Awareness of what is on the local discount formulary may save the patient hundreds of dollars in prescription costs and increase compliance. Factors likely to lead to poor adherence include a drug that is expensive in relation to a patient's finances, a drug that must be taken daily as part of a complex regimen, and a drug that is not covered by insurance.

Where Is the Information to Answer These Questions?

Nurses have always evaluated sources of drug information and learned which ones to trust. For an NP, the sources of drug information expand to include the drug company representative who visits the clinic, the medical literature that ranges from the well-reputed *Annals of Internal Medicine* to what some NPs refer to as "throw-away" literature that can fill the NP's mailbox, the multitude of computerized drug databases (Micromedex, Lexicomp), information from the U.S. Food and Drug Administration, formula programs that can be loaded onto a personal digital assistant (PDA), and the Internet. These resources are further discussed in Chapter 11.

The prescriber needs to evaluate how reliable the information is. How can reliability be determined? Is the information source written by someone who may benefit from presenting biased information? Is the information source up to date? Today's "wonder drug" may be removed from the market tomorrow. Is the information relevant to the specific patient for whom the drug will be prescribed? If the information is a research report, what type of research design was used? Are there questions about the validity and reliability of the data? To prescribe drugs appropriately, NPs must be able to answer these questions; and to answer them, they must master sources of information and use them on a regular basis.

The legal aspects of prescription writing and how to write a prescription are covered in Chapter 4.

COLLABORATION WITH OTHER PROVIDERS

No one member of the health-care team can provide high-quality care without the collaboration of other team members. The NP most often collaborates with physicians; pharmacists; and other primary care providers including APNs who are not NPs, PAs, and other nurses.

Physicians

Collaboration with physicians has been something of a roller-coaster ride for NPs. Early in NP role development, physicians were the teachers in the NP programs and accepted NPs as physician-extenders. As the role of the NP evolved to clearly indicate that it was advanced nursing practice, and as legislation made autonomy of practice possible, the relationship became more adversarial, with the American Medical Association (AMA) making statements regarding NP and PA scope of practice (American Medical Association, 2009), often for economic reasons. A recent AMA document, *AMA Scope of Practice Series: Nurse Practitioner,* stated, "It is the AMA's intention that these Scope of Practice Data Series modules provide the background information necessary to challenge the state and national advocacy campaigns of limited licensure health care providers who seek unwarranted scope-of-practice expansions that may endanger the health and safety of patients" (American Medical Association, 2009, p. 4). Although this struggle still continues at the national level (Partin, 2008; Pearson, 2009), NPs and physicians must work together on an individual basis. In an era of managed care and health-care reform, our joint concerns about patient care decisions require us to be allies. Physicians have a history as prescribers and can offer suggestions from their experience. Their focus related to pharmacology is on understanding biochemistry and prescribing for a given pathophysiology. Their emphasis is on the disease and the drug, with less emphasis on the impact on the patient. Patient education by physicians is limited or left to the nurse or pharmacist. NPs will always approach prescribing drugs in a slightly different manner from that of physicians. As NPs prescribe a drug for a given pathophysiology, their nursing background leads them to place equal emphasis on understanding the impact the drug will have on the patient. Patient education is a central focus of NP practice. Knowledge and clinical experience shared from these two perspectives are mutually beneficial to the providers and the patient. The NP can benefit from the in-depth knowledge about the drugs in the physician's specialty area and from the power base that physicians have established in dealing with drug companies. The physician can benefit from NPs' focus on the impact of the drug on the patient and from their patient education skills. In the age of managed care, increasing emphasis is being placed on these latter issues.

Pharmacists

Collaboration with pharmacists requires an understanding of the educational preparation and evolution of roles of the Doctor of Pharmacy (PharmD). The profession of pharmacy requires graduate-level preparation for all pharmacists with the granting of a practice doctorate, the PharmD. PharmDs have extensive knowledge about pathophysiology and take an active role in determining the best drug to prescribe. They can provide the necessary information, such as available dosage forms, potential adverse reactions, and drug interactions, for the NP to choose a drug and write a valid prescription. Like the physician, the PharmD can add clinical knowledge to the drug choice.

Both physicians and NPs increasingly consult PharmDs for their knowledge of pharmacokinetics and pharcotherapeutics when prescribing for complex patients.

Other Nurse Practitioners and Advanced Practice Nurses Who Are Prescribers

Collaboration with other NPs and APNs who have prescriptive privileges has two major advantages. On a one-to-one basis dealing with individual patient issues, NPs and APNs can share "clinical pearls" from their knowledge base and practice experience to improve the care of the patient and expand the knowledge of both of them. On a bigger scale, there is power in numbers. Collaboration on issues related to scope of practice and prescriptive privilege at the state and national level is critical to obtaining and maintaining the autonomy of practice needed to provide optimal patient care.

Other Advanced Practice Nurses Who Are Not Prescribers

Because they cannot prescribe drugs, these APNs have often had to develop creative nonpharmacological strategies to deal with patient problems. Prescribing a drug is not the only or even always the best therapy. Collaboration at this level can increase the expertise of NPs in a wide range of therapies and make these therapies available to patients. Those APNs who currently cannot prescribe may want to add prescriptive privilege to their practice. The same power of numbers related to scope of practice and prescriptive privilege issues applies here. It is in the interest of all APNs to work together to foster the optimal scope of practice for both prescribing and nonprescribing APNs.

Physician Assistants

The focus of the PA's practice is similar to that of the physician, so both the NP and the PA can benefit from interaction with each other in much the same way as the interaction with physicians. Many PAs desire more autonomy in their practice, and the experience of NPs in developing autonomy may be helpful. It is necessary to remember that, at this time, such autonomy does not exist and so it is important to know the laws that govern the practice of the PA as well as the NP in each state to determine how collaboration can best occur.

Nurses Not in Advanced Practice Roles

NPs also regularly collaborate with other nurse colleagues who are not in advanced practice roles. These nurses and their assistants carry out the prescriptive orders of the NP. For each of these care providers, it is important to remember their preparation and knowledge level and their legal responsibility in carrying out the NP's orders. RNs and licensed practical/vocational nurses function under their own licenses. Their preparation and responsibility are defined by the nurse practice act in each state. Whether they can legally take orders from an NP is also delineated in these statutes. When prescribing drugs that others will administer, NPs must know these parameters. Medical assistants, who often have a role in clinics, may have certification in the state that delineates their preparation, but generally they are not licensed. Their knowledge of drugs is very limited, if they have had any formal education in the area of pharmacology at all. When prescribing drugs to be administered by medical assistants, NPs must take care to ensure that they clearly understand what they are to do; careful supervision is critical.

CANADIAN NURSE PRACTITIONER PRACTICE

As in the United States, where NP scope of practice and regulation vary from state to state, NP scope of practice and regulation in Canada vary from province to province. NPs practice independently in most of the provinces with the exception of Prince Edward Island, where NPs must practice with a collaborating physician. The scope of practice for NPs also varies from province to province, as well as by practice setting. For example in Ontario, an RN with extended class (EC) licensure or an NP can prescribe independently in primary care, long-term care, and outpatient clinics, but does not have independent prescriptive authority in an acute care hospital (Forchuck & Kohr, 2009). Adding to the varying scope of practice and regulation is the fact that the title *nurse practitioner* only recently became a protected title in Canada, so nurses without the required education could call themselves an NP (Forchuck & Kohr, 2009). There are now pediatric, family practice, adult, and anesthesia NPs who can prescribe in Canada. Mental health NPs are working on prescriptive authority and currently must qualify as a prescribing NP in either adult, pediatric, or primary care.

CURRENT ISSUES AND TRENDS IN HEALTH CARE AND THEIR EFFECT ON PRESCRIPTIVE AUTHORITY

Autonomy and Prescriptive Authority

The growth in autonomy and prescriptive authority for NPs and other APNs is a source of pride. APNs have now successfully overcome the "cannot prescribe," "cannot diagnose and treat," and "cannot admit" prohibitions to practice that have required so much time and energy in the past. More states are broadening and expanding the legal, reimbursement, and prescriptive authority to practice for all APNs, including NPs. By January 2004, all states had recognized the NP title, scope of practice, and prescriptive authority in legislation. In 2009, 22 states reported an expanded legislative or regulatory NP scope of practice

(Pearson, 2009). Other APNs also have this recognition, although the scope of practice and prescriptive authority is often more restricted. These gains are not written in stone, however, and can be reversed. Despite continuing research studies (Newland, 2009; Pearson, 2009) that demonstrate the effectiveness of the role of the APN in improving patient outcomes, barriers remain. Major concerns related to prescriptive authority must continue to be addressed. Not all states have legislation that permits NPs to prescribe independently of any required physician involvement (Pearson, 2009; Phillips, 2009). Turf battles continue between NPs and physicians at national and many state levels over physician supervision requirements and cosignatures on prescriptions (Partin, 2008). The advent of the Doctorate of Nursing Practice (DNP) degree with its comparable level of education to other health-care providers and a focus on independent practice may address some of these issues about supervision. However, the American Medical Association continues to stress the need for physician supervision and final authority for the patient, even for NPs who hold the DNP (Partin, 2008). This push for physician control occurs despite data from malpractice and malfeasance ratios that clearly show that the rationale for physician supervision is unfounded (Pearson, 2009).

Interdisciplinary Teams

In a study by Kaplan and Brown (2004), the top three barriers to effective prescriptive authority for NPs all related to interactions with physicians. Among the top 12, two related to interactions with pharmacists. It is time to put this battle behind us and work together to create teams of health-care professionals who work together to foster excellent health care for every patient. Such teams would provide care of higher quality with better patient outcomes if the strengths of each team member were fully utilized. Research comparing care given by such teams with that given by physicians alone supports this assertion (Scisney-Matlock, Makos, Saunders, Jackson, & Steigerwalt, 2004). The Institute of Medicine Committee on Health Professions Education (2003) states, "All health professionals should be educated to deliver patient-centered care as members of an interdisciplinary team, emphasizing evidence-based practice, quality improvement approaches and informatics" (p. 45).

Level of Education of Team Members

One of the issues to be addressed in interdisciplinary teams is the level of education of the various providers. When the level of education is different, issues of collegiality, collaboration, and, especially, supervision arise. Pharmacists have "stepped up to the plate" to move the education of their profession to the practice doctorate. Medicine has been at the practice doctorate level for over 50 years. NPs are now addressing this issue. Recognizing that gaps exist between what is taught in master's level education programs and the knowledge that is needed for practice, in 2004 the American Association of Colleges of Nurses (AACN) in collaboration with National Organization of Nurse Practitioner Faculties (NONPF) formed a task force to develop the practice doctorate and publish core content and competencies for such educational preparation. As stated in the *Position Statement on the Practice Doctorate in Nursing*, the practice-focused doctorate provides a "distinct model of doctoral education that provides an additional option for attaining a terminal degree in the discipline" (p. 8). The practice doctorate, to use the title DNP, was presented in a position statement in March 2004. In October 2004, AACN published a position statement on the practice doctorate (http://www.aacn.nche.edu) and in October 2006, the organization published *The Essentials of Doctoral Education for Advanced Nursing Practice* (http://www.aacn.nche.edu). In April 2006, NONPF published the entry-level competencies for the graduate of a DNP program (http://www.nonpf.com). These competencies are in addition to the ones in the existing *Domains and Core Competencies of Nurse Practitioner Practice* document produced by NONPF. They include the following:

a) a strong emphasis on independent and interprofessional practice;
b) a focus on evidenced-based practice based on a strong scientific foundation;
c) excellent information technology skills, including the development and use of clinical information systems;
d) application of investigative skills for evaluation of health outcomes and the translation of new knowledge into practice; and
e) a leadership role in the health-care delivery system, including influencing health policy and managing risk.

A date of 2015 has been set for the educational preparation of all APNs, including Certified Registered Nurse Anesthetists, Certified Nurse Midwives, Clinical Nurse Specialists, and Nurse Practitioners, to be at the doctoral level. As of May 2009, more than 90 DNP programs are accepting students (http://www.nonpf.com). This move to the same level of education as other members of the health-care provider team will address some of the issues surrounding the interdisciplinary team. The content in this book is consistent with the recommendations of both AACN and NONPF related to the knowledge base in pharmacotherapeutics for DNP prepared nurses.

Reimbursement

The passage of legislation and the adoption of regulations related to reimbursement are infrequently reported (Phillips, 2009), yet the reimbursement by third-party payers continues to be a practice barrier for many nurses in advanced practice. With the current focus at the federal level on restructuring the health-care delivery system, this issue takes a front-and-center place in the future of advanced practice.

The potential transfer of accountability for Medicaid from the federal government to the states also has the potential to jeopardize implementation of federal mandates for services and access to NPs as providers, especially if NPs are seen as primary care providers only to underserved populations that are financially undesirable for physicians. NPs must be careful that they are not seen as physician-substitutes or physician-extenders, but rather as APNs; otherwise, the current autonomy we enjoy and the level of autonomy we hope to attain may disappear as the number of family practice and other primary care physicians increase.

Private-sector and government restructuring of health care with a focus on cost control and for-profit groups has both positive and negative potential for the autonomy of the NP. Negatively, this means treatment options and decision making about their use are often transferred to the corporation or the government. This can limit the NP's ability to determine treatment options, and the extra time the NP takes to educate and counsel patients may be seen as a liability rather than as an asset. Positively, NPs have demonstrated their ability to control costs and improve patient outcomes (Pearson, 2009). We must continue to conduct research on the ability of NPs to provide competent, cost-effective, high-quality services to improve the health of our patients, whether in NP-only practices or in collaborative practices, and to share the findings of that research with the decision makers in the changing world of health care. Better yet, we must become decision makers.

NPs and other providers must address these challenges and take control of the future in health care so that preferred outcomes are achieved rather than having the outcomes designed and implemented by others. This requires a commitment of time and energy from each NP, APN, and PA to work together with other providers and other nurses to deal with these issues at local, state, and national levels. Keeping current on new knowledge in pharmacology and on the latest drugs and their clinical applications is only part of the role of the health-care provider as prescriber. NPs, APNs, and PAs should join and support their professional organizations and engage in positive political activity to maintain the prescriptive authority already gained in each state and to extend autonomous prescriptive authority to all states.

REFERENCES

American Academy of Physician Assistants. (2008). *Summary of state laws for physician assistants: Abridged version*. Retrieved, May 13, 2009, from http://www.aapa.org

American Association of Colleges of Nursing. (2004). *Position statement on the practice doctorate in nursing*. Retrieved May 13, 2009, from http://www.aacn.nche.edu

American Association of Colleges of Nursing. (2006). *The essentials of doctoral education for advanced nursing practice*. Retrieved May 13, 2009, from http://www.aacn.nche.edu

American Medical Association. (2009). *AMA scope of practice series: Nurse practitioner.* American Medical Association. AE13:08-0424rev: pdf:10/09.

Blair, K. (2004, April 22–25). *Report of the faculty practice committee*. Paper presented at the 30th Annual Meeting of the National Organization of Nurse Practitioner Faculties.

Forchuck, C., & Kohr, R. (2009). Prescriptive authority for nurses: The Canadian perspective. *Perspectives in Psychiatric Care, 45*(1), 3–8.

Institute of Medicine Committee on Health Professions Education. (2003). *Health professions education: A bridge to quality*. Washington, DC: The National Academies Press.

Kaplan, L., & Brown, M. (2004). Prescriptive authority and barriers to NP practice. *Nurse Practitioner, 29*(3), 28–35.

National Organization of Nurse Practitioner Faculties (NONPF). (2006). *Practice doctorate nurse practitioner entry-level competencies*, 2006. Retrieved May 7, 2009, from http://www.nonpf.com/NONPF 2005/ Practice Doctorate Resource Center/Competency Draft Final April 2006.pdf

Newland, J. (2009). NPs: The cornerstone of healthy patients. *Nurse Practitioner, 34*(5), 5.

Partin, B. (2008). Advocacy in practice: Unite to fight AMA resolutions. *Nurse Practitioner, 33*(12), 11.

Pearson, L. (2009). The Pearson report: A national overview of nurse practitioner legislation and healthcare issues. *American Journal for Nurse Practitioners, 13*(2), 8–82.

Phillips, S. (2009). 21st annual legislative update. *Nurse Practitioner, 3*(1), 19–41.

Scisney-Matlock, M., Makos, G., Saunders, T., Jackson, F., & Steigerwalt, S. (2004). Comparison of quality-of-hypertensive-care indicators for groups treated by physician versus groups treated by physician-nurse team. *Journal of the American Academy of Nurse Practitioners, 16*(1), 17–23.

CHAPTER 2

REVIEW OF BASIC PRINCIPLES OF PHARMACOLOGY

Teri Moser Woo

Chapter Outline

Pharmacology is one of the cornerstones of drug discovery. Pharmacology is defined as the study of drugs and drug actions, derived from the Greek **pharmakos**, "medicine" or "drug," and logos, "study" (Adams & Koch, 2010). With the help of biochemistry and medicinal chemistry, new compounds are discovered. However, the science of pharmacology will define the potential benefits of new compounds. Oswald Schmiedeberg (1838–1921) is generally recognized as the founder of modern pharmacology. Until recently, most drugs were impure mixtures of only vaguely known composition, and primarily of plant and animal origin. Health-care providers were required to know only the therapeutic benefits of the drugs when these agents were administered. How these agents produce these effects was beyond the knowledge of the day.

Today, health-care providers are required to know the therapeutic benefits, indications, contraindications, adverse effects, drug interactions, and precise mechanism by which beneficial effects are observed. Rational drug selection may require choosing among several similar drugs with similar effects and different mechanisms of action.

Rational drug therapy for any patient requires adequate knowledge of the disease states, comorbid conditions, pharmacodynamic properties of the selected drug, drug and drug interactions and pharmacokinetics of the drug (the individual patient's ability to absorb, distribute, metabolize, and eliminate the drug).

The objective of drug therapy is to deliver and maintain therapeutic levels of a drug in the target tissues. To achieve this goal, the clinician must have basic knowledge of onset of action, intensity of drug effect, and duration of drug effect. These factors are controlled by absorption, distribution, metabolism, and excretion of the drug. First, drug absorption permits entry of the drug into plasma. Second, the drug may then leave the bloodstream and distribute into the interstitial and intracellular fluids. The drug is metabolized and then eliminated, most commonly via the kidneys.

Understanding drug effects is based on knowledge of the relationship between drug concentration and pharmacodynamic action. Drugs act by affecting biochemical and physiological processes in the body. Most drugs act at specific receptors but may produce multiple effects because of the location of the receptor in various organs. Knowledge of drug-receptor interaction helps to predict the behavior of a drug in the body and is an important guide in the selection of appropriate doses and dosage intervals.

A complete review of pharmacological principles is beyond the scope of this book. This chapter assumes users have had a basic pharmacology course in their initial education, so the chapter focuses on reviewing critical basic principles for being a safe prescriber.

PHARMACODYNAMICS

Pharmacodynamics is the study of the effects of drugs on the body. Drug effect is the result of an interaction between the drug and a target cell or receptor to produce a therapeutic effect. Most medications are thought to interact with a receptor at the site of action. These receptors are found in cell membranes, enzymes, cellular proteins, and constituents of the cells, such as nucleic acids. The combination of the receptor and the drug is the action, and the results are considered the effect of the drug. Drug effects can be momentary or can last for days.

Drug-Receptor Interaction

A fundamental hypothesis of pharmacology is that a relationship exists between a beneficial or a toxic effect of a drug and the concentration of the drug at the site of action as measured by the concentration in the blood. This hypothesis has been confirmed for many drugs and is the basis for the determination of effective or toxic concentrations reported in the literature and followed clinically by serum drug level testing. Knowing the relationship between drug concentration and effects allows the clinician to take into account the various pathological and physiological features of a particular patient that make that patient different from the "average" individual, based on clinical trials and mean statistical data. See Figure 2–1.

Drug-Receptor Activity

Drugs have an affinity for certain portions of a cell or tissue, known as the cell receptor that can be occupied to cause a certain effect. If the drug is an agonist, the drug combines with the receptor that stimulates the target organ. The drug agonist–cell receptor relationship is like a lock and key; it must be a perfect fit to get a pharmacological response (Figure 2–1). If the drug is an antagonist, the drug combines with the receptor but interferes with the naturally occurring agonist or other drug agonists that may be present. The antagonist is not capable of producing a biological effect. Antagonists are often called "blockers," as in **beta blockers**. The different drug-receptor relationships are depicted in Figure 2–2.

In general, the larger the drug dose, the higher the drug concentration will be at the receptors at the site of action. The higher concentration then leads to a greater drug effect, up to a maximum effect. Further increases in drug dose will not cause further effects because all possible receptor sites are being stimulated by the drug and the maximum response has been attained.

A variety of natural agonists of many different receptors have been identified. These *receptor* subtypes have been noted for a number of therapeutic agents that have selectivity for subtype receptors so that effects can be specific and adverse reactions minimized. For example, several histamine receptors, H_1 and H_2, and catecholamine receptors, $alpha_1$, $alpha_2$, $beta_1$, and $beta_2$, have been identified.

Natural agonists interact with receptors to regulate the functioning of the body. If receptors are continually stimulated by drugs, their responsiveness may be decreased, which is referred to as *down-regulation*, or *desensitization*. This can be due to a decrease in the number of receptors or a change in the existing receptors. Severe down-regulation may result in *refractoriness*, or a lack of response to the drug.

If a receptor's activity is chronically reduced by antagonists, a state of *up-regulation*, or *hypersensitization*, may occur. If the drug is rapidly withdrawn, the receptors react strongly to the natural agonists, resulting in exaggerated response because of the exaggerated response of the supersensitive receptors to the normal amounts of natural agonist. For example, rapid withdrawal of **antihypertensives** may result in hypertensive episodes.

In most cases, the interaction between a drug and a receptor is temporary, with the drug action ending when the drug leaves the receptor site. This drug-receptor relationship is termed a *reversible agonist*. This principle provides for the relationship between drug concentration and drug effect. When a high concentration of drug is present, the receptors are frequently stimulated; and as

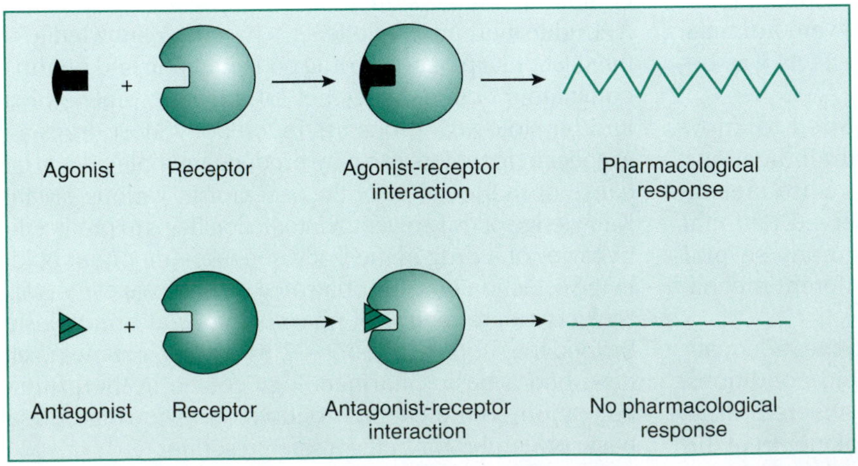

Figure 2–1. Drug-receptor activity. *(From Kuhn, M. A. [1998]. Pharmacotherapeutics: A nursing process approach [4th ed., p. 46]. Philadelphia: F. A. Davis, with permission.)*

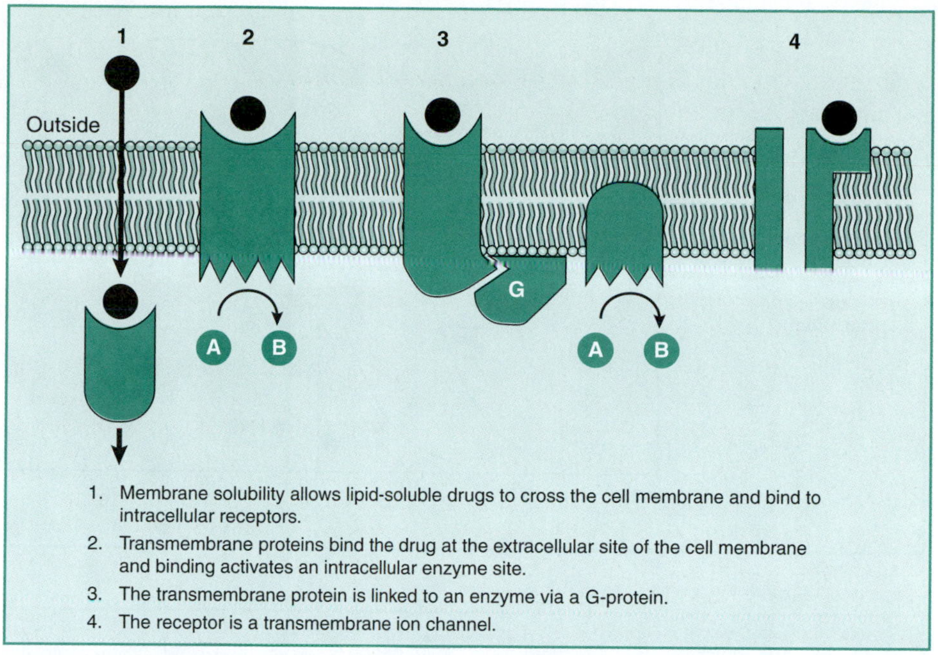
1
2
3
4
Outside
G
A
B
A
B
1. Membrane solubility allows lipid-soluble drugs to cross the cell membrane and bind to intracellular receptors.
2. Transmembrane proteins bind the drug at the extracellular site of the cell membrane and binding activates an intracellular enzyme site.
3. The transmembrane protein is linked to an enzyme via a G-protein.
4. The receptor is a transmembrane ion channel.

Figure 2–2. Drug receptors.

the concentration goes down, fewer receptors are filled, and the drug effect dissipates with time. If a drug occupies a receptor permanently, then the interaction is termed *irreversible.*

The same is true if the drug acts as an antagonist; if the binding of drug and antagonist is reversible, the antagonist is called a *competitive antagonist.* This refers to the fact that the effect of the antagonist can be overcome by higher doses of the agonist competing for the receptor site with the antagonist, with the blocking of the receptor overcome by higher concentrations of the drug. If the receptor is irreversibly blocked by the antagonist, then the effect of the antagonist cannot be overwhelmed by the agonist, and the antagonist is a *noncompetitive inhibitor* of the receptor A *partial agonist* is a drug agonist that acts to compete with a full *agonists* for drug receptors. The end result is a decrease of effect on the receptor over what is seen with an *agonist* alone.

In summary, these are the key concepts related to drug-receptor binding:

- Drugs that bind to receptors may be agonists, partial agonists, or antagonistic.
- Drug-receptor binding is usually reversible.
- Drug-receptor binding is selective.
  - Very specific
  - If the key doesn't fit . . .
- Drug-receptor binding is graded.
  - The more receptors filled, the greater the pharmacological response will be.

Therapeutic Index

The relationship between a drug's desired therapeutic effects and its adverse effects is called its therapeutic index (see Fig. 2–3). The therapeutic index is the ratio of the doses required to produce death or serious toxicity in 50 percent of subjects compared with the doses required for effective treatment of 50 percent of subjects. If the difference is wide, several orders of magnitude, then the therapeutic index is wide, the drug is safe, and close therapeutic monitoring is not usually required. If the difference is small, less than 10-fold, then the index is narrow, and close monitoring of doses is needed to prevent adverse reactions in a patient.

Dose-Response Relationship

Once a drug is administered and absorption begins, blood levels of the drug start to rise. However, no measurable response will occur until a minimum effective concentration of free drug molecules in the blood is reached. The onset of action is the time needed for the drug concentration to reach this minimum level. While blood concentration and the intensity of the response are rising toward the peak, absorption rates are greater than elimination rates. The onset of action can be shortened by administering drugs in a manner to eliminate or shorten absorption time such as IV or IM. The time to peak is the time required for the maximum effect to occur after administration. The fall of blood levels and decreased response reflect metabolism and excretion at rates faster than absorption and distribution. The duration of action is the time during which the blood levels are above the minimum effective concentration and is not affected by the route of administration. The point at which the drug level drops below the minimum effective concentration is the termination of action. Figure 2–4 depicts the dose-response relationship.

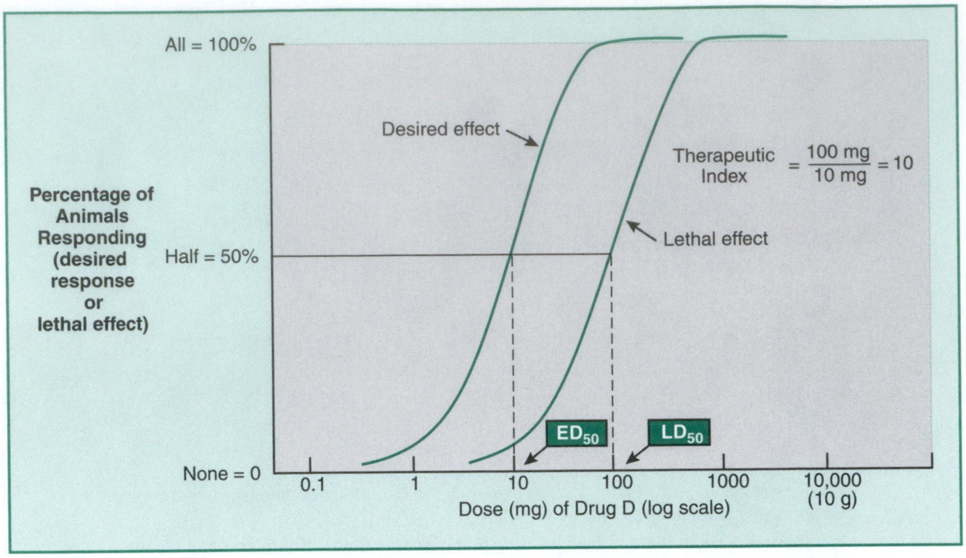

Figure 2–3. The therapeutic index. *(From Shlafer, M. [1993]. The nurse, pharmacology, and drug therapy: A prototype approach [2nd ed., p. 82]. Redwood City, CA: Addison-Wesley Nursing, with permission.)*

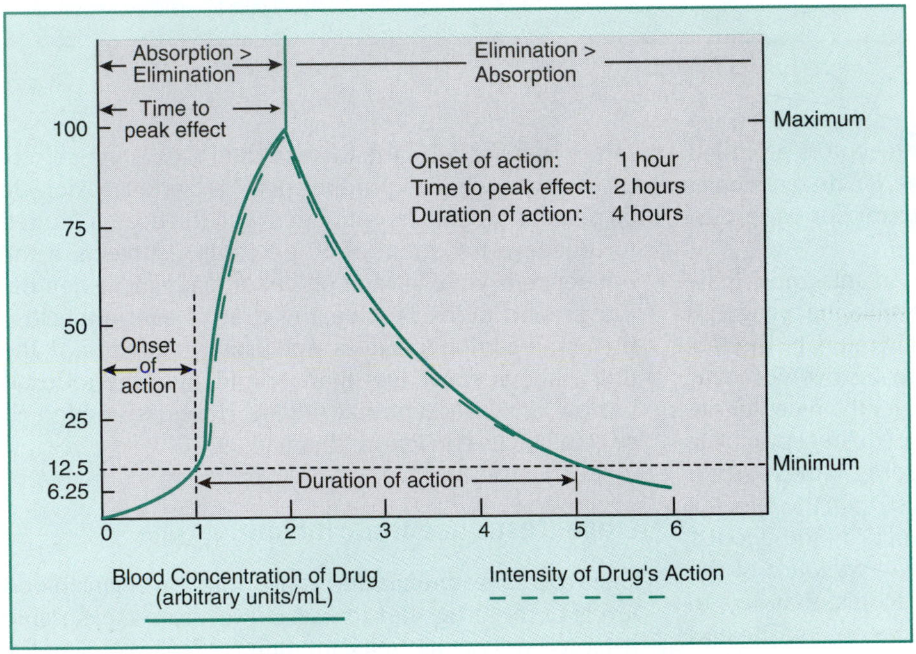

Figure 2–4. The dose-response relationship. *(From Shlafer, M. [1993]. The nurse, pharmacology, and drug therapy: A prototype approach [2nd ed., p. 82]. Redwood City, CA: Addison-Wesley Nursing, with permission.)*

The prescriber needs to be aware of the dose-response curve of a drug to determine how soon the medication will take effect (reach minimum concentration), how long the drug will be effective (in the therapeutic range), and when the drug effect will terminate. A clinical example is the administering of the antihistamine **diphenhydramine** (**Benadryl**). If a rapid onset of action is required, then IV or IM administration is preferred, whereas if slower onset is acceptable to the therapeutic goal, oral administration can be used. When the duration of action is complete and **diphenhydramine** enters the termination phase ("wears off"), the allergic symptoms will often recur.

Drug Potency and Efficacy

The dose response of a drug has two important properties, efficacy and potency. Efficacy is measured by the maximum effect that the drug can achieve. Potency of a drug is a relative measure that compares the doses of two different drugs that are required to achieve the same effect. A drug is said to be potent when it possesses a high intrinsic activity at low unit doses. Potency is influenced by absorption, distribution, metabolism, and excretion. When similar drugs with different potencies are switched, the ratio of equally effective doses needs to be considered (see Fig. 2–5).

For clinical use, distinguishing between a drug's potency and its maximum effect is helpful. The clinical effectiveness of a drug depends not on its potency but on its maximum efficacy and its ability to reach relevant receptors. In deciding which of two drugs to prescribe, the provider must consider their relative maximum effectiveness rather than their relative potency.

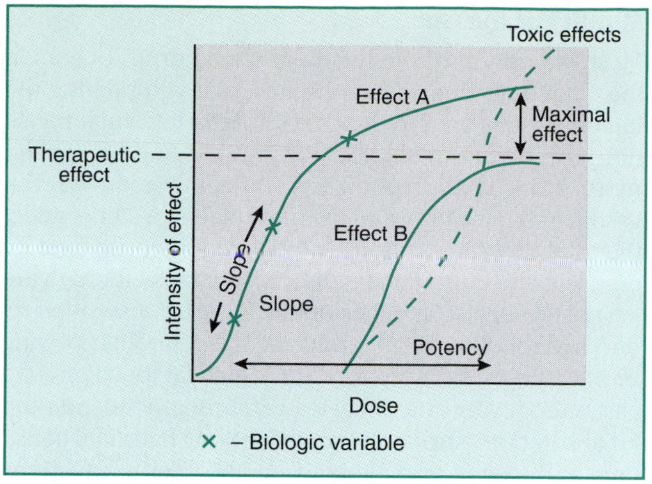

Figure 2–5. Drug potency and maximum effect. *(From Kuhn, M. A. [1998]. Pharmacotherapeutics: A nursing process approach [4th ed., p. 48]. Philadelphia: F. A. Davis, with permission.)*

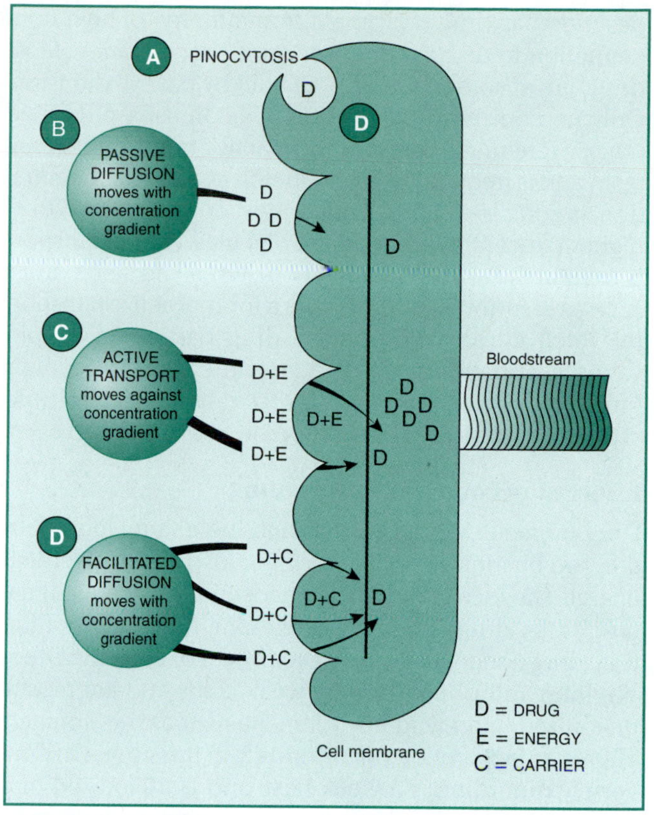

Figure 2–6. Mechanisms of drug absorption. *(From Kuhn, M. A. [1998]. Pharmacotherapeutics: A nursing process approach [4th ed., p. 39). Philadelphia, F. A. Davis, p. 39, with permission.)*

PHARMACOKINETICS

Pharmacokinetics is the study and analysis of the time course of the drug in the body. The ease with which drugs pass through membranes is the key to assess the rates of absorption and extent of distribution throughout the many body compartments. Drugs are transported throughout the circulatory system and end up at tissues and organs where their presence is beneficial and also at some areas where their presence may be detrimental. Drugs are usually metabolized in the liver either before they travel to the site of action ("first pass") or after they have been to the site of action. Drugs are eliminated from the body most commonly via the kidneys.

Drug Absorption

The first stage of pharmacokinetics is drug absorption. Drug absorption includes all the chemical and biological processes during a drug molecule's progress from the pharmaceutical dosage form to the systemic circulation. To reach the site of action, the drug must be absorbed from the dosage form into the body.

Many basic pharmacological principles pertain to drug absorption including passive diffusion, active transport, and facilitated diffusion. Passive diffusion refers to the simple diffusion of drug from areas of high concentration to areas of lower concentration. Facilitated diffusion occurs where the drug molecule combines with another molecule to facilitate absorption. Active transport occurs where the molecule is actively transported across the cell membrane, often via the ATP pump. The mechanisms of drug absorption are shown in Figure 2–6.

Parenteral Drug Absorption

Parenteral drug formulations are commonly clear solutions of a drug, designed for direct injection. These drug solutions have few absorption problems because they are in solution when given. Drugs injected directly into the venous circulation (IV) begin distribution throughout the body immediately. This is the unique property and advantage of IV administration.

However, drugs for IM or subcutaneous (SC) administration do undergo absorption from the injection site and are subject to some of the factors affecting oral drug absorption. Although they do not have to dissolve and diffuse through the gastrointestinal (GI) membrane and are not affected by the first-pass effect, they are affected by blood flow to the site of injections. Some IM preparations are formulated in oil or as a suspension to prolong absorption and provide a prolonged drug effect. These preparations cannot be given IV because of the risk of pulmonary emboli with the insoluble drugs and ingredients.

Oral Drug Absorption

Oral drug absorption is the most common type of drug absorption, and oral dosage forms make up most of the medications given to patients. Active drugs must dissolve in liquid and be available in solution because the body cannot absorb solids. In most cases, drug absorption across membranes occurs in the same manner as nutrient absorption from foods. Passive diffusion includes simple diffusion, convective absorption, and carrier-mediated diffusion; requires no energy expenditure; and can be described as drug movement from an area of high concentration to an area of lower drug concentration. Most drugs are absorbed from the GI tract by passive diffusion. Only nonionized, lipid-soluble drugs diffuse well. Active transport requires energy and an active transport mechanism and is frequently demonstrated against a concentration gradient—that is, from a low concentration to a higher concentration of drug molecules. Active transport is used in the absorption of **electrolytes** and some drugs such as **levodopa.** Pinocytosis is a form of active transport in which the cell engulfs the drug particle in a lipid vacuole and transports it across the cell membrane. Pinocytosis is commonly used to transport **fat-soluble vitamins** across the cell membrane. See Figure 2–6.

Effect of pH on Oral Absorption

Drug molecules can pass through the cell membrane if they are un-ionized; that is, they do not have an electrical charge. The local pH of the GI tract and the chemical nature of the drug (pK_a) will determine how much of the total drug concentration is un-ionized. For example, **theophylline** and **phenytoin** are weak acids and are mostly un-ionized in an acid environment such as the stomach. Therefore, absorption occurs mostly in the stomach. Conversely, **quinidine** is a weak base and is un-ionized in a basic environment such as the intestine, where most of its absorption occurs. For example, a weak base ($pK_a = 5.7$) in the low-pH environment of the stomach is highly ionized, with a ratio of ionized to un-ionized of 5,000:1. Most of the drug cannot be absorbed. In the higher-pH environment of the intestine, the ratio of ionized to un-ionized changes to 1:10. In this situation, 90 percent of the drug is available for absorption in the intestine. The site of absorption determines which factors, such as gastric emptying time and intestinal motility, will have an effect on a specific drug's absorption (Fig. 2–7).

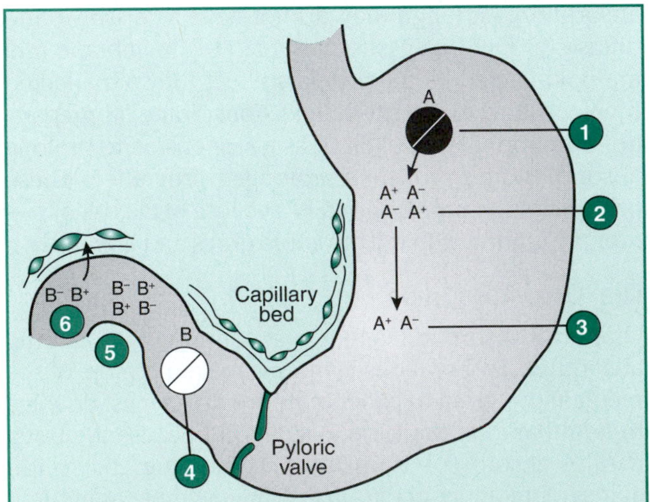

Figure 2–7. Effect of pH on oral absorption. *(From Kuhn, M. A. [1998]. Pharmacotherapeutics: A nursing process approach [4th ed., p. 39]. Philadelphia, F. A. Davis, with permission.)*

Motility of the Gut

Most absorption of orally administered drugs occurs in the small intestine, where the mucosal villi provide the largest surface area in the GI tract. If the intestinal transit time is reduced or sections of the intestine have been removed, drug absorption is significantly reduced. The gastric emptying time and the intestinal transit time affect the total drug absorption by changing the drug contact time with the intestinal mucosa. Rapid transit through the part of the GI tract most favorable for drug absorption reduces absorption, and prolonged contact through slowing transit increases absorption. Solid, high-fat foods prolong gastric emptying and delay drug delivery to the intestine for absorption. **Anticholinergics** prolong intestinal transit time and may increase total drug absorption. **Laxatives** decrease intestinal transit time, thereby decreasing drug absorption.

Blood Flow

Drug absorption depends on normal blood flow past the absorptive surface. For oral administration, food stimulates gastric blood flow and absorption, and physical exercise, by diverting blood to the muscles, decreases GI blood flow and lowers absorption. If blood flow is reduced as in cardiac disease, then IM medications are absorbed more slowly from the injection site. Blood flow to the skin affects the absorption of topical medications, with vasoconstriction causing decreased absorption.

First-Pass Metabolism

The metabolism of a part of the administered dose of a drug before it reaches the systemic circulation is referred to as the first-pass metabolism. Orally administered drugs are absorbed in the stomach or small intestine and move through the portal vein into the liver before passing into the general circulation. For some drugs, a clinically significant portion of the drug taken is metabolized during this first trip through the liver, so that the oral dose required for a given effect is much higher than for other routes that do not use the portal circulation (parenteral or sublingual). For example, **propranolol** has a recommended oral dose of 40 to 120 mg and an equivalent IV dose of 1 to 3 mg because of the first-pass metabolism of portal circulation. Drugs with clinically significant first-pass metabolism include **dopamine, lidocaine, propranolol, imipramine, morphine, reserpine, nitroglycerin, isoproterenol,** and **warfarin.** Drugs with significant first pass effect require either increased dosing or administered via an alternative route such as IV, IM, rectal, or sublingual.

Enterohepatic Recycling

After being absorbed, drugs move through the bloodstream and return to the liver for metabolism. Some drugs leave the liver circulation and enter the biliary tract to be excreted in bile, eventually returning to the intestine and becoming available for reabsorption through the intestinal wall back into the bloodstream. Each day, 80 percent of bile is reabsorbed, so the active drug or metabolites recirculate for a long time. Some of the drug may go to the kidney for renal elimination. This process is defined as enterohepatic recycling (Fig. 2–8).

Bioavailability

The combination of inert ingredients determines the disintegration, dissolution, and drug availability in the body, and different combinations can result in different clinical effects among products of the same labeled potency. The amount of the drug dose that reaches the systemic circulation determines its bioavailability. A product that is not completely absorbed or is eliminated by the liver in its first pass has low bioavailability. Differences in bioavailability may be evident between two products that contain the same amount of drug but result in two different plasma concentrations. The total amount of drug reaching the systemic circulation is reflected by the area under the curve (AUC) of a plasma concentration versus the time curve. Comparisons of the AUCs of various dosage forms of a drug compare their bioavailabilities. Note that bioavailability does not take into account the rate of absorption; it only estimates the extent of absorption. Although rate of absorption can be important when rapid effects are required, it is usually not important when a drug is administered chronically.

Drug Distribution

After a drug reaches the bloodstream or is absorbed into the body, the drug molecules are distributed throughout the body in several phases. The initial phase distributes medication to high-flow areas such as the heart, liver, kidney, and brain. The second phase occurs to areas of slower blood flow such as fat, bone, and skin. The rate and extent of distribution of a drug throughout the body determine how much of the drug will be available to exert the pharmacological actions in the body and how soon the drug will be eliminated. Drug distribution to various body tissues and compartments is affected by many factors, such as body composition, cardiac output, regional blood flow, and binding propensities. Drug diffusion is also dependent on protein binding and lipid solubility.

Plasma Protein Binding

A drug's affinity for aqueous or lipid tissue and its degree of binding to proteins determine where a drug goes and whether it reaches a therapeutic drug level at the site of desired action. During distribution throughout the body, the drug comes in contact with plasma carrier proteins, storage tissue, or receptor protein. Drugs bound to protein are called the drug-protein complex. Bound drugs cannot cross over the plasma membrane to leave the vascular space. The drug that is bound to protein becomes inactive and is unavailable for binding to receptor sites and exerting therapeutic activity. An unbound drug is called a free drug. A free drug is able to cross the plasma membrane and bind to receptor sites at the site of action. Equilibrium is achieved when a stable ratio of drug is found within all body compartments. However, a bound drug can rapidly free itself from binding to restore the equilibrium between bound and free drug in the body.

The percentage of free drug is constant for a single drug but differs between drugs. For example, about 90 percent of the total **gentamicin** in the plasma is free, whereas only about 1 percent of the total **warfarin** in the plasma remains unbound. Administering a single dose of **aspirin** to a patient on **warfarin** therapy causes competition for protein binding between the two drugs. As a result, the amount of free **warfarin** in the plasma is increased from 1 to 2 percent, as some of the **warfarin** is replaced by **aspirin** on the plasma protein and becomes unbound. Although the 1 percent increase seems unimportant, the

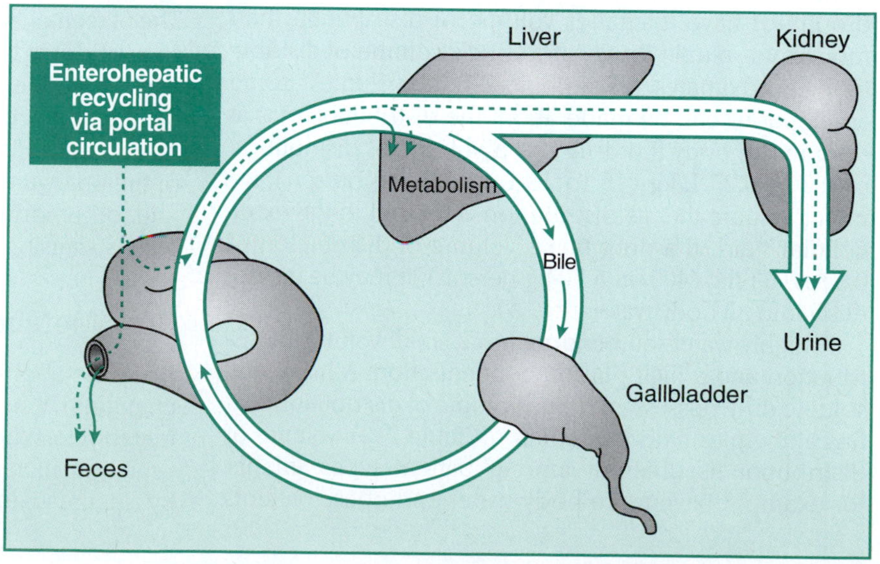

Figure 2–8. Enterohepatic recycling. *(From Kuhn, M. A. [1998]. Pharmacotherapeutics: A nursing process approach [4th ed., p. 45]. Philadelphia:, F. A. Davis, with permission.)*

amount of free **warfarin** available to exert anticoagulant effects is doubled, with possible serious consequences.

The percentage of drug that remains free and available for binding depends on the amount of plasma protein available, which differs among patients, depending on their medical condition. For example the patient with hypoalbuminemia may demonstrate exaggerated pharmacological response because of excess free drug. The affinity of a drug for protein and the percentage of bound plasma protein and tissue are usually constant for an individual drug. This is usually called the percentage protein bound or protein binding of the drug. Only free drugs can cross membranes to enter body tissues or to be eliminated, and only free drugs can interact with receptors to produce therapeutic effects. Clinical laboratories usually report the total serum concentration, which includes both free and bound drug. For most patients, this is a good indicator of drug effect; in some circumstances, however, free drug concentration must be obtained.

Table 2–1 **Example of Volume of Distribution Calculation**

Type of Drug	Water Soluble	Fat Soluble
Percentage in tissue (30% of body)	10%	90%
Percentage in fluids (70% of body)	90%	10%
Dose given	100 mg	100 mg
Amount found in fluids (blood)	90 mg	10 mg
Serum concentration	1.29 mg/mL	0.14 mg/mL
V_d calculation	100 mg 1.29 mg/mL	100 mg 0.14 mg/mL
Volume of distribution	78 mL	714 mL

Volume of Distribution

Volume of distribution (V_d) is a mathematically determined measure of the size of a compartment that would be filled by the amount of a drug in the same concentration as that found in the blood or plasma. In reality, the amount of drug in the body is constantly changing because of elimination, making it difficult to calculate the volume in which a drug distributes. One way to calculate the apparent volume distribution is to administer an IV dose and measure the serum concentration right away, before elimination has had much of an effect. The concentration just after IV administration is known as C_0, and the amount of drug given is X_0 or V_d 5 X_0/C_0. This volume is not real, but it is useful in expressing the affinity of a drug to tissue and storage sites and in calculating a drug's clearance from the body. A larger volume of distribution indicates that a larger dose should be administered to achieve a target concentration. It is not useful in determining the drug's effectiveness or duration of action.

In the example in Table 2–1, water-soluble drugs (hydrophilic) have a smaller volume of distribution than more lipid-soluble drugs. If a drug's volume of distribution approximates physiological fluid volumes, some assumptions can be made about the distribution of that drug in the body. If a drug has a volume of distribution of 0.2 to 0.25 L/kg (15 to 18 L in a 70-kg person), we might assume that its distribution is limited to the extracellular fluid. If a drug has a volume of distribution of 0.5 to 0.6 L/kg (40 L in a 70-kg person), it may be distributing into all body water.

A highly water-soluble drug has a small volume of distribution and a high plasma concentration. A highly fat-soluble drug possesses a large volume of distribution and has a low plasma concentration (Table 2–2). Volume of distribution is different among patient types. Infants, for example, have more body water and obese patients have more body fat, both of which affect the volume of distribution of drugs. Variable drug concentrations among different organs and tissues can complicate drug distribution. For example, **antibiotics** do not distribute to abscesses and exudates. The distribution of a drug can also be affected by the drug's ability to cross various barriers like the blood–brain barrier or placental barrier.

The Blood–Brain Barrier

The blood–brain barrier refers to a network of capillary endothelial cells in the brain. These cells have no pores and are surrounded by a sheath of glial connective tissue that makes them impermeable to water-soluble drugs. This barrier excludes ionized drug molecules, like **dopamine**, from the brain and allows un-ionized drug molecules, such as **barbiturates**, to pass readily and enter the brain. Usually, only medications that are lipid soluble, such as **atropine**, **general anesthetics**, and **psychotropics**, cross this barrier.

The Placental Barrier

The placental barrier is a lipid membrane that allows passage of drugs by simple diffusion. The fetus is generally exposed to the same drug concentrations as the mother. Smaller molecule drugs pass across the placental barrier more easily. Placental transfer is responsible for many of the untoward effects of **alcohol**, cigarettes, **narcotics**, and other drugs. Some drugs may have teratogenic effects, causing physical defects in the developing fetus.

Drug Metabolism

Drug metabolism refers to the process of chemically changing a drug to a different compound called a metabolite. When drugs are metabolized, the change is usually an increase in water solubility, often accompanied by a decrease in lipid solubility. The resulting compounds

Table 2–2 **Examples of Physiological Tissues and Approximate Volumes of Distributions of Various Drugs**

Compartment	Volume (L/kg)	Type of Drug	Example
Total body water	0.6	Water soluble	Ethanol
Extracellular water	0.2	Higher molecular weight, water soluble	Mannitol
Plasma	0.04	Highly protein bound	Heparin
Fat	0.2–0.35	Highly fat soluble	Chlorpromazine Imipramine
Bone	0.07	Some ions	Fluoride Calcium

can be more readily excreted in the urine. The metabolites formed are usually less active than the parent compound. Many other drugs are active per se but also have active metabolites whose pharmacokinetic and pharmacological profiles differ from that of the parent drug. The pharmacological effects seen in the patient are the result of the parent compound and all of its metabolites. Some drugs, such as **angiotensin-converting enzyme (ACE) inhibitors**, are administered as an inactive prodrug that must be metabolized to an active metabolite to have any effect. Drug metabolism occurs mainly in the liver (see the discussion of the first-pass effect), but other tissues such as lungs, kidneys, placenta and the gut wall may also metabolize drugs.

Although many different types of chemical reactions are seen in drug metabolism, the most important are the **phase 1** reactions such as oxidation, reduction, and hydrolysis. **Oxidation** reactions typically insert an oxygen atom into the drug molecule. The most clinically significant oxidation enzymes include **cytochrome P450 (CYP450). Phase 2** reactions, called synthetic or **conjugation** reactions, involve the attachment of another chemical group to the drug, resulting in a chemical with greater water solubility needed for renal elimination. Drugs may undergo one or both of the phases during their metabolism to produce a metabolite that will be easily excreted in the urine.

Drug Interactions Due to Changes in Metabolism

Alcohol, a variety of drugs, and cigarette smoke stimulate the synthesis of drug-metabolizing enzymes. This process is called enzyme induction and is clinically significant for many drug products. Other drugs inhibit the metabolism of another drug and are called enzyme inhibitors. These changes in drug metabolism can result in drug interactions, clinically significant changes in drug dose, and adverse effects. Coadministration of drugs where one is an inducer or inhibitor of CYP450 enzymes will predictably affect the therapeutic level of the other drug. A few common drugs that cause drug interactions through induction or inhibition of metabolism are listed in Table 2–3.

Table 2–3 **Common Drugs That Cause Drug Interactions Through the Effect on Metabolism**

Drugs That Inhibit Enzymes	Drugs That Inhibit Metabolism
Erythromycin	Amphetamines
Cimetidine	Ephedrine
Sodium valproate	Phenylephrine
Oral contraceptives	Digoxin
Propranolol	Warfarin
Some sulfonamides	Theophylline
	Carbamazepine
	Propranolol
Drugs That Induce Enzymes	**Drugs That Accelerate Metabolism**
Rifampin	Theophylline
Phenytoin	Imipramine
Carbamazepine	Pentazocine
Primidone	Chlorpromazine
Griseofulvin	Diazepam
Cigarette smoke	Dexamethasone Prednisone Methadone

Patient Variation in Drug Metabolism

Much of the observed difference in drug effects from one patient to the other is due to differences in drug metabolism caused by a variety of factors that determine the ability of a specific patient to metabolize a specific drug at a specific time:

1. Genetic influences: Some acetylation and oxidative reactions have ethnic and familial patterns.

2. Age: Neonates and older adults may have reduced drug metabolism.
3. Pregnancy: Drug metabolism may be increased or decreased during pregnancy.
4. Liver disease: The rate of elimination of high-clearance drugs may be reduced.
5. Time of day: Circadian rhythm has some effect on drug metabolism.
6. Environment: Smoking, air pollution, and exposure to industrial chemicals may affect drug metabolism.
7. Diet: Drug metabolism may be affected by food–drug interactions or by malnutrition.
8. Alcohol: **Alcohol** may cause induction of drug metabolism.
9. Drug interactions: The concentration or function of various hepatic enzymes may change.

Drug Elimination

Drug elimination refers to the excretion of drugs and their transport outside the body. Some drugs are excreted unchanged, and others are metabolized by the body. In excretion, a drug is removed from tissues and circulation. Most drugs and drug metabolites are excreted by the kidney through active and passive mechanisms. The biliary route of excretion is important for some drugs, such as **ampicillin** and **rifampin**, and is the beginning of enterohepatic recirculation, which is important for a few drugs, such as **digoxin** and the **estrogens**. Drugs can also be excreted by the lungs and skin, and via breast milk and sweat.

Renal Excretion

Renal excretion is by far the most common method of excretion from the body. The kidney usually removes a drug that is unbound and free in the plasma. Renal excretion is the net effect of three different mechanisms within the kidney: (1) glomerular filtration, (2) tubular secretion, and (3) tubular reabsorption.

Glomerular Filtration

In glomerular filtration, blood flows into the glomeruli in the kidney; and the diffusion of fluids and solutes across the glomerular membrane is passive. In a healthy adult, up to 130 mL/min of fluid crosses this membrane. Three factors determine whether a drug will be filtered: molecular size, protein binding, and glomerular integrity and function. Drugs dissolved in plasma can cross the membrane, whereas drugs that are protein bound or have a molecular weight higher than 60,000 are not filtered. Renal disease alters glomerular function and drug excretion.

Tubular Secretion

Some drugs undergo tubular secretion, during which they are actively secreted from the proximal tubule into the urine. These drugs, primarily weak acids, are secreted by processes that may be subject to competition from other drugs or chemicals in the body that are also actively secreted. For example, **probenecid** and **penicillin** are both secreted from the tubule; if given together, they compete, and **penicillin** is secreted more slowly in the presence of **probenecid**. In this particular case, the drug interaction can be used to prolong the effect of **penicillin**.

Tubular Reabsorption

Most drugs undergo tubular reabsorption passively in the distal tubules for drugs that are lipid soluble or not highly ionized. Tubular reabsorption is dependent on the physical and chemical properties of the drug and the pH of the urine. Drugs that are ionized at urine pH have less tubular reabsorption and tend to be excreted. Any change in the pH of the urine influences the excretion process. It is the ionized portion of the drug molecule that is water soluble and can be excreted by the kidney. Weak acids are excreted more rapidly in alkaline urine; weak bases are excreted more rapidly in acid urine. The rate of excretion can be changed for these drugs by changing the pH of the urine with other drugs. For example, an overdose of a weak base such as **amphetamine** can be eliminated from the body more quickly by acidifying the urine with ammonium chloride.

Biliary Excretion

Many drugs are actively transported by the liver cells from blood to bile. These drugs, or a conjugated metabolite of a drug, are excreted in the bile and enter the GI tract, where they are excreted in the feces. Some of these conjugates can be broken down by enzymes in the gut bacteria to liberate the original drug, which may be reabsorbed into the body through intestinal absorption. This enterohepatic reabsorption may be interfered with by oral **antibiotics** that remove the gut bacteria; this is the mechanism of the interaction between **oral contraceptives** and **antibiotics**. Biliary excretion may serve as an alternative route of elimination of some drugs, such as **digoxin** and **oxazepam**, in patients with renal impairment.

Other Routes of Excretion

Drugs are eliminated through the lungs, skin, saliva, tears, and, in lactating women, the mammary glands. Pulmonary excretion occurs commonly with drugs administered by inhalation or drugs in a vapor state. The pulmonary excretion of **alcohol**, for example, is the basis of the **alcohol** breath test that is correlated to blood **alcohol** levels. Drugs can also be excreted by the skin, sweat, saliva, and tears. Although these routes seldom result in significant loss of drug concentration, they may be important to some patients if an adverse drug reaction occurs such as a skin rash caused by skin excretion. Excretion in the saliva is the reason patients will experience a metallic taste with some medications; the medication is excreted in the saliva and passes into the GI system when swallowed.

Biological Half-Life

The half-life of a drug is the amount of time it takes to eliminate one-half of the drug from the body and is depicted in Figure 2–9. The half-life of a drug ultimately determines how often a drug is administered. The half-life is usually not dose dependent; therefore, doubling the dose does not double the half-life. The half-life for a given drug generally remains the same for a given patient, but a patient with renal or hepatic disease may have increased drug half-life. Generally it takes 4 to 5 half-lives for a drug to reach steady state when given continuously and 4 to 5 half-lives to be totally eliminated from the body when a drug is discontinued. Half-life is an important variable to consider for solving problems concerning time:

1. Estimating the time needed to reach steady-state plasma concentration after the change of a maintenance dose.
2. Estimating the time required to eliminate all or a portion of a discontinued drug from the body.
3. Predicting the plasma levels following the initiation of therapy.
4. Determining the dose interval needed to provide a desired fluctuation in plasma concentration during that interval.
5. Determining the fluctuation in plasma concentrations, given a specific dosing interval.

SUMMARY

An understanding of pharmacodynamic and pharmacokinetic principles is critical to the safe prescribing of medications. The prescriber needs to understand the developmental and disease-related differences in pharmacokinetics that may affect the choice of medications for a specific patient.

Box 2–1 contains a glossary of common pharmacological terms the prescriber needs for Unit II and Unit III of this text.

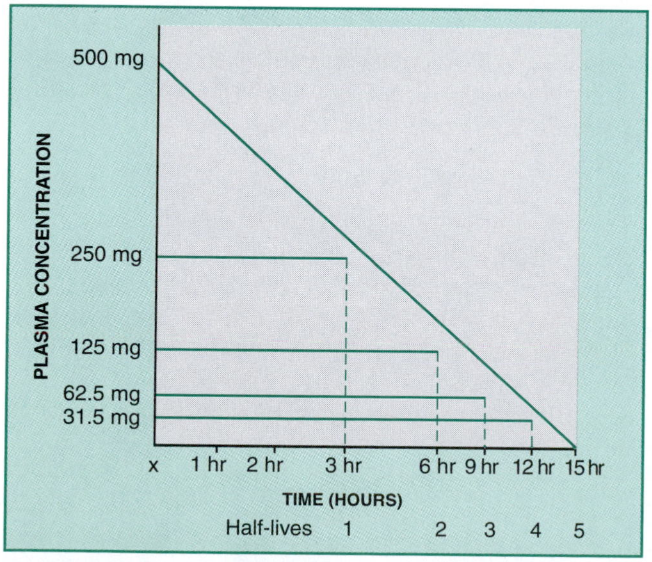

Figure 2–9. Elimination half-life determination. *(From Kuhn, M. A. [1998]. Pharmacotherapeutics: A nursing process approach [4th ed., p. 43]. Philadelphia: F. A. Davis, with permission.)*

BOX 2–1 GLOSSARY OF COMMON PHARMACOLOGY TERMS

Pharmacodynamic Terms

Receptor agonist: drug is a "perfect fit" on the receptor site
Receptor antagonist: drug blocks or competes for the receptor site
Tolerance: drug produces decreased physiological response after repeated doses of a drug
Tachyphylaxis: patient has quickly developing tolerance; initial response cannot be repeated, higher doses needed
Cumulative effect: there is a buildup of a drug
Idiosyncrasy: patient has abnormal or peculiar response to a drug
Drug dependence: patient has a physiological withdrawal syndrome if the drug is stopped
Drug interaction: effects of drug are modified by another drug
Drug antagonism: combined effect of two drugs is less than sum of two drugs given separately
Summation: AKA Additive effect—combining two drugs produces effect that is the sum of the individual drugs
Synergism: AKA synergistic effect—combining two drugs produces an effect that is greater than the sum of the two drugs
Potentiation: concurrent administration of drugs increases effect of another drug

Pharmacokinetic Terms

Absorption: the movement of a drug from it site of administration into the blood. Variables that influence absorption: Nature of the cell membrane; Blood flow at site of administration; Solubility of drug; pH; Molecular weight; Drug concentration
Distribution: the movement of absorbed drug in bodily fluids throughout body to target tissues
Metabolism: the enzymatic alteration of drug structure to

1. Enhance excretion
2. Inactivate the drug
3. Increase therapeutic action
4. Activate a prodrug
5. Increase or decrease toxicity

Elimination: removal of the drug from the body by organs of elimination

REFERENCES

Adams, M. P., & Koch, R. W. (2010). *Pharmacology: Connections to nursing practice*. Upper Saddle River, NJ: Pearson.

Burton, L., Lazo, J., & Parker, K. (2005). *Goodman & Gilman: The pharmacological basis of therapeutics* (11th ed.). New York: McGraw-Hill.

Rakhmanina, N. Y., & van den Anker, J. N. (2006). Pharmacological research in pediatrics: From neonates to adolescents. *Advanced Drug Delivery Reviews, 58,* 4–14.

Ulbricht, W. (2005). Sodium channel inactivation: Molecular determinants and modulation. *Physiology Review, 85*(4), 1271–1301.

Whitebread, S., Hamon, J., Bojanic, D., Urban, L., Whitebread, S., & Hamon, J., et al. (2005). Keynote review: In vitro safety pharmacology profiling: An essential tool for successful drug development. *Drug Discovery Today, 10,* 1421–1433.

CHAPTER 3

RATIONAL DRUG SELECTION

Teri Moser Woo

Chapter Outline

The process of prescribing medication requires a thoughtful, evidence-based approach to drug selection. The World Health Organization (WHO) definition of rational drug selection is that "patients receive medications appropriate to their clinical needs, in doses that meet their own individual requirements, for an adequate period of time, and at the lowest cost to them and their community" (WHO, 2010). WHO states that irrational use of medication is a "major problem" worldwide with an estimated 50 percent of drugs prescribed, dispensed, or sold inappropriately (2010). This chapter discusses the process of rational drug selection and the drug factors that influence drug selection as well as influences on rational prescribing.

THE PROCESS OF RATIONAL DRUG PRESCRIBING

Thoughtful prescribing requires a systematic process that is used every time a prescription is written. The WHO model for rational drug prescribing is one approach a provider can use (de Vries, Henning, Hogerzeil, & Fresle, 1994). The first step in the WHO process is an accurate diagnosis and a determination of the therapeutic objective, for example, treating an infection. The appropriate treatment is chosen with these factors in mind. It is critical that the provider collaborates with and educates the patient regarding the therapy. The chosen therapy then needs to be monitored to determine the effectiveness of the regimen (Box 3–1).

BOX 3–1 WORLD HEALTH ORGANIZATION'S SIX-STEP MODEL OF RATIONAL PRESCRIBING

Step	Description
Step 1	Define the patient's problem.
Step 2	Specify the therapeutic objective.
Step 3	Choose the treatment.
Step 4	Start the treatment.
Step 5	Educate the patient.
Step 6	Monitor effectiveness.

Source: de Vries, T. P., Henning, R. H., Hogerzeil, H. V., & Fresle, D. A. (1994). *Guide to good prescribing.* WHO/DAP/94.11. Geneva, Switzerland: World Health Organization.

Define the Patient's Problem

The process of prescribing begins with the assessment of the patient and formulation of a working diagnosis and possible differential diagnosis. Is there a clear indication for drug therapy after the diagnosis? What drugs are effective in treating this disorder? Differential diagnosis is not within the scope of this book, but the reader will find the diagnostic criteria and pathophysiology of common diseases treated with medications discussed in the chapters in Unit III.

Specify the Therapeutic Objective

Before deciding what medication to prescribe, it is important to clarify the therapeutic objective (de Vries et al, 1994). Is the goal to cure the disease? Relieve symptoms of disease? Replace deficiencies (i.e., insulin or iron)? Long-term prevention? Or is the goal treating the combination of two outcomes such as treating pain and inflammation. Sometimes the goal is to make the patient comfortable with palliative therapy. Maxwell suggests that the provider clarifies whether the treatment goals are curative, symptom relieving, or preventive (2009). The WHO model recommends that the provider include the patient in this stage of the process so the patient is a partner in the treatment regimen (de Vries et al, 1994). Eliciting patient beliefs and preferences regarding the drug therapy is essential to successful drug therapy, especially in chronic diseases, such as diabetes, that require long-term drug treatment (Latter et al, 2010). When the goal is long-term therapy for a chronic disease, it is necessary to look at costs and how well the drug fits into the patient's lifestyle. Factors that influence positive medicine-taking behavior are discussed in depth in Chapter 6.

Choose the Treatment

Determining the drug treatment is actually a two-step process of first determining what would be the appropriate therapy based on evidence-based guidelines, then individualizing the drug choice for the specific patient (Richir, Tichelaar, Geijtemann, & de Vries, 2007). Individualizing the drug choice includes consideration of other drugs that the patient may be taking and potential interactions with the drug treatment choice being made. Richir and colleagues (2007) describe two types of reasoning used when choosing drug therapy: analytical and nonanalytical. Novice providers use an analytical approach, which is slow, time consuming, systematic, and evidence-based. More experienced providers use their experience and pattern recognition to carry out a nonanalytical process in a faster, subconscious manner (Richir et al, 2007). When experienced providers are confronted with a complex patient situation, they will use a more analytical, systematic approach to prescribing.

Individualizing drug therapy requires examining the suitability of the drug for the patient. WHO recommends that the provider examine the drug and the dose, the dosage schedule, duration of treatment, effectiveness, and safety (de Vries et al, 1994). The criteria for examining a drug for appropriate prescribing is discussed later in this chapter. A mnemonic that new prescribers can use when learning to prescribe is proposed by Iglar, Kennie, and Bajcar (2007) and is summarized in Box 3–2. Table 3–1 provides an example of the use of the mnemonic.

Start the Treatment

Once the appropriate drug has been chosen, a prescription is written, and the patient must have the prescription dispensed at a pharmacy. The legal requirements for writing a prescription are discussed in Chapter 4.

Care should be taken when writing a prescription to make sure that the drug, dose, and schedule are accurate. At the time of writing the prescription, drug costs need to be addressed with the patient. If patients cannot afford to fill the prescription, they will not take the medication, regardless of how appropriate the drug is for the disease process. The pharmacoeconomic aspects of prescribing are discussed in depth in Chapter 12.

Educate the Patient

Up to 50 percent of patients do not take their medications as prescribed or they do not take them at all (de Vries et al, 1994). Poor medication adherence leads to worsening disease and death, as well as increased health-care costs; 33 to 69 percent of medication-related hospital admissions are related to poor adherence, at a cost of $100 billion per year (Osterberg & Blaschke, 2005). Patient education regarding the purpose of the medication, instructions for administration, and potential adverse drug effects will improve adherence to the medication regimen. Patient education should be tailored to the patient and presented at the appropriate health literacy level (fifth- or sixth- grade reading level), with an understanding

BOX 3–2 THE I CAN PRESCRIBE A DRUG MNEMONIC

Indication
Contraindications
Precautions
Cost/**C**ompliance
Efficacy
Adverse effects
Dose/**D**uration/**D**irection

Source: Iglar, K., Kennie, N., & Bajcar, J. (2007). I can PresCribE a Drug: Mnemonic-based teaching of rational prescribing. *Family Medicine, 39*(4), 236–240.

Table 3–1 **Example of the Use of the I Can PresCribE a Drug Mnemonic**

Case: A 23-yr-old female presents to the clinic with symptoms of a urinary tract infection (UTI). Urine analysis confirms initial diagnosis of UTI and a urine culture is pending.	
Indication	Antibiotics are indicated in UTI treatment. Treatment guidelines for UTIs are found in Chapter 47. Sulfamethoxazole and trimethoprim (SMZ-TMP, Septra, Bactrim) is the recommended first-line drug in most patients.
Contraindications	SMZ-TMP is contraindicated in patients who are allergic or who have allergies to drugs with known cross-sensitivity to sulfa drugs (discussed in Chapter 24), porphyria, megaloblastic anemia due to folate deficiency.
Precautions	SMZ-TMP is Pregnancy Category C. Use cautiously in patients with G-6-PD deficiency, impaired renal function, or hepatic function. Potential drug–drug interactions should be evaluated.
Cost/Compliance	SMZ-TMP is on the $4 list of many retail pharmacies. It is dosed twice a day for 3 d for UTI. Fewer doses and shorter treatment length have higher compliance.
Efficacy	*E. coli* is the most common pathogen in UTI and is usually sensitive to SMZ-TMP. Culture results will need to be followed to determine sensitivity.
Adverse effects	Adverse effects of SMZ-TMP are discussed in Chapter 24.
Dose/Duration/Direction	Dose: 1 double-strength tablet twice a day. Duration: 3 d Direction: Drink plenty of fluids while taking SMZ-TMP.

that 9 out of 10 adults have difficult reading health information (Centers for Disease Control and Prevention [CDC], 2010). Appropriate patient education is discussed for each drug category in the chapters in Unit II.

Monitor Effectiveness

Once the patient begins taking the prescribed medication, the chosen drug needs to be monitored for effectiveness. The WHO model describes two types of monitoring: passive and active (de Vries et al, 1994). Passive monitoring occurs when the patient is educated on the expected outcome of the drug therapy and is instructed to contact the provider if the treatment is not effective or if adverse drug effects occur. This is common when short-term treatment, such as an antibiotic, is prescribed, and no test of cure is required. Active monitoring occurs when the provider schedules a follow-up examination to determine the effectiveness of the drug therapy (de Vries et al, 1994). Active monitoring may include evaluating therapeutic blood levels and making dosage adjustments, as is needed in anticoagulant therapy or patients taking an antiseizure medication. Active monitoring may also include adding or subtracting medications from the treatment regimen based on the effectiveness of the treatment. Monitoring parameters are often published for a drug, but may need to be adjusted based on age or concurrent disease processes.

CLINICAL PEARL

Drugs don't work in patients who don't take them.
—C. Everett Koop, MD

At the follow-up visit, the provider will determine whether to continue the medication. If the treatment has been effective and the disease has been cured, the drug can be stopped. The treatment can also be effective but not curative, as in the case of chronic disease management. If the drug is working well for the patient, then it should be continued. If the medication is not effective or if the patient experiences significant adverse effects, the drug may need to be changed. Even an appropriately chosen medication will not work in every patient; therefore, evaluating the effectiveness of therapy and making adjustments as needed are essential.

DRUG FACTORS INFLUENCING DRUG SELECTION

Evidence-based guidelines are the gold standard for initial drug selection, but providers need to examine the drugs recommended in the guideline for their clinical utility with the individual patient. Selecting the appropriate drug treatment requires that the provider consider multiple factors regarding the drug and the patient who will be receiving the medication: pharmacokinetics, pharmacodynamics, therapeutic issues, safety, and cost (Spector & Vesell, 2002). Additionally, individual patient and provider factors may influence drug choice. The nurse practitioner should review and consider all seven of these criteria prior to prescribing (Spector & Vesell, 2002).

Pharmacodynamic Factors

The pharmacodynamics of a drug must be specific and selective to the target tissues affected by the disease to have the greatest therapeutic effect with the least adverse effects (Spector & Vesell, 2002). The ease of titration is influenced by the dose-response curve of the drug (Maxwell, 2009). The relationship between a drug's desired therapeutic effects and its adverse effects is called its therapeutic index (see Chap. 2). Drugs with a low or narrow therapeutic index may require close monitoring for toxicity or adverse effects, whereas drugs with a wide therapeutic index are fairly safe and require less monitoring. **Antibiotics**, for example, tend to have fairly wide therapeutic indices. **Propranolol (Inderal)** has such a wide therapeutic index that doses safely range from 20 mg to 320 mg.

Pharmacokinetic Factors

When deciding what drug in a class to prescribe, the pharmacokinetic properties of a drug may influence drug selection. For example the bioavailability (BA) of different formulations may influence prescribing (Maxwell, 2009). For instance, the bioavailability of **digoxin** varies between 60 and 100 percent depending on the formulation used. Because this drug has a very narrow therapeutic index, this difference in BA is critical in formulation choice. Another consideration is metabolism. Different drugs in a class may use different cytochrome P450 (CYP450) enzymes, which may influence metabolism or drug interactions. Drugs that are excreted almost exclusively by the kidney may not be appropriate for a patient with decreased renal function, such as the older adult. Therefore, a patient's renal function and the pharmacokinetics of the drug need to be evaluated during the drug selection process. Additionally, the dose-concentration curve and half-life will determine the dosing schedule, with fewer doses per day encouraging adherence to the drug regimen (Maxwell, 2009; Spector & Vesell, 2002). Pharmacokinetics are discussed in depth in Chapter 2.

Therapeutic Factors

The therapeutic impact of a drug is reviewed in the literature and observed in the individual patient. A nurse practitioner examines the evidence for the therapeutic impact of a selected drug, using evidence from clinical trials, clinical practice guidelines, and systematic reviews (including *Cochrane Reviews* or *Clinical Evidence Reviews*) to determine the impact of a drug. The effect of a drug on decreasing morbidity, mortality, and hospitalization is examined (Spector & Vesell, 2002) as well as the drug's ability to relieve symptoms and treat the disease process (Maxwell, 2009). Extrapolating results from randomized controlled trials (RCTs) should be done with caution because RCTs usually recruit patients who are relatively healthy with few comorbidities, whereas most patients are more complex (Maxwell, 2009).

Safety

The safety profile of a drug is taken into consideration and weighed against other factors when prescribing. Safety is initially determined in clinical trials and is outlined in the precautions and contraindications in the drug monograph. Safety may vary with the population; for example, a drug may be safe in a healthy elder but also be a teratogen; thus, it would be unsafe in pregnant women (Iglar et al, 2007). Safety may also vary with the disease process; for example, some drugs have safety concerns in patients with liver or renal dysfunction. Contraindications to a drug in a specific patient population or allergy to the drug eliminate it from the potential drugs that can be prescribed for the patient.

The U.S. Food and Drug Administration (FDA) collects information on and monitors the safety of drugs via postmarketing surveillance by the MedWatch program (http://www.fda.gov/Safety/Medwatch). The FDA has a tiered system of safety announcements to promote drug safety. The agency gathers initial reports via MedWatch; then, it issues an early communication about an "Ongoing Safety Review" while it collects and analyzes data (http://www.fda.gov). The FDA issues a "Public Health Advisory" when there is drug safety information that needs to be conveyed to patients or caregivers. When new drug information affects safe prescribing, the FDA may issue a "Letter to Health Care Professionals" or an "Information for Health Care Professionals" information sheet to provide specifics about the safety issue and factors to consider when making treatment decisions. When drugs are determined by the FDA to have serious safety issues, particularly ones that may lead to serious injury or death, the FDA may require a warning to be displayed prominently on the drug monograph, often referred to as a "Black Box" warning. Prescribers are responsible for keeping up to date on the latest drug safety information.

Cost

When prescribing, the nurse practitioner must consider the costs to the patient and the cost to the health-care system or to society at large. The cost to patients may be so high that they cannot afford prescriptions, and cost then becomes a barrier to adherence. Many insurance policies do not cover the cost of drugs, and patients must therefore pay out of pocket for their medications. Medicare patients with Part D coverage may reach the "donut hole," the coverage gap between $2,250 and $5,100 in drug costs where the proportion of out of pocket costs goes up to 50%. This coverage gap will slowly be decreased to 25% for generic drugs by 2020, but

Medicare patients will still pay 50% of brand name drug costs while in the coverage gap.

Increasingly, as soon as the patent on a brand-name drug expires, that drug is made in a generic form. Prescribing generics when possible and knowing what drugs are on the $4 retail pharmacy prescription lists assists in keeping costs reasonable for the patient. For example, **albuterol** nebulizer solution (20 mL) is on the Walmart $4 list, whereas generic albuterol nebulizer solution (20 mL bottle) is $20.60 at www.drugstore.com. Knowing the approximate costs of medications and discussing with clients their out-of-pocket costs will improve adherence. Drug costs are shown in the Available Dosage Forms tables for each drug category in the chapters in Unit II.

Prescription drug spending has increased significantly over the past few years, from $239.9 billion in 2004 to $291.5 billion in 2008 (IMS Health, 2009). Although the out-of-pocket costs to patients may be acceptable to them, providers still need to consider the actual costs of the medications to the health system. Each prescriber plays a part in controlling prescription drug expenditures through thoughtful prescribing of the most cost-effective drug for the patient. The pharmacoeconomics of prescribing are discussed in depth in Chapter 12.

Patient Factors

Patient factors that may affect prescribing include drug adverse effects that influence adherence, health beliefs, values, and current drug therapy that may interfere with the new drug (Maxwell, 2009; Spector & Vesell, 2002). In addition to interference with the new drug, unnecessary duplications with other drugs being taken may occur. Any time a regimen can be simplified by reducing duplication, adherence is more likely. Other patient factors that affect prescribing are the patient's age (children and older adults), pregnancy, mental health diagnosis, or another disease. **Beta blockers,** for example, have adverse drug reactions (ADRs) that include anxiety, depression, and mental status changes. The drugs in this class that have higher central nervous system (CNS) penetration are more likely to have these ADRs. If a **beta blocker** is to be prescribed for a patient with a mental health diagnosis, it is best to use the ones that are less lipophilic because this subset of the drug class is less likely to exhibit these ADRs.

Previous Adverse Drug Reactions

ADRs can be a significant factor in nonadherence. Some patients, such as those with renal dysfunction, are at higher risk of experiencing ADRs. Exploration of previous experiences with medications will identify those at risk for ADRs (Maxwell, 2009). Listening to the patient and noting unusual responses is a proactive approach to prescribing. Remembering each patient's response to a medication may differ and taking the time to carefully choose a medication that has the fewest ADRs will promote adherence. Chapter 5 provides an extensive discussion of ADRs.

Health Beliefs

Health beliefs and patient attitudes both affect the medication regimen. Patients who believe the medication is going to help them feel better or prevent long-term harm are more likely to adhere to the drug regimen and to have positive outcomes from taking the drug. For example, in patients taking mood-stabilizer medication, beliefs about themselves and control over the disorder had more influence on adherence than did adverse drug reactions (Scott, 2002). Belief that one does not have asthma when symptoms are absent is more common among older asthmatics with poor health literacy, leading to nonadherence in use of asthma medications (Federman, Wisnivesky, Wolf, Leventhal, & Halm, 2010). Assessment of beliefs and attitudes is critical to medication adherence.

Current Drug Therapy

A patient's current drug therapy may affect the drug selected or the dosage prescribed because of the potential for drug interactions (Maxwell, 2009). Throughout this text potential drug interactions are listed for each drug category, with suggested alteration in therapy if needed. If a patient is on a complex medication regimen, consultation with a pharmacist or PharmD who has access to drug interaction software is warranted for patient safety.

Patient Age

Patients at the extremes of age, either the very young or the very old, have developmental pharmacokinetic differences that warrant careful prescribing. Infants have immature liver and renal function that place them at risk for toxicity and ADRs, and may require dosage adjustments based on age. Likewise, the elderly population has decreased liver and renal functions related to the physiological changes associated with aging, placing them at risk for increased ADRs. Prescribing for children is discussed in Chapter 50 and prescribing for geriatric patients is discussed in Chapter 51.

Pregnancy

Pregnant patients pose a challenge to the prescriber. Early in pregnancy, there is a risk for drugs being teratogenic to the fetus. The FDA assigns a pregnancy category to prescription drugs, rating them as Pregnancy Category C, D, or X, known to cause fetal harm (U.S. Food and Drug Administration, 2009). Later in pregnancy, drugs may cause fetal adverse effects, such as tachycardia or stroke, or may cause the fetus to abort during premature labor. The National Library of Medicine TOXNET Developmental and Reproductive Toxicology Database (DART) is a Web-based databank of the latest information on the developmental and reproductive effects of drugs (http://toxnet.nlm.nih.gov). Drugs in pregnancy are discussed in the Precautions and Contraindications sections for each drug class and in Chapter 48.

Provider Factors

Ease of Prescribing or Monitoring

Providers often develop a personal formulary of drugs with which they are familiar and that they are comfortable prescribing (Maxwell, 2009). Unfamiliar medications require the provider to research the drug and educate themselves in order to prescribe the drug safely. The amount of provider follow-up required, whether it is titrating doses or therapeutic monitoring may influence prescribing decisions (Maxwell, 2009; Spector & Vesell, 2002).

Formularies

Many health insurance plans have restricted formularies and the provider must prescribe from the formulary or the patient may have significant additional out-of-pocket costs. The restricted formulary of many health plans requires that nurse practitioners move away from their personal formulary. Nurse practitioners need to be familiar with the formulary of medications they are allowed to prescribe from and to keep themselves updated as formularies change (Spector & Vesell, 2002).

INFLUENCES ON RATIONAL PRESCRIBING

Pharmaceutical Promotion

In 2008 the pharmaceutical industry was one of the top three most profitable industries on *FORTUNE* magazine's FORTUNE 500 list (CNNMoney/FORTUNE 500, 2008). Pharmaceutical companies fund many academic research studies. There have been reports of some of these studies not publishing negative results of industry-sponsored clinical trials (Institute of Medicine, 2009). Pharmaceutical companies also offer free dinners, gifts, and free drug samples to providers to raise awareness of their product and to influence prescribing (Wilkes & Hoffman, 2001). Gifts range from small items such as pens and coffee mugs to medical textbooks and equipment (Wilkes & Hoffman, 2001). The Institute of Medicine issued a report in 2009 regarding the conflicts of interest and noted the influence of meals and gifts on physician prescribing, stating, "Data suggest that these relationships may influence physicians to prescribe a company's medicines even when evidence indicates another drug would be more beneficial" (p. 3).

There has been little research regarding the influence of pharmaceutical marketing on nurse practitioner (NP) prescribing practice. Blunt (2005) surveyed NPs ($N = 393$) regarding the influence of pharmaceutical company education and gifts, and 80 percent of respondents reported that they changed their prescribing practices after pharmaceutical company education or interaction with a drug representative. In focus groups of geriatric nurse practitioners (GNP) exploring prescriptive decision making, the GNPs reported skepticism regarding the information provided by pharmaceutical representatives. They noted that the studies presented to them often excluded their geriatric patients in the sample, thus making the information provided of little use for their practice (Mahoney & Ladd, 2010). Mahoney and Ladd noted that the participants of their focus groups felt their nursing background influenced their prescribing, and that GNPs have a more holistic approach to prescribing than do physicians. More research is needed regarding the influence of pharmaceutical marketing and education on NP prescribing.

In light of the influence that pharmaceutical marketing has on prescribing, professional organizations have issued statements regarding such marketing. The Institute of Medicine recommends conflicts of interest and financial relationships be disclosed by those providing education and that providers limit the use of drug samples to patients who do not have financial access to medication (Institute of Medicine, 2009). The Pharmaceutical Research and Manufacturers of America (PhRMA) has developed its Code on Interactions with Healthcare Professionals, stating a commitment to high ethical standards in the marketing of pharmaceutical products (PhRMA, 2010). NP prescribers need to be aware of the influences of all aspects of pharmaceutical marketing on their prescribing.

When Prescribing Recommendations Change

The approach of expert providers may serve them well most of the time, but when guidelines change or new evidence becomes available, expert providers may need to be coached or reeducated regarding appropriate prescribing. Prior to the 1990s antibiotics were widely prescribed for upper respiratory infections. The excessive and inappropriate use of anti-infectious agents became a major factor in drug resistance (Bishai, Morris, & Scanland, 2004; CDC, 2009; Linares, Ardanuy, Pallares, & Fenoll, 2010).

The emergence of antibiotic resistance due to antibiotic over-prescribing led to a need to shift attitudes and prescribing patterns. The CDC developed the "Get Smart" campaign, with a similar STAR (Stemming the Tide of Antibiotic Resistance) campaign conducted in the United Kingdom (Bekkers et al, 2010; CDC, 2009). The CDC employed an intervention of collaboration with the medical professional organizations and intensive education regarding appropriate prescribing of antibiotics. The STAR program used Social Learning Theory, online-learning, and context bound learning to change attitudes about prescribing antibiotics (Bekkers et al, 2010; Simpson et al, 2009). Changing engrained prescribing behavior is essential to reducing antibiotic resistance and each prescriber is responsible for thoughtful prescribing of antibiotics to prevent resistance.

The changing recommendations regarding prescribing antibiotics is just one example of how prescribing recommendations may change and the necessity that prescribers keep up-to-date on the current guidelines for prescribing.

REFERENCES

Bekkers, M. J., Simpson, S. A., Dunstan, F., Hood, K., Hare, M., Evans, J., et al, and the STAR study team. (2010). Enhancing the quality of antibiotic prescribing in primary care: Qualitative evaluation of a blended learning intervention. *BMC Family Practice, 11*(24). Retrieved from http://www.biomedcentral.com/1471-2296/11/34

Bishai, W., Morris, C., & Scanland, S. (2004). Treatment of community acquired pneumonia. *Clinician Reviews,* New York: Jobson Publishing. Retrieved November 29, 2010 from http://www.clinicianreviews.com/index.asp?page=/courses/3061/disclaimer.htm

Blunt, E. (2005). Do "pharma" perks sway patient care? *Holistic Nursing Practice, 19*(5), 242.

Centers for Disease Control and Prevention (CDC). (2009). Get smart: Know when antibiotics work. Treatment guidelines for upper respiratory tract infections. Retrieved from http://www.cdc.gov/getsmart/campaign-materials/treatment-guidelines.html

Centers for Disease Control and Prevention (CDC). (2010). Call to action to improve health literacy. Retrieved from http://www.cdc.gov/features/healthliteracy/

CNNMoney/FORTUNE (2008). FORTUNE 500: Our annual ranking of America's largest corporations. Top industries: Most profitable. *CNN Money.com.* Retrieved from http://money.cnn.com/magazines/fortune/fortune500/2008/performers/industries/profits/

de Vries, T. P., Henning, R. H., Hogerzeil, H. V., & Fresle, D. A. (1994). *Guide to good prescribing.* WHO/DAP/94.11. Geneva, Switzerland: World Health Organization.

Federman, A. D., Wisnivesky, J. P., Wolf, M. S., Leventhal, H., & Halm, E. A. (2010). Inadequate health literacy is associated with suboptimal health beliefs in older asthmatics. *Journal of Asthma: Official Journal of the Association for the Care of Asthma, 47*(6), 620–626.

Iglar, K., Kennie, N., & Bajcar, J. (2007). I can PresCribE a Drug: Mnemonic-based teaching of rational prescribing. *Family Medicine, 39*(4), 236–240.

IMS Health. (2009). Channel distribution by U.S. sales. IMS National Sales Perspectives. Retrieved from http://www.imshealth.com/deployedfiles/imshealth/Global/Content/StaticFile/Top_Line_Data/2008_Channel_Distribution_by_U.S._Sales.pdf

Institute of Medicine. (2009). Conflict of interest in medical research, education, and practice. Report brief. Retrieved from http://www.iom.edu/~/imedia/Files/Report%20Files/2009/Conflict-of-Interest-in-Medical-Research-Education-and-Practice/COI%20report%20brief%20for%20web.pdf

Latter, S., Sibley, A., Skinner, T. C., Cradock, S., Zinken, K. M., Lussier, M. T., et al. (2010). The impact of an intervention for nurse prescribers on consultation to promote medicine-taking in diabetes: A mixed methods study. *International Journal of Nursing Studies, 47,* 1126–1138.

Linares, J., Ardanuy, C., Pallares, R., & Fenoll, A. (2010). Changes in antimicrobial resistance, serotypes and genotypes in *Streptococcus pneumoniae* over a 30-year period. *Clinical Microbiology and Infection, 16,* 402–410.

Mahoney, D. F., & Ladd, E. (2010). More than a prescriber: Gerontological nurse practitioners' perspectives on prescribing and pharmaceutical marketing. *Geriatric Nursing, 31,* 17–27.

Maxwell, S. (2009). Rational prescribing: The principles of drug selection. *Clinical Medicine, 9*(5), 481–485.

Osterberg, L., & Blaschke, T. (2005). Drug therapy: Adherence to medication. *New England Journal of Medicine, 353*(5), 487–497.

Pharmaceutical Research and Manufacturers of America (PhRMA). (2010). Code on interactions with healthcare professionals. Retrieved from http://www.phrma.org/code_on_interactions_with_healthcare_professionals

Raebel, M. A., Carroll, N. M., Kelleher, J. A., Chester, E. A., Berca, S., & Macid, D. J. (2007). Randomized trial to improve prescribing safety during pregnancy. *Journal of the American Medical Informatics Association, 14,* 440–450.

Richir, M. C., Tichelaar, J., Geijtemann, E. C. T., & de Vries, T. P. G. M. (2007). Teaching clinical pharmacology and therapeutics with an emphasis on therapeutic reasoning of undergraduate medical students. *European Journal of Clinical Pharmacology, 64*(2), 217–224.

Scott, J. (2002). Using health belief models to understand the efficacy-effectiveness gap for mood stabilizer treatments. *Neuropsychobiology, 46*(Suppl. 1), 13–15.

Simpson, S. A., Butler, C. C., Hood, K., Cohen, D., Dunstan, F., Evans, M. R., and the STAR Study Team. (2009). Stemming the Tide of Antibiotic Resistance (STAR): A protocol for a trial of a complex intervention addressing the "why" and "how" of appropriate antibiotic prescribing in general practice. *BMC Family Practice, 10*(20). Retrieved from http://www.biomedcentral.com/1471-2296/10/20

Spector, R., & Vesell, E. S. (2002). A rational approach to the selection of useful drugs for clinical practice. *Pharmacology, 65,* 57–61.

U.S. Food and Drug Administration. (2009). Pregnancy and lactation labeling. Retrieved from http://www.fda.gov/Drugs/DevelopmentApprovalProcess/DevelopmentResources/Labeling/ucm093307.htm

Waller, D. G. (2005). Rational prescribing: The principles of drug selection and assessment of efficacy. *Clinical Medicine, 5,* 26–28.

Wilkes, M. S., & Hoffman, J. R. (2001). An innovative approach to educating medical students about pharmaceutical promotion. *Academic Medicine, 76,* 1271–1277.

World Health Organization (WHO). (2010). Rational use of medicines. Retrieved from http://www.who.int/medicines/areas/rational_use/en/index.html

CHAPTER 4

LEGAL AND PROFESSIONAL ISSUES IN PRESCRIBING

Tracy Klein

Chapter Outline

FEDERAL DRUG LAW

History

The Food, Drug, and Cosmetic Act of 1906 was the first federal law designed to protect the public by restricting the manufacture and distribution of drugs. The law designated that drugs must meet official standards for strength and purity, and prohibited "the manufacture of adulterated or misbranded or poisonous or deleterious foods, drugs, medicines, and liquors" (U.S. Food and Drug Administration [FDA], 2010). Focusing primarily on how drugs were ultimately labeled or branded, it did not broadly prevent the manufacturing of unsafe or ineffective medications.

In 1937, a manufacturer marketed an elixir of **sulfanilamide** that used di-ethylene glycol as a solvent for the new antibiotic. Because its pharmacological effects were not tested, its toxicity went unnoticed until reports of more than 100 patient deaths were collected. The public outcry for new laws resulted in the federal Food, Drug, and Cosmetic Act of 1938 (FDA, 2010). This act has three basic principles that restrict drug adulteration, misbranding, and the interstate commerce of an unapproved drug. It also created the U.S. Food and Drug Administration (FDA). As a regulatory agency, the FDA was initially charged with enforcing new laws requiring that drugs were checked before they went to market. From 1938 to 1962, the approval of new drugs was based on safety. In the early 1960s, the use of **thalidomide** by women in the early stages of pregnancy resulted in the birth of hundreds of deformed babies in Europe. A tragedy of this scale was avoided in the United States because the drug was not approved for marketing here. This situation spurred the passage of the Kefauver-Harris amendments in 1962 (FDA, 2010). These amendments required that both safety and efficacy of a drug be proven before it is marketed. In addition, the act required that all drugs marketed from 1938 to 1962 be evaluated for efficacy. This study was performed by the National Academy of Sciences/National Research Council and called the Drug Efficacy Study Implementation (DESI). Thousands of drugs were studied, and ineffective drugs were withdrawn from the market.

Two additional acts have had considerable influence on improving drug availability and benefiting patients with rare diseases. The Orphan Drug Act of 1983 fosters orphan drug development for diseases so rare that the usual approval process would take decades to complete (FDA, 2010). The Drug Price Competition and Patent Term Restoration Act of 1984 expanded the number of generic drugs suitable for an abbreviated new drug application (ANDA). This makes it possible for generic drug companies to market generic versions of drugs by proving bioequivalence rather than duplicating the clinical trials needed for initial drug approval.

Another significant legislative act was the Pediatric Research Equity Act passed in 2003 (FDA, 2010). This act, referred to as the "Pediatric Rule," authorized the FDA to request pediatric studies of already marketed drugs, or to require studies by others if the manufacturer refuses. Since the passage of the Pediatric Rule, several drugs in common use for children were removed from the market, because their safety and efficacy had never been tested in pediatric subjects.

U.S. Food and Drug Administration Regulatory Jurisdiction

The FDA regulatory jurisdiction over drugs encompasses the standardization of nomenclature, the approval process for new drugs and new indications, official labeling, surveillance of adverse drug events, and methods of manufacture and distribution (FDA, 2009). The classification of a drug as a prescription or nonprescription medication is a matter of federal law. Products labeled with the legend "Caution: Federal law prohibits dispensing without a prescription" are regulated by the FDA and are referred to as *legend drugs*.

The FDA also regulates medical devices that meet criteria under the 1976 Medical Devices Amendment of the Food, Drug and Cosmetic Act (FDA, 2009). Examples of medical devices include ultrasound imaging equipment, artificial joints, and HIV testing kits.

Prior to 1997, the FDA strictly limited direct to consumer advertisements (FDA, 2010). However, such advertising is now commonplace, and studies show it holds increasing influence on consumer and prescriber decision making regarding medications. The federal Food, Drug, and Cosmetic Act provides that the advertising of prescription drugs must conform to the labeling. Any advertisement that describes a drug's use must contain the generic name and amount of active ingredient, the name and address of the manufacturer, and a brief summary of the prescribing information. A prescription drug advertisement that implies incorrectly that a drug is the treatment of choice or is useful for an off-labeled indication is unlawful. Drug manufacturers are increasingly marketing prescription drugs to patients through print and electronic media, which has increased the demand on practitioners to prescribe advertised drug products.

The New Drug Approval Process

The U.S. system of new drug approvals is perhaps the most rigorous in the world. On average, it costs a company $897 million to get one new medicine from the laboratory to the pharmacist's shelf, according to a 2003 Tufts University analysis for its Center for the Study of Drug Development, which included costs for drugs that were never marketed as well as postmarketing research (DiMasi, Hanson, & Grabowski, 2003). It takes 8.5 years on average for an experimental drug to travel from laboratory preclinical trials to FDA approval (Duke Clinical Research Institute, 2010).

Preclinical Research

The process of synthesis and extraction identifies new molecules with the potential to produce a desired change in a biological system (e.g., to inhibit or stimulate an important enzyme, to alter a metabolic pathway, or to change cellular structure). The process may require research on the fundamental mechanisms of disease or biological processes, research on the action of known therapeutic agents, or random selection and broad biological screening. New molecules can be produced through artificial synthesis or extracted from natural sources (plant, mineral, or animal). The number of active pharmaceutical ingredients that can be produced based on the same general chemical structure runs into the hundreds of millions.

Biological screening and pharmacological testing use nonhuman studies to explore the pharmacological activity and therapeutic potential of compounds. These tests involve the use of animals, isolated cell cultures and tissues, enzymes, and cloned receptor sites, as well as computer models. If the results of the tests suggest potential beneficial activity, related compounds are tested to see which version of the molecule produces the highest level of pharmacological activity and demonstrates the most therapeutic promise, with the smallest number of potentially harmful biological properties.

Pharmaceutical dosage formulation and stability testing make up the process of turning an active compound into a form and strength suitable for human use. A pharmaceutical product can take any one of a number of dosage forms (for example, liquid, tablets, capsules, ointments, sprays, patches) and dosage strengths.

Toxicology and safety testing determines the potential risk a compound poses to people and the environment. These studies use animals, tissue cultures, and other test systems to examine the relationship between factors such as dose level, frequency of administration, and duration of exposure to both the short- and the long-term survival of living organisms. Tests provide information on the dose-response pattern of the compound and its toxic effects. Most toxicology and safety testing is conducted on new molecular entities prior to their human introduction, but companies can choose to delay long-term toxicity testing until after the therapeutic potential of the product is established.

Clinical Studies

An investigational new drug (IND) application is filed with the FDA prior to human testing. The IND application is a compilation of all known information about the compound. It also includes a description of the clinical research plan for the product and the specific protocol for phase I study. Unless the FDA says no, the IND is automatically approved after 30 days, and clinical tests can begin. The FDA has formulated IND regulations for the clinical study of a new drug's safety and efficacy and has divided this evaluation into three phases:

1. Phase I clinical evaluation is the first testing of a new compound in subjects, for the purpose of establishing the tolerance of healthy human subjects at different doses, defining its pharmacological effects at anticipated therapeutic levels, and studying its absorption, distribution, metabolism, and excretion patterns in humans.
2. Phase II clinical evaluation is controlled studies performed on patients with the target disease or disorder to determine a compound's potential usefulness and short-term risks. A relatively small number of patients, usually no more than several hundred subjects, are enrolled in phase II studies.
3. Phase III trials are controlled and uncontrolled clinical trials of a drug's safety and efficacy in hospital and outpatient settings. Phase III studies gather precise information on the drug's efficacy for specific indications, determine whether the drug produces a broader range of adverse effects than those exhibited in the small study populations of phases I and II studies, and identify the best way of administering and using the drug for the purpose intended. If the drug is approved, this information forms the basis for deciding the content of the product label. Phase III trials verify that the acceptable risk/benefit ratio seen in phase II persists under conditions of anticipated usage and in groups of patients large enough to identify statistically and clinically significant responses.

Conferences between the sponsor and the FDA are held during all three phases of development. While an IND is in effect, the sponsor must report in writing to the FDA within 10 working days any serious and unexpected adverse reactions that may be drug related. The treatment IND program is part of the FDA's efforts to facilitate the development of significant new therapies. Under this program, treatment protocols using an investigational drug can be approved for life-threatening illnesses for which there is no comparable alternative therapy. Information on the availability of an investigational drug under a treatment IND is published in the *Journal of the American Medical Association* and other public means. Patients and families can learn about clinical trials and access to investigational drugs for cancer treatment through the National Cancer Institute's PDQ database available online. The National Institute of Health Clinical Center (NIH CC) Pharmacy Department Pharmaceutical Development Section maintains a database of investigational drugs, accessible at http://www.cc.nih.gov/phar.development.html and the NIH CC also sponsors an extensive database of clinical trials for a wide range of medical conditions that can be accessed online at http://clinicalstudies.info.nih.gov/.

Bioavailability Studies

Healthy volunteers are used to document the rate of absorption and excretion from the body of a compound's active ingredients. Companies conduct bioavailability studies both at the beginning of human testing and just prior to marketing to show that the formulation used to demonstrate safety and efficacy in clinical trials is equivalent to the product that will be distributed for sale. Companies also conduct bioavailability studies on marketed products whenever they change the method used to administer the drug (for example, from injection or oral dose form), the composition of the drug, the concentration of the active ingredient, or the manufacturing process used to produce the drug.

Regulatory Review: New Drug Application

To market a new drug for human use, a manufacturer must have a new drug application (NDA) approved by the FDA. All information about the drug gathered during the drug discovery and development process is assembled in the NDA. During the review period, the FDA may ask the company for additional information about the product or seek clarification of the data contained in the application. The FDA must review the NDA within 180 days. Usually, the FDA requests additional information, and the manufacturer needs from 1 to 5 years to complete any additional well-controlled trials necessary to support the claimed indications or prove the drug's safety.

Accelerated Approval of a New Drug Application

The timely availability of new drugs remains the subject of considerable debate. In December 1991, the FDA published new regulations to accelerate approval of certain new drugs that provide therapeutic benefit to patients with serious or life-threatening illnesses (FDA, 2010). The FDA can approve these drugs based on well-controlled clinical trials establishing that the product has an effect on a therapeutic end point that is likely to predict clinical benefit. The applicant is required to conduct postmarketing studies.

Postapproval Research

Clinical experience with a new drug may include no more than 1,000 to 2,000 patients. The detection of rare (less than 1 in 1,000) adverse drug reactions is not reliable until hundreds of thousands of patients have taken the drug. Clinical trials conducted after a drug is marketed (referred to as phase IV studies in the United States) are an important source of information on as-yet undetected adverse outcomes, especially in populations not included in the premarketing trials (e.g., children, the elderly, pregnant women), and the drug's long-term morbidity and mortality profile. Regulatory authorities can require companies to conduct phase IV studies as a condition of market approval. An important source of postapproval information is data collected and submitted by practitioners in the field through programs such as MedWatch through the FDA's safety and adverse effect reporting system (http://www.fda.gov/Safety/MedWatch). Although this system is voluntary, it is relied on to obtain postmarketing information that may lead to further trials or even drug withdrawal from the market.

Official Labeling

The legal distinction between a legend drug and an over-the-counter (OTC) drug is not founded on relative safety per se but rather involves a regulatory decision on whether adequate directions for the drug's proper use can be written for the layperson. If the FDA determines that adequate directions can be written, the manufacturer is not allowed to identify the drug with a prescription legend.

Conversely, for a prescription drug, the manufacturer's directions or FDA-approved labeling (the package insert) is intended for the prescriber, pharmacist, or nurse and provides a summary of information about the chemical and physical nature of the product, pharmacological indications and contraindications, means of administration, dosages, side effects and adverse reactions, how the drug is supplied, and any other information pertinent to safe and effective use. This summary, or official labeling, is developed by discussion between the FDA and the drug manufacturer. The material in the *Physician's Desk Reference* (PDR) is a verbatim presentation of the official labeling.

The FDA's jurisdiction over the uses of marketed drugs and doses extends only to what the manufacturer may recommend and must disclose in its labeling. The FDA is not charged with dictating how a prescriber should practice. The FDA is concerned with the marketing and availability of drugs that have demonstrated substantial evidence of an acceptable risk/benefit ratio for labeled indications. The proper and efficacious therapeutic use of these drugs is the responsibility of the prescriber.

Off-Labeled Use

The prescription of an FDA approved drug for an off-labeled (unlabeled) indication may be initiated by patient need. Clinical support can be demonstrated for off-labeled use if the proposed use is based on rational scientific theory or controlled clinical studies. The FDA has made it clear that it neither has nor wants the authority to compel prescribers to adhere to FDA-approved use in all clinical situations. An example of off-labeled use is that of **trazodone**, which is an **antidepressant**, for sleep. In this example, a side effect of the medication (drowsiness) has been shown to have clinical efficacy for patients with difficulty sleeping whether or not they are clinically depressed. Although not FDA approved for insomnia, **trazodone** is commonly prescribed for this indication.

Nurse practitioners (NPs) are responsible for knowing the FDA indication and approval status of any drug they prescribe. However, a prescribing decision on how to use a drug must be based on what is best for the patient and then supported by available evidence. In professional liability suits, FDA-approved drug labeling may have evidentiary weight, but drug labeling is not intended to set the sole standard for what is good clinical practice.

Controlled Substance Laws

The most comprehensive federal drug legislation is the Controlled Substances Act of 1970 (FDA, 2010). This law was designed to improve regulation of the manufacturing, distribution, and dispensing of drugs identified as "controlled" drugs by providing a closed system for legitimate providers of these substances. Every person who manufactures, distributes, prescribes, procures, or dispenses any controlled substance must register and obtain a registration number with the U.S. Drug Enforcement Administration (DEA). The *Practitioner's Manual: An Informational Outline of the Controlled Substances Act*, published in 2006, outlines regulations and requirements for controlled drug prescribing. This pamphlet is available from the DEA or can be viewed online (http://www.deadiversion.usdoj.gov/pubs/manuals/pract/index.html). All those who regularly dispense and administer controlled substances during the course of their practice must maintain and keep on file for 2 years accurate records of drugs they purchase, distribute, administer, and dispense.

Many states have controlled substance acts patterned after federal law. Because differences are allowed in the scheduling of drugs among states (a state may be more restrictive but not less restrictive), NPs must become acquainted with the provisions of the regulations in the state in which they are licensed. NPs wanting authority to prescribe controlled substances must apply for state prescriptive authority prior to application for a federal DEA number. Applications for a DEA number may be obtained online through the DEA or though the regional office for your state. Before applying, it is important to verify with your state board of nursing or pharmacy if a state-issued prescribing number or certificate is also issued separately from your NP license.

For many years the DEA number was inappropriately used for other than controlled substances by pharmacies, primarily to bill insurance or track medications under a provider-unique identifier. Concern over this as well as the plethora of separate numbers used for Medicaid and Medicare billing led to development and use of the National Provider Identifier number (NPI). The NP should obtain an NPI as soon as it is feasible. Application is free and available online. This number is provider unique and will be used for all prescriptions that are billed through insurance, as well as for other billing services.

In an effort to control drug distribution, a classification system was developed to categorize drugs as "controlled" according to their abuse, accepted medical use, and diversion potential. NPs must know the different classifications and schedules of controlled drugs as well as the associated prescribing rules and regulations. Controlled drugs are placed into different schedules to which different regulations apply. There are five different schedules: I, II, III, IV, and V. Controlled substance authority for NPs varies from state to state regarding ability and autonomy of practice.

Table 4–1 presents the schedules, controls required, and examples of drugs.

Controlled Substance Prescribing Precautions

Prescribers should take precautions with controlled drug prescription pads and information included on the controlled substance prescription to minimize the chance for fraud and diversion of these drugs. The prescription pad (or blanks) should be stored in a locked area. Prescriptions should never be signed in advance or used as notepads. The prescriber's name, NPI number, address, and telephone number should be printed on the pads to allow verification by the dispensing pharmacist. The DEA registration number should be designated on all controlled substance prescriptions. The prescription should be dated on the day it is written, indicating any authorized refills as allowed and clinically appropriate. It is helpful to spell out the quantity dispensed as well giving an Arabic numeral (e.g., "forty [40]") to discourage alterations in the intended quantity.

A prescription for a controlled substance may be directly faxed to the pharmacy as an additional precaution, with the exception of Schedule II controlled substances. A fax cannot be considered the original for Schedule II drugs unless the drug in question is (1) for a nursing home, (2) for a hospice, or (3) parenteral medication for home IV administration.

As of 2009, tamper-proof prescription pads are required for prescriptions written for patients under Medicaid payment plans. State law incorporates the federal guidelines for what constitutes a tamper-proof prescription into any additional state-specific requirements for controlled substances, such as duplicate prescription pads. A practitioner may find the use of tamper-proof prescription pads to be advisable for all written prescriptions, because many drugs are not currently controlled that have abuse potential. Such drugs include **tramadol**, **carisoprodol**, and **pseudoephederine**.

Table 4–1 **Controlled Drug Schedules**

Schedule	Controls Required	Drug Examples
I	No accepted medical use No legal use permitted For registered research facilities only	Heroin, LSD, mescaline, peyote,* marijuana
II	No refills permitted No telephone orders unless true emergency and followed up by written prescription within 7 days Electronic prescribing permitted as of 2011 with specific software and secure identification processes	Narcotics (morphine, codeine, meperidine, opium, hydromorphone, oxycodone, oxymorphone, methadone, fentanyl) Stimulants (cocaine, amphetamine, methylphenidate) Depressants (pentobarbital, secobarbital)
III	Prescription must be rewritten after 6 mo or 5 refills Telephone or fax prescription okay	Narcotics (codeine in combination with non-narcotic ingredients not to exceed 90 mg/tab; hydrocodone not to exceed 50 mg/tab) Stimulants (benzphetamine, chlorpheniramine, diethylpropion) Depressants (butabarbital)
IV	Same as Schedule III Penalties for illegal possession are different	Pentazocine, propoxyphene, phentermine, benzodiazepines, meprobamate
V	Same as all prescription drugs May be dispensed without a prescription unless regulated by the state	Loperamide, diphenoxylate

*Marijuana may be classified under individual state law as a Schedule II drug and used for medical purposes. It may not be "prescribed," however.

A few medications have such high abuse potential or potential for serious adverse effects that they should be prescribed very cautiously and with increased monitoring. The medications with high abuse potential that fall into this category include **methadone, amphetamine,** and scheduled diet pills. Medications with especially problematic adverse-effect profiles include **propoxyphene, meperidine,** and **butalbital.** Medications with exceptionally narrow safety margins include **secobarbital, pentobarbital, meprobamate, methadone,** and **ethchlorvynol.** Medications with little established efficacy include **propoxyphene, carisoprodol, butalbital,** and scheduled diet pills.

Opioids such as **morphine** have legitimate clinical usefulness, and the practitioner should not hesitate to prescribe them when indicated for patients who require analgesia or symptomatic relief not provided by other **analgesics. Methadone** is also used for chronic pain management due to its cost and long half-life. However, as noted, **methadone** also has an extremely variable half-life (7 to 60 or more hours) that differs for individuals based on their metabolism. It therefore should not be a first-line therapy for pain management, especially for the less experienced practitioner. **Methadone** is legal to prescribe for pain management provided that an NP has his or her own Schedule II authority. It is not legal for an NP to prescribe **methadone** or **buprenorphine** for narcotic addiction, and such patients should be referred to an MD or a state-registered clinic that specializes in addiction treatment. A specific clinical challenge regarding controlled drug prescribing is the patient who has a history of drug or alcohol abuse or dependence and who needs management of pain, anxiety, and insomnia. Special attention should be given to patients with current dependence on **opioids** or other central nervous system depressants such as **benzodiazepines.** If a genuine symptomatic need is established by adequate diagnostic confirmation, evaluation, and periodic reevaluation and other analgesics or nondrug treatments are ineffective, then it is the practitioner's responsibility to prescribe **opioids** or refer to a specialized pain management clinic. In this situation, evaluation must be made of the patient using clinically available tools that have been validated, such as SOAPP (Screener and Opioid Assessment for Patients in Pain) or SOAPP-R (Screener and Opioid Assessment for Patients in Pain—Revised) (Butler, Fernandez, Benoit, Budman, & Jamison, 2008). In developing a pain treatment plan, it is important to consider that the effective dose will vary according to the degree of tolerance that the patient has developed. For any patient, abrupt discontinuation can precipitate a withdrawal syndrome if the patient undergoes major surgical or medical trauma while dependent on the drug. Drug dependence can be maintained until the patient begins to recover from the intervening illness, or patients can be instructed in planned withdrawal or taper in conjunction with their surgical or hospital team.

The practitioner must caution any patient for whom an antianxiety or hypnotic is prescribed about the potentiating effects of **alcohol.** Practitioners should also be aware that **benzodiazepines** in particular have associated cautions due to their clinical effects and potential for abuse that contraindicate them for patients on **methadone** or with a current substance use disorder.

CONTROLLED SUBSTANCE MISUSE: PRESCRIBER EDUCATION

In standard clinical practice there are many opportunities for individuals to obtain excessive quantities of controlled drugs, either intentionally or as a result of duplicate prescribing, often by different prescribers. The problems and costs associated with misuse of controlled prescription drugs may have an impact on patients and their prescribers.

Principles for prescribers related to prescription drug misuse assessment include the following:

1. Acquisition and wide use of chemical dependence screening skills.
2. Early and firm limit setting regarding indications for controlled drug prescribing.
3. Careful documentation of a confirmed diagnosis and the ruling out of chemical dependence before initiating a controlled prescription or drug subject to misuse.
4. Practice in "just saying no" and feeling comfortable in being firm without escalating the discussion into an argument with the patient.

Further discussion of pain medication abuse is found in Chapter 53.

Behavioral Red Flags

Almost every practice experiences the chemically dependent patient who uses dishonest mechanisms to obtain increasing supplies of controlled prescriptions. There are certain behaviors that are "red flags" for patients who may be addicted or diverting their controlled medications. Passik and colleagues (1998) provides a list of behaviors that providers should be aware of that are predictive of addiction (Table 4–2).

Once a scam has worked in a given practice, that scam will continue to surface periodically in that office practice until the provider ceases to reinforce the scam. Drug enforcement investigators and prescription drug–abusing patients commonly observe that the greater the ease patients find when practicing scams and drug-seeking behavior in a provider's practice, the higher the prevalence of prescription drug–abusing patients there will be in that practice. Dealing with scams consists of the following steps:

1. Learn to recognize the common ones.
2. Refuse to give in to them.
3. Practice the skill of turning the tables on the scammer.

Table 4–2 **Behaviors More and Less Predictive of Addiction**

Probably More Predictive	Probably Less Predictive
Prescription forgery	Drug hoarding during periods of reduced symptoms
Selling prescription drugs	Aggressive complaining about need for higher doses
Stealing or borrowing another patient's drugs	Requesting specific drugs
Injecting oral formulation	Unapproved use of drug to treat another symptom
Obtaining prescription drugs from nonmedical sources	Obtaining similar drugs from other medical sources
Concurrent use of illicit drugs	Reporting psychic effects not intended by the provider
Unsanctioned dose escalations	Unsanctioned dose escalations one or two times
Recurrent prescription losses	Resistance to change in therapy associated with tolerable adverse effects, with expressions of anxiety related to return to severe symptoms
Evidence of deterioration in the ability to function at work, in the family, or socially, which appears to be related to drug use	
Repeated resistance to changes in therapy despite clear evidence of adverse physical or psychological effects from the drug	

Passik et al (2006).

Scams are generally reasons for more medications, indications for more potent or higher dosage formulations, indications for higher-street-value brands of drugs, ways to obtain a controlled drug without a chart or visit note, or reasons to avoid noncontrolled alternatives. Most scams produce discomfort in providers, and patients using scams are often willing to push the practitioner if they encounter resistance to the scam. Patient-generated pressure to prescribe in the face of clinician hesitancy is one classic sign of a scam. Patients rarely argue pharmacology with providers unless the issue of prescribing controlled drugs is being contested. The clinical phenomenon of an initial no (refusal to prescribe by the practitioner) becoming a yes (eventual willingness to prescribe) if the patient brings the right pressure to bear on the practitioner is pathognomonic of prescription drug misuse.

Prescription altering and forging are a frequently encountered scams. Variations include stealing prescriptions, forging blank prescriptions, photocopying prescriptions, and rewriting prescriptions. Additional prescription alteration strategies that are more common include changing the strength of drug prescribed, the number of pills prescribed, the number of refills indicated, or the date of the prescription. Patients and staff members who have substance misuse issues may also call in prescriptions with the NP's DEA number, as current law permits phoned in prescriptions for Schedules III–V.

Pressure to Prescribe

Another factor that increases the demand for controlled substances is the pressure to prescribe at every visit and the expectation that patients deserve a prescription for something at each visit or for each symptom offered. This process results in two well-known adverse situations: (1) overprescribing of antibiotics and resulting antibiotic resistance and (2) polypharmacy, especially of the elderly. It also may result in a tendency on the part of practitioners to prescribe higher-potency noncontrolled substances and then ultimately controlled drugs when patients persist with vague somatic complaints.

Enabling

Enabling refers to the powerful instinct in practitioners to do anything medically possible to enable patients with present or potential disability to live at a higher level of function. Unfortunately, the disease of chemical dependence has a bottomless appetite for enabling, also defined as behaviors on the part of a friend, family member, or health-care provider that shelter the chemically dependent individual from the adverse consequences of the disease. When the practitioners' enabling instincts interact with chemically dependent patients, the patients are often able to manipulate the practitioners to avoid the consequences of their disease process, thus permitting that disease to progress to further, more pathological levels. This is especially true when controlled drug prescribing is involved. A common statement from practitioners who have been manipulated into enabling and overprescribing to patients is "I was only trying to help." Chemical dependence is one disease process in which practitioners must strive against enabling tendencies, especially when prescribing controlled drugs.

When You Suspect a Patient Is Misusing Medications

Communication Barriers

Newer curricula in training programs over the past two decades have led to an emphasis on the clinical interview and practitioner–patient relationship-building skills. Skill building involves active learning strategies in the areas of verbal and nonverbal communication, empathy, and rapport building. Nursing socialization further emphasizes therapeutic patient advocacy, sometimes without the counterbalance of coaching nurses on how to say no and enforce boundary limitations. Therefore, many NPs feel acutely uncomfortable with conflict and interpersonal confrontation. It is obvious how the practitioners' fear and avoidance of confrontation play into the hands of chemically dependent patients, who have a stronger relationship with the prescription than they do with the practitioners.

Communication Skills

Practitioners must be able to identify common scams and defuse them efficiently and effectively. One strategy is to just say no and mean it. Chemically dependent patients have learned that the practitioners' enabling instincts and confrontation discomfort are so great that when NPs initially say no, it usually ultimately can be turned into a yes if enough pressure is applied. Thus, it is important to be able to mean no and to stick with it. A higher-level clinical skill is initially to say no and then to turn the tables on a patient who demands the prescription. This strategy is based on the clinical fact that patients who demand controlled drugs generally have a pathological relationship with that prescription because of underlying chemical dependence. By making the statement "I am feeling pressured by you to write a prescription today that is not clinically indicated. Because of this I am really concerned about you, and we need to talk about your use of alcohol or other substances," the NP can often effectively turn the tables and shift the discomfort to the patient while still refusing to prescribe.

> **CLINICAL PEARL**
>
> **Prescribing Tips**
>
> A few prescribing tips can help the practitioner reduce environmental facilitation of prescription misuse. First, collect and document a complete history and examination before prescribing controlled substances. Do not rely on patient-supplied history, x-rays, or medical records to confirm your assessment—obtain this information directly from the primary source. Prescribe limited quantities without refills on a first visit, allowing additional time for patient assessment and confirmatory documentation. Educate medical and assistive staff in reinforcement of consistent clinic policies and procedures related to scheduling, forms, urine drug screening, records review and release, and refills. It is not uncommon for patients who do misuse substances to quickly identify the "weak link" among the treatment team and focus their energies on this person or process. Standardize expectations regarding after-hours calls, use of multiple providers, and weekend or early refills and post them where they are readily available.
>
> Patients covered by insurance plans, including Medicaid and Medicare, can be limited to one pharmacy or one prescriber through their payment plan. Case managers can often be utilized to help review and manage medication use and advocate for access to additional options for pain management and control. Other tips include prescribing generic, longer-acting formulations of drugs that have less street value and writing out the quantity prescribed rather than using only numerals, which can be altered.

Systemic Solutions to Problems of Controlled Substance Prescribing

Law enforcement and legislative efforts have produced few solutions to the problem of imbalance in controlled drug prescribing. Until recently, these approaches have targeted diversion of drugs and overprescribing. Results of duplicate and triplicate prescription policies, as well as stricter investigation and enforcement, led to decreased prescribing of controlled drugs across the board, even to patients in need of them for legitimate medical reasons. The development of more permissive policies and pain management guidelines by state legislatures and health regulatory boards increased prescribing for pain management; however, a concurrent 65 percent increase in hospitalizations in the United States for poisonings from prescription drugs (**opioids**, **sedatives**, and **tranquilizers**) ensued from 1999–2006 (Coben et al, 2010). Coben and colleagues report a 400 percent increase in admissions for **methadone** overdose. This increase is possibly due to inappropriate dosing and use of **methadone** for pain management, as well as by diversion of legitimately prescribed medications from the patient for whom it was originally prescribed.

Careful charting and documentation habits are essential for prescribing controlled drugs. Document clearly in a progress note (1) physical evaluation of the patient, (2) the diagnosis, (3) the clinical indications for treatment, (4) the written treatment plan, (5) the expected symptom outcomes, (6) informed consent and agreement for treatment from the patient, and (7) consultation and/or collaboration necessary to meet treatment goals and objectives. These strategies reduce, but do not eliminate, the risk of controlled drug diversion from one's practice.

Medication Agreements

One tool for defining and implementing treatment objectives is the medication agreement. This written tool can be incorporated into treatment of chronic pain, particularly if long-term management with **opioids** is indicated. The agreement is not limited to **opioid** prescribing practice, however. A pain agreement can be used for treatment of pain or other conditions with medications that are not **opioids** but still have potential for patient misuse such as **benzodiazepines**, **tramadol**, or other adjunctive medications. Formats can be found in the links at the end of this chapter and in Chapter 53. These may be modified for individual clinic setting and client population. It is advisable to treat pain agreements under a "universal precaution" model of care, meaning that the NP develops and uses agreements that are expected of all patients diagnosed with chronic cancer or noncancer pain. It is inequitable and a potential legal liability to pick and choose patients who will be asked to sign a pain agreement based on their age, income status, use of other controlled or illicit substances, or other personal characteristics. NPs are advised to familiarize themselves with urine drug and alcohol screens and their availability, cost, sensitivity, and specificity. In-office rapid screenings are now available that can be done quickly and without prior notice in order to confirm adherence to pain agreement criteria. An example of a pain medication use agreement is found in Chapter 53.

Prescription Drug Monitoring Programs

As of July 2010, 34 states had prescription drug monitoring programs in place and 7 more were in the process of considering or introducing legislation according to the U.S. Drug Enforcement Administration (DEA, 2010). A prescription drug–monitoring program enables practitioners to query a confidential database of controlled substances statewide to evaluate whether a patient is currently receiving a prescription elsewhere. Some states also have regulations that permit cross-state sharing of this information, which has reduced the ability of patients who misuse controlled substances to obtain multiple prescriptions from multiple providers. For more information regarding these programs and how to access them, contact your local DEA office or state board of pharmacy.

STATE LAW

Jurisdiction

Federal law establishes whether a drug requires a prescription but does not dictate who may prescribe. The authority to prescribe is a function of state law. Unlike the uniform nature of federal law, prescriptive authority varies from state to state. The states have the authority to license health-care professionals. Although a state may sign a compact agreement permitting cross-state practice, as is the case with the Nurse Licensure Compact, there are no currently implemented cross-state agreements that cover NP practice.

Regulation of nursing education and practice is relatively recent. The NP role originated in the 1960s as an extension of the registered nurse (RN) role. States thereafter implemented a variety of methods for recognizing NP practice. Although the National Council of State Boards of Nursing recommends licensure as the appropriate level of regulation for the autonomy and authority of the NP role, some states still recognize NPs with certification, endorsement, or through delegated authority from a physician. States have authority under the states' "police power" to take regulatory action to protect public health, welfare, and safety including emergency suspension or revocation of practice authority. The courts have consistently upheld professional licensing laws as legitimate use of this power. The purpose of these laws is to ensure that those who provide health-care services for a fee have demonstrated a minimum level of competency.

A license is always required for practice as an NP. The state Nurse Practice Act specifies the exact title that must be used for practice and on a prescription. NPs working in federal facilities such as the Veterans Administration or Indian Health Services need to have a state-based license that governs their scope of practice in that facility, but may practice in a facility different from the state of origin under the same license. Persons practicing in a federal facility are also exempt from fees for DEA registration.

Each state has practice acts that set forth licensing requirements for health professionals, define the scope of practice, and prohibit unauthorized practice. These laws usually provide for a state board that governs each profession and establishes administrative rules of conduct for each profession. Prescriptive authority may be granted to a variety of types of health-care providers in a state, including optometrists, naturopaths, and clinical psychologists. Some states grant prescriptive authority to NPs solely through the board of nursing (plenary authority), whereas others require a joint process through a board of medicine or pharmacy. Some states require only involvement of a board or authority other than the board of nursing when controlled substances will be part of prescriptive authority.

Prescriptive authority exists as dependent and independent authority. Independent authority permits the prescriber to exert autonomous judgment. Dependent authority exists when the primary prescriber delegates the authority to another through a collaborative or supervisory agreement. These agreements usually involve written guidelines and/or a protocol for treatment. Some states limit authority by restricting prescribing to a written formulary. Other restrictions may apply, including limits on the geographic locations of the clinical site or limits on the number of doses or refills that may be authorized, or requiring written agreements with a practicing NP that spell out the scope of the prescribing authority. Dispensing, which means the release of a prescription from other than a pharmacy for a patient to take home, is an authority that some states grant to prescribing practitioners with varying degrees of requirements. All states permit NPs some degree of prescribing and all permit receipt of samples with appropriate prescriptive authority.

Discussion of the laws across states occurs in Chapter 1. Each year, the January issues of *Nurse Practitioner* and *The Journal for Nurse Practitioners* contains a review of the current state laws regarding prescriptive authority for advanced practice nurses. This review is useful in determining the current status of prescribing in each state.

Writing and Transmitting the Prescription

The Prescription Format

A number of directions need to be communicated in writing or verbally to the dispensing pharmacist to complete a prescription properly. Tools such as the Institute for Safe Medication Practice's (ISMP) *List of Error-Prone Abbreviations, Symbols and Dose Designations* (2007) can help prescribers decrease transmission errors. The following are suggestions to provide a complete safe prescription:

1. Use preprinted prescription pads that contain the name, address, and telephone number and NPI number of the prescriber. This will allow the pharmacist to contact the prescriber if there are any questions about the prescription.
2. Write the complete drug name, strength, dosage, and form.
3. Write the date of the prescription.
4. Use metric units of measure such as milligrams and milliliters; avoid apothecary units of measure.
5. Avoid abbreviations.
6. Avoid the use of "as directed" or "as needed."
7. Include the general indication, such as "for infection."
8. Write "Dispense as Written" if generic substitution is not desired.
9. Include the patient weight, especially if pediatric or elderly.
10. Indicate if a safety cap is not required, as medications will be dispensed with them by default.

Examples of prescriptions are found in Figures 4–1 and 4–2.

As of April 1, 2008, all written prescriptions for covered outpatient drugs paid for by Medicaid must be written on a tamper-proof prescription pad. The required elements are adopted into state pharmacy law, and include specific inks and papers. Contact your board directly regarding your state-specific prescription pad requirements.

The appropriate amount of drug and the refill authorization benefit the patient in convenience and may reduce the cost of therapy. For acute therapies, the amount prescribed should be enough to cure the illness or maintain therapy until the next patient visit. Overprescribing is costly, permits inappropriate self-treatment with leftover doses, and contributes to the risk of accidental overdose.

Health and Wellness Clinic
5000 N. Willamette Blvd.
Portland, Oregon
503-555-1111

Anita Lee Wynne PhD, FNP-C **Teri Woo, CPNP**

Jane Doe DOB: 4/18/01 Wt. 48lbs

Amoxicillin 250 mg per 5 mL
Disp: 300 mL. Give pediatric dosing spoon.
Sig: 15 mL po bid X 10 days for otitis media.
No refills
Teri Woo, CPNP Date: ____________

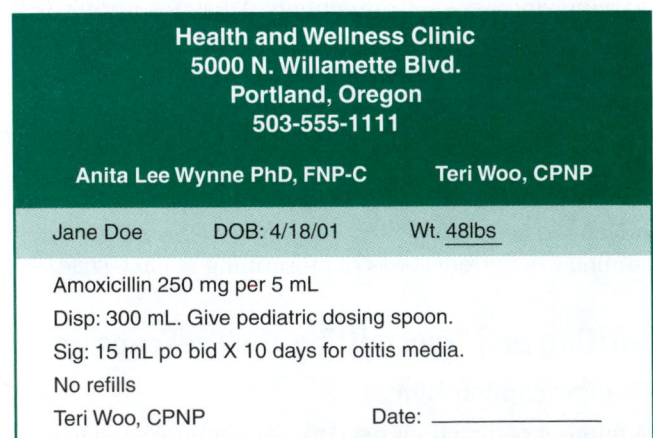

Figure 4–1. Sample prescription.

Health and Wellness Clinic
5000 N. Willamette Blvd.
Portland, Oregon
503-555-1111

Anita Lee Wynne PhD, FNP-C **Teri Woo, CPNP**

John Doe DOB: 6/5/51 Date: ____________

Oxycodone 5mg
Disp: 30 (thirty)
Sig: 1 tablet q4–6h prn back pain.
Do not drive or use hazardous machinery until response is known. May produce drowsiness. Do not exceed 6 tablets per day.
No refills
Anita Lee Wynne, FNP-C DEA # on file in pharmacy

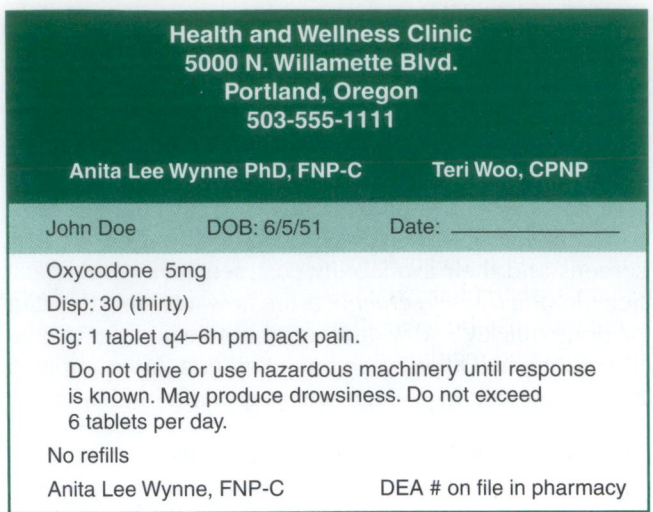

Figure 4–2. Sample prescription for controlled substance.

Patients cannot return unused drugs to the pharmacy for credit or disposal. Conversely, for the treatment of chronic illness, it is more economical to obtain a supply of medication for 1 to 3 months instead of repeated refills of smaller quantities. Mail-order pharmacies and insurance plans may require that a 3-month supply is dispensed with each prescription. It is judicious to prescribe small initial trial supplies until patient dosage and compliance can be determined, followed by larger refill quantities for chronic therapy.

Schedule II drugs may not be refilled, and require a new prescription for each dispensed quantity. However, it is legal and acceptable to write 3 months' worth of prescriptions at one visit for established and stable patients. This is done by writing 3 separate prescriptions, each with the current visit date, and a statement "do not fill until__". The dates for the next 2- and 3-month refills can be filled in on each prescription, and these can be given to the patient in one visit, mailed, or left for pick up and signature.

What May Be Prescribed

Prescriptions are required for all legend and the majority of controlled drugs (state laws may permit the sale of Schedule V controlled substances without a prescription in limited quantities). They are also required for some medical devices, home-health and home-testing equipment, durable medical equipment, needles and syringes, and sometimes for Medicaid or Medicare coverage of OTC medications that are required for patient health. Prescriptions are required in order to compound medications for patient administration in strengths or formulas not otherwise available.

State-Specific Elements

State pharmacy law determines the required format for a prescription. A few states require duplicate or triplicate copy pads for controlled substances. NPs who prescribe in a state with mandated collaboration or supervision may need to indicate the name and information of this person on their prescription pads. A state can also designate that a drug is controlled and requires a DEA number or other special authority, even if the federal government does not. This is becoming true of **pseudoephederine**, which is used for methamphetamine manufacturing. A state may pass laws regarding medications that are more restrictive, but may not pass laws more permissive than federal law. NPs must verify prescribing laws through their state board of nursing and pharmacy. Less commonly, a board of medicine may also be legally involved in an NP's prescribing practices and regulations.

Electronic Prescribing and Secure Prescribing

The days of "writing" a prescription may soon be over. Electronic prescribing is enjoying support and institutional funding as a method to decrease medication error and increase drug tracking and accountability. Electronic prescribing has been implicated, however, in medication errors as well. Prescribers may become exceedingly reliant on prepopulated protocols and dosages that may not apply to the individual patient's clinical circumstances. Most electronic health record systems have override features that are easy to implement, and this can be a benefit, but it can also be a danger in the wrong hands. It is critical that NPs who prescribe take responsibility for individually verifying appropriate doses and treatments. If in doubt, a pharmacist may be consulted directly, and many large universities run free consulting services for this purpose.

In March 2010 the Office of the Federal Register published an Interim Final Rule titled "Electronic Prescriptions for Controlled Substances" that revises DEA regulations to provide practitioners with the option of writing prescriptions for controlled substances electronically (DEA, 2010). By the date of publication of *Pharmacotherapeutics for Nurse Practitioner Prescribers* (this book), it is assumed this rule will become final. NPs will need to be aware of this emerging issue, carefully follow state and federal legislation related to the area of electronic prescribing, and follow all DEA instructions regarding the software to purchase to meet DEA specifications for electronic prescribing of controlled substances.

ETHICAL ASPECTS OF PRESCRIBING

Informed Consent

The notion of informed consent is shorthand for the doctrine of informed decision making, which proposes that each patient has the right to make informed decisions about those things that will affect herself or himself. Although some question whether consent to medical procedures can ever be truly informed, the doctrine has been assimilated into American society's concept of what clinical practice should include. Informed consent should be obtained from a patient before all medical interventions, diagnostic as well as therapeutic. A patient may either agree to or refuse a proposed intervention; in both situations, the patient is making her or his own informed decision.

The provider who performs a specific service is responsible for obtaining consent to that specific service. The consent usually is given to the identified individual, as well as others working with him or her to perform the specific procedure or associated procedures. In general, a referring provider is not responsible for getting consent for a procedure performed by another provider. Some exceptions may apply, however, and practitioners who send patients for tests or consultations should inform them generally about the procedure and their clinical recommendations for requiring it.

Informed consent has four critical features: (1) a competent patient (2) who is provided adequate information with which to make a decision (3) and who voluntarily (4) consents to a proposed intervention. Although legal opinions tend to merge the concepts, it is helpful to consider competence as two related but distinct areas: legal competence and clinical competence. A patient must be both legally and clinically competent to give informed consent. In general, an adult is presumed to be legally competent unless declared incompetent in formal legal proceedings. To be clinically competent for medical decision making, a patient must be able to comprehend information that is provided, formulate a decision about a proposed intervention, and communicate that decision to the health-care team. Patients may be deemed legally competent to make certain types of decisions or give consent but unable to be legally responsible for all decision making.

Clinical competence is also not an all-or-none phenomenon. A patient may be competent to make some choices but not others. Clinical competence may vary over time and is affected by the course of an individual's illness and therapies currently in use. Assistive devices and environmental modification may be important to maintaining and enhancing clinical competence. Hearing aids, interpreters, and communication boards may be key assistive devices to certain patients. Examples of environmental factors that affect clinical competence include sedative medications, presence of background noise for a patient with a hearing disability, and the side of approach to a patient with a visual field loss.

A medication agreement, as discussed in this chapter, may also outline informed consent for initial and ongoing treatment with medications that have the potential for side effects and habituation. Mental health medications have specific consent regulations due to the vulnerability of their target population. Other areas that may have specific consent procedures include prescribing medications for elderly or minor patients. Parental or partner involvement in prescribing determinations related to sexually transmitted infections, family planning, and birth control may be limited under specific state law, and a minor may give informed consent for some surgical or medical procedures even if a parent is not informed. These are sensitive areas of law that require specific study. Advice of an attorney may be required.

Prescribing for Self, Family, or Friends

State law varies regarding whether an NP can prescribe for family or friends. In order for a prescription to be clinically legitimate, a patient must be assessed and have a record of his or her assessment. It is clearly unethical to prescribe for oneself, and many states punish this with significant fines or board action. Although it may be technically legal to prescribe for family or friends, an NP needs to consider whether it is ethical. If the clinical circumstance requires a controlled substance, the judicious prescriber will refer a friend or family to a colleague for confidential assessment and treatment. It is never considered ethical for a mental health provider to engage a family member or close friend in a clinically therapeutic relationship, whether or not prescribing is involved.

Sale of Pharmaceuticals and Supplements

It is illegal to sell pharmaceuticals that are designated as samples and provided to a clinic for free distribution to patients. Depending on the dispensing laws of your state, it may be permissible to stock and sell limited amounts of commonly prescribed medications within your practice setting. It may also be permissible to sell supplements such as **prenatal vitamins** or **fish oil**, especially if the prescriber is able to order them at a discount and pass the savings on to the patient. It may not be technically illegal but can be ethically questionable if the prescriber is selling medications with a broad profit margin to patients perceived as vulnerable.

NURSE PRACTITIONER ROLE OUTSIDE THE UNITED STATES

The NP role is expanding to health systems outside of the United States. As an example, in 2004–2006 the Canadian government funded the Nurse Practitioner Initiative to promote recognition, education, and utilization of NPs as primary care providers. Similar to U.S. states, Canadian provinces have individual practice acts that designate the parameters and autonomy of prescriptive authority. Prior to legislative recognition of the NP role, many provinces, such as Ontario, had provisions for a class of RN with expanded or extended practice permitting limited diagnosis and prescribing.

One significant difference in Canada, which is also true of the UK and their Nurse Practitioner movement, is that prescribing is supported by a national pharmacy system. Nationally adopted core competencies outlined in *The Canadian Nurse Practitioner Core Competency Framework* (Canadian Nurses Association, 2005) clearly articulate preparation of an NP who will be competent to select, prescribe, monitor and dispense prescription medications. A national expert advisory committee (CEDAC) reviews and recommends drugs for provincial formularies based on efficacy and evidence-based review. Provinces develop formularies for prescribing, which may be further modified based on scope of practice for individual health professions. A provincial pharmacy network, known as PharmaNet, records all community prescriptions in a central database, which facilitates checking for duplication, contraindications, and interactions.

NPs have controlled substance prescribing ability in many Canadian provinces. They may also order laboratory tests, blood products, and other therapeutic interventions and diagnostics. Both NPs and pharmacists in the UK have prescribing ability, based on formularies or standards adopted based on national guidelines. The NP role is expanding in other countries such as Australia and New Zealand to address primary care needs.

BOX 4–1 WEB RESOURCES FOR LEGAL AND ETHICAL ISSUES IN PRESCRIBING

National Cancer Institute Clinical Trials: http://www.cancer.gov/clinicaltrials
National Institute of Health Clinical Trials: http://clinicaltrials.gov/ct2/home
FDA MedWatch: http://www.fda.gov/Safety/MedWatch/default.htm
U.S. Drug Enforcement Administration: http://www.dea.gov
National Provider Identifier Number application: http://www.cms.hhs.gov/nationalprovidentstand/03_apply.asp
National Council of State Boards of Nursing: www.ncsbn.org
Institute for Safe Medication Practices: www.ismp.org
Opioid Assessment and Management Tools: http://www.painedu.org/soap.asp
Pain Agreement Sample Tools: http://www.ohsu.edu/ahec/pain/form.html

REFERENCES

Barton, J. H., Emanuel, E. J. (2005). The patents-based pharmaceutical development process: Rationale, problems, and potential reforms. *Journal of the American Medical Association, 294,* 2075–2082.

Butler, S. F., Fernandez, K., Benoit, C., Budman, S. H., & Jamison, R. N. (2008). Validation of the Revised Screener and Opioid Assessment for Patients with Pain (SOAPP-R). *Journal of Pain, 9*(4), 360–372.

Canadian Nurses Association. (2005). *The Canadian nurse practitioner core competency framework.* Retrieved from http://www.cno.org/for/rnec/pdf/CompetencyFramework_en.pdf

Corbin, J. H., Davis, S. M., Furbee, P. M., Sikora, R. D., Tollitson, R. D., & Bossarte, R. M. (2010). Hospitalizations for poisoning by prescription opioids, sedatives, and tranquilizers. *American Journal of Preventive Medicine, 38*(5), 517–524.

DiMasi, J. A., Hansen, R. W., & Grabowski, H. G. (2003). The price of innovation: New estimates of drug development costs. *Journal of Health Economics, 22,* 151–185.

Duke Clinical Research Institute. (2010). New drug development timeline. Clinical Trials Network Best Practices. Retrieved from https://www.ctnbestpractices.org/

Hsu, J., Price, M., Huang, J., Brand, R., Fung, V., Hui, R., et al. (2006). Unintended consequences of caps on Medicare drug benefits. *New England Journal of Medicine, 354,* 2349–2359.

Institute for Safe Medication Practices. (2010). ISMP's List of Error-Prone Abbreviations, Symbols, and Dose Designations. Retrieved from http://www.ismp.org/tools/errorproneabbreviations.pdf

Labby, D., Koder, M., & Amann, T. (2004). *Opioids and chronic nonmalignant pain: A clinician's handbook.* Retrieved from http://www.ohsu.edu/ahec/pain/home.html

Oregon State Board of Nursing. (2009). *Prescriptive authority in Oregon for nurse practitioners and clinical nurse specialists.* Retrieved from http://www.oregon.gov/OSBN

Passik, S., & Portenoy, R. (1998). Substance abuse issues in palliative care. In A. Berger (Ed.), *Principles and practices of supportive oncology* (pp. 513–530). New York: Lippincott-Raven.

Portenoy, R. K. (1996). Opioid therapy for chronic nonmalignant pain: Clinicians' perspective. *Journal of Law and Medical Ethics, 24*(4), 296–309.

U.S. Drug Enforcement Administration (DEA). (2006). *A practitioner's manual: An informational outline of the Controlled Substances Act.* Retrieved from http://www.deadiversion.usdoj.gov/pubs/manuals/pract/index.html

U.S. Drug Enforcement Administration (DEA). (2010). State prescription drug monitoring programs. Retrieved from http://www.deadiversion.usdoj.gov/faq/rx_monitor.htm#4

Use of opioids for the treatment of chronic pain: A consensus statement from the American Academy of Pain Medicine and the American Pain Society. (1997). *Clinical Journal of Pain, 13,* 6–8.

U.S. Food and Drug Administration (FDA). (2009). What FDA regulates. Retrieved from http://www.fda.gov/AboutFDA/WhatWeDo/WhatFDARegulates/default.htm

U.S. Food and Drug Administration (FDA). (2010). Milestones in food and drug law history. Retrieved from http://www.fda.gov/AboutFDA/WhatWeDo/History/Milestones/default.htm

CHAPTER 5

ADVERSE DRUG REACTIONS

Teri Moser Woo

Chapter Outline

In general, when drug products are administered, the benefit should outweigh the risk. However, every drug product has certain risks. The World Health Organization (WHO) defines an adverse drug reaction (ADR) as "harmful, unintended reactions to medicines that occur at doses normally used for treatment" and notes that ADRs are among the leading cause of death in many countries (2008). *Pharmacovigilance* is preventing and detecting adverse effects of medicines (WHO, 2008). This chapter describes the various types of ADRs and how providers can anticipate and prevent ADRs whenever possible.

The terms *adverse drug event* and *side effect* describe the potential unwanted effects that patients experience as a result of medication therapy. ADRs include symptoms that are uncomfortable for the patient but may be tolerable, such as nausea, vomiting, fatigue, dizziness, and hypotension. ADRs may also include syndromes that require immediate termination of therapy, such as anaphylaxis, thrombocytopenia, and lupus.

ADRs may occur within minutes of drug exposure (e.g., anaphylaxis), days (e.g., gastrointestinal [GI] bleeding), or weeks (e.g., renal failure). Alternatively, important reactions can develop insidiously over a prolonged period (e.g., corticosteroid-induced cataracts). Other reactions may be apparent only after the drug has been discontinued (e.g., cancer related to immunosuppressants). It is even possible that the adverse effect will affect the offspring of the patient, without affecting the patient at all (e.g., congenital abnormalities caused by drug therapy).

INCIDENCE OF ADRS

Pharmacovigilance

The need to address drug safety emerged after the **thalidomide** disaster in 1961 led to a resolution at the World Health Assembly in 1963 that addressed the need for early and rapid dissemination of information on adverse drug reactions (WHO, 2002). From this initial meeting, WHO developed the International Drug Monitoring Programme. The science of pharmacovigilance emerged from the early work of the program, with pharmacovigilance agencies developed in member countries. As of September 2010 there were 99 countries with national pharmacovigilance centers participating in the WHO Drug Monitoring Programme (Box 5–1), including the U.S. Food and Drug Administration (FDA) Adverse Events Reporting System (AERS) and Health Canada's Canada Vigilance Program. The European Union has developed a similar system, the EU Pharmacovigilance System, and Great Britain has the Yellow Card Scheme, which is housed in the Medicines and Healthcare Products Regulatory Agency. Each of these agencies has an online reporting system where providers, patients, or manufacturer can

BOX 5–1 SELECTED PHARMACOVIGILANCE CENTERS

U.S. Food and Drug Administration Adverse Events Reporting System (AERS)
Medwatch reporting system (www. fda.gov/Safety/MedWatch)

Health Canada MedEffect Canada
Canada Vigilance Program (http://www.hc-sc.gc.ca/dhp-mps/medeff/index-eng.php)

European Union
EU Pharmacovigilance System (http://ec.europa.eu/health/human-use/pharmacovigilance/index_en.htm)

Great Britain Medicines and Healthcare Products Regulatory Agency
Yellow Card Scheme (http://www.mhra.gov.uk)

World Health Organization International Drug Monitoring System
The Uppsala Monitoring Centre (http://www.who-umc.org)

report adverse events related to drugs, allowing for early emergence of new knowledge regarding ADRs of drugs.

In spite of the ease of reporting ADRs, underreporting of ADRs is common. Hazell and Shakir (2006) conducted a review of 37 studies from 12 countries and determined the median underreporting rate was 94 percent. Clearly there is work to be done educating providers and the public about the importance of reporting ADRs, because only through reporting will significant trends in ADRs be discovered.

ADR Prevalence

The prevalence of adverse drug reaction is difficult to determine. The FDA AERS keeps statistics on the number of postmarket adverse events related to drugs reported to the Medwatch reporting system. The statistics are grouped by whether the report is domestic (U.S.) or foreign in origin. In 2009, a total of 490,836 adverse events were reported (300,910 domestic and 178,406 foreign) (U.S. Food and Drug Administration [FDA], 2010). Health Canada maintains a similar database as part of the MedEffect Canada system, Canada Vigilance Program. The Canadian program reported 27,469 adverse reaction reports in 2009 (Canada Health, 2010).

Another method of determining prevalence of ADRs is to monitor events that occur related to patient ambulatory care visit, hospitalization, or death. In the 2006 National Ambulatory Medical Care Survey, adverse effects of medical care, a combination of adverse drug reactions, and surgical complications accounted for 5.9 million visits (Cherry, Hing, Woodwell, & Rechtsteiner, 2008). In a retrospective review of hospital admissions for ADRs, McDonnell and Jacobs (2002) found 80 percent of ADRs were related to toxic drug concentration or abnormal laboratory value. In a study of over 12 million Medicare patients admitted to hospitals in 1998, the overall ADR rate was 1.73 percent (Bond & Raehl, 2006). In a random review of deaths in three Swedish counties, 8.3 percent were determined to be fatal adverse drug reactions; the most common drugs associated with the fatal ADRs were antithrombotic drugs (63%), **NSAIDs** (18%), **antidepressants** (14%), and **cardiovascular drugs** (8%) (Wester, Jonsson, Spigset, Druid, & Hagg, 2007).

Populations at Higher Risk for ADRs

ADRs are more likely to occur in females, patients with renal impairment, and patients taking multiple medications, although the highest risk groups are children and the elderly. The proposed theories for why women have more ADRs than men include differences in body water, muscle mass and body fat ratio, physiological differences such as pregnancy and menopause, and differences in pharmacokinetics between genders (Zopf et al, 2008). Patients with renal dysfunction have decreased drug elimination, leading to risk for drug accumulation and toxicity. Likewise, patients who are on more medications have a greater likelihood of drug interactions causing ADRs.

Infants and children are at increased risk of ADRs for multiple reasons related to developmental pharmacology and off-labeled prescribing of medications to children. First, as discussed in depth in Chapter 50, neonates and infants have immature liver and kidney function, which places them at risk of ADRs. In addition, many drugs prescribed for neonates, infants, children, and adolescents lack safety and efficacy studies in this population, and there may be differences in the pharmacokinetic and pharmacodynamics of drugs in children not picked up in adult studies. The drug class reported to cause the most pediatric hospital admissions for ADRs in one study are the **antiepileptic drugs** (Le, Nguyen, Law, & Hodding, 2006). The reported rate of ADRs in hospitalized children is 0.85 to 1.6 percent, although this number is thought to be low because of underreporting (Temple, Robinson, Miller, Hayes, & Nahata, 2004; Le et al, 2006). **Antidepressants** create an increased risk of suicide ideation in adolescents, leading to a black box warning regarding their use in adolescents. An unknown is the ADR rate of over-the-counter (OTC) drugs given to children. The safety and efficacy of OTC **cough and cold medications** have been questioned after a number of reports of deaths of infants taking **cold medications**, leading to an FDA recommendation that these medications not be used in children younger than 4 years (Centers for Disease Control and Prevention [CDC], 2007; FDA, 2008). Clearly children are at risk for ADRs and prescribers need to be cognizant of these risks.

The elderly are at increased risk for similar reasons to children: alterations in pharmacokinetics as they age and lack of studies regarding safety and efficacy of medications in the elderly. As people age, the liver decreases in size and enzymes decrease in number, leading to reduced ability to metabolize medications. Esophageal peristalsis is reduced, placing the older adult at risk for tablets remaining in the esophagus, especially if they are not swallowed with enough water. Distribution of drugs in older adults is affected by cardiac output, decreased plasma proteins, and decreased body water (Merle, Laroche, Dantoine, & Charmes, 2005). The blood–brain barrier is more permeable in the elderly, leading to increased sensitivity and ADRs to drugs that work in the central nervous system. An age-related decrease in renal function places older patients at risk for drug accumulation and toxicity. In addition, older patients are at risk for decompensation if anything upsets their physiological balance, such as increased sodium in their diet or a fever affecting their fluid balance (Merle et al, 2005). The elderly tend to take more medications than do other age groups, increasing their risk for ADRs from drug interactions. The frail elderly need to be monitored closely for ADRs, as they are at increased risk due to their physical condition. In a study of ADRs in frail elderly posthospital discharge, Hanlon and colleagues (2006) found a 33 percent of frail elderly experienced ADRs after discharge. Prescribing for elderly and chronically ill patients is discussed in depth in Chapters 51 and 52.

Drug–Drug Interactions Causing ADRs

There is some temptation to add drugs to existing treatments, especially if the current regimen was prescribed by someone else. The nurse practitioner (NP) may feel that the earlier prescriber knew more about the clinical situation. Even if this is true, it is important to review all of the patient's medications, including OTC medications and herbal remedies, before adding new medications to the treatment regimen. Software packages are available to assess risk of drug interactions if considering adding a new medication to a treatment regimen.

Dose-Related ADRs

Some drug effects are dose related. Because of individual differences in pharmacokinetics, a dose tolerated by one patient may cause adverse effects in another. Medication errors may lead to an excessive amount of the drug being given or taken, as may a change of products of the same drug entity (changing from depot or sustained-release forms to regular forms of the same drug product). Any alteration in dose or delivery system requires monitoring for ADRs.

Disease-Related ADRs

The presence of disease can markedly influence the incidence and occurrence of ADRs. Diseases of the kidney and liver increase the risk of ADR. Table 5–1 presents examples of ADRs associated with diseases.

CATEGORIES OF ADVERSE DRUG REACTIONS

The World Health Organization Adverse Reaction Terminology (WHO-ART) was developed to give a standardized way of describing ADRs. Adverse reactions are classified into six categories (Edwards & Aronson, 2000):

Type A reactions are dose dependent, common, and related to the pharmacological effects of the drug.

Type B reactions are allergic or idiosyncratic reactions; they are not dose dependent and are usually not predictable or preventable.

Type C reactions are related to the cumulative dose of the medication; they are dose and time related, and they are relatively uncommon.

Table 5–1 **Examples of Adverse Drug Reactions Associated With Disease**

Disease	Drug	Possible Adverse Drug Reaction
Renal failure	Aminoglycosides Digoxin Furosemide	Nephrotoxicity, ototoxicity Digitalis toxicity Ototoxicity
Hepatic precoma	Morphine	Precipitate encephalopathy
Peptic ulcer disease	Corticosteroids, NSAIDs	Increased risk of GI bleeding
Heart failure	High-dose beta blockers, NSAIDs	Aggravate or precipitate heart failure
Epilepsy	Phenothiazines, tricyclic antidepressants	May aggravate seizures
Hyperthyroidism	Digoxin	Digitalis toxicity

Type D reactions are delayed reactions that become apparent some time after the use of a drug; they are time related and uncommon.

Type E reactions are associated with the withdrawal of a drug and may be predictable or unpredictable.

Type F reactions are unexpected failure of therapy, are often caused by drug interactions, and are quite common.

Table 5–2 presents the categories of ADRs.

Type A Adverse Drug Reactions

Type A ADRs are the result of an unwanted but otherwise normal pharmacological action of a drug given in the usual therapeutic doses. Type A reactions are predictable from a drug's known pharmacological properties. They are usually dose dependent, and their incidence and morbidity are generally well known. Their mortality rate is usually low. When a group of individuals receives a drug, a spectrum of response is observed. This variability manifests itself as needing different doses to achieve the desired therapeutic effects or differing responses to the same dose. Type A reactions are likely to occur when the therapeutic index is low, as in the case of **digoxin**. In some instances, the type A reaction occurs as an exaggeration of the primary pharmacological effect. Examples include bleeding with **anticoagulants**, hypoglycemia with **insulin**, and hypotension with **antihypertensives**. In other circumstances, the type A reaction is the result of the drug's secondary reactions. Examples include **tricyclic antidepressants**' anticholinergic properties, which are unrelated to the effects that mediate the drug's therapeutic action. At times, reduction of the dose may be sufficient to lessen or stop these reactions; otherwise, the drug has to be discontinued.

Causes

Type A reactions develop in individuals who are at the extremes of the dose-response curves for pharmacological and secondary drug effects. There are three basic reasons for unexpected type A reactions: (1) defects in drug quality, (2) abnormal pharmacokinetics, and (3) altered sensitivity of the target receptors because of disease or individual genetics. If the drug product is of poor quality, there can be more actual drug than the amount stated or the release of the drug from the dosage form can be much faster than desired, which will result in an adverse reaction. Changes in the individual pharmacokinetic parameters of adsorption, distribution, or elimination may result in high concentrations of the drug in the body and an exaggerated effect in the body. Many ADRs result from abnormal pharmacokinetic handling of the drug in an individual patient. ADRs may also be due to differences in target organ sensitivity to the drug. These differences may be due to genetic differences in the number of receptors among individuals, the presence of other drugs in the body, or the effect of diseases on various physiological systems in the body. Any or all of these factors may result in unwanted adverse effects on the administration of a drug. Table 5–3 presents the causes of type A ADRs.

Table 5–2 **Categories of Adverse Drug Reactions**

Type of Reaction	Features	Examples
Type A	• Augmented effect • Dose related • Related to the pharmacological action of the drug • Predictable • Common	Toxic effects from elevated serum levels or ADRs such as anticholinergic effects of medications
Type B	• Bizarre effect • Not dose related • Unpredictable • Not related to pharmacological action of drug	Allergic reactions or idiosyncratic reactions such as malignant hyperthermia
Type C	• Dose related and time related • Related to cumulative dose of drug • Chronic effects	Hypothalamic-pituitary-adrenal axis suppression by corticosteroids
Type D	• Time related • Delayed • Becomes apparent after the use of a drug	Teratogens or carcinogens
Type E	• Withdrawal • Occurs when the medication is stopped	Opiate withdrawal syndrome or beta blocker withdrawal
Type F	• Unexpected failure of therapy • May be caused by a drug interaction	CYP450 enzyme interactions

Source: Derived from Edwards, I. R., & Aronson, J. K. (2000). Adverse drug reactions: Definitions, diagnosis and management. *Lancet,* 356, 1255–1259.

Table 5–3 **Causes of Type A Adverse Drug Reactions**

Cause of Reaction	Mechanism of Reaction	Examples
Drug quality	Drug overdose	Mislabeled drug has more active ingredient than shown on the label or differences in bioavailability between brands or generic drugs.
	Release rate too fast	Long-acting dosage form releases all of the drug at once instead of over several hours.
Pharmacokinetics	Unexpectedly high drug levels cause an enhanced pharmacological response	Reduced elimination in renal disease causes drug to accumulate and cause toxicity. Reduced protein binding causes more free drug to be available.
Receptor sensitivity	Exaggerated or secondary pharmacological effects of a drug	Anticholinergic effects in some patients at very low doses. Cardiac failure may be unmasked in some patients by beta blockers.

Type B Adverse Drug Reactions

Type B ADRs are allergic or idiosyncratic effects that are not dose dependent or expected from the pharmacological actions of the drugs. They are usually unpredictable and unavoidable. Examples include anaphylactic reactions, serum sickness, lupus erythematosus, urticaria, hemolytic anemia, and photosensitivity. The development of type B ADRs usually requires discontinuation of the therapy.

Allergic Causes

Drug allergies range from very mild (e.g., urticaria) to very severe (e.g., anaphylactic shock) reactions. Patients who report drug allergies need to be evaluated carefully, even though often the events reported are type A reactions such as nausea and vomiting rather than true allergic reactions.

Drugs are usually extremely small molecules and have no antigenic activity. The drug combines with a carrier molecule or protein and forms a drug–protein complex. This drug–protein complex possesses antigenic activity and invokes specific antibody formation, thereby sensitizing the body to the drug. This synthesis of antibodies usually occurs after a period of 1 to 2 weeks. When subsequent exposure to the drug occurs, an antigen–antibody interaction results in the typical allergic manifestations. Extremely small quantities of antigen are required to provoke an allergic reaction. Drug allergies may manifest themselves over a full spectrum of immediate and delayed reactions. As an example, skin reactions may extend from mild rash to severe exfoliative dermatitis.

Drug allergies are classified into five types of reactions (Riedl & Casillas, 2003):

1. In type I reactions, called immediate hypersensitivity reactions, the drug–protein complex binds with immunoglobulin E (IgE) on the surface of basophils and mast cells, which causes the release of mediators such as histamine, prostaglandins, and leukotrienes. These substances cause the clinically apparent symptoms of urticaria, bronchospasm, or anaphylactic shock. Drug-induced skin reactions such as urticaria or angioedema can occur as isolated reactions or can be accompanied by other types of allergic reactions.
2. In type II reactions, called cytotoxic hypersensitivity reactions, the IgG or IgM antibody reacts with the drug–protein complex on the wall of blood cells. This destruction of the formed elements of the blood results in drug-induced thrombocytopenia, neutropenia, hemolysis, or anemia.
3. In type III allergic reactions, called immune complex hypersensitivity, the drug–protein complex combines with IgG and IgM to trigger the release of complement and cause local vascular damage. This is seen clinically as serum sickness; fever, joint, and muscle pain; and lymphadenopathy. Such reactions may take the form of fever only or involve generalized lymphadenopathy and joint swellings accompanied by urticaria and angioedema. In the initial exposure to the drug, the symptoms develop after significant amounts of antibody are synthesized by the body, usually in about a week. Symptoms may appear 3 weeks after the drug has been discontinued. **Penicillin** and **sulfa drugs** have been associated with these adverse reactions.
4. Type IV allergic reactions, called delayed hypersensitivity reactions, occur if the drug–protein complex is recognized by T lymphocytes, which causes a direct cytotoxicity and activation of macrophages to the cell. Clinically, this is seen as fixed drug eruptions or topical contact dermatitis to topical drug preparations.
5. Another type of allergic reaction is the autoimmune reaction. In this case, the drug-protein complex puts

into effect changes in the immune system that result in increased cytotoxic T-cell proliferation and formations of immunoglobulins that produce conditions such as systemic lupus erythematosus, glomerulonephritis, and certain types of granulocytopenia.

Idiosyncratic Causes

Individual patients vary widely in their reactions to drugs. Some patients have reactions that are not expected from the known pharmacological actions of a drug. The patient's unique genetic makeup contributes to the variability. When given an average and safe dose of a drug, some patients experience no effects, and others have severe adverse reactions. The cause of these bizarre effects may be pharmaceutical, pharmacokinetic, or genetic in origin.

Three potential sources of idiosyncratic type B adverse reactions are due to problems with the drugs themselves: (1) decomposition of the active ingredients, (2) effects of additives placed in the dosage form for pharmaceutical reasons, and (3) effects from the by-products of the manufacturing of the drug.

The administration of decomposed product is most likely to produce a therapeutic failure; however, the decomposed compounds may be toxic. An example is **tetracycline**, which can degrade into compounds that can cause renal failure (Fanconi's syndrome). It is well known that tartrazine dye in some products causes allergic reactions and bronchospasm. **L-tryptophan** was withdrawn from the market when certain brands contained a manufacturing by-product that caused eosinophilia and myalgia. When patients exhibit bizarre adverse reactions to common drugs, it is useful to keep drug product problems in mind as a possible cause.

Patients can also react to drugs in an unexpected way if they have an abnormality of metabolism of the drug that creates a toxic substance that causes direct organ damage. Examples of these reactions are hepatotoxicity with **tacrine** and **halothane**, agranulocytosis with **clozapine**, and hypersensitivity with **carbamazepine**. Why a very few individuals develop these reactions is unknown. These patients may have overactive activation pathways, underactive protective pathways, or immunological systems that are more responsive to allergic stimuli.

The final source of idiosyncratic reactions is some qualitative or quantitative abnormal response by the patient. Many of these abnormal responses are genetic in origin. For example, the patient with hemophilia may bleed excessively if given **aspirin**, the patient with glucose-6-phosphate dehydrogenase (G6PD) deficiency may develop hemolytic anemia if given **primaquine**, or the patient with excess aminolevulinic acid may develop porphyria if given drugs such as **barbiturates** or **estrogens**.

Type C Adverse Drug Reactions

Type C ADRs are the cumulative effects of a drug seen with chronic use of medications and are dose related and time related. A classic example of type C ADRs occurs when the hypothalamic-pituitary-adrenal axis is suppressed by chronic **corticosteroid** therapy (Edwards & Aronson, 2000). The treatment for type C ADRs is to reduce the dose or a slow withdrawal.

Type D Adverse Drug Reactions

Type D reactions or delayed ADRs become apparent some time after the medication is administered; examples include teratogenesis (congenital malformation) and carcinogenesis.

Teratogenesis (Congenital Malformation)

The possibility that a drug may cause teratological changes is well known. These ADRs are type A, being dose related and predictable. Congenital malformations are defined as irreversible functional or morphological defects present at birth and can be caused by genetic or environmental (including drug) factors. A teratogen is generally defined as an exogenous agent that has the ability to produce congenital malformations during fetal development. Major congenital malformations occur in 3 percent of all live births (CDC, 2008), and it is important to understand this background risk in evaluating the prevalence of drug-induced malformations. Associations of congenital malformations with drugs have been described in case reports and case series. Although these are important in drawing attention to a suspected teratogen, they do not prove teratogenicity. Epidemiological studies, which correct for confounding factors and have appropriate statistical analyses, are needed to detect associations between drug therapy and adverse outcomes.

The FDA's use-in-pregnancy rating system (Table 5–4) weighs the degree to which available information has ruled out risk to the fetus against the drug's potential benefit to the patient. All drugs available are not rated, and the list is not inclusive. If a drug is not rated, there may be pregnancy precautions listed in the prescribing information and postmarketing collection of pregnancy exposures are conducted, often with a toll-free number supplied by the manufacturer.

In general, the decision to use a drug for therapy in any patient is made by evaluating the benefits versus the risks to the patient. The situation is more complex in treating the pregnant patient because this evaluation must be made for two patients, the mother and the unborn child, and the ADRs in the fetus are usually irreversible. Unfortunately, many new drugs' risks to the fetus are unknown.

The identification of a drug or chemical as a teratogen is hampered by the fact that all exposed fetuses do not show congenital malformations. Even with drugs such as **thalidomide** and **retinoids**, the occurrence is 20 to 40 percent. Other substances, such as **carbamazepine** and **valproic acid**, cause malformations in only 1 to 2 percent of prenatal exposures. In addition, the use of animal models is not very helpful. There are known teratogens that do not cause malformations in some animals, and some substances that cause malformations in animals are

Table 5–4 **FDA Use-in-Pregnancy Ratings**

FDA Rating (Category)	Criteria for Rating
Contraindicated in Pregnancy	
X	Studies in animals or humans have shown fetal risk that clearly outweighs any possible benefit to the patient.
Positive Evidence of Risk	
D	Investigational or postmarketing data show risk to the fetus. Nevertheless, potential benefits may outweigh the potential risk.
Risk Cannot Be Ruled Out	
C	Human studies are lacking, and animal studies are either positive for risk or are lacking as well. However, potential benefits may outweigh the potential risk.
No Evidence of Risk in Humans	
B	Either animal findings show risk, whereas human findings do not, or, if no adequate human studies have been done, animal findings are negative.
Controlled Studies Show No Risk	
A	Adequate, well-controlled studies in pregnant women have failed to show risk to the fetus.

FDA = U.S. Food and Drug Administration.

not teratogens for humans. Given that the expected rate of malformation is 3 percent, an agent that is given frequently during pregnancy will be associated with some malformations. Rational drug selection for pregnant patients depends on careful examination of available information on the drugs being used and of the risks to both mother and child of withholding treatment.

Principles of Teratogenicity

No teratogenic drug compound causes malformations with every exposure. Some patients can take drugs without any apparent ill effects on the fetus. The specific malformations induced by a given drug are often similar but may be seen with a spectrum of severity. The presence and severity of malformations depend on three main factors: genetic susceptibility, developmental stage during the exposure, and dose of the drug.

A complicating factor in teratogenicity is the large differences between species in the adverse effects of drugs on the fetus. All human teratogens have been found to cause malformations in at least one animal; however, some drugs (e.g., **aspirin**) can induce malformations in animals but do not produce them in humans. Interpatient variation in susceptibility is found in humans as well. Only a small percentage of exposed fetuses demonstrate malformations, and some of this resistance is due to resistance to the effects of the drug.

The damage drugs cause is highly dependent on the time of exposure. The fetus's stage of development at the time of exposure—blastogenesis (2 weeks), embryogenesis (2 to 8 weeks), or fetogenesis (8 to 32 weeks)—determines whether the malformation will be seen. Malformations are not induced during the first 2 weeks after conception. Embryogenesis is the period of greatest susceptibility to malformations, a period when some women do not know they are pregnant.

During fetogenesis, the major risk is to the development of the central nervous system. Functional and behavioral defects have been associated with exposure while the brain is still growing and developing. Knowledge of fetal milestones and specific drug exposure is clinically important for making treatment decision in pregnant patients. Most drugs have a window of opportunity for malformations, which may allow their use outside these periods if drug therapy is essential. For example, **carbamazepine** causes neural tube defects only during the blastogenesis stage, the first 2 weeks after conception.

Teratogenic effects depend on the dose of the teratogen. This dose dependency may have a steep dose-response curve, giving a clear threshold of teratogenicity. Because of wide differences between patients in placental function and fetal and maternal metabolism of drugs, there is wide variability in toxic doses from one patient to another. This makes identification of a safe dose of a teratogen impossible. Teratogens may cause spontaneous abortion, fetal malformations, growth retardation, mental retardation, carcinogenesis, and mutagenesis. Factors that influence the teratogenicity of a drug include the fetus's gestational age, the type of malformation induced, and simultaneous exposure to other drugs or environmental agents.

Often, a patient has already taken a drug before seeking advice about the teratogenic risk. In this situation, it is important to accurately determine the drug(s), dose, route of administration, exact gestational age at exposure, and other drugs taken concurrently. The patient's general health and previous obstetrical history may be helpful. The practitioner can then provide all the information available about the teratogenic risk.

Mechanisms of teratogenicity are poorly understood, and drug therapy is to be avoided if at all possible in pregnant patients. Occasionally, however, the mother's treatment is essential for both mother and child. Rational drug selection is then determined by carefully examining the dose, timing, and functional effects of the drug on both patients.

Carcinogenesis

Today, we know that certain drugs and environmental agents are capable of inducing cancer. Carcinogenesis may arise from genetic damage that is dose related; this may be due to activation of oncogenes or inactivation of suppresser genes. It may also occur as the result of some potentially neoplastic tissue in the patient; a preneoplastic cell may be transformed into cancer by the administration of a drug, such as an **estrogen** or **androgen**, given for an unrelated condition.

The American Cancer Society lists all known carcinogens at its Web site, http://www.cancer.org. Drugs that are known carcinogens include but are not limited to **antineoplastics, immunomodulators (azathioprine, tracrolimus)**, and **oral contraceptives**. Drugs that are probably carcinogenic include **androgens, corticosteroids, estrogens, metronidazole, nitrites**, and **progestins. Ethanol** in alcoholic beverages is a known carcinogen. Patients need to be informed of the potential carcinogenic ADRs of any drug prescribed.

Chemicals and other substances that are known or potentially carcinogenic include asbestos, benzene, carbon tetrachloride, chloroform, dioxin, herbicides, nitrosamines, pesticides, tobacco smoke, and TRIS (a flame retardant).

Type E Adverse Drug Reactions

Type E reactions are seen at the end of drug therapy, with a physiological withdrawal seen after a medication is discontinued. The classic example is **opiate** withdrawal, although withdrawal symptoms will be seen with **amphetamines**, chronic **benzodiazepine** therapy, and **alcohol**. Abrupt discontinuation of **beta blockers** may cause rebound hypertension and tachycardia. Drugs with type E ADRs will need to be slowly tapered when discontinuing, observing for symptoms of withdrawal. If withdrawal symptoms occur, the patient may need a temporary increase in dose and a slower taper.

Type F Adverse Drug Reactions

Unexpected failure of therapy is classified as a type F ADR. The most common reason for a type F ADR is a drug–drug interaction. As more is learned about how the CYP450 enzymes and their ability to induce or inhibit the metabolism of drugs, the reason for unexpected failures may be explained. For example, some patients are CYP2C19 poor metabolizers and may need higher doses of **clopidogrel** to have the desired effect on platelet aggregation. Type F ADRs are also seen with **oral contraceptive** failure from drug interactions or when patients have **clopidogrel** treatment failure when they take it with **omeprazole**, a CYP2C19 inhibitor. A more complete discussion of the CYP enzymes and their impact on drug ADRs is found in Chapters 2 and 8.

CONCLUSION

Recent evidence suggests that adverse drug events are a significant and growing problem in health care. The risk/benefit ratio of each drug therapy decision must be carefully weighed, and the why, how, and when of therapy, including the risks, must be explained to the patient.

REFERENCE

American Cancer Society. (n.d.). Known and probable human carcinogens. Retrieved from http://www.cancer.org

Bond, C. A., & Raehl, C. L. (2006). Adverse drug reactions in United States hospitals. *Pharmacotherapy, 26*(5), 601–608.

Canada Health. (2010). Adverse reaction and incident reporting—2009. Canada Vigilance Program. *Canada Adverse Reaction Newsletter, 20*(2). Retrieved from http://www.hc-sc.gc.ca/dhp-mps/medeff/bulletin/carn-bcei_v20n2-eng.php#_Adverse_reaction_and

Centers for Disease Control and Prevention (CDC). (2007). Infant deaths associated with cough and cold medications—two states, 2005. *Morbidity and Mortality Weekly, 56*(1), 104.

Centers for Disease Control and Prevention (CDC). (2008). Update on overall prevalence of major birth defects—Atlanta, Georgia, 1978–2005. *Morbidity and Mortality Weekly, 57*(1), 1–5.

Cherry, D. K., Hing, E., Woodwell, D. A., & Rechtsteiner, E. A. (2008). National Ambulatory Medical Care Survey: 2006 summary. *National Health Statistics Report, 3*. Retrieved from http://www.cdc.gov/nchs/data/nhsr/nhsr003.pdf

Edwards, I. R., & Aronson, J. K. (2000). Adverse drug reactions: Definitions, diagnosis and management. *Lancet, 356*, 1255–1259.

Hanlon, J. T., Pieper, C. F., Hajjar, E. R., Sloane, R. J., Lindblad, C. I., Ruby, C. M., & Schmader, K. E. (2006). Incidence and predictors of all and preventable adverse drug reactions in frail elderly persons after hospital stay. *Journal of Gerontology, 61A*(5), 511–515.

Hazell, L., & Shakir, S. A. W. (2006). Under-reporting of adverse drug reactions: A systematic review. *Drug Safety, 29*(5), 385–396.

Le, J., Nguyen, T., Law, A. V., & Hodding, J. (2006). Adverse drug reactions among children over a 10-year period. *Pediatrics, 118*, 555–562.

McDonnell, P. J., & Jacobs, M. R. (2002). Hospital admissions resulting from preventable adverse drug reactions. *The Annals of Pharmacotherapy, 36*(9), 1331–1336.

Merle, L., Laroche, M. L., Dantoine, T., & Charmes, J. P. (2005). Predicting and preventing adverse drug reactions in the very old. *Drugs Aging, 22*(5), 375–392.

Reidl, M. A., & Casillas, A. M. (2003). Adverse drug reactions: Types and treatment options. *American Family Physician, 68*(9), 1781–1791.

Temple, M. E., Robinson, R. F., Miller, J. C., Hayes, J. R., & Nahata, M. C. (2004). Frequency and preventability of adverse drug reactions in pediatric patients. *Drug Safety, 27*(11), 819–829.

U.S. Food and Drug Administration (FDA). (2008). FDA releases recommendation regarding use of over-the-counter cough and cold products. Retrieved from http://www.fda.gov/NewsEvents/Newsroom/PressAnnouncements/2008/ucm116839.htm

U.S. Food and Drug Administration (FDA). (2010). AERS domestic and foreign reports by year (as of March 31, 2010). Retrieved from http://www.fda.gov/Drugs/GuidanceComplianceRegulatoryInformation/Surveillance/AdverseDrugEffects/ucm070441.htm

Wang, X., Chen, C., Wang, L., Chen, D., Guang, W., & French, J. (2003). Conception, early pregnancy loss, and time to clinical pregnancy: A population-based prospective study. *Fertility and Sterility, 79*(3), 577–584.

Wester, K., Jonsson, A. K., Spigset, O., Druid, H., & Hagg, S. (2007). Incidence of fatal adverse drug reactions: A population based study. *British Journal of Clinical Pharmacology, 65*(4), 573–579.

World Health Organization (WHO). (2002). *The importance of pharmacovigilance: Safety monitoring of medicinal products.* Geneva, Switzerland: World Health Organization. Retrieved from http://apps.who.int/medicinedocs/pdf/s4893e/s4893e.pdf

World Health Organization (WHO). (2008). Medicines: Safety of medicines—adverse drug reactions. Retrieved from http://www.who.int/mediacentre/factsheets/fs293/en/index.html

Zopf, Y., Rabe, C., Neubert, A., Gassmann, K. G., Rascher, W., Hahn, E. G., et al. (2008). Women encounter ADRs more often than do men. *European Journal of Clinical Pharmacology, 64*, 999–1004.

CHAPTER 6

FACTORS THAT FOSTER POSITIVE OUTCOMES

Anita Lee Wynne

Chapter Outline

Health-care providers' goal is to help patients become healthier. When the patient does not or cannot follow recommendations or instructions that lead to this goal, the provider may become frustrated. Multiple clinical studies have revealed that even though providers expect adherence and positive outcomes, in reality it may not happen.

OVERVIEW OF NONADHERENCE

The problem of poor adherence to drug therapy is widespread (Bartels, 2004). In the United States, the National Cholesterol Education Program (2002, 2004) estimated that only about 50 percent of patients adhere to their drug regimen at 6 months and 30 to 40 percent at 1 year. Other studies report similar data (National High Blood Pressure Education Program [NHBPEP], 2003; Osterberg & Blaschke, 2005), and Benner et al (2002) found nonadherent rates (less then 20% of drug being taken as prescribed) as high as 56 percent after 60 months. One study of Medicaid claims data from 1990 to 1994 revealed that only 39 percent of patients with type 2 diabetes who were prescribed a **sulfonylurea** obtained a 6-month or greater supply of the drug (Bartels, 2004). Similar rates have been found in other studies and other countries. Those at highest risk include patients who have asymptomatic conditions, chronic conditions (Hayes, McCahon, Panahi, Hamre, & Pohlman, 2008; Mahat, Scoloveno, & Donnelly, 2007), cognitive impairment, psychiatric illness, or disorders requiring significant lifestyle changes (e.g., smoking cessation) (Myung, McDonnell, Kazinets, Seo, & Moskowitz, 2009), and those who are on complex regimens with multiple daily dosing and significant adverse reactions (Luthy, Peterson, & Wilkinson, 2008; Sarver & Murphy, 2009). When patients' interactions with the provider include poor communication (Zagaria, 2008), the risk of nonadherence is even higher.

The health-care provider–patient relationship is not a parent–child relationship; it is one of setting and working toward realistic mutual goals (Hayes & McCahon, 2008; Horne, 2004; Osterberg & Blaschke, 2005). Providers cannot expect compliance. Compliance implies an involuntary act of submission. What is expected is adherence or positive outcomes, which implies a voluntary act of negotiation and joint acceptance of a treatment regimen. Horne (2004) points out that "typically, over 30% of patients harbor strong concerns" about the need for their medication and the risk involved in taking it. What is more, the patient tends to overestimate the risk. If these issues are not addressed by open communication, surreptitious nonadherence is likely to result. Because of the change in attitude from compliance to adherence, the provider now has an increased responsibility to educate patients about their diseases and the drugs used to treat them.

Nonadherence to pharmacological regimens can compromise the efficacy of a drug and lead to failure of the desired treatment goal, which may be very costly. Sipkoff (2005) reports a recent 3-year study by the University of Michigan School of Medicine in which patients who stopped using their drugs because of cost issues had more complications from their disease that resulted in total increased cost for themselves and the health-care system. As the number of uninsured or underinsured patients in the United States continues to rise, cost has become an increasingly important issue (Luthy et al, 2008). The pharmacoeconomics chapter (Chapter 12) addresses this issue in more detail.

Although the previous discussion has focused on issues concerning interaction of patient and provider, the health-care system itself creates barriers to adherence by limiting access to health care; using restricted formularies; and having prohibitively high costs for drugs, co-payments, or both. A cost-benefit analysis reported in a National Bureau of Economic Research publication (Lozada, 2005) showed a cost for complications of type 2 diabetes that far exceeded any cost savings by increasing co-payments for drugs. Providers need to work to remove potential barriers to adherence within the system as well as within themselves and their patients.

Why do patients not adhere to instructions about taking their medications? What occurs outside the office setting to sabotage the best of intentions? What is the patient's responsibility, and what is the provider's? This chapter discusses the major issues in nonadherence and ways to foster positive outcomes.

ADVERSE DRUG REACTIONS

Adverse drug reactions can take many forms. Some of them are real; some are the patient's perceptions about a drug learned from well-meaning friends. One telephone survey (Wysocke & Davis, 1999) contacted approximately 700 women regarding their use of **oral contraceptives.** Half of those women surveyed thought that **oral contraceptives** caused most women to gain weight, and about one-fourth of those women reported never using **oral contraceptives** because of the fear of gaining weight. Studies comparing **oral contraceptive** use and weight gain revealed that weight gain could not always be attributed to **oral contraceptive** use. More often, the weight gain was attributed to other causes such as increase in eating out in restaurants. The providers' education regarding the real side effects of **oral contraceptives** provided women with greater choices. Real or perceived adverse reactions directly affect the outcome of a prescribed drug regimen. If a patient perceives that a prescribed drug is causing a reaction, then the provider should explore alternative options to treating the problem. This response assures patients that the provider is willing to listen and work with them until the right drug or right dosage is prescribed. Patients might think that their skepticism about a drug will be interpreted as lack of confidence in the provider (Horne, 2004). It may be difficult for patients to tell providers that they have a different view of the drug. Encouraging open communication about these concerns and perceptions is important. Communication is discussed further below.

Certain adverse reactions are more likely to produce nonadherence than others. Oddly enough, serious adverse reactions such as severe hypotension or anaphylaxis are not among them. The ones most likely to produce nonadherence are the "irritating" ones that interfere with the patient's ability to carry out activities of daily living, including what he or she may do for a living. These reactions include headache, dizziness, anorexia, nausea and vomiting, constipation, and diarrhea. Unfortunately, these are also the most common adverse reactions. For **angiotensin-converting enzyme inhibitors**, the most common reason given for nonadherence is the dry, hacky, "tickle" cough that affects up to 15 percent of those taking these drugs.

What is a problematic adverse reaction for one person may not be for another. When looking for potential nonadherence, it is important to look for the adverse reactions that commonly cause nonadherence and talk to patients about them, but it is also important to ask which ones would be a problem for the individual patient and take these into consideration in making a drug choice.

ASYMPTOMATIC CONDITIONS

A variety of disease states are essentially asymptomatic until their later stages. Some of these can be treated with drugs in their early stages to prevent their progression. However, it may be difficult to convince a patient that he or she has a serious disease when there is no overt indication of the disorder except the provider's word about it. It is even more problematic when the drugs given to treat this "invisible" disorder produce "disease symptoms" themselves. One of the most common of these asymptomatic disorders is hypertension.

Intermittent adherence to **antihypertensive** drugs is one of the major reasons for uncontrolled hypertension and presumably persistent left ventricular hypertrophy (NHBPEP, 2003). Patients may realize through education that control of hypertension is very important to their health but may not adhere to the regimen secondary to the adverse reactions they experience to the drugs given to treat this disease. **Antihypertensive** drugs that have a rapid onset and short duration of action are not very desirable in long-term therapy secondary to possible large variations in blood pressure. These drugs lower the blood pressure quickly; however, if the patient misses one dose, the **antihypertensive** effect disappears, creating a possible rebound or adverse reaction. Since most of the drugs used to treat hypertension have those "irritating" adverse reactions, nonadherence (including missed doses) is likely. Selecting a more "forgiving" drug that either does not depend on half-life or has a longer half-life will produce limited effect on the efficacy of the drug if doses are delayed or missed (Osterberg & Blaschke, 2005). **Antihypertensives** that require several dose titrations (e.g., **alpha-adrenergic blockers**) can be particularly troublesome (e.g., severe orthostatic hypotension) if the patient misses some doses and then restarts the drug, even if it is not at the full dose.

Erectile dysfunction is a highly publicized medical problem affecting a significant number of men. The cause of erectile dysfunction may be an adverse reaction to **antihypertensive** therapy. **Antihypertensives** and **psychotropic** drugs have been implicated as the cause of this particular problem related to their predicated pharmacological action. The provider must explore possible drug actions prior to prescribing. Remember, a drug expresses all its actions, not just the ones desired to treat the disease. Understanding all the drugs actions helps to predict probable adverse reactions.

Many different classes of drugs are available for control of hypertension. Recognizing that these drugs have several possible adverse reactions, the provider looks at the tolerability profile of each drug and discusses it in selecting drugs for a particular patient. Tolerability is directly linked to patient adherence for both short- and long-term therapy and ultimately to the overall success of treatment. Chapter 40 discusses the problems with adherence found in drugs used to treat this largely asymptomatic, chronic condition.

Other diseases that are asymptomatic in their early stages include diabetes (see Chapter 33), HIV (see Chapter 37), hyperlipidemia (see Chapter 39), and some sexually transmitted infections (see Chapter 44). Adherence issues are covered related to each of these specific diseases in the chapter that focuses on that disease.

CHRONIC CONDITIONS

Some chronic conditions are also asymptomatic in their early stages and they are addressed previously. There are other conditions, however, that have overt symptoms that persist over time. These chronic conditions are often treated with complex drug regimens as discussed later, but they have an additional issue: the length of time over which the drugs must be taken. Everyone has experienced times when they had a short course of drugs for an acute condition and yet were unable to take those drugs exactly as prescribed even for that short space of time. Consider if those drugs had to be taken every day for years.

Ideally, the patient develops a pattern of taking the drugs consistent with her or his activities of daily living, for example, take the white pill before breakfast and the blue one at dinner. But life is often not consistent in these routines. Weekends, vacations, visiting family, and unexpected events alter the pattern. In addition, some days it may just seem like too much trouble to get the pill out, especially if the patient feels better on that day. Many chronic diseases have exacerbations and remissions. When feeling bad, the drug seems very important, but what about when the patient feels good (for a change) and the pill has adverse reactions that make him or her feel "less good"? Building support mechanisms and setting up monitoring of drug taking for patients with chronic disease is critical to their adherence to their regimens, including their drugs. Kutzleb and Reiner (2006), for example, found significantly improved symptom control and disease self-management in patients with heart failure who received weekly telephone follow-up by nurse practitioners. Early phone contacts enable the provider to determine if the information shared in the clinic has been clearly understood and is being followed. Similar results were found with Web-based collaborative care for type 2 diabetes patients (Ralston et al, 2009). Such follow-up contacts not only help with adherence, but also contribute to building a stronger patient–provider relationship. Patients feel special when their provider contacts them about their plan of care outside the formal clinic visit. Chapter 11 has a section on "telehealth" that discusses the use of automated provider phone messages and calls as well as the use of Web-based communication to enhance adherence.

KNOWLEDGE DEFICIT AND PATIENT PERCEPTION

"Just teach them what they need to know and they will take their drugs as prescribed. The problem is lack of education." Understanding the disease state and the treatment regimen plays a role in adherence. Providing educational material alone, written or oral, cannot ensure that the patient will not have a knowledge deficit regarding the drug regimen or that she or he will be adherent. In this era of managed care, providers may feel pressured into having shorter visits with the patient. A greater length of time spent with a patient, however, is not the only component related to increased patient adherence. The quality of the communication and interaction that occur during that time is most important. Patients report greater adherence to a drug regimen if they feel that their concerns and specific points of knowledge deficit are addressed.

Keys to Patient Education

To be effective, patient education must:

- Be simple and focus on the critical points. What does the patient need to know to take this drug safely?
- Use language that is clear and understandable to the patient. This does not just mean "English versus Spanish," for example; it means reduced "medicaleze." It is important, however, not to talk down to people who do understand the medical terms. Never assume patients do or do not understand terms used.
- Be in a form the patient can refer to as needed after the contact with the provider. Herein lies the problem with literacy (Zagaria, 2008). Studies that looked at the reading level of many prepackaged materials found that they are written at least at the 12th grade reading level. Most patients read at or below the 6th grade reading level, and some do not read at all and are too embarrassed to tell the provider.
- Include aids, such as colored bottles and calendars, to help the patient know when to take which drug. The more complex the regimen, the more important these aids are.
- If steps are required to take a drug, present information on the steps in the order they will be used.
- Where children are involved, inclusion of the family is essential. Health behaviors are learned and reinforced with the family, so a family-centered approach (Mahat et al, 2007; Tyler & Horner, 2008) that engages and supports parents and children has a better chance of improving adherence.

Assess other issues that may interfere with adherence, such as social support and the ability to purchase the drugs. Patients may understand what you taught, but not be able to follow through even when they want to do so. Some of these other issues are discussed later.

Health and Cultural Beliefs

Other influences regarding a patient's knowledge deficit include health beliefs the patient holds, cultural beliefs (see Chapter 7), and the relationship between the patient and the provider (Castro & Ruiz, 2009). Some patients do not want to share in the decision-making process. Because of health beliefs or cultural beliefs, they perceive that they need to do what the health-care provider tells them to do. The idea of having to share the control of taking care of themselves is very foreign. Patients who expect the provider to tell them what to do perceive that the decision-sharing provider does not know what she or he is doing and may not return to that provider. Conversely, the patient who wants to be in control and has a provider who presents information in an authoritarian manner can also create a mismatch.

Medical Terminology Literacy

Using language that the patient understands increases the chances of reversing knowledge deficit. Listen actively to patients' terminology when they refer to their body parts or disease processes. When a provider refers to "cystitis," the patient may not understand; if the provider says, instead, "urinary tract infection," usually the patient understands. By using biomedical terminology, the provider is putting up a barrier that may unintentionally create a greater knowledge deficit. Using the patient's terminology can reduce the possible trial-and-error period that may result when the provider attempts to communicate the physiological findings. Finding common terminology with the patient will increase the patient's confidence in the provider's desire to help.

Certain populations are especially at risk for low health literacy. They include adults 65 years of age and older, minority populations, low-income individuals (who may read below the 5th grade level), and immigrant populations whose English proficiency may be limited (Zagaria, 2008). Some resources that may help the provider understand the health-literacy issue and assist in dealing with it include the following:

- http://www.npsf.org/askme3/. This is a program sponsored by the Partnership for Clear Health Communication, a coalition of organizations working to promote awareness of and solutions to health-literacy problems.
- http://www.healthliteracy.com/. A health-literacy consulting group.
- http://www.nifl.gov. A Washington, DC–based national literacy institute.

- http://www.healthlit.fcm.arizona.edu. A self-learning module for assisting older adults with health-literacy problems.
- http://www.sph.emory.edu/WELLNESS/reading.html. A resource to check reading levels of patient materials.

Written Handouts

Do not hand out written material without taking the time to explain it. The inclusion of a drug insert may make patients anxious as they read how many adverse reactions may occur. Certainly, the information about interactions may prevent serious complications, but what about patients who are sure they have every possible complication that might develop? In this situation, the provider and pharmacist must work closely together to provide patients with correct information while reassuring them about the degree of risk for any given adverse reaction and the ability to prevent or treat it should it occur. Having open communication with patients and using their terminology can enhance the positive outcomes from the drug regimen. Enhanced, clear communication forms a positive relationship between patient and provider. In an atmosphere of shared values, shared language (Castro & Ruiz, 2009), and mutual respect, adherence and positive patient outcomes occur.

COGNITIVE IMPAIRMENT AND PSYCHIATRIC ILLNESS

Communicating effectively with patients who have cognitive impairments (e.g., Alzheimer's disease) can be a challenge. Providers need to be able to count on the patient's ability to understand and remember education presented about the drug if adherence is to occur. Each person with cognitive impairment is unique, having a different constellation of abilities and needs for support in understanding and remembering. Assessing the abilities of each patient is important to maximizing adherence. This may involve working with a caregiver or guardian (see later). The Alzheimer's Association has written materials to assist in this assessment and to provide tips for fostering adherence. They may be reached at http://www.alz.org.

Patients with psychiatric illnesses are notorious for not adhering to their drug regimen. Half of the patients with major depression for whom antidepressants are prescribed will not be taking the drugs 3 months after the initiation of therapy (Osterberg & Blaschke, 2005). Rates of adherence among patients with schizophrenia are between 50 and 60 percent (Lacro, Dunn, Dolder, Leckbane, & Jeste, 2002; Perkins, 2002), and among those with bipolar disorder, the rates are as low as 35 percent (Colom et al, 2000). Three major factors are involved here: (1) Psychiatric illness has a social stigma. When symptoms are no longer present (because of the drugs being taken), the patient may be tempted to think that the diagnosis was wrong and he or she is not really mentally ill. (2) The presence of symptoms may result in thoughts and behaviors that do not foster adherence—for example, paranoia, agitation, or depression. Finally, (3) the adverse effects with **psychotropics**—for example, dizziness, orthostatic hypotension, blurred vision, decreased central processing, and confusion—are effects commonly associated with nonadherence. Those adverse effects and others, such as agitation, constipation, and urinary retention, are especially problematic for older, cognitively impaired adults in whom these drugs may be used for behavior control (Bulat, Castle, Rutledge, & Quigley, 2008).

Longer-Acting Drugs

As with hypertension, selecting drugs with longer half-lives may reduce the likelihood of drug withdrawal symptoms and return of illness. For example, **fluoxetine (Prozac)**, a **serotonin reuptake inhibitor** used to treat depression, has a 2-week duration of action so that missing doses or stopping the drug altogether produces a long taper and gives the provider time to discover the problem and work to correct it. **Fluphenazine (Prolixin)** is in a parenteral formulation that also lasts 2 weeks and is very helpful in patients with schizophrenia. Other drugs are also being developed in depot formulations that are long acting and can be given IM. These agents combine better efficacy and tolerability with improved adherence.

Use of Reinforcements

Osterberg and Blaschke (2005) suggest the use of reinforcements such as monetary rewards or vouchers, frequent contact with the patient, and personalized reminders Educational approaches appear to be most effective when combined with behavioral techniques and supportive services, including reinforcements.

Regardless of the diagnosis, mental health patients require careful monitoring related to their adherence to drug therapy that may include help from family, friends, and other providers. Monitoring adherence is discussed later.

CAREGIVER'S ROLES

When the patient is a child, an adult with cognitive deficits or disabilities, or a person with mental illness, the patient's caregiver must be involved in the educational process. The caregiver can provide valuable information regarding the patient's responses to drugs or difficulties in adhering to the prescribed medication regimen. If the provider detects that the caregiver may be having difficulty in adhering to the drug regimen, it is possible that the caregiver may need to be provided one-on-one interventions to help foster positive outcomes for the patient.

The Pediatric Patient

Achieving full adherence in pediatric patients requires the cooperation not only of the child but also of a devoted, persistent, and adherent parent or caregiver (Mahat et al, 2007; Tyler & Horner, 2008). Adolescent patients create even more challenges, given the unique developmental, psychosocial, and lifestyle issues implicit in adolescence. Adherence rates in children and adolescents are similar to those seen in adults, with rates of adherence to drug regimens averaging about 50 percent. Special interventions for children are discussed in the chapter on pediatric patients (Chapter 50).

Caregiver's Quality of Life

The caregiver's quality of life has a huge impact on the patient's quality of life. By exploring with the caregiver the psychological, physical, and social impact of giving care, the provider is acknowledging the difficulties the caregiver must face every day. Try to help the caregiver find ways to "take a break" for herself or himself. Showing concern for the caregiver as well as the patient will foster a positive relationship with the provider. By understanding the impact the caregiver has on the patient, greater adherence and positive outcomes can occur.

Behavioral Therapy

Behavioral therapy can empower the caregiver to provide appropriate interventions. Discuss situations in which the patient does not cooperate with his or her care, including drug therapy. Help the caregiver to remember the times the patient did cooperate and try to determine what the characteristics of the situation were that elicited that cooperation. Techniques to elicit cooperation can then become part of the routine care.

Behavioral changes for the caregiver and patient are best identified early in the disease process. It may be that an interdisciplinary approach is the best intervention for caregivers of patients having a multitude of complicating factors. The caregiver has a huge role in communicating to the provider and the patient the possibility of adverse reactions.

Always include the caregiver when providing education to the patient. Acknowledgment of the caregiver's roles in the patient's outcome is a powerful intervention. The thoughtful provider realizes this impact and considers its potential outcome in every encounter.

COMPLEXITY OF DRUG REGIMEN AND POLYPHARMACY

Drugs are being increasingly used to treat a wide range of disorders. Many of these disorders require multiple drugs to treat them. It is generally accepted that few hypertensive patients will meet their target blood pressure on fewer than two drugs, and they often require three or four. This is assuming that they do not have concurrent diseases, and patients with hypertension commonly have them. The same can be said of diabetes, heart diseases, asthma, and many other diseases. These complex drug regimens are also more likely in older adults with multiple chronic illnesses (Bartels, 2004). An increased number of drugs used to manage multiple complex disease processes increases the possibility of nonadherence and the chances of a decreased positive outcome for the patient. Deciding what to do and when to do it can be complex and frustrating for all involved, patient and provider alike.

Education for the patient, written and oral, regarding the importance of following a daily schedule is the gold standard. Points to consider are discussed previously. However, this is only one of the components in solving the dilemma of complex drug regimens or polypharmacy.

Personalized Drug Schedules

Helping patients set up a personalized drug schedule devised only for them is one possible solution. Working with nursing staff at the clinic, a matrix of activities of daily living can be devised into which drug schedules can be fit. Because the schedule is specific to that individual patient's life, it is easier for the patient to follow and to remember.

Simplifying the Regimen

Multiple studies have been done relating adherence to the number of times a drug must be taken each day and the total number of drugs being taken daily. One study of diabetics (Morris, Brennan, MacDonald, & Donnan, 2000) found that for each increase in daily dosing frequency, there was a 22 percent decrease in adherence. A systematic review of 38 hypertension drug adherence trials involving 15,519 patients (Schroeder, Fahey, & Ebrahim, 2004) found that simplification of dosing regimens improved adherence between 8 and 19.6 percent. A literature review of 76 publications by Claxton, Cramer, and Pierce (2001) showed that adherence to once-daily dosing was 79 percent, twice a day was 69 percent, three times a day was 65 percent, and four times a day was 51 percent. The data on short-term use of **antibiotics** for respiratory infections are even more impressive, with nearly 100 percent adherence for once-daily dosing. When given an **antibiotic** dosing schedule of twice daily, at least one-third of patients missed one or more doses. As the number of doses increased, so did the nonadherence (Carlson, Stool, & Stutman, 2005). The ideal drug, it appears, would be taken once daily. Interestingly, anything other than daily dosing seems to result in decreased, rather than increased, adherence.

Cues as Reminders

A variety of things can be used as cues. Pill containers can be purchased with compartments from daily dosing to multiple times/day dosing and from weekly to monthly schedules. These containers not only serve as cues to take a drug but also help to monitor when a drug is or is not taken. Daily calendars with sections for each hour of the day can be marked with the name of the drug to be taken. Monthly calendars are sometimes needed for drugs taken on a less-frequent-than-daily basis. New technologies include reminders through cell phones, person digital assistants, and pillboxes with paging systems. For pediatric patients, stickers, which can be applied to a reminder board or chart, are also helpful. Good locations to place these reminders include the refrigerator or bathroom mirror.

Matching Drugs to Clinic Scheduling

Patients who miss appointments are often those who need the most help to improve their ability to adhere to a drug regimen. Such patients often benefit from clinical scheduling that matches their drug regimen. If a drug is prescribed for 2 weeks, the next appointment should be on the day after the drug should be completed. For chronic illness, clinic scheduling around the time for drawing any laboratory work or doing physical assessments such as blood pressure can also include consideration for the time to fill the prescriptions. Initial prescription may be given for short time intervals until the patient has time to fit the drugs into their daily routine and demonstrate adherence. Then longer intervals with larger amounts of drug dispensed can occur. These follow-up appointments also give the provider the opportunity to assess for adverse reactions in the drug regimen.

Another method that fosters adherence and positive outcomes with complex drug regimens or polypharmacy is the anticipatory guidance framework. This method anticipates what education and guidance will be needed at different intervals of the patient's learning process. The provider who chooses to utilize this method must have knowledge of the physiological, psychological, and developmental concerns of the individual patient. A child, teenager, young adult, and older adult are in definite stages of development. Interventions designed for a child certainly are not appropriate for other age levels unless a cognitive deficiency is present. The theme of individualized assessment and education is repeated, but its importance cannot be stressed enough. Patient management can utilize multidisciplinary team members to help achieve the most positive outcomes.

FINANCIAL IMPACTS

Pharmacological interventions are costly. This cost can have a huge impact on the ability and willingness of the patient to adhere to drug regimens. Even if the patient has access to financial assistance (e.g., Medicaid, insurance coverage for drugs), this does not ensure that the patient will view drugs as a primary financial need. Basic needs (e.g., food, housing) may take precedence over drugs in planning a monthly budget. This is especially true for older adults who are frequently on fixed incomes and yet are the highest users of prescription and over-the-counter drugs.

Cost Versus Complications

Sipkoff (2005) reports a recent 3-year study by the University of Michigan School of Medicine that measured the medical effect of nonadherence on 8,000 people with chronic conditions, including hypertension, diabetes, and depression. Researchers found that study subjects who said they cut back on their prescriptions because of cost were 75 percent more likely to have suffered a significant decline in their overall health and 50 percent were more likely to have had a heart attack, stroke, or chest pain episode than those who filled their prescriptions.

For newly diagnosed patients with chronic illnesses, high cost-sharing—that is, having a large co-payment for each prescription or having to pay up to a certain dollar amount before insurance pays the rest—has been shown to delay the initiation of drug therapy. For example, a study of patients with hypertension found that 54.8 percent of the patients delayed initiating therapy when cost-sharing was doubled (Solomon, Goldman, Joyce, & Escarce, 2009).

Out-of-Pocket Versus Insurance

Having an adequate payment system to cover the cost of medications does not in itself guarantee appropriate utilization of this benefit. Certainly, those patients who have to cover the cost of drugs out of pocket are at greater risk for inadequate adherence to costly drugs. Lozada (2005) reports a cost-benefit study done by Dor and Encinosa on a sample of 27,057 patients with type 2 diabetes. They estimated that the cost saved by increasing a co-payment for their drugs as little as $6 would also increase the rate of diabetic complications related to increased nonadherence by $360 million per year, far exceeding the savings of $31.2 million incurred by the co-payment increase.

An increasing number of patients are either uninsured or underinsured. Drug costs should be considered when encouraging patient adherence in the uninsured and underinsured (Luthy et al, 2008).

Family Versus Self

Patients who have several family members to support may view drugs taken for themselves as somehow being selfish. The child who has a chronic disease also affects the financial stability of the family, which may cause resentment from parents or siblings.

Generic Versus "New and Improved" Brand Name

The patients see them advertised on TV and the provider hears it from the drug representative: "This new drug is so much better than the old one" or "This brand-name drug is so much better than a generic." There are times when a new drug has characteristics that make it better than anything else on the market, and generic drugs that are not bioequivalent are not a good idea. However, choosing a new or nongeneric formulation that is very expensive requires careful consideration. Throughout this book, tables that show available dosage forms attempt to give both the brand-name and the generic drug costs. Sometimes the difference is almost unbelievable. A brand-name drug may cost *hundreds* of times as much as the generic. For example, **Atenolol**, a **beta blocker**, costs $16 for 100 tablets in the generic form and $177 for 100 tablets in the brand name **Tenormin**. Providers need to discover this information before prescribing a drug, even if the patient or the insurance provider appears to be able to cover the cost.

Public Assistance

The issue of public assistance is certainly a complex and difficult one. Having an awareness of possible public programs available to assist financially is only a part of the whole picture. The provider also has to have knowledge of the patient and whether that patient will accept public assistance. All the public assistance in the world will not work if the patient or family views it as a social or cultural stigma that is unacceptable.

COMMUNICATION DIFFICULTIES

Communication difficulties exist not only in finding common terminology but also in speech, hearing, and language barriers. Such difficulties can cause considerable frustration for the provider and patient. Cooperation between the provider and the patient is a must for any positive outcome, but this becomes a very clear problem with those patients who cannot hear, cannot speak, or do not understand the language that is predominantly spoken.

Non–English Speakers and Interpreters

Language barriers are a difficulty in adhering to a drug regimen. Federal law requires that clinics provide an interpreter if the primary language is different from the provider's. Clinics are able to contact interpreters for a number of different languages. The difficulty that arises is whether the interpreter is repeating exactly what the provider is saying and, in return, whether the interpreter is saying exactly what the patient is saying. A certain amount of trust must be exhibited between the interpreter and the provider.

Professional interpreters are preferable. A patient may not want to share certain information with the family member who is the interpreter, and the family interpreter may not wish to give the provider certain information about the patient. Cultural norms play a major role here. When a professional interpreter is not accessible, every effort must be made to find a reliable interpreter. The provider can be held liable for poor outcomes if she or he suspects an unreliable interpreter and does nothing to correct the situation.

Speech and Hearing Issues

Patients with hearing or speech difficulties present their own challenges. Patients with hearing difficulties may have learned to compensate by reading lips. If this is the case, the provider must stand directly in front of the patient and speak clearly, looking directly at the patient's face. Presbycusis (aging hearing loss) is commonly associated with decreased ability to hear higher-pitched tones, often those within the range of the human voice. Speaking in low tones or finding a provider with a lower voice may improve the patient's hearing ability.

Patients with speech difficulties include those who are deaf and, therefore, have never heard speech and those who have had strokes or laryngectomies or other surgical procedures that reduce their ability to produce speech. Sometimes, these patients have learned coping mechanisms or had speech therapy to enable them to communicate, and the provider must discover what tools the patient uses/needs to communicate and use these to the patient's advantage. For patients who use American Sign Language, an interpreter should be provided. Patients using speech-enhancing devices usually bring such items with them. In any case, special attention should be paid to ensure that these patients communicate effectively with the provider and vice versa.

COMMUNICATION BETWEEN PROVIDERS

It can be disconcerting and exasperating when attempting to coordinate health care for a patient who sees several different providers. Open lines of communication are a must between the patient and his or her provider(s) and among health-care providers. If a patient sees a specialist for whatever reason, ask the patient to request that the records of each visit be sent to the coordinating primary-care provider. However, the patient or the specialist's staff does not always follow through on this request. A congenial call by the primary-care provider will do much toward receiving the reports; coordinating care, regimens, and appointments; letting patients know the provider thinks they are important; and letting the specialists know who is the primary-care provider, thus also enhancing the visibility and credibility of primary-care practice.

Patients who see several health-care providers or who do not consistently have the same provider show greater problems with adherence to treatment therapy. Encouraging repeat visits to the same provider increases communication and knowledge between the patient and the provider.

Coordination by one primary-health-care provider also alleviates part of the problem between multiple providers.

Communication in identifying the patient's major concerns and meeting expectations is extremely important. If the patient must be referred to a specialist, making a follow-up appointment that does not interfere with the specialist's appointments informs the patient that their primary-care provider believes the patient and the specialist are important. Patients may feel abandoned if follow-up appointments are not made or at least suggested when the patient must be turned over to a specialist. Primary-care providers can enable a positive outcome by creating open communication between themselves and other providers to whom the patient has been referred.

PATIENT'S RESPONSIBILITIES

Providers have responsibilities for determining the best plan of care for a patient and for working with the patient to actualize that plan of care. However, the plan of care should be mutually arrived at with the patient, and the patient carries some of the responsibility for its actualization. Not taking a drug, not taking it as prescribed, or premature discontinuance of a drug are common forms of nonadherence. Failure to fill the prescription is another form of nonadherence. All of these are within the control and responsibility of the patient.

Antibiotic resistance has increasingly become a concern for health-care providers. The responsibility for overuse and misuse of antibiotics lies in part with the public, which is uneducated or undereducated about the appropriate use of antibiotics. A patient who presents with a cold may demand an antibiotic to "fix" the situation. Many health-care consumers do not know the difference between viruses and bacteria. Explaining why an antibiotic does not work on a viral infection must be done in terminology that the patient understands. The health-care provider has the ultimate responsibility to protect patients from resistant organisms. Chapter 24 discusses the issue of antibiotic resistance in more detail.

Chronic illnesses create some of the greatest problems for the patient who has to adhere to ongoing therapy. Time, finances, and a desire to be perceived as healthy appear to have the greatest impact. Tuberculosis is one chronic illness that has begun to increase in prevalence, and part of the reason is related to nonadherence to drug therapy. Public health departments attempted to control the increasing epidemic of tuberculosis in several ways, one of which was creating directly observed therapy programs. Directly observed programs were more effective than self-administration programs; however, many patients delayed treatment to avoid mandatory therapy or detainment. The patients who had adherence to the drug regimen were those who had a personal desire to be free of the symptoms associated with tuberculosis. This personal investment is one of the keys to successful long-term management of any chronic disease. Chapter 45 discusses in more detail the issues of nonadherence with tuberculosis drugs.

Self-monitoring has been shown to have positive effects on outcomes of drug regimens. For the patient with asthma, self-monitoring of peak expiratory flow rates can improve disease awareness and predict asthma flare-ups (see Chapter 30). Patients demonstrated better adherence after the first follow-up visits but gradually tapered off unless the use of the drugs was reiterated in follow-up visits. This technique can be utilized with other chronic diseases (e.g., diabetes, chronic obstructive pulmonary disease, cardiac disease, hypertension, depression) by reviewing whatever device is utilized for home management. Sarver and Murphy (2009) stress the importance of patient-centered versus disease-centered management strategies that include comprehensive patient and caregiver education and "solid partnerships between healthcare providers and patients."

Do not assume that the patient with a history of homelessness or substance abuse will not follow a treatment plan or that the well-educated, affluent patient will. The provider must find out if the patient actually wants to take the drug and is committed to adhere to a drug regimen. Patients have the responsibility to try to adhere to pharmacotherapeutics, but it is also the provider's responsibility to attempt to discover the barriers that are impeding a positive outcome.

MEASURING ADHERENCE

Adherence can rarely be measured by only one method. Methods that may be used include patient reports, clinical outcomes, pill counts, refill records, and biological and chemical markers.

Patient Reports

Keeping in mind that most patients want to please the provider, patient reports are the easiest monitoring tool. Just ask the patient:

- Did you fill your prescription?
- How often have you taken your drug in the past [number of days or weeks]?
- Have you missed any scheduled times to take the drug? If so, what was the reason? The answer to this question may give the provider insight into ways to improve adherence by removing barriers to it.
- Are there things we could do together to help you take your drugs?

Have the patient keep a drug diary to help him or her answer these questions honestly.

Clinical Outcomes

Most drugs have a clear clinical outcome that is attempting to be achieved. Did the drug actually lower their blood pressure or their blood glucose? Did the patient have fewer asthma attacks or trips to the emergency room? Matching the patient's clinic visit time for assessment of a clinical outcome with the time to refill a prescription helps to address issues that may be adherence related. If the clinical outcome was not met, adherence may be part of the answer. Remember, it is rarely the whole answer.

Pill Counts

Pill counts can be helpful in determining if the correct number of pills was taken between visits. Some new technologies dispense only one pill at a time, thereby reducing the risk that the patient may pour out pills to avoid being "caught." This type of dispensing can also be tied to reminders to take the pills. Bubble packs are cheap pill-counting methods that do not require fancy technology. If the patient has a caregiver, the caregiver can do the pill counts.

Refill Records

Such records can be kept in the patient's chart or can be obtained from the pharmacy if the patient uses only one pharmacy to refill his or her prescriptions. This technique is discussed in Chapter 53 as it relates to pain contracts, but it may be useful in other instances.

Biological and Chemical Markers

These markers usually are laboratory tests or other diagnostic markers. Their use is similar to the clinical outcomes discussed previously.

SUMMARY

Patient education, enhanced communication between patient and provider and between providers, and consideration of multiple complicating social factors all contribute to fostering adherence and positive outcomes. Identifying patients at risk for nonadherence or those who actually are nonadherent, determining the cause of the nonadherence, facilitating the removal of the cause or barriers to adherence, and developing partnerships with patients to produce adherence and positive clinical outcomes are important roles for the prescribing provider.

REFERENCES

Bartels, D. (2004). Adherence to oral therapy for type 2 diabetes: Opportunities for enhancing glycemic control. *Journal of the American Academy of Nurse Practitioners, 16*(1), 8–16.

Benner, J., et al. (2002). Long-term persistence in use of statin therapy in elderly patients. *Journal of the American Medical Association, 288*, 455–461.

Bulat, T., Castle, S., Rutledge, M., & Quigley, P. (2008). Clinical practice algorithms: Medication management to reduce fall risk in the elderly—Part 4, anticoagulants, anticonvulsants, anticholinergics/bladder relaxants and antipsychotics. *Journal of the American Academy of Nurse Practitioners, 20*(4), 181–190.

Carlson, L., Stool, S., & Stutman, F. (2005). Adherence and dosing. *Sound Advice, 1*(12), 1–12.

Castro, A., & Ruiz, E. (2009). The effects of nurse practitioner cultural competence on Latina patient satisfaction. *Journal of the American Academy of Nurse Practitioners, 21*(5), 278–286.

Claxton, A., Cramer, J., & Pierce, C. (2001). A systematic review of the association between dose regimens and medication compliance. *Clinical Therapeutics, 23*, 1296–1310.

Colom, F., Vieta, E., Martinez-Aran, A., Reinares, M., Benabarre, A., & Gasto, C. (2000). Clinical factors associated with treatment noncompliance in euthymic bipolar patients. *Journal of Clinical Psychiatry, 61*, 549–555.

Hayes, E., McCahon, C., Panahi, N., Hamre, T., & Pohlman K. (2008). Alliance not compliance: Coaching strategies to improve type 2 diabetes outcomes. *Journal of the American Academy of Nurse Practitioners, 20*(3), 155–162.

Horne, R. (2004). Non-adherence with drugs more likely if patients' beliefs are ignored. *The Pharmaceutical Journal, 273*(7320), 525.

Kardas, P. (2002). Patient compliance with antibiotic treatment for urinary tract infections. *Journal of Antimicrobial Chemotherapy, 49*, 897–903.

Kutzleb, J., & Reiner, D. (2006). The impact of nurse-directed patient education on quality of life and functional capacity in people with heart failure. *Journal of the American Academy of Nurse Practitioners, 18*(3), 116–123.

Lacro, J., Dunn, L., Dolder, C., Leckbanc, S., & Jeste, D. (2002). Prevalence of and risk factors for medication nonadherence in patients with schizophrenia: A comprehensive review of recent literature. *Journal of Clinical Psychiatry, 63*, 892–909.

Lozada, C. (2005). Effects of co-payment on prescription drug demand. *National Bureau of Economic Research.* Retrieved October 20, 2005, from http://www.nber.org/digest/apr05/w10738.html

Luthy, K., Peterson, N., & Wilkinson, J. (2008). Cost-efficient treatment options for uninsured or underinsured patients for five common conditions. *Journal for Nurse Practitioners, 4*(8), 577–584.

Mahat, G., Scoloveno, M., & Donnelly, C. (2007). Written educational materials for families of chronically ill children. *Journal of the American Academy of Nurse Practitioners, 19*(9), 471–476.

Morris, A., Brennan, G., MacDonald, T., & Donnan, P. (2000). Populations-based adherence to prescribed medication in type 2 diabetes: A cause for concern. *Diabetes Care, 23*, 1278–1283.

Myung, S., McDonnell, D., Kazinets, G., Seo, H., & Moskowitz, J. (2009). Effects of web- and computer-based smoking cessation programs: Meta analysis of randomized controlled trials. *Archives of Internal Medicine, 169*(10), 929–937.

National Cholesterol Education Program. (2002). Third report of the expert panel on detection, evaluation, and treatment of high blood cholesterol in adults (Adult Treatment Panel III): Final report. *Circulation, 106*, 3143–3421. Also available at http://www.nhlbi.nih.gov/guidelines/cholesterol

National Cholesterol Education Program. (2004). *ATP III update 2004: Implications of recent clinical trails for the ATP III guidelines.* Retrieved June 1, 2009, from http://www.nhlbi.nih.gov/guidelines/cholesterol

National High Blood Pressure Education Program (NHBPEP). (2003). *The seventh report of the Joint National Committee on Prevention, Detection, Evaluation, and Treatment of High Blood Pressure*. Rockville, MD: National Institutes of Health, National Heart, Lung, and Blood Institute.

Osterberg, L., & Blaschke, T. (2005). Adherence to medication. *New England Journal of Medicine, 353*(5), 487–497.

Ralston, J., Hirsch, I., Hoath, J., Mullen, M., Cheadle, A., & Goldberg, H. (2009). Web-based collaborative care for type 2 diabetes: A pilot randomized trial. *Diabetes Care, 32*(2), 234–239.

Perkins, D. (2002). Predictors of noncompliance in patients with schizophrenia. *Journal of Clinical Psychiatry, 63*, 1121–1128.

Sarver, N., & Murphy, K. (2009). Management of asthma: New approaches to establishing control. *Journal of the American Academy of Nurse Practitioners, 21*(1), 54–65.

Schroeder, K., Fahey, T., & Ebrahim, S. (2004). How can we improve adherence to blood pressure lowering medication in ambulatory care? Systematic review of randomized controlled trials. *Annals of Internal Medicine, 164,* 722–732.

Sipkoff, M. (2005). Generics linked to improved compliance due to lower cost. *Drug Topics: The Online Newsmagazine for Pharmacists.* Retrieved October 20, 2005, from http://www.drugtopics.com/drugtopics/article/articleDetail.jsp?id=152724

Solomon, M., Goldman, D., Joyce, G., & Escarce, J. (2009). Cost sharing and the initiation of drug therapy for the chronically ill. *Archives of Internal Medicine, 169*(8), 740–748.

Tyler, D., & Horner, S. (2008). Family-centered collaborative negotiation: A model for facilitating behavioral change in primary care. *Journal of the American Academy of Nurse Practitioners, 20*(4), 194–203.

Wysocke, S., & Davis, A. J. (1999). *Clinical challenges in women's health: A handbook for nurse practitioners.* Jamesburg, NJ: NP Communications.

Zagaria, M. (2008). Health literacy: Striving for effective communication. *The American Journal for Nurse Practitioners, 12*(9), 23–26.

CHAPTER 7

CULTURAL AND ETHNIC INFLUENCES IN PHARMACOTHERAPEUTICS

Diane Vines

Chapter Outline

The United States has been named a melting pot of races and cultures. In the 2000 census, the total population in the United States was 281,421,906. The 2000 census data indicates that the U.S. population is 12.5 percent Hispanic or Latino, 12.3 percent black or African American, 0.9 percent Alaska Native or American Indian, 3.6 percent Asian, 0.1 percent Native Hawaiian and other Pacific Islander. The U.S. Census Bureau (2008) predicts that, by 2042, minorities as a group will be a majority of the population; among children, the current "minorities" will be the majority by 2023. Hispanics are the fastest growing group, followed by the Asian population. A growing percentage of Americans are those born in another country.

In the past, census respondents could choose only a single racial category. The 2000 census is the first time that respondents could choose more than one racial category, with 2.4 percent of the population indicating they were of two or more races. The U.S. Census Bureau (2006) predicts that this mixed-race group will more than triple by 2050. The shifting of the U.S. population away from a Western European racial majority (U.S. Census Bureau, 2008) has an impact on every decision the provider makes when caring for a diverse population of patients.

Equally important is consideration of cultural factors. Who makes the decisions in the family about health care? Does this person support the use of the prescribed drug? How well does the patient's view of health and illness and the way both should be managed match the provider's view? Will this attitude create problems with adherence? Although each person with a specific cultural heritage is a unique individual who may not subscribe to all or even most of the health beliefs and health practices of that cultural group, it is important to know what is common among members of the group. Cultural heritage plays an important role in helping to explain attitudes, beliefs, and health practices.

Another factor only recently being incorporated into pharmacotherapeutic decision making is that of ethnopharmacology, a study of racial differences in drug metabolism and response. Practitioners may know and guidelines may sometimes specify that certain drugs are less or more efficacious or may have different side effects with certain racial groups. Research is increasingly demonstrating the underlying genetic reasons for these differences in efficacy. Research with the cytochrome P450 (CYP450) enzyme system has been especially fruitful in this area, but it is not the only source of racial differences. As research samples are broadened to reflect the diversity of the population, more information is gained in the area of ethnic differences in drug pharmacokinetics. The pharmacokinetic factors that can be expected to potentially exhibit these differences are (1) bioavailability for drugs that undergo gut or hepatic first-pass metabolism, (2) protein binding, (3) volume of distribution, (4) hepatic metabolism, and (5) renal tubular secretion. Absorption, filtration at the glomerulus, and passive tubular reabsorption would not be expected to exhibit racial differences. Because relatively few drugs have research evidence of racial differences, it is often necessary to predict whether these differences might exist. For example, a drug that is eliminated entirely by the kidney through filtration and reabsorption and is not highly protein bound is highly unlikely to exhibit racial differences. Conversely, a drug that undergoes significant hepatic first-pass metabolism and is highly protein bound is more likely to exhibit pharmacokinetic differences between racial groups.

This chapter focuses on both cultural and ethnopharmacological factors that influence the choice of drugs that practitioners prescribe. Pharmacogenetics also influences prescribing and is described in Chapter 8. The data provided are based both on evidence derived from drug research and on identifying those drugs most likely to exhibit differences in their pharmacokinetics. In using this information, it is important to keep in mind that most Americans are not of any "pure" cultural or racial background and that patients must be treated as unique individuals.

The American Anthropological Society (AAS) has raised several pertinent issues related to both racial and cultural heritage in the United States. Although the U.S. Census Bureau collects data based on five distinct groupings, the AAS states that the United States is home to at least 26 different and distinct racial and cultural groupings; the U.S. Census Bureau lists 184 ethnic groups. It is not possible within this chapter to delineate all of these groupings, so the 5 groups delineated by the census are used. Readers should understand, however, that these are artificial groupings and that people listed within a specific group may be very divergent from one another; for example, Japanese, Chinese, Vietnamese, and Koreans are all grouped under the umbrella category "Asian," yet differences have been found within these ethnic groups in the manner in which they metabolize certain drugs (Purnell and Paulanka, 2005).

Socioeconomic factors also influence prescription choices and may supersede cultural and racial differences. For this reason, discussion of cultural factors includes such socioeconomic data as demographics, education, and employment (many patients obtain health insurance through their employment), and health-care utilization. This information is based on data from the 2000 U.S. census (U.S. Census Bureau, 2006).

Cultural awareness allows the provider to be aware of and open to the differences between patients, regardless of their culture. Leininger, in her Culture Care Sunrise model, focuses on assessing the patient in his or her environmental context, which includes seven major areas: technological; religious; social and kinship; cultural values; political/legal; economic and educational factors (Leininger, 2004). The provider considers all these factors to provide culturally congruent care for clients regardless of racial or ethnic group. For example, the provider would assess the patient's economic resources and education as well as culture before planning care for the patient. Another example is provided by Steinman, Sands, and Covinsky (2001) in a study of African American and Latino Veterans Administration patients age 70 and older. They found that the Latinos who lacked prescription benefits were more likely than white older adults to not take the prescribed medications because of cost. In providing transcultural care, Leininger states that the provider must decide which preservation/maintenance, accommodation/negotiation, or repatterning/restructuring actions should be undertaken. For example, when a Latino is newly diagnosed with diabetes, the provider structures care to preserve relevant values that are important to the patient while negotiating changes in behavior, such as food choices. The client will need to change or greatly modify some behaviors in order to have optimal health outcome, which in the example of the Latino diabetic, may be taking medication. Using a framework such as Leininger's allows the provider to provide individualized, culturally appropriate care regardless of ethnic or cultural group.

STANDARDS OF CULTURAL COMPETENCY

A term that has gained popularity in use among health-care practitioners is *cultural competency,* implying more than an awareness of cultural differences; it includes the knowledge and skills to provide culturally competent care as well. Purnell and Paulanka (2008) add categories to be considered, including health-care practices and practitioners, and high-risk health behaviors.

In 2001 in response to a 1994 Federal law, the U.S. Office of Minority Health (2006) proposed the National Standards of Culturally and Linguistically Appropriate Services

(CLAS) for all organizations receiving federal funds. CLAS has 14 standards grouped under culturally competent care, language access services, and organizational supports for cultural competence. There are three types of standards: mandates, guidelines, and recommendations. The standards call for the provision of professional language assistance services rather than the use of family and friends for translation. The standards encourage education and training of staff members and the provision of culturally appropriate and easily understood teaching materials, including those for adults with low literacy levels. They encourage collaboration with the communities served by the organization and stringent assessment practices. Other organizations have proposed strategies for CLAS implementation and in 2007 the Joint Commission that accredits health-care organizations "cross-walked" the CLAS standards to the Joint Commission standards.

One of the nursing education professional bodies, the American Association of Colleges of Nursing (2008), proposed that the cultural competency standards be adapted for baccalaureate nursing education; the rationale included concern for disparities in health and health care, social justice, and globalization. These competencies include having nursing students "explain the relationship among cultural, physiological, ecological, pharmacologic, and genetic factors" (p. 3) among other relevant competencies. They also expect that baccalaureate nursing students explain the "effect of drugs on specific groups of patients" (p. 6). Competency 4 is also relevant to this discussion; it states that nursing students should advocate for social justice, be committed to the health of vulnerable populations and to the elimination of health disparities (p. 6).

AFRICAN AMERICANS

Cultural Factors

Demographics

According to the U.S. Office of Minority Health, in July 2008 African Americans made up about 13.5 percent of the population, and their numbers are increasing faster than the overall population. The National Center for Health Statistics (2010) predicts that, by 2035, African Americans will make up 14.3 percent of the population. As a group, they are younger (35% under age 20) and more likely to be unmarried (61%), urban (81%), and female (53%). The majority of African Americans (56%) live in the South. The proportion below the poverty line in 2007 was 24.5 percent, compared with 8.2 percent for white Americans. The mean household income was $33,916 compared to $54,920 for white families. Almost 25 percent lived at poverty level compared to 8.2 percent for white Americans.

Education and Employment

Fewer African Americans complete high school (80%) and a four-year college (15%) than do white Americans. More black women than black men earn a college degree. The unemployment rate is more than twice that of white Americans and higher than that of any other ethnic group except American Indian–Alaska Natives, and African Americans are more likely to be employed in hazardous occupations.

Family Relationships

Although over half are raised in single-parent homes, a strong kinship bond among family members still exists. Ever alert for signs of discrimination, they may see health care providers as "outsiders" in health decisions. The female is the dominant family force, and the grandmother is often the major decision maker. Sickness can bring families together (Purnell and Paulanka, 2005, p. 33) and extended and nuclear family members take care of one another.

Health-Care Utilization

In 2007, 49 percent of African Americans compared to 66 percent of whites had employer-sponsored health insurance and 19.5 percent of African Americans compared to 10.4 percent of whites were uninsured. African Americans were also at higher risk of misdiagnosis of mental illness, and then receive the wrong medication for their illness (Purnell and Paulanka, 2005, p. 25). Beal and colleagues (2007) found that more African Americans (21%) than whites had no usual source of health care, and that cost considerations for prescribing drugs are especially important. African Americans use hospital clinics and emergency rooms as their care providers more than did any other ethnic group, perhaps in part because of their urban residence.

In addition to lacking health insurance, many African Americans have a long-standing distrust of the modern health-care system because of the Tuskegee experiment. In that decades-old study, treatment for syphilis was withheld for many years from African American males in order for the federal government to learn more about syphilis's long-term effects. Despite public apologies from the U.S. government, many African Americans still harbor a suspicion of government-provided health care.

Moreover, there is a dearth of African American providers, and there may be a feeling that pain is inevitable and should be endured. Some African Americans may use folk practitioners. For African American patients, nurses are generally seen as having less importance than physicians (Purnell and Paulanka, 2005, p. 35).

Health Status

The gap in life expectancy between African Americans and white Americans is narrowing but still exists (National Centers for Health Statistics, 2008, p. 5). African Americans' life expectancy is shorter than the average American by 4.7 years (National Center for Health Statistics, 2010). According to the U.S. Office of Minority Health (OMH) maternal mortality rates are almost three times higher than other ethnic groups or whites and the infant mortality rate is 2.3 times that of whites. Infants have a lower birth weight. These statistics are related to the high teen pregnancy rate (Purnell and Paulanka, 2005, p. 24).

The patterns of illness in the African American population include a higher prevalence of coronary heart disease, cancer, and stroke. The prevalence and age-adjusted mortality rate for diabetes is twice that of whites, and prevalence of hypertension is more than twice that of whites. They have a lower rate of immunizations for influenza and pneumococcus. Cigarette smoking is more prevalent; 26 percent of men and 17 percent of women smoke. Thirty-six percent of men are obese and 53 percent of women. About 39 percent of men and 43 percent of women have hypertension. They have greater bone density than other ethnicities so suffer less osteoporosis (Purnell, 2005, p. 25). About 50 percent of all new HIV/AIDS infections are in the African American population (National Center for Health Statistics, 2008). In 2008, the percent of African Americans of all ages who reported their health as fair or poor was 13 percent (CDC, 2008).

African Americans respond differently to **alcohol**, psychotropic drugs, and **caffeine** than do whites; they have higher blood levels, faster therapeutic response, and a higher rate of extrapyramidal effects than do whites (Purnell and Paulanka, 2005, p. 25).

Health Beliefs and Practices

For a significant portion of the African American population, health is a gift from God, and illness and suffering are God's will or are caused by evil influences. Because God's will is the source of the illness, they rely heavily on the healing powers of religious ritual and the advice of their religious leader. They take their religion seriously and practice prayer for many requests. Folk healers and folk medicine—such as cod liver oil to prevent colds, sulfur and molasses in the spring to promote health, and copper or silver bracelets to protect from harm—are often used. Herbal remedies are also used. Allopathic health care is not considered for prevention.

The U.S. Office of Minority Health attributes the poor health outcomes for African Americans to, among other things, "discrimination, cultural barriers, and lack of access to health care" (National Center for Health Statistics, 2010, p. 2).

Regional differences are often a factor for all ethnic groups, including African Americans. Those who were raised in the southeastern part of the United States are more likely to subscribe to health beliefs and practices common to that region than are African Americans raised elsewhere, for example.

Racial Differences in Drug Pharmacokinetics and Response

African Americans have been studied more than other ethnic groups in relation to ethnopharmacology, which has resulted in a larger body of knowledge about racial differences in pharmacokinetics for this group. This intense interest in ethnic pharmacology led to the first drug being approved by the U.S. Food and Drug Administration (FDA) in 2005 specifically for adjunctive treatment of heart failure in patients who self-identify as African American. **BiDil** is a fixed-dose combination of two generic drugs, **hydralazine** and **isosorbide dinitrate**, the first drug labeled exclusively for a specific race.

In establishing ethnic differences, Johnson and Burlew (1996) used **metoprolol** as a prototype drug to look at metabolism of drugs by the CYP450 2D6 isoenzyme group. This particular isoenzyme group is responsible for several important drug groups, including **antiarrhythmics**, **antidepressants**, and **neuroleptics**. They concluded that drugs primarily metabolized by this isoenzyme system will not exhibit racial differences between African Americans and whites.

Bertilsson (1995) studied CYP450 2C19 in relation to the difference between Asian Americans and whites (see discussion later). Because the separation of whites from Asians is fairly recent in the evolutionary process and the separation of Africans from whites and Asians occurred much earlier, it might be expected that African Americans will show even greater differences in drugs metabolized by CYP450 2C19 than do Asian Americans.

Differences have also been demonstrated between African Americans and whites in plasma protein binding (Johnson & Livingston, 1997). The study found increased unbound fractions of drugs bound to albumin, a common binding site for many drugs. The researchers were careful to point out, however, that differences in protein concentrations might also explain the racial differences. Further study is needed in this area, because a large number of drugs could be affected by this racial difference if it can be replicated.

Hypertension has a high prevalence in African Americans. One reason behind this phenomenon appears to be salt sensitivity (Weinberger, 1993), which is often cited as the reason to use **diuretics** as first-line therapy for this ethnic group. In a study looking at the use of **beta-adrenergic blockers** to treat hypertension in African Americans, a practice that is not usually recommended, Prisant and Mensah (1996) found that not all African Americans are salt sensitive. When salt sensitivity was controlled for, there was no racial difference in efficacy when **beta-adrenergic blockers** were used with **diuretics** as combination therapy for hypertension. This study suggests that **beta-adrenergic blockers** should be given to some African Americans for certain indications, such as myocardial infarction prophylaxis.

A study by Weir and colleagues (1998) also demonstrated that controlling for salt sensitivity affected response to two other classes of drugs (**angiotensin-converting enzyme [ACE] inhibitors** and **calcium channel blockers**). **Calcium channel blockers** are recommended second-line therapy for African Americans. African Americans who were salt sensitive had more blood pressure lowering with **isradipine** (a **calcium channel blocker**) than with **enalapril** (also a **calcium channel blocker**). The differences appear to be not only between drug classes but also within them.

To further confuse the issue of **beta-adrenergic blockers**, studies have been done related to racial differences in nucleotide-mediated smooth muscle relaxation (vasodilation) in response to nitric oxide. Studies by Cardillo, Kilcoyne, Cannon, and Panza (1998, 1999) support a difference between African Americans and whites in vasodilation response. The vasodilation effect of **beta-adrenergic blockers** stems from the combination of direct smooth muscle stimulation and endothelial nitric oxide release.

Other drugs dependent on nitric oxide for their action include the **nitrates.** Both drug classes may not be efficacious or may require dosage alterations to achieve efficacy in African Americans.

ACE inhibitors are also useful in treating hypertension, but African Americans appear to have less renin-dependent hypertension, and these drugs are less useful with that group. A study by Mitchell and colleagues (1997) confirmed racial differences in the renal hemodynamic response to chronic use of ACE inhibition that was independent of diuretic use and the magnitude of blood pressure lowering.

A serious adverse reaction to **ACE inhibitors** that contraindicates their use is angioedema. It is thought to be related to the reduced breakdown of bradykinin in patients taking this class of drugs. A study by Gainer, Nadeau, Ryder, and Brown (1996) concluded that African Americans show racial differences in the kallikrein-kinin system and are more sensitive to bradykinin, placing them at increased risk of ACE inhibitor–associated angioedema, independent of dose or concurrent drugs.

Diabetes mellitus has a higher prevalence in African Americans. The Bogalusa Heart Study Twentieth Anniversary Symposium (1995) suggested that elevated insulin levels observed in African American adolescents, especially girls, may be attributed to their decreased hepatic insulin clearance. This suggests consideration of drugs that affect hepatic insulin clearance (e.g., **metformin [Glucophage]**) for treating African Americans with type 2 diabetes. Stephens, Gillapsy, Clyne, Mejia, and Pollack (1990) also found racial differences in the incidence of end-stage renal disease associated with diabetes, which suggests that more aggressive management may be needed to prevent this complication.

Cryer and Feldman (1996) studied racial differences in gastric function among African Americans and whites. Gastric bicarbonate secretion was significantly higher in African Americans, making their gastric pH also higher. This might be a factor in the absorption of drugs that require highly acid media for absorption. Mucosal biopsies demonstrated a much higher prevalence of *Helicobacter pylori* infection and chronic active superficial gastritis in African Americans. Even those who were negative for this infection had differences in gastric bicarbonate secretion. Drug combinations used to treat *H. pylori* infection include those that have pH-raising drugs. Are these the best ones for African Americans?

Finally, a study by Carmel (1999) looked at racial differences in cobalamin and homocysteine levels among African Americans and whites. Concern was raised about potential underreporting and undertreatment of pernicious anemia because African Americans have significantly higher serum cobalamin levels than do whites. They also have significantly lower homocysteine levels, metabolize homocysteine more efficiently, and do not show the same benefit from vitamin therapy in treating this anemia. A further question raised related to the prescription of folate: "Given their lower rate of neural tube defects, possibly lower homocysteine levels, more efficient homocysteine metabolism, and lesser impact of vitamin therapy on it, does the untargeted promotion of high folate intake provide less benefit to blacks than to whites while exposing them to an equal risk for adverse effects because of unrecognized pernicious anemia?" (Carmel, 1999, p. 90).

AMERICAN INDIAN–ALASKA NATIVE GROUPS

Cultural Factors

Demographics

American Indian (Native American) and Alaska Native peoples are a diverse group with more than 560 different tribes recognized by the federal or state governments and others that are not so recognized. The census records that this group represents 1.6 percent of the population and that their numbers are increasing faster than the growth in the overall population. As a group, they are young (30% under the age of 15), less educated, and poorer than the rest of the United States. The median household income is $33,627, and 25 percent live below the poverty level (U.S. Census Bureau, 2008). In fact, they have the highest poverty level of all Americans. They are divided in residence, with 50 percent living in urban areas.

One problem in reporting the actual numbers of American Indians is the tendency of this population group to avoid being counted as American Indians and the requirement by many tribal groups that an individual be at least a certain percentage American Indian to be recorded as a member of that tribe. Interracial marriages are also common, and the children are often documented as being of the race of the non-Indian parent. A shift to recognition and pride in American Indian heritage has occurred. The 2000 census permitted individuals to list more than one race, allowing for children of mixed-race couples not to have to choose to be identified as one race or another.

Education and Employment

About 76 percent of American Indian adults have at least a high school diploma and 14 percent have a bachelor's degree. In fact, the proportion of American Indians completing college is less than half that of all races in the United States, and the unemployment rate is twice as high as all other races combined. American Indians are about twice as likely to be unemployed as whites. Since employment is often the method most Americans have access to health insurance, it should be no surprise that, in 2006, only 36 percent of American Indians had private health insurance (U.S. Census Bureau, 2008).

Family Relationships

The average American Indian family household has four to five members, making it the largest family size of any of the ethnic minority groups. Women head 25 percent of the households. The family is extended, including relatives from both sides. Elder members assume leadership roles. Some tribal groups are matriarchal and some are patriarchal, with the leadership and the health decision making coming from the sex that matches the leadership orientation, often with the help of spiritual leaders or medicine people.

Health-Care Utilization

Since 1849 and under treaty agreements, the federal government has provided the health-care services for the federally recognized tribes. The U.S. Indian Health Service has provided no-cost comprehensive health care to these tribes and Alaska Natives, and approximately 70 percent of all members of this group who claim American Indian heritage receive that care. Some tribes have chosen to take over the provision of health care from the Indian Health Service (IHS) under the provisions of the 1975 Indian Self-Determination and Education Assistance Act, often because of the long-held deep suspicion of the federal government. Since 1972, IHS has attempted to provide health services off the reservations because only 20 percent live on the reservations or trust lands.

Many people live in remote areas, where the ratio of providers to patients is half the national average. The main reason for utilization of health-care services is obstetric care. In 2007, 33 percent of Native Americans had no health-care coverage.

Health Status

Life expectancy is 73.2 years, compared with about 79 years for white females. The five top causes of mortality are not that different from the general population: heart disease, injury, cancer, diabetes, and stroke. Other causes, in descending order, are chronic liver disease (associated with high rates of alcohol abuse), cerebrovascular disease, pneumonia and influenza, and suicide. Among young males, accidents, suicide, and assault are the leading killers.

The higher the percentage of American Indian or Alaska Native genetic heritage that a person has, the more likely that individual is to manifest diabetes, almost exclusively type 2. This may be correlated with the increased obesity found in this group with new research finding a possible genetic marker for obesity and type 2 diabetes, specifically in the Pima Indian men (Ma et al, 2005). As more research is done regarding genetics, obesity, and type 2 diabetes in the Indian population, there will be an ever-increasing level of evidence to guide the care of this population.

High-risk behaviors among Indians include alcoholism and its associated problems—probably related to alcohol metabolism issues—and high smoking rates for both men and women. The infant mortality rate is 1.5 times that of whites, and they have twice the rate of infant death syndrome. Because of isolation, they may have no infectious disease immunity, and some tribes have high tuberculosis (TB) rates. Native Americans have high rates of prostate cancer and low rates of breast cancer; 79 percent have lactose intolerance. Eskimos also have high rates of enzyme deficiencies in lactose and sucrose.

Health Beliefs and Practices

For these populations, health is harmony with nature and oneself. Illness is disharmony and may be caused by a supernatural force or by violation of a restriction or prohibition. The illness is seen as an imbalance of mind, body, and spirit. Because the cause of the illness is external, illness prevention practices that relate the cause of illness to the behavior of the patient are questioned. This is an interesting conflict, because self-control is considered to be a central attribute to maintaining harmony, and each person is accountable for his or her own health.

Theology and medicine are strongly interwoven. They have a belief in a Supreme Being but, at the same time, witchcraft is feared, and medicine bags may be worn or carried to protect a person from witchcraft or to promote wellness and harmony. "Medical" care is often sought from a member of the family or tribe who has the ability to use her or his powers of healing in conjunction with herbs and rituals in a purely positive way to heal; therefore, providers need to determine which herbal remedies a patient is using before prescribing modern medicines. The medicine person may use negative force powers, but only against the sick person's enemies. Singing is often part of the healing ritual.

Allopathic medicine is accepted but not seen as able to heal except when used with native healing practices. Because the hospital is considered the place to die, the patient may resist hospitalization. Pain is supposed to be borne, so they often do not request pain medication when needed.

Racial Differences in Drug Pharmacokinetics and Response

Although a large portion of this ethnic group has health care provided by the U.S. Indian Health Service, little research has been done related to racial considerations in pharmacokinetics or other therapies. The few studies in the literature were related to metabolism of alcohol, which were contradictory (Bennion & Li, 1976; Chan, 1986), and to lipoprotein levels. A study related to lipoproteins (Harris-Hooker & Sanford, 1994) reported that American Indians have a lower prevalence of coronary heart disease related to lower low-density lipoprotein (LDL)–cholesterol and higher high-density lipoprotein (HDL)–cholesterol levels. Few studies were found related to diabetes and its treatment, despite a prevalence of 50 percent in Pima Indians and a lower but still elevated prevalence in other American Indian groups. Clearly, this ethnic group requires more study.

ASIAN AMERICANS/PACIFIC ISLANDERS

Cultural Factors

Demographics

Asian Americans, people originating from the Far East, Southeast Asia, or the Indian continent, and Pacific Islanders made up 5 percent of the population in the 2008 Census studies. Like the American Indian–Alaska Native group, they are extremely diverse, with more than 100 languages and dialects and 20 different subgroupings; generalizations are quite difficult. In fact, in recognition of this diversity, the 2000 census counted this group as two groups—one the "Asian American" group and the other the "Hawaiian and Other Pacific Islanders" group. Most of the combined group (92%) live in urban areas, and the majority live in California. Thirty percent of Hawaiian and other Pacific Islanders are under age 18. In the 2007 census study, the median household income for the combined group was $15,600 higher than for all households (U.S. Census Bureau, 2008). However, as a reminder of the diversity of this group, the poverty levels range from 6 percent for Filipinos and 64 percent among the Hmongs; although the averages look good, this group represents both extremes of health and socioeconomic indicators.

Education and Employment

Asian Americans are better educated and better paid than the general U.S. population. The unemployment rate is lower than that of the general population, with 6.3 percent of Asians unemployed in the 2000 census, compared with an overall unemployment rate of 7.2 percent. About 45 percent were employed in highly skilled, high-wage jobs compared to 34 percent of the total population. The Vietnamese are the poorest and least well-educated of these groups.

In 2007 (National Center for Health Statistics, 2010), 86 percent of Asian American adults had at least a high school diploma, which is similar to the total population but 50 percent of Asian Americans compared to 28 percent of the total American population had at least a bachelor's degree.

A high percentage of this population does not speak English at home: 62 percent of Vietnamese; 50 percent of Chinese families; 24 percent of Filipino families; 23 percent of Asian Indians; and 42 percent of Hawaiian/Pacific Islanders (CDC, 2008).

Family Relationships

Family relationships are strong, with extended (multigenerational) families and an expectation of family loyalty from all members. Families are a source of strength. In Japanese families, the father is away from the home on business a great deal of the time, so the mother–eldest son relationship is very strong. Before the eldest son is of age, the mother is the dominant person in the home. They include the nuclear and extended families in decision making. In all Asian American groups, respect for elders is taught at an early age. Males are more "valued" than females. Females are submissive to males. Individuals' wishes and needs are subordinated to the needs of the group. Spector (2004) says that adherence to Buddhism, Confucianism, and Taoism leads these Asian American families to avoid admitting physical or mental illness. Conflicts are handled within the family, and there is kinship solidarity in which the individual is subservient to family and kin.

The average family size for Hawaiian/Pacific Islanders is four and may be matriarchal. Taboos and modesty are important.

Health-Care Utilization

Visits to health-care providers are less frequent, with Asian Americans over age 65 making about half as many visits to health-care providers as their white counterparts. Asians are also well insured, with only 18 percent of U.S. Asians uninsured in the years 2002 to 2004, the lowest of all the minority groups (U.S. Census Bureau, 2005). Recent immigrants are likely not to have health-care coverage.

Health Status

The health status of this group as a whole is excellent. They have a longer life expectancy and lower death rates from all causes than does the general population. The illnesses that are experienced at higher levels than those in the general population include stomach cancer (among Japanese) and suicide (among elderly Chinese women). Southeast Asian refugees have a higher incidence of intestinal parasites, positive tuberculin tests, and presence of hepatitis B antigen and more anemia than other Asian Americans or the general population. Overall the leading causes of death are cancer, heart disease, stroke, accidents, and diabetes. They have the highest rate of TB of any cultural group and twice the rate of the hepatitis B virus than white Americans (although this is decreasing). Sudden infant death syndrome is the fourth leading cause of infant mortality. They have a high rate of chronic obstructive pulmonary disease (COPD). Asian American women have a low smoking rate.

Hawaiian and Pacific Islanders have a high rate of smoking, alcohol consumption, and obesity; the leading causes of death are cancer, heart disease, accidents, stroke, and diabetes. They have a high infant mortality rate and, in 2007, the TB rate was 21 times higher than that for whites. The Chinese have high smoking rates in men and teenagers, leading to high rates of lung disease. The Chinese diet is high in peanuts and soybeans. They have a rare Rh-negative blood group.

Health Beliefs and Practices

Health beliefs and practices vary among different Asian American subgroups. Chinese and Vietnamese people have a fatalistic attitude and believe that health is a result of forces that rule the world: yin (cold) and yang (hot). Illness results when there is an imbalance in these forces. Illness is diagnosed by pulses (there are seven different ones), color and texture of the tongue, and other means not commonly used by allopathic medicine. Treatment is provided with the opposing force to achieve balance. For example, a "cold" illness (e.g., colic, diarrhea, or edema) is treated with "hot" herbs and foods. "Hot" illnesses (e.g., hypertension, blood diseases, or a cough) are treated with "cold" herbs and foods. Healers within the group are skilled at diagnosis and prescription of therapy. Such therapy may include acupuncture, acupressure, tai chi, moxibustion, or medicinal herbs. Chapter 10 discusses herbal therapy, with the important caveat that one must understand and subscribe to a totally different view of health and illness to prescribe these herbs appropriately. "Chi" is innate energy, and lack of it results in fatigue and long illnesses. They may call on their ancestors for help and the Vietnamese may use cupping with a heated cup or glass jar that is placed on the skin to create a vacuum. This practice leaves bruising and may be misinterpreted in children as child abuse.

These populations may believe that mental illness and physical disabilities should be hidden. Women usually seek care from female providers. Older clients may appear willing to comply with prescribed therapies but then don't follow them; their respect for the provider prohibits them from discussing their unwillingness to follow the regime.

Japanese beliefs are influenced by Shinto, a religious orientation. They believe that humans are inherently good and that evil is caused by outside spirits. Both Japanese and Vietnamese people believe that pleasing good spirits and avoiding evil ones help to maintain harmony and health. Evil is removed by purification, and there are rituals for this purpose. Mental illness is taboo and often translates into acceptable somatic symptoms, and addictions are shameful (Purnell and Paulanka, 2005, p. 306). Alcoholism and family violence are hidden but serious problems.

Filipinos also subscribe to the concept of yin and yang, but believe that God's will and supernatural forces govern the universe and determine health and illness. Illness is punishment for violations of God's will. Amulets and religious medals may be worn as a shield from witchcraft or as a good-luck charm. Filipinos often have healing rituals and may perform sacrifices. The "evil eye" may be considered as a reason for illness in infants and children.

Filipinos are the most likely of the Asian American group to be obese. They have high alcohol consumption and smoking rates.

All of these groups use combinations of allopathic and ethnically defined health and illness care. The allopathic approach, however, is often chosen last or to supplement ethnically defined care. In a study (Horne et al, 2004, p. 1307) of college students who identified themselves as having an Asian or European background, Asian students had more negative views of medications than European students. Asian students were more likely to view medicines as "intrinsically harmful, addictive substances" and were less likely to believe in the benefits of modern medicine. All the students viewed taking prescribed medications more favorably if they had taken prescribed medications before.

Racial Differences in Drug Pharmacokinetics and Response

Bertilsson (1995) compared Asian Americans and whites on the basis of drug metabolism by the CYP450 2D6 and 2C19 isoenzyme systems. The 2D6 isoenzyme system is responsible for metabolism of **antiarrhythmics, antidepressants**, and **neuroleptics**, among others. The mean activity of 2D6 extensive metabolizers is lower in Asian Americans and is the molecular genetic basis for slower metabolism of **antidepressants** and **neuroleptics** in Asian Americans. This difference in metabolism requires lower doses of these drugs. The 2C19 system is involved in the metabolism of acids (e.g., **mephenytoin**), bases (e.g., **imipramine** and **omeprazole**), and neutral drugs (e.g., **diazepam**). **Diazepam (Valium)** is partially demethylated by 2C19, and the high frequency of mutated alleles in Asian Americans is probably the reason that such populations have slower metabolism and are treated with lower doses of **diazepam** than are whites. Although other drugs in this same class have not been studied, it is likely that they have similar metabolic fates as **diazepam. Omeprazole (Prilosec)** is hydroxylated to a major extent by 2C19, and there is an approximately 10-fold difference in oral clearance between Asian Americans and whites. Hence, a lower dose for this drug is required among Asian Americans.

McSweeney and Zhan (1994) stated that many Asians have a deficiency of the active form of dehydrogenase, an enzyme used in the metabolism of **alcohol**. In these people, a "flushing" may appear after they ingest only a small amount of alcohol. Chan (1986) also reported this "atypical" dehydrogenase, which he stated is present in 85 to 90 percent of Asian Americans.

Asians have also been described as "fast acetylators." Recent studies have determined that Asian subgroups that originate in eastern Asia (Bangladesh, Thailand, Malaysia, China, Hong Kong, Korea, and Japan) have a higher percentage of fast acetylators than those from western Asia (Turkey, Russia, and Saudi Arabia.) Researchers have determined an East–West geographic longitude, termed the Asian "fast acetylator longitude," which allows for prediction of acetylator status (Zaid et al, 2004). Hepatic acetylation is responsible for metabolism of many drugs, including **cardiac** and **psychotropic drugs**, and 78 to 93 percent of Asians are "fast acetylators" (Lin, Poland, Smith, Strickland, & Mendoza 1991). This faster metabolism may require a more frequent or higher dose of drugs metabolized by acetylation to achieve efficacy.

Frackiewicz, Srmek, Herrera, Kurtz, and Culter (1997) did a MEDLINE search of articles from 1966 to 1996 that identified racial differences in response to **antipsychotic** drugs. Their studies suggest that Asians may respond to lower doses of **antipsychotics** because of pharmacokinetic and pharmacodynamic differences. Confounding the issue, however, Lee, Yang, and Hu (1998) found lack of racial differences in **lithium** pharmacokinetics between Taiwanese Chinese bipolar patients and whites. In a recent study from Australia, ethnic Chinese required significantly lower doses of **sertraline (Zoloft)** to achieve clinical efficacy than white patients (Hong Ng et al, 2006). "Despite controlling for weight, gender and dietary factors (**alcohol, nicotine** and **caffeine**) because of their possible influence on the metabolism of **sertraline**, the difference observed between ethnic groups remained statistically significant [$F(2,34) = 4.15, P < .05$]" (Hong Ng et al, 2006). This study may indicate that **selective serotonin reuptake inhibitors** need to be dosed lower in Asian patients.

A class of drugs used to treat Parkinson's disease is **dopaminergics**. Filipinos require lower doses of **levodopa** than do whites, and they develop dyskinesia more readily at comparable doses. This difference appears to be related to racial differences in erythrocyte catechol-o-methyltransferase (Rivera-Calimlim & Reilly, 1984).

In comparing Asian American children with African Americans, Hispanics, and whites, Liu and Levinson (1996) found a higher prevalence of elevated blood pressure in Asian Americans. This suggests a need to consider racial differences in **antihypertensive** drug metabolism and responses. Studies do appear to support such differences, including the need for lower doses of **beta-adrenergic blockers** (Hui & Pasic, 1997; Matthews, 1995), and **ACE inhibitors** and **calcium channel blockers** (Hui & Pasic, 1997), based in part on increased adverse drug reactions at doses used for whites.

HISPANICS/MEXICANS

Cultural Factors

Demographics

The federal government considers race and language to be two separate things so "Hispanic Americans" may be of any race. For these purposes, individuals of Hispanic descent in the United States include Mexicans (58.5%), Puerto Ricans (9.6%), Cubans (3.5%), and people from Central and South America (U.S. Census Bureau, 2006). Hispanics of all races make up 15 percent of the U.S. population, not including the 4 million Puerto Rican residents. Hispanics are the second-largest minority group, although they are predicted to surpass African Americans and become the largest minority group in the United States, making up 30 percent of the population by 2050 (National Center for Health Statistics, 2010). This group is young, with 34.3 percent under age 18 compared to 22.3 percent for whites (CDC, 2010). Most live in urban areas, with the highest percentage living in the southwestern states (Arizona, California, Colorado, New Mexico, and Texas). The mean household income in 2002 to 2004 was $34,200, and the percentage of families below the poverty line was 21.5 percent compared to 8.2 percent of whites (CDC, 2010). Twelve percent of the total population spoke Spanish at home in 2007 (CDC, 2010).

Education and Employment

Sixty-one percent of Latino adults compared to 89 percent of the total population in 2007 (OMH, 2010) had a high school education, 12.5 percent compared to 30.5 percent had at least a bachelor's degree, and 3.8 percent had advanced degrees. The unemployment rate for Hispanics in 2004 was 6.5 percent (U.S. Department of Labor Statistics, 2006), but this may not accurately reflect the migrant farm worker population nor undocumented workers.

Family Relationships

The family is the most important unit, and strong kinship bonds include godparents, who are established by ritual kinship and are a major source of support. The family is usually large and home centered. Respect for parents and elders is taught early and the family is the major source of support for the elderly infirm. Many live in extended family situations and there is a respect for collective rather than individual achievement (Giger and Davidhizar, 2008, pp. 230–231). Religious leaders are also a source of support for families (Purnell and Paulanka, 2008) and food is used to maintain family ties. Males and females have clearly differentiated roles. The father is the main decision maker in the family, but women, who are considered the primary healers in the group, decide health-related issues and provide health advice and remedies. Native healers *(curanderas)* are usually women.

Health-Care Utilization

The combination of unemployment and lack of documentation of farm workers means that this group has the highest percentage of people without health insurance (between 30% and 33% in 2008), and therefore a lack of access to preventive care and health promotion (National Center for Health Statistics, 2010). Public health clinics and emergency departments are often the sites for health care.

Health Status

The National Center for Health Statistics (2008) data indicate that, in 2008, 9.5 percent of Hispanics/Latinos were reported to be in fair or poor health. Obtaining accurate health statistics on Hispanics is difficult because their data are often included with those of whites or go unreported owing to undocumented status. What is known is that the prevalence of type 2 diabetes is one-third more prevalent than it is in whites (9.1% vs. 6.6%), a gap that is narrowing owing to increased diabetes in non-Hispanic whites (Geiss et al, 2006). Nonetheless, obesity is a significant problem in the Hispanic population, with 69 percent of women and 70 percent of men over age 20 self-reporting being overweight (National Center for Health Statistics, 2006b).

The strong religious traditions and connection with the Roman Catholic Church mean that they are the least likely minority group to use contraception, which increases their risk for pregnancy and sexually transmitted infections. The leading causes of mortality are cardiovascular disease, cancer, accidents, stroke, and diabetes (CDC, 2008). The suicide rate is the lowest among the ethnic groups although Hispanic adolescents had more suicide ideation and attempts than whites (U.S. Department of Health and Human Services, 2010). They have high rates of obesity; however, being overweight may be viewed as attractive and a sign of wealth in that the family or individual can afford enough food to be overweight (Purnell and Paulanka, 2008). Pain is often expressed with verbal moaning and crying (Purnell & Paulanka, 2008). Other health disparities include the following: Puerto Ricans living on the mainland have six times the national average of HIV/AIDS; there is a low rate of individuals who receive the flu vaccine; Puerto Ricans have the highest rate of diabetes; and in the total group there is more than twice the death rate from asthma than is seen in whites (CDC, 2008). Many pregnant women do not seek prenatal care until late in their pregnancy; however, the low birth weight rate is lower than whites except for a high rate in Puerto Ricans (OMH, 2010). Puerto Ricans have low rates of prostate and breast cancer but a high rate of stomach and liver cancer.

Health Beliefs and Practices

Similar to the Asian concept of yin and yang, Hispanic peoples subscribe to the concept of hot and cold but also consider wet and dry. Illness results from an imbalance of these forces. Illness may also be caused by *mal ojo* ("evil eye") that results from the look or gaze of an individual thought to possess evil intention and evil powers. Health-care providers can be imagined as inadvertently giving this look. Health beliefs often have a strong religious association, with health a gift from God as a reward for good behavior. Eating proper foods, working the proper amount of time, wearing religious medals, and sleeping with relics in the home are thought to prevent illness. Hispanics typically consult both traditional healers and allopathic providers and may or may not follow the modern medicine prescribed. For example, in one study only 53 percent of Latinos with high blood pressure were taking antihypertensive medications. Hispanics underuse preventive services and health promotion activities (Fordyce, 2003) and, in 2006, compared to 15 percent of whites, 43 percent of Hispanics had no medical home (Beal et al, 2007). Curanderas ("healers") treat illness with a variety of herbs, teas, visits to shrines, medals, candles, and promises to God to change behavior. Understanding the herbs used and considering them when prescribing other drugs will reduce the risk for drug interactions. As with Asian medicinal therapies, it is important to understand that illness conditions are defined differently and that there are illnesses that have no correlate in allopathic medicine.

Racial Differences in Drug Pharmacokinetics and Response

An interracial comparison of the pharmacokinetics of 3-hydroxy-3-methylglutaryl **coenzyme A (HMG-CoA) reductase inhibitors** (Muck, Unger, Kawano, & Ahr, 1998) was undertaken because these drugs are extensively metabolized by the liver and, therefore, are in a class at risk for racial differences. The results of this study showed no evidence of any clinically relevant interethnic difference in their metabolism among white, African American, Hispanic, and Japanese subjects. Studies of other drugs in a class at risk for racial differences that included Hispanic patients (Jamerson & DeQuattro, 1996) reported a similar lack of difference between Hispanic Americans and whites.

Asthma is the most common chronic illness among all children, with around 10 percent of children afflicted, but Puerto Ricans have a much higher rate of asthma, with 25 percent afflicted. Conversely, only 8 percent of Mexican American children are reported to have asthma. Similar statistics are found between Puerto Rican and Mexican adults in the United States (National Center for Health Statistics, 2002). This difference among these Latino groups may be due to genetic differences between Puerto Ricans and Mexican Hispanics. Choudhry and colleagues (2005) studied the differences in response to the drug **albuterol** between Puerto Ricans and Mexicans with asthma and found that for Puerto Ricans with asthma with baseline forced expiratory volume at 1 second (FEV_1) less than 80 percent of predicted, but not in those with FEV_1 greater than 80 percent, there was a very strong association between the Arg16 genotype and greater **bronchodilator** responsiveness. This association was not seen in the Mexican study participants, indicating that not all Hispanics respond to asthma medications in a similar fashion.

Despite preliminary evidence of racial differences in insulin secretion and glucose metabolism and in factors associated with cardiovascular risk, evidence of differences in drug pharmacokinetics and response to drugs is lacking. This may be related to the genetic variability among persons classified as Hispanic or to a lack of studies.

NONHISPANIC WHITES

Limited discussion is required about this segment of the population because most allopathic health care is currently directed at this group. Within this group, however, are some subgroups that bear a short discussion.

Whites of various ethnic backgrounds may hold to beliefs in the "evil eye" and to the curative powers of folk medicine. German, Polish, and Italian Americans also see stress and environmental changes as sources of illness. Along with Irish Americans, they have strong family ties, with the male as the dominant force and decision maker. Polish and Italian Americans may use folk remedies and native healers. All four groups have strong religious ties, with Polish, Irish, and Italian Americans having Roman Catholicism as their main religion. Religious medals and rituals are often used to promote health, prevent illness, and heal. An increasing percentage of the population are seeing alternative sources of health care or are self-medicating with herbal remedies; this is discussed in Chapter 10.

One interesting study by Gaskin and colleagues (2008) seems to defy the widely held belief that, in the United States, minorities receive poorer care than white Americans. Gaskin and colleagues found that "when whites and minorities were admitted to the hospital for the same reason or to receive the same hospital procedure, they receive the same quality of care."

SUMMARY

Consideration of demographic, socioeconomic, and cultural factors is important in prescribing appropriate drugs for patients and in recognizing the potential for drug interactions with herbs or foods that may be used in culture-specific healing practices. Becoming culturally sensitive requires recognizing that cultural diversity exists, identifying and exploring one's own cultural beliefs, and being willing to modify health-care delivery to be more congruent with the patient's cultural background.

As can be seen from the research and other articles discussed, the study of ethnopharmacology often presents conflicting data. It is incumbent on prescribers to keep current in the literature and to take the time to review research studies for the validity and reliability of the methods and statistics used in the research and for the appropriateness of application to their patients. Box 7–1 describes sources of information for providers. Studies that report differences without stating a specific metabolic or biochemical relationship should be especially suspect. It is also important to look at articles in journals with reputations for peer review and careful selection of their research reports.

BOX 7–1 RESOURCES FOR CULTURALLY COMPETENT CARE

Center for Cross-Cultural Research

Western Washington University

Housed within and an integral part of the Department of Psychology at Western Washington University, the Center for Cross-Cultural Research was started in response to the Euro-American bias in psychological theory, research, and practical applications. http://www.ac.wwu.edu/~culture/overview.htm

Cross Cultural Health Care Program

The mission of the Cross Cultural Health Care Program is to serve as a bridge between communities and health-care institutions to ensure full access to quality health care that is culturally and linguistically appropriate.http://www.xculture.org

Diversity Rx

Diversity Rx promotes language and cultural competence to improve the quality of health care for minority, immigrant, and ethnically diverse communities. http://www.diversityrx.org

Madeline Leininger Theory of Culture Care

Dr. Madeleine Leininger is the founder of the worldwide Transcultural Nursing movement. She is one of nursing's most prolific writers and the world's foremost authority on cultural care. http://www.madeleine-leininger.com/

National Center for Cultural Competence

The mission of the National Center for Cultural Competence (NCCC) is to increase the capacity of health and mental health programs to design, implement, and evaluate culturally and linguistically competent service delivery systems. http://gucchd.georgetown.edu/nccc/

Transcultural Nursing Society

The mission of the Transcultural Nursing Society (TCNS) is to enhance the quality of culturally congruent, competent, and equitable care that results in improved health and well-being for people worldwide. The TCNS seeks to provide nurses and other health-care professionals with the knowledge base necessary to ensure cultural competence in practice, education, research, and administration.www.tcns.org

Many racial differences in drugs relate to their metabolism by the CYP450 enzyme system. One quick way to review the literature in ethnopharmacology related to this system is a relatively new Web site (http://www.mhc.com)

sponsored by Mental Health Connections, Inc. that is devoted exclusively to CYP450 drug interactions. It includes a full discussion of the cytochrome enzymes and gives clinically relevant information and recommendations (including racial differences) in one window while showing the data used to arrive at these conclusions in another window.

REFERENCES

Afzal, A., Brar, J., Ali, A., Jafri, S., Goldstein, A., & Khaja, F. (1997). Racial difference in patients with chest pain syndrome and abnormal coronary angiography. *Chest, 112*(3S), 24.

American Association of Colleges of Nursing. (2008). Cultural competency in baccalaureate nursing education. Washington, DC.

Aronoff, S., Bennett, P., Rushforth, N., Miller, M., & Unger, R. (1976). Arginine-stimulated hyperglucagonemia in diabetic Pima Indians. *Diabetes, 25*(5), 404–407.

Beal, H. C., Doty, M. M., Hernandez, S. E., Shea, K. K., & Davis, K. (2007). Closing the divide: how medical homes promote equity in health care. The Commonwealth Fund.

Bell, R. (1994). Prominence of women in Navajo healing beliefs and values. *Nursing and Health Care, 15*(5), 232–240.

Bennion, L., & Li, T. (1976). Alcohol metabolism in American Indians and whites: Lack of difference in metabolic rate and liver alcohol dehydrogenase. *New England Journal of Medicine, 294*(1), 9–13.

Bertilsson, L. (1995). Geographic and interracial differences in polymorphic drug oxidation: Current state of knowledge of cytochromes P450 (CYP) 2D6 and 2C19. *Clinical Pharmacokinetics, 29*(3), 192–209.

Bogalusa Heart Study Twentieth Anniversary Symposium. (1995). *American Journal of Medical Science, 310,* S1–S138.

Cardillo, C., Kilcoyne, C., Cannon R., III, & Panza, J. (1998). Racial differences in nitric oxide–mediated vasodilator response to mental stress in forearm circulation. *Hypertension, 31*(6), 1235–1239.

Cardillo, C., Kilcoyne, C., Cannon R., III, & Panza, J. (1999). Attenuation of cyclic nucleotide-mediated smooth muscle contraction in blacks as a cause of racial differences in vasodilator function. *Circulation, 99*(1), 90–95.

Carmel, R. (1999). Ethnic and racial factors in cobalamin metabolism and its disorders. *Seminars in Hematology, 36*(1), 88–100.

Centers for Disease Control and Prevention (CDC). (2008). FASTSTATS. Retrieved on August 20, 2010 from www.cdc.gov/nchs.

Chan, A. (1986). Racial differences in alcohol sensitivity. *Alcohol, 21*(1), 93–104.

Choudhry, S., Ung, N., Avila, P. C., Ziv, E., Nazario, S., Casal, J., et al. (2005). Pharmacogenetic differences in response to albuterol between Puerto Ricans and Mexicans with asthma. *American Journal of Respiratory and Critical Care Medicine, 171*(6), 563–570.

Cryer, B., & Feldman, M. (1996). Racial differences in gastric function among African-Americans and Caucasian Americans: Secretion, serum gastrin and histology. *Professional Association of American Physicians, 108*(6), 481–489

Cubeddu, L., Arnada, J., Singh, B., Klein, M., Brachfeld, J., Freis, E., et al. (1986). A comparison of verapamil and propranolol for the initial treatment of hypertension: Racial differences in response. *Journal of the American Medical Association, 256*(16), 2214–2221.

Dries, D., Exner, D., Gersh, B., Cooper, H., Carson, P., & Domanski, M. (1999). Racial difference in the outcome of left ventricular dysfunction. *New England Journal of Medicine, 340*(8), 609–616.

Flaws, J., & Bush, T. (1998). Racial differences in drug metabolism: An explanation for higher breast cancer mortality in blacks? *Medical Hypotheses, 50*(4), 327–329.

Fordyce, M. (2003). Culture, ethnicity, and medications. *Aging Today,* xxiv(1), 9–12.

Frackiewicz, E., Srmek, J., Herrera, J., Kurtz, N., & Culter, N. (1997). Ethnicity and antipsychotic response. *Annals of Pharmacotherapeutics, 31*(11), 1360–1369.

Friday, K., Srinivasan, S., Elkasabany, A., Dong, C., Wattigney, W., Dalferes E., Jr., et al. (1999). Black-white differences in postprandial triglyceride response and postheparin lipoprotein lipase and hepatic triglyceride lipase among young men. *Metabolism, 48*(6), 749–754.

Gainer, J., Nadeau, J., Ryder, D., & Brown, N. (1996). Increased sensitivity to bradykinin among African-Americans. *Journal of Allergy and Clinical Immunology, 98*(2), 283–287.

Gaskin, D. J., Spencer, C. S., Richard, P., Anderson, G. F., & Powe, N. R. (2008). Do hospitals provide lower-quality care to minorities than to whites? *Health Affairs, 27*(2), 518–527.

Geiss, L. S., Pan, L., Cadwell, B., Gregg, E. W., Benjamin, S. M., & Engelgau M. M. (2006). Changes in incidence of diabetes in U.S. Adults, 1997–2003. *American Journal of Preventive Medicine, 30*(5), 371–377.

Giger, J. N., & Davidhizar, R. E. (2008). *Transcultural nursing: Assessment and intervention.* St. Louis, MO: Mosby Elsevier.

Harris-Hooker, S., & Sanford, G. (1994). Lipid, lipoproteins and coronary heart disease in minority populations. *Atherosclerosis, 108*(Suppl.), 83–104.

Hong Ng, C., Norman, T. R., Naing, K. O., Schweitzer, I., Kong Wai Ho, B., Fan, A., et al. (2006). A comparative study of sertraline dosages, plasma concentrations, efficacy and adverse reactions in Chinese versus Caucasian patients. *International Clinical Psychopharmacology, 21*(2), 87–92.

Horne, R., Graupner, L., Frost, S., Weinman, J., Wright, S. M., & Hankins, M. (2004). Medicine in a multicultural society: The effect of cultural background on beliefs about medications. *Social Science and Medicine,* 59(6), 1307–1313.

Hui, K., & Pasic, J. (1997). Outcome of hypertension management in Asian Americans. *Archives of Internal Medicine, 157*(12), 1345–1348.

Jamerson, K., & DeQuattro, V. (1996). The impact of ethnicity on response to antihypertensive therapy. *American Journal of Medicine, 101*(3 Supplement 1), 22S–32S.

Johnson, J. (1997). Influence of race or ethnicity on pharmacokinetics of drugs. *Journal of Pharmacology Science, 86*(12), 1328–1333.

Johnson, J., & Burlew, D. (1996). Metoprolol metabolism via cytochrome P450 2D6 in ethnic populations. *Drug Metabolism Disposition, 24*(3), 350–355.

Johnson, J., & Livingston, T. (1997). Differences between blacks and whites in plasma binding of drugs. *European Journal of Clinical Pharmacology, 51*(96), 485–488.

Kountz, D. S. (2004). Hypertension in ethnic populations: Tailoring treatments. *Clinical Cornerstone, 6*(3), 39–48.

Koup, J., Abel, R., Smithers, J., Eldon, M., & de Vries, T. (1998). Effect of age, gender, and race on steady state procainamide pharmacokinetics after administration of Procanbid sustained-release tablets. *Therapeutic Drug Monitoring, 20*(91), 733–737.

Lannin, D., Mathews, H., Mitchell, J., Swanson, M., Swanson, F., & Edwards, M. (1998). Influences of socioeconomic and cultural factors on racial differences in late-stage presentation of breast cancer. *Journal of the American Medical Association, 279,* 1801–1807.

Lee, C., Yang, Y., & Hu, O. (1998). Single-dose pharmacokinetic study of lithium in Taiwanese/Chinese bipolar patients. *Australia and New Zealand Journal of Psychiatry, 32*(1), 133–136.

Lee, S. S. J. (2005). Racializing drug design: Implications of pharmacogenomics for health disparities. *American Journal of Public Health, 95*(12), 2133–2138.

Leininger, M. (2004). Leininger's Sunrise Enabler to Discover Culture Care. Retrieved April 24, 2006, from http://www.madeleine-leininger.com.

Leininger, M. (2006). Madeline M Leininger's Theory of Culture Care Diversity and Universality. In M. E. Parker (Ed.), *Nursing theories and nursing practice* (2nd ed.). Philadelphia: F.A. Davis.

Lin, K., Poland, R., Smith, M., Strickland, T., & Mendoza, R. (1991). Pharmacokinetic and other related factors affecting psychotropic responses in Asians. *Psychopharmacology Bulletin, 27*(4), 427–437.

Liu, K., & Levinson, S. (1996). Comparisons of blood pressure between Asian-American children and children from other racial groups in Chicago. *Public Health Reports, 111*(Suppl. 2), 65–67.

Liu, K., Ruth, K., Flack, J., Jones-Webb, R., Burke, G., Savage, P., et al. (1996). Blood pressure in young blacks and whites: Relevance of obesity and lifestyle factors in determining differences: The CARDIA study. *Circulation, 93,* 60–66.

Ma, L., Tataranni, P.A., Hanson, R. L., Infante, A. M., Kobes, S., Bogardus, C., et al. (2005). Variations in peptide YY and Y2 receptor genes are associated with severe obesity in Pima Indian men. *Diabetes, 54,* 1598–1602.

Matthews, H. (1995). Racial, ethnic and gender difference in response to medicines. *Drug Metabolism and Drug Interaction, 12*(2), 77–91.

McSweeney, E., & Zhan, L. (1994). Cultural and pharmacologic considerations when caring for Chinese elders. *Journal of Gerontological Nursing, 30*(10), 11–16.

Mitchell, H., Smith, R., Cutler, R., Sica, D., Videen, J., Thompsen-Bell, S., et al. (1997). Racial differences in the renal response to blood pressure lowering during chronic angiotensin-converting enzyme inhibition: A prospective double-blind randomized comparison of fosinopril and lisinopril in older hypertensive patients with chronic renal insufficiency. *American Journal of Kidney Diseases, 29*(6), 897–906.

Moskowitz, W., Schwartz, P., & Schieken, R. (1999). Childhood passive smoking, race, and coronary artery disease risk: The Medical College of Virginia Twin study. *Archives of Pediatric Adolescent Medicine, 153*(5), 446–453.

Muck, W., Unger, S., Kawano, K., & Ahr, G. (1998). Inter-racial comparisons of the pharmacokinetics of the HMG-CoA reductase inhibitor cervistatin. *British Journal of Clinical Pharmacology, 45*(6), 583–590.

Munoz, C., & Hilgenberg, C. (2005). Ethnopharmacology. *American Journal of Nursing, 105*(8), 40–48.

National Center for Health Statistics. (2002). A demographic and health snapshot of the U.S. Hispanic/Latino population: 2002 National Hispanic Health Leadership Summit. Retrieved April 26, 2006, from http://www.cdc.gov/NCHS/data/hpdata2010/chcsummit.pdf

National Center for Health Statistics. (2006a). Health of Hispanic/Latino population. Retrieved April 26, 2006, from http://www.cdc.gov/nchs/fastats/hispanic_health.htm

National Center for Health Statistics. (2006b). Health of Mexican American population. Retrieved April 26, 2006, from http://www.cdc.gov/nchs/fastats/mexican_health.htm

National Center for Health Statistics. (2010). Health, United States, 2008. Washington, DC. Retrieved on August 20, 2010 from http://www.cdc.gov/nchs.

O'Hara, E., & Zhan, L. (1994). Cultural and pharmacologic considerations when caring for Chinese elders: Knowledge of traditional Chinese medicine is necessary. *Journal of Gerontological Nursing, 30*(10), 11–16.

O'Malley, P. (2005). Ethnic pharmacology: Science, research, race and market share. *Clinical Nurse Specialist, 19*(6), 291–293.

Prisant, L., & Mensah, G. (1996). Use of beta-adrenergic receptor blockers in blacks. *Journal of Clinical Pharmacology, 36*(10), 867–873.

Purnell, L. D., & Paulanka, B J. (2005). *Culturally competent care.* Philadelphia: F.A. Davis Company.

Purnell, L. D., & Paulanka, B. J. (2008). *Transcultural health care: A culturally competent approach.* (3rd ed.). Philadelphia: F.A. Davis Company.

Rivera-Calimlim, L., & Reilly, D. (1984). Difference in erythrocyte catechol-o-methyltransferase activity between Orientals and Caucasians: Difference in levodopa tolerance. *Clinical Pharmacology and Therapeutics, 35*(6), 804–809.

Siriwardena, A. N. (2004). Specific health issues in ethnic minority groups. *Clinical Cornerstone, 6*(1), 34–42.

Spector, R. E. (2004). *Cultural diversity in health and illness.* Upper Saddle River, NJ: Pearson Prentice Hall.

Steinman, M.A., Sands, L. P., & Covinsky, K. E. (2001). Self-restriction of medications due to cost in seniors without prescription coverage. *Journal of Internal Medicine, 16*(12), 793–799.

Stephens, G., Gillapsy, J., Clyne, D., Mejia, A., & Pollack, V. (1990). Racial differences in the incidence of end-stage renal disease in types I and II diabetes mellitus. *American Journal of Kidney Diseases, 15*(6), 562–567.

Summerson, J., Bell, R., & Konen, J. (1995). Racial differences in the prevalence of microalbuminuria in hypertension. *American Journal of Kidney Diseases, 26*(4), 577–579.

Thompson, J., & Wilson, S. (1996). *Health assessment for nursing practice.* St. Louis, MO: Mosby.

Tortolero, S., Goff, D., Jr., Nichaman, M., Labarthe, D., Grunbaum, J., & Harris, C. (1997). Cardiovascular risk factors in Mexican-American and non-Hispanic white children: The Corpus Christi heart study. *Circulation, 96,* 418–423.

U.S. Census Bureau. (2005). *Income, poverty and health insurance coverage in the United States: 2004. Current population reports.* Publication P60-229. Washington, DC: U.S. Government Printing Office.

U.S. Census Bureau. (2006). 2000 Census: Race and ethnicity. Retrieved from http://factfinder.census.gov/

U.S. Census Bureau. (2008). *Income, poverty and health insurance coverage in the United States: 2007. Current population reports.* Publication P60-235. Washington, DC: U.S. Government Printing Office.

U.S. Department of Health and Human Services. (2010). Office of the Surgeon General, SAMHSA. *Mental health: Culture, race, ethnicity.* Retrieved on January 22, 2010 from http://mentalhealth.samsa.gov/cre.

U.S. Department of Labor Statistics. (2006). Employment status of foreign born and native born populations. Retrieved from http://www.bls.gov/news.release/forbrn.t01.htm

U.S. Office of Minority Health (OMH). (2006). Closing the health gap 2005 [Fact sheet]. Retrieved from http://www.healthgap.omhrc.gov/2005factsheet.htm

Weaver, C. (1998). Calcium requirements: The need to understand racial differences. *American Journal of Clinical Nutrition, 68,* 1153–1154.

Weinberger, M. (1993). Racial differences in renal sodium excretion: Relationship to hypertension. *American Journal of Kidney Diseases, 21*(4), 41–45.

Weir, M., Chrysant, S., McCarron, D., Canossa-Terris, M., Cohen, J., Gunter, P., et al. (1998). Influence of race and dietary salt on the antihypertensive efficacy of an angiotensin-converting enzyme inhibitor or a calcium channel antagonist in salt-sensitive hypertensives. *Hypertension, 31*(5), 1088–1096.

Winkleby, M., Kraemer, H., Ahn, D., & Varady, A. (1998). Ethnic and socioeconomic differences in cardiovascular disease risk factors: Findings for women from the Third National Health and Nutrition Examination Survey, 1988–1994. *Journal of the American Medical Association, 280,* 356–362.

Winkleby, M., Robinson, T., Sundquist, J., & Kraemer, H. (1999). Ethnic variations in cardiovascular disease risk factors among children and young adults. *Journal of the American Medical Association, 281*(11), 1006–1013.

Wood, A. (1998). Ethnic differences in drug disposition and response. *Therapeutic Drug Monitoring, 20*(5), 525–526.

Zaid, R. B., Nargis, M., Neelotpol, S., Hannan, J. M., Islam, S., Akhter, R., et al. (2004). Acetylation phenotype status in a Bangladeshi population and its comparison with that of other Asian population data. *Biopharmaceutics & Drug Disposition, 25*(6), 237–241.

CHAPTER 8

PHARMACOGENOMICS

Elizabeth Farrington

Chapter Outline

Advances in health care have led to a significant improvement in patient survival in the past three decades. Introduction of more selective and potent therapeutic agents and optimal patient-care services has affected patient survival and quality of life significantly, with life expectancy rising from 70.9 years in 1970 (U.S. Department of Health, Education, and Welfare, 1974) to 77.7 years in 2006 (Arias, 2010). Drug therapy is often the most challenging aspect of care. Optimal drug treatment requires selection of the best possible agents with close monitoring of pharmacokinetics, pharmacodynamics, adverse drug reactions, and cost of different agents. This chapter focuses on the pharmacogenomic influences on drug therapy. Adverse drug reactions (ADRs) are discussed in depth in Chapter 5, although this chapter will discuss ADRs related to genetic polymorphisms.

Pharmacogenetics and pharmacogenomics seek to identify patterns of genetic variation that will guide design of optimal medication regimens in individual patients. Historically, approach to drug therapy has been largely empiric and based on clinical studies that determined the maximally tolerated dose and reasonable toxicity in a narrowly defined population. This approach typically leads to the safe and effective administration of drugs for most individuals. However, with empiric therapy, inter-individual variation in drug response occurs. The differences will vary from a lack of therapeutic effect to potentially life-threatening ADRs. Genetic variations may explain some of the well-documented variability in response to drug therapy. Obviously, many factors other than genetics—such as age, sex, other drugs administered and underlying disease states—also contribute to variation in drug response. However, inherited differences in the metabolism and disposition of drugs and genetic polymorphisms in the targets of drug therapy (i.e., receptors) can have an even greater influence on the efficacy and toxicity of medications.

The Human Genome Project mapped the human genome, identifying single-nucleotide polymorphism (SNP) that may be responsible for the differences in response seen in pharmacotherapy (Howe, 2009). With the identification of the individual SNPs, our understanding of pharmacogenetics and pharmacogenomics has exploded.

GENETICS REVISITED

An individual's genetic makeup (or genotype) is derived as a result of the mixing of genetic materials from that individual's parents. Interestingly, even though two unrelated people share about 99.9 percent of the same DNA sequences, the less than 0.1 percent difference between them translates into a difference of 3 million nucleotides. These variants are the SNPS (pronounced "snips") (Howe, 2009). The variability of the genome at these various SNPs accounts for nearly all of the phenotypic differences we see in each other. The Human Genome Project has sought not only to identify and correlate SNPs with phenotypic differences but also to record and map haplotypes as well (Nebert, Zhang, & Vesell, 2008). Haplotypes are large portions of genetic material (around 25,000 base pairs) that tend to travel together. Understanding how SNPs and haplotypes make humans genetically unique is the current focus of much genetic research

(Nebert et al, 2008). The completion of the Human Genome Project, as well as the mapping of SNPs and haplotypes, has allowed the field of pharmacogenomics to understand the variability of drug metabolism seen across individuals and populations. Box 8–1 provides definitions of terms used in pharmacogenetics and pharmacogenomics.

HISTORY OF PHARMACOGENETICS

Pythagoras, the Greek philosopher and mathematician, recorded the first inter-individual difference of drug administration in 510 BCE when he noted that some patients developed hemolytic anemia after ingesting the fava bean (Nebert et al, 2008). The term pharmacogenetics was first coined by Vogel in 1959 but not until1962 was pharmacogenetics defined as the study of heredity and the response to drugs by Kalow (Nebert et al, 2008). Since 1962, the term pharmacogenetics has been used to refer to the effects of genetic differences on a person's response to drugs.

Interest in pharmacogenetics emerged in the 1950s in response to the discovery of an abnormal butyrylcholinesterase enzyme in psychiatric patients who exhibited prolonged muscular paralysis after administration of **succinylcholine** before electroconvulsive therapy (Meyer, 2004). Also in the 1950s the connection was established between the development of hemolysis in African American males treated for malaria with **primaquine** due to glucose-6-phosphate dehydrogenase deficiency (Beutler, 1959). Other seminal pharmacogenetic findings include the identification of the proportion of slow acetylators in certain ethnic groups, including 10 percent of Japanese and Eskimos; 20 percent of Chinese; and 60 percent of whites, blacks, and South Indians (Ellard, 1976), and attribution of peripheral neuropathy to slow acetylation of **isoniazid** in some patients treated for tuberculosis due to genetic diversity in the enzyme *N*-acetyltransferase (Fig. 8–1) (Yamamoto, Subue, Mukoyama, Matsuoka, & Mitsuma, 1999).

BOX 8–1 DEFINITIONS

Genetics: the study of heredity and its variations
Genomics: the study of the complete set of genetic information present in a cell, an organism, or species
Pharmacogenetics: the study of the influence of hereditary factors on the response of individual organisms to drugs (Venes, 2005); the study of variations of DNA and RNA characteristics as related to drug response (U.S. Food and Drug Administration, 2010b)
Pharmacogenomics: the study of the effects of genetic differences among people and the impact that these differences have on the uptake, effectiveness, toxicity, and metabolism of drugs
SNP: single-nucleotide polymorphism
Genetic polymorphism: multiple differences of a DNA sequence found in at least 1 percent of the population

Source: Venes, D. (2005). *Taber's cyclopedic medical dictionary* (21st ed.). Philadelphia: FA Davis; U.S. Food and Drug Administration. (2010b). Table of valid genomic biomarkers in the context of approved drug labels. Retrieved from http://www.fda.gov/RegulatoryInformation/Guidances/ucm129286.htm

PHARMACOGENOMICS

The ultimate promise of pharmacogenomics is the possibility that knowledge of the patient's DNA sequence might be used to enhance drug therapy to maximize efficacy, to target drugs only to those patients who are likely to respond, and to avoid ADRs. Increasing the number of patients who respond to a therapeutic regimen with a concomitant decrease in the incidence of ADRs is the promise of pharmacogenomic information. The long-term expected benefits of pharmacogenomics are selective and potent drugs, more accurate methods of determining appropriate drug dosages, advanced screening for disease, and a decrease in the overall cost of health-care system in the United States caused by ineffective drug therapy.

GENETIC DIFFERENCES IN DRUG METABOLISM

Genetic differences in metabolism were first realized by the observation that sometimes very low or very high concentrations of drug were found in some patients despite their having been given the same amount of drug. Most genetic differences in drug metabolism have been found to be "monogenic" genetic polymorphisms, meaning that they arise from the variation in one gene (Nebert et al, 2008).

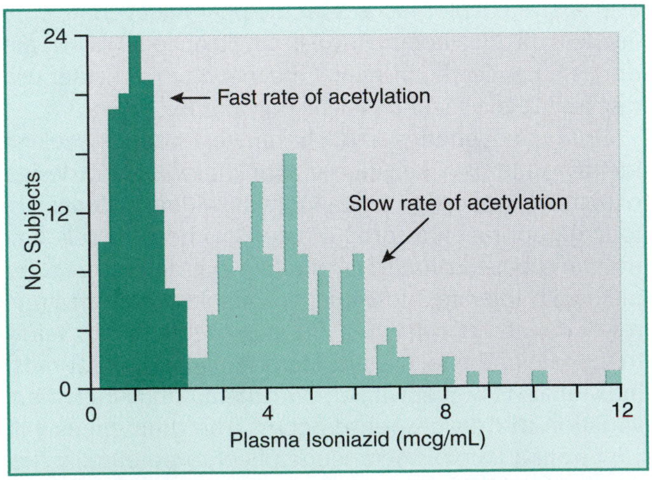

Figure 8–1. Pharmacogenomics of acetylation in isoniazid. Plasma isoniazid concentrations in 267 patients measured 6 hours post-dose. The bimodal distribution shows the effect of an NAT-2 genetic polymorphism.

Genetic Polymorphism

A genetic polymorphism occurs when a difference in the allele(s) responsible for the variation is a common occurrence. An allele is an alternative form of a gene. A gene is called polymorphic when allelic variations exist stably throughout a given population at a rate of less than 1 percent (Howe, 2009). Under such circumstances, mutant genes will exist somewhat frequently alongside wild-type genes. The mutant genes will encode for the production of mutant proteins in these populations. The mutant proteins will, in turn, interact with drugs in different manners, sometimes slight, sometimes significant. Monogenic traits cannot explain the complexity of drug metabolism by themselves (Nebert et al, 2008). Genes interact on a complex level, yielding different responses depending on which genes are wild type and which show mutant phenotypes. Sometimes these interactions can be very difficult to elucidate and may in fact be the source of seemingly unexplainable drug reactions. Figure 8–2 illustrates the relationship between genetic polymorphisms in drug metabolism and at drug receptors.

Four different phenotypes categorize the effects that genetic polymorphisms have on individuals: Poor metabolizers (PMs) lack a working enzyme; intermediate metabolizers (IMs) are heterogeneous for one working, wild-type allele and one mutant allele (or two reduced function alleles); extensive metabolizers (EMs), with two normally functioning alleles; and ultrarapid metabolizers (UMs), with more than one functioning copy of a certain enzyme (Belle & Singh, 2008). See Table 8–1 for the clinical implications of genetic polymorphisms.

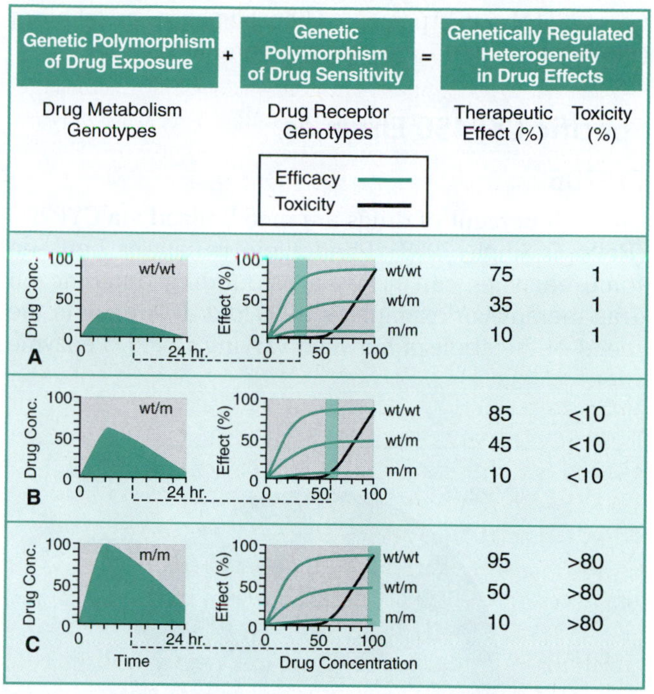

Figure 8–2. Genetic polymorphisms and drug metabolism/receptors.

Phase I and Phase II Metabolism

Drug metabolism generally involves the conversion of lipophilic substances and metabolites into more easily excretable water-soluble forms. Drug metabolism takes place mostly in the liver and is divided into two major categories, phase I (oxidation, reduction, and hydrolysis reactions) and phase II metabolism (conjugation reactions). A hallmark experiment in pharmacogenomics, diagramed in Figure 8–2, illustrates how differences in the rates of the phase II metabolizing enzyme *N*-acetyltransferase (NAT-2) can affect the half-life and plasma concentration of drugs that are subject to NAT-2 metabolism (Meyer, 2004).

Phase I metabolism enzymes are responsible for approximately 59 percent of the adverse drug reactions cited in the literature (Phillips, Veenstra, Oren, Lee, & Sadee, 2001). The high genetic variability of the cytochrome P450 (CYP450) enzymes constitutes the most important of the phase I metabolizing enzymes, with a total of 57 genes encoding for CYP450 enzymes. Of these, CYP2D6, CYP2C9, and CYP2C19 are the most highly polymorphic and account for

Table 8–1 **Clinical Implications of Genetic Polymorphisms**

Metabolizer Phenotype	Effect on Drug Metabolism	Clinical Implications
Poor to intermediate metabolizers	Slow	Prodrug will be metabolized slowly into active drug metabolite. May have accumulation of prodrug. Active drug will be metabolized slowly into inactive metabolite. Potential for accumulation of active drug. Patient requires lower dosage of medication.
Ultra rapid metabolizers	Fast	Prodrug rapidly metabolized into active drug. No dosage adjustment needed. Active drug rapidly metabolized into inactive metabolites leading to potential therapeutic failure. Patient requires higher dosage of active drug.

upward of about 40 percent of hepatic phase I metabolism (Phillips et al, 2001). See Figure 8–3 and Table 8–2.

Specific CYP450 Enzymes

CYP2D6

Up to 25 percent of drugs are metabolized via CYP2D6 (Belle & Singh, 2008). Phenotypic variations between some enzymes can have an astounding outcome on drug therapy. For example, a 1,000-fold difference in the speed of metabolism between varying CYP2D6 enzyme phenotypes has been observed! Figure 8–4 illustrates this difference within the European population and the CYP2D6 substrate nortriptyline.

CYP2D6 is a well-studied polymorphism and acts on many common prescription drugs (Table 8–3), including the selective **serotonin reuptake inhibitors (SSRIs)** such as **fluoxetine, tricyclic antidepressants (TCAs), beta blockers (metoprolol), calcium channel blockers**

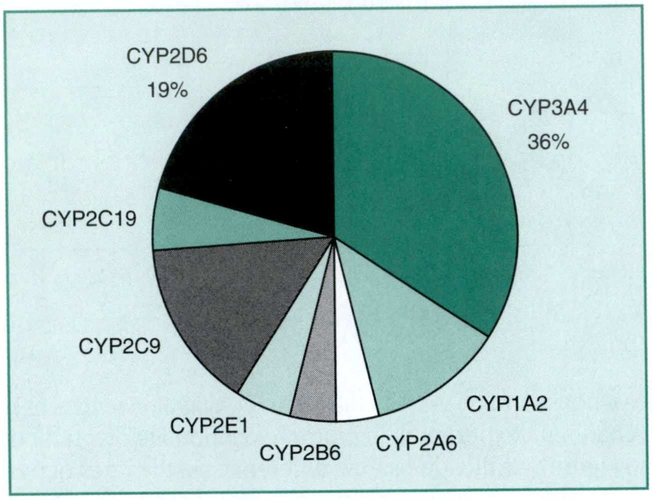

Figure 8–3. Proportion of drugs metabolized by CYP450 isoenzymes.

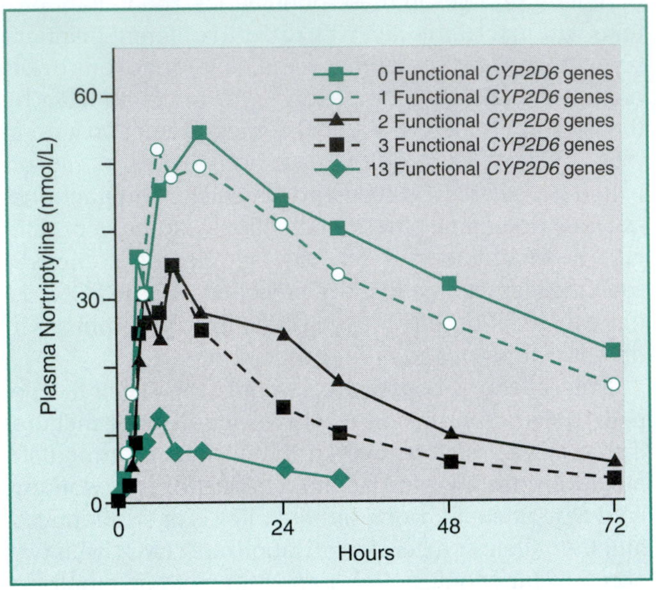

Figure 8–4. European population and the CYP2D6 substrate nortriptyline.

Table 8–2 **Medications and Their Receptors**

Gene	Medications	Drug Effect Linked to Polymorphism
Drug-Metabolizing Enzymes		
CYP2C9	Tolbutamide, warfarin, phenytoin, NSAIDs	Anticoagulant effect of warfarin
CYP2D6	Beta blockers, antidepressants, antipsychotics, codeine, debrisoquine, dextromethorphan, encainide, flecainide, guanoxan, methoxyamphetamine, *N*-propylajmaline, per- hexiline, phenacetin, phenformin, propafenone, sparteine	Tardive dyskinesia from antipsychotics; narcotic side effects, efficacy, and dependence: imipramine dose requirement; beta blocker effect
Dihydropyrimidine dehydrogenase	Fluorouracil	Fluorouracil neurotoxicity
Thiopurine methyltransferase	Mercaptopurine, thioguanine, azathioprine	Thiopurine toxicity and efficacy; risk of second cancers
Drug Targets		
ACE	Enalapril, lisinopril, captopril	Renoprotective effects, cardiac indices, blood pressure, immunoglobulin A nephropathy
Potassium channels	Quinidine	Drug-induced long QT syndrome
HERG	Cisapride	Drug-induced torsade de pointes
KvLQT1	Terfenadine, disopyramide, mefloquine	Drug-induced long QT syndrome
hKCNE2	Clarithromycin	Drug-induced arrhythmia

Table 8–3 **CYP 2D6**

Substrate	Inhibitors	Inducers
Codeine	Amiodarone	Carbamazepine
Dextromethorphan	Fluoxetine	Phenytoin
Metoprolol	Labetalol	Phenobarbital
Paroxetine	Paroxetine	Rifampin
Haloperidol	Propafenone	
Propranolol	Quinidine	
Risperidone	Sertraline	
Timolol	Cimetidine	
Amitriptyline		
Nortriptyline		
Clozapine		
Morphine		
Methadone		

(diltiazem), and **theophylline** (Phillips et al, 2001). Research has shown that approximately 10 percent of the white population has the poor metabolizer phenotype of this enzyme (Belle & Singh, 2008). Up to 7 percent of blacks and 4.8 percent of Asians have the poor metabolizer phenotype (Belle & Singh, 2008). Five percent of the white and 4.9 percent of the black population have the ultrarapid metabolizer phenotype (Belle & Singh, 2008). Up to 21 percent of Asians are ultrarapid 2D6 metabolizers, leading to therapeutic failure or increased dosages needed of drugs such as the **SSRIs** (Belle & Singh, 2008). Thirty-five percent of the population carries a nonfunctional 2D6 allele. This nonfunctional allele may increase the risk of ADRs, especially in patients with polypharmacy.

Opioid analgesics such as **codeine** rely on CYP2D6 enzymes to convert them to their active form, **morphine** (Belle & Singh, 2008). Genetic polymorphisms of the CYP2D6 enzyme can greatly alter the effect that codeine has on patients with PM or UM types. UM types may not experience the analgesic effects of the drug at normal therapeutic doses. While PMs may not be able to convert **codeine** to its active metabolite **morphine** thus experience little or no clinical benefit. Other **narcotics** that are active when administered to patients may experience the effects of excess drug at even the lower end of therapeutic dosing. See Table 8–3.

CYP2C9

CYP2C9 is the primary route of metabolism for warfarin and antiepileptic drugs **(phenytoin)**, **glipizide**, and other common drugs (Belle & Singh, 2008). The presence of CYP2C9 mutations is associated with a reduction in the metabolism of S-warfarin. Clinically, **warfarin** maintenance dosing requirements are lower in patients with CYP2C9*2 polymorphisms, and further reduced in patients with CYP2C9*3 variants (Gulseth, Grice, & Dager, 2009). In addition, patients with homozygous presentation of a CYP2C9 mutation appear to have a greater reduction in dosing requirement than do heterozygotes. Approximately one-third of the population are carriers of at least one allele for the slow-metabolizing form of CYP2C9 (U.S. Food and Drug Administration, 2009). The clinical implications of altered **warfarin** metabolism can be significant; the clinical implications of pharmacogenomic variants are found later in this chapter. See Table 8–4.

CYP3A4

The CYP3A group of isoenzymes is responsible for up to 50 percent of drug metabolism (Howe, 2009). CYP3A4 isoenzyme is responsible for metabolism of several important classes of drugs that are commonly used in primary care (see Table 8–1). Examples of these classes include **azole antifungals, calcium channel blockers, antihistamines, anticonvulsants, antimicrobials,** and **corticosteroids.** Both drug-related induction or inhibition of CYP450 3A4 isoenzyme may complicate drug therapy in patients (Howe, 2009). Predicting the onset and offset of these effects is very difficult. The time to onset and offset of drug–drug interactions is closely related to each drug's half-life and the half-life of enzyme production. Clinically significant drug interactions in this setting may increase the risk of toxicity. For example, **amiodarone** has a half-life close to 60 days and requires months to reach steady state and inhibit the CYP450 enzyme system effectively (Table 8–5). Conversely, it takes less than 2 days for **rifampin**, which is

Table 8–4 **CYP 2C (9 and 19)**

Substrate	Inhibitors	Inducers
S-warfarin	Amiodarone	Carbamazepine
Losartan	Cimetidine	Phenytoin
Diazepam	Chloramphenicol	Rifampin
Imipramine	Fluconazole	
Amitriptyline	Isoniazid	
Phenytoin	Ketoconazole	
Rosiglitazone	Zafirlukast	
	Fluoxetine	
	Fluvoxamine	
	Sertraline	
	Rosiglitazone	

Table 8–5 **CYP 3A4**

Substrate	Inhibitors	Inducers
Cyclosporine, FK 506	Erythromycin	Carbamazepine
Corticosteroids	Clarithromycin	Phenobarbital
Erythromycin	Diltiazem	Rifampin
Felodipine, isradipine	Ketoconazole	Rifabutin
Nifedipine	Fluconazole	Phenytoin
Nisoldipine	Itraconazole	Corticosteroids
Nitrendipine	Quinidine	INH
Digoxin, quinidine	Grapefruit juice	St. John's wort
Verapamil	Cimetidine	
Warfarin	Indinavir	
Sildenafil	Fluoxetine	
Astemizole	Zileuton, zafirlukast	
Terfenadine	Verapamil	
Pioglitazone	Amiodarone	
R-warfarin	Corticosteroids	
	Fluvoxamine	

a nonspecific CYP450 inducer with a shorter half-life, to decrease blood concentrations of many drugs to a subtherapeutic level and significantly increase the risk of therapeutic failure. Close monitoring is required when prescribing drugs that induce or inhibit CYP3A4 enzymes. See Table 8–5 for further information.

P-GLYCOPROTEIN

P-glycoprotein is a membrane-bound transport system responsible for drug transport across cell membranes (Howe, 2009). P-glycoprotein is a member of adenosine triphosphate (ATP)-binding proteins, which also act as gastrointestinal barriers for absorption of many xenobiotics. P-glycoprotein at the site of the gastrointestinal (GI) tract effluxes hydrophilic drugs out of the cell and inhibits drug absorption through the GI tract (Howe, 2009) As drugs passively diffuse through the GI tract, P-glycoprotein pumps intercept a drug's penetration into the cell or move drugs from cytoplasmic areas to extracellular media. Substrates of P-glycoprotein include **carvedilol, diltiazem,** and **digoxin** (Howe, 2009). In the case of **digoxin,** P-glycoprotein affects the level of **digoxin** available for absorption and elimination (Howe, 2009). P-glycoprotein inhibitors include **verapamil, quinidine, cyclosporine,** and **ketoconazole** (Howe, 2009). If an inhibitor of P-glycoprotein is administered, then blood levels of substrates will rise, as seen if **quinidine** is administered with **digoxin.**

Drugs can be categorized as reversible or suicidal inhibitors or P-glycoproteins. For example, **calcium channel blockers** and **high-dose steroids** are considered as reversible inhibitors of both P-glycoproteins and CYP450. However, grapefruit and **ritonavir** are suicidal agents for both P-glycoprotein and CYP450, meaning the effect of grapefruit juice will be prolonged, perhaps up to 24 hours. See Figure 8–5.

CLINICAL IMPLICATIONS OF PHARMACOGENOMICS

Adverse Drug Reactions

One benefit of understanding pharmacogenomics is the possibility of a decrease in the number of ADRs. The CYPP450 enzymes in families 1 to 3 mediate 78 to 80 percent of all phase I–dependent metabolism of clinically used drugs (Spatzenegger & Jaeger, 1995). The polymorphic forms of CYPP450s are responsible for the development of idiosyncratic ADRs (Kalgutkar, Obach, & Maurer, 2007). According to Phillips and Van Bebber (2005), 56 percent of drugs cited in ADR studies are metabolized by polymorphic phase I enzymes, of which 86 percent are P450s.

Warfarin

In 2008 the package insert for **warfarin** was updated by the U.S. Food and Drug Administration (FDA) to include application of pharmacogenomics to the dosing of **warfarin.** Previous work had identified variable metabolism by CYP2C9 as a major contributor to the variable response to the drug. In 2004, coding-region mutations in VCORC1, encoding a subunit of the vitamin K epoxide reductase complex (the pharmacologic target for the drug), were found to cause a rare syndrome of **warfarin** resistance. Subsequently, the variants in VCORC1 have been found to account for a much greater fraction of variability in warfarin response (21%) than do variations in CYP2C9 (6%) (Gulseth et al, 2009). Although genetic testing prior to prescribing has not yet been required by the FDA, numerous **warfarin** dosing calculators exist on the Web where a clinician can insert clinical information

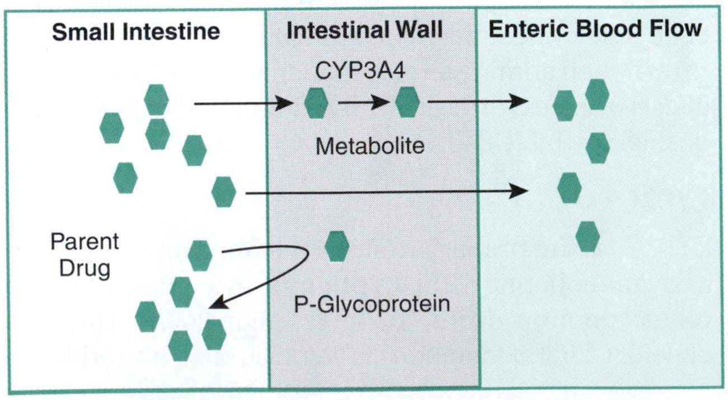

Figure 8–5. Drug–metabolism interactions.

about the patient, including genetic test results and indications, and a dosing regimen will be calculated or "individualized" for that patient (http://www.warfarindosing.com; http://www.globalrph .com/warfarin.htm).

Pharmacogenetic Testing Prior to Prescribing

The FDA now requires additional pharmacogenomic information on several drug package inserts (Table 8–6). The pharmacogenetic tests mentioned on drug labels can be classified as "test required," "test recommended," and "information only." Currently, four drugs are required to have pharmacogenetic testing performed before they are prescribed: **cetuximab**, **trastuzumab**, **maraviroc**, and **dasatinib**. **Cetuximab** treatment needs a confirmation of epidermal growth factor receptor (*EGFR*) expression. **Trastuzumab** therapy requires testing for *HER2/NEU* overexpression. Infection with *CCR-5*-tropic HIV-1 should be confirmed before initiation of therapy with **maraviroc** (an antiretroviral). **Dasatinib** is used for the treatment of patients with Philadelphia chromosome-positive acute lymphoblastic leukemia resistant to or intolerant of prior therapy (U.S. Food and Drug Administration, 2010b).

In December 2007, the FDA added a black-box warning on the **carbamazepine** label, recommending testing for the *HLA-B*1502* allele in patients with Asian ancestry before initiating **carbamazepine** therapy because these patients are at high risk of developing **carbamazepine**-induced Stevens-Johnson syndrome (SJS) or toxic epidermal necrolysis (TEN). Interestingly, although Asians or patients with Asian ancestry have been reported to have a strikingly high frequency (10 times higher than whites) of **carbamazepine**-induced SJS or TEN if they carry an *HLA-B*1502* allele; other races carrying the allele do not seem to have the increased risk (U.S. Food and Drug Administration, 2007).

The anticancer agent **irinotecan** is a prodrug used for the treatment of colorectal cancer, small-cell lung cancer, and other solid tumors. The active metabolite of **irinotecan** is SN-38, a topoisomerase I inhibitor, and uridine diphosphate glucuronosyltransferase 1A1 (UGT1A1) plays a critical role in inactivating SN-38 (McLeod & Hoskins, 2007). The low activity of the UGT1A1 enzyme may increase the risk for adverse events associated with **irinotecan** therapy (e.g., neutropenia) by increasing serum concentrations of the active metabolite. A polymorphism in the promoter region of the UGT1A1 gene determines patient exposure to SN-38 (McLeod & Hoskins, 2007). Patients homozygous for the polymorphism (UGT1A1*28) are at a 5-fold greater risk of **irinotecan**-related toxicity compared with patients with one or two normal alleles. Additionally, the FDA has approved a test for detection of the UGT1A1*28 genotype for **irinotecan** dosing. Additional genotype tests approved by the FDA and their implications are summarized in Table 8–7.

SUMMARY

We live in remarkable times, in which multiple therapeutic options are available for most common diseases. However, the selection of the optimal medication for an individual patient is still problematic. Practitioners still pick the "right" initial medication only half the time and ADRs are still unpredictable. In addition, the expense of new biological agents is such that even wealthy countries such as the United States cannot afford to treat all patients.

The completion of the Human Genome Project has enabled the development of clinical tools for patient evaluation. Pharmacogenomics may allow identification

Table 8–6 **U.S. Food and Drug Administration Positions on Necessity of Pharmacogenetic Testing as Indicated on Drug Labeling**

Pharmacogenetic Biomarker	Drug
Test Required	
EGFR expression	Cetuximab
HER2/NEU overexpression	Trastuzumab
CCR-5-tropic HIV-1	Maraviroc
Presence of Philadelphia chromosome	Dasatinib
Test Recommended	
HLA-B*1502	Carbamazepine
HLA-B*5701	Abacavir
CYP2C9 variants	Warfarin
VKORC1 variants	Warfarin
Protein C deficiency	Warfarin
TPMT variants	Azathioprine, mercaptopurine, thioguanine
UGT1A1 variants	Irinotecan
G6PD deficiency	Rasburicase
Urea cycle disorders	Valproic acid
Information Only	
c-KIT expression	Imatinib
CYP2C19 variants	Voriconazole
CYP2C9 variants	Celecoxib
CYP2D6 variants	Atomoxetine, tamoxifen, fluoxetine
DPD deficiency	Capecitabine, fluorouracil
EGFR expression	Erlotinib
G6PD deficiency	Rasburicase, primaquine
NAT variants	Isoniazid, rifampin

Continued

Table 8–6 U.S. Food and Drug Administration Positions on Necessity of Pharmacogenetic Testing as Indicated on Drug Labeling—cont'd

Pharmacogenetic Biomarker	Drug
Philadelphia chromosome deficiency	Busulfan
PML/RAR gene expression	Tretinoin

EGFR = epidermal growth factor receptor; HER2/NEU = v-erb-b2 erythroblastic leukemia viral oncogene homolog 2; CCR-5 = chemokine C-C motif receptor; HLA = human leukocyte antigen; CYP2C9 = cytochrome P-450 isoenzyme 2C9; VKORC1 = vitamin K epoxide reductase complex subunit 1; TPMT = thiopurine *S*-methyltransferase; UGT1A1 = uridine diphosphate-glucuronosyltransferase 1A1; c-KIT = v-kit Hardy-Zuckerman 4 feline sarcoma viral oncogene homolog; CYP2C19 = cytochrome P-450 2C19; CYP2D6 = cytochrome P-450 isoenzyme 2D6; DPD deficiency = dihydropyrimidine dehydrogenase; G6PD = glucose-6-phosphate dehydrogenase; NAT = *N*-acetyltransferase; PML/RAR = promyelocytic leukemia/retinoic acid receptor.cytochrome P-450 isoenzyme 2D6; DPD deficiency = dihydropyrimidine dehydrogenase; G6PD = glucose-6-phosphate dehydrogenase; NAT = *N*-acetyltransferase; PML/RAR = promyelocytic leukemia/retinoic acid receptor.

Source: Derived from U.S. Food and Drug Administration. (2010b). Table of valid genomic biomarkers in the context of approved drug labels. Retrieved from http://www.fda.gov/Drugs/ScienceResearch/ResearchAreas/Pharmacogenetics/ucm083378.htm

Table 8–7 FDA Approved Diagnostic Test Commercially Available for Commonly Prescribed Pharmacologic Therapies

Genetic Test	Drug	Benefit of Genetic Test
CYP2C9/ VCORC1	Warfarin	Reduce time to target INR; possibly decrease bleeding episodes
CYP2D6	Tamoxifen Codeine Oxycodone Tricyclic antidepressants	Reduce therapeutic failure Reduce GI toxicities/ improve pain control Reduce GI toxicities/ improve pain control Reduce therapeutic failure
TMPT	Azathiaprine 6-mecaptopurine	Reduce myelosuppression Reduce myelosuppression
UGT1A1	irinotecan	Reduce neutropenia

Source: Derived from McLeod, H. L., & Hoskins. J. M. (2007). Personalized drug therapy: The era of pharmacoeconomics. Retrieved from http://www.ipit.unc.edu/files/1233076125-one.pdf

of patients most likely to benefit from a given therapy and those patients for whom the cost and risk outweigh the benefits. Both the safety and efficacy of drug therapy may improve. In the future, genotyping may be used to personalize drug treatment for vast numbers of patients, decreasing the cost of drug treatment and increasing the efficacy of drugs and health in general.

REFERENCES

Arias, E. (2010). United States life tables, 2006. *National Vital Statistics Reports, 58*(21). Retrieved from http://www.cdc.gov/nchs/data/nvsr/nvsr58/nvsr58_21.pdf

Belle, D. J., & Singh, H. (2008). Genetic factors in drug metabolism. *American Family Physician, 77*(11), 1553–1560.

Beutler, E. (1959). The hemolytic effect of primaquine and related compounds: A review. *Blood, 14*(2), 103–139.

Ellard, G. A. (1976). Variations between individuals and populations in the acetylation of isoniazid and its significance for the treatment of pulmonary tuberculosis. *Clinical Pharmacology and Therapeutics, 19* (5, Pt. 2), 610–625.

Evans, W. E., & Relling, M. V. (1999). Pharmacogenomics: Translating functional genomics into rational therapeutics. *Science, 286,* 487–491.

Gulseth, M. P., Grice, G. R., & Dager, W. E. (2009). Pharmacogenomics of warfarin: Uncovering a piece of the warfarin mystery. *American Journal of Health Systems Pharmacists, 66,* 123–133.

Howe, L. A. (2009). Pharmacogenomics and management of cardiovascular disease. *The Nurse Practitioner, 34*(8), 28–35.

Kalgutkar, A. S., Obach, R. S., & Maurer, T. S. (2007). Mechanism-based inactivation of cytochrome P450 enzymes: Chemical mechanisms, structure-activity relationships and relationship to clinical drug-drug interactions and idiosyncratic adverse drugs reactions. *Current Drug Metabolism, 8,* 407–447.

McLeod, H. L., & Hoskins. J. M. (2007). Personalized drug therapy: The era of pharmacoeconomics. Retrieved from http://www.ipit.unc.edu/files/1233076125-one.pdf

Meyer, U. A. (2004). Pharmacogenetics—five decades of therapeutic lessons from genetic diversity. *Nature Reviews, Genetics, 5*(9), 669–676.

Nebert, D. W., Zhang, G., & Vesell, E. S. (2008). From human genetics and genomics to pharmacogenetics and pharmacogenomics: Past lessons, future directions. *Drug Metabolism Reviews, 40,* 187–224.

Penny, M. A., & McHale, D. (2005). Pharmacogenomics and the drug discovery pipeline: When should it be implemented? *American Journal of Pharmacogenomics, 5*(1), 53–62. Review.

Peters, G. J., Smorenburg, C. H., & Van Groeningen, C. J. (2004). Prospective clinical trials using a pharmacogenetic/pharmacogenomic approach. *Journal of Chemotherapy, 16*(Suppl. 4)2, 5–30. Review.

Phillips, K. A., & Van Bebber, S. L. (2005). Measuring the value of pharmacogenomics. *Nature Reviews Drug Discovery, 4*(6), 500–509.

Phillips, K. A., Veenstra, D. L., Oren, E., Lee, J. K., & Sadee, W. (2001). Potential role of pharmacogenomics in reducing adverse drug reactions: A systematic review. *Journal of the American Medical Association, 286*(18), 2270–2279.

Spatzenegger, M., & Jaeger, W. (1995). Clinical importance of hepatic cytochrome P450 in drug metabolism. *Drug Metabolism Reviews, 27,* 397–417.

Suarez-Kurtz, G. (2005). Pharmacogenomics in admixed populations. *Trends in Pharmacology Science, 26*(4), 196–201.

U.S. Department of Health, Education, and Welfare. (1974). *Vital statistics of the United States, 1970* (Vol. 2, Sec. 5) (DHEW Publication No. HRA 74-1104). Retrieved from http://www.cdc.gov/nchs/data/lifetables/life70.pdf

U. S. Food and Drug Administration. (2007). Information on carbamazepine (marketed as Carbatrol, Equetro, Tegretol and generics) with FDA alerts. Retrieved from http://www.fda.gov/Drugs/DrugSafety

U.S. Food and Drug Administration. (2009). Critical path initiative—warfarin dosing. Retrieved from http://www.fda.gov/ScienceResearch/SpecialTopics/CriticalPathInitiative/FacesBehindCriticalPath/ucm077473.htm

U.S. Food and Drug Administration. (2010a). E15 definitions for genomic biomarkers, pharmacogenomics, pharmacogenetics, genomic data and sample coding categories. Retrieved from http://www.fda.gov/RegulatoryInformation/Guidances/ucm129286.htm

U.S. Food and Drug Administration. (2010b). Table of valid genomic biomarkers in the context of approved drug labels. Retrieved from http://www.fda.gov/Drugs/ScienceResearch/ResearchAreas/Pharmacogenetics/ucm083378.htm

Vermes, A., & Vermes, I. (2004). Genetic polymorphisms in cytochrome P450 enzymes. Effect on efficacy and tolerability of HMG0CoA Reductase inhibitors. *American Journal of Cardiovascular Drugs, 4*(4), 247–255.

Walgren, R. A., Meucci, M. A., & McLeod, H. L. (2005). Pharmacogenomic discovery approaches: Will the real genes please stand up? *Journal of Clinical Oncology, 23*(29), 7342–7349.

Yamamoto, M., Subue, G., Mukoyama, M., Matsuoka, Y., & Mitsuma, T. (1999). Demonstration of slow acetylator genotype of *N*-acetyltransferase in isoniazid neuropathy using an archival hematoxylin and eosin section of a sural nerve biopsy specimen. *Journal of Neurological Sciences, 135*(1), 51–54.

CHAPTER 9

NUTRITION AND NUTRACEUTICALS

Teri Moser Woo

Chapter Outline

Eating is a part of daily life. The use of nutrition as therapy is beginning to take its rightful place in health promotion, disease prevention, and disease treatment. We have significant knowledge about the importance of nutrition as a key factor in health promotion, disease prevention, and treatment. We know that nutrition therapy can provide effective and efficient treatment when the medical condition affects nutritional needs or the diet affects the medical condition. When nutritional considerations are part of the plan of care, the health-care provider helps patients feel better; improves management of their health-care problems; and avoids complications that affect quality of life, productivity, and health-care costs. This chapter examines the role nutrition plays in pharmacotherapy, including the role of food intake on drug pharmacokinetics and the use of nutraceuticals (foods that claim to have a medicinal effect).

NUTRIENT–DRUG INTERACTIONS

Drugs do not create new bodily functions but rather interact with cellular function. Key to adequate cell function is the supply of needed nutrients. Because drugs are designed to improve altered cell function, it seems logical to conclude that nutritional factors can, in turn, affect pharmacological therapy. Clinically, health-care providers are concerned about the effect of drugs on the absorption, transport, metabolism, cellular uptake, and excretion of nutrients and the effect of nutrients on the pharmacokinetics of drugs. Additionally, some foods contain chemicals that may directly compete with medications; for example, foods high in **vitamin K** compete with **warfarin.** Therefore, drug–nutrient interactions must be considered to utilize drugs effectively in the prevention and treatment of disease. Patient education must be provided about drug–food interactions, especially if there is a potential for adverse patient outcomes.

Influence of Diet on the Pharmacokinetics of Drugs

Drug Absorption

The most frequent type of drug–food interaction is the effect that food has on the gastrointestinal (GI) absorption of drugs. Drug absorption can be decreased, delayed, accelerated or increased by food (Singh, 1999; Singh & Malhotra, 2004). Drug absorption takes place across the mucosa of the GI tract. The proximal part of the small intestine plays a significant role in drug and nutrient absorption, secondary to its large surface area.

Drugs utilize the same transport mechanisms as nutrients: passive and facilitated diffusion, endocytosis, and active transport. Several physiological factors affect drug absorption during the transport process: bioavailability, presystemic metabolism, gastric emptying time, concentration gradient, and absorptive surface area. Food in the GI tract at the time of drug administration affects absorption and bioavailability of the drug by changing the gastric emptying time, through interaction within the GI lumen and by competitive inhibition.

Bioavailability—the percentage of drug available to produce a pharmacological effect—is influenced by the presence of food within the GI tract. Therefore, absorption of drugs can be increased or decreased, depending of the presence of food (Singh, 1999). Food decreases the amount of fluid in the GI tract, thus slowing down drug dissolution. Lack of food for an extended period—fasting for a day, for example—can decrease absorption secondary to vasoconstriction. Gastric emptying time also can influence drug absorption. However, the effect varies, depending on the type of drug preparation and the need for presystemic metabolism or dissolution. A drug that requires interaction in the stomach for disintegration and dissolution would have reduced absorption owing to the rapid gastric emptying time that might accompany a fasting state. Delayed gastric emptying that might occur with a meal high in fat would facilitate drug absorption because the drug is given more time for maximal disintegration and dissolution. Clearly, a change in gastric emptying can affect drug absorption, but the impact of the change is related to the dosage form and dissolution characteristics of the drug. A change in the drug form or time of administration can potentially affect bioavailability. Questioning the food intake of a patient who has had a change in the effectiveness of a pharmacological therapy can be an important part of the clinical decision-making process.

In addition, the effect of food on the pH of the stomach can change bioavailability. The degree of ionization that occurs when a drug is taken into the stomach is a function of GI pH. If a drug is a weak acid with best absorption in the nonprotonated (nonionized) state, then the low pH of the stomach is essential to drug absorption to allow the acid to remain nonionized and absorbable.

Chemical and physical changes in the drug can also occur as a result of interaction with food. These changes affect the absorption of the drug. Every nurse is aware of the need to advise patients to take **tetracycline** on an empty stomach or with foods that are not high in calcium, aluminum, iron, and magnesium because of decreased absorption, as the drug chelates with these minerals. The binding of **phenytoin** with enteral nutrition products that results in fluctuation of **phenytoin** levels has provided the impetus for the development of protocols that stop enteral nutrition before, during, and after delivery of this medication when the patient is tube fed.

Additional physiological factors that may change a drug's absorption from the GI tract include food-induced changes in splanchnic blood flow, resulting in variation of drug absorption. As pointed out earlier, use of the same cellular transport proteins could result in competition for transport systems. **Levodopa** absorption is thought to be reduced with high-protein diets because of competition for the same transport system.

The potential for change in drug absorption by food or nutrients in the GI system is quite high. Drugs that have decreased absorption with food may need to be administered on an empty stomach, unless that is the desired effect, as when **griseofulvin** is given with a high-fat meal. When food has no effect on drug bioavailability, then the drug may be administered without regard to food intake. Patient education regarding the coordination of medication administration and food intake should be integral to the prescribing process.

Drug Metabolism

The rate of drug metabolism in both the GI tract and the liver is affected by nutrient intake. A low-carbohydrate, high-protein diet may increase drug-metabolizing enzymes. Increasing intake of antioxidant cruciferous vegetables may increase the activity of drug-metabolizing enzymes. Clinically, we see examples of the effect of foods on metabolism daily, as unexplained variability in drug response or therapeutic drug levels.

The cytochrome P450 (CYP450) system is the major enzyme group responsible for the metabolism of foreign chemicals that come into the body. Information is expanding about the clinically significant interactions between nutrients and drugs utilizing the CYP450 enzyme system. In addition, the CYP450 system has a significant amount of polymorphism associated with it; that is, there are between-individuals differences in the presence and/or function of a particular enzyme group. This difference reinforces the need to understand the nutrient effect on metabolizing enzymes. A more detailed discussion of the CYP450 system is provided in Chapter 8 including the genetic issues surrounding this system.

Grapefruit Juice and CYP3A4

Grapefruit juice influences the metabolism of many drugs because it contains components that inhibit CYP3A4, leading to alterations in the metabolism of drugs. Studies have determined that it is the furanocoumarins in the grapefruit juice that have been identified as CYP3A4 inhibitors, decreasing first-pass metabolism of drugs (Gertz, Davis, Harrison, Houston, & Galetin, 2008; Mertens-Talcott, Zadezensky, DeCastro, Derendorf, & Butterweck, 2006; Paine et al, 2006). Ingestion of grapefruit juice leads to increased levels of **calcium channel blockers, cyclosporine, tacrolimus**, and the **statins** (Kuypers, 2009; Vaquero et al, 2010). The maximum inhibitory effect occurs if the grapefruit juice is ingested at the same time or within 4 hours of a drug (Gertz et al, 2008).

Foods and CYP1A2

Other foods or beverages that influence drug oxidation or conjugation reactions include indolic compounds in vegetables (cruciferous), **methylxanthine**-containing beverages (**caffeine**), and charcoal broiling. Cruciferous vegetables induce CYP1A2, an enzyme responsible for the metabolism of many drugs including **theophylline**. Patients who consume large amounts of cruciferous vegetables may have therapeutic failure if they are being treated with drugs that are metabolized by CYP1A2 (Schein, 1997). Tobacco smoking and charcoal-broiled meat induce CYP1A2 due to their high concentrations of olycyclic aromatic hydrocarbons (Larsen & Brosen, 2005). Patients will need to be educated regarding intake of foods that induce CYP1A2.

Drug Excretion

Certain foods can change urinary pH, which then increases or decreases the amount of the ionized form of a drug or metabolite. The half-life of some medications may be changed by altering urine pH (Ishmail, 2009). For example, **gentamicin** as a basic drug would be more likely to be reabsorbed in the renal tubule when there is an alkaline pH. Foods that alkalinize the urine include milk, vegetables, and citrus fruits. Foods that acidify the urine include meat, fish, cheese, and eggs (Ishmail, 2009).

Drug-Induced Nutrient Depletion

Another mechanism of interaction between drugs and nutrients is the affect drugs can have on nutrient absorption, synthesis, transport, storage, metabolism, and excretion. The side effect profile of a drug taken over a period of time can be related to the effect of that drug on nutrient depletion. The number of potential drug-induced nutrient deficiencies is large and growing, and research in this area continues.

The mechanisms of action for drug-induced nutrient deficiencies are varied. As discussed previously, the GI changes due to dietary factors that affect drug absorption can also be induced by drugs and thus affect nutrient absorption. The alterations in gastric emptying time, changes in pH, mucosal irritation (enteropathy), and formation of complexes that can result from drug therapy often have an impact on nutrient absorption. For example, changes in the pH from antacid therapy or potassium therapy can reduce absorption of **folic acid**, **iron**, and **vitamin B_{12}**. Drugs can induce or inhibit metabolic processes and, as a result, affect nutrient metabolism and bioavailability. For example, **phenytoin** reduces the level of **folic acid** by inhibition of intestinal enzymes needed for **folic acid** absorption. Many metabolic pathways rely on specific nutrient availability; therefore, a deficiency results in cellular dysfunction. For example, the synthesis of vitamins, coagulation factors, and neurotransmitters can be affected by reduction in nutrient substrates.

Just as the nutrient can affect excretion of drugs, drugs can affect urinary secretion, reabsorption, and elimination of nutrients. For example, the commonly seen depletion of sodium, calcium, and potassium with **loop diuretic** use is the result of interference with renal reabsorption. Thus, drug-induced nutrient malabsorption, maldigestion, and vitamin antagonism are potential adverse reactions to commonly prescribed drugs.

Outcomes of Nutrient–Drug Interactions

The physiological and cellular basis for nutrient–drug interactions is strong. However, it is the outcome of the interaction that takes the spotlight. Does the interaction cause a change in the expected outcome of drug therapy or a nutrient deficiency that enhances the potential for adverse reactions or disease progression? Clinically, practitioners often overlook this area. If the expected outcome of drug therapy is not occurring or the adverse reaction profile is enhanced, the practitioner must know the key questions to ask to determine what is happening. It should be clear that a piece of the data needed is related to food and nutrient intake. Could the patient who became pregnant on the **low-estrogen birth control pill** have a reduction in drug bioavailability owing to food intake? Is the **antidepressant** not working secondary to high **caffeine** intake? Is the **digoxin (Lanoxin)** serum level low because of an aggressive bowel care program with high-fiber intake? And even more important, did the change in dietary fiber intake contribute to the **digoxin** toxicity the patient is experiencing?

An example of a food–drug interaction is one that occurs between **warfarin** and **vitamin K**–containing foods. Patients who are taking **warfarin** should not ingest foods high in **vitamin K**, as the combination may lead to therapeutic failure. Patients taking **warfarin** need to be educated regarding the **vitamin K** content of foods (Table 9–1). **Warfarin** and **vitamin K** interactions are further discussed in Chapter 18.

A high intake of food containing tyramine can result in enhanced **norepinephrine** synthesis—which can be problematic if the same patient is taking drugs that increase **norepinephrine** availability at the neurological synapse. For example, the adverse effect of acute hypertension associated with the use of **monoamine oxidase inhibitors (MAOIs)** is enhanced by intake of foods high in tyramine. The inhibition of aldehyde dehydrogenase by **metronidazole** results in a **disulfiram-like** reaction—flushing, headache, nausea, and abdominal or chest pain—when it is taken with alcohol or **alcohol**-containing products because of alteration in the alcohol metabolism.

Food contains many highly interactive ingredients that can have an impact on drug therapy. For example, the use of **caffeine** with known central nervous system (CNS) effects is problematic for patients utilizing **psychotropic** medications. The ability to manage the mental health problem becomes a challenge when high or variable levels of **caffeine** are consumed. Sorbitol, a common ingredient in sugar-free foods, has a significant effect on GI transit time and thus can influence the absorption of both drugs and nutrients.

Table 9–1 **Vitamin K Content in Common Foods**

Food	Serving Size	Daily Value (%)
Foods High in Vitamin K (more than or equal to 200% DV)	**Eat No More Than 1 Serving per Day**	
Kale, fresh, boiled	½ cup	660
Spinach, fresh, boiled	½ cup	560
Turnip greens, frozen, boiled	½ cup	530
Collards, fresh, boiled	½ cup	520
Swiss chard, fresh, boiled	½ cup	360
Parsley, raw	¼ cup	300
Mustard greens, fresh, boiled	½ cup	260
Foods Moderately High in Vitamin K (60% to 199% DV)	**Eat No More Than 2 Servings per Day**	
Brussels sprouts, frozen, boiled	½ cup	190
Spinach, raw	1 cup	180
Turnip greens, raw, chopped	1 cup	170
Green leaf lettuce, chopped	1 cup	125
Broccoli, raw, chopped	1 cup	110
Endive lettuce, raw	1 cup	70
Romaine lettuce, raw	1 cup	70

Source: Warren Grant Magnuson Clinical Center, National Institutes of Health Drug-Nutrient Interaction Task Force, 2003.

Alcohol consumption is also associated with significant drug interaction problems. Alcohol can either induce or inhibit the CYP450 system enzymes, depending on the ingestion pattern. Chronic low levels cause enzymatic induction, whereas high binge intake or high chronic use, resulting in hepatic failure, inhibits the metabolizing enzymes. Therefore, the provider needs to know the patient's specific level of alcohol consumption to better understand the potential for interaction with drugs.

Clinical Decision Making

What can providers do to improve their skill in recognizing nutrient–drug interactions? The provider should consider the following:

1. Use up-to-date resources to evaluate the potential for drug–food interactions.
2. Seek out educational materials that can provide accurate and appropriate drug information to patients.
3. Consult with other practitioners, pharmacists, and registered dietitians to identify drug–nutrient interactions.
4. Get a complete patient profile in terms of drug, herb, and nutrient intake. Knowing all of the medications taken—prescribed, over the counter, herbs, vitamins, alcohol, nutrient supplements—is key to the identification of interaction potential.

The nurse practitioner must understand how the medication is taken in relation to food and fluids. How stable is food intake in terms of the substances known to affect drug absorption, such as fiber, protein, and fat? Clearly communicate to the patient the best routine for medication administration. The nurse practitioner needs to ensure that he or she and the patient read warning labels for instructions about mixing with food, using with nutritional supplements, and taking with fluid.

NUTRITIONAL MANAGEMENT

Consumers have shown increased interest and awareness of the importance of nutrition and nutrients in staying healthy. An outcome of this knowledge is increased use of nutrient supplementation. Nutritional supplementation is the use of vitamins, minerals, or other food factors to support health and prevent or treat disease. There are approximately 50 essential nutrients that must be acquired in the diet to maximize health. Although all nutritionists will explain that the interplay of these nutrients is significant to their role in the body, many still will recommend supplementation of specific nutrients or combinations of nutrients for individuals at risk. It is vital that providers include recommendations about how to utilize diet as part of the plan of care, but it is not uncommon that the ability to accomplish the recommendation by diet alone is difficult for given individuals. In addition, recommended diet alterations might not be best in consideration of other health problems. Therefore, the provider must become skilled in accurately advising patients about the benefits of nutraceuticals in maintaining health, preventing disease, and treating disease. Those individuals who might be on drug therapy that can induce nutrient deficiencies need specific recommendations about diet and nutrient supplementation to avoid additional drug adverse reactions.

A complete or focused nutritional assessment should be part of the information gathered during the patient interaction. Data from the diet history, anthropometric measurement, physical examination, and laboratory findings are useful for pharmacological decision making. Team members such as a pharmacist and a registered dietitian are especially important in the care of patients with complex medical problems or pharmacological treatment plans. Disease-specific nutritional therapy is beyond the scope of this chapter; the American Dietetic Association (ADA) has developed medical nutrition therapy protocols for a variety of diagnoses (http://www.eatright.org) and the American Society of Parenteral and Enteral Nutrition (ASPEN) has developed clinical guidelines to reflect current, evidence-based approaches to the practice of nutrition support (http://www.nutritioncare.org).

Although much of the research surrounding use of supplements is not conclusive in terms of randomized clinical trials and is even sometimes contradictory, patients' use of nutritional supplementation is not waiting for conclusive outcomes. To partner with the patient who is interested in nutritional supplementation, nurse practitioners must have a clear understanding of the patient's philosophy surrounding nutritional supplementation and the recommendations of experts in the area. The ADA has developed a position statement about vitamin and mineral supplementation that provides a solid foundation for assisting patients with their nutrient supplementation decisions. The ADA supports obtaining nutrients through a wide variety of foods as the best way to promote health and reduce risk of disease (ADA, 2009).

However, the ADA also defines clearly in their position statement the circumstances in which supplementation is indicated. The following are populations that may warrant supplementation (ADA, 2009):

- Infants and children, including adolescents, need supplementation with 400 IU of **vitamin D** daily.
- Women of childbearing age who may become pregnant need 400 mcg/day of **folic acid.**
- Pregnant women need **folic acid** 600 mcg/day, a **multivitamin/mineral** supplement, 27 mg/day of **iron** (60 mg/d if patient is anemic), and **vitamin B_{12}** if the patient is vegan or lacto-ovo-vegetarian.
- Older adults over age 50 need **vitamin B_{12}** 2.4 mcg/day, and need to ensure adequate intake of **vitamin D** and **calcium.**
- Patients at risk for suboptimal **vitamin D** levels (older patients, patients with dark skin, patients who are not exposed to sufficient sunlight) should consume **vitamin D**-fortified foods and/or supplements.

The need to utilize nutritional supplementation is individualized and the nurse practitioner must guide patients to understand their need. Most important in this interaction between patient and practitioner is an open, honest discussion of the nutritional supplementation decision. Although **vitamin** supplementation is often inexpensive and unlikely to cause harm, the same cannot be said for many other nutrients for which there is no recommended daily allowance (RDA) and no established standard for supplementation. If you do recommend or prescribe a multiple vitamin and mineral supplement for an at-risk individual, it is important to frame the dosage needed around the RDA and recommended vitamin and mineral intake ranges.

NUTRACEUTICALS

As noted previously, nutraceuticals are foods that claim to have a medicinal effect on health. There are five major categories of nutraceuticals used routinely in primary care: dietary fiber; vitamins and minerals; bioactive substances; fatty acids; and pre-, pro-, and symbiotics. Some nutraceuticals may also be called functional foods or dietary supplements.

The nutraceuticals reviewed here are not an exhaustive list and are limited to those for which there are adequate safety and efficacy data to recommend their use. For a more expansive list of nutraceuticals with the current evidence, the reader is referred to the National Institutes of Health Office of Dietary Supplements (ODS) (http://ods.od.nih.gov/). The ODS Web site contains extensive information for both providers and patients regarding nutraceuticals, including nutrient recommendations, a clinical trials database, and consumer safety information.

Fiber

Fiber is the term used to describe the substances in plants that the body cannot digest. According to the Institute of Medicine (2002), there are two types of fiber: dietary fiber and functional fiber. Dietary fiber is the nondigestible carbohydrates and lignin parts of the plant that are intrinsic and intact, whereas functional fiber is the nondigestible carbohydrates that have beneficial effects in human beings. Total fiber is the sum of the two types of fiber.

There are over 2.5 million visits per year to providers for constipation. Adequate fiber intake is necessary to prevent constipation. There have been controlled trials in chronically ill children (Daly, Johnson, & MacDonald, 2004), pregnant women (Jewell & Young, 2001), and women in the Nurses' Health Study (Dukas, Willett, & Giovanucci, 2003) that demonstrate a decrease in constipation with an increase in fiber in the diet. The American College of Gastroenterology recommends increased fiber intake to prevent constipation (Ward, 2010).

Dietary fiber intake may also lower cholesterol, improve cardiovascular health, and provide a feeling of fullness that may aid in weight loss. The National Health and Nutrition Examination Survey (NHANES) demonstrated a reduced risk of coronary heart disease with increased fiber intake (ADA, 2008). The American Heart Association (AHA) and the ADA both recommend increased fiber intake (at least 25 g/d) for cardiovascular health (ADA, 2008; AHA, 2010c).

Increased soluble fiber intake has been associated with a number of additional benefits, including better glucose control in diabetics and improved blood lipid levels (Aleixandre & Miguel, 2008; Vuksan, Rogovik, Jovanovski, & Jenkins, 2009). Evidence that dietary fiber decreases cancer risk is inconsistent. Recommended fiber intake is found in Table 9–2.

Vitamins and Minerals

Vitamins and minerals are the most widely used supplements. When ingested as part of food sources, vitamins may be considered nutraceuticals. Evidence regarding recommended dosages and the preventive health properties of vitamins and minerals is constantly evolving. The most commonly recommended vitamins are discussed here and are found in Table 9–3. Iron is discussed in Chapters 18 and 27. More extensive information of vitamins and minerals may be found at the ODS Web site (http://ods .od.nih.gov).

Vitamin A

Vitamin A plays a critical role in vision, bone growth, reproduction, immune function, cell division and differentiation (ODS, 2010b). There are two types of **vitamin A**: preformed vitamin A, which is derived from animal sources, and provitamin A carotenoid, which is derived from plant sources. A healthy diet should contain a variety of carotenoid-rich fruits and vegetables.

Vitamin A deficiency is rare in the United States, but deficiencies may be found in developing countries. **Vitamin A** deficiency can lead to night blindness and decreased immune function. **Vitamin A** may reduce the severity and duration of diarrheal episodes in malnourished children but not in well-nourished children (ODS, 2010b). **Vitamin A** supplementation has also been found to decrease bronchopulmonary dysplasia in extremely low-birth-weight infants with no increase in mortality or neurodevelopmental disorder (Ambalavanan et al, 2005). Chronic alcoholism may lower **vitamin A** levels, and patients with chronic alcoholism may require supplementation. Caution should be used with excessive **vitamin A** supplementation as toxicity may occur. Levels above recommended amounts may be teratogenic in pregnant women; **vitamin A** is labeled Pregnancy Category X if intake is greater than recommended amounts.

Table 9–2 **Recommended Fiber Intake**

Gender/Age	Fiber (g/d)
1–3 yr	19
4–8 yr	25
Female 9–13 yr	26
Male 9–13 yr	31
Female 14–18 yr	29
Male 14–18 yr	38
Female 19–50 yr	25
Male 19–50 yr	38
Female 51 yr or older	21
Male 51 yr or older	30

Vitamin B_1

Vitamin B_1 (thiamine) is a water-soluble vitamin critical for many body functions and is widely available in fortified breads and cereals. Deficiency of **thiamine** can lead to beriberi or Wernicke's encephalopathy. Alcoholic patients develop **thiamine** deficiency at 8 to 10 times the rate of the nonalcoholic population (Agabio, 2005). Wernicke's encephalopathy is a serious neurological illness in alcoholic patients and requires immediate high-dose levels of **thiamine** (100 mg IV, then 50 to 100 mg/d). Treatment for beriberi in children is IV **thiamine** 10 to 25 mg daily or 10 to 50 mg daily for 2 weeks and in adults 5 to 30 mg IM/IV or 5 to 30 mg/day for a month.

Vitamin B_2

Vitamin B_2, also known as **riboflavin**, is a water-soluble vitamin. **Riboflavin** deficiency is rare, but may be seen in alcoholics, anorexic patients, and those with lactose intolerance who cannot drink milk or consume other dairy products. **Riboflavin** has been found to decrease headaches and migraines in some patients (Taylor, 2009). **MigreLief**, an over-the-counter product that contains **feverfew, riboflavin, magnesium**, and other vitamins, is a commonly used preventive headache medication. Doses of 25 to 400 mg of **riboflavin** daily are used for migraine prevention.

Vitamin B_3

Vitamin B_3, or **niacin**, is a water-soluble vitamin and antilipidemic. Niacin deficiency or pellagra results from inadequate intake. Pellagra is treated with 50 to 100 mg **niacin** three times daily. Use of **niacin** in the treatment of hyperlipidemia is discussed in Chapter 39.

Vitamin B_6

Vitamin B_6, also known as **pyridoxine**, is a water-soluble vitamin needed for protein and red blood cell metabolism, as well as glucose regulation. Vitamin B_6 deficiency may be drug induced by use of **isoniazid (INH)**, **cycloserine**, or **hydrazine**, or caused by a diet that is deficit in vitamin B_6–containing foods (fortified cereals,

Table 9–3 Recommended Reference Intakes of Vitamins and Minerals

Nutrient	Age	RDA	Food Sources
Folate	Children:		Enriched cereal grains, dark leafy vegetables, enriched and whole-grain breads and bread products, fortified ready-to-eat cereals
	1–3 yr	150 mcg/d	
	4–8 yr	200 mcg/d	
	Adolescents aged 9-13 yr	300 mcg/d	
	Adults	400 mcg/d	
	Pregnancy	600 mcg/d	
Riboflavin (Vitamin B_{12})	Children:		Organ meats, milk, bread products and fortified cereals
	1–3 yr	0.5 mg/d	
	4–8 yr	0.6 mg/d	
	Adolescents aged 9–13 yr	0.9 mg/d	
	Adults	1.3 mg/d	
	Pregnancy	1.4 mg/d	
Thiamin (Vitamin B_1)	Children:		Enriched, fortified, or whole-grain products; bread and bread products, mixed foods whose main ingredient is grain, and ready-to-eat cereals
	1–3 yr	0.5 mg/d	
	4–8 yr	0.6 mg/d	
	Adolescents aged 9–13 yr	0.9 mg/d	
	Adults males	1.2 mg/d	
	Adult females	1.1 mg/d	
	Pregnancy	1.4 mg/d	
Vitamin A	Children:		Liver, dairy products, fish, darkly colored fruits and leafy vegetables
	1–3 yr	300 mcg/d	
	4–8 yr	400 mcg/d	
	Adolescents aged 9–13 yr	600 mcg/d	
	Adults males	900 mcg/d	
	Adult females	700 mcg/d	
	Pregnancy	770 mg/d	
Vitamin B_6	Children:		Fortified cereals, beans, meat, poultry, fish, and some fruits and vegetables (bananas, spinach, avocados)
	1–3 yr	0.5 mg/d	
	4–8 yr	0.6 mg/d	
	Adolescents aged 9–13 yr	1.0 mg/d	
	14–18 yr male	1.3 mg/d	
	14–18 yr female	1.2 mg/d	
	Adults males 19–50 yr	1.3 mg/d	
	Adult males >50 yr	1.7 mg/d	
	Adult females 19-50 yr	1.3 mg/d	
	Adult females >50 yr	1.5 mg/d	
	Pregnancy	1.9 mg/d	
Vitamin C	Children:		Citrus fruits, tomatoes, tomato juice, potatoes, Brussels sprouts, cauliflower, broccoli, strawberries, cabbage, and spinach
	1–3 yr	15 mg/d	
	4–8 yr	25 mg/d	
	Adolescents aged 9–13 yr	45 mg/d	
	14–18 yr male	75 mg/d	
	14–18 yr female	65 mg/d	
	Adults males	90 mg/d	
	Adult females	75 mg/d	
	Pregnancy	85 mg/d	
Vitamin D	Children:		Fish liver oils, flesh of fatty fish, liver and fat from seals and polar bears, eggs from hens that have been fed vitamin D, fortified milk products, and fortified cereals
	1–3 yr	400 IU/d	
	4–8 yr	400 IU/d	
	Adolescents aged 9–18 yr	400 IU/d	
	Adults	400 IU/d	
	Pregnancy	200 IU/d	

Continued

Table 9–3 **Recommended Reference Intakes of Vitamins and Minerals—cont'd**

Nutrient	Age	RDA	Food Sources
Calcium	0–6 mo	210 mg	Milk, yogurt, cheese and other dairy products. Nondairy sources: Chinese cabbage, kale, broccoli, sardines.
	7–12 m	270 mg	
	1–3 yr	500 mg	
	4–8 yr	800 mg	
	9–13 yr	1,300 mg	
	14–18 yr	1,300 mg	
	19–50 yr	1,000 mg	
	50+ yr	1,200 mg	
Iron	0–6 mo	0.27 mg/d	Chicken liver, oysters, beef, clams, turkey dark meat. Legumes, dark green vegetables. Fortified breads and cereals. Iron-fortified infant formula.
	7–12 mo	11 mg/d	
	1–3 yr	7 mg/d	
	4–8 yr	10 mg/d	
	9–13 yr	8 mg/d	
	14–18 yr male	11 mg/d	
	14–18 yr female	15 mg/d	
	19–50 yr male	8 mg/d	
	19–50 yr female	18 mg/d	
	19 to 50 yr pregnant	27 mg/d	
	50+ yr	8 mg/d	

potatoes, bananas, meat). **Pyridoxine (vitamin B_6)** 25 mg/day should be added to the regimen in pregnant patients to decrease the incidence of peripheral neuropathy associated with INH (American Thoracic Society, 2003). **Pyridoxine** (adults 100 to 200 mg/d in divided doses) may also be given prophylactically to patients on **isoniazid**, **cycloserine**, or **hydrazine** to prevent drug-induced neuritis.

Vitamin B_{12}

Vitamin B_{12} is a water-soluble vitamin that is essential for red blood cell formation and neurological function. **Vitamin B_{12}** deficiency will lead to megaloblastic anemia, fatigue, loss of appetite, and neurological changes (numbness and tingling in hands and feet). A complete discussion of **Vitamin B_{12}** replacement is found in Chapter 27 under the discussion of anemia.

Vitamin C

Vitamin C, also known as **ascorbic acid**, is a water-soluble vitamin that humans do not have the ability to synthesize so they must get adequate amounts of it in their diet. Patients with inadequate **vitamin C** intake may develop scurvy, with symptoms of fatigue, malaise, and gum inflammation or bleeding. Scurvy is rare in developed countries, but may occur in cases of limited intake or limited food variety. Smokers and persons who are heavily exposed to secondary smoke have decreased **vitamin C** levels; therefore, it is recommended they take 35 mg more **vitamin C** per day than nonsmokers (ODS, 2010c). Other groups at risk of **vitamin C** deficiency are infants fed evaporated milk or boiled milk without additional supplementation of **vitamin C**, patients with malabsorption disorders, and patients with end-stage renal disease who are on hemodialysis (ODS, 2010c).

Vitamin C therapy has been studied for its effects on health because of its antioxidant and immune function action. **Vitamin C** has been touted as prevention or treatment of the common cold since the 1970s, when Linus Pauling published his landmark study. A *Cochrane Review* in 2007 of 30 trials did not find that **vitamin C** decreases the incidence of colds in the general population (Douglas, Hemiliä, Chalker, & Treacy, 2007).

The role of **antioxidants** in reducing the risk of cardiovascular disease has been studied extensively with mixed results. The Nurses' Health Study found an inverse relationship of coronary heart disease with **vitamin C** intake (Osganian et al, 2003). In the Physicians' Health Study, **vitamin C** supplementation for a 5.5-year period did not decrease risk for cardiovascular disease mortality (Muntwyler, Heenekens, Manson, Buring, & Gaziano, 2002). However, a large (N = 20,649 men and women) study in Great Britain found those who had the highest **vitamin C** concentrations at baseline had a 42 percent lower risk of stroke, when controlling for age, sex, lifestyle, and other risk factors (Myint et al, 2008).

Vitamin C has been studied as an antioxidant to prevent cancers with mixed results. In a long-term (10-year), large (N = 77,721) study of the effect of **vitamin C** supplementation on the development of lung cancer, there was no decreased risk of cancer in the group taking **vitamin C** (Slatore, Littman, Au, Satia, & White, 2007). A large, multiethnic study of Hispanic and non-Hispanic white women did not find any protective effects against breast cancer in women who took dietary antioxidants including **vitamin C** (Wang et al, 2009). Decreased cervical cancer was found in a smaller study (*N* = 144) of women who had higher intakes of the antioxidant **vitamins** A, C, and E; the isolated effects of **vitamin** C are not known (Kim et al, 2010). The Nurses' Health Study and examined breast cancer risk in relation to **vitamin** C intake found a 63 percent reduced risk of breast cancer in premenopausal women with a positive family history if they consumed an average of 205 mg per day of **vitamin** C (Zhang et al, 1999). Because of the mixed results, there is no strong recommendation for **vitamin** C supplementation, beyond the recommended daily amounts, as prevention for cancer.

Table 9–3 lists the recommended **vitamin** C intake levels for all ages.

Vitamin D

Vitamin D is a fat-soluble vitamin that is available in some foods such as egg yolks and fatty fish (salmon and mackerel). The body synthesizes **vitamin** D when sunlight strikes the skin and triggers **vitamin** D synthesis. **Vitamin** D supplements, food sources, and the **vitamin** D synthesized from sunlight must be converted to an active form of drug in the liver and kidneys. The liver converts **vitamin** D into 25-hydroxyvitamin D, or calcidiol. The kidneys convert **vitamin** D into 1,25-dihydroxyvitamin D, or calcitriol. **Vitamin** D is critical to bone health as it is required for absorption of **calcium** from the intestinal tract and, when converted to calcitriol, regulates serum calcium and phosphate levels. It is a critical component in bone growth and remodeling. **Vitamin** D deficiency will lead to brittle bones that may become misshapen, a condition known as rickets in children and as osteomalacia in adults (ODS, 2010d). Serum levels of 25(OH)D can be drawn to determine whether the patient is **vitamin** D deficient. Table 9–4 lists ranges of 25(OH)D associated with deficiency and toxicity. **Vitamin** D is added to milk, most milk substitutes, infant formula, and dry cereal, and is available in supplements as either **vitamin** D_2 or D_3. The use of **vitamin** D in the prevention and treatment of rickets, osteomalacia, and osteoporosis is discussed in depth in Chapter 38.

Vitamin K

Vitamin K, a critical component of blood clotting, is found in many foods and is synthesized by intestinal bacteria. **Vitamin** K deficiency is rare beyond the newborn period. Newborns are at risk for early **vitamin** K deficiency bleeding of the newborn and the American Academy of Pediatrics recommends that all newborns receive **vitamin** K within the first two weeks of life (American Academy of Pediatrics [AAP] Committee on Fetus and Newborn, 2003). The AAP reaffirmed the 2003 statement in 2009. The dose of **vitamin** K (**phytonadione**) recommended by the AAP is 0.5 mg to 1.0 mg IM, ideally given within the first hour of life (AAP Committee on Fetus and Newborn, 2003). Oral **vitamin** K is used by some countries and by some providers in the United States. The AAP notes that several countries have reported an increase in late-onset, vitamin K–deficiency bleeding in newborns who received oral **vitamin** K. The AAP recommends IM administration until further study of oral administration is conducted.

Warfarin interferes with the **vitamin** K–dependent clotting factors (II, VII, IX, and X), leading to decreased formation of clots. **Vitamin** K (**phytonadione**) is prescribed for patients who develop critically high INRs while on **warfarin**.

Folate

Folate is a water-soluble vitamin that is critical to the production and maintenance of new cells. **Folate** is found in foods such as green leafy vegetables, citrus fruits, and dried legumes. **Folic acid**, the synthetic form of **folate**, is added to breads, flours, pastas, rice, and other grain products (ODS, 2010a). **Folate** deficiency occurs in time of increased demand such as occurs in pregnancy and lactation, or when loss increases (malabsorption, alcohol abuse, dialysis, liver disease). Medications may interfere with **folate** utilization, leading to deficit (Box 9–1). **Folic acid** supplementation is recommended for all women of childbearing age (400 mcg/d), with extra given when a woman is pregnant (600 mcg/d) to prevent neural tube

Table 9–4 Serum 25-Hydroxyvitamin D [25(OH)D] Concentrations and Health*

ng/mL**	nmol/L**	Health Status
<10–11	<25–37.5	Associated with vitamin D deficiency, leading to rickets in infants and children and osteomalacia in adults
<10–15	<25–37.5	Generally considered inadequate for bone and overall health in healthy individuals
≥15	≥37.5	Generally considered adequate for bone and overall health in healthy individuals
Consistently >200	Consistently >500	Considered potentially toxic, leading to hypercalcemia and hyperphosphatemia, although human data are limited. In an animal model, concentrations ≤400 ng/mL (≤1,000 nmol/L) demonstrated no toxicity

* Serum concentrations of 25(OH)D are reported in both nanograms per milliliter (ng/mL) and nanomoles per liter (nmol/L).
** 1 ng/mL = 2.5 nmol/L
Source: Office of Dietary Supplements, 2010

defects in the fetus (ODS, 2010a). Lactating women should take 500 mcg/day.

Folate is necessary for the normal maturation and functioning of red blood cells. **Folate** deficiency produces a macrocytic-normochromic anemia. Patients with folic acid–deficiency anemia commonly complain of glossitis, stomatitis, nausea and anorexia, and diarrhea, and a systolic ejection murmur may be heard. Oral **folic acid** is well absorbed, and doses of 1 to 2 mg/day result in correction of the deficiency in 4 to 5 weeks. Hemoglobin (Hgb) levels begin to rise within the first week, and anemia is completely corrected in 1 to 2 months.

Calcium

Calcium is a critical mineral in the function of the body, required for muscle contraction, blood vessel health, bone health, and normal nerve conduction. Maintaining calcium balance is a complex relationship between adequate intake of **calcium** and **vitamin D**, and endocrine system function. Populations at risk for **calcium** deficiency include postmenopausal women, amenorrheic women, women with female athlete triad, patients with lactose intolerance who cannot tolerate dairy products, and vegans. In the 2003–2006 NHANES study, the population groups with inadequate dietary calcium intake were females aged 9 to 13 years, 14 to 18 years, 51 to 70 years, and those over age 70 (Bailey et al, 2010). **Calcium supplements** were used by 43 percent of the NHANES 2003–2006 study population, leading to an adequate total **calcium** intake for all groups except for females in the 9- to 13-year-old and 14- to 18-year-old groups (Bailey et al, 2010). Recommended daily amounts of **calcium** are found in Table 9–3. The use of **calcium** for osteoporosis prevention is discussed in Chapter 38.

Iron

Iron is an essential mineral required for the regulation of cell growth and differentiation, as well as a component of oxygen transport. Patients with **iron** deficiency will develop microcytic-hypochromic anemia and have red blood cells that are small in size, pale, and low in hemoglobin. Iron-deficiency anemia (IDA) reduces the oxygen-carrying capacity of the blood, leading to fatigue and decreased immunity. Too much **iron** can lead to **iron** toxicity; therefore, patients should be advised to take only the recommended amount for their age and condition (Table 9–3). The use of **iron** for the treatment of IDA is discussed in depth in Chapter 27.

BOX 9–1 MEDICATIONS INTERFERING WITH FOLATE UTILIZATION

- Antiepileptic drugs (phenytoin, primidone)
- Metformin
- Sulfasalazine
- Triamterene
- Methotrexate
- Barbiturates
- Trimethoprim
- Pyrimethamine
- Isoniazid
- Oral contraceptives

Fatty Acids

The **fatty acids** are also called essential fatty acids. **Fatty acids** need to be consumed in food or via supplements, as the body cannot make them. The polyunsaturated fatty acid alpha-linolenic acid (ALA) is ingested in the diet and is an **omega-3 fatty acid** and linoleic acid (LA) also from the diet is an **omega-6 fatty acid. Omega-3** is converted to the fatty acids eicosapentaenoic acid (EPA) and docosahexaenoic acid (DHA) in the body. Most Americans consume more **omega-6** than **omega-3 fatty acids**, although it is recommended that more **omega-3** than **omega-6** should be consumed (ODS, 2010e). Dietary sources of ALA are nuts, vegetable oils, and leafy green vegetables, whereas LA is found in vegetable oils and meat. Dietary sources of EPA and DHA are fish and organ meats.

The ODS conducted extensive evidence-based reviews to determine the best science regarding **fatty acid** supplementation. There is extensive evidence for the use of **omega-3 fatty acids**, either via the diet or supplementation, for its cardiovascular effects (ODS, 2010e). **Omega-3 fatty acid** and its derivatives DHA and EPA have well-documented vascular protective effects, as well as anti-inflammatory effects.

Fish oil might have antiarrhythmic effects (ODS, 2004a) and consumption of **omega-3 fatty acids**, whether from fish or from supplements, reduces mortality and improves outcomes in patients with cardiovascular disease (Lee, O'Keefe, Lavie, Marchioli, & Harris, 2008; ODS, 2004b). In patients with diabetes **omega-3 fatty acids** reduced triglyceride levels, but have no significant effect on total cholesterol, high-density lipoprotein (HDL) cholesterol, low-density lipoprotein (LDL) cholesterol, fasting blood sugar, or glycosylated hemoglobin (ODS, 2004d).

Omega-3 fatty acids have received attention as a possible treatment for autism and attention deficit-hyperactivity disorder (ADHD). The theory is that either deficiency in **omega-3** or an imbalance in the **omega-3** to **omega-6** fatty acid ratio is affecting neurocognitive development in children. It is clear that sufficient amounts of the **essential fatty acids** are crucial in central nervous development, with deficiency or imbalance found in multiple observational studies of children with neurocognitive issues (Schuchardt, Huss, Stauss-Grabo, & Hahn, 2009). This has led to commercial infant formulas adding **DHA** and **ARA** (Enfamil LIPIL) to meet the need in the key developmental period of infancy. In an extensive review of new and novel treatments for autism spectrum disorder, Rossingnol (2009) rates **omega-3 fatty acids** with a C for supportive evidence (A to D scale; C indicates either one low-quality, randomized controlled trial or two case series reports). In another study by Meiri, Buchovsky, and Belmaker (2009) autistic children administered 1 gram of **omega-3 fatty acids** daily demonstrated a 33 percent improvement on the Autism Treatment Evaluation Checklist. Numerous studies of the use of **omega-3 fatty acids** in children with ADHD demonstrate improvement in ADHD scores (Schuchardt et al, 2009). With these findings and the understanding of the need for **essential fatty acids** in neurological development, ensuring a diet that is rich in essential fatty acids throughout infancy and childhood is critical, with trial of supplemental **omega-3 fatty acids** in children with autism or ADHD warranted.

Not all health claims for **essential fatty acids** have evidence to support their use. The evidence does not support the use of **omega-3 fatty acids** in the care of asthma (ODS, 2004b), prevention of cancer or treatment after tumor removal (ODS, 2005a), or mental health disorders (including schizophrenia) (ODS, 2005b). Inconsistent findings in organ transplant patients warrant that **omega-3 fatty acids** be studied further in this population (ODS, 2005c). The effects of **omega-3 fatty acids** were studied in patients with rheumatoid arthritis, with no reported improvement in patient report of pain, swollen joint count, erythrocyte sedimentation rate (ESR), and patient global assessment (ODS, 2004d). Research regarding the use of **omega-3s** in adult patients with cognitive decline was inconclusive (ODS, 2010e).

Recommended amounts of **omega-3 fatty acids** can be ingested in the diet by eating fatty fish or by taking fish oil capsules. The American Heart Association recommends two servings a week of fatty fish such as salmon, mackerel, herring, lake trout, sardines, and albacore tuna for heart health (2010a). The recommended amount of **omega-3 fatty acid** from fish per day is 500 mg/day if there is no history of coronary heart disease (CHD), 1 g per day if there is a documented history of CHD, and 2 to 4 g/day to lower triglycerides (American Heart Association, 2010a; Covington, 2004; Lee et al, 2008). It may take 2 to 3 weeks for the effects of **omega-3** to be seen. There are no recommendations for **omega-3** intake in children (Brulotte, Bukutu, & Vohra, 2009). The studies of **omega-3** for the treatment of ADHD and autism used 500 mg to 1 g/day.

Plant Sterols

Plant sterols are found in all plant-based foods, as part of the structural components of the cell membrane (Ellegard, Andersson, Normen, & Andersson, 2007). **Plant sterols** are similar in structure to cholesterol, but contain an extra methyl or ethyl group. When consumed in the diet, **plant sterols** compete with cholesterol in the intestine, reducing the amount of cholesterol that is absorbed (Devaraj & Jialal, 2006). Intake of 2 g/day of **plant sterols** has an associated 6 to 10 percent reduction in LDL cholesterol (Devaraj & Jialal; Ellegard et al, 2007). Combining **plant sterols** with cholesterol-lowering medications results in an additional 16 to 20 percent reduction in LDL (Berger, Jones, & Abumweis, 2004; Katan et al, 2003). The only adverse effect of **plant sterols** is reduced beta-carotene levels, which can be treated with an increased intake of carotene-containing fruits and vegetables (Berger et al, 2004; Devaraj & Jialal, 2006).

Plant sterols are present in edible oils (corn oil and canola oil have the highest amount), seeds and nuts (Ellegard et al, 2007). There are many commercial food products available with added **plant sterols**, including margarine (Promise active 1 g/serving, Benecol spread 0.85 g/serving, Smart Balance HeartRight 1.7 g/serving), orange juice (Minute Maid Heart Wise 1 g/serving), and milk (Smart Balance HeartRight 400 mg/serving). The recommended amount of **plant sterols** for LDL reduction is up to 2 g/day (Devaraj & Jialal, 2006). **Plant sterols** may be combined with a low saturated fat and cholesterol diet, dietary fiber, and/or lipid-lowering drugs for an additive effect on reducing LDL cholesterol (Devaraj & Jialal, 2006). Children older than age 5 years may use **plant sterol** products, but should have increased intake of foods containing beta-carotene (Berger et al, 2004).

Pre-, Pro, and Symbiotics

Probiotics are nonpathogenic bacteria normally found in the intestinal microflora, the most common of which are *Lactobacillus acidophilus* and the *Bifidobacterium* species. **Prebiotics** are nondigestible food ingredients that stimulate growth of probiotic organisms, and symbiotics are a mixture of probiotics and prebiotics. **Probiotics** are used to restore the normal balance of gut flora that is disturbed with antibiotics, immunosuppressive medications, and other conditions (Williams, 2010).

Probiotics have been used for many years and have been studied extensively for their health benefits and their effects on diarrhea. A *Cochrane Review* of the use of **probiotics** in rotavirus-associated acute diarrhea in children found **probiotics** reduced diarrhea severity and duration by 1 to 3 days (Allen, Okoko, Martinez, Gregorio, & Dans, 2004). **Probiotics** also reduce antibiotic-associated diarrhea in adults (D'Souza, Rajkumar, Cooke, & Bulpitt, 2002; Safdar, Barigala, Said, & McKinley, 2008; Tong, Ran, Shen, Zhang, & Xiao, 2006) and in children (Johnston, Supina, Ospina, & Vohra, 2007). It is reasonable to prescribe **probiotics** for patients with infectious or antibiotic-associated diarrhea.

Probiotics may also improve inflammatory bowel disorders and necrotizing enterocolitis (NEC). Premature infants have sterile guts when they are born and are at risk for bowel problems, including NEC. Multiple studies and reviews have found **probiotics** beneficial in preventing

BOX 9–2 RESOURCES

American Dietetic Association
http://www.eatright.org

Drugs.com Drug Interaction Checker
http://www.drugs.com/drug_interactions.php

Food and Medication Interactions
http://www.foodmedinteractions.com

Medscape Drug Interaction Checker
www.medscape.com

National Institutes of Health Office of Dietary Supplements
http://ods.od.nih.gov/Health_Information/Health_Information.aspx

NEC and death in preterm infants (AlFaleh & Bassler, 2008; Deshpande, Rao, Patole, & Bulsara, 2010; Lin et al, 2008). Use of **probiotics** improved Symptom Severity Scores in patients with irritable bowel syndrome (Williams et al, 2008). **Probiotics** have also been found to improve eradication rates in patients being treated for ***Helicobacter pylori*** (Tong et al, 2006).

REFERENCES

Agabio, R. (2005). Thiamine administration in alcohol-dependent patients. *Alcohol and Alcoholism, 40*(2), 155–156.

Aleixandre, A., & Miguel, M. (2008). Dietary fiber in prevention and treatment of metabolic syndrome: A review. *Critical Reviews in Food Science and Nutrition, 48,* 905–912.

AlFaleh, K. M., & Bassler, D. (2008). Probiotics for prevention of necrotizing enterocolitis in preterm infants. *Cochrane Database of Systematic Reviews, 1,* CD005496.

Allen, S. J., Okoko, B., Martinez, E. G., Gregorio, G.V., & Dans, L. F. (2004). Probiotics for treating infectious diarrhea. *Cochrane Database of Systematic Reviews, 2,* CD003048.

Ambalavanan, N., Tyson, J. E., Kennedy, K. A., Hansen, N. I., Vohr, B. R., Wright, L. L., et al. (2005). Vitamin A supplementation for extremely low birth weight infants: Outcome at 18 to 22 months. *Pediatrics, 115*(3), e249–e254.

American Academy of Pediatrics Committee on Fetus and Newborn. (2003). Controversies concerning vitamin K and the newborn. Committee on Fetus and Newborn. *Pediatrics, 112*(1), 191–192.

American Dietetic Association. (2008). Position of the American Dietetic Association: Health implications of dietary fiber. *Journal of the American Dietetic Association, 108*(10), 1716–1731.

American Dietetic Association. (2009). Position of the American Dietetic Association: Nutrient supplementation. *Journal of the American Dietetic Association, 109,* 2073–2085.

American Heart Association. (2010a). Fish and omega-3 fatty acids. Retrieved from http://www.americanheart.org/presenter.jhtml?identifier=4632

America Heart Association. (2010b). Frequently asked questions about "better" fats. Retrieved from http://www.heart.org/HEARTORG/GettingHealthy/NutritionCenter/Frequently-Asked-Questions-About-Better-Fats_UCM_305985_Article.jsp

American Heart Association. (2010c). Whole grains and fiber. *American Heart Association.* Retrieved from http://www.americanheart.org/presenter.jhtml?identifier=4574

American Thoracic Society. (2003). American Thoracic Society/Centers for Disease Control and Prevention/Infectious Diseases Society of America: Treatment of tuberculosis. *American Journal of Respiratory and Critical Care Medicine, 167,* 603–662.

Bailey, R. L., Dodd, K. W., Goldman, J. A., Gahche, J. J., Dwyer, J. T., Moshfegh, A. J., et al. (2010). Estimation of total calcium and vitamin D intakes in the United States. *Journal of Nutrition, 140*(4), 817–822.

Berger, A., Jones, P. J. H., & Abumweis, S. S. (2004). Plant sterols: Factors affecting their efficacy and safety as functional food ingredients. *Lipids in Health and Disease, 3*(5). Retrieved from http://www.lipidworld.com/content/3/1/5

Brulotte, J., Bukutu, C., & Vohra, S. (2009). Complementary, holistic, and integrative medicine: Fish oils and neurodevelopmental disorders. *Pediatrics in Review, 30*(4), e29–e33.

Covington, M. B. (2004). Omega-3 fatty acids. *American Family Physician, 70*(1), 133–140.

Daly, A., Johnson, T., & MacDonald, A. (2004). Is fibre supplementation in paediatric sip feeds beneficial? *Journal of Human Nutrition and Dietetics, 17*(4), 365–370.

Deshpande, G., Rao, S., Patole, S., & Bulsara, M. (2010). Updated meta-analysis of probiotics for preventing necrotizing enterocolitis in preterm neonates. *Pediatrics, 125,* 921–930.

Devaraj, S., & Jialal, I. (2006). The role of dietary supplementation with plant sterols and stanols in the prevention of cardiovascular disease. *Nutrition Reviews, 64*(7), 348–354.

Douglas, R. M., Hemilä, H., Chalker, E., & Treacy, B. (2007). Vitamin C for preventing and treating the common cold. *Cochrane Database of Systematic Reviews, 3,* CD000980.

D'Souza, A. L., Rajkumar, C., Cooke, J., & Bulpitt, C. J. (2002). Probiotics in prevention of antibiotics associated diarrhea: Meta-analysis. *BMJ: British Medical Association, 324,* 1361–1364.

Dukas, L., Willett, W. C., & Giovannucci, E. L. (2003). Association between physical activity, fiber intake, and other lifestyle variables and constipation in a study of women. *American Journal of Gastroenterology, 98*(8), 1790–1796.

Ellegard, L. H., Andersson, S. W., Normen, A. L., & Andersson, H. A. (2007). Dietary plant sterols and cholesterol metabolism. *Nutrition Reviews, 65*(1), 39–45.

Gertz, M., Davis, J. D., Harrison, A., Houston, J. B., & Galetin, A. (2008). Grapefruit juice-drug interaction studies as a method to assess the extent of intestinal availability: Utility and limitations. *Current Drug Metabolism, 9,* 785–795.

Institute of Medicine, Food and Nutrition Board. (2002). *Dietary reference intakes: Energy, carbohydrates, fiber, fat, fatty acids, cholesterol, protein and amino acids.* Washington, DC: National Academies Press.

Ishmail, M. Y. M. (2009). Drug-food interactions and role of pharmacist. *Asian Journal of Pharmaceutical and Clinical Research, 2*(4), 1–10. Retrieved from http://ajpcr.com/Vol2Issue4/226.pdf.

Jefferson, J. (1999). Drug and diet interactions: Avoiding therapeutic paralysis. *Journal of Clinical Psychiatry, 59*(Suppl. 16), 31–39.

Jewell, D., & Young, G. (2001). Interventions for treating constipation in pregnancy. *Cochrane Database of Systematic Reviews, 2.* Edited Issue 1, 2009.

Johnston, B. C., Supina, A. L., Ospina, M., & Vohra, S. (2007). Probiotics for the prevention of pediatric antibiotic-associated diarrhea. *Cochrane Database of Systematic Reviews, 2,* CD004827.

Katan, M. B., Grundy, S. M., Jones, P., Law, M., Miettinen, T., & Paoletti, R. (2003). Efficacy and safety of plant sterols and sterols in the management of blood cholesterol levels. *Mayo Clinic Proceedings, 78*(8), 965–978.

Kim, J., Kim, M. K., Lee, J. K., Kim, J. H., Son, S. K., Song, E. S., et al. (2010). Intakes of vitamin A, C and E and beta-carotene are associated with risk of cervical cancer: A case-control study in Korea. *Nutrition and Cancer, 62*(2), 181–189.

Kuypers, D. R. J. (2009). Immunotherapy in elderly transplant recipients: A guide to clinical significant drug interactions. *Drugs and Aging, 26*(9), 715–737.

Larson, J.T., & Brosen, K. (2005). Consumption of charcoal-broiled meat as an experimental tool for discerning CYP1A2-mediated drug metabolism in vivo. *Basic & Clinical Pharmacology & Toxicology, 97*(3), 141–148.

Lee, J. H., O'Keefe, J. H., Lavie, C. J., Marchioli, R., & Harris, W. S. (2008). Omega-3 fatty acids for cardioprotection. *Mayo Clinic Proceedings, 83*(3), 324–332.

Lin, H. C., Hsu, H. C., Chen, H. L., Chung, M., Hsu, J. F., Lien, R., et al. (2008). Oral probiotics prevent necrotizing enterocolitis in very low birth weight preterm infants: A multicenter, randomized, controlled trial. *Pediatrics, 122,* 693–700.

Meiri, G., Bichovsky, Y., & Belmaker, R. H. (2009). Omega 3 fatty acid treatment in autism. *Journal of Child and Adolescent Psychopharmacology, 19*(4), 449–451.

Mertens-Talcott, S. U., Zadezensky, I., DeCastro, W. V., Derendorf, H., & Butterweck, V. (2006). Grapefruit-Drug Interactions: Can Interactions With Drugs Be Avoided? *Journal of Clinical Pharmacology, 46,* 1390–1416.

Muntwyler, J., Hennekens, C. H., Buring, J. E., & Gaziano, J. M. (2002). Vitamin supplement use in a low-risk population of U.S. male physicians and subsequent cardiovascular mortality. *Archives of Internal Medicine, 162,* 1472–1476.

Myint, P.K., Luben, R. N., Welch, A. A., Bingham, S. A., Wareham, N. J., & Khaw, K.T. (2008). Plasma vitamin C concentrations predict risk of incident stroke over 10 y in 20,649 participants of the European Prospective Investigation into Cancer Norfolk prospective population study. *American Journal of Clinical Nutrition, 8,* 64–69.

Office of Dietary Supplements. (2004a). Health effects of omega-3 fatty acids on arrhythmogenic mechanisms in animal and isolated organ/cell culture studies. Retrieved from http://www.ahrq.gov/clinic/tp/o3arrtp.htm#Report

Office of Dietary Supplements. (2004b). Health effects of omega-3 fatty acids on asthma. Retrieved from http://www.ahrq.gov/clinic/tp/o3asthmtp.htm#Report

Office of Dietary Supplements. (2004c). Health effects of omega-3 fatty acids on cardiovascular disease. Retrieved from http://www.ahrq.gov/clinic/tp/o3cardtp.htm#Report

Office of Dietary Supplements. (2004d). Health effects of omega-3 fatty acids on lipids and glycemic control in type II diabetes and the metabolic syndrome and on inflammatory bowel disease, rheumatoid arthritis, renal disease, systemic lupus erythematosus and osteoporosis. Retrieved from http://www.ahrq.gov/clinic/tp/o3lipidtp.htm

Office of Dietary Supplements. (2005a). Effects of omega-3 fatty acids on cancer. Retrieved from http://www.ahrq.gov/clinic/tp/o3cantp.htm#Report

Office of Dietary Supplements. (2005b). Effects of omega-3 fatty acids on mental health. Retrieved from http://www.ahrq.gov/clinic/tp/o3menttp.htm#Report

Office of Dietary Supplements. (2005c). Effects of omega-3 fatty acids on organ transplantation. Retrieved from http://www.ahrq.gov/clinic/tp/o3organtp.htm#Report

Office of Dietary Supplements. (2010a). Folate: Health professionals fact sheet. Retrieved from http://ods.od.nih.gov/factsheets/folate.asp

Office of Dietary Supplements. (2010b). Vitamin A: Health professional fact sheet. National Institutes of Health. Retrieved from http://ods.od.nih.gov/factsheets/vitamina

Office of Dietary Supplements. (2010c). Vitamin C: Health professional fact sheet. National Institutes of Health. Retrieved from http://ods.od.nih.gov/factsheets/VitaminC.asp#en78

Office of Dietary Supplements. (2010d). Vitamin D: Health professional fact sheet. National Institutes of Health. Retrieved from http://ods.od.nih.gov/factsheets/vitamind.asp

Office of Dietary Supplements (2010e). Omega-3 fatty acids and health. National Institutes of Health. Retrieved from http://ods.od.nih.gov/factsheets/Omega3FattyAcidsandHealth/

Osganian, S. K., Stampfer, M. J., Rimm, E., Spiegelman, D., Hu, F. B., Manson, J. E., et al. (2003). Vitamin C and risk of coronary heart disease in women. *Journal of the American College of Cardiology, 42,* 246–252.

Paine, M. F., Widmer, W.W., Hart, H. L., Pusek, S. N., Beavers, K. L., Criss, A. B., et al. (2006). A furanocoumarin-free grapefruit juice establishes furanocoumarins as the mediators of the grapefruit juice-felodipine interaction. *American Journal of Clinical Nutrition, 83*(5), 1097–1105.

Rossignol, D. A. (2009). Novel and emerging treatments for autism spectrum disorders: A systematic review. *Annals of Clinical Psychiatry, 21*(3), 213–236.

Safdar, N., Barigala, R., Said, A., & McKinley, L (2008). Feasibility and tolerability of probiotics for prevention of antibiotic-associated diarrhea in hospitalized U.S. military veterans. *Journal of Clinical Pharmacy and Therapeutics, 33,* 663–668.

Schein, J. R. (1997). Cruciferous vegetables and drug metabolism. *European Journal of Drug Metabolism and Pharmacokinetics, 22*(1), 85–86.

Schuchardt, J. P., Huss, M., Stauss-Grabo, M., & Hahn, A. (2009). Significance of long-chain polyunsaturated fatty acids (PUFAs) for the development and behavior of children. *European Journal of Pediatrics, 169,* 149–164.

Singh, B. N. (1999). Effects of food on clinical pharmacokinetics. *Clinical Pharmacokinetics, 37*(3), 213–255.

Singh, B. N., & Malhotra, B. K. (2004). Effects of food on the clinical pharmacokinetics of anticancer agents: Underlying mechanisms and implications for oral chemotherapy. *Clinical Pharmacokinetics, 43*(15), 1127–1156.

Slatore, C. G., Littman, A. J., Au, D. H., Satia, J. A., & White, E. (2007). Long-term use of supplemental multivitamins, vitamin C, vitamin E, and folate does not reduce the risk of lung cancer. *American Journal of Respiratory and Critical Care Medicine, 177*(5), 524–530.

Taylor, F.R. (2009). Headache prevention with complementary and alternative medicine. *Headache, 49*(6), 966–968.

Tong, J. L., Ran, Z. H., Shen, J., Zhang, C. X., & Xiao, S. K. (2006). Meta-analysis: The effect of supplementation with probiotics on eradication rates and adverse events during *Helicobacter pylori* eradication therapy. *Alimentary Pharmacology & Therapeutics, 25,* 155–168.

Vaquero, M. P., Sanchez Muniz, F. J., Jimenez Redondo, S., Prats Olivan, P., Higueras, F.J., & Bastida, S. (2010). Major diet-drug interactions affecting the kinetic characteristics and hypolipidaemic properties of statins. *Nutrición Hospitalaria: Organo Oficial de la Sociedad Española de Nutrición Parenteral y Enteral, 25*(2), 193–206.

Vuksan, V., Rogovik, J., Jovanovski, E., & Jenkins, A. L. (2009). Fiber facts: Benefits and recommendations for individuals with type 2 diabetes. *Current Diabetes Reports, 9,* 405–411.

Wang, C., Baumgartner, R. N., Yang, D., Slattery, M. L., Murtaugh, M. A., Byers, T., et al. (2009). No evidence of association between breast cancer risk and dietary carotenoids, retinols, vitamin C and tocopherols in southwestern Hispanic and non-Hispanic white women. *Breast Cancer Research Treatment, 114,* 137–145.

Ward, A. (2010). Constipation and defecation problems. The American College of Gastroenterology, Retrieved from http://www.acg.gi.org/patients/gihealth/constipation.asp

Warren Grant Magnuson Clinical Center, National Institutes of Health Drug-Nutrient Interaction Task Force. (2003). Important information to know when you are taking: Coumadin and vitamin K. Retrieved from http://ods.od.nih.gov/Health_Information/Vitamin_and_Mineral_Supplement_Fact_Sheets.aspx

Williams, et al. (2008). Probiotics have also been found to improve eradication rates in patients being treated for Helicobacter pylori (Tong, et al. (2006)

Williams, N. T. (2010). Probiotics. *American Journal of Health-System Pharmacy, 67,* 449–458.

Yetley, E. A. (2008). Assessing the vitamin D status of the U.S. population. *American Journal of Clinical Nutrition, 88,* 558S–564S.

Zhang, S., Hunter, D. J., Forman, M. R., Rosner, B. A., Speizer, F.E., Colditz, G. A., et al. (1999). Dietary carotenoids and vitamins A, C, and E and risk of breast cancer. *Journal of the National Cancer Institute, 91,* 547–556.

CHAPTER 10

HERBAL AND COMPLEMENTARY THERAPIES

Fujio McPherson

Chapter Outline

Phytomedicine, defined as "the practice of using plants or plant parts to achieve a therapeutic cure" (Fetrow & Avila, 1999), is the oldest form of known medicine. Originally herbs were considered only for their nutritional value, but awareness of their planting cycles, the influence of astrological and environmental changes on planting outcomes, and the effects of specific herbs to create or remove various symptoms in the human body led to the medicinal use of herbs as well as their use in mystical and spiritual ceremony. In many cultures, herbal traditions provide a history that extends well beyond the scientific dissection of their cellular components.

This chapter serves as an introduction to phytomedicine. Because this is a relatively new area of study for western health practitioners, definitions of terms are necessary, as is knowledge of the various principles involved in prescribing and using herbal medicines in North America. The purpose of this chapter is not to train the reader to be an herbalist but rather to introduce the reader to some of the major herbal theories used in the prescription of herbs. The chapter is meant to be used in an informative way rather than as a prescriptive resource.

HISTORY OF HERBAL MEDICINE

Determining precisely when humans first discovered the medicinal use of any given plant is difficult, but through time and observation every culture developed a pharmacopoeia of herbal remedies. The Egyptians were widely respected for their written record and use of herbal remedies, and many remedies—including **opium**, cannabis, myrrh, frankincense, and fennel—are still used today. Greek and Roman use of herbs based on the principles of the four humors was derived from cultures in India and China. The use of herbs such as **opiates** to heighten the healing power of Asclepian healing temples in Greek medicine survived for centuries as myth and ritual. And one of the oldest forms of herbal medicine comes from the shamans who sought the spiritual power of plants to discover their healing properties.

The use of herbal medicine in the United States has grown significantly since the early 1990s, which may be a reflection of the growth in the use of complementary and alternative medicine (CAM) therapies. In a 2005 study that looked at herbal use in the U.S. adult population, 57.3% said that they had used herbs or supplements during the previous 12 months (Kennedy, 2005).

As mainstream medicine has diverged from a predominantly plant-based pharmacopoeia to a synthesized chemically based pharmacopoeia accompanied by a myriad of harmful side effects, a belief that herbal medicines are safer and have less harmful side effects has begun to evolve. With limited regulation by the U.S. Food and Drug Administration (FDA), the availability of herbal formulas and products, classified as food sources, has expanded exponentially, as has their use. In 1997, an estimated 15 million adults (18.4% of all prescription users) took prescription medications concurrently with herbal remedies and/or high-dose vitamins (Eisenberg, Davis, & Ettner, 1998). A 2005 study of herbal and supplemental use in the U.S. adult population showed an estimated 38.2 million adults had used herbs and supplements, and more than half of all users felt the herbs and supplements were important to their health and well-being. However, only 33.4 percent of them told their physician about their use of herbs and supplements (Kennedy, 2005).

Thus, allopathic providers are now faced with the challenge and need to consider herbal use among their patients and to consider the impact those herbs may have on medical and pharmaceutical management of a condition. In many cases, herbal therapy has proved to be very effective at enhancing medical management of a disease, reducing the need for stronger pharmaceutical management and, in some cases, successfully replacing more harmful pharmaceutical drugs while at the same time achieving the same efficacy without the harmful side effects. For example, it has been the practice for many years in Asia to use the root bark of *Hibiscus syriacus* as an antipyretic, antihelminthic, and antifungal agent, and the results of a study in 2008 indicated a significant and dose-dependent antiproliferative effect on lung cancer cells in vitro and in vivo (Cheng, Lee, Harn, Huang, & Chang, 2008).

At the same time, many studies identifying potentially harmful effects of herbal therapy exist. Buettner, Mukamal, Gardiner, and Davis (2009) found lead levels to be 10 percent higher among women who used **St. John's wort**, ayurvedic herbs, and some traditional Chinese herbs. **Coenzyme Q10**, a commonly used supplement to improve memory and cardiovascular function, was found to reduce the effectiveness of **warfarin** and evidence is still inconclusive regarding its effect in reducing cardiovascular conditions such as exercise-induced angina. When taken in doses of more than 3,000 mg a day for a prolonged period of time, **coenzyme Q10** can cause elevated liver enzymes.

However, many of these studies may better support the argument for further research or regulations and testing guidelines instead of being used as a true evaluation of how safe or efficacious the actual herb is in the treatment of a specific disorder. Every pharmaceutical prescription has side effects that range from mild to life threatening, so to use side effects of an herb as the lone criterion for exclusion from use is not only misguided but fails to consider the difference between herbal side effects and pharmaceutical side effects. Using side effects for exclusion also fails to recognize the theories and long traditions used by trained herbalists in diagnosing conditions that may benefit from herbal therapy and how these theories are applied to specific herbs.

OVERVIEW OF HERBAL MEDICINE

Readers should remember that herbal therapy by definition encompasses any plant source; therefore, herbal therapy also includes food. Only when the plant or a constituent of the plant is identified as a specific treatment for a disease or symptom is it often referred to as an herb. And the designation of an herb as a medicine lies in the definition of how it is used. Herbs have long been considered one of the safest medicines to take, and, like foods, can be classified as having mild, strong, or toxic effects on the body.

Most herbalists rely mainly on the mild herbs. However, the way herbs are used to treat diseases, based on theories of herbal medical practice, and the way herbal preparations are made or manufactured can influence their effects. Therefore, nurse practitioners and other allopathic providers need to understand not only the name, the ingredients, and the source of a particular herb but also the various theories used in herbal medicine. And they should consult with clinicians and CAM providers trained in herbal medicine when caring for a patient who chooses to use herbal remedies.

DEFINITIONS

Medicinally, an herb is any plant part or plant used for its therapeutic value. Yet, many of the world's herbal traditions also include mineral and animal substances as well. Herbal medicine, with a written history more than 5,000 years old, is the art and science of using herbs for promoting health and preventing and treating illness. Although the use of herbs in the United States has been overshadowed by dependence on modern medications during the past 100 years, 75 percent of the world's population relies primarily on traditional healing practices, most of which is herbal medicine.

Pharmacognosy is the branch of pharmacology that uses the chemicals from plants, molds, fungi, insects, and marine animals for their medicinal value. Today, most pharmaceutical drugs are single chemical entities from plant sources that have been highly refined, purified, and synthesized into a single active component of the plant. Many of the drugs used in allopathic medicine were derived from plants in this way, including **digitalis** from foxglove, **ephedrine** from *Ephedra*, and **ergotamine** from *Claviceps purpurea*.

In 1987 about 85 percent of modern drugs were derived from plants. However, today only about 15 percent of all drugs are derived from plants because of advancements in synthetic reproduction and purification of plant constituents. In contrast, herbal medicines are prepared only from living or dried plants and contain hundreds to thousands of interrelated compounds, creating a type of synergy between the many constituents which science is now considering the reason for the safety, effectiveness, and lower incidence of side effects of herbs (Farnsworth, 1993).

COMMON HERBS USED FOR MEDICINE

By examining the many herbal traditions practiced in the world today, the reader can better understand the concepts and theories of herbal medicine. For this text, three traditions are examined: western herbal medicine, ayurvedic herbal medicine, and traditional Chinese herbal medicine. Other traditions of herbal medicine worthy of exploring include Unani medicine, homeopathic, Native American traditional medicine, and shamanic herbal medicine, to name a few.

Western Herbal Medicine

The science-based herbal medicine can be traced back to Europe during the Renaissance, when political independence from the church and advances in science contributed greatly to the study of medicine. William Turner (1510–1568), the father of British botany, was the first to study plants scientifically. John Gerrard (1545–1612), a surgeon and the author of *Gerard's Herbal,* studied more than 1,000 plants and recorded his observations of their behavior and uses. One of the most interesting scientists of this era was Nicolas Culpepper (1616–1654), who studied the relationship of herbs to astrology. Although he was ostracized by his peers at the time for his theories, his understanding of herbs from an energetic perspective—influenced by factors other than the physical components of nutrients—was very similar to the eastern interpretation of plant-based medicine. Yet he fared much better than those who used herbal medicine to heal outside of the scientific community. Such healers were mostly women and were branded as witches during the Inquisition. Witch hunts effectively suppressed and denigrated the efforts of lay healers. However, many of these traditions have survived and are practiced today.

In western herbology, herbs are primarily classified according to their therapeutic properties and constituents of the plant. For example, categories such as **diuretics**, diaphoretics, and tonics allow western herbalists to group herbs with similar qualities and then use them accordingly. This system is primarily based on examination of the chemical constituents of the plant, which remains the basis of western pharmacology as well the basis of some herbal therapies used by many naturopath physicians (ND) and other herbalists who base their practice on scientific examination of the plant. For example, **bromelain**, a sulfhydryl proteolytic enzyme obtained from the pineapple plant, which activates proteolytic activity at sites of inflammation, is commercially used as a natural anti-inflammatory agent (Pizzorno & Murray, 2006). Another example is the use of herbs for a specific purpose like a tonic such as ginger root *(Zingiber officinale),* which contains sesquiterpenes that have significant antirhinoviral activity and may be used to combat colds (Mills & Bone, 2000), and golden seal *(Hydrastis canadensis),* which contains isoquinoline alkaloids found to inhibit microbial adherence and reduce infections (Mills & Bone, 2000).

The same plant is commonly used in several different herbal theories, and although the principle actions are the same, how the plant is used and which parts of the plant are used are different. One example is cinnamon. Cinnamon *(Cinnamomum zeylanicum)* is often referred to as "true cinnamon" or Ceylon cinnamon. However, commercially a related species known as cassia *(C. aromaticum),* or Saigon cinnamon *(C. loureirii),* and *C. burmannii* are labeled as cinnamon. True cinnamon *(Cinnamomum zeylanicum)* comes from the thin inner bark, is finer and less dense, has a more crumbly texture, and is considered to be less strong than cassia. Cassia is derived from the entire bark layer so it is thicker and has a much stronger, harsher flavor than does cinnamon. This distinction is important because of a moderately toxic component called coumarin, which can cause liver and kidney damage in high concentration; it is found in higher doses in cassia than it is in Ceylon cinnamon, in which the levels of coumarin are negligible. Often used for its oil, cinnamon contains primarily cinnamic aldehyde but also has ethyl cinnamate, eugenol (found in the leaves), beta-caryophyllene, linalool, and methyl chavicol. It is used to cure colds, treat diarrhea, and other problems of the digestive system. Cinnamon has been reported to be effective in treating type 2 diabetes mellitus (Khan et al, 2003). In traditional Chinese medicine, cinnamon (gui zhi) is used to treat colds but is defined by its ability to release excess, wind-cold conditions; warm and open channels and collaterals; and warm yang. Gui zhi is identified as being contraindicated in patients with yin deficiency (excess heat) and in patients with blood disorders because cinnamon stimulates blood circulation (Chen & Chen, 2001).

Traditional Chinese Herbs

The origins of Traditional Chinese Medicine (TCM) are difficult to date. However, one of the oldest surviving texts that forms the basis of TCM is the *Huangdi Neijing*. The work is composed of two texts each with 81 chapters or treatises and is primarily a written record of questions and answers between the mythical Huangdi (Yellow Emperor) and six of his ministers. The first text, the *Suwen*, covers the theoretical foundation of Chinese medicine and its diagnostic methods, and the second text, the *Spiritual Pivot*, discusses acupuncture therapy.

The Huangdi Neijing not only departed from the shamanic beliefs of the past but elaborated on the concepts of Daoist theory from which TCM is practiced and distinguishes itself from western medicine. This theory is based on the concept that the human is a microcosm of nature's larger macrocosm. Thus, for humans to stay healthy or "in balance," humans must have an intimate respect and understanding for the laws of nature and how to apply those laws in such a way that the body is able to benefit from it and sustain health. According to TCM theory, health is sustained by having a free flow of energy (qi). If Qi flows smoothly, and is nourished by what is consumed and perceived, it will allow the body to achieve a form of balance in the mind, body and spirit and enhance the ability of the body to heal itself. Just as in nature, when water, nutrients, and sunlight are adequate, a plant will flourish and grow. Of course, knowing how to determine imbalance and how to achieve balance is the principle science of TCM. By understanding the basic principles of yin and yang theory (a concept of balance between two opposing forces); the five elements (a concept of the interrelationship, and connection among all things); the influence of environmental factors (wind, damp, hot, and cold, dry, wet); the effects of diet, lifestyle, age, and emotions, the practitioner can develop a specific TCM diagnosis regarding the cause of imbalance. And by using herbal therapy along with other treatment modalities, such as acupuncture, diet, counseling, movement, and massage specific to the individual, balance can be restored and self healing can occur. One of the biggest differences between the origins of western and eastern medicine is the reliance on a scientific evaluation of the human body and health and the Daoist perspective of viewing the body as a microcosm of nature (or macrocosm) with a reliance on observation and response. Treatments in TCM are nature based and not science based. And the principles of herbal therapy are based on a focus of the plants cycle of growth, the characteristics of the plant (according to taste and expression), and the underlying condition of the individual consuming the herb and not specifically on the chemical properties found among the constituent parts of the plant.

The second important text in Chinese herbal medicine is the *Shang Hang Lun*, "Treatise on the Treatment of Acute Diseases Caused by Cold," written by Zhang Zhong-Jing (142–220). The *Shang Hang Lun* decribes the six stages of acute disease as an approach to the diagnosis and treatment of acute illness and is composed of classical herbal formulas that can be used to treat them. Today, formulas contained in the *Shang Hang Lun* such as Ge-Gen tang, Shao Yao Gan Cao tang, and Xiao Qing Long tang, are still commonly used among TCM practitioners.

In TCM herbology, herbs are classified by their energies, quality, season, tastes, directions, and actions on the body (e.g., moving blood, reducing dampness or heat, breaking up stagnation). The Chinese traditionally also add animals and minerals to their formulas with the same properties. Based on a broader overview of the body, Chinese herbology considers not only the energies of the herb, for example, yin (cooling) versus yang (warming), but also the constitution of the person consuming the herb which assumes a more holistic approach to healing and the role of herbs. For example, menopause in TCM is often considered a time of yin deficiency (loss of cold balance with excess heat), so herbs that are yin in nature (e.g., cooling) and clear heat arising from deficient yin such as mountain peony bark (mu dan pi) and phellodendron bark (huang bai), or formulas which contain each are often recommended (Liu & Tseng, 2003). In contrast to the few herbs discussed above that are used by western herbologists, TCM would not consider any of them to be a true tonic but rather would subclassify them by their properties: golden seal as having cooling energies and ginger as having warming energy. In doing so, TCM recognizes that if these herbs are applied inappropriately—for example, if a cooling herb is given as a tonic to a person with a cold condition—then the tonic could make the condition worse. A more appropriate recommendation by the provider would be to give ginger to a person with a cold condition (no fever) and golden seal to a person with a heat (fever) condition. Remember that TCM does not isolate treatment to single herbal therapy: The principles of the Tao and concepts of change indicate that the treatment and prevention of disease include nutrition (in which herbal therapy is included); activities for the spirit; and the practice of acupuncture, energy movements (tai chi), and massage (tui nai); and practices to balance the body, mind, and spirit.

Ayurvedic Herbs

Ayurvedic medicine was developed in ancient India and is defined as the study of life; ayur means "life" and veda means "to study." Based on original text derived from Vedic scriptures that date from 1500 BCE to 1200 BCE, ayurvedic is considered the world's oldest form of medicine. Evidence of its influence and spread from India can be seen in several systems of medicine: traditional

Chinese, Japanese, Unani, and the humoral medicine practiced by Hippocrates. Although many of the teachings originate from knowledge handed down through generations of healers, many believe ayurveda is of divine origin received from the meditation of sages. Similar to TCM, ayurvedic medicine encompasses a myriad of therapies based on the constitution of the individual and nature of that person's disease.

But the use of herbal medicine in ayurveda is somewhat broader because it is used in a number of medas and delivery systems that go beyond an oral route. Herbs are used in body massage oils, in food preparations, and aromatherapy, as well as taken orally. However, the choice of herbal therapy is still based on an individual and is linked to the patient's constitution and level of imbalance.

In ayurvedic herbology, herbal therapy is interchangeable with food and spices, which are viewed as a sequence of herbal therapies ranging from mild (food) to moderate (spices) to strong (herb). Their use depends on a person's constitution, classified according to a tridosha theory and the nature of the diseases. In the tridosha system, within all entities of matter, including people and plants, three doshas exist: *vata* (air/ether), which corresponds to the nervous system and movement; *pitta* (fire/water), representing transformation, circulation, warmth, and digestion; and *kapha* (water/earth) representing nourishment, solidity, and the formative aspects of tissue, fluid, and bone (Tiwari, 1995a,b). Although all three doshas exist together, often plants and people are classified by the one that is most dominant in them and referred to as the person's prakriti, which is specific to the individual. Treatment is then based on balancing the specific constitutional type, as each dosha is aggravated or pacified by certain therapies, herbs, and foods. Therefore, in ayurvedic medicine (similar to TCM) herbal therapy begins with the foods and spices consumed daily to maintain the balance of a given doshic constitution. An example of this theory is treating a person with a vata constitution with a vata disorder. Vata means "wind" and conceptually is made up of the elements of ether and air. Ether (space) affects the ability of air to gain momentum, and if unrestricted, air can gain momentum and become forceful. If balanced, a vata type person will have free movement and flow (e.g., breathing will be strong, movement of the muscle and bones easy and light, movement of blood smooth, movement of thought and emotions easy, movement of the colon unimpeded). If unbalanced and either is in an excess or deficient condition, the person may experience an excessive movement (manic behavior, diarrhea, nervousness, etc.) or deficient movement (e.g., constipation, depression, asthma). Therefore, the goal of therapy is to counter the excess or deficiency first with food and spice and then support it with specific herbal therapy. One ayurvedic principle similar to the one used in homeopathic medicine is that "like increases like." Consequently, substances of similar doshas will increase those qualities in the body. A person experiencing an excess vata imbalance tends to be intolerant of dry or bitter substances (which are considered vata in nature); therefore, treatment is to avoid foods that are dry and bitter and incorporate foods such as honey and rose hips and herbs such as calamus or marshmallow root in the diet (Tiwari, 1995a). Similar to TCM, ayurvedic treatment of imbalances within the tridoshic theory is not limited to herbal therapy; treatment also includes the five purification therapies (*panchakarma*—diet, aromatherapy, massage (*abyanga*), meditation, daily routine (*dinacarya*)—plus the practice of yoga.

In most traditional cultures throughout the world, herbal therapy is applied according to the herbs' energetic effects on the body and not on the individual constituents found in a plant. This in part is a result of a recognition that the synergistic effects of the plant are more important than are its individual components. The conceptual model upon which clinical decisions and herbal recommendations are made is remarkably different from western allopathic medicine, yet in the west, herbal medicines are often used strictly for their actions, with disregard for the energetic composition of the herb or the person consuming it. This practice in the short term may result in a positive effect, but in the long and/or short term it can often lead to poor or harmful effects. Therefore, the western clinician who has an interest in herbal medicine or has a patient who is taking herbal medicine needs to be aware of the different systems used to classify and use herbal therapy and to recognize the importance of consulting with providers trained in a particular system. In doing so, a provider can employ herbs efficiently and effectively and avoid improper applications, possibly either resulting in no effect or creating an opposite and undesired effect.

HERBAL SAFETY

Today, practitioners of TCM and ND must meet national standards and certification requirements for licensure to prescribe herbal therapy; however, state requirements may vary. In addition, herbal certification programs are now available, and guidelines for safe herbal practice have been established by the American Herbal Guild (AHG). The AHG is a nonprofit, educational organization founded in 1989 to represent the goals and voices of herbalists; it is the only peer-review organization in the United States for professional herbalists specializing in the medicinal use of plants. Herbalists, from any tradition, with sufficient education and clinical experience, who demonstrate advanced knowledge in the medicinal use of plants, and who pass the AHG credentialing process (a careful review by a multidisciplinary admissions board) receive professional status and the title, Registered Herbalist, AHG. The AHG has also developed a code of ethics, continuing education programs, and specific standards for professional members as well as establishing curriculum guidelines for herbal educational programs. The AHG Educational

Guidelines recommend a curriculum with a minimum of 1,600 hours of total study, 400 of which should be in actual clinical work (AHG, 2006).

When considering herbal medicines, providers need to understand that the development and preparation of medicines from plant and animal products can introduce wide variations, based on the conditions of growth, harvesting, processing, storing, and shipping. Plants grown in the wild may be quite different from the same plants grown agriculturally. Methods of harvesting and weather variations in nature inevitably are different from plants harvested under controlled environments. In addition, variations in how plants are processed based on the drying and sterilizing techniques used have an effect on the potency of the herb. If products are not stored carefully, the inherent quality of the herb may be further compromised and be less effective.

In the United States, pharmaceuticals must meet a strict standard established by the FDA, not only in the research and development stages, but also in processing stages to maintain consistent standards of quality. Herbs, however, are regarded as food sources and do not fall under the drug and pharmaceutical standards established by the FDA. However, many herbal manufacturers, particularly those in the United States, have adopted the FDA Good Manufacturing Practice (GMP) criteria for manufacturing, packing, and handling human food standards in the preparation of herbal medicines. The GMP establishes federal guidelines for plant management, disease control, harvesting, storage, and distribution of foods and herbs. Those foods and herbs meeting the standards are authorized to display the GMP label on their products. Herbal products also provide supplement facts, active ingredients, and serving recommendations.

In addition, the federal Dietary Supplement Health and Education Act (DSHEA) requires dietary supplements (of which herbs are included) to carry on the label this statement: "This product has not been evaluated by the FDA. This product is not intended to diagnose, treat, cure, or prevent any disease." These measures have been taken to ensure the safety of herbal products and should be reviewed with each patient and practitioner who recommends or reviews a patient's use of herbs.

EVIDENCE FOR THE USE OF HERBS

Evidence Grading

In an effort to evaluate herbal therapy, several systems have been developed to provide clinicians with methods to understand the mechanism, use and potential harmful effects of herbal therapy using an evidence-based system.

Natural Standard

Natural Standard (http://www.naturalstandard.com) is a complementary medicine grading system founded by clinicians and researchers from more than 100 academic institutions. It is designed to provide clinicians with the latest scientific data and expert opinion on complementary therapies including herbal therapies and is based on the Jadad scoring system of study quality (Jadad et al, 1996). A Jadad score of 0 to 5 is given, with 5 being the highest quality study.

In addition, a "magnitude of benefit" score is given to evaluate how strong a study is able to show the benefit of a therapy. Natural Standard determines magnitude of benefit by subtracting the mean of the treatment group from the mean of the placebo group.

Natural Standard takes the Jadad score, the magnitude of benefit, and other factors and grades the treatment. Grades reflect "the level of available scientific evidence in support of the efficacy of a given therapy for the specific indication." Treatments are also graded based on "evidence of harm." The Natural Standard evidence rating method is graded on a scale from A to F. A grade of A indicates strong scientific evidence of the benefit of the therapy, whereas an F suggests strong negative scientific evidence (Blum, n.d.).

Healthnotes™

Healthnotes' *The Natural Pharmacy* (Gaby, 2006) was designed as a reference for both practitioners and consumers. It evaluates the current state of evidence regarding herbs and nutritional supplements. This text is a culmination of the research of 25,000 articles and more than 600 peer reviewed journals. In addition, a team of medical doctors, pharmacists, naturopaths, and chiropractors, all of whom have been in clinical practice, contribute the chapters in the text. New editions of this manual are updated continually with the latest evidence-based information and recommendations.

The *Natural Pharmacy* (2006) is notable for providing evidence based almost solely on human studies, as well as information that specifically addresses contraindications to any herb or supplement. In addition, each recommendation is based on evidence derived from clinical, double-blind, meta-analyses or traditional empirical studies.

Rakel's Evidence Versus Harm Scale©

The *Rakel Evidence Versus Harm Scale* (Rakel, 2007) utilizes the Strength of Recommendation Taxonomy (SORT) (Ebell, Siwek, & Weiss, 2004) to rate the scientific evidence of a variety of integrated medicine treatments. The scale includes strength of the evidence along with the evidence of potential harm. The evidence of benefit is graded from A to C, with A indicating that the evidence is "based on consistent, good quality, patient-oriented evidence." Potential harm of a therapy is graded from 1 (little or no risk of harm) to 3 (potential to result in death or permanent disability). A grade A rating represents evidence culled from systematic reviews or meta-analysis. It also incorporates *Cochrane Reviews* of high-quality, randomized controlled trials that resulted in clear recommendations.

Cochrane Database of Systematic Reviews

Cochrane Database of Systematic Reviews (Cochrane Collaboration, n.d.) was created to help health-care providers keep up with and evaluate relevant scientific evidence. The Cochrane Collaboration produces reviews of evidence, and creates a database of health-care interventions. The quality of the studies included in a review is evaluated using specific predefined criteria. Most *Cochrane Reviews* are based on randomized controlled trials and are statistically summarized into meta-analyses, showing a more thorough validation of clinical effect. Cochrane is considered one of the best sources of reliable evidence for and against specific treatments for specific conditions.

German Commission E Monographs

The German Federal Institute for Drugs and Medical Devices Commission E is a federal organization formed in 1978 to determine the efficacy and safety of herbs and supplements sold in Germany (National Institutes of Health, National Cancer Institute, n.d.). The commission is a multidisciplinary team of scientists, physicians, pharmacists, and herbal medicine experts who review and analyze available data, and form clinical recommendations based on the current evidence. To date, more than 300 herbs have been included in the recommendations and have been approved for clinical use in Germany.

Recommendations are published as monographs for each herb. Monographs include all pertinent botanical data, explanation of mechanism (pharmacodynamic and pharmacokinetic action), and a complete therapeutic index (indications, contraindications, side effects, drug interactions, dosing, and duration). Additionally, the monographs include traditional uses, unapproved uses, and a summary of evidence. Commission E monographs are considered authoritative by experts in the field, and have been reviewed for completeness and accuracy by the American Botanical Council (American Botanical Council [ABC], 2009).

American Botanical Council

The ABC is a nonprofit educational and research organization dedicated to the science of herbal medicine (ABC, 2009). They look at evidence from both modern scientific and traditional perspectives. The ABC comprises an advisory council of experts, and is affiliated with several natural medicine health science institutions and organizations. The ABC maintains comprehensive databases and publishes a peer-reviewed journal, *Herbalgram*. The ABC provides commentary, additions, and in some cases editor's notes for correction on all Commission E monographs. Although not a true evidence-graded system, specific herbal indications by Commission E will be considered as having strong supported evidence for inclusion within the context of this work (ABC, 2009).

The two systems that may be the most valuable to the primary care provider are *Natural Standards* and *Rakel* because they provide a broad approach to recommended interventions for a given condition. *Healthnotes*, however, provides the most comprehensive data on individual supplements and serves as an expert source for clinical investigation of an herbal product. The *Cochrane Database of Systematic Reviews* contains high-quality data review but it is clinically the least useful for CAM evaluation because of its specificity in regards to what is reviewed.

Challenges to Using an Evidenced–Based Model

Evidenced-based medicine (EBM) is currently considered the gold standard of care for practice. However, using blinded, randomized controlled trials (RCTs) based on a statistical analysis to validate and determine efficacy of a particular medication or medical procedure may not be the most effective way to evaluate a holistic approach to care, particularly when the statistical analysis is deemed the only acceptable basis for health outcomes. The value and role of the health provider are undermined, the psychological and social aspects of medicine are neglected, and sole reliance on EBM is in danger of creating a utilitarian orthodoxy (Williams & Garner, 2002).

Three factors become problematic when evaluating CAM therapies, particularly herbal therapy. First, the western scientific method applied to drug-based or pharmaceutical research is designed to measure single chemical components in relation to outcome. This is the drug-based, or pharmaceutical, model used in the evaluation of western herbs but it does not reflect the philosophy and treatment parameters used in ayurvedic or TCM, which use the synergistic properties of the whole plant with the symptoms of the patient consuming it. Second, definitions used in CAM pose a unique problem for EBM researchers. The scientific method cannot be used to measure ideas and practices that have yet to be physically defined by western science. The concepts of qi and prana, representing universal energy or life force, are one example, but other concepts such as yin (cooling, feminine, etc.) and yang (heating, masculine, etc.), vatta (ether and air), kapha (earth and water), and pitta (fire and water) also serve to illustrate the complexity of analyzing concepts that do not have equivocal biomedical definitions. Third, the outcomes in TCM and ayurvedic medicine are determined largely by empirical rather than experimental diagnostic measures. Changes in a person's tongue coat and pulse, or changes in symptoms often are enough to satisfy clinical management and evaluate the efficacy of an herbal formula.

Diabetes mellitus type 2 presents a good example for looking at the fundamental differences between these systems (pharmaceutical and whole plant) in disease-diagnostic and treatment criteria. In biomedicine, diabetes is seen as a specific set of characteristics and laboratory markers. A fasting blood glucose greater than 126 mg/dL on more than one occasion would validate a diagnosis of this disease (Joslin Diabetes Center and Joslin Clinic,

2007). In eastern medicine, diabetes is made up of seven possible patterns, none of which would be called "diabetes" (Bob Flaws, 2005).

The differences in the two systems become particularly problematic around the selection of herbal medicines. In traditional CAM modalities, herbs are prescribed based on the phenotypical manifestation of the disease and the constitutional expression of the patient. This is in direct opposition to the drug model of herbal prescription currently being used by biomedicine. This model is based solely on the pharmacological understanding that relies on "perhaps erroneously, a preference for empirical evidence gained from controlled clinical trials regardless of the underlying theory of disease and healing" (Tonelli & Callahan, 2001). The drug-based model of herbal medicine is a reductionist view and it purposely ignores thousands of years of empirical evidence that has been validated within many traditional medical models.

In a review of 19 randomized controlled trials that utilized ginseng (serving as a hypothesis), the authors of one study found that no traditional patterns were used to determine the appropriateness of herb selection (Yan, Engle, He, Jiao, & Gu, 2009). Ginseng, specifically *Panax ginseng,* or ren shen, is an herb used traditionally to support specific symptom manifestations of qi deficiency, characterized by fatigue, gas or bloating and loose stools, weakness, cold, sweating, bleeding, and prolapsed organs (Kaptchuk, 2000). In addition, several of the 19 trials utilized a different species of ginseng, each of which traditionally has different properties and applications (Yan, et al, 2009). Analyzing the results as if looking at them through an eastern medicine theory lens, the reviewer found that positive results of ginseng use were seen only in the conditions that corresponded to the traditional Chinese concept of qi deficiency (Yan, et al, 2009). This demonstrated that biomedical evidence-based research, directed by traditional theory, may have a totally different outcome. Research that can employ these concepts can both improve study design and help validate traditional theory within a biomedical context.

Another challenge to herbal therapy is the use of polyherbal formulations common to traditional medical systems. Using the example of diabetes for a single herb, the criteria for a polyherbal formula take into account numerous factors based on a traditional medicine model. Thus, the patient who wants to take an herbal formula for a particular problem without the assistance of a trained herbalist has an ongoing dilemma: how to decide what herbal remedy(s) is best suited for him or her.

HERBAL THERAPY

Today most grocery or health supplement stores throughout the United States carry a variety of herbal remedies. These remedies are available without prescription or guidance, except what is printed on the label. Of course, consumers may consult other sources that may or may not be reliable. Therefore, nurse practitioners, nurses, and other health professionals must have an awareness of herbal therapy and how it might be used.

The purpose of this chapter is not to teach any particular style of herbal medicine but rather to use examples of TCM and ayurvedic medicine to illustrate the differences in herbal therapy and to encourage practitioners to consult an appropriate herbalist, naturopath, or Traditional Chinese Medicine or ayurvedic practitioner whenever herbal therapy is considered. This section is not a recommendation for prescribing to clients but rather a guideline and reference.

Western Herbs

Mental Health Symptoms

The most common symptoms for which people use herbs are anxiety, insomnia, depression or dysphoria, and forgetfulness and confusion. As with pharmaceutical drugs, some herbs may be beneficial across similar symptoms.

Anxiety

Kava, mugwort, wormwood, pill-bearing spurge, and **passion flower** are commonly used for relief of anxiety. **Kava** and **mugwort** are exemplars in this category. **Kava (ava, awa, kava-kava, kawa, kew, tonga)** comes from the dried root of *Piper methysticum,* a member of the black pepper family. This shrub is native to the Pacific Islands and commonly used by the Hawaiians as a celebratory drink as **alcohol** is used in the West. But unlike **alcohol, kava** does not stimulate aggression and is not associated with hangovers. It is prepared as a drink from the pulverized root but also comes in tablet, capsule, and extract forms. This herb has been studied in humans and appears to have more than one active component to produce the effects. One component acts as a local anesthetic when chewed, and it produces intense muscle relaxation. It appears to act on the limbic system to suppress emotional excitability and produce mild euphoria without affecting memory or cognition. In therapeutic drug trials, **kava** seems to act on the gamma-amino butyric acid (GABA) receptor, like the benzodiazepines. Like the benzodiazepines, **kava** can reduce seizure activity and can be used for sedation. Dose varies, depending on the form and the amount of active components retained in the preparation, and studies indicate 70 to 240 mg daily as the adult dose. Pharmacokinetics are unavailable for **kava,** but it seems to be preferred in divided doses, usually three times a day. Unlike the **benzodiazepines,** it does not seem to produce dependence, but the studies are very limited. When used short term, it seems to have few adverse reactions, including decreased motor reflexes, diminished judgment, and visual disturbances. Chronic use may decrease platelet count and may cause dry, flaky skin, reddened eyes, shortness of breath, pulmonary hypertension, and weight loss. Liver failure has been reported. Because it seems to act like the **benzodiazepines,** it may potentiate **alcohol,** other **sedatives,** and **GABA-ergic**

drugs such as **phenobarbital** and **benzodiazepines**. At higher doses, **kava** seems to block dopamine receptors, and therefore to improve psychotic levels of anxiety as well as interact with **antipsychotic drugs**. It should not be used in pregnancy or when breastfeeding because its safety is uncertain during pregnancy (Volz, 1997).

Mugwort (felon herb, wild wormwood, St. John's plant) comes from the root of the *Artemisia vulgaris* plant. It should not be confused with **St. John's wort**, which comes from a different plant. The name maybe derived from its common use of flavoring beer before the use of hops to do so. It is available as dried leaves and roots, fluid extract, tincture, or a tea infusion but only the root is used for its active constituents, thought to come from its volatile oil and acrid resin and tannins. It is a very versatile herb, but its medicinal use is more for its value as a nervine and emmenagogue (hastening menstrual flow when combined with pennyroyal and southernwood). When taken for anxiety and sedation, the usual dose is 5 mL of tincture 30 minutes before bedtime, although few studies support this use. It does have an anticholinergic effect observed in animal studies. In a recent study of **mugwort**, elements of alkaloids, coumarins, flavonoids, saponins, sterols, tannins and terpenes were found with concentration-dependent (0.3 to 10 mg/mL) relaxation of spontaneous jejunum contractions, and a combination of anticholinergic and Ca(2+) antagonist mechanisms supporting its use in hyperactive gut and airway disorders such as abdominal colic, diarrhea, and asthma (Khan & Gilani, 2009). This accounts for its use in the treatment of gastrointestinal problems and menstrual cramps.

One of the unique uses of **mugwort** actually comes from TCM, where it is used topically and burned to treat pain and tonify deficient conditions. It is used extensively in Japanese acupuncture as well as TCM, in several different forms and in a variety of methods (e.g., as a stick; directly on the skin; or by using a medium of holder, box, ginger; by holding it over acupuncture points, or pain locations, with or without needles).

Adverse reactions to **mugwort** when taken internally include anaphylaxis and induction of premature birth or miscarriage, and if used topically, contact dermatitis. It should not be used during pregnancy or breastfeeding or by anyone who has a clotting abnormality or allergy to hazelnuts. Because no controlled studies on **mugwort** have been conducted, no therapeutic claims can be made.

Insomnia

In addition to **mugwort**, **melatonin**, **valerian**, **passion flower**, and **chamomile** are used for sedation. **Melatonin** and **valerian** are used here as exemplars. **Melatonin** is not an herb but rather a hormone produced by the pineal gland. Because it is a hormone, exogenous consumption over extended periods of time may act as negative feedback and suppress normally secreted **melatonin**.

Melatonin is produced when serotonin is broken down in the pineal gland with the help of two enzymes: arylakylamine N-acetyltransferase (AA-NAT) and hydroxyindole-O-methyltransferase (HIOMT). It is the AA-NAT that seems to be a regulating enzyme because when it is elevated, **melatonin** is elevated. Unfortunately, AA-NAT is rapidly destroyed and production of melatonin is reduced by light. Under certain physiological conditions, melatonin is released during the fourth stage of sleep along with prolactin and growth hormone. It is used to induce sleep via the same GABA-ergic mechanism as benzodiazepine sedatives and is widely used to prevent and treat jet lag. A single study identified the utility of melatonin in elderly people to help induce and maintain sleep, probably because the elderly usually have some degree of melatonin deficiency under normal circumstances. Used long term, it can increase prolactin secretion, which can decrease luteinizing hormone, progesterone, and estradiol levels. Long-term use can also reset the sleep-wake cycle and contribute to disturbed sleep cycling.

Melatonin is available in tablets, capsules, extended-release capsules, and liquid form. For difficulty in getting to sleep, 1 to 5 mg taken at bedtime is the usual dosage, but it should not be used more than three nights a week. In the elderly, the dosage is usually 1 to 2 mg taken 2 hours before bedtime.

Adverse reactions include altered sleep patterns, confusion, headache, tachycardia, and hypothermia. **Melatonin** potentiates **benzodiazepines**. It also potentiates **succinylcholine**, thereby increasing the blocking action, which can be dangerous. Its content of active drug may vary widely in commercial **melatonin**, making it difficult to determine correct dosages (Brzezinski, 1997; Fetrow & Avila, 1999).

Valerian (all-heal, amantilla, setewale, capon's tail, herba benedicta) is derived from the roots of *Valeriana officinalis*. It seems to inhibit uptake and increase presynaptic release of GABA; however, it is not readily absorbed, is highly unstable, and readily decomposes. Therefore, availability of the active drug is minimal when it is taken orally. German Commission E suggests **valerian root** for anxiety, restlessness, and difficulty in getting to sleep. Because of the instability, dosages are difficult to determine, especially among different brands. Usually 400 to 900 mg of extract at bedtime or 1 teaspoon of dried herb in tea several times a day is useful in inducing sleep. Commercial **valerian** tea at bedtime acts as a relaxant and permits a person to fall asleep spontaneously.

Valerian has no adverse reactions when used at the recommended level; however, over dosage at 2.5 g or more can cause cardiac disturbance, excitability, headache, insomnia, and nausea. It can potentiate **alcohol** and other **central nervous system (CNS) depressants** if taken in large amounts. Because clinical trial studies are limited, it should not be used by pregnant or breastfeeding women, children, or patients with impaired liver function.

Depression

The popular media have touted the benefits of **St. John's wort** for depression, contributing to its popularity.

Additionally, **kava**, **mugwort**, and **dehydroepiandrosterone (DHEA)** have been used to treat mild depression. **St. John's wort** and **DHEA** are used as exemplars here.

St. John's wort is obtained from the tops and flowers of the *Hypericum perforatum* plant, which is common all over Europe, Asia, and the United States. The exact mechanism of action is still unknown but assumed to be related to inhibition of serotonin presynaptic uptake. Early studies show inhibition of monoamine oxidase (MAO) type A and minimally type B; however, this was later attributed to contaminants. In studies to determine effective dosages, **St. John's wort** was effective at blocking serotonin reuptake at much higher doses than could be achieved. **St. John's wort** also seems to act on the **benzodiazepine** receptor of GABA, norepinephrine reuptake inhibition, and acetylcholine blocking, as well as inhibiting stress-induced corticotropin-releasing hormone, adrenocorticotropic hormone (ACTH), and cortisol and increasing nighttime release of **melatonin**. Some reports have also indicated antiviral activity, including retroviruses (Chavez, 1997). With such a wide range of receptor activity, it is not surprising that **St. John's wort** is used to treat depression, enuresis, gastritis, hypothyroidism, insomnia, kidney disorders, scabies, hemorrhoids, wound healing, HIV infection, and Kaposi's sarcoma.

Most commonly, **St. John's wort** is used to relieve mild to moderate depression, less than would meet the criteria for major depressive episode or dysthymia. Therefore, the herb seems most effective for individuals who have sadness and lesser degrees of depression. When used for clinically diagnosed depression, **St. John's wort** is relatively ineffective and may dishearten or demoralize the person who is trying to avoid using more potent antidepressants.

For standardized, commercially prepared **St. John's wort**, the usual dosage is 300 mg taken three times daily; because of the delayed neuroreceptor response, 4 to 6 weeks may be needed to determine effectiveness. When **St. John's wort** is used as a tea, the amount needed is 2 to 4 g of tea steeped in 1 to 2 cups of boiling water for 10 minutes and taken daily to be effective within 4 to 6 weeks. The few adverse reactions, attributable to the anticholinergic blockade, include constipation, dry mouth, dizziness, gastrointestinal (GI) upset, restlessness, and insomnia. **St. John's wort** interacts with **MAO inhibitors (MAOIs)**, **tricyclic antidepressants**, **serotonin reuptake inhibitors**, **over-the-counter (OTC) cold** and **flu medications**, **narcotics**, and **sympathomimetics**. Because no adequate studies are available, **St. John's wort** should not be taken by children or pregnant or breastfeeding women. The primary care provider who determines that the patient meets the *Diagnostic and Statistical Manual of Mental Disorders,* 4th ed. (1994) criteria for depression might advise the client to consider taking another kind of **antidepressant** if results are minimal in 3 to 4 weeks.

DHEA is a steroid precursor found in plants of the yam family and secreted by primate adrenal glands. Physiologically, DHEA is converted into androgens and estrogens (depending on the person's gender) and may raise the blood level of a precursor of the human growth hormone. Many benefits are attributed to **DHEA**, including immune enhancement, prevention of osteoporosis, prevention of the development of malignant cells (acting as an antineoplastic), and acting as an antiaging agent, as well as being an antidepressant. Because few studies on humans are available, exact pharmacokinetics and pharmacodynamics are not known, but **DHEA** does not seem to be readily absorbed through the GI tract.

The lack of studies of **DHEA** also makes determining dosage difficult. At present, 50 mg daily is commonly used, but serum levels should be checked, with an expected level of 3600 ng/mL for men and 3000 ng/mL for women. Because **DHEA** is a hormone-like drug, it may cause negative feedback to the adrenal glands, thereby reducing production of endogenous hormones. Adverse reactions to be expected with an androsteroid include aggressiveness, hirsutism, insomnia, and irritability. Patients with hormone-sensitive cancers should be discouraged from using **DHEA**, as should pregnant and breastfeeding women. **DHEA** is likely to interact with other hormone therapy, such as estrogen replacement therapy. When used for depression, **DHEA** may have a 4-week lag time before an effect on depression is seen (Wolkowitz, 1997).

Confusion and Forgetfulness

Confusion and forgetfulness, along with other cognitive impairments, are often seen in dementia, depending on the root cause of the dementia. Additionally, people who are concerned about benign forgetfulness take herbs both to improve their cognitive abilities and to prevent memory problems. Common herbs used include **ginkgo**, **ginseng**, and **chaparral**, **Ginseng** and **ginkgo** are used here as exemplars, and they are often taken together or combined in a single preparation.

Ginseng (**American ginseng**, **Asian ginseng**, **Chinese ginseng**, **five-fingers**, **Japanese ginseng**, **Korean ginseng**, **seng and sang**, **schinsent**) is from the *Panax quinquefolius* plant, especially the root. **Asian ginseng** should not be confused with **Siberian ginseng**, which seems to bind with estrogen receptors. **Asian ginseng** is usually dried or cured and is highly valued, whereas **American ginseng** has less processing but is not as widely sought. Several compounds have biological activity, producing different effects. The mechanisms of action are not understood, but ginseng is said to have differing effects depending on the involved active component: anticonvulsant, analgesic, and antipsychotic effects; CNS-stimulating, antifatigue, hypertensive, and stress ulcer exacerbation; improvement of cardiac function; depression of cardiac function; antiarrhythmic activity; reduction of cholesterol and triglycerides; decrease in platelet adhesiveness; impaired coagulation; and increased fibrinolysis. The presumed focus of action is in the adrenal gland, although popular literature claims **ginseng** decreases thymus gland activity. Consequently, **ginseng** is used as a sedative, aphrodisiac, antidepressant, hypnotic, and diuretic. It is also used to improve stress resistance, stamina, work efficiency, concentration, mental performance and general feelings of well-being. Some studies found **ginseng** decreased fasting blood sugar and hemoglobin to such a degree that some diabetics no longer needed insulin.

Ginseng comes in capsules, tea bags, and extract, and in some Asian markets **ginseng** root can be bought in bulk. In processed form, however, it is difficult to standardize. Used for illness, **ginseng** is usually taken at 0.5 to 2 g a day of dry root or 200 to 600 mg of extract daily in divided doses. For dementia in frail elderly people, it is usually taken at 0.4 to 0.8 g of dry root daily. Achieving maximum effectiveness may take up to 90 days for full results.

Ginseng seems to have minimal and mild adverse reactions, including dizziness, drowsiness, headache, and insomnia, although chest pain, diarrhea, hypertension, impotence, nervousness, agitation, palpitations, nausea, and vomiting have also been reported. **Ginseng** may potentiate **insulin** and **oral hypoglycemics**, and it interacts with **MAOIs** to cause headaches, tremors, and mania. Studies have been conducted on ginseng to identify its effectiveness, yet the pharmacodynamics are elusive. The German Commission E considers **ginseng** to be an effective drug (Sorensen & Sonne, 1996; Wesnes et al, 2009).

Ginkgo (**ginkgo biloba, ginkogink**) is an extract from the leaves of the ginkgo tree, with the toxic ginkgolic acid removed. It is available in many forms, including tablets, capsules, sublingual sprays, and even included in juices and foods. **Ginkgo** is thought to stimulate prostaglandin synthesis, and thereby cause vasodilatation, increasing tissue perfusion and cerebral blood flow. **Ginkgo** has been used for centuries in Asian countries to improve mental alertness and today is used in the treatment of cerebrovascular disease and peripheral vascular disease. Additionally, it is popularly taken to improve thinking ability, concentration, and memory.

Dosage for confusion and dementia symptoms is 120 to 240 mg daily in two or three divided doses. For vascular disease, 120 to 320 mg daily has been used, but 4 to 6 weeks are needed before maximum effect is obtained.

Adverse reactions include diarrhea, headache, nausea, vomiting, bruising, excessive bleeding, and seizures in overdose. Trying to use ginkgo leaves to make a home remedy is potentially dangerous because of the ginkgolic acid and the difficulty in determining the quantity of active ingredients. Because it reduces platelet-activating factor and erythrocyte aggregation, **ginkgo** should not be taken with **anticoagulants** or **antiplatelet** medications. The German Commission E approved ginkgo for the treatment of dementia and peripheral arterial occlusive disease (Fetrow & Avila, 1999).

Gastrointestinal Problems

Probably the most common use of home remedies is for GI upset, such as constipation, diarrhea, indigestion, and nausea. Because the underlying causes of these complaints are also common, the herbal medications used for them overlap. The herbs most often used for constipation are also incorporated into commercial OTC medications: **cascara, castor bean,** and **senna. Cascara sagrada** is dried bark from the *Rhamnus purshiana* tree (found primarily in the Pacific Northwest and from Canada to California) that has been dried and aged for at least 1 year and up to 3 years. **Cascara** acts by increasing the smooth muscle tone of the large intestine and thus peristalsis. The FDA approved **cascara** as a safe and effective laxative to be sold OTC. It is available as an extract or extract capsules. Although **cascara** is very safe, it may produce such adverse reactions as abdominal cramping, diarrhea, fluid and electrolyte imbalance, steatorrhea, vomiting, and vitamin and mineral deficiencies in long-term use. **Cascara** can be used in pregnancy but should not be used by breastfeeding women because it is excreted in milk and may cause serious diarrhea in the infant. Because a person can become dependent on **cascara**, it should be limited to short-term use.

Senna comes from the leaves and pods of the *Cassia* shrub and is the active ingredient in OTC medications such as **Senokot, Senokot-S,** and **Senolax** and comes in capsules, tablets, and syrup. Dried **senna** leaves can also be made into a tea by adding 100 g of leaves to a liter of boiling water and steeping it for 10 minutes. Sliced ginger or crushed coriander leaves make the tea more palatable. When it enters the intestinal tract, bacteria convert it into a biologically active agent. **Senna** increases peristaltic action in the lower bowel. **Senna** is excreted in breast milk and should not be taken by the breastfeeding woman.

The usual adult dosage is about 340 mg taken at bedtime or 0.5 to 1 dr of syrup. Adverse reactions are similar to those of **cascara**: abdominal cramping, diarrhea, hypokalemia, and clubbing of the fingers with chronic use. **Calcium channel blockers** or **indomethacin** blocks the diarrheal effects. A patient with irritable bowel, hemorrhoids, GI inflammatory conditions, or prolapsed rectum should not use **senna**; it can be overused and create a laxative dependency.

Indigestion and heartburn plague Americans, as evidenced by the large amounts of antacids sold each year. In addition to these antacids, common household herbs can be used effectively and safely. **Caraway** oil distilled from dried seeds of the *Carum carvi* herb or **caraway** water made from soaking 1 oz of crushed **caraway** seeds in a pint of cold water for 6 hours can be used for indigestion, flatulence, constipation, and menstrual cramps. Because of its mild action, **caraway** can be given to infants for colic. The usual dosage for adults is 1 to 4 drops of oil in a teaspoon of sweetened water; and for infants 1 to 3 tsp of caraway water. The only adverse reactions reported are diarrhea and mucous membrane irritation.

Licorice root has also been used for gastric irritation and dyspepsia. **Licorice** comes from the dried root of the *Glycyrrhiza glabra* shrub and is available in capsules, tablets, liquid extracts, chewing gum, tea, and candy. Studies indicate that glycyrrhetic acid is the active element that potentiates endogenous steroids and stimulates gastric mucus synthesis. **Licorice** is a soothing and mild expectorant, mild laxative, and antispasmodic. Additionally, it has antiarrhythmic effects and lowers cholesterol and triglyceride levels; it may cause immunosuppression.

The usual dose of **licorice** is in 200- to 600-mg tablets taken daily for 4 to 6 weeks or **licorice** tea simmered for 5 minutes and taken three times a day after eating. Reported adverse reactions include mineralocorticoid effects of headache, lethargy, sodium and water retention, hypokalemia, and hypertension; in overdose the adverse reactions include muscle weakness, heart failure, and cardiac arrest.

Licorice interacts with many medications such as **antihypertensives, diuretics, corticosteroids, digoxin, loratadine, procainamide, quinidine,** and **spironolactone.** A patient who is taking **licorice** regularly should be warned against excessive and chronic use, especially when it is combined with **diuretics.** Licorice candy does not actually contain the herb but rather licorice flavoring, usually from anise oil.

Papaya enzymes, available in tablets and chewable tablets, are frequently used to prevent or treat common heartburn, although it is not effective for gastroesophageal reflux. **Papaya** is a proteolytic enzyme in the leaves, seeds, pulp, and latex of the *Carica papaya* tree. The clinical trials with humans have mostly focused on treating inflammation from trauma and surgery. **Papaya** also has been used effectively as a debriding agent and for intradisk injections in patients with herniated disks. The dosage of **papaya** for inflammation is 10 mg four times a day for 1 week. Dosage for dyspepsia is variable and not standardized, but usually 4 to 5 tablets are taken immediately after eating.

Adverse reactions to **papaya** are uncommon and limited to dermatitis, hypersensitivity, decreased heart rate and CNS activity, and perforation of the esophagus with excessive ingestion. No drug interactions have been reported. No studies have been conducted with pregnant and breastfeeding women, so avoiding use during pregnancy and breastfeeding is safest.

Pain

Joint pain, soft tissue pain, and headache are problems that people often treat with herbal and home remedies. The medications to treat each of these kinds of pain overlap. Two products currently in health food stores are **glucosamine** and **chondroitin,** both of which are not herbal. **Glucosamine** is an amino acid found in mucopolysaccharides and chitin. Most of the **glucosamine** sold in the United States, however, is synthetically made and is sold under such names as **Arth-X Plus, Glucosamine Mega, Joint Factors,** and **Nutri-Joint,** in capsules or tablets in a range of dosages. **Glucosamine** is thought to stimulate cartilage production and enhance rebuilding of damaged cartilage. Some European studies in people with osteoarthritis demonstrated good relief of pain and rapid restoration of mobility and range of motion.

The dose used in the studies was 500 mg three times a day. Adverse reactions were benign: Constipation, diarrhea, drowsiness, headache, heartburn, nausea, and rash were the most common. No drug interactions reported. Frequently, **glucosamine** is combined with **chondroitin** for greater efficacy.

Chondroitin is extracted from the cartilage of cow trachea and is available in 200- and 400-mg capsules. **Chondroitin** seems to stimulate chondrocyte metabolism and synthesis of collagen, improving the formation of cartilage. Other studies identified stimulation of hyaluronic acid in synovial cells in patients with rheumatic disease, resulting in increased viscosity and amount of synovial fluid. When **chondroitin** was used for up to 4 months, patients were able to reduce pain medication and were doing weight-bearing exercises comfortably.

The dosage of **chondroitin** depends on a patient's weight: For patients under 120 lb, the dosage is 1,000 mg of **glucosamine** and 800 mg of **chondroitin;** for patients 120 to 200 lbs, the dosage is 1,500 mg of **glucosamine** and 1,200 mg of **chondroitin.** Both are taken in either divided doses or a single dose.

Adverse reactions include dyspepsia, headache, motor restlessness, euphoria, nausea, and risk of internal bleeding. **Chondroitin** may potentiate **anticoagulants.** Because no studies of **glucosamine** and **chondroitin** have been conducted with pregnant or breastfeeding women, **glucosamine** and **chondroitin** should not be used by this population.

Wintergreen oil and **liniments** have been deemed effective in relieving pain from muscle strains, inflamed muscles, ligaments, and joints. Usually the oil is a combination of oil extracted from the leaves and bark of *Gaultheria procumbens* and methyl salicylate. Although no studies on the efficacy of **wintergreen** have been conducted, **wintergreen** likely acts through counterirritation—which masks pain—or through the analgesic and anti-inflammatory effects of the salicylate.

Ten percent **wintergreen oil** is applied to the skin no more often than three to four times a day. Overgenerous application can result in salicylate poisoning from absorption into the bloodstream. People who are allergic to **aspirin** or who are taking oral **anticoagulants** should not use **wintergreen oil.**

Feverfew is an interesting herb used most often to treat headache and migraines. It has also been used for toothache, joint pain, asthma, stomachache, menstrual problems, and threatening miscarriage. **Feverfew (bachelors' button, featherfoil, Santa Maria, midsummer daisy)** is extracted from the leaves of the **feverfew** plant, *Chrysanthemum parthenium*. The assumed mechanism of action is the inhibition of serotonin release from platelets.

Feverfew is available in capsules, liquid, tablets, and dried leaves for tea. Research with feverfew shows a decrease in the number, duration, and severity of migraines in a double-blind, crossover study (Murphy, Heptinstall, & Mitchell, 1988). The average dose for the treatment of migraines is 543 mcg of **parthenolide** (the active component of **feverfew**) daily; for migraine prevention, the dose is 25 mg daily of freeze-dried leaf extract. The most common adverse reactions are mouth ulcerations, hypersensitivity, and a withdrawal syndrome characterized by moderate to severe pain and joint and muscle stiffness.

Traditional Chinese Herbs

The use of herbal medicine in TCM is not often isolated to a single remedy but rather as a part of a holistic approach to healing that is most effective when combined with other TCM therapies that include; acupuncture, manipulative therapies (tui na), food, and movement (qigong and tai ji). Yet, contemporary practitioners will often prescribe single herbs or herbal formulas for a particular disorder in the same way that western clinicians prescribe medicines. But the primary difference is in how the herb is applied.

The application of herbs specifically is based on the nature and capabilities of the herb and the energies, flavors, movement, and meridian.

The Four Energies

The four energies in herbal medicine are cold, hot, warm, and cool and are derived from years of empirical research and observation of the direct effect of taking an herb over time. If an herb is effective in the treatment of a heat condition, it is classified as having a cooling energy. In the most basic sense, herbs can be divided into yin (cooling) and yang (heating) energies. But because temperature can be a matter of interpretation, many TCM practitioners refer to the herbal energy as extremely warm or slightly warm and extremely cold or slightly cold.

The Five Flavors

The five flavors refer to the effect that the herb has on a person's sense of taste and are classified as being pungent (or acrid), sweet, sour, bitter, and salty. Not only do the five flavors describe taste but they also exhibit properties that are used medically. Pungent herbs can disperse and promote the flow of energy; sour herbs can constrict and obstruct; sweet herbs can slow down, tone up, and harmonize; bitter herbs can harden, dry up, and cause diarrhea; and salty herbs can soften up and promote downward movement. Often questions arise about things that are tasteless. Tasteless is considered a flavor and tends to be classified with sweet and can help disperse dampness and promote urination.

The Four Movements

The four movements of herbs are upward, downward, floating, and sinking. To push upward means that the herb has the capacity of lifting something that can no longer be supported, for example, prolapsed organs such as the uterus or rectum. To push downward means that the herb is capable of suppressing a rebellious symptom, for example, the hiccups or a cough. To float means that the herb is capable of dispersing outward, such as inducing perspiration or a purging action. And to sink means that the herb is capable of promoting diarrhea and directing excess energy downward. Often the movement of an herb is combined. Herbs that push upward and those that can float have the common function of moving upward and outward, by inducing perspiration and vomiting and elevating the yang energy. The herbs that can push downward and those that can sink have the common function of moving downward and inward and relieving symptoms such as vomiting or excess perspiration or diarrhea.

Meridian Routes

Meridian routes refer to the meridians (or pathway of energy identified in TCM that corresponds to the 12 organ systems) that the herb can enter and move through. Two herbs with the same energy and flavor can display two different actions because their meridian routes are different (for example, two heating herbs may have different actions; one may be better for cold lung conditions, whereas the other may work better for cold spleen conditions).

Actions of Chinese Herbs

All Chinese herbs or herbal formulas have several common actions but they are expressed differently from western medication. A western medication will be classified as an antihistamine because it blocks the effects of histamine, but a Chinese herb will be classified by its action to clear heat, stop wind, or reduce fire. A formula will have multiple actions that are designed specifically for the patient's condition; for example, one herb will clear lung heat, the other may transform phlegm, and the other may cool blood. In this way, the formula can be changed as the patient's symptoms change. This is one argument against the prolific use of standardized formulas.

Chinese Herbal Formulas

In most cases, a syndrome will have more than one symptom and cannot be treated with a single herb. Thus, the primary method of herbal therapy used in TCM is the herbal formula. Although many practitioners will use their own formulas to treat patients, most will use established classic formulas with one or two modifications. The general format for herbal formulas is the use of three or more specific herbs. The primary herb, which treats the major symptom, is called the king herb; the second herb will reinforce the action of the king herb as well as treat the concurrent symptoms and is called the subject herb. Other herbs are then added to control undesirable effects of the first. These last are two called the assistant herbs. The fourth herb may be one that can direct the formula to the affected region and harmonize the herbs in the formula; it is called the servant herb.

How to Take Chinese Herbs

TCM formulas are commonly taken three ways: as a decoction, as a powder or in granular form, or by tablet. A decoction is considered the best method, although it is often not practical for many patients. Decoctions are made from raw herbs that are placed in a pot of water and cooked/boiled for an average of 20 minutes. The benefit of a decoction is that it is readily absorbed by the body, takes effect more quickly, and can produce the best therapeutic effect.

Powders or granules can be dissolved in water. However, the quantity will depend on a patient's weight. The disadvantage of a powder is similar to that of most powdered drinks: They are difficult to dissolve completely and absorption by the body is slower.

The most common method of taking herbs is in tablet form, normally made by a manufacturer, not by the individual consumer. The advantage of tablets is the ease of taking the medication and convenience but they have slow absorption rates and cannot be adjusted. The quality of the product depends on the manufacturing process.

Rules for Taking a Formula

In general, taking Chinese herbal formulas is guided by three rules: timing, temperature, and not accompanying the herbal formula with a tea. To get the most beneficial effect from an herbal formula, when and how to take the herb must be understood. Some herbs are better absorbed with food, others without. In addition, in accordance with TCM theory, during certain times of the day the energy of a certain organ system is highest and depending on the action of the herb and the organ's condition, taking the herb during those times will improve the effect that the herb has on the organ.

Next, the temperature of the herbal formula should be considered, depending on the condition being treated. If a cold condition is being treated, the temperature of the herbal formula should be hot, and if a heat condition is being treated, the herb is best taken cold.

Finally, the patient should refrain from taking herbal formulas with tea for three reasons. First, tea can obstruct the movement of the herb and reduce its effect. Second, tea is also cold in nature and can interfere with warming herbs. And third, tea contains caffeine and can excite the nervous system, cancelling the effect of calming herbs.

Insomnia

Depending on the source, according to TCM insomnia can be caused by several conditions: heart–spleen deficiency, heart–kidney disconnect, heart–gallbladder deficiency, phlegm fire, or indigestion from eating too late in the evening. For the purpose of illustration, one of these differential diagnoses (heart–spleen deficiency) is presented to show the rationale behind the herbal formula selection and how each ingredient can be modified (added or removed) depending on the patient's clinical presentation.

CLINICAL PEARL

TCM Diagnosis

Although this text does not cover TCM diagnosis or an explanation of the disorder mentioned (e.g., spleen deficiency or heart fire), the general purpose of including a differential diagnosis is to demonstrate how diverse TCM diagnosis is and how it applies to the choice of herbal medicine prescribed. Please refer to TCM textbooks to understand TCM diagnosis.

Heart–Spleen Deficiency

In TCM, insomnia is often associated with the heart because it is considered to be the place where the mind (shen) resides, and disturbances of the shen often result in the symptom of insomnia. Symptoms of a heart–spleen deficiency include sleeplessness and waking often, abdominal swelling, watery thin stools, poor appetite, fatigue, impotence, night sweats, and palpitations. The treatment principle is to tone the heart and spleen and calm the mind (shen).

Herbal Formula for Insomnia: Gui-Pi-Tang

Gui-Pi-Tang (decoction to restore the spleen) is used for spleen qi deficiency with heart blood and yin deficiency, and used to tonify qi and blood, nourish the heart, and strengthen the spleen. Therefore, the indications for its use are similar to those of heart–spleen deficiency: fatigue, palpitations, insomnia, poor sleep or dream-disturbed sleep, night sweats, but also include anxiety, phobias, poor appetite, sallow complexion, poor memory, withdrawal, and early menstrual periods with loss of excess blood, continuous spotting, blood in the stool, and metrorrhagia.

Gui Pi Tang—Ingredients

1. Bai Zhu 5 to 10 g (Rhizoma Atractylodis Macrocephalae) properties include aromatic, slightly acrid, nontoxic, sweet, and warm; supplements the spleen and qi; dries dampness; enters the spleen and stomach channels; and is used in the treatment of indigestion and stomach disorders.
2. Dang gui 12 g *(Angelica sinensis)* properties are warm, bitter, sweet, slightly pungent, and it supports the liver and spleen. It is used as a tonic for female deficiencies and to enrich blood, promote circulation, stimulate appetite, improve muscle tone, stimulate the immune system, and moisturize dryness.
3. Fu-shen 12 g *(Poria cocos)* is a mushroom. Its properties include a sweet taste; used to calm the liver and heart and quiet the spirit; enters the heart, spleen, and lung channel; and is used for palpitations, fearfulness, and bad memory due to a frightful experience. Considered a superb yin tonic.

4. **Gan cao** 6 g *(Radix glycyrrhizae)* or licorice root; its properties are sweet, neutral; tonifies the spleen and strengthens the qi; improves symptoms such as fatigue, lack of appetite, loose stools, and shortness of breath. Enters all 12 primary channels but particularly the lung, heart, spleen, and stomach. Used to lessen the harsh and toxic nature of other herbs and protect the middle jiao (the primary source of digestion) and enhance the overall effects of a formula. Often used with honey to treat drug poisoning or Xing Ren (Semen Armeniacaae Amarum) for lead poisoning.
5. **Huang qi** 20 g (Radix Astragali Membranacei) or astragalus; its properties are sweet, slightly warm; enters the lung and spleen channels, tonifies qi and blood, and is used to treat symptoms of spleen deficiency; can raise yang, tonify the wei qi (protective qi), treat spontaneous sweating, promote urination, and expel pus.
6. **Long yan rou** 15 g (Arillus Euphoriae Longanae) is flesh of the longan fruit and translated as "dragon eye flesh." Properties are sweet and warm; it enters the heart and spleen channel. Actions are primarily to tonify the blood.
7. **Suan zao ren** *(Ziziphus jujuba)* is commonly called sour jujube seed; the temperature and taste are neutral, sweet, and sour; and it supports several channels (gallbladder, heart, liver, spleen). It nourishes heart yin, nourishes blood, calms the spirit, and inhibits sweating. It is used to treat insomnia, irritability, dream-disturbed sleep due to yin, and blood deficiency, as well as wind-damp bi syndrome, and wind-heat skin rashes and itching. It is given in doses of 10 to 18 g or 1.5 to 3 g in powder form at bedtime. Suan zao ren is also given as a nourishing sedative.
8. **Yuan Zhi** 6 g (Radix Polygalae Tenuifoliae) or Chinese senega root; its properties are bitter, spicy, slightly warm; it enters the heart, lung, and liver channels. It is used to nourish the heart and calm the shen.

Single Herbs to Add to Formula

Bai zi ren *(Biota orientalis)* and others can be added to a formula. Commonly called arbor vitae seed, the temperature and taste are neutral and sweet, and it supports several channels (heart, kidney, large intestine, and spleen). Therefore, it is used to nourish the heart, and calm the spirit as well as moisten the intestine and unblock the bowels. Indications for its use include the treatment of insomnia, irritability, palpitations, anxiety, and forgetfulness due to heart blood deficiency. It is also used to treat constipation due to yin and blood deficiency and night sweats due to yin deficiency. Dosages are usually 10 to 18 g every day.

Yin Tonic Herbs

1. **Bai he.** Commonly called lily bulb, its temperature and taste are cold, bitter, and sweet, and it supports the heart and lung channel. It is used to moisten the lungs, clear the heat, calm the spirit and the heart, and stop cough. It is often used to treat menopause and also to treat dry cough and sore throat, insomnia, restlessness, and irritability. It is also used to treat qi and yin deficiency after a febrile disease. Often given in doses of 10 to 30 g daily.
2. **Bai mu er.** Its common name is fruiting body of tremella. Its temperature is neutral, sweet, and bland, and it supports the lung and stomach channel. It is used to tonify the lung and stomach, nourish yin, and generate fluids. It is also used to treat dry cough from lung heat and night sweats. The dosage is 3 to 10 g of herb, soaked for 1 to 2 hours in soup until it is soft.

Herbal Considerations

The example presented is just one herbal therapy for one of the several differential diagnoses causing insomnia according to the theories of TCM. It demonstrates the complexity of TCM herbal medicine and the diversity of choices and considerations available to a TCM herbal practitioner when treating a patient and attending disease. For this reason, TCM practitioners often question the value of standardized TCM formulas commonly found on the market. They also question the use of granules and raw herbs. Yet, consumer behavior may ultimately determine the outcome because raw herbs are difficult to prepare and take. Also, because of the herbs' unpleasant taste, consumers are more apt to take a pill than a preparation.

Ayurvedic Herbs

Ayurvedic herbology is based on the tridoshic theory that six basic tastes exist (sweet, sour, salty, pungent, astringent, and bitter). When used correctly, these tastes (associated with all plants, herbs, and food) can be used to balance or counter an excess or deficient condition. Therefore, the first and basic principle in ayurvedic medicine is the use of food, spices, and herbs not only to prevent and maintain good health but also to treat diseases. In general, sweet, sour, and salty tastes reduce vata, whereas bitter, pungent, and astringent tastes enhance it. Astringent, bitter, and sweet taste reduces pitta while sour, salty and pungent taste enhances it. Bitter, pungent, and astringent foods reduce kapha, whereas sweet, salty, and sour tastes enhance it. Using this formula, food, spices, and herbs with these specific effects are used to balance disharmonies in vata, pitta, and kapha conditions depending on the existence of an excess or deficient condition.

In women's health, for example, ayurvedic medicine considers women to possess a greater amount of vata characteristics than do men (women have a tendency to be cold, dry, and light), which increases with age (old age is considered to be vata dominant). Therefore, emphasis on foods, spices, and herbs possessing sweet, sour, and salty tastes are often prescribed. However, in recognizing the uniqueness in all people, ayurveda also recognizes that, as different as body types are, so too are peoples' nutritional requirements. For example, if a person is thin framed, always cold, with dry skin, the person is considered to have a vata constitution and should eat a vata-balanced diet as a lifetime program. However, if the person starts to retain water, feel sluggish, and have excess mucus, the person is demonstrating a kapha imbalance, and should avoid a sweet, sour, and salty diet and change to a bitter, astringent, and pungent diet until the body is back in balance.

Additional Approach

Although using tridoshic theory to individualize herbal therapy is the primary method used by ayurvedic practitioners, using herbs and herbal formulas that target specific disorders is a common approach when recommending commercial ayurvedic herbs and herbal formulas.

Common Ayurvedic Herbs

Digestive Disorders

In ayurvedic theory, most digestive disorders are a result of poor digestive *Agni,* fire, which is responsible for absorbing nutrients in food, destroying pathogens, and converting food that is acceptable to the digestive system. If Agni fire is weak, then the body will not be able to perform these functions and food can become a negative pathogen for the body, creating toxins and reducing the immune system.

Herbs that enhance Agni fire are generally pungent, sour, or salty (for example, black pepper, cayenne, or ginger). However, recommendations should be based on the condition of Agni fire. If it is too high, herbs such as aloe, barberry, and gentian are appropriate, and if variable, spices such as ginger, cumin, or rock salt are recommended. Generally, sustaining digestive fire is done with mild herbs (e.g., cardamom, turmeric, coriander, and fennel).

Selected Ayurvedic Formulas

Triphala

Triphala is a blend of herbs or three fruits: **amla** *(Emblica officinalis),* **bibitaki** *(Terminalia belerica),* and **haritaki** *(Terminalia chebula).* The fruits are dried, powdered, and mixed together and given as a general tonic and detoxifier. **Triphala** is taken every day to help balance all three doshas—amla controls pitta; bibitaki controls kapha; and harataki controls vata. **Triphala** has traditionally been used to treat gastrointestinal disorders and restore bowel health; however, most research has been isolated to animal trials. In 2007, a study evaluated the inhibitory activities of triphala against common bacterial isolates from HIV-infected patients. The study results supported an antibacterial activity by triphala against the bacterial isolates (Srikumar, Parthasarathy, & Shankar, 2007).

Trikatu is a blend of three herbs: ginger *(Zingiber officinale),* black pepper *(Piper nigrum),* and Indian long pepper *(Piper longum).* Used for its bitter taste, it rejuvenates digestive fire as well as the respiratory tract.

Rejuvenative Disorders

In ayurvedic theory, disorders that include symptoms of low energy, fatigue, lack of sexual motivation, anxiety, and impotence are often caused by vata (air) conditions. Therefore, tonification therapy will include an anti-vata diet including foods such as dairy products, ghee (clarified butter), nuts, okra, and meat. However, tonics such as **shatavari, chyavanprash,** and **ashwagandha** are commonly prescribed as well.

Shatavari Root

Shatavari root (Asparagus racemosus), in Sanskrit translates to "she who possesses a hundred husbands" and is the main women's ayurvedic tonic, with a role similar to that of the Chinese tonic dong quai. But it can also be used by men to treat impotence because it has a role similar to that of ginseng. **Shatavari** is a woody climber with pine-like needles, white flowers, and small spikes. **Shatavari** belongs to the Liliaceae family. By taste it is sweet and bitter, and it is cooling in nature. It is used as a nutritive and calming agent to regulate menstrual flow and boost hormonal triggers, making it valuable in treating menopausal complaints such as vaginal atrophy and in increasing female sexuality. Research on **shartavari** has found it to have multiple influences on the body, and it acts as an adaptogen, antitussive, antioxidant, antibacterial, immune-modulator, digestive, cyto-protective, galactogogue, anti-oxytocic (preventing the stimulation of involuntary muscles of the uterus), antispasmodic, antidiarrheal, and sexual tonic (Thomas, 2002).

Amla Fruit

Amla fruit (*Emblica officinalis,* Indian gooseberry) is a small, very sour fruit that is the most widely used as a general rejuvenate herb in ayurveda. This fruit is particularly high in vitamin C, having 20 to 30 times the amount found in oranges. The vitamin C in amla is also heat stable, surviving the cooling and drying process and making it an extremely powerful antioxidant. Amla is the principle ingredient in the jelly chyavanprash, which has been used for over a thousand years to help rejuvenate the body and fortify the mind.

Ashwagandha

Ashwagandha *(Withania somnifera),* or "Indian ginseng," has been used for hundreds of years for its ability to restore vitality and strength. It translates from Sanskrit as "the smell of a horse" and has traditionally been used as a male tonic. Classified as an adaptogen, **ashwagandha** contains steroidal lactones, alkaloids, choline, fatty acids, amino acids, and a variety of sugars.

Herbs for Common Disorders

Table 10–1 presents additional information on herbal medicines for common health problems. Although many

Table 10–1 **Selective Herbal Agents Used for Common Conditions**

Condition	Treatment
Candida	Garlic Berberine-containing herbs: Oregon grape, goldenseal, scutellaria, gentian, grapefruit seed extract Ginseng, astragalus, red clover, dandelion root, burdock root, asafetida, cumin
Constipation	Psyllium seeds, fennel, fenugreek, olive oil, cannabis seeds For constipation due to heat: turmeric, gentian, dandelion, Oregon grape, yellow dock Ayurvedic herb: triphala or rhubarb
Diarrhea	Blackberry root, raspberry leaf, agrimony, bayberry bark, oak bark, yarrow Spleen qi tonics: ginseng, *Codonopsis*, white atractylodes, and *Dioscorea* Cinnamon, ginger, or cardamom
Pain	
Headaches	Chinese herbs: Ligusticum (chuan xiong) or Chinese lovage Feverfew, chamomile, willow bark Western herbs: angelica Bupleurum, *Artemisia annua* (Sweet Annie) Menstrual headaches:, black cohosh, dandelion, chrysanthemum, and feverfew or the formula of dang gui, cooked rehmannia, white peony, and Ligusticum
Arthritis	Borage, capsicum, chondroitin, evening primrose oil, ginger glucosamine, turmeric
Insomnia	Chamomile, skullcap, valerian, or kava kava, passion flower, hops, ashwagandha to calm the nervous system, St. John's wort, lemon balm, *Schisandra*, jujube dates
Benign prostatic hypertrophy	Nettle, pumpkin seed, saw palmetto
Menorrhagia	Shepherd's purse tincture, 3 to 6 drops every 2 h or a combination of cattail pollen, agrimony, mugwort, yarrow, shepherd's purse, raspberry, and blackberry leaves Building blood with iron floradix or blackstrap molasses, along with Chinese herbs dang qui, lycii, cooked rehmannia, and white peony
Dysmenorrhea	Combination of equal parts of vitex, wild yam, block cohosh, dang qui, sassafras, and licorice with ½ part ginger
Urinary tract infections	Cornsilk tea, parsley, dandelion, horsetail, cranberry, and for extreme burning, use goldenseal, gentian, gardenia

Source: Adapted from Tierra, L. (2003). *Healing with the herbs of life.* Berkeley, CA: Crossing Press; Fetrow, C.W., & Avila, J. R. (1999). *Professional's handbook of complementary and alternative medicines.* Springhouse, PA: Springhouse.

other herbs may be used for these disorders, the ones listed have all been studied in human trials. Those not listed have been used and reported in case or anecdotal reports only.

HERBAL PREPARATIONS

The proper preparation of herbs ensures that they are used to their maximum effect. The following is a summary of several of the most common preparations and their proper use.

Bolus

Bolus refers to a suppository inserted into the rectum. Common herbs used are astringents such as white oak bark or bayberry bark; demulcents such as comfrey root or slippery elm; and antibiotics such as garlic, echinacea, chaparral, and golden seal.

Compress and Fomentation

Compress and fomentation are two different terms that refer to the same treatment, applying herbs externally to the body. This treatment is especially effective for herbs that are too strong to take internally but can be absorbed slowly in small amounts. Compresses are used to treat many superficial ailments such as swelling and pain and to stimulate circulation of blood or lymph in the area where applied.

Liniments

Liniments are warming herbal extracts rubbed in the skin. They are commonly used to relieve sore or strained muscles and to treat conditions such as arthritis or itchy skin.

Oils

Oils are concentrated extracts used for massaging the body. Oil preparations come in two types: soothing emollients that use herbs such as calendula flower, lavender, and lemon balm; and warming and stimulating oils that use herbs such as ginger, peppermint, and eucalyptus. Oils are usually infused for a particular herb with consideration given to the moistening capacity of the oil: nondrying oils include jojoba, cocoa butter, and avocado; semidrying oils include safflower and sunflower; drying oils include soybean and linseed (flax).

Capsules or Pills

Capsules or pills are the most popular preparations used in herbal therapy today because they are convenient and mimic western medicine. Prepared entirely with herbs, however, capsules generally have twice the concentration of pills.

Poultices and Plasters

Poultices and plasters are topical applications of herbs that have been powdered, crushed, or mashed and are usually applied moist, either hot or warm, and left on an area on the body for 12 to 20 hours. Caution must be taken to avoid skin reactions and burns.

Mixtures for Smoking

Mixtures for smoking are herbs, such as datura leaf, that patients smoke for the treatment of asthma. Smoking of herbs should be done only occasionally, and patients should be warned about the risk of lung disease, as with any smoking habit.

Teas

Teas are the most well-known method for taking herbs. Although tea is generally taken as beverage, it can have the strongest medicinal effect of any preparation, making it suitable for the most serious illnesses. To be effective, the proportion of herbs to water must be greater than usual.

Tinctures

Tinctures are an extract of herbs preserved in alcohol or vinegar. The advantage to a tincture is that it has long shelf life when stored in cool, dry place, whereas dried herbs begin to lose potency after the first year. Tinctures tend to make herbals energetically "hotter," and affect the circulatory system. Consideration of other chemical constituents found in alcohol such as glycosides and sugars must be taken into account.

CONSIDERATIONS FOR THE ADVANCED PRACTICE NURSE PRESCRIBER

People use herbal remedies instead of conventional medicines for many reasons. Sometimes these reasons are not consistent with those of western medicine or supported by evidence-based studies; however, health-care providers have to respect a consumer's right to choose and acknowledge that consumers are using herbs at an ever-growing rate. Therefore, nurse practitioners, physicians, physician's assistants and other health-care providers should be prepared to educate patients about the many different concepts and herbal traditions used and help guide them to an appropriate resource. In addition, providers need to educate themselves about the herbs commonly used by their patients and be aware of the growing amount of research that is being conducted to evaluate interactions with herbal therapy and allopathic medicines.

Because a product is natural, does not mean it is risk free. In the late 1980s a particular brand of **L-tryptophan** tablets resulted in several cases of fatal eosinophilia myalgia, and from 1993 to 1997 several hundred cases of serious adverse effects were documented from **ephedra** in diet and weight-loss supplements. However, some herbal preparations, such as **astragalus** and **dong quai** for the treatment of infections and menopause, have been accepted and found to be relatively safe when used in combination with western medication.

What is seriously overlooked, though, when consumers and nonherbalists speak either positively or negatively about any given herb is an acknowledgment of the many different herbal traditions and of those practitioners who are either certified in herbal therapy or trained in a given medical discipline that has a history of using herbal therapy but do not fall within the definitions of western medicine. Often a failure of consulting or evaluation of a specific herbal theory or with herbal medicine practitioners is what leads to the adverse effects cited in clinical research and by consumers.

Health-care professionals need to keep an open mind to all the possible ways to treat health problems, and that ultimately may require the inclusion or consideration of medical systems that are not commonly practiced by western culture. Primary care providers may need to explore the resources available to the public at large, critique the

BOX 10–1 WEB-BASED RESOURCES FOR HERBS AND ALTERNATIVE THERAPIES

American Botanical Council http://www.herbalgram.org
American Herbalist Guild http://www.americanherbalistsguild.com
Biofeedback Certification Institute of America http://www.bcia.org
National Center for Complimentary and Alternative Medicine http://nccam.nih.gov
Natural Standard: The Authority on Integrative Medicine http://www.naturalstandard.com/
Cochrane Database of Systematic Reviews http://www.cochran.org

information, and assist patients in finding practitioners that can meet their needs for non–western-based treatments. However, professionals must also recognize their scope of practice and not venture into prescribing or recommending without adequate knowledge and training in the area.

HERBS IN SELECTED MEDICAL CONDITIONS

Hypertension

Evidence supports the inclusion of mixed fish oil, **coenzyme Q10**, and probably calcium in the treatment of both essential and primary hypertension. Clinical consideration should also be given to incorporation of both acupuncture and mind–body techniques, in addition to diet modification and exercise. Because of the broad systemic effects and safety profile of these interventions, supplemental therapy should be used to help control hypertension, prevent progression to advanced stages, and potentially decrease polypharmacy use. Table 10-2 and Table 10-3 discuss the comparison grading criteria for the evidence related to the use of CAM in the treatment of hypertension and hyperlipidemia

Hyperlipidemia

Diet and lifestyle modifications, combined with appropriate supplementation, have strong evidence for treating high cholesterol. **Psyllium** husk as fiber and mixed

BOX 10–2 **HERBAL RESOURCES**

Banyan Botanical
6705 Eagle Rock Ave, NE
Albuquerque, NM 87113
1-800-953-6424
http://www.banyanbotanicals.com
Good source for ayurvedic herbs

East West School of Herbology
P.O. Box 275
Ben Lomond, CA 95005
1-800-717-5010
herbcourse@planetherbs.com or http://wwww.planteherbs.com
Sponsor of planetary herbal formulas; supplies western, eastern, and ayurvedic herbs

Herb Pharm
Box 116
Williams, OR 97544
1-800-348-4372
http://www.herb-pharm.com
Specializing in herbal tinctures

Mountain Rose Herbs
P.O. Box 50220
Eugene, OR 97405
1-800-879-3337
http://www.mountainroseherbs.com
Large selection of bulk organic herbs, spices, teas, essential oils, and bulk ingredients

Spring Wind Herb Company
2325 4th Street #6
Berkeley, CA 94710
Good source for Chinese herbs

The Tao of Tea
3430 SE Belmont Street
Portland OR 97214
1-503-736-0198
http://www.taooftea.com
Good selection of herbal teas

Table 10–2 **Comparison of Grading Criteria: Hypertension**

CAM Therapy*	Natural Standard,™	Healthnotes,™	Rakel©	WHO	Commission- E
Acupuncture	Grade C			Category 1 (essential & primary HTN)	
Diet/exercise	Grade B (qi gong/yoga)		A1		
Mind–body	Grade B		B1		
Coenzyme Q10	Grade B	3 Star	B2		
Fish oil(mixed EPA/DHA)	Grade A	3 Star	A2		Approved component
Calcium	Grade B	2 Star			

continued

Table 10–2 **Comparison of Grading Criteria: Hypertension—cont'd**

CAM Therapy*	Natural Standard,™	Healthnotes,™	Rakel©	WHO	Commission- E
Magnesium		2 Star			
Garlic	Grade C	2 Star			Approved
Hawthorn (*Crataegus* spp.)	Grade D	1 Star		B1	Approved

Cochrane Summary:

- Review of calcium demonstrated positive effects but reviewers concluded data were insufficient because of poor study design and lack of heterogeneity between trials, leading to bias.
- Garlic review for peripheral arterial occlusion was inconclusive. No statistical significance in walking distances was seen.
- EPA/DHA are essential fatty acids; eicosapentaenoic acid and docosahexaenoic acid.

*Table not inclusive.

Table 10–3 **Comparison of Grading Criteria: Hyperlipidemia**

CAM Therapy	Natural Standard,™	Healthnotes,™	Rakel©	WHO	Commission- E*
Acupuncture				Category 2	
Diet/exercise	Grade B (Yoga)		A1		
Mind–body	Grade C				
Plant sterols	Grade A	3 Star	A2		
Psyllium	Grade A	2 Star	A2		Approved as fiber for constipation and diarrhea
Fish oil (Mixed EPA/DHA)	Grade A	3 Star	A2		Approved component
B vitamins	Grade A	3 Star (niacin—B_3)	A2		
Guggul *(Commifora mukul)*	Grade C	3 Star			Not approved
Fenugreek *(Trigonella foenum-graecum)*	Grade C	2 Star			Approved as appetite stimulator and digestive aid
Red yeast rice *(Monascus purpureus)*	Grade A	2 Star			
Garlic	Grade B		2 Star		Approved

Cochrane Summary:

- Omega-3 fatty acids (fish oils) have strong evidence for lowering triglycerides and Very –low-density lipoprotein (VLDL) a type of lipoprotein made by the liver and one of the five major groups of lipoproteins.
- No conclusive data on dietary intervention for familial hyperlipidemia.
- Plant sterol review currently pending.
- Garlic protocol currently pending.

*Table not inclusive: Commission E approval is specific per condition unless otherwise noted.

EPA/DHA fish oil should be considered as standard treatment because of the impact they have on both cholesterol and blood pressure. **Niacin** (vitamin B_3) is available by prescription. **Red yeast rice**, **garlic**, and **guggul** can be considered as adjuncts, as these herbs also affect blood glucose levels and hematological clotting parameters. The cholesterol-lowering properties of **red yeast rice** are largely due to fungal metabolites known as monacolins, one of which, monacolin K, is identical to **lovastatin** and has been found to be effective at lowering cholesterol with minimal side effects (Becker, Gordon, Halbert, & French, 2009). However, **guggul** has been associated with elevated liver function test and acute hepatitis (Geico, Miete, Pompili, & Biolato, 2009). Therefore, the practitioner should still screen the patient for liver abnormalities prior to starting these herbs and monitor him or her during therapy. Although the risks are lower, product uniformity, purity, labeling, and safety cannot be guaranteed, and it is the responsibility of the provider to solicit information from a particular company regarding production process to ensure patient safety. Implications for practice are discussed in Table 10-4 and Table 10-5.

Table 10–4 Clinical Implications for Practice: Hypertension Example

Herb/Supplement	Indications	Contraindications	Dose	Rakel Harm Scale©
Coenzyme Q10	HTN	None	90–150 mg/qd	2
Fish oil (mixed EPA/DHA)	HTN	Coagulation (bleeding) disorders	3 g/qd	2
Calcium	HTN	Hypercalcemia, Constipation, kidney stones, prostate cancer	800–1,500 mg/qd	
Magnesium	HTN	Caution in renal insufficiency	250–350 mg/qd	
Garlic	Hyperlipidemia	Allergy Caution with warfarin (WHO)	1–3 g/qd	
Hawthorn (*Crataegus* spp.)	Cardiac insufficiency/heart failure	Allergy	Varies with form: Tincture 35% ETOH 406 mL/tid Tea: 5–10 g/tid	1

*Dosing recommendation compiled from Healthnotes,™, Natural Standards,™, ABC Clinical recommendations, and Bastyr University clinical monographs.

Table 10–5 Hyperlipidemia Example

Herb/Supplement	Indications	Contraindications	Dose	Rakel Harm Scale©
Plant sterols	Hyperlipidemia	None (Caution in estrogen receptor + neoplasms)	2–3 g/qd	2
Psyllium	Hyperlipidemia	Caution in IBS	10–30 g/qd	
Fish oil (mixed EPA/DHA)	Hyperlipidemia HTN	Coagulation (bleeding) disorders	3 g/qd	2
Niacin (B_3)	Hyperlipidemia Depression	Active liver disease, active ulcer or arterial bleeding	1 g/tid	2
Guggul *(Commifora mukul)*	Hyperlipidemia	Allergy, coagulation (bleeding) disorders, and pregnancy/ lactation	25 mg/bid (standardized extract guggulsterone)	
Fenugreek *(Trigonella foenum-graecum)*	Poor digestion Hyperlipidemia Type 1 and 2 diabetes	Early pregnancy, hyperchlorhydria/gastroesophageal reflux disease (GERD) and active peptic ulcer	Tincture: 30% ETOH, 3–5 mL/tid	
Red yeast rice *(Monascus purpureus)*	Hyperlipidemia	Pregnancy and lactation	1,200 mg/bid	
Garlic	Hyperlipidemia	Allergy Caution with warfarin (WHO)	1–3 g/qd	

*Dosing recommendation compiled from Healthnotes,™, Natural Standards,™, ABC Clinical recommendations, and Bastyr University clinical monographs.

BOX 10–3 SUGGESTED READING

Western Herbs

Bach, Phyllis A. *Prescription for Herbal Healing*. New York: Avery Books, 2002.

Kushi, Michio. *The Book of Macrobiotics: The Universal Way of Health, Happiness, and Peace*. New York: Japan Publications, 1977.

Pitchford, Paul. *Healing With Whole Foods: Asian Traditions and Modern Nutrition* (3rd ed.). Berkeley, CA: North Atlantic Books, 2002.

Tierra, Michael. *Planetary Herbology*. Santa Fe: Lotus Press, 1988.

Weil, Andrew. *Health and Healing: The Philosophy of Integrative Medicine and Optimum Health*. New York: Houghton Mifflin, 2004.

Chinese Medicine

Beinfield, Harriet, & Efrem Korngold. *Between Heaven and Earth: A Guide to Chinese Medicine*. New York: Ballantine Books, 1992.

Chen, John K., & Tina T. Chen. *Chinese Herbal Formulas and Applications*. City of Industry, CA: Art of Medicine Press, 2008.

Chen, John K., & Tina T. Chen. *Chinese Medical Herbology and Pharmacology*. City of Industry, CA: Art of Medicine Press, 2001.

Maciocia, Giovanni. *The Foundations of Chinese Medicine*. New York: Churchill Livingstone, 1989.

Ayurvedic Medicine

Lad, Vasant. *Ayurveda: A Practical Guide: The Science of Self-Healing*. Twin Lakes, WI: Lotus Press, 1984.

Lad, Vasant. *The Complete Book of Ayurvedic Home Remedies*. New York: Three Rivers Press, 1999.

Tiwari, Maya, *Ayurveda Secrets of Healing*. Twin Lakes, WI: Lotus Press, 1995.

Tiwari, Maya. *A Life of Balance: The Complete Guide to Ayurvedic Nutrition and Body Types with Recipes*. Rochester, VT: Healing Arts Press, 1995.

General Recommendations

Blome, Gotz. *Advanced Bach Flower Therapy: A Scientific Approach to Diagnosis and Treatment*. Rochester, VT: Healing Arts Press, 1999.

Buhner, Stephen Harrod. *The Lost Language of Plants: The Ecological Importance of Plant Medicines to Life on Earth*. White River Junction, VT: Chelsea Green, 2002.

Cowan, Eliot. *Plant Spirit Medicine*. Columbus, NC: Swan-Raven, 1995.

Pollan, Michael. *The Omnivore's Dilemma: A Natural History of Four Meals*. New York: Penguin, 2007.

Tierra, L. *Healing With the Herbs of Life*. Berkeley, CA: Crossing Press, 2003.

REFERENCES

Adams, K., Lindell, K., Kohlmeier, M., & Zeisel, S. H. (2006). Status of nutrition education in medical schools. *American Journal of Clinical Nutrition, 83*(Suppl.), 941S–944S.

American Botanical Council (ABC). (2009). Commission E monographs. Retrieved February 24, 2009, from http://www.herbalgram.org

American Herbalist Guild (AHG). (2007). *American Herbalist Guild—An Association of Herbal Practitioners*. Retrieved February 1, 2009, from http://www.americanherbalistsguild.com

Barnes P.M., & Bloom, B. (2008, December). The Use of Complementary and Alternative Medicine in the United States. National Institute of Health. Retrieved April 17, 2009, from http://nccam.nih.gov/news/camstats/2007/camsurvey_fs1.htm

Barnes, P.M., Bloom, B., & Nahim, R. L. (2008). Complementary and alternative medicine use among adults and children: United States, 2007, *National Health Statistics Report, 12*, 1–23.

Bastyr University. (2008). Bastyr University catalog 2008–2009 [Brochure]. Kent, WA: Author.

Becker, D. J., Gordon, R.Y., Halbert, S. C., & French, B. (2009). Red yeast rice for dyslipidemia in statin-intolerant patients: A randomized trial. *Annals of Internal Medicine, 150*(12), 830–839.

Biofeedback Certification Institute of America. (n.d.). Entry level general biofeedback certification information. Retrieved April 28, 2009, from http://www.bcia.org

Biomedical Acupuncture Institute. (2005). Biomedical acupuncture course descriptions. Retrieved May 30, 2009, from www.biomedicalacupuncture.com

Blum, R.L. (n.d.) Essays, retrieved December 2010 from; http://www.bobblum.com/ESSAYS/MEDICINE/EVIDENCE.html

Bob Flaws, P.S. (2005). *The treatment of modern western diseases with Chinese medicine: A textbook and clinical manual* (2nd ed.). Boulder, CO: Blue Poppy Press.

Brzezinski, A. (1997). Melatonin in humans. *New England Journal of Medicine, 336*, 186–195.

Buettner, C., Mukamal, K. J., Gardiner, P., & Davis, R. B. (2009). Herbal supplement use and blood levels of United States adults. *Journal of General Internal Medicine, 24*(11), 1175–1182.

Centers for Disease Control and Prevention, National Center for Health Statistics. (2008). Americans make nearly four medical visits a year on average. Retrieved November 17, 2008, from http://www.cdc.gov/nchs/about.htm

Chavez, M. L. (1997). Saint John's wort. *Hospital Pharmacy, 32*, 1621–1632.

Chen, J. K., & Chen, T.T. (2001). *Chinese medical herbology and pharmacology*. City of Industry, CA: Art of Medicine Press.

Cheng, Y. L., Lee, S. C., Harn, H. J., Huang, H. C., & Chang, W. L. (2008). The extract of *Hibiscus syriacus* inducing apoptosis by activating p53 and AIF in human lung cancer cells. *American Journal of Chinese Medicine, 36*(1), 171–184.

Cochrane Collaboration. (n.d.). *The Cochrane database of systematic reviews*. Retrieved January 15, 2009, from http://www.cochran.org.

Demory-Luce, D., & McPherson, R. S. (1999). Nutritional knowledge and attitudes of physician assistants. *Topics in Clinical Nutrition, 14*(2), 71–82.

Dietary Supplement Health and Education Act of 1994. (1994). Retrieved February 1, 2006, http://www.cfsan.fda.gov/dms/dietsupp.html

Ebell, M. H., Siwek, J., & Weiss, B. D. (2004). Strength of Recommendations Taxonomy (SORT): A patient centered approach to grading evidence in the medical literature. *American Family Physician. 69*, 548–556.

Eisenberg, D. F., Davis, R. B., & Ettner, S. L. (1998). Trends in alternative medicine use in the United States, 1990–1997. *Journal of the American Medical Association, 280*(18), 1569–1575.

Farnsworth, N. (1993). Relative Safety of Herbal Medicine. *Herbalgram*, 29, 36A–36H.

Fetrow, C.W., & Avila, J. R. (1999). *Professional's handbook of complementary & alternative medicines*. Springhouse, PA: Springhouse.

Forgues, E. (2009). Methodological issues pertaining to the evaluation of the effectiveness of energy-based therapies, avenues for a methodological guide. *Journal of Complementary and Integrative Medicine, 6*(1), 1–19.

Fortin, M., Bravo, G., Hudon, C., Vanasse, A., & Lapointe, L. (2005). Prevalence of multimorbidity among adults seen in family practice. *Annals of Family Medicine, 3,* 223–228.

Gaby, A. R. (2006). *The natural pharmacy: Complete A–Z reference to natural treatments for common health conditions* (3rd ed.). New York: Three Rivers Press.

Geico, A., Miele, L., Pompili, M., & Biolato, M. (2009). Acute hepatitis caused by a natural lipid-lowering product: When "alternative" medicine is no "alternative" at all. *Journal of Hepatology, 50*(6), 1273–1277.

Hamilton, J. L., Roemheld-Hamm, B., Young, D. M., Jalba, M., & DiCicco-Bloom, B. (2008). Complementary and alternative medicine in U.S. family medicine practices: A pilot qualitative study. *Alternative Therapies in Health & Medicine, 14*(3), 22–27.

Hayes, M., Buckley, D., & Judkins, D. Z. (2007). Are any alternative therapies effective in treating asthma? *Journal of Family Practice, 56*(5), 385–389.

Hirschkorn, K. A., & Bourgeault, I. L. (2008). Structural constraints and opportunities for CAM use and referral by physicians, nurses, and midwives. *Health: An Interdisciplinary Journal for the Social Study of Health, Illness & Medicine, 12*(2), 193–213.

Hoffer, J. L. (2003). Complementary or alternative medicine: The need for plausibility. *Journal of the Canadian Medical Association, 168*(2), 180–182.

Institute for Functional Medicine. (2006). *Textbook of functional medicine.* Gig Harbor, WA: Author.

Institute for Functional Medicine. (2009). *Functional medicine certification program* [Brochure]. Gig Harbor, WA: Author.

Jadad, A. R., Moore, R. A., Carroll, D., Jenkinson, C., Reynolds, D. J., Gavaghan, D. J., et al. (1996). Assessing the quality of reports of randomized clinical trials: Is blinding necessary? *Controlled Clinical Trials, 17*(1), 1–12.

Jenkins, J. J., Jonkman, E., Leonard, J. H., Petrini, J. O., & van Lier, J. J. (1997). The cognitive, subjective, and physical effects of a ginkgo biloba/panax ginseng combination in health volunteers with neurasthenic complaints. *Psychopharmacology Bulletin, 33*(4), 677–683.

Joslin Diabetes Center and Joslin Clinic. (2007, January). *Joslin Diabetes Center clinical guideline for pharmacological management of type 2 diabetes.* Boston: Joslin Diabetes Center; Publication Department.

Kaptchuk, T. (2000). The web that has no weaver: understanding Chinese medicine. Chicago: Contemporary Books.

Kennedy, J. (2005). Herb and supplement use in the U.S. adult population. *Clinical Therapists, 27*(11), 1847–1858.

Khan, A. U., & Gilani, A. H. (2009). Antispasmodic and bronchodilator activities of *Artemisia vulgaris* are dedicated through dual blockade of muscarinic receptors and calcium influx. *Journal of Ethnopharmacology, 126*(3), 480–486.

Khan, A. Safdar, M. Mohammad, M.A.K., Khan, N. K., & Anderson, R. A. (2003). Cinnamon improves glucose and lipids of people with type 2 diabetes. *Diabetes Care, 26*(12), 3215–3218.

Kleronomos, C. A. (2009). *Complementary and alternative medicine course development: Evidence for primary care.* Unpublished scholarly project submitted in partial fulfillment of the requirements for MSN, Seattle University.

Lad, V. (2002). *Textbook of ayurveda: Fundamental principles.* Albuquerque, NM: Ayurvedic Press.

Lino, M., Dinkins, J., & Bente, L. (1999). Household expenditures on vitamins and minerals by income level. *Family Economics and Nutrition Review,* 1–6.

Liu, C., & Tseng, A. (2003). *Chinese herbal medicine: Modern applications of traditional formulas.* Boca Raton, FL: CRC Press.

Ma, Y. (2007). Biomedical acupuncture: An evidence based acupuncture model. *Medical Acupuncture, 19*(4), 217–223.

Macciocia, G. (2005). *The foundations of Chinese medicine* (2nd ed.). Philadelphia: Churchstone Livingstone.

Mills, S., & Bone, K. (2000). *Principles and practice of phytotherapy: Modern herbal medicine.* Philadelphia: Churchill Livingstone.

Mind–body medicine in primary care. (2003). *Journal of the American Board of Family Practice, 16*(2), 131–147.

Murphy, J. J., Heptinstall, S., & Mitchell, J. R. (1988). Randomized, double-blind, placebo-controlled trial of feverfew in migraine prevention. *Lancet, 2,* 189–192.

National Center for Complementary and Alternative Medicine. (2008). The use of complementary and alternative medicine in the United States. Retrieved January 19, 2009, from http://nccam.nih.gov/

National Institutes of Health, National Cancer Institute. (n.d.). Definition: German Commission E. Retrieved March 14, 2009, from http://www.cancer.gov

Natural Standard. (2009). Natural Standard integrative medicine database. Retrieved from http://www.naturalstandard.com/

Pizzorno, J. E., & Murray, M. T. (2006). *Textbook of natural medicine* (3rd ed.). St. Louis, MO: Churchill Livingstone Elsevier.

Porter, S., & O'Halloran, P. (2009). The postmodernist war on evidence-based practice. *International Journal of Nursing Studies, 46*(5), 740–748.

Prout, L. (2000). *Live in the balance.* New York: Marlowe.

Rakel, D. (2007). *Integrative Medicine* (2nd ed.). Philedelphia: Saunders Elsevier.

Rakel, D. P., Guerrera, M. P., Bayles, B. P., Desai, G. J., & Ferrara, E. (2008). CAM education: Promoting a salutogenic focus in health care. *Journal of Alternative and Complementary Medicine, 14*(1), 87–93.

Rotblatt, M., & Ziment, I. (2002). *Evidence-based herbal medicine.* Philadelphia: Hanley & Belfus.

Schwartz, L. (2000). Evidence-based medicine and traditional Chinese medicine: Not mutually exclusive. *Medical Acupuncture, 12*(1).

Sorensen, H., & Sonne, J. (1996). A double-masked study of the effects of ginseng on cognitive function. *Current Therapy Research, 57,* 959–968.

Srikumar, R., Parthasarathy, N. J., & Shankar, E. M., (2007). Evaluation of the growth inhibitory activities of triphala against common bacterial isolates from HIV infected patients. *Phytotherapy Research, 21*(5), 476–480.

Thomas, M. (2002). Shatavari–*Asparagus racemosus.* Retrieved from http://www.Phytomedicine.com

Tierra, M. (1989). *Planetary herbology.* Twin Lakes, WI: Lotus Press.

Tiwari, M. (1995a). *Ayurveda: A life of balance.* Rochester, VT: Healing Arts Press.

Tiwari, M. (1995b). *Ayurveda: Secrets of healing.* Twin Lakes, WI: Lotus Press.

Tonelli, M., & Callahan T. (2001). Why alternative medicine cannot be evidence-based. *Academic Medicine, 76*(12), 1213–1220.

University of Arizona, Arizona Center for Integrative Medicine. (2009). Fellowship. Retrieved April 7, 2009, from http://www.integrativemedicine.arizona.edu

U.S. Food and Drug Administration. (2009). Quality systems regulation. Retrieved from http://www.fda.gov/cdrh/comp/gmp.html

Viskoper, R., Shapira, I., Priluck, R., Mindlin, R., Chornia, L., Laszt, A., et al. (2003). Non-pharmacological treatment of resistant hypertensives by device-guided slow breathing exercises. *American Journal of Hypertension, 16,* 484–487.

Volz, H. P. (1997). Kava-kava extract WS-1490 versus placebo in anxiety disorders: A randomized placebo-controlled 25-week outpatient trial. *Pharmacopsychiatry, 30,* 1–5.

Wesnes, K. A., Faleni, R. A., Hefting, N. R., Hoogsteen, G., Houben, J. J., & Weisfeld, V. (2009). Summit on integrated medicine and health of the public: Issue background and overview. *Institute of Medicine Summit on Integrative Medicine and the Health of the Public,* 1–16.

Williams, D. D. R., & Garner, J. (2002). The case against "the evidence": A different perspective on evidence-based medicine, *British Journal of Psychiatry, 180,* 8–12.

Wolkowitz, O. M. (1997). Dehydroepiandrosterone treatment of depression. *Biological Psychiatry, 41,* 311–318.

World Health Organization. (2003). Acupuncture: Review and analysis of reports on controlled clinical trials. Retrieved December 28, 2008, from http://www.who.int/en/

Yan, J., Engle, V., He, Y., Jiao, Y., & Gu, W. (2009). Study designs of randomized controlled trials not based on Chinese medicine theory are improper. *Chinese Medicine, 4*(1).

CHAPTER 11

INFORMATION TECHNOLOGY AND PHARMACOTHERAPEUTICS

Danita Lee Ewing

Chapter Outline

Several dramatic changes are occurring in health-care informatics. One is a change in emphasis from the information technology (IT) itself—something only a small number of people knew how to use—to how IT can support the processes of prescribing. A second change is acknowledging that there is an urgent need for adopting and integrating information systems into care. A third change is the convergence of technology into such devices as smart phones. Finally, patients, who are more familiar with forms of IT, expect to see it used as part of their health care.

Increasingly, health-care providers are expected to master the use of various information technologies in their clinical practice. This chapter explores ways IT and informatics (a blending of information science and technology) can help advanced practice nurses and other health-care providers fulfill their prescriptive roles efficiently and safely. The first section of the chapter provides an overview of current technology issues and the uses, strengths, and limitations of various forms of IT. The second section focuses on ways IT can assist the advanced practice nurse before, during, and after a patient encounter. Each of these areas is not without controversy and contradictions, which will be discussed.

First is a brief discussion of hardware and software that can form a foundation to support providers' prescribing role. Interested readers can find additional information in journals such as those in the reference list, online, and in books such as *Computers for Nurses*.

OVERVIEW

The American Nurses Association has a set of informatics competencies expected of nurses (Bickford & Humes, 2008). Experienced nurses are expected to be skillful information managers who are able to use IT to manage data, knowledge, and information in their specialty; search for information effectively; and secure the safety and integrity of health information. Nurses are expected to be able to serve as content experts in developing, implementing, and evaluating systems and act as champions in the adoption of health IT. Skillful documentation and analysis of data are also expected. Being knowledgeable about IT and how it may be used in clinical practice is an important aspect of a nurse's competence.

Process Versus Task

Currently, most health IT is designed with a task focus. For example, computerized provider order entry (CPOE) is one of the most researched and used forms of health IT. CPOE designers view entering orders as a discrete, linear task, without examining and integrating the nonlinear aspects. CPOE is a seen as one person generating orders. The reality of practice is quite different. Prescribing is a task requiring communication among multiple people and based on a particular set of reasons or decisions. Medication errors most often occur when communication breaks down. Providers may need to change their prescribing processing patterns. For example, instead of reaching for a hard-copy drug book, the prescriber may use a system such as Micromedix to look up the needed drug information. Some electronic health record (EHR) systems have drug databases of information embedded in the ordering screens. Prescribers can click on a highlighted link and look up information without having to find a book or open other software. Web browsing can also be used to look up a current guideline or new drug. Getting into the habit of bookmarking and organizing sites can also help the provider manage and process needed information quickly when making prescribing decisions.

Additionally, while decision support systems may give alerts, they rarely say *why* a particular option is important or take the unique context of the patient's situation into account (Berner & Moss, 2005; Walker & Carayon, 2009). Providers weigh contextual information in a dynamic process of decision making when prescribing. Decision support systems are more generic and static. Reimagining ways to use health IT to support the provider care is critical to maximizing benefits while minimizing negatives (Walker & Carayon, 2009). This shift in focus from task to process requires changes in policy, system design, and user education. Budgets for system design and education of staff are often stretched thin after the initial outlay for the expensive hardware and software setup. Such monetary concerns make it difficult to attend to process rather than isolated tasks. Examination of processes takes time and attention to detail but can result in more effective, safer systems.

The promise of a safer, more efficient, less costly healthcare system because of the use of IT is one of the driving forces in its adoption. However, several barriers and concerns exist before the goals of safe and efficient IT system implementation can be realized. Table 11–1 summarizes pros and cons of IT system use from patient/consumer and provider standpoints.

Unclear Definitions, Regulations, and Standards

The federal government plans to link Medicare and Medicaid reimbursement for services with electronic health record (EHR) implementation. Beginning in 2011, federal stimulus money from Centers for Medicare & Medicaid Services (CMS) will be available to facilitate EHR implementation over the course of 5 years. The qualifying EHR system must be used in a meaningful way. On July 13, 2010, the U.S. Department of Health and Human Services (DHHS) announced final rules to support "meaningful use" of EHR. One regulation defines the "meaningful use" objectives that providers must meet and provides the framework for the incentives program using stimulus money, and a second regulation identifies the technical

Table 11–1 **Advantages and Disadvantages of Computers as Information Sources**

	Advantages	Disadvantages
From the patient's view	• Convenience of access to information on demand • Ability to individualize the information search • Access at distant sites, in rural areas, and to patients with mobility issues • Provision of emotional support, especially from peers • Anonymity and perceived objectivity of information	• Cost, especially of initial investment • Potential for misinformation • Confidentiality risks • Lack of access to the technology • Lack of access to information on how to use the technology
From the provider's view	• Convenience of access to information on demand • Access to highly skilled experts • Access at distant sites in rural areas • Access to evidence-based guidelines and recommendations • Point of care access	• Cost, especially of initial investment • Compatibility between systems • Frequent system updates required • Patient confidentiality risks • Time needed to learn to use versus time it saves • Data fatigue

capabilities required for EHR technology to be certified. Information on these regulations and the incentive program is found at http://cms.gov/EHRincentive and http://healthit.hhs.gov/standardsandcertification. If EHR is not implemented by 2014, beginning in 2015 providers will have Medicare reimbursement rates cut by up to 3 percent ("EMR: One Hospital That Got It Right," 2009). At present, only about 1.5 percent of acute care hospitals have fully implemented EHR and only 8 percent have a basic EHR system in operation.

Electronic health records have drawbacks. Table 11–2 lists the advantages and disadvantages of these types of records.

Financial Issues

Costs, which range from $20 to $200 million for hospitals, have been identified as a major barrier to implementation of EMR ("EMR: One Hospital That Got It Right," 2009). Roughly 3 percent of operating expenses are dedicated to IT (Doyle, 2009). For small private or solo practices, the costs can be prohibitive. Many vendors do not focus on small or solo practices at present. Rural hospitals face cost issues because of small size, limited resources and high risk for being at the "last mile" or slower end of the information highway. The references at the end of the chapter provide several articles for those in solo or small group practices making decisions about going paperless (Doyle, 2009; Torda, Han, & Scholle, 2010; Torres, 2010).

One resource to help defray costs is General Electric's no-interest loans with deferred payments so that users of IT can get access sooner without the upfront costs (DeSilva, 2009). Whether other organizations will take advantage of this market and federal stimulus monies remains to be seen. Another option is to contact professional organizations to find other small or solo practices, and then join forces to meet with vendors to gather data and select an EHR that is appropriate for the providers' practice.

Lagging Implementation

Implementation of a health IT system can take months to years, depending on the degree of implementation, number and skills of users, and the complexity of the system. Support is crucial at all levels of the organization, including adequate technical support and staff development (Larkin, 2009). Without thoughtful planning, large numbers of IT implementations fail. Although no single set of implementation strategies that result in failure has been supported by researchers (Gurber, Cummings, Leblanc, & Smith, 2009), the highest failure rates were at the "go live" stage. End-user input into the system development and support throughout implementation is a key factor in determining successful implementation.

Interoperability of Systems

The time and effort necessary to learn to use a system can be considerable. Providers may be required to use

Table 11–2 **Advantages and Disadvantages of Electronic Health Records**

Advantages	Disadvantages
• All patient data are in one centralized location • Data from multiple sources are unified • Data are accessible to multiple providers • Data are accessible when a patient travels (e.g., smart cards or Web-based EHR) or has an emergency • Reliance on patient and family recall of medications and drug regimen is no longer necessary • Data are kept current • Guidelines, drug and allergy alerts, and decision supports can be integrated into system and prescribing process • Problems with legibility are eliminated • Data are entered once and distributed to multiple points (e.g., prescription to pharmacy, corollary laboratory orders to laboratory) • Data and results from entire medical records can be shown in the graphical format to indicate trends over time • Research and data mining can aid care, particularly in underserved populations • Macros and templates can address patients' common health conditions, prescribing or teaching needs, and discharge summaries • Ability to translate information into multiple languages exists	• Cost is high, especially initial outlay • Time is needed to learn new system and keep updated on changes • Providers can become too comfortable with macros and templates; as a result, care is no longer as individual as it was • Data entry errors can have rapid negative effects and may go undetected • Off-the-shelf EHR systems may not be a good fit with providers' practice but the systems are cheaper then customized ones • Customized EHR systems take time to set up and cost more than off-the-shelf systems, but customized systems are usually better fits with the local provider's practice • Privacy and data security are concerns • Who owns data and is responsible for their upkeep have not been decided • Multiple users with multiple information needs or specialty data can result in a cumbersome system with many fields in which to enter data or read to find needed information • Lack of standardized hardware, software, platforms, and standards make interoperability between systems difficult

multiple systems as no single standard system or platform is currently in use. Some organizations have been waiting for a standard to be implemented before making the outlay needed for a complex implementation. The marketplace, however, has not developed such an umbrella standard. Institutions may have several systems in place, some for the pharmacy department, some for laboratory, and another for direct care providers. The systems may have difficulty communicating or have different technology requirements. That is not just within a large, integrated system but also between health-care systems.

The goal of patients being able to take their health information anywhere is possible only with interoperability in which there are standards and cross-platform compatibility. In short, providers need to be entering similar data, using the same language into a computer system that can "talk" with other computer systems. Standardized taxonomies and classification methods are critical for such systems to function.

Languages and taxonomies such as the National Drug Code (NDC) (Simonaitis & McDonald, 2009) can help bridge part of the communication gap effectively. Simonaitis and McDonald (2009) found that the NDC covered all but 0.11 to 0.21 percent of their outpatient prescriptions and 1.7 to 7.4 percent of the inpatient prescriptions. Use of standardized nomenclatures such as North American Nursing Diagnosis Association (NANDA), Nursing Intervention Classification (NIC), and Nursing Outcomes Classification (NOC) in EHR systems facilitates system communication as well as communication between providers (Klehr, Hafner, Spelz, Steen, & Weaver, 2009). Nurses play a crucial role in design, evaluation and implementation of the systems as content experts as well as end-users. Table 11–3 contains information about the NDC.

Investment of Provider's Time

Providers also are concerned about the time it takes to use an electronic system as opposed to a paper one and there have been several studies, usually using a time and motion observational method, that have investigated this. The results are not consistent. Hakes and Whittington (2008) found that the time spent on nursing documentation before and after EHR implementation was not different. Hollingworth and colleagues (2007) found that the implementation of an e-prescribing system in an ambulatory care setting required less time in writing but took more time in performing increased computer tasks. Overall, e-prescribing took 12 seconds longer with each prescription than handwriting the prescription did, and slightly more staff nursing time was needed with the computer system was needed. Similarly, Lo and colleagues' (2007) findings had a slight but not statistically significant

Table 11–3 **National Drug Code Database**

Name	Organization	Description
NDC Directory	Food and Drug Administration, Rockville, MD	Entire formulary of current prescription drugs and partial OTC drugs.
Rebate Drug Product Data	Health Care Financing Administration, Baltimore, MD	Entire formulary of drugs that are used in Medicaid and Medicare drug rebate programs. Includes prescription and OTC drugs.
Veterans Affairs Drug File	Department of Veterans Affairs, Washington, DC	Entire formulary of drug products used in VA hospitals.
Redbook	Medical Economics Data, Inc., Montvale, NJ	Entire formulary of drug products from major drug companies. Includes all active and obsolete prescription and OTC drugs.
National Drug Data File	Hearst Corporation, First Data Bank, San Bruno, CA	Entire formulary of drug products from major drug companies. Includes all active and obsolete prescription and OTC drugs.
Medi-Span Electronic Drug File	Medi-Span Inc., Indianapolis, IN	Entire drug products from major drug companies. Includes all active and obsolete prescription and OTC drugs.
Bergen, Durr-Fillauer Drug File	Bergen Brunswig, Durr-Fillauer Medical Inc., Montgomery, AL	Entire formulary of drug products from major drug companies in a regional wholesaler. Includes all active prescription and OTC drugs.
Medicaid Drug File	Alabama Medicaid Agency, Montgomery, AL	Entire list of drug products in Medicaid drug formulary. Includes all active prescription and OTC drugs.

OTC = over-the-counter.

increase in provider time in an ambulatory setting. However, an earlier systematic review (Poissant, Pereira, Tamblyn, & Kawasumi, 2005) found that CPOE increased physicians' documentation time from 98.1 percent to 328.6 percent. Documentation time for staff nurses was less. If time were the only consideration, EHR would have mixed reviews.

Data Security and Privacy

Keeping sensitive health information secure and ensuring that only those who need to access the information can do so has long been a major concern. The consequences of the disclosure of someone's health information can be devastating. It can result in loss of health insurance or employment and embarrassment, and may have a negative impact on social relationships. El Emam and colleagues (2010) compared the risk of financial information disclosure and health information disclosure in peer to peer file sharing in Canada and the United States. The authors found that 0.4 percent of Canadian and 0.5 percent of U.S. peer-to-peer file sharing networks contained private health information. More financial information was available: 1.7 percent of Canadian and 4.7 percent of U.S. Internet protocol (IP) addresses. While only a small percentage of the search terms would return PHI and PFI files from these networks, there were people who were actually searching these files for PHI and PFI.

However, the goal of keeping patient information confidential can be in direct conflict with proposed benefits to sharing health information. These benefits include (1) access of the most current information by all providers anytime, anywhere (see the Interoperability of Systems section); and (2) collection of aggregated health information for quality evaluation, research, and policy uses.

The Health Insurance Portability and Accountability Act (HIPPA) requirements carry stiff penalties for breaches in patient data security. Data privacy and security of personal health information rely on several factors. One factor is the technology itself. Software needs to be designed in such a way that only those who need the information can gain access. Multiple layers of protections must be used to create a robust system and protocols to update those protections in a timely fashion are necessary ("EMR: One Hospital That Got It Right," 2009). Physically restricting access can be another protective factor. Clinicians have to be consistent about maintaining data security. A major vulnerability arises when clinicians do not log off before they leave the computer or system or who do not protect their login and password information.

One of the ways in which data can be secured is through a unique patient identifier (UPI). Ideally, a UPI could reduce errors and improve systems interoperability. RAND Corporation studies found that UPIs did not increase security or privacy breaches and that although it would be more expensive to implement, the improvements in patient safety, system efficacy, and improved privacy protection outweighed the cost (Brook, 2009). RAND estimated savings of $77 billion a year because of system efficiencies in using an UPI alone. The 1996 HIPPA mandated the creation of a UPI to enable data sharing. However, the U.S. Congress has banned the DHHS from funding UPI development. Currently, these efforts are stalled while privacy concerns are addressed.

Finally, public health informatics is an emerging field whose practitioners can use EHR for data mining and other techniques to access information about traditionally underserved or underresearched groups. The findings generated could affect practice and health policy in ways more responsive to the needs of the health of the general public. New health concerns could be identified proactively. The data, in theory, would be aggregated so no patient identities are compromised and patients do not need to consent when data are aggregated. However, the ability of many people to gain access to an individual's private health information increases the risk of a security breach and raises legal and ethical questions. The system would become one in which patients would have to opt out rather than opt in to be part of a study. If they did opt in, would consent be needed for every study? Some underrepresented groups have an understandable wariness because in the past, their rights were violated in health-care research.

Data Fatigue

Another barrier to the adoption of IT and EHR is the sheer volume of information providers are expected to know and manage. The rate at which health information doubles is astounding (Chung, 2009; Dawes et al, 2007), and providers are expected to keep up with new information, particularly in relation to medications and guidelines for practice. Ideally, using IT can help the provider access relevant information to answer clinical questions at the point of care in a timely fashion. Sometimes, however, IT gives providers too much information instead of too little. The overload can be seen in several ways when examining prescribing by advanced practice nurses.

IT is rarely organized and salient to the unique patient situation at hand, and wading through information that is not relevant takes time. Having accurate and complete information is important (Berner & Moss, 2005), but too much information at once can obscure relevant clinical data needed to make prescribing decisions or to avoid medication errors or adverse drug events (ADEs).

Not all information in an IT system is accurate. Data are entered by someone and subject to human entry error. Alternately, the information in the EHR may be more accurate. Clark and colleagues (2009) studied the difference between self-reported mammography rates in black women, paper charting rates, and EHR rates concerning whether the women had actually had mammography screening. Paper charts had the lowest prevalence of documented mammography (58%), whereas self-reporting and EHR rates were more similar with 88 percent at sites with continuous access to EHRs and 61 percent at sites without EHR access.

Another way in which data fatigue can affect prescribers is with a misalignment of clinician and patient expectations. Patients expect that providers will have reviewed their EHR data prior to the visit. Particularly for the complex, chronically ill patient, such information may be voluminous. Should providers be expected to review all the information, some of it (and if so which), or only summaries? What is essential for safe, high-quality patient care (Berner & Moss, 2005)?

Prescriber interaction with EHR system alerts are another way in which data fatigue can be exhibited. Galanter, Didomenico, and Poikaitis (2005) studied the interaction between physicians and contraindicated medication alerts. Use of decision support systems such as alerts to medications that might not be appropriate for that patient because of allergies, patient history, laboratory values, other mediations, clinical guidelines, or other factors is heralded as a key factor in reducing medication errors and ADEs. Although alerts did decrease administration of contraindicated medications (from 89% before to 47% after implementation of the alert system), clinicians often ignored them or turned them off. Clinicians report varied reasons for turning off alerts, including excessive numbers of alerts, clinically unhelpful alerts, and alert settings that are too sensitive for every potential drug allergy or drug to drug interactions and for dose-limit checks (Kuperman, Reichley, & Bailey, 2006).

Excessive alerts also decrease the provider's confidence that the system contains accurate information and lead to ignoring clinically relevant alerts, thus diluting or negating the entire purpose of the medication alert system. Hunteman, Ward, Jolly, and Heckman (2009) found that allergy medication alerts were overridden because of the patient's having previously tolerated the medication (47%), benefit outweighing the risk (29%), or the medication was therapeutically appropriate (24%). In total, 97 percent of alerts were overridden by the prescriber.

Prompting systems can integrate information on risk, morbidity, medication use, laboratory data, and needed preventive services for each patient. This advantage is nullified however, when providers turn off alerts. Turning off alerts raises safety and legal issues. Another reason that providers need to be integral parts of designing and evaluating these systems is to reduce the likelihood of generating spurious or unnecessary alerts while increasing the alerts that are clinically significant.

TECHNOLOGY AND FUNCTION

Devices

Computers

Computers, including stationary and handheld devices, have become familiar to most health-care providers; therefore, this section will be brief. Computers perform various functions that are useful in prescribing including calculation, data storage, information retrieval, Web browsing, and access to guidelines. Stationary devices tend to have greater storage capacity than handheld devices such as smart phones and personal digital assistants (PDAs) but lack portability for providers. Handheld computer devices such as Tablet PCs, the iPad, or laptops can have similar capabilities as stationary computers. Computers may be stand-alone or they may be linked to other computers via a network.

Stand-alone computer data are usually more secure than data shared via linked computers, as a user must physically interact with that computer. Some computers have wireless capability to collect or disseminate data or to communicate with others. All computers are subject to file corruption, viruses, malware, and worms.

Data Storage Devices

Flash (or thumb drives) and CD-ROMs are common data storage and transfer devices. They are also useful for backing up a computer system's data files. The number of gigabytes each device is capable of storing varies. CD-ROMs can be rewritable and handle larger volumes of information than flash drives but are less easily portable and more easily damaged. Data storage devices should be scanned before opening documents as the devices can also become infected with viruses or other damaging programs. Providers must be diligent about protecting the quality of the data by scanning for viruses, worms, malware, and phishing programs. Protective software that automatically updates itself and scans the system is necessary in a safe system.

Services exist to back up data automatically at secure sites. Providers are responsible for keeping patient records secure, current, and readable. In addition to backing up data off site (in the event of fire or other disaster), computers can be set to back up to a local network or main server at preset intervals.

Communication Devices

Computers can be used for communication purposes such as e-mail, video conferencing, or instant messaging—usually over the Internet. Adequate bandwidth and 3G and 4G networks have sped up data transfer time and allow for more real-time applications for communication. A smartphone is an example of one communication device on which multiple applications exist. Using one, a provider might receive a call or text from a patient, respond, and then e-mail or log onto a remote access pharmacy clinical information system and order a prescription via phone. Although such IT may increase timeliness and convenience, increased accessibility means that providers have less private or uninterrupted time unless they take steps to manage chosen communication technology.

Internet

The best known part of the Internet is the World Wide Web (www) or Web. The Web is a network of hypertext documents that are accessed via the Internet (http://encyclopedia.thefreedictionary.com/WWW2, April 2010). Although most Web pages are in English, more than 75 languages are currently used on the Web. Growth in the number of Web pages has been rapid, with estimates in excess of 11.5 billion Web pages on the publicly indexable Web as of 2005 and over 63 billion Web pages as of June 2008. As more software and cheap services or applications to build a Web page have come available, more people have their own Web pages.

The letters *www* are not required as a prefix from a technical standpoint, but many use it as the choice for the site's host name. Some browsers (Internet Explorer, Firefox, Safari, Opera, Google Chrome) automatically add *www* or *.com* to Web site Uniform Resource Locators (URLs) if the Control and Enter keys on the computer are pressed simultaneously. This keyboard shortcut can save the user keystrokes and, therefore, time. File transfer protocols (ftp) are used to access, upload, and download files from databases or sites and are an example of documents or files that are not located on the Web. Table 11–4 shows four Web types.

The Web has a number of advantages and disadvantages. These include benefits and barriers in the areas of access, currency of data, and support tools.

Access

Access has been growing since the 1996 Telecommunications Act by which schools and libraries became sites to increase public access to the Internet regardless of location or income. Access comes in a variety of speeds and may be via a landline or cable system or wireless as well as satellite.

Poverty is still a barrier to access in some areas, although computers in public libraries have improved free access. Smartphones are equipped with wireless access, and services such as Google's Gmail are free, so access is becoming less of a concern. Providers need to support continued free computer access in schools and libraries.

In addition, older adults may have other barriers to access, and this group often requires health-care services. Cresci, Yarandi, and Morell (2010) found that the 27 percent of older adults were using a computer. Users were

Table 11–4 **Internet Web Types**

Name	What Is It and What Does It Do?
Visible Web; also called www, Web, or Shallow Web	This is the traditional Web, part of the first construction of the Internet. This Web is searchable and indexed. Public Web pages are available through Web browsers/search engines to any user. Current estimates of size are 167 terabytes. As an example, the Library of Congress, which is attempting to make copies of all published information available online, contains 11 terabytes of data.
Deep Web; also called the Invisible or Hidden Web or Deepnet	Not all Web sites are visible to the public. Secure databases or pay-for-service applications are an example of content that is not registered with a search engine. The current size is estimated at 91,000 terabytes of data. Content on the Deep Web may be unlinked to other pages, require passwords and logins, and may not allow search engines to access these Web pages. Content that is not HTML or text, such as video or graphics files, and certain file formats may not be handled by the traditional Web. Federally based search engines—such as Science.gov—are one way to find the information online. Human Web crawlers find interesting links (example: StumbleUpon's service).
www2; also called Web2	www2 is of particular interest to businesses and researchers. Designed to enhance creativity and information sharing capacity, Web2 is designed for the creation and dialectic growth of Web-based communities and hosted services. Although the technology is the same as the traditional Web, the way users interact and the software used can be different. The goal is to use the Web's features and capabilities to build applications and services that are a good match rather than to use the Web only as a platform to post things onto Web pages. Web2 pages are often a form of open source and developed by individuals with a focus on innovation and design. Examples include Skype, Wikipedia, eBay, and Craigslist, as well as Flickr (photosharing) and iTunes (music files).
www3	www3 is a term used to describe anything referring to the future of the Web. Definitions and views of what www3 will be are varied. Some of the possible futures being posited include the Web as a giant database, a form of artificial intelligence, or the development of the semantic Web. That www3 might be individually responsive and offer an array of services for users to select from is part of the vision.

evenly divided between male and female, were more educated, and wealthier than nonusers. The percentage of older adults using computers is increasing, up from 21 percent in a previous study. Of interest is that computer users were significantly healthier than nonusers and less likely to be recently hospitalized. Computer users were also the most likely to have an active social and leisure life. Nonusers are at risk for health problems and social isolation and could benefit from computer and Internet access. Lack of use may mean they may not be effectively reached.

Providers must ask patients about the availability of a computer and their level of comfort in using a computer before recommending computer use or Internet-based activities or materials. Seniornet.org and other Web sites or businesses provide tutorials on how to use computers, software, and the Internet. Knowing about these sites may be beneficial when making recommendations to patients if knowledge or comfort with technology is a barrier to use.

Currency and Ability to Update

The Internet's content can be updated frequently. It can provide a source of downloadable material to update other devices such as PDAs with the latest drug information or guidelines. A user's computer device can be preprogrammed to access the Internet at times of low levels of use (such as when the user is sleeping) to hotsync and download new information.

The same dynamism that makes the Web such an accessible source of information also means that Web pages and hyperlinks may disappear; pages may relocate so that the hyperlink no longer points to the content the searcher is seeking; and content is changed, updated, deleted, or replaced ("Web rot"). The resulting dead links make finding information difficult, unlike paper systems or discs, which are physically present and can retain information in an unchanged format. Providers can bookmark the main page of large, stable sites such as healthfinder.gov that are vetted for content, searchable, and regularly updated.

Support Tools

Free tools exist online to support providers. Google has an entire suite of programs that allow sharing of calendars, documentation, and other information online (http://docs.google.com). Google Voice, a telecommunications phone forwarding service, is now available to the public. Providers can give out a telephone number selected from Google to colleagues and patients for them to use as a "communication hub." Options can be set with Google Voice to forward calls to cell phone, home phone, or voicemail. Calls can be transcribed and sent to e-mail, a particularly useful feature for handling and documenting patient calls (Perry, 2010).

Tools such as Pageflakes (http://pageflakes.com) that serve as personal, online notebooks to help gather information are not free. However, another program, Zotero, is free, although it runs only on the browser Firefox (http://www.firefox.com) but is compatible with Linux, Windows, and Macintosh operating systems. The program has many features including automatic citation capture, backing up and synchronizing your library remotely, capturing and storing (portable document format [pdf]) and image formats, taking notes in any language, and interfacing in more than 30 languages. Citations can be exported in common reference formats. Searching features are advanced and allow data mining (Perry, 2009).

Online Drug Information

A wealth of drug information is available online. Table 11–5 provides information on a selected number of these Web sites.

Table 11–5 **Selected Drug-Related Internet Sites**

Site	Address	Comments
	.gov sites	
Agency for Health Research and Quality	*www.ahrq.gov*	Access to AHRQ clinical guidelines, including those that have drug treatment protocols. Information is as current as latest guidelines, but some guidelines are several years old, and the number of guidelines is limited. Maintained by AHRQ. No charges or fees.
Centers for Disease Control and Prevention	*www.cdc.gov/travel/html*	Current CDC recommendations for screening and treatment of communicable disease and immunizations for travel. Updated frequently with new guidelines, often before they appear in written publications. Maintained by CDC. No charges or fees.
Food and Drug Administration	*www.fda.gov/* *www.fda.gov/medbull/contents.html*	Access to information about drugs, foods, and devices regulated by FDA. Medical bulletin with information on drugs, foods, and devices and the MedWatch program.

Table 11–5 **Selected Drug-Related Internet Sites—cont'd**

Site	Address	Comments
National Institutes of Health	*www.nih.gov* *www.nih.gov/database/alerts/clinical_alerts.html*	NIH guidelines for treatment of specific diseases, including drug therapies for these diseases. Current research on drugs and drug therapies. Site has search engine to help locate information. Each institute has a separate address that includes the NIH link. Some of these documents require an Adobe Acrobat Reader to print and read. The reader is available via free download from most large servers. Updated frequently. No charges or fees. Highly recommended site. Clinical alerts provide latest results of clinical trials on a variety of therapies, including drugs. Includes information on upcoming information releases, making it extremely current. Links to other sites. Maintained by NIH. No charges or fees. Highly recommended site.
	www.nlm.nih.gov	Access to data from National Library of Medicine. Provides access to premier databases and search engines, including MEDLINE, that can be searched at no cost. Excellent site.
	.com sites	
American Academy of Neurology	*www.aan.com/*	Patient and provider information on neurological diseases, with links to other sites and internet search engine. Includes data on drug therapies. Maintained by AAN. Co-charges or fees. Excellent site.
Internet Mental Health	*www.mentalhealth.com/*	Primary care provider- and patient-oriented information regarding 52 of the most common psychiatric disorders, with guidelines for treatment and diagnosis. Comprehensive information on 65 of the most frequently used psychiatric drugs. Includes American and European information. Extensive links to other mental health–related Internet sites. Highly recommended site.
Medicinenet	*http://medicinenet.com/*	Patient- and provider-oriented information regarding drugs, side effects, and related material. Drugs listed in alphabetical order by brand and generic name. Listing of clinical trials and poison control centers. Source is network of physician educators. Links to other sites. Adding chat feature. Limited depth of information. No charges or fees.
MDConsult	*www.MDConsult.com*	Reliable, comprehensive medical information service. Integrated collection of trusted resources: 35 medical texts, 48 medical journals, and >600 peer-reviewed clinical practice guidelines searched. Simplifies searches to answer clinically based questions quickly. Uses common terms, so no need to learn search language. Has 2,500 patient education handouts that can be individualized with practitioners' special instructions. Regularly updated prescribing information on >300,000 drugs. Has fee for use, but allows 10-day free trial before subscribing.
RXList: The Internet Drug Index	*www.rxlist.com/*	Full package-insert information for >4,000 prescription products and simplified listing for OTC drugs. Can be searched by entering brand or generic names or therapeutic category. Also can search by imprint codes, important to identification of generic drugs. Information similar to PDR. Checked by PharmD who works for major pharmaceutical distributor. Lists top 200 prescribed drugs. No charges or fees.
Pharmaceutical Information Network	*http://pharminfo.com*	Drug information available by brand and generic names with limited information at the site itself. Has search engine and links to other sites with more detailed information. Has received Internet awards. Latest information on this site was almost 1 year old. Supported by advertising.

Continued

Table 11–5 **Selected Drug-Related Internet Sites—cont'd**

Site	Address	Comments
	.edu sites	
HIV Insite Home Page	*http://hivinsite.ucsf.edu/*	Up-to-date research findings and clinical information regarding effectiveness of treatment strategies, risk analysis, and prognoses. Latest treatment protocols and guidelines. Source is University of California San Francisco AIDS Research Institute, University of California San Francisco AIDS project at San Francisco General Hospital, and the Center for AIDS Prevention Studies. Links to other sites. Excellent site.
Oncolink: University of Pennsylvania	*http://cancer.med.upenn.edu*	Disease-specific therapies including drug therapies. Clinical trials in progress and results of completed trials.
Oregon Health Science University Cliniweb	*www.ohsu.edu/cliniweb/wwwv1*	Includes pharmacy site with multiple links to other Web sites. Up-to-date information on drug therapy. Has disease-specific and drug-specific search engines. Source is Oregon Health Science University. Originally designed to provide access to the expertise available on that campus for providers in rural areas. No charges or fees. Excellent site.
	.org sites	
American Academy of Allergy, Asthma and Immunology	*www.aaaai.org*	Patient- and provider-oriented information on allergic disorders, asthma, and immunologic disorders, including drug therapies. Includes frequently asked questions (FAQ). Sponsored by unrestricted grant from Schering/Key Pharmaceuticals.
American Cancer Society	*www.cancer.org*	Information on all aspects of cancer; links to other sites. Cancer treatment guidelines, including drug therapies. Patient and family information, including alternative treatments. Highly recommended site for cancer information.
American Heart Association	*www.amhrt.org/*	One of the most comprehensive reference sources on Internet. Patient- and provider-oriented information, including prevention and treatment protocols. Visit home page to see all that is available. Excellent site.
United States Pharmacopeia	*www.usp.org*	Different subsites for health-care providers, pharmaceutical manufacturers, patients, and distributors of book form of USPDI. Information on drugs and botanicals, anonymous medication error reporting (MER) program (MedMARx), and drug products problem reporting (DPPR) program. Has search engine and links to many other sites. Data on current MedWatch alerts. Updated frequently. Subscribes to HON code. Highly recommended site.

Specialty organizations may offer services as well. Prescribers can subscribe to receive scheduled and emergent updates automatically. *Facts and Comparisons* (http://www.factsandcomparisons.com) allows subscribers to sign up for an array of drug and guideline information delivered via computer or wirelessly, including patient education handouts. Facts & Comparisons Mobile provides point of care access. Additional information can be found in resources such as the *Physician's Desk Reference* and at individual drug company Web sites. None of the references given here are intended as a product endorsement. The benefit of such systems is that they are more quickly updated with new information than hard copy materials such as books or journals.

Resources for Prescribers

Even the most skillful users of information technology find themselves in need of assistance from time to time. Two excellent resources for assistance related to nursing and pharmacotherapeutics information are informaticists and technical support.

Informaticists

Informaticists are experts in organizing and synthesizing information as well as using or creating systems to make information as accessible and comprehensible as possible. Nursing informatics draws on nursing, informatics, and computer science to manage and process information of interest to nursing. This is an emerging science in nursing but more programs are offering preparation in informatics. As information becomes both more plentiful and complex and as evidence-based practice evolves, nurse practitioners need to be more sophisticated users of information and information technologies. Knowledge and experience are related to the quality of assessment, diagnosis or clinical inference, and planning of care. Information technology can provide access to a variety of information resources—such as knowledge bases and decision support systems—to increase the nurse practitioner's knowledge level. Structured patient assessment forms with links to knowledge bases have the potential to improve patient assessment quality and diagnosis accuracy or clinical inference.

Nurse practitioners often deal with complex tasks in which there are several options, each of which is potentially appropriate. Model-based decision support applications such as decision analysis and multi-attribute utility theory can assist them and patients to analyze and compare the treatment alternatives in a systematic manner. Informaticists are an excellent resource for practice, research and education information needs. Informaticists practice in a variety of settings including larger hospitals, universities, and in private practice. They can also be located through professional organizations such as the nursing informatics organization (http://www.ania-caring.org).

Technical Support

Determining what technical support is available from the technology provider/vendor and the practitioner's own system or network, and what might be available from other sources such as online help or help applications within the program is key to capitalizing on technical support. The user needs to know ahead of time where to find assistance and the costs and limitations of that assistance. Ideally, this knowledge should be considered as part of the information technology purchase. Providers should experiment with the computer program's Tutorial and Help functions before trying to use the program with patients. Also, they should have a backup plan when using information or telehealth technologies in case a problem arises. Keeping current with the latest software or system can be difficult. Fortunately, updating a system with each new version is rarely necessary or cost effective.

Using the Internet as an information source has advantages and disadvantages such as issues of confidentiality and privacy, and the time needed to learn and use the technology effectively and efficiently as well as initial and upgrading costs, all of which are similar to those discussed in the Computers section.

INFORMATION TECHNOLOGY IN A BUSY PRACTICE

Face-to-face visits and phone communication are not the only ways in which patients and providers may interact. Other technologies, such as e-mail and video streaming, are becoming more common. Therefore, the word *encounter* is used in the next section, which discusses how IT can support a prescriber's patient care.

Nurse practitioners are undergoing unwanted pressure to shorten the time spent with each patient. So time-saving measures that can be instituted in areas other than in patient contact are welcome. Information technology can provide those time-saving measures if it is used appropriately.

Time-Savers

The following are eight suggestions for making information technology a help:

1. Separate professional and personal searching. Personal searching, even for material that might be useful to patient care in general, is best done outside office hours.
2. Prioritize what is needed information, and how much time you have for your search.
3. Be systematic with your search. Avoid spending time reading "interesting" information that is not central to the problem at hand. Quickly determine whether information is relevant and needed, nice to know but not immediately relevant, or marginally relevant. Move past the last two categories unless you have a lot of time.
4. Automate computer tasks such as virus scanning and file backup.
5. Do not check e-mail frequently. Establish a routine such as a check first thing in the morning and early to mid-afternoon. Set aside time to handle e-mail. Many practitioners already do this for telephone messages. Use a similar strategy with information technology.
6. Use a separate account for personal and professional e-mail. Give your professional e-mail address to professional or close personal contacts and check it more frequently than your personal account. You can also use your personal account address for trying out new sites or listservs that you might later want to unsubscribe to or to avoid spending a lot of work time going through spam.
7. If you have a slow modem or connection, or are just not interested in graphics, you can turn off the default browser setting to download graphics.
8. Set your default browser home page to a blank page or set it to your most frequently used site such as a favorite search engine or a page of links to drug sites.

Pre-encounter and Postencounter

Because many of the same functions can be used for both pre- and postencounter (patient contact), the two will be discussed together here with exceptions noted. Access to an EHR can enable the advanced practice nurse to review records and have a picture of the patient before or between visits. How much providers need to review depends on the setting.

For example, before seeing a patient in an urgent care clinic, providers may want to review only a patient's current diagnoses/history, what medications the patient is taking, allergies, recent laboratory work-ups, and whether the patient has been seen recently for the admitting problem (for example, a patient was seen for knee pain a week ago and is coming in with the same concern). Knowing how the previous encounter went and what steps were taken helps the provider make treatment and prescribing decisions. Patients can then feel that the provider knows them better and thus cares more about them.

Other functions/interactions that can occur outside the face-to-face patient encounter include screening, sharing data with other providers, and communication that is not face-to-face. The idea that patients will think the provider does not care about them if they are not seen face-to-face is not borne out in research. Data collected from patients outside of the face-to-face encounter prior to or between visits when the patient is not acutely ill, anxious, or away from their medication bottles may be more accurate and complete and result in a more efficient face-to-face encounter.

Screening

Patients can be screened in several ways using IT. For example, in a study by Persell, Dunne, and Baker (2009), patients being tracked via their EHR in a primary care practice (n = 23,111 adults) were screened using automated assessments of cardiovascular risk factors. The EHR system identified patients in need of cholesterol-lowering therapy (9.2%), and patients eligible for anticoagulants (8%). The medication needs of these patients had been unmet. The system results were very accurate and resulted in improved patient care.

Another way to screen patients using IT is a population-based method, as done by Kesman, Rahman, Lin, Barnitt, and Chaudhry (2010). The researchers conducted the study, which was designed to raise screening rates in at-risk patients in a primary care setting. Female patients in at-risk age groups who had not been screened were divided into a usual care group and an intervention group. The intervention group received letters indicating the need for screening. Patients were tracked via databases to determine who had responded to the letter and completed screenings. Patients who received letters had a 7.4 percent higher rate of screenings than those receiving usual care.

Another way IT can assist providers with screening is for providers to receive automatic alerts about specific treatment-related data such as HbA_{1c} levels. For example, in a 2009 study to improve patient's HbA_{1c} levels and provider adherence to diabetic care guidelines in a primary care practice, HbA_{1c} summary reports were automatically sent to providers whenever levels were greater than 7 percent (Howard, Sommers, Gould, & Mancuso, 2009). The patients with the poorest glycemic control benefited most from the IT alerts. After 5 years, the positive results continued.

Patient–Provider Information Sharing

An emerging trend, especially in chronic illness populations, is for patients and providers to become partners in data collection and analysis. IT's function in that collaboration is being studied. Patient acceptance and satisfaction with such collaborations are high. The areas of highest patient satisfaction reported were medication refill services (96%), patient–provider messaging (93%), and getting medical test results (86%) (Ralston et al, 2007).

In many cases, patients may actually be more satisfied and feel that they are receiving higher quality care when IT systems are incorporated into their care. For example, patients do not want to answer the same questions over and over. Answering the questions once is possible with EHR systems. Patients or caregivers can fill out a form and mail or e-mail it back to the clinic or other setting if the encounter is planned rather than emergent. Data can be scanned or manually entered depending on the situation. Patients or caregivers can also enter data at the clinical site in urgent situations or routine visits. In a 2005 study by Porter, Kohane, and Goldman, parents of children with asthma used a data-entry kiosk in an emergency department to enter information about their children's medications. Parents using the kiosk provided accurate, relevant information. The information provided proved more accurate than the physician or nurse medication histories taken verbally.

Patients (or family caregivers) can collect a variety of data either to bring to a visit or to update the provider between visits. Having a system designed to flag such information for providers so they can check it is necessary to avoid missing critical data. The system can be designed to provide alerts for critical values or other information that the provider needs to prioritize for a particular patient. Providers may be able to obtain greater quantity and higher quality information when patients use IT systems to collect health data to manage their own illness in partnership with providers. For example, in a 2009 study, Vallee-Smejda, Hahn, Aubin, and Rosmus compared paper record-keeping with e-journaling in a group of hemophiliac patients and found that more mandatory information was recorded with the electronic format and that patients collected nearly twice the information providers needed. Record-keeping of patients' home infusions and treatments was more accurate. Data were transferred to providers via phone lines or secure, encrypted Internet connection, which meant providers could access the information from a central server or online at any time. Patients in the study found the e-journals more useful and more organized than paper record-keeping but the electronic version required more time.

While the Vallee-Smejda and colleagues' study (2009) was of young patients from a pediatric clinic, data collection and sharing can be used effectively with older adult patients as well. In one study, older adult patients with COPD were able to use a Web-based system for self-monitoring of their exercise activities and symptoms (Johnson, Nguyen, & Wolpin, 2009). Users of the system were highly satisfied and learned to use the system with minimal difficulty and errors.

Using IT, patients can also provide information about the effects and problems of medications, information that can help providers make prescribing decisions. For example, patients receiving chemotherapy walk a fine line between effective therapy and toxicities. In 2007, Basch and colleagues compared an online system for collecting patient data about chemotherapy toxicities with a paper system. The electronic system included alerts to patients to e-mail providers about serious toxicities. Patients and providers reported higher than 95 percent satisfaction with the system. Patient attrition in the use of the system over 16 months was insignificant. During an 8-week period, 57 alerts were generated on 25 toxicities. Based on these reports, providers chose to delay chemotherapy, to adjust dosages, and to make scheduling changes.

E-Mail Communication Visits

Providers have raised several concerns about electronic communications with patients: data security, timeliness of response/workflow, documentation, legal/liability issues, and reimbursement. For more information on data security, see the Data Security and Privacy section. As for e-mail communications, providers are concerned about patients deliberately or accidentally misusing such communications and the liabilities that may arise from using e-mail (Sands, 2004). E-mail does have several advantages over traditional phone contacts. Time and text of the interaction is documented with e-mail, whereas phone calls are not well documented. Therefore, e-mail may actually reduce liability and improve documentation of patient health issues. Only a small percentage of physicians regularly e-mail patients, despite patient desire for and satisfaction with such communication.

When one study analyzed e-mail communications between patients and providers, the researchers found that patients usually communicated around one issue per message (White, Moyer, Stern, & Katz, 2004). Updates to the provider (41.4%), prescription renewals (24.2%), health questions (13.2%), and test results (10.9%) were major categories. The e-mails were directed first to a triage nurse, who determined if the provider needed to be contacted. Some features, such as asking about test results or prescriptions, could be automated and communicated directly to patients, without the need for contact, if the provider chooses to set up a patient's file in that manner.

Discharge Summaries

Discharge summaries are a special postencounter case. Many EHR systems include standardized discharge summaries or have a system in which the provider can generate such summaries from a template for particular conditions or patient populations. These forms can be adapted by the provider and individualized when text is entered. The file can then be saved as part of the patient's chart. A printed copy with instructions can be given to the patient during discharge teaching. In addition, Web sites can be entered into the instructions or can be visited with the patient at discharge. Patients may forget oral discharge instructions and having something to read once they are home can facilitate adherence to instructions.

Follow-Up on Prescription Use

A significant percentage of patients never fill the prescriptions, and others do not take drugs as prescribed for a variety of reasons. Chapter 6 discusses these reasons, which may include cost or needed further teaching on a medication regimen. Some pharmacy systems can now send automated alerts to let providers know if and how often prescriptions are filled. Such notification can cue the prescriber that a problem requires follow-up. The notification can help the prescriber make decisions about changing medications, helping locate additional resources such as drug company discounts or free medications, or providing additional teaching to clarify unclear information.

Adjuncts to Pharmacotherapy

Prescribing decisions do not occur in a vacuum. Such decisions are part of providing care for a patient but not the entirety. Other forms of care, particularly online resources or programs and telehealth, may benefit patients. Providers need to be aware of trends in new ways of providing care, including prescribing. A few examples are discussed here. First, treatments may be delivered online. Reasons for doing so include a lack of resources or provider experts in a particular local. Another reason is that the patient lives in a rural, frontier, or isolated area. For example, women with alcoholism in rural Missouri have been treated with a 90-day online program (Finfgeld-Connett, 2009). Satisfaction with the components of the program, including (1) reference and decision-making modules, (2) synchronous and asynchronous communication, and (3) communication with the researcher, has been high. Communication between researchers and participants and among participants included widely varied content.

Online support groups are available for patients with a variety of illnesses or conditions. These groups can share information in addition to providing social support. For instance, McCormack (2010) found that an online social support group was effective, easily accessible, and inexpensive for persons with eating disorders.

Finally, the IT system may be set up so that providers can examine quality indicators such as adherence with guidelines and targeted patient outcomes to determine strengths and limitations of their practice. Getting feedback from the system should be part of the routine use of any EHR.

Encounter Use of Information Technology

Provider Information Needs

During a clinical encounter, providers have unmet needs for information to make clinical decisions more than half the time (Ely, Osheroff, Maviglia, & Rosenbaum, 2007). Knowledge of how to use information technology during a clinical encounter and how to phrase questions that are answerable via IT are key factors to being able to rapidly answer clinical questions at point of care. For more information, see the article, in the Reference section, by Stillwell, Fineout-Overholt, Melnzk, and Williamson (2010) on how to frame a clinical question to best use evidence.

Handheld devices such as PDAs represent one way to use IT at the point of care. Such devices need software to support searching activities and wireless capability. The devices may be inappropriate if used in settings where bandwidth is narrow, where wireless coverage is lacking, or where the device could interfere with medical equipment. A recent study (Hauser et al, 2007) conducted with residents using handhelds during rounds to answer clinical questions found that the average time to answer a clinical question was less than 4 minutes, and roughly one-third of queries were successfully answered using the system. Therefore, the clinicians did not have to take as much time from the patient's bedside to seek information. Nor did they need to make the decisions without the desired information. Westbrook, Coiera, and Gosling (2005) found that using an online information retrieval system helped clinicians answer questions and resulted in significant improvement in the quality of their answers in response to typical clinical problems.

In addition to answers to clinical questions, information systems can be used to gather data needed at the start of an encounter, resulting in time savings and having information to review before seeing the patient. Utilizing IT with standardized screening or data collection tools during the patient encounter increases the consistency and quality of data gathered. Data can more easily be compared between encounters as well. Patients, for example, in a rheumatology practice were studied using the American College of Rheumatology Patient Assessment Questionnaire (Williams, Templin, & Mosley-Williams, 2004). The data were collected during office visits. Costs and labor efforts were reduced with a data capture rate of 83.5 percent, which was compared to a preintervention rate of 13.5 percent; therefore, using the system saved time and money. Questionnaires completed using the computer had no missing data compared to paper questionnaires, which were only 33 percent completed.

Working With Informed/Proactive Patients

Providers may feel uncomfortable with patients who are very knowledgeable about their disease. Such patients may use the Internet to acquire information about their disease and its treatment. The time it takes to go over this information, which may or may not be relevant to the patient's situation, and may be something the provider is unfamiliar with, can be perceived as a negative. If patients arrive with information that they found online, however, then the provider can use that information as an excellent opportunity to build rapport, assist in self-management, and teach patients (if needed) how to evaluate the quality of health information found online. Access to computers and the Internet at point of care provides opportunities to show patients material directly related to their care.

Advanced practice nurses should be prepared to discuss health information that a patient may have found on the Internet. Some suggestions for interacting with such a patient include asking open-ended questions, identifying what problem or concern led the patient to search for information, discussing how the information applies or does not apply to the patient's situation, and identifying reliable sources of information and quality standards. Interacting with a patient presents a more collaborative model of care than does dismissing the patient's efforts.

Because the quality of online material can be questionable, providers can help patients and their families become savvy consumers of health-care information by teaching how to identify high-quality Web sites as well as how to identify those with content or features that should raise red flags. A site with high standards, for example, is one that has the Geneva, Switzerland, Health on the Net Foundation code applied to it. Box 11–1 lists the principles on which this code is based. The code is voluntary and if a site visitor finds the site violating the code, the organization can be notified and the code removed.

BOX 11–1 HEALTH ON THE NET: STATEMENT OF PRINCIPLES

- Information must come from medically/health-trained professionals or state that it does not.
- The information is supplemental to the patient–provider relationship.
- Confidentiality of data related to individual patients and visitors to the site is respected.
- Wherever possible, source of the information is supported by clear references and HTML links to the data. The date the site was last updated is displayed.
- Balanced evidence—pro and con statements—is provided.
- Information is provided in the clearest possible manner, and the Webmaster displays his or her e-mail address throughout the site.
- Support for any advice or data given (e.g., financial, commercial) is identified.
- If advertising is a source of funding, it is clearly stated. Advertising is presented in a manner and context so that the viewer can clearly differentiate it from the original material created by the operator of the site.

Patient Teaching

One of IT's strengths, besides providing prescribing information, is patient and family teaching, which can be adapted to meet the needs of patients with varied learning styles. For a visual learner, for example, an animation or graphic of how medication is supposed to work or be administered can be invaluable. Children and those with low literacy levels or language barriers can also benefit from visual additions to patient and family education. Plus, providers can find materials online that they can print out to distribute as handouts. Other IT aids include translation software and educational software packages in multiple languages.

Incorporating IT into a patient encounter takes skill and tact. Showing a patient, and if appropriate or permitted, family members, what is on the computer screen builds trust and makes the patient part of the decision-making process.

IT can assist with health promotion, along with patient teaching, if the IT system includes automatic alerts. For example, just-in-time reminders about mammography or colorectal screening can aid the provider in explaining the need for such health promotion. Some other benefits of using IT during patient encounters include ordering services or durable medical equipment, making referrals, or adapting patient education materials to the unique needs of a patient.

Decision Support Systems

Guidelines

One of the first aspects of prescribing is determining whether a prescription is needed. Screening data and having access to an EHR to analyze laboratory values or other findings can assist the prescriber. Chapter 4 discusses legal and professional issues related to prescribing. Rational drug selection can be facilitated by access to guidelines, prompts for corollary orders, and decision support.

Practice guidelines, including medication therapeutics, can be found in many places. One source of regularly updated guidelines that are vetted for quality is the Agency for Healthcare Research and Quality (AHRQ, http://www.ahrq.gov). The AHRQ also houses the National Guideline Clearinghouse (http://www.guideline.gov), a repository of guidelines from many organizations. Guidelines can be downloaded for free in pdf format and other formats to computers and handheld devices such as PDAs (http://www.guideline.gov/resources/pda.aspx). Professional specialty organization guidelines are included on the Web site but each organization can have its own guidelines posted. Sometimes, guidelines offer conflicting information. Chapter 33 has an example of the difference between two professional organization recommendations about the use of **roziglitazone**. Guidelines are, by their nature, generic and each prescriber must judge the appropriateness of a selected treatment for a patient, given that patient's circumstances and unique characteristics.

The National Guideline Clearinghouse is one source that examines multiple guidelines. Another is the Cochrane Collaboration (http://www.cochrane.org). The Cochrane Collaboration conducts and provides access to the latest in randomized control trials, state of science reports, and systematic reviews. Sometimes a fee is charged for this information. The Cochrane Collection has an international reputation for accuracy and currency.

Guidelines can also be integrated into decision support systems in several ways. The provider can receive prompts when entering medication orders. Certain disease states, laboratory values, or other data can bring up an automatic selection of usually ordered medications when following a particular set of guidelines. For example, if a guideline calls for a patient to be started on **furosemide**, the drugs may show up on the screen with usual doses and the prescriber need only click on the selected drug and dose. Given how quickly evidence changes, the system needs to be regularly updated. In a similar fashion, corollary orders such as ordering a potassium supplement and/or potassium laboratory value for the patient on **furosemide** are also aspects of decision support.

Accessing data and receiving alerts about updates can be handled in multiple ways. However, a systematic review conducted by Moxley and colleagues (2010) found that seven major areas could be barriers or facilitators to use of decision support systems.

- Access was an issue both in terms of too few computers as well as the location of hardware.
- Technology problems could cause users to lose confidence in the system or become frustrated.
- Users were more likely to accept the system when technical support was rapid and effective.
- Systems that were slow or had lots of glitches were barriers.
- Systems must be integrated with other computer systems in order for providers to work effectively. If the system did not integrate with the prescribers' own system, then it was not accepted.
- Endorsement of the system by respected members of the prescribers' community—what change theory refers to as "champions"—was effective in getting prescribers to use the systems.
- Prescribing is not a linear task. If others who need information are out of the communication loop because of the system, then the system will not be accepted.

Listservs

Listservs, or mailing list managers, are another way that providers can receive e-mails or tweets from Twitter about current medications or prescribing practices. For example, journal@healthorbit.ca provides research updates from the United States, Canada, and the UK, with a heavy focus on pharmacology.

Listservs automatically deliver e-mail directly to a subscriber's e-mail account. Listservs use abbreviations such as *.majordomo*, *.listserv*, or *.listproc* in the URL. They are either one-way listservs, in which the editor or person who controls the list is the one who posts to members or two-way listservs that have the ability for members to communicate with one another. Listservs are often used for discussion groups and as a teaching strategy for courses, such as those provided by universities. Nurse practitioner groups have formed listservs for discussion of clinical problems.

News Groups

News groups also post to sites on the Web. They are unmoderated forums for discussion. Although useful information may be provided, they must be used cautiously, because material presented is not routinely monitored for accuracy except by those involved in the group. News groups differ from listservs in that the newsgroup site has to be visited periodically to see new postings. Information is not automatically delivered.

Computerized Provider Order Entry

Decision support systems are usually part of computerized provider order entry (CPOE). Entering orders into a system using CPOE has multiple advantages. First, the orders are legible and complete. Medication errors due to illegible or incomplete orders are common in handwritten prescriptions. Second, orders are sent to the pharmacy and other departments automatically, saving time for the prescriber, pharmacist, and patient. Being able to click on corollary orders at the same session can improve quality of care and means that providers do not have to search for that field to enter into the system. Data to analyze prescribing patterns and quality of care can be extracted from the system readily for Continuous Quality Improvement and peer review.

CPOE with or without decision support has been presented as a way to decrease medication errors and detect adverse drug events (ADE). Devine and colleagues (2010), in examining ways that patient safety was improved by avoiding medication errors and ADEs, found that medication errors declined by an adjusted odds of 70 percent (from 18.2% to 8.2%). Error reduction was attributed to elimination of illegibility (97%), use of inappropriate abbreviations (94%), and missing information (85%). Also a 57 percent reduction of benign ADEs was seen, although not enough harmful ADEs occurred in the sample to draw conclusions about CPOE system effects. A computerized system was able to detect ADEs at a rate 3.6 times greater than a noncomputerized system for voluntary reporting at the university hospital studied and at 12.3 times that of the community hospital (Kilbridge, Campbell, Cozart, & Mojarrad, 2006). Using data from automated surveillance, prescribers can look for patterns and improve practice and patient safety.

CPOE can have unintended consequences (Campbell, Sittig, Ash, Guappone, & Dykstra, 2006). Campbell and colleagues (2006) categorized 79 unintended consequences they had identified in previous work. In descending order, they identified nine categories of consequences. The top three are reported here. First was creation of more or new work for clinicians (19.8%). Clinicians reported that although they got a better overview of their patients with the computerized systems, it was harder to gather the information for that overview. Second was an unfavorable impact on workflow (17.6%). A computerized system is an ideal version of clinical practice and can be a mismatch with the realities of practice. Third were the never-ending system demands (14.8%). The persistence of paper, resulting in duplication of effort and documentation issues; changes in communication patterns and processes; feelings about the system; new types of errors; power structure changes; and overdependence on the technology were the remaining categories. Incorporation of IT into a clinical environment is not without consequences, some readily identifiable and some known only when the system goes live. Being flexible and having contingency plans for problems can help maximize benefits and minimize drawbacks.

Finally, the decision support system must address providers' concerns about liability and privacy issues, as covered in the Technology and Function section. Used properly and consistently, decision support systems can have positive impacts on patients' care. For example, in a study to examine how decision support in the EHR affected lipid management in a primary care setting, Gill, Chen, Glutting, Diamond, and Lieberman (2009) found some improvement in outcomes, but only up-to-date lipid testing for high-risk patients showed statistically significant improvement.

SUMMARY

Like any other tool, IT is no substitute for the prescribers' knowledge and judgment. IT can be useful to advanced practice nurse prescribers in a variety of ways. The provider must, however, be knowledgeable about the benefits and limitations of the technology as well as ways to use it.

Nurse practitioners can play an important role as information facilitators or guides rather than being the sole or main source of health- or illness-related information. In the facilitator role, nurse practitioners might consider maintaining a list of Web sites or having a CD-ROM library and computer access at their practice for patient use. That way, the quality and quantity of patient education can be improved through the judicious use of information technology.

How nurse practitioners use IT in relation to pharmacotherapeutics is changing. Information technologies can catch potential problems, such as drug interactions, before they happen by providing rapid access to the latest information on specific drugs and practice guidelines, and by enabling the practitioner to gain access to the current medication records of patients. Problems caught early often are easier to manage, take less time to manage, and result in fewer complications later in care.

In the information age, particularly in health care, there is an abundance of information to sift through. Determining what is relevant and useful and what is extraneous can be challenging. The time and expense of acquiring and learning new systems or system upgrades and the potential for "information overload" are all very real problems. Careful selection of information technologies that fit the nurse practitioner's practice can address these issues. It is important to stress, however, that no information technology alone can replace the judgment and skill of the nurse practitioner. These technologies are intended to supplement rather than supplant the nurse practitioner's knowledge and patient contact.

REFERENCES

Basch, E., Artz, D., Iasonos, A., Speakman, J., Shannon, K., Lin, K., et al. (2007). Evaluation of an online platform for cancer patient self-reporting of chemotherapy toxicities. *Journal of the American Medical Informatics Association, 14*(3), 264–268.

Berner, E. S., & Moss, J. (2005). Informatics challenges for the impending patient information explosion. *Journal of the American Medical Informatics Association, 12*(6), 614–617.

Bickford, C. J., & Humes, Y. D. (Eds.). (2008). *Nursing informatics: Scope and standards of practice*. Silver Springs MD: American Nurses Association.

Brook, R. (2009). Identity crisis? Approaches to patient identification in a national health information network. *Clinical Scholars Review RAND Health Research Highlights, 2*(1), 10–12.

Campbell, E. M., Sittig, D. F., Ash, J. S., Guappone, K. P., & Dykstra, R. H. (2006). Types of unintended consequences related to computerized provider order entry. *Journal of the American Medical Informatics Association, 13*(5), 547–556.

Chung, G. (2009). Sentence retrieval for abstracts of randomized controlled trials. *BMC Medical Informatics and Decision Making, 9*(10), 1–13.

Clark, C. R., Baril, N., Kunicki, M., Johnson, N., Soukup, J., Lipsitz, S., et al. (2009). Mammography use among black women: The role of electonic medical records. *Journal of Women's Health, 18*(8), 1153–1162.

Cresci, M. K., Yarandi, H. N., & Morrell, R. W. (2010). The digital divide and older urban adults. *Computers, Informatics, Nursing, 28*(2), 88–94.

Dawes, M., Pulye, P., Shea, L., Grad, R., Greenberg, A., & Nie, J. (2007). The identification of clinically important elements within medical journal abstracts: Patient-population-problem, exposure-intervention, comparison, outcome, duration and results (PECODR). *Informatics in Primary Care, 15,* 9–16.

DeSilva, B. (2009). GE program could boost EMR adoption. *Healthcare Benchmarks and Quality Improvement,* 16(9), 103–104.

Devine, E. B., Hansen, R. N., Wilson-Norton, J. L., Lawless, N. M., Fisk, A. W., Blough, D. K., et al. (2010). The impact of computerized provider order entry on medication errors in a multispecialty group practice. *Journal of the American Medical Informatics Association, 17*(1), 78–84.

Doyle, M. J. (2009). Open source will help drive EHR costs down. *Health Management Technology,* 30(9), 10–11.

El Emam, K., Neri, E., Jonker, E., Sokolova, M., Peyton, L., Neisa, A., et al. (2010). The inadvertent disclosure of personal health information through peer to peer file sharing programs. *Journal of the American Medical Informatics Association, 17*(2), 148–158.

Ely, J. W., Osheroff, J. A., Maviglia, S. M., & Rosenbaum, M. E. (2007). Patient-care questions that physicians are unable to answer. *Journal of the American Medical Informatics Association, 14*(4), 407–414.

EMR: One hospital that got it right. (2009). *Health Management Technology, 30*(8), 14–17.

Finfgeld-Connett, D. (2009). Web-based treatment for rural women with alcohol problems. *Computers, Informatics, Nursing, 27*(6), 345–353.

Galanter, W. L., Didomenico, R. J., & Poikaitis, A. (2005). A trial of automated decision support altert for contraindicated medications using computerized physician order entry. *Journal of the American Medical Informatics Association, 12*(3), 269–274.

Gill, J. M., Chen, Y. X., Glutting, J. J., Diamond, J. J., & Lieberman, M. I. (2009). Impact of decision support in electronic medical records on lipid management in primary care. *Population Health Management, 12*(5), 221–226.

Gurber, D., Cummings, G. G., Leblanc, L., & Smith, D. L. (2009). Factors influencing outcomes of clinical information systems implementation: A systematic review. *Computers, Informatics, Nursing, 27*(3), 151–163.

Hakes, B., & Whittington, J. (2008). Assessing the impact of an electronic medical record on nurse documentation time. *Computers, Informatics, Nursing, 26*(4), 234–241.

Hauser, S. E., Demner-Fushman, D., Jacobs, J. L., Humphrey, S. A., Ford, G., & Thoma, G. R. (2007). Using wireless heldheld computers to seek information at the point of care: An evaluation by clinicians. *Journal of the American Medical Informatics Association, 14*(6), 807–815.

Hollingworth, W., Devine, E. B., Hansen, R. N., Lawless, N. M., Comstock, B. A., Wilson-Norton, J. L., et al. (2007). The impact of e-prescribing on prescriber and staff time in ambulatory care clinics: A time-motion study. *Journal of the American Medical Informatics Association, 14*(6), 722–730.

Howard, J. A., Sommers, R., Gould, O. N., & Mancuso, M. (2009). Effectiveness of an HbA_{1c} tracking tool on primary care management of diabetes mellitus: Glycaemic control, clinical practice and usability. *Informatics in Primary Care, 17,* 41–46.

Hunteman, L., Ward, L., Jolly, M., & Heckman, M. (2009). Analysis of allergy alerts within a computerized prescriber-order-entry system. *American Journal of Health System Pharmacy, 66,* 373–377.

Johnson, S. K., Nguyen, H. Q., & Wolpin, S. (2009). Designing and testing a web-based interface for self-monitoring of exercise and symptoms with older adults with chronic obstructive pulmonary disease. *Computers, Informatics, Nursing, 27*(3), 166–174.

Kesman, R. L., Rahman, A. S., Lin, E. Y., Barnitt, E. A., & Chaudhry, R. (2010). Population informatics-based system to improve osteoporosis screening in women in a primary care practice. *Journal of the American Medical Informatics Association, 17,* 212–216.

Kilbridge, P. M., Campbell, U. C., Cozart, H. B., & Mojarrad, M. G. (2006). Automated surveillance for adverse drug events at a community hospital and an academic medical center. *Journal of the American Medical Informatics Association, 13*(4), 372–377.

Klehr, J., Hafner, J., Spelz, L., Steen, S., & Weaver, K. (2009). Implementation of standardized nomenclature in the electronic medical record. *International Journal of Nursing Terminologies and Classifications, 20*(4), 169–180.

Kuperman, G. J., Reichley, R. M., & Bailey, T. C. (2006). Using commercial knowledge bases for clinical decision support: Opportunities, hurdles and recommendations. *Journal of the American Medical Informatics Association, 13*(4), 369–371.

Larkin, H. (2009). The sooner, the better. *Hospitals and Health Networks,* 44–46. Retrived December 17, 2010, from http://www.hhnmag.com/hhnmag_app/jsp/articledisplay.jsp?dcrpath=HHNMAG/Article/data/OSMAY2009/0905HHW_FEA_mostwired&domain=HHNMAG

Lo, H. G., Newmark, L. P., Yoon, C., Volk, L.A., ,Carlson, V. L., Kittler, A. F., Lippincott, M., et al. (2007). Electronic health records in specialty care: A time-motion study. *Journal of the American Medical Informatics Association, 14*(5), 609–615.

McCormack, A. (2010). Individuals with eating disorders and the use of online support groups as a form of social support. *Computers, Informatics, Nursing, 28*(1), 12–19.

Moxley, A., Robertson, J., Newby, D., Hains, I., Williamson, M., & Pearson, S.-A. (2010). Computerized clinical decision support for prescribing: Provision does not guarantee uptake. *Journal of the American Medical Informatics Association, 17*(1), 25–33.

Perry, W. (2009). Notes from the Net Nomad. *Computers, Informatics, Nursing, 27*(3), 129.

Perry, W. (2010). Notes from the Net Nomad. *Computers, Informatics, Nursing, 28*(1), 3.

Persell, S. D., Dunne, A. P., & Baker, D. W. (2009). Electronic health record-based cardiac risk assessment and identification of unmet preventative needs. *Medical Care, 47*(4), 418–424.

Poissant, L., Pereira, J., Tamblyn, R., & Kawasumi, Y. (2005). The impact of electronic health records on time efficiency of physicians and nurses: A systematic review. *Journal of the American Medical Informatics Association, 12*(5), 505–516.

Porter, S. C., Kohane, I. S., & Goldman, D. A. (2005). Parents as partners in obtaining the medication history. *Journal of the American Medical Informatics Association, 12*(3), 299–305.

Ralston, J. D., Carrell, D., Reid., R., Anderson, M., Moran, M., & Hereford, J. (2007). Patient web services integrated with a shared medical record: Patient use and satisfaction. *Journal of the American Medical Informatics Association, 14,* 798–806.

Sands, D. Z. (2004). Help for physicians contemplating use of e-mail with patients. *Journal of the American Medical Informatics Association, 11*(4), 268–269.

Simonaitis, L., & McDonald, C. J. (2009). Using National Drug Codes and drug knowledge bases to organize prescription records from multiple sources. *American Journal of Health System Pharmacy, 66,* 1743–1753.

Stillwell, S. B., Fineout-Overholt, E., Melnzk, B. M., & Williamson, K. M. (2010). Asking the clinical question: A key step in evidence-based practice. *American Journal of Nursing, 110*(3), 58–61.

Torda, P., Han, E. S., & Scholle, S. H. (2010). Easing the adoption and use of electronic health records in small practices. *Health Affairs, 29*(4), 668–675.

Torres, C. (2010). Focus on electronic health records. *National Medicine, 16*(3), 251.

Vallee-Smejda, S., Hahn, M., Aubin, N., & Rosmus, C. (2009). Recording practices and satisfaction of hemophiliac patients using two different data entry systems. *Computers, Informatics, Nursing, 27*(6), 372–378.

Walker, J. M., & Carayon, P. (2009). From tasks to processes: The case for changing health information technology to improve health care. *Health Affairs, 28*(2), 467–477.

Westbrook, J. I., Coiera, E. W., & Gosling, A. S. (2005). Do online information retrieval systems help experienced clinicians answer clinical questions? *Journal of the American Medical Informatics Association, 12*(3), 315–321.

White, C. B., Moyer, C. A., Stern, D. T., & Katz, S. J. (2004). A content analysis of e-mail communication between patients and their providers: Patients get the message. *Journal of the American Medical Informatics Association, 11*(4), 260–267.

Williams, C. A., Templin, T., & Mosley-Williams, A. D. (2004). Usability of a computer-assisted interview system for the unaided self-entry of patient data in an urban rheumatology clinic. *Journal of the American Medical Informatics Association, 11*(4), 249–259.

CHAPTER 12

PHARMACOECONOMICS

Teri Moser Woo

Chapter Outline

Today more than ever, third-party payers, health-care providers, government regulators, and patients are demanding that new drug treatments not only be clinically more effective but also be cost effective. Angiography, stent placement, transplantation, and use of monoclonal antibodies for the treatment of oncological disorders have become relatively routine treatment. After transplantation, patients who were dialysis dependent are restored to relatively normal lives and are able to contribute to society. These accomplishments do not come without cost to the patient or society.

Pharmacoeconomics provides a framework for evaluating drug treatments in terms of comparing one treatment against another and whether the treatment is providing "value for the money" spent (Hay, 2008). Pharmacoeconomic evaluations of medical and surgical procedures have very seldom taken into account factors other than the actual cost of pharmaceutical agents to the health-care system (Berger & Teutsch, 2005). This underestimates the real cost of drug treatment, which depends on adherence, efficacy of therapeutic agents, hospitalizations and treatment for adverse drug reaction, and finally productive life years. Also, a disturbing trend in modern medicine is to achieve excellent short-term benefits but have relatively little long-term impact on comorbid conditions, drug toxicities, or drug nonadherence. This misleading information about the actual cost of drug therapy is seen through introduction of "me-too drugs" (similar drugs developed by multiple drug companies) and the number of highly promoted drugs.

Prescription drug spending increased significantly over the past few years from $239.9 billion in 2004 to $291.5 billion in 2008 (IMS Health, 2009a). Health-care organizations and pharmacy benefits managers have tried to control drug costs by using generic drugs and strict formularies. The sale of generic drugs was reported to be $9.2 billion in 1995 and was $58 billion in 2007 (Generic Pharmaceutical Association, 2009), with 14 of the top 15 dispensed prescriptions being generic formulas in 2008 (IMS Health, 2009b). Although the use of generic drugs has a place in health care, the decision to use them should be more than just a cost-cutting issue. However, with today's cost-conscious health-care delivery, quality of care may be compromised in trade for cost cutting. Health care has become more a business with a bottom line. Medicine cannot be just a business. Now, more than any time in history, we are responsible for distinguishing between excellent care and inappropriate cost cutting. Factors that influence pharmacoeconomics are found in Table 12–1.

PHARMACOECONOMIC STUDIES

Pharmacoeconomic studies were originally designed to study the cost of drug therapy to the health-care system. Clinical studies evaluated the safety and efficacy of a

Table 12–1 **Factors Influencing Pharmacoeconomic Outcomes**

Research Type
Clinical outcomes
Efficacy
Safety
Adverse drugs reaction
Drug–drug reaction
Hospital admission, clinic visits
Humanistic outcomes
Patient satisfaction with care
Quality of life measured by validated instrument
Economic outcomes
Cost associated with immunosuppressive therapy
Cost to treat adverse drug reactions
Cost to treat drug–drug interactions
Cost to treat long-term toxicity (nephrotoxicity, hypertension)
Cost of laboratory work-ups

drug therapy, whereas pharmacoeconomic studies investigated the dollar value of patient care. Pharmacoeconomic studies are an increasing trend in the all fields of health care, and studies should focus primarily on clinical and humanistic outcomes and secondarily on economic factors. Unfortunately, most pharmacoeconomic drug studies have been conducted solely on economic outcomes, with little attention paid to clinical efficacy, safety, and humanistic outcomes. All health-care providers must understand the limitations of these pharmacoeconomic studies. Methods, which are routinely used for the study of pharmacoeconomics, include cost minimization, cost benefit, and cost effectiveness. The information obtained from a well-designed, on-site (local) pharmacoeconomic study should help health-care providers make important decisions regarding which protocol, treatment, services, and drugs should be used. A well-designed study should include several components (Table 12–2):

Components of Well-Designed Studies

Pharmacoeconomics is the analysis of the costs and consequences of any given health care–related treatment or service. When working with pharmacoeconomic analysis, several different studies may be performed, and each is specific for answering a different type of question. For any given analysis, knowing the *point of view*—whether a third-party payer, hospital, or government determining the cost to society—is critical. Along with point of view, one should have a good understanding of the various *types of costs* and which are included in each type of analysis.

Direct costs are those that can be directly attributed to the treatment or disease state in question. They can include factors such as the acquisition price of medications, health-care provider time, or the cost of diagnostic tests. Direct, nonmedical costs must also be considered. This latter category includes transportation to the medical facility or child-care expenses incurred while receiving treatments. Direct costs can further be divided into fixed and variable costs, but as fixed costs are usually associated with overhead and are not influenced by the treatment or disease state, they are often excluded in a pharmacoeconomic analysis.

Table 12–2 **Commonly Used Pharmacoeconomic Research Methodologies**

Method	Outcome	Examples
Cost minimization	Outcome must be clinically identical in similar patient population All social costs should be considered	Adalat CC vs Procardia XL Generic azathioprine vs brand name azathioprine
Cost-effectiveness	Different clinical outcome Justify the incremental cost increase for the therapeutic benfit from extra costs associated with treatment	Antilymphocyte induction vs no induction
Cost benefit	Expressing clinical outcome purely in monetary units Assigns a dollar value to specific disease state Unethical and should be avoided	10 mm Hg reduction in blood pressure worth $100

Besides direct costs, *indirect costs* associated with the therapy must be considered in an analysis. These costs derive from morbidity and mortality and include things such as loss or reduction of wages owing to illness or the costs associated with premature death. Indirect costs can be calculated by two different methods, each having its own inherent flaws. The human capital method assumes losses based on an individual's capacity to earn money and is therefore skewed against the elderly, homeless, and unemployed. The second method is the willingness to pay method. In this method, the patient is asked how much money he or she would be willing to spend to reduce the likelihood of a particular illness. This method tends to have a wide range of answers and is often not realistic.

Intangible costs are very difficult to measure. They are related to nonfinancial outcomes and are hard to express monetarily. Included here are things such as inconvenience, pain and suffering, and grief. These costs are included in the willingness to pay calculation, but not the human capital calculation.

Cost-of-Illness Analysis

Cost of illness identifies the costs of a specific disease in a given population. It is a good baseline number when looking at different treatment or prevention strategies. The total for the cost of illness evaluation includes the cost for the medical resources used to treat the specified illness; the cost of nonmedical resources; and the loss of productivity by the patient. Intangible costs, such as pain and suffering, are difficult to quantify and thus are not included in this calculation. For many disease states, including diabetes and certain cancers, this number has already been calculated. According to the American Diabetes Association (2009), the cost of diabetes in the United States was estimated at $174 billion in 2007. Note: This strictly provides an estimate of economic burden and does not determine treatment options.

Cost-Minimization Analysis

Cost minimization is a very straightforward analysis. It looks at two or more treatment alternatives that are considered equal in efficacy and compares the cost of each alternative in dollars. It assumes that evidence supporting the efficacy of each alternative already exists, and strictly looks at which would be the least costly to administer. An example of this is a comparison between two or more generic medications in the same therapeutic class for treatment of the same condition. Note: The costs are not just related to acquisition of the product, but include costs for any preparation, administration, or monitoring needed. A comparison of **heparin** and its counterpart, the **low-molecular-weight enoxaprin** is a good example. **Heparin** is inexpensive, but patients receiving it have associated laboratory costs, technician time, and pharmacist dosage adjustments that must be figured into the cost. Although **enoxaprin** is more expensive to acquire, the lack of laboratory monitoring may help to bring the overall cost of **enoxaprin** to about equal to that of **heparin**. Therefore, when doing cost minimization with pharmaceuticals, generics are not necessarily always the least costly alternative.

Cost-Effectiveness Analysis

Unlike cost-minimization analysis, cost-effectiveness analysis compares two or more treatments or programs that are not necessarily therapeutically equivalent. This type of analysis compares various treatment costs with a specific therapeutic outcome. The outcome is usually a nondollar unit, such as mm Hg drop in blood pressure or number of cases cured. One of the following three conditions must be met to be considered cost effective: The cost-effective alternative may be less expensive and at least as effective as its comparator; it may be more expensive but provide an additional benefit worth the cost; or it may be less expensive and less effective in a situation in which the extra benefit is not worth the extra cost.

This method aims to find and promote the most efficient therapy for the given problem and finds the best health care for each dollar spent. An example of this analysis is a comparison of two different regimens for treating hypertension. Regimen A might consist of three medications and decrease systolic blood pressure by an average of 35 points. Regimen B, consisting of two medications that cost significantly less per month than Regimen A, lowers systolic blood pressure by 20 points. To determine which is more cost effective, the analysis team must decide if the extra drop in blood pressure is worth the added cost of regimen A. For example, one cost-effectiveness model for long-acting **risperidone** examined the cost of the longer-acting formula versus increased compliance with a simpler dosing schedule, factoring in the economic implications of poorly managed schizophrenia (Haycox, 2005).

Cost-Benefit Analysis

In cost-benefit analysis, the costs of a specific treatment or intervention are calculated and then compared with the dollar value of the benefit received. One way to think about this analysis is whether or not a given benefit will exceed the cost needed to implement it. Many cost-benefit analyses (CBAs) will look at two separate interventions or programs and determine which produces a greater benefit for the money. The two benefits may or may not be similar. The results of a CBA can be described in two different formats. The first is a ratio and the second is the dollar difference between the two. If a specific treatment is valued at $5,000 and the benefit is determined to be $50,000, one could determine that the cost-benefit ratio was 10:1

(benefit divided by cost) or the benefit of this specific treatment is $45,000 (benefit minus cost). Seeing the net benefit (or cost) is more common than seeing a ratio, as a 10:1 ratio could imply numbers with vastly different benefits (i.e., $1,000,000 to $100,000 vs. $40 to $4).

One of the challenges of this type of analysis is that the benefits are often perceived; thus, it is difficult to quantify them. A common use of CBA is for budgeting purposes. A pharmacy can determine whether an existing anticoagulation program is worth keeping or whether that money would be better spent on a new hypertension clinic or diabetes education program.

Cost-Utility Analysis

In cost-utility analysis, the costs of the treatment choice are in dollars and the outcomes are expressed in terms of patient preference or quality-adjusted life years (QALY). A full year at full health is considered 1 QALY, whereas various diseases and their treatments bring about a lower number (0.01–0.99). These QALY values are quite subjective, and agreement on a scale to measure utility is lacking. The best use for this analysis is when quality of life is the most important factor to be considered and the analysis is commonly used in situations in which the treatment option can be life extending but have significant side effects. Cancer treatment options are often reviewed with CBA. A chemotherapy treatment regimen, for example, may bring about a 6-month extension of life expectancy, but if the patient is too nauseated to get out of bed or eat, it may not be worth the extra 6 months.

IMPACT OF GENERIC DRUGS ON DRUG THERAPY

Drug pricing in today's health-care system is complex. The goal is to reduce acquisition drug costs to the lowest possible amount without affecting quality of care. Most pharmacies can control acquisition costs by purchasing generic drugs. However, in some situations, brand-name drugs are less expensive than generic drug products owing to internal bidding, group purchasing, and negotiations with vendors. The cost of generic drugs and single-source, brand-name drugs to pharmacies and patients differs and is driven by market-force competition for the limited pool of dollars. Although most drugs are sold for 15 to 20 percent less than the average wholesale price (AWP), AWP is routinely used for comparison of different agents. A common method for determining reimbursement and controlling health-care system costs used by the Federal Health Care Financing Administration (HCFA) and private payers is the maximum allowable cost (MAC). Although drug pricing is complex in most pharmacy benefits groups, they are still businesses seeking profit. According to the MAC list prices, most pharmacy benefits groups select a drug with the lowest acquisition cost regardless of generic or brand-name status to reduce the cost of drug therapy. The estimated cost savings for the average pharmacy benefits group for dispensing generic drugs is approximately 37 to 50 percent. In most cases, pharmacy benefits groups pass this cost savings on with substantially lower co-payments for generic drugs to the patients. Many benefit plans have a two- or three-tiered benefit, in which the patient pays a greater co-payment for brand-name drugs than for generic equivalent prescriptions. Most pharmacy benefits groups have maximum annual benefits for brand-name drugs, ranging from $1,500 to $2,000 per year. The generic drug benefit is unlimited and the purchase of generic drugs will not count against the $2,000 annual ceiling. For many generic drugs, the AWP is at least 50 percent that of the brand-name drug. Therefore, in general, co-payments are usually 50 percent of the wholesale price for single-source, brand-name drugs. Patients may also take advantage of the numerous prescription programs offered by many large retail pharmacies where patients can get a month's supply of a list of generic drugs for $4, and not have to be concerned about their prescription coverage. The availability of less costly generic drug products for expensive agents would ease financial burdens for most patients, enabling them to comply with their treatments. Increased compliance may decrease health-care utilization in these patients, allowing greater access to health care for other patients. In addition, most patients can easily be stabilized on a generic drug product with narrow therapeutic index as well as on an innovator brand.

Generic Substitution

As health-care system costs continue to escalate, accountability in health-care spending and patient outcomes as a measure of effectiveness of health-care delivery has become crucial. Decreasing the total cost of drug therapy while improving outcomes has become a challenging responsibility for health-care providers. Today, generic substitution for brand-name drugs is a common practice in most health-care organizations in order to decrease the total cost of pharmacotherapy (Almarsdottir & Traulsen, 2005). In 2008, 69 percent of all prescriptions were filled with generic drugs in the United States, yet generic accounted for only 16 percent of dollars spent on prescriptions (IMS Health, 2009a). The practice of generic drug substitution has been an emotional issue for health-care providers, payers, and patients. Health-care providers are under increasing pressure from both innovator companies and payers. Innovator companies that have supported the field of medicine over the past two decades through educational grants and clinical drug studies have recently intensified the pressure on health-care providers to continue to prescribe brand-name drugs only. Insurance companies, health-care payers (private and government), pharmacy benefits groups, policy makers, and some patients are requesting the use of generic drugs to reduce drug costs (Shrank et al, 2006). The critical issue in using generic drugs involves justifying conversion from a brand-name drug to a generic agent in stable patients or using the drug de novo in terms of safety, efficacy, and economics. To help address this issue, the generic bioequivalence standards and different methods of studying pharmacoeconomics should be considered.

Generic Bioequivalence

The U.S. Food and Drug Administration (FDA) regulates the manufacturing of generic drugs by setting rigorous standards for bioequivalence and is responsible for protecting patients and assuring prescribers that generic drug products truly are "equivalent" to those of the innovator pharmaceutical companies. The FDA's requirements, standards, and definitions have been published elsewhere. In a report using FDA bioequivalence standards, the observed mean bioavailability difference between generic drugs and innovator products has been only 3.5 percent in 224 approved drugs since 1962. Several closely related terms may confuse clinicians, but these terms are really quite distinct and specific.

Pharmaceutical Equivalents

Drug products are considered pharmaceutical equivalents when both agents contain identical amounts of active ingredients in the same salt or ester form, dosage form, and route of administration and possess identical disintegration times and dissolution rates.

Therapeutic Equivalents

Drug products are considered therapeutically equivalent when the generic drugs are pharmaceutical equivalents and show the same efficacy and safety profile as that product whose efficacy and safety has been established.

Bioequivalence

Bioequivalence is defined as pharmaceutical equivalents that display the same rate and extent of absorption. Biological equivalence means delivering the same amount of active drug moiety to the site of action when generic and innovator drugs are administered at the same molar dose under similar conditions. Only therapeutically equivalent drug products are safe and should be considered for generic substitution in most patients. However, both health-care providers and patients should be informed regarding generic substitution and true potential cost savings.

APPLYING PHARMACOECONOMICS TO PRACTICE

Generic drug versus brand-name drug prescribing is discussed in this section, demonstrating clinical examples of and rationales for generic substitution. An explanation of Medicare Part D will demonstrate why prescribers need to be familiar with their patients' prescription drug coverage, as it may affect compliance.

Prescribing Generic Versus Brand-Name Medications

Generic drugs that are considered therapeutic equivalents may be exchanged for brand-name drugs with confidence. Pharmacists may substitute a generic equivalent for brand name unless the prescriber specifies "Dispense as Written" on the prescription. In a study of pharmacy claims for 5,399 new prescriptions, 23.4 percent were originally filled as generics and an additional 14.9 percent switched to a generic drug in the first year of therapy (Shrank et al, 2007). The researchers noted patients residing in high-income zip codes were more likely to initiate treatment with a generic drug and those with a three-tier pharmacy benefit were 2.5 times more likely to switch from brand-name to generic drugs (Shrank et al, 2007). It is critical to discuss pharmacy benefit coverage with the patient before prescribing to determine if a generic drug could be the drug of choice.

Many retail stores offer prescription programs in which a select list of generic drugs are offered for $4 for a 30-day supply and $10 for a 90-day supply. This may be a substantial savings for patients, especially those without prescription drug coverage or with a high co-payment for their medications. For example, generic **metformin** 500-mg tablets are $4 for a 30-day supply, whereas the retail price for the brand-name **Glucophage** is $70 for the same 30-day supply. The caveat is that the patient must live near or have transportation to one of the retail pharmacies that have retail drug programs, such as Walmart, Target, Kroger, and Sam's Club stores.

Medicare Part D

In 2004 Congress added a prescription drug benefit to the Medicare program called Medicare Part D. Part D was enacted to assist seniors with the high cost of their medications, but the implementation has been confusing for many. For Medicare beneficiaries, Part D covers 75 percent of drug costs once the patient pays a deductable of $250 per year. Prescription costs between $250 and $2,250 cost the patient 25 percent of the price of the medication. Once the patient's medications costs reach $2,250, the patient pays 100 percent of the costs of the medication until the total reaches $5,100. The coverage gap between $2,250 and $5,100 is often referred to as the "donut hole" point of coverage. Once the patient reaches $5,100 in drug costs, Part D covers the prescriptions 100 percent. Part D has increased the use of essential drugs such as **statins, warfarin,** and **clopidogrel** among elders who did not have drug coverage before the prescription benefit plan was implemented (Schneeweiss et al, 2009). Schneeweiss and colleagues noted a 5 percent decline in the proportion of patients filling their **clopidogrel** prescription when patient drug costs reached the coverage gap. Similarly, a 4.8 percent decline in **warfarin** and 6.3 percent decline **statin** prescription refills were noted (Schneeweiss et al,

2009). With the federal health-care reform of 2010, changes have been made to gradually decrease the amount paid by Medicare recipients in the "donut hole." In 2011, Medicare enrollees will get a 50 percent discount on brand-name drugs during the gap in coverage period and drug costs in the gap will be gradually reduced from 100 percent to 25 percent by 2020. Medicare patients will still pay 50 percent for brand-name drugs, but patients will only have to pay 25 percent for generic drugs. Providers must work with patients to determine if less expensive, but equally as effective prescriptions can be used to prevent patients with limited means from reaching the point of having to pay the full amount for their prescriptions, as paying the full amount may decrease compliance.

CONCLUSION

Pharmacoeconomics is the study of appropriate application of drug utilization for the treatment of specific disease. Pharmacoeconomic studies characterize the improved outcomes while justifying additional drug expenditures. Because the value and economics of many approved drugs are unknown at the time, the true impact of new drug substitution on the cost and care of most patients with complicated conditions is also unknown. In theory, if a therapeutically equivalent and less expensive product is available, it should be substituted and this may substantially affect the cost of drug therapy and overall health-care cost. Applying pharmacoeconomics to prescribing practice involves understanding the impact of drug costs on patients and making an educated prescribing decision to ensure the best outcome.

REFERENCES

Almarsdottir, A., & Traulsen, J. (2005). Cost-containment as part of pharmaceutical policy. *Pharmacy World Science, 27,* 144–148.

American Diabetes Association. (2009). The direct and indirect costs of diabetes in the United States. American Diabetes Association. Retrieved from http://www.diabetes.org/diabetes-statistics/cost-of-diabetes-in-us.jsp

Berger, M. L., & Teutsch, S. (2005). Cost-effectiveness analysis: From science to application. *Medical Care, 43*(Suppl. 7), II 49–II 53.

Choudhry, N. K., & Detsky, A. S. (2005). A perspective on U.S. drug reimportation. *Journal of the American Medical Association, 293*(3), 358–362.

Drummond, M., & Sculpher, M. (2006). Better analysis for better decisions: Has pharmacoeconomics come of age? *Pharmacoeconomics, 24,* 107–108.

Generic Pharmaceutical Association. (2009). About generics: Facts at a glance. Generic Pharmaceutical Association. Retrieved from http://www.gphaonline.org/about-gpha/about-generics/facts

Gregson, N., Sparrowhawk, K., Mauskopf, J., & Paul, J. (2005). Pricing medicines: Theory and practice, challenges and opportunities. *National Review of Drug Discovery, 4,* 121–130.

Hay, J. (2004). Evaluation and review of pharmacoeconomic models. *Expert Opinion in Pharmacotherapy, 5,* 1867–1880.

Hay, J. W. (2008). Using pharmacoeconomics to value pharmacotherapy. *Clinical Pharmacology & Therapeutics, 84*(2), 197–200.

Haycox, A. (2005). Pharmacoeconomics of long-acting risperidone: Results and validity of cost-effectiveness models. *Pharmacoeconomics, 23*(Suppl. 1), 3–16.

Hill, S. (2005). Transparency in economic evaluations. *Pharmacoeconomics, 2,* 967–969.

Hoffman, J., Shah, N., Vermeulen, L., Schumock, G., Grim, P., Hunkler, R., et al. (2006). Projecting future drug expenditures—2006. *American Journal of Health Systems Pharmacy, 63,* 123–138.

IMS Health. (2009a). Channel distribution by U.S. sales. IMS National Sales Perspectives. Retrieved from http://www.imshealth.com/deployedfiles/imshealth/Global/Content/StaticFile/Top_Line_Data/2008_Channel_Distribution_by_U.S._Sales.pdf

IMS Health. (2009b). Top 15 U.S. pharmaceutical products by dispensed prescriptions. IMS National Sales Perspectives. Retrieved from http://www.imshealth.com/deployedfiles/imshealth/Global/Content/StaticFile/Top_Line_Data/2008_Top_15_Products_by_U.S._RXs.pdf

Jacobs, P., Ohinmaa, A., & Brady, B. (2005). Providing systematic guidance in pharmacoeconomic guidelines for analyzing costs. *Pharmacoeconomics, 23*(2), 143–153.

Kozma, C. (2005). Perspective and pharmacoeconomic analyses. *Management Care Interface, 18,* 53–54.

Lyles, A. (2004). Pharmaceutical economics and health policy research using administrative data. *Clinical Therapies, 26,* 1122–1123.

Malone, D. (2005). The role of pharmacoeconomic modeling in evidence-based and value-based formulary guidelines. *Journal of Managed Care Pharmacy, 11,* S7–S10.

Schneeweiss, S., Patrick, A. R., Pedan, A., Varasteh, L., Levin, R., Liu, N., et al. (2009). *Health Affairs, 28*(2), w305–w316.

Shrank, W., Hoang, T., Ettner, S., Glassman, P., Nair, K., Delapp, D., et al. (2006). The implications of choice: Prescribing generic or preferred pharmaceuticals improves medication adherence for chronic conditions. *Archives of Internal Medicine, 166,* 332–337.

Shrank, W. H., Stedman, M., Ettner, S. L., DeLapp, D., Dirstine, J., Brookhard, A., et al. (2007). Patient, physician, pharmacy, and pharmacy benefit design factors related to generic medication use. *Journal of General Internal Medicine, 22,* 1298–1304.

Vogel, R. (2004). Pharmaceutical pricing, price controls, and their effects on pharmaceutical sales and research and development expenditures in the European Union. *Clinical Therapies, 26,* 1327–1340.

CHAPTER 13

OVER-THE-COUNTER MEDICATIONS

Teri Moser Woo

Chapter Outline

Patients are now taking a more active and informed role in their own health care. Thousands of self-help books, articles, Web sites, and television commercials demonstrate the rapidly growing trend in self-care. Surveys consistently show that consumers are increasingly self-medicating with nonprescription drugs. Over-the-counter (OTC) retail drug sales were $16.8 billion in 2008 (excluding Walmart sales), an amount that has increased every year since 2000 (Consumer Healthcare Products Association, 2009). A survey of 2,976 U.S. individuals ages 57 to 85 years revealed 42 percent of the respondents reported using at least one OTC medication and 49 percent reported dietary supplement use (Qato et al, 2008). This trend must be taken into account by health-care providers when assessing for medication use and when prescribing

An OTC drug has the following characteristics: (1) it must be safe (the benefit must outweigh the risks), (2) it has low potential for misuse or abuse, (3) it can be labeled, (4) the patient must be able to self-diagnose the condition for which the drug is being taken, and (5) it must be for a condition that the patient can manage without supervision by a licensed health professional (U.S. Food and Drug Administration Center for Drug Evaluation and Research [FDA CDER], 2010). The U.S. Food and Drug Administration Center for Drug Evaluation and Research is responsible for ensuring that OTC drugs are properly labeled and that their benefits outweigh their risks. New OTC drug ingredients must undergo the New Drug Application process, just as prescription drugs do (FDA CDER. 2010). The FDA CDER is reviewing older OTC drugs to evaluate ingredients and labeling to develop an OTC drug monograph for each, with a goal to improve overall safety of OTC medication use.

There are more than 80 therapeutic categories of OTC drugs and over 100,000 OTC drug products (FDA CDER,

2010). In addition, in the past 10 years, there has been a dramatic increase in the number of prescription medications that have moved to OTC status, for a variety of reasons. Cohen, Paquette, and Cairns (2005) propose three motives for moving prescription drugs to OTC: "pharmaceutical firms' desire to extend the viability of brand names; attempts by healthcare funders to contain costs; and the self care movement" (p. 39). A blockbuster drug such as the **proton pump inhibitor Prilosec** or the **antihistamine Zyrtec** can continue to reap large profits by moving OTC. Insurers often drop drugs from coverage when they move to OTC status and so have pushed for drugs to become OTC, as in the case of Well-Point's petitioning the FDA to move three antihistamines (**loratadine, cetirizine**, and **fexofenadine**) to OTC status (Cohen et al, 2005). Clearly, when drugs are close to reaching the end of their patent, pharmaceutical firms and insurers have a motivation to move the drug to OTC status.

Sales of OTC medications reported by the Consumer Healthcare Products Association can be used to determine the common physical complaints patients self-treat with OTC medications. Over $4 billion was spent on cough and cold medications in 2008, representing the highest sales category (Consumer Healthcare Products Association, 2009.) Internal analgesics represented $2.4 billion in 2008 sales, indicating acute and chronic pain were common self-treated conditions. Self-treatment of heartburn led to $1.2 billion in sales of heartburn remedies in 2008, but with the addition of **Nexium** to the market in late 2009, these sales are likely to increase. Other conditions commonly treated by OTC medications include constipation ($809 million), acne ($333 million), and diarrhea ($173 million). **Nicotine** replacement products are used for tobacco cessation and represented $491 million in sales in 2008. Clearly, patients are diagnosing and self-treating for a variety of common complaints.

Because patients are likely to treat many symptoms and conditions first with nonprescription drugs, the practitioner should assume that some therapy has been started when patients present for care and therefore should ask about OTC medication use. Patients are more likely to self-treat themselves or their children when they feel their illnesses are not serious enough to require medical care. Table 13–1 presents conditions for which OTC drugs are marketed.

Nonprescription drug therapy should not be undervalued or underestimated in the current health-care environment. OTC medications are powerful drugs that should be considered just like prescription drugs with respect to their pharmacology, toxicology, contraindications, precautions, adverse effects, and drug interactions. As many former prescription drugs have recently been converted to nonprescription (OTC) status, the same care and thought needed to monitor prescription drugs use are necessary for nonprescription drugs.

This chapter discusses in general terms OTC drugs that patients commonly use. For more specific information on these drugs, see the appropriate chapters in this book.

ANALGESICS AND ANTIPYRETICS

The OTC analgesics and antipyretics available in the United States are **aspirin** and other **salicylates, acetaminophen, ibuprofen, naproxen**, and **ketoprofen.**

Aspirin and Other Salicylates

Aspirin (acetylsalicylic acid) was patented in 1900 and was a popular OTC analgesic until the development of **acetaminophen** in the 1960s. **Aspirin**'s use waned until the 1990s when aspirin's role as an antiplatelet drug in the prevention of heart attacks and strokes led to its wide use as a standard preventive medication. **Aspirin** is a cyclooxygenase (COX) 1 and COX 2 inhibitor, leading to its activity as an analgesic, antipyretic, antiplatelet, and anti-inflammatory drug. **Aspirin**'s inhibition of COX also creates issues with adverse drug reactions (ADRs) such as bleeding problems and gastrointestinal irritation. Patients need to be educated on the correct use and dosage of **aspirin** to ensure safe use of this common OTC drug.

Certain patients should not take **aspirin. Aspirin** acetylates platelets, causing irreversible inhibition of platelet aggregation. This effect provides a unique advantage in preventing thrombus, but it increases the risk of bleeding. **Aspirin** is contraindicated in those with hemophilia, vitamin K deficiency, or a history of peptic ulcer disease.

Table 13–1 **Conditions for Which OTC Drugs Are Marketed**

Most frequently treated conditions	Acne, athlete's foot, cold sores, colds, cough, cuts, dandruff, headache, heartburn, indigestion, insomnia, premenstrual, sinusitis, sprains
Other conditions	Abrasions, aches and pains, allergic rhinitis, anemia, arthralgia, asthma, bacterial infection (superficial), boils, burns, candidal vaginitis, canker sores, chapped skin, congestion, conjunctivitis, constipation, contact lens care, contraception, corns, dental care, dermatitis (contact), diaper rash, diarrhea, dysmenorrhea, dyspepsia, feminine hygiene, fever, gastritis, gingivitis, hair loss, halitosis, head lice, impetigo, insect bites, jet lag, motion sickness, nausea, obesity, otitis (external), periodontal disease, pharyngitis, pinworms, prickly heat, psoriasis, ringworm, seborrhea, smoking cessation, sty, sunburn, swimmer's ear, teething, toothache, vomiting, warts, xerostomia

OTC = over-the-counter.

Likewise, **aspirin** and other **salicylates** can affect uric acid secretion and reabsorption. Doses of 1 to 2 g per day increase plasma uric acid levels. All **salicylates** should be avoided in patients with a history of gout or hyperuricemia. **Aspirin** produces local gastrointestinal (GI) damage by penetrating the gastric mucosa and leading to cellular and vascular erosion by stomach acid. This can happen in two ways: a local effect from the drug coming in contact with the stomach lining and via COX 1 inhibition, which affects the mucoprotective layer in the stomach. Ulceration can be asymptomatic until it is advanced. Older patients, patients with a history of gastric ulceration or bleeding, and those with alcoholic liver disease are at increased risk for gastric bleeding and should avoid **aspirin**.

Since 1988, the U.S. Food and Drug Administration (FDA) has required that labels of nonprescription drugs containing **aspirin** warn that children and teenagers with flu or chickenpox should not use the medication because of the association of **aspirin** (or salicylate) use with Reye syndrome. Reye syndrome is a potentially fatal illness characterized by vomiting, liver damage, encephalopathy, and hypoglycemia. The syndrome occurs in children and usually follows a viral infection with influenza or chickenpox. The Centers for Disease Control and Prevention (CDC) and the American Academy of Pediatrics have confirmed an association with those viral infections, **aspirin** ingestion, and Reye syndrome. The use of **aspirin** as a pediatric antipyretic has all but ceased in the United States over the past 20 years, as have reports of Reye syndrome.

A more detailed discussion of **aspirin** in its antiplatelet role is found in Chapter 18. Its role as an anti-inflammatory is discussed in Chapter 25 and its role in pain management is found in Chapter 53.

Acetaminophen

Acetaminophen is a nonnarcotic analgesic and antipyretic widely used for more than 40 years to treat pain and fever. **Acetaminophen** is available OTC as a single product **(Tylenol, Panadol)** and in combination with other drugs, as in cough and cold remedies **(Tylenol Cold, Nyquil)** or products for dysmenorrheal **(Midol, Pamprin)**. **Acetaminophen** is also available in prescription form in combination with opioid agonists **(Tylenol #3, Percocet)**.

Although **acetaminophen** taken at recommended dosage is safe and effective, the use of combination products and lack of patient understanding regarding maximum safe dosage has lead to a concern for liver toxicity due to unintentional overdose. Patients should be taught that **acetaminophen** is toxic to the liver in doses higher than 4 g per day in adults. Patients taking large doses of **acetaminophen** or who have liver disease should have liver function monitored. Because **acetaminophen** does not have strong COX 1 or COX 2 activity, the clinical problems noted for **aspirin** or **NSAIDs** are not seen. **Acetaminophen** has no effect on platelets, urinary excretion of uric acid, bleeding time, GI mucosa, or renal function.

Appropriate dosing of **acetaminophen** is critical for safe administration. Patients should be encouraged to read labels for "hidden" **acetaminophen**, especially in cough and cold products. Likewise, parents administering **acetaminophen** to children should be educated regarding the different strengths of liquid and chewable forms of the drug. Accidental overdose may occur if parents are inaccurately measuring liquid forms of **acetaminophen** or giving full-strength adult forms to children. Dosing and use of acetaminophen are discussed in later chapters.

Ibuprofen, Ketoprofen, and Naproxen

Ibuprofen, ketoprofen, and **naproxen** are very similar and share the properties of other **NSAIDs.** NSAIDs are cyclooxygenase (COX) 1 and COX 2 inhibitors, leading to their activity as analgesic, antipyretic, antiplatelet, and anti-inflammatory drugs. **Ibuprofen** is the most widely used OTC **NSAID.**

Similar to **aspirin,** the most frequent adverse effects of **ibuprofen** affect the GI tract: Heartburn, nausea, and epigastric pain are common complaints. **Ibuprofen** produces less GI bleeding than does aspirin and less gastric erosion with chronic therapy. Although **ibuprofen** inhibits platelet aggregation, the effect is reversible, lasting about 24 hours.

Ibuprofen may decrease renal blood flow as a result of inhibiting prostaglandin synthesis. This effect is important in patients with congestive heart failure or chronic renal impairment. Patients with those conditions should not take **ibuprofen. Ibuprofen** and prescription **NSAIDs** may increase the risk of cardiovascular disease and should be used at the lowest effective dose for the shortest duration, consistent with individual patient treatment goals. Some patients with asthma may experience bronchospastic symptoms with **ibuprofen.**

As with **acetaminophen, ibuprofen** is combined with other drugs in OTC cough and cold medications, sleep remedies, and dysmenorrhea products. Appropriate use and accurate dosing of OTC **ibuprofen** and **ibuprofen**-containing products **(Advil Cold & Sinus, Children's Motrin Cold, Advil PM, Pamprin IB)** should be discussed with patients. The anti-inflammatory effects of NSAIDs are discussed in detail in Chapter 25 and the use of NSAIDs for pain is discussed in Chapter 53.

ANTIHISTAMINES AND DECONGESTANTS

Antihistamines

Antihistamines are first-line agents for the prophylaxis and treatment of allergic symptoms such as rhinitis or urticaria. **Antihistamines** competitively compete with one of the mediators of allergic reaction (histamine), and their effectiveness depends on the timing and dosage of the drug. Histamine is the primary mediator for sneezing and itching, and **antihistamines** are very effective with these symptoms, but much less effective for rhinorrhea and congestion.

There are two generations of **antihistamines.** First generation **antihistamines** are highly lipophilic and cross the blood–brain barrier to cause significant sedation, whereas second generation **antihistamines** are less sedating. **Antihistamines** may have significant anticholinergic effects (dry mouth, eyes, and nose; urinary retention; blurred vision). Both generations of **antihistamines** are available OTC; many second-generation drugs have moved from prescription to OTC during the past few years.

Patients require guidance and education regarding the appropriate use of OTC antihistamines. A *Cochrane Review* found no evidence that **antihistamines** improve symptoms of the common cold when used alone, but a slight improvement of symptoms in adults may be seen when **antihistamines** are combined with **decongestants** (De Sutter, Lemiengre, & Campbell, 2003). **Antihistamines** alone or in combination with a **decongestant** are not effective in relieving cold symptoms in small children (De Sutter et al, 2003). In addition, adults should be advised not to drive while taking sedating **antihistamines,** as some states consider this "driving under the influence."

Full prescribing information for **antihistamines** is found in Chapter 17.

Decongestants

Decongestants are sympathomimetic, vasoconstrictive drugs that reduce nasal congestion. They are frequently given in combination with **antihistamines** as they have no effect on histamine or other mediators of allergy.

Decongestants are available for either oral or nasal administration. Topical **decongestants** are minimally absorbed, and their side effects tend to be minimal. Rebound congestion is a common problem when nasal preparations are administered for more than 5 days. The provider should include the possibility of rebound congestion when educating patients regarding safe short-term use of topical **decongestants.**

Systemic **decongestants** constrict vascular beds and stimulate the central nervous system (CNS). This action causes increased blood pressure, insomnia, and increased heart rate. Stimulation of alpha-adrenergic receptors may cause urinary sphincter constriction in men with benign prostatic hyperplasia (BPH) and increase intraocular pressure in patients with glaucoma.

Multiple combinations of **antihistamines, decongestants,** and **analgesics** are available in products for patients to select for self-medication. Table 13–2 lists the most commonly available national brand names. As a general rule, it is best to suggest that patients use single agents directed at specific symptoms rather than combinations. Rarely does a patient have all the symptoms that a combination drug can treat and the more drugs being used the more the risk for adverse effects.

Concern over the use of decongestant medications has been expressed in recent years. For example, the Combat Methamphetamine Epidemic Act, which is part of the 2006 US Patriot Act, restricts the sales of all cough and cold

Table 13–2 **Common Antihistamines, Decongestants, and Combination OTC Products**

Brand-Name Product	Generic Name/Contents	Dosage Forms
	Antihistamines	
Benadryl, Benadryl Allergy Ultratab, Benadryl Dye Free	Diphenhydramine HCl	Syrup, tablet, capsule, thin strips
Chlor-Trimeton 4-Hour Allergy	Chlorpheniramine maleate	Tablet
Claritin	Loratadine	Elixir, tablet, quick-dissolve tablets
Contac 12-Hour Allergy	Clemastine fumarate	Tablet
PediaCare Children's Allergy	Diphenhydramine	Liquid
Tavist-1	Clemastine fumarate	Tablet
Triaminic	Diphenhydramine	Thin strips
Zyrtec	Ceterizine	Syrup, tablet, chewable tablet
	Decongestants	
Afrin 12-Hour, Afrin 12-Hour Pediatric, Afrin Extra Moisturizing, Afrin Sinus	Oxymetazoline HCl	Nasal spray, drops, pump, nasal drops
Allerest 12 Hour Nasal Spray	Oxymetazoline HCl	Nasal spray
Benzedrex (Menthol)	Propylhexedrine	Nasal inhaler
Dristan 12-Hour	Oxymetazoline HCl	Nasal spray

Table 13–2 **Common Antihistamines, Decongestants, and Combination OTC Products—cont'd**

Brand-Name Product	Generic Name/Contents	Dosage Forms
4-Way Fast Acting	Phenylephrine HCl and naphazoline HCl	Nasal spray
4-Way Long Lasting	Oxymetazoline HCl	Nasal spray
Neo-Synephrine Mild, Neo-Synephrine Regular	Phenylephrine HCl	Nasal spray
Neo-Synephrine Nighttime	Oxymetazoline HCl	Nasal spray
PediaCare Children's Decongestant	Phenylephrine	Liquid
Sinex Long Acting	Oxymetazoline HCl	Nasal spray
Sinex Regular	Phenylephrine HCl	Nasal spray
Sudafed, Sudafed 12-Hour, Sudafed 24-Hour, Sudafed Children's	Pseudoephedrine HCl	Tablet, time-release tablet, liquid
Sudafed PE	Phenylephrine HCl	Tablet, liquid
Vicks Sinex VapoSpray 4 Hour	Phenylephrine HCl	Nasal spray
Vicks Sinex VapoSpray 12-Hour	Oxymetazoline HCl	Nasal spray
Vicks Vapo Inhaler	Levmetamfetamine	Nasal inhaler
Combination Products	*Decongestant/Antihistamine*	
Actifed Cold & Allergy	Chlorpheniramine/phenylephrine	Tablet
Allerest Maximum Strength	Pseudoephedrine/chlorpheniramine	Tablet
Benadryl D Allergy Plus Sinus	Phenylephrine/diphenhydramine	Tablet, Fastmelt tablets
Chlor-Trimeton 12-Hour Allergy Decongestant, Chlor-Trimeton 4-Hour Allergy Decongestant	Pseudoephedrine/chlorpheniramine	Tablet
Dimetapp Cold & Allergy	Phenylephrine/brompheniramine	Chewable tablet, liquid
Dristan Cold Multiformula	Acetaminophen/chlorpheniramine/ phenylephrine	Tablet
Dimetapp Nighttime Cold & Congestion	Diphenhydramine/phenylephrine	Liquid
Pediacare Children's Allergy & Cold	Phenylephrine/diphenhydramine	Liquid
Sudafed PE Sinus and Allergy	Phenylephrine/chlorpheniramine	Tablet
Triaminic Cold & Allergy	Phenylephrine/chlorpheniramine	Syrup
Triaminic		

OTC = over-the-counter.

products (including combination products) that contain the methamphetamine precursor chemicals **ephedrine**, **pseudoephedrine**, or **phenylpropanolamine**. The law specifically includes a daily and 30-day limit on retail store and Internet purchases of known methamphetamine precursors. All potential precursors are to be stored behind the counter in retail stores and retailers are required ask for identification and keep a log of who is purchasing the drugs. Some states have additional restrictions; for example, Oregon has listed **pseudoephedrine** as a Schedule III drug under state law. Internationally, countries including Mexico, Australia, New Zealand, and the United Kingdom are limiting unrestricted OTC sales of **pseudoephedrine**.

Another concern with **decongestant** medications is the use of cough and cold medications in young children, specifically children under age 5 years. Safety and efficacy of these medications have been questioned after a number of reports of deaths of infants taking cold medications (Centers for Disease Control and Prevention, 2007). In October 2007, an FDA panel met and recommended that all pediatric cough and cold medications be relabeled as not indicated for use in children under age 4 years. In October 2007, manufacturers voluntarily removed all infant drop formulas of cough and cold medications from the market. Use of **decongestants** in children is discussed in Chapters 17 and 50.

ANTACIDS, HISTAMINE$_2$ ANTAGONISTS, AND PROTON PUMP INHIBITORS

The OTC treatment of dyspepsia and acid reflux has evolved significantly over the past 15 years. Prior to the mid-1990s, the only OTC treatment available for dyspepsia or acid reflux was antacids. **Cimetadine (Tagamet)** moved from prescription to OTC status in the mid-1990s soon after the patent on **Tagamet** expired, leading to the multiple **histamine$_2$ receptor-antagonists (H_2RAs)** currently on the OTC shelves. **Omeprazole (Prilosec)** was the **first proton pump inhibitor** (PPI) and in 2003 was also the first PPI to move to OTC status. This section of the chapter will focus on the use of OTC acid reflux medications; more complete information regarding prescribing these medications and their use in the treatment of gastroesophageal reflux disease is found in Chapter 20.

Antacids

Antacids consist of a cation and an ion compound that neutralize gastric acid secreted by the parietal cells of the stomach. **Antacids** neutralize the existing acid; they do not affect the amount of acid being secreted. **Antacids** do not neutralize the gastric pH but raise it to about 4 to 5. At this level, gastric pepsin is inhibited.

Antacid potency is expressed as acid-neutralizing capacity (ANC), the amount of acid buffered per dose. The formulation of an **antacid** is important for neutralizing capacity, as well as for patient acceptance and compliance. Only dissolved **antacids** can react with stomach acid, and the size of **antacid** particle is the determinant of neutralizing capacity. **Antacid** suspensions are already in a form to react with acid, whereas tablets must be chewed so that they will dissolve and react with the acid. Many patients prefer tablets, but they should be instructed to chew them well and take them with a glass of water.

All **antacids** are basic compounds that react with gastric acid to form a salt and water. Four primary compounds are found in today's products: sodium bicarbonate, calcium carbonate, aluminum hydroxide, and magnesium hydroxide. Most commercially available products contain a mixture of aluminum and magnesium hydroxide (Table 13–3). Because constipation from aluminum and diarrhea from magnesium are dose-related, combining these two agents allows potent ANC with lower doses of each agent. Theoretically, the two effects would balance out, but diarrhea appears to be the predominant effect. Up to 75 percent of patients taking combination products experience diarrhea, whereas constipation is rarely encountered. Patients with poor renal function may experience hypermagnesemia, hyperaluminumemia, or metabolic alkalosis.

Antacids interact with most medications and may decrease the absorption of any other medication. Most interactions can be avoided by separating the antacids by at least 2 hours from the dosing of the other oral medications. Intraluminal interactions occur in the stomach when an **antacid** chelates another drug or adsorbs another drug onto its surface.

The best-known interaction is with **tetracycline. Aluminum hydroxide** and **magnesium hydroxide** have a strong affinity for **tetracycline** and form an insoluble and inactive chelate. This interaction can reduce bioavailability of **tetracycline** by 90 percent and result in clinical failures. This chelation occurs with all other forms of **tetracycline**, including **doxycycline** and **minocycline**. Patients should not take any **antacid** until at least 2 hours after **tetracycline** administration. A similar interaction exists with the **quinolone antibiotics**, such as **ciprofloxacin** and **ofloxacin. Antacids** are discussed in Chapter 20.

Histamine$_2$ Receptor-Antagonists

The introduction of **histamine$_2$ (H_2) receptor-antagonists** (H_2RAs) in 1977 completely changed the treatment of

Table 13–3 **Combination Antacids**

Combinations of Antacids	Brand-Name Product	Dosage Forms	Other Compounds
Aluminum hydroxide and magnesium hydroxide	Gelusil Maalox Maalox Antacid Plus AntiGas Maalox Extra Strength Plus Mylanta (Regular & Double Strength)	Tablet Suspension, tablet Tablet Suspension Gelcap, chewable tablet, suspension	Simethicone Simethicone Simethicone Simethicone
Aluminum hydroxide and magnesium carbonate	Gaviscon ESR, Gaviscon ESRF	Chewable tablet, suspension	Alginic acid (ESR)
Aluminum hydroxide, magnesium trisilicate, and sodium bicarbonate	Gaviscon, Gaviscon-2	Chewable tablet	Alginic acid
Calcium carbonate and magnesium hydroxide	Di-Gel Rolaids Calcium & Magnesium	Chewable tablet, liquid Tablet	Simethicone

acid peptic disorders. Today, all of these products are now available in OTC tablet formulations: **cimetidine** (Tagamet HB), **ranitidine** (Zantac 75 and 150), **nizatidine** (Axid AR), and **famotidine** (Pepcid AC and Mylanta AR).

The H_2RAs inhibit gastric acid secretion by blocking the histamine$_2$ receptors. Although all phases of acid production are inhibited, baseline and nocturnal acid secretions are inhibited to a greater extent. An effect begins within 1 hour and continues for 6 to 12 hours. Both the degree and the duration of acid suppression are dose dependent, so the reduction in acid and duration of effect are significantly lower with nonprescription-strength products.

As a class, the H_2RAs are among the most studied drugs. More than 60 million patients have taken these agents, which have rarely caused severe side effects. This safety profile suggests that the lower OTC doses are safe. The most common side effects are headache, nausea, and diarrhea, at rates (less than 10%) that are usually the same as they are with a placebo.

Cimetidine has the greatest potential to interact with other drugs because it binds to cytochrome P450 enzymes to impair hepatic metabolism of drugs that are normally cleared by the liver. The inhibition is dose dependent, with very little effect at doses lower than 400 mg a day. However, the potential for adverse clinical consequences exists, particularly in older patients with declining renal function and multiple medications. **Famotidine** and **nizatidine** do not bind appreciably to the system and, therefore, do not inhibit the metabolism of other drugs.

A major concern with OTC H_2RAs is that patients with angina, cancer, or gastroesophageal reflux disease (GERD) will self-medicate and delay appropriate treatment. The potential for undertreatment of peptic ulcer disease (PUD) also exists because the H_2RAs treats pain without healing the ulcer. Because of these concerns, these OTC products are not recommended to be taken for longer than 2 weeks.

Despite the fact that these drugs may cause problems for certain patients and have the possibility of interacting with prescription drugs, the nonprescription strengths of H_2RAs offer convenient self-care for patients. The overall safety record of these drugs supports their OTC availability. Providers can minimize the risks by recognizing and triaging patients who are at risk for serious GI disorders, by recognizing patients at risk for **cimetidine** drug interactions, and by taking a careful history for their OTC use. H_2RAs are discussed in detail in Chapter 20.

Proton Pump Inhibitors

Proton pump inhibitors (PPIs) suppress gastric acid secretion by inhibition of the H+/K+/ATPase in the gastric parietal cell. A single daily dose of **omeprazole** or **lansoprazole** can suppress gastric acid for up to 24 hours. The OTC form of **omeprazole (Prilosec OTC)** or **lansoprazole (Prevacid)** are indicated for short-term (14 days) treatment of frequent heartburn.

PPIs may alter the absorption of pH-dependant drugs (**digoxin, iron, ketoconazole**) and may potentiate the effects of **warfarin** and **diazepam**. The adverse drug reactions associated with **PPIs** are usually mild and include diarrhea, constipation, headache, and abdominal pain. The main concern with the OTC use of **PPIs** is patients' self-diagnosing and treating chronic acid reflux. Patients should be educated regarding using **PPIs** in the short term unless under the supervision of their provider.

LAXATIVES

Extensive advertising suggests that bowel movements somehow enhance physical well-being and mood. **Laxatives** are widely used and are a common part of a nonprescription medication history. By definition, a **laxative** facilitates the passage and elimination of feces from the colon and rectum. **Laxative** drugs have been classified by their mechanism of action: bulk forming, stimulants, surfactants, and the osmotic laxative polyethylene glycol (PEG) 3350. Full prescribing information can be found in Chapter 20.

Bulk-Forming Laxatives

Bulk-forming laxatives cause water to be retained in the small and large intestines. This water helps produce formed stools. **Bulk-forming laxatives** are the best choice for the initial treatment of constipation. They are made from natural sources such as semisynthetic hydrophilic polysaccharides and cellulose derivatives, most of which are not absorbed by the body. They produce bulk in the form of a gel that passes easily through the intestines. **Bulk-forming laxatives** generally take 12 to 24 hours to work, but they can take as long as 72 hours. Patients need to drink a large glass (8 oz) of water when taking these **laxatives**. Not only does the water promote stool formation, but also it prevents obstruction in the intestines or esophagus. If **bulk-forming laxatives** are taken in dry form or the tablets are chewed and swallowed, esophageal obstruction may occur. **Bulk-forming laxatives** are the safest form of **laxatives** for long-term use.

The main ingredients in **bulk-forming laxatives** are methylcellulose, polycarbophil, tragacanth, and psyllium. Polycarbophil is the calcium salt of a polyacrylic resin and has a large capacity for binding water. The calcium content of this product is approximately 150 mg per tablet, which may increase the risk of hypercalcemia in susceptible patients.

Psyllium products are not absorbed and do not seem to interfere with nutrient absorption. The dose of psyllium can be titrated up to achieve effects.

Stimulant Laxatives

Stimulant laxatives are classified according to their chemical structure and pharmacological activity. These

laxative products stimulate secretion of water and electrolytes in either the small or large intestine, or both, depending on the specific **laxative.** Intensity of action is proportional to dosage, but individually, effective doses vary. All **stimulant laxatives** may produce gripping, colic, increased mucus secretion, and, in some people, excessive evacuation of fluid. **Stimulant laxatives** are most commonly used to empty the colon prior to rectal and bowel examinations and before surgical procedures involving the GI tract. They should never be used routinely. Because they act fairly quickly, they are often abused. Abuse can lead to dehydration, loss of protein, loss of potassium, severe cramping, or a dysfunctional colon. Because these products do have a quick onset of action, they are best not used at certain times (e.g., at bedtime).

Bisacodyl

A commonly used stimulant laxative is **bisacodyl. Bisacodyl,** administered in a combination of tablets and suppositories or tablets and enemas, has been recommended for cleaning the colon before GI surgery, endoscopy, or radiography. **Bisacodyl** is effective in patients with colostomies, and it may reduce or eliminate the need for irrigation. **Bisacodyl** acts in the colon on contact with the mucosal nerve plexus. Its action is independent of intestinal tone, and the drug is minimally absorbed systemically (approximately 5%). Action on the small intestine is negligible. A soft, formed stool is usually produced 6 to 10 hours after oral administration and 15 to 60 minutes after rectal administration. Adverse effects, which come with chronic, regular use (abuse), include metabolic acidosis or alkalosis, hypocalcemia, tetany, loss of enteric protein, and malabsorption. The suppository form may produce a burning sensation in the rectum. No adverse effects on the liver, kidney, or hematopoietic system have been observed after administration. **Enteric-coated bisacodyl** tablets prevent irritation of the gastric mucosa and therefore should not be broken, crushed, chewed, or administered with agents that increase gastric pH, such as **antacids, H_2RAs,** or **proton pump inhibitors.**

Anthraquinone Stimulant Laxatives

Anthraquinone stimulant laxatives include **aloe, cascara sagrada, casanthranol, senna, aloin, danthron, rhubarb,** and **frangula.** The drugs of choice in this group are the **cascara, casanthranol,** and **senna** (Senokot, Ex-lax) compounds. The cathartic activity of **anthraquinones** is limited primarily to the colon. **Anthraquinones** usually produce their action 8 to 12 hours after administration but may require up to 24 hours. Preparations of **senna** are more potent than those of **cascara** and can produce considerably more abdominal cramping. Patients should be educated regarding the misuse of stimulant laxatives and to discuss chronic abdominal pain or constipation with their provider to determine the cause of their symptoms.

Surfactant Laxatives

Surfactant laxatives such as **docusate (Colase)** are anionic surfactants that, when taken orally, increase the wetting efficiency of intestinal fluid and soften fecal mass. These **laxatives** are considered "stool softeners." They work best to prevent rather than cure constipation. They are best for people who should not strain while having a bowel movement, such as new mothers, patients who have had rectal or vaginal surgery, and those with heart disease or high blood pressure. **Surfactant laxatives** do not stimulate bowel movements when used alone and are usually effective after 1 to 2 days. These **laxatives** are nonabsorbable, nontoxic, and inert; however, their detergent properties may facilitate the absorption of other substances in the GI tract, including prescription drugs.

Osmotic Laxatives

PEG 3350 (MiraLAX) is a laxative that increases fecal water content by osmosis, thus softening the stool. **PEG 3350** is not habit forming and can be used to treat chronic constipation. **PEG 3350** powder is mixed with 8 oz of water, juice, or other fluid and taken once a day. **PEG 3350** is safe and usually well tolerated. Adverse drug reactions, including abdominal bloating, flatulence, or diarrhea, are usually relieved by decreasing the dose.

Magnesium hydroxide (Milk of Magnesia) works as an antacid when taken at low dose (0.5 to 1.5 g/dose) and acts as an osmotic saline laxative when a 2- to 3-g dose is administered. As mentioned above, magnesium-containing laxatives have an adverse effect of diarrhea, whereas the intended effect when treating constipation is to loosen the stool. **Milk of Magnesia** is well tolerated by most patients, except the elderly and patients with decreased renal function who may develop hypermagnesemia. If diarrhea occurs, patients can decrease the daily dose of **Milk of Magnesia** until the stool is of soft consistency, titrating between 1 and 3 tablespoons daily. Patients should be encouraged to drink 8 oz of water with their **Milk of Magnesia** dose.

Table 13–4 presents common OTC **laxatives.** These drugs are discussed further in Chapter 20.

ANTIDIARRHEAL PRODUCTS

In the United States, most acute nonspecific diarrhea is self-limiting in nature. Some health-care providers recommend **loperamide** or adsorbents in acute diarrhea. With the exception of **loperamide** and **bismuth subsalicylate** in traveler's diarrhea, however, scientific evidence is lacking to prove that pharmacological agents reduce stool frequency or duration of disease. Nevertheless, when used according to labeling, nonprescription antidiarrheals may provide relief.

Table 13–4 **Common OTC Laxatives**

Brand-Name Product	Active Ingredient	Dosage Forms
Bulk-Forming Laxatives		
Citrucel (Regular and Sugar Free)	Methylcellulose	Powder
Equalactin	Polycarbophil	Chewable tablet
Fibercon	Polycarbophil	Tablet
Fiberall	Polycarbophil	Tablet
Fiberall (Oatmeal Raisin)	Psyllium	Wafer
Fiberall (Orange)	Psyllium	Powder
Konsyl	Psyllium	Powder
Konsyl Fiber	Polycarbophil	Tablet
Metamucil Fiber (Apple Crisp)	Psyllium	Wafer
Metamucil (Original and Sugar Free)	Psyllium	Packet
Metamucil (Original Texture; Smooth Texture-Orange, Regular; Smooth Texture-Sugar Free, Citrus)	Psyllium	Powder
Perdiem Fiber	Psyllium	Granule
Stimulant Laxatives		
Alophen	Phenolphthalein	Tablet
Dulcolax	Bisacodyl	Suppository, tablet
Evac-U-Gen	Phenolphthalein	Chewable tablet
Ex-Lax Chocolate, Regular, or Maximum	Phenolphthalein	Tablet
Ex-Lax Gentle Nature	Sennosides	Tablet
Fleet	Bisacodyl	Suppository, tablet, enema
Fletcher's Castoria	Senna	Liquid
Fletcher's, Fletcher's Children's Cherry	Phenolphthalein	Liquid
Kellogg's Tasteless Castor Oil	Castor oil	Liquid
Milk of Magnesia Cascara	Cascara sagrada	Suspension
Modane	Phenolphthalein	Tablet
Nature's Remedy	Cascare sagrade, aloe	Tablet
Senokot	Senna	Tablet
Surfactant Laxatives		
Colace	Docusate sodium	Capsule, liquid, syrup
Correctol Stool Softener Laxative	Docusate sodium	Soft gel
Ex-Lax Stool Softener	Docusate sodium	Caplet
Surfak	Docusate sodium	Liqui-gel
Osmotic Laxative Products		
Miralax (PEG 3350)	Polyethylene glycol	Powder
Milk of Magnesia	Magnesium hydroxide	Liquid, caplets

OTC = over-the-counter.

Antidiarrheals

The most commonly used nonprescription antidiarrheal medication currently available is **loperamide.** It is the drug of choice for treating uncomplicated diarrhea. It is used for traveler's diarrhea, nonspecific acute diarrhea, and chronic diarrhea associated with inflammatory bowel disease, and it possesses a more favorable side effect profile than do opiate and opiate-like agents. It not only reduces the frequency of stool loss but also helps relieve the cramping that often accompanies diarrhea. It slows intestinal motility and produces a positive movement of electrolytes and water through the gut. Like other antiperistaltic drugs, **loperamide** should be used for no more than 48 hours in acute diarrhea and is usually not recommended for the treatment of infectious viral gastroenteritis in children. **Loperamide** should be stopped if no improvement in diarrhea is seen after 48 hours at maximum dose.

Bismuth Subsalicylate

Most OTC antidiarrheal products used to contain **kaolin pectin**, but since 2003 the main ingredient in OTC antidiarrheals is **bismuth subsalicylate (Pepto Bismol)**, including the product currently called **Kaopectate**. The exact mechanism of action of **bismuth subsalicylate** is not known, but the drug may stimulate the absorption of water and electrolytes across the intestinal wall, and when subsalicylate is converted to salicylate, it has anti-inflammatory activity on the intestinal wall. **Bismuth subsalicylate** is used for travelers' diarrhea prophylaxis because it binds toxins produced by *Escherichia coli* and the byproducts, bismuth oxychloride and bismuth hydroxide, are believed to have bactericidal action. **Bismuth subsalicylate** may also be used in the treatment of mild dyspepsia, nausea, and indigestion.

The adverse effects of **bismuth subsalicylate** are minimal if it is taken as directed. Because salicylate is a byproduct, **bismuth subsalicylate** should not be taken concurrently with aspirin, as toxicity could occur. Likewise, to guard against Reye syndrome, children with a viral illness such as influenza should not be given **bismuth subsalicylate.** Harmless black-stained stool may occur while taking the drug, which should not be confused with melena, and harmless darkening of the tongue may occur as well. Mild tinnitus is a side effect that may be associated with moderate to severe salicylate toxicity. If diarrhea is seen with high fever or continues beyond 24 hours, the patient should seek medical care. **Bismuth** is radiopaque and may interfere with radiographic intestinal studies.

Anti-diarrheal products are discussed further in Chapter 20.

ANTIFUNGAL PREPARATIONS

The most common types of fungal infections that affect the skin are tinea pedis (athlete's foot), tinea cruris (jock itch), tinea capitis, tinea corporis (ringworm), tinea versicolor, and candidiasis (vaginal yeast infection and thrush). These infections respond well to topical OTC antifungal medications.

Tinea pedis, or athlete's foot, is the most commonly encountered type of fungal infection involving the skin. Multiple, effective OTC antifungal products are marketed for athlete's foot. Treatment consists of using a topical azole such as **clotrimazole (Lotrimin AF), miconazole (Micatin)**, or an allylamine **terbinafine (Lamisil AT)** or **tolnaftate (Tinactin).** These same products are effective against tinea cruris or tinea corporis, although the length of treatment varies with the site of the fungal infection.

Topical antifungals used for tinea are well tolerated if used as directed, with topical dermatitis the main adverse reaction in sensitive patients. The patient should be educated regarding the correct use of the drug, including the extended length of treatment (up to 4 weeks) required for some topical antifungals to work for tinea pedis. The OTC topical antifungals are clearly labeled to indicate length of treatment for each condition.

Tinea capitis is treated with systemic antifungals (prescription) and bi-weekly shampoo with sporicidal shampoo to reduce the spread of the fungus. OTC antifungal shampoos **selenium sulfide (Selsun Blue, Head & Shoulders Intensive Treatment)** and **ketoconazole (Nizoral A-D)** are used as directed by the manufacturer twice weekly for the duration of treatment. Close contacts to the patient are empirically treated with sporicidal shampoo. Seborrhoeic dermatitis on the scalp and dandruff are treated with shampoos containing **selenium sulfide, ketocolazole**, or **pyrithione zinc (Head & Shoulders).**

Recommended initial therapy for candidal vulvovaginitis is with an azole product. Four topical imidazole derivatives are currently available in the United States for treating candidal vulvovaginitis: **butoconazole (Femstat), clotrimazole (Gyne-Lotrimin), miconazole (Monistat)**, and **tioconazole (Vagistat).** These products are available as vaginal creams, suppositories, and tablets. Studies have shown the **imidazoles** to be equally effective and without major toxicities; effectiveness rates are approximately 85 to 90 percent.

Side effects from topical therapy are minimal. Topical **imidazoles** are associated with vulvovaginal burning, itching, and irritation. These side effects are more likely to occur with the initial application of the vaginal preparation and are similar to symptoms of the vaginal infection. Abdominal cramps, headache, penile irritation, and allergic reactions are rare. The vaginal antifungals can be used during menses, and women should be instructed to continue therapy if menses begin during the course of therapy. Relief of symptoms can occur as early as several hours after initiation of therapy, but relief of symptoms is not synonymous with cure. The provider should also emphasize the importance of continuing therapy despite early symptomatic relief.

Table 13–5 presents common topical OTC antifungal products. Antifungal care is available in oral as well as topical preparations. Oral formulations are discussed in

Table 13–5 **Common Topical OTC Antifungal Products**

Brand-Name Product	Active Ingredient	Dosage Forms	Use
Betadine First Aid	Povidone-iodine	Cream, spray	
Betadine	Povidone-iodine	Gel, douche, ointment	
Cruex Antifungal	Undecylenate	Spray-powder, cream	Tinea cruris, pedis
Desenex Antifungal	Tolnaftate	Spray-liquid	Tinea pedis, cruris, corporis, versicolor
Desenex Antifungal Aerosol	Undecylenate	Spray-powder	Tinea pedis, cruris
Desenex Antifungal	Undecylenate	Cream, ointment, powder	Tinea pedis, cruris
Desenex Foot & Sneaker Deodorant Powder Plus	Undecylenate	Powder	Tinea pedis
Femstat-3	Butoconazole	Cream, prefilled applicators	Candidiasis
Gyne-Lotrimin (Vaginal)	Clotrimazole	Vaginal inserts, cream	Candidiasis
Lotrimin AF	Clotrimazole	Cream	Tinea pedis, cruris, corporis, versicolor
Lotrimin AF Jock Itch	Clotrimazole	Spray-powder, lotion	Tinea cruris
Micatin Athlete's Foot	Miconazole nitrate	Cream	Tinea pedis
Monistat 7 (Vaginal)	Miconazole nitrate	Vaginal inserts, cream	Candidiasis
Monistat 3 (Vaginal)	Miconazole nitrate	Vaginal cream	Candidiasis
Tinactin Cream	Tolnaftate	Cream	Tinea pedis
Tinactin Powder	Tolnaftate	Powder	Tinea pedis
Vagistat-1	Tioconazole	Ointment	Candidiasis
Zeasorb-AF	Miconazole nitrate	Powder	Tinea pedis, cruris, corporis, versicolor

OTC = over the counter.

more detail in Chapter 24. Topical formulations are also discussed in Chapter 23.

SLEEP AIDS

Insomnia is one of patients' most common complaints, listed third after the common cold and headache; therefore, it is very common for sleep aids to appear in a patient's OTC drug history. Currently, only two active ingredients are available in OTC sleep-aid medications: the antihistamines **diphenhydramine (Sominex, Nytol)** and **doxylamine (Unisom)**. They are not used here for their primary antihistaminic action, but for their side effect of drowsiness.

Additional sleep products combine a nonnarcotic analgesic, **acetaminophen** (**Tylenol PM**) and **ibuprofen** (**Advil PM**), with a sleep aid (**diphenhydramine**). If mild pain symptoms are present or more pronounced at bedtime, these combination medications can be quite effective.

The primary adverse effects of **diphenhydramine** and **doxylamine** are anticholinergic, such as dry mouth, constipation, blurred vision, and tinnitus. Older male patients may have difficulty in urinating. These effects may be additive with the anticholinergic effects of other drugs that are being taken. Older patients may develop delirium from modest doses of **diphenhydramine**. All of these issues must be considered if a patient is taking these OTC drugs.

Table 13–6 presents common OTC sleep aids. **Antihistamines** are discussed related to their primary uses in treating allergic reactions and their role as a sleep aid in Chapter 17.

CONTRACEPTIVES

OTC contraceptives are an essential aspect of patient-centered birth control and sexually transmitted infection prevention. OTC contraceptives are divided into three categories: barrier (male and female condom), spermicidal, and emergency contraception. Clients may need guidance as to the appropriate OTC contraceptive to meet their needs. Full prescribing information is found in Chapter 31.

Barrier Methods

Condom use to prevent pregnancy has been reported for more than 300 years. Condoms remain an effective method of preventing pregnancy and sexually transmitted

Table 13–6 **Common OTC Sleep Aids**

Brand-Name Product	Antihistamine	Analgesic	Dosage Forms
Doan's P.M.	Diphenhydramine	Magnesium salicylate	Tablet
Excedrin P.M.	Diphenhydramine	Acetaminophen	Caplet, tablet, soft gel
Nytol (Regular & Extra Strength)	Diphenhydramine	—	Caplet, tablet
Sleepinal (Regular & Maximum Strength)	Diphenhydramine	—	Capsule
Sominex	Diphenhydramine	—	Caplet, tablet
Sominex Pain Relief	Diphenhydramine	Acetaminophen	Caplet, tablet, gelcap
Tylenol P.M. (Regular & Extra Strength)	Diphenhydramine	Acetaminophen	Caplet, tablet, gelcap
Unisom	Doxylamine	—	Tablet
Unisom Sleepgels (Maximum Strength)	Diphenhydramine	—	Softgel

OTC = over-the-counter.

infections (STIs) and are available in two types: male and female. Male condoms are made of latex, lambskin, or polyisoprene for latex-sensitive persons. Some condoms contain a spermicide as a lubricant. The advantages to male condoms are that they are readily available in multiple settings and when used properly and consistently are quite effective in preventing pregnancy and infection.

Female condoms (Reality, F.C.2) are polyurethane pouches with flexible rings at each end. One ring sits deep in the vagina and the other is outside the body. Female condoms collect the semen so pregnancy is prevented. Female condoms are also an effective method to prevent STIs. Female condoms are available via drugstores and online pharmacies, but are not as readily available as male condoms.

Spermicides

Spermicides are inserted into the vagina just before intercourse to immobilize the sperm and prevent pregnancy. **Nonoxynol-9** is the most commonly used spermicide and is available as a cream, jelly, foam, or suppository, as well as in the lubricant on male condoms. The vaginal sponge **(Today Sponge)** combines the barrier and absorbability of a sponge that is inserted into the vagina with a spermicidal **(nonoxynol-9)** to prevent pregnancy. **Nonoxynol-9** is the spermicide used with diaphragms to prevent pregnancy. Some patients are sensitive to **nonoxyl-9** and may not tolerate the use of the spermicide.

Emergency Contraception

The **emergency contraception** drugs **Plan B One-Step** and **Next Choice** are available for women or men age 17 years or older to purchase OTC. **Plan B One-Step** consists of one 1.5-mg **levonorgestrel** tablet and **Next Choice** consists of two 0.75-mg tablets taken 12 hours apart. Both **emergency contraceptive** drugs are indicated to prevent pregnancy after known or suspected contraceptive failure and must be taken no longer than 72 hours after unprotected intercourse. Nausea is the most commonly reported adverse reaction, reported in 23 percent of women who take **emergency contraception** drugs. If a patient vomits within 2 hours of taking **emergency contraception,** the dose should be repeated. Patients may experience menstrual irregularities (lighter, heavier, or irregular bleeding) after using **emergency contraception.** Patients under age 17 need a prescription for either **emergency contraception** drug. More complete prescribing information is found in Chapter 31.

SUMMARY

The provider must keep in mind that the prescription drug history, although very important, is usually not the only part a patient's drug use. A careful history of both OTC medications and herbals is needed to avoid overlooking important aspects, such as adverse drug effects and drug interactions, caused by these drugs and herbal products in tandem with any prescription drugs. Many people diagnose their own symptoms, select a nonprescription drug product, and monitor their own therapeutic response. This process is not often reliably reported when, during a routine health history, a patient is asked, "Do you take any medications?" Specific questions need to be asked.

Properly used, OTC medications are useful in self-care to relieve minor complaints and transient conditions. If used improperly or in combination with other medications, these medications can cause a multitude of problems, adverse drug events, and drug interactions.

REFERENCES

Armstrong, S., & Cozza, K. (2003). Antihistamines. *Psychosomatics, 44*(5), 430–434.

Brass, E. (2001). Changing the status of drugs from prescription to over-the-counter availability. *New England Journal of Medicine, 345,* 810–816.

Centers for Disease Control and Prevention. (2007). Infant deaths associated with cough and cold medications—two states, 2005. *Morbidity and Mortality Weekly, 56*(1), 104.

Cohen, J. P., Paquette, C., & Cairns, C. P. (2005). Switching prescription drugs to over the counter. *BMJ: British Medical Association, 330,* 39–41.

Consumer Healthcare Products Association. (2009). OTC facts and figures. Retrieved from http://www.chpa-info.org/pressroom/OTC_FactsFigures.aspx

De Sutter, A. I. M., Lemiengre, M., & Campbell, H. (2003). Antihistamines for the common cold. *The Cochrane Database of Systematic Reviews,* Issue 1. Chichester, England: The Cochrane Collaboration: John Wiley & Sons.

Marsh, T. (1997). Nonprescription H2-receptor antagonists. *Journal of the American Pharmacists Association, 5,* 552–556.

Qato, D. M., Alexander, G. C., Conti, R. M., Johnson, M., Schumm, P., & Lindau, S. T. (2008). Use of prescription and over-the-counter medications and dietary supplements among older adults in the United States. *Journal of the American Medical Association, 300*(24), 2867–2878.

Sullivan, P., Nair, K., & Patel, B. (2005). The effect of the Rx-to-OTC switch of loratadine and changes in prescription drug benefits on utilization and cost of therapy. *American Journal of Managed Care, 6,* 374–382.

U.S. Food and Drug Administration Center for Drug Evaluation and Research (FDA CDER). (2010). Regulation of nonprescription products. Retrieved from http://www.fda.gov/AboutFDA/CentersOffices/cder/ucm093452.htm

Winkelman, J., & Pies, R. (2005). Current patterns and future directions in the treatment of insomnia. *Annals of Clinical Psychiatry, 1,* 31–40.

UNIT II

Pharmacotherapeutics With Single Drugs

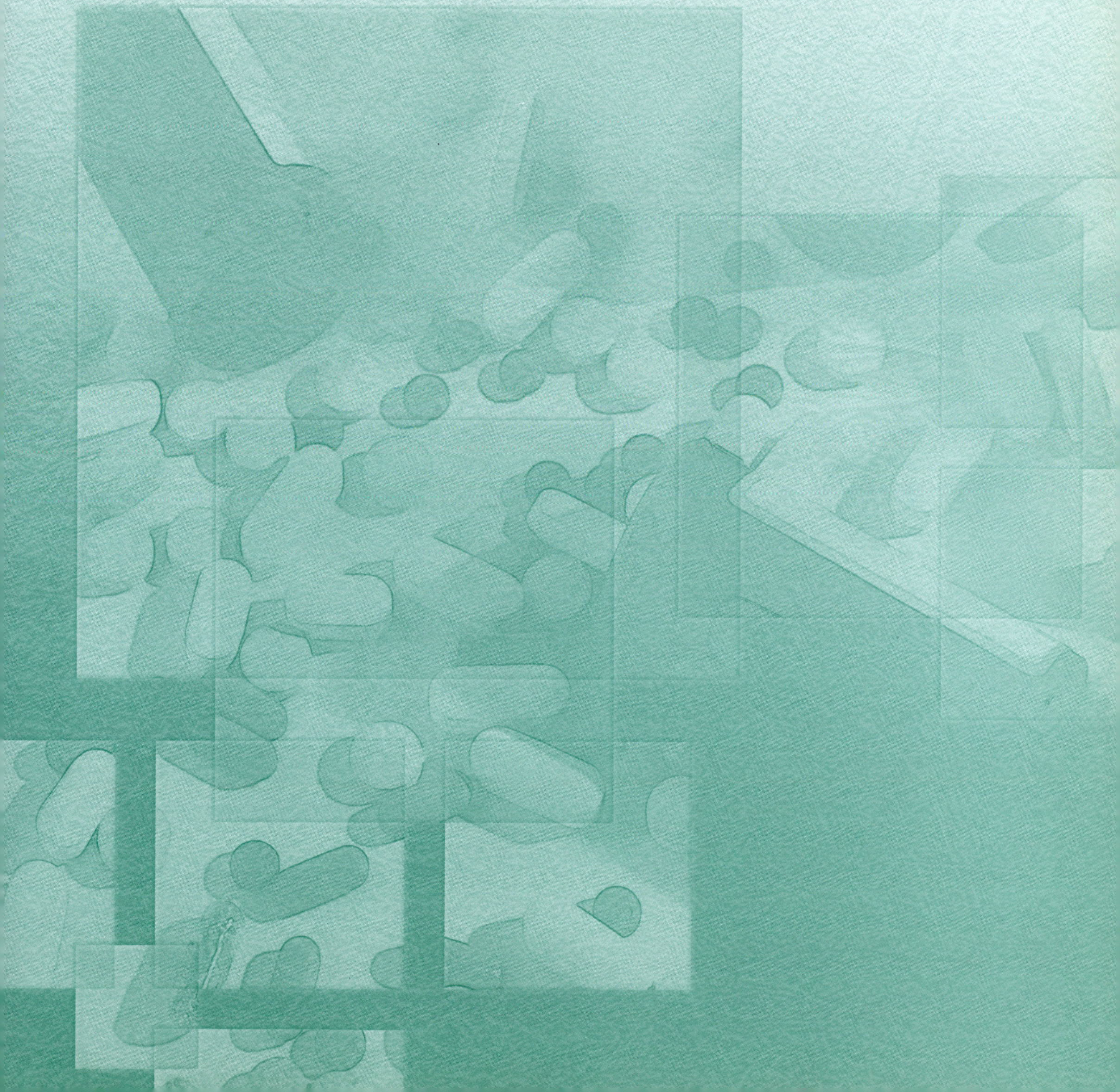

CHAPTER 14

DRUGS AFFECTING THE AUTONOMIC NERVOUS SYSTEM

Anita Lee Wynne

Chapter Outline

The resting activity of most organs is maintained by opposing influences from the parasympathetic nervous system (PNS) and its neurotransmitter, acetylcholine (ACh), and the sympathetic nervous system (SNS) and its neurotransmitters, epinephrine, norepinephrine, and dopamine. Changes in resting activity can occur by increasing the activity of either the PNS or the SNS or by decreasing the activity of the opposing system (Fig. 14–1).

Because these drugs are not organ-specific, when one organ is targeted for therapeutic reasons, the drug simultaneously produces effects in other organs. The targeted organ effects become the desired drug action and the other organ effects become the adverse drug effects.

Drugs that produce these effects are used for a wide variety of diseases and in settings from intensive care to primary care. This chapter focuses on the drugs used in

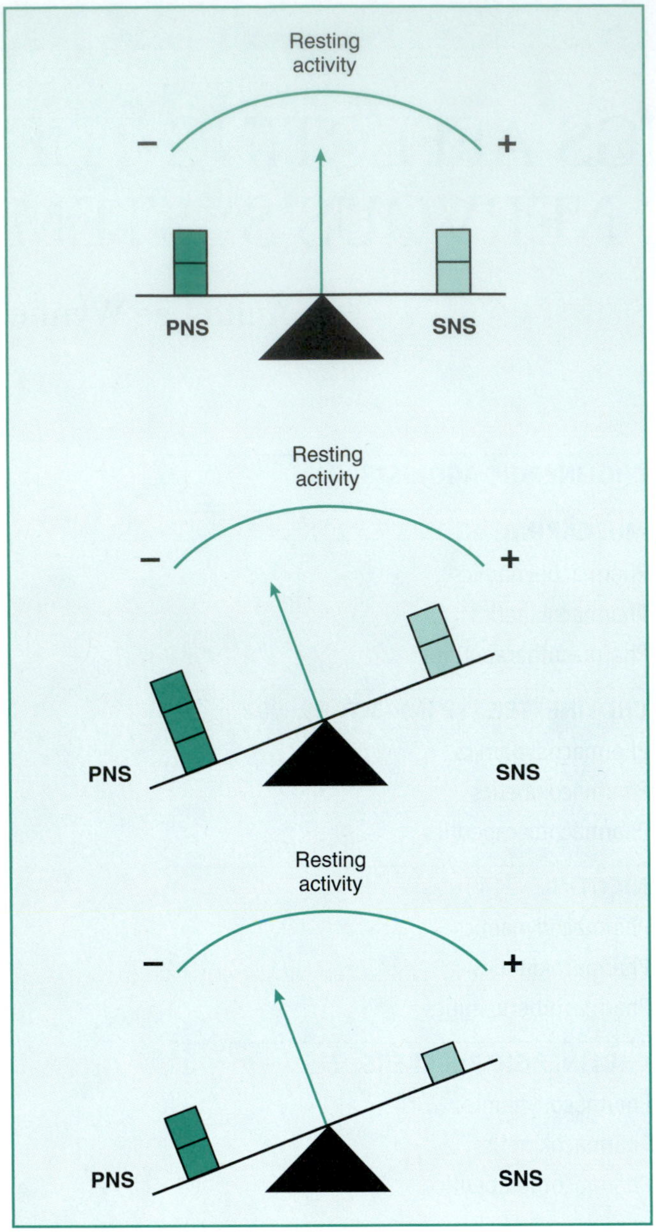

Figure 14–1. Resting activity and the autonomic nervous system.

primary care to treat conditions usually managed by nurse practitioners (NPs). IV forms of the drugs are generally not used in primary care and are not discussed. **Dopamine** and drugs affecting dopamine are discussed in Chapter 15. **Alpha$_1$ agonists** acting peripherally are used mainly as **decongestants**, and **beta agonists** are used mainly for their bronchodilating effects. These drugs are discussed in Chapter 17.

ADRENERGIC AGONISTS

Adrenergic agonists act directly on the SNS by direct receptor binding to organs or tissues, promotion of norepinephrine release, or mimicking the action of norepinephrine or epinephrine. Four main receptor types are involved: alpha$_1$, alpha$_2$, beta$_1$, and beta$_2$. Recently a third beta receptor has been identified. Alpha$_1$ receptors are mostly associated with excitation or stimulation and are found mainly in the eye, salivary glands, arterioles, post-capillary venules, and gastrointestinal (GI) and genitourinary (GU) sphincters. They act by formation of IP3 (inositol1,4,5-triphosphate) and DAG (diacylgylcerol) to ultimately increase intracellular calcium. Alpha$_2$ receptors are mostly associated with relaxation or with inhibition of norepinephrine release and are located mainly in the presynaptic nerve terminals of smooth muscles, and in platelets, and lipocytes. They inhibit adenylyl cyclase resulting in decreased cAMP production via G$_1$ G-protein-coupled receptors. Beta$_1$ receptors, found mostly in the heart, brain, kidney, and lipocytes, are associated with stimulation of adenylyl cyclase via G$_5$ G-protein coupled receptors to increase cAMP production. Beta$_2$ receptors are located in the smooth muscle of the eye, arterioles, venules, bronchioles, liver, pancreas, and GI and GU tracks. They stimulate adenylyl cyclase, increase cAMP, and activate cardiac G$_1$ under certain conditions. Norepinephrine stimulates all alpha and beta$_1$ receptors. Epinephrine stimulates all four types of receptors. Centrally acting alpha$_2$ agonists are the relevant agonist drugs, and they are discussed here (Table 14–1).

Table 14–1 **Actions of Autonomic Nervous System Based on Receptor**

Organ or Tissue	Receptor	Adrenergic Effect	Receptor	Cholinergic Effect
Eye (radial muscle)	Alpha$_1$	Contraction (mydriasis)	M$_3$	None
Eye (ciliary muscle)	Beta$_2$	Relaxation for far vision	M$_3$	Contraction for near vision
Eye (sphincter muscle)	—	None	—	Contraction (miosis)
Lacrimal glands	—	None	—	Secretion
Nasopharyngeal glands	—	None	—	Secretion
Salivary glands	Alpha$_1$	Secretion of potassium and water	—	Secretion of potassium and water
Heart (SA node)	Beta$_1$	Increases heart rate	M$_2$	Decreases heart rate; vagus arrest

Table 14–1 Actions of Autonomic Nervous System Based on Receptor—cont'd

Organ or Tissue	Receptor	Adrenergic Effect	Receptor	Cholinergic Effect
Heart (atria)	Beta$_1$	Increases contractility and conduction velocity	M$_2$	Decreases contractility; shortens action potential duration
Heart (AV junction)	Beta$_1$	Increases automaticity and propagation velocity	—	Decreases automaticity and propagation velocity
Heart (ventricles)	Beta$_1$	Increases contractility	—	None
Arterioles (coronary)	Alpha$_1$	Constriction	—	Dilation
	Beta$_2$	Dilation	—	
Arterioles (skin and mucosa)	Alpha$_1$ and alpha$_2$	Constriction	—	
Arterioles (skeletal muscle)	Alpha$_1$	Constriction	M$_3$	Dilation
	Beta$_2$	Dilation	—	
Arterioles (cerebral)	Alpha$_1$	Constriction (slight)	—	None
Arterioles (pulmonary)	Alpha$_1$	Constriction	—	None
	Beta$_2$	Dilation	—	
Arterioles (renal)	Alpha$_1$	Constriction	—	None
	Beta$_1$ and beta$_2$	Dilation	—	
Veins (systemic)	Alpha$_1$	Constriction	—	None
	Beta$_2$	Dilation	—	
Platelets	Alpha$_2$	Aggregation	—	None
Lungs (bronchial muscle)	Beta$_2$	Relaxation	M$_3$	Contraction
Lungs (bronchial glands)	Alpha$_1$	Decreases secretion	—	Stimulation
	Beta$_2$	Increases secretion	—	
GI (motility)	Alpha$_1$ and beta$_2$	Decrease	M$_1$	Increase
GI (sphincters)	Alpha$_1$	Contraction	M$_3$	Relaxation
GI (secretion)	—	M$_3$	Stimulation and increased secretion	
Liver	Alpha$_1$, alpha$_2$, and beta$_2$	Glycogenolysis and gluconeogenesis	—	Glycogen synthesis
Pancreas (islet cells)	Alpha$_2$	Decreases secretion	—	None
	Beta$_2$	Increases secretion	—	
Adrenal medulla	—		N and M$_3$	Secretion of epinephrine and norepinephrine (nicotinic effect)
Kidney	Alpha$_1$	Decreases renin secretion	—	None
	Beta$_1$	Increases renin secretion	—	
Ureter (motility and tone)	Alpha$_1$	Increases	—	Increases

Continued

Table 14–1 **Actions of Autonomic Nervous System Based on Receptor—cont'd**

Organ or Tissue	Receptor	Adrenergic Effect	Receptor	Cholinergic Effect
Urinary bladder (detrusor)	$Beta_2$	Relaxation	—	Contraction
Urinary bladder (trigone and sphincter)	$Alpha_1$	Contraction	M_3	Relaxes
Uterus	$Beta_2$	Promotes smooth muscle relaxation	—	None
Male sex organs	$Alpha_1$	Ejaculation	M	Erection
Fat cells	$Alpha_2$	Inhibition of lipolysis	—	
	$Beta_1$	Stimulation of lipolysis	—	
Endothelium	—		M_3	Releases EDRF

M = muscarinic receptors.

ALPHA$_2$ AGONISTS: CENTRAL

Pharmacodynamics

Activation of central alpha$_2$ receptors results in inhibition of cardioacceleration and vasoconstriction centers in the brain. This action causes a decrease in peripheral outflow of norepinephrine, leading to decreases in peripheral resistance, renal vascular resistance, heart rate, and blood pressure. Because they lower blood pressure by reducing sympathetic function, they can produce compensatory effects on blood pressure, resulting in retention of sodium and expansion of blood volume through mechanisms that are not dependent on adrenergic nerves. For this reason, they may be given in combination with a diuretic. The drugs in this class, commonly used to treat hypertension, are **clonidine** (Catapres), **guanabenz** (Wytensin), **guanfacine** (Tenex, Intuniv), and **methyldopa**. Centrally activating alpha$_2$ agonists are used largely as second-line drugs in the treatment of mild to moderate hypertension. **Clonidine** also has several off-labeled uses including treatment of withdrawal symptoms from heroin, alcohol, and nicotine, based on its ability to lower the adrenergic stimulation that is associated with this withdrawal. Other off-labeled uses are shown in Table 14–4.

Clonidine activates alpha$_2$ receptors in the medulla of the brain, reducing sympathetic tone and increasing parasympathetic tone, which results in lower blood pressure and bradycardia, particularly when patients are upright. It also directly stimulates peripheral presynaptic alpha$_2$ receptors in arterioles, resulting in vasodilation and decreased renal vascular resistance with maintenance of renal blood flow. This combination of actions rarely results in postural hypotension. **Clonidine** also binds to a nonadrenergic receptor, the imidazoline receptor, which is considered to be part of the final common pathway for sympathetic vasomotor outflow. Orthostatic effects are mild and transient and the drug does not alter normal hemodynamic responses to exercise. **Clonidine** also reduces plasma renin activity and excretion of aldosterone and catecholamines.

Guanabenz and **guanfacine** also reduce sympathetic outflow by activating alpha$_2$ receptors in the brain but do not directly stimulate peripheral receptors, so that blood pressure is reduced in both the supine and standing positions without alterations in normal postural mechanisms. Postural hypotension has been observed in only 15 percent of patients taking **guanfacine** and it is dose related. Pulse rates are reduced by about 5 beats per minute (bpm).

Methyldopa is an analogue of **L-dopa.** Because the pathways for its metabolism directly parallel the synthesis of norepinephrine (NE), its metabolite alpha-methylnorepinephrine is stored in adrenergic nerve vesicles where it replaces NE. Stimulation of central alpha$_2$ receptors by this active metabolite produces a decrease in sympathetic outflow to the heart, kidney, and blood vessels. The end result is a decrease in blood pressure, peripheral resistance, and heart rate with a slight decrease in cardiac output. It also produces reduction in renal vascular resistance. **Methyldopa** also produces a net reduction in tissue concentrations of serotonin (5-HT), dopamine, norepinephrine (NE), and epinephrine.

Pharmacokinetics

Absorption and Distribution

Absorption following oral administration varies among the drugs. **Clonidine** is easily absorbed from the GI tract and the skin and is lipid soluble so that it rapidly enters the brain from the circulation. **Guanabenz** and **guanfacine** are also well absorbed (70% to 80%), but **methyldopa** is incompletely absorbed (50%) from the GI tract and enters the brain via an aromatic amino acid transporter. All of the drugs are widely distributed in body tissues. Both **clonidine** and **methyldopa** cross the placenta and are found in breast milk.

Metabolism and Excretion

The liver in varying degrees metabolizes each of these drugs. **Guanfacine** has a significant first-pass effect. The drug is conjugated on the aromatic ring, possibly by CYP3A4 with about 50 percent of the oral dose metabolized to inactive sulfate metabolites and 50 percent eliminated unchanged in the urine. **Methyldopa** is also extensively metabolized by the liver to inactive metabolites, with only approximately 17 percent of the active drug appearing in the plasma. The kidney is the organ of excretion for each of these drugs. **Methyldopa** and its metabolites accumulate in renal failure resulting in prolonged hypotensive action and increased adverse effects in these patients. Fifty percent of the **clonidine** dose is hepatically metabolized to inactive metabolites and the remaining 50 percent excreted unchanged in the urine. Table 14–2 shows the pharmacokinetics of these drugs.

Pharmacotherapeutics

Precautions and Contraindications

Cautious use is recommended in the presence of severe coronary insufficiency, recent myocardial infarction (MI), and renal function impairment. Because they cross the blood–brain barrier, **methyldopa** and **clonidine** are used cautiously in the presence of cerebrovascular disease. **Clonidine** should not be given to patients who are at risk for mental depression, and it should be discontinued if depression occurs. Because they affect cognitive function, **centrally acting alpha$_2$ agonists** should be avoided or used with extreme caution with older adults and others for whom this adverse response creates a significant problem.

Both **guanabenz** and **clonidine** are Pregnancy Category C. No adequate human studies have been done on **guanabenz**; skeletal anomalies were found in the offspring of mice that were given the drug. **Clonidine** crosses the placenta and no well-controlled studies have been done in pregnant women. Both **guanfacine** and **methyldopa** are listed as Pregnancy Category B. **Guanfacine** should be used only when clearly needed because of the lack of adequate, well-controlled studies in pregnant women. **Methyldopa** has a long record of safety and efficacy and is recommended for use in pregnant women. Even though **methyldopa** crosses the placenta, no adverse reactions or teratogenic effects have been observed.

The American Academy of Pediatrics considers **methyldopa** compatible with breastfeeding. All of the

Table 14–2 ▶ **Pharmacokinetics: Selected Centrally Acting Alpha$_2$ Agonists**

Drug	Onset	Peak	Duration	Protein Binding	Bioavailability	Half-Life	Elimination
Clonidine	Oral: 30–60 min	Oral: 3–5 h	Oral: 8 h	20%–40%		12–16 h: up to 41 h in impaired renal function	40%–60% unchanged in urine 50% metabolized in liver
	Trans-dermal: 2–3 days	Transderma: unknown	Trans-dermal: 7 days (8 h of effect after patch is removed)				
Guanabenz	60 min (onset of anti-HTN action)	2–5 h	12 h	90%		6 h: prolonged in renal impairment	<1% unchanged in urine
Guanfacine	1 h	1–4 h	24 h	70%	80%	*Adults:* 17 h *Younger adults:* 13–14 h *Older adults:* 17–18 h	50% unchanged in urine 70% in urine unchanged or as metabolites
Methyldopa	2–3 h	2–6 h	12–24 h	>20%	50%	1.8 h: blood pressure reduction is pronounced and prolonged in renal failure	Extensively metabolized in liver 70% in urine as metabolites

other drugs are not recommended for nursing mothers. **Methyldopa** and **clonidine** have pediatric doses. **Methyldopa** can be safely used in children younger than 12 years and sources vary regarding the safe use of **clonidine** in this age group.

Adverse Drug Reactions

The major adverse reactions are related to the action of the drug on organs other than the targeted organ. They include drowsiness, dry mouth, constipation, urinary retention, and impotence. Nightmares and insomnia have been associated with **clonidine.** Cardiac symptoms include hypotension, chest pain, and bradycardia. GI symptoms are more commonly associated with **guanabenz** and additionally include abdominal pain, vomiting, anorexia, and altered taste. Gynecomastia has also been associated with **guanabenz** and **clonidine.** All drugs in this class have also been associated with life-threatening rebound hypertension mediated by increased SNS activity after sudden withdrawal of these drugs. **Clonidine** and **methyldopa** have especially been noted to have this adverse reaction, which is exacerbated if the patient is also taking **beta-adrenergic blockers** (Table 14–3). All patients given these drugs should be warned about this possibility. If the drug must be withdrawn, it should be done gradually. All of the drugs in this class may result in pruritic rashes. The transdermal form of **clonidine** has been associated with a rash that is an allergic reaction to the adhesive on the patch.

Table 14–3 ■ **Drug Interactions: Centrally Acting Alpha$_2$ Agonists**

Drug	Interacting Drug	Possible Effect	Implications
Clonidine	Alcohol, antihistamines, phenothiazines, barbiturates, benzodiazepines	Additive sedation	Avoid concurrent use
	Beta-adrenergic blockers	Attenuation or reversal of antihypertensive effect of clonidine; may result in life-threatening hypertension (HTN)	Avoid concurrent use; if patient is taking both drugs and withdrawal is required, withdraw beta-adrenergic blocker first to prevent excessive unopposed alpha stimulation that may lead to malignant HTN within 12 h
	Nitrates, other antihypertensives	Additive hypotensive effects	Avoid concurrent use
	Prazosin	Decreased antihypertensive effect of clonidine	Choose alternative drug
	TCAs	Block antihypertensive effects of clonidine and may result in life-threatening HTN	Choose alternative antidepressant
	Verapamil	Synergistic pharmacological and toxic effects; may result in atrioventricular block and severe hypotension	Choose alternative calcium channel blocker or antihypertensive
Guanabenz, guanfacine	Alcohol, antihistamines, phenothiazines, barbiturates, benzodiazepines	Additive sedative effects	Avoid concurrent use or choose alternate antihypertensive
	Alcohol, nitrates, other antihypertensives	Additive hypotension	Avoid concurrent use or monitor blood pressure closely
Methyldopa	Alcohol, antihistamines,	Additive sedation	Avoid concurrent use
	Beta-adrenergic blockers	May result in life-threatening HTN	Less likely with beta$_1$ selective agents; see clonidine above for implications
	Haloperidol	Potentiate antipsychotic effects or may produce psychosis	Choose different antipsychotic
	Levodopa	Potentiate antihypertensive effects of methyldopa and central effects of levodopa in Parkinson's disease	Avoid concurrent use; choose alternative antihypertensive

Table 14–3 ■ **Drug Interactions: Centrally Acting Alpha$_2$ Agonists—cont'd**

Drug	Interacting Drug	Possible Effect	Implications
Methyldopa (cont'd)	Lithium	Increased risk for lithium toxicity	Choose alternative antihypertensive
	Monoamine oxidase inhibitors (MAOIs)	Metabolites of methyldopa stimulate release of endogenous catecholamines that are usually metabolized by MAOIs; result is excessive SNS stimulation	Avoid concurrent use
	Nitrates, other antihypertensives	Additive hypotension	Avoid concurrent use
	Phenothiazines, sympathomimetics, barbiturates, amphetamines	May result in serious HTN	Avoid concurrent use
	Tolbutamide	Tolbutamide metabolism may be impaired, resulting in enhanced hypoglycemic effects	Choose alternative hypoglycemic
	TCAs	Attenuation or reversal of antihypertensive effect of methyldopa	Avoid concurrent use; choose alternative drugs for depression or HTN
	Herbals: Licorice Yohimbe, ginseng	May affect electrolyte levels May decrease efficacy of methyldopa	Monitor blood pressure and inform patient

Methyldopa has been associated with development of a positive Coombs' test, usually between 6 and 12 months after initiation of therapy. Rarely, this is associated with hemolytic anemia. The lowest incidence of this problem has been reported with doses of less than 1 g. Perform baseline hemoglobin and hematocrit levels, and repeat them at 6 and 12 months after initiation of therapy.

Drug Interactions

All centrally acting alpha$_2$ agonists have additive sedative effects with central nervous sytem (CNS) depressants and additive hypotension with other drugs that also reduce blood pressure. Table 14–3 gives the specific drugs. **Tricyclic antidepressant (TCA)** agents decrease the antihypertensive effects of all centrally acting alpha$_2$ agonists. Several other drugs used to treat psychoses interact with **centrally acting alpha$_2$ agonists,** resulting in toxicity, psychoses, or excessive SNS stimulation. Careful selection of the drugs to treat each condition is required. **Beta-adrenergic blockers** interact with **clonidine** and **methyldopa** to produce potentially life-threatening hypertension if either **clonidine** or **methyldopa** is abruptly discontinued. They should not normally be used concurrently, but there are occasions, such as when **beta-adrenergic blockers** are used for MI prophylaxis, when use of both drugs is necessary. If withdrawal of one or both of these drugs is required because of adverse effects, the **beta-adrenergic blocker** is always withdrawn first to prevent excessive unopposed stimulation of alpha$_2$ receptors that can result in a hypertensive crisis in as little as 12 hours. **Methyldopa** enhances the hypoglycemic effects of **tolbutamide (Orinase)**, which may result in serious hypoglycemia. There are a variety of oral hypoglycemics so that an alternative oral hypoglycemic can be chosen.

Clinical Use and Dosing

Hypertension

Centrally acting alpha$_2$ agonists are used to treat mild to moderate hypertension and are second-line drugs usually chosen when other drugs are not effective in achieving blood pressure control. The exception is **methyldopa,** which is first-line therapy for pregnant patients. These drugs are not well suited for monotherapy because they produce troublesome adverse reactions in almost all patients who take them. **Methyldopa** and **clonidine** can be used effectively when combined with a **diuretic** to address the problems with sodium and water retention. **Clonidine** is now available in a combination tablet with **chlorthalidone,** a **thiazide diuretic (Clorpres).**

Doses vary with each drug, but adverse reactions occur at higher doses and with older adults. Beginning with the lowest dose recommended for each drug, the dose is increased at weekly intervals until blood pressure control or the maximum dose is reached. To minimize the sedation, which is more common with **clonidine** and **methyldopa,** the dose may be divided, with a higher dose in the evening than in the morning. Smaller doses are required in renal impairment. Use of the low end of the dose range of **guanfacine** produces the least problems for patients with renal insufficiency.

Chapter 40 provides detailed discussion of the management of hypertension. It includes further discussion of the use of these drugs.

Unlabeled Uses of Clonidine

Clonidine has been evaluated for many off-labeled uses. It lowers the adrenergic stimulation associated with **alcohol** and **nicotine** withdrawal and lessens the unpleasant symptoms of withdrawal. Attention deficit-hyperactivity disorder is associated with decreased stimulation of certain centers in the brain, and the stimulation of central $alpha_2$ receptors by **clonidine** has resulted in improved concentration and reduced behavioral symptoms in some children. Dosage schedules for these and other unlabeled uses are presented in Table 14–4.

Guanfacine has also been evaluated for off-labeled use in children and young adults (ages 4–20) with ADHD and also those with Tourette syndrome. Both of these uses are based on relatively small studies with some benefit shown. Dosing is shown in Table 14–4.

Table 14–4 **Schedule: Centrally Acting $Alpha_2$ Agonists**

Drug	Indication	Initial Dose	Maintenance Dose
Clonidine	Hypertension	*Adults:* 0.1 mg bid PO (older adults may need lower dose)	*Adults:* Increase in increments of 0.1 mg PO in weekly intervals; maintenance dose 0.1–0.3 mg bid; max dose: 1.2 mg bid
		Transdermal: Catapres-TTS 1 (0.1 mg)	After 1–2 wk, if desired blood pressure (BP) is not achieved, increase in increments of 0.1 mg/wk (Catapres-TTS comes in 2 [0.2 mg] and 3 [0.3 mg] patches)
		Children (12 yr and older): 0.1 mg bid	*Children:* Increase in 0.1-mg increments at weekly intervals; maintenance dose 0.1–0.3 mg bid. Max dose: 2.4 mg/d
	Unlabeled uses:		
	Alcohol withdrawal		0.3–0.6 mg q 6 h
	ADHD		0.005 mg/kg/d
	Nicotine withdrawal		0.15–0.4 mg/d or 0.2 mg/24 h patch
	Postherpetic neuralgia		0.2 mg/d
	Restless legs syndrome		0.1–0.3 mg/d; up to 0.9 mg/d
	Ulcerative colitis		0.3 mg tid
	Hot flashes		0.05–0.4 mg twice daily
	Tourette syndrome		0.0025–0.015 mg/kg/d for 6 wk to 3 months
Clonidine HCl and Chlorthalidone (Clorpres) (B)	Hypertension	0.1 mg clonidine plus 15 mg chlorthalidone once or twice daily	Max dose 0.6 mg clonidine plus 30 mg chlorthalidone
Guanabenz	Hypertension	4 mg bid	Increase in increments of 4–8 mg/d every 1–2 wk until target BP achieved; max dose 32 mg bid
Guanfacine	Hypertension	1 mg daily at bedtime	May increase to 2 mg qd after 3–4 wk if target BP not achieved; 2-mg dose may be given as 1 mg bid; max dose 3 mg qd
	ADHD (extended release only) (off-labeled use; trials ongoing)	0.5 mg every 3–4 d or 0.25–0.5 mg every 5–7 d as needed or tolerated	Majority managed on 1.5 mg/d
	Tourette syndrome (extended release only) (off-labeled; trials ongoing)	0.5 mg/d	Titrate slowly based on response. Max dose 4 mg/d in 3 divided doses
Methyldopa	Hypertension	*Adults:* 250 mg bid or tid for first 48 h	Increase in increments of 250 mg every 2 d until target BP is achieved: to minimize sedation, increase dose in evening; smaller doses should be used in renal impairment; maintenance dose 500–2,000 mg/d in 2–4 divided doses
		Children: 10 mg/kg/d in 2–4 divided doses	*Children:* max dose is 65 mg/kg or 3,000 mg, whichever is less

Both drugs are used as adjunctive therapy and mainly to treat comorbid problems such as insomnia caused by ADHD drugs or the tics associated with Tourette syndrome.

Rational Drug Selection

Age

Only **clonidine** and **methyldopa** have pediatric doses and are approved for use with children. **Clonidine** works better in older adults. Dosage reductions may be required for **methyldopa** and **clonidine** when prescribed for older adults because of the risk for fluid retention and orthostatic hypotension.

Concomitant Disease Processes

Because it does not affect the renin-angiotensin-aldosterone (RAA) axis, **clonidine** works well for patients with decreased renal function. It also does not affect glucose metabolism and is useful for patients with diabetes.

Pregnancy

The National High Blood Pressure Education Program, in its Seventh Report of the Joint National Committee on Prevention, Detection, Evaluation, and Treatment of High Blood Pressure (2003), recommends **methyldopa** as the drug of choice for pregnant women.

Route of Administration

Patients who have difficulty taking pills, who have trouble remembering more frequent doses, or who for other reasons would have better adherence to the treatment regimen with a transdermal system can be given **clonidine.** This drug is the only **antihypertensive** currently available in a transdermal formulation (Table 14–5). Because the transdermal form of the medication results in lower serum levels (lack of a peak associated with oral administration), this dosage form may minimize many of the drug's bothersome adverse effects.

Table 14–5 ◆ **Available Dosage Forms: Selected Centrally Acting Alpha$_2$ Agonists**

Drug	Dosage Form	Package	Cost
Clonidine (G) (Catapres)(B)	Tablets: 0.1 mg (Catapres is scored)	In bottles of 100, 500, 1,000 tablets and in UD 100	0.1 mg = $20/100 (G) $147/100 (B)
	0.2 mg (Catapres is scored)	In bottles of 100, 500, 1,000 tablets and in UD 100	0.2 mg = $22/100(G) $212/100 (B)
	0.3 mg (Catapres is scored)	In bottles of 100 tablets and in UD 100	0.3 mg = $22/100 (G) $247/100 (B)
CloNIDine (G)	Transdermal: 0.1-mg patch 0.2-mg patch 0.3-mg patch	In boxes of 4 for all strengths	$166/box of 4 $180/box of 4 $246/box of 4
(Catapres-TTS)	Transdermal: Catapres-TTS 1: 0.1 mg/24 hr Catapres-TTS 2: 0.2 mg/24 hr Catapres-TTS 3: 0.3 mg/24 hr	In packages of 4 and 12 In packages of 4 and 12 In packages of 4	$128/box of 4 $201/box of 4 $276/box of 4
Clonidine and chlorthalidone (Clorpres) (B)	Tablets: (scored) Clonidine 0.1 mg + Chlorthalidone 15 mg Clonidine 0.2 mg + Chlorthalidone 15 mg Clonidine 0.3 mg + Chlorthalidone 15 mg	In bottles of 100 tablets for all strengths	$131/100 $167/100 $201/100
Guanabenz (G) (Wytensin) (B)	Tablets: 4 mg 8 mg (scored)	In bottles of 100, 500 tablets (Wytensin in Redipak 100s) In bottles of 100, 500 tablets (Wytensin in bottles of 100)	$157/100
Guanfacine (G) (Tenex) (B)	Tablets: 1 mg 2 mg	In bottles of 100 tablets for both strengths	$68/100 (G) $262/10 (B) $84/100 (G) $354/100 (B)

Continued

Table 14–5 ◆ **Available Dosage Forms: Selected Centrally Acting Alpha_2 Agonists—cont'd**

Drug	Dosage Form	Package	Cost
Intuniv (B)	Tablets (extended-release): 1 mg 2 mg 3 mg 4 mg	In bottles of 100 tablets for all strengths	
Methyldopa (G)	Tablets: 250 mg	In bottles of 100, 500, 1,000 tablets and in UD100	$22/100
	500 mg	In bottles of 100, 500 tablets and in UD100	$43/100
Methyldopa/ hydrochlorothiazide	Tablets: 250 mg methyldopa/ 25 mg hydrochlorothiazide	In bottles of 60 and 100 tablets	$38/100

Monitoring

Clinical monitoring of blood pressure is appropriate for all drugs in this class as with any other antihypertensive drug. Baseline blood pressure should be taken before initiating therapy and with each change in dosage. Weight and other indicators of fluid status should also be monitored. See Chapter 40 for further discussion of blood pressure monitoring.

For patients who have or are at risk for renal impairment, dosage alterations are required. Assess serum creatinine prior to initiation of therapy and regularly thereafter for up to 1 year.

Methyldopa is associated with a risk for development of hemolytic anemia. A forewarning of this development is a positive Coombs' test between 6 and 12 months after initiation of therapy. Patients receiving this drug should have a baseline Coombs' test and complete blood count (CBC) done prior to initiation of therapy and at 6 and 12 months of therapy. Although only about 5 percent of patients who develop the positive Coombs' test go on to develop hemolytic anemia, the drug is withdrawn in the presence of a positive test. Hemolytic anemia resolves soon after the withdrawal, even though the Coombs' test may remain positive for several months.

Liver function studies are also done prior to therapy and at 6 and 12 months. **Methyldopa** has been associated with hepatotoxicity. Liver function usually returns to normal after withdrawal of the drug.

Patient Education

Administration

The drug should be taken exactly as prescribed, at the same time each day, even if the patient is feeling well. Missed doses are taken as soon as they are remembered unless it is almost time for the next dose. Doses are not doubled. If more than one oral dose of any of these drugs is late or if the **clonidine transdermal system** is changed 3 or more days late, report the occurance to the health-care provider. These drugs must be withdrawn slowly over 2 to 3 days to prevent rebound hypertension, and missed doses increase the risk for the occurrence of rebound hypertension. To prevent missing doses, patients should make certain they have enough medication available for weekends, holidays, and vacations.

Methyldopa has known interactions with several herbals; therefore, prescribers should ask patients about herbal use and be aware that drug interactions may occur. Drug–herbal interactions are listed in Table 14–3.

Instruct patients who are on the transdermal **clonidine** system in proper application of the patch. Apply the patch to a hairless area of intact skin on the upper arm or torso once every 7 days. Use a different site from the previous application. They should not cut or trim the patch. It can remain in place during bathing and swimming.

Adverse Reactions

Hypotension is the most common adverse reaction. Changing positions slowly, not exercising in hot weather, avoiding **alcohol**, and drinking more than 2 L of noncaffeinated fluid per day will decrease these reactions. For patients with heart failure, not increasing fluid intake by this amount may be clinically important.

Drowsiness and dry mouth are also common. Avoid activities requiring mental alertness until the patient's individual response to the drug is known. Drowsiness frequently subsides after 7 to 10 days of continuous therapy. Dry mouth can be minimized by practicing good oral hygiene, chewing sugarless gum, or sucking on hard candy.

Concurrent use of **alcohol** or other CNS depressants should also be avoided. **Centrally acting alpha_2 agonists** can produce additive sedation with these drugs.

Fluid retention is indicated by weight gain and swelling in the feet and ankles. Report any weight gain of more than 2 lb (1 kg) in 1 day to the health-care provider. Fluid retention may be treated by the addition of a **diuretic** to the treatment regimen.

Methyldopa has some unique adverse reactions. Jaundice may indicate hepatotoxicity and should be reported to the health-care provider. Decreased energy levels may indicate anemia. In the absence of another explanation for decreased energy, this symptom should also be reported to the health-care provider. Warn the patient that urine left standing may darken or turn red black. This does not indicated hematuria.

Lifestyle Management

Drugs control hypertension, but they do not cure it. Encourage patients to adhere to other interventions for management of hypertension such as weight loss, aerobic exercise, a low-sodium diet, smoking cessation, and stress management. See Chapter 40 for more detailed discussion of lifestyle management for patients with hypertension.

ADRENERGIC ANTAGONISTS

Adrenergic antagonists act directly by blockade of adrenergic receptors or indirectly by decreasing norepinephrine release within SNS terminals. Most of the clinically useful actions of these drugs result from blockade of $alpha_1$ receptors in blood vessels, $beta_1$ receptors in the heart, and $alpha_1$ receptors in the bladder neck and prostate gland. **Adrenergic antagonists** are categorized on the basis of receptors that are blocked and include drugs that block only one receptor and those that block more than one receptor. The following section discusses antagonist drugs whose major effect is on $alpha_1$ and beta receptors outside the CNS (peripherally acting).

$ALPHA_1$ ANTAGONISTS

Alpha 1 antagonists include nonselective and selective types. Following are their differences and the drugs in each category.

Nonselective Alpha Antagonists

Nonselective alpha antagonists include **phentolamine** (Regitine) and **phenoxybenzamine** (Dibenzyline). These drugs have approximately equal affinities for both the postsynaptic $alpha_1$ receptors and the presynaptic $alpha_2$ receptors. **Phenoxybenzamine** blocks the receptors irreversibly, whereas the blockade by **phentolamine** is reversible. These drugs will result in lowered blood pressure as a result of the blockade of the postsynaptic $alpha_1$ receptor. In addition, blockade of the presynaptic $alpha_2$ receptors results in reflex cardiac stimulation because the negative feedback inhibition of neurotransmitter release is being blocked. For this reason, these drugs are not used in the treatment of hypertension. They do have a role in the treatment of pheochromocytoma in which they are used to prophylax against hypertensive crisis as a result of release of norepinephrine from the tumor. Additionally, given by the intradermal route, they have a role in the treatment of extravasation of vasopressor drugs. Because these drugs are used almost exclusively by specialists, they are not discussed further here.

Selective $Alpha_1$ Antagonists

The **$alpha_1$ antagonists** reversibly block the effects of catecholamines at the postsynaptic $alpha_1$ receptors in vascular smooth muscle and in the smooth muscle of the bladder neck and prostate. These drugs are useful in lowering blood pressure as well as relieving outflow obstruction secondary to benign prostatic hypertrophy (BPH). Six drugs in this class are used clinically: **doxazosin** (Cardura), **prazosin** (Minipress), **terazosin** (Hytrin), **tamsulosin** (Flomax), **alfuzosin** (Uroxatral), and **silodosin** (Rapaflo). **Doxazosin**, **prazosin**, and **terazosin** can be used to treat both hypertension and BPH. **Tamsulosin**, **alfuzosin**, and **silodosin** have increased selectivity for the $alpha_1$ receptors in the prostate and as a result these drugs have little effect on blood pressure while relieving symptoms associated with BPH.

Pharmacodynamics

Reversible **$alpha_1$ antagonists** block postsynaptic $alpha_1$ receptors in the vasculature, resulting in a decrease in both arterial and venous vasoconstriction. Because arteriole and venous tone are determined largely by the stimulation of $alpha_1$ receptors in vascular smooth muscle, the result is a decrease in peripheral vascular resistance and lowered blood pressure. Both supine and standing blood pressures are lowered, with the most pronounced effect on diastolic blood pressure. Orthostatic hypotension may result from their action on receptors in venous smooth muscle. Reflex tachycardia may result from compensatory mechanisms but is minimal with **prazosin** (5.3%), **terazosin** (1.4%), and **doxazosin** (0.95). Since the remaining **$alpha_1$ antagonists** are more specific for the receptors found in the prostate, they do not cause reflex tachycardia. **Prazosin** and **terazosin** rarely produce reflex tachycardia. Chronic use of **$alpha_1$ antagonists** may result in compensatory increases in blood volume but at a fairly low rate of incidence (1% to 4%). The newer selective blockers have no mention of edema. **Tamsulosin**, **silodosin**, and **alfuzosin** have not been approved for treatment of hypertension.

The reduction in symptoms and improved urine flow rates in patients with BPH is related to relaxation of smooth muscle produced by blockade of the $alpha_1$ receptors, which are densely located in the bladder neck and prostate gland. Blockade of these receptors decreases urethral resistance and may relieve the obstruction and improve urine flow and BPH symptoms. Because there are few $alpha_1$ receptors in the body of the bladder, these drugs are able to reduce bladder outflow obstruction without affecting bladder contractility. Three subtypes of the $alpha_1$ receptors have been pharmacologically identified and cloned: $alpha_{1a}$, $_{1b}$, and $_{1d}$. Approximately 70 percent of the $alpha_1$ receptors in the prostate are subtype 1a and are also localized to the prostatic stroma. Presumably, if the efficacy of the selective **alpha$_1$ blockers** is mediated by the relaxation of the prostate smooth muscle, then the development of a selective **alpha$_{1a}$ receptor antagonist** would be advantageous. This would also result in fewer adverse drug reactions, which are theoretically mediated by the alpha$_{1b}$ and $_{1d}$ receptor subtypes. However, there is evidence that the selective **alpha$_{1a}$ receptor antagonists** relieve the lower urinary tract symptoms (LUTS) by a mechanism that is unrelated to prostate smooth-muscle relaxation. Therefore, an **alpha$_1$ antagonist** that does not demonstrate selectivity for subtypes may still be useful in the treatment of BPH. This premise is born out when looking at the available **alpha$_1$ antagonists** with indications for BPH. **Tamsulosin** is about ten times more selective for the alpha$_{1a}$ versus the alpha$_{1b}$ subtype. This selectivity is probably not enough to result in a clinical advantage. **Alfuzosin** demonstrates high affinity for the alpha$_1$ receptor but does not demonstrate selectivity for any one of the receptor subtypes. Last, **silodosin** demonstrates a 583-fold selectivity for the alpha$_{1a}$ receptor subtype and 56-fold selectivity for the alpha$_{1d}$ receptor subtype.

Pharmacokinetics

Absorption and Distribution

Five of the drugs in this class are well absorbed after oral administration (Table 14–6); **silodosin** is the exception. **Tamsulosin** is the most slowly absorbed. The absorption of **alfuzosin** was reduced by 50 percent when taken in a fasting state and it should be administered with food. Taking **tamulosin** in a fasting state increases bioavailability by 30 percent and increases C_{max} by 40 percent to 70 percent. Given the risk for adverse effects when given in a fasting state, however, the dose should be administered 30 minutes following the same meal each day. Despite the fact that the bioavailability for **silodosin** is about 32 percent, the package insert recommends administering the drug with a meal. All drugs in this class are widely distributed in the body and all are highly protein bound. **Doxazosin** accumulates in breast milk with a concentration 20 times that in maternal plasma. **Prazosin** is found in small amounts in breast milk, and it is not known if **terazosin** is excreted in breast milk. No information about breast milk concentration is provided for **tamsulosin, alfuzosin,** or **sildosin,** which would not be given to female patients.

Metabolism and Excretion

Extensively metabolized by the liver, reversible **alpha$_1$ antagonists** are excreted in both feces and urine. **Doxazocin** has significant first-pass metabolism and enterohepatic recycling of this drug causes plasma elimination to be biphasic. After morning dosing, the area under the curve (AUC) was 11 percent less than after evening dosing and the time to peak concentration after evening dosing occurred significantly later than after morning dosing. **Doxazocin** is primarily eliminated in the feces.

Prazosin undergoes demethylation and conjugation in the liver, and a majority of the dose is eliminated via biliary excretion in the feces. **Prazosin** has four active metabolites that have approximately 10 to 15 percent activity of the parent drug and may contribute to the pharmacological effect of the drug. Elimination of **prazosin** is slower in patients with congestive heart failure (CHF) than in normal individuals. In the presence of renal failure, elimination half-life of this drug may be prolonged, protein binding decreased, and peak plasma levels increased.

Terazosin has minimal hepatic first-pass metabolism to one active and three inactive metabolites. Nearly all of the circulating dose is in the form of parent drug. **Tamsulosin** is extensively metabolized by CYP 450 enzymes; less

Table 14–6 Selected Alpha$_1$-Adrenergic Antagonists

Drug	Onset	Peak	Duration	Protein Binding (%)	Bioavailability (%)	Half-Life	Elimination
Alfuzosin	UK	8 h	UK	82–90	49 (with food)	10 h	69% in feces; 24% in urine
Doxazosin	60–120 min	2–3 h	24 h	98	65	22 h	63% in bile/ feces; 9% in urine
Prazosin	120–130 min	1–3 h	6–12 h	92–97	48–68	2–3 h	90% in bile/ feces; 10% in urine
Silodosin	Unknown	2.6 h	Unknown	97	32	13.8 h	35.5% in urine; 55% in feces
Tamsulosin	Unknown	5 days	Unknown	94–99	>90	9–15 h	<10% unchanged in urine
Terazosin	15 min	1–2 h	12–24 h	90–94	90	9–12 h	60% in bile/ feces; 40% in urine

than 10 percent of the dose is eliminated unchanged, but the specific isoenzymes have not been identified. The resulting metabolites undergo conjugation with glucuronide or sulfate and then are eliminated in the urine.

Alfuzosin is extensively metabolized to inactive metabolites via CYP 3A4, and only about 11 percent of the administered drug is eliminated unchanged in the urine. The metabolites are eliminated primarily in the feces.

Silodosin is metabolized by hepatic CYP 3A4, along with glucuronidation and alcohol and aldehyde dehydrogenase. **Silodosin** has an active metabolite that has a half-life of approximately 24 hours.

Pharmacotherapeutics

Precautions and Contraindications

All the "azosin" drugs are contraindicated in the presence of volume depletion and CHF. Peripheral vasodilation caused by these drugs decreases venous return to the heart and may precipitate significant heart failure. Several of the drugs are associated with fluid retention that may exacerbate CHF.

The dosing for **prazosin, doxazosin, terazosin,** and **tamsulosin** does not need to be adjusted in renal or hepatic impairment. However, since each of these drugs is extensively metabolized by the liver and has significant potential for hypotensive events, it is prudent to start with the lowest dose and adjust based on clinical response. This approach is especially true for **doxazocin** because of the enterohepatic recycling discussed previously. With creatinine clearance (CrCl) of less than 30 mL/min, limited safety data are available for **alfuzosin**; therefore, the drug should be used cautiously.

Alfuzosin should not be given to patients with mild to moderate hepatic impairment (Childs-Pugh classes B and C). **Silodosin** requires no adjustment of dose in patients with mild to moderate hepatic impairment but is not recommended in those patients with severe hepatic impairment (Childs-Pugh score equal to or greater than 10). For patients with CrCl greater than or equal to 50 mL/min no dose adjustment is required for **silodosin**; for patients with CrCl 30 to 49 mL/min, the dose should be halved and when the CrCl falls below 30 mL/min, the use of **silodosin** is not recommended.

Doxazosin, prazosin, and **terazosin** are Pregnancy Category C. Teratogenicity and reduced fertility have been demonstrated in animal studies. There are no adequate and well-controlled studies in pregnant women. Because of its high concentration in breast milk, **doxazosin** should not be given to nursing mothers. **Prazosin** has also been found in breast milk. Exercise caution when administering **prazosin** or **terazosin** to nursing mothers, and do so only when benefits clearly outweigh risks to the baby. **Tamsulosin, alfuzosin,** and **silodosin** are not prescribed to female patients. Safety and efficacy for use with children have not been established.

Adverse Drug Reactions

Each of these drugs carries a risk for significant first-dose orthostatic hypotension that may result in syncope that tends to occur within 30 to 90 minutes of drug administration. This adverse reaction is decreased with continued doses, but returns if therapy is interrupted for even a few doses, if the dosage is increased, or if another antihypertensive is added to the treatment regimen. The first dose should be given in the clinic or taken at bedtime. The "first-dose" reaction may be minimized by starting with a 1-mg dose and slowly increasing the dosage at 2-week intervals (Table 14–7). **Terazosin** exhibits this reaction most often, **prazosin** is average, and it occurs least with **doxazosin**.

Table 14–7 ● Dosage Schedule: Selected Alpha$_1$-Adrenergic Antagonists

Drug	Indication	Initial Dose	Maintenance Dose
Doxazosin	Hypertension	1 mg daily at bedtime	2–16 mg daily. Depending on standing blood pressure (BP), increase dose in 2-mg increments until target BP is achieved. Doses >4 mg increase risk of postural hypotension
	BPH	1 mg daily at bedtime Extended-release form is 4 mg taken once daily at breakfast	1–8 mg daily. Depending on the urodynamics and BPH symptoms the dose is increased to 2 mg and then to 4 mg and 8 mg/daily. The recommended maximum dose is 8 mg. The titration interval is 1–2 wk
	Ureteral stones (off-labeled)	4 mg daily at bedtime	Give for up to 1 month or until expulsion of stone
Prazosin	Hypertension	Adults: 1–2 mg bid or tid; take first dose at bedtime	Adults: 6–15 mg/daily in 2–3 divided doses. Depending on standing BP, increase dose in 1-mg increments, with the larger dose being given at bedtime until target BP is achieved. Doses >20 mg/d usually do not increase efficacy

Continued

Table 14–7 ● **Dosage Schedule: Selected Alpha$_1$-Adrenergic Antagonists—cont'd**

Drug	Indication	Initial Dose	Maintenance Dose
Silodosin	BPH	8 mg once daily with a meal	No data are published about increasing dosage. Depending on standing BP, the starting dose may be 4 mg with increases to 8 mg as tolerated
Tamsulosin	BPH	0.1 mg daily 30 min prior to the same meal	May be increased after 2–4 wk to 0.8 mg daily
	Ureteral stones (off-labeled)	0.4 mg daily 30 min prior to the same meal	Give for up to 6 wk or until expulsion of stone
Terazosin	Hypertension	1 mg daily at bedtime	1–5 mg daily. Depending on standing BP, increase dose in 1-mg increments until target BP is achieved. Doses >20 mg/daily not increase efficacy
	BPH	1 mg daily at bedtime	Increased in a stepwise fashion to 2, 5, and then 10 mg. Doses at 10 mg are usually required for clinical effect. Dose may be 10–20 mg daily. Four to 6 wk are required to assess for beneficial response, so this is the interval for dosage adjustment
	Ureteral stones (off-labeled)	2 mg–5 mg daily at bedtime	Give for up to 1 month or until expulsion of stone
Alfuzosin	BPH	10 mg daily after the same meal	10 mg daily after the same meal

Fluid retention that results in peripheral edema occurs in several of these drugs. Close monitoring of weight changes may be needed, especially early in therapy, and the addition of a **diuretic** to the therapy regimen may be required.

Other adverse reactions are associated with alpha$_1$-adrenergic blockade (nasal congestion, blurred vision, dry mouth, constipation, impotence, and urinary frequency). Hypotension (dizziness, headache, fatigue, tachycardia, and nausea) is also a potential adverse effect.

Drug Interactions

The major drug interactions result in decreased antihypertensive effects with the interacting drug or in additive hypotension, with increased risk for postural hypotension. All six drugs have increased risk for postural hypotension when administered with acute **alcohol** ingestion, other **antihypertensives**, or **nitrates**. **Doxazosin** has the fewest published drug interactions and **prazosin** has the most. **Cimetidine** interacts with **tamsulosin** to decrease **tamsulosin's** effects. **Alfuzosin** is predominately metabolized by the CYP 3A4 isoenzyme systems, and other drugs also metabolized by this subsystem present a risk of interaction. Table 14–8 depicts the common drug interactions.

Clinical Use and Dosing

Hypertension (HTN)

Alpha$_1$-adrenergic antagonists (except **alfuzosin, tamsulosin**, and **silodosin**, which are not approved to treat HTN) are the drugs of choice for treating hypertension (HTN) in older men with concomitant BPH. Their actions simultaneously improve both conditions. They are also effective for African Americans, although not the first-line drugs. All drugs in this class reduce total cholesterol and triglycerides and raise high-density lipoprotein levels. **Doxazosin** and **terazosin** also lower low-density lipoprotein levels. This class of drugs is useful for patients with HTN who also have altered lipoprotein levels. They also enhance **insulin** sensitivity, cause regression of left ventricular hypertrophy, and improve the activity of the fibrinolytic system, making them useful for patients with diabetes and heart failure. Because they do not aggravate bronchospastic disease, they are useful for patients with asthma. **Alpha$_1$-adrenergic antagonists** are usually not used for monotherapy because they cause troublesome adverse reactions in almost all patients who take them. They can be used effectively in combination with other drugs that address these adverse reactions.

The Antihypertensive and Lipid-Lowering Treatment to Prevent Heart Attack (ALLHAT) trial was recently reevalutated considering information from new clinical trials, meta-analyses, and recent subgroup and explanatory analyses from ALLHAT. The reevaluation included special focus on studies related to the consequences of cardiovascular disease. Findings in the initial study and supported in the reevaluation show **alpha$_1$-adrenergic antagonists** are surpassed by thiazide-type **diuretics** as initial therapy for reduction of cardiovascular and renal risk associated with hypertension (Wright et al, 2009). In the initial ALLHAT study, the drug used was **doxazosin**; this part of the study was discontinued early because so many subjects dropped out because of adverse effects

Table 14–8 ■ **Drug Interactions: Selected $Alpha_1$-Adrenergic Antagonists**

Drug	Interacting Drug	Possible Effect	Implications
Alfuzosin	Ketoanazole, itraconazole, ritoniver	Decrease metabolism and increase effects of alfuzosin	Avoid concurrent use
	Cimetidine, atenolol, dilitiazem	Increases level of alfuzosin and may increase effects of atenolol and dilitiazem	Monitor blood pressure and heart rate
	Antihypertensives, calcium channel blockers, nitrates, and alcohol	Increased hypotension risk	Monitor blood pressure or avoid concurrent use
Prazosin	Beta-adrenergic blockers	May enhance acute postural hypotension following first dose of $alpha_1$-adrenergic blocker	Select different $alpha_1$-adrenergic blocker. No adverse reaction seen with doxazosin or terazosin
	Clonidine	May decrease antihypertensive effect of clonidine	Avoid concurrent use
	Indomethacin	Antihypertensive action of prazosin may be decreased	Select different $alpha_1$-adrenergic blocker or different NSAID. No adverse reaction with doxazosin or other NSAIDs
Silodosin	Calcium channel blockers and thiazides	Increased incidence of dizziness and orthostatic hypotension	Exercise caution and monitor for adverse effects
	Azole antifungals, clarithromycin and other strong CYP3A4 inhibitors	Ketoconazole increased Cmax and AUC	Concomitant use with strong CYP3A4 inhibitors contraindicated
	Diltiazem, erythromycin, verapamil, and other moderate CYP3A4 inhibitors	May increase plasma levels	Exercise caution and monitor for adverse effects
	Phosphodiesterase type 5 inhibitors (e.g., sildenafil, tadalafil)	Increased incidence of orthostatic hypotension	Exercise caution and monitor for adverse effects
Tamsulosin	Cimetidine	May increase blood levels of tamsulosin, with increased risk for hypotension and toxicity	Select different $histamine_2$ blocker if one must be used
Terazosin	NSAIDs, sympathomimetics, estrogens	May decrease antihypertensive effects of terazosin	Avoid concurrent use or select doxazosin or another drug class for antihypertensive therapy
	Verapamil	Increases serum terazosin levels and may increase sensitivity to terazosin-induced postural hypotension	Avoid concurrent use
	Finasteride	Increase in peak plasma concentration and AUC of finasteride	Clinical significance unknown; monitor for adverse effects of finasteride
Doxazosin, prazosin, tamsulosin, terazosin, alfuzosin	Alcohol, antihypertensives, nitrates	Additive hypotension	Avoid concurrent use or administer first dose in the office and monitor blood pressure response closely

and because the blood pressure lowering effect was the least. Given these data, it seems appropriate that this class of drugs be used mainly when a primary goal is treatment of BPH symptoms rather than hypertension.

To reduce "first-dose" postural hypotension, the dose is begun at 1 mg qd to bid, depending on the drug (Table 14–7). The dose is then gradually increased until target blood pressure is achieved or the maximum dose reached. When the dose is increased, the first larger dose is always given at bedtime to reduce orthostatic hypotension effects. **Doxazosin** has once-daily dosing. Postural hypotension effects are most commonly seen 2 to 6 hours after taking a dose. Measure the blood pressure at this time interval for the first dose and when increasing the dose to determine if the target blood pressure is being reached. **Prazosin** has a bid or tid dosing schedule. Measure blood pressure 2 to 3 hours after dosing to see when maximum and minimum benefits in blood pressure lowering result. If the response is substantially diminished at 24 hours on bid dosing, consider increasing the dose or using a tid regimen. Measure blood pressure 2 to 3 hours after dosing for **terazosin** as well. Although **terazosin** usually has once-daily dosing, if the response is diminished, consider bid dosing. When a **diuretic** is added to the treatment regimen of any of these drugs, the dose of the **alpha$_1$-adrenergic antagonist** is reduced for 2 to 3 days and then retitrated to control the blood pressure.

Benign Prostatic Hyperplasia

Tamulosin, **alfuzosin**, and **silodosin** have all been approved for treatment of symptoms of benign prostatic hyperplasia. The recommended dose of **tamulosin** is 0.4 mg once daily administered approximately 30 minutes following the same meal each day. If the patient fails to respond to this dose after 2 to 4 weeks, the dose is increased to 0.8 mg once daily. **Alfuzosin** is recommended at 10 mg of the extended-release tablet daily to be taken immediately after the same meal each day. **Silodosin** starting dose is 8 mg given once daily with a meal (*Drug Facts and Comparisons*, 2009).

Ureteral Stones

Doxazosin, **tamsulosin**, and **terazosin** have off-labeled use as adjunct treatment to promote ureteral stone expulsion. These drugs do so by reducing ureteral pressure, peristaltic frequency and ureteral contractions. American Urological Association and European Association of Urology guidelines for the management of ureteral calculi indicate that the administration of these drugs can effectively accelerate the spontaneous passage of these stones (*Drug Facts and Comparisons*, 2009).

Rational Drug Selection

Cost

Prazosin is the least expensive of this drug class. **Terazosin** is the most expensive, and **doxazosin** is in the middle for cost. **Doxazosin** is less likely than the other two drugs to produce postural hypotension and fluid retention, however, and may be used as monotherapy. The overall cost of the treatment regimen is reduced if an additional drug is unnecessary.

Convenient Dosing and Tolerability

Terazosin and **doxazosin** are both longer acting alpha$_1$-receptor antagonists, but both need to be titrated to the target dose because of hypotension issues. **Tamsulosin** is also a longer acting **alpha$_1$-receptor antagonist**, but it produces a response without dose titration. **Tamsulosin's** disadvantage is an increased incidence of ejaculatory dysfunction. **Alfuzosin** is marketed as a slow-release formulation, and thus has relatively low adverse drug reactions. It also does not require dose titration and has the advantage of not causing ejaculatory dysfunction. **Silodosin** does not require dose titration but has an increased incidence of ejaculatory dysfunction when compared with tamsulosin.

Both **doxazosin** and **terazosin** offer once-daily dosing (Table 14–9) and **doxazosin** is now available in an extended-release formulation for treating BPH. **Prazosin** requires bid or tid dosing. **Doxazosin** is scored to allow the tablet to be broken in half so that dosages can be easily increased without a change in tablet size.

Tachycardia

Although all drugs in this class may exhibit reflex tachycardia due to their antihypertensive effects, **prazosin** is especially noted for this problem and frequently requires increased dosages over time. **Prazosin** can be mixed with concomitant administration of a diuretic.

Indications

Doxazosin, **prazosin**, and **terazosin** are all approved to treat hypertension. Treatment of BPH symptoms is Food and Drug Administration (FDA) approved only for **doxazosin**, **tamsulosin**, **alfuzosin**, **silodosin**, and **terazosin**, although dosage data for this indication are published for **prazosin**.

Monitoring

Clinical monitoring of symptoms according to guidelines for HTN (see Chapter 40) and for BPH is the main monitoring parameter. Fluid retention is monitored by weekly weighing and patient education about signs and symptoms of fluid overload to report (e.g., peripheral edema, weight gain of more than 1 kg in a 24-hour period). Reduced white blood cell (WBC) counts of 1 to 2.4 percent have been noted, although no patients became symptomatic with these lower counts. A baseline WBC is drawn prior to initiation of therapy and as part of regular physical examinations. This class of drugs is heavily metabolized by the liver, so baseline liver function tests are also recommended.

Cancer of the prostate gland and BPH often coexist and have the same symptoms. Patients who are to begin

Table 14–9 **Available Dosage Forms of Selected Alpha$_1$-Adrenergic Antagonists**

Drug	Dosage Forms	Package	Cost
Alfuzosin (Uroxatral) (B)	Tablet: 10 mg extended-release	In bottles of 30 and 100 and UD 100	$112/30
Doxazosin (G) (Cardura) (B)	Tablets: 1 mg, 2 mg, 4 mg, 8 mg	In bottles of 100, 500, and 1,000 tablets for the generic and bottles of 100 and UD 100 for the brand name	Generic: 1 mg = $53/100 2 mg = $49/100 4 mg = $67/100 8 mg = $70/100 Brand: 1 mg = $53/100 2 mg = $151/100 4 mg = $153/100 8 mg = $171/100
Cardura XL (B)	Tablets: (extended-release) 4 mg, 8 mg	In bottles of 30 tablets for both strengths	4 mg = $56/30
Prazosin (G) (Minipress) (B)	Generic capsules: 1 mg, 2 mg, 5 mg	In bottles of 100, 500, and 1,000 capsules	Generic: 1 mg = $30/100 2 mg = $38/100 5 mg = $57/100
	Minipress capsules: 1 mg, 2 mg, 5 mg	In bottles of 250 capsules	Brand: 1 mg = $49/100 2 mg = $105/100 5 mg = $166/100
Silodosin (Rapaflo)	Capsules: 4 mg 8 mg	In bottles of 30 and 100 In bottles of 30, 90, and 1,000	Brand: 8 mg = $120/30
Tamsulosin (Flomax) (B)	Capsules: 0.4 mg	In bottles of 100 and 1,000 capsules	$335/90
Terazosin (G) (Hytrin) (B)	Generic tablets: 1 mg, 2 mg, 5 mg, 10 mg	In bottles of 100 and 1,000 tablets	$38/100 for all strengths
	Generic capsules: 1 mg, 2 mg, 5 mg, 10 mg	In bottles of 100 and 500 capsules	$38/100 for all strengths
	Hytrin capsules: 1 mg, 2 mg, 5 mg, 10 mg	In bottles of 100 capsules and UD 100	

on **alpha$_1$-adrenergic antagonist** therapy for BPH should first have digital rectal examinations and prostate-specific antigen (PSA) levels drawn to rule out prostate cancer. Research has indicated that **doxazosin** and **terazosin** do not affect PSA levels in patients treated for less than 3 years (*Drug Facts and Comparisons,* 2009).

Patient Education

Administration

The drug should be taken exactly as prescribed, at the same time each day, even if the patient is feeling well. The first dose at initiation of therapy and the first dose each time the dosage is increased should be taken at bedtime to minimize the first-dose effect (potential hypotension and syncope). Missed doses are taken as soon as they are remembered unless it is almost time for the next dose. Doses are not doubled. Drugs in this class that may be taken without regard to food intake are **doxazosin, prazosin,** and **terazosin. Alfuzosin** should be taken with food or after food intake and **tamsulosin** should be taken 30 minutes after food intake. **Silodosin** should be administered with a meal.

NSAIDs decrease the antihypertensive effects of most drugs in this class. Over-the-counter (OTC) medications that contain NSAIDs should be avoided. Advise the patient to consult the health-care provider before taking any OTC drug, especially cough, cold, and allergy remedies.

If the drug is given for BPH, teach the patient the signs and symptoms of BPH to monitor (urinary frequency, a feeling of incomplete bladder emptying, interruption of urinary stream, decreased size and force of stream, terminal urinary dribbling, and straining to start the flow of urine). Improvement in these symptoms may take 4 to 6 weeks.

Adverse Drug Reactions

Hypotensive reactions are the most common. In addition to taking the first dose at bedtime, teach patients to rise slowly from a supine position and to dangle their feet over the side of the bed before arising. Not exercising in hot weather and maintaining a fluid intake of 2 L per day of noncaffeinated fluids can also decrease these reactions.

Larger volumes of fluid may exacerbate another common adverse reaction: fluid retention. The best assessment of excessive fluid is weight gain. Report gains of more than 2 lb (1 kg) in 1 day or swelling of the ankles to the health-care provider.

Nasal congestion and/or rhinitis may occur. It should not be treated with OTC **antihistamines** or other cold remedies without first consulting with the health-care provider. Drowsiness and dry mouth are also common. The patient should avoid activities requiring mental alertness until the patient's individual response to the drug is known. Drowsiness frequently subsides after 7 to 10 days of continuous therapy. Dry mouth can be minimized by practicing good oral hygiene, chewing sugarless gum, or sucking on hard candy.

The leading cause of nonadherence to a treatment regimen with **alpha$_1$-adrenergic antagonists** is inhibition of ejaculation and impotence. These reactions should be reported to the health-care provider, who may choose a different drug to treat the disorder or change the dosage.

Lifestyle Management

If the drug is being given for HTN, encourage the patient to adhere to additional interventions for reduction of blood pressure, such as weight loss, low-sodium diet, smoking cessation, regular exercise, and stress management. Further discussion of patient education related to HTN is found in Chapter 40. BPH is discussed in the Men as Patients chapter (Chapter 49).

BETA-ADRENERGIC ANTAGONISTS (BLOCKERS)

Beta-adrenergic antagonists (blockers) are mainstays in the treatment of hypertension and cardiac disorders. They are also useful in a variety of other disorders, including glaucoma, migraine headache prophylaxis, and hyperthyroidism. They act by occupying beta-receptor sites and competitively preventing occupancy of these sites by **catecholamines** and other **beta agonists**. A major difference among these drugs is their selectivity for beta$_1$- and beta$_2$-receptor sites, and this difference has important clinical implications. Initially this partial agonist activity was thought to be useful in situations such as bronchospastic diseases or CHF where it would not block the beta receptor entirely. However, intrinsic sympathetic activity (ISA) has not been shown to have any clinical significance.

The action of these drugs is through blockade of beta-adrenergic receptors, and they are usually referred to in health-care literature as **beta blockers**. Because this term is easily recognized, **beta blocker** is used throughout this text to denote **beta-adrenergic antagonists**.

> **CLINICAL PEARL**
>
> Patients may have difficulty understanding how best to determine changes in force of urine stream. Try asking male patients if they have to stand closer to the toilet when voiding.

Pharmacodynamics

Blockade of beta-adrenergic receptors produces clinically significant action on the cardiovascular, renal, and respiratory systems and on the eye. This blockade also results in metabolic and endocrine effects.

Cardiovascular Effects

The heart has mainly beta$_1$ receptors. Blockade of these receptors acts at the sinoatrial (SA) node to decrease heart rate (negative chronotropism), in the atria and ventricles to decrease contractility (negative inotropism) and conduction velocity (negative dromotropism), and at the atrioventricular (AV) junction to slow conduction. Taken together, these effects decrease the incidence of angina, decrease cardiac rhythm disturbances associated with rapid rhythms, decrease both supine and standing blood pressure, and reduce reflex orthostatic tachycardia. In patients whose severely damaged hearts require sympathetic stimulation for adequate ventricular function, beta blockade may worsen the condition.

In the vascular system, beta blockade opposes beta$_2$-mediated vasodilation and may initially result in a rise in peripheral vascular resistance, but chronic drug administration leads to a fall in peripheral resistance through a possible central effect that causes reduced sympathetic outflow to the periphery. These effects are central to the use of these drugs in the treatment of hypertension.

Renal Effects

Blockade of the beta$_1$ receptors in the juxtaglomerular apparatus of the kidney reduces the release of renin. This effect on the rennin-angiotensin-aldosterone (RAA) system leads to less angiotensin II–mediated vasoconstriction and aldosterone-mediated volume expansion, resulting in decreases in blood pressure.

Respiratory Effects

Beta$_2$ receptors are located throughout the body. In the lungs, blockade of these receptors interferes with endogenous adrenergic bronchodilator activity, which results in passive bronchial constriction. This increase in airway resistance is particularly problematic for patients with reactive airway diseases such as asthma.

Ocular Effects

Although $beta_2$ stimulation results in changes in pupil size and accommodation, **beta blockers** administered topically as ophthalmic solutions have little or no effect on pupillary muscles. The exact mechanism by which these drugs reduce intraocular pressure is not established but is thought to be achieved by reduction in the production of aqueous humor. Some studies have shown a slight increase in acqueous humor outflow via Schlemm's canal with **timolol (Timoptic)**. Topical use of **beta blockers** is discussed in Chapter 26.

Metabolic and Endocrine Effects

$Beta_2$-blockade effects on the liver lead to inhibition of lipolysis, resulting in increased triglycerides and cholesterol and decreased high-density lipoproteins. For patients with hyperlipidemia, $beta_2$ blockade may worsen the condition.

Effects on the liver also lead to inhibition of gluconeogenesis. **Beta blocker** action on the pancreas results in impaired insulin release that leads to hyperglycemia in patients with type 2 diabetes. Taken together, these actions may also impair recovery from hypoglycemia in patients with diabetes. $Beta_1$-selective drugs are less likely to cause these problems.

Effects on Other Systems

The effect of beta blockade on other body systems is the source of the adverse drug reactions that may cause nonadherence to the drug regimen. The vascular effects on the male sex organs may result in impotence. Increased GI motility may contribute to diarrhea. Fatigue, dizziness, and depression are also common adverse effects related to the effects on other body systems.

Pharmacokinetics

Absorption and Distribution

All **beta blockers** are well absorbed when given orally and are widely distributed in body tissues (Table 14–10). All cross the placenta and enter breast milk. CNS penetration varies, based on lipid solubility, with minimal penetration for **acebutolol, atenolol, nadolol,** and **pindolol** and moderate penetration for **timolol** and **metoprolol**, with **propranolol** having the highest CNS penetration. **Nebivolol** is

Table 14–10 ▶ **Pharmacokinetics: Selected Beta Blockers**

Drug	Onset	Peak	Duration	Protein Binding (%)	Bioavailability (%)	Half-Life	Elimination
Acebutolol*	60 min	4–6 h	24–30 h	26	<50	3–4 h; (18–13 h for diacetolol, the active metabolite)	30%–40% in urine; 50%–60% in feces/bile
Atenolol	60 min	2–4 h	24 h	6–16	50–60	6–9 h	50% unchanged in urine; rest in feces
Metoprolol	15 min	90 min	13–19 h	12	50–77	3–7 h	<5% unchanged in urine
Nadolol	5 days†	3–4 h	17–24 h	30	30–50	20–40 h	Unchanged in urine
Nebivolol	15 min	1.5–4 h	UK	98	UK	12–19 h based on genetic differences	38%–67% in urine; 13%–44% in feces
Pindolol*	7 days†	1 h	24 h	40	100	3–4 h	60%–65% metabolites and 35%–40% unchanged drug in urine
Propranolol	30 min	60–90 min	6–12 h	90	30	3–5 h	<1% unchanged in urine
Propranolol ER	UK	6 h	24 h	90	9–18	8–11 h	<1% unchanged in urine
Timolol	UK	1–3 h	12–24 h	10	75	4 h	Metabolites and unchanged drug in urine

UK = unknown.
*Intrinsic sympathomimetic activity. Pindolol more than acebutolol.
†Onset of cardiovascular effects.

highly lipophilic and has CNS penetration, but the exact degree of penetration is not clear.

Metabolism and Excretion

Most **beta blockers** are metabolized extensively by the liver and eliminated via the bile and feces. Dosages of most of these agents may need to be decreased in patients with hepatic impairment. **Nebivolol**, a new third generation **beta blocker**, has several routes of metabolism and a metabolic fate that is heavily genetically based. Most of the population are extensive metabolizers (EM) of the drug and about 10 percent are poor metabolizers (PM). Metabolism includes glucuronidation and hydroxylation by CYP2D6 and to a lesser extent dealkylation and oxidation via this same isoenzyme system. It has two active sterospecific isomers. The d-isomer is the most active and PMs attain a 5-fold higher maximal drug concentration (Cmax) and a 10-fold higher AUC of this isomer than EMs (*Drug Facts and Comparisons*, 2009).

Several **beta blockers (acebutolol, atenolol, nadolol,** and **nebivolol)** require dosage adjustment in patients with renal impairment. The dose of **acebutolol** should be decreased by 50 percent when CrCl is less than 50 mL/min and by 75 percent if CrCl is less than 25 mL/min. Because approximately 40 percent of **atenolol** is excreted unchanged in the urine, the dose of this drug will need to be adjusted if creatinine clearance falls below 35 mL/min. Because **nadolol** is excreted unchanged in the urine, dosing must be adjusted in renal impairment. The recommendation for dosing **nadolol** in this situation involves extending the dosing interval. Last, with CrCl less than 30 mL/min, **nebivolol** dosing should be started at 2.5 mg daily and titrated.

Pharmacotherapeutics

Precautions and Contraindications

Beta blockers are contraindicated for patients with respiratory conditions that include a bronchospastic component. Although there are $beta_1$-selective drugs that have less effect on the $beta_2$ receptors in the lungs, to date no **beta blocker** is sufficiently selective to $beta_1$ to completely reduce the risk of $beta_2$ blockade. Even $beta_1$-selective drugs show $beta_2$ effects at higher doses. Because of their relative $beta_1$ selectivity, *Drug Facts and Comparisons* (2009) suggests that low doses of **acebutolol, atenolol, betaxolol, bisprolol,** and **metoprolol** may be cautiously used for patients with bronchospastic disease who do not respond to any other hypertensive treatment. **Nebivolol** is also $beta_1$ selective, but no recommendation about its use has yet been made.

These drugs are also contraindicated for patients with AV block, where their actions to decrease heart rate and myocardial contractility result in increased reduction in cardiac output and worsened failure. Decreased cardiac output and the initial vasoconstrictive action of these drugs may also worsen peripheral vascular diseases. Recognition that beta-adrenergic stimulation is a factor in heart failure has resulted in the use of **beta blockers** in congestive heart failure, where it was formerly contraindicated. Chapter 36 discusses their use for this indication in more detail.

Older adults often have limited cardiac and renal reserves. **Beta blockers** are used to treat conditions common to older adults, but care must be taken with dosing, and closer monitoring of cardiac and renal status is required. Based on meta-analyses of previous studies, **beta blockers** are less efficacious than other first-line therapies for cardiovascular disorders in patients who are 60 years or older, especially for stroke prevention (Institute for Clinical Systems Improvement [ICSI], 2008). Use of these drugs as initial therapy for older adults should be restricted to situations in which there is another indication for their use.

Beta blockers may precipitate or exacerbate type 2 diabetes (American Association of Clinical Endocrinologists [AACE], 2006). Because of their effects on carbohydrate metabolism and their ability to mask the common symptoms of hypoglycemia, **beta blockers** must be used cautiously in patients with diabetes. **Beta blockers** have proved to be effective in the management of the ischemic and congestive cardiac disorders that are more common in patients with diabetes, so they do have a role. If **beta blockers** must be used, $beta_1$-selective drugs, including the new third generation drug **nebivolol**, are less likely to produce those problematic diabetes effects.

Beta blockers may also mask clinical signs of developing or continuing thyrotoxicosis, and abrupt withdrawal may precipitate hyperthyroidism, including thyroid storm. They are used with caution in patients at risk for developing or having hyperthyroidism. In contrast, **propranolol** may be useful in decreasing the symptoms of thyrotoxicosis and has been used for this purpose, although it is not FDA approved.

Beta blockers vary in Pregnancy category. **Atenolol** is Pregnancy Category D; administering **atenolol** starting in the second trimester has been associated with small-for-gestational-age infants. **Betaxolol, metoprolol, nadolol, nebivolol, timolol,** and **propranolol** are Pregnancy Category C. All cross the placenta and can cause fetal or neonatal bradycardia, hypotension, hypoglycemia, or respiratory depression. If these drugs must be used, avoid use during the first trimester, use the lowest dose that produces a therapeutic effect, and discontinue the drug at least 2 to 3 days prior to delivery. **$Beta_1$-selective drugs** appear to be somewhat less problematic in this regard. **Acebutolol, sotalol,** and **pindolol** are listed as Pregnancy Category B. Note, however, that neonates of mothers who received these latter drugs had reduced birth weight and decreased blood pressure and heart rate at birth.

Propranolol is excreted in breast milk, but with a concentration too low to have any significant effect. **Metoprolol** is excreted in very small quantities. All other **beta blockers** are excreted in larger amounts. Although adverse effects to infants have not been demonstrated, nursing mothers should be given these drugs only when benefits clearly outweigh risks. Studies in rats have shown that **nebivolol** is excreted in breast milk. It is not known if it is excreted in human milk, but it is not recommended during breast feeding.

Safety and efficacy in children have not been established for some **beta blockers**. **Atenolol** and **propranolol** have pediatric dosing schedules for children with hypertension. **Toprol XL** was studied with pediatric hypertensive patients ages 6 to 16 years old. It did not meet the primary endpoint of the study, but some study endpoints demonstrated effectiveness. Dosage schedules for hypertension are posted on http://www.fda.gov.

Adverse Drug Reactions

Beta blockade affects target organs and nontarget organs and tissues alike. This wide range of effects results in many adverse reactions for these drugs, although most adverse reactions have been mild and transient and have rarely required withdrawal of therapy. The discussion here focuses on the adverse reactions on each organ system.

Cardiovascular

Bradycardia, CHF with concomitant pulmonary edema, and hypotension are the most common cardiovascular adverse reactions. They have been discussed here in the Precautions and Contraindications section.

Central Nervous System and Psychiatric

Fatigue, weakness, and dizziness are associated with reduced oxygen transport to the brain secondary to excessive hypotension. Anxiety, depression, drowsiness, insomnia, nightmares, and mental status changes are more common in those drugs that have higher CNS penetration and in older adults. These adverse reactions may disappear when a less lipophilic **beta blocker** is substituted.

Endocrine

Alterations in carbohydrate metabolism resulting in hyperglycemia, hypoglycemia, or unstable diabetes have been discussed in the Precautions and Contraindications section.

> **CLINICAL PEARL**
>
> For patients with diabetes who must take a **beta blocker,** the diaphoresis associated with hypoglycemia is not masked by these drugs. Patients should be taught to recognize this indication of possible hypoglycemia and test their blood glucose levels whenever unexplained diaphoresis occurs.

Gastrointestinal

Dry mouth is uncommon, but may occur. It may be reduced by practicing good oral hygiene, chewing sugarless gum, or sucking on hard candy. Changes in GI motility may result in anorexia, nausea, vomiting, flatulence, and constipation or diarrhea.

Genitourinary

One of the most likely reasons for nonadherence to a treatment regimen that includes **beta blockers** is the risk for impotence and decreased libido, based on the action of the drugs on the male sexual organs.

Respiratory

Bronchospasm and dyspnea have been discussed in the Precautions and Contraindications section. Nasal stuffiness may also occur.

Others

Less common adverse reactions include muscle and joint pain, pruritic rashes, and facial swelling. These are not directly related to the actions of these drugs.

Drug, Food, and Laboratory Test Interactions

Drug Interactions

Many drug interactions occur with **beta blockers**, and before they are prescribed, Table 14–11 should be consulted. Common problems include additive hypotension with other antihypertensives, acute ingestion of **alcohol** or **nitrates**, bradycardia with **digitalis**, and altered effectiveness of hypoglycemic drugs. Concurrent use of several drugs found in OTC cold remedies (**ephedrine**, **phenylephrine**, **pseudoephedrine**) may result in unopposed alpha-adrenergic stimulation, causing excessive hypertension and tachycardia. **Metoprolol**, **nebivolol**, and **propranolol** have drug interactions in addition to those found with other **beta blockers**. The drug in this category with the fewest interactions is **atenolol**.

Life-threatening and fatal increases in blood pressure have been observed in patients taking **clonidine** and a **beta blocker** concurrently when the **clonidine** was withdrawn or when both the **clonidine** and the **beta blocker** were withdrawn. It is best to avoid using these drugs together, but if they are both given and withdrawal of one or both becomes necessary, taper the **beta blocker** first to avoid unopposed alpha stimulation and significant hypertension.

Food Interactions

Food enhances the bioavailability of **metoprolol** and **propranolol**. This effect is not noted with **nadolol**, **nebivolol**, or **pindolol**.

Laboratory Test Interactions.

Beta blockers may cause increased blood urea nitrogen (BUN), serum lipoprotein, potassium, triglyceride, and uric

Table 14–11 ■ **Drug Interactions: Selected Beta Blockers**

Drug	Interacting Drug	Possible Effect	Implications
All beta blockers	Aluminum salts, barbiturates, calcium salts, cholestyramine, colestipol, NSAIDs, ampicillin, rifampin, salicylates	Decrease bioavailability and plasma levels of beta-adrenergic antagonists, possibly resulting in decreased pharmacological effect	Avoid concurrent use. Separate administration of cholestyramine or colestipol from administration of beta-adrenergic antagonist by 4 h
	Calcium channel blockers	Potentiate effects of beta-adrenergic antagonists	Do not administer within 24 h of each other. If must give both, monitor for heart failure and decreased peripheral perfusion
	Ciprofloxacin and other quinolones, cimetidine	Bioavailability of beta-adrenergic antagonists metabolized by CYP450 may be increased	Select different antibiotic or different beta-adrenergic antagonist
	Digoxin	Additive bradycardia	Avoid concurrent administration. If must give both, monitor closely for digitalis toxicity. May need to adjust doses of one or both
	Antihypertensives, alcohol, nitrates	Additive hypotension	Avoid acute ingestion of alcohol. Monitor blood pressure (BP) closely
	Amphetamines, cocaine, ephedrine, epinephrine, norepinephrine, phenylephrine, pseudoephedrine	Concurrent use may result in unopposed alpha adrenergic stimulation, resulting in excessive hypertension and bradycardia	Avoid concurrent use. Warn patients because many of these are included in OTC cold remedies
	Prazosin	Concurrent administration may potentiate postural hypotension	Avoid concurrent administration
	Sulfonylureas	Hypoglycemic effects of sulfonylureas may be attenuated	Select different hypoglycemic or antihypertensive. If they must be given together, monitor blood glucose closely
	Clonidine	Life-threatening and fatal increases in BP have resulted after discon-tinuance of clonidine in patients also receiving beta-adrenergic antagonist or after simultaneous withdrawal	
Metoprolol, propranolol	Ranitidine	May increase bioavailability of metoprolol; other beta-adrenergic antagonists not affected	Select different histamine$_2$ blocker, but avoid cimetidine (see above)
	Hydralazine	Additive pharmacological effect	Avoid concurrent use or closely monitor effects
	MAOIs	Bradycardia may develop	Avoid concurrent use or use within 14 days of MAOI
	Propafenone	Plasma levels of metoprolol increased	Avoid concurrent use
	Benzodiazepines (BDZ)	Effects of BDZ increased by lipophilic beta-adrenergic antagonist	Change to atenolol. It does not interact
	Seratonin reputake inhibitors (SRIs)	Certain SRIs may inhibit metabolism (CYP2D6) of these beta blockers leading to exessive beta blockades	Avoid concurrent use. Select different beta blocker

Table 14–11 ■ **Drug Interactions: Selected Beta Blockers—cont'd**

Drug	Interacting Drug	Possible Effect	Implications
	Thyroid hormone	Decrease actives of these beta blockers when patient is convented to euthyroid state	Monitor for decreased effects. Increase beta-blocker dose if needed
Propranolol only	Acetaminophen	Decreased acetaminophen clearance	Avoid concurrent use or reduce dose
	Gabapentin	Increased gabapentin adverse responses	Avoid concurrent use
	Haloperidol	Hypotensive episodes	Select different antipsychotic
	Loop diuretics	Propranolol plasma levels and cardiovascular effects enhanced	Atenolol not affected. Use atenolol instead
	Phenothiazines	Propranolol bioavailability and phenothiazine plasma levels increased, with potential toxicity	Selected different beta-adrenergic antagonist
	Warfarin	Increased anticoagulant effect	Select different beta-adrenergic antagonist
Nebivolol only	CYP2D6 inhibitors (e.g., fluoxetine, paroxetine, propafenone, quinidine)	Increased inhibition of CYP2D6 leading to increased plasma levels of nebivolol	Dose of nebivolol may need to be reduced
	Histamine 2 blockers (e.g., cimetidine)	Increased plasma levels of Nebivolol metabolite by 23%	Avoid concurrent use
	Disopyramide	Clearance of disopyramide decreased leading to hypotension and sinus bradycardia	Avoid concurrent use or use caution and monitor closely if must coadminister
	Sildenafil	Decreased AUC and Cmax of sildenafil by 21% and 23%, respectively	May require dosage adjustment

acid levels. They may also increase antinuclear antibody (ANA) titers and blood glucose levels.

Clinical Use and Dosing

Regardless of the indication for which a **beta blocker** is given, there is no simple correlation between dose or plasma level and therapeutic effect. The dose-sensitivity range in clinical practice is wide because sympathetic tone and first-pass metabolism varies widely among individuals. Proper dosing requires titration.

Angina

Atenolol, metoprolol, nadolol, and **propranolol** are indicated for long-term management of angina (*Drug Facts and Comparisons,* 2009; Gibbons et al., 2003). **Beta blockers** lower blood pressure; reduce symptoms of angina; improve mortality; and reduce cardiac output, heart rate; and AV conduction. Both **beta$_1$-selective** and **nonselective** drugs affect the myocardial oxygen supply-demand equation on the demand side by decreasing the force of myocardial contractility, heart rate, and conduction velocity (National High Blood Pressure Education Program [NHBPEP], 2003). Nonselective agents, by a mechanism that is not clearly understood, decrease systemic vascular resistance and blood pressure, reducing afterload. Because they reduce myocardial oxygen demand, **beta blockers** are the drugs of choice for exertional angina. They are especially useful for patients with exertional angina whose lifestyle involves frequent vigorous activity, for patients with resting tachycardia, and for patients who have concomitant disease that might benefit from beta blockade (e.g., hypertension, post-MI migraine headaches). They do not improve myocardial oxygen supply, and **propranolol** has been reported to increase the risk for coronary artery vasospasm in some patients. Additional discussion of their use in patients with angina is found in Chapter 28.

To reduce the risk for adverse drug reactions, doses are started low and increased slowly, usually at no shorter than weekly intervals, based on resolution of symptoms. Dosage adjustment based on hepatic impairment and renal function is discussed in the metabolism and excretion section.

Hypertension

Initial drug therapy for hypertension is with a **diuretic** or a **beta blocker** in combination with a **diuretic** because they have been shown to reduce morbidity and mortality in numerous randomized controlled trials (RCT) (NHBPEP, 2003). **Propranolol** is now available in a combination form that includes **hydrochlorothiazide. Beta blockers** are also chosen because of reduced cost. They may be used in combination with other antihypertensives, largely to mitigate the adverse effects associated with these drugs. **Atenolol, metoprolol, nadolol**, and **propranolol** are the drugs most commonly chosen. **Nebivolol** is relatively new on the market (approved in 2007), so the amount of its use remains to be seen. Because of their relatively long half-lives, these drugs can be administered once daily, improving adherence. **Pindolol** and **acebutolol** have fewer myocardial depressant effects and do not increase cholesterol and triglyceride levels. Consideration of renal function is again important for dosing of some **beta blockers**. Additional discussion of the use of **beta blockers** in hypertension management is found in Chapter 40.

Heart Failure

A variety of neurohormonal systems may be activated in heart failure, most commonly the renin-angiotensin-aldosterone system and the sympathetic nervous system. Such activation leads to abnormal ventricular remodeling, left ventricular (LV) enlargement, and reduced cardiac contractility. This progression can be significantly reduced by effective therapy with **angiotensin-converting enzyme (ACE) inhibitors, beta blockers**, and **diuretics** (Dickstein et al, 2008; Hunt et al, 2005). **Beta blockers** have favorable effects on survival and disease progression in heart failure and treatment should be initiated as soon as LV dysfunction is diagnosed. Early treatment should begin even when symptoms are mild or have responded to other therapies (Hunt et al, 2005).

In stage B heart failure (New York Heart Association [NYHA] class I) and in stage C (NYHA classes II–III), **ACE inhibitors** and **beta blockers** are recommended. For Stage C, Hunt et al (2005) recommend the use of one of the three **beta blockers** that have proven to reduce mortality: **bisoprolol, carvedilol** (a combined alpha-beta drug), and **sustained-release metoprolol succinate.**

The European Society of Cardiology (ESC) (2008) recommends that all patients with symptomatic heart failure and a left ventricular ejection fraction (LVEF) of less than 40 percent should take **ACE inhibitors** and **beta blockers** unless they are contraindicated. **Beta blockers** should be started in patients who are clinically stable on an **ACE inhibitor** and have no recent changes in dose for any **diuretic** they may be taking.

Blood pressure targets have not been firmly established in heart failure, but one trial demonstrated benefits of beta blockade in improving heart failure symptoms in patients with systolic blood pressure (SBP) as low as 85 mm Hg (Packer et al, 2001). In most trials, however, the SBP were lowered to the range of 110 to 130 mm Hg. Chapter 36 discusses heart failure management in more detail.

Postmyocardial Infarction Prophylaxis

Use of **beta blockers** in post-MI prophylaxis has been shown to decrease mortality by 30 to 40 percent. They are most effective for patients who have had severe anterior MIs. The mechanism of action in MI prophylaxis appears to be related to limitation of infarct size, prevention of primary arrhythmic events, protection from subsequent ischemia, and prevention of recurrent coronary occlusion. In comparing benefits versus adverse reaction profiles, the most benefits go to older adults and those with tachycardia. These drugs are less beneficial for young patients and those with small MIs. **Atenolol, metoprolol, propranolol**, and **timolol** have been shown to be effective for this indication.

Migraine Headache Prophylaxis

Propranolol in doses of 160 to 200 mg/day has proved effective in reducing the incidence of migraine headache in some patients. The mechanism of action is related to prevention of beta receptor–induced vasodilation and promotion of increased extracellular levels of serotonin. **Timolol** with initial doses of 10 mg bid and maintenance doses of 10 to 30 mg/day has also been effective for this indication. For **propranolol**, if a satisfactory response to the maximum dose is not obtained in 4 to 6 weeks, the drug should be gradually withdrawn because a longer trial is not associated with any better outcome. For **timolol**, the trial should be 6 to 8 weeks. **Atenolol** (50–100 mg/day), **metoprolol** (50–100 mg/day), and **nadolol** (40–80 mg/day) have also been tried. The trial time is similar to that for **propranolol.**

Arrhythmias

Propranolol, pindolol, and **acebutolol** have indications for the treatment of supraventricular arrhythmias, suppression of premature ventricular contractions, and tachycardia. These indications are useful mainly for inpatients and are not discussed here.

Glaucoma

Topical application of **beta blockers** in the treatment of glaucoma is discussed in Chapter 26.

Unlabeled Uses

Unlabeled indications for which some evaluation of effectiveness has been made include the following:

1. Alcohol withdrawal syndrome: **atenolol** 50 to 100 mg/day.
2. Aggressive behavior: **metoprolol** 200 to 300 mg/ day and **propranolol** 80 to 300 mg/day.
3. Antipsychotic drug–induced akathisia: **nadolol** 40 to 80 mg/day, **pindolol** 5 mg/day, **propranolol** 20 to 80 mg/day, and **metoprolol** more than 100 mg/ day.

4. Essential tremor: **metoprolol** 50 to 300 mg/day, **nadolol** 120 to 240 mg/day, and **timolol** 10 mg/day.
5. Situational anxiety (stage fright): **propranolol** 40 mg and **nadolol** 20 mg. **Propranolol** 40 to 320 mg/day has been used for acute panic syndromes.

Withdrawal of Beta Blockers

For all **beta blockers**, abrupt withdrawal can be life threatening. It can result in severe angina, MI, ventricular arrhythmias, and death. To withdraw any of these drugs, taper the dose by one-half every 4 days. Patients at high risk for serious consequences to rapid withdrawal include those with angina, coronary artery disease, and migraines. Low-risk patients include those with hypertension and supraventricular tachycardia.

Rational Drug Selection

Beta Selectivity

In selecting the most appropriate **beta blocker**, first consideration is usually given to $beta_1$ selectivity. **Atenolol, acebutolol,** and **metoprolol** are $beta_1$-selective drugs. **Nadolol, pindolol, propranolol,** and **timolol** are nonselective drugs. The new third generation drug, **nebivolol**, is $beta_1$ selective in extensive metabolizers (EMs) and nonselective in poor metabolizers (PMs).

The clinical significance of selectivity relates to the relative lack of action of $beta_1$-selective drugs on the $beta_2$ receptors. This relative lack of action makes **$beta_1$-selective blockers** more appropriate than nonselective agents for patients with chronic obstructive pulmonary diseases, asthma, peripheral vascular diseases such as Raynaud's syndrome, or diabetes mellitus. Among the $beta_1$-selective blockers, **atenolol** has greater selectivity than does **metoprolol**, which has greater selectivity than **acebutolol**.

Pharmacokinetics

The best choice of drug based on pharmacokinetics would be one with a long enough half-life to permit once-daily dosing, consistent bioavailability and limited interpatient variability in dosing, limited CNS penetration to reduce adverse reactions, and an excretion mechanism that does not require dosage adjustments, so that extensive laboratory testing prior to initiation of therapy is not required. No one drug meets all these requirements, but several come close.

Atenolol, metoprolol, nadolol, and **nebivolol** have longer half-lives that permit once-daily dosing regimens, although **metoprolol** frequently has its best effects with bid dosing. All other **beta blockers** have half-lives that require at least bid dosing, with **propranolol** requiring bid and tid dosing. **Propranolol** is sometimes used to treat anxiety symptoms in depressed patients specifically because it clears the system quickly in cases of overdose.

Atenolol and **nadolol** do not have significant hepatic first-pass effects. **Acebutolol, metoprolol,** and **propranolol** have significant first-pass effects and increased interpatient variability in the amount of drug that enters the patient's bloodstream. They also have short half-lives and require more frequent dosing. **Timolol** has some first-pass effects but the drug is about 75 percent bioavailable so the first-pass effect is less significant. **Pindolol** does not have a significant first-pass effect.

Timolol has the least CNS penetration, but it is a nonselective agent. **Acebutolol** and **atenolol** have minimal CNS penetration. The drug with the most CNS penetration is **propranolol**.

Beta blockers that are excreted primarily by the kidney have increased half-lives in renal failure. Dosage adjustments are necessary. **Atenolol, nebivolol,** and **nadolol** fall into this category (Table 14–12). Although

Table 14–12 ◉ Dosage Schedule: Selected Beta Blockers

Drug	Indication	Initial Dose	Maintenance Dose
Acebutolol (Sectral)	Hypertension	*Adults:* 400 mg/d in slingle or 2 divided doses *Older adults:* 200 mg/d in single or 2 divided doses	If target blood pressure (BP) not achieved in 1–2 wk, increase to 800 mg daily. Max dose is 1200 mg. Reduce dosage by 50% if creatinine clearance (CCr) <50 mL/min; by 75% if CCr <25 mL/min
	Ventricular arrhythmias	200 mg bid	Increase to 600–1,200 mg/d as needed to control arrhythmia
	Angina	300 mg tid	May increase to 400 mg tid if needed
Atenolol (Tenormin) (Canadian drug name: Apo-atenolol)	Hypertension	*Adults:* 25–50 mg daily *Children:* 0.8 mg/kg/d	If target BP not achieved in 1–2 wk, increase to 100 mg daily for adults and 1.5 mg/kg/d for children. Max dose for children is 2 mg/kg/d. Higher doses not likely to help in adults. Reduce dosage to 50 mg if creatinine clearance (CCr) 15–35 mL/min; 50 mg qod if CCr <15 mL/min

Continued

Table 14–12 ◉ **Dosage Schedule: Selected Beta Blockers—cont'd**

Drug	Indication	Initial Dose	Maintenance Dose
	Angina	50 mg daily	If symptoms continue, increase to 100 mg daily. Some patients may need 200 mg. Reduce dosage to 50 mg if CCr 15–35 mL/min; 50 mg qod CCr <15 mL/min
	MI (prophylaxis)	50 mg daily	50–100 mg daily (see note above re CCr)
Metoprolol (Lopressor) (Canadian drug names: Apo-Metoprolol, Betaloc)	Hypertension	*Adults*: 50–100 mg/d in single or divided doses (extended-release tablets: 50–100 mg daily) *Older adults:* 25 mg/d in single or divided doses	If target BP not achieved, increase at weekly intervals. Maintenance dose usually 100–450 mg/d. Does better in divided doses (extended-release tablets: 100–400 mg daily)
	Angina	100 mg/d in two divided doses (extended-release tablets: 100 mg daily)	If symptoms continue, increase in weekly intervals up to 400 mg/d in two divided doses (extended release: up to 400 mg daily)
	MI (prophylaxis)	100 mg/d in two divided doses	100 mg/d in two divided doses
Nadolol (Corgard)	Hypertension	40 mg daily	Increase in doses of 40–80 mg/d until target BP achieved. Maintenance dose usually 40–80 mg/d. Max dose 320 mg/d in divided doses. Increase dosage interval in renal impairment: CCr >50 = q 24 h; CCr 31–50 = q 24–36 h; CCr 10–30 = q 24–48 h; CCr <10 = q 40–60 h
	Angina	40 mg daily	If symptoms continue, increase in 3–7 d intervals to 80–160 mg/d. Max dose is 240 mg/d. Increase dosage interval in renal impairment: CCr >50 = q 24 h: CCr 31–50 = q 24–36 h; CCr 10–30 = q 24–48 h; CCr <10 = q 40–60 h
Nebivolol (Bystolic)	Hypertension	5 mg daily CCr <30 or moderate hepatic impairment = reduce dose to 2.5 mg daily	May increase dose at 2 wk intervals up to max dose of 40 mg/d. CCr <30 or moderate hepatic impairment = cautious upward titration
Propranolol (Inderal) (Inderal LA) (InnoPran XL) (Canadian drug name: Apo-pranolol and Novopranolol)	Hypertension	*Adults:* 40 mg bid (SR = 80 mg daily) *Children:* 0.5 mg/kg/d in 2 divided doses	*Adults:* Usual maintenance dose is 120–240 mg bid or tid (SR = 120–160 mg daily); max dose = 640 mg/d *Children:* Max dose 16 mg/kg/d
	Angina	80–320 mg in 2, 3, or 4 divided doses (SR = 80 mg daily)	If symptoms continue; give 160-mg SR tablet; max dose, 320-mg SR
	MI (prophylaxis)	180–240 mg/d in 2–3 divided doses	
	Migraine prophylaxis	80 mg/d (SR)	160–240 mg/d in divided doses
Timolol (Blocadren)	MI (prophylaxis)		10 mg bid
	Migraine prophylaxis	10 mg bid	Maintenance dose 10–30 mg. May take up to 8 wk of maximum daily dose

SR = sustained release.

acebutolol has some excretion through the GI tract, its active metabolite is excreted through the kidneys, and the daily dose must be reduced in renal failure. Poor renal function has only minor effects on **pindolol** clearance, and the half-life of **metoprolol** is essentially unchanged.

Cost

Generic **propranolol** is the least expensive of the **beta blockers,** followed by **metoprolol** and **atenolol.** Many **beta blockers** are now available in generic form. All **beta blockers** are significantly more expensive in their brand name formulation.

With all of these parameters taken together, the most cost-effective and convenient **beta blocker** for angina management, hypertension, and post-MI prophylaxis is **atenolol,** which has once-daily dosing, low CNS penetration, a low adverse reactions profile, and $beta_1$ selectivity (Table 14–13).

Concurrent Disease States

Disease processes that contraindicate use of **beta blockers** or require cautious use have been discussed: diseases with a bronchospastic component, AV block, and diabetes mellitus. Because these drugs produce decreased

Table 14–13 ◆ **Available Dosage Forms: Selected Beta Blockers**

Drug	Dosage Form	Package	Cost
Acebutolol (G) (Sectral) (B)	Capsules: 200 mg	In bottles of 100 and 1,000 capsules (G). In bottles of 100 and Redipak 100s (B)	200 mg = $55/100 (G) $300/100 (B)
	Capsules: 400 mg	In bottles of 100 and 1,000 capsules (G). In bottles of 100 (B)	400 mg = $64/100 (G) $405/100 (B)
Atenolol (G) (Tenormin) (B)	Tablets: 25 mg, 50 mg, 100 mg	In bottles of 30, 60, 90, 100, and 1,000 tablets (G). In bottles of 100 (B)	Generic: 25 mg = $16/100 50 mg = $20/100 100 mg = $22/100 Brand: 25 mg = $177/100 50 mg = $182/100 100 mg = $252/100
Atenolol/ Chlorthalidone (G) (Tenoretic) (B)	Tablets: 50 mg atenolol/ 25 mg chlorthalidone, 100 mg atenolol/25 mg chlorthalidone	In bottles of 30, 90, 100 tablets	50/25 mg = $37/100 (G) $189/100 (B) 100/25 mg = $34/100 (G) $276/100 (B)
Metoprolol tartrate (G) (Lopressor) (B)	Tablets: 25 mg, (G) 50 mg, 100 mg	In bottles of 30, 9, 100, and 1,000 tablets In bottles of 100, and 1,000 tablets (G) In bottles of 100 and 1,000 and UD 100 (B) scored tablets	Brand: 50 mg = $167/100 100 mg = $227/100 Generic: 25 mg = $18/100 50 mg = $21/100 100 mg = $26/100
Metoprolol succinate (G) (Toprol-XL) (B)	Tablets, extended release: 25 mg, 50 mg, 100 mg, and 200 mg	In bottles of 100 and 1,000 tablets (G); (B) in bottles of 100 scored tablets (G) and (B) in bottles of 100 tablets In bottles of 100 1,000, and UD 100 (G) and in bottles of 100 (B)	Generic: 25 mg = $73/90 50 mg = $86/90 100 mg = $116/90 200 mg = $204/90 Brand: 25 mg = $100/90 50 mg = $100/90 100 mg = $146/90 200 mg = $243/90

Continued

Table 14–13 ◆ **Available Dosage Forms: Selected Beta Blockers—cont'd**

Drug	Dosage Form	Package	Cost
Metoprolol/ hydrochlorothiazide (G) (Lopressor HCT) (B)	Tablets: 50 mg metoprolol/ 25 mg HCTZ, 100 mg metoprolol/ 25 mg HCTZ 100 mg metoprolol/ 50 mg HCTZ	In bottles of 100 tablets all strengths	50/25 mg = $100/100 (G) $183/100 (B) 100/25 mg = $144/100 (G) $177/100 (B) 100/50 mg = $156/100 (G) $250/100 (B)
Nadolol (G) (Corgard) (B)	Tablets: 20 mg	In bottles of 100 tablets and UD 100 (G). In bottles of 100 scored tablets and *Unimatic* 100 (B)	Brand: 20 mg = $266/100 40 mg = $302/100 80 mg = $333/100 120 mg = $322/100 160 mg = $370/100 Generic: 20 mg = $22/100 40 mg = $33/100 80 mg = $44/100 160 mg = $70/100
	40 mg (G)	In bottles of 100, 1,000 tablets, and UD 100	
	80 mg (G)	In bottles of 30, 100, 500, 1,000, and UD 100 tablets	
	120 mg	In bottles of 100, 500, and 1,000 tablets (G). In bottles of 100 and 1,000 scored tablets (B)	
	160 mg	In bottles of 100, 500, and 1,000 tablets (G). In bottles of 100 scored tablets (B)	
Pindolol (G) (Visken) (B)	Tablets: 5 mg, 10 mg	In bottles of 100, 500, and 1,000 tablets (G). In bottles of 100 tablets (B)	Generic: 5 mg = $27/100 10 mg = $28/100
Propranolol (G)	Tablets (G): 10 mg, 20 mg, 40 mg, 80 mg	In bottles of 100, 500, and 1,000 tablets and UD 100	10 mg, 20 mg and 40 mg = $14/100 80 mg = $18/100 $46 for 480 mL
	Tablets (G): 60 mg, 90 mg	In bottles of 100 and 500 tablets	
	Solution: 20 mg/ 5 mL	In bottles of 240 mL and 480 mL	
Propranolol CR extended release (G) (Inderal LA) (B)	Capsules: 60 mg, 80 mg, 120 mg, 160 mg	In bottles of 100 and 1,000 capsules (G) In bottles of 100 and 1,000 and UD 100 (B)	Generic 60 mg = $100/100 80 mg = $116/100 120 mg = $140/100 160 mg = $183/100 Brand: 60 mg = $364/90 80 mg = $354/90 120 mg = $442/90 160 mg = $565/90
(InnoPran XL)(B)	Capsules: 80 mg, 120 mg	In bottles of 30, 100, 500 and UD 100	80 mg = $202/90 120 mg = $200/90
Propranolol/ Hydrochloro-thiazide (G) (Inderide) (B)	Tablets: 40 mg, 25 mg	In bottles of 100 tablets	Generic: 40/25 mg = $28/100 80/25 mg = $37/100 Brand: 40/25 mg = $154/100 80/25 mg = $196/100
	80 mg/25 mg	In bottles of 100 and 1,000 tablets	
Timolol (G) (Blocadren) (B)	Tablets: 5 mg, 10 mg (G only), 20 mg	In bottles of 100 tablets for both (G) and (B) 20-mg (B) tablets are scored	Generic: 5 mg = $38/100 10 mg = $43/100 20 mg = $65/100

perfusion as a result of decreased cardiac output and a relative increase in the $alpha_1$ stimulation, which can produce some vasoconstriction, they are also poor choices for patients with peripheral vascular disease and Raynaud's syndrome.

Beta blockers are good choices to treat patients who have more than one of the disease processes for which they are indicated. Hypertensive patients who also have angina or who have had a previous MI, for example, are excellent candidates for **beta blockers. Atenolol, metoprolol,** and **propranolol** are useful for all of these indications.

Indications for Specific Drugs

Specific agents have been demonstrated to work with specific disorders. Other drugs in the class may not work as well. For example, **propranolol** is the only one proven useful in managing exertional or other stress-induced angina associated with idiopathic hypertrophic subaortic stenosis. The drug chosen should have research to support its use.

Monitoring

Monitoring parameters for **beta blockers** are essentially those used to monitor the disease process they are being used to treat (e.g., number of anginal attacks, lowering of blood pressure). For the drugs requiring dosage adjustments based on renal function, serum creatinine and/or creatinine clearance testing should be done prior to initiation of therapy. For drugs with significant first-pass effects, it may be appropriate to assess liver function before beginning therapy. Because almost 50 percent of people with diabetes are unaware that they have this condition, and the management of diabetes may be compromised by the addition of a **beta blocker**, a HbA1C level should also be drawn prior to therapy.

Patient Education

Administration

The patient should take the drug exactly as prescribed, at the same time each day, even if feeling well. Do not skip or double doses. If a dose of **atenolol, metoprolol,** or **nadolol** is missed, it should be taken up to 8 hours before the next dose is due. **Pindolol, propranolol,** and **timolol** should be taken up to 4 hours before the next dose. Abrupt withdrawal may precipitate life-threatening arrhythmias, hypertension, and myocardial ischemia. Be certain there is enough drug on hand to cover weekends or traveling. The patient should wear identification describing the disease process and the medication regimen at all times.

Food may enhance the bioavailability of **propranolol** and **metoprolol.** They should be taken consistently either with food or on an empty stomach. **Propranolol** can be crushed and mixed with food, including oral solutions and semisolids, if it is consistently given with food. Food intake does not affect other **beta blockers.**

Consult with the health-care provider before taking any OTC drugs, especially cold remedies, while taking a **beta blocker.** Several drugs common in these preparations have drug interactions that result in hypertension and excessive bradycardia.

If these drugs are being taken for angina, **beta blockers** cannot relieve acute anginal attacks. If acute chest pain occurs, the patient should contact the health-care provider immediately or go to the nearest hospital.

Adverse Reactions

Hypotensive reactions and bradycardia are the most common adverse reactions. Arising slowly from a supine position and dangling the feet over the side of the bed before standing will reduce postural hypotension. No exercise in hot weather and intake of at least 2,000 cc of noncaffeinated fluid a day will also reduce these problems. Assessment of blood pressure and pulse is necessary on a biweekly basis for those taking these drugs. Teach the patient home blood pressure and pulse monitoring and advise contacting the health-care provider if the pulse is less than 50 bpm or if the blood pressure changes suddenly.

Beta blockers may exacerbate diseases with a bronchospastic component. Teach patients to report wheezing or difficulty in breathing to the health-care provider immediately. Dizziness and drowsiness may occur with the drugs. Avoid driving or other activities that require mental alertness until response to the drug is known. Insomnia can be reduced by not taking the last dose of the day late in the evening. Dry mouth responds to practicing good oral hygiene, chewing sugarless gum, or sucking on hard candy.

Depression and confusion have been associated with the **beta blockers** that have significant CNS penetration. The patient should report such problems, and a different **beta blocker** or a different class of drugs may be tried.

For diabetics, these drugs may mask the signs and symptoms of hypoglycemia and impair recovery from a hypoglycemic episode. **$Beta_1$-selective** drugs are less likely to cause this problem. The one indication of hypoglycemia that is not masked is diaphoresis. In the event of unexplained diaphoresis, the patient should check the blood glucose level immediately.

Beta blockers are contraindicated in the first trimester of pregnancy and must be withdrawn before delivery. Women of childbearing age should have this warning discussed with them. Other pregnancy considerations relate to the specific pregnancy category of the **beta blocker** being considered.

Nonadherence to a treatment regimen with a **beta blocker** is often caused by inhibition of ejaculation and impotence. If these occur, the patient should report them to the health-care provider, who may choose a different drug to treat the disorder or change the dosage.

Lifestyle Management

If the drug is being given for hypertension, encourage the patient to adhere to additional interventions for reduction of blood pressure, such as weight loss, a low-sodium diet, smoking cessation, regular exercise, and stress management. Further discussion of patient education is found in Chapter 40. Further discussion of patient education about angina is found in Chapter 28 and discussion of heart failure is found in Chapter 36.

COMBINED ALPHA- AND BETA-ADRENERGIC ANTAGONISTS

Drugs that exhibit blockade at both alpha and beta receptors have effects that would be expected from a combination of an alpha and a beta blocker. Because the alpha blockade predominates, however, they are less likely to produce significant reductions in heart rate or cardiac output. Alpha blockade also balances the tendency of **beta blockers** to produce reflex vasoconstriction.

There are two drugs in this class: **carvedilol (Coreg)** and **labetalol (Normodyne)**. Both are used to treat hypertension, and **carvedilol** is also used to reduce progression of CHF and to treat left ventricular dysfunction following an MI. This section focuses on aspects of these drugs that are different from **alpha-adrenergic antagonists** and **beta blockers**. Similar aspects of these drugs to the other two classes are discussed only briefly.

Pharmacodynamics

These two drugs combine selective alpha$_1$-adrenergic and nonselective beta blockade. The alpha and beta blockades decrease blood pressure; standing blood pressure is more affected than supine. They also decrease peripheral resistance by peripheral vasodilatation (**carvedilol** more than **labetalol**). These combined effects decrease myocardial oxygen demand and lower cardiac workload. Single doses of **labetalol** have no significant effect on sinus rate, intraventricular conduction, or QRS duration. AV conduction time is only modestly prolonged. No significant change in cardiac output occurs. **Labetalol** has been associated with rare orthostatic hypotension because of standing blood pressure is lowered more than supine. **Carvedilol** reduces orthostatic hypotension and exercise-induced reflex tachycardia. In hypertensive patients with normal renal function, it also decreases renal vascular resistance. Neither of these drugs demonstrates a significant effect on serum lipoproteins.

Although beta blockade is useful in angina and hypertension, sympathetic stimulation is vital in some situations. For example, in patients with severely damaged hearts, adequate ventricular function may depend on sympathetic drive (*Drug Facts and Comparisons*, 2009).

Pharmacokinetics

Absorption and Distribution

Both drugs are rapidly absorbed (Table 14–14). **Carvedilol** is more protein bound than **labetalol**. Both drugs are widely distributed in body tissues.

Metabolism and Excretion

Both drugs undergo rapid hepatic first-pass metabolism resulting in bioavailabilities between 25 and 35 percent. **Carvedilol** is metabolized by CYP2D6 and 2C9 and **labetolol** undergoes glucoronidation and sulfation, which are not CYP meditated. **Carvedilol** undergoes more excretion in bile and feces than does **labetalol.**

Pharmacotherapeutics

Precautions and Contraindications

Because they include nonselective beta blockade, **alpha-beta blockers** are contraindicated for patients with respiratory conditions that include a bronchospastic component. They are also contraindicated in overt, New York Heart Association (NYHA) class IV heart failure, greater than first-degree AV block, and severe bradycardia due to their negative inotropic effects. However, **carvedilol** has been shown to be effective in the management of NYHA class II and III heart failure because of its limited effects on heart rate and myocardial contractility while improving hemodynamics and cardiac performance.

Cautions related to diabetes and thyroid disease and problems with withdrawal are similar to those of **beta blockers**. Although they produce less reflex vasoconstriction, caution is still required when these drugs are administered to patients with peripheral vascular disease.

Table 14–14 ▶ **Pharmacokinetics: Combined Alpha-Beta Blockers**

Drug	Onset	Peak	Duration	Protein Binding	Bioavailability	Half-Life	Elimination
Carvedilol	1 h	1–2 h	12 h	>98%	25%–35%	7–10 h	Primarily in bile and feces: <2% unchanged in urine
Labetalol	20 min	1–4 h	8–12 h	50%	25% (increased by food and in older adults)	3–8 h	In bile and feces; 50%–60% as conjugates in urine

Hepatic impairment creates issues for both drugs. Like many **beta blockers**, they are heavily metabolized by the liver, and use in patients with clinically manifested liver disease is not recommended. Hepatic injury has occurred rarely with both drugs, and onset of jaundice or hepatic dysfunction indicated by symptoms or elevations of liver function tests necessitates withdrawal of the drug.

Both drugs are also Pregnancy Category C for the same reasons as **beta blockers**. Small amounts of **labetalol** (0.004%) are excreted in breast milk, and the amount of **carvedilol** excreted in breast milk is unknown. Caution should be exercised in giving these drugs to nursing mothers, with careful consideration of benefits versus risks.

Plasma levels of **carvedilol** average 50 percent higher in older adults than in young adults. Although there was no notable difference in adverse reactions in study subjects, it is advisable to monitor older patients more closely for adverse reactions such as dizziness, which places them at risk for falls.

Safety and efficacy in children younger than 18 years of age have not been established for either drug. In a double-blind study discussed by the FDA on their pediatric exclusivity site, children ages 2 months to 17 years with chronic heart failure showed no significant effect of treatment with **carvedilol** on clinical outcomes after 8 months follow up. Despite this FDA report, **caevedilol** is being used off-label to treat idiopathic cardiomyopathy in children.

Adverse Drug Reactions

Adverse drug reactions are essentially the same as those seen with **beta blockers**, with the exception of fewer cardiac-related reactions (e.g., bradycardia, decreased contractility) and a lower incidence of CNS-related reactions. The risk for orthostatic hypotension is higher than with **beta blockers** and is related to the alpha$_1$-adrenergic blockade.

Drug, Food, and Laboratory Test Interactions

Drug Interactions

Drug interactions are similar to those for **beta blockers**, with a few additions (Table 14–15). As with some of the other **beta blockers**, drugs that inhibit the CYP450 2D6 system increase plasma levels of **carvedilol.**

Food Interactions

When **carvedilol** is taken with food, its rate of absorption is slowed, but the bioavailability is not affected. Taking it with food minimizes the risk for postural hypotension. Food slows the rate of absorption of **labetalol** but increases the absolute bioavailability. As a result, **labetalol** should be taken consistently with regard to food.

Laboratory Test Interactions

The presence of a **labetalol** metabolite in the urine may falsely increase urinary catecholamine levels measured by a nonspecific trihydroxyindole reaction. There have also been reversible increases in serum transaminases (4% of patients) and, rarely, reversible increases in BUN. **Labetalol** has also produced a false-positive test for amphetamine in a patient whose urine was screened for the presence of drugs.

Table 14–15 ■ Drug Interactions: Combined Alpha-Beta Blockers

Drug	Interacting Drug*	Possible Effect	Implications
Carvedilol	Inhibitors of CYP-450 2D6 (e.g., cimetidine, ciprofloxacin and other quinolones, quinidine, fluoxetine, paroxetine, propafenone)	Increased blood level of carvedilol	Avoid concurrent use
	Rifampin	Plasma concentration of carvedilol reduced by 70%	Avoid concurrent use
	Diphenhydramine	Inhibits metabolism of carvedilol leading to increased plasma concentrations and effects	Avoid concurrent use Wam patients related to OTC antihistamine
Labetalol	Beta agonists, theophylline	Labetalol can blunt the bronchodilator effect	A greater than normal dose of beta agonist may be required
	Cimetidine	Increases bioavailabity of labetalol	Avoid concurrent use

*Other drug interactions that are the same as for beta blockers: antihypertensives, alcohol, calcium channel blockers, clonidine, digoxin, MAOIs, nitrates, and sulfonylureas. See Table 14–11.

Clinical Use and Dosing

Hypertension

Both drugs are used to treat essential hypertension. They are used alone or in combination with other antihypertensive agents, especially **thiazide-type diuretics.** Cost considerations remove them from first-line choices. Both drugs are begun at a low dose, and dosage is increased until target blood pressure is achieved (Table 14–16). **Carvedilol** begins at 6.25 mg bid. Adjustments are made at 7- to 14-day intervals, based on standing systolic blood pressure. **Labetalol** is initiated at 100 mg bid and increased in 100-mg increments every 2 to 3 days until target blood pressure is achieved.

Congestive Heart Failure

Carvedilol has an indication for treatment of heart failure in a narrow group of patients: mild to moderate (NYHA class II or III) heart failure of ischemic or cardiomyopathic origin, in conjunction with **diuretics** and **(ACE) inhibitors**, to reduce the progression of disease and increase survival (*Drug Facts and Comparisons,*

Table 14–16 ◉ **Dosage Schedule: Combined Alpha-Beta Blockers**

Drug	Indication	Initial Dose	Maintenance Dose
Carvedilol	Hypertension	6.25 mg bid; if dose is tolerated using standing systolic blood pressure (BP) measured 1 h after the dose, maintain this dose for 7–14 d	After initial dose, increase to 12.5 mg bid if needed, based on trough BP using same standing systolic BP. Maintain this dose for 7–14 d before increasing to 25 mg if needed. When increasing dose, give first larger dose at bedtime or give with food to slow or to avoid orthostatic hypotension. Full antihypertensive effect seen in 7–14 d. Maximum dose is 50 mg
	CHF	3.125 mg bid for 2 wk	Individualize dose and closely monitor during up-titration. If initial dose is tolerated, increase to 6.25 mg bid. Dose can then be doubled every 2 wk to the highest level tolerated by the patient. Maximum dose is 25 mg bid for <85 kg; 50 mg bid for >85 mg. Transient worsening of CHF may be treated by increasing diuretic or reducing carvedilol dose
	LV dysfunction following MI	6.25 mg bid	Increased after 3–10 days, based on tolerability, to 12.5 mg bid, then again to target dose of 25 mg bid
	Off-labeled: Chronic stable angina	12.5 mg bid	Increase as needed/tolerated to 25–50 mg bid for 2–12 wk
	Idiopathic cardiomyopathy (Adults)	6.25 mg daily	Increased as needed/tolerated. Max dose 75 mg/d. Continue for at least 6–8 mo
	Idiopathic cardiomyopathy (Children <62.5 kg)	0.05 mg/kg bid	Increase dose twice at 2-wk intervals to 0.1 and 0.2 mg/kg bid. Max dose: 0.4 mg/kg
	(Children > 62.5 kg)	3.125 mg bid	Increase twice at 2-wk intervals to 6.25 mg bid and 12.5 mg bid. Max dose 25 mg bid
Labetalol	Hypertension	*Adults:* 100 mg bid alone or added to a diuretic	If target BP is not achieved in 2–3 d, increase in increments of 100 mg bid every 2–3 d. Maintenance dose is usually 200–400 mg bid. Full antihypertensive effect seen within first 1–3 h of initial dose. Maximum dose 2,400 mg/d
		Older adults: 100 mg bid	Maintenance dose is usually 100–200 mg bid
	Off-labeled: Hypertension (Children 1–17 yrs of age)	0.5–2 mg/kg every 12 h	

Table 14–17 ◆ **Available Dosage Forms: Combined Alpha-Beta Blockers**

Drug	Dosage Form	Package	Cost
Carvedilol (G) (Coreg) (B)	Tablets: 3.125 mg, 6.25 mg, 12.5 mg, 25 mg	In bottles of 28, 30, 100, 500, and 1,000 tablets and UD 100 and blister packs 100 for all strengths of the generic. In bottles of 100 tablets for all strengths of the brand name.	Generic: 3.125 mg = $50/100 6.25 mg = $44/100 12.5 mg = $44/100 25 mg = $50/100 Brand: 3.125 mg and 6.25 mg = $230/100 12.5 mg and 25 mg = $238/100
Coreg CR	Capsules: (extended-release) 10 mg, 20 mg, 40 mg, 80 mg	In bottles of 30 and 90 capsules for all strengths	$365/90 for all strengths
Labetalol HCl (G)	Tablets: 100 mg, 200 mg, 300 mg	In bottles of 30, 100, 250, 500, and 1,000 tablets	100 mg = $35/100 200 mg = $48/100 300 mg = $65/100
Labetalol (Trandate) (B)	Tablets: 100 mg, 200 mg, 300 mg	In bottles of 100, 500 scored film-coated tablets and UD 100	100 mg = $71/100 200 mg = $85/100

2009; Packer et al, 2001). Treatment is begun at one-half the hypertension dosage (3.125 mg bid), with increases at 2-week intervals. Maximum dose is based on patient weight.

It should be noted that neither the ACC/AHA (Hunt et al, 2005) nor the ESC (Dickstein et al, 2008) practice guidelines for diagnosis and management of chronic heart failure mention the use of **carvedilol.** Perhaps this is because of the narrow group of patients for which it is useful and the lack of sufficient numbers of randomized controlled trials to date with this drug in this indication.

Off-Labeled Uses

Labetalol has been used to treat the withdrawal hypertension associated with **clonidine** withdrawal, using the maintenance dose for treating hypertension. **Carvedilol** appears to be beneficial in treating angina (25 to 50 mg bid) and idiopathic cardiomyopathy (6.25 to 25 mg bid). Other off-labeled uses are shown in Table 14–16.

Withdrawal of the Alpha-Beta Blockers

As with **beta blockers**, abrupt withdrawal can be life threatening. Angina has not been observed, but withdrawal can result in MI, ventricular arrhythmias, and death. To withdraw either of these drugs, taper the dose by one-half every 4 days over a period of 1 to 2 weeks. Patients at high risk for serious consequences due to rapid withdrawal include those with angina, coronary artery disease, and migraines. Low-risk patients include those with hypertension but no coronary artery disease.

Rational Drug Selection

Rational drug selection is largely related to cost and indications. See the discussion in the Clinical Use and Dosing section.

Race and Ethnicity

For hypertension, **alpha-beta blockers** are effective in the African American population when lifestyle modification and **diuretics** are not sufficient to reach the target blood pressure.

Age

Because of the risk for orthostatic hypotension, these drugs should be used with caution in older adults.

Concomitant Diseases

Carvedilol may be chosen when the patient has concomitant mild to moderate heart failure. **Labetalol** may be chosen when the patient cannot tolerate changes in heart rate but needs beta blockade (e.g., post-MI prophylaxis).

Cost

Both **Carvedilol** and **Labetalol** are available in generic form, which reduces their cost (Table 14–17).

Monitoring

Liver function tests should be performed before initiating therapy, when adjusting dosage, and at the first indication of liver dysfunction (pruritus, dark urine, persistent anorexia, jaundice, upper-right quadrant tenderness, or unexplained flu-like syndrome). If the patient has laboratory evidence of liver injury, stop the drug and do not restart it.

Renal function tests should be performed prior to initiating therapy and at regular intervals for any patients with a concomitant disease process that may impair renal function.

Clinical monitoring of the disease process for which the drug was prescribed is also indicated. Discussion of such monitoring for hypertension is discussed in Chapter 40.

Patient Education

Administration

The patient should take the drug exactly as prescribed, at the same time each day, even if feeling well. Do not skip or double doses. If a dose is missed, for **labetalol**, it should be taken up to 8 hours before the next dose is due. For **carvedilol**, it should be taken up to 4 hours before the next dose. Abrupt withdrawal may precipitate life-threatening arrhythmias, hypertension, and myocardial ischemia. Be certain there is enough drug on hand to cover weekends or traveling. The patient should wear identification describing the disease process and the medication regimen at all times.

Take **carvedilol** with food. This slows absorption and reduces the chance of orthostatic hypotension.

The patient should consult with the health-care provider before taking any OTC drugs, especially cold remedies, while taking an **alpha-beta blocker**. Several ingredients common in these preparations cause drug interactions that result in hypertension and excessive bradycardia.

Adverse Reactions

Hypotensive reactions and bradycardia are the most common adverse reactions. Arising slowly from a supine position and dangling the feet over the side of the bed before standing will reduce postural hypotension. No exercise in hot weather and liquid intake of at least 2,000 mL of non-caffeinated fluids a day will also reduce these problems. Intake of this quantity of fluid is not advisable for patients with heart failure, however. Assessment of blood pressure and pulse is necessary on a biweekly basis for patients taking these drugs. Teach patients home blood pressure and pulse monitoring, and advise them to contact the health-care provider if their pulse is less than 50 bpm or if their blood pressure changes suddenly.

Alpha-beta blockers may exacerbate diseases with a bronchospastic component. Teach patients to report wheezing or difficulty in breathing to the health-care provider immediately.

Dizziness and drowsiness may occur with these drugs. Patients should avoid driving or other activities that require mental alertness until their response to the drug is known.

For diabetics, these drugs may mask the signs and symptoms of hypoglycemia and impair recovery from a hypoglycemic episode. **$Beta_1$-selective** drugs are less likely to cause this problem and neither of these drugs is $beta_1$ selective. The one indication of hypoglycemia that is not masked is diaphoresis. In the event of unexplained diaphoresis, patients should check their blood glucose levels immediately.

Because **alpha-beta blockers** have **beta blocking** activity, they are contraindicated in the first trimester of pregnancy and must be withdrawn before delivery. Women of childbearing age should have this topic discussed with them. A leading cause of nonadherence to a treatment regimen with an **alpha-beta blocker** is inhibition of ejaculation and impotence. If these occur, report them to the health-care provider, who may change the dosage or choose a different drug to treat the disorder.

Lifestyle Management

Lifestyle management is the same as for **beta blockers**.

CHOLINERGIC AGONISTS

Cholinergic agonists, also known as parasympathomimetics or muscarinic agonists, promote or mimic the action of acetylcholine (ACh). These effects may be achieved either by direct agonist effect or indirectly by preventing the breakdown of ACh by acetylcholinesterase (AChE). As with **adrenergic agonists**, these drugs are not organ specific; when one organ is targeted for therapeutic reasons, the drug simultaneously produces effects in other organs. The targeted organ effects become the desired drug action, and the other organ effects become the adverse drug effects.

There are three categories of drugs in this class: **muscarinic agonists**, **cholinesterase inhibitors**, and **ganglionic stimulants**. Each category is discussed separately. The prototypic drug among **ganglionic stimulants** is **nicotine**, which is the only drug discussed in this category.

MUSCARINIC AGONISTS

Pharmacodynamics

Muscarinic receptors are located in the eye, heart, blood vessels, lung, GI tract, urinary bladder, and sweat glands. The results of stimulation of these receptors are depicted in Table 14–1. Their activation by **muscarinic agonists** modifies organ function by release of ACh from PNS nerves: (1) to activate muscarinic receptors on target organs to alter organ function and (2) to activate muscarinic receptors on nerve terminals to inhibit the release of their neurotransmitters.

There are five drugs in this group, each with a different susceptibility to breakdown by cholinesterase and different degrees of action at muscarinic and nicotinic receptors. **ACh (Miochol)** is highly susceptible to cholinesterase and very active at both types of receptors. **Carbachol (Isopto Carbachol)**, **pilocarpine (Isopto Carpine)**, and **bethanechol (Urecholine)** have negligible susceptibility to cholinesterase, and all three act at muscarinic receptors. **Carbachol** also acts at nicotinic receptors. **Methacholine (Provocholine)** has little susceptibility to cholinesterase and is very active at muscarinic receptors only.

Muscarinic agonists are used clinically to treat glaucoma and to improve GI and urinary bladder tone. **ACh** lacks selectivity to target tissues and is so rapidly destroyed by cholinesterase that its half-life is too short for most clinical applications. Its use is restricted to dilation of the pupil for ophthalmic surgery. **Methacholine** is used only for diagnosis of bronchial airway hyper-reactivity by specialists familiar with its use for this purpose. Neither of these drugs is discussed here.

Carbachol and **pilocarpine** are used to treat glaucoma. This use is discussed in Chapter 26. **Pilocarpine** comes in an oral form that can be used to increase salivary gland secretion for the management of xerostomia in patients who have undergone radiation therapy of the neck. This use is too restricted for discussion in this text. The only remaining drug in this category is **bethanechol**, and the remainder of this section discusses that drug.

Bethanechol increases the tone of the detrusor urinae muscle, and produces contraction strong enough to initiate micturation and empty the bladder. It stimulates gastric motility as well, increasing gastric tone and often restoring rhythmic peristalsis. Doses that stimulate micturation and increase peristalsis do not usually stimulate ganglia or voluntary muscles.

Pharmacokinetics

Absorption and Distribution

Bethanechol can be given orally or subcutaneously (SC). Effects appear in 30 to 90 minutes after oral administration and 5 to 15 minutes after SC administration. The effects peak in 60 minutes for the oral dose and 15 to 30 minutes for the SC dose. Duration of action is approximately 1 to 6 hours for the oral dose and 2 hours for the SC dose. The dose required to produce a therapeutic effect is significantly different by these two routes because **bethanechol** is a quaternary ammonium compound carrying a positive charge, which greatly impedes absorption from the GI tract. Because **bethanechol** is not destroyed by cholinesterase, its effects are more prolonged than those of ACh. Because of its selective nature, nicotinic symptoms of cholinergic stimulation are usually absent or minimal while the muscarinic effects are prominent.

Metabolism and Excretion

The metabolic fate and mode of excretion of **bethanechol** have not been elucidated. The drug does not cross the blood–brain barrier.

Pharmacotherapeutics

Precautions and Contraindications

Bethanechol is contraindicated in the presence of many diseases. It is contraindicated in peptic ulcer disease because at the usual therapeutic doses it can cause excessive secretion of gastric acid that could intensify gastric erosion and precipitate gastric bleeding and possible perforation. It is contraindicatedin patients with intestinal obstruction because of its ability to increase GI peristalsis. Because of its ability to contract the bladder and increase pressure within the urinary tract, it is also contraindicated in the presence of urinary tract obstruction or weakness of the bladder wall. Stimulation of the muscarinic receptors in the lungs may result in bronchoconstriction, and therefore it is contraindicated in patients with latent or active bronchospastic disorders. **Bethanechol** can rarely cause hypotension and bradycardia especially when given subcutaneously. However, more typically, therapeutic doses have very little effect on heart rate, blood pressure, or peripheral circulation. It is contraindicated for patients with preexisting hypotension, bradycardia, or cardiovascular disease.

Bethanechol is also contraindicated in patients with hyperthyroidism. When initially given **bethanechol**, patients with hyperthyroidism react similarly to other patients by experiencing hypotension and bradycardia. However, the body reacts to the hypotension with the release of increased amounts of norepinephrine from sympathetic nerves, resulting in increased heart rate. Because the heart tissue of patients with hyperthyroidism is highly sensitive to norepinephrine levels, even small increases in the amount of norepinephrine can produce cardiac arrhythmias.

It is not known whether **bethanechol** can cause fetal harm when given to pregnant women or if it can affect reproductive capacity. It is Pregnancy Category C and should be used only when the benefits clearly outweigh the potential risk to the fetus. Whether **bethanechol** is excreted in breast milk is also unknown.

Adverse Drug Reactions

Adverse reactions are rare following oral administration but more common after SC administration. GI, respiratory, and cardiac reactions were discussed in the Precautions and Contraindications section. Additional GI symptoms include abdominal pain, nausea, belching, and diarrhea. Other adverse reactions include increased tearing and miosis of the pupils and flushing that produces a feeling of warmth and a sensation of heat about the face.

Toxicity

Muscarinic poisoning can occur from overdosage and from ingestion of certain poisonous mushrooms. Early symptoms of poisoning are abdominal cramps, salivation, flushing, nausea, and vomiting. **Atropine** is the specific antidote. The preferred route of administration is SC to provide a rapid response. The recommended dose for adults is 0.6 mg repeated every 2 hours, based on clinical response. The recommended dose for children under the age of 12 is 0.01 mg/kg repeated every 2 hours, based on clinical response. The maximal single dose in children should not exceed 0.4 mg.

Drug Interactions

Additive drug interactions may occur with **cholinesterase inhibitors**. A critical fall in blood pressure may occur with **ganglionic blockers**. **Quinidine**, **procainamide**, and older **phenothiazines** such as **chlorpromazine** and **thioridazine** and **histamine$_1$ blockers** such as **diphenhydramine** and **promethazine** all have antimuscarinic activity. As a result, these drugs may antagonize the effects of **bethanechol**. Avoid concurrent administration of these drugs.

Clinical Use and Dosing

Urinary Retention

Bethanechol is used in primary care for neurogenic atony of the urinary bladder with retention. Oral dosing begins at 10 to 50 mg tid or qid. The minimum effective dose is determined by giving 5 to 10 mg initially and repeating the dose every hour until a satisfactory response occurs or 50 mg is reached. SC dosing begins with 2.5 mg. The minimum effective dose is determined by injecting 2.5 mg initially and repeating every 15 to 30 minutes until satisfactory response is obtained or adverse reactions appear, but the maximum number of doses is four. The minimum effective dose is then given tid or qid as needed. The dosage for children is 0.2 mg/kg or 0.6 mg/m^2 tid.

Reflux Esophagitis

Bethanechol has been used on an investigational basis for the treatment of gastroesophageal reflux. The drug is given orally in a dose of 25 mg qid for adults. In infants and children, the oral dose is 3 mg/m^2 tid. However, for this indication, it has been replaced with newer agents.

Patient Education

Administration

To avoid nausea and vomiting, the patient should take the drug 1 hour before or 2 hours after a meal. The SC form is intended for subcutaneous use only and should never be given intramuscularly (IM) or IV because the resultant high drug levels can cause severe toxicity, evidenced by bloody diarrhea, bradycardia, profound hypotension, and cardiovascular collapse.

Adverse Reactions

This drug may cause abdominal discomfort, salivation, sweating, or flushing. Teach the patient to notify the health-care provider if these occur. The dose may be reduced or the drug discontinued.

Dizziness or lightheadedness may occur when the patient arises from a lying or sitting position. The probable cause is hypotension. Arising slowly from a supine position and dangling the feet over the side of the bed before standing will reduce postural hypotension. No exercise in hot weather and a daily fluid intake of at least 2,000 cc of noncaffeinated liquids will also reduce these problems.

Bethanechol is contraindicated in patients with asthma and other diseases with a bronchospastic component. Teach the patient to report wheezing or breathing difficulties to the health-care provider immediately.

CHOLINESTERASE INHIBITORS

This class of drugs prevents the degradation of ACh by AChE, thereby enhancing the activity of ACh at cholinergic receptors. These drugs act as indirect cholinergic agonists. These inhibitors can intensify ACh activity at all cholinergic junctions (muscarinic, ganglionic, and nicotinic) and so have a wide range of responses and adverse reactions.

There are two basic categories of **cholinergic inhibitors**. (1) Reversible inhibitors produce effects of moderate duration. They include **ambenonium (Mytelase)**, **demecarium (Humorsol)**, **donepezil (Aricept)**, **galantamine (Reminyl)**, **neostigmine (Prostigmin)**, **pyridostigmine (Mestinon)**, **physostigmine (Antilirium)**, **rivastigmine (Exelon)**, and **tacrine (Cognex)**. (Drugs in this group that are used for clinical diagnosis or for treatment of glaucoma are not discussed in this chapter.) (2) Irreversible inhibitors are highly toxic and, although they can be split from AChE, the split takes place extremely slowly, and effects exist until new cholinesterase can be generated. They contain a phosphate atom and are referred to as **organophosphate cholinesterase inhibitors**. Because they are highly lipid-soluble, they can be absorbed even through the skin. Because of their systemic toxicity, they have only one clinical indication, as a treatment for glaucoma. The irreversible drugs are not discussed in this chapter.

Although it is not a **cholinesterase inhibitor**, **memantine (Namenda)** is used to treat Alzheimer's disease and has off-labeled uses for vascular dementia, attention deficit-hyperactivity disorder (ADHD), postherpetic neuralgia, and prevention of migraine in adults. It does this by a novel mechanism of N-methyl-D-aspartate receptor inhibition. Because several of the reversible AChE inhibitors mentioned above are also used to treat Alzheimer's disease, **memantine** will also be discussed in this section.

Pharmacodynamics

The **reversible AChE inhibitors** act as poor substrates for AChE. The process by which AChE breaks down ACh into choline and acetic acid takes place in two steps: (1) binding ACh to the active center of AChE and (2) splitting of the ACh, which regenerates free AChE. This reaction is rapid so that one molecule of AChE can break down a large amount of ACh in a relatively short time. The **reversible AChE inhibitors** follow this same process, except that the process takes place slowly; the drug is bound to the active center of AChE for a relatively long time, preventing the regeneration of free AChE, and preventing AChE from catalyzing the breakdown of more ACh. The slowing down of the inactivation of ACh results in an increased intrasynaptic concentration of ACh and intensified neural transmission at virtually all junctions where ACh is the neurotransmitter. In doses higher than the usual therapeutic doses, **neostigmine** and **pyridostigmine** can produce skeletal muscle stimulation and activation of muscarinic, ganglionic, and nicotinic receptors in the CNS. In therapeutic doses, they usually affect only muscarinic and nicotinic receptors at the myoneural junction without altering CNS function.

Tacrine, donepezil, rivastigmine, and **galantamine,** which are used to treat Alzheimer's disease (AD), are designed to alter CNS function. AD is associated with profound cholinergic depletion. All of these agents increase the availability of ACh in the brain by competitively inhibiting AChE but are all structurally dissimilar.

Tacrine is an acridine AChE inhibitor. Inhibition of AChE by **tacrine** is short lived. In addition, the drug has more cholinergic activity in the periphery than do the other agentshas and, therefore, may have more peripheral cholinergic adverse drug reactions (ADR) associated with it. It may also act as a partial agonist at muscarinic receptors by blocking reuptake of dopamine, serotonin, and norepinephrine.

Donepezil is a piperidine type AchE inhibitor with increased affinity for the CNS and, thus, a decreased number of peripheral ADRs. It has a longer duration of inhibitory action than **tacrine.**

Rivastigmine is a potent, selective inhibitor of AChE in the cortex and hippocampus. The selectivity of this drug for the brain, like **donepezil,** accounts for the decreased number of peipheral cholinergic ADRs. Because of its carbamate structure, after binding to the esteratic site, the drug dissociates much more slowly from AChE than does ACh. Thus, the drug is considered to be a pseudo-irreversible inhibitor of the enzyme. This action also helps explain why that enzyme is inhibited for a much longer time frame than the plasma half-life would suggest.

Galantamine is a natural tertiary alkaloid that reversibly inhibits AChE. Some evidence suggests that along with the AChE inhibition, the drug may enhance the effect of ACh on nicotinic receptors by binding at an allosteric site. But whether this effect results in increased clinical efficacy has not been demonstrated. Because these agents work to increase levels of ACh released from cholinergic neurons, as AD progresses and the patient has fewer functional cholinergic neurons, these drugs may have less effect.

Persistent stimulation of the N-methyl-D-aspartate (NMDA) receptors by the excitatory amino acid glutamate may contribute to the symptomatology of Alzheimer's disease. **Memantine** is a low to moderate noncompetitive antagonist at NMDA receptors. It binds preferentially to the receptor-operated cation channels. The drug has low to negligible affinity for gamma-aminobutyric acid (GABA), benzodiazpine, dopamine, adrenergic, histamine, and glycine receptors. It does show antagonistic effects at the 5-HT3 (serotonin) receptor and blocks nicotinic ACh receptors but with less potency. It does not effect the inhibition of AChE by **donepezil, galantamine,** or **tacrine.**

Pharmacokinetics

Absorption and Distribution

Each of the **AChE inhibitors** differs in its pharmacokinetics (Table 14–18). **Neostigmine** and **pyridostigmine** carry a positive charge. This charge results in poor absorption from the GI tract, and oral doses must be much greater

Table 14–18 ▶ **Pharmacokinetics: Selected Acetylcholinesterase Inhibitors**

Drug	Onset	Peak	Duration	Protein Binding (%)	Bioavailability	Half-Life	Elimination
Donepezil	Within 6 wk*	4 h	24 h	94–96	100%	60–100 h	57% in urine; 15% in feces
Galantamine	Within 6 wk*	1 h; delayed 90 min by food	UK	18	90%	7 h	95% in urine; 5% in feces
Memantine	Within 6 wk*	3–7 h	UK	45	UK	60–80 h	82% unchanged in urine. Urine pH increase decreases elimination
Neostigmine	45–75 min	UK	2–4 h	15–25	1%–2%	40–60 min	By enzymatic degradation
Pyrido-stigmine PO	30–35 min	UK	3–6 h	UK	11%–17%	3.7 h	By enzymatic degradation

Continued

Table 14–18 ▶ **Pharmacokinetics: Selected Acetylcholinesterase Inhibitors—cont'd**

Drug	Onset	Peak	Duration	Protein Binding (%)	Bioavailability	Half-Life	Elimination
Pyrido-stigmine SR	30–60 min	UK	6–12 h	UK	UK	3.7 h	By enzymatic degradation
Rivastigmine	Within 6 wk*	1 h; delayed 90 min by food	UK	40	36%	1.5 h	97% in urine as metabolites
Tacrine	Within 6 wk*	1–2 h	4–8 h	55	5%–30%; food reduces BA by 30%–40%	2–4 h	1% as unchanged drug in urine

UK = unknown.
*Observable reduction in clinical symptoms.

than SC doses to produce a therapeutic effect. Once absorbed, these drugs distribute to sites of action in the myoneural junction and at peripheral muscarinic receptors, and have limited ability to cross the blood–brain barrier.

Tacrine is rapidly absorbed following oral administration, but then undergoes extensive first-pass metabolism, resulting in an absolute bioavailibility of 5 to 30 percent. Absorption is significantly reduced when the drug is taken with food, and a 30 to 40 percent decrease in bioavailability results; therefore, it should be given on an empty stomach. Because it is lipid soluble, it crosses the blood–brain barrier, and its drug concentration is highest in the brain. Women tend to have concentrations that are 50 percent higher than those of men, even when they take the same dose.

Food has no effect on the absorption of **donepezil**; the distintegrating tablets and the solution are bioequivalent to its regular tablets. Total **galantamine** absorption is also not affected by food, but Cmax is decreased by 25 percent and T_{max} is delayed 90 minutes when the drug is taken with food. Both **donepezil** and **galantamine** are well absorbed following oral administration, with a bioavailability of greater than or equal to 90 percent. Unike **tacrine**, **donepezil** is concentrated in the CNS, with very little peripheral activity. Both drugs exhibit linear pharmacokinetics.

Rivastigmine is completely absorbed following oral administration; however, its bioavailibility is only 36 percent, indicating a significant first pass effect. When taken with food, the absorption of **rivastigmine** is delayed and C_{max} is decreased by 30 percent. However, the AUC increases by about 30 percent. Thus this drug should be taken with food to maximize bioavailibility. It also has nonlinear pharmacokinetics, and doubling the dose from 3 to 6 mg twice daily results in a 3-fold increase in AUC.

Memantine is highly absorbed following oral administration. Food has no effect on absorption. It has linear pharmacokinetics over the dosage range.

Metabolism and Excretion

Neostigmine and pyridostigmine are degraded by AChE and metabolized by hepatic microsomal enzymes to inactive products, but only to a small extent. Both drugs are eliminated largely as unchanged drug in the urine: for neostigmine 50 to 70 percent of the dose is unchanged; pyridostigmine is mainly eliminated unchanged. Both drugs will potentially require dosing adjustment in renal impairment.

Tacrine is extensively metabolized by CYP 1A2 isoenzymes in the liver. The higher concentrations of drug in women may be related to decreased CYP 1A2 isoenzyme activity in women. Cigarette smoking also reduces this isoenzyme, and smokers have higher concentrations than nonsmokers. The relatively high first-pass effect in the metabolism of **tacrine** is dependent on the dose administered. The CYP 1A1 system can be saturated at low doses. Once in the plasma, elimination is not dose dependent. Although studies in patients with liver disease have not been done, it is reasonable to expect that hepatic dysfunction reduces clearance of this drug. Dosing of this drug does not require adjustment in elderly patients or in patients with renal impairment.

Donepezil is extensively metabolized by CYP 2D6 and 3A4 isoenzyme systems in the liver to two active and two less active metabolites. Approximately 57 percent of it is excreted in the urine and 15 percent in feces. Hepatic impairment has been shown to decrease clearance by 20 percent. Dosing of this drug does not require adjustment in elderly patients or in patients with renal impairment.

Galantamine is extensively metabolized by CYP 2D6 and 3A4 isoenzymes. Approximately 20 percent of the dose is excreted as unchanged drug in the urine. Total renal elimination is 95 percent, with 5 percent eliminated in feces. Approximately 7 percent of the population has a genetic variation that leads to reduced levels of activity of CYP 2D6. However, there are no AUC changes seen in these individuals and no dosage adjustments are required. **Galantamine** clearance is decreased by about 25 percent in patients with moderate hepatic impairment, and these patients, as well as those with moderate renal impairment, probably should not have a dosage exceeding 16 mg/d.

Rivastigmine is rapidly and extensively metabolized primarily by cholinesterase-mediated hydrolysis to one active metabolite. Evidence suggests that there is minimal involvement of the CYP450 system. Most of the drug is excreted as its metabolite in the urine. Moderate renal impairment reduces clearance by 64 percent, and moderate hepatic impairment reduces it by 60 percent. Dosage adjustment is not required in either scenario because the drug is usually titrated to tolerability. **Nicotine** use increases the clearance of this drug.

Memantine undergoes little metabolism with the majority (57% to 82%) of an administered dose excreted unchanged in the urine. The remainder is converted primarily to three polar metabolites that possess minimal N-methyl-D-aspartate (NMDA) receptor antagonism. The CYP450 enzymes system does not play a significant role in its metabolism. Renal clearance involves active tubular secretion moderated by a pH-dependent tubular reabsorption. Although data on the effect of renal impairment are limited, based on its renal excretion, it is very likely that patients with moderate to severe renal impairment will have higher levels of the drug (*Drug Facts and Comparisons*, 2009).

Pharmacotherapeutics

Precautions and Contraindications

The only absolute contraindications for **neostigmine** and **pyridostigmine** are mechanical intestinal and urinary obstruction. The reasons are the same as those given for **bethanechol**. A relative contraindication is a history of reaction to bromides. **Neostigmine** and **pyridostigmine** are Pregnancy Category C because they may cause uterine irritability, and neonates may display muscular weakness. Use these drugs only when clearly needed and the benefits clearly outweigh the risks to the fetus. **Neostigmine** is ionized at physiological pH and is not expected to be excreted in breast milk. **Pyridostigmine** is excreted in breast milk and should not be used by breastfeeding women. Safety and efficacy have not been established for children.

Tacrine has been associated with hepatotoxicity. It is contraindicated for patients who have previously been treated with the drug and developed jaundice, and for patients with abnormal transaminase levels or clinical jaundice with a serum bilirubin above 3 mg/dL. Patients who are unwilling or unable to avoid drinking alcohol should also not have this drug prescribed because concurrent use may have additive toxic effects on the liver. Unlike **tacrine, donepezil, galantamine,** and **rivastigmine** are not associated with hepatotoxicity. **Memantine** has been temporally associated with hepatic failure, but data are insufficient to document causality.

Both **tacrine** and **donepezil** are Pregnancy Category C. There are no data to support findings that either of these drugs causes harm to the fetus. Safety has not been established in pregnancy. For **rivastigmine**, animal studies did not demonstrate teratagenicity with doses two to four times the maximal dose used in humans. Animal studies also showed that at doses three to six times the amount used for treatment, **galantamine** caused a slight delay in fetal development and some skeletal variations. Both **rivastigmine** and **galantamine** are Pregnancy Category B. **Memantine** is Pregnancy Category B because no adequate and well-controlled studies in pregnant women have been conducted.

Drug clearance of **rivastigmine** and **galantamine** decreases in the presence of hepatic impairment and renal impairment. However, recommendations for both these drugs are to titrate to response and tolerability rather than specific dose recommendations. Administration of **galantamine** to patients with severe hepatic impairment or CrCl less than 9 mL/min is not recommended. In patients with renal impairment, no dosage adjustments are recommended for **donepezil** or **tacrine**. However, in patients with hepatic impairment **donepezil** should be titrated to response and tolerability, and **tacrine** should be discontinued when the transaminase levels are greater than five times the upper limit of normal (ULN).

Because **memantine** undergoes little metabolism, no dosing adjustment is required in patients with hepatic impairment. No dosing adjustment is required in mild to moderate renal impairment, but with CrCl between 5 and 29 mL/min, the dosage should not exceed 5 mg bid. There are no specific recommendations for CrCl less than 5 mL/min.

Cholinergic agonists are thought to have some potential to cause generalized seizures. **Tacrine** is also contraindicated for patients with a history of stroke, subdural hematoma, hydrocephalus, or CNS tumor because they are at increased risk for this adverse reaction.

Cholinergic agonists and **cholinesterase inhibitors** tend to increase gastric acid secretion because of increased cholinergic activity. Monitor patients closely for indications of active or occult GI bleeding, especially patients at increased risk for developing ulcers.

All of these drugs should be used with caution for patients with a history of bronchospastic disorders, peptic ulcer disease, cardiovascular diseases that may worsen in the presence of hypotension or bradycardia, and hyperthyroidism. The reasons are the same as for **muscarinic agonists** and are based on the increased activity of ACh.

Adverse Drug Reactions

Each of these drugs differs in adverse reactions; however, all except **memantine** are associated with the adverse reactions common to all **cholinergic agonists**. (See precautions above.) In addition, muscle weakness, fasciculations, cramps, and spasms have been noted. **Memantine** has been associated with syncope, bradycardia, and hypotension; vertigo and ataxia; dyspnea and bronchospasm; and emotional lability and paranoid reactions in a small percentage of patients.

Donepezil, **galantamine**, and **rivastigmine** are well tolerated, with few adverse reactions. The most common are headache, nausea, diarrhea, and insomnia. Patients with a history of frequent GI complaints may be prone to recurrence of these problems while taking these drugs. Because of their effects on the SA and AV nodes of the heart, bradycardia has been observed. As with **tacrine**, cholinergic-associated adverse reactions are usually dose dependent and can be treated by temporarily reducing the dose or by taking the drug with meals, although the latter reduces bioavailability.

Toxicity

The warning signs of overdose are very similar to common adverse reactions, and there is a narrow margin between the first appearance of adverse reactions and serious toxic effects. Adverse reactions such as excessive GI stimulation, excessive salivation, miosis, and fasciculations of voluntary muscles should be reported to the health-care provider immediately, and the drug will be temporarily discontinued. **Atropine** 0.5 to 1 mg IV may be required.

Hepatotoxicity

Tacrine has been associated with hepatotoxicity and it has been demonstrated that metabolites of **tacrine** are cytotoxic. A significant number of patients develop elevated serum transaminases (aspartate transaminase [AST], and alanine aminotransferase [ALT]). If the drug is promptly withdrawn, clinical evidence of liver injury is rare. To prevent liver injury in patients on this drug, monitor their liver function frequently. This topic is discussed in the Monitoring section.

Drug Interactions

Synergistic effects occur between these drugs and other **cholinergic agonists**. Antagonistic effects occur with **anticholinergic** drugs. **Neostigmine** and **pyridostigmine** have increased risks for neuromuscular blockade with **aminoglycoside antibiotics** and **succinylcholine**. With the latter drug, respiratory support may be needed. These combinations should be avoided. **Atropine** and **belladonna** derivatives suppress many of the early warning symptoms of **neostigmine** and **pyridostigmine** overdose and toxicity. Given the narrow margin between therapeutic dose and overdose, this increased risk is unacceptable, and these drugs should not be given together. **Corticosteroids** and magnesium also interact with these drugs. Their interactions are presented in Table 14–19.

Many drug interactions for **donepezil**, **galantamine**, and **tacrine** occur because they undergo significant

Table 14–19 ■ **Drug Interactions: Selected Acetylcholinesterase Inhibitors**

Drug	Interacting Drug	Possible Effect	Implications
Donepezil	Anticholinergics	Donepezil antagonizes activity of anticholinergics	Avoid concurrent administration
	Bethanechol, succinylcholine	Synergistic cholinergic activity	Reduce bethanechol dose if they must be given concurrently
	NSAIDs	Donepezil increases gastric acid secretion	Monitor for active or occult bleeding
	Furosemide, digoxin, warfarin	At concentrations of 0.3–10 mg/mL did not affect binding or these drugs	
	Ketoconazole, quinidine, other drugs metabolized by CYP-450 2D6 and 3A4 isoenzymes	Potentially inhibit donepezil metabolism	Choose alternative "azole" or antiarrhythmic
	CYP2D6 and 3A4 inducers: carbamazepine, dexamethasone, phenobarbital, phenytoin, rifampin	Potentially increase rate of elimination	Avoid concurrent administration
Galantamine	Succinylcholine, bethanechol	Synergistic effect when combined	Memantine does not have this effect
	Cimetidine	Increased bioavailability of galantamine by 16%	Ranitidine does not have this effect
	Ketoconazole	Increased galantamine AUC by 30%	Select different antifungal

Table 14–19 ■ **Drug Interactions: Selected Acetylcholinesterase Inhibitors—cont'd**

Drug	Interacting Drug	Possible Effect	Implications
	Paroxetine	Increased bioavailability of galantamine by 40%	Avoid concurrent use
	Erythromycin	Increased galantamine AUC by 10%	Select different antibiotic
	Other inhibitors of CYP3A4: Amitriptyline, fluoxetine, fluvoxamine, quinidine	Clearance of galantamine decreased by 25%–33%	Select different antidepressant or antiarrhythmic
	NSAIDs	Galantamine increases gastric acid secretion	Monitor for active or occult bleeding
Memantine	Amantidine, ketamine, dextromethorphan	Interaction not evaluated, but also NMDA antagonists	Use with caution
	Hydrochlorothiazide, cimetidine, ranitidine, quinidine, nicotine, triamterene	Potential altered plasma levels of both drugs since both use same renal cationic system for elimination	Avoid concurrent use or monitor for increased drug effects
	Drugs, diet, and clinical states that make urine alkaline	Clearance of memantine reduced by 80% under alkaline urine concentrations at pH 8. Can lead to accumulation of drug with increased adverse effects	Use memantine with caution under these conditions
Neostigmine, pyridostigmine	Succinylcholine	Increase neuromuscular blocking; prolonged respiratory depression with extended periods of apnea	Provide respiratory support as needed or avoid concurrent use
	Aminoglycoside antibiotics	Aminoglycosides have mild but definite nondepolarizing blocking action that may accentuate neuromuscular block	Choose different antibiotic or monitor closely for increased blockade
	Local and general anesthetics, antiarrhythmics	Decreased effects of neostigmine	Increase dose of neostigmine while patient is taking these drugs
	Atropine, belladonna derivatives	Suppress muscarinic symptoms of excessive GI stimulation, leaving only more serious symptoms of fasciculation and paralysis of voluntary muscles as signs of overdose	Avoid concurrent use. Margin of safety is already quite narrow, and this makes it narrower
Corticosteroids	Decrease anti-AChE effects of neostigmine or pyridostigmine. Anti-AChE effects may increase after stopping steroids	Avoid concurrent use or provide respiratory support as needed. Monitor respiratory status closely after stopping steroid	
	Magnesium	Has direct depressant effect on skeletal muscle; may antagonize beneficial effects of neostigmine or pyridostigmine	Avoid concurrent use
	Methocarbamol	A single case report indicates this drug may impair effect of pyridostigmine	Only one case report. Monitor for possible effect

Continued

Table 14–19 ■ **Drug Interactions: Selected Acetylcholinesterase Inhibitors—cont'd**

Drug	Interacting Drug	Possible Effect	Implications
Rivastigmine	No drug interactions based on no CYP 450 activity		
	Anticholinergics	Rivastigmine may interfere with their activity	Avoid concurrent use. (See note below related to tacrine)
	Cholinomimetics and other cholinesterase inhibitors	Synertistic effects	Avoid concurrent use
Tacrine	All drugs metabolized by CYP-450 1A2 isoenzymes	May inhibit metabolism of tacrine	Avoid concurrent use, or monitor effects and adjust doses as needed
	Anticholinergics	Tacrine interferes with anticholinergic activity	Monitor for anticholinergic activity if they must be given together. *Note*: Many drugs have anticholinergic-like effects even if not anticholinergic drugs. These should also be watched
	Cimetidine	Increases the peak plasma level of tacrine by 54% and the AUC by 64%	Choose different histamine$_2$ blocker
	Bethanechol, succinylcholine	Synergistic effects. Can cause bladder outlet obstruction	Avoid concurrent use
	Theophylline	Coadministration doubles theophylline elimination half-life and average plasma level	Monitor plasma theophylline levels and reduce theophylline dose if they must be given together
	NSAIDs	Increased risk for GI bleed	Monitor for occult bleeding with serial stool guaiac tests and hemoglobin determinations. May need to take antacids while on tacrine therapy

AUC = area under curve.

metabolism by the CYP enzyme systems of the liver. Any drug metabolized by the CYP 1A2 isoenzymes has interactions with **tacrine**, and those metabolized by 2D6 and 3A4 have interactions with **donepezil** and **galantamine.** The number of drugs metabolized by the 1A2 isoenzymes is relatively small, but the number metabolized by 2D6 and 3A4 is large. To date, these drug interactions have largely been in vitro and theoretical, but as these drugs are prescribed for larger numbers of patients, the interactions are likely to occur. **Donepezil** does not interact with **furosemide, digoxin,** and **warfarin,** drugs often prescribed for older adults who are also likely candidates for **donepezil.** The bioavailability of **galantamine** increases when given with **erythromycin** due to inhibition of CYP3A4 by **erythromycin.** Because of its inhibition of both CYP 3A4 and 2D6**paroxetine** increases the AUC of **galantamine. Cimetidine** increases the bioavailability of **galantamine**, but **ranitidine** does not.

Memantine interacts with other **NMDA receptor antagonists** such as **amantadine, ketamine,** and **dextromethorphan.** Drugs that make urine alkaline reduce renal clearance of this drug and many drugs that use the same renal cation exchange system also interact with this drug to decrease its renal clearance.

Clinical Use and Dosing

Myasthenia Gravis

Neostigmine and **pyridostigmine** are used to treat myasthenia gravis. In this disorder, an autoimmune process occurs in which the patient's immune system produces antibodies directed against nicotinic receptors on skeletal muscle, reducing the number of receptors by 70 to 90 percent, resulting in muscle weakness. **Reversible cholinesterase inhibitors** are the mainstay of treatment, preventing ACh inactivation and intensifying the effects of ACh on motor neurons. These drugs do not cure the disorder, but manage its symptoms, so treatment is life long.

Establishing an optimal dose for treatment can be a challenge because these drugs produce widespread effects, not just at selected target organs. A small initial dose is administered, followed by other small doses until an optimal dose is reached. Signs of improvement that indicate optimal dosage include improved ability to swallow and to raise the eyelids.

The initial adult dose of **neostigmine** is usually 15 mg/day, and for children it is 2 mg/kg daily in divided doses given every 3 to 4 hours. The interval between dose increases is highly individualized. The average adult dose is 150 mg/day, but the maximum dose may approach 375 mg/day. Larger portions of the daily dose may be given 30 to 60 minutes prior to activities that produce greater fatigue, such as eating or shopping. For **pyridostigmine**, the initial adult dose is 60 mg/day, and for children it is 7 mg/kg divided into five or six doses daily (Armstrong & Schumann, 2003). Sustained-release tablets are available that require once- or twice-daily dosing. Regular tablets or syrup may be administered with extended-release tablets for optimal control of symptoms. Both of these drugs can be given parenterally if the patient has difficulty swallowing, but it is important to remember that, because of their first-pass effects, oral doses are 30 to 40 times greater than parenteral doses.

Reversal of Nonpolarizing Neuromuscular Blockade

By producing increased ACh at the myoneural junction, **neostigmine** and **pyridostigmine** can reverse the effects of nondepolarizing blocking agents. They cannot be used to counter the effects of **succinylcholine** because it is a depolarizing neuromuscular blocker. The most common application of this role is immediately postoperative and is determined by the anesthesiologist. Because it would probably not be used in primary care or by a nurse practitioner, this use is not discussed further.

Alzheimer's Disease (AD)

This disease is associated with a significant deficiency in brain levels of choline acetyltransferase, the enzyme responsible for the synthesis of ACh. In addition, cholinergic neurons in the brain's basal ganglia degenerate, resulting in a loss of cholinergic input to the muscarinic receptors in the frontal and temporal lobes of the cerebral cortex (Lai et al, 2001; Minger et al, 2000). Enhancing cholinergic activity with drugs is designed to counteract the decreased stimulation of the remaining cholinergic neurons. **Donepezil, galantamine, rivastigmine,** and **tacrine** are all used to treat AD by preventing the degradation of ACh by AChE. Another mechanism thought to contribute to AD symptoms is persistent stimulation of NMDA receptors by glutamate. **Memantine** relieves symptoms by blocking this stimulation.

Tacrine is a centrally active, noncompetitive, reversible AChE inhibitor. Approximately 30 to 40 percent of AD patients who were able to complete their drug trials demonstrated modest improvement in cognitive and functional measures. Unfortunately, these improvements were not noted to last longer than 30 weeks, and many patients did not complete the trials because of the adverse reactions associated with this drug. The response was dose related, and adverse reactions increase as the dose increases.

Dosing usually begins with 10 mg given four times daily between meals. Taking the drug with meals makes it more tolerable, but the bioavailability is decreased by 30 to 40 percent, requiring higher doses for the same effect. Doses are increased at 6-week intervals, based on liver function studies, to a maximum of 160 mg/day. The monitoring requirements are discussed later. An adequate response is defined as the lack of apparent disease progression for 6 months, and it requires at least 8 weeks at doses greater than 120 mg/day. The highest-tolerated dose is the most efficacious.

Tacrine was the first drug to show some success in treating AD. Because it has many adverse reactions and requires extensive monitoring because of its hepatotoxicity, **tacrine** is the least used of the drugs to treat AD today.

Donepezil is a piperidine-based derivative dissimilar from other AChE inhibitors in its pharmacokinetics and tolerability. It is also a centrally active, noncompetitive, reversible AChE inhibitor, but its duration of inhibitory action is longer than **tacrine.** This longer duration of action permits once-daily dosing, which is a major advantage for this drug. Another advantage for this drug is its better adverse reactions profile. The most problematic adverse reaction is digestive complaints, and this may require dosage reduction.

Clinical trials (Pratt, 2002; Salloway, Pratt, & Perdomo, 2003; Winblad et al, 2001) showed improvement in cognitive function for as long as 2 years, but after this period there were indications that the drug did not prevent further long-term disease progression. The improvement was dose related, and adverse reactions also increased with the increased dose.

The mean age of patients in clinical trials was 73 years; 80 percent of the patients were between 65 and 84 years of age and 49 percent were 75 years or older. Although there was no clinically significant difference in response compared to other age groups, the most adverse reactions were reported by patients 65 to 75 years of age and younger than 65 years of age (*Drug Facts and Comparisons,* 2009).

The recommended starting dose of **donepezil** is 5 mg daily at bedtime. Doses are increased at 4- to 6-week intervals to reduce adverse reactions. The maximum dose is 10 mg daily. The higher dose should be used if tolerated because it is more efficacious, especially for severe disease. Unlike **tacrine, donepezil** is not likely to cause hepatotoxicity and does not require assessment of liver function in order to increase the dose or frequent monitoring of liver function throughout therapy. Patients are monitored for indications of active or occult bleeding because of the potential for **anticholinesterase inhibitors** to increase gastric acid secretion (*Drug Facts and Comparisons,* 2009).

Galantamine is administered twice daily, preferably with morning and evening meals. The initial dose is 4 mg bid. After a minimum of 4 weeks of treatment, if the drug is well tolerated, the dose may be increased to 8 mg bid. A further increase to 12 mg bid should be attempted only after a minimum of 4 weeks at the previous dose. If therapy is interrupted for several days or longer, the dose must be reinitiated at 4 mg bid and increased based on the same titration as above. The usual maintenance dose is 8 to 12 mg bid. Based on the reduced clearance seen in patients with moderate hepatic or renal impairment, the dose for these patients generally should not exceed 16 mg/d.

Razadyne, the brand name form of **galantamine**, is also available in an extended-release formulation allowing for once-daily dosing. The initial dose for this formulation is 8 mg. The dosage is increased at 4-week intervals, as with the regular formulation. The ususal maintenance dose is 16 to 24 mg daily. This formulation also carries a dosage restriction for hepatic and renal impairment.

Rivastigmine is also administered twice daily, in the morning and evening with food. The starting dose is 1.5 mg bid. If the dose is well tolerated, it may be increased to 3 mg bid after 2 weeks of treatment. Subsequent increases to 4.5 and 6 mg bid also require a 2-week interval. Treatment interrupted for several doses is reinstitued at the 1.5-mg bid dose and titrated as above. The most effective dose in clinical trials (*Drug Facts and Comparisons*, 2009) was 3 to 6 mg bid.

For patients who have difficulty swallowing, **Exelon**, the brand name formulation of **rivastigmine**, is available in an oral solution and in a transdermal patch. Dosing regimens for these two forms are shown in Table 14–20.

Memantine is started at 5 mg once daily with a target dose of 20 mg daily. The dose is increased in 5-mg increments: 10 mg/day is given as 5 mg bid; then 15 mg is given 5 mg and 10 mg in two doses; then 20 mg is given 10 mg bid. The minimal recommended interval between dosage increases is 1 week. Dosages may need to be reduced in patients with moderate renal impairment. The drug is not recommended for patients with severe renal impairment.

Table 14–20 shows the clinical use and dosing schedules for all of these drugs. Only uses associated with primary care are presented. Several of these drugs have off-labeled uses. Those with some degree of supportive evidence are also presented in Table 14–20.

Rational Drug Selection

Formulation

For **neostigmine** and **pyridostigmine**, formulation is a consideration (Table 14–21). Difficulty in swallowing is a common problem for patients with myasthenia gravis. **Pyridostigmine** is available in a syrup form that can be used by many patients with this problem without having to resort to an injectable form. In addition, the syrup can be used for children to administer their individualized doses based on body weight.

For patients with Alzheimer's disease, **rivastigmine** has an oral-solution dosing formulation that permits it to be taken directly from the syringe or mixed with juice or

Table 14–20 ● Dosage Schedule: Acetylcholinesterase Inhibitors

Drug	Indication	Initial Dose	Maintenance Dose
Donepezil	AD	5 mg daily at bedtime for 4–6 wk	May increase to 10 mg daily after 4–6 wk. The higher dose should be used if tolerated because it is more efficacious, especially for severe AD
	Off-labeled: Autism	2.5 mg/d for 1 wk	Increase by 2.5 mg until maximal tolerated dose or 10 mg/d
Galantamine (G) (Razadyne) (B)	AD	4 mg twice daily with morning and evening meals	Increase dose to 8 mg twice daily after 4 wk of therapy if drug well tolerated. Titration to 12 mg twice daily only after another 4-wk interval. Maintenance dose 8–12 mg bid. If therapy interrupted for several days or longer, reinitiate at 4 mg and follow same titration. Dose should not exceed 16 mg/d for patients with moderate renal of hepatic impairment
(Razadyne) ER (B)		8 mg once daily in the morning	Increase to 16 mg daily after minimum of 4 wk. May increase to 24 mg daily after another 4-wk interval. Maintenance dose 16–24 mg daily. See above for renal and hepatic impairment
Memantine (Namenda)	AD	5 mg once daily	Target dose is 20 mg daily. Titrate up in 5 mg increments/d: go to 5 mg twice daily (10 mg/d), then 5 mg in one dose and 10 mg in another dose (15 mg/d), then 10 mg twice daily (20 mg/d). Minimal interval for titration is 1 wk. Dosages may need to be reduced if moderate renal impairment. Not recommended for severe renal impairment

Table 14–20 ● **Dosage Schedule: Acetylcholinesterase Inhibitors—cont'd**

Drug	Indication	Initial Dose	Maintenance Dose
	Off-labeled: ADHD in children 6–12 years	4.8 mg daily	Titrate up (as above) to 20 mg/d
	Postherpetic neuralgia (adults 20–78 yrs)	20 mg daily in divided doses	Max dose 55 mg/d in divided doses for up to 9 wk
	Prevention of migraine headaches (adults 14–78 yrs)	5 mg daily	May increase to 20 mg daily. Use for at least 2 months
Neostigmine	Myasthenia gravis	*Adults:* Oral: 15 mg/d divided and given every 3–4 h. Increase dose in 15-mg increments at daily intervals until optimal response is achieved	Usual dose is 150 mg/d divided and given every 3–4 h. Maximum dose is 375 mg/d
		SC/IM: 0.5 mg every 2–3 h	Usually needed short-term, and dose is 5 mg every 2–3 h
		Children: Oral: 2 mg/kg/d in 6–8 divided doses	Same maintenance dose
		SC/IM: 0.01–0.04 mg/kg every 2–3 h	Usually needed short term. Same dose
Pyridostigmine (G) (Mestinon) (B)	Myasthenia gravis	*Adults:* Oral: 60 mg/d divided and given every 3–4 h Increase dose in 60-mg increments at daily intervals until optimal dose is achieved	Usual dose is 600 mg/d divided and given every 3–4 h. Maximum dose is 1,500 mg/d
		IM: one-third the oral dose	
		Children: Oral: 7 mg/kg/d divided into 5–6 doses	Same maintenance dose
		IM: 0.05–0.15 mg/kg/dose every 2–3 h	Usually needed short term. Same dose
Mestinon ER (B)		180 mg daily	Usual dose 180–540 mg daily or bid with dosing interval of at least 6 hrs
Rivastigmine (G) (Exelon) (B) Exelon oral solution (B)	AD and dementia associated with Parkinson's disease	1.5 mg twice daily in the morning and evening with food	Increase dose to 3 mg twice daily after 2 wk, if well tolerated. Titration to 4.5 mg and 6 mg twice daily also requires 2-wk interval. If several doses missed, reinitiate at 1.5 mg and follow same titration. Most effective dose for AD is 3–6 mg twice daily; for PD is 1.5–6 mg bid
Exelon transdermal patch		Initiate with the 4.6 mg/24 h patch applied once daily	After a minimum of 4 weeks, and, if well tolerated, increase to 9.5 mg/24 h patch applied once daily. If adverse reactions cause intolerance, therapy should be discontinued for several days and restarted at the next lower dose. If treatment is interrupted for longer than several days, reinitiate with the lowest daily dose
Tacrine (Cognex)	AD	10 mg qid between meals for 4 wk; may be given with food, but bioavailability is decreased 30%–40%	If ALT remains unchanged, increase by 40 mg/d every 4 wk up to a maximum of 40 mg qid. Usual maintenance dose is 120 mg/d. Elevated ALT requires detailed dosing adjustments

ALT = alanine amino-transferase.

Table 14–21 ◆ **Available Dosage Forms: Acetylcholinesterase Inhibitors**

Drug	Dosage Form	Package	Cost
Donepezil (Aricept)	Tablets: 5 mg, 10 mg	In bottles of 30 and 90 tablets; unit dose blister packs of 100 tablets	Tablet: 5 mg = $214/30 10 mg = $223/30
(Aricept ODT)	Orally disintegrating tablets: 5 mg, 10 mg	In UD blister packs of 30 ODTs	ODT: 5 mg = $221/box of 30
	Oral solution: 1 mg/mL	In 300 mL	
Galantamine (G) (Razadyne) (B)	Tablets: 4 mg, 8 mg, 12 mg	In bottles of 60 and 1,000 (G); 60 and 100 film-coated tablets (B)	Generic: 8 mg = $156/60 Brand: 4 mg = $302/100 8 mg = $323/100 12 mg = $323/100
Razadyne (B)	Oral solution: 4 mg/mL	In 100 mL with calibrated pipette	
Galantamine ER (G) Razadyne ER (B)	Capsules (extended release): 8 mg, 16, mg, 24 mg	In bottles of 30 and 500 capsules and UD 30 (G). In bottles of 30 capsules (B)	Brand: $203/30 for all strengths
Memantine (Namenda)	Tablets: 5 mg, 10 mg	In bottles of 60, 200, and 2,000 and unit dose 100s and titration packs	5 mg = $181/60 10 mg = $180/60
	Oral solution: 2 mg/mL	In 360 mL	
Neostigmine (Prostigmin)	Tablets: 15 mg	In bottles of 100 scored tablets	15 mg = $55/60
Pyridostigmine (G) (Mestinon) (B)	Tablets: 60 mg	In bottles of 100, 500 tablets	60 mg = $53/100 (G) $183/100 (B)
Mestinon (B)	SR tablets: 180 mg	In bottles of 30 tablets	180 mg = $95/30
Mestinon (B)	Syrup: 60 mg/5 mL	In 480-mL bottles of raspberry-flavored syrup (5% alcohol, sorbitol)	$135/480 mL
Rivastigmine (G) (Exelon) (B)	Capsules: 1.5 mg, 3 mg, 4.5 mg, 6 mg	In bottles of 60, 100, 500 and unit dose 100s	Brand: 1.5 mg = $385/100 3 mg = $370/100 4.5 mg = $373/100 6 mg = $371/100
Exelon (B)	Oral solution: 2 mg/mL	In 120-mL bottles	
Exelon (B)	Transdermal patch: 4.6 mg/24 h	In 30 patches	4.6 mg = $211 for 1 box of 30
	9.5 mg/24 h	In 30 patches	9.5 mg = $214 for 1 box of 30
Tacrine (Cognex)	Tablets: 10 mg, 20 mg, 30 mg, 40 mg	In bottles of 120 tablets; unit dose packs of 100 tablets	10 mg = $263/100 20 mg = $258/100 40 mg = $260/100

water for those who have difficulty in swallowing tablets. Once mixed, the drug is stable for 4 or fewer hours. **Rivastigmine** is also available in a transdermal patch. **Donepezil** is available in an oral solution and in orally disintegrating tables. **Galantamine** and **memantine** are also available in an oral solution.

Cost

There is not a significant cost differentiation between **neostigmine** and **pyridostigmine**. The cost differential between **tacrine** and **donepezil** is largely related to the monitoring costs. **Donepezil** does not produce hepatotoxicity and requires only routine monitoring of blood chemistries. **Tacrine**, which does produce hepatotoxicity, requires frequent monitoring of liver function. The monitoring guidelines are presented later. The cost associated with frequent and long-term testing is high. **Galantamine** and **rivastigmine** are available in less expensive generic formulations. **Donepezil** and **memantine** are available only in brand name formulations.

Dosing Schedule

The dosing schedules of **neostigmine** and **pyridostigmine** are similar. Those of the drugs used to treat Alzheimer's disease are quite different. **Donepezil** has a once-daily dosing regimen. **Galantamine, rivastigmine,** and **memantine** are all bid doses, but **galantamine** is available in extended-release capsules that are dosed once daily. **Rivastigmine** can also be dosed once daily in the transdermal patch form. **Tacrine** requires four daily doses, and is most effective on an empty stomach, which results in the doses being adjusted for meals. For patients who are older adults and who have a disease process that includes memory problems, or for patients whose caregivers are also older adults, this complex regimen may present adherence problems.

Adverse Reactions Profile

Neostigmine and **pyridostigmine** have similar adverse reaction profiles. Among the drugs used to treat Alzheimer's disease, **tacrine** and **rivastigmine** have the worst adverse reaction profiles and **donepezil** has the best.

Time to Recurrence of Disease Progression

Tacrine has been associated with loss of beneficial effects after about 30 weeks. **Donepezil, galantamine, memantine,** and **rivastigmine** have shown positive effects for at least 2 years.

Monitoring

Monitoring parameters for **tacrine** are complex and, at a minimum, continue for 9 months. Baseline liver function tests (total bilirubin, AST, and ALT) should be done prior to initiation of therapy. ALT levels, the ones most likely to indicate hepatotoxicity, should be monitored every other week for the first 16 weeks of therapy, then monthly for 2 months, and then every 3 months. If the ALT level remains less than double the upper limit of normal, then the dose may be left unchanged or titrated upward as needed. If the ALT level is more than double the upper limit of normal, weekly monitoring of liver function is required. If the ALT level is three to five times the upper limit of normal, then weekly monitoring of liver function is required, and the dose must be decreased by 40 mg/day. If the ALT level returns to the normal range with the reduced dose, then every other week monitoring of ALT levels is sufficient. Treatment is discontinued if the ALT concentration is more than five times the upper limit of normal.

Donepezil requires routine monitoring of blood chemistries and hematology. Baseline liver function studies seem advisable for **galantamine** and **rivastigmine**, but they are not required. Assessment of renal function is advisable for **galantamine** and **memantine**; dosage adjustments are based on renal function. **Neostigmine** and **pyridostigmine** do not have monitoring parameters beyond those of the disease process they are used to treat.

Patient Education

Administration

Administration education differs for the two groups of drugs. For all of the drugs, the drug should be taken exactly as prescribed. Doses should not be skipped or doubled up.

For **neostigmine** and **pyridostigmine**, patients may need to set a backup alarm to remind them to take a dose when the doses are every 3 to 4 hours. Taking the dose late may cause myasthenic crisis, and taking it early may result in cholinergic crisis. Because drug therapy is life long, it is important to establish a regimen that the patient can follow over time.

For **donepezil**, missed doses should be skipped and the schedule resumed the next day. Missed doses of **galantamine, rivastigmine,** and **memantine** should be skipped and the next dose taken as scheduled. Patients taking **tacrine** should deal with missed doses by taking them as soon as possible unless it is within 2 hours of the next dose. For all of these drugs, increasing the dose may not improve the symptoms but it does increase the risk for adverse reactions. Abruptly discontinuing the drug may cause a decline in cognitive function, with varying "washout" times.

The oral solution dose of **donepezil** is measured in teaspoons; a 5-mg dose equals 1 teaspoon. Dosing teaspoons used to measure children's liquid medications are available at most pharmacies. **Donepezil** orally disintegrating tablets should be allowed to dissolve on the tongue and then followed with water.

Rivastigmine oral solution comes with a dosing syringe kept in a protective case. Push down and twist the child-resistant closure to open the bottle of drug. Insert the tip of the syringe into the opening in the white stopper. Invert the bottle and while holding the syringe, pull the plunger out to the appropriate markings on the side of the syringe that indicates the dose. Teach the patient how to remove any large bubble from the syringe to avoid an inaccurate dose. The drug may be taken directly from the syringe or mixed in a small glass of water, cold fruit juice, or soda. Do not mix it with other liquids. The syringe should be stored in its protective case.

Memantine and **galantamine** are also available in oral solutions. Both of these also have oral dosing devices. Instructions are enclosed with the product.

The **rivastigmine** transdermal patch is applied once daily (24 hours apart) to a clean, dry area of skin that does not have hair. Although no recommendation is made by the drug manufacturer, it is probably advisable to rotate the site used.

Adverse Reactions

All of these drugs have in common the adverse reactions associated with an increased amount of ACh: dizziness, miosis, lacrimation, excessive secretions in the respiratory and GI tracts, bronchospasm, bradycardia, abdominal cramps, nausea, vomiting, diarrhea, and excessive salivation. Because they have fewer peripheral effects, drugs used to treat Alzheimer's disease have fewer of the peripheral adverse reactions and more of those associated with the CNS. Patients and their caregivers should observe safety precautions related to the dizziness.

Administration of **neostigmine** or **pyridostigmine** with food or milk helps to minimize adverse GI reactions. Patients with myasthenia gravis often have difficulty with swallowing. Sustained-release tablets must be swallowed whole. Immediate-release tablets may be crushed, and syrup forms of **pyridostigmine** are available to facilitate administration in this situation. The mottled appearance of the sustained-release form of **pyridostigmine** does not affect its potency.

Administration with food may reduce GI complaints for **donepezil** and does not affect its bioavailability. Although **tacrine** can also be administered with food, this decreases its bioavailability by 30 to 40 percent and may necessitate increased dosage. However, higher doses are associated with increased risk for adverse reactions. For patients with difficulty in swallowing, **tacrine** capsules can be dissolved in any aqueous solution. Orange juice masks the bitter taste best. **Memantine** and **galantamine** can be administered without regard to food. **Rivastigmine** should be given with food.

Tacrine has adverse reactions associated with hepatotoxicity. Patients who experience jaundice, rash, or fever should contact the health-care provider immediately. The drug will be discontinued.

Lifestyle Management

No specific lifestyle modifications are directly related to these drugs. Patients with myasthenia gravis should at all times wear identification describing the disease and the medication regimen.

NICOTINE

The major source of **nicotine** use is tobacco products. Although tobacco contains many hazardous products (carbon monoxide, hydrogen cyanide, ammonia, nitrosamines, and tar), the one of major concern and the one associated with the addictive mechanism of tobacco products is **nicotine**. The focus of this chapter is on **nicotine** as a drug and on **nicotine replacement**. Chapter 43 discusses smoking cessation.

Pharmacodynamics

The actions of **nicotine** are based on their effects on nicotinic receptors. The chief alkaloid in tobacco products, **nicotine** binds stereoselectively to ACh receptors in the autonomic ganglia, in the adrenal medulla, at neuromuscular junctions, and in the brain.

Cardiovascular Effects

Cardiovascular effects result from stimulation of the sympathetic ganglia and the adrenal medulla, promoting the release of epinephrine and norepinephrine. These catecholamines produce vasoconstriction, accelerated heart rate, and increased force of ventricular contraction. The end result is increased blood pressure and increased cardiac output.

Gastrointestinal Effects

The GI effects result from stimulation of the nicotinic receptors in the parasympathetic ganglia, resulting in increased secretion of gastric acid and increased tone and motility of the GI smooth muscle. **Nicotine** can also induce vomiting, based on a complex process that involves the receptors in the aortic arch and the CNS. Vomiting often follows tobacco ingestion by infants and children.

Central Nervous System Effects

Two types of CNS effects may account for **nicotine**'s addictive properties. A stimulating effect, mainly on the locus ceruleus, makes the person increasingly alert and improves cognitive performance. The "pleasure center" in the limbic system is also stimulated. At low doses the stimulant effects predominate; at high doses the pleasure center effects predominate. **Nicotine** also facilitates the release of dopamine at the pleasure center, producing the same effects as other highly addictive drugs, such as cocaine, amphetamines, and opioids.

Acute and chronic tolerance develops rapidly (less than 1 hour), but at different rates from the physiological effects. Withdrawal symptoms, such as cigarette craving, can be reduced in some persons by plasma levels of **nicotine** lower than those attained by smoking. Most of the **nicotine** in smoked tobacco products is destroyed by burning or escapes in sidestream smoke so that the dose is relatively low. For cigarette, cigar, and pipe smokers, **nicotine** stimulates nicotinic receptors at all the locations above.

The replacement therapy formulations produce similar but lesser effects because the dose of **nicotine** is lower and the pharmacokinetics are different. Depending on the formulation used, the stimulation of the pleasure centers may be significantly different.

Pharmacokinetics

Absorption and Distribution

Four forms of replacement therapy for **nicotine** addiction exist: chewing gum, transdermal patches, oral inhalation, and nasal spray (Table 14–22). Each of these systems is labeled by the actual amount of **nicotine** absorbed.

The **nicotine** in the gum is bound to an exchange resin and released only during chewing. The blood level depends on the vigor and duration of the chewing. The trough level of **nicotine** obtained by smoking one cigarette/hour is approximately twice that of chewing one 2-mg piece of gum. Approximately 68 percent of the **nicotine** in patches is absorbed via the skin. Both of these formulations raise blood levels of **nicotine** slowly, producing

Table 14–22 ▶ **Pharmacokinetics: Selected Nicotine Replacement Systems**

Drug	Onset	Peak	Duration	Protein Binding	Percent Absorbed	Half-Life	Elimination
Nicorette gum	Rapid	15–30 min	UK	<5%	UK	3–4 h	10% unchanged in urine. Up to 30% with high urine flow rates and pH 5
Nicoderm patch*	Rapid	2–12 h	24 h	<5	68	3–4 h	10% unchanged in urine. Up to 30% with high urine flow rates and pH 5
Nicotrol patch	Rapid	6–12 h	24 h	<5	68	3–4 h	10% unchanged in urine. Up to 30% with high urine flow rates and pH 5
Nicotrol nasal spray	Rapid	4–15 min	UK	UK	93	1–2 h	10% unchanged in urine. Up to 30% with high urine flow rates and pH 5
Nicotrol Inhaler	Rapid	15 min	UK	UK	UK	3 min	10% unchanged in urine. Up to 30% with high urine flow rates and pH 5

*Steady-state concentrations 25% to 30% higher are achieved following the second daily application.
UK = unknown.

less pleasure than cigarettes, but relieve withdrawal symptoms. Approximately 93 percent of the **nicotine** in the nasal spray is absorbed through the nasal mucosa, and blood levels rise rapidly, much the same as with smoking, producing some subjective pleasure while suppressing withdrawal symptoms. Most of the **nicotine** released from the inhaler is deposited in the mouth with less than 5 percent reaching the lower respiratory tree. Taking eight deep inhalations over 20 minutes releases an average 4 mg of **nicotine** from each cartridge, which results in 2 mg systemically absorbed. Intermittent use of the inhaler typically produces **nicotine** plasma levels of 6 to 8 ng/mL, which equates to about 33 percent of that achieved with cigarette smoking.

Nicotine replacement therapy (NRT) by any formulation is widely distributed in the body, crosses the placenta, and enters the breast milk.

Metabolism and Excretion

Nicotine is metabolized mainly by the liver and, to a lesser extent, by the kidney and lung. There is no significant skin metabolism. More than 20 metabolites have been identified, all of which are believed to be less active than the parent compound. The half-life of **nicotine** is 3 to 4 hours, but the half-life of its primary metabolite (cotinine) is 15 to 20 hours, and its concentrations exceed **nicotine** by 10-fold. The activity of the metabolite, however, is only 25 percent of the activity of **nicotine.**

Ten to 20 percent of **nicotine** is excreted unchanged in the urine. As high as 30 percent may be excreted with high urine flow rates and urine acidity below pH 5. Following removal of the patch, plasma levels of **nicotine** drop exponentially with a mean half-life of 3 to 4 hours. Nonsmoking patients will have no detectable **nicotine** concentrations in 10 to 12 hours.

Table 14–22 describes the pharmacokinetics of selected **nicotine replacement systems.**

Pharmacotherapeutics

Precautions and Contraindications

The effects on the various body systems determine the contraindications. In each case, the decision to use or not to use NRT is based on the likelihood of smoking cessation and its benefits versus the potential adverse effects.

Cardiovascular effects result in contraindicated use of NRT for patients with severe cardiovascular disease, life-threatening arrhythmias, severe or worsening angina, or vasospastic diseases and during the immediate post-MI period. NRT is used in the presence of hypertension only when the benefits of smoking cessation clearly outweigh the risk for perpetuating the hypertension.

The actions of **nicotine** on the adrenal medulla require cautious use of NRT for patients with hyperthyroidism, pheochromocytoma, or type 1 diabetes mellitus. **Nicotine** is extensively metabolized by the liver, and its total clearance is dependent on liver blood flow. NRT should be used with caution in the presence of hepatic impairment. Only severe renal impairment is expected to affect the clearance of nicotine or its metabolites. Less severe renal impairment does not preclude the use of NRT.

Nicotine delays healing in esophagitis and peptic ulcer disease and should be used for patients with active disease only when the benefits clearly outweigh the risks. **Transdermal systems** are usually well tolerated by patients with normal skin but may be irritating for patients with some skin disorders.

Administration of **nicotine** during pregnancy can cause fetal harm. It is associated with decreased fetal breathing movements and with decreased placental perfusion, resulting in infants who are small for gestational age. Some forms are Pregnancy Category X (**nicotine polacrilex**), and some are Pregnancy Category D (**transdermal nicotine**). Pregnant women should use them only if the likelihood of smoking cessation justifies the potential risk to the fetus.

Nicotine passes freely into breast milk and has the potential for serious harm to the nursing infant. **Replacement therapy** should be undertaken only if the likelihood of smoking cessation justifies the potential risk to the nursing infant.

The amount of **nicotine** that can be tolerated by an adult can produce poisoning or be lethal in children. The systems used for **replacement therapy** are contraindicated for children. Adults using these systems should take every precaution to keep them out of the reach of children.

Adverse Drug Reactions

Adverse reactions are largely based on the actions of nicotine on the various body systems. CNS adverse effects include headache, insomnia, and dizziness. Cardiovascular adverse effects include tachycardia and hypertension. GI system effects include abnormal taste, dry mouth, and dyspepsia.

Nicorette gum may produce pharyngitis, belching, increased salivation, hiccoughs, and nausea and vomiting. **Nicotrol nasal spray** may produce nasopharyngeal irritation, rhinitis, sneezing, and watery eyes. **Transdermal systems** may produce burning, erythema, and pruritus at the patch site. Applying the patch to different sites each day may reduce these symptoms. **Nicotine patch** pharmacokinetics findings are similar for all sites of application on the upper body and upper outer arm.

Drug Interactions

Smoking cessation, with or without NRT, may alter the patient's response to a number of drugs for which smoking is known to increase the metabolism and lower the blood levels. Table 14–23 lists these drugs and the changes in patient response.

Table 14–23 ■ **Drug Interactions: Nicotine Replacement Therapy or Smoking Cessation**

Interacting Drug	Patient Response With Smoking	Patient Response With Nicotine Replacement Therapy or Smoking Cessation	Implications
Acetaminophen, caffeine, imipramine, labetalol, oxazepam, pentazocine, prazosin, propranolol and other beta blockers, theophylline	Increased metabolism and lowered blood levels of these drugs	Reversal of increased metabolism	Dosage reduction at cessation of smoking and onset of nicotine replacement therapy may be necessary
Catecholamines, cortisol	Increased circulating catecholamines and cortisol	Return to normal levels	Dosage of adrenergic agonist andantagonists may need to be adjusted
Furosemide	Reduced diuretic effects and decreased cardiac output	Increased diuretic effects	Dosage reduction may be needed
Insulin		Increased SC insulin absorption	Monitor blood glucose levels and adjust dosage of insulin
Propoxyphene	Increased first-pass metabolism	Decreased first-pass metabolism	Dosage adjustments may be needed

Effective absorption of **Nicorette gum** requires slightly alkaline saliva. Coffee, tea, cola, and other drinks and foods may reduce salivary pH. It may be beneficial for patients not to ingest food or drink while using the gum or within 15 minutes of using it.

Clinical Use and Dosing

The only indication for **NRT** is smoking cessation. Choice of route and dose are dependent on patient preferences, cost, and smoking history (Table 14–24).

Nicorette gum comes in two strengths: 2 mg/piece and 4 mg/piece (Table 14–24). Patients with low to moderate nicotine dependence use the 2-mg/piece strength; patients with high dependence use the 4-mg/piece strength. The average dosage is 9 to 12 pieces of gum/day. The maximum dose is 30 pieces of the 2-mg/piece strength and 20 pieces of the 4-mg/piece strength. Dosing on a fixed schedule (e.g., one piece every 2 to 3 hours) is more effective than as-needed dosing. After 3 months, the patient should discontinue **nicotine** use. Withdrawal should be gradual. Gradual reduction is accomplished over 2 to 3 months by decreasing the daily dose by one or more pieces every 4 to 7 days and decreasing the chewing time with each piece from 30 minutes to 10 to 15 minutes every 4 to 7 days. The gum may be discontinued when one or two pieces per day are sufficient to control the craving for nicotine. Use of this product beyond 6 months is not recommended.

Patches are applied every morning to clean, dry, hairless skin of the upper body or upper arm and worn for 16 (**Nicotrol**) to 24 (all other patches) hours each day. The site is changed daily and not reused for at least 1 week. Most patients begin with the largest dosage patch and gradually decrease the dose. Patients with cardiovascular disease, those who weigh less than 100 lb, or those who smoke less than one-half pack per day should begin treatment with a smaller patch.

> **CLINICAL PEARL**
>
> Substituting one or more pieces of sugarless gum for pieces of **Nicorette** gum and increasing the number of substitutions may help in reducing the dose during withdrawal.

Nicoderm patches come in 21-mg/day, 14-mg/day, and 7-mg/day doses. The 21-mg/day patch is worn for 6 weeks (step 1), and then the 14-mg/day dose (step 2) and the 7-mg/day dose (step 3) are worn for 2 weeks each. The entire course of therapy is 8 to 10 weeks.

Nicotrol patches come in 15-mg/day, 10-mg/day, and 5-mg/day doses. The 15-mg/day patch is worn for 6 weeks (step 1), and then the 10-mg/day (step 2) and 5-mg/day (step 3) patches are worn for 2 weeks each. The entire course of therapy is 8 to 10 weeks.

Persons who smoke 10 or fewer cigarettes per day do not use step 1. These patients start with step 2 for 6 weeks and then progress to step 3 for 2 weeks. The entire course of therapy is 8 weeks.

Nicotine transdermal patches have an off-labeled indication in Tourette syndrome. One 7-mg or one 10-mg patch is worn each day for 2 days. Research on this use shows fair results. Trials are underway to determine a potential use in ulcerative colitis.

Nicotrol NS nasal spray device delivers 0.5 mg of **nicotine** per activation. Two sprays (one in each nostril) constitute one dose and are equivalent to the **nicotine** in one cigarette. Initial dosing is 1 to 2 doses per hour but never more than 5 doses per hour or 40 doses per day.

Table 14–24 ◆ **Available Dosage Forms: Nicotine Replacement Therapy**

Drug	Dosage Form	Package
Nicotine gum (G) (Nicorette) (B)	Gum: 2 mg per square	In packs of 48 and 108 (G) and 48, 108, and 168 (B)
Nicotine gum (G) Nicorette DS (B)	Gum: 4 mg per square	In packs of 48 and 108 (G) and 48, 108, and 168 (B)
Committ (B)	Lozenge: 2 mg and 4 mg	In packs of 72
Nicoderm CQ (B)	Transdermal: 21 mg, 14 mg, 7 mg	In 7 and 14 systems per box for step 1 and 14 for steps 2 and 3
Nicotine transdermal system (G)	Transdermal: 21 mg, 14 mg, 7 mg	In 7 and 30 systems per box
Nicotrol (B)	Transdermal: 15 mg, 10 mg, 5 mg	In 7 and 14 systems per box
Nicotrol NS	Nasal spray: 10 mg/mL (0.5 mg nicotine per spray)	In 10-mL bottles (100 doses)
Nicotrol inhaler	Inhaler: 4 mg delivered (10-mg cartridge)	Each kit contains 6 cartridges. In 42 and 168 kits

After 4 to 6 weeks, the doses are gradually reduced and then stopped completely.

Nicotrol inhaler delivers 4 mg of nicotine if the patient takes eight deep inhalations over 20 minutes. Only 2 mg of this dose are systemically absorbed. Patients self-titrate to the dose they require. Most patients who successfully quit smoking use between 6 and 16 cartridges per day. The recommended duration of treatment is 3 months, with gradual withdrawal over the next 6 to 12 weeks.

Rational Drug Selection

Cost

If cost is calculated on a daily basis, assuming the recommended dose of the patches and the midrange use of the gum, the average daily cost for the gum is about $6.25 per day for **Nicoderm**, and for **Nicotrol**, about $4 per day. Among the patches, the daily cost is about the same. The total cost for the entire course of therapy is higher for **Nicorette gum** at $562 for 3 months of therapy. Total cost for **Nicoderm** is about $278, and for **Nicotrol** it is $360.

Convenience

The patches are often the preferred method of **NRT** because they provide relatively constant concentrations of serum **nicotine** and they are convenient to use. A new patch is applied on a daily basis. All formulations are now available OTC (in a locked cabinet that is accessed by the pharmacist) and do not require a prescription or the cost of a visit to a health-care provider.

Success Rates

According to some studies, **nicotine gum** improves smoking cessation rates by 40 to 60 percent at 12 months. **Transdermal** patches approximately double the 6- to 12-month abstinence rates of a placebo. There is "good news, bad news" for abstinence with the **nasal spray.** Nearly 50 percent of users avoided smoking for 1 year, but many of these people continued to use the spray and were unwilling or unable to give it up. The same was true for the **inhaler.**

Concomitant Diseases

Gum is more likely to produce GI adverse reactions and should be avoided for patients with esophagitis and active peptic ulcer disease. **Patches** are well tolerated by patients with normal skin but may cause problems for patients with certain skin disorders. Patients who have sinus problems, allergies, or asthma should avoid the sprays.

Monitoring

No specific monitoring is required.

Patient Education

Administration

Nicorette gum is not swallowed. It is chewed for a few seconds until a peppery taste or tingling sensation occurs. It is then "parked" between the cheek and gum until the sensation is almost gone (about 1 minute), and the process of chewing and parking the gum is repeated for approximately 30 minutes. Rapid, vigorous chewing is more likely to result in adverse reactions and is to be avoided. Dosing on a fixed schedule (e.g., one piece every 2 to 3 hours) is more effective than as needed dosing. Eating or drinking acidic beverages should be avoided 15 minutes before or during the use of the gum. Gradual reduction of the dose can be accomplished by decreasing the daily dose by one or more every 4 to 7 days, by decreasing chewing time to 15 minutes, or by substituting sugarless gum for one or more of the daily doses.

Transdermal patches (Nicoderm, Nicotrol) are applied at the same time each day to clean, dry, hairless skin of the upper torso or upper arm. Sites are rotated daily, and the same site should not be used again for at least 1 week. The patch is kept in its sealed pouch until it is applied. It is then pressed firmly in place with the palm for 10 seconds to be sure there is good contact. The patch remains in place while the patient is showering, bathing, or swimming. **Nicotrol patches** remain in place for 16 hours. All others remain in place for 24 hours. Wash hands with plain water after handling the patches because soap increases the absorption of nicotine. To prevent children from exposure to the drug in the patch, fold them in half and wrap them in aluminum foil before disposal.

Nicotrol NS nasal spray is used much like other nasal sprays. Tilt the head back slightly and spray once into each nostril. Do not sniff, swallow, or inhale through the nose as the spray is administered. Replace the child-resistant cap after using and before disposal. Gradual reduction of the dose is accomplished by using one spray at a time, using the spray less frequently, or skipping a dose. A date for stopping the spray should be set.

The **Nicotrol inhaler** has a mouthpiece that is attached to the cartridge. Best effect is achieved by frequent continouous puffing for about 20 minutes. After using the inhaler, the mouthpiece is separated and should be thrown away out of the reach of children or pets. The mouthpiece has about 6 mg of its initial drug content when discarded, enough to be lethal to small children or pets. The mouthpiece should be stored in its plastic case for further use and cleaned regularly with soap and water.

Adverse Reactions

The most common adverse reactions vary with the route of administration. For **Nicorette gum,** the most common are increased salivation, sore mouth, and pharyngitis. Substituting sugarless gum for some doses of **Nicorette** not only aids in dosage reduction but also can improve these symptoms. Good oral hygiene and adequate fluid intake are also helpful.

For the **transdermal patches,** burning, erythema, and itching at the application site may occur. These usually subside within 1 hour. Allergic reactions can occur, including reactions to the adhesive. Teach the patient to report rash or other symptoms of an allergic reaction or failure of these symptoms to resolve. A different brand or a different route of administration may be required.

For the **nasal spray**, nasopharyngeal irritation, sneezing, rhinitis, and watery eyes may occur. This route should be avoided in patients with sinus problems or asthma.

Lifestyle Management

Successful smoking cessation is dependent on more than NRT. It often involves counseling and support groups and may involve other drugs such as **antidepressants** concomitantly. Lifestyle changes associated with addictive substances are never easy. Chapter 43 provides more data on smoking cessation.

CHOLINERGIC BLOCKERS

Cholinergic blockers are also referred to as parasympatholytics, muscarinic antagonists, and **anticholinergics.** The term *anticholinergic* can be deceiving because it implies blockade of all cholinergic receptors. In reality, **cholinergic blockers** produce selective muscarinic blockade against the actions of ACh. Because muscarinic receptors are found in many organs of the body (the eye, heart, blood vessels, lung, GI tract, urinary bladder, and sweat glands), and these drugs cannot be targeted at a single organ, they have many adverse reactions. Throughout this section, **cholinergic blocker** will be synonymous with muscarinic blockade unless otherwise stated.

There are several subtypes of **cholinergic blockers** based on the organs they are likely to target. **Atropine** is the prototype drug in this class and affects most muscarinic receptors. Its main use orally is as an adjunct to treatment of GI disorders. Other uses are more related to hospital-based care. Its oral use is discussed in this section. **Scopolamine** has actions similar to **atropine** except for increased CNS depression and ability to suppress motion sickness and emesis. It is also covered in this section. The antispasmodic group of drugs is indicated for reduction of GI motility and urinary tract smooth muscle spasm. They are covered in this section. **Ipratropium bromide (Atrovent)** is used to treat acute exacerbations asthma and other respiratory diseases such as chronic obstructive pulmonary disease (COPD). It is discussed in Chapter 17. **Mydriatic cycloplegics** are used for ophthalmic procedures. This use is covered in Chapter 26. **Centrally acting cholinergic blockers** are used to treat Parkinson's disease and to counteract the extrapyramidal adverse reactions associated with some psychotropic drugs. They are briefly discussed here, but their uses for this indication are covered in Chapter 15.

Pharmacodynamics

Cholinergic blockers competitively block the actions of ACh at muscarinic receptors. They have no direct effect on the receptor. Their actions are based on preventing interaction of endogenous neurotransmitters from activating the receptor and thereby blocking the action associated with stimulation of these receptors. The results of the stimulation of these receptors are depicted in Table 14–1. Blockade produces clinically significant action on the cardiovascular, respiratory, urinary, GI, and central nervous systems; on exocrine glands; and on the eye. Different drugs in the class affect these systems to differing degrees.

The actions of these drugs are, to some extent, dose dependent. Some muscarinic receptors can be blocked at relatively low doses, and some require higher doses for blockade to occur. Doses that block receptors in the stomach and bronchial smooth muscle are higher, for example, than those required to block receptors at other locations. Because treatment with higher doses results in more adverse reactions, and other drugs are more effective, this class of drugs is not used as primary agents to suppress gastric acid secretion or to dilate the bronchi.

Cardiovascular Effects

The sinoatarial node is very sensitive to muscarinic stimulation. Because stimulation of muscarinic receptors decreases heart rate, blockade increases heart rate. In the presence of high vagal tone, muscarinic blockade can significantly reduce the PR interval of the electrocardiogram (ECG) by blocking receptors in the AV node, increasing AV node conduction and decreasing the refractory period of the AV node. The effect on contractility and automaticity is minimal because control of these is primarily via the sympathetic nervous system. Blood vessels have no direct innervation from the parasympathetic nervous system (PNS); however, PNS stimulation does dilate coronary arteries.

Respiratory Effects

Both smooth muscle and secretory glands of the respiratory tract have vagal innervation and contain muscarinic receptors. Blockade of muscarinic receptors relaxes bronchial muscle resulting in bronchodilation, whereas blockade of receptors in the bronchial glands decreases bronchial secretions.

Exocrine Gland Effects

Muscarinic blockade is very effective in the salivary glands, resulting in dry mouth. It is used for this purpose preoperatively, but it is an unwanted effect in patients taking these drugs for such conditions as Parkinson's disease or urinary incontinence. Gastric acid secretions are less effectively blocked. The volume and amount of acid, pepsin, and mucin are reduced. Basal secretion is more affected than stimulated secretion. Sympathetic cholinergic fibers innervate eccrine sweat glands and many of these have muscarinic receptors. Cholinergic (muscarinic) blockers suppress thermoregulatory sweating. This is minimally problematic for adults, but even ordinary doses of atropine, for example, can produce fevers in infants and children.

Urinary and Gastrointestinal Effects

Blockade of muscarinic receptors has extensive effects on smooth muscle in the gut and the urinary system. Gastrointestinal smooth muscle is affected from the stomach to the colon. In muscarinic blockade, the visceral walls are relaxed and both tone and peristalsis are diminished. This prolongs gastric emptying time and intestinal transit time. Smooth muscle of the ureters and bladder wall is relaxed with muscarinic blockade. This action is useful in treatment of urinary tract spasms, but it can precipitate urinary retention, especially in older adult males with benign prostatic hyperplasia.

Central Nervous System Effects

At therapeutic doses, muscarinic blockade produces mild CNS excitation. At higher doses, scopolamine, and to a lesser extent atropine, can produce agitation, hallucinations, and delirium. The relative excess of cholinergic activity in parkinsonian tremor and extrapyramidal symptoms associated with antipsychotic drugs can be partially corrected by muscarinc blockade, especially if combined with a dopamine precursor.

Optic Effects

The papillary constrictor depends on muscarinic receptor stimulation. Blockade of muscarinic receptors results in unopposed sympathetic dilator activity, producing mydriasis. Blockade of receptors on the ciliary muscle produces cycloplegia, which results in loss of the ability to accommodate for near vision.

Pharmacokinetics

Absorption and Distribution

Cholinergic blockers in the belladonna alkaloid group (**atropine, scopolamine**) are well absorbed from the gut and cross the conjunctival membrane (Table 14–25). When applied in a suitable vehicle, **scopolamine** is absorbed from the skin. In contrast, only about 10 to 30 percent of a dose of the drugs in the quaternary group (**propantheline** [Probanthine]) is absorbed after oral administration because these drugs have a positive charge, which decreases their ability to move across membranes. **Benztropine** (Cogentin), **darifenacin** (Enablex), **fesoterodine** (Toviaz), **oxybutynin** (Ditropan), **solifenacin**

Table 14–25 ▶ Pharmacokinetics: Selected Cholinergic Blockers

Drug	Onset	Peak	Duration	Half-Life	Elimination
Atropine PO	30 min	30–60 min	4–6 h	3 h	77%–94% in urine
Benztropine PO	1–2 h	Several days	6–10 h	Unknown	Unknown
Dicyclomine PO	1–2 h	60–90 min		9–10 h	80% in urine; 10% in feces
Darifenacin PO (extended-release tablets)	Unknown	7 h	Unknown	12–13 h for EM; 19 h for PM	60% in urine and 40% in feces
Fesoterodine PO (extended-release tablets)	Unknown	5 h	Unknown	7 h	70% in urine as active metabolite and 7% in feces
Propantheline	30–60 min	2–6 h	6 h	3–4 h	Inactivated in upper small intestine
Oxybutynin (tablets and syrup)	30–60 min	3–6 h	6–10 h	2–3 h	Unknown
Oxybutyin transdermal and gel	Within 24 h	36 h	3–4 d	7–8 h	<0.1% unchanged drug in urine
Oxybutynin XL	30–16 min	2–6 h	24 h	Unknown	<0.1% unchanged drug in urine
Scopolamine PO	30 min	1 h	4–6 h	8 h	Mostly metabolized by liver
Scopolamine transdermal	4 h	Unknown	72 h	9.5 h	Mostly metabolized by liver
Solifenacin PO	Unknown	3–8 h	Unknown	45–68 h	69% in urine; 23% in feces
Tolterodine	Unknown	1–2 h	12 h	1.9–3.7 h	77% in urine; 17% in feces

Table 14–25 ▶ **Pharmacokinetics: Selected Cholinergic Blockers—cont'd**

Drug	Onset	Peak	Duration	Half-Life	Elimination
Tolterodine (LA)	Unknown	2–6 h	24 h	2.9–3.1 h	77% in urine; 17% in feces
Trihexyphenidyl	1 h	2–3 h	6–12 h	5.6–10.2 h	In urine
Trospium PO	Unknown	5–6 h	Unknown	20 h	85% in feces; 5.8% in urine Active tubular secretion is a major factor in renal excretion

EM = extensive metabolizers and PM = poor metabolizers.

(Vesicare), **tolterodine** (Detrol), and **trihexyphenidyl** (Trihexy) are all well absorbed following oral administration and **oxybutynin** is also well absorbed from the skin. Less than 10 percent of **trospium** (Sanctura) is absorbed following oral administration.

The belladonna alkaloid group is widely distributed, with significant levels reaching the CNS within 30 to 60 minutes after administration. The quaternary group is widely distributed except to the CNS, where it is poorly taken up. The distribution of **benztropine** and **trihexyphenidyl** is not clearly known. **Darifenacin** (Enablex), **fesoterodine** (Toviaz), **Oxybutynin**, **solifenacin** (VESIcare), and **tolterodine** are highly bound to plasma proteins and have large volumes of distribution. **Trospium** (Sancture, Sanctura XR) has lower protein binding (50% to 85%),

Metabolism and Excretion

Both the belladonna alkaloids and the quaternary groups are metabolized mostly by the liver and excreted in urine. **Oxybutynin** and **solifenacin** are metabolized by the CYP 3A4 isoenzyme system and **tolterodine** is metabolized by the CYP 2D6 isoenzyme system. **Darifenacin** and **fesoterodine** metabolized by both 3A4 and 2D6 systems. The metabolism of **trospium** is not clearly known but early studies suggest that the CYP isoenzyme systems are not inhibited in clinically relevant concentrations.

Pharmacotherapeutics

Precautions and Contraindications

Absolute contraindications to these drugs are few and based on their effects on various body systems. **Cholinergic blockers** are contraindicated in glaucoma, particularly angle-closure glaucoma, because of their ability to produce mydriasis and cycloplegia, thereby impeding the flow of aqueous humor. Cautious use is necessary in obstructive disorders of the GI and urinary tracts, including bladder outlet obstruction and BPH, based on the ability of these drugs to decrease tone and motility in these systems. Patients with hypertension and tachycardia or other cardiac arrhythmias require cautious use, based on the potential for these drugs to increase heart rate.

Older adults are particularly susceptible to the CNS effects of **cholinergic blockers**, with an increased risk for cognitive impairment and falls. Other drugs should be chosen when possible, or **cholinergic blockers** should be used with caution.

All drugs in this class except **dicyclomine** and **oxybutynin** are Pregnancy Category C. There are no well-controlled studies in pregnant women, and these drugs should be used only when potential benefits clearly outweigh the risk to the fetus. **Dicyclomine** and **oxybutynin** are Pregnancy Category B. No risk to the fetus has been shown in animal or human studies.

The quaternary group of drugs is not widely distributed in the body and is the least problematic for lactating women. All other **cholinergic blockers** either have wide distribution including breast milk, or their distribution is not known. They should be avoided in nursing mothers unless clearly needed.

Safety and efficacy of many of these drugs have not been established in children. **Atropine** has safe dosing schedules down to infants weighing 7 pounds. **Oxybutynin** has safe dosing schedules (Food and Drug Administration, 2009) for children older than 6 years of age with detrusor overactivity associated with a neurological condition. **Tolterodine** has been shown in studies to increase aggressive, abnormal, and hyperactive behavior and attention disorders in children (Food and Drug Administration, 2009) and should not be used in children.

Adverse Drug Reactions

Adverse reactions to **cholinergic blockers** are based on their actions on tissues other than the target tissue or organ. The discussion here focuses on the adverse reactions on each organ system.

Cardiovascular

Cholinergic blockade eliminates the parasympathetic influence on the heart, resulting in tachycardia. This action can be used therapeutically to treat patients with bradycardia below 50 bpm. The belladonna alkaloids have the highest incidence of this adverse reaction.

Respiratory

Cholinergic blockers are sometimes used to produce relaxation of bronchial smooth muscle for patients with an acute exacerbation of asthma and with COPD, but their tendency to thicken and dry bronchial secretions can result in ineffective airway clearance and make patients more at risk for respiratory infection.

Exocrine Glands

Blockade of muscarinic receptors on sweat glands can produce anhidrosis. Because sweating is necessary for cooling the body, patients are at risk for hyperthermia. The effect on salivary glands produces xerostomia (dry mouth). This can be irritating and can impair swallowing. Practicing good oral hygiene, chewing sugarless gum, and using other methods to reduce this problem should be taught to patients.

Gastrointestinal and Urinary

Decreased tone and motility in the GI tract can lead to constipation, especially when the secretory function of the intestine is also reduced. Patients are taught to increase their intake of fluids and dietary fiber. Blockade of muscarinic receptors in the urinary tract reduces contractile force and pressure in the urinary bladder and increases tone in the urinary sphincter. These combined effects produce urinary hesitancy and urinary retention and increase the risk for urinary tract infection. Impotence has also been reported.

Eye

Mydriatic and cycloplegic action of **cholinergic blockers** results in increased intraocular pressure, blurred vision, and photophobia.

Central Nervous System

Cholinergic blockers that cross the blood–brain barrier produce varied adverse reactions, from mild excitation to dizziness and confusion and, in the case of scopolamine, CNS depression. These adverse reactions are more common in older adults.

Drug Interactions

Many drugs that are not **cholinergic blockers** can produce significant muscarinic blockade. These drugs include **antihistamines, disopyramide, quinidine, phenothiazine antipsychotics,** and **TCAs**. Additive or synergistic antimuscarinic effects occur when these drugs are given with **cholinergic blockers.** Additive CNS depression can occur with **alcohol, antidepressants, opioids,** and **sedative-hypnotics.**

Because **cholinergic blockers** alter transit time through the GI tract, they may alter the absorption of any orally administered drug. For drugs with a narrow therapeutic range or drugs that can reach toxic levels if retained too long in the GI tract, concurrent administration is not recommended. **Antacids** and **adsorbent antidiarrheals** decrease the absorption of **cholinergic blockers.**

Drug interactions specific to each drug are presented in Table 14–26.

Clinical Use and Dosing

Parkinson's Disease

First-line management of Parkinson's disease is usually accomplished with **dopaminergics** and **dopamine**

Table 14–26 ■ Drug Interactions: Selected Cholinergic Blockers

Drug	Interacting Drug	Possible Effect	Implications
Atropine, dicyclomine, propantheline, scopolamine	Other drugs with cholinergic blocking effects: antihistamines, disopyramide, quinidine, phenothiazines, TCAs, MAOIs	Additive cholinergic blocking adverse effects; antipsychotic effects of phenothiazines decreased	Avoid concurrent use or select drug in each category with the fewest cholinergic blocking properties. Adjust phenothiazine dose
	Orally administered drugs	Atropine may alter absorption by slowing GI motility	Separate administration or select drugs that do not have narrow therapeutic ranges for which altered absorption would create a problem
	Antacids	Decrease the absorption of the cholinergic blocker	Separate administration. Give cholinergic blocker first and then antacid at least 30 min later
	Amantadine	Coadministration may result in increased cholinergic blocking adverse effects	Consider decreasing the dose of the cholinergic blocker
	Atenolol	Pharmacological effects of atenolol may be increased	Metoprolol and propranolol not affected. Substitute one of these if possible
	Oral potassium	May increase GI mucosal lesions	Take with food and at least 8 oz water

Table 14–26 ■ **Drug Interactions: Selected Cholinergic Blockers—cont'd**

Drug	Interacting Drug	Possible Effect	Implications
Benztropine, trihexyphenidyl	Other drugs with cholinergic blocking effects: antihistamines, disopyramide, quinidine, phenothiazines, TCAs	Additive cholinergic blocking adverse effects; antipsychotic effects of phenothiazines decreased	Additive cholinergic blocking adverse effects. Antipsychotic effects of phenothiazines decreased. Adjust phenothiazine dose
	Bethanechol	Counteracts the cholinergic effects of bethanechol	Avoid concurrent use
	Antacids and antidiarrheals	May decrease absorption	Separate administration. Give cholinergic blocker first and then antacid or antidiarrheal at least 30 min later
	Haloperidol	Worsens schizophrenic symptoms, increases risk for tardive dyskinesia, decreases blood levels of haloperidol	Avoid concurrent use for schizophrenic patients. Increase dose of haloperidol for others*
	Levodopa	Decreased GI motility, increased deactivation of levodopa, and reduced intestinal absorption	Effectiveness of levodopa is reduced. May need to alter dose of levodopa if both must be given
Darifenacin	Strong inhibitors of CYP3A4 (e.g., clarithromycin, azole antifungals, nefazone, and protease inhibitors)	Darifenacin levels may be increased	Dose of darifenacin should not exceed 7.5 mg when coadminsitered with these drugs
	Moderate CYP3A4 inhibitors (e.g., diltiazem, erythromycin, fluconazole, verapamil)	Darifenacin levels may be increased	No dosage adjustments recommended
	CYP2D6 substrates (e.g., felcainide, thioridazine, despiramine, imipramine)	Mean Cmax and AUC of interacting drug may increase	Use caution when darifenacin is given with drugs metabolized by CYP2D6 and that have a narrow therapeutic window
	Digoxin	Increased in digoxin levels (16%)	If must coadminister, monitor digoxin levels closely
Fesoterodine, solifenacin	CYP3A4 inhibitors (e.g., clarithromycin, erythromycin, itraconazole, ketoconazole)	Increases the active metabolite of fesoterodine	For fesoterodine doses >4 mg/d and for solifenacin doses >5 mg/d are not recommended in patients taking these inhibitors
	CYP3A4 inducers (e.g., rifampin)	Coadministration decreases Cmax and AUC of fesoterodine by 70% and 75%, respectively	No dosing adjustments recommended at this time
Oxybutynin	CNS depressants: alcohol, antihistamines, antidepressants, opioids, sedative-hypnotics	Additive CNS depression	Avoid concurrent administration or monitor closely for CNS effects. May need to alter dosage
	Other drugs with cholinergic blocking effects: antihistamines, disopyramide, quinidine, phenothiazines, TCAs, MAOIs	Additive cholinergic blocking adverse effects; antipsychotic effects of phenothiazines decreased	Additive cholinergic blocking adverse effects. Antipsychotic effects of phenothiazines decreased. Adjust phenothiazine dose
	Haloperidol	Worsens schizophrenic symptoms, increases risk for tardive dyskinesia, decreases blood levels of haloperidol	Avoid concurrent use for schizophrenic patients. Increase dose of haloperidol for others*

Continued

Table 14–26 ■ **Drug Interactions: Selected Cholinergic Blockers—cont'd**

Drug	Interacting Drug	Possible Effect	Implications
	Atenolol	Bioavailability of atenolol increased; increased effects	Metoprolol and propranolol not affected. Substitute one of these if possible
	Nitrofurantoin	Increased blood levels and bioavailability of nitrofurantoin	Choose different antibiotic to treat urinary tract infection if patient already on oxybutynin
Scopolamine	Alcohol, meperidine	Additive CNS depression	Unless desired therapeutic effect, may need to alter dose of one or both
Tolterodine	Erythromycin, ketoconazole, itraconazole, miconazole	May inhibit metabolism and increase effects of tolterodine	Avoid concurrent use
Trospium	Drugs that are eliminated by active renal tubular secretion (e.g., digoxin, procainamide, morphine, vancomycin, metformin, tenofovir)	May increase the serum concentration of trospium and/or the competing drug	If must coadminister, carefully monitor for adverse effects. For digoxin, monitor drug levels carefully

*Administration of these drugs may be a therapeutic choice with phenothiazines to reduce extrapyramidal adverse reactions associated with phenothiazines.

agonists. Rather than as direct treatment of the disorder, **cholinergic blockers** are useful early in the course of the disease to control tremor by relaxing smooth muscle. They are also useful for middle-age patients who have tremor but little rigidity or bradykinesia and for control of salivation and drooling.

Trihexyphenidyl is one **cholinergic blocker** currently used as an adjunct to therapy with **carbidopa/levodopa.** The initial dose is 1 to 2 mg the first day, increased by 2-mg increments at 3- to 5-day intervals until a total of 6 to 10 mg are given daily (Table 14–27). Many patients receive maximum benefits at this dose, but postencephalitic patients often require doses of 12 to 15 mg/day. The drug is best tolerated when the daily dose is divided into three doses and taken at mealtimes. High doses may be divided into four doses and taken at mealtimes and bedtime. Because of the relatively high dosage of sustained-release capsules, they are not used for initial

Table 14–27 ◉ **Dosage Schedule: Selected Cholinergic Blockers**

Drug	Indication	Initial Dose	Maintenance and Maximum Dose
Atropine	Irritable bowel syndrome, peptic ulcer disease	*Adults:* 400 mg q 4–6 h	May increase to 600 mcg if needed
	(In children also used for frequent urination and bed-wetting)	*Children:* 7–16 lb = 0.1 mg; 17–24 lb = 0.15 mg 24–40 lb = 0.2 mg 40–65 lb = 0.3 mg 65–90 lb = 0.4 mg >90 lb = 0.4 mg q 4–6 h	Not to exceed 400 mcg, Use lowest effective dose
Benztropine	Parkinson's disease	1–2 mg/d For postencephalitic patients: 2 mg/d	Increase in increments of 0.5 mg/d gradually at 5- or 6-d intervals until symptom relief. Use smallest dose that achieves effect. Maximum dose is 6 mg/d. Older adults and thin patients may not tolerate higher doses. Giving dose at bedtime is preferred
	Drug-induced EPS	1–2 mg daily or bid PO or IM	1–2 mg PO provides relief in 1–2 d and prevents recurrence. If inadequate relief in that time, may increase to 2 mg tid. 1–2 mg IM provides rapid relief. Maximum dose by either route is 6 mg/d

Table 14–27 ◉ **Dosage Schedule: Selected Cholinergic Blockers—cont'd**

Drug	Indication	Initial Dose	Maintenance and Maximum Dose
Darifenacin	For overactive bladder with symptoms of incontinence, urgency and frequency	7.5 mg once daily	May increase to 15 mg once daily as early as 2 weeks after starting therapy. In moderate hepatic impairment or when coadministered with strong CYP3A4 inhibitor, daily dose should not exceed 7.5 mg. Maximum dose: 15 mg/d
Fesoterodine	For overactive bladder with symptoms of incontinence, urgency and frequency	4 mg once daily	May increase to 8 mg once daily based on individual response and tolerability. In severe renal insufficiency or when coadministered with strong CYP3A4 inhibitor, dose should not exceed 4 mg/d. This drug should not be given to patients with severe hepatic impairment
Dicyclomine	Irritable bowel syndrome	80 mg/d in 4 equally divided doses	Increase to 160 mg/d in 4 divided doses
Oxybutynin	Antispasmodic for bladder instability and overactive bladder	*Adults*: 5 mg bid or tid immediate-release The XL formulation is recommended for overactive bladder and is given once daily Transdermal formulation is used only in adults. Dose is 3.9 mg system applied twice weekly (every 3–4 d) *Frail elderly:* 2.5 mg bid or tid	*Adults:* 5 mg qid or 10 mg bid of the XL formulation
		Children >5 years of age: 5 mg bid	*Children >5 years of age:* Maximum doses of 5 mg tid of immediate release and 20 mg/d of extended release
	Detrusor overactivity associated with a neurological condition	*Children 6 years of age and older:* 5 mg once daily of extended-release tablets	*Children 6 years of age or older:* Dosage adjustments in 5 mg increments to achieve a balance of efficacy and tolerability up to a maximum of 20 mg/d
		Children >5 years of age: 5 mg bid of immediate-release tablets or syrup	*Children >5 years of age:* Dosage adjustments in 5 mg increments to achieve a balance of efficacy and tolerability up to a maximum of 5 mg tid
Propantheline	Peptic ulcer	15 mg 30 min before meals and 30 mg at bedtime	Same as initial dose
Scopolamine	Prevention of nausea and vomiting associated with motion sickness	One transdermal disk applied to postauricular skin 4 h before antiemetic effect is desired	One disk delivers 0.5 mg/d for 3 days. If effect needed for >3 d, remove and replace with new disk
Solifenacin	For overactive bladder with symptoms of incontinence, urgency and frequency	5 mg once daily	May increase to 10 mg once daily based on patient response and tolerability. In severe renal impairment, moderate hepatic impairment or when coadministered with strong CYP3A4 inhibitor, daily dose should not exceed 5 mg mg. This drug should not be given to patients with severe hepatic impairment
Tolterodine (Detrol)	Antispasmodic for bladder instability	1 mg bid	Usual dose 2 mg daily. Adult with impaired hepatic or renal function or on concurrent enzyme inhibitors may require dose reduction to 1 mg bid

Continued

Table 14–27 ◉ **Dosage Schedule: Selected Cholinergic Blockers—cont'd**

Drug	Indication	Initial Dose	Maintenance and Maximum Dose
Detrol LA		2–4 mg daily	Usual dose 4 mg daily. Adult with impaired hepatic or renal function or on concurrent enzyme inhibitors may require dose reduction to 2 mg bid
Trihexy phenidyl	Parkinson's disease Drug-induced EPS	1–2 mg/d tablets or elixir. Initial therapy usually not begun with sustained release	Increase in increments of 2 mg at 3- to 5-d intervals until 6–10 mg/d. Postencephalitic patients may require 12–15 mg/d. All doses tolerated better when given in 3 divided doses with meals. Higher doses given in 4 divided doses with meals and at bedtime. After dosage is stabilized, sustained-release forms may be used. Total daily dose is same as other forms but can be given daily at breakfast or in 2 divided doses 12 h apart
Trospium (Sanctura)	For overactive bladder with symptoms of incontinence, urgency and frequency	20 mg bid Take at least 1 h before meals or on an empty stomach	May increase to a total daily dose of 60 mg. In severe renal impairment (CrCl <30 ml/min) dose is 20 mg once daily at bedtime
Sanctura XR		60 mg daily in the morning. Take at least 1 h before morning meal or on an empty stomach	Not recommended for patient with severe renal impairment (CrCl <30 mL/min)

EPS = extrapyramidal symptoms.

therapy. Once patients have been stabilized on regular formulations, they may be switched to sustained release. Sustained-release capsules are administered in a once-daily dose after breakfast or in bid doses 12 hours apart.

When given concurrently with **levodopa**, the usual dose may need to be reduced. Conversely, **trihexyphenidyl** decreases the total bioavailability of **levodopa**. Careful adjustment of the doses of the two drugs is required, depending on adverse reactions and degree of symptom control.

Benztropine is also used for this indication. The dose is 1 to 2 mg/day with a range of 0.5 to 6 mg/day. Therapy is initiated with a 0.5- to 1-mg dose and increased in 0.5-mg increments until optimal benefits are achieved. Postencephalitic patients begin with 2 mg/day in one or more doses, which are increased by 0.5 mg/day until optimal benefits are reached.

The long duration of action of this drug makes it especially suitable for a bedtime medication, and some patients experience greatest relief by taking the entire dose at bedtime. Others do better with divided doses, bid to qid.

Management of Extrapyramidal Symptoms (EPS) Secondary to Drug Therapy

Cholinergic blockers are the drugs of choice for treating akathisia arising from antipsychotic drugs. Both **benztropine** and **trihexyphenidyl** are used for this indication. Size and frequency of dosing are determined empirically within usual dosing recommendations.

The initial dose of **trihexyphenidyl** for this indication is 1 mg in a single dose. If symptoms are not controlled within a few hours, the dose is gradually increased until control is achieved. Daily dosages range from 5 to 15 mg, although symptoms have been controlled on as little as 1 mg/day. An elixir form is available for patients who have difficulty with swallowing tablets. Control can be more rapidly achieved by temporarily reducing the dose of the antipsychotic drug when **trihexyphenidyl** therapy is initiated and then adjusting both drugs until the desired effects are achieved without EPS reactions.

Benztropine therapy is initiated with 1 to 2 mg daily or bid. Dosage titration is in 0.5-mg increments at 5- or 6-day intervals so that the smallest amount required for symptom relief is used. A dose of 1 to 2 mg bid or tid usually provides symptom relief within 1 to 2 days. The maximum dose is 6 mg/day. Older adults and thin patients often cannot tolerate the higher doses. **Benztropine** also comes in an injectable form that can be used for patients with severe dystonic reactions or for those who cannot swallow a pill. The intramuscular dose is 1 to 2 mg, and relief of symptoms is rapid.

For both of these drugs, after several weeks of therapy, the drug may be withdrawn to see if symptoms return and to determine the need for continued therapy. Some patients' symptoms will not return, and some drug-induced EPS reactions do not respond to these two drugs.

Antispasmodic for Bladder Instability and Overactivity

Overactive bladder and urinary incontinence prevalence ranges from 10 to 50 percent in the general population (Parazzini, Lavezzari, & Artibani, 2002). **Darifenacin, fesoterodine, oxybutynin, solifenacin, tolterodine,** and **trospium** treat these disorders by exerting direct antispasmodic effects and inhibiting the muscarinic action of ACh on smooth muscle. **Oxybutynin** exhibits only one-fifth the cholinergic blocking activity of **atropine** but has 4 to 10 times the antispasmodic activity. No cholinergic blocking effects occur at the myoneural junction for any of these drugs. This combination of effects makes them especially useful to treat bladder spasms. Patients with conditions characterized by involuntary bladder contractions experience increased bladder capacity, diminished frequency of urination, and reduced urgency related to voiding. These effects are strongest for patients with uninhibited neurogenic bladder, including children with detrusor overactivity associated with a neurological condition. They are also extremely effective for patients who experience incontinence and are well tolerated in long-term administration (more than 2 years). Because **oxybutynin** increases blood levels and bioavailability of **nitrofurantoin**, a different **antibiotic** should be chosen to treat any concurrent urinary tract infection that may be associated with urinary retention. Assessment for bladder outlet obstruction should be done prior to prescribing because obstruction contraindicates the use of this drug.

For adults, the initial dose of **oxybutynin** is 5 mg bid or tid of the regular formulation or the syrup and 5 to 10 mg daily for the extended-release (XL) formulation (Table 14–28). For frail elderly, the initial dose is 2.5 mg given bid or tid because of a prolongation of the elimination half-life from 2 or 3 hours to 5 hours. Symptom response usually occurs with the first dose but may require up to a week for the full effect. If the desired effects have not occurred in 1 week, the dose is increased. Both the regular and extended-release formulations are similarly effective and tolerable (Diokno et al, 2003). The maximum dose is 20 mg/day for immediate release and 30 mg/day for extended release. For children, the initial dose is 5 mg bid for immediate-release tablets or syrup (for children more than 5 years of age) and 5 mg once daily for extended-release tablets (for children more than 6 years of age), with a maximum dose of 15 mg/day of immediate release and 20 mg/day of extended release. Adverse reactions are more likely with higher doses, and lifestyle modifications should be made concurrently to keep the dose as low as possible. For children and adults who have difficulty swallowing pills, the drug is available in syrup form. There is also a transdermal formuation that is used only in adults. The 3.9-mg system is applied twice weekly.

Table 14–28 ◆ Available Dosage Forms: Selected Cholinergic Blockers

Drug	Dosage Form	How Supplied	Cost
Atropine PO (Canadian drug name: Atropair)	Tablets: 400 mcg	In bottles of 100 tablets	
Benztropine (G) (Cogentin) (B) (Canadian names: Apo-Benztropine; PMS Benztropine)	Tablets: 0.5 mg, 1 mg, 2 mg (Cogentin in 0.5 mg tablets only) Injection: 1 mg/mL	In bottles of 100 tablets and UD 100s Cogentin: In bottles of 100 tablets that are scored In 2-mL ampules	Generic tablets: 0.5 mg and 1 mg = $20/100 2 mg = $26/100
Darifenacin (Enablex) (B)	Tablets, extended release: 7.5 mg	In bottles of 30, 90, and UD 100	$414/90
	15 mg	In bottles of 30, 90 and UD 100	$427/90
Dicyclomine (G), Bentyl (B), Byclomine (B), Di-Spaz (B) (Canadian names: Bentylol, Formulex, Lomine, Protylol)	Tablets: 10 mg	In bottles of 30, 100, 120, 1,000, and UD 100s (G) In bottles of 100, 500, and UD 100 for Bentyl In bottles of 100, 250, 1,000 and UD 100 for Byclomine In bottles of 1,000 for Di-Spaz	
	Tablets: 20 mg	In bottles of 15, 20, 30, 100, 120, 250, 1,000, and UD 100s (G) In bottles of 100, 500, 1,000, and UD 100 for Bentyl In bottles of 100, 250, 1,000, and UD 100 for Byclomine	Generic: 20 mg = $22/100 Bentyl: $73/100

Continued

Table 14–28 ◆ **Available Dosage Forms: Selected Cholinergic Blockers—cont'd**

Drug	Dosage Form	How Supplied	Cost
	Capsules: 10 mg and 20 mg	In bottles of 100 and 1,000 (G)	Generic: 10 mg = $18/100 Bentyl: 10 mg = $48/100
	Syrup: 10 mg/5 mL	In 118-mL, 250-mL, 480-mL bottles (G)	Generic solution = $46/480 mL Bentyl syrup: $54/480 mL
Fesoterodine (Toviaz) (B)	Tablets, extended release: 4 mg	In bottles of 30, 90, and UD 100	$388/90
	8 mg	In bottles of 30, 90, and UD 100	$388/90
Oxybutynin (G), (Ditropan) (B)	Tablets: 5 mg (G) Syrup: 5 mg/5 mL	In bottles of 100, 500, 1,000, blister pack 25 and UD 100s (G) In 480 mL (G) and 300 mL (B)	Ditropan: 5 mg = $105/100 tablets Generic: 5 mg = $23/100 Syrup (G)= $70/ 480 mL
Oxybutynin XL (G) and (Ditropan XL) (B)	XL tablets: 5 mg, 10 mg, 15 mg	In bottles of 100, 500 (G); 100 (B) In bottles of 100 (G) and (B)	Ditropan syrup: $71/300 mL XL (G) 5 mg = $289/100, 10 mg = $292/100, 15 mg = $308/100 Ditropan: 5 mg = $104/100
(Oxytrol) (B) (Gelnique) (B)	Transdermal: 3.9 mg/d Topical gel 10%: In 1 g sachets	In patient calendar boxes of 8 systems In carton of 30 sachets	Transderm = $148/8 patches $130/30 sachets
Propantheline (G) (ProBanthine) (B)	Tablets: 7.5 mg (B)	In bottles of 100 sugar-coated tablets	
(Canadian name: Propanthel)	Tablets: 15 mg	In bottles of 100, 500, 1,000, and UD 100s (G); 100, 500, and UD 100 (B)	Generic: $53/100
Scopolamine	Transderm-Scop: 1.5-mg disk	In 10- and 24-unit blister packs	$18.48/4 patches
Solifenacin (VESIcare) (B)	Tablets: 5 mg	In bottles of 30, 90, and UD 100	$488/90
	10 mg	In bottles of 30, 90, and UD 100	$437/90
Tolterodine (Detrol)	Tablets: 1 mg, 2 mg	In bottles of 60, 500; and unit dose 140s	1 mg = $238/100 2 mg = $253/100
Detrol LA	Capsules (extended release): 2 mg, 4 mg	In bottles of 30, 90, 500 and blister packs of UD 100	2 mg = $360/90 4 mg = $388/90
Trihexy-phenidyl (G) (Artane) (B) (Canadian names: Aparkane, Apo-Trihex)	Tablets: 2 mg, 5 mg Sequels (sustained release) (Artane brand only): 5 mg Elixir: 2 mg/5 mL	In bottles of 30, 100, 250, 1,000, and UD 100s; Artane tablets are scored In bottles of 100, 250 and 1,000 and UD 100 In bottles of 60 sequels In 480-mL bottles, lime-mint flavor	Generic: 2 mg = $26/100 5 mg = $37/100
Trihexy	Tablets: 2 mg and 5 mg	In bottles of 100 and 1,000 tablets	
Trospium (Sanctura) (B)	Tablets: 20 mg	In bottles of 60 and 500 tablets and blister packs of14 tablets	$242/90
(Sanctura XR) (B)	Capsules, extended release: 60 mg	In bottles of 30	$439/90

The remaining drugs are used only in adults and have no dosages for children. **Darifenacin, festerodine,** and **solifenacin** are extended-release formulations and are taken once daily. The initial dose of **darifenacin** is 7.5 mg. If the desired effects do not occur in 2 weeks, the dose can be increased to 15 mg once daily. **Fesoterodine** is started at 4 mg once daily. It may be increased to 8 mg once daily based on patient response and tolerability. **Solifenacin** is initiated at 5 mg once daily with an increase to 10 mg once daily if symptoms require. The initial dose of **trospium** depends on its formulation. The immediate-release formulation dose is 20 mg bid. The extended-release formulation is initiated at 60 mg daily in the morning. Administration with a high-fat meal resulted in reduced absorption, with AUC and Cmax values 70 and 80 percent lower that those obtained while fasting. All doses should be taken at least 1 hour before meals or on an empty stomach.

Renal function is a factor in dosing most of these drugs. The dose should not exceed the initial dose in the case of severe renal impairment (CrCl less than 30 mL/min) for **fesoterodine** and **solifenacine.** No dosage adjustments are recommended in moderate renal impairment. Only the immediate-release formulation of **trospium** can be used in patients with severe renal impairment and the dose must not exceed the initial dose (20 mg).

Hepatic function is a dosing factor in all of these drugs. Doses should not exceed the initial dose for **darifenacin** and **solifenacin** in patients with moderate hepatic impairment. Cautious use in moderate hepatic impairment is recommended for **fesoterodine.** The metabolic pathway for **trospium** has not been fully defined and there is no information regarding the effect of severe hepatic impairment on exposure to this drug. Although caution should be used when administering **trospium** to moderate or severe hepatic impairment, the drug is not contraindicated in this situation. All of these drugs except **trospium** are contraindicated in the presence of severe hepatic impairment. The initial dose of **tolterodine** is 1 mg bid with a usual dose of 2 mg daily for maintenance. Doses of 2 to 4 mg once daily of the extended-release capsules are used with a usual maintenance dose of 4 mg daily. Adults with impaired hepatic or renal function often require the lower dose both initially and for maintenance. Symptom relief is similar to **oxybutynin.**

Prevention of Nausea and Vomiting Associated With Motion Sickness

Scopolamine in a transdermal form is used for this indication. One disk is applied to the clean, dry postauricular skin at least 4 hours before the antiemetic effect is desired. Over a space of 3 days, 0.5 mg is delivered. If therapy is required for more than 3 days, the original disk is removed and replaced with a new one. Only one disk is worn at a time. After application of the disk, the hands are washed with soap and water to prevent any traces of the drug from coming into direct contact with the eyes.

Adjunct Therapy in Management of Irritable Bowel Syndrome and Peptic Ulcer Disease

Atropine is used for both indications. **Dicyclomine** is used for the management of irritable bowel syndrome in patients who do not respond to the usual interventions with sedation and diet. **Propantheline** is indicated for its antisecretory activity in the management of peptic ulcer disease.

The initial adult dose of **atropine** for both indications is 400 mcg every 4 to 6 hours. Doses may be increased, if necessary, to 600 mcg. For children, the dose is 10 mcg/kg every 4 to 6 hours. The dose is not to exceed 400 mcg. Children are especially sensitive to the adverse reactions associated with atropine, and every effort should be made to keep the dose as low as possible.

Symptoms of poisoning in infants and children differ from adult symptoms. They include burning sensations in the mouth, difficulty in swallowing; rash; blurred vision; tachycardia; tachypnea; fever up to 109.8°F; muscle incoordination; and eventually seizure, respiratory paralysis, and death. The antidote for **atropine** poisoning is **physostigmine.**

The only oral dose of **dicyclomine** shown to be effective is 160 mg/day in four equally divided doses. However, because of adverse effects, the initial dose is 80 mg/day in four equally divided doses. The dose is then increased if tolerated. For patients who have difficulty with swallowing, a syrup form is available with the same dosage range. A formulation for IM administration is also available. The dose is 80 mg/day in four equally divided doses.

The oral dose of **propantheline** for adults is 15 mg 30 minutes before meals and 30 mg at bedtime. For patients with mild manifestations, older adults, and patients of small stature, the dose is 7.5 mg tid. The safety and efficacy of this drug for treating peptic ulcer in children have not been established. There is a dosage schedule published for antisecretory and antispasmodic use in children, but it is an unlabeled use. The dose for children is 1.5 mg/kg a day in three or four divided doses for antisecretory indications and 2 to 3 mg/kg a day in four to six divided doses given every 4 to 6 hours for antispasmodic indications.

Other Uses

Both **atropine** and **scopolamine** are used as part of preoperative medication to reduce secretions and facilitate induction of anesthesia. **Atropine** is also used in acute care to treat bradyarrhythmias and anticholinesterase poisoning. These indications are not commonly part of primary care and are not discussed here.

Rational Drug Selection

Aside from clinical indications, there are few parameters that assist in deciding which is the best drug to choose. Some are associated with slightly fewer adverse reactions, but all have several reactions that cause patients not to adhere to treatment regimens.

Cost

Each indication has a limited number of drugs to choose from, and their costs often vary significantly. Generic drugs are, as usual, less expensive than brand names, and oral forms are less expensive than injectables. In the case of **trihexyphenidyl (Artane)** and **benzotropine (Cogentin)**, however, only the brand-name tablets are scored to enable titrating doses more closely. According to the cost index in *Drug Facts and Comparisons* (2009), **atropine** tablets produced by Lilly Pharmaceutical are significantly less expensive than other brands. This source also lists **benztropine** as less expensive than **trihexyphenidyl**.

The older drugs used to treat overactive bladder are less expensive than the newer ones: **oxybutinin** (5-mg generic tablets cost $23 for 100 tablets) is less expensive than **tolterodine** (1-mg immediate-release brand-name tablets cost $238 for 100 tablets). The extended-release formulation of **tolterodine** costs about $360 for 90 tablets, which is nearly the same as the cost of the extended-release formulations of the newer drugs. The newer drugs vary from $242 for 90 tablets for the immediate-release formulation of **trospium**, to $388 **(fesoterodine)** to $488 **(solifenacin)** for 90 tablets for the extended-release formulations.

Formulation

In addition to these cost data, formulation can be an issue when speed is a major concern (e.g., severe dystonic symptoms in a patient who is taking an antipsychotic) or when the patient has difficulty in swallowing for any of a variety of reasons, including the progression of a disease process itself. Several drugs come in injectable or syrup forms. **Oxybutynin** has a transdermal formulation that may also address this issue. Extended-release formulations may improve adherence by simplifying the treatment regimen.

Monitoring

No specific monitoring parameters are required for **cholinergic blockers** beyond monitoring for adverse reactions and the monitoring parameters that are appropriate for the disease being treated.

Patient Education

Administration

Instruct the patient to take the drugs exactly as prescribed. If a dose is missed, take it as soon as remembered unless it is almost time for the next dose. Do not double doses. **Benztropine** is administered with food or immediately after meals to minimize gastric irritation. The tablet may be crushed and administered with food if the patient has difficulty in swallowing. **Atropine, dicyclomine**, and **propantheline** are administered 30 to 60 minutes before a meal; **oxybutynin** is administered on an empty stomach (may be given with food to minimize GI irritation); and **trihexyphenidyl** is administered after a meal (may be given before a meal for patients with dry mouth or with the meal if GI distress occurs). Extended-release formulations must be swallowed whole and not crushed or chewed. Calibrated measuring instruments such as medicine cups or syringes should be used with liquid formulations to make certain the dose is accurate.

The **scopolamine disk** has specific instructions for its application. The disk is applied to clean, dry skin behind the ear at least 4 hours before the antiemetic effect is desired. It is left in place for up to 3 days. Only one disk at a time is worn. If longer effects are required, the disk is removed and replaced. Hands are washed with soap and water after application to make sure no trace of the drug comes in contact with the eyes. The same procedure is followed when removing the disk.

Adverse Reactions

Cholinergic blockers have many adverse reactions because their actions are not organ specific. Cardiovascular reactions include tachycardia. Teach patients to take their own pulses and report heart rates above 100 bpm. Dosage adjustments may be required. This adverse effect is especially problematic for patients who concurrently have coronary artery disease and for older adults.

Cholinergic blockers tend to thicken and dry respiratory secretion. Advise the patients to drink at least 2 quarts of noncaffeinated fluid daily to maintain adequate hydration.

Fluid and fiber intake are also important because these drugs may cause constipation and difficulty in voiding. Dry mouth can be relieved by practicing good oral hygiene, consuming cold drinks, sucking on hard candy, or chewing sugarless gum.

The therapeutic goal for many of these drugs is to reduce gastric secretion. Substances that increase gastric acid secretion such as **alcohol, tobacco, caffeine,** and **aspirin** should be avoided.

Activities that require visual acuity, mental alertness, and vigorous activity in warm weather can create problems. **Cholinergic blockers** may result in blurred vision, photophobia, and dizziness, and they reduce the sweating necessary to cool the body during exercise.

Lifestyle Management

Several of the disease processes for which these drugs are prescribed require lifestyle modifications. Incontinence can also be treated with a variety of therapies besides drugs. Bladder retraining, Kegel exercises, biofeedback, and other nonpharmacological therapies should also be used in treating many of these disorders.

REFERENCES

American Association of Clinical Endocrinologists (AACE). (2006). American Association of Clinical Endocrinologists medical guidelines for clinical practice for the diagnosis and treatment of hypertension. *Endocrinology Practice, 12*(2), 193–222.

Armstrong, S., & Schumann, L. (2003). Myasthenia gravis: Diagnosis and treatment. *Journal of the American Academy of Nurse Practitioners, 15*(2), 72–78.

Dickstein, K., Cohen Solai, A., Filippatos, G., McMurray, J., Ponikowski, P., Poole-Wilson, P., et al, and ESC Committee for Practic Guidelines. (2008). ESC guidelines for the diagnosis and treatment of acute and chronic heart failure 2008: The task force. *European Heart Journal, 29*(19), 2388–2442.

Diokno, A., Appell, R., Sand, P., Dmochowski, R., Gburek, B., Klimberg, I., Kell, S., and the OPERA Study Group.. (2003). Prospective, randomized, double-blind study of the efficacy and tolerability of the extended-release formulations of oxybutynin and tolterodine for overactive bladder: Results of the OPERA trial. *Mayo Clinic Proceedings, 78,* 687–695.

Food and Drug Administration. (2009). Pediatric exclusivity labeling changes. Retrieved June 22, 2009, from http://www.fda.gov/Drugs/DevelopmentApproval Process/DevelopmentResources

Gibbons, R., Abrams, J., Chatterjee, K., Daley, J., Deedwania, P., Douglas, J., et al. (2003). ACC/AHA 2002 guideline update for the management of patients with chronic stable angina–summary article: A report of the American College of Cardiology/American Heart Association Task Force on Practice Guidelines. *Journal of the American College of Cardiology, 41,* 159–168.

Hunt, S., Abraham, W., Chin, M., Feldman, A., Francis, G., Ganiats, T., et al. (2005). ACC/AHA 2005 guideline update for the diagnosis and management of chronic heart failure in the adults: A report of the American College of Cardiology/American Heart Association Task Force on Practice Guidelines. American College of Cardiology Foundation: Bethesda (MD). 82 p.

Institute for Clinical Systems Improvement (ICSI). (2008). Hypertension diagnosis and treatment. Institute for Clinical Systems Improvement: Bloomington (MN). 59 p. Retrieved on June 16, 2009, from http://www.guideline.gov/summary/aspx

Lai, M., Lai, O., Keene, J., Esiri, M., Francis, P., Hope, T., and Chen, P. (2001). Psychosis of Alzheimer's disease is associated with elevated muscarinic M2 binding in the cortex. *Neurology, 57*(5), 805–811.

Minger, S., Esiri, M., McDonald, B., Keener, J., Carter, J., Hope, T., and Francis, P. (2000). Cholinergic deficits contribute to behavioral disturbance in patients with dementia. *Neurology, 55*(10), 1460–1467.

National High Blood Pressure Education Program (NHBPEP). (2003). *The seventh report of the Joint National Committee on Prevention, Detection, Evaluation, and Treatment of High Blood Pressure.* Rockville, MD: National Institutes of Health, National Heart, Lung, and Blood Institute.

Nhi-Ha, T., Hobllyn, J., Mohanty, S., & Yaffe, K. (2003). Efficacy of cholinesterast inhibitors in the treatment of neuropsychiatric symptoms and functional impairment in Alzheimer's disease. *Journal of the American Medical Association, 289*(2), 210–216.

Packer, M., Coasts, A., Fowler, M., Katus, H., Krum, H., Mohacsi, P., et al. (2001). Effect of carvedilol on survival in severe heart chronic heart failure. *New England Journal of Medicine, 344,* 16.

Parazzini, F., Lavezzari, M., & Artibani, W.; on behalf of the Gruppo Interdisciplinare di Studio Incontinenza Urinaria. (2002). Prevalence of overactive bladder and urinary incontinence. *Journal of Family Practice, 51,* 1072–1075.

Pratt, R. (2002). Patient populations in clinical trials of the efficacy and tolerability of donepezil in patients with vascular dementia. *Journal of Neurological Science, 203–204,* 57–65.

Salloway, S., Pratt, R., & Perdomo, C. (2003, April). A comparison of the cognitive benefit of donepezil in patients with cortical versus subcortical vascular dementia: A subanalysis of two 24-week, randomized, double-blind, placebo-controlled trials. Oral presentation of abstract at the annual meeting of the American Academy of Neurology, Honolulu, Hawaii.

Winblad, B., Engedal, K., Soininen, H., Verhey, G., Waldemar, A., Wimo, A., et al. (2001). A one-year, randomized, placebo-controlled study of donepezil in patients with mild to moderate AD. *Neurology, 57*(3), 489–495.

Wolters Kluwer Health. (2009). *Drug facts and comparisons.* St. Louis: Wolters Kluwer Health.

Wright, J., Probstfield, J., Cushman, W., Pressel, S., Cutler, J., Davis, B., et al, for the ALLHAT Collaborative Research Group. (2009). ALLHAT findings revisited in the context of subsequent analyses, other trials and meta-analyses. *Archives of Internal Medicine, 169*(9), 832–842.

CHAPTER 15

DRUGS AFFECTING THE CENTRAL NERVOUS SYSTEM

Margaret Scharf

Chapter Outline

This chapter addresses drugs that affect the central nervous system in two broad ways: to treat psychiatric conditions and to treat other neurological conditions. Traditionally, drugs to treat psychiatric conditions were developed serendipitously and identified with the psychiatric diagnosis associated with the responsiveness. As the neurophysiology of psychiatric symptoms has been researched more deliberately, it has become clear that drugs affect specific neuroreceptors and neurotransmitters in different parts of the brain to bring about a response. The response is not limited to a psychiatric diagnosis because the diagnoses are based not on neurophysiology but on behavioral presentations. Therefore, this chapter will try to bridge the traditional reference to drugs based on diagnoses (e.g., antidepressants) and on their pharmacological mechanism of action (e.g., serotonin reuptake inhibitors). Similarly, because some drugs that originally were used to treat a nonpsychiatric neurological condition have since been found to be useful in treating psychiatric conditions with similar neuropathological mechanisms (e.g., anticonvulsants used to treat mood lability), these drugs may be discussed in more than one section. This is because the brain functions in a very complex fashion but also has neurological redundancy, permitting efficiency in responsiveness.

This chapter focuses on drugs that affect the central nervous system. In addition, Chapter 29 focuses on drugs to treat anxiety and depressive disorders in greater depth. Some redundancy is necessary.

ANOREXIANTS

Anorexiants are short-term adjuncts to calorie-limiting, cognitive-behavioral weight loss programs for severely obese individuals. The anorexiants commonly in use today are nonamphetamine appetite suppressants that are chemically and pharmacologically related to amphetamines. These drugs include **phentermine (Adipex-P, Banobase, Fastin, Ionamin, Obenix, Oby-Cap, Phentercot, Phentride, T-Diet, Teramine, Zantryl)**, **benzphetamine (Didrex)**, **diethylpropion HCL (Tenuate)**, **phendimetrazine tartrate (Bontril, Prelu-2, Plegine, Rexigen Forte, X-Trazine)**, and **sibutramine (Meridia)**. Two formerly used drugs, **fenfluramine (Pondimin)** and **dexfenfluramine (Redux)**, were removed from the market by the U.S. Food and Drug Administration (FDA) in 1997 because of potentially fatal cardiac and pulmonary adverse reactions. In October 2010 the FDA asked that the manufacture voluntarily withdraw **sibutramine** from the U.S. market due to cardiovascular side effects.

Pharmacodynamics

Anorexiants are sympathomimetic amines and are thought to exert their action by stimulation of satiety centers in the hypothalamus and limbic region. They act through noradrenergic, dopaminergic, or serotonergic pathways.

Pharmacokinetics

Absorption and Distribution

After oral administration, **anorexiants** are absorbed in the stomach and small intestine, depending on whether they are in regular or extended-release form. They are lipid soluble, widely distributed, and cross the blood–brain barrier. **Diethylpropion** and its metabolites cross the placental barrier and are Pregnancy Category C.

Metabolism and Excretion

Anorexiants are metabolized in the liver and excreted through the kidneys. Duration of action is 4 to 6 hours in the regular form and longer in extended-release forms. Half-lives vary from 8 to 20 hours.

Table 15–1 presents the pharmacokinetics of anorexiants.

Pharmacotherapeutics

Precautions and Contraindications

Anorexiants carry a high risk of tolerance and dependence, both physical and psychological, and use in patients with known histories of **alcohol** or drug dependence should be cautious because of the high risk of cross-tolerance. Actively drinking alcoholics taking **anorexiants** have experienced depression, paranoia, and psychosis. Use of **anorexiants** should be limited to a maximum period of 6 months and discontinued at any sign of tolerance. **Anorexiant** use is contraindicated in patients who abuse substances such as cocaine, phencyclidine, and methamphetamine because of the potential for excessive adrenergic stimulation. Patients with diabetes may experience altered **insulin** or oral hypoglycemic dosage requirements.

Adverse Drug Reactions

Adverse reactions to **anorexiants** include central nervous system (CNS) overstimulation and agitation, confusion, insomnia, dizziness, hypertension, headache, palpitations and arrhythmias, dry mouth, mydriasis, dysuria, constipation, vomiting, diarrhea, and impotence. Patients taking high doses of **anorexiants** over a long period may experience

Table 15–1 ▶ **Pharmacokinetics: Anorexiants**

Drug	Onset	Peak	Duration	Half-Life	Excretion
Phendimetrazine tartrate	—	—	4–6 h	1.9–9.8 h	Urine
Benzphetamine	—	—	4–6 h	—	Urine
Diethylpropion HCI	—	—	4–6 h	—	Urine
Phentermine	—	—	4–6 h	—	Urine
Sibutramine	—	3–4 h	—	1.1 h	Urine

dizziness, fatigue, and depression if the drug is suddenly withdrawn.

Drug Interactions

The potential for hypertensive crisis with coadministration of **anorexiants** and **MAO inhibitors** exists. **Anorexiants** may elevate serotonin levels and should not be prescribed to patients on other **serotonergic agents** because of the increased risk of serotonin syndrome (hyperthermia, agitation, restlessness, confusion, ataxia, myoclonus, tremor, rigidity, tachycardia, hypotension or hypertension, diaphoresis). The actions of **adrenergic blockers, insulin, sulfonylureas,** and **phenothiazines** may be antagonized during concomitant administration of **anorexiants.** Table 15–2 presents drug interactions.

Clinical Use and Dosing

Anorexiants are indicated for the treatment of morbid exogenous obesity in conjunction with a calorie-restrictive diet. The course of treatment should last no longer than 6 months. An alternative method of dosing is to use the drug for a few weeks followed by no drug for a period, suggested to be half the length of time with the drug, followed by reinstitution of the drug for a few more weeks. Evening dosing should be avoided because of the likelihood of insomnia. Table 15–3 presents the dosage schedule and available dosage forms for **anorexiants.**

Rational Drug Selection

Significant increases in blood pressure, palpitations, and arrhythmias can occur with **phentermine;** thus, use is not advisable in hypertensive clients or those with cardiovascular disease. **Diethylpropion** causes less insomnia than does **phentermine. Diethylpropion** is considered one of the safest noradrenergic appetite suppressants and may be used in patients with mild to moderate hypertension or angina pectoris.

Table 15–2 ■ **Drug Interactions: Anorexiants**

Drug	Interacting Drug	Possible Effect	Implications
All anorexiants	MAOIs	Hypertensive crisis	Do not prescribe during or within 14 d of use of MAOI
	Alcohol	CNS depression	Abstain from alcohol use
	Phenothiazines	Psychosis	Monitor for increased psychotic symptoms
	Insulin, sulfonylureas	Altered requirements	Monitor blood glucose
	Guanethidine	Antagonization of effect	Monitor for increased blood pressure
	Furazolidone	Serotonin syndrome	Monitor for symptoms of syndrome

Table 15–3 ● **Dosage Schedule: Anorexiants**

Drug	Indications	Dosage	Available Dosage Forms
Benzphetamine (Didrex)	Short-term adjunctive treatment of exogenous obesity	25–50 mg daily; max 50 mg tid Not approved for children	Tablets: 50 mg, scored tablets
Diethylpropion (Tenuate, Tenuate Dospan)	Short-term adjunctive treatment of exogenous obesity	25 mg tid ac* or prn if needed; sustained-release: 75 mg q a.m.	Tablets: 25 mg Sustained-release: 75 mg
Phendimetrazine tartrate (Bontril PDM, Prelu-2)	Short-term adjunctive treatment of exogenous obesity	35 mg bid or tid 1 h ac; sustained-release: 105 mg daily 30–60 min before breakfast *Not for children*	Tablets: 35 mg Capsules: 35 mg Sustained-release: 105 mg
Phentermine (Zantryl, Adipex-P, Ionamin)	Short-term adjunctive treatment of exogenous obesity	*Adults*: 8 mg tid, 30 minutes ac or 15–37.5 mg daily before breakfast or 10–14 h before bedtime	Tablets: 8 mg, 30 mg, 37.5 mg Capsules: 15 mg, 30 mg, 37.5 mg
Sibutramine HCL (Meridia)	Short-term adjunctive treatment of exogenous obesity	10 mg daily to 15 mg daily max (after 4 weeks) *(use for age 16 and up)*	Capsules: 5, 10, 15 mg Note: sibutramine was withdrawn from the market in October 2010.

*ac = *ante cibum* (before meals).

ANTICONVULSANTS

Seizures are the result of the abnormal discharge of neurons. Anything that disrupts the stability of the neuron may trigger abnormal activity and seizures. Many factors can precipitate seizures including hyperventilation, sleep deprivation, sensory stimuli, emotional stress, and hormonal changes. Some drugs with anticonvulsant properties are increasingly being used in the treatment of mood disorders and will be discussed in that section of this chapter (e.g., **valproates, gabapentin, lamotrigine**). **Phenobarbital**, used to treat seizure disorders, will be discussed with **sedative-hypnotics** later in this chapter. **Benzodiazepines**, also used to treat seizures, will be discussed with **anxiolytic drugs**. Three major classes of anticonvulsant drugs, the **hydantoins, iminostilbenes**, and **succinimides**, are discussed here.

Hydantoins

The **hydantoins, phenytoin** (Dilantin), **ethotoin** (Peganone), and **fosphenytoin** (Cerebyx), are the first-line treatment of choice for tonic-clonic and partial complex seizures and the least sedating drugs used to treat seizure disorders of any type. **Phenytoin** is the most commonly used.

Pharmacodynamics

Hydantoins inhibit and stabilize electrical discharges in the motor cortex of the brain by affecting ion exchanges during depolarization and repolarization, thus limiting seizure propagation. They also affect the brainstem's contribution to grand mal seizures and have antiarrhymic properties.

Pharmacokinetics

Absorption and Distribution

The usual route of administration is oral. Absorption occurs in the small intestine and is slow, although the rate varies with the form of the drug. **Hydantoins** enter the brain quickly, and are then redistributed to other body tissues including saliva and breast milk. The rate and degree of absorption from intramuscular (IM) administration is erratic, generally resulting in lower plasma levels than the oral route. **Hydantoins** are 87 to 93 percent protein bound. The therapeutic plasma level range is 10 to 20 mcg/mL and correlates well with treatment effect.

Metabolism and Excretion

Metabolism of **hydantoins** takes place in the liver; excretion, via the kidneys. Plasma half-lives range from 6 to 24 hours.

Table 15–4 presents the pharmacokinetics of hydantoins.

Pharmacotherapeutics

Precautions and Contraindications

Hydantoins are contraindicated in hypersensitivity. **Phenytoin**-induced hepatitis is a common hypersensitivity reaction. Other hypersensitivity reactions include fever,

Table 15–4 ▶ **Pharmacokinetics: Antiepileptic Drugs**

Drug	Onset	Peak	Duration	Half-Life	Excretion
Hydantions					
Ethotoin (Peganone)	—	—	—	3–9 h	Urine
Fosphenytoin (Cerebyx)	—	—	—	12–29 h	Urine
Phenytoin (Dilantin)	slow	4–12 h (extended) 1.5–3 h (rapid)	5 h	22 h	Urine
Iminostilbenes					
Carbamazepine		4 to 8 h Chronic use: 1.5 h		25 to 65 h Multiple dosing *Children:* 8 to 14 h *Adults:* 12–17h	Urine
Oxcarbazepine		4.5 h		2 hr Metabolite 9 h	Urine
Succinimides					
Ethosuximide		2 to 4 h		Children 30h *Adults:* 50-60h	Urine Small amounts in feces
Methsuximide	Rapid	1 to 4h		2.6 to 4h	Urine

Table 15–4 ▶ **Pharmacokinetics: Antiepileptic Drugs—cont'd**

Drug	Onset	Peak	Duration	Half-Life	Excretion
Drugs That Affect GABA					
Gabapentin	—	2 to 2.5 h		*Adults:*: 2.5 to 3.5 hrs Children 9 mo to 12 y: 2.4 h Neonates: 2.4 h	80% to 90% excreted unchanged in urine
Tiagabine	Rapid Food slows absorption	45 min		7 to 9 h Patients on enzyme-inducing AEDs: 2 to 5 h	Urine 25% Feces 63%
Topiramate	Rapid	2 h		Urine	
Levetiracetam	Rapid			6 to 8 h	Renal
Lamotrigine		1.7–2.2		25.4 to 35.8h	Renal

rash, arthralgias, and lymphadenopathy. **Phenytoin** may cause insulin demands to be altered, and death has resulted from too-rapid IV administration. **Phenytoin** is contraindicated in sinus bradycardia, sinoatrial block, second- and third-degree atrioventricular block, and Stokes-Adams syndrome. It should be used cautiously in patients with hepatic or renal disease. **Ethotoin** is contraindicated in the presence of hepatic or hematological disorders.

Although fetal defects have been associated with use of **hydantoins** during pregnancy and it is classified as Pregnancy Category D, the majority of fetuses exposed in utero have been born defect free. Pregnant women who take **phenytoin** can decrease the risks to the fetus by taking **folic acid** 400 international units (IU) per day. Some women with epilepsy have fewer seizures during pregnancy; in others, the risks to the woman who goes without the drug may outweigh any risks to the fetus. **Hydantoins** are present in breast milk; their safety during lactation has not been established.

Rebound status epilepticus may result from abrupt discontinuation of these drugs. **Phenytoin** has a narrow therapeutic range and older adults or those with impaired liver function may manifest signs of toxicity at lower-than-usual doses. Use cautiously in patients with myocardial insufficiency and hypotension.

Adverse Drug Reactions

Possible adverse effects are multiple and may include CNS effects such as agitation, ataxia, confusion, dizziness, drowsiness, headache, and nystagmus; cardiovascular effects such as hypotension and tachycardia; gastrointestinal effects such as nausea, vomiting, anorexia, altered taste, constipation, dry mouth, and gingival hyperplasia; and genitourinary effects such as urinary retention and reddish-brown discoloration of the urine. Other possible adverse effects include skin rashes, hyperglycemia, tinnitus, gynecomastia, coarsening of facial features and enlargement of the lips, hematopoietic changes, photophobia, and polyarthropathy.

Drug Interactions

Drug interactions consist of those that either increase or decrease the effect of the **hydantoin** and those that decrease the effect of the other drug. Interactions that increase **hydantoin's** effect because of increased metabolism, competition for binding sites, or for unknown reasons occur with **benzodiazepines, cimetidine, disulfiram,** acute **ethanol** use, **tricyclic antidepressants, salicylates,** and **valproic acid.** Conversely, interactions that decrease **hydantoin's** effect include **barbiturates,** chronic **ethanol** use, **rifampin, theophylline, influenza vaccine, pyridoxine,** and **antacids.**

Concurrent administration causes the decreased effect of **carbamazepine, estrogens, corticosteroids, haloperidol, methadone, levodopa, sulfonylureas, oral contraceptives,** and **cardiac glycosides.**

Table 15–5 presents drug interactions.

Clinical Use and Dosing

Table 15–6A presents the indications and dosage schedules of **hydantoins** and Table 15–6B presents the available dosage forms and approximate costs for **hydantoins.**

Rational Drug Selection

Hydantoins are used for the treatment of grand mal and psychomotor seizures. **Phenytoin,** however, may worsen absence seizures. **Hydantoins** are not the first-line treatment of status epilepticus, but IV **phenytoin** can be used for the control of grand mal types of seizures. **Fosphenytoin** is used for short-term (less than 5 days) management of seizures when oral use is not feasible.

Table 15–5 ■ **Drug Interactions: Hydantoins (Anticonvulsants)**

Drug	Interacting Drug	Possible Effect	Implications
All hydantoins	Allopurinol, cimetidine, diazepam, disulfiram, alcohol (acute intake), phenacemide, succinimides, valproic acid	Increased plasma level of hydantoins	May need to decrease hydantoin dose; monitor plasma level
	Barbiturates, carbamazepine, alcohol (chronic use), theophylline, antacids, calcium	Decreased plasma level of hydantoins	May need to increase hydantoin dose; monitor plasma level
	Corticosteroids, dicumarol, digitoxin, doxycycline, haloperidol, methadone, oral contraceptives, dopamine, furosemide, levodopa	Decreased effect of interacting drug	Monitor plasma levels where possible; monitor signs and symptoms
Iminostilbenes			
Carbamazepine	CYP 3A4 inhibitors: cimetidine, danazol, diltiazem, macrolides, erythromycin, troleandomycin, clarithromycin, fluoxetine, fluvoxamine, nefazodone, trazodone, loxapine, olanzapine, quetiapine, loratadine, terfenadine, omeprazole, oxybutynin, dantrolene, isoniazid, niacinamide, nicotinamide, ibuprofen, propoxyphene, azoles (e.g., ketaconazole, itraconazole, fluconazole, voriconazole), acetazolamide, verapamil, ticlopidine, grapefruit juice, protease inhibitors, valproate	CYP 3A4 inhibitors inhibit carbamazepine metabolism and can thus increase plasma carbamazepine levels	
	CYP 3A4 inducers: cisplatin, doxorubicin HCl, felbamate†, fosphenytoin, rifampin, phenobarbital, phenytoin, primidone, methsuximide, theophylline, aminophylline	CYP 3A4 inducers can increase the rate of carbamazepine metabolism leading to decreased plasma carbamazepine levels	
Oxcarbazepine	Carbamazepine, phenobarbital, phenytoin, valproic acid	Decreased oxcarbazepine levels	
Succinimides			
Ethosuximide	Phenytoin Valproic acid	Elevated phenytoin levels Increased or decreased ethosuximide levels	
Methsuximide	Carbamazepine, hydantoins (e.g., phenytoin), Lamotrigine Phenobarbital, primidone	Methsuximide plasma concentrations may be reduced Plasma concentrations of the active metabolite of primidone, phenobarbital, may be elevated by methsuximide	
Drugs That Affect GABA			
Gabapentin	No significant drug interaction		
Tiagabine	Bupropion, gemfibrozil Enzyme-inducing antiepileptic drugs (e.g., carbamazepine, phenobarbital, phenytoin, primidone)	Tiagabine plasma concentrations may be increased Tiagabine clearance may be increased	

Table 15–5 ■ **Drug Interactions: Hydantoins (Anticonvulsants)—cont'd**

Drug	Interacting Drug	Possible Effect	Implications
Topiramate	Phenytoin Carbamazepine	Decreased plasma concentrations of Topiramate	
	Ethinyl estradiol	Decreased ethinyl estradiol levels	
	Carbonic anhydrase inhibitors (e.g., zonisamide, acetazolamide or dichlorphenamide)	May increase the severity of metabolic acidosis and may also increase the risk of kidney stone formation	If Topiramate is given concomitantly with another carbonic anhydrase inhibitor, the patient should be monitored for the appearance or worsening of metabolic acidosis
Levetiracetam	No significant drug interactions		
Lamotrigine	Estrogen-containing oral contraceptive preparations containing 30 mcg ethinylestradiol and	Decreased lamotragine levels	Decreased Lamotrigine levels approximately 50%.
	150 mcg levonorgestrel,	Decreased levonorgesterel levels	Decrease in levonorgestrel component by 19%.
	Carbamazepine, Phenobarbital/Primidone, Phenytoin, Rifampin	Decreased lamotragine levels	Decreased Lamotrigine concentration approximately 40%
	Valproate	Increased lamotragine levels	Increased Lamotrigine concentrations slightly more than 2-fold

Table 15–6A ◉ **Dosage Schedule: Selected Anticonvulsants**

Drug	Indications	Dosage
Ethotoin	Generalized tonic-clonic or psychomotor seizures	*Adults:* initially 1 g/d or less in 4–6 divided doses, spaced as evenly as possible, taken after food; increase gradually to usual maintenance dose of 2–3 g/d
		Children: initial maximum dose of 750 mg/d in divided doses as with adult; usual maintenance dose of 500–1,000 mg/d
Fosphenytoin	Status epilepticus	IV loading dose: 15–20 mg PE/kg diluted in 5% dextrose or 0.9% saline solution at rate of 100–150 mg PE/min (PE: phenytoin sodium equivalent units)
		Other measures such as IV diazepam will be needed
		Nonemergent loading dose and maintenance: loading dose 10–20 mg PE/kg IV or IM; maintenance 4–6 mg PE/kg/d at rate of 150 mg PE/min or less
		Children: usual range 100–400 mg/d
Phenytoin	Generalized tonic-clonic, psychomotor, and simple partial seizures; status epilepticus	*Adults:* initial PO dose 1 g in 3 divided doses, then after 24 h, 300 mg/d in 1 dose (extended-release); IV loading dose of 10–15 mg/kg at rate of 50 mg/min; maintenance dose of 100 mg PO or IV every 6–8 h
		Children: 4–8 mg/kg/d PO in divided doses; 15–20 mg/kg IV at rate of 50 mg/min
Drugs That Affect GABA		
Gabapentin	Epilepsy	*Adults and children > 12 yrs:* The starting dose is 300 mg tid. The dose may be increased using 300 or 400 mg capsules, or 600 or 800 mg tablets tid up to 1,800 mg/day. Dosages up to 2,400 mg/day have been well tolerated in long-term clinical studies. The maximum time between doses in the TID schedule should not exceed 12 hours.

Continued

Table 15–6A ◉ **Dosage Schedule: Selected Anticonvulsants—cont'd**

Drug	Indications	Dosage
		Children 3–12 years: The starting dose should range from 10-15 mg/kg/day in 3 divided doses, and the effective dose reached by upward titration over a period of approximately 3 days. The effective dose of gabapentin in patients 5 years of age and older is 25–35 mg/kg/day and given in divided doses (tid). The effective dose in pediatric patients ages 3 and 4 years is 40 mg/kg/day and given in divided doses (tid). Dosages up to 50 mg/kg/day have been well-tolerated in a long-term clinical study. The maximum time interval between doses should not exceed 12 hours.
	Postherpetic Neuralgia	*Adults:* Therapy is initiated as a single 300-mg dose on Day 1,600 mg/day on Day 2 (divided BID), and 900 mg/day on Day 3 (divided TID). The dose can subsequently be titrated up as needed for pain relief to a daily dose of 1,800 mg (divided TID).
Tiagabine	Adjunctive therapy in adults and children 12 years and older in the treatment of partial seizures	*Enzyme-induced adults and adolescent > 12 yrs:* Week 1: 4 mg q day Week 2: Increase dose by 4 mg/d, to 8 mg divided bid Week 3: increase dose by 4 mg/d, to 12 mg/d divided tid Week 4: increase dose by 4 mg/day to 16 mg/day divided bid or qid Week 5: increase dose by 4 to 8 mg/day, to 20 to 24 mg/day divided bid or qid Week 6: increase dose 4 mg/d, to 24 to 32 mg/d divided bid or qid Usual adult maintenance dose in induced patients: 32 to 56 mg/day divided bid or qid
Topiramate	Monotherapy for Epilepsy	*Adults and children ≥ 10 years:* Week 1: 25 mg bid Week 2: 50 mg bid Week 3: 75 mg bid Week 4: 100 mg bid Week 5: 150 mg bid Week 6: 200 mg bid
	Adjunctive Therapy for Epilepsy, partial seizures, Lennox-Gastaut Syndrome	*Adults age ≥ 17 yrs:* Initial dose: 25 to 50 mg/day, titrate dose in 25 to 50 mg/day increments in weekly intervals to a dose of 200 to 400 mg/day *Pediatric Patients (age 1 to 16 yrs):* Initial dose of 1 to 3 mg/kg/day (max 25 mg) for a week. Dosage is increased by 1 to 3 mg/kg/day in 1 to 2 week intervals. The dose is divided in bid dosing. The total recommended daily dose is 5 to 9 mg/kg/day. Dose titration is guided by clinical response.
	Migraine prophylaxis	Week 1: 25 mg in PM Week 2 25 mg bid Week 3: 25 mg in AM, 50 mg in PM Week 4: 50 mg bid The recommended dosage for migraine prophylaxis is 100 mg/day.
Levetiracetam	Partial onset seizures	*Adults and adolescents ≥ 16 yrs*: Initial dose 500 mg bid. Increase dose in increments of 1,000 mg/day every 2 weeks until to a maximum of 3,000 mg/day divided bid. *Children 4 yrs to < 16 yrs:* Initial dose 20 mg/kg in 2 divided doses (10 mg/kg bid). Increase dose every 2 weeks by 20 mg/kg to the recommended daily dose of 60 mg/kg/day.
	Myoclonic Seizures in Patients ≥12 yr With Juvenile Myoclonic Epilepsy	Initial dose of 1,000 mg/dau (500 mg bid). Increase dose by 1,000 mg/day every 2 weeks to the recommended dose of 3,000 mg/day.
	Primary generalized tonic-clonic seizures	*Adults > 16 yr:* Initial dose 1,000 mg/day divided bid (500 mg bid). Increase dose 1,000 mg/day every 2 weeks to the recommended dose of 3,000 mg/day.

Table 15–6A ◉ **Dosage Schedule: Selected Anticonvulsants—cont'd**

Drug	Indications	Dosage
		Pediatric patients age 6 yr to < 16 yr: Initial dose 20 mg/kg/day divided bid (10 mg/kg bid). Increase dose 20 mg/kg/day every 2 weeks to the recommended daily dose of 60 mg/kg/day divided bid.
Lamotrigine	Epilepsy therapy in patients not taking enzyme-inducing AEDs	*Adults and children ≥12 yr:* Week 1 and 2: 25 mg/day Weeks 3 and 4: 50 mg per day Week 5: 100 mg/day Increase dose by 50 mg per day every 1 to 2 weeks until the usual maintenance dose of 225 mg to 375 mg per day in two divided doses. *Children 2 yr to 12 yr:* Weeks 1 and 2: 0.3 mg/kg per day in one or two divided doses. The dosage should be rounded down to the nearest whole tablet and tablets should not be cut. Weeks 3 and 4: 0.6 mg/kg per day in two divided doses rounded down to the nearest whole tablet. Starting in week 5 the dose is increased every 1 to 2 weeks by calculating 0.6 mg/kg/day, round this amount down to the nearest whole tablet and add this amount to the previously administered daily dose. The dose is titrated to to effect, with an average daily dose of 4.5 to 7.5 mg/kg per day. Maintenance dose may need to be increased by as much as 50 percent in children who weigh less than 30 kg.
	Patients Taking Enzyme-Inducing AEDs (not valproate)	*Adults and children ≥ 12 years:* Weeks 1 and 2: 50 mg per day. Weeks 3 and 4: 100 mg per day in 2 divided doses. Beginning in week 5 the dose is increased by 100 mg/day every 1 to 2 weeks to the usual maintenance dose of 300 to 500 mg per day in two divided doses. *Pediatric patients 2 yr to 12 yr:* Weeks 1 and 2: 0.6 mg/kg/day in 2 divided doses, rounded down to the nearest whole tablet. Weeks 3 and 4: 1.2 mg/kg/day in 2 divided doses, rounded down to the nearest whole tablet. Beginning in week 5 the dose is increased by 1.2 mg/kg/day, rounded down to the nearest whole tablet and added to the previously administered daily dose. The usual daily maintenance dose is 5 to 15 mg/kg per day, with a maximum of 400 mg per day in two divided doses. The maintenance dose of lamotrigine may need to be increased by as much as 50 percent in children who weight less than 30 kg.
	Patients Taking Valporate	*Adults and children > 12 yrs:* Weeks 1 to 4: 25 mg per day Beginning in week 5 the dosage is increased 25 to 50 mg per day every one to two weeks. The usual maintenance dose of lamotrigine in patients taking valproate alone is 100 to 200 mg per day. If patients are taking valproate and other drugs that induce glucuronidation the usual maintenance dose is 100 to 400 mg per day. *Children age 2 yr to 12 yr:* Weeks 1 and 2: 0.15 mg/kg/day in 1 or 2 divided doses rounded down to the nearest whole tablet. Children that weigh more than 6.7 kg and less than 14 kg 2 mg every other day Weeks 3 and 4: 0.3 mg/kg/day in 1 or 2 divided doses, rounded down to the nearest whole tablet. Week 5: calculate 0.3 mg/kg/day and round this amount down to the nearest whole tablet and add this amount to the previously administered daily dose. The usual maintenance dose in children taking valproate is 1 to 5 mg/day with a maximum of 200 mg/day. The maintanence dose of lamotrigine may need to be increased by as much as 50 percent in children who weigh less than 30 kg.

Continued

Table 15–6A ◉ **Dosage Schedule: Selected Anticonvulsants—cont'd**

Drug	Indications	Dosage
	Bipolor Disease	*Adult patients with bipolar disorder not taking enzyme-inducing AEDs or valproate:* Weeks 1 and 2: 25 mg daily Weeks 3 and 4: 50 mg/day Week 5: 100 mg/day. Week 6: 200 mg/day, which is the maintenance dose of lamotrigine. *Adults taking enzyme-inducing AEDs (carbamazepine, phenytoin, phenobarbital or primidone) and not taking valproate:* Weeks 1 and 2: 50 mg/day Weeks 3 and 4: 100 mg/day in divide doses. Week 5: 200 mg/day Week 6: 300 mg/day divided bid Week 7: 400 mg per day in divided doses *Adults with bipolar disease valproate:* Week 1 and 2: 25 mg every other day Weeks 3 and 4: 25 mg daily Week 5: 50 mg per day Week 6: increase to the maintenance dose of 100 mg daily.
	Women Taking Oral Contraceptives	Oral estrogen-containing contraceptives decrease lamotrigine levels by approximately 50 percent. If the patient is already taking lamotrigine and an oral contraceptive is started the lamotrigine dose is increased 50 mg per day weekly. The lamotrigine dose may need to be twice the normal dose.

Table 15–6B ◈ **Available Dosage Forms of Antiepileptic Drugs**

Drugs	Dosage Form	How Supplied	Cost (per 100 Units)
Phenytoin sodium	Chewable tablets	50 mg	
	Oral suspension	125 mg/5 mL	$29/237 mL
Phenytoin sodium, extended-release	Capsules	30, 100 mg	100 mg = $32/90
Phenytoin sodium with phenobarbital	Capsules	100 mg/16 mg or 100 mg/32 mg	
Carbamazepine (Tegretol [T], Carbatrol [C])	Chewable tablets Tablets Tablets extended Capsules Oral suspension	Tablets: (Chewable) 100 mg, 200 mg (G), 100 mg (T) Tablets: 100, 200, 300, 400 mg (G), 200 mg (T) Tablets, extended-release: 100 mg (T & G), 200 mg (T & G), 400 mg (T & G) Capsules, extended-release: 100 mg (C), 200 mg (C), 300 mg (C) Oral suspension: 100 mg/5 mL (G), 100 mg/5 mL (T),	100 mg chew = $15/60 200 mg = $14/90 200 mg XR = $96/100 400 mg XR = $76/100 $62/450 mL

Monitoring

Patients should be assessed for **phenytoin** hypersensitivity syndrome (fever, skin rash, lymphadenopathy), which usually occurs at 3 to 8 weeks. Baseline blood count, urinalysis, and liver function tests should be assessed prior to onset of treatment, with frequent reassessment during the first few months of treatment.

Plasma levels should be monitored, especially when drugs that increase plasma **hydantoin**, such as **ibuprofen**, are used. Conversely, other drugs negatively affected by concurrent administration with **hydantoins** may need plasma level monitoring. **Phenytoin** may alter thyroid hormone demand, which may require monitoring.

Patient Education

The patient should be instructed to take the medication exactly as directed and to avoid missing doses. Abrupt withdrawal may lead to status epilepticus. Advise the patient to wear a medical identification bracelet, to avoid hazardous situations if drowsiness occurs, and to report adverse effects to the clinician. Advise the patient to maintain good oral hygiene to prevent tenderness, bleeding, and gingival hyperplasia. Inform the patient that **phenytoin** may color the urine pink, red, or reddish brown, but this color change is not a cause for alarm. Advise diabetic patients to monitor blood glucose levels and report significant changes to the clinician.

Iminostilbenes

Carbamazepine (Tegretol) is an iminostilbene derivative structurally related to **tricyclic antidepressants** (TCAs). It is used to treat epilepsy, bipolar affective disorder, aggressive and assaultive behavior, and some neuralgias.

Pharmacodynamics

Carbamazepine exerts its effect by depressing transmission in the nucleus ventralis anterior of the thalamus. This area is associated with the spread of seizure discharge. Seizure spread is believed to occur through inhibition of voltage-gated sodium channels.

Absorption and Distribution

Carbamazepine is absorbed through the stomach, the suspension being absorbed more quickly than the tablet form. Absorption from immediate-release tablets is slow and erratic because of its low water solubility. The drug is highly lipophilic, resulting in high body tissue binding.

Metabolism and Excretion

Carbamazepine is metabolized in the liver and has the unique ability to induce its own metabolism (autoinduction). Due to autoinduction, initial concentrations within a therapeutic range may later fall despite good compliance. It also induces the metabolism of many CYP450 enzymes and other substrates. Excretion is through urine and feces.

Onset, Peak, and Duration

Average peak blood levels of **carbamazepine** occur approximately 6 hours after administration. Half-life can be as long as 65 hours with initial dosing, but is typically 12 to 17 hours as administration continues. It is noteworthy that the half-life after a single dose is much longer than the half-life after long-term use. Steady state is attained in 2 to 4 days.

Pharmacotherapeutics

Precautions and Contraindications

Contraindications include hypersensitivity to **carbamazepine** or **TCAs**, history of bone marrow suppression, and concurrent administration with **monoamine oxidase inhibitors** (MAOIs). **Carbamazepine** is Pregnancy Category D; teratogenic defects have occurred, including spina bifida. It is excreted in human milk but is not contraindicated during lactation.

Carbamazepine has a black box warning regarding serious dermatological reactions (Stevens-Johnson syndrome and toxic epidermal necrolysis) and the risk of developing aplastic anemia and agranulocytosis. Use with caution in patients with increased intraocular pressure because of its mild anticholinergic effects. Caution is also advised in patients with a history of previous adverse hematological reactions to any drugs in those with cardiac, renal, or hepatic impairment.

Adverse Drug Reactions

Carbamazepine has a black box warning due to its potential to cause blood dyscrasias, some potentially lethal. Although a transient decrease of the white blood cell count can occur and is manageable, **carbamazepine** can depress the bone marrow and lead to leukopenia, thrombocytopenia, agranulocytosis, and aplastic anemia. For that reason, a baseline blood screen that includes a complete blood count (CBC), chemistry, liver function tests, and thyroid-stimulating hormone (TSH) test should be obtained, followed by periodic monitoring. Follow-up studies should be more frequent initially, decreasing to every 3 to 4 months if the results remain normal or the CBC and differential are only minimally lowered.

Other adverse reactions to **carbamazepine** include hepatic damage and impaired thyroid function. Less serious early adverse events may include drowsiness, dizziness, blurred vision, ataxia, nausea and vomiting, dry mouth, diplopia, and headache.

Drug Interactions

The interactions of most significance are those that increase the plasma level of **carbamazepine** to potentially toxic levels, such as the concurrent administration of **propoxyphene, hydantoins, cimetidine**, some **antibiotics** (**erythromycin, clarithromycin**), **isoniazid**, and **verapamil**. Interactions that can result in hepatic damage occur with coadministration of some **anesthetics** and with **isoniazid**. Interactions that decrease plasma levels of the other drug occur with **beta blockers, succinimides, valproic acid, warfarin, haloperidol, doxycycline,** and **nondepolarizing muscle relaxants**. Grapefruit juice increases serum levels and effects of **carbamazepine**.

Table 15–7 presents drug interactions.

Clinical Use and Dosing

Table 15–8 presents the indications, dosage schedules, and available dosage forms of **carbamazepine**.

Rational Drug Selection

Carbamazepine is indicated in the treatment of partial complex seizures. It is also useful for generalized tonic-clonic seizures. Its relative lack of side effects compared to

Table 15–7 ■ **Drug Interactions: Carbamazepine and Oxcarbazepine (Anticonvulsants)**

Drug	Interacting Drug	Possible Effect	Implications
Carbamazepine	Anesthetics	Hepatic or renal damage	Ensure anesthetist is aware of carbamazepine use
	Cimetidine, propoxyphene, isoniazid, calcium channel blockers, fluoxetine, valproic acid, erythromycin, paroxetine, fluvoxamine, danazol, grapefruit juice, influenza vaccine, olanzapine, loxapine, ritonavir, nicotinamide	Increased plasma level of carbamazepine	Monitor plasma level
	Hydantoins, barbiturates, primidone, felbamate, rifampin, cisplatin, theophylline	Decreased plasma level of carbamazepine	Monitor level for possible dosage increase; monitor for seizure activity
	MAOIs	Hyperpyretic crisis	Do not give during or within 14 d of MAOI use
	Doxycycline, anticoagulants, warfarin, theophylline, haloperidol, acetaminophen, alprazolam, clozapine, anticonvulsants, clomipramine, phenytoin, primidone	Decreased effect of interacting drug	Monitor plasma levels when able; monitor for signs and symptoms of condition for which interacting drug was prescribed
	Lithium	Increased risk of neurotoxicity	Monitor plasma levels of both drugs; monitor for CNS-related adverse events
	Oral contraceptives	May decrease ethinyl estradiol and levonorgestrel availability	Use other birth control measures

Table 15–8 ◉ **Dosage Schedule: Carbamazepine and Oxcarbazepine (Anticonvulsants)**

Drug	Indications	Dosage	Available Dosage Forms
Carbamazepine	Partial complex seizure disorder	*Adults and children >12 yr:* initially 200 mg bid; increase by 200 mg/d at weekly intervals to maximum of 1,000 mg/d for children 12–15 yr; maintenance range: 800–1,200 mg/d 3–4 times/d	Tablets: 100, 200, 300, 400 mg
		Children <12 yr; initially 100 mg bid; increase by 100 mg/d tid-qid at weekly intervals to maximum of 1,000 mg/d: may also give at 20–30 mg/kg/d tid-qid; maintenance range 400–800 mg/d	Chewable tablets: 100, 200 mg Suspension: 100 mg/5 mL
	Trigeminal neuralgia	*Adults:* 100 mg bid on first day; increase by 200 mg/d at 100 mg every 12 h to maximum of 1,200 mg/d; maintenance range 200–1,200 mg/d, usually 400–800 mg/d: decrease dosage or discontinue every 3 mo	
	Bipolar disorder, aggressive/assaultive behavior	Same dosage guidelines as above until severe mood swings are stabilized and plasma level is within therapeutic range	
Oxcarbazepine	Monotherapy or adjunctive therapy of partial seizures	*Adults PO:* 300 mg bid increased by 600 mg/d weekly up to 1,200 mg bid PO children (4–16 yr) 4–5 mg/kg bid, increased over 2 wk	Tablets 150, 300, 600 mg Oral suspension 300 mg/5mL

phenytoin and phenobarbital has resulted in increased use for a variety of seizure disorders. The drug is also used as a third-line mood stabilizer for bipolar patients who have not responded to lithium or divalproex (Depakote) and for patients unable to tolerate either of the others. Carbamazepine, in a dosage range of 100 to 300 mg at bedtime, can be used to treat restless legs syndrome. Carbamazepine is sometimes used to relieve the pain of trigeminal neuralgia.

Monitoring

Plasma carbamazepine levels should be monitored on a regular basis. The therapeutic range is 4 to 12 mcg/mL. Higher levels can lead to toxic symptoms consisting of the initial adverse effects and also hypertension, tachycardia, electrocardiogram (ECG) changes, stupor, agitation, nystagmus, urinary retention, respiratory depression, seizures, and coma. Children and elderly patients may develop toxicity at levels below 12.

Patient Education

Patients taking carbamazepine should be instructed to report to the clinician any symptoms such as skin lesions, bruising, fever, or sore throat. Carbamazepine should then be discontinued and another drug substituted. Tell the patient that administration with food may increase absorption, and because carbamazepine can be sedating, care should be exercised in situations in which mental and physical alertness is required for safety. Advise the patient that it is important to take the medication exactly as directed. If a dose is missed, the patient should take it as soon as possible but not just before the next scheduled dose; do not take double doses. Advise the patient to carry medical identification of the seizure disorder.

Succinimides

The succinimides are used for the treatment of absence seizures in children and adults. The succinimides include ethosuximide (Zarontin), and methsuximide (Celontin).

Pharmacodynamics

The succinimides exert their anticonvulsant effects by decreasing nerve impulses and transmission in the motor cortex. This produces a variety of effects, including an increase in the seizure threshold and reducing the electroencephalogram (EEG) spike-and-wave pattern of absence seizures.

Pharmacokinetics

Absorption and Distribution

Succinimides are administered orally and are thoroughly absorbed from the GI tract.

Metabolism and Excretion

Succinimides are metabolized in the liver and excreted through the urinary tract, although a small amount of phensuximide is excreted in bile.

Onset, Peak, and Duration

There is a wide difference in half-lives, ranging from 30 hours in children and 60 hours in adults for ethosuximide, and 2.6 to 4 hours for methsuximide. Peak plasma levels are reached in 1 to 4 hours for methsuximide, and in 3 to 7 hours for ethosuximide. Methsuximide has an onset of action of 15 to 30 minutes and a duration of 3 to 4 hours.

Pharmacotherapeutics

Precautions and Contraindications

Anticonvulsants in general are associated with fetal defects but the succinimides, with careful monitoring of plasma levels, appear to be safe for use during pregnancy and are Pregnancy Category C. They are contraindicated, as are other anticonvulsants, during lactation.

Although uncommon, succinimides have caused blood dyscrasias and use should be preceded by a CBC with differential repeated at frequent intervals initially and less often as the patient continues on the medication without adverse effects. Liver function tests should also be obtained prior to instituting treatment.

Adverse Drug Reactions

The most common adverse reactions to the succinimides are gastrointestinal (GI) distress, which can be relieved by taking the medication with food or milk, and CNS depression, characterized by sedation, ataxia, and lethargy. Other adverse reactions may include headache, rash, pruritus, and mood changes. Symptoms of toxicity are a worsening of these adverse reactions.

Drug Interactions

The most significant drug interactions are those that increase CNS depression, such as alcohol, opioid agonists, benzodiazepines, and CNS depressants. Succinimides may be given concurrently with other anticonvulsants but may antagonize the other and contribute to tonic-myoclonic breakthrough seizures, therefore requiring the need for a higher dose of the other anticonvulsant.

Avoid concurrent use with TCAs and phenothiazines because an antagonistic effect on succinimides may lower the patient's seizure threshold. Haloperidol may change the pattern or frequency of seizures, necessitating an adjustment in dosage of the anticonvulsant.

Succinimides may decrease the effectiveness of oral contraceptives; thus, the patient should be advised to use a backup birth control method.

Clinical Use and Dosing

Table 15–9 presents the indications, dosage schedules, and available dosage forms of succinimides.

Rational Drug Selection

Succinimides are the treatment of choice for childhood absence seizure disorders. They are sometimes used for the treatment of absence seizures in adults, but valproic

Table 15–9 ◉ **Dosage Schedule: Succinimides (Anticonvulsants)**

Drug	Indications	Dosage	Available Dosage Forms	Cost (per 100 Units)
Ethosuximide (Zarontin)	Absence seizures (petit mal)	*Adults and children >6 yr:* 500 mg daily or 250 mg bid; may increase by 250 mg every 4–7 d to maximum of 1.5 g/d	Capsules: 250 mg	$104 *Now also generic*
		Children <6 yr: 250 mg daily or 125 mg bid; optimal dose 20 mg/kg/d; maximum dose 1.5 g/d	Syrup: 250 mg/5 mL	$109/480 mL
Methsuximide (Celontin)	Absence seizures (petit mal); second choice	*Adults and children:* initially 300 mg/d; may increase by 300 mg/d increments at weekly intervals to maximum of 1.2 g/d in divided doses	Capsules: 150, 300 mg	$102

acid becomes the primary treatment in adults. **Methsuximide** is equally effective as **ethosuximide** but may have more adverse reactions.

Monitoring

Plasma levels should be monitored. The normal therapeutic range of **ethosuximide** is 40 to 100 mcg/mL. In addition to monitoring seizure activity, evaluate liver, renal, and hematological studies periodically for adverse effects on these systems. The therapeutic range for **methsuximide** is 10 to 40 mcg/mL, with levels greater than 40 mcg/mL considered toxic.

Patient Education

Advise the patient to avoid alcohol and, if sedation occurs, to avoid hazardous activities. To decrease stomach distress, take **succinimides** with milk or food. Because adverse mood changes can occur while taking these medications, advise the client to report any behavioral changes to the clinician. Caution the client that withdrawal of the medication may precipitate absence seizures. Inform the client taking **phensuximide** that harmless changes in urine color may occur.

Drugs That Affect GABA

The AEDs that affect gamma aminobutyric acid (GABA) include **gabapentin (Neurontin)**, **topiramate (Topamax)**, and **tiagabine (Gabitril)**. The AEDs that affect the inhibitory neurotransmitter GABA, are also used for pain, including neuropathic pain (**gabapentin**) and migraine (**topiramate**).

Pharmacodynamics

The mechanism of action of the drugs that affect GABA are not well understood. **Gabapentin** is thought to be a GABA analogue that binds to unknown receptors in the brain, it does not bind to GABA receptors, nor does it mimic GABA. **Topiramate** may block sodium channels or potentiate GABA. **Tiagabine** may potentiate the action of GABA by blocking GABA reuptake into presynaptic neurons, allowing for more GABA to be available to bind to postsynaptic neuronal receptors.

Pharmacokinetics

Absorption and Distribution

All the AEDs that affect GABA are rapidly absorbed after oral administration. **Gabapentin** peaks in 2 to 3 hours after oral administration. Food increases absorption of **gabapentin** 14 percent. **Topiramate** peaks 2 hours after oral administration and is not affected by food intake. **Tiagabine** peaks 45 minutes after ingestion if taken on an empty stomach. The drugs that affect GABA are widely distributed, including into the central nervous system and into breast milk. Pharmacokinetics of drugs that affect GABA are found in Table 15–10.

Metabolism and Excretion

Gabapentin is not metabolized. It is excreted unchanged in the urine (75 percent to 80 percent) and the feces (10 percent to 20 percent). **Topiramate** is not extensively metabolized, with minor amounts metabolized in the liver via hydroxylation, hydrolysis and glucuronidation. The percentage of **topiramate** metabolized in the liver increases when co-administered with drugs that are enzyme inducers. **Tiagabine** is extensively metabolized in the liver, primarily by CYP 3A4 and undergoes enterohepatic recirculation.

Gabapentin is excreted 75 to 80 percent unchanged in the urine and 10 to 20 percent unchanged in the feces. The half-life of **gabapentin** is 4.7 hours in infants and children, and 5.3 hours in adults. Adults with renal

Table 15–10 ▶ **Pharmacokinetics: Tricyclic Antidepressants**

Drug	Onset	Peak	Duration	Half-Life	Excretion
Amitriptyline HCl	45 min	2–12 h	Long-acting	31–46 h	Urine, feces
Amoxapine	90 min	2–4 wk	Long-acting	8–30 h	Urine
Clomipramine	4, 7 h	2–4 wk	Long-acting	19–37 h	Urine
Desipramine HCl	2–5 d	2–3 wk	Long-acting	12–24 h	Urine
Doxepin HCl	2–8 d	2–4 wk	Long-acting	8–24 h	Urine
Imipramine HCl	2–4 h	2–4 wk	Long-acting	11–25 h	Urine, feces
Nortriptyline HCl	—	2–4 wk	Long-acting	18–44 h	Urine
Protriptyline HCl	8–12 h	24–30 h	Long-acting	67–89 h	Urine
Trimipramine maleate	—	—	Long-acting	9–11 h	Urine

insufficiency (CrCl less than 30 mL/min) may have a half life of 52 hours.

Topiramate is eliminated 70 percent unchanged in the urine. The half life of **topiramate** in adults is 21 hours and in adults with renal impairment the half life is 59 hours.

Tiagabine is eliminated as metabolites, 25 percent in the urine and 63 percent in the feces. The half life of **tiagabine** in adults is 7 to 9 hours. In children age 3 to 10 years the mean half life is 5.7 hours. In children who are on enzyme-inducing AEDs the half life of **tiagabine** is 3.2 hours and in adults on enzyme-inducing AEDs the half life is 2 to 5 hours.

Pharmacotherapeutics

Precautions and Contraindications

Gabapentin

Gapapentin is contraindicated in patients who are hypersensitive to **gabapentin. Gabapentin** should not be abruptly discontinued as it may precipitate status epilepticus, decrease dose over at least a week.

Neuropsychiatric events such as behavior problems, hostility, aggressive behavior, thought disorder including changes in school performance and hyperkinesias have been reported in pediatric patients age 3 to 12 years taking **gabapentin.**

AEDs including **gabapentin** increase the risk of suicidal behavior and ideation, patients should be monitored for emergence or worsening of depression, suicidal thoughts or changes in behavior.

Gabapentin is Pregnancy Category C. **Gabapentin** is excreted in breast milk and nursing infants may be exposed to up to 1/mg/kg/day. **Gabapentin** should be used in nursing women only if the benefits outweigh the risks. Monitor the infant for lethargy or other neurological effects.

Safety and effectiveness of **gabapentin** has not been established in children younger than age 3 years.

Topiramate

Patients taking **topiramate** may have decreased serum bicarbonate concentrations due to ihibitionof carbonic anhydrase and increased renal bicarbonate loss, leading to hyperchloremic metabolic acidosis. In adults doses of a low as 50 mg per day of **topiramate** may result in low serum bicarbonate, with the incidence of decreased serum bicarbonate 30 percent in clinical trials when **topiramate** dosage was 400 mg per day. Low serum bicarbonate levels in children 2 to 16 years of age were reported in up to 67% of children receiving 6 mg/kg/day. Severe metabolic acidosis has been reported in infants receiving a **topiramate** dose of 5 mg/kg/day. Serum bicarbonate should be monitored at baseline and periodically throughout therapy.

An ocular syndrome consisting of acute myopia and angle closure glaucoma has been reported in adults and children taking **topiramate**. Symptoms usually occur within one month of starting **topiramate**. Patients who have eye pain or blurred vision should contact their provider immediately. Treatment is to discontinue **topiramate** as soon as possible.

A rare adverse effect of **topiramate** is oligohidrosis (decreased sweating) and hyperthermia. Most cases were reported in children and were associated with vigorous exercise and/or high environmental temperatures. Patients, especially children should be monitored for decreased sweating and hyperthermia, especially in warm weather. Use caution when prescribing drugs that predispose patients to heat-related disorders (**anticholinergic drugs** and **carbonic anhydrase inhibitors**).

AEDs including **topiramate** increase the risk of suicidal behavior and ideation, patients should be monitored for emergence or worsening of depression, suicidal thoughts or changes in behavior.

Topiramate should not be abruptly discontinued as it may precipitate status epilepticus, withdraw gradually.

Topiramate is Pregnancy Category D and has been found to be teratogenic in animal studies. There is an increased risk of cleft lip and/or cleft palate in infants born to women who take **topiramate** during pregnancy. **Topiramate** is excreted in breastmilk, with infant plasma concentrations of 10 percent to 20 percent of maternal concentrations. Infants ingesting **topiramate** via breast milk should be monitored for drowsiness, weight gain and developmental milestones (Toxnet, 2011).

Tiagabine

Tiagabine is contraindicated in patients who are hypersensitive to **tiagabine** or any component.

Post-marketing reports have shown that patients without epilepsy that are prescribed **tiagabine** may have seizure or status epilepticus. Seizures have been reported in doses as low as 4 mg per day. Most patients were taking other medications concomitantly, such as **antidepressants, antipsychotics, stimulants** or **narcotics**. It is thought the concomitant drug lowered the seizure threshold. Seizures occurred soon after a dosage increase.

Dosing recommendations for **tiagabine** are based on a study sample that were also taking enzyme-inducing **AEDs**, such as **carbamazepine, phenytoin, primidone** and **phenobarbital**, leading to lower plasma **tiagabine** levels.

AEDs including **tiagabine** increase the risk of suicidal behavior and ideation, patients should be monitored for emergence or worsening of depression, suicidal thoughts or changes in behavior.

Tiagabine should not be abruptly discontinued as it may precipitate increased seizure activity, withdraw gradually.

Tiagabine is Pregnancy Category C. It has been found to be teratogenic in fetal rats. There are not adequately well controlled studies in pregnant women. **Tiagabine** is excreted in breast milk and its use is not recommended in lactating women unless there are no other options for maternal treatment. Infants should be monitored for adequate weight gain and developmental milestones.

Tiagabine has been minimally studied in children and it is not labeled for use in children younger than age 12 years.

Adverse Drug Reactions

The most common central nervous system (CNS) adverse effects of **gapapentin** include somnolence (28 percent in clinical trials) and dizziness (21 percent). Less common CNS effects include ataxia (3.3 percent) and abnormal thinking (2.7 percent). In children 3 to 12 years of age neuropsychiatric adverse effects of **gabapentin** include emotional lability (6 percent), hostility (5.2 percent), hyperkinesias (4.7 percent) and thought disorder, including problems with concentration and school performance (1.7 percent).

Peripheral edema occurred in 8.3 percent of patients taking **gabapentin** in clinical trials versus 2.2 percent in the control group.

The central nervous system (CNS) adverse effects of **topiramate** include ataxia, parathesia, dizziness, somnolence and difficulty concentrating. Patients in the treatment group also reported anorexia, difficulty with memory, confusion, depression, mood problems, and psychomotor slowing. In children the most common CNS adverse effects are somnolence and fatigue. Weight loss was reported in 6 percent of patients taking 50 mg/day and 16 percent of patients taking 400 mg/day of **topiramate**.

There is an increase in incidence of kidney stones (2 to 4 percent greater than expected in clinical trials) in patients taking **topiramate**. Kidney stones were more prevalent in men and also occurred in children during clinical trials.

Hyperammonemia with and without encephalopathy has been observed in in clinical trials and in post-marketing reports in patients who were taking **topiramate** both with and without concomitant **valproic acid** use. **Topiramate** inhibits carbonic anhydrase leading to renal bicarbonate loss and may cause metabolic acidosis.

The adverse drug reactions most commonly reported for **tiagabine** were related to the central nervous system, including difficulty with concentration or attention, dizziness, light-headedness, somnolence, confusion, asthenia or lack of energy and nervousness or irritability. Suicidal thinking has been reported, as previously mentioned.

Drug Interactions

Gabapentin does not interfere with the metabolism of commonly coadministered **AEDs**. Coadministration of **naproxen** increases absorption of **gabapentin** 12 to 15 percent. **Gabapentin** may increase the effects of **alcohol** and other CNS depressant drugs.

Gabapentin may cause a false positive urinary protein level with N-Multistik SG® test.

Clinical Use and Dosing

Dosing of **gabapentin** for seizures in children older than age 12 years and adults is 300 mg three times a day. Doses are titrated upward to the usual dose of 900 to 1,800 mg three times a day. Dosages up to 2,400 mg per day have been tolerated in long-term studies. Initial **gabapentin** dosing for children 3 to 12 years is 10 to 15 mg/kg/day divided into 3 doses per day, the dose is titrated up to a usual dose of 40 mg/kg/day in children 3 to 4 years, and 25 to 35 mg/kg/day in children 5 to 12 years. Neuropathic pain is treated in adults with a starting dose of 100 mg three times a day, with the dose titrated upward 300 mg per day at weekly intervals, to a dose of at least 900 mg per day. The usual **gabapentin** dosage range for neuropathic pain is 1,800 to 2,400 mg per day, divided three times a day. The dose of **gabapentin** to treat post-herpetic neuralgia in adults is an initial dose of 300 mg per day, on day two the dose is 300 mg twice a day and on day three the dose is 300 mg three times a day. The dose is titrated up to 600 mg three times a day as needed to relieve pain. Dosage adjustment of **gabapentin** is required in patients with renal failure.

When **topiramate** is used as monotherapy for epilepsy in children age 10 years or older and adults the recommended dose is 400 mg per day in two divided doses. Patients should be titrated up to the recommended dosage. The **topiramate** starting dose is 25 mg twice a day for a week, then the dose is increased to 50 mg twice a day for a week. In week three the dose is 75 mg twice a day and in week four the dose is 100 mg twice a day. In week five the **topiramate** dose is increased to 150 mg twice a day and in week six the goal dosage of 200 mg twice a day is achieved. The recommended total daily dose in patients with partial onset seizures or Lennox-Gastaut Syndrome is 200 to 400 mg daily. In pediatric patients age 2 years to16 years with partial onset seizures, primary generalized tonic-clonic seizures, or seizures associated with Lennox-Gastaut syndrome the **topiramate** dose is approximately 5 to 9 mg/kg/day in two divided doses. Pediatric dosing is started at 1 to 3 mg/kg/day (maximum 25 mg/day) in two divided doses and titrated up by 1 to 3 mg/kg/day at one to two week intervals to achieve clinical response. Usual maintenance dose of **topiramate** in children is 5 to 9 mg/kg/day, divided into twice a day dosing. In patients with renal impairment, half the usual dosage is recommended.

Tiagabine dose depends on whether a patient is concurrently taking an enzyme-inducing AED. Use of **tiagabine** in patients not taking enzyme-inducing AEDs may result in serum concentration up to twice that of patients on enzyme-inducing AEDs. **Tiagabine** dosage adjustment is needed if an enzyme-inducing drug is added, discontinued or has a dosage change. Avoid loading doses or rapid escalation of dose. The initial dose of **tiagabine** in adolescents age 12 years to 18 years is 4 mg once daily for a week, then in week two the dose is 4 mg twice a day (8 mg/day total). Dosage in increased by 4 to 8 mg daily at weekly intervals until clinical response is achieved. The maximum dose of **tiagabine** in adolescents is 32 mg per day. The dosage for adults on enzyme-inducing AEDs is 4 mg once daily week one, then increased by 4 to 8 mg per day increments until the maximum daily dose of 32 to 56 mg per day divided in 2 to 4 doses is achieved. If a dose is missed, the patient should skip that dose and administer the next dose at the regularly scheduled time. Patients should not double the dose to catch up. If multiple doses of **tiagabine** have been missed, possible retitration may be required.

Rational Drug Selection

Drug selection of drugs that affect GABA is based on the type of seizure and possible drug interactions that may affect therapy.

Monitoring

Seizure frequency, duration and severity are monitored with all AEDs. Mood changes, signs of depression, anxiety, and suicidal thoughts should be monitored with all AEDs.

Patients taking **gabapentin, topiramate** and **tiagabine** do not require routing monitoring of serum drug levels.

Patients taking **topiramate** should have serum electrolyte including sodium bicarbonate monitored at baseline and periodically. Weight is monitored in all patients on **topiramate.** Body temperature is monitored in patients taking **topiramate**, as well as ability to sweat especially in warm weather. Serum ammonia levels should be drawn in any patient taking **topiramate** who exhibit any change in level of consciousness, unexplained lethargy or vomiting.

Patient Education

Administration

Patients taking **AEDs** that affect GABA should take the medication exactly as prescribed to maintain consistent therapeutic levels. Missing doses may cause an increase in seizures. Withdrawal seizures may occur if any of these medications is abruptly discontinued, therefore patients need to be warned to take their medication as scheduled and to not stop taking it without discussing with their provider.

Adverse Reactions

Patients and family members of patients taking **AEDs** should be warned about the potential neuropsychiatric ADRs, including suicidal thoughts and action, and behavioral changes. Any changes should be reported to the prescriber immediately.

Patients should also be warned about the possibility of somnolence, dizziness or balance issues when starting on AEDs that affect GABA.

Patients taking **topiramate** will need to monitor their ability to sweat and monitor their temperature in warm weather.

Any signs of confusion, unexplained vomiting or mental status change in patients taking **topiramate** requires investigation for elevated ammonia levels or metabolic acidosis.

Lifestyle management

Patients who have seizures should get adequate sleep and exercise and avoid stressful situations that may trigger seizures.

Levetiracetam

Levetiracetam (Keppra) is an antiepileptic indicated as an adjunct drug in the treatment of partial onset seizures. It is its own unique drug class, as it is chemically unrelated to other AEDs.

Pharmacodynamics

The exact mechanism of action of **levetiracetam** is not known. It does not appear to inhibit or affect GABA, nor does it effect calcium or sodium currents or channels. *In vitro* and *in vivo* recordings of epileptiform activity during clinical trials have shown that **levetiracetam** inhibits burst firing without affecting normal neuronal excitability, suggesting that levetiracetam may prevent epileptiform burst firing and spread of seizure activity.

Pharmacokinetics

Absorption and Distribution

Levetircetam is almost completely absorbed after oral administration. Time to peak concentration is 1 hour in immediate-release tablets and 3 hours in extended relese **levetiracetam**. Intake of high calorie, high fat meal before administration delays time to peak in the extended-release **levetiracetam** by up to 2 hours. It is less than 10% protein bound.

Metabolism and Excretion

Levetiracetam is not extensively metabolized and does not use the cytochrome P450 enzymes. It is metabolized by hydrolysis of the acetamide group, which produces an inactive carboxylic acid metabolite.

Levetiracetam is 68% eliminated renally. The half-life of **levetiracetam** is 7 hours. Renal clearance is impaired in patients with renal dysfunction.

Pharmacotherapeutics

Precautions and Contraindications

The only absolute contraindication to the use of **levetiracetam** is sensitivity to the drug.

Patients taking AEDs, including **levetiracetam** are at increased risk for suicidal thoughts, depression and unusual changes in mood and behavior. The mood changes can occur as early as one week from the onset of therapy and persist throughout the duration of therapy. Patients and caregivers should be informed of the risk for neuropsychiatric changes while taking **levetiracetam** and to report any changes in mood, suicidal thoughts or behavior changes.

There is a potential for withdrawal seizures if **levetiracetam** is abruptly stopped. **Levetiracetam** should be withdrawn slowly to prevent seizures.

Levetiracetam may cause somnolence, fatigue, dizziness and muscle coordination difficulties. Patients should be warned not to drive or operate heavy machinery until they know the effects of **levetiracetam.**

Levetiracetam may cause a transient decrease in white blood count (WBC), with 3.2% of patients in the clinical trials experiencing a decreased WBC and 2.4% experiencing a decreased neutrophil count. Neutrophil counts returned to normal after continued use.

Levetiracetam is Pregnancy Category C, although there are no well controlled trials in pregnant women. Administration of **levetiracetam** to rats lead to minor fetal skeletal abnormalities. Altered pharmacokinetics during pregnancy may affect **levetiracetam** serum concentrations; with decreased serum concentration reported during pregnancy. Discontinuing AEDs during pregnancy may be harmful to the mother, so consultation with a perinatologist is warranted. Pregnant women who take **levetiracetam** during pregnancy should be reported and enrolled in North American Antiepileptic Drug Pregnancy Registry (888-233-2334).

Levetiracetam is FDA approved for use in children age for years or older as adjunct therapy in partial seizures and as adjunctive therapy in children age 6 years and older with primary generalized tonic-clonic seizures.

Adverse Drug Reactions

The most common ADR reported in clinical trials of **levetiracetam** was somnolence, reported in 15% of patients. Dizziness is another common ADR (9% of patients).

Behavioral changes are an uncommon but significant in patients taking **levetiracetam**, including nervousness (4% of patients), anxiety (2%), hostility (2%), and emotional liability.

As previously mentioned, suicidal thinking or behavior may occur in patients taking **AEDs**. In clinical trials, of 11 different **AEDs**, patients randomized to one of the **AEDs** had approximately twice the risk of suicidal thoughts or behavior of the controls.

Alopecia has been reported in post-marketing surveillance of **levetiracetam**, with recovery reported once the drug was discontinued.

Drug Interactions

Levetiracetam is mostly unbound and does not use CYP 450 enzymes for metabolism, thereby decreasing the likelihood of drug interactions.

Levetiracetam does not interact with **phenytoin, valproate, carbamazepine, gabapentin, lamotrigene** or **phenobarbital.** It has also been studied and does not interact with oral **contraceptives** or **warfarin.**

Clinical Use and Dosing

Levetiracetam is prescribed as adjunct therapy in patients with refractory partial seizures. **Levetiracetam** is added to a stable dosing regimen of an AED.

Rational Drug Selection

Levetiracetam is the only drug in its class and is used as adjunct therapy in patients with partial seizures. There are two forms available, immediate-release and extended-release (**Keppra XR**) tablets. The extended release formula is FDA approved for age 16 years and older. There is a significant cost difference between generic **levetiracetam** and the brand name **Keppra**, with 60 tablets of 250 mg generic costing $24 and 60 tablets of 250 mg **Keppra** costing $260 (www.drugstore.com).

Monitoring

Routine laboratory monitoring of patients on **levetiracetam** is not necessary. Efficacy is determined by a decreased in the mean weekly frequency of partial onset seizures.

Patient Education

Administration

Patients should take **levetiracetam** exactly as prescribed. Missing doses may cause an increase in seizures. Withdrawal seizures may occur if **levetiracetam** is abruptly discontinued, therefore patients need to be warned to take their medication as scheduled and to not stop taking it without discussing with their provider.

Adverse Reactions

Patients and family members of patients taking **levetiracetam** should be warned about the potential neuropsychiatric ADRs, including suicidal thoughts and action, and behavioral changes. Any changes should be reported to the prescriber immediately.

Patients should also be warned about the possibility of somnolence, dizziness or balance issues when starting on **levetiracetam.**

Lifestyle Management

Patients who have seizures should get adequate sleep and exercise and avoid stressful situations that may trigger seizures.

Lamotrigine

Pharmacodynamics

The exact mechanism of action of **lamotrigine** is not known. It is thought that **lamotrigine** affects voltage-sensitive sodium channels and inhibits presynaptic release of glutamate and aspartate in the neuron. The mechanism of action of **lamotrigine** in the treatment of bipolar disorder is not known.

Pharmacokinetics

Absorption and Distribution

Lamotrigine is well absorbed after oral administration. **Lamotrigine** chewable tablets have the same rate of absorption whether chewed or dissolved in water. Orally disintegrating tablets and regular tablets taken with water have the same rate and extent of absorption. Immediate release **lamotrigine** peaks in 2 hours. Some patients may have a second peak at 4 to 6 hours due to enterohepatic recirculation. Extended release **lamotrigine** peaks in 4 to 11 hours.

The mean volume of distribution of **lamotrigine** is 0.9 to 1.3 L/kg after oral administration. **Lamotrigine** is 55 percent protein bound. It crosses the placenta and is excreted in breastmilk.

Metabolism and Excretion

Lamotrigine is metabolized extensively in the liver via glucuronic acid conjugation. When **lamotrigine** is given alone, after multiple doses it induces its own metabolism resulting in a 25 percent decrease in half-life.

Ninety-four percent of **lamotrigine** is excreted as metabolites in the urine and 2 percent is excreted in the feces.

Pharmacotherapeutics

Precautions and Contraindications

Lamotrigine is contraindicated in patients hypersensitive to the drug or its ingredients. Life-threatening hypersensitivity reactions have occurred. Reactions include multiorgan failure or dysfunction, hepatic abnormalities and disseminated intravascular coagulation. Early symptoms of hypersensitivity, such as fever or lymphadenopathy require evaluation and **lamotrigine** discontinued if reason for symptoms cannot be established.

Lamatrigine has a Black Box warning regarding life-threatening rashes that may occur, including Stevens-Johnson syndrome, toxic epidermal necrolysis and rash-related death. Pediatric patients are more likely to have serious rash than adults. Coadministration with **valproate** may increase the risk of rash. Exceeding recommended initial doses or exceeding recommended dosage escalation of **lamotrigine** increases risk of rash. **Lamotrigine** should be discontinued at the first sign of rash, unless clearly not drug related.

Multiorgan failure has been reported in patients taking **lamotrigine**.

Blood dyscrasias, including neutropenia, leukopenia, anemia, thrombocytopenia, pancytopenia and aplastic anemia have been reported in patients taking **lamotrigine.**

Patients taking AEDs, including **lamotrigine** are at increased risk for suicidal thoughts, depression and unusual changes in mood and behavior. The mood changes can occur as early as one week from the onset of therapy and persist throughout the duration of therapy. Patients taking **lamotrigine** for bipolar disorder may experience worsening of depression and emergence of suicidal ideation. Patients and caregivers should be informed of the risk for neuropsychiatric changes while taking **lamotrigine** and to report any changes in mood, suicidal thoughts or behavior changes.

There is a potential for withdrawal seizures if **lamotrigine** is abruptly stopped. **Lamotrigine** should be withdrawn slowly (over at least 2 weeks) to prevent seizures.

Lamotrigine is Pregnancy Category C. Although not specifically found to be teratogenic, **lamotrigine** decreases folate levels in animals studies. **Lamotrigine** should only be prescribed to pregnant women if the benefit outweighs the risk. Pregnant women who take **lamotrigine** during pregnancy should be referred to enroll in the North American Antiepileptic Drug Pregnancy Registry (888-233-2334). Providers may enroll patients in the **Lamotrigine** Pregnancy Registry by calling 1-800-336-2176.

Lamotrigine is excreted in breast milk. Breastfed infants of women taking **lamotrigine** have measurable serum levels of **lamotrigine.** Infant serum levels of **lamotrigine** may be 30 to 50 percent of maternal levels. Neonates have limited ability to metabolize **lamotrigine**

placing them at higher risk of exposure. If there are no other therapeutic options to maternal **lamotrigine** use, then the infant should be monitored closely for drowsiness, poor suck, apnea and rash. Consider measuring serum **lamotrigine** levels and platelet count in the infant. Infants may exhibit withdrawal symptoms if breastfeeding is abruptly discontinued.

Lamotrigine is FDA approved for use in children age 2 years or older for the treatment of generalized tonic-clinic seizures, partial seizures and Lennox-Gastaut syndrome. Safety and effectiveness in the treatment of bipolar disorder in patients younger than 18 years of age has not been established.

Adverse Drug Reactions

As discussed in the Precautions and Contraindications section, **lamotrigine** has a Black Box warning regarding serious, possibly life-threatening rashes including Stevens-Johnson. The incidence in pediatric patients age 2 to 16 years of age is 0.8 percent (8 in 1,000) and 0.3 percent in adults taking **lamotrigine** as adjunctive therapy. Any unexplained rash requires discontinuation of **lamotrigine** and investigation.

Multiorgan failure has been reported in patients taking **lamotrigine**, including hepatic failure.

Blood dyscrasias may occur in patients taking **lamotrigine**. Reported abnormalities include neutropenia, anemia, thrombocytopenia and pancytopenia. Rare reactions include aplastic anemia and red cell aplasia.

Patients taking **lamotrigine** for any reason may have increased suicidal thoughts or behavior. Monitor patients for mood changes or suicidal thoughts, especially those taking **lamotrigine** for bipolar disorder.

Abruptly discontinuing **lamotrigine** may cause withdrawal seizures. Patients may exhibit withdrawal seizures if they are taking **lamotrigine** for bipolar disorder also. To avoid withdrawal seizures, **lamotrigine** should be tapered off over 2 weeks.

Lamotrigine may cause increased seizures, including status epilepticus.

Drug Interactions

There are many drug interactions with **lamotrigine** due to enzyme induction that affect drug levels of both **lamotrigine** and the concurrently administered drugs. For example the enzyme inducers **carbamazepine, phenytoin, phenobarbital**, and **primidone** decrease **lamotrigine** concentrations by approximately 40 percent.

Oral estrogen-containing contraceptives decrease **lamotrigine** levels by approximately 50 percent. If the patient is already taking **lamotrigine** and an **oral contraceptive** is started the **lamotrigine** dose may need to be twice the normal dose. **Lamotrigine** decreases **levonorgestrel** levels by 19 percent when taken with combined **oral contraceptives**.

Rifampin decreases **lamotrigine** concentrations by 40 percent when taken concurrently.

The most concerning interaction with **lamotrigine** is with **valproate**. When **valproate** is administered concurrently with **lamotrigine** there is an increased risk of life-threatening rash such as Stevens-Johnson developing. **Valproate** also increases **lamotrigine** levels by more than 2-fold.

Clinical Use and Dosing

Dosing of **lamotrigine** is dependant on the concurrent medications the patient may be taking. It is critical to follow recommendations for initial dosing and the escalation schedule to avoid the development of life-threatening rashes. There are **Lamictal** starter kits and **Lamictal ODT** Patient Titration kits available for the first 5 weeks of treatment if adherence to escalation schedule is a concern.

Tablets should not be crushed or chewed. There is a chewable tablet that may be dissolved in water or juice if needed. Do not prescribe partial tablets of either regular or chewable tablets.

Dosing in Treating Seizures

Patients Not Taking Enzyme-Inducing AEDs

Patients age 12 years of age or older and adults who are not taking enzyme-inducing **AEDs** (**carbamazepine, phenytoin, primidone** or **valproate**) are started on 25 mg every day for two weeks. In weeks 3 and 4 the dosage is increased to 50 mg per day. In week 5 the **lamotrigine** dosage is increased 50 mg per day and dosage increases by 50 mg per day every 1 to 2 weeks until the usual maintenance dose of 225 mg to 375 mg per day in two divided doses.

The dosage for children age 2 years to 12 years of age with epilepsy who are not taking an enzyme-inducing **AED** begins with 0.3 mg/kg per day in one or two divided doses in weeks 1 and 2. The dosage should be rounded down to the nearest whole tablet and tablets should not be cut. In weeks 3 and 4 the dosage is 0.6 mg/kg per day in two divided doses rounded down to the nearest whole tablet. Starting in week 5 the dose is increased every 1 to 2 weeks by calculating 0.6 mg/kg/day, round this amount down to the nearest whole tablet and add this amount to the previously administered daily dose. The dose is titrated to to effect, with an average daily dose of 4.5 to 7.5 mg/kg per day. Maintenance dose may need to be increased by as much as 50 percent in children who weight less than 30 kg.

Patients Taking Enzyme-Inducing AEDs

For patients age 12 years an older taking **carbamazepine, phenytoin, phenobarbital** or **primidone** and not taking **valproate** the dose for the initial 2 weeks is 50 mg per day. In weeks 3 and 4 the dose is 100 mg per day in two divided doses. Beginning in week 5 the dose of **lamotrigine** is increased by 100 mg/day every 1 to 2 weeks to the usual maintenance dose of 300 to 500 mg per day in two divided doses.

The dosage in pediatric patients age 2 years to 12 years taking **carbamazepine, phenytoin, phenobarbital**, or **primidone** and not taking **valproate** is 0.6 mg/kg/day in

2 divided doses, rounded down to the nearest whole tablet for the first two weeks. In weeks 3 and 4 the dose is 1.2 mg/kg/day in 2 divided doses, rounded down to the nearest whole tablet. Beginning in week 5 the dose of **lamotrigine** is increased by 1.2 mg/kg/day, rounded down to the nearest whole tablet and added to the previously administered daily dose. The usual daily maintenance dose is 5 to 15 mg/kg per day, with a maximum of 400 mg per day in two divided doses. The maintenance dose of **lamotrigine** may need to be increased by as much as 50 percent in children who weight less than 30 kg.

Patients Taking Valporate

Valproate inhibits glucuronidation and decreases clearance of **lamotrigine**, therefore the escalation schedule is slower. The initial dose of **lamotrigine** in patients older than age 12 years is 25 mg per day for the first 4 weeks. Beginning in week 5 the dosage is increased 25 to 50 mg per day every one to two weeks. The usual maintenance dose of **lamotrigine** in patients taking **valproate** alone is 100 to 200 mg per day. If patients are taking **valproate** and other drugs that induce glucuronidation the usual maintenance dose is 100 to 400 mg per day.

In children age 2 years to 12 years taking **valproate** are started on 0.15 mg/kg per day of **lamotrigine** in 1 or 2 divided doses rounded down to the nearest whole tablet for the first two weeks. Children that weigh more than 6.7 kg and less than 14 kg are given 2 mg of **lamotrigine** every other day for weeks 1 and 2. The dose for weeks 3 and 4 is 0.3 mg/kg/day in 1 or 2 divided doses, rounded down to the nearest whole tablet. Beginning in week 5 calculate 0.3 mg/kg/day of **lamotrigine** and round this amount down to the nearest whole tablet and add this amount to the previously administered daily dose. The usual maintenance of **lamotrigine** in children taking **valproate** is 1 to 5 mg/kg per day with a maximum of 200 mg per day. The maintanence dose of **lamotrigine** may need to be increased by as much as 50 percent in children who weigh less than 30 kg.

Dosing in Bipolor Disease

The dosage of **lamotrigine** in adult patients with bipolar disorder who are not taking enzyme-inducing AEDs or **valproate** the initial dose is 25 mg daily for the first two weeks. During weeks 3 and 4 the dose is increased to 50 mg per day. Week 5 the dose of **lamotrigine** is increased to 100 mg per day. Week six the dose is increased to 200 mg per day, which is the maintenance dose of **lamotrigine**.

For patients taking **carbamazepine**, **phenytoin**, **phenobarbital** or **primidone** and not taking **valproate** the dose to treat bipolar disease for the initial 2 weeks is 50 mg per day. In weeks 3 and 4 the dose is 100 mg daily in divide doses. In week 5 the dose increases to 200 mg per day. The dose is increased to 300 mg per day in week 6, with the dose divided into two doses per day. In week 7 the **lamotrigine** dose is increased up to 400 mg per day in divided doses.

In bipolar patients taking **valproate** the initial dose of **lamotrigine** is 25 mg every other day for the first two weeks. In weeks 3 and 4 the dose is increased to 25 mg daily. The **lamotrigine** dose is increased to 50 mg per day in week 5. In week 6 the **lamotrigine** is increased to the maintenance dose of 100 mg daily.

Patients Taking Oral Contraceptives

Oral estrogen-containing contraceptives decrease **lamotrigine** levels by approximately 50 percent. If the patient is already taking **lamotrigine** and an **oral contraceptive** is started the **lamotrigine** dose is increased 50 mg per day weekly. The **lamotrigine** dose may need to be twice the normal dose.

Rational Drug Selection

Lamotrigine is the only drug in its class. Its use is determined by the type of seizures, concurrent medications and patient profile. Consultation with a neurologist is warranted when prescribing **lamotrigine**.

Monitoring

Patients should be monitored closely for any newly occurring rash and for hypersensitivity reactions. Complete blood count and differential should be monitored, as well as renal and hepatic function.

Patients need to be instructed to monitor seizure activity. Concurrent AED levels should be monitored.

Monitor for signs of suicidality or mood changes. Bipolar patients should be monitored for worsing depressive symptoms.

Patient Education

Administration

Patients need to be instructed to take **lamotrigine** exactly as prescribed. Patients should follow escalation schedule exactly. Tablets should not be crushed or chewed. Chewable tablets are chewed and washed down with a small amount of juice or water. Chewable tablets may be dissolved in a small amount of water or juice.

Adverse Reactions

Any rash needs to be reported to the provider immediately and the patient examined.

Patients and family members of patients taking **levetiracetam** should be warned about the potential neuropsychiatric ADRs, including suicidal thoughts and action, and behavioral changes. Any changes should be reported to the prescriber immediately.

Lifestyle Management

Patients who have seizures should get adequate sleep and exercise and avoid stressful situations that may trigger seizures.

ANTIDEPRESSANTS

The **antidepressants** are usually identified in five classes: **tricyclics (TCAs), selective serotonin reuptake inhibitors (SSRIs), monoamine oxidase inhibitors (MAOIs), serotonin-norepinephrine reuptake inhibitors (SNRIs), norepinephrine reuptake inhibitors (NRIs)**, and some miscellaneous drugs that do not easily fit one of the other categories.

As of 2007, all categories of **antidepressants** carry an FDA black box warning regarding increased risk of suicidal thought and behavior. This is most likely to occur in children, adolescents, and young adults to age 24 and is most likely to occur in the first 2 months of treatment. It is emphasized that depression and other serious psychiatric illnesses are themselves important causes of suicide. Providers and patients and their families must weigh benefits versus risks and if prescribed, monitor closely for suicidal ideation and behavior.

Tricyclic Antidepressants

The development of **TCAs** grew out of work with phenothiazines, to which they are structurally related. Prior to **TCAs'** availability in the 1960s, depression had been treated with **stimulants** and **tranquilizers**, both of which had some utility but left the basic mood disorder essentially unchanged. They were not overshadowed until the late 1980s, when the new **SSRIs** began to be widely marketed.

Although now used less frequently than in the past, **amitriptyline (Elavil), nortriptyline (Pamelor, Aventyl), imipramine (Tofranil), doxepin (Sinequan), trimipramine maleate (Surmontil), amoxapine (Asendin), desipramine (Norpramin, Pertofrane), protriptyline HCL (Vivactil)**, and **clomipramine (Anafranil)** still have their individual usefulness. Essentially, the **TCAs** are equally efficacious as the newer drugs in treating depression, cost less, but have much more troublesome side effects. Also the **TCAs** are less safe in treating depression in those who are at high risk for suicide because overdose can be fatal, whereas the newer **antidepressants** are much less likely to be fatal.

Pharmacodynamics

The **TCAs** act on the neurotransmitters serotonin and norepinephrine by inhibiting their reuptake at the presynaptic neuron. However, they also act on histamine (contributing to drowsiness and weight gain) and acetylcholine. **Loxapine**, an active metabolite of **amoxapine**, acts as an **antipsychotic** by blocking the dopamine receptor.

Pharmacokinetics

Absorption and Distribution

All the **TCAs** are administered orally, thoroughly absorbed, and highly lipophilic and protein bound. They have a fairly long half-life of elimination; therefore, steady state is achieved in approximately 5 days. There is a lag timeof 2 to 4 weeks before remission of depressive symptoms become apparent. Half-life ranges from 8 to 90 hours but averages 24 to 36 hours. Table 15–10 includes the pharmacokinetics of **TCAs**.

Metabolism and Excretion

The **TCAs** undergo first-pass metabolism by the liver and are excreted by the kidneys. At least two (**amitriptyline** and **imipramine**) of the **TCAs** are metabolized into active metabolites that further extend the half-life and contribute to the difficulty in overdosage.

Pharmacotherapeutics

Precautions and Contraindications

Due to their direct alpha-adrenergic blocking effect and **quinidine**-like effect on the myocardium, **TCAs** are contraindicated with cardiovascular disorders. Similarly, due to their acetylcholine blocking effect they should be used with caution in those who have glaucoma, prostatic hypertrophy, or urinary incontinence. They should not be prescribed in combination with **MAOIs**, or to individuals who have demonstrated hypersensitivity in this class.

Safety of use in pregnancy is unclear. **TCAs** are Pregnancy Category C and are excreted in low doses in breast milk.

Although rare, tardive dyskinesia and neuroleptic malignant syndrome have been reported, and are more likely with **amoxapine** use due to its dopaminergic effect.

As with any drug that affects the CNS, the **TCAs** should be titrated gradually in either direction. Nausea, headache, vertigo, malaise, and nightmares have been noted following abrupt discontinuance of the drug or after large dose decreases.

The most significant risks related to TCA use are cardiac conduction disorder. At highest risk are children and the elderly; therefore, baseline ECG and periodic monitoring should be performed. The most common cardiovascular effect is sinus tachycardia due to the inhibition of norepinephrine reuptake and anticholinergic action. In addition, **TCAs** contribute to slowing of depolarization of the cardiac muscle contributing to prolongation of the QRS complex and the PR/QT intervals.

TCAs can lower the seizure threshold of those with a seizure disorder or those taking medications that also decrease the seizure threshold. Because the index between therapeutic and toxic levels is narrow, great care needs to be taken when prescribing for a person who is depressed and has suicidal ideas. When treating such a person, the nurse practitioner needs to be alert for an energizing effect that precedes depressive symptom remission as this may contribute to sufficient activation to follow through with a suicidal plan. Such patients need to be monitored on a weekly basis, especially regarding suicidal thoughts and behaviors, and medication should be dispensed in only small amounts until suicidal risk decreases.

Finally, **TCAs** should be used with extreme caution if at all with the elderly. Due to their anticholinergic and norepinephrine effects, they can contribute to confusion, orthostatic hypotension, and falls.

Adverse Drug Reactions

Anticholinergic adverse effects are common and can include dry mouth, constipation, urinary hesitancy or retention, blurred vision, sedation, orthostatic hypotension, weight gain, nausea and vomiting, gynecomastia, and changes in libido. Patients newly prescribed a TCA should be cautioned about safety in a situation in which mental alertness is required until the full effect of the drug has been determined.

Drug Interactions

The most significant drug interactions are those that increase the plasma level of the TCA and thereby increase the risk of cardiotoxicity, such as can occur with the concurrent use of **SRIs**, **cannabis**, and **sympathomimetics**. Hyperpyrexia can occur with **MAOIs** and **TCAs**. Table 15–11 presents drug interactions.

Clinical Use and Dosing

The **TCAs** have shown efficacy in a variety of clinical conditions including depression, panic disorder, enuresis, and chronic neuropathic pain. Due to their serotonergic and noradrenergic effects, they are especially helpful with anxiety disorders such as obsessive-compulsive disorder (**clomipramine**) and panic disorder (**imipramine**). Some TCAs, especially secondary and tertiary amines, contribute to significant drowsiness as a side effect; therefore, they are more commonly used for insomnia than they are for depression. Most notable of the TCAs used for insomnia include **doxepin (Sinequan)**, **amitriptyline (Elavil)**, and **trazodone (Desyrel)**. **Amitriptyline** and **imipramine** are useful for neuropathic pain. Dosages are shown in Table 15–12.

Rational Drug Selection

Indications for the use of TCAs are depression, anxiety with sleep disturbance, enuresis in children 6 years or older, obsessive-compulsive disorder, and eating disorders. Prior to prescribing, the nurse practitioner needs to obtain a patient and family history of suicide and cardiovascular disease, as these are risk factors for adverse events. These drugs should be avoided with the elderly and used with caution with children.

Monitoring

A preliminary ECG should be done with QT correction and repeated after 3 weeks. Plasma levels can be assessed to assure delivery of an adequate dosage and to support patient adherence. Drugs with secondary active metabolites

Table 15–11 ■ **Drug Interactions: Tricyclic Antidepressants**

Drug	Interacting Drug	Possible Effect	Implications
All TCAs	SSRIs, anorexiants, cimetidine, oral contraceptives, charcoal, calcium channel blockers, protease inhibitors, propoxyphene, methylphenidate	Increased plasma level of TCA and increased risk of cardiotoxicity	Use with caution; monitor plasma levels of TCA
	Narcotics, barbiturates, antihistamines, alcohol, benzodiazepines, antipsychotics	Increased CNS depression; increased TCA plasma level; increased risk of cardiotoxicity	Use with caution; monitor plasma level of TCA
	Anticholinergics	Increased anticholinergic adverse reactions	Avoid concurrent use if possible
	Dicumarol	Increased prothrombin time	Monitor
	Carbamazepine, phenytoin	Increased plasma level of anticonvulsant	Monitor blood levels of anticonvulsants
	MAOIs	Hyperpyretic crisis, convulsions	Avoid concurrent use
	Guanethidine	Hypotension	Monitor blood pressure
	Clonidine	Hypertension	Monitor BP
	Levodopa	Hypertension, dyskinesia	Use different type of antidepressant
	Tamoxifen, nicotine, rifampin	Decreased TCA effect	May require higher dose
	Sympathomimetics	Hypertension, risk of arrhythmias	Avoid if possible
	Cannabis	Increased risk of cardiotoxicity, tachycardia, light-headedness, confusion, mood lability, delirium	Avoid

Table 15–12 ◉ **Dosage Schedule: Tricyclic Antidepressants**

Drug	Indications	Dosage	Available Dosage Forms	Cost (per 100 Units)
Amitriptyline (Elavil)	Depression, insomnia	*Adult:* 75 mg/d in divided doses to maximum of 150 mg/d; may give entire dose at bedtime; hospitalized patients may require 200–300 mg/d.	Tablets: 10, 25, 50, 75, 100, 150 mg	$10/any dose
		Adolescents and older adults: 10 tid or 25 mg at bedtime maximum 100 mg/d.	Syrup: 10 mg/5 mL	
Amoxapine (Asendin)	Depression, psychotic depression	*Adults and children >16*: 50 mg bid-tid, gradually increasing to 200–300 mg/d/ if needed; maximum 400 mg/d. If total dose equals 300 mg or more, give in divided doses. *Older adults:* 25 mg bid-tid; may gradually increase to maximum of 300 mg/d	Tablets: 25, 50, 100, 150 mg	$37/30 mg $46/50 mg $72/100 mg
Clomipramine	OCD	*Adults:* 25 mg/d initially, increase over 2 wk to maximum or 250 mg/d. Give with food to minimize GI distress. May divide dose initially, give at bedtime for maintenance.	Capsules: 25, 50, 75 mg	$17/25 mg $20/50 mg $31/75 mg
		Children and adolescents: 25 mg/d initially; may gradually increase over 2 wk to maximum of 3 mg/kg/d or 100 mg, whichever is smaller, or for adolescents, to maximum of 3 mg/kg/d or 200 mg, whichever is smaller.		
Desipramine HCl (Norpramin)	Depression	*Adults:* 100–200 mg/d in single or divided dose; maximum 300 mg/d *Adolescents and older adults:* 25–100 mg/d maximum 150 mg/d.	Tablets: 10, 25, 50, 75, 100, 150 mg	$23/10 mg $28/25 mg $45/50 mg $50/75 mg $65/100 mg
Doxepin HCl (Sinequan)	Depression, insomnia	*Adults*: 75–150 mg/d, preferably at hs; maximum 300 mg/d. Dilute concentrate with 120 mL of milk, water, or juice.	Capsules: 10, 25, 50, 75, 100, 150 mg Concentrate; 10 mg/mL	$11/25 mg $14/50 mg $16/75 mg $19/100 mg $38/150 mg
Imipramine HCl (Tofranil, Tofranil PM)	Depression, enuresis in children >6 yr	*Adults:* 50–150 mg/d at hs; maximum 200 mg/d. Hospitalized patients may require 250–300 mg/d.	Tablets: 10, 25, 50, 75,	
		Adolescents and older adults: 30–40 mg/d to maximum of 100 mg/d.	Capsules: 75, 100, 125, 150	
		Children: 1.5 mg/kg/d tid to maximum of 5 mg/kg/d. Increase by increments of 1–15 mg/kg/d at 3- to 5-d intervals.		

Table 15–12 ● **Dosage Schedule: Tricyclic Antidepressants—cont'd**

Drug	Indications	Dosage	Available Dosage Forms	Cost (per 100 Units)
Nortriptyline HCl (Pamelor, Aventyl)	Depression	*Adults:* 25 mg tid-qid to maximum of 100 mg/d.	Capsules: 10, 25, 50, 75 mg	$47/10 mg (Aventyl)
		Adolescents and older adults: 30–50 mg/d in divided doses.	Solution: 10 mg/5 mL	
Protriptyline HCl (Vivactil)	Depression	*Adults*: 100–200 mg/d in single or divided dose; maximum 60 mg/d. Make increase in a.m.	Tablets: 5, 10 mg	$95/5 mg
		Adolescents and older adults: 25–100 mg/d: maximum 150 mg/d.		$136/10 mg
Trimipramine maleate (Surmontil)	Depression	*Adults:* 75–150 mg/d in divided doses; maximum 200 mg/d. Hospitalized patients may require 250–300 mg/d. *Adolescents and older adults:* 50–100 mg/d.	Capsules: 25, 50, 100 mg	$107/25 mg $175/50 mg $254/100 mg

will show the plasma level in terms of each metabolite as well as a total level. Again, suicidal ideation must be monitored carefully during the first month after initiation, then periodically if residual depressive symptoms remain.

Patient Education

Advise the patient to avoid engaging in hazardous activities or using heavy machinery if drowsy or sedated. If the patient develops dry mouth, advise him or her to use sugarless candy or gum. If constipation develops, advise patient to increase fluid and fiber intake and to use a bulking agent or stool softener.

Monoamine Oxidase Inhibitors

MAOIs are infrequently used in mental health nursing and psychiatry today because safer drugs that are equally efficacious are available. If the nurse practitioner decides to prescribe these drugs, it is advisable to do so with expert consultation. These drugs are primarily reserved for the treatment of refractory unipolar depression. There are four MAOIs available: **phenelzine** (Nardil), **isocarboxazid** (Marplan), **tranylcypromine** (Parnate), and **selegiline** (Emsam), a transdermal preparation.

Pharmacodynamics

The MAOIs exert their effect by irreversibly inactivating the enzymes that metabolize norepinephrine, serotonin, and dopamine, thereby increasing the bioavailability of these neurotransmitters. In addition, they prevent the breakdown of tyramine found in many foods that are aged or fermented. Because tyramine is toxic to humans, contributing to rapid extreme hypertension, these drugs require careful dietary restrictions. **Selegiline transdermal** (Emsam) requires dietary restriction only for doses above 9 mg in 24 hours.

Pharmacokinetics

Absorption and Distribution

The MAOIs are administered orally, and are rapidly and thoroughly absorbed from the GI tract.

Metabolism and Excretion

There is a major first-pass effect of liver metabolism, and most of these drugs have P450 2D6 as a substrate. They are excreted by the liver. Half-life is variable within 1 to 3 hours. They are excreted by the kidneys.

Onset, Peak, and Duration

Whereas SRIs and TCAs have long half-lives, requiring 3 to 4 weeks before full therapeutic benefits are evident, patients taking MAOIs may begin to experience relief of their depressive symptoms immediately or within approximately 14 days. Onset is 1 to 2 weeks; the peak for **isocarboxazid** and **tranylcypromine** is 0.7 to 3 hours and 1 to 2 hours for **phenelzine**.

Pharmacotherapeutics

Precautions and Contraindications

Contraindications include liver or kidney disease, hypersensitivity, congestive heart failure or arteriosclerotic disease, and age over 60 years. They should not be used with patients who are impulsive, cognitively impaired, or cannot follow the necessary dietary restrictions.

These drugs are rated Pregnancy Category C. They are excreted in breast milk, and safety has not been established. They have not been approved for use with children.

Postural hypotension and suppression of myocardial pain may occur.

Adverse Drug Reactions

Initial adverse effects may include insomnia, anxiety, and agitation as a result of the delayed metabolism of dopamine. In addition, dry mouth, blurred vision, urinary retention, and constipation occur due to anticholinergic activity. Most common side effects include dizziness, headache, insomnia, restlessness, and hypotension.

Clinical Use and Dosing

Because safer and more convenient drugs are available, the MAOIs are reserved for drug-resistant, refractory depressions.

Drug and Food Interactions

Because **MAOIs** inhibit the metabolism of norepinephrine, hypertensive crisis can occur if they are administered concurrently with other drugs or foods that raise blood pressure, including anticholinergics, sympathomimetics, stimulants, and foods containing tyramine. Tyramine is a precursor to dopamine, norepinephrine, and epinephrine. Foods that have been aged or fermented are rich in tyramine; therefore, dietary restrictions apply during use or within 14 days following discontinuance of the **MAOI**.

Symptoms of hypertensive crisis include headache, heart palpitations, stiff or sore neck, chest tightness, tachycardia, sweating, and dilated pupils. The crisis needs to be managed immediately, and the patient should remain standing until it is. Usual treatment is **phentolamine (Regitine)** 5 mg IV and then 0.25 to 0.5 mg IM every 4 to 6 hours.

The prolonged metabolism of norepinephrine and the pressor effect of other drugs can lead to interactions resulting in hypotension and heart failure.

The 14-day restriction discussed previously also applies to initiating **SRI** or **SNRI** drug treatment. The increased amount of serotonin available due to inhibition of its metabolism by the **MAOI** leads to a risk of the potentially fatal serotonin syndrome.

As a result of other drug interactions, particularly with meperidine, CNS depression can also occur. Table 15–13 presents drug interactions.

Rational Drug Selection

Use of **MAOIs** should be limited to conditions that are resistant to other forms of pharmacotherapy. Most notably, **MAOIs** have been used with treatment-resistant unipolar depression, panic disorder, and atypical depression associated with borderline personality disorder.

Monitoring

Periodic liver function tests should be performed and the drug discontinued if any abnormalities are found.

Patient Education

Advise the patient that strict dietary restrictions need to be followed. Provide a written list of foods to be avoided, including cheese, yogurt, sour cream, aged meat and meat products, dried fish and herring, alcoholic beverages, fermented vegetables such as sauerkraut, soy sauce, miso

Table 15–13 ■ Drug Interactions: Monoamine Oxidase Inhibitors

Drug	Interacting Drug	Possible Effect	Implications
All MAOIs	Anorexiants, venlafaxine, SSRIs, bupropion, bromocriptine, L-dopa, L-tryptophan, MAO-B inhibitor, sumatriptan	Increased serotonergic effect, possible serotonin syndrome	Avoid
	CNS depressants, meperidine, antipsychotics	Increased CNS depression	Use cautiously in hazardous situations
Amphetamines	Buspirone, L-dopa, reserpine, tetrabenazine, guanethidine, meperidine	Increased blood pressure and possible hypertensive crisis	Monitor blood pressure; avoid if possible
	Antihypertensives, propoxyphene, meperidine, diuretics, nitroglycerin, dextromethorphan	Hypotension agitation diaphoresis, vascular collapse	Monitor blood pressure; avoid concurrent administration if possible
	Insulin, sulfonylureas	Hypoglycemia	Monitor blood glucose and for signs and symptoms of hypoglycemia
	Carbamazepine	Increased carbamazepine level	Monitor level; use alternative anticonvulsant if possible
	TCAs and SSRIs	Seizures and delirium	Avoid

soup, bean curd, fava beans, avocados, bananas, raisins, caffeine, chocolate, and ginseng.

Selective Serotonin Reuptake Inhibitors

The SSRIs were first approved by the FDA in 1985 with the introduction of **fluoxetine (Prozac)** and quickly followed by **paroxetine (Paxil)**, **sertraline (Zoloft)**, **fluvoxamine (Luvox)**, **citalopram (Celexa)**, and most recently **escitalopram (Lexapro)**. Because of their safety and equitable efficacy, they have exceeded the prescriptions for TCAs and MAOIs.

Pharmacodynamics

All the SRIs affect the serotonin neurotransmitter in the synaptic cleft by blocking the serotonin transporter from returning remaining serotonin to the presynaptic cell. Although traditionally these drugs are referred to as *selective* serotonin reuptake inhibitors, each one has different effects on other neurotransmitters. For example, **fluoxetine** significantly affects dopamine that contributes to the development of side effects. **Citalopram** and **escitalopram** are probably the closest to serotonin selective reuptake inhibitor. Through this mechanism, more serotonin is available to bind with the postsynaptic receptors.

Pharmacokinetics

Absorption and Distribution

All of the SRIs are given orally and thoroughly absorbed through the gastrointestinal tract. They are all highly protein bound with variable biodistribution ranging from 12 to 40 L/kg. Peak plasma levels range from 1 to 8 hours, and have a positive correlation with parent half-life.

Metabolism and Excretion

The SRIs have a significant first-pass effect in the liver and are metabolized predominantly by the CYP450 system. Consideration of the half-life requires consideration of active metabolites as well as the possibility of inhibiting its own metabolism. For example, **fluoxetine** as the parent drug has a half-life of 1 to 3 days and its first metabolite, norfluoxetine, has an additional half-life of 4 to 16 days, resulting in an overall half-life of 4 to 16 days. Similarly, **sertraline** has a half-life of 24 to 26 hours but inhibits the P450 2D6 enzyme that is also the substrate for metabolism. Table 15–14 presents the pharmacokinetics of SSRIs.

Excretion of the SSRIs is primarily by the kidneys.

Pharmacotherapeutics

Precautions and Contraindications

Contraindications to use are limited to hypersensitivity to any of the drugs and concurrent or within 14 days of the administration of an MAOI. They should be used cautiously in patients with severe hepatic or renal impairment and should be avoided in the first and last trimesters of pregnancy. Although safety of use during pregnancy has not been definitively established, **sertraline** in particular has been used without adverse consequences. Risk versus benefit needs to be carefully considered, as it does during lactation as well. Caution is recommended. **Fluvoxamine** is Pregnancy Category C, and the others are Category B. Children generally require smaller doses than do adolescents or adults, although some of these agents have not been tested specifically with children. Elderly patients generally are prescribed the same doses as younger patients.

Although clinical drug trials do not substantiate a link between SRIs and suicidal thinking, there is clearly a greater risk of suicide within the first 3 weeks of taking SRIs and other **antidepressants**. This is related to the lag time in receiving full therapeutic effect while there is an increase in neurocognitive activation early in initiation of

Table 15–14 ▶ **Pharmacokinetics: SNRIs, SRIs, and Other Antidepressants**

Drug	Peak	Duration	Half-Life	Excretion
Trazodone	1–2 h	Long-acting	3–9 h	Urine, feces
Fluoxetine HCl	6–8 h	Long-acting	1–384 h	Urine
Fluvoxamine maleate	3–8 h	Long-acting	16 h	Urine
Nefazodone HCl	1 h	Long-acting	2–18 h	Urine, feces
Mirtazapine	12 h	Long-acting	20–40 h	Urine, feces
Bupropion HCl	2 h	Long-acting	21–37 h	Urine
Paroxetine HCl	5.2 h	Long-acting	21–33 h	Urine
Sertraline HCl	4.5–8 h	Long-acting	26 h	Urine
Venlafaxine	1–3 h	Long-acting	5–11 h	Urine
Citalopram	4 h	Long-acting	35 h	Urine
Escitalopram	5 h	Long-acting	27–32 h	Urine

the drug. Therefore, patients have greater energy to act on suicidal thoughts.

Adverse Drug Reactions

Adverse reactions to this group of drugs depend on which receptors are affected but are usually relatively minor and transient. Most common are nausea and sometimes vomiting, headache, light-headedness, dizziness, dry mouth, increased sweating, weight gain or loss, exacerbation of anxiety, and agitation. Sexual side effects may occur in up to 35 percent of patients and manifests as diminished, delayed, or absent orgasm; premature ejaculation; and decreased libido. A patient may not experience the same sexual side effects with other **SRIs** and it is reasonable to decrease the dosage or change to another medication if they develop.

A significant adverse effect is serotonin syndrome, which occurs in the presence of excessive serotonergic activity. Therefore, maximum recommended doses must be adhered to, adjunctive combinations of serotonergic agents must be avoided, and adequate time for titration when changing from one serotonergic to another must be provided. A safe guideline when making such a change is to allow five half-lives per dose decrease, so that titrating off a 20-mg dose of **paroxetine** would need 5 days at 10 mg before starting another serotonergic drug. Symptoms of serotonin syndrome are nausea, diarrhea, chills, sweating, hyperthermia, hypertension, myoclonic jerking, tremor, agitation, ataxia, disorientation, confusion, and delirium. It can progress to coma and death.

Several years after the **SSRIs** had been on the market, it became apparent that some have a significant withdrawal syndrome that can be very disturbing to patients. In fact, the shorter half-life drugs such as **paroxetine, sertraline, citalopram,** and **escitalopram** can show withdrawal symptoms with just one missed dose. These symptoms are nausea, dizziness, and paresthesias such as electric shock sensations or visual tracers with eye movements. **Fluoxetine** is the only **SSRI** that does not require gradual and slow tapering because of its long half-life and active metabolites. In fact, a single dose of **fluoxetine** as the last step in tapering off other **SSRIs** is helpful in avoiding withdrawal symptoms.

Drug Interactions

Significant drug interactions may occur. As previously mentioned, the most significant are with **MAOIs** and other serotonergic drugs. With **MAOIs** there needs to be at least a 14-day washout period before initiating an **SSRI** and at least 21 days washout of **fluoxetine** before initiating an **MAOI**. Drugs that inhibit the P450 2D6 will increase the effects of the **SRI** and many **SRIs** inhibit the 2D6 and 3A3/4 and will interact with drugs that use these enzymes as substrates. CNS depression can occur with **alcohol, antihistamines**, and **opioid analgesics**. Concomitant use of **St. John's wort** and/or **SAMe** (S-adenosylmethionine) may contribute to serotonin syndrome. **SSRIs** should not be prescribed with **TCAs** and require washout between drugs. The **SSRI** may increase the plasma level of the **TCA**, which increases the risk of cardiac conduction complications. Table 15–15 includes the drug interactions with the **SRIs**.

Clinical Use and Dosages

Table 15–16 includes the indications, dosages, and available forms for the **SRIs** and **non-TCA antidepressants**.

Table 15–15 ■ **Drug Interactions: Selective Serotonin Reuptake Inhibitors (SSRIs)**

Drug	Interacting Drug	Possible Effect	Implications
All (SSRIs)	Anorexiants, ergotamine, tryptophan	Serotonin syndrome	Avoid; or use with caution
	MAOIs	Hypertensive crisis	Contraindicated
	Valproate carbamazepine	Increased level of anticonvulsant	Monitor plasma levels
	TCAs	Increased level of TCA, increased risk of cardiotoxicity	Monitor blood levels of TCA; use with caution
	Benzodiazepines	Increased plasma level of benzodiazepines with sedation and psychomotor/cognitive impairment	Avoid long-term use of benzodiazepines
	Beta blockers	Bradycardia, syncope, increased serum levels of SSRI	Warn patient
	Insulin	Increased insulin sensitivity	Monitor blood glucose
	Neuroleptics	Increased plasma level of neuroleptic	Monitor for adverse reactions
	Zolpidem	Hallucinations and delirium	Avoid
	Aspirin, NSAIDs	Risk of bleeding increased	Caution
	Alcohol	May potentiate alcohol effects	Avoid

Table 15–16 ◉ **Dosage Schedule: Non-TCA Antidepressants**

Drug	Indications	Neurotransmitters Affected	Dosage	Available Dosage Forms
Bupropion (Wellbutrin, Wellbutrin SR, Wellbutrin XL)	Depression, Seasonal Affective disorder	Dopamine, norepinephrine	*Adolescents and adults:* 75–450 mg/d; give 2–3 times/d with 6-h intervals in between; no single dose to exceed 150 mg; increase at 3- to 4-d intervals Wellbutrin XL 150–300 mg qAM	Tablets: 75, 100 mg Sustained-release tablets: 75, 100 mg Extended release: 150, 300 mg
Citalopram (Celexa)	Depression, anxiety (off-labeled)	Primary: serotonin Secondary: norepinephrine and dopamine	*Adults:* 20 mg qd; may increase in 20-mg increments at weekly intervals; maximum 60 mg/d *Older adults:* 20 mg/d	Tablets: 10, 20, 40 mg
Desvenlafaxine (Pristiq)	Depression	Serotonin, Norepinephrine	*Adults:* 50 mg qam, max 100 mg/d	Tabs, extended-release 50, 100 mg
Duloxetine (Cymbalta)	Depression, diabetic neuropathy, fibromyalgia, anxiety	Serotonin and norepinephrine	*Adults*: 40–60 mg/d max 60 mg 60 mg for neuropathy and fibromyalgia	Tablets: 20, 30, 60 mg
Escitalopram (Lexapro)	Depression, anxiety	Serotonin	*Adults:* 10 mg qam, Max 20 mg qd *Children 12 and up:* 10 mg, may increase to 20 mg after 3 weeks	5, 10, 20 mg tabs Oral solution 1 mg/mL
Fluoxetine (Prozac)	Depression, OCD, bulimia, panic disorder	Primary: serotonin Secondary: norepinephrine	*Adolescents and adults:* 20–80 mg/d; may increase slowly at 5-d intervals after 3- to 4-wk trial at lower dose; OCD may require a higher dose *Children 8–17:* 10 mg qd, increase by 10 mg in 1 wk. Slower titration with lower weight children *Older adults:* half dose	Capsules: 10,0 mg, 40 Liquid: 20 mg/5 mL Delayed-release capsules: 90 mg
Fluvoxamine (Luvox)	OCD, social anxiety disorder, Depression (off-labeled)	Primary: serotonin Secondary: norepinephrine	*Adults:* 50–300 mg/d; dose >100 mg should be divided; increase in 50-mg increments every 4–7 d *Older adults:* half dose	Tablets: 50, 100 mg
Mirtazapine (Remeron, Remeron Soltabs)	Depression	Primary: histamine Secondary: serotonin and norepinephrine	*Adults:* 15–45 mg/d, preferably at bedtime Disintegrating Soltab: 15, 30, 45 mg Lower doses may increase sedation	Tablets: 15, 30, 45 mg
Nefazodone	Depression	Primary: serotonin Secondary: adrenergic	*Adults:* 200–600 mg/d in 2 divided doses; increase in 100- to 200-mg/d increments at weekly intervals	Tablets: 50, 100, 150, 200, 250 mg
Paroxetine (Paxil, Paxil CR)	Depression, OCD, panic disorder, social phobia, PTSD, anxiety, PMDD (CR)	Primary: serotonin Secondary: norepinephrine	*Adolescents and adults:* 20–60 mg/d; panic disorder and OCD may require higher doses; taper off slowly *Older adults:* half dose	Tablets: 10, 20, 30, 40 mg Control-release: 12.5, 25 Oral suspension: 10 mg/5 mL

Continued

Table 15–16 ● **Dosage Schedule: Non-TCA Antidepressants—cont'd**

Drug	Indications	Neurotransmitters Affected	Dosage	Available Dosage Forms
Sertraline (Zoloft)	Depression, OCD, GAD, PMDD, PTSD, Social anxiety disorder	Primary: serotonin Secondary: norepinephrine	*Adolescents and adults:* 50–200 mg/d; increase at weekly intervals *Older adults:* half dose	Tablets: 25, 50, 100 mg Concentrate: 20 mg/mL
Trazodone (Desyrel)	Depression, Off label for sleep	Primary: serotonin Secondary: adrenergic	*Adults:* 50–400 mg/d; increase in 50-mg increments every 3–4 d; take with food	Tablets: 50, 100, 150, 300 mg
Venlafaxine (Effexor)	Depression, PTSD, GAD, social anxiety, panic disorder	Primary: serotonin Secondary: norepinephrine	*Adults:* 75–375 mg/d in divided doses. When discontinuing, taper off over a 2-wk period; increase in 75-mg increments at 4-d intervals; take with food Extended-release: 37.5, 75, 150 mg	Tablets: 25, 37.5, 50, 75, 100 mg

Rational Drug Selection

The SRIs, with the exception of **fluvoxamine**, are indicated for the treatment of depressive, anxiety, and panic disorders; obsessive-compulsive disorder (OCD); and bulimia. **Fluvoxamine** is FDA-approved for the treatment of OCD, although it is likely to be as effective as the others for the listed disorders. More recently the FDA has approved the indication for premenstrual dysphoric disorder, post-traumatic disorder, generalized anxiety disorder, and social phobia.

Off-labeled uses include the treatment of anorexia, depressive phase of bipolar disorder, chronic headaches and other types of pain, impulse control disorders, and trichotillomania.

The patient needs to be monitored closely during the first 2 to 3 weeks of initiation of **SRIs** including regular assessment of suicidal thinking. There should be at least telephone contact on a weekly basis with an agreement to notify the prescriber immediately if suicidal thoughts occur or persist.

Monitoring

No specific monitoring is required.

Patient Education

Advise the patient that these drugs may take as long as 3 to 4 weeks until their full therapeutic benefits become evident and that the initial adverse reactions, commonly including nausea, intermittent light-headedness, sedation, muscle restlessness, and sleep disruptions, should be minor and transient. Also, tell the patient to assess the level of sedation the drug can initially cause before engaging in hazardous activities. Patients also need to be reminded not to miss a dose or let their prescription run out before seeking a refill because of the withdrawal syndrome.

Serotonin-Norepinephrine Reuptake Inhibitors (SNRIs)

In the United States there are three **SNRIs** that have been approved by the FDA: **venlafaxine (Effexor and Effexor XR)**, **desvenlafaxine (Pristiq)**, and **duloxetine (Cymbalta)**. Although **venlafaxine** has been available since 1996, **duloxetine** and **desvenlafaxine** were approved more recently. **Nefazodone** is a serotonin antagonist and reuptake inhibitor that also inhibits the reuptake of norepinephrine. It is available only in generic form. In 2004, the FDA added a black box warning to **nefazodone** related to liver toxicity in 1 out of 250,000 cases of those taking **nefazodone** and 21 deaths related to liver failure. It will not be discussed in detail in this chapter.

Pharmacodynamics

Venlafaxine and **duloxetine** both block the serotonin and norepinephrine transporters, thereby inhibiting the reuptake of the neurotransmitter and increasing the availability to bind with the postsynaptic receptors. At lower doses (75 mg), **venlafaxine** predominantly affects serotonin reuptake, contributing to greater anxiety reduction more so than depressive symptom reduction. **Duloxetine**, however, appears to be a more potent and equal serotonin and norepinephrine reuptake inhibitor than **venlafaxine** is.

In contrast, **nefazodone** blocks the serotonin and norepinephrine transporters as well as occupies the serotonin 2 (5-HT_2) receptor. By blocking the 5-HT_2 receptor, there are significantly less sexual side effects and less weight gain.

Pharmacokinetics

Absorption and Distribution

These drugs are rapidly absorbed after oral intake and metabolized extensively in the liver. Time needed to reach maximum plasma concentration is 2 hours for both venlafaxine and duloxetine. **Venlafaxine** has only 30 percent protein binding whereas **duloxetine** is greater than 90 percent.

Metabolism and Excretion

Venlafaxine is metabolized by CYP450 2D6 with one active metabolite (O-desmethylvenlafaxine) and two less active metabolites. **Duloxetine** is metabolized by CYP450 2D6 and 1A2. **Venlafaxine** has a half-life of 5 hours and the active metabolite is 11 hours. Steady state is achieved in 3 to 4 days. **Duloxetine** has a half-life of 12 hours, reaching steady state in 3 days. Both drugs are excreted mostly in the urine.

Pharmacotherapeutics

Precautions and Contraindications

As with other drugs used to treat depression, a major precaution is increased suicidal thinking during the first few weeks of initiation and change in dosage of the medication. The patient must be monitored at least weekly and assessed for suicide risk each time. In addition, hypersensitivity to **venlafaxine** or **duloxetine** contraindicates its use. Similarly, there needs to be patient monitoring for mood lability and switching into a manic or hypomanic state.

Both **venlafaxine** and **duloxetine** are rated as Pregnancy Category C for pregnant and lactating women. A recent study, however, showed that the use of **venlafaxine** during pregnancy did not increase the incidence of fetal malformations or low birth weight infants (Einarson et al, 2001). **Duloxetine** has been tested only in animal studies and there is insufficient information regarding pregnancy in humans to evaluate the risk of use during pregnancy. Both **venlafaxine** and **duloxetine** has been found in breast milk.

Duloxetine may exacerbate narrow-angle glaucoma and should be used cautiously with these patients. **Duloxetine** has also shown increased serum transaminase levels and should not be used with patients with liver disorders.

Adverse Drug Reactions

The most common side effects with both **venlafaxine** and **duloxetine** include headache, somnolence, dizziness, insomnia, nervousness, nausea, dry mouth, constipation, and abnormal ejaculations. Appetite and weight decreases may occur. At higher doses, both drugs may contribute to elevated blood pressure. There was no effect shown to the QTc interval with either of these drugs.

Drug Interactions

Drugs that inhibit CYP450 2D6 will interact with both **venlafaxine** and **duloxetine** including **fluoxetine** and **quinidine**. With **duloxetine**, drugs that inhibit 1A2 will also interact, especially **fluvoxamine** and some **quinolone antibiotics**. There seems to be no interaction with **alcohol** and either **venlafaxine** or **duloxetine**; however, frequent use of **alcohol** may affect the liver function and therefore **duloxetine** should not be used with patients who abuse or are dependent on **alcohol**.

Clinical Use and Dosing

These drugs are indicated in treating major depressive disorders and bipolar mood disorders. **Venlafaxine** is also approved for treating anxiety disorders such as generalized anxiety disorder, social phobia, and post-traumatic stress disorder. **Duloxetine** is also approved to treat neuropathic pain and overactive bladder. It is likely that **duloxetine**, due to its neurophysiological action, will eventually be approved for treating anxiety disorders as well.

Venlafaxine is available in extended-release (XR) form as well as immediate release. The immediate release must be taken at least twice a day and has uncomfortable discontinuation symptoms if doses are missed, including paresthesias, dizziness, nausea, and vomiting. The initial dose for **venlafaxine XR** is 75 mg/day and increased to 150 to 300 mg/day in increments of 75 mg every 4 days. Severely depressed patients may require a higher dosage of 375 to 450 mg/day in divided doses to prevent side effects.

The initial dose of **duloxetine** is 20 mg/day and increased to 60 mg/day in increments of 20 mg every 4 days. There is no evidence that doses higher than 60 mg/day produces better results than 60 mg/day. **Desvenlafaxine (Pristiq)**, an active metabolite of **venlafaxine**, is available only in extended-release capsules.

Rational Drug Selection

Initially, it was thought that **duloxetine** would be especially effective for patients with melancholic depressions or the type of depressions with low energy, hypersomnia, low motivation, and social withdrawal. However, the results have been inconclusive about this selective and difficult-to-treat population. Both **venlafaxine** and **duloxetine** are more activating than the SSRIs and therefore are first-line drugs to use with patients who have the more sluggish types of depression. **Venlafaxine** also seems effective with adults who have both depression and attention deficit-hyperactivity disorder.

Monitoring

No specific serum level monitoring is available for either of these drugs. With **duloxetine**, liver function should be monitored once weekly, once monthly, biannually, and finally annually. All patients taking **antidepressants** need to be carefully monitored for suicidal risk as well as activation of hypomanic or manic symptoms.

Patient Education

Patients should be given written descriptions of side effects and ways to relieve them. Women of childbearing age need to be told to report if pregnant and should be tapered off medication, especially in the third trimester. As with the SSRIs, sudden discontinuation frequently results in uncomfortable withdrawal symptoms; and patients need to request refill prescriptions in an adequate amount of time to avoid running out.

ANTIPSYCHOTICS

Since 1952, when **chlorpromazine** (Thorazine) was first used to treat psychosis, there has been substantial growth in the types of **antipsychotic** agents available. **Antipsychotic drugs** (APs) are generally divided into two major categories of drugs, although numerous specific classes exist. The older **APs** are variably termed conventional, traditional, or typical **antipsychotics**. They are also referred to as **neuroleptics** or major **tranquilizers**. The newer APs are generally termed **atypical antipsychotics**. In this chapter, the older **APs** will be termed **typical APs** and the newer agents will be termed **atypical APs**. The specific classes of APs and examples of these include the **benzisoxazoles** (**risperidone, ziprasidone**), **butyrophenones** (**haloperidol**), **dibenzoxazepines** (**loxapine**), **dibenzodiazepines** (**clozapine**), **dibenzothiazepines** (**quetiapine**), **dihydroindolones** (**molindone**), **diphenylbutylpiperidines** (**pimozide**), **phenothiazines** (**chlorpromazine**), **quinolinones** (**aripiprazole**), **thienobenzodiazepines** (**olanzapine**), and **thioxanthenes** (**thiothixene**).

Traditionally, it was believed that overstimulation of dopamine (D) receptors was at the heart of schizophrenia. This theory, called the dopamine hypothesis, formed the basis for understanding the effect of **typical APs** in reducing the positive symptoms of schizophrenia such as hallucinations and delusions. A more current hypothesis is that schizophrenia involves overactivity of D_2 receptors in the basal ganglia, hypothalamus, limbic system, brainstem, and medulla, and underactivity of D_1 receptors in the prefrontal cortex. The overactivity of these D_2 receptors is thought to contribute to the positive symptoms of schizophrenia, whereas the underactivity of D_1 receptors explains the negative symptoms of schizophrenia such as lack of motivation and social isolation. As new knowledge of the brain evolves, it is apparent that it is not a simple question of too much or too little of a neurotransmitter (NT), but where is there too much, too little, or an imbalance of neurotransmitters.

Typical Antipsychotics

The **phenothiazine** group of **typical APs** includes **chlorpromazine** (**Thorazine**), **thioridazine** (**Mellaril**), **fluphenazine** (**Prolixin**) and **fluphenazine decanoate**, **perphenazine** (**Trilafon**), and **trifluoperazine** (**Stelazine**). Nonphenothiazine **typical APs** include **haloperidol** (**Haldol**) and **haloperidol decanoate**, **thiothixene** (**Navane**), **loxapine** (**Loxitane**), and **molindone** (**Moban**).

Pharmacodynamics

The **typical APs** block D_2 receptors in the basal ganglia, hypothalamus, limbic system, brainstem, and medulla and reduce the positive symptoms of schizophrenia. **Typical APs**, however, are less effective in treating the negative symptoms of schizophrenia such as flat affect, decreased motivation, withdrawal from interpersonal relationships, and poor grooming and hygiene. Clinical effectiveness occurs when 60 to 70 percent of D_2 receptors are blocked. Too much dopamine blockade, however, leads to symptoms resembling those of parkinsonism. Prolactin elevation appears beyond 72 percent D_2 occupancy. As D_2 occupancy nears 78 percent, extrapyramidal symptoms (EPSs) are more prominent.

Pharmacokinetics

Absorption and Distribution

Typical APs are usually administered orally, although parenteral versions and long-acting decanoate forms of **haloperidol** and **fluphenazine** are available. The drugs are absorbed rapidly and distributed widely to adipose tissue. Onset of action varies among agents. Onset of oral agents is generally within 1 to 2 hours, IM injections within 10 to 30 minutes, and decanoate forms within 1 to 9 days.

Metabolism and Excretion

Typical APs are metabolized in the liver and excreted in the urine. Half-life varies widely among agents and types of agents. Because of their lipid solubility, several weeks may be required before their antipsychotic benefits become evident.

Table 15–17 presents the pharmacokinetics.

Pharmacotherapeutics

Precautions and Contraindications

Typical APs may be grouped according to whether they are high or low potency. High-potency drugs such as **haloperidol** and **fluphenazine** carry an increased risk of causing EPSs, whereas low-potency drugs such as **chlorpromazine** and **thioridazine** carry less risk of EPSs, but more risk of anticholinergic adverse reactions (dry mouth, constipation, urinary retention, blurred vision) and antiadrenergic effects (orthostatic hypotension).

Contraindications for use may include narrow-angle glaucoma, bone marrow depression, and severe liver or cardiovascular disease. These agents should be used cautiously in the presence of CNS tumors, epilepsy, diabetes mellitus, respiratory disease, and prostatic hypertrophy. Safety is not established in pregnancy and lactation.

All **antipsychotic** medications now have an FDA black box warning regarding increased mortality in elderly patients with dementia-related psychosis and are not approved for the treatment of such patients.

Adverse Drug Reactions

Typical APs have many adverse effects that make compliance a common issue. A life-threatening adverse reaction is neuroleptic malignant syndrome (NMS) characterized by fever up to 107°F, elevated pulse, diaphoresis, rigidity, stupor or coma, and acute renal failure. EPSs are among the most troublesome side effects and include pseudoparkinsonism (shuffling, pill-rolling, cog-wheeling, tremors, drooling,

Table 15–17 ▶ **Pharmacokinetics: Typical Antipsychotics**

Drug	Onset	Peak	Duration	Half-Life	Excretion
Chlorpromazine HCl	Erratic	2–4 h	Up to 6 mo	10–30 h	Urine
Fluphenazine	1 h	—	6–8 h	4.7–15.3 h	Urine
Fluphenazine decanoate	1 h 1–3 d	2–4 h: 2–3 d	6–8 h; up to 4 wk	6.8–14.3 d	Urine
Perphenazine	Erratic	2–4 h	6 h	12–24 h	Urine
Trifluoperazine	Erratic	2–4 h	4–6 h	13 h	Urine and feces equally
Thioridazine HCl	Erratic	2–4 h	4–6 h	24–36 h	Urine
Thiothixene	Slow	2–8 h	Up to 12 h	34 h	Urine
Loxapine	20–30 min	2–4 h	12 h	5–19 h	Urine
Pimozide	—	6–8 h	—	55 h	Urine
Haloperidol	2 h	2–6 h	8–12 h	21–24 h	Urine
Haloperidol decanoate	3–9 d	—	Up to 4 wk	12–36 h; 3 wk	Urine, bile
Molindone HCl	Erratic	1.5 h	24–36 h	10–20 h	Urine and feces equally

rigidity), akathisia (restlessness), dystonia (involuntary, painful movements), and tardive dyskinesia (involuntary buccolingual movements, difficulty speaking and swallowing, which may be irreversible). Antiparkinson, antihistamine, and anticholinergic drugs are given to counter EPSs. Other side effects of **typical APs** include sedation, weight gain, anticholinergic effects, photosensitivity, reduction of seizure threshold, orthostatic hypotension, sexual dysfunction, galactorrhea, and amenorrhea.

Drug Interactions

Drug interactions are many and varied, the most serious of which is CNS depression with concomitant use of CNS depressants. There may be additive hypotension with **antihypertensives. Lithium** in combination with a **phenothiazine** increases the risk of EPSs and masks the early signs of **lithium** toxicity. There is an increased risk of anticholinergic effects with other agents having anticholinergic properties.

Table 15–18 presents drug interactions.

Clinical Use and Dosing

Typical APs are more effective in reducing the positive than they are the negative symptoms of schizophrenia. **Typical APs** may be more effective than **atypical APs** in treating very severe psychosis. Patients who need rapid

Table 15–18 ■ **Drug Interactions: Typical Antipsychotics**

Drug	Interacting Drug	Possible Effect	Implications
	Alcohol, antihistamines, barbiturates, hypnotics, narcotics, benzodiazepines	CNS depression	Avoid; monitor for adverse reactions
	Lithium	Increased risk of neurotoxicity and EPS	Monitor lithium levels and signs and symptoms of toxicity
	Lithium, antacids, cimetidine	Decreased antipsychotic effect	May require increased antipsychotic dose
	Anticholinergics	Increased anticholinergic effect; increased risk of hyperthermia	Monitor temperature
	Beta blockers	Increased effect of both drugs	Monitor for adverse reactions
	Dopaminergics	Antagonize antipsychotic effect	Avoid concurrent use
	Hypoglycemics	Decreased diabetic control	Monitor blood glucose closely

Continued

Table 15–18 ■ Drug Interactions: Typical Antipsychotics—cont'd

Drug	Interacting Drug	Possible Effect	Implications
	Phenytoin	Increased toxicity of phenytoin	Monitor blood level of phenytoin; lower dose of antipsychotic may be needed
	Trazodone	Increased hypotension	Monitor postural hypotension; warn patient to change position slowly
	Diazoxide	Hyperglycemia	Monitor blood glucose
	TCAs	Increased sedation, risk of seizures, anticholinergic effect, serum levels of TCA, risk of arrhythmias	Use SSRI
	SSRIs	Increased antipsychotic levels	Monitor dose of antipsychotic
	Nicotine	Decreased antipsychotic levels	Monitor dose of antipsychotic

control of agitation and dangerous psychosis can be treated with IV **haloperidol**. IM **chlorpromazine** also provides rapid sedation.

Table 15–19 presents the indications and dosage schedules of typical **APs**. Table 15–20 presents available dosage forms.

Rational Drug Selection

The choice of a specific agent can be guided by past response to the medication, initial response, family history, and side effect profile of the medication. Usually EPSs can be decreased or eliminated by the addition of drugs such as **benztropine** (Cogentin), **diphenhydramine** (Benadryl), **trihexyphenidyl** (Artane), **atenolol** (Tenormin), or **amantadine** (Symmetrel). A decrease in the dose or a change to a different type of **antipsychotic** may also counter these effects. Some anticholinergic effects, such as constipation, can be addressed by nonpharmacological measures such as increased fluid intake and dietary bulk.

The depot or decanoate form of medication may be used if compliance is an issue. It is usually administered every 2 to 4 weeks.

Monitoring

Motor function of individuals taking **typical antipsychotics** should be routinely assessed with the use of the Abnormal Involuntary Movement Scale (AIMS), which rates various movements such as joint rigidity and balance on a numerical scale, thereby enabling the clinician,

Table 15–19 ● Dosage Schedule: Typical Antipsychotics

Drug	Indications* Not for Dementia-Related Psychosis in Elderly	Dosage
Chlorpromazine HCl (Thorazine)	Psychosis; acute severe agitation	*Adults:* PO: 25 mg tid to maximum of 40 mg/d IM: 25 mg initially; may repeat with 25–50 mg in 1 h: maximum 400 mg IM every 4–6 h; substitute with oral as soon as possible; give concentrate with 60 mL or more of diluent *Children:* PO: 0.5 mg/kg every 4–6 h as needed Rectal: 1 mg/kg every 6–8 h as needed IM: 0.5 mg/kg every 6–8 h as needed
Fluphenazine (Prolixin)	Psychosis; acute severe agitation	*Adults:* PO: 0.5–10 mg/d in divided doses at 6- to 8-h intervals IM: 5 mg every 6 h to maximum of 30 mg/d *Older adults:* PO 1–2.5 mg/d: IM one-third to one-half oral dose starting with 1.25 mg Decanoate: 12.5–25 mg deep IM every 1–3 wk

Table 15–19 ◉ Dosage Schedule: Typical Antipsychotics—cont'd

Drug	Indications* Not for Dementia-Related Psychosis in Elderly	Dosage
Perphenazine (Trilafon)	Psychosis; acute severe agitation	*Adults:* 8–16 mg 2–4 times daily to maximum of 64 mg/d. Older adults: one-third to one-half adult dose *Children >12 yr:* lowest adult dose possible
Trifluoperazine (Stelazine)	Psychosis; acute severe agitation	*Adults:* 15–20 mg/d in divided doses to maximum of 40 mg/d IM: 1–2 mg every 4–6 has needed *Older adults:* low end of adult dose *Children >6 yr:* 1 mg 1–2 times daily; adjust according to weight
Thioridazine (Mellaril)	Psychosis; acute severe agitation	*Adults:* 50–100 mg tid to maximum of 800 mg/d *Children >2 yr:* 0.5 to maximum of 3 mg/kg/d
Thiothixene (Navane)	Psychosis; acute severe agitation	*Adults:* 6–60 mg/d in divided doses; maximum 60 mg/d
		IM: 16–20 mg 2–4 times/d to maximum of 30 mg/d
Loxapine (Loxitane)	Psychosis; acute severe agitation	*Adults and children >15 yr:* 10 mg bid initially; may increase rapidly to maintenance of 20–60 mg/d
		IM: 12.5–50 mg every 4–6 h until desired response; then start oral
Pimozide (Orap)	Psychosis; acute severe agitation	*Adults and children >12 yr:* 30 mg/d in divided doses; range 20–60 mg/d
		Older adults: 10–15 mg/d in divided doses or single hs dose
Haloperidol (Haldol)	Psychosis; acute severe agitation	*Adults:* 0.5–5 mg 2–3 times daily to maximum of 100 mg/d IM: 2–5 mg; may repeat after 60 min; substitute with oral as soon as feasible. First oral dose should be administered 12–24 h following last IM dose Decanoate: deep IM every 4 wk; initial dose 10–15 times oral dose; not to exceed 100 mg *Older adults:* lower doses and slower titration *Children:* 0.05–15 mg/kg/d, may give in divided doses
Molindone HCl (Moban)	Psychosis; acute severe agitation	*Adults and children >12 yr:* 50–75 mg/d to maximum of 225 mg/d Maintenance of nonsevere case: 5–15 mg 3–4 times daily

Table 15–20 ◈ Available Dosage Forms: Typical Antipsychotics

Drug	Dosage Form	How Supplied	Cost (per 100 Units)
Chlorpromazine	Tablets Concentrate	10, 15, 25, 50, 100, 150, 200 mg 30, 100 mg/mL	$20/10 mL $30/25, 50, 100 $45/200
Fluphenazine	Tablets Elixir Concentrate Injection Decanoate/ethanoate (SC)	1, 2.5, 5, 10 mg 2.5 mg/5 mL 5 mg/mL 2.5 mg/mL 25 mg/mL	$12/1 mg $15/2.5 mg $19/10 mg
Perphenazine	Tablets Concentrate Injection	2, 4, 8, 16 mg 16 mg/5 mL 5 mg/mL	$25/2 mg $30/4 mg $38/8 mg $50/16 mg
Trifluoperazine	Tablets Concentrate Injection	1, 2, 5, 10 mg 10 mg/mL 2 mg/mL	

Continued

Table 15–20 ◈ **Available Dosage Forms: Typical Antipsychotics—cont'd**

Drug	Dosage Form	How Supplied	Cost (per 100 Units)
Thioridazine	Tablets Suspension Concentrate	10, 15, 25, 50, 100, 150, 200 mg 25, 100 mg/5 mL 30, 100 mg/mL	$19/10 mg $39/15 mg $23/25 mg $27/50 mg $35/100 mg $50/150 mg $91/200 mg
Thiothixene	Capsules Concentrate Injection	1, 2, 5, 10, 20 mg 5 mg/mL 2 mg/mL	$15/1 mg $18/2 mg $20/5 mg $32/10 mg
Loxapine succinate/HCIs	Capsules Concentrate Injection	5, 10, 25, 50 mg 25 mg/mL 50 mg/mL	$62/5 mg $82/10 mg $122/25 mg $157/50 mg
Pimozide (Orap)	Tablets	2 mg	$87/1 mg $116/2 mg
Haloperidol	Tablets Concentrate Decanoate	0.5, 1, 2, 5, 10, 20 mg 2 mg/mL 5, 50, 100 mg/mL	$12/0.5 mg $16/1 mg $19/2 mg $22/5 mg $112/10 mg $217/20 mg
Molindone HCI (Moban)	Tablets Concentrate	5, 10, 25, 50, 100 mg 20 mg/mL	$122/5 mg $175/10 mg $260/25 mg $346/50 mg

All costs are generic unless noted.

over time, to detect changes that represent early EPSs. Table 15–21 presents an AIMS checklist that the nurse practitioner may use to evaluate patients.

Typical APs may elevate prolactin levels because dopamine, which inhibits prolactin, is blocked. Patients should be monitored for the consequences of chronic prolactin elevation such as galactorrhea, gynecomastia, amenorrhea, and sexual dysfunction.

Patient Education

Anticipate the need for refills before the patient runs out of medication. Teach the patient to avoid sudden withdrawal of the medication because EPSs can occur. Emphasize that it is important to take the medication as prescribed, because noncompliance is the leading cause of increased symptoms and hospitalization. Advise the patient to report any side effects of EPSs, TD, or NMS. Advise

Table 15–21 **Abnormal Involuntary Movement Scale (AIMS) Checklist**

Instructions: Rate on a scale from 1 to 5, with 1 being none and 5 being severe. Rate at each appointment initially, then decrease frequency unless patient is a male under age 25 or a female over age 70.

Abnormal Involuntary Movement	Scale	Notes
Holding arms outstretched to sides		
Arms outstretched to front with hands flat and parallel		
Walking in a straight line		
Fluidity of shoulder and elbow joints		
Touching each finger with thumb of both hands		
Sticking tongue out straight		
Rolling head laterally, front and back		

the patient to rise slowly to minimize orthostatic hypotension. Caution the patient to avoid taking **alcohol** or other CNS depressants concurrently with these drugs. Caution the patient to avoid driving or other activities requiring alertness, because medication may cause drowsiness. Advise the patient to wear sunscreen and protective clothing because photosensitivity and changes in skin pigmentation may occur.

Atypical Antipsychotics

A number of **atypical APs** have been marketed since 1990. These drugs include **aripiprazole** (Abilify), **clozapine** (Clozaril), **olanzapine** (Zyprexa, Zyprexa Zydis, IM), **quetiapine** (Seroquel), **risperidone** (Risperdal, Risperdal M-Tabs, Risperdal Consta), **ziprasidone** (Geodon), **paliperidone** (Invega, Invega Sustenna), **asenapine** (Saphris), and **iloperidone** (Fanapt). **Atypical APs** address both the positive and negative symptoms of schizophrenia. Some of the superiority, as compared to **typical APs**, in treating negative symptoms may be related to less interference with cognitive functioning. Because there is better patient tolerability than with the **typical APs**, patients are more likely to continue taking the **atypical APs**. These newer agents are characterized by less risk for EPSs, TD, and elevation of prolactin levels. The **atypical APs**, however, are associated with unhealthy weight gain, which leads to a metabolic syndrome (abdominal obesity, high blood pressure, high cholesterol levels, and insulin resistance). Schizophrenia itself, as well as the **atypical APs**, increases the risk of diabetes. Before starting any **atypical antipsychotic**, patients should be assessed for waist circumference, body mass index (BMI), blood pressure (BP), fasting plasma glucose, and lipid profile. The practitioners should recheck BMI monthly and laboratory work-ups at 3 months. After 3 months, the BMI should be checked quarterly and BP, laboratory work-ups, and waist circumference annually.

Pharmacodynamics

Although the mechanism of action for these **APs** is not precisely understood, the **atypical APs** are thought to block serotonin receptors in the cortex, which blocks the usual ability of serotonin to inhibit the release of dopamine. Thus, more dopamine is released to the prefrontal cortex, which reduces the negative symptoms of schizophrenia. All drugs with antipsychotic properties block dopamine D_2 receptors, but atypical **APs** generally have less D_2 blockade than the typical **APs**. Drugs with the least D_2 blockade (**clozapine, olanzapine**) have the lowest incidence of EPSs. Most of the **atypical APs** also variously affect adrenergic, histaminic, and cholinergic receptors. Drugs that are potent histamine H_1 receptor antagonists (**olanzapine, clozapine**) produce more weight gain and sedation. Drugs that block noradrenergic receptors (**clozapine**) produce more hypotension.

Pharmacokinetics

Absorption and Distribution

These drugs are commonly administered orally and are rapidly and completely absorbed. Parenteral or long-acting decanoate forms of **olanzapine, risperidone**, and **ziprasidone** also exist. Orally disintegrating tablets of **olanzapine** and **risperidone** are available, and helpful when "cheeking" of medication is suspected.

Metabolism and Excretion

All are metabolized in the liver and primarily excreted through the renal system.

Onset, Peak, and Duration

Onset of action is within a few days to a few weeks. These drugs reach their peak activity in approximately 1 to 6 hours and steady state within a few days. Half-lives vary widely. For example, **clozapine** peaks in 2.5 hours and has a half-life of 8 to 12 hours, whereas **olanzapine** peaks in 6 hours and has a half-life of 21 to 54 hours.

Pharmacotherapeutics

Precautions and Contraindications

Atypical APs are not recommended in pregnancy (Pregnancy Category C), lactating women, or young children. They should be prescribed cautiously in the presence of hepatic or renal disease. Analysis of risk versus benefit is indicated in individuals who have hepatic or renal disease, but who also have poor quality of life without treatment with an **antipsychotic**. Because of liver function decline, the geriatric population generally requires smaller doses. An additional contraindication is hypersensitivity.

Adverse Drug Reactions

Although the risk of developing EPSs, tardive dyskinesia, and neuroleptic malignant syndrome exists with any antipsychotic, it is significantly less with the **atypical APs** than it is with the **typical APs. Atypical APs** do have other negative side effects including seizures, weight gain, diabetes, hyperprolactinemia, dizziness, orthostatic hypotension, tachycardia, sleep disturbance, constipation, and rhinitis.

Specific adverse reactions may occur with individual agents. Because of the risk of potentially fatal agranulocytosis, clozapine is reserved for the treatment of severe schizophrenia refractory to complete trials of at least two different types of **antipsychotics. Clozapine** is available only through a patient management system in which a clinician and patient are both registered. A baseline CBC with differential is obtained prior to treatment, then monitored weekly or biweekly, depending on the length of time the patient has been taking **clozapine**, before the next week's medication is dispensed by the pharmacy. Monitoring should be continued for 4 weeks after **clozapine** is discontinued. The clinician must be aware of the indications of a falling white blood count (WBC) (fever, lethargy, bruising, sore throat, flu-like symptoms). A precipitous onset of agranulocytosis is potentially lethal within 24 to 72 hours and requires immediate attention.

The dosage of **risperidone** should be titrated up slowly over a few days or longer to minimize adverse side effects. Adverse effects may include orthostatic hypotension, bradykinesia, akathisia, agitation, and elevation of prolactin levels. Weight gain with **risperidone** is generally less than it is with **clozapine** or **olanzapine**.

The most problematic side effects of long-term use of **olanzapine** are sedation and weight gain. This weight gain appears to be associated with increased appetite, with much of the weight gain occurring in the first 6 months of drug therapy. **Olanzapine** is very sedating and should be taken at bedtime if possible. **Olanzapine** has a low incidence of EPSs.

The most common side effects of **quetiapine** are dizziness and somnolence. Other side effects may be weight gain and orthostatic hypotension.

Ziprasidone appears to be well tolerated in general. It is unique among the **atypical APs** in that it does not cause significant weight gain, and may even result in weight loss and reduced triglyceride levels. **Ziprasidone** has a low incidence of EPS. The most common side effects are drowsiness, dyspepsia, dizziness, constipation, and nausea. One concern with **ziprasidone** is that it is associated with mild to moderate QT interval prolongation in about 5 percent of patients taking this drug. Patients with a known history of arrhythmia should have a baseline and repeat ECG.

Aripiprazole is relatively weight neutral and lacks any significant effect on QT intervals. It has good **antidepressant** properties, but may be unpleasantly activating to some patients. Side effects include agitation, akathisia, nausea, tremor, insomnia, and headache.

Drug Interactions

Concurrent use with **fluvoxamine** (1A2 inhibitor) may increase **atypical AP** levels. Use with **alcohol** and other CNS depressants results in increased sedation and orthostasis. Use with **antihypertensives** may increase orthostasis. **Carbamazepine** decreases serum levels of **olanzapine** and is contraindicated with **clozapine. Ciprofloxacin (Cipro)** is a potent 1A2 inhibitor and increases **atypical antipsychotic** levels. Smoking increases the rate of metabolism of **APs**, thereby potentially decreasing their effect. Combinations of **APs** may increase the risk of TD and NMS.

Table 15–22 presents drug interactions.

Table 15–22 ■ Drug Interactions: Atypical Antipsychotics

Drug	Interacting Drug	Possible Effect	Implications
All atypical antipsychotics	Antihypertensives CNS depressants Ciprofloxacin (Cipro)	Hypotension Increased CNS depression Potent 1A2 inhibitor	Monitor blood pressure, orthostasis Warn patient about drowsiness Increase atypical antipsychotic levels
Clozapine	Anticholinergics	Increased anticholinergic effect	Increase fluid intake; use hard candies for dry mouth; stool softener if needed; monitor for urinary retention
	Caffeine	Increased effect of clozapine	Monitor CNS depression, WBC
Lithium	Increased risk of neurotoxicity and agranulocytosis	Monitor lithium level, WBC, and for signs and symptoms of neurotoxicity	
	Carbamazepine	Decreased serum levels of olanzapine	Contraindicated with clozapine
Quetiapine	Glucocorticoids	Decreased effect of quetiapine	Avoid concurrent use
Clozapine, quetiapine	Phenytoin	Increased toxicity of phenytoin; decreased antipsychotic effect	Monitor phenytoin blood levels and for increased psychotic symptomatology
	Erythromycin, ketoconazole, itraconazole, fluconazole	Increased effect of antipsychotics	Monitor for increasing CNS depression
Olanzapine, quetiapine	Rifampin, SSRIs	Decreased effect of antipsychotics	Monitor for increased psychotic symptomatology
Olanzapine, quetiapine, risperidone	Carbamazepine	Increased toxicity of carbamazepine	Monitor plasma levels of carbamazepine

Table 15–22 ■ Drug Interactions: Atypical Antipsychotics—cont'd

Drug	Interacting Drug	Possible Effect	Implications
	Dopaminergic	Antagonistic to effect of antipsychotics	Do not use if possible; increased dose may be required
Olanzapine, quetiapine, clozapine	Cimetidine	Increased effect of antipsychotics	Monitor for increasing CNS depression
Aripiprazole	Ketoconazole or other CYP3A4 inhibitors	Decreases metabolism and increases effects of antipsychotic	Reduce aripiprazole dose by 50%
Ziprasidone	Drugs that prolong QT interval	Potentially life threatening cardiac changes	ECG monitoring

Clinical Use and Dosing

Table 15–23 presents the indications, dosages, and available dosage forms of atypical APs.

Rational Drug Selection

Indications for use of the atypical APs include schizophrenia, schizoaffective disorder, depression or mania with psychotic features, and severe agitation and delusions with dementia. Selecting one atypical antipsychotic over another may be based on specific patient risk factors, history of response to specific medications, or adverse effects experienced by the patient. Change from one AP to another should be accomplished by slowly titrating off the first medication and onto the second, with a washout period in between if possible. If the presence of psychotic symptoms makes a washout period unfeasible, overlap of medications should be at the lowest doses and for the shortest period of time possible.

Monitoring

No specific blood tests are available to determine the plasma level of these medications. Dosages are adjusted based on subjective information provided by the patient and the clinician's objective observations of the client.

Table 15–23 ● Dosage Schedule: Atypical Antipsychotics

Drug	Indications	Dosage	Available Dosage Forms	Cost (per 100 Units)
Aripiprazole (Abilify)	Schizophrenia, psychotic disorders, acute agitation, acute mania, bipolar maintenance, adjunct to antidepressant treatment for major depression	*Adult dose:* 10–15 mg/d single dose, may increase dose at 2-wk intervals up to 30 mg/d Bipolar: 15 mg q d initially Depression adjunct: 2–5 mg/d, may increase by 5 mg q wk to max 15 mg *Children:* Schizophrenia age 12–17 yrs 2 mg/d, increase to 5 mg after 2 d, then to target dose of 10 mg after 2 d, then 5 mg q d if needed to max 30 mg Bipolar age 10–17: 2 mg/d, increase to 5 mg after 2 d, then in 2 d, if needed to max of 10 mg. Abilify injection: 9.75 mg IM, may repeat in 2 h, max 30 mg/d	Tablets: 2 mg 5 mg 10 mg 15 mg 20 mg 30 mg Oral solution 1 mg/mL Dose equivalent to tabs until 30 mg tab = 2 5 mg liquid Discmelt 10, 15 mg Injection 7. 5 mg/mL (IM)	$296/30 $296/30 $296/30 $417/30 $417/30
Asenapine (Saphris)	Schizophrenia, acute bipolar mania	*Adults:* 5 mg bid, max 10 mg bid For acute mania: initial 10 mg bid	Oral disintegrating tablets, 5, 10 mg	

Continued

Table 15–23 ● **Dosage Schedule: Atypical Antipsychotics—cont'd**

Drug	Indications	Dosage	Available Dosage Forms	Cost (per 100 Units)
Clozapine (Clozaril)	Refractory severe schizophrenia	*Adults:* Initial dose: 25–50 mg/d increasing by 25-mg increments/d until target range of 300–450 mg/d; maximum dose 900 mg/d; can give once daily or in divided doses; do not increase dose until adequate time for response has been provided, usually a few weeks. See pharmacy titration schedule	Tablets: 25 100 mg	$54 (G) $123 $41
		Maintenance: lowest dose possible to resolve psychotic symptoms	25 mg (G) 100 mg (G)	$160 $411
		Discontinuation: taper slowly over 1–2 wk		
Iloperidone (Fanapt)	Schizophrenia	*Adults:* start with 1 mg bid, increase to 2 mg bid on second day, then by 2 mg bid q day to target dose of 12–24 mg bid on day 7	1-, 2-, 4-, 6-, 8-, 10-, 12-mg tabs	
Olanzapine (Zyprexa, Zyprexa Zydis (oral disintegrating form) Zyprexa IM)	Psychotic disorders, severe agitation, acute mania, bipolar maintenance	Schizophrenia: 5–10 mg daily in single dose; dosage adjustment should occur no less often than once weekly; 5 mg/d in debilitated patients or those with predisposition to hypotension Bipolar: initially 10–15 mg qd, may increase by 5 mg/d to target dose 20 mg/d Bipolar maintenance: 5–20 mg/d Acute agitation: IM 2.5–10 mg/dose deep IM, 3 doses 2–4 h apart up to 3 in 24 h	Tablets: 2.5 5 mg 7.5 mg 10 mg 15 mg 20 mg Zydis: 5 mg 10 mg 15 mg 20 mg IM: 10-mg vial (before reconstitution)	$311 $367 $447 $552 $828 $1,102 $308 $446 $583
Paliperidone (Invega, Invega Sustenna)	Schizophrenia, Schizoaffective disorder	*Adults:* 6 mg qam, increase by 3 mg q 4–5 days to max of 12 mg. (Lower doses for renal impairment) Invega Sustenna (IM) First establish tolerability with oral treatment, deep deltoid 234 mg day 1, in one wk, 156 mg. Maintenance injection: deltoid or gluteal 117 mg monthly (range 39–234 mg. (Lower doses for renal impairment)	Tabs (extended-release): 3, 6, 9 mg Invega Sustenna extended-release injection: 39, 78, 117, 156, 234 mg	
Risperidone (Risperdal) (Risperidal M-TAB) (orally disintegrating form) Risperdal Consta (IM)	Psychotic disorders, severe agitation, acute mania, autism related irritability in children	Schizophrenia: *Adults:* Initial dose: 1 mg bid; increase (q 24 h), by 1 mg per dose to target dose of 4–8 mg/d most efficacious in range of 4–6 mg/d;	Tablets: 0.25 mg 0.5 mg 1 mg 2 mg 3 mg 4 mg	$173/60 $189/60 $201/60 $314/60 $368/60 $493/60

Table 15–23 ◉ **Dosage Schedule: Atypical Antipsychotics—cont'd**

Drug	Indications	Dosage	Available Dosage Forms	Cost (per 100 Units)
		Children 13–17: 0.5 mg qd, increase by 0.5 mg q 24 h to target of 3 mg/d. Divide dose is somnolence occurs (debilitated patients should begin with 0.5 mg bid and the dose increased in 0.5-mg increments) For bipolar I maintenance or adjunct to Lithium or valproate: *Adult:* range 1–6 mg/d *Children 10–17:* target 2.5 mg/d, max 6 *For irritable autism symptoms age 5–16:* <20 kg, 0.25 mg/d increase in 4 d to 0.5 mg. Remain for 14 d, then may increase 0.25 mg q 2 wk. >20 kg 0.5 mg, may increase in 4 d to 1 mg. Remain for 14 d then may increase 0.5 mg q 2 wk Risperdal Consta for adults: After trial with oral only, give IM deep gluteal or deltoid. Give injection with oral dose for 3 wk, then stop oral. Every 2 wk, 25 mg IM adjust q 4 wk if needed to max 50 mg q 2 wk injection.	Solution: 1 mg/1 mL M-TAB: 0.5 mg 1 mg 2 mg Consta: Long-acting injectable, 25 mg 37.5 mg 50 mg	$113/30 $100/30 $116/30 $174/28
Quetiapine (Seroquel, Seroquel XR)	Psychotic disorders, severe agitation, schizophrenia acute mania, bipolar maintenance, bipolar depression, adjunct to major depressive disorder antidepressant treatment	*Adults:* Schizophrenia Seroquel-Initially 25 mg bid, day 1 and increase q d by 25–50 mg in divided doses to target of 300–400 mg/d (divided) by day 4. Then increase by 25–50 mg in 2-d intervals to max 800 mg; lower in the elderly or with hepatic impairment. XR formulation: Initially 300 mg in pm (3–4 h before hs), increase by 300 mg/d to range 400–800/d. Mania: 100 mg/d divided, increase by 100 mg/d (divided) to 400 mg by day 4, then 200 mg increments to 800 mg (divided) by day 6. Depression: 50 mg day 1 at hs, then increase by 100 mg qhs until 300 mg on day 4. May increase to 400 mg day 5 and 600 mg day 8 if needed.	Tablets: 25 mg 100, 200, 300, 400 mg XR tablets: 50, 150, 200, 300, 400 mg	$169 $295 $554 $437/60

Continued

Table 15–23 ◉ **Dosage Schedule: Atypical Antipsychotics—cont'd**

Drug	Indications	Dosage	Available Dosage Forms	Cost (per 100 Units)
		XR formulation: Mania— 300 mg in PM, day 1, then 600 mg in PM day 2. Day 3 titrate to effective dose (range 400–800) Depression—50 mg day 1, 100 mg day 2, 200 mg day 3, and 300 mg day 4 Give evening dose 3–4 h before hs.		
Ziprasidone (Geodon)	Schizophrenia, severe agitation, Mania	*Adults*: must be taken with full meal for proper absorption. *Schizophrenia:* Initial dose: 20 mg bid may increase at 2-d intervals up to 80 mg bid Mania: Initial dose 40 mg bid, day 2 60–80 mg bid Injection: severe agitation 10–20 mg IM to max 40 mg per day (10 mg q 2 h or 40 mg q 4 h), not to exceed 3 days	Capsules: 20 mg 40 mg 60 mg 80 mg IM: 20-mg vial (before reconstitution)	$264/60 $264/60 $287/60 $287/60

G = generic; B = costs are brand for 60 units.

Patient Education

Patients need to be informed of the possible adverse reactions that may be associated with individual agents. Patients taking **clozapine**, for example, need to be knowledgeable of the signs and symptoms of agranulocytosis so that these symptoms can be promptly reported to the clinician. Advise the patient to change position slowly to prevent orthostatic hypotension. Provide the patient with safety instructions for driving and other activities that require alertness. Sugarless gums, candies, or ice chips may be used to alleviate symptoms of dry mouth. Alert the patient to avoid the use of **alcohol** or other CNS depressants. Advise the patient of the potential for significant weight gain and increase in triglycerides, and assist the client in modifying diet and exercise regimes to counter these undesirable effects.

DOPAMINERGICS

The **dopaminergics**, also known as **dopamine agonists**, are the pharmacological treatment of choice for Parkinson's disease. These agents include **amantadine (Symmetrel)**, **bromocriptine (Parlodel)**, **carbidopa-levodopa (Sinemet)**, **selegiline hydrochloride (Eldepryl)**, **pramipexole (Mirapex)**, and **ropinirole (Requip)**. **Amantadine** is occasionally used to treat the parkinsonism-like EPS of the antipsychotic drugs, but to give a dopamine-enhancing drug to a patient with schizophrenia might cause psychotic symptoms to increase.

Pharmacodynamics

Dopamine and acetylcholine are the neurotransmitters primarily responsible for balance and coordinated musculoskeletal functioning, and each needs to balance the other for smooth functioning to take place. When dopamine depletion occurs, either idiopathically as in Parkinson's disease or because of inadequate synthesis or impaired storage, transmission, or reuptake, the classic signs of muscular rigidity, tremors, and psychomotor retardation appear. Excessive amounts of dopamine are thought to produce the positive symptoms of schizophrenia, such as hallucinations and delusions.

Amantadine is effective because it releases dopamine from storage, whereas the dopamine precursors levodopa and carbidopa-levodopa increase dopamine synthesis. **Bromocriptine** and **pergolide** act as dopamine agonists at the postsynaptic receptor sites. **Selegiline** inactivates monoamine oxidase (MAO), which then leads to increased amounts of dopamine available in the CNS. **Pramipexole** and **ropinirole** act by stimulating dopamine receptors in the brain.

Pharmacokinetics

Absorption and Distribution

Dopaminergics are administered orally and are relatively rapidly and completely absorbed. These agents are widely distributed and enter breast milk.

Metabolism and Excretion

Variations occur in metabolism; for example, **bromocriptine** is metabolized in the liver, but **amantadine** is excreted unchanged in the urine. **Selegiline** has three active metabolites, including **amphetamine** and **methamphetamine**, and deaths have occurred when selegiline has been taken concurrently with **meperidine**. **Dopaminergics** are excreted through urine and feces.

Table 15–24 presents the pharmacokinetics of dopaminergics.

Pharmacotherapeutics

Precautions and Contraindications

These agents are contraindicated in hypersensitivity and should be used cautiously in patients with a history of cardiac, psychiatric, or ulcer disease. **Dopaminergics** are Pregnancy Categories B and C; their safety of use during lactation and in children has not been determined. **Selegiline** is contraindicated with concurrent administration of meperidine. Renal impairment should be carefully assessed before using **amantadine** because it is excreted unchanged through the kidneys. Patients with underlying cardiac arrhythmias who have taken pergolide have experienced bradycardia and sinus tachycardia. **Ropinirole** and **pramipexole** should be used cautiously in geriatric patients because of the increased risk of hallucinations. Carbidopa-levodopa is contraindicated in narrow-angle glaucoma and malignant melanoma.

Adverse Drug Reactions

Pharmacotherapeutics

Adverse effects may include nausea and vomiting, dizziness, postural hypotension, abdominal pain, dyspepsia, constipation, dry mouth, depression, insomnia, confusion, and hallucinations. **Pramipexole** and **ropinirole** may cause sleep attacks in which the patient has unexpected episodes of falling asleep.

Drug Interactions

Drug interactions among the **dopaminergic agents** are many and varied. For example, administration with **MAO inhibitors** may cause hypertensive crisis. Concurrent use with **antihypertensives** may increase hypotension. Concurrent use with **antihistamines, phenothiazines, quinidine**, and **tricyclic antidepressants** may increase anticholinergic effects. **Phenothiazines, haloperidol**, and **phenytoin** may decrease the effect of **levodopa**. Concurrent use of **levodopa** with **pramipexole** increases the risk of hallucinations and dyskinesia. Ropinirole is extensively metabolized by the liver's CYP450 CYP1A2 enzyme systems; thus, drugs that alter the activity of these enzyme systems may affect the activity of **ropinirole**.

Table 15–25 presents drug and food interactions.

Table 15–24 ▶ **Pharmacokinetics: Dopaminergics**

Drug	Onset	Peak	Duration	Half-Life	Excretion
Amantadine (Symmetrel)	48 h	4 h	—	18–24 h	Urine
Bromocriptine mesylate (Parlodel)	—	1–3 h	4–8 h	3–8 h	Feces (85%–98%) Urine
Carbidopa-levodopa (Sinemet)	—	1–3 h	4–6 h	—	Urine
Selegiline HCI (Eldepryl)	—	0.5–2 h	—	18–20 h	Urine
Pergolide (Permax)	—	—	—	—	Urine
Pramipexole (Mirapex)	—	2 h	8 h	8 h	Urine
Ropinirole (Requip)	—	—	8 h	6 h	Urine

Table 15–25 ■ **Food and Drug Interactions: Dopaminergics**

Drug	Interacting Drug or Food	Possible Effect	Implications
All dopaminergics	Antihypertensives	Increased antihypertensive effect	Monitor for postural hypotension, blood pressure
	Oral contraceptives	Decreased effectiveness of oral contraceptives	Use backup contraception
	MAOIs, TCAs, opioids	Hypertensive crisis	Avoid concurrent use
Carbidopa-levodopa	Food	Increased plasma level of carbidopa-levodopa with sustained-release form	Avoid taking with food

Continued

Table 15–25 ■ **Food and Drug Interactions: Dopaminergics—cont'd**

Drug	Interacting Drug or Food	Possible Effect	Implications
	Anticholinergics	Increased adrenocorticotropic hormone (ACH) adverse effects and decreased effect of levodopa	Monitor eye pain/vision; effect of dopaminergic
	Haldol, hydantoins	Decreased effect of levodopa	Monitor eye pain/vision; effect of dopaminergic
Pramipexole Ropinirole	Levodopa	May increase effect of levodopa	Monitor for hallucinations, dyskinesia (may allow dosage reduction of levodopa)

Clinical Use and Dosing

Table 15–26 presents the indications and dosage schedule of **dopaminergics.** Table 15–27 presents the available dosage forms of dopaminergics.

Rational Drug Selection

Treatment with a **dopamine agonist** such as **bromocriptine, pergolide, pramipexole,** or **ropinirole** is recommended as the first-line therapy for patients with mild to moderate parkinsonism symptoms. As symptoms worsen over time, **levodopa** may be introduced. Combinations such as **levodopa** with **amantadine** or **carbidopa-levodopa** with **selegiline** may provide improved response over a single drug or in cases of deterioration in status. In late-stage therapy, a controlled-release preparation (**Sinemet CR**) may relieve "wearing off," the recurrence of severe symptoms hours after the dose of medication. Patients who take **levodopa** for several years may experience a decrease in the effectiveness of the drug and require a drug holiday to restore effectiveness. Some newer **dopamine agonists,** such as **pramipexole,** have been used in the treatment of resistant depression.

Table 15–26 ■ **Dosage Schedule: Dopaminergics**

Drug	Indications	Dosage
Amantadine	Parkinson's disease; drug-induced EPS; parkinsonism syndrome following carbon monoxide poisoning	*Adults:* 100–200 mg bid; may increase to maximum of 400 mg/d in divided doses after several weeks without response after lower dose In conjunction with levodopa: 100 mg qd-bid
Bromocriptine mesylate	Parkinson's disease	*Adult:* initial dose 1.25 mg bid with meals; if dosage increase needed after 2 weeks, increase by 2.5 mg/d in divided doses with meals; maintain at lowest dose producing optimal response; usual range 10–40 mg/d
Carbidopa-levodopa	Parkinson's disease; parkinsonism syndrome following carbon monoxide or manganese poisoning	*Adult:* 1 tab (25 mg carbidopa and 100 mg levodopa) tid or 1 tab (10 mg carbidopa and 100 mg levodopa) tid-qid; may increase by 1 tab daily or every other day until maximum of 8 tabs/d. Tablets of various ratios may be used but maintain 70–100 mg carbidopa/d
		CR form: 1 tab bid with minimum of 6 h between doses; increase as above; do not crush or chew tabs
Selegiline HCl	Adjunctive treatment of Parkinson's disease with carbidopa-levodopa	*Adult:* 5 mg bid with breakfast and lunch; after 2–3 d, decrease dose of carbidopa-levodopa
Pramipexole	Parkinson's disease	*Adult:* 0.125 mg tid initially, may increase 5–7 d up to 1.5–4.5 mg/d in 3 divided doses
Ropinirole	Parkinson's disease	*Adult:* 0.25 mg tid for 1 wk, then 0.5 mg tid for 1 wk, then 0.75 mg tid for 1 wk, then 1 mg tid for 1 wk; then may increase by 1.5 mg/d each wk up to 9 mg/d; then may increase by up to 3 mg/d each wk up to 24 mg/d

CR = controlled release.

Table 15–27 ◆ **Available Dosage Forms Dopaminergics**

Drug	Dosage Form	How Supplied	Cost (per 100 Units)
Amantadine	Capsules	100 mg	$35
	Syrup	50 mg/5 mL	
Bromocriptine	Tablets	2.5 mg	$206
	Capsules	5 mg	
Carbidopa-levodopa	Tablets	10 mg carbidopa/100 mg levodopa 25 mg carbidopa/100 mg levodopa 25 mg carbidopa/250 mg levodopa	$72 $81 $103
	Sustained-release tablets	50 mg carbidopa/200 mg levodopa	$175
		25 mg carbidopa/100 mg levodopa	$91
Selegiline	Tablets	5 mg	$14/60
Pramipexole	Tablets	0.125, 0.25, 0.5, 1,1.5 mg	
Ropinirole	Tablets	0.25, 0.5, 1, 2, 4, 5 mg	

Monitoring

Monitor the effectiveness of the drug in managing parkinsonism symptoms. Assess for "on-off" phenomenon in which symptoms suddenly worsen or improve. Monitor hepatic and renal function in patients on long-term therapy. Monitor patients on **pramipexole** and **ropinirole** for the occurrence of drowsiness and sleep attacks.

Patient Education

Advise the patient to exercise care when changing position to prevent postural hypotension and to avoid hazardous activities if drowsy or dizzy. Explain that gastric irritation may be decreased by taking medication with food, but that high-protein meals may impair **levodopa's** effects. Caution patient to monitor skin lesions for any changes, because **carbidopa-levodopa** may activate malignant melanoma. Advise the patient that large amounts of **vitamin B (pyridoxine)** may interfere with the action of **levodopa.**

ANXIOLYTICS (ANTIANXIETY) AND HYPNOTICS

Drugs used to treat anxiety can be divided into three groups based on their pharmacological action: serotonergics, gaba-ergics, and dopaminergics. Traditionally, however, **anxiolytics** were seen as the **benzodiazepines** such as **diazepam** or **alprazolam.** The **benzodiazepines** affect the gamma amino butyric acid (GABA) receptors at a particular site within the receptor, whereas other gaba-ergics affect the receptor more globally. The net effect of inhibiting GABA is to slow down the neurotransmission and thereby produce reduction in anxiety. Serotonin as a neurotransmitter has a calming effect as well, due to the areas of the brain where there are high concentrations of these pathways. Finally **dopaminergics** have an anxiolytic effect in a fashion similar to that of serotonin but in more specific areas of the brain. Therefore, the prescriber needs to select a drug based not only on the general class of drugs but also on the specific symptomatology produced by the neurophysiology.

Because the **SSRIs** and **serotonin-dopamine antagonists** are discussed elsewhere in this chapter, this section focuses on the gaba-ergics, including the **benzodiazepines.** There is one exception and that is **buspirone** (BuSpar), which is a partial serotonin receptor agonist. For greater depth of discussion regarding the treatment of anxiety, see Chapter 30.

Benzodiazepines

Benzodiazepines have been frequently prescribed to treat anxiety and insomnia. However, because of the increased potential for tolerance and dependence on the newer variations, the CNS depressant-related adverse effects, and the development of buspirone, many clinicians are more cautious in assessing risks versus benefits for their patients than they might have been previously. The drugs in this class include the following:

- Alprazolam (Xanax, Xanax XR)
- Chlordiazepoxide (Librium)
- Clonazepam (Klonopin)
- Diazepam (Valium)
- Halazepam (Paxipam)
- Lorazepam (Ativan)
- Prazepam (Centrax)
- Oxazepam (Serax)

Benzodiazepines have also been extensively used as a muscle relaxant and for preanesthesia sedation, prevention and treatment of panic attacks, acute agitation and dystonia, emergency treatment of uncontrollable seizures, and treatment of restless leg syndrome.

Pharmacodynamics

Benzodiazepines are thought to exert their anxiolytic and sedative effects by increasing the action of GABA, an inhibitory neurotransmitter, thereby decreasing the effect of neuronal excitation. Within the GABA receptor is an area which the **benzodiazepines** bind to, referred to as the **benzodiazepine** receptor.

Pharmacokinetics

Absorption and Distribution

Benzodiazepines are rapidly and widely distributed following oral administration and reach their peak levels within 30 minutes to 6 to 8 hours. **Chlordiazepoxide (Librium)** and **diazepam (Valium)** are slowly and inconsistently absorbed after intramuscular administration but **lorazepam (Ativan)** and **midazolam** are rapidly absorbed and widely distributed after IM injection.

These drugs are lipid soluble and highly protein bound, which means that they may have prolonged activity in obese people and compete with other protein-bound drugs for receptor sites.

Metabolism and Excretion

Benzodiazepines are metabolized in the liver and biotransformed by oxidation. Some (**lorazepam** and **temazepam**) are biotransformed by conjugation. These two mechanisms may influence the patient's reaction to the drug. **Benzodiazepines** that are metabolized by conjugation are better tolerated by patients with impaired liver function or who are elderly or are smokers, whereas those drugs metabolized by oxidation may have a prolonged effect in the elderly.

Duration of effect is influenced by the lipid solubility and the half-life of the active metabolites more than the parent drug. Half-lives and active metabolites are included in Table 15–28.

Pharmacotherapeutics

Precautions and Contraindications

The development of dependence, which can be psychological as well as physical, is of concern with the **benzodiazepines**. Although dependence is usually related to dose (high) and duration of use (more than a few weeks), it can occur in the absence of these parameters. It is thought that **alprazolam (Xanax)** and **lorazepam (Ativan)** are more likely to cause dependence because of their high potency and rapid, short-term action but **clonazepam (Klonopin)** is less likely because of its long action.

Symptoms of withdrawal, which usually occur 1 to 2 days after the last dose of short-acting **benzodiazepines** and 5 to 10 days after the last dose of the long-acting compounds, resemble withdrawal symptoms of other CNS depressants. Use of the drug should be gradually tapered rather than abruptly discontinued because of the risk of severe withdrawal symptoms.

One strategy for tapering is to decrease the dose by 0.5 mg per week, and then by 0.25 mg per week for the last few weeks. Another is to substitute in an equivalent dose a long-acting **benzodiazepine** such as **clonazepam** for a short-acting one and then titrate down.

Benzodiazepines are contraindicated in pregnancy and lactation and in the presence of hepatic and renal disease, and they are not recommended for children less than 6 years. Other contraindications include hypersensitivity to **benzodiazepines** and acute narrow-angle glaucoma.

Geriatric patients generally should not be prescribed **benzodiazepines** and if they are prescribed, they should be in very low doses due to their decreased rate of metabolism and consequent potential accumulation of the drug.

These drugs are not the treatment of choice for depression or psychosis or in the absence of anxiety signs and symptoms.

Adverse Drug Reactions

Major adverse effects are due to the drug's action as CNS depressants. The same concerns as with other CNS depressants apply to their use: excessive sedation, particularly initially, in a situation requiring mental and physical alertness, and the potential for cardiac and respiratory depression, especially in combination with other CNS depressants.

Paradoxical anxiety, agitation, and acute rage may occur with **benzodiazepines. Clonazepam** may increase

Table 15–28 ▶ **Pharmacokinetics: Benzodiazepines**

Drug	Onset	Peak	Duration	Half-Life	Excretion
Alprazolam	Intermediate	1–2 h	Intermediate	8–37	Urine
Chlordiazepoxide	Intermediate	0.5–4 h	Long	5–30 h	Urine
Clonazepam	Intermediate	1–4 h	Long	30–40	Urine
Clorazepate	Fast	1–2 h	Long	40–50 h	Urine
Diazepam	Very fast	0.5–2 h	Long	20–80 h	Urine
Lorazepam	Intermediate	2–4 h	Intermediate	10–20 h	Urine
Oxazepam	Slow	2–4 h	Intermediate	5–20 h	Urine

salivation. Other common side effects include dizziness, confusion, blurred vision, and hypotension.

Drug Interactions

Drug interactions of greatest concern are those involving other CNS depressants, such as **barbiturates**, **alcohol**, **antihistamines**, and **neuroleptics**, because of their additive effects. **Benzodiazepines** also increase the blood levels of **TCAs** and **digitalis** preparation. Table 15–29 includes drug interactions and possible effects.

Clinical Use and Dosing

Benzodiazepines are indicated for the short-term treatment of anxiety and anxiety-related disorders. Additional uses include muscle relaxants, emergency treatment of status epilepticus, irritable bowel syndrome, chemotherapy-induced nausea and vomiting, and restless legs syndrome. Because they have cross sensitivity with **alcohol** and act as an **anticonvulsant**, the **benzodiazepines** are especially useful in **alcohol** withdrawal and delirium tremens. Table 15–30 includes dosages and available dose forms for the **benzodiazepines**.

Rational Drug Selection

Diazepam is the treatment of choice for status epilepticus, administered by a parenteral route, preferably IV because of the rapidity of absorption and effect.

In acute **alcohol** withdrawal, care must be exercised so that cross-tolerance does not develop. Because dependence has occurred after as little as 4 to 6 weeks of use, these drugs should be not be used beyond the acute **alcohol** withdrawal and should be slowly tapered to avoid withdrawal symptoms.

All of the **benzodiazepines** are equally efficacious and drug selection depends on the patient's and prescriber's

Table 15–29 ■ **Drug Interactions: Benzodiazepines**

Drug	Interacting Drug	Possible Effect	Implications
All benzodiazepines	Digoxin	Increased level of digoxin	Monitor level; take pulse before giving digoxin
	TCAs	Increased plasma level of TCAs	Monitor level of TCA
	Barbiturates, nefazodone, fluoxetine, fluvoxamine, MAOIs, sertraline, antihistamines	Increased CNS depression	Avoid concurrent administration
	Clozapine	Increased sedation, salivation, hypotension, delirium, respiratory arrest	Avoid concurrent administration
Alprazolam	Cimetidine oc, disulfiram, omeprazole, Macrolide antibiotics		Warn of increased effects
	Grapefruit juice	Decreased metabolism and increased effect of alprazolam	Use alternative juice
	Ketoconazole		Concurrent use contraindicated
Alprazolam, clonazepam	Carbamazepine	Decreased plasma level of benzodiazepines	Use alternative anticonvulsant
Clonazepam	Lithium	Increased sexual dysfunction	Warn of possible adverse effects
Clonazepam, diazepam, chlordiazepoxide	Phenytoin	Decreased plasma level and toxicity of phenytoin	Use alternative anticonvulsant
		Decreased clinical effect of BZD	Monitor phenytoin blood level; may need lower dose
Clonazepam, lorazepam	Valproate	Decreased metabolism and increased effect of benzodiazepines	May require lower dose of benzodiazepine
Diazepam	Phenobarbital	Additive CNS depression; increased metabolism of diazepam	May affect treatment of status epilepticus

Table 15–30 ◆ **Available Dosage Forms: Benzodiazepines**

Drugs	Dosage Form	How Supplied	Cost	
Alprazolam (Xanax)	Tablets	0.25 mg	$54/30 (Xanax)	$12/30 (generic)
		0.5 mg	$61/30	$12/30
		1 mg	$76/30	$12/30
		2 mg	$124/30	$15/30
	Orally disintegrating tablets	0.25 mg	$44/30	
	Intensol solution	1 mg/mL concentrated solution to be mixed with liquid or semisolid food, using only the provided calibrated dropper		
	Extended-release tablets (Xanax XR)	0.5 mg		$97/30
		1 mg		$116/30
		2 mg		$152/30
		3 mg		$216/30
Chlordiazepoxide (Librium)	Tablets	10 mg		$101
		25 mg		$9.50
		5 mg		$10
	Capsules	10 mg		
	Powder for injection	25 mg		
		100 mg		
Clonazepam (Klonopin)	Tablets	0.5 mg	$8 (generic)	$10.3 (Klonopin)
		1 mg	$8.50	$11.7
		2 mg	$10	$16.1
Diazepam (Valium)	Tablets	2 mg	$99 (Valium)	$9.50 (generic)
		5 mg	$152	$10
		10 mg	$225	$10.50
	Oral solution	5 mg/5 mL		
	Intensol solution	5 mg/mL		
	Injection	5 mg/mL		
Lorazepam (Ativan)	Tablets	0.5 mg	$88 (Ativan)	$12 (generic)
		1 mg	$165	$13
		2 mg		$16
	Intensol solution	2 mg/mL		
	Injection	2 or 4 mg/mL		
Oxazepam (Serax)	Tabs & caps Capsules	10 mg		$33
		15 mg		$52
		30 mg		$105

preference and the patient's side effect profile. For long-term treatment of anxiety, other classes of drugs should be considered first (e.g., **buspirone** or **SSRIs**); and if the **benzodiazepine** is necessary, then **clonazepam** is preferred due to its long half-life and daily dosing ability.

Monitoring

Increased blood levels of **TCAs** and **digitalis** may occur with concurrent use of **benzodiazepines** and should be monitored. In long-term use, periodic assessment of liver function and complete blood cell counts should be performed.

Patient Education

Advise the patient to avoid **alcohol.** Because drowsiness and impaired cognition may be an adverse effect, tell the patient to avoid taking a **benzodiazepine** before or during situations in which mental or physical alertness is required to maintain safety. Patients should also be advised to report ocular pain or changes in vision immediately.

Serotonergic Anxiolytics

Neurophysiologically, it makes sense that enhancing serotonin would contribute to relief of anxiety because of the areas of the brain that are heavily innervated by serotonin. However, there are 15 subtypes of serotonin receptors, some of which may actually contribute to anxiety. **Buspirone** is a serotonergic that is a member of the azapirones, a relatively new group of **anxiolytics**. Other drugs in this group are **ipsapirone** and **gepirone**, neither of which is approved for use in the United States for treatment of anxiety. These drugs exert their effects without the CNS depression and sedation of **barbiturates** and **benzodiazepines** but also without the anticonvulsant or muscle-relaxant qualities. **Buspirone** has little risk of dependence and few drug interactions, and it is considered relatively safe, even in high doses.

Pharmacodynamics

Buspirone has a similar chemical structure to butyrophenone **antipsychotics** such as **haloperidol** (Haldol) and was thought to be an **atypical antipsychotic** similar to **clozapine** (Clozaril) without the extrapyramidal side effects. However, further human studies showed that it had greater efficacy as an anxiolytic, through its action on the serotonin-1A (5-HT 1a) presynaptic and postsynaptic receptors. At the presynaptic 5-HT 1a receptor, **buspirone** is a full agonist, that is, it contributes to the channel's opening and permitting serotonin binding, thereby inhibiting neuron firing. **Buspirone** also is a partial agonist at the postsynaptic 5-HT 1a receptors. When there is an excess of serotonin, **buspirone** acts as an antagonist, but in a deficit state such as is presumed in anxiety and depression, it acts as an agonist.

Remembering that **buspirone** was originally thought to be an **atypical antipsychotic**, it is not surprising that **buspirone** inhibits the increase in dopamine D_2 receptors. However, the dopaminergic action is minor compared to the serotonergic effects. **Buspirone** has no effect on the GABA receptor and cannot be used as a substitute for **benzodiazepines** in withdrawal treatment.

Pharmacokinetics

Absorption and Distribution

When taken with food, **buspirone** has a reduced first-pass effect, allowing for more active drug going directly into circulation. It has many metabolites that have no effect on anxiety symptoms, but at least one metabolite has noradrenergic effects, which may explain why **buspirone** is contraindicated in panic attacks (Schatzberg & Nemeroff, 2009). It has a short half-life ranging from 1 to 10 hours but a slow onset of action (up to 6 weeks); therefore, it requires multiple dosing during the day. It is highly protein bound and lipid soluble, therefore having broad distribution in brain and adipose tissue.

Metabolism and Excretion

Buspirone is metabolized by oxidation in the liver and is a substrate for the CYP450 3A4 enzyme. It does not inhibit any of the CYP450 enzymes; therefore, it has few drug interactions. It is excreted in the urine and feces.

Onset, Peak, and Duration

For unknown reasons it takes 1 to 2 weeks for onset of anxiolytic effects and up to 6 weeks for maximum effects. It peaks in circulation in 0.7 to 1.5 hours and has an intermediate duration.

Pharmacotherapeutics

Precautions and Contraindications

Buspirone is contraindicated in patients with known hypersensitivity or in those with severe hepatic or renal disease. As mentioned previously, it is contraindicated in the treatment of panic disorder both because of its prolonged onset and possibility of exacerbating panic.

Buspirone is considered Pregnancy Category B. The extent of excretion in breast milk is not clear and use during lactation should be avoided. Although **buspirone** is not commonly thought to be sedating, as with other **anxiolytics**, drowsiness should be assessed prior to use in situations requiring cognitive or motor alertness in order to maintain safety.

Adverse Drug Effects

Adverse effects are few and usually resolve with continued use. Most common are light-headedness, headache, insomnia, nausea, nervousness, and dry mouth. Akathisia and involuntary movements are possible although rare.

Drug Interactions

Interactions between **buspirone** and other serotonergic drugs such as **MAOIs** and **SSRIs** have the potential to cause serotonin syndrome with symptoms of nausea, diarrhea, chills, sweating, elevated temperature and blood pressure, agitation, ataxia, coma, and death.

Interactions with **antipsychotic drugs**, especially **haloperidol**, contribute to increased serum levels of **haloperidol** due to competition for metabolism. When combined with **trazodone**, there may be an increased ALT (alanine transaminase).

Clinical Use and Dosing

Used primarily for anxiety, **buspirone**'s usual dose is 15 mg per day in two or three doses. Initially the patient takes 5 mg two or three times a day for 4 days, then the dose is increased by 5 mg each dose to a maximum dose of 60 mg per day. It is available in 5-, 10-, and 15-mg tablets bisected or trisected for easy titration. The tablets are small and may be difficult to handle for those with hand mobility problems.

Rational Drug Selection

Although **buspirone** can be used as the sole pharmacotherapeutic modality for anxiety, it is frequently used adjunctively with **SSRIs** in treatment-resistant depression because of the combined serotonergic mechanisms, that is, postsynaptic reuptake inhibition and receptor agonism. **Buspirone** is indicated in treating generalized anxiety disorder, depression with an overlay of anxiety, and situational anxieties that are long lasting. It is essential, however, that the drug be taken daily and cannot be used on an as-needed basis.

A positive response may begin within 7 to 10 days of starting the drug, but maximum benefits may not become evident for 3 to 6 weeks. It may be necessary to add a **benzodiazepine** in very low doses initially to relieve the patient's anxiety and fear about the anxiety.

Monitoring

No monitoring other than periodic reassessment of the drug's continued effectiveness is required.

Patient Education

To maintain safety, advise the patient to try the medication and observe the effects, especially drowsiness, before engaging in activities requiring mental or physical alertness. The patient also needs to be told of the prolonged onset and be offered nonpharmacological strategies for anxiety management during this time.

Barbiturates

Before the **benzodiazepines** became standard treatment, anxiety was treated with a variety of drugs with different mechanisms of action. **Barbiturates** have been used historically as **anxiolytics**, **sedative-hypnotics**, and **anticonvulsants**. Because of tolerance and dependence problems associated with their use, the indications for short-acting **barbiturates** are limited to preanesthesia sedation, short-term treatment of insomnia, and uncomfortable seizure activity, such as status epilepticus. Long-acting **phenobarbital (Solfoton, Mebaral)** is the drug of choice for some types of epilepsy, the only indication for its long-term use.

Pharmacodynamics

Barbiturates are CNS depressants and can be short (30 minutes to 4 hours), intermediate (6 to 8 hours), or long acting (10 to 12 hours). They produce sedation and sleep by decreasing sensitivity to stimuli in the reticular formation, a primitive area deep in the brainstem through which all the sensorimotor nerve tracts pass. They bind to $GABA_A$ receptors at a site other than the **benzodiazepines**, and contribute to prolonged opening of the chloride ion channel. With a prolonged activation of the GABA in the reticular activating system, decreased motor stimulation and increased sleep would be expected.

Pharmacokinetics

Absorption and Distribution

Barbiturates are administered by oral, parenteral, and rectal routes. Their rate of absorption depends on the route of administration, but generally, salts are absorbed more rapidly than are acid forms. They are widely distributed, particularly to brain, kidney, and liver tissue and fluid.

Metabolism and Excretion

Barbiturates are metabolized in the liver by CYP450 2C19 enzymes. They induce their own metabolism thereby increasing the rate of their metabolism and increasing the potential for tolerance. They are excreted in the urine, although up to 50 percent is eliminated unchanged. Table 15–31 includes the pharmacokinetics of the **barbiturates**.

These drugs are FDA Pregnancy Category D and should be avoided during pregnancy. Infant sedation has occurred when the lactating mother has used barbiturates. When used with women of childbearing age, care is needed to maintain birth control to prevent unwitting teratogenicity in the first trimester.

Table 15–31 ▶ **Pharmacokinetics: Barbiturates**

Drug	Onset	Peak	Duration	Half-Life	Excretion
Pentobarbital	10–15 min	—	3–4 h	15–50 h	Urine, feces
	IV immediate				
Secobarbital	10–15 min IV immediate	—	3–4 h	15–40 h	Urine, feces
Amobarbital	45–60 min	—	6–8 h	16–40 h	Urine, feces
Butabarbital	45–60 min	—	6–8 h	66–140 h	Urine, feces
Phenobarbital	30 min or more IV: less than 5 min	IV: 15 min or more	10–16 h	53–118 h	Urine, feces

Pharmacotherapeutics

Precautions and Contraindications

Barbiturates combined with **alcohol** have contributed to many deaths, whether suicide or accident, because of the additive depressive effect each has on the other. Caution should be exercised in prescribing them for patients with a history of depression, suicide attempts, or alcoholism. If the clinician has any doubts about the patient's safety and there is no other medication option, no more than a week's worth of the drug should be supplied at a time and for as short a period as possible.

Because of the anxiolytic effect of the short-acting **barbiturates**, known as downers on the street, they are drugs of choice for abuse. In addition to the hazard associated with the narrow therapeutic index and the risk for combining them with other CNS depressants, particularly **alcohol**, the short-acting barbiturates **secobarbital (Seconal)** and **pentobarbital (Nembutal)** can cause physiological dependence quickly. Tolerance leads the individual to increase the dose. One gram can cause toxic adverse effects, and 2 to 10 grams can be fatal.

Withdrawal and detoxification are potentially fatal and should be accomplished extremely slowly. Withdrawal symptoms usually begin 8 to 12 hours after the last dose and can include nausea and vomiting, confusion, and tremors to delirium and seizures, with the latter beginning approximately 16 hours after the last dose. If untreated, symptoms can last for several days.

Barbiturates are not recommended for children less than 6 years. Other contraindications include **barbiturate** sensitivity, severely impaired liver function, nephritis, impaired pulmonary function with dyspnea or obstruction, and history of dependence on **barbiturates, hypnotics,** or **alcohol.** They should not be administered subcutaneously or intra-arterially.

Adverse Drug Reactions

Adverse reactions are due to the CNS depressant effects of the drug and can consist of persistent sedation and drowsiness, leading to safety concerns for patients in situations requiring alertness. Although respiratory depression and cardiac depression are dose related, they are always a concern, especially in combination with other CNS depressants.

Other adverse reactions may include agitation, particularly in young children and older adults, confusion, headache, insomnia, ataxia, skin rash, nausea and vomiting, bradycardia, dyspnea, and somnolence.

Rebound status epilepticus may follow abrupt withdrawal of barbiturates during daily administration for treatment of seizure disorders.

Drug Interactions

As discussed earlier, CNS depression may occur with concurrent use of drugs such as **antihistamines, alcohol, benzodiazepines, valproic acid,** and **MAOIs.** Table 15–32 includes the drug interactions with **barbiturates.**

Barbiturates may also decrease the efficacy of **beta blockers, steroids, hormones, doxycycline, theophylline, protease inhibitors, dicumarol, exogenous corticosteroids,** and **vitamins K** and **D**, due to the P450 enzyme induction of 2C19.

Clinical Use and Dosing

Phenobarbital and **mephobarbital** are effective in the treatment of some types of epilepsy, primarily tonic-clonic, simple partial, and complex partial seizures, because the reduction of response to stimuli raises the threshold of seizure activity.

In addition to epilepsy, other indications for use include preanesthetic sedation and short-term treatment of insomnia. The latter indication, however, is last resort because of the risk of dependence and the comorbidity of

Table 15–32 ■ Drug Interactions: Barbiturates

Drug	Interacting Drug	Possible Effect	Implications
Barbiturates	Anticoagulants	Induces metabolism of anticoagulants and rebound bleeding when barbiturate stopped	Monitor bleeding times
	Antihistamines, alcohol, benzodiazepines	Increases CNS depression	Avoid concurrent administration
	Neuroleptics	Decreases effect of neuroleptic	Monitor for increase in psychotic symptoms
	Beta blockers, steroids, estrogen, doxycycline, protease inhibitors, valproate, theophylline, griseofulvin, quinidine, phenylbutazone	Induces metabolism and decreases effectiveness of drugs	Monitor blood levels where appropriate and assess effectiveness if concurrent administration unavoidable
	Caffeine	Antagonizes sedation and increases insomnia	Avoid coffee, tea, cola, and chocolate

sleep disturbance and depression, raising the risk for suicide.

Other than parenteral administration of **phenobarbital** in medical emergencies such as eclampsia and status epilepticus, **barbiturates** are generally given orally. The short-, intermediate-, and long-acting forms have an onset of action ranging from 10 to 60 minutes, a duration of action from 3 to 16 hours, and half-lives from 24 to 100 hours. Table 15–33 includes the indications, dosage schedules, and available dose forms for the **barbiturates**.

Rational Drug Selection

Although efficacious in the treatment of partial, tonic-clonic, and cortical focal seizures, **phenobarbital** and **mephobarbital** are not considered the first-line treatment of the medical emergencies mention previously, which also include seizures associated with meningitis and tetanus. The first choice in such situations is intravenous **diazepam (Valium)**.

Phenobarbital for the treatment of epilepsy is usually prescribed in low doses so that dependence and tolerance are not significant concerns. Adults are treated with 50 to 100 mg two to three times per day, and children are prescribed 3 to 5 mg/kg per day. For uses other than treatment of tonic-clonic seizures and focal epilepsy, safer drugs are available.

Short-acting **barbiturates** are Schedule II controlled drugs and therefore may not be available to some nurse practitioners. **Phenobarbital** is Schedule IV and may be included on a state nurse practitioner formulary, depending on the individual state's rules and regulations.

Table 15–33 ● **Dosage Schedule: Barbiturates**

Drug	Indications	Dosage
Amobarbital sodium	Sedation, hypnotic, preanesthetic, acute convulsive episodes	Sedative: 30–50 mg bid to tid Hypnotic: 65–200 mg IM: 65–500 mg IV: do not exceed 50 mg/min *Children 6–12 yr:* 65–500 mg Single dose not to exceed 1 g
Butabarbital sodium	Sedation, hypnotic, preanesthetic, acute convulsive episodes	Sedation: 15–30 mg tid to qid Hypnotic: 50–100 mg hs Preoperative sedation: 50–100 mg 60–90 min before surgery *Children:* 2–6 mg/kg/d; not to exceed 100 mg
Pentobarbital sodium	Sedation, hypnotic, preanesthetic	IV: Initial dose of 100 mg in adult with proportional decrease of dose for children or debilitated adults. Wait for a full minute to assess effect before adding more. Not to exceed 200–500 mg for healthy adult. IM: Usual adult dose is 150–200 mg *Children:* 2–6 mg/kg as single injection; not to exceed 100 mg
Phenobarbital	Sedation, hypnotic, preanesthetic, treatment of partial and generalized tonic-clonic and cortical focal seizures status epilepticus	Epilepsy *Adults:* 60–100 mg/d *Children:* 3–6 mg/kg/d Acute convulsions *Children:* 200–320 mg IM/IV, repeat q6h prn *Children:* 4–6 mg/kg/d IM/IV for 7–10 d to blood level of 10–15 mcg/mL
		Sedation *Adults:* 30–120 mg/d in divided doses; not to exceed 400 mg/24 h *Children:* 8–32 mg Hypnotic *Adult:* 100–200 mg *Children:*dose based on age and weight Preoperative sedation *Adults:* 100–200 mg IV 60–90 min before surgery *Children:* 1–3 mg/kg IM or IV Status epilepticus 15–20 mg/kg IV over 10–15 min; may require 15 min or more to achieve peak

Table 15–33 ● **Dosage Schedule: Barbiturates—cont'd**

Drug	Indications	Dosage
Secobarbital sodium	Sedation, hypnotic, preoperative sedation, status epilepticus	Preoperative sedation *Adult:* 200–300 mg 1–2 h before surgery or 1 mg/kg IM 10–15 min before surgery *Children:* 2–6 mg/kg not to exceed 100 mg or 4–5 mg/kg IM Hypnotic *Adult:* 100 mg at bedtime, 100–200 mg IM, or 50–250 mg IV Status epilepticus *Children:* 15–20 mg/kg IV over 15 min

*hs = *hora somni* (at bedtime).

Monitoring

The difference between therapeutic and toxic plasma levels is not wide, and levels should be monitored frequently. The therapeutic range is 15 to 40 mcg/mL. It is necessary to closely monitor blood levels when prescribing **barbiturates** with other drugs metabolized by CYP450 2D19.

Sedative-Hypnotics

Insomnia can be either a symptom within a syndrome or a specific type of sleep disorder. However, it should not be treated as an illness by itself. When patients complain about difficulty sleeping, it is necessary to further assess the kind of difficulty, that is, is the difficulty falling asleep (initial or onset insomnia), difficulty staying asleep (sleep maintenance insomnia), waking up too early and not being able to return to sleep (late or terminal insomnia), or waking up tired and not rested? Each of these components indicates different problems and is treated differently. Onset insomnia frequently is a symptom of anxiety or agitated depression and better treated by sleep hygiene measures. Terminal insomnia again is common in depression and improves when the depression remits. Waking up tired and waking up several times during the night may be depression, pain, or other physical problem such as overactive bladder. Finally, other medical conditions (e.g., fibromyalgia, chronic obstructive pulmonary disease [COPD], cardiac arrhythmias) or medications (e.g., beta blockers, corticosteroids, bronchodilators) may contribute to sleep disturbances.

Insomnia may occur transiently, lasting only a few days; short term, lasting 2 to 3 weeks; or chronic, lasting longer than 3 weeks and even years. Transient and short-term insomnia can often be treated with sleep hygiene only. Chronic insomnia should be treated with medication for a few months, then the patient should be tapered off the medication. If the problem persists, however, the practitioner should refer the patient for a sleep laboratory study before continuing with treatment.

Whatever the cause of the insomnia, sleep disturbance can contribute to other health problems and requires attentive decision making. Prior to considering medication, sleep hygiene measures should be the first resort. This includes limiting the bedroom and bed to purposes of sleep and sex only. Working in bed, watching television, eating in bed are all activities that disturb sleep and contribute to the perception that the bed is a battleground on which to fight sleep. In addition, the patient may be advised to establish a bedtime routine that includes comforting and relaxing measures an hour before going to bed. These may include a hot bath, a warm noncaffeine drink or high tryptophan snack, light reading, and relaxation or mild stretch exercises. More vigorous exercise should be avoided within 4 hours of going to bed, as should eating. If not asleep within 30 minutes, the patient should get up and read, or do some simple tasks and return to bed when sleepy.

Benzodiazepine Hypnotics

If sleep is still a problem that treating the underlying problem does not help, the most common sedatives or hypnotics include **benzodiazepines** and **nonbenzodiazepine gabaergics**. The **benzodiazepines** most commonly used for sleep include the rapid-onset, slow-acting **triazolam (Halcion)**; delayed-onset, intermediate-acting **temazepam (Restoril)** and **estazolam (Prosom)**; and rapid-onset, long-acting **flurazepam (Dalmane)** and **quazepam (Doral)**. They all have the potential for dependence and tolerance and should not be used more than 3 weeks at a time of daily dosing and no more than three times a week for no more than 3 months. The pharmacodynamics and pharmacokinetics are the same as the **benzodiazepine anxiolytics** shown in Table 15–28.

Nonbenzodiazepine Hypnotics

Pharmacodynamics

This class of drugs also act at the GABA receptor but not at the benzodiazepine site. There are four drugs in this class including: **zolpidem (Ambien)**, **zaleplon (Sonata)**, and **eszopiclone (Lunesta)** (**zopiclone** is not available in the United States).

Pharmacokinetics

Absorption and Distribution

These drugs are rapidly absorbed through oral administration and are protein bound differentially; that is, **zaleplon** is minimally protein bound but zolpidem is 92 percent protein bound. They have short half-lives ranging from 1 hour (**zaleplon**) to 5.8 hours (**eszopiclone**) and short duration. Peak onset occurs in 0.5 to 1 hour.

Metabolism and Excretion

All three are extensively metabolized by aldehyde oxidase and the CYP450 3A4 isoenzymes. They are excreted by the kidneys.

Pharmacotherapeutics

Precautions and Contraindications

All of these drugs are within Pregnancy Category C and should not be used during pregnancy or lactation. Although there has been no clinical evidence of dependence or abuse, no sleeping medication should be used acutely beyond 3 weeks or chronically beyond 3 months without careful evaluation of the treatment plan.

Adverse Drug Reactions

The most common side effects include headache, mild transient anterograde amnesia, dizziness, somnolence, and nausea. There appears to be minimal rebound effect, that is, difficulty sleeping after cessation of drug therapy, but there may be daytime drowsiness, especially if taken 4 hours or less before it is necessary to awaken.

Drug Interactions

These drugs have an additive effect with CNS depressants including **benzodiazepines** and **alcohol**. Drugs that induce CYP450 3A4 will decrease the blood levels of these hypnotics including **cimetidine, phenytoin, rifampin,** and **carbamazepine**. Drugs that inhibit CYP450 3A4 will increase the blood levels of these hypnotics including **ketoconazole, clarithromycin, erythromycin,** and **protease inhibitors.**

Clinical Use and Dosing

The primary use of the **nonbenzodiazepine gaba-ergics** in this class is for sedation during episodes of insomnia. **Zaleplon** is available in 5- and 10-mg capsules, **zolpidem** is available in 5- and 10-mg tablets, and **eszopiclone** is available in 1-, 2-, and 3-mg tablets. Lower doses should be used with the elderly.

Rational Drug Selection

There is little to distinguish between these drugs other than individual response. Care must be taken with patients who have a drug or **alcohol** abuse history that may contribute to psychological dependence.

Monitoring

No drug monitoring is needed or available.

Patient Education

Patients should be advised to take these immediately before bedtime and to get at least 4 hours of sleep. They should be advised to use caution if driving a vehicle or operating hazardous machinery until they know what effect the drug has for them. Patients should not combine these drugs with **over-the-counter sleeping aids** or **alcohol.**

MOOD STABILIZERS

Mood stabilizers are used with patients who have bipolar disorders with evidence of depressive and manic or hypomanic episodes. Bipolar disorders are distinctive from unipolar depression by virtue of mood swings and require medication not just for depression but to restore balance in the moods. Neurophysiologically, this is achieved by maintaining a regularity to nerve firing as opposed to the erratic firing characterized by changes in behavior and mood. An oversimplified analogy is that bipolar disorder is like epilepsy, but the erratic firing occurs between the limbic system and the frontal cortex as opposed to the motor strip in clonic seizures. The most direct way to achieve regularity is by affecting the calcium channel on the nerve axon that permits influx of ions and stimulates the release of GABA.

Traditionally, bipolar disorder has been treated with **lithium salts** first introduced in the mid-19th century and reintroduced in 1960. Although at the time it was not understood how it worked, more recently theories focus on **lithium** exchanging with sodium ions to propel the nerve impulse along the cell membrane. Currently, the theory underlying neuromodulation is that the catecholaminergic, indolaminergic, cholinergic, and gamma aminobutric acid systems interact to alter the pre- and postsynaptic receptors and postsynaptic activity. The most direct manner of affecting these systems is with the anticonvulsant drug classes; therefore, this section will focus on the anticonvulsants used in mood stabilization. Chapter 30 addresses additional approaches to the prominent depressive episodes.

Although traditionally medications to stabilize mood in bipolar disorders included **lithium** and **anticonvulsants,** more recently the **atypical APs** demonstrate mood stabilization through the combination neurotransmitter effects on dopamine and serotonin. A product released in 2003 departs from the standard because it combines **fluoxetine** and **olanzapine** in the brand-name form of **Symbyax** to provide mood stabilization. Because this drug is predominantly used in patients with mixed bipolar disorder, it will be discussed in greater detail in Chapter 30 with anxiety and depression.

Lithium

Lithium's stabilizing effect on manic individuals was discovered in the mid-1940s, making it the earliest psychotropic drug available for use. Until recently it was considered the treatment of choice for classic bipolar mood disorder and is used as an adjunct for treatment-resistant unipolar depression.

Pharmacodynamics

Lithium carbonate (Lithobid, Eskalith) is a naturally occurring substance, similar to sodium in its lack of metabolism, its excretion through the renal system, and its affinity for the same binding sites. Both are widely distributed and interchangeable.

The relationship between sodium, **lithium**, and body fluid is inverse in that when sodium and fluids are depleted, as can occur during severe vomiting, prolonged heavy sweating, and **diuretic** use, the level of **lithium** is increased. The opposite also occurs, for example, as a result of water intoxication, which has the effect of decreasing the **lithium** level. Such variations in **lithium** concentration can also be the product of abrupt dietary changes or seasonal weather changes.

Lithium's mechanism of action is not completely understood but, because of the two substances' ability to substitute for each other, it is believed that **lithium** replaces sodium during depolarization in neuronal pathways, effectively stopping the transmission of electrical impulses. Additionally, it is suspected that **lithium** acts on the second messenger system postsynaptically to inhibit either the inositol monophosphatase enzyme to modulate the G-proteins or the messenger RNA to alter the protein kinase C (Stahl, 2009).

Pharmacokinetics

Absorption and Distribution

Lithium is quickly absorbed through the GI tract after oral administration and shows no protein binding. Ingestion of food does not affect absorption. It is widely distributed throughout the body according to water volume. Distribution across the blood–brain barrier is slow.

Metabolism and Excretion

Lithium is one of the few psychopharmacological agents that is not metabolized by the liver and is essentially excreted into the urine unchanged. Because it is excreted by the kidneys, kidney function is critical in the use of **lithium** in treatment. The excretion half-life is between 10 and 50 hours.

Onset, Peak, and Duration

Lithium reaches maximum blood level within 0.5 to 3 hours and has a half-life of 17 to 36 hours. Steady state is achieved in 5 to 7 days.

Pharmacotherapeutics

Precautions and Contraindications

Because **lithium** is almost completely excreted through the renal system, it is essential that the presence of kidney disease be assessed before starting **lithium**. Baseline blood chemistry, including creatinine, blood urea nitrogen (BUN), and TSH levels, should be obtained. In the event of positive findings, a different drug should be used.

Lithium is contraindicated in children less than 12 years because of insufficient clinical trials with young children. **Lithium** is rated Pregnancy Category C and should not be used with pregnant or lactating women without serious balancing of risks and benefits. When taken in the first trimester there is a 10 percent chance of fetal abnormalities including Epstein's cardiac anomaly and tricuspid valve prolapse. When taken in the third trimester, there is a significant risk for neonatal **lithium** toxicity, hypertonicity, congenital hypothyroidism, and congenital goiter (Williams & Oke, 2000).

Extreme caution should be used when prescribing **lithium** to patients with sodium depletion or to those taking **diuretics.** Hypothyroidism and kidney failure may occur with long-term administration.

Adverse Drug Reactions

Early, transient adverse reactions may occur, including most commonly fine tremors of the fingers, nausea, dry mouth, headache, and drowsiness. **Lithium** may be taken with food to minimize GI distress, and the form of the drug may be changed to sustained release to minimize adverse effects associated with dosage peaks. Even at therapeutic blood levels, some patients may have ECG changes that are not necessarily indicative of underlying cardiac disease but should be monitored.

The index between therapeutic and toxic levels is narrow at the upper end, requiring frequent monitoring initially and in the event of significant changes in fluid balance, as often as daily if necessary. The therapeutic range is 0.5 to 1.5 mEq/L.

Indicators of toxicity, which can also occur at therapeutic levels, are coarse tremors of the hands that impair function, nausea and vomiting, diarrhea, confusion, stupor, polydipsia and polyuria, muscle weakness, and ataxia. If the **lithium** level is elevated enough, coma and death can result. Treatment for overdose is supportive, including ensuring adequate hydration and even dialysis. Because lithium overdose may contribute to arrhythmias, ECG monitoring is necessary.

Drug Interactions

Because the liver does not metabolize **lithium**, drug interactions due to the CYP450 system are not an issue. However, drug interactions associated with altering fluid balance and **lithium** concentrations may increase the risk for **lithium** toxicity. **Diuretics** may increase sodium excretion and increase **lithium** concentrations. **NSAIDs** reduce renal elimination and elevate serum **lithium** levels. **Lithium** prolongs the effects of neuromuscular-blocking agents used before surgery and during electroconvulsive treatments (ECT). Table 15–34 includes the drug interactions with **lithium.**

Decreased **lithium** levels may result with **theophylline**, concurrent use of sodium salts and bulking agents such as **Metamucil.** Concurrent administration with **anticonvulsants** may increase toxicity of both drugs.

Table 15–34 ■ **Drug Interactions: Lithium**

Drug	Interacting Drug	Possible Effect	Implications
Lithium	Angiotensin-converting enzyme (ACE) inhibitors, antibiotics (ampicillin, doxycycline, tetracycline, spectinomycin), antihypertensives, metronidazole, NSAIDs, antimicrobials, diuretics, fluoxetine	Increased lithium level	Monitor lithium blood levels and for signs and symptoms of toxicity Avoid NSAIDs
	Caffeine, psyllium, urinary alkalizers, theophylline	Decreased lithium level	Monitor lithium blood level and recurrence of manic signs and symptoms for need to increase dose
	Anticonvulsants, calcium channel blockers, phenothiazines, haloperidol, methyldopa	Increased neurotoxicity	Avoid coadministration
	Benzodiazepines	Sexual dysfunction	Avoid
	SSRIs	Serotonin syndrome	Keep SSRI dose low
			Monitor for signs and symptoms of serotonin excess
	Acetazolamide, osmotic diuretics, theophyllines, urinary alkalizers	Increased renal excretion	Monitor PT response and lithium blood levels, adjust lithium dose
	Neuromuscular blocking agents, TCAs	Increased pharmacological effects of additive drugs	Adjust dosage accordingly

Clinical Use and Dosing

Table 15–35 includes the indications, dosage schedule and available dose forms for **lithium**.

Rational Drug Selection

Because of its long half-life, **lithium** takes 10 to 14 days to reach maximum efficacy; therefore, it is not indicated in the treatment of acute mania. Rather, it is indicated for maintenance of mood stability and prevention of mania or hypomania. A strategy for responding to acute mania would be to start a patient on **lithium** supplemented initially with a **dopaminergic** or **serotonergic-dopaminergic drug** such as **haloperidol** or **risperidone** and to discontinue the neuroleptic, if possible, when the required length of time for **lithium** to be become efficacious has elapsed and the mania has abated.

Some clinicians raise the dosage initially to achieve a serum level of 1.2 mEq/L during an acute stage and back down to 0.8 mEq/L for maintenance. As a patient achieves and maintains stability, levels need not be obtained as frequently.

Lithium is also prescribed for patients who have been resistant to adequate trials of the usual **antidepressants** based on the theory that the resistance is due to an underlying bipolar pathology. Adjunctive doses of **lithium** are frequently lower than they would be for bipolar disorder, with concomitantly lower risks.

Monitoring

Because signs and symptoms of toxicity may occur even at subtoxic blood levels, patients should always be assessed for tremors, nausea, and drowsiness. Lowering the dose will usually be sufficient to resolve the problems.

Blood levels should be obtained 14 days after beginning treatment and 14 days after every dosage change. Generally, routine blood levels are obtained every 3 to 6 months after stability is achieved. In the event of patient illness involving severe vomiting, diarrhea, prolonged high fever, or heatstroke, more frequent monitoring is needed and would also be the case in a planned dietary change or weight loss plan.

The procedure for obtaining an accurate **lithium** level is to have the sample drawn 12 hours after the last dose, usually the bedtime dose, before any morning dose has been taken. The patient need not be fasting, but the timing needs to be accurate within an hour to ensure standardization of interpretation of the results.

Routine blood counts with differential, chemistry screens, and thyroid panels should be obtained yearly. In addition, there should be a baseline ECG and annual ECG to ascertain arrhythmias.

Table 15–35 ● **Dosage Schedule: Lithium**

Drug	Indications	Dosage	Available Dosage Forms	Cost
Lithium (Lithobid, Eskalith, lithium carbonate, Lithotabs)	Treatment of manic phase of bipolar disorders and prevention of manic episodes	Acute mania; 600 mg tid or 900 mg bid extended-release Maintenance: 300 mg tid-qid or 450 mg bid Controlled-release	Capsules (G): 150 mg 300 mg 600 mg Tablets: 300 mg Controlled-release tablets: 300 mg and 450 mg Syrup: 300 mg/15 mL Slow-release capsules 150 and 300 mg	 $19/90 $26/90 $34/90 $18/30

Refractory unipolar depression = 300–600 mg daily.

G = generic.

Patient Education

Patients should be informed of the procedure for obtaining an accurate **lithium** level as described above. Advise the patient to report any illness involving severe vomiting, diarrhea, or prolonged fever. Also tell patients engaging in activities that produce copious sweating to increase their water intake and maintain an adequate salt intake. Women of childbearing age need to be advised of contraceptive strategies and that unplanned pregnancies may result in congenital malformations.

Valproates

Although **valproate** (Depakote) was approved for treatment of seizures in the 1960s, the FDA did not approve its use in mania until 1995. It is currently seen as the first- or second-choice drug in the treatment of bipolar disorder, especially in acute mania and maintenance for bipolar, manic disorder.

Pharmacodynamics

Although the exact mechanism is unknown, **valproate** blocks GABA uptake into presynaptic neurons without affecting the **benzodiazepine** binding site. It appears to enhance GABA function thereby slow down repolarization and reduce glutamate functioning at the sodium and calcium channels.

Pharmacokinetics

Absorption and Distribution

Valproate is administered orally and rapidly absorbed by the GI tract. It has also been approved for IV administration for immediate treatment of seizures but this route has not been used in rapid treatment of mania. It is 100 percent bioavailable with high protein binding. It reaches peak levels in 1 to 4 hours and has a half-life of 6 to 16 hours. **Valproate** may be displaced by **carbamazepine** and **warfarin** contributing to toxic side effects.

Metabolism and Excretion

Valproate is metabolized by the liver with several active metabolites. It is metabolized by P450 2C9, 2C19, and 2A6; possibly induces 2C9 and 2C19; and inhibits 2C9, 2D6, and 3A4. Such a complicated metabolism contributes to many drug interactions, as described below. It is excreted by the kidneys.

Onset, Peak, and Duration

Peak plasma levels occur within 1 to 4 hours, although when administered by syrup, the drug peaks sooner. Conversely, the enteric-coated version delays absorption and peaking.

Pharmacotherapeutics

Precautions and Contraindications

Contraindications include hypersensitivity and hepatic disease.

Use of these drugs during the first trimester of pregnancy is associated with neural tube defects including spina bifida. They are Pregnancy Category D. Their use should be restricted to cases in which the woman's life would be endangered without them and then only beyond the first trimester. They should be used with caution during lactation.

The plasma level range is 50 to 100 mcg/mL. Levels above 100 mcg/mL are thought to be toxic, although symptoms of toxicity can occur at blood levels within the normal range, and patients have been maintained on levels above 100 mcg/mL without apparent toxicity. Therefore, **valproate** has a wider safety margin than **lithium.** Symptoms of toxicity include dizziness, hypotension, tachycardia or bradycardia, drowsiness, visual hallucinations, and respiratory depression. Coma and death may result.

Although relatively uncommon, **valproate** may impair platelet aggregation so that bleeding time may be prolonged, and it may suppress bone marrow production. For this reason, a CBC with differential and platelets should precede use and be repeated with regularity initially and less frequently beyond the first 3 months as the patient continues to take the medication without adverse events.

Rare cases of hepatotoxicity and liver failure have occurred, primarily in children less than 2 years who have been on combination **antiepileptic drug therapy.** Because bipolar disorder has not yet been diagnosed in children less than 2 years, valproate has not been used for mood stabilization in this population.

Patients with diabetes taking **valproate** may show falsely positive ketone urine tests because the drug is partially excreted in the urine as a ketone metabolite. Any patient may have initially elevated liver enzymes, but this is usually transitory.

Adverse Drug Reactions

Valproate is well tolerated, and most adverse effects, such as GI distress, heartburn, and CNS depression, are mild and transient. Safety in situations requiring mental alertness are of concern initially, and the patient should be instructed to avoid potentially dangerous situations until the effect of the drug can be assessed. Alopecia has also been reported and the hair usually grows back although of a different texture.

Drug Interactions

Many common drug interactions have to do with the competition with protein-binding sites and the P450 enzyme involvement. **Valproates** in combination with other CNS **depressants** can lead to an additive depressant effect. Bleeding time can be increased in combination with **anticoagulants.** Combinations of **TCAs** and **valproates** can lead to increased risk of cardiotoxicity. Combinations of **valproates** with **carbamazepine** or **hydantoins** may result in increased levels of these drugs and reduced efficacy of valproate. **Chlorpromazine, cimetidine, erythromycin, rifampin,** and **salicylates** may increase **valproate** serum levels. Table 15–36 includes the drug interactions with the **valproates.**

Clinical Uses and Dosages

Table 15–37 includes the indications, dosage schedule, and available dose forms for the **valproates.**

Rational Drug Selection

Valproate psychiatric indications include the treatment of bipolar disorder, particularly the rapid cycling or mixed

Table 15–36 ■ **Drug Interactions: Valproates**

Drug	Interacting Drug	Possible Effect	Implications
Valproic acid and derivatives	CNS depressants	Increased sedation and disorientation	Warn patient about safety issues; avoid if possible
	Anticoagulants	Increased bleeding time	Monitor bleeding time
	Anticonvulsants	May increase plasma level of anti decrease valproate efficacy	Monitor plasma levels
	TCAs, barbiturates, diazepam, ethosuximide	Increased blood level and increased risk of cardiotoxicity	Monitor blood level
	Clonazepam	Increased risk of absence seizure	
	Lithium	Increased tremors	Decrease lithium dose
	Typical antipsychotics	Increased risk of neurotoxicity, sedation, EPS	Monitor for signs and symptoms of toxicity
	Antiviral	Decreased valproate level	Monitor plasma level of valproate
	Cimetidine, salicylates, rifampin, erythromycin	Increased plasma level and half-life of valproate	Monitor plasma level of valproate
	Lamotrigine	Decreased valproic levels, increased lamotrigine levels	Monitor plasma levels

Table 15–37 ◉ **Dosage Schedule: Valproates**

Drug	Indications	Dosage	Available Dosage Forms	Cost
Valproic acid (Depakote, Depakene; Depacon)	Complex partial, simple (petit mal), absence seizure epilepsy; mania; migraine headache	*Adults:* 750 mg daily in divided doses; may increase rapidly to control acute mania to maximum of 60 mg/kg/d For migraine headache: 250 mg bid *Children and older adults:* reduce dose Sprinkle capsule should not be chewed and not stored for future use once opened; take with food to prevent GI distress For acute mania: 60-mg IV infusion (20 mg/min or less) at same frequency as oral dose	Depakene: 250 mg capsule 250 mg/5 mL syrup Generic: 250 mg capsules 250 mg/5 mL syrup Depakote enteric coated tablet: 125 mg 250 mg 500 mg 125 mg sprinkle capsule Extended-release Depakote 250 mg and 500 mg Depacon: 5 mg injection	$90/30 capsules $103/150 mL $15/30 capsules $19/150 mL $74/60 $137/60 $243/60 $70/60 $68/30 $112/30

types, both for acute mania and prevention. It can be given in large doses in an acute state with minimal concern for toxicity.

Other uses include treatment of mood stability associated with borderline personality disorder or post-traumatic stress disorder (PTSD), anger and aggression, and adjunctive treatment for drug resistant unipolar depression.

The usual adult dose is 750 to 3,000 mg/day taken initially in divided dose then can be taken once daily at bedtime if side effects are tolerable. Because it inhibits its own metabolism after reaching steady state, the drug begins to maintain a consistent blood level sufficient for single daily dosing.

Monitoring

Plasma levels should be assessed to help guide dosage adjustments. CBCs and chemistries should be obtained prior to onset of treatment and then every 3 months for 1 year. After 1 year, monitoring can be done annually.

Patient Education

Patients should be advised about the side effects, especially the possibility of bruising and delayed clotting initially. Patients who are prone to falls should especially be advised to tell their primary care provider and family members. Patients should be advised to avoid hazardous activities until their level of sedation is determined. Also, advise patients not to abruptly discontinue the drug.

Nonclassified Mood Stabilizers

The **nonbenzodiazepine gaba-ergics** used in the treatment of epilepsy have shown effectiveness in treating bipolar states as might be expected based on the data about **valproates.** These include **lamotrigine (Lamictal), gabapentin (Neurontin),** and **topiramate (Topamax).** Only **lamotrigine** has been approved by the FDA for this use.

Pharmacodynamics

All of these drugs act in some way on GABA as well as other mechanisms. **Lamotrigine** also acts as a 5-HT_3 blocker and glutamate modulator as well as inhibiting the sodium channels to slow down depolarization. **Gabapentin** does not act directly on GABA but instead seems to act as a GABA transporter inhibitor, thereby increasing the availability of GABA. As with **lamotrigine, gabapentin** decreases the excitatory amino acid neurotransmitter, glutamate. Finally, **topiramate** acts in a manner similar to **gabapentin** to enhance GABA functioning and interfere with glutamate by means of the sodium and calcium channels.

Pharmacokinetics

Absorption and Distribution

All three of these drugs are readily absorbed through the GI tract and between 80 to 90 percent bioavailability. **Gabapentin's** bioavailability decreases as the dose increases, however. **Lamotrigine** has the longest half-life at 25 hours, **topiramate** at 21 hours, and gabapentin at 5 to 8 hours. Food does not alter absorption for any of these drugs.

Metabolism and Excretion

Lamotrigine is metabolized by glucuronidation; however, all three drugs are essentially excreted by the kidneys relatively unchanged. Neither **gabapentin** nor **topiramate** undergoes metabolism at all.

Pharmacotherapeutics

Precautions and Contraindications

All three of these drugs are rated Pregnancy Category C. Based on the pregnancy registry, there is no evidence of harm to the fetus; however, there is an insufficient database to determine the risk. The prescriber would need to balance the risks and the benefits of treating a pregnant woman with these drugs. If it is necessary to use the drugs, it serves the fetus best to wait until the second trimester. Although no detrimental effects have been reported to the breastfeeding newborn, each of these drugs is excreted in breast milk and exposes the healthy neonate unnecessarily to the drug.

These drugs have not been tested in children and should not be used to treat children less than 2 years. There are no age-related differences in safety; however, dosages may need to be changed in the elderly to accommodate to the changes in renal clearance.

Topiramate has shown hyperchloremic non-anion gap metabolic acidosis and should be used cautiously with patients with eating disorders.

Adverse Drug Reactions

These drugs have relatively few side effects. Most commonly seen are somnolence, dizziness, ataxia, and fatigue. **Gabapentin** has weight gain associated with it, whereas **topiramate** and to a lesser extent **lamotrigine** have weight loss associated with them. In addition, diplopia, blurred vision, nausea, and rhinitis are not uncommon. **Lamotrigine** and **topiramate** have a rare incidence (0.8% in children; 0.3% in adults) of Stevens-Johnson syndrome occurring within the first 2 to 8 weeks of therapy that can be fatal. **Topiramate** has a 1 percent occurrence of renal calculi.

Drug Interactions

Because these drugs are minimally metabolized by the liver, there are few drug interactions. When given in conjunction with other **antiepileptic drugs**, such as **carbamazepine**, or **phenytoin**, the half-life of **lamotrigine** is decreased, but with **valproate** the half-life is increased. **Gabapentin** reduces the bioavailability of antacids, but **cimetidine** increases the bioavailability of **gabapentin**. **Gabapentin** also increases the serum levels of **contraceptives**. **Topiramate** decreases the effectiveness of **oral contraceptives** and **carbonic anhydrase inhibitors** may increase the risk of kidney stones.

Clinical Use and Dosing

The primary use of these drugs is for epilepsy; however, **lamotrigine** has been approved for use in acute mania, maintenance and prophylaxis of mood lability, and may even reduce the incidence of depression in bipolar disorders. **Gabapentin** and **topiramate** have not been approved to treat bipolar disorders; however, indication for this is likely to be approved in the near future.

Rationale Drug Selection

Currently these three drugs are seen as third line for the treatment of bipolar disorder and are often used in conjunction with other therapies for treatment resistant bipolar conditions. They are safe and easy for patients to maintain treatment.

Monitoring

No routine serum levels are necessary. Patients should monitor skin appearances and report any rashes within the first 2 months of therapy, especially if blisters form. Weight monitoring is important, especially with **gabapentin**.

Patient Education

Patients must be informed of the risks and benefits of these drugs as well as the possible side effects. Patients taking topiramate need to be advised to drink plenty of water due to the risk of kidney stones. Advise patients of the potential for Stevens-Johnson syndrome and what to do if a rash appears.

OPIOID ANALGESICS AND THEIR ANTAGONISTS

When nonopioid agents are ineffective for pain relief, **opioids** are a next logical step in the treatment of pain. These agents alter the perception of and response to painful stimuli. This group of drugs includes natural opium alkaloids, synthetic agents, and a combination of the two. Most of this group of drugs are schedule II narcotics under federal law. Many states allow prescription of these agents by nurse practitioners, but state laws may vary.

Opioids are generally classified as agonists, mixed agonist-antagonists, or partial agonists. Agonists include **codeine (Tylenol #3 or #4)**, **fentanyl (Sublimaze, Duragesic)**, **hydrocodone (Vicodin, Lortab)**, **hydromorphone (Dilaudid)**, **levorphanol (Levo-Dromoran)**, **meperidine (Demerol)**, **methadone (Dolophine)**, **morphine (MSIR, Roxanol, MS Contin, Oramorph, Kadian)**, **oxycodone (Percocet, Percodan, Roxicodone, OxyContin)**, and **propoxyphene (Darvon, Darvocet)**. Some of these agents such as **hydrocodone** and **codeine** are typically combined with **acetaminophen** or an **NSAID**.

Mixed agonist-antagonists include **butorphanol (Stadol)**, **nalbuphine (Nubain)**, and **pentazocine (Talwin)**. Partial agonists include **buprenorphine (Buprenex)** and **dezocine (Dalgan)**.

Opiate antagonists include **naloxone HCL (Narcan)**, **naltrexone HCL (Revia)**, and **nalmefene HCL (Revex)**.

Pharmacodynamics

Narcotic analgesics are active at various opioid receptor sites and act as agonists, partial agonists, or mixed agonist-antagonists of endogenously occurring opioid peptides (eukephalins, endorphins). **Opioids** interact with mu, kappa, delta, or sigma receptors producing both the desired and adverse effects of **opioids.** The primary receptors associated with analgesia are the mu and kappa receptors. Activation of these receptors is thought to create an analgesic effect by inhibiting adenyl cyclase activity, which results in a reduction in intracellular cyclic adenosine monophosphate. In addition to an analgesic effect, activation of mu receptors may cause euphoria, physical dependence, and respiratory depression. Activation of kappa receptors may cause miosis, sedation, and respiratory depression. Activation of delta and sigma receptors accounts for many of the adverse effects of **opioids** such as dysphoria, hallucinations, and respiratory and vasomotor stimulation. Mixed **agonist-antagonists** can cause withdrawal symptoms when given to narcotic-dependent individuals because of their preference at specific opioid receptor sites.

Narcotic antagonists block or reverse opioids by competing at their receptor sites and reverse respiratory depression, hypotension, and sedation. Indications for use are **narcotic** overdose and prolonged surgical use of **narcotics.**

Pharmacokinetics

Absorption and Distribution

Opioid analgesics are available in oral, parenteral, rectal, sublingual, and transdermal routes. Rate of absorption depends on the route used. Oral drugs are convenient and have a slower onset of action, delayed peak time, and a longer duration of action than drugs administered parenterally. Overall, onset of action of **opioid analgesics** is rapid and varies from 2 or 3 minutes up to 60 minutes, depending on the route of administration. Half-life is generally up to 6 hours, although some are longer, for example, **levorphanol** with a half-life of 12 to 16 hours and methadone with a half-life of 15 to 30 hours. **Meperidine** has an active metabolite, normeperidine, whose half-life is 15 to 30 hours.

The **opioid antagonists nalmefene HCL, naloxone** HCL, and **naltrexone** HCL are indicated for acute crises and are given parenterally. Their onset of action is within 2 to 15 minutes, with duration of action 1 to 4 hours. Because their half-lives can be shorter than the **narcotic** they are reversing, patients must be closely monitored for symptoms of a recurrence of respiratory depression.

Metabolism and Excretion

Opioid analgesics and **antagonists** are metabolized in the liver and excreted in urine. Table 15–38 presents the pharmacokinetics.

Pharmacotherapeutics

Precautions and Contraindications

Because of the respiratory depressant effect of these drugs, compromised pulmonary function is a contraindication.

Table 15–38 ▶ **Pharmacokinetics: Opioid Analgesics and Antagonists**

Drug	Onset	Peak	Duration	Half-Life	Excretion
Alfentanil	Immediate	—	—	1–2 h	Urine
Codeine	10–30 min	0.5–1 h	4–6 h	3 h	Urine
Fentanyl IM transdermal	7–15 min 6 h	20–30 min 12–24 h	1–2 h 72 h	1.5–6 h	Urine
Hydromorphone	15–30 min	0.5–1 h	4–5 h	2–3 h	Urine
Levorphanol	30–90 min	0.5–1 h	6–8 h	1–16 h	Urine
Meperidine	10–45 min	0.5–1 h	2–4 h	3–4 h	Urine
Methadone	30–60 min	0.5–1 h	4–6 h	15–30 h	Urine
Morphine	15–60 min	0.5–1 h	3–7 h	1.5–2 h	Urine
Oxycodone	15–30 min	1 h	4–6 h	—	Urine
Oxymorphone	5–10 min	0.5–1 h	3–6 h	—	Urine
Propoxyphene	30–60 min	2–2.5 h	4–6 h	6–12 h	Urine
Sufentanil	1.3–3 min	—	—	2.5 h	Urine
Nalmefene	5–15 min	1.5–2.3 h	—	1–10.8 h	Urine
Naloxone	2 min	—	1–4 h	30–81 min	Urine
Naltrexone	Rapid	Within 1 h	—	4–13 h	Urine
Buprenorphine	15 min	60 min	6 h	2.2–3.5 h	Urine
Butorphanol	<10 min	30–60 min	3–4 h	2.5–4 h	Urine

Continued

Table 15–38 ▶ **Pharmacokinetics: Opioid Analgesics and Antagonists—cont'd**

Drug	Onset	Peak	Duration	Half-Life	Excretion
Dezocine	<15–30 min	30–150 min	2–4 h	2.4 h	Urine
Nalbuphine	15–30 min	30–60 min	3–6 h	5 h	Urine
Pentazocine	15–30 min	15–60 min	3 h	2.2–3.5 h	Urine

Cautious use is indicated in the case of head injury, increased intracranial pressure, and acute abdominal conditions because of the drugs' capacity to mask symptoms of pain and to increase cerebrospinal fluid pressure.

Safety of use in pregnant and nursing women is not established, and they are classified as Pregnancy Category C. Infants born to addicted mothers suffer sedation, respiratory depression, and withdrawal. **Oxycodone, propoxyphene, methadone, oxymorphone,** and **hydromorphone** should not be used in children.

Narcotic analgesics carry the risk of physical tolerance and dependence, as well as having street value. Thus, the prescribing clinician needs to obtain a clear history of current substance use because of the dangers of cross-tolerance and additive CNS depression. These agents have been implicated in suicide or accidental death, particularly in combination with **alcohol.** As indicated previously, **mixed agonist-antagonists** should not be prescribed for **narcotic**-addicted individuals because of the risk of physical withdrawal. Patients wishing treatment of **narcotic** addiction with **methadone** should be referred to an appropriate treatment facility.

Careful titration of **opioid antagonists** is required, because the blockade of **opioids** by antagonistic action means that the individual may experience withdrawal symptoms, called acute abstinence syndrome, at about the time the next **narcotic** dose would be due. Achieving a balance between reversing CNS depression and preventing acute withdrawal is delicate and requires careful titration in small increments. This situation applies equally to the drug-affected neonate. In addition to these concerns, attention is also needed in postoperative situations in which the antagonist's action may leave the patient in severe, acute pain.

Adverse Drug Reactions

Adverse reactions to **opioids** include respiratory depression, hypotension, confusion, sedation, nausea, vomiting, dizziness, visual disturbances, hallucinations, euphoria, lethargy, uncoordinated movements, constipation, agitation, depression of cough reflexes, and paresthesias.

Adverse reactions to **antagonists** include nausea, vomiting, tachycardia, hypertension, fever, and dizziness. **Naltrexone** is particularly hepatotoxic and can be injurious to the liver when used in high doses. Individuals with impaired liver function should be assessed carefully for signs of further damage.

Drug Interactions

Some interacting drugs such as **alcohol, sedative-hypnotics, barbiturates, antihistamines,** and **antipsychotics** can create additive CNS-depressant effects. Others, such as **cimetidine, hydantoins, nicotine,** and **droperidol,** can interfere with **narcotic** effects. Other drug interactions, for example, with **carbamazepine** and **warfarin,** may decrease the effect of the interacting drug. Use with extreme caution with **MAOIs** because severe, even fatal, reactions may occur.

Table 15–39 presents drug interactions.

Table 15–39 ■ **Drug Interactions: Opioid Analgesics and Antagonists**

Drug	Interacting Drug	Possible Effect	Implications
Opioids	CNS depressants, alcohol, hypnotics, barbiturates, benzodiazepines, antipsychotics	Additive CNS depression	
	Cimetidine, hydantoins, rifampin, droperidol, charcoal, nicotine	Decreased effect of opioid	Increased doses of opioid may be required
	Carbamazepine, warfarin, MAOIs, furazolidone, nitrous oxide	Decreased effect of interacting drug	Monitor blood levels when possible
Nalmefene	Flumazenil	Seizures	Use with caution
Naltrexone	Thioridazine	Decreased effect of thioridazine	Higher dose may be required

Clinical Use and Dosing

Table 15–40 presents the indications and dosage schedules of **opioid analgesics** and **antagonists**.

Rational Drug Selection

Indications for the use of **opioid analgesics** are the control of pain, primarily acute pain as in the case of postoperative, cancer, and obstetric pain. **Opioid analgesics** are also used in the treatment of chronic pain, which is not alleviated with nonopioid agents. In selecting among available agents, the degree and duration of pain must be considered as well as the patient variables of subjective therapeutic response to an agent and adverse effects experienced. **Morphine** is the standard against which other **opioids** are measured, and is considered the drug of choice for cancer pain (Gordon, 2003). **Roxanol** is a convenient method of receiving **oral morphine.**

For the treatment of mild to moderate pain not alleviated by **non-opioids**, treatment can start with a lower potency **opioid** as **codeine**, often given in combination

Table 15–40 ◉ Dosage Schedule: Opioid Analgesics and Antagonists

Drug	Indications	Dosage
Alfentanil HCl (Alfenta)	Anesthetic adjunct only	—
Codeine	Mild to moderate pain; coughing	*Adults:* PO, IM, IV, SC: 15–60 mg every 4 h to maximum of 360 mg/24 h; usual dose is 30 mg *Children >1 yr:* PO, IM, SC: 0.5 mg/kg every 4–6 h
Fentanyl (Sublimaze, Duragesic, Oralet)	Anesthesia; postoperative analgesia; management of chronic pain	*Adults:* Postoperative analgesia: 0.05–0.1 mg IM every 1–2 h Transdermal: 25, 50, 75, 100, 125, 150, 175, 200, 225, 250, 275, and 300 mcg/h system; change once every 72 h Titrate dose upward first time only in 3 d, thereafter at 6-d intervals
Hydromorphone HCl (Dilaudid)	Moderate to severe pain	*Adults:* PO: 2–4 mg every 4–6 h Parenteral: 1–4 mg every 4–6 h; slow IV over 1–5 min Rectal: 3 mg every 6–8 h
Levorphanol tartrate (Levo-Dromoran)	Management of opioid dependence	*Adults:* PO, SC: 2–3 mg
Meperidine (Demerol)	Moderate to severe pain; preoperative sedation	*Adults:* PO, IM, SC: 50–150 mg every 3–4 h *Children:* PO, IM, SC: 1–1.8 mg/kg (0.5–0.8 mg/lb) every 3–4 h
Methadone (Dolophine)	Severe pain; management of opioid dependence	*Adults:* PO, IM, SC: 2.5–10 mg every 3–4 h; oral dose is half of parenteral
Morphine sulfate (Astramorph PF, Duramorph, Infumorph, MSIR, MS Contin, Oramorph SR, Roxanol, OMS concentrate, MS/L, RMS)	Moderate to severe acute and chronic pain; preanesthetic sedation	*Adults:* PO: 10–30 mg every 4 h Controlled-release: 30 mg every 8 h; do not crush or chew SC/IM: 5–20 mg/70 kg every 4 h IV: 2.5–15 mg/70 kg in 4–5 mL water for injection over 4–5 min Continuous IV pump infusion: 0.1–1 mg/mL in 5% dextrose Rectal: 10–20 mg every 4 h *Children:* SC, IM: 0.1–0.2 mg/kg to maximum of 15 mg every 4 h
Oxycodone (Roxicodone, OxyContin)	Moderate to moderately severe pain	*Adults:* 5 mg or 5 mL every 6 h
Oxymorphone (Numorphan)	Moderate to severe pain; preanesthetic sedation; relief of anxiety/dyspnea in pulmonary edema and left ventricular failure	*Adults:* SC, IM: 1–1.5 mg every 4–6 h IV: 0.5 mg Rectal: 5 mg every 4–6 h
Propoxyphene HCl (Darvon)	Mild to moderate pain	*Adults:* 65 mg every 4 h to maximum of 390 mg/d
Propoxyphene napsylate (Darvon-N)	Mild to moderate pain	*Adults:* 100 mg every 4 h to maximum of 600 mg/d

Continued

Table 15–40 ● **Dosage Schedule: Opioid Analgesics and Antagonists—cont'd**

Drug	Indications	Dosage
Buprenorphine (Buprenex)	Moderate to severe pain	*Adults and children >13:* IM, IV: 0.3 mg every 6 h; may repeat once 30–60 min later if needed; compatible with most IV solutions
Butorphanol tartrate (Stadol)	Pain; preanesthesia sedation	*Adults:* IM: 1–4 mg every 3–4 h to nonambulatory patients IV: 0.5–2 mg every 3–4 h Nasal: 1 mg = 1 spray in each nostril; may repeat if needed in 60–90 min; may repeat 2 dose sequences in 3–4 h
Dezocine (Dalgan)	Pain management	*Adults:* IM: 5–20 mg every 3–6 h; usual dose 10 mg IV: 2.5–10 mg every 2–4 h; usual dose 5 mg
Nalbuphine (Nubain)	Moderate to severe pain; preoperative sedation	*Adults:* SC, IM, IV: 10 mg/70 kg every 3–6 h to maximum of 20 mg/dose or 160 mg/24 h
Pentazocine (Talwin, Talwin NX)	Moderate to severe pain; preoperative sedation	*Adults:* PO: 50–100 mg every 3–4 h to maximum of 600 mg/24 h; initial dose 50 mg IM, SC, IV: 30 mg every 3–4 h to maximum of 360 mg/24 h
Pentazocine combinations	Mild to moderate pain	*Adults:* 12.5 mg with 325 ASA (Talwin compound caplets): 2 tabs tid—qid 25 mg with acetaminophen 650 mg (Talacen caplets): 1 tab every 4 h to maximum of 6 tabs/24 h
Nalmefene (Revex)	Reversal of opioid effects	Opioid-dependent patients: Initial challenge dose of 0.1 mg/70 kg. If no signs or symptoms of withdrawal within 2 min, use following guidelines: Non–opioid-dependent patients: Initial dose of 0.25 mg/kg followed by 0.25 mcg/kg doses at 2–5 min intervals until degree of opioid reversal is attained Give IV; if no IV access is available, give 1 mg SC or IM as single dose
Naloxone (Narcan)	Reversal of opioid depression	*Adults:* IV, IM, SC For overdose: 0.4–2 mg IV; may repeat at 2- to 3-min intervals Postoperative: 0.1–0.2 mg IV at 2- to 3-min intervals; may repeat in 1- to 2-h intervals if needed *Children:* For overdose: 0.01 mg/kg IV; may follow with 0.1 mg if needed; if no IV access, give IM or SC in divided doses Postoperative: initial dose of 0.005–0.01 mg IV repeated at 2- to 3-min increments if needed
Naltrexone (ReVia)	Blocks effects of opioids; treatment of alcohol dependence	Alcoholism: 100 mg PO once daily Opioid dependence: do not give until patient has been abstinent for 10 d, then give challenge dose of 25 mg once; if no withdrawal signs and symptoms occur, continue with maintenance dose; if signs and symptoms occur, repeat challenge in 24 h Maintenance: 50 mg every 24 h; dosing may be flexible (e.g., 100 mg on Mon and Wed; 150 mg on Fri)

with **acetaminophen**. If pain is not alleviated by **codeine**, the derivatives of **codeine, oxycodone** and **hydrocodone**, are approximately eight times more potent. These drugs are available in combination with **aspirin** and **acetaminophen**, which limit the overall dose of the **opioid** that can be given.

For patients with moderate to severe pain who have not been treated with **opioids**, treatment can begin with a short half-life agonist (**morphine, hydromorphone, oxycodone**). These drugs are easier to titrate than those with a longer half-life such as **methadone** or **levorphanol**.

Morphine is the drug of choice for severe pain. Sustained-release preparations such as **MS Contin** and **Oramorph SR** provide pain relief for 8 to 12 hours. **Morphine** has the advantage of a wide range and flexibility of dosing.

Chronic stable pain may be managed with sustained-release **morphine, oxycodone, methadone,** or **transdermal fentanyl. Methadone** has an advantage of low cost and oral efficacy, but it can cause excessive sedation. **Methadone** has the ability to antagonize NMDA (N-methyl-D-aspartate) receptors and is particularly useful in the treatment of chronic and neuropathic pain. **Fentanyl** is a potent **opioid,** available as a transdermal patch, that provides up to 3 days of continuous analgesia. **Fentanyl** must be titrated carefully, however, to avoid oversedation. **Meperidine** is not recommended for chronic pain because it has a short half-life and has a toxic metabolite, normeperidine, that causes central nervous system excitability manifested by dysphoria, tremors, seizures, and irritability.

Partial agonists and mixed agonist-antagonists are limited by a dose-related ceiling effect, but are effective in treating moderate to severe pain. These agents are useful for patients who are intolerant of **morphine** or **meperidine. Mixed agonist-antagonists** are contraindicated in patients receiving full **agonist opioids** because they reverse some of the pain control provided by the full agonist. These agents may cause less respiratory depression than **morphine,** however, which is a consideration for patients with compromised pulmonary function.

In addition to selecting an **opioid** for pain relief, some of these agents may be utilized for other purposes such as antitussive or antidiarrheal effects. For example, **camphorated tincture of opium (paregoric)** is used in the treatment of diarrhea. **Codeine** possesses both antitussive and antidiarrheal properties.

Further discussion of pain management is found in Chapter 42.

Monitoring

It is important to monitor for adverse reactions, as discussed previously. It is also important to monitor for **opioid** withdrawal. Symptoms of **opioid** withdrawal resemble a flu-like syndrome manifested by muscle cramps, dilated pupils, lacrimation, rhinorrhea, yawning, sneezing, anxiety, anorexia, nausea, vomiting, diarrhea, and gooseflesh.

Patient Education

Patients should be warned about the potential for physical dependence and advised that these agents should primarily be used for relief of acute, severe pain. Long-term use for chronic pain can result in tolerance and hypersensitivity to pain. Patients should be instructed to avoid the concurrent use of **alcohol** and other **CNS depressants. Opioid analgesics** may cause drowsiness and, for safety reasons, should not be used when mental or physical alertness is required. Advise the patient to change position slowly to minimize postural hypotension. Because these agents may cause constipation, patients should be advised to increase daily intake of fluid and fiber. **Opioids** may be taken with food to prevent nausea. Because **opioids** are controlled substances, patients should be cautioned to prevent use or theft of these agents by unauthorized persons.

STIMULANTS

The FDA approved the use of **stimulants** in treating attention deficit-hyperactivity disorder (ADHD), narcolepsy, and weight reduction. In therapeutic ranges these drugs improve alertness, mood, attention, wakefulness, vigilance, psychomotor performance and have an anorexiant effect. The prototype stimulant drug is **amphetamine,** which was developed more than 100 years ago. It has been used to treat depression, obesity, narcolepsy, and respiratory depression and as an energizer during World War II. Because of these same foci, **amphetamines** possess notoriety as street drugs of abuse.

The **stimulants amphetamine, dextroamphetamine, methylphenidate,** and, less commonly, **methamphetamine (Desoxyn)** are used in the treatment of ADHD and narcolepsy. Primarily **methylphenidate (Ritalin, Methylin, Metadate, Concerta, Focalin, Daytrana patch), Adderall,** a combination of **dextroamphetamine (Dexedrine)** and **amphetamine salts,** are used. In addition, **atomoxetine (Strattera)** a norepinephrine reuptake inhibitor is available as an alternative to **stimulants** for ADHD.

Other **stimulants** such as caffeine and phenylpropanolamine found in over-the-counter **cold medicines** are significant because of the additive stimulant effects they have in combination with other **stimulants.**

Pharmacodynamics

The CNS **stimulants** are sympathomimetic amines that act as dopamine agonists and indirectly release and prevent the reuptake of dopamine, serotonin, and norepinephrine in presynaptic nerve endings. This action stimulates the cerebral cortex, brainstem, and reticular activating system and appears to stimulate the reward center in the brain that consists of the nucleus accumbens, the amygdale, and the ventral tegmentum. The dopamine and norepinephrine (and to a lesser extent the serotonin) nerve fibers connect these regions of the brain to the prefrontal cortex to coordinate thinking, feeling, and responding to emotional stimuli. When receptors in the reward center are occupied, there is a sense of well-being; it is because of this response that these drugs have considerable abuse potential.

Pharmacokinetics

Absorption and Distribution

Taken orally, these drugs are quickly and thoroughly absorbed, with a rapid onset of action. Depending on the formulation, peak plasma levels occur in less than 1 to

4 hours. Their half-lives are from 1 to 12 hours. Although biodistribution is unknown for **methylphenidate, atomoxetine** is highly protein bound.

Metabolism and Excretion

Dextroamphetamine and **methylphenidate** are metabolized in the liver by de-esterification without the influence of the P450 system, whereas **atomoxetine** is metabolized by 2D6 and 2C19 predominantly. In addition, **atomoxetine** has an equally potent metabolite that circulated in a lower concentration. All three are excreted by the kidneys. Urine acidity affects the rate of excretion of **amphetamine** in that increased alkalinity increases its half-life, a fact that can be important in drug overdose. Table 15–41 presents pharmacokinetics.

Pharmacotherapeutics

Precautions and Contraindications

Contraindications to use include arteriosclerotic and symptomatic heart disease, hypertension, hyperthyroidism hypersensitivity to sympathomimetic amines, glaucoma, motor tics, agitation, history of drug abuse, and during or within 14 days of use of an MAOI.

Stimulants are contraindicated for pregnant (Pregnancy Category C) and lactating women. **Methylphenidate** is found in high concentrations in breast milk. **Stimulants** may cause insomnia and should therefore be taken no closer than 6 hours before bedtime. **Concerta** should be used cautiously in patients with esophageal motility disorders, as there is an increased risk of obstruction.

Adverse Drug Reactions

Undesirable effects include insomnia, undesired weight loss, growth retardation in children, tachycardia, palpitations, restlessness, irritability, euphoria, headache, blurred vision, tremor, increased libido with impaired ability, hypertension, and arrhythmias. Some individuals may experience a paradoxical drowsiness.

Drug Interactions

Various undesirable drug interactions may occur, perhaps the most significant being the risk of hypertensive crisis if stimulants are taken within 14 days of an **MAOI**. Additive sympathomimetic effects occur if these agents are taken concurrently with other adrenergics, including **vasoconstrictors** and **decongestants**. Metabolism of **warfarin, anticonvulsants**, and **tricyclic antidepressants** may be decreased and their effects increased.

Due to the P450 involvement, **atomoxetine** has a different interaction profile than **methylphenidate** or **dextroamphetamine**. CY2D6 inhibitors (e.g., **fluoxetine**) will increase the plasma levels of **atomoxetine**, and **pressor agents** will contribute to increased effects on blood pressure. **Atomoxetine** needs to be used with caution with **albuterol** due to the potentiation of the cardiovascular effects of albuterol.

Table 15–42 presents drug interactions.

Table 15–41 ▶ **Pharmacokinetics: Stimulants**

Drug	Onset	Peak	Duration	Half-Life	Excretion
Dextroamphetamine	30 min	1–3 h	4–20 h	10–30 h	Urine
Methamphetamine HCl	30 min	1–3 h	3–6 h	4–5 h	Urine
Methylphenidate HCl	30–60 min	1.9–4.7 h	4–6 h	1–3 h	Urine
Atomoxetine	—	1–2 h		5–22 h	Urine

Table 15–42 ■ **Drug Interactions: Stimulants**

Drug	Interacting Drug	Possible Effect	Implications
All stimulants	MAOIs	Increased risk of hypertensive crisis and stroke	Avoid
	CNS depressants, alkalinizing agents	Decreased effect of stimulant	Dosage may need adjustment
	Antidepressants	Increased effect of antidepressant, especially with TCAs; increased risk of cardiotoxicity in children	Avoid use of TCAs
	Guanethidine	Increased hypotensive effect	Warn patient about dizziness and syncope
	Hypoglycemic agents	Increased glucose lability and decreased control	Monitor blood glucose

Table 15–42 ■ **Drug Interactions: Stimulants—con'td**

Drug	Interacting Drug	Possible Effect	Implications
	Acidifying agents	Decreased effect of stimulant	Dosage adjustment may be required
	Phenytoin	Increased plasma level of phenytoin	Monitor plasma level
Atomoxetine	Fluoxetine, paroxetine, and quinidine	Increased plasma level of atomoxetine	Increase dosage only after 4 wk

Clinical Use and Dosing

Table 15–43 presents the indications, dosage schedules, and available dosage forms of **stimulants**.

Rational Drug Selection

With the exception of **atomoxetine**, **stimulants** are DEA Schedule II and can be prescribed only by nurse practitioners whose state permits Schedule II prescribing. Because they are Schedule II drugs, the pharmacy requires a new hard copy of the prescription every month. **Stimulants** can be prescribed only without refills, although states may have a mechanism for providing more than one month's prescription at a time. Providers should check with the state's regulatory authorities.

Table 15–43 ◉ **Dosage Schedule: Stimulants**

Drug	Indications	Dosage	Available Dosage Forms	Cost
Dextroamphetamine (DextroStat, Dexedrine ER)	ADHD, narcolepsy, exogenous obesity	*Adults:* 10 mg daily; may increase by 10-mg increments every week to maximum of 30 mg/d; give individual doses at 4- to 6-h intervals *Children age 3–5*: 2.5 mg/d; increase by 2.5 mg daily at weekly intervals to range of 0.1–0.5 mg/kg/d; give in morning *Children >5 yr:* 5 mg 1–2 times/d; may increase in 5-mg increments weekly to maximum of 40 mg/d; usual range 0.1–0.5 mg/kg/d *Extended-release: Adult and child 6 and older:* 5 mg qam, increase by 5mg/d qwk. Max 40 mg/d	Tablets: 5 mg, 10 mg Sustained-release spansules: 5 mg, 10 mg, 15 mg	*Generic:* 5 mg = $18/30 10 mg = $27.69/30 *Generic extended release:* 5 mg = $62/30 10 mg = $85/30 15 mg = $99/30
Methamphetamine HCl (generic)	ADHD, narcolepsy, exogenous obesity	*Adults and children >12 yr:* 5 mg 1–2 times/d; may increase at 5-mg increments weekly to maximum of 25 mg/d may be twice-daily dosing	5-mg tab 10 mg tab 20 mg tab	5 mg = $45/30 10 mg = $24/30 20 mg = $31.49
Amphetamine and dextroamphetamine (Adderall, Adderall XR)	ADHD Narcolepsy XR for ADHD only	*Age 3-5:* 2.5 mg qd, increase by 2.5 mg/wk *Age 6 and up:* 5 mg qd or bid, then increase by 5 mg q wk. Not to exceed 40 mg *Narcolepsy: Children 6–12 yr:* 5 mg daily up to 60 mg/d max *Sustained-release for age 6 and up only:* 6–12, 10–30 mg qd *Age 12–18:* 10–20 mg qd *Adults:* 20 mg qd	Adderall: 5-, 7.5-, 10-, 12.5-, 15-, 20-, 30-mg tabs Adderall XR: 5-, 10-, 15-, 20-, 25-, 30-mg caps	5 mg = $124.48/30 10 mg = $116.98/30 15 mg = $113.98/30 20 mg = $122.97/30 30 mg = $123 5 mg = $235.49/30 10 mg = $237.39/30 15 mg = $237.39/30 20 mg = $237.39/30 25 mg = $237.39/30 30 mg = $237.39/30

Continued

Table 15–43 ● **Dosage Schedule: Stimulants—cont'd**

Drug	Indications	Dosage	Available Dosage Forms	Cost
Lisdexamfetamine (Vyvanse)	ADHD	*Age 6 and up:* 30 mg qam, increase by 10-20 mg/d every 7 days. Not to exceed 70 mg total qd for any patient. May dissolve contents in water, drink immediately, do not subdivide caps	20-, 30-, 40-, 50-, 60-, 70-mg caps	20 mg = $178/30 30 mg = $190/30 40 mg = $171/30 50 mg = $171/30 60 mg = $176/30 70 mg = $171/30
Methylphenidate HCl (Ritalin, Ritalin SR, Ritalin LA, Methylin, Methylin ER, Daytrana patch)	ADHD, narcolepsy (Ritalin and Ritalin SR)	*Ritalin and Methylin: Adults:* 10–30 mg/d in 2–3 divided doses; maximum 60 mg/d in divided doses.	Ritalin tablets: 5, 10, 20 mg	5 mg = $62/30 10 mg = $42/30 20 mg = $64/30
		Children >6 yr: 5 mg bid before breakfast and lunch, with increase of 5–10 mg at weekly intervals; maximum 60 mg/d in divided doses. Stop drug if no improvement in 4 wk	Methylin tabs: 5, 10, 20 mg Methylin chews: 2.5, 5, 10 mg	5 mg = $21/30 10 mg = $21/30 20 mg = $21/30
		All ages: Ritalin SR tabs taken in morning may be supplemented with afternoon regular tablets if needed, no later than 6pm.	Methylin oral solution: 5 mg/ 5ml, 10 mg/5 ml. Ritalin SR Sustained-release tablets: 20 mg	20 mg SR = $86/30
		Ritalin LA: age 6 and up: whole or sprinkled in applesauce, 20 mg qam, increase by 10 mg weekly to max 60 mg/d	Ritalin LA: Extended-release caps 10, 20, 30, 40 mg (half immediate-release, half extended-release beads)	10 mg LA = $151/30 20 mg LA = $151/30 30 mg LA = 151/30 40 mg LA = $151/30
		Methylin ER: child age 6 and up: 10 mg qam, increase weekly by 10 mg/d to max 60 mg in divided doses. Adults: 10–20 mg qam, increase by 10 mg weekly to max of 60 mg in divided doses.	Methylin ER: 10-, 20-mg tabs	10 mg ER = $30/30 20 mg ER = $39/30
		Daytrana patch: 6–12 yr: 10-mg patch to hips 2 h before desired effect. Remove 9 h after application, earlier if shorter duration needed. Titrate dose q week. Rotate application site.	Daytrana patch: 10, 15, 20, 30 mg delivered over 9 h	10 mg = $186/30 15 mg = $188/30 20 mg = $182/30 30 mg = $187/30
Methylphenidate (Concerta)	ADHD	*Age 6-12:* start at 18 mg qd, Max 54 mg/d *Age 13–17:* start at 18 mg/d Max 72 mg/d *Adults:* 18–36 mg/d, Max 72 mg/d For patients already on methylphenidate: 5 mg bid/tid = 18 mg 10 mg bid/tid = 36 mg 15 mg bid/tid = 54 mg 20 mg bid/tid = 72 mg/d	18, 27, 36, 54 mg extended-release	18 mg = $180/30 27 mg = $201/30 36 mg = $196/30 54 mg = $212/30
Metadate ER	ADHD, Narcolepsy	*Metadate ER: Age 6 and up:* swallow whole, 10 mg qam, increase by 10 mg q week. Max 60 mg/d in divided doses	Metadate ER:10-, 20-mg tabs	10 mg ER = $48/30 20 mg ER = $55/30

Table 15–43 ● **Dosage Schedule: Stimulants—cont'd**

Drug	Indications	Dosage	Available Dosage Forms	Cost
Metadate CD	ADHD	*Metadate CD: Age 6 and up:* swallow whole or sprinkle on applesauce: 20 mg before breakfast, increase weekly by 10–20 mg/d. Max 60 mg once daily	Metadate CD: 10-, 20-, 30-, 40-, 50-, 60-mg caps (immediate-release and extended-release beads)	10 mg CD = $145/30 20 mg CD = $149/30 30 mg CD = $148/30 60 mg CD = $240/30
Dexmethylphenidate (Focalin, Focalin XR)	ADHD	*Age 6 and up:* 2.5 mg bid, increase by 2.5 mg at weekly intervals. Max 20 mg/d *Extended-release:* once daily in a.m. swallow whole or sprinkle onto applesauce. *Age 6 and up:* 5 mg/d, may increase by 5 mg/wk. *Adults:* start at 10 mg/d, increase by 10 mg weekly. Max dose for adults and children 20 mg/d	2.5-, 5-, 10-mg tablets XR: 5, 10, 15, 20 caps. (contains immediate- and extended-delayed release beads)	5 mg = $43/30 10 mg = $55/30 5 mg XR = $165/30 10 mg XR = $169/30 15 mg XR = $165/30 20 mg XR = $181/30 30 mg XR = $162/30
Atomoxetine (Strattera)	ADHD Drug-resistant depression	*PO Adults and Children >70 kg:* start w/40 mg/d; and increase dose every 3 days to target 80 mg. After 2–4 wk dose may be increased to 100 mg/d	Capsules: 10, 18, 20, 25, 40, 60, 80, 100 mg	10 mg = $1777/30 18 = $188/30 25 mg = $177/30 40 mg = $189/30 60 mg = $186/30 80 mg = $203/30 100 mg = $206/30
Modafinil (Provigil)	Narcolepsy, and excessive sleepiness due to sleep apnea and shift work	*Age 16 and up:* 200 mg qd in am. Max 400 mg/d in divided doses. For shift work, take dose 1 h before work.	100-, 200-mg tabs	100 mg = $464/30 200 mg = $656/30

ER, XR = extended release,
CD = continuous release, SR = sustained release.

To prevent anorexia and growth retardation in children, providers should maintain records of growth and weight and consider drug holidays on weekends or in summertime to permit the child to catch up on growth. Some children may exhibit symptoms of ADHD as the drug begins to wear off and may do better on a sustained-release formulation, especially if they must complete homework in the afternoon or early evening. If symptom coverage with extended release is not adequate, a short-acting formulation after school may be needed.

Central nervous system **stimulants** are indicated for the treatment of ADHD, narcolepsy, and exogenous obesity refractive to other forms of treatment. The use of **stimulants** in the treatment of adolescent and residual adult ADHD is a matter of some controversy, given the street value of these drugs, the increase in societal abuse of these drugs, and the association of these agents with violent behavior. Because **atomoxetine** seems to stimulate the reward center less so than do other agents and has a delayed onset of action, it is less useful as a drug of abuse, but may also be less effective therapeutically.

These agents should be given cautiously to emotionally unstable patients, including those with a history of drug or **alcohol** abuse, because such patients may be more likely to increase their doses unnecessarily.

Monitoring

It is important to monitor for adverse reactions as discussed previously. The clinician should monitor that the amount of drug used is consistent with the amounts prescribed and dispensed.

Patient Education

These agents may cause insomnia so patients should not take them within 6 hours of bedtime. Abrupt cessation of **stimulants** may cause extreme fatigue and mental depression. These agents may cause dizziness or blurred vision, so caution patients to avoid driving or other hazardous activities until response to medication is known. To reduce anorexia and growth retardation in children, these agents should be given with or after meals. Parents should notify the school nurse of medication regime. Parents need to be aware that these drugs have street value and should be stored safely in the home. Children and teens require an explanation of why these drugs are appropriate for their disorder as distinctive from drugs of abuse, and assistance in handling peers' responses to their use of these medications.

REFERENCES

Detke, M. J., Lu, Y., Goldstein, D. J., Hayes, J. R., & Demitrack, M. A. (2002). Duloxetine, 60 mg once daily, for major depressive disorder: A randomized double-blind placebo-controlled trial. *Journal of Clinical Psychiatry, 63*(4), 308–15.

Drug facts and comparisons. (2010). Philadelphia: Wolters Kluwer Health.

Dubovsky, S. (2005). *Clinical guide to psychotropic medications.* New York: W.W. Norton.

Einarson, A., Fatoye, B., Sarkar, M., Voyer Lavigne, S., Brochu, J., Chambers, C., et al. (2001). Pregnancy outcome following gestational exposure to venlafaxine: A multicenter prospective controlled study. *American Journal of Psychiatry, 158,* 1728–1730.

Gordon, D. B. (2003). Multiple uses and misconceptions about addiction. *Oncology Issues,* July/August, 41–42.

Janicak, P. G., Davis, J. M., Preskorn, S.H., & Ayd, F. J. (2006). *Principles and practice of psychopharmacology* (4th ed.). Philadelphia: Lippincott Williams & Wilkins.

Keltner, N. L., & Folk, D. G. (2005). *Psychotropic drugs* (4th ed.). Philadelphia: Elsevier.

Meltzer, H. Y., Arvanitis, L., Bauer, D., & Rein, W., Meta-Trial Study Group. (2004). Placebo-controlled evaluation of four novel compounds for the treatment of schizophrenia and schizoaffective disorder. *American Journal of Psychiatry, 161,* 975–984.

Pies, R. (2005). *Handbook of essential psychopharmacology* (2nd ed.). Washington, DC: American Psychiatric Publishing.

Sadock, B. J., Sadock, V. A., & Ruiz, P. (2009). *Kaplan and Sadock's comprehensive textbook of psychiatry* (9th ed.). Philadelphia: Lippincott Williams & Wilkins.

Schatzberg, A., Cole, J., & DeBattista, C. (2007). *Manual of clinical psychopharmacology* (6th ed.). Washington, DC: American Psychiatric Publishing.

Schatzberg, A. F., & Nemeroff, C. B. (2009). *The American Psychiatric Press textbook of psychopharmacology* (4th ed.). Washington, DC: American Psychiatric Publishing.

Stahl, S. (2009). *Essential psychopharmacology: The prescriber's guide.* New York: Cambridge University Press.

Toxnet (2011). Topiramate. LactMed National Library of Medicine: Bethesda MD. Retrieved June 7, 2011 from http://toxnet.nlm.nih.gov/cgi-bin/sis/search/f?./temp/~fKnb74:1

Williams, K., & Oke, S. (2000). Lithium and pregnancy. *The Psychiatrist, 24,* 229–231.

Wynn, G., Oesterheld, J., Cozza, K., & Armstrong, S. (2008). *Clinical manual of drug interaction principles for medical practice.* Washington DC: American Psychiatric Press.

CHAPTER 16

DRUGS AFFECTING THE CARDIOVASCULAR AND RENAL SYSTEMS

Anita Lee Wynne and Sharon Maxey

Chapter Outline

ANGIOTENSIN-CONVERTING ENZYME INHIBITORS AND ANGIOTENSIN II RECEPTOR BLOCKERS

Angiotensin-converting enzyme inhibitors (ACEIs) and **angiotensin II receptor blockers (ARBs)** have multiple uses related to the cardiovascular system. Their action on the renin-angiotensin-aldosterone (RAA) system lowers blood pressure (BP), improves oxygenation to heart muscle, decreases inappropriate remodeling of heart muscle after myocardial infarction (MI) or with heart failure (HF), and reduces the adverse affects of diabetes on the kidney. Their mild and usually transient adverse effects and their ease of dosing make them popular drugs. ARBs have similar roles in the treatment of hypertension (HTN), and HF. Their roles in angina and diabetic nephropathy prevention are evolving.

Pharmacodynamics

As shown in Figure 16–1, inhibition of ACE activity (ACEIs) results in decreased production of both angiotensin II

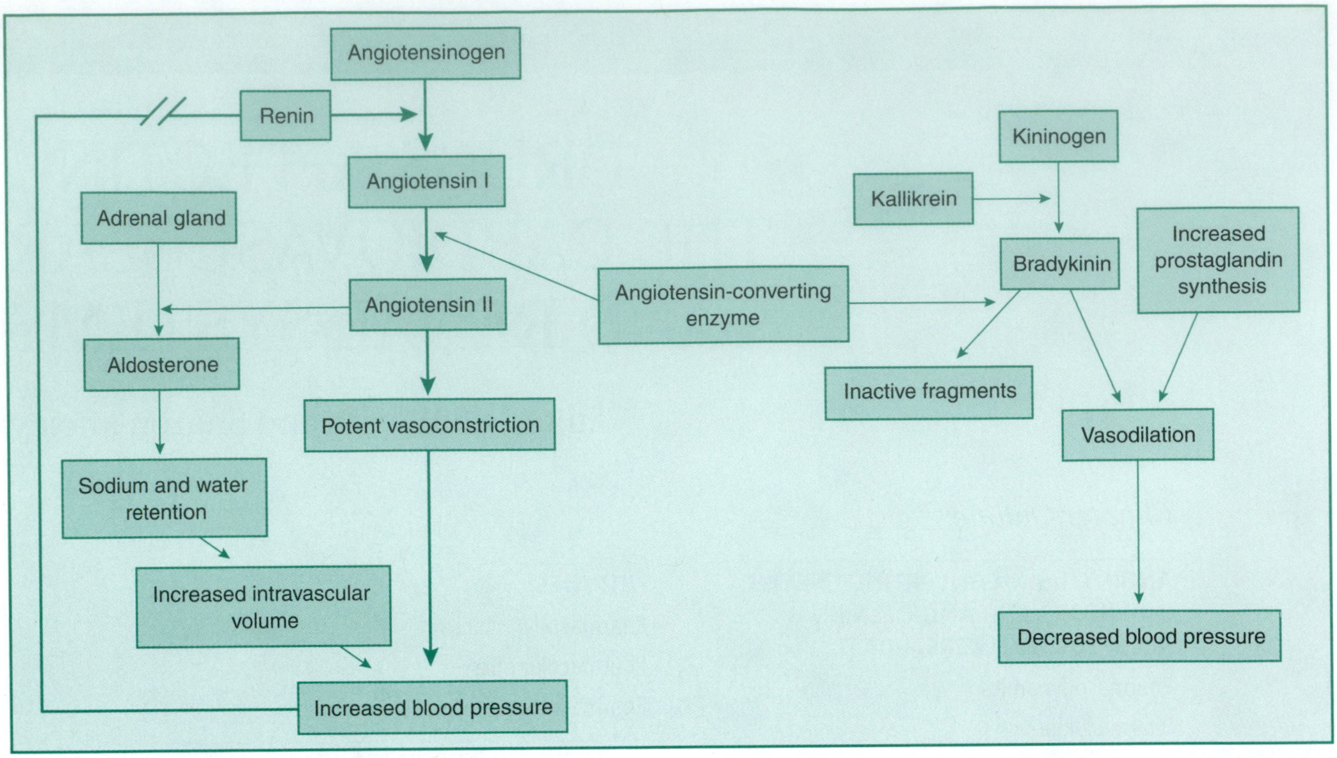

Figure 16–1. Renin-angiotensin-aldosterone system. Renin acts on angiotensinogen to create the inactive decapeptide angiotensin I. Angiotensin I is then converted, primarily in the lung, to angiotensin II, a potent vasoconstrictor, through the activity of angiotensin-converting enzyme (ACE). Angiotensin II stimulates aldosterone secretion, causing retention of sodium and water and loss of potassium by the kidney. ACE is also involved in the inactivation of bradykinin, a vasodilator. Together, these systems help to control blood pressure.

(AT II) and aldosterone. AT II has multiple roles in the cardiovascular system. It increases vasomotor tone by direct stimulation of vascular smooth muscle contraction and through the inhibition of endothelial nitric oxide and prostaglandin release, raising BP and decreasing blood flow through arteries, including the coronary arteries. AT II increases intravascular volume through its stimulation of sodium and water retention (with aldosterone), shifting of the pressure-natriuresis relationship, and altering glomerular hemodynamics. It is also produced in response to tissue injury. This latter action results in stimulation of smooth muscle cell and fibroblast proliferation with thickening of the vessel wall (remodeling). This action, combined with its inhibition of the endothelium's ability to resist monocyte and platelet adhesion, promotes intravascular inflammation and clotting and contributes to the atherosclerotic process. Finally, in the heart, AT II also causes remodeling, resulting in hypertrophy and fibrosis of myocardial tissue after ischemic injury or in response to persistent afterload. This is a primary mechanism in HF.

ACE also has a role in the kinin-kallikrein-bradykinin system. Bradykinin in low doses causes dilation of vessels and acts with prostaglandin to produce pain and cause extravascular smooth muscle contraction, increased vascular permeability, and increased leukocyte chemostaxis. Bradykinin has a primary role in inflammation. ACE facilitates the breakdown of bradykinin into inactive fragments, thus reducing these actions. High levels of bradykinin are thought to be a factor in the cough associated with ACEI use.

ARBs do not affect ACE activity but rather act by blocking the AT II receptor. They have similar action to ACEIs on vasoconstriction and aldosterone secretion but no activity related to bradykinin. ACEIs and ARBs do not affect cardiac output and so do not produce reflex tachycardia.

The effectiveness of ACEIs in preventing diabetic nephropathy probably results from decreased glomerular efferent arteriolar resistance and a reduction in intraglomerular capillary pressure, which causes improved renal hemodynamics, diminished proteinuria, retarded glomerular hypertrophy, and a slower rate of decline in glomerular filtration rate (GFR). These drugs do not affect glucose metabolism or raise serum lipid levels, but they do improve insulin sensitivity; all of these are important issues in type 2 diabetes mellitus. ARBs are also useful in preventing diabetic nephropathy.

Pharmacokinetics

Absorption and Distribution

The ACEIs and ARBs are well absorbed orally, with some variation in bioavailability based on the presence of food in the gut (Table 16–1). **Captopril (Capoten)**, the prototype drug for the ACEI class, is rapidly absorbed, with a bioavailability of about 70 percent when taken on

Table 16–1 ▶ **Pharmacokinetics: Angiotensin-Converting-Enzyme Inhibitors and Angiotensin II Receptor Blockers**

Drug	Onset(h)	Peak (h)	(Duration (h)	Protein Binding	Bioavailability (BA)	Effect of Food on Absorption	Active Metabolite	Half-Life (h)	Elimination
ACE Inhibitors									
Benazepril	1	2–4	24	95%	37%	Slows	Benazeprilat	NRF: 10–11 IRF: prolonged	20% in urine; 11–12% in bile
Captopril	0.25	0.5–1.5	6–12	25%–30%	75%	Reduced by 30%–40%	—	NRF: <2 IRF: 3.5–32	>90% in urine
Enalapril	1	4–6	24	50%–60%	60%	None	Enalaprilat	NRF: 1.3 IRF: nd	Total: 94% in urine and feces Unchanged: 54% in urine
Enalaprilat	0.25	1–4	6	UK	NA	NA	NA	UK	>90% in urine
Fosinopril	1	2–6	24	95%	36%	Slows	Fosinoprilat	NRF: 12 IRF: prolonged	Total: 50% in urine and feces Unchanged: 54% in urine
Lisinopril	1	6	24	none	25%	None	—	NRF: 12 IRF: prolonged	Total: nd Unchanged: 100% in urine
Moexipril	1	3–6	24	50%	15%	Markedly reduced	Moexiprilat	NRF: 2–9 IRF: prolonged	Total: 13% in urine; 50% in feces Unchanged: negligible
Perindopril	UK	3–7	24	60%	75%	Reduced BA of metabolite	Perindoprilat	0.8–1	In urine
Quinapril	1	2–4	24	97%	60%	Reduced	Quinaprilat	NRF: 2 IRF: prolonged	Total: 60% in urine; 37% in feces Unchanged: trace
Ramipril	1–2	4–6.5	24	73%	50%–60%	Reduced	Ramiprilat	NRF: 13–17 IRF: prolonged	Total: 60% in urine; 40% in feces Unchanged: <2%
Trandolaparil	1	4–8	24	80%	10% (70%) metabolite	Slows	Trandolaprilat	6	33% in urine; 66% in feces

Continued

Table 16–1 ▶ **Pharmacokinetics: Angiotensin-Converting-Enzyme Inhibitors and Angiotensin II Receptor Blockers—cont'd**

Drug	Onset(h)	Peak (h)	(Duration (h)	Protein Binding	Bioavailability (BA)	Effect of Food on Absorption	Active Metabolite	Half-Life (h)	Elimination
ARBs									
Candesartan	2–4	6–8	24	99%	15%	None	Inactive metabolite	9	33% in urine; 66% in feces
Eprosartan	1	2	24	98%	13%	Decreased by 25%	Inactive	5–9	7% in urine; 90% in feces
Irbesartan	2	3–14	24	90%	60%–80%	None	Inactive metabolite	11%–15%	20% in urine; 80% in feces
Losartan	Varies	1 parent; 6 metabolites	24	98%	33%	Decreased by 10%	5-carboxylic acid	1 parent; 6–9 metabolites	35% in urine; 60% in feces
Olmesartan	1	2	24	99%	26%	None	None	13	35% in urine; 65% in feces
Telmisartan	3	UK	24	99.5%	42% (40 mg)/ 58% (160 mg)	Reduced 6% (40 mg)/20% (160 mg)	Active; less potent	24	0.5% in urine; >97% in feces
Valsartan	2	4–6	24	95%	25%	Decreased by 40%–50%	Metabolite significantly less potent	6	13% in urine; 83% in feces

NRF = normal renal function; IRF = impaired renal function; nd = no data; UK = unknown.

an empty stomach. Bioavailability is decreased to 30 to 40 percent if taken with food. **Losartan (Cozaar)**, the prototype drug for the ARB class, undergoes extensive first-pass metabolism, resulting in 33 percent bioavailability. It may be taken without regard to food.

Distribution is to most body tissues except the central nervous system (CNS). **ACEIs** and **ARBs** cross the placenta and are found in breast milk.

Metabolism and Excretion

Except for **captopril** and **lisinopril (Zestril, Prinivil)**, all **ACEIs** are prodrugs converted to active metabolites by hydrolysis, primarily in the liver. **Losartan** has both an active drug and an active metabolite (5-carboxylic acid) hydrolyzed by the liver. **Captopril** is metabolized by the liver to inactive compounds. The kidney is the primary organ of excretion for all **ACEIs** except **fosinopril (Monopril)** and **moexipril (Univasc)**, and impaired renal function can significantly prolong their half-lives. **ARBs** have significant excretion in feces. The percentage excreted in feces varies from 50 percent to more than 97 percent. **Captopril**, with a half-life of less than 2 hours, is the only short-acting ACEI. It requires bid or tid administration, with steady state achieved in 2 to 3 days. All other members of the class have 6- to 12-hour half-lives and require more time to achieve steady state but can be given daily. **Losartan** has a 2-hour half-life, and its active metabolite has a 6- to 9-hour half-life. Dosing may be daily or in two divided doses. Steady state is achieved in 3 to 6 weeks.

Losartan is significantly inhibited by inhibitors of cytochrome P450 (CYP450) 3A4 and 2C9. **Irebesartan** has a similar problem with CYP450 2C9. Clinical significance of these inhibitions is negligible, however, because the active metabolite is unaffected.

Pharmacotherapeutics

Precautions and Contraindications

Only three absolute contraindications to the use of ACEIs exist: bilateral renal artery stenosis, angioedema, and pregnancy. In bilateral renal artery stenosis, increased vascular pressure and vasoconstriction appear to be required to sufficiently overcome the stenotic blood flow to perfuse the kidney. The vasodilating effect of an ACEI or an ARB prevents the kidney from maintaining its perfusion, and ischemic renal failure may develop. Angioedema occurs in approximately 0.2 percent of patients taking **ACEIs** and can be life threatening. The physiological reason for this adverse response appears to be related to an increase in bradykinin level associated with inhibition of ACE. It usually occurs with the first dose or within the first month of therapy and is more common in the longer-acting agents. Because this is a class phenomenon, the **ACEI** must be discontinued, and no other drug in this class may be used. **ARBs** do not affect the bradykinin system and should not cause this adverse response. Angioedema is a very serious adverse response, so administration of an **ARB** in a patient who exhibited angioedema with an **ACEI** is still a questionable clinical practice.

ACEIs and **ARBs** should be used cautiously with patients who have impaired renal function, *especially older adults.* Dosage adjustment may be required for all **ACEIs**. Hypovolemic or hyponatremic states also require cautious use. Adequate hydration is required to maintain an appropriate GFR and must be adequate before starting these drugs to prevent renal dysfunction. Inadequate hydration can produce hypovolemia based on the vasodilating effects of **ACEIs** and **ARBs**. Hyperkalemia contraindicates use because reduced aldosterone secretion may worsen this electrolyte imbalance. Hyperkalemia risk increases for patients with chronic heart failure (CHF) because of the reduced blood flow to the kidneys. Patients should have their serum potassium level checked prior to initiating therapy and within 1 week to note trends.

Hepatic impairment also requires cautious use. For **ACEIs**, **fosinopril** metabolism is cut in half, the maximum concentration (C_{max}) was cut in half and the area under the curve (AUC) increased 300 percent for **moexipril**, plasma concentrations were 50 percent higher for **perindopril**, and plasma concentrations were reduced for **quinapril**. For **ARBs**, **losartan** total plasma clearance was about 50 percent lower and bioavailability was twice as high, the AUC was increased 60 percent for **olmesartan**, AUC was twice that for **valsartan** and increased 40 percent for **eprosartan**.

Because **ACEIs** and **ARBs** can cause fetal and neonatal morbidity and mortality, they are **Pregnancy Category C** in the first trimester of pregnancy and **Pregnancy Category D** in the second and third trimesters and during lactation.

Safety and efficacy in children has been established for **enalapril** and **lisinopril** only. *Drugs Facts and Comparisons* (Wolters Kluwer Health, 2009) does mention use of **captopril** in infants and children, but it is an unlabeled use.

Adverse Drug Reactions

Adverse reactions for both **ACEIs** and **ARBs** are usually transient, mild, and more common in longer-acting agents. Most common are those associated with hypotension (dizziness, headache, fatigue, orthostatic hypotension). Tachyphylaxis frequently occurs with continued therapy. Also common and often cited as the reason for discontinuance of **ACEIs** is a dry, hacking cough that usually occurs in the first week of therapy. This is a class phenomenon for **ACEIs**, but changing to a different **ACEI** has been associated with less cough in some patients. Because the action of bradykinin may be responsible for the adverse reactions of cough and angioedema, **ARBs** do not produce these effects (Wolters Kluwer Health, 2009). Changing to an **ARB** provides benefits similar to those of the **ACEI** with less likelihood of cough. Less common adverse reactions with ACEIs include a rash that is most common with **captopril** and not a class phenomenon, and neutropenia that increases with high doses, renal impairment, and concomitant collagen diseases.

Drug Interactions

Additive hypotensive effects occur with **diuretics**, and this drug interaction is sometimes used clinically. Additive hypotension may also occur with other **antihypertensives**, **nitrates**, **phenothiazines**, and acute **alcohol** ingestion. Because of the interference with aldosterone secretion, the concurrent use of **potassium supplements**, **potassium-sparing diuretics**, or **cyclosporine** may result in hyperkalemia. The antihypertensive response is reduced by **NSAIDs** because of their effect on prostaglandins. CYP 2C9 and 3A4 isoenzymes are involved in the metabolism of **losartan**; 2C9 for **irebsartan.** Drugs that inhibit this system (e.g., **cimetidine**) may cause increased levels of free drug. Other specific drug interactions and the appropriate actions to prevent them are given in Table 16–2.

Table 16–2 ■ Drug Interactions: Angiotensin-Converting-Enzyme Inhibitors and Angiotensin II Receptor Antagonists

Drug	Interacting Drug	Possible Effect	Implications
All ACEIs	Lithium	Increased serum lithium levels and symptoms of toxicity	Monitor lithium levels more closely.
	Diuretics	Hypotension and renal dysfunction	Discontinue 2–3 days before initiating therapy with ACEI or initiate with low dose. Ensure adequate hydration prior to first dose and warn about potential for dizziness.
	Antihypertensives, nitrates, alcohol, phenothiazines	Hypotension	Warn patient. Avoid concurrent use if possible. Avoid or reduce alcohol use.
	Potassium supplements, potassium-sparing diuretics	Hyperkalemia	Avoid concurrent use. Teach patient that salt substitutes often are high in potassium. Read label and check with provider before using.
	NSAIDs	Blunted antihypertensive effects	Avoid concurrent use or monitor for need to increase ACEI dose. Teach patient not to take over-the-counter drugs (OTCs) without informing provider.
	Antacids	Decreased absorption of ACEI; increased risk for digitalis or lithium toxicity	Avoid use or separate doses by at least 1 h.
	Allopurinol	Increased risk of hypersensitivity reactions	Avoid concurrent use.
	Capsaicin	Increased incidence of cough	
Captopril	Probenecid	Decreased elimination and increased levels of captopril	Avoid concurrent use.
Enalapril	Rifampin	Decreased effectiveness of enalapril	Monitor for need to increase dose of enalapril or select a different ACEI.
Losartan	Fluconazole	May inhibit metabolism of losartan causing increased antihypertensive and adverse effects	Fluconazole does not affect eprosartan. Select difference antifungal or use eprosartan.
	Indomethacin	Reduced hypotensive effects of losartan	Avoid concurrent use. Select different ARB.
Telmisartan	Digoxin	Median increase in digoxin peak concentration (49%) and trough concentration (20%)	Avoid concurrent use. Select different ARB.

Table 16–2 ■ **Drug Interactions: Angiotensin-Converting-Enzyme Inhibitors and Angiotensin II Receptor Antagonists—cont'd**

Drug	Interacting Drug	Possible Effect	Implications
All ARBs	Cimetidine	Increased effects of ARB	Select different histamine$_2$ blocking agent.
	Phenobarbital	May decrease effects of ARB	If use is necessary, monitor for need to change ARB dose.
	Diuretics, especially thiazide diuretics	Hypotension	Same as for ARBs.

Clinical Use and Dosing

Hypertension

Because primary HTN has no identifiable cause, the treatment necessarily depends on interfering with normal physiological mechanisms that regulate BP. **ACEIs** and **ARBs** act on the RAA system to reduce pressure by decreasing sodium and water retention (aldosterone action), by decreasing vasoconstriction (angiotensin direct action), and by increasing vasodilation (bradykinin action). **ACEIs** and **ARBs** are the drugs of choice for patients who are young and white and for patients with diabetes, HF, or MI, for whom they are most effective and have the lowest incidence of adverse reactions. They are generally not as effective for black patients, however, the interracial differences in BP-lowering observed with any drug class are abolished when the drugs is combined with a **diuretic**. Despite noted differences in BP response at the population level, race alone is a poor predictor of BP response to any particular class of drugs if they are given in adequate doses and with sufficient time to work.

Racial differences in adverse responses may occur. African Americans and Asians, for example, have a 3- to 4-fold higher risk of angioedema (ALLHAT Officers and Coordinators for the ALLHAT Collaborative Research Group, 2002), and more cough has been attributed to ACE than in whites (Elliot, 1996). Unfortunately, insufficient numbers of Mexican Americans and other Hispanic Americans, Native Americans, or Asian/Pacific Islanders have been included in most of the major clinical trials to make strong recommendations about their responses.

No specific difference related to gender has been shown (National High Blood Pressure Education Program [NHBPEP], 2003). Doses for HTN vary with each drug, but adverse reactions increase with higher doses. The first dose may cause a steep drop in BP, especially for patients taking diuretics. **Diuretics** should be stopped for 2 to 3 days to allow rehydration before starting an ACEI. **ACEIs** and **ARBs** increase in effectiveness when given with a **diuretic**, and **diuretics** should be reintroduced after the ACEI or ARB dose has been stabilized, since data suggest that all patients with HTN should be on a diuretic unless it is specifically contraindicated. Because reduced aldosterone secretion may result in potassium retention, **thiazide diuretics** make an excellent combination owing to their tendency to foster potassium loss. The best approach is to start low and go slow. Begin with the lowest dose recommended for the ACEI or ARB and increase the dose at 1- or 2-week intervals until BP is controlled. Table 16–3 provides dosage schedules for each of the drugs based on their indications. For further information, see Chapter 40 on drugs used to treat HTN.

Hypertensive Proteinuric Diabetes

To prevent diabetic nephropathy or slow its progression, **ACEIs** or **ARBs** should be used to treat the HTN (AACE Hypertension Task Force, 2006; American Diabetes Association, 2009). In patients with type 1 diabetes, with or without HTN, **ACEIs** have been demonstrated to significantly delay the progression of diabetic nephropathy. In patients with type 2 diabetes, HTN, and microalbuminuria, **ACEIs** and **ARBs** have been shown to delay the progression to macroalbuminuria. In patients with type 2 diabetes, HTN, macroalbuminuria, and renal insufficiency, **ARBs** have been shown to delay the progression to nephropathy (AACE Hypertension Task Force, 2006; American Diabetes Association, 2009; Brenner et al, 2001; Remuzzi, Schieppati, & Ruggenenti, 2003). Dual blockade by combining an ACEI and an ARB has been shown to provide statistically significant reduction in albuminuria and BP. While it requires additional monitoring for hyperkalemia, it is safe (Remuzzi et al, 2003; Wade & Gleason, 2004). Dosages generally used for HTN are appropriate for this indication. Further discussion is found in Chapters 33 and 40.

Angina and Ischemic Heart Disease

Angina is largely a problem of imbalance between myocardial oxygen supply (MOS) and myocardial oxygen demand (MOD). ACEIs affect both the MOS and the MOD sides of the equation. Their prevention of formation of AT II decreases peripheral-vascular resistance (PVR) and, thereby, MOD; decreases the thickening of coronary artery walls, resulting in increased MOS; and decreases the thickening of ventricular walls, resulting in decreased MOD. Their reduced secretion of aldosterone decreases

Table 16–3 ◉ **Dosage Schedules: Angiotensin-Converting-Enzyme Inhibitors and Angiotensin II Receptor Blockers**

Drug	Indication	Initial Dose	Maintenance Dose	Maximum Dose
ACEI Benazapril	HTN (Not recommended for children <6 years of age)	10 mg daily (If not on a diuretic; 5 mg if on diuretic or older adult) 5 mg daily (For Ccr <30 mL/min) *Children:* 0.2 mg/kg once daily (up to 5 mg)	20–40 mg daily in a single or divided dose	80 mg/d 40 mg/d *Children:* 0.6 mg/kg (up to 40 mg)
Captopril	HTN	25 mg bid or tid (6.25–12.5 mg bid if older adult)	Increase to 50 mg bid to tid after 2 weeks if BP not controlled. If BP still not controlled add 25 mg/d HCTZ	450 mg/d (300 mg if older adult)
	Heart failure	6.25–12.5 mg tid (If previous or concurrent diuretic or older adult) 25 mg tid (adult)	Titrate every 2 weeks Increase to 50 mg tid in 2 weeks if no improvement	450 mg/d (see above)
	Diabetic Nephropathy	25 mg tid	25 mg tid	450 mg/d (see above)
	LVD/post-MI	6.25 mg for one dose (3 d post-MI)	12.5 mg tid, the increase to 25 mg tid with a target of 50 mg tid over several weeks	450 mg/d
Enalapril	HTN (May use for children 1 month–16 yrs of age)	5 mg daily (if not on diuretic) *Children:* 0.08 mg/kg (up to 5 mg) once daily	Increase at 4-day intervals to 10–40 mg/d as single or two divided doses.	40 mg/d *Children:* 0.58 mg/kg (up to 40 mg)
		2.5 mg daily (If serum creatinine >1.6 mg/dL)	Increase by 2.5 mg/d at 4-day intervals.	40 mg/d
	Heart failure	2.5 mg/d	Increase to 40 mg/d over wks.	40 mg/d
	LVD (no symptoms)	2.5 mg bid	Increase over wks to 20 mg/d in divided doses	40 mg/d
Fosinopril	HTN *Children:* Not recommended for children <50 kg	10 mg daily	20–40 mg/d	80 mg/d
	Heart failure	10 mg daily	Increase over wks to 20–40 mg/d	40 mg/d
Lisinopril	HTN *Peds:* Not recommended for children <6 yrs of age	10 mg daily 5 mg daily (If Ccr ≥10 <30 mL/min) 2.5 mg daily (If Ccr <10 mL/min or older adult) *Children:* ≥6 years old: 0.07 mg/kg/d (up to 5 mg)	20–40 mg/d 20–40 mg/d 20–40 mg/d	80 mg/d 40 mg/d 40 mg/d *Children:* 0.61 mg/kg/d (up to 40 mg/d)

Table 16–3 ◉ **Dosage Schedules: Angiotensin-Converting-Enzyme Inhibitors and Angiotensin II Receptor Blockers—cont'd**

Drug	Indication	Initial Dose	Maintenance Dose	Maximum Dose
	Heart failure Post-MI	5 mg daily 5 mg within 24 h of MI followed by 5 mg 24 h later, then 10 mg after 48 h	5–20 mg 10 mg daily	20 mg/d 20 mg/d
Moexipril	HTN	7.5 mg prior to meal once daily	7.5–30 mg/d in single or divided doses; 1 h prior to meal	60 mg/d
		3.75 mg (If Ccr <40 mL/min)	7.5–15 mg/d	15 mg/d
Perindopril	HTN	4 mg daily	4–8 mg in single or divided doses	8 mg/d
Quinapril	HTN	10–20 mg/d	20–80 mg/d in single or divided doses Increase at 2-wk intervals	80 g/d
	Heart failure	5 mg daily	20–40 mg in divided doses. Increase at 2-wk intervals	40 mg/d
Ramipril	HTN	2.5 mg daily	2.5–20 mg/d in single or divided doses 1.25 mg bid	20 mg/d
		1.25 mg daily (If Ccr < 40 mL/min)		5 mg/d
	Heart failure and post-MI	2.5 mg bid 1.25 mg bid (If Ccr < 40 mL/min)	Increase in 1 wk to 5 mg bid 1.25 mg bid	10 mg/d 2.5 mg bid
Trandolapril	HTN	1 mg/d (2 mg/d in blacks) 0.5 mg/d (If Ccr < 40 mL/min)	Increase dose at 1-wk intervals to 2–4 mg/d	8 mg/d
	Heart failure, post-MI or LVD	1 mg/d	Increase dose at 1-wk intervals to 4 mg/d	8 mg/d
Candesartan	HTN	40 mg daily	20–80 mg/d. Increase dose at 2-wk intervals	80 mg/d
Esprosartan	HTN	600 mg daily	400–800 mg. Increase dose at 2-wk intervals	800 mg/d
Irbesartan	HTN Diabetic nephropathy	150 mg daily Adults and children 13–16 years old: 150 mg daily	150–300 mg/d in single dose 300 mg/d in single dose	300 mg/d 300 mg/d
Losartan	HTN *Children:* Not recommended for children <6yrs of age	50 mg daily *Children:* 0.7 mg/kg (up to 50 mg) once daily	25–100 mg in single or divided doses	100 mg/d *Children:* 1.4 mg/kg (up to 100 mg)
		25 mg/d (if volume depleted or diuretics)	Increase dose at 1-wk intervals	
	HTN with LVD	50 mg/d	Add HCTZ 12.5 mg/d and increase dose at 1-wk intervals to 100 mg/d	100 mg/d

Continued

Table 16–3 ◉ **Dosage Schedules: Angiotensin-Converting-Enzyme Inhibitors and Angiotensin II Receptor Blockers—cont'd**

Drug	Indication	Initial Dose	Maintenance Dose	Maximum Dose
	Diabetic nephropathy	50 mg/d	Increase at 1-wk intervals to 100 mg/d	100 mg/d
			May be given with insulin or oral antidiabetic agents	
Olmesartan	HTN	20 mg/d	20–40 mg/d. Increase dose at 2-wk intervals	40 mg/d
Telmisartan	HTN	40 mg/d	20–80 mg/d. Increase dose at 2-wk intervals	80 mg/d
Valsartan	HTN *Children:* Note recommended for children <6 yrs of age	80 mg/d *Children:* 1.3 mg/kg (up to 40 mg) once daily	80–160 mg/d. Increase dose at 2-wk intervals. Adding diuretic has greater effect than doses above 80 mg/d	320 mg/d *Children:* 2.7 mg/kg (up to 160 mg)

LVD = left ventricular dysfunction.
All maintenance doses are titrated to target blood pressure. Lowest dose that meets target is used.

the retention of sodium and water, thereby reducing extracellular fluid (ECF) volume and preload.

ACEIs are recommended by the American College of Physicians (Snow et al, 2004) for all symptomatic patients with chronic stable angina to prevent MI or death and to reduce symptoms. American College of Cardiology/American Heart Association (Hunt et al, 2005) and the Veterans Health Administration/Department of Defense (VA/DoD, 2003) also recommend this drug class, but limit it to coronary artery disease (CAD) patients who also have diabetes or left ventricular (LV) dysfunction. They recommend that **ACEIs** be considered in CAD patients even without LV dysfunction. The Institute for Clinical Symptoms Improvement (ICSI, 2007 with a 2009 update) also states that **ACEIs** and **ARBs** are appropriate treatment options for stable CAD. Ample evidence exists for basing the use of both **ACEIs** and **ARBs** for long-term use in patients with CAD even without other comorbidities (Kaiser Permanente Care Management Institute, 2006). Doses are found in Table 16–4. Further discussion is found in Chapter 28.

Postmyocardial Infarction

Survivors of acute MI have a risk for subsequent morbidity and mortality that is 1.5 to 15 times greater than the general population. A combination of an **ACEI**, a **beta blocker** (BB), antiplatelet therapy, and lipid-lowering therapy after MI is appropriate. The reduced morbidity and mortality owing to the use of **ACEIs** results from reduced AT II after myocardial injury and its prevention of ventricular remodeling in noninfarcted myocytes, its alteration of ventricular mass, and its hemodynamic effects on BP and fluid and electrolyte balance. **ARBs** are also extremely effective here because they affect not only AT II but also AT I receptors. In addition, bradykinin has cardioprotective effects and a combination of an **ACEI** and an **ARB** provides complete inhibition of AT II and increased levels of bradykinin, which may be more beneficial than either class alone (Forclaz, Maillard, Nussberger, Brunner, & Burnier, 2003; Veverka, 2004).

ACEIs, with or without **ARBs**, should be started early after MI in stable, high-risk patients (anterior MI, previous MI, Killip class II). They should be continued indefinitely for all patients with LV dysfunction (ejection fractions less than 40%) or symptoms of HF and used as needed to manage BP or symptoms in all other patients (Hunt et al, 2005; Veverka, 2004). Dosages usual for treating HTN are used unless HF is present (see Table 16–3).

Heart Failure

CAD is the underlying cause in about two-thirds of patients with LV dysfunction, which begins with some injury to the myocardium and progresses even in the absence of additional myocardial insults. The principal mechanism relates to remodeling. **ACEIs** and **ARBs** are useful in treating heart failure related to CAD, primarily for their role in reducing remodeling. Another underlying cause for HF is chronic HTN. **ACEIs** and **ARBs** are also effective in treating this underlying cause.

ACEIs, a cornerstone of therapy for HF in all the guidelines (Flather et al, 2000; Hunt et al, 2005; ICSI, 2004; National Collaborating Centre for Chronic Conditions [NCCCC], 2003), are recommended for patients with a history of atherosclerotic vascular disease, diabetes mellitus,

Table 16–4 ◆ **Available Dosage Forms: Angiotensin-Converting-Enzyme Inhibitors and Angiotensin II Receptor Blockers**

Drug	Dosage Form	How Supplied	Cost	Combinations
ACEI				
Benazapril (Lotensin)	(G) (B)	In bottles of 90, 100, and UD 100 all doses	(G) $6 for all strengths (B) 5 mg, 10 mg, and 20 mg = $20; 40 mg = $24	Combined with amlodipine (Lotrel) and with HCTZ (Lotensin HCT) Cost: $44
Captopril (Capoten)	Tablets: 12.5 mg (G)	In bottles of 100, 500, 1,000, 5,000, UD 100, and blister 600	$4	Combined with HCTZ
	12.5 mg (B)	In bottles of 100, 1,000, and UD 100	$97	(Capozide)
	25 mg (G)	In bottles of 100, 500, 1,000, 5,000, UD 100, and blister 600	$4	
	25 mg (B)	In bottles of 100, 1,000, and UD 100	$105	
	50 mg (G)	In bottles of 100, 500, 1,000, 5,000, UD 100, and blister 600	$6	
	50 mg (B)	In bottles of 100, 1,000, and UD 100	$270	
	100 mg (G)	In bottles of 100, 500, 1,000, UD 100, and blister 600		
	100 mg (B)	In bottles of 100	$251	
Enalapril (Vasotec)	Tablets: 2.5 mg (G)	In bottles of 100 and 1,000	$6	Combined with HCTZ
	2.5 mg (B)	In bottles of 100, 1,000, 10,000, and UD 90 and 100	$41	(Vaseretic)
	5 mg (G)	In bottles of 100 and 1,000	$7	Combined with felodipine
	5 mg (B)	In bottles of 100, 1,000, 10,000, and UD 90 and 100	$54	(Lexxel)
	10 mg (G)	In bottles of 100 and 1,000	$11	
	10 mg (B)	In bottles of 100, 1,000, 10,000, and UD 90 and 100	$119	
	20 mg (G)	In bottles of 100 and 1,000	$11	
	20 mg (B)	In bottles of 100, 1,000, 10,000, and UD 90 and 100	$144	
Fosinopril (Monopril)	Tablet: 10 mg, 20 mg	In bottles of 90 and 1,000	$11 (G) $43 (B)	Combined with HCTZ
	40 mg (all B)	In bottles of 90	$112	
Lisinopril (Prinivil, Zestril)	Tablet: 2.5 mg (G)	In bottles of 100, 500, and 1,000		Combined with HCTZ (Prinzide) and (Zestoretic) Cost: (G) $9; (B) $49

Continued

Table 16–4 ◆ **Available Dosage Forms: Angiotensin-Converting-Enzyme Inhibitors and Angiotensin II Receptor Blockers—cont'd**

Drug	Dosage Form	How Supplied	Cost	Combinations
	2.5 mg (P)	In bottles of 30, 1,000, and UD 100	$63	
	2.5 mg (Z)	In bottles of 100	$72	
	5 mg (G)	In bottles of 100 and 1,000	$6	
	5 mg (P)	In bottles of 1,000; 10,000; UD 90 and 100; blister 31	$39	
	5 mg (Z)	In bottles of 100 and UD 100	$39	
	10 mg (G)	In bottles of 100 and 1,000	$7	
	10 mg (P)	In bottles of 1,000; 10,000; UD 30, 90, and 100; blister 31	$40	
	10 mg (Z)	In bottles of 100 and UD 100	$40	
	20 mg (G)	In bottles of 10 and 1,000	$8	
	20 mg (P)	In bottles of 1,000; 10,000; UD 30, 90, and 100; blister 31	$43	
	20 mg (Z)	In bottles of 100 and UD 100	$43	
	30 mg (G)	In bottles of 100, 500, and 1,000		
	30 mg (Z)	In bottles of 100		
	40 mg (G)	In bottles of 100, 500, 1,000, and UD 100	$9	
	40 mg (P)	In UD 100	$63	
	40 mg (Z)	In bottles of 100	$63	
Moexipril (Univasc)	Tablets: 7.5 mg (G)	In bottles of 100	$46	Combined with HCTZ (Uniretic)
	7.5 mg (B)	In bottles of 100 and UD 90		
	15 mg (G)	In bottles of 100	$48	
	15 mg (B)	In bottles of 100 and UD 90		
Perindopril (Aceon)	Tablets: 2 mg, 4 mg, 8 mg (all B)	In bottles of 100 (all doses)	4 mg = $60 8 mg = $73	
Quinapril (Accupril)	Tablets: 5 mg, 10 mg, 20 mg 40 mg (both G and B)	In bottles of 90 and UD 100 In bottles of 90	$9 for all doses (G); $50 for all doses (B)	Combined with HCTZ (Accuretic) Cost: $50
Ramipril (Altace)	Tablets: 1.25 mg (B) 2.5 mg (B) 5 mg (B) 10 mg (B)	 In bottles of 100 and UD 100 In bottles of 100, 500, 1,000; UD 100 and bulk 5,000 In bottles of 100, 500, 1,000; UD 100 and bulk 5,000 In bottles of 100, 500, and 1,000	 $54 $57 $67	

Table 16–4 ◆ Available Dosage Forms: Angiotensin-Converting-Enzyme Inhibitors and Angiotensin II Receptor Blockers—cont'd

Drug	Dosage Form	How Supplied	Cost	Combinations
Trandolapril (Mavik)	Tablets: 1 mg, 2 mg, 4 mg (both G and B)	In bottles of 100 and UD 100 (all doses)	$21 for all doses (G); $38 for all doses (B)	
ARB				
Candesartan (Atacand)	Tablets: 4 mg, 8 mg	In UD 30	4 and 8 mg = $47;	Combined with HCTZ
	16 mg, 32 mg (all B)	In UD 30, 90, and 100	16 mg = $57; 32 mg = $77	Combined with HCTZ 12.5 mg. Cost $77 and $79
Esprosartan (Teveten)	Tablets: 400 mg (B) 600 mg (B)	In bottles of 100 In bottles of 100	$65 $82	Combined with HCTZ Cost: $87
Irbesartan (Avapro)	Tablets: 75 mg (B) 150 mg (B) 300 mg (B)	In bottles of 30 and 90 In bottles of 30, 90, 500, and UD 100 In bottles of 30, 90, and 500	$45/30 and $130/90 $46/30 and $136/90 $56/30 and $164/90	
Losartan (Cozaar)	Tablets (all B): 25 mg 50 mg 100 mg	In bottles of 90, 100 and UD 100 In bottles of 1,000 and UD 30, 90, and 100 In UD 30, 90, and 100	$60 $81 $119	Combined with HCTZ (Hyzaar) Cost: $61 and $84
Olmesartan (Benicar)	Tablet: 5 mg (B) 20 mg, 40 mg (B)	In bottles of 30 In bottles of 30, 90, and blister card 100	$45/30 $45/30	Combined with HCTZ Cost: $68, $76, and $86
Telmisartan (Micardis)	Tablets: 20 mg, 40 mg, 80 mg (all B)	In blister pak 28 (all doses)	$45/28 and 48/28 $52/28	Combined with HCTZ Cost: $64, $70, and $79
Valsartan (Diovan)	Tablets: 40 mg, 80 mg, 160 mg, 320 mg (all B)	In bottles of 30 and UD 100 In bottles of 100 and UD 100	$42/30 (40 mg) $64/30 (80 mg) and $69/30 for 160 mg	Combined with HCTZ 12.5 mg Cost: $69 for 80 mg and $75 for 160 mg

(G) = generic; (B) = brand; (P) = Prinivil; (Z) = Zestril.
All costs are for 100 tablets unless otherwise noted (e.g., $45 for 30 tablets = $45/30).

or HTN and associated cardiovascular risk factors. They have been shown to improve symptoms, decrease morbidity, and increase life expectancy. Because they are the only drugs that address all of the pathological mechanisms that produce HF, they are appropriate for all subsets of patients unless these patients have an absolute contraindication. They are also useful for preventing the development of HF in patients with ventricular dysfunction but no overt symptoms. **ACEIs** are superior to all other drugs and drug combinations used to treat HF. The NCCC (2003) recommends that "all patients with heart failure due to left ventricular systolic dysfunction should be considered for treatment with an **ACE inhibitor**" (p. 39) and that such therapy should be started before other drug classes are tried. In addition, it is noted that they should be started immediately without waiting for symptoms to worsen.

For symptomatic HF, the dose is about half that used for HTN. Start low and go slow also applies here. A common problem is the parameters given for systolic blood pressure (SBP) in patients with CHF. In patients with CHF and low ejection fractions (less than 40%), the vasodilating effect of **ACEIs** provides adequate perfusion even with SBP below 90 mm Hg. For patients who cannot tolerate an ACEI, **hydralazine**, in combination with a **long-acting**

nitrate, has been shown to be equally effective in reducing morbidity and mortality from CHF. Further discussion of HF is found in Chapter 36.

Rational Drug Selection

Short-Acting versus Long-Acting

Adverse reactions such as angioedema and renal dysfunction usually occur within the first few doses. Instituting therapy with **captopril**, a short-acting form, enables rapid onset of action, assessment of patient tolerance, and the ability to clear the drug quickly should an adverse reaction occur. **Captopril** requires frequent dosing, and adherence is less likely with this treatment regimen in the long term. Other **ACEIs** have the advantage of once-daily dosing, and as soon as patient tolerance is determined, patients should be converted to these other agents to improve adherence. **ARBs** also allow once-daily dosing.

Cost

ACEIs and **ARBs** are expensive. Several have recently become generic, which has significantly reduced their cost. Initiate therapy with **captopril** for the reasons given previously, and then change to the least expensive long-acting form or to an **ARB**. Cost information on individual **ACEIs** and **ARBs** is provided in Table 16–4.

Difficulty in Swallowing

For patients who have difficulty in swallowing, **ramipril (Altace)** may be a good choice. The capsules may be opened and sprinkled on applesauce, added to apple juice, or dissolved in 4 oz water with no change in the effectiveness of the drug. **Captopril** may be crushed but may have a sulfurous odor and requires bid or tid dosing. Available dosage forms are listed in Table 16–4.

Monitoring

Baseline BP and pulse reading should be taken before initiating therapy, within 1 hour of first dose (when a steep drop in BP may occur), and with each change in dosage. Weight and other indicators of fluid status should also be monitored. See Chapter 40 for further BP monitoring guidelines and other related chapters for monitoring guidelines for the various disease processes for which these drugs are used.

During administration of **ACEIs** and **ARBs**, monitoring renal function is important. Serum creatinine levels should be drawn before beginning therapy, after the first week of therapy, monthly during the first 3 months, and when increasing the dose. The **ACEI** dose should be reduced if serum creatinine is more than 2.5 mg/dL (NHBPEP, 2003).

For patients with renal impairment or receiving an **ACEI** or **ARB** that requires dosage adjustments for renal impairment, assess urine protein prior to initiation, every 2 to 4 weeks for the first 3 months of therapy, and regularly thereafter for up to 1 year. Increased proteinuria suggests reevaluation of **ACEI** therapy. For patients on **ARBs**, no change in dosage is required based on renal impairment. Initial **ARB** doses may be lower for patients with impaired hepatic function. Liver function tests (LFTs) should be performed prior to initiating therapy. The dose may be increased as tolerated. According to drug company literature, no patient has had to discontinue an **ARB** because of increased LFT values.

For **ACEIs**, the white blood cell (WBC) count with differential should be monitored prior to initiation of therapy, monthly for the first 3 to 6 months, and periodically for up to 1 year for patients at risk for neutropenia (renal impairment, collagen vascular disease, high doses). Therapy should be discontinued if the neutrophil count is less than 1,000/mm^3.

Patient Education

Patient education focuses on administration of the drug, adverse reactions to expect and appropriate responses to each, and concomitant lifestyle management.

CLINICAL PEARL

If you hear an abdominal bruit in a patient known to have vascular disease, give **captopril,** a short-acting **ACEI,** and measure serum creatinine prior to the dose and within 1 or 2 days after the dose. A rapid rise in the creatinine level suggests renal artery stenosis. A slower rise probably indicates a problem with poor hydration that can be corrected by rehydrating the patient and discontinuing or lowering the dose of any **diuretics** the patient is taking.

CLINICAL PEARL

Many **ACEIs** have the same cost for different strengths. It is possible to prescribe a high strength of the drug and have the patient halve it to achieve the desired dose, resulting in considerable cost savings.

CLINICAL PEARL

Patients should be monitored for indications of angioedema. Suspect angioedema in any patient who calls the next morning after taking the first dose and complains of voice changes or swollen tongue. Stop the drug immediately. The symptoms recede as the drug is eliminated. Protection of the airway is rarely needed, but careful assessment of airway status is required.

Administration

The drug should be taken exactly as prescribed, at the same time each day, even if the patient is feeling well. Missed doses should be taken as soon as remembered unless it is almost the time for the next dose. Doses should not be doubled. The ACEIs vary on whether food alters absorption (see Table 16–1). ARBs may be administered without regard to food intake.

Drug interactions occur with some over-the-counter (OTC) and prescription drugs. The patient should consult the health-care provider before taking any OTC drugs, especially **cold remedies**. Because they affect prostaglandins, **NSAIDs** may counteract the effects of ACEIs. Salt substitutes often contain potassium and should be avoided unless approved by the health-care provider.

Adverse Reactions

Hypotensive reactions are the most common. Changing position slowly, not exercising in hot weather, and keeping fluid intake at more than 2 L/day (noncaffeinated) will decrease these reactions. Fluid intake at this level is not practical in patients with heart failure who need to limit their fluid intake, but ACEIs are not contraindicated in this situation (see Chap. 36). There is no effective treatment to date for the cough. Changing to another ACEI or to an ARB may help. For the few patients who experience impairment in taste, this generally resolves in 8 to 12 weeks, even with continued therapy. Rash is rare and mostly occurs with **captopril**. It should be reported, and a different ACEI may be prescribed.

Serious adverse reactions include angioedema and renal failure. If flushing or pallor of the face; hoarseness; swelling of the face, eyes, lips, or tongue; or difficulty in swallowing or breathing occurs, the patient should discontinue the drug and notify the health-care provider immediately. Swelling of the feet and ankles and decreased urine output should also be reported.

ACEIs and ARBs are contraindicated in pregnancy. In women of childbearing age, this topic should be discussed and effective contraception instituted prior to prescription.

Lifestyle Management

A cardiac-healthy lifestyle includes weight loss, aerobic exercise, tobacco avoidance, decreased dietary saturated fats, and moderation in alcohol and dietary sodium. Stress management is also important.

CALCIUM CHANNEL BLOCKERS

Calcium is a vital component in the excitation-contraction process in muscles, in electrical excitation, and in facilitating myocardial relaxation. Calcium enters cells via three types of voltage-dependent calcium channels (L-type, N-type, and T-type). The L-type, or long-lasting, channels are predominant in cardiac and smooth muscle and the ones blocked by most **calcium channel blockers (CCBs)**. CCBs have multiple indications, including angina, HTN, and selected tachyarrhythmias. Unlabeled indications include migraine headache prophylaxis, Raynaud's syndrome, cardiomyopathy, and esophageal spasm. Laboratory evidence indicates that CCBs may interfere with platelet aggregation and reduce the development of atherosclerotic lesions; however, clinical studies have not yet firmly established roles in blood clotting and atherosclerosis in humans.

Pharmacodynamics

As shown in Figure 16–2, contraction of smooth muscles is triggered by an influx of calcium through transmembrane calcium channels. CCBs directly block the influx of calcium at the onset of the cycle, like the sodium channel blockade in local anesthetics. The drugs act from the inner side of the membrane and bind to channels in depolarized membranes, converting the mode of operation of the channel from frequent openings to rare openings. The result is a marked decrease in transmembrane calcium content and prolonged vascular smooth muscle relaxation.

The blocking action of CCBs occurs via three different receptors: diphenylalkylamine-based and benzothiazepine-based (both type 1 receptors) and dihydropyridine-based (type 2 receptors). The physiological response in the calcium channel is different for these two receptor types, and these differences are important in the clinical choice of CCB. All CCBs relax arterial smooth muscle but have little effect on venous beds. This results in significant reduction in afterload but limited effect on cardiac preload. In cardiac muscle, reduction in contractility (negative inotropism) and decreases in sinoatrial (SA) and atrioventricular (AV) nodal conduction velocity also occur. Although this is true of all classes of CCBs, the greater degree of vasodilation seen in the **dihydropyridines** causes sufficient reflex increase in sympathetic tone to overcome the negative inotropic effects. The effect of a CCB on nodal conduction depends on whether it delays slow calcium channel recovery. **Nifedipine (Adalat, Procardia)** and the other **dihydropyridines** do not affect the rate of recovery of these channels. At doses used clinically, they do not affect conduction through the AV node. In contrast, **verapamil (Calan, Isoptin)** not only affects openings of calcium channels but also decreases the rate of recovery, resulting in depression of the SA node firing rate and slowing of AV nodal conduction. This is the basis of its use in treating supraventricular tachycardias. **Verapamil** also has a direct negative inotropic effect.

Pharmacokinetics

Absorption and Distribution

All CCBs are well absorbed orally, but there is variance in bioavailability among them (Table 16–5). **Verapamil** and

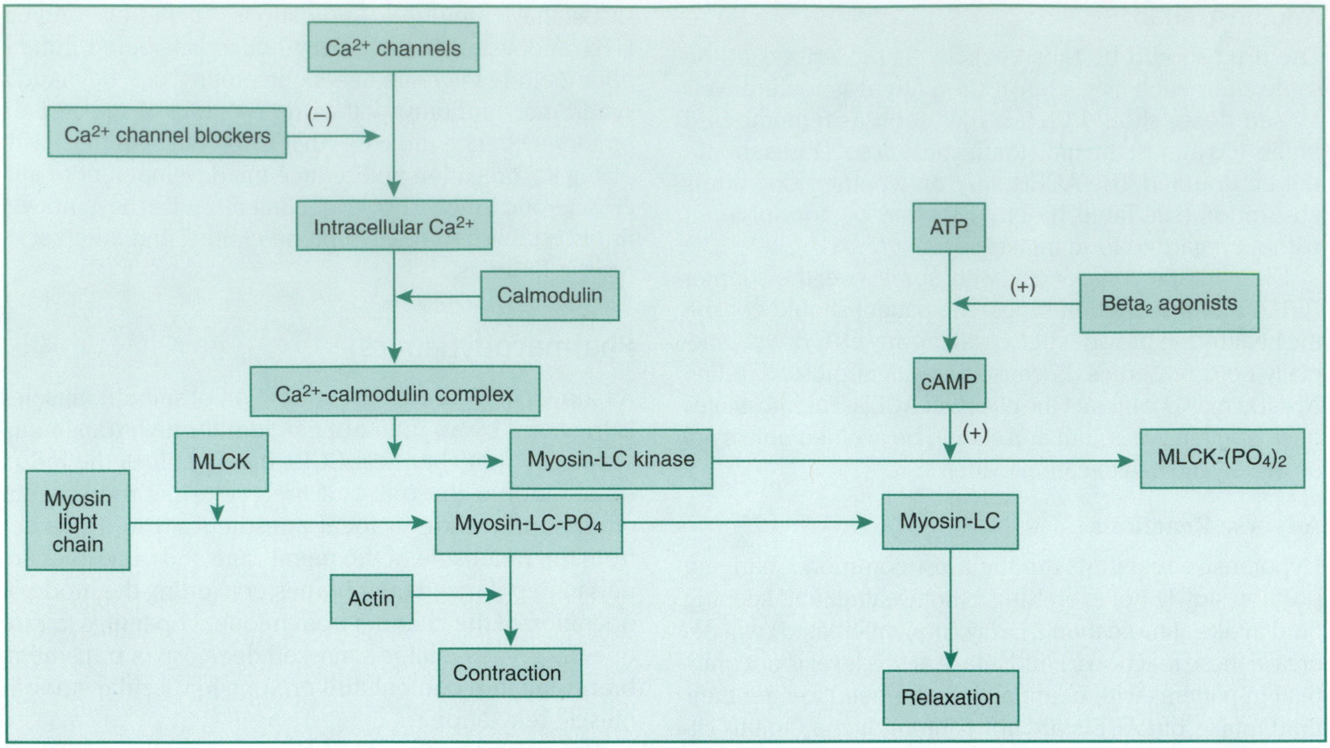

Figure 16–2. Control of smooth muscle contraction. Contraction is triggered by influx of calcium (Ca) through transmembrane calcium channels. The calcium combines with calmodulin to form a complex that converts the enzyme myosin light-chain kinase (MLCK) to its active form. The latter phosphorylates the myosin light chains, initiating the interaction of myosin with actin that produces contraction. Relaxation begins with the reabsorption of calcium, removing it from interaction with the myosin system. Substances that increase cyclic adenosine monophosphate (cAMP), including beta agonists, may cause relaxation in smooth muscle by accelerating the inactivation of MLCK.

diltiazem (Cardizem), prototype type 1 CCBs, are rapidly absorbed but rapidly metabolized to yield bioavailabilities of 20 to 35 percent and 40 to 65 percent, respectively. The **dihydropyridines (type 2 CCBs)** are absorbed at varying rates, and their bioavailabilities vary from 65 to 90 percent for **amlodipine** (Norvasc) to 15 percent for **isradipine** (DynaCirc). The presence of food in the gut does not affect bioavailability in any of these drugs. In the past, **nifedipine** was sometimes administered sublingually. This practice led to serious adverse reactions and has been discontinued. IV forms are available for some **CCBs**. This latter form is not used in primary care and is not discussed in this chapter.

Distribution is to most body tissues, with only **nimodipine** (Nimotop) crossing the blood–brain barrier. Because **nimodipine** has only one very restricted application in the acute-care setting, it is not discussed further. All cross the placenta. **Verapamil, diltiazem,** and **nicardipine** (Cardene) are excreted extensively in breast milk. **Nifedipine** is excreted at less than 5 percent in breast milk, making it the drug of choice during lactation.

Metabolism and Excretion

All **CCBs** are extensively metabolized by the liver. CYP 3A4 has a major role is the metabolism of all **CCBs**, and inducers and inhibitors of that isoenzyme can affect their metabolism. This is more of a problem for type 1 **CCBs** than for **dihydropyridines**. Many **CCBs** have elimination routes in both the urine and the feces (see Table 16–5). Dosage reduction based on renal impairment is recommended only for **nicardipine**.

Most **CCBs** have short-acting forms with half-lives between 2 and 8 hours and sustained-release forms with half-lives of 12 to 24 hours. **Amlodipine** is the exception, with a half-life of 30 to 50 hours. Reduced adverse reactions are seen with the use of sustained-release forms. Table 16–5 depicts the pharmacokinetics of **CCBs.**

Pharmacotherapeutics

Precautions and Contraindications

Verapamil has the strongest negative inotropic effect and should be avoided in CHF, in which this effect can worsen the disorder. It also has the strongest effect on nodal conduction and can significantly worsen bradycardia. **Diltiazem** also affects nodal conduction and can worsen or cause bradycardia, although less than **verapamil.** None of the **CCBs** are drugs of choice immediately after MI, but **diltiazem** has shown some benefit in reducing mortality in non–Q-wave MI for a selected group of patients whose ejection fractions are above 40 percent. For those with ejection fractions below 40 percent and for all other patients early after MI, **type 1 CCBs** are contraindicated

Table 16–5 ▶ Pharmacokinetics: Calcium Channel Blockers

Drug	Onset (h)	Peak (h)	Duration (h)	Protein Binding	Oral Bioavailability	Half-Life (h)	Elimination
Dihydropyridines							
Amlodipine	1 h	6–12	24 +	>93%	65%–90%	30–50 (56 in hepatic impairment)	10% drug and 60% metabolite in urine
Felodipine	1 h	2.5–5	24	>99%	15%–20%	11–16	70% in urine; 10% in feces
Isradipine	<2 h	1.5	12	95%	15%–24%	8	60%–65% in urine; 25%–30% in feces
Isradipine CR	2	7–18	24	95%	15%–24%	8	60%–65% in urine; 25–30% in feces
Nicardipine IR	20 min	1–2	8	95%	35%	2–4	<1% unchanged in urine
Nicardipine SR	UK	1–4	12	>95%	35%	2–4	60% in urine; 35% in feces
Nifedipine IR	20 min	0.5–1	6–8	90%	45%–70%	2–5	60%–80% in urine; 15% in feces
Nifedipine XL	20 min	6–8	24	92%–98%	85%–90%	2–5	60%–80% in urine; 15% in feces
Nisoldipine	UK	6–12	24	99%	5%	7–12	60%–80% in urine
Type 1							
Diltiazem IR	30 min	2–3	6–8	70%–80%	40%–65%	4.5	2%–4% unchanged in urine
Diltiazem ER	UK	10–14	24	70%–80%	40%	4–9.5	2%–4% unchanged in urine
Diltiazem SR/CD	30–60 min	6–11	24	70%–80%	67%	5–7	2%–4% unchanged in urine
Verapinil IR	30 min	0.5–1	3–7	90%	20–35%	4.5–12	70% in urine; 16% in feces
Verapamil SR	1.2	5–7	24	88%–92%		4–12	70% in urine; 16% in feces
Verapamil ER	UK	11	24	>90%	20%–35%	4.5–12	70% in urine; 16% in feces

IR = immediate release; UK = unknown; SR = sustained release; CR = controlled release; ER = extended released; CD = continuous dosing.

because of their negative inotropic and bradycardic effects. Patients with ventricular dysfunction, SA or AV nodal conduction disturbances, and SBPs below 90 mm Hg should not be treated with type 1 **CCBs** because of the high risk for induction of HF and significant hypotension. The **dihydropyridines** are less dependent on the heart for their effects, but they are still not the drugs of choice after MI. **Dihydropyridines** should also be avoided for patients with significant peripheral edema. Their strong peripheral vasodilating effects result in peripheral pooling of blood and may lead to reflex tachycardia. They are also contraindicated in unstable angina because of their potential to cause tachycardia. Short-acting forms more commonly cause these problems, and the short-acting form of **nifedipine** resulted in increased morbidity and mortality when used to treat patients post-MI and with CHF. The short-acting form of this drug is no longer used. If it is necessary to give a **dihydropyridine** to a patient who has peripheral edema or a tachyrhythm disturbance, the sustained-release forms are preferred. All **CCBs** should be used cautiously in severe hepatic impairment, with dosage reduction recommended for most agents.

All **CCBs** relax smooth muscle contractions of the esophagus and have been used (off-labeled) to treat esophageal spasm. This relaxation makes gastroesophageal reflux disease (GERD) worse, and **CCBs** should be avoided for patients with this disorder.

Teratogenic and embryotoxic effect have been demonstrated in small animals. There are no adequate and well-controlled studies in pregnant women. These drugs are Pregnancy Category C. Female patients capable of childbearing should be made aware of the risks of these drugs, and contraception should be instituted before **CCBs** are prescribed. They should be used only when benefits clearly outweigh risks.

Verapamil, **diltiazem**, **nifedipine**, and **nicardipine** are all found in breast milk. They should not be given to nursing mothers. It is not known if **amlodipine**, **isradipine**, **nislodipine (Sular)**, or **felodipine (Plendil)** is excreted in breast milk. For these drugs, the determination to continue nursing is based on the importance of the drug for the mother and the presence or absence of acceptable alternatives. Safety and efficacy of these drugs have not been established in children.

Adverse Drug Reactions

The more common adverse reactions of **CCBs** are extensions of their actions. Reduction in BP secondary to vasodilation may result in dizziness, headache, hypotension, and syncope. These reactions occur less often in long-acting formulations. Decreased myocardial contractility may lead to HF with congestion, shortness of breath, cough, and palpitations. Gastrointestinal (GI) symptoms are especially disturbing to patients and include dry mouth, nausea, vomiting, and constipation.

Although not common, sexual dysfunction and gynecomastia may occur. Hyperglycemia is also uncommon but may affect the choice of the drug in patients with diabetes. Other common adverse reactions, such as peripheral edema, dysrhythmias, and HF, are discussed in the Precautions and Contraindications section.

The highest rate of adverse reactions is found in the **short-acting dihydropyridines** (17%), with the lowest rate for this group being in **amlodipine** (less than 4%). All adverse drug reactions for **CCBs** are less common with sustained-release forms because the amount of drug in the system at any given time is more stable.

Drug Interactions

Additive hypotensive effects are major concerns with all **CCBs** given concurrently with other **antihypertensives**, **nitrates**, **quinidine**, or **alcohol**. Antihypertensive effects may be decreased with concurrent use of **NSAIDs**. **Verapamil**, **diltiazem**, and some **dihydropyridines** have an additive bradycardic effect with **BBs** or **digoxin**. Serum **digoxin** levels may be increased with risk of toxicity when it is concurrently used with **verapamil**, **diltiazem**, or **nifedipine**. **Verapamil** may decrease the effectiveness of **rifampin**, and the effectiveness of **verapamil** may be decreased by concurrent administration of **vitamin D** and calcium. **Verapamil** may also alter serum **lithium** levels. CYP3A4 isoenzymes are involved in the metabolism of all **CCBs**. Drugs that inhibit this system, including grapefruit juice, may increase free drug levels. Food interactions also occur for several of the **CCBs**. Specific drug and food interactions and appropriate actions to prevent them are found in Table 16–6.

Clinical Use and Dosing

Chronic Stable Angina

Both type 1 and type 2 **CCBs** are effective in the treatment of stable and exertional angina (Table 16–7). They act on both sides of the supply–demand equation: Peripheral vasodilation and negative inotropism reduce oxygen demand; dilation of coronary arteries increases oxygen supply.

Among the **dihydropyridines**, **nifedipine**, **nicardipine**, and **amlodipine** are drugs of choice. The long-acting form of **nifedipine (Procardia XL)** is the most often prescribed. Combining this drug with **propranolol (Inderal)**, **a BB**, has proved more effective than either agent given alone, possibly because the BB suppresses the reflex tachycardia that may occur with **type 2 CCBs**.

Nicardipine is structurally similar to **nifedipine** but less likely to cause hypotension and LV dysfunction. It is useful for patients with angina who also have mild HF or

CLINICAL PEARL

Amlodipine can also be crushed and put down a nasogastric (NG) tube, which is not possible with sustained-release preparations. This provides the clinical advantage of acting as if **amlodipine** were sustained release with less venous pooling, less reflex tachycardia, and once-daily dosing.

CLINICAL PEARL

Constipation is especially common with **verapamil,** with almost 100 percent of patients experiencing significant constipation. Patients taking this drug should be encouraged to increase the fiber in their diet and may need to have a stool softener ordered.

Table 16–6 ■ **Drug Interactions: Selected Calcium Channel Blockers**

Drug	Interacting Drug	Possible Effect	Implications
All CCBs	Histamine$_2$ blockers	Serum concentrations of CCB may increase	Monitor cardiovascular status closely. May need to adjust dose
	Fentanyl, nitrates, antihypertensives, acute alcohol ingestion, quinidine	Additive hypotension	Monitor for orthostatic changes. Warn patient. Reduce or avoid alcohol use
	NSAIDs	Decreased antihypertensive effects	Warn patient. Avoid concurrent use or monitor therapeutic response and adjust CCB dose.
Diltiazem and Verapamil	Benzodiasepines; buspirone; carbamazepine	Serum concentrations of psychotropics increased	Monitor serum levels closely and adjust dose as needed
	HMG-Co-A reductase inhibitors (statins)	Serum concentrations of statin may be elevated, except lovastatin which may be reduced	Monitor clinical response and adjust dose as needed if concurrent use cannot be avoided
Verapamil, diltiazem, nifedipine	Digoxin	Increased serum digoxin levels	Monitor for digoxin toxicity. Teach signs and symptoms to report to provider.
	CYP-450 3A4 inhibitors (including grapefruit juice)	Decreased hepatic clearance of CCB with increased risk of toxicity to CCB	Monitor for orthostatic changes, rate and rhythm changes
	Calcium salts, vitamin D	Reduced response to CCB	Avoid concurrent use. If use is necessary, monitor therapeutic response and adjust CCB dose.
	Cyclosporine, prazosin, quinidine, theophylline, carbamazepine	Decreased metabolism of these drugs and increased toxicity risk	Monitor therapeutic levels and signs and symptoms of toxicity
Verapamil, diltiazem, felodipine, isradipine, nicardipine, nifedipine, nimodipine	Beta-adrenergic blockers, digoxin, disopyramide, phenytoin	Myocardial depression, bradycardia, conduction defects, CHF	Do not administer within 24 h of each other. If you must give both, monitor for heart failure and decreased peripheral perfusion.
Diltiazem	Phenobarbital, phenytoin	Increased metabolism and decreased effect of diltiazem	Avoid concurrent use. Select different anticonvulsant.
	Cyclosporine	Enhanced action of cyclosporine	Monitor renal function with blood urea nitrogen (BUN) and creatinine levels. Monitor cyclosporine levels.
Verapamil	Rifampin	Decreased effect of rifampin	Avoid concurrent use. Select different CCB if rifampin is needed to treat tuberculosis.
	Lithium	Altered serum lithium levels with increased toxicity risk	Avoid concurrent use. Select different CCB.
Dihydropyridines	Azole antifungals	Increased concentrations of CCB	Monitor cardiovascular effects and adjust dose if concurrent use cannot be avoided

Continued

Table 16–6 ▣ **Drug Interactions: Selected Calcium Channel Blockers—cont'd**

Drug	Interacting Drug	Possible Effect	Implications
Food Interactions			
Felodipine, nifedipine, nislodipine, verapamil, amlodipine	Grapefruit juice	Increased serum concentrations of CCB	Avoid concurrent use
Diltiazem, felodipine, nislodipine	High-fat or high-carbohydrate meal	Drug taken with this kind of meal has increased AUC and C_{max} of CCB	Avoid taking drug and eating this type of meal concurrently
Nicardipine	High-fat meal	Taken together results in decreased AUC and C_{max} for CCB	Avoid taking drug and eating this type of meal concurrently

Table 16–7 ◉ **Dosage Schedule: Selected Calcium Channel Blockers**

Drug	Starting Dose	Maintenance Dose	Maximum Dose
Amlodipine *Peds:* Not recommended for children <6 yrs of age.	5 mg daily	5–10 mg daily	10 mg qd
Diltiazem PO	30 mg q6–8h	30–90 mg q6–8h	240 mg/d
Diltiazem CD	120 mg daily	120–180 mg daily	300 mg/d
Diltiazem SR	60 mg q12h	60–120 mg q12h	240 mg/d
Felodipine	2.5 mg daily	2.5–5 mg daily	20 mg/d
Isradipine	2.5 mg q12h	2.5–5 mg q12h	20 mg/d
Nicardipine PO	60 mg tid	60 mg tid	120 mg/d
Nicardipine SR	60 mg q12h	60 mg q12h	120 mg/d
Nifedipine (Adalat CC)	30 mg	30–60 mg daily	90 mg/d
Nifedipine (Procardia XL)	30 mg	30–60 mg daily	120 mg/d
Verapamil PO	80 mg tid	80–160 mg tid	480 mg/d
Verapamil SR	120 mg daily or q12h	120–240 mg daily or q12h	480 mg/d

borderline HTN. **Amlodipine** is well tolerated, with less venous pooling and minimum reflex tachycardia, and is safe to use for patients with significant ventricular dysfunction. In addition, its long half-life means it acts like a sustained-release form. Although sustained-release forms of the other drugs cannot be crushed, **amlodipine** can be crushed so that patients who have difficulty in swallowing or who have nasogastric (NG) tubes can use this drug and still benefit from the reduced adverse effects associated with sustained release. The dose is 5 mg initially, with a maximum dose of 10 mg. Doses higher than 10 mg have not demonstrated any increase in benefit. **Amlodipine** has been used in combination with several BBs to produce improved response. The long-acting form of each of these drugs offers once-daily dosing, which improves adherence.

Diltiazem, also effective in angina therapy, is less likely to cause hypotension and other adverse responses associated with peripheral vasodilation (reflex tachycardia) than **nifedipine**, and it has less negative inotropic activity than **verapamil**. The reduction in average daily heart rate associated with this drug improves coronary artery filling time and myocardial oxygen supply. Of the type 1 drugs, it is most often chosen because of its low adverse drug response profile. **Diltiazem** is a good choice for patients who need to reduce their heart rate. **Verapamil** is more often prescribed for treatment of arrhythmias because it has the most potent negative inotropic effect and significantly slows AV nodal conduction. It is not used for patients with compromised LV function, bradycardia, or AV block. **Verapamil** might be chosen for patients with supraventricular tachycardia who also have angina.

Vasospastic (Variant, Prinzmetal's) Angina

CCBs that produce more coronary artery vasodilation and reduce vasospasm are the drugs of choice. **Diltiazem, long-acting nifedipine,** and **amlodipine** are the most commonly used.

Unstable Angina

Medical therapy for unstable angina involves **nitrates, BBs,** and **heparin,** which are effective in controlling pain, and **aspirin,** which reduces mortality. When vasospasm is a component of this angina, CCBs may offer an additional treatment. There is insufficient evidence at this time, however, to indicate whether this addition decreases mortality. When a CCB is chosen, **verapamil** is the drug of choice. Type 2 CCBs are contraindicated because they tend to increase heart rate and have less vasospastic protection. Because **verapamil** is often given in combination with other drugs that lower BP, hypotension is a serious potential adverse response.

Hypertension

Initial drug therapy for HTN is monotherapy. Because **ACEIs, ARBs, diuretics,** and **BBs** have been shown to reduce cardiovascular morbidity and mortality in controlled trials, these classes of drugs are preferred as initial therapy (NHBPEP, 2003). CCBs are equally effective in reducing BP, but there is insufficient research to date to demonstrate their efficacy in reducing morbidity and mortality, and they should be reserved for special indications or used when the drugs discussed previously have proved ineffective. Special indications include black patients, who, as a group, are more responsive to **diuretics** and **CCBs** than they are to **BBs** or **ACEIs.** CCBs would also be appropriate for patients with certain concomitant pathologies such as asthma, in which **BBs** are contraindicated. CCBs are also indicated for both severe (BP greater than 160/110) and nonsevere hypertension (BP 140–159/90–109) in pregnancy. **Nifedipine** capsules and PA tablets are useful for both disorders (Magee, Helewa, Moutquin, von Dadelszen, & Hypertension Guideline Committee, Society of Obstetricians and Gynaecologists of Canada, 2008; University of Michigan Health System, 2009).

When a CCB is chosen, **amlodipine** is especially good for patients with LV dysfunction and CHF. **Long-acting nifedipine, diltiazem,** or **verapamil** may be used for patients with CAD. **Long-acting nifedipine** is a good choice as well for patients who also have peripheral-vascular disease (PVD) because of its peripheral vasodilating effect.

> **CLINICAL PEARL**
>
> The delivery system for **nifedipine (Procardia XL)** is excreted in the feces as a whole orange capsule. This does not mean that the liquid drug inside the capsule was not absorbed. To avoid alarm, the patient should be warned about this.

For all CCBs, older adults usually require a starting dose about half the usual dose, and increases in dosage should be gradual to reduce adverse drug responses. (See Chap. 40 for further discussion.)

Supraventricular Tachycardia and Atrial Fibrillation

Type 1 CCBs are useful in treating selected supraventricular tachycardias because they slow AV nodal conduction. **Verapamil** (80–120 mg orally) can be used to terminate the rhythm. Conversion usually occurs in about 1 hour. **Diltiazem** (40–80 mg orally) can also be tried. Prophylaxis with **verapamil** (240–480 mg/d) is effective for patients with paroxysmal supraventricular tachycardia (PSVT). It is important to be certain that the rhythm is not ventricular; **verapamil** may worsen ventricular rhythm disturbances because of its negative inotropic effects. **Verapamil** is also used as an alternative to digoxin to slow a rapid ventricular response in the treatment of atrial fibrillation through its direct effect on the AV node, prolonging its refractory period and conduction time. Doses are similar to those used for PSVT. If it must be used concurrently with **digoxin,** then the **digoxin** level must be evaluated frequently because **verapamil** slows the clearance of **digoxin** and may increase the risk of toxicity.

Patients with Wolff-Parkinson-White syndrome who also have atrial fibrillation can have ventricular responses that are dangerously rapid. Drugs commonly used to control ventricular response such as **diltiazem, verapamil,** and **digoxin** are ineffective in this situation and can facilitate conduction through the accessory pathway, increasing the risk for ventricular fibrillation (Institute for Clinical Symptoms Improvement [ICSI], 2008a).

Migraine Headache Prophylaxis

Migraine prophylaxis is an unlabeled indication for CCBs. Of patients with frequent migraines for whom CCBs are prescribed, 30 percent report a 30 percent reduction in migraines. The CCB used most often is **verapamil** (240–480 mg/d). To facilitate adherence, it is best to use the sustained-release form to permit once-daily dosing. The trial to determine effectiveness should last at least 3 months. Failure to give an adequate dose or an adequate trial time is a common reason for failure of migraine prophylaxis.

Raynaud's Syndrome

Raynaud's syndrome is also an unlabeled indication. **Type 2 CCBs** are the CCB choice for this disorder because of their peripheral vasodilating effects and some platelet inhibition. The drug most studied and the first choice is **long-acting nifedipine**. The initial dose is 10 mg orally given in the office to assess the effect on BP. If the patient does not experience a drop in SBP more than 20 mm Hg below baseline or a drop below 90 mm Hg, then 10 mg orally tid is prescribed. The dose may be increased by 10 mg/d every 3 to 4 days to a maximum of 30 mg tid to achieve the desired effect. Monitoring every 2 to 4 months is necessary because the initial response may be transient. If **nifedipine** does not work, **diltiazem** may be tried, beginning at 30 mg qid and increasing every 3 to 4 days until a maximum of 120 mg qid is reached. **Felodipine** and **isradipine** are also powerful vasodilators and may be tried. Research is absent on their use. Raynaud's syndrome symptoms are often present only during exposure to cold temperatures. Drugs may be stopped during the summer months.

Esophageal Spasm

Although this is an unlabeled indication, **CCBs** may offer transient improvement for patients with mild spasm. **Diltiazem** (90 mg qid) has been used. Because this drug makes GERD worse, this disorder must be ruled out before a CCB is prescribed.

Rational Drug Selection

Short-Acting versus Long-Acting Forms

Short-acting forms of **CCBs** have been associated with more adverse drug reactions. In several trials, the short-acting form of **nifedipine** was associated with increased mortality in post-MI patients. All **type 2 CCBs** cause vasodilation that results in reflex tachycardia and peripheral pooling of blood. These actions are greatly reduced in the long-acting forms. To reduce adverse drug reactions and improve adherence, long-acting forms should be used.

Indication

Specific drugs are more appropriate for specific indications. Any CCB should be chosen with the indications clearly in mind.

Cost

CCBs are expensive; some are generic and less expensive. **Verapamil** is the least expensive, but its adverse reaction profile includes significant constipation in almost 100 percent of patients. Although this reaction can be mitigated by the concurrent prescription of a **stool softener**, the cost advantage is lost by the additional cost of the **stool softener**. The sustained-release forms of **diltiazem** are the most expensive **CCBs** and must be given bid. The remaining drugs fall between these two. Cost may be a factor in choosing to use a CCB, but it is not a major factor in choosing among them. Cost data are provided in Table 16–8.

Difficulty in Swallowing or Nasogastric Tube Placement

Only **amlodipine** can be crushed and mixed with food for patients who have difficulty swallowing; it can also be put down an NG tube.

Monitoring

Liver function should be evaluated prior to initiating therapy. Dosage reductions for most **CCBs** are recommended with severe hepatic impairment because of the extensive metabolism of these drugs by the liver.

Table 16–8 ◆ Available Dosage Forms: Selected Calcium Channel Blockers

Drug	Dosage Form	How Supplied	Cost
Amlodipine (G) (Norvasc) (B) (also combined with benazepril [Lotrel])	Tablets: 2.5 mg	In bottles of 90 and 100	$13 for 5 mg/30 (G) and $17 for 10 gm/30 (G)
	5 mg	In bottles of 90, 100, 300, and UD 100	$134/90 $134/90
	10 mg	In bottles of 90, 100, and UD 100	$184/90 Lotrel: (G) $65, (B) $90
Diltiazem (Cardizem)	Tablets: 30 mg (G), 60 mg (G), 90 mg (G), 120 mg (G)	In bottles of 100, 500, and 1,000 (all doses)	30 mg = $7.50; 60 mg = $10; 90 mg = $14
	30 mg (B), 60 mg (B), 90 mg (B), 120 mg (B)	In bottles of 100, 500, and UD 100 (all doses)	30 mg = $53; 60 mg = $81; 90 mg = $114

Table 16–8 ◆ **Available Dosage Forms: Selected Calcium Channel Blockers—cont'd**

Drug	Dosage Form	How Supplied	Cost
	Capsules (ER): 60 mg (G), 90 mg (G)	In bottles of 100	
	120 mg (G)	In bottles of 30, 90, 100, 500, and 1,000	
	180 mg (G)	In bottles of 30, 90, 100, 500, and 1,000	
	240 mg (G)	In bottles of 30, 90, 100, 500, and 1,000	
	300 mg (G)	In bottles of 30, 90, 500, and 1,000	
	Capsule (CD): 120 mg	In bottles of 30, 90, and UD 100	$119/90
	180 mg, 240 mg,	In bottles of 30, 90, and UD 100	240 mg = $200/90
	300 mg,	In bottles of 30, 90, and UD 100	$259/90
	360 mg	In bottles of 90	$281/90
	Capsule (SR): 60 mg,	In bottles of 100	$36
	90 mg, 120 mg	In bottles of 100	90 mg = $44; 120 mg = $61
Diltiazem (Cartia XT) All (B)	Capsules: 120 mg, 180 mg, 240 mg, 300 mg	In bottles of 30, 90, 500, and 1,000 (all doses)	120 mg = $72; 180 mg = $87; 240 mg = $122; 300 mg = $164
Diltiazem (Dilacor XR) All (B)	Capsules: 120 mg, 180 mg, 240 mg	In bottles of 100 and 500 (all doses)	120 mg = $47; 180 mg = $54; 240 mg = $54
Diltiazem (Diltia XT) All (B)	Capsules: 120 mg, 180 mg, 240 mg	In bottles of 100, 500, and 1,000 (all doses)	
Diltiazem (Tiazac) All (B)	Capsules (extended release): 120 mg, 180 mg, 240 mg, 300 mg, 360 mg, 420 mg	In bottles of 7, 30, 90, and 1,000 (all doses)	120 mg = $73/90 180 mg = $75/90 240 mg = $105/90 300 mg = $168/90 360 mg = $139/90
Felodipine (Plendil) (also combined with enalapril [Lexxel])	Tablets: 2.5 mg (B), 5 mg (G), 5 mg (B); 10 mg (G) and 10 mg (B)	In bottles of 30, 100, and UD 100 (all doses)	2.5 mg = $132; 5 mg (G) = $37/30; 5 mg (B) = $46/30; 10 mg (G) = $66/30, 10 mg (B) = $82/30
Isradipine (G) (DynaCirc) (B)	Capsules: 2.5 mg (G), 5 mg (G), 5 mg (B)	In bottles of 60 and 100	2.5 mg = $132; 5 mg (G) = $102; 5 mg (B) = $197
	Tablets (CR): 5 mg (B),	In bottles of 30 and 100	$172
	10 mg (B)	In bottles of 30 and 100	$272
Nicardipine (Cardene)	Capsules:		
	20 mg (G)	In bottles of 90 and 500	$15
	30 mg (G)	In bottles of 90 and 500	$19
	Capsules:		
	20 mg (B)	In bottles of 100 and 500	$61
	30 mg (B)	In bottles of 100 and 500	$96
	Capsules (SR):		
	30 mg	In bottles of 60 and 200	$57
	45 mg	In bottles of 60 and 200	$90
	60 mg	In bottles of 60	$107
Nifedipine	Tablets: 30 mg (G),	In bottles of 100 and 300	$25/30
	60 mg (G)	In bottles of 100 and 300	$43/30
	90 mg (G)	In bottles of 100	$67/30

Continued

Table 16–8 ◆ Available Dosage Forms: Selected Calcium Channel Blockers—cont'd

Drug	Dosage Form	How Supplied	Cost
(Adalat)	30 mg (B) 60 mg (B) 90 mg (B) Capsules: 10 mg (G) 20 mg (G)	In bottles of 100 and UD 100 In bottles of 100 and UD 100 In bottles of 100 and 300 In bottles of 100 and 300	$42/30 for 30 mg; $75/30 for 60 mg; $87/30 for 90 mg.
(Adalat)	10 mg (B) 20 mg (B)	In bottles of 100, 300 and UD 100 In bottles of 100, 300 and UD 100	
(Procardia)	10 mg (B) 20 mg (B)	In bottles of 100 and 300 In bottles of 100	$77
Nifedipine (Procardia XL)	Tablets: 30 mg 60 mg 90 mg	In bottles of 100, 300, 500 and UD 100 In bottles of 100 and UD 100	30 mg = $152; 60 mg = $262 90 mg = $302
Nislodipine (Sular) All (B)	Tablets (extended release): 10 mg, 20 mg, 30 mg 40 mg	In bottles of 100 and UD 100 In bottles of 100 and UD 100 In bottles of 100	10 mg = $132; 20 mg = $132 $178 $178
Verapamil (Calan)	Tablets: 40 mg (G) 40 mg (B) 80 mg (G) 80 mg (B) 120 mg (G) 120 mg (B) Tablet (SR): 120 mg 180 mg 240 mg	In bottles of 30, 100, 500, and 1,000 In bottles of 100 In bottles of 100, 250, 500, 1,000, 7,000, and UD 100 In bottles of 100, 500, and 1,000 In bottles of 100, 250, 500, 4,000, and UD100 In bottles of 100 and 1,000 In bottles of 100 and UD 100 In bottles of 100 and UD 100 In bottles of 100, 500, and UD 100	$16 $54 $10 $76 $13 $102 $141 $179 $204
Verapamil (Covera-HS) (Isoptin-SR)	Tablets (extended release): 120 mg (G) 180 mg (G) 240 mg (G) Capsules (extended release): 120 mg, 180 mg 240 mg Tablets: 180 mg, 240 mg Tablets: 120 mg, 180 mg 240 mg	In bottles of 100 In bottles of 100 and 500 In bottles of 100 and 500 In bottles of 100 and UD 100 In bottles of 100, 500, and UD 100 In bottles of 100 and UD 100 In bottles of 100 In bottles of 100 and 500	$56 $41 $42 120 mg = $54; 180 mg = $57 $68 180 mg = $140; 240 mg = $196
(Verelan PM)	Capsules (extended release): 100 mg, 200 mg, 300 mg	In bottles of 100 (all doses)	100 mg = $136 200 mg = $174 300 mg = $252
(Verelan)	Capsules (sustained release): 120 mg, 180 mg, 240 mg, 360 mg	In bottles of 100 (all doses)	120 mg = $197 180 mg = $205 240 mg = $232 360 mg = $340

(G) = generic; (B) = brand;
(ER), (CD), (HS), (XL), (XT), and (XR) = extended release; (SR) = sustained release; (CR) = controlled release.
All of these formulations are brand name drugs. All costs are for 100 units unless otherwise stated.

Patient Education

Administration

The drug should be taken exactly as prescribed, at the same time each day, even if the patient is feeling well. Sustained-release drugs taken once daily are best taken in the morning for therapeutic effect. Missed doses should be taken as soon as remembered unless it is almost the time for the next dose. Doses should not be doubled. Sudden withdrawal may precipitate myocardial ischemia, so withdrawal is gradual. **CCBs** cannot relieve acute anginal attacks. If acute chest pain occurs, the health-care provider should be contacted immediately or the patient should go to the nearest hospital. For patients taking **isradipine** or **nifedipine**, anginal attacks sometimes occur 30 minutes after administration because of reflex tachycardia. This is usually temporary and not necessarily an indication for stopping the drug, but this symptom should be reported to the health-care provider.

Several of the **CCBs** come in more than one form, from short-acting drugs requiring multiple doses daily to long-acting drugs with once-daily dosing (see Table 16–8). The patient has to read the label carefully and follow the appropriate dosing schedule. This is especially important if a different form or a different CCB is prescribed.

Some **CCBs** have food interactions, especially with high-fat or high-carbohydrate meals and with grapefruit juice. The patient should be informed so that the interactions can be avoided.

Drug interactions occur with some OTC and prescription drugs and with **alcohol**. The patient should consult the health-care provider before taking any OTC drugs, especially cold remedies.

Adverse Reactions

Hypotensive reactions are the most common. Changing position slowly, not exercising in hot weather, and keeping intake of noncaffeinated fluids above 2 L/d will decrease these reactions. Adding fluid is not practical for patients with heart failure who must limit their fluid intake. A more appropriate approach for those patients is to lower the dose if hypotensive reactions occur. Bradycardia is also possible, especially for patients on **type 2 CCBs**. Patients should learn how to monitor their own pulse rate and contact the health-care provider if the rate is less than 50 beats per minute (bpm) or has irregular beats. HF may also develop. Report dyspnea, pronounced dizziness, or nausea. **Type 1 CCBs** more commonly exhibit peripheral edema. Report swelling of hands and feet or ankles and decreased urine output.

Constipation is especially a problem for **verapamil** but may occur with other **CCBs**. The patient should increase dietary fiber and report this adverse response to the health-care provider. **Stool softeners** may be prescribed prophylactically with **verapamil** and for treatment with other **CCBs**.

Wearing protective clothing and using sunscreen will prevent photosensitivity reactions.

Lifestyle Management

See the section Angiotensin-Converting Enzyme Inhibitors and Angiotensin II Receptor Blockers.

CARDIAC GLYCOSIDES

Cardiac glycosides (**CGs**) are among the oldest known drugs. They have been medically recognized in the treatment of HF since 1785. Although there are three main **glycosides** available, **digoxin** is by far the most commonly prescribed because of its convenient pharmacokinetics, the alternative routes of administration, and the techniques for monitoring its serum level. This section focuses on **digoxin** and its use in treating supraventricular tachycardias and HF.

Pharmacodynamics

Mechanical Effects on Heart Muscle

All **CGs** are strong and highly selective inhibitors of the sodium-potassium-adenosine triphosphatase (ATPase) system: the "sodium pump." The preferential binding of **CGs** to ATPase occurs following phosphorylation of the alpha subunit of the enzyme. Extracellular potassium promotes dephosphorylation of the enzyme and decreases the affinity of the enzyme for the **CG**. This may explain why increased extracellular potassium reverses some of the toxic effects of these drugs.

The sodium pump is the major determinant of the concentration of sodium in the cell. As shown in Figure 16–3, inhibition of this pump results in sodium and calcium buildup inside the cell. The combination of the changes in sodium and calcium results in increased velocity of the shortening of cardiac muscle, with a shift upward and to the left in the ventricular function curve, causing an increase in stroke work for a given filling volume or pressure (positive inotropism).

Electrical Effects on Heart Muscle

A mixture of direct and autonomic actions produces the electrical effects (negative chronotropism) seen with **CGs**. At therapeutic levels, **CGs** decrease automaticity and conduction velocity through the AV node via central vagal stimulation and facilitation of muscarinic transmission at the cardiac muscle cell. Because cholinergic innervation is more prevalent in the atria, these actions affect atrial and AV nodal function more than Purkinje or ventricular function.

Other Effects

Several studies suggest that **digoxin** may also decrease plasma renin activity, reduce plasma norepinephrine levels, and restore baroreceptor sensitivity, all of which are factors in HF pathology. **CGs** affect all smooth excitable tissues, including smooth muscle and the CNS. These actions on other tissues explain many of their adverse responses.

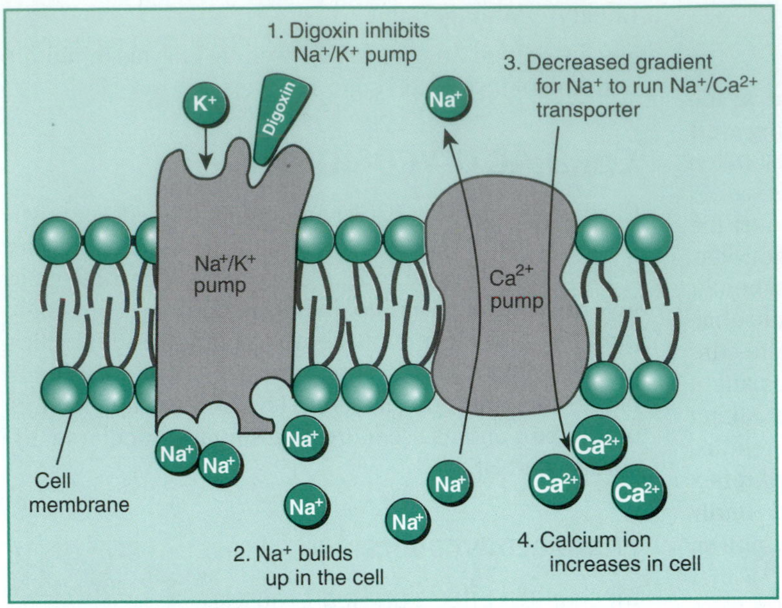

Figure 16–3. Effects of digoxin on the sodium–potassium pump. The sodium pump is the major determinant of the concentration of sodium in the cell. Inhibition of this pump results in sodium buildup inside the cell. The resultant decrease in sodium gradient reduces the sodium–calcium transport mechanism and calcium ions also increase inside the cell. The influx of sodium through voltage-gated channels is a major determinant in cardiac action potentials. This influx is reduced when the sodium gradient is decreased. Ultimately, contraction of cardiac muscle results from the interaction of calcium with the actin–myosin system. Reduced extracellular calcium levels decrease this contraction.

Pharmacokinetics

Absorption and Distribution

Digoxin is well absorbed orally (Table 16–9). Taking digoxin with food or after meals results in slower absorption. Taking it with a high-bran meal results in reduced total absorption of the drug. Approximately 10 percent of individuals have intestinal bacteria that inactivate digoxin in the gut, greatly reducing bioavailability and requiring higher-than-average doses to produce a therapeutic response. Treatment of these individuals with **antibiotics** can cause a sudden increase in bioavailability, which results in toxicity. Product formulation may also be a factor in bioavailability. Generic tablet preparations have a bioavailability of 70 to 80 percent; the bioavailability is 90 to 100 percent for **digoxin** elixir and encapsulated gel. The narrow safety margin between therapeutic effect, loss of effect, and toxicity means that even small variations in bioavailability can have serious consequences. It is best to prescribe by brand.

Once absorbed, **CGs** are widely distributed to tissues, including the CNS. **Digoxin's** volume of distribution is large (4–7 L/kg) and dependent on plasma protein-binding capacity. Its highest tissue concentration (10–50 times that

Table 16–9 ▶ **Pharmacokinetics: Cardiac Glycosides**

Drug	Onset	Peak	Duration	Protein Binding	Oral Bioavailability	Half-Life	Time to Steady State	Volume of Distribution	Elimination
Digoxin PO	1–2 h	6–8 h	2–4 d	20%–40%	Tablets: 60%–80% Capsules: 90%–100% Elixir: 75%–85%	NRF: 36–48 h IRF: prolonged	1 wk or 4 doses	6.3 L/kg	Unchanged by kidney
Digoxin IM	30 min	4–6 h	2–4 d	20%–40%	50%–75%	NRF: 36–48 h IRF: prolonged	1 wk or 4 doses	6.3 L/kg	Unchanged by kidney
Digitoxin	30 min–2 h	4–12 h	2–3 wk	>90%	>90%	NRF: 4–6 d IRF: not prolonged	0.6 L/kg	Metabolized by liver excreted into gut via bile	

NRF = normal renal function; IRF = impaired renal function.

in plasma) is found in the heart, kidney, and liver. The principal tissue reservoir is skeletal muscle, so dosing is based on lean muscle mass. Neonates and infants tolerate and seem to require higher doses to achieve a therapeutic effect than do older children and adults.

Digoxin crosses the placenta, and drug levels in maternal and umbilical vein blood are similar.

Metabolism and Excretion

Digoxin is not extensively metabolized and is excreted largely unchanged by the kidneys. Its half-life is 36 to 48 hours with normal or near-normal renal function. In the absence of oral or IV loading doses, steady state is achieved in about 4 half-lives or 1 week. Its clearance rate is proportional to the GFR and is similar for neonates, infants, children, and adults. For patients with elevated serum creatinine levels, drug clearance closely parallels creatinine clearance. Improvement in cardiac output and renal blood flow through therapy with a variety of agents may increase renal **digoxin** clearance and require dosage adjustments. Several drugs (most notably **quinidine, amiodarone, verapamil,** and **diltiazem**) reduce clearance and can double the serum concentration, resulting in toxicity unless the dose of **digoxin** is reduced.

Pharmacotherapeutics

Precautions and Contraindications

CGs are contraindicated in AV blocks and uncontrolled ventricular arrhythmias because their action on the AV node may worsen the arrhythmia. Patients with idiopathic hypertrophic subaortic stenosis (IHSS) may develop worsening outflow tract obstruction with CG use because of the action of **CGs** on myocardial contractility. Their use in cor pulmonale is questionable. Although they may be beneficial for some patients, toxicity risk increases in the presence of hypoxia.

Because **digoxin** is excreted essentially unchanged by the kidneys, renal impairment effectively contraindicates its use. Patients with chronic renal disease have very labile creatinine levels, which can be easily disturbed, so it is difficult to monitor these patients closely enough to prevent catastrophe. Hypothyroidism and chronic renal failure decrease **digoxin's** volume of distribution, necessitating a decrease in both loading and maintenance doses. **Digoxin** may be used safely in renal impairment as long as renal function and necessary dosage adjustments are made.

CGs are used cautiously for patients with electrolyte abnormalities because the concentrations of potassium, calcium, and magnesium in the extracellular compartment affect sensitivity to **CGs** and may result in digitalis toxicity. **Digoxin** may exacerbate atrial fibrillation due to Wolff-Parkinson-White syndrome by facilitating conduction through the bypass tract and shortening its refractory period. It should not be used to treat this disorder (ICSI, 2008a).

Older adults are particularly at risk for toxic effects because of altered renal clearance; they require slower digitalization and careful monitoring.

Because 20 to 30 percent of **digoxin** is bound to plasma proteins, diseases that lower serum albumin may require alterations in loading doses.

Digoxin is a Pregnancy Category C drug. Although safety has not been formally established, **digoxin** has been used safely in pregnancy for many years without adverse effects to the fetus. The volume of distribution (Vd) of this drug, however, suggests that it will use fetal tissue as a distribution site. Blood volume also changes throughout pregnancy, and this may affect both maternal and fetal levels of **digoxin.** Blood levels should be monitored carefully during this time to avoid toxicity, and pregnant women who require **digoxin** are probably best managed by a specialist.

Studies have shown that concentrations of **digoxin** in the mother's serum and milk are similar. However, the actual amount of drug the infant gets while nursing is relatively small, so no pharmacological effect is usually seen in the infant. Nonetheless, care should be taken in this case.

Newborns and premature and immature infants are particularly sensitive to the effects of **digoxin.** The dose must be highly individualized. There are children's doses for this drug. Once again, consultation or referral is suggested in these instances.

Adverse Drug Reactions

The GI tract is the most common site of adverse drug reactions, including anorexia, nausea, vomiting, and diarrhea. These result from CNS actions, including chemoreceptor trigger zone stimulation. Other CNS-based adverse responses include fatigue, disorientation, depression, and hallucinations, especially in older adults, and visual disturbances, including yellow vision and green halos around lights. The visual disturbances are considered classic signs of toxicity but actually occur rarely. Atrial arrhythmias and atrial tachycardia with AV block are the most common signs of toxicity in children. Cardiac adverse reactions are extensions of the therapeutic action of these drugs (bradycardia, junctional and AV block arrhythmias, premature ventricular contractions [PVCs], and bigeminy). Gynecomastia is a rare adverse reaction reported in some men.

Toxicity

Toxicity is commonly caused by excessive administration of a **CG**, by too much diuresis resulting in hypokalemia, by concurrent development of renal insufficiency, or by administration of drugs that interfere with excretion of **digoxin** (see the section Drug Interactions). It is especially common in older adults. Each of these common etiologies and the patient's calcium and magnesium levels should be considered in the differential diagnosis.

Diagnosis of toxicity is based on both clinical and laboratory data. Serum levels alone are insufficient to

> **CLINICAL PEARL**
>
> A full neutralizing dose of **Digibind** is relatively expensive ($2,000–$3,000). This cost should be considered in deciding to treat patients with suspected or non–life-threatening toxicity. It should also be remembered that **Digibind** has a half-life of 2 to 6 hours, and during that time the rhythm disturbance for which the **CG** was given may recur and cannot be treated with a **CG.**

diagnose toxicity because there is considerable overlap in serum concentrations between those with and without evidence of toxicity (see the Monitoring section for times to draw serum levels). Toxicity commonly occurs with serum levels greater than 2 ng/mL. Recognition of CG toxicity is an important differential diagnosis of arrhythmias and neurological and GI symptoms for patients taking CGs. The more common arrhythmias were listed previously.

Treatment of toxicity depends on the problem. AV junctional and first-degree block rhythms, ventricular ectopic beats, or an excessively slow ventricular response to atrial fibrillation often requires CG dosage adjustment and careful monitoring. **Potassium** administration should be considered to reduce automaticity, even when serum potassium is in the normal range, unless a high-grade AV block is also present. **Lidocaine** has minimum effects on the AV node and may be used to treat ventricular ectopic beats that threaten hemodynamics. Bradycardia and second- or third-degree AV block usually respond to **atropine**. When toxicity is severe or life threatening, the antidote for CG toxicity is antidigoxin immunotherapy, **digoxin immune fab (Digibind)**. Patients who require this medication are hospitalized so that cardiopulmonary resuscitation equipment and medications are available when it is administered.

Any patient who becomes toxic to a CG should have the indications for that drug carefully reviewed. In some cases, it is possible to stop the drug altogether. Several studies, however, have shown negative consequences for withdrawal of **digoxin**, so the decision should be carefully made.

Drug Interactions

Any drug that may cause hypokalemia, hypercalcemia, or hypomagnesemia increases the risk of toxicity. Several antiarrhythmic drugs (**quinidine, amiodarone, verapamil, diltiazem,** and **propafenone**) increase serum CG levels and toxicity risk. Drugs that can have an adverse response of bradycardia can exhibit additive bradycardia when given with CGs. This is especially a concern with **BBs. Antacids** and **kaolin-pectin** interfere with absorption.

Interactions with Potassium, Calcium, and Magnesium

Potassium and CGs interact by inhibiting each other's binding to sodium-potassium-ATPase. Hyperkalemia reduces the enzyme-inhibiting actions of CGs, and hypokalemia facilitates these actions. Hyperkalemia, however, inhibits the abnormal cardiac automaticity seen in excessive doses of CGs so that moderately increased extracellular potassium reduces toxic effects of CGs. Calcium facilitates the toxic actions of CGs by overloading the intracellular calcium stores. Hypercalcemia increases the risk of CG-induced arrhythmias. Magnesium has the opposite effects to calcium. Hypomagnesemia is a risk factor for arrhythmias. Specific drug interactions and the appropriate actions to prevent them are given in Table 16–10.

Table 16–10 ■ Drug Interactions: Cardiac Glycosides

Drug	Interacting Drug	Possible Effect	Implications
CGs	Phenobarbital, phenytoin, rifampin	Decreases the effect of digitoxin	Increase dose of digitoxin or change to digoxin
	Thiazide and loop diuretics, mezlocillin, piperacillin, ticarcillin, amphotericin B, glucocorticoids	May cause hypokalemia and increase risk of CG toxicity	Monitor serum potassium levels, and teach patient signs and symptoms of hypokalemia to monitor for and report. Administer potassium supplement prn and encourage diet high in potassium. Where possible, choose alternative drug, especially antibiotic.
	Calcium preparations	Facilitates toxicity by accelerating overloading of intracellular calcium stores	Monitor for indications of toxicity. Avoid concurrent administration. Separate administration of CG and milk intake by at least 30 min.
	Spironolactone	Increases digoxin half-life	Reduce dose of digoxin or increase dosing interval

Table 16–10 ■ **Drug Interactions: Cardiac Glycosides—cont'd**

Drug	Interacting Drug	Possible Effect	Implications
	Beta-adrenergic blockers, quinidine, disopyramide	Additive bradycardia	Avoid concurrent use or teach patient to monitor pulse rate and report pulse <60 bpm. Monitor electrocardiogram (ECG) regularly.
	Antacids, colestipol, kaolin-pectin, cholestyramine	Decreases absorption of CG if given concurrently	Separate administration by at least 1 h and give CG first
	Thyroid hormones	May decrease therapeutic effects and cause arrhythmias	Monitor for effectiveness. Monitor ECG at regular intervals.
Digitalis	Quinidine, cyclosporine, amiodarone, verapamil, diltiazem, propafenone, diflunisal	Increases serum levels of digitalis and risk of toxicity	Avoid concurrent use or monitor serum levels 5–7 d after adding one of these drugs. Consider reducing digitalis dose by half if patient has signs of toxicity or a high normal digitalis level at initiation of interacting drug.
	Aminoglycosides (oral), colestipol, rifampin, St. John's wort, sulfasalazine	Decrease digitalis serum levels	Avoid concomitant use
	Benzodiazepines, clarithromycin, diphenoxylate, erythromycin, indomethasone, itraconazole, tetracyclines, verapamil	Increases serum levels of digitalis and risk of toxicity	Avoid concurrent use or monitor serum levels 5–7 d after adding one of these drugs. Consider reducing digitalis dose by half if patient has signs of toxicity or a high normal digitalis level at initiation of interacting drug
	Calcium channel blockers	Additive effects on AV node may result in complete heart block	Monitor patient carefully if both are chose with HF
Food Interaction			
Digitalis	High-bran meal	Taking with this meal results in reduced absorption of digitalis	Take 30 min prior to meal

Clinical Use and Dosing

Atrial Fibrillation, Paroxysmal Supraventricular Tachycardia

Treatment is aimed at slowing the rate and converting to sinus rhythm if possible. Asymptomatic or mildly symptomatic patients with a rapid ventricular response should be treated with a CG, with a goal of a resting ventricular rate between 70 and 80 bpm (Table 16–11). **Digoxin** is preferred because it slows AV nodal conduction, resulting in a slower ventricular rate. It does not convert to sinus rhythm directly. Slowing heart rate yields greater diastolic filling time, permitting improved myocardial oxygenation. Cardiac muscle with an improved supply-demand ratio may return to sinus rhythm. **Digoxin** is less effective at slowing heart rate when vagal tone is low and adrenergic stimulation is high, such as during exercise, and in maintaining sinus rhythm or reducing the incidence of PSVT. Additional **antiarrhythmic drugs** may need to be added for these purposes.

For asymptomatic and mildly symptomatic patients, a loading dose is rarely required. Treatment is started with a maintenance dose if the ventricular response is less than 120 bpm. For young patients and those with normal renal function, the maintenance dose is 0.25 mg to 0.5 mg daily. For older adults and those with renal impairment, the maintenance dose is 0.125 mg daily.

If the ventricular rate is between 120 and 150 and still well tolerated, outpatient digitalization with a loading dose is reasonable. The dose is 10 to 15 mcg/kg in divided doses over 24 hours. The usual pattern is 50 percent of the digitalizing dose orally and the remainder in divided doses over 4 to 8 hours. If creatinine clearance is less than 20 mL/min, give one-half the loading dose and start with 0.125 mg daily for maintenance. Patients who are not

Table 16–11 ◉ **Dosage Schedule: Cardiac Glycosides**

Drug	Indication	Patient Status	Digitalizing or Loading Dose	Maintenance
Digoxin	Atrial fibrillation with ventricular response <120 bpm *or* stable CHF	Young adult *or* normal renal function	None	0.25–0.5 mg/d for atrial fibrillation; 0.25 mg/d for CHF
		Older adult *or* impaired renal function	None	0.125 mg/d
	Atrial fibrillation with ventricular response 120–150 bpm *or* less stable CHF	Young adult or normal renal function	1–1.5 mg/d in four divided doses 6 h apart	0.25–0.5 mg/d for atrial fibrillation; 0.25 mg/d for CHF
		Older adult *or* impaired renal function	If creatinine clearance <20 mL/min, give half the loading dose in four divided doses 6 h apart	0.125 mg/d
Digoxin (tablets)	Atrial fibrillation with rapid ventricular response or heart failure	Adult with normal renal function	0.75–1.25 mg (10–15 mcg/kg) given as 50% of dose initially and additional fractions at 4–8 h intervals	0.063–0.5 mg/d as tablets or 0.035–0.5 mg/d as gelatin capsules. Dose is based on lean body mass and Ccr.* Usual dose is 0.25 mg/d in morning.
		Older adult or impaired renal function	Same as adult	Same calculation. Usual dose is 0.125 mg in morning
(capsules)		Children with normal renal function based on lean body weight: 2–5 yr	25–35 mcg/kg given as 50% of dose initially and additional fractions at 4–8 h intervals	25%–35% of digitalizing dose given daily in two divided doses
		5–10 yr	15–30 mcg/kg given as above	Same as above
		>10 yr	8–12 mcg/kg given as above	Same as above except in single dose
Digoxin (elixir)	Heart failure	Children with normal renal function based on lean body weight: Premature infant Full-term 1–24 mo 2–5 yr 5–10 yr >10 yr	20–30 mcg/kg given as 50% of dose initially and additional fractions at 4–8 h intervals 25–35 mcg/kg given as above 35–60 mcg/kg given as above 30–40 mcg/kg given as above 20–35 mcg/kg given as above 10–15 mcg/kg given as above	20%–30% of oral digitalizing dose given daily in two divided doses 25%–35% of oral digitalizing dose for full term to >10 yr All in two divided doses except for >10 yr

*Maintenance dose = loading dose × (14 + Ccr/5). Ccr should be corrected to 70 kg body weight.
Therapeutic serum level of digoxin: atrial fibrillation, 1.5–2 ng/mL; CHF, 0.8–1.2 ng/mL.

hemodynamically stable require rapid digitalization in a hospital.

Drug levels may be drawn at steady state (5–7 days), but the best indication of appropriate dosing is an acceptable heart rate. An adequately digitalized patient has a serum level of 1.5 to 2 ng/dL when atrial fibrillation is being treated.

Heart Failure

Although no longer the first-line drug for treatment of HF, **digoxin** is still central to treatment for patients with severe systolic dysfunction (ejection fractions less than 40 percent and with an audible S_3 heart sound). In fact, the presence of S_3 is a potent predictor of response to CG therapy. **Digoxin** is also beneficial in HF resulting from uncontrolled HTN or severe aortic stenosis, although BP reduction and valve surgery are the mainstays of therapy in these disorders. **CGs** are less beneficial with ejection fractions of more than 40 percent or in HF secondary to hypertrophic cardiomyopathies. They have no benefit in HF due to recurrent transient ischemia. The primary mechanism of action in HF is through its positive inotropic action, increasing ejection fraction at a given preload and afterload.

Doses are calculated based on lean body weight and creatinine clearance (Ccr). Specific dosages and calculations are given in Table 16–11. Patients who are hemodynamically stable are often treated with an initial dose of 0.125 mg, increasing to 0.25 mg. The American College of Cardiology/American Heart Association (ACC/AHA) (Hunt et al, 2005) and ICSI (2004) guidelines suggest, however, that patients with mild-to-moderate HF often become asymptomatic on optimal doses of **ACEIs** and **diuretics** and usually do not require **digoxin.** For less stable patients, the treatment regimen includes a loading dose similar to that used to treat atrial fibrillation and a usual maintenance dose of 0.25 to 0.5 mg/d. **Diuretics** are the first drugs in treating patients with HF to reduce ECF volume and thereby afterload. Vasodilators may be added to reduce preload and afterload. **ACEIs** are the drugs of choice for vasodilation because of their proven beneficial effects on mortality risk and functional status (see the section Angiotensin-Converting Enzyme Inhibitors and Angiotensin II Receptor Blockers). **Digoxin** is usually added to this treatment regimen for those patients with severe HF whose symptoms persist despite optimal doses of **ACEIs** and **diuretics.** See Chapter 36 for further discussion.

Therapeutic levels usually occur in 5 to 7 days. An adequately digitalized patient has a serum level of 0.8 to 1.2 ng/mL, lower than that needed to treat atrial fibrillation.

Rational Drug Selection

Formulation

Digoxin is well absorbed orally, with a bioavailability of 60 to 80 percent for tablets. **Digoxin elixir** in capsules and encapsulated gel form (**Lanoxicaps**) has a 90 to 100 percent bioavailability and may be useful when careful titration of the dose is important. Pediatric elixir has a bioavailability of 70 to 85 percent. Tablets are not generally used for children, but children's digitalizing and maintenance doses are provided for both the capsule and the elixir (see Table 16–11).

Brand

The best choice of CG is the purified glycoside, **digoxin.** It is well absorbed, can be used parenterally if needed, and has an intermediate duration of action, with a half-life of 36 to 48 hours. Even in the presence of renal failure, it can be used if the dose is adjusted.

Cost

Digoxin is available in a generic form that reduces the cost.

Monitoring

Routine monitoring of **digoxin** levels is generally overdone. Monitoring should occur in addition to clinical judgment, rather than as a substitute for it. In general, testing should be done when any of the following occurs:

1. The patient is taking other drugs that may alter the pharmacokinetics of **digoxin** (see the section Drug Interactions).
2. Steady state has been achieved (4–5 half-lives or 1–2 weeks after starting dose).
3. Toxicity is suspected.
4. Confirmation of adequacy of maintenance dose is needed in situations of poor therapeutic response.
5. A reference point is needed in adjusting a dose.
6. Patient adherence to the treatment regimen is questioned.
7. The patient has unstable renal function.

To avoid sampling during the distribution phase of the drug response curve, levels should be drawn at least 6 hours after the last dose. Therapeutic levels vary, based on the reason for treatment, but generally range from 0.8 to 2 ng/mL.

Because of their critical role in sensitivity to toxicity, serum electrolytes (potassium, calcium, magnesium) should be monitored on a regular basis, especially for patients who are taking concurrent **diuretics.** Renal function status is also critical to dosing of **CGs**; therefore, serum creatinine levels should be evaluated periodically and prior to any dosage change.

Patient Education

Administration

The patient should take the drug exactly as prescribed, at the same time each day. The long half-life means that taking it at different times each day would be permissible, but the narrow therapeutic range means that missing a dose or doubling a dose could result in toxicity. Taking the drug at the same time each day lessens the likelihood

CLINICAL PEARL

1. **CGs** should not be used unless there is clear evidence of severe chronic systolic dysfunction or atrial fibrillation. In older adults, ankle edema is more often due to venous insufficiency than to heart failure. Even if it is related to heart failure, it is more often caused by diastolic dysfunction and better treated with **diuretics** or **ACEIs.**
2. **Digoxin** should not be discontinued unless a reversible cause of the heart failure has been completely corrected or there was no basis for the drug in the first place. Patients who respond appropriately to **digoxin** therapy have a chronic problem and need the drug chronically.
3. ST-T wave changes on the ECG do not correlate directly with serum drug levels and should not be used as an indication of toxicity. Serum drug levels are needed.

of nonadherence to the appropriate regimen. When the drug is prescribed on an eccentric schedule (e.g., 0.25 mg Monday, Wednesday, Friday [MWF] and 0.125 mg Tuesday, Thursday, Saturday, Sunday [TTSS]), taking at the same time each day reduces the complexity of the schedule. Placing the appropriate dose in a pill container with compartments for each day of the week also reduces the chance of nonadherence. If one dose is missed but remembered within 12 hours, it should be taken. If two doses are missed, the health-care provider should be contacted for instructions. The drug should not be stopped or the dosage altered without first contacting the health-care provider.

Although the presence of food in the gut does not alter absorption of CGs, the ingestion of a high-fiber meal may decrease absorption. Tablets can be crushed and administered with food for patients who have difficulty swallowing. Patients should eat a diet high in potassium (bananas, orange juice, tomato juice, spinach, melons, dates, raisins, soybeans, prunes, potatoes, and molasses), unless also taking a **potassium-sparing diuretic** or an ACEI, and eat moderate amounts of calcium (800–1,000 mg/d).

Do not alternate between dosage forms (Table 16–12). Each form has a different bioavailability, and changing forms may result in toxicity. For the same reason, the patient should check with the pharmacist during each drug refill to make certain the drug comes from the same manufacturer.

Store the drug in its original, tightly covered, light-resistant container. The patient who uses a pillbox for weekly dosing should not mix the digoxin with other drugs in the same compartment. Drugs often look alike and can be mistaken for one another.

CGs interact with many prescription and OTC drugs. Patients should avoid concurrent use of other drugs without first consulting the health-care provider and should not take **antacids** or antidiarrheal drugs within 1 hour of taking the CG. Milk may have the same effect on absorption, and doses should also be separated by 1 hour.

Adverse Reactions

Patients should learn to take their own pulse and then contact the health-care provider before taking the drug if the pulse rate is less than 60 or more than 100 bpm. Signs and symptoms of toxicity include nausea, vomiting,

Table 16–12 ◆ **Available Dosage Forms: Oral Cardiac Glycosides**

Drug	Dosage Form	How Supplied	Cost
Digoxin (Lanoxin) (Digitek)	Tablets:		
	0.125 mg (G)	In bottles of 100 and 1,000	$13
	0.125 mg (L)	In bottles of 30, 100, 1,000, 5,000, and UD 100	$23
	0.125 mg (D)	In bottles of 100, 1,000, and 5,000	
	Tablets:		
	0.25 mg (G)	In bottles of 1,000	$13
	0.25 mg (L)	In bottles of 30, 100, 1,000, 5,000, and UD 100	$23
	0.25 mg (D)	In bottles of 100, 1,000, and 5,000	
	Capsules:		
	0.05 mg (L)	In bottles of 100	$25
	0.1 mg (L)	In bottles of 100	$27
	0.2 mg (L)	In bottles of 100	$31
	Pediatric elixir:		
	0.05 mg/mL (G)	In 60 mL and UD 2.5 and 5 mL	
	0.05 mg/mL (L)	In 60 mL with calibrated dropper	

(G) = generic; (L) = Lanoxin; (D) = Digitek.
Cost for all is in 100 units.

diarrhea, confusion, depression, irregular pulse, yellow vision, and green halos around lights. Pulse changes and these symptoms should be reported to the health-care provider immediately. Some patients can tolerate heart rates as low as 50 bpm without other symptoms and can be taught mainly to report symptoms of toxicity or worsening HF. Signs and symptoms of worsening HF include persistent cough; shortness of breath; weight gain of more than 2 lb in 1 day or 5 lb in 1 week; swelling of ankles, legs, or hands; and sensation of fullness in the abdomen. Follow-up appointments are also critical to evaluate the effectiveness of these drugs and to monitor for toxicity.

Lifestyle Management

Cardiac-healthy lifestyle is discussed in the section **Angiotensin-Converting Enzyme Inhibitors** and **Angiotensin II Receptor Blockers**. At all times, patients should carry identification or wear a medical information bracelet or necklace that describes the disease process and drug regimen.

ANTIARRHYTHMICS

Cardiac rhythm disturbances range from benign and asymptomatic to malignant and life threatening. For some arrhythmias, definitive drug therapy has research support; for many arrhythmias, there is no demonstrated correlation between a particular rhythm disturbance and a particular class of antiarrhythmic drug. Selection of a specific drug is often arbitrary and largely based on adverse responses, interactions with other drugs being taken, and concurrent clinical problems. Unfortunately, **antiarrhythmic drugs** can paradoxically cause lethal arrhythmias in some patients. Choosing not to treat may be a better choice, especially in asymptomatic or minimally symptomatic patients. Debate continues about the relative merits of invasive versus noninvasive testing to assist in the selection of a specific **antiarrhythmic**. Given these variables, it is probably best to refer to a cardiologist any patients with rhythm disturbances for which there is no clearly demonstrated appropriate drug choice. When the drug is chosen by the specialist, management in the primary care setting requires understanding both the beneficial effects and the adverse effects of these drugs, the monitoring required, and appropriate patient education. The six classes of **antiarrhythmics** are discussed here with that management approach in mind. To be practical in a primary care setting, the drug must be available in oral form and have an effective half-life of at least 6 hours. Drugs that do not meet these criteria are not discussed.

Pharmacodynamics

Arrhythmias are caused either by abnormal pacemaker activity or by abnormal impulse conduction. The goal of therapy with an **antiarrhythmic** is to reduce ectopic pacemaker activity or alter abnormal conduction. The major mechanisms by which **antiarrhythmics** act to do this are (1) sodium channel blockade, (2) blockade of sympathetic nervous system (SNS) effects on the heart, (3) prolongation of the effective refractory period, and (4) blockade of the calcium channel. Different classes of **antiarrhythmics** act in one or more of these ways, and drugs in one class may have significant actions associated with a different class. Placement in a given class is based on predominant action.

All pacemakers in the heart, normal and ectopic, depend on appropriate phase 4 diastolic depolarization. Increasing the phase 4 slope may result in accelerated pacemaker discharge. Figure 16–4 depicts the cardiac action potential with slope phases. Potential causes of this increased slope include hypokalemia, beta-adrenergic stimulation, fiber stretch, acidosis, and partial depolarization by currents of injury. Blockade of sodium channels (**class I antiarrhythmics**) or **calcium channels** (**class IV antiarrhythmics**) reduces the permeability ratio of these ions to potassium, making the threshold more negative and reducing the phase 4 slope. **BBs** (**class II antiarrhythmics**) indirectly reduce the slope by blocking the chronotropic action of norepinephrine. Hyperkalemia stabilizes the membrane potential and also reduces the rate of pacemaker firing. Vagal discharge also reduces phase 4 slope and makes the potential more negative (CG activity).

Disturbances in impulse conduction are either (1) simple blocks related to severely depressed conduction that may sometimes be relieved by the parasympathetic action of atropine or (2) reentry conduction, in which one impulse reenters and excites areas of the heart more than once. Reentry requires (1) an obstacle to normal conduction, (2) unidirectional block in the circuit, and (3) conduction time around the circuit timed so that the impulse does not enter refractory tissue (Table 16–13). Too slow an impulse results in bidirectional block or the impulse collides with the next normal impulse; too fast results in bidirectional conduction or the impulse reaches tissue that is still refractory. Slowing conduction by depressing the sodium current (**class I**) or calcium current (**class IV**) abolishes reentry arrhythmias. Lengthening or shortening the refractory period also makes reentry less likely. Converting unidirectional block to bidirectional block (**class III**) also decreases reentry.

Effective **antiarrhythmics** act more on cardiac tissue being abnormally stimulated than on normal cardiac tissue. These drugs decrease the automaticity of ectopic pacemakers more than the SA node, and they reduce conduction or increase the refractory period more in depolarized tissue than in normally polarized tissue.

Class I

Class I antiarrhythmic drugs are sodium channel blockers. **Class IA** lengthens the duration of the action potential, **class IB** shortens it, and **class IC** has no effect or may minimally increase action potential duration. **Class IB**

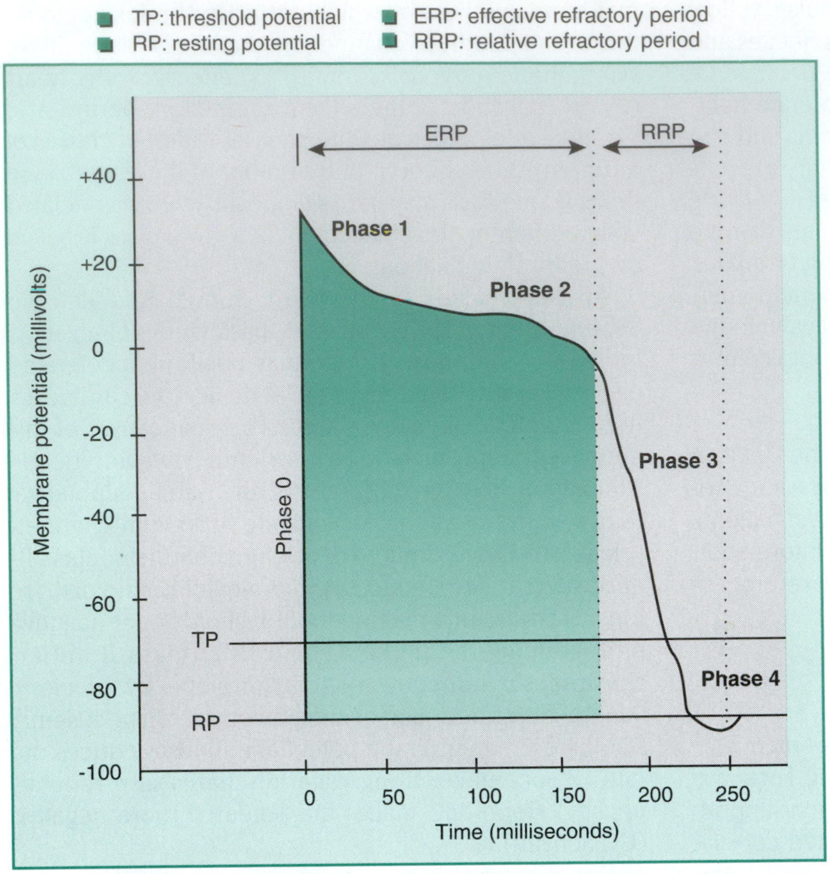

Figure 16–4. Cardiac action potential: ventricles.

Table 16–13 **Mechanism of Action of Selected Antiarrhythmics**

Drug	Effect on Sinoatrial Rate	Effect on Atrioventricular Node Refractory Period	Effect on PR Interval	Effect on QRS Duration	Effect on QT Interval	Sinoatrial Node Automaticity
Amiodarone	–	+	+	+	++	–
Disopyramide	± (2)	± (2)	± (2)	+	++	±
Flecainide	0	0	+	++	0	–
Mexiletine	0 (1)	±	0	0	0	–
Procainamide	±	± (2)	± (2)	+	+	±
Propafenone	0	+	+	+	0	0
Quinidine	± (2)	± (2)	± (2)	+	+	±
Sotalol	—	++	++	0	++	–
Tocainide	0 (1)	–	0	0	0	0/–

– = suppresses or slows; + = stimulates or increases speed or duration; (1) = may suppress diseased sinus nodes; (2) = anticholinergic effect and direct depressant action.

interacts rapidly with sodium channels, **class IC** acts slowly, and **class IA** is intermediate.

Class IA drugs reduce the rate of firing of ectopic foci, increase the effective refractory period (ERP), and reduce the speed of conduction. They also block parasympathetic nervous discharge, resulting in increased conduction rate at the AV node. This anticholinergic activity can produce serious increases in ventricular rate in the presence of rapid atrial activity, such as that found in atrial fibrillation. **Class IB** drugs block both activated and inactivated sodium channels. The effect is extremely limited in normally polarized tissue but highly effective in depolarized and injured tissue. They do not affect the automaticity of the SA node or conductivity through the AV node. Their shortening effect on the ERP eliminates unidirectional block and may trigger reentry arrhythmias. **Class IC** drugs primarily block the sodium fast channel during phase 0 of the action potential. Because of their propensity for severe exacerbation of arrhythmias, even in normal doses with post-MI patients they are reserved for patients with severe ventricular tachycardias for whom other drugs have not worked.

Class II

Class II drugs (BBs) reduce adrenergic activity in the heart. Blockade by these drugs increases threshold potential and prolongs ERP, thereby decreasing heart rate and conduction velocity. These effects probably convert unidirectional block to bidirectional. They also exert a significant negative inotropic effect, reducing force of contraction. This class includes $beta_1$ selective drugs that act mainly on cardiac muscle and nonselective $beta_1$ and $beta_2$ drugs that also act on lung, arteriole, pancreatic, kidney, adipose, and liver tissues, resulting in a wide range of adverse responses. BBs are discussed more thoroughly in Chapter 14.

Class III

Class III drugs prolong the ERP by some mechanism other than sodium channel blockade, often by blocking potassium channels, which results in a decreased rate of automaticity of ventricular ectopic beats. They may also convert unidirectional block to bidirectional block in reentry arrhythmias but have little effect on depolarization. Most of the drugs in this class also have significant actions associated with other classes.

Class IV

CCBs constitute **class IV.** They were discussed in more detail, including their role in arrhythmia management, earlier in this chapter.

Pharmacokinetics

Absorption and Distribution

All classes of **antiarrhythmics** are well absorbed orally, with sustained-release forms and **amiodarone (Cordarone)** having slower absorption times (Table 16–14). Bioavailabilities vary greatly depending on protein binding, with **propafenone (Rhythmol)** having the lowest at 3 percent bioavailability, with 97 percent protein binding, and **sotalol (Betapace)** having the highest (90%), with no protein binding. The presence of food in the gut does not affect bioavailability except for **sotalol**; food may reduce its absorption by as much as 20 percent.

Distribution is to most body tissues. **Amiodarone** exhibits high levels of drug in fat, muscle, lung, and spleen

Table 16–14 ▶ **Pharmacokinetics: Selected Antiarrhythmics**

Drug	Onset	Peak	Duration	Bioavailability	Protein Binding	Half-Life	Active Metabolite	Elimination
Amiodarone	1–3 wk	UK	wk–mo	35%–65%	95%	26–107 d	Yes (DEA)	99% in bile
Disopyramide PO	0.5–3.5 h	2.5 h	1.5–8.5 h	50%	35%–95%	4–10 h increased in hepatic, renal impairment	No	10% unchanged in feces, 50% unchanged in urine
Disopyramide CR	0.5–3.5 h	4.9 h	12 h	50%	35%–95%	4–10 h increased in hepatic, renal impairment	No	10% unchanged in feces, 50% unchanged in urine
Flecainide	Days	d–wk	12 h	>80%	40%	20 h	No	30% unchanged in urine
Mexiletine	0.5–2 h	2–3 h	8–12 h	>80%	60%–75%	12 h	No	10% unchanged in urine
Procainamide PO	0.5 h	1–1.5 h	3–4 h	75%	15%–20%	3–4 h increased in renal impairment	Yes (NAPA)	40%–70% unchanged in urine
Procainamide SR	0.5 h	1–1.5 h	6 h	75%	15%–20%	3–4 h increased in renal impairment	Yes (NAPA)	40%–70% unchanged in urine

Continued

Table 16–14 ▶ **Pharmacokinetics: Selected Antiarrhythmics—cont'd**

Drug	Onset	Peak	Duration	Bioavailability	Protein Binding	Half-Life	Active Metabolite	Elimination
Propafenone	UK	4–5 d	UK	3%–11%	97%	7 h (90% of patients); 10–32 h in slow metabolizers (10%)	Yes	<1% excreted unchanged
Quinidine PO (sulfate)	0.5 h	1–1.5 h	6–8 h		80%	6–8 h increased in CHF and severe liver impairment	Yes	20% unchanged in urine; urinary excretion enhanced in acid urine
Quinidine PO (sulfate-ER)	0.5 h	4 h	8–12 h		80%	6–8 h increased in CHF and severe liver impairment	Yes	20% unchanged in urine; urinary excretion enhanced in acid urine
Quinidine PO (gluconate)	0.5 h	3–5 h	6–8 h		80%	6–8 h increased in CHF and severe liver impairment	Yes	20% unchanged in urine; urinary excretion enhanced in acid urine
Sotalol	Hours	2–3 d	UK	90%	Not bound	7–12 h	No	90% unchanged in urine

UK = unknown; CHF = congestive heart failure.
Class II (beta blockers) are covered in Chapter 12; **class IV (CCBs)** are covered earlier in this chapter.

tissues. Cardiac tissue concentration is about 30 times higher than plasma concentration. **Amiodarone** and **quinidine** easily cross the placenta. **Disopyramide (Norpace), quinidine,** and **sotalol** are all found in breast milk, and **mexiletine (Mexitil)** is found in breast milk in concentrations similar to those found in plasma. **Disopyramide** has an unusual protein-binding curve, with binding sites becoming saturated at increasing dosages, leading to a nonlinear rise in free drug and misleading measurements of plasma concentration.

Metabolism and Excretion

All **antiarrhythmics** are metabolized by the liver. Half-lives of these drugs vary from 3 to 4 hours for **procainamide** to 26 or more days for **amiodarone.** As the only short-acting **antiarrhythmic, procainamide** requires frequent dosing administration, with steady state achieved in 2 to 3 days. Other **antiarrhythmics** have longer half-lives and require more time to achieve steady state. Hepatic impairment increases half-life in those drugs eliminated totally or partially in feces. Renal impairment significantly increases half-life in those drugs eliminated all or largely in the urine. Reduced dosages of **procainamide** and **quinidine** are required for patients with CHF or renal impairment that decreases volumes of distribution of these drugs. Many cardiac patients who need **antiarrythmics** have either decreased systolic function or renal impairment. Because of these concerns, **quinidine** and **procainamide** are infrequently used for such patients. Approximately 10 percent of patients are slow metabolizers of **propafenone,** resulting in an increase in half-life from 7 hours to 10 to 32 hours. Because this drug has been associated with proarrhythmia and increased mortality post-MI, the trend is away from its use.

Pharmacotherapeutics

Precautions and Contraindications

Because their mechanisms of action differ, the various classes also have different precautions and contraindications.

Class IA

Antimuscarinic actions in the heart common to this class inhibit vagal effects and may lead to increased sinus rate and AV conduction. Use cautiously for patients with cardiac problems, for whom increased heart rate might worsen the condition.

Class IB

Use cautiously for patients with HF related to the potential for hypotension secondary to decreased myocardial contractility. This occurs mainly with large doses and in fewer than 10 percent of patients. The major extracardiac adverse effects of these drugs are neurological and occur most frequently in older adults, so patients with neurological conditions and older adults should be carefully monitored for these adverse responses.

Class IC

No muscarinic effects are present with this class, but severe exacerbations of arrhythmia have occurred in patients with preexisting ventricular tachyarrhythmias and previous MI, even with normal doses of the drugs. These drugs should be reserved for patients unresponsive to less toxic drugs, especially if these patients have CHF, sinus nodal dysfunction, or heart block.

Class II

BBs are generally contraindicated for patients with bronchospastic disorders such as asthma. They are used with caution for patients with diabetes because they decrease insulin secretion and may mask many of the signs of hypoglycemia. Because of their peripheral vasoconstrictive effects, they are a poor choice for patients with PVD and Raynaud's syndrome.

Abrupt withdrawal of **BBs** may result in rebound beta stimulation resulting in tachycardia; therefore, they should be tapered by half every 4 hours. Patients at high risk for serious exacerbation of their disease related to abrupt withdrawal include those with angina, CAD with ventricular arrhythmias, and migraines. Hypertensive patients are at lower risk. **BBs** are discussed in more detail in Chapter 14.

Class III

Sotalol is the major **class III** drug used in primary care. It is a nonselective BB that also prolongs action potential. Its precautions are similar to those for class II. **Amiodarone**, also a **class III** drug, has significant properties of several other classes as well. The muscarinic effects associated with sodium channel blockade suggest cautious use for patients with SA or AV nodal dysfunction, bradycardia, or CHF. **Amiodarone** inhibits the enzyme that converts T4 to T3, and iodine is a major component of this drug; therefore, about 5 percent of patients with underlying predisposition to thyroid disease may develop thyrotoxicosis or hypothyroidism. If this drug must be used to treat the rhythm disturbance, careful monitoring and treatment of the thyroid disorder must be undertaken. Potentially fatal pulmonary fibrosis occurs in 5 to 15 percent of patients, and use for patients with pulmonary disease is questioned. At-risk patients should have thyroid and pulmonary function studies done before **amiodarone** therapy is initiated.

> **CLINICAL PEARL**
>
> For patients with diabetes who must take a **beta blocker,** the diaphoresis associated with hypoglycemia is not masked by these drugs, and diabetics should be taught to recognize this indication of hypoglycemia.

Class IV

CCBs have been discussed earlier in this chapter.

All **antiarrhythmics** are Pregnancy Category C, except **amiodarone,** which is Pregnancy Category D.

Adverse Drug Reactions

The more common adverse reactions of **antiarrhythmics** are extensions of their actions. Reduction in BP may result in dizziness, hypotension, fatigue, and syncope. Decreased myocardial contractility may result in CHF. Each class has the potential to produce rhythm disturbances, often exaggerations of or the reverse of the one being treated. **Class IC drugs** are especially proarrhythmic. GI symptoms, which are especially disturbing to patients, include nausea, vomiting, diarrhea, and constipation. GI symptoms are especially prevalent in **class IA** drugs, occurring in 33 to 50 percent of patients. Although not common, sexual dysfunction and urinary retention may occur in **classes I** and **III.** The **atropine**-like activity of **disopyramide** (urinary retention, dry mouth, and constipation) may require discontinuance of the drug. Adverse neurological reactions of **antiarrhythmics** include tremor, blurred vision, and nervousness. **Amiodarone** has several adverse drug effects not common to other **antiarrhythmics,** including extrapyramidal syndrome (EPS) effects, hepatitis, epididymitis, corneal and skin deposits, peripheral neuropathy, and photosensitivity. These effects increase with cumulative doses and limit its utility for long-term therapy. Adverse effects associated with beta blockade in **class II** drugs and **sotalol** are discussed in Chapter 14. Those relevant to **CCBs** have been discussed earlier in this chapter.

Drug Interactions

Cross-class and intraclass increases in cardiac effects are common between antiarrhythmics, increasing serum levels and toxicity risks. Several drugs increase or decrease the metabolism of **antiarrhythmics: cimetidine** (Tagamet), **phenobarbital, rifampin** (Rifadin), and **phenytoin** (Dilantin), which also has **class IB antiarrhythmic** activity, resulting in alterations in effectiveness and toxicity risk. The anticoagulation effects of **warfarin (Coumadin)** are increased by many antiarrhythmics, particularly **amiodarone.**

Additive anticholinergic effects occur as an interaction between several **antiarrhythmics** and other drugs that have anticholinergic properties. The metabolism and excretions of several class I drugs are significantly affected by urine pH, resulting in altered serum levels and toxicity risk. The CYP 3A4 system is involved in the metabolism of **quinidine.** Drugs that inhibit this system, including grapefruit juice, may increase free drug levels. CYP 2D6 is involved in **flecainide (Tambocor)** and **propafenone** metabolism. Drugs that inhibit this system may similarly increase free drug levels. Selected **antiarrhythmics** may potentiate the hypotensive effects of **antihypertensives, nitrates,** and **alcohol. BBs** may alter the effectiveness of **insulin** and **oral hypoglycemics.** Specific drug interactions and the appropriate actions to prevent them are given in Table 16–15.

Table 16–15 ■ **Drug and Food Interactions: Selected Antiarrhythmics**

Drug	Interacting Drug/Food	Possible Effect	Implications
Amiodarone*	Digoxin	Increases blood levels and toxicity risk	Decrease dose of digoxin by 50%. Monitor for toxicity
	Class I antiarrhythmics	Increases blood levels and toxicity risk	Decreases of these drugs by 30%–50%
	Phenytoin	Increases blood levels of phenytoin; may decrease amiodarone blood levels	Avoid concurrent use: If they must be given together monitor serum levels of both drugs
	BBs, CCBs	Increases risk for bradyrhythms, sinus arrest, and AV block	Monitor for dizziness and ortho-static and mental status change. Safety issues
	Cholastyramine	May decrease amiodarone blood levels	Separate doses by 1 h and give amiodarone first
	Antihypertensives	May produce profound hypotension	Monitor BP. Safety issues
Disopyramide*, †, ‡	Phenytoin, phenobarbital	Decreases blood levels and effectiveness	Monitor pulse, ECG for effectiveness
	Other antiarrhythmics	Additive cardiac toxic effects (prolonged conduction, decreased cardiac output)	Avoid using disopyramide for 48 h before or 24 h after verapamil
	Drugs with anticholinergic properties	Additive anticholinergic effects	Monitor for dry mouth, wheezing, urinary retention, orthostatic hypotension
Flecainide†	CCBs, Disopyramide,	Increases arrhythmia risk	
	BBs, verapamil	Additive myocardial depression	Combination should be avoided or given cautiously
	Amiodarone	Doubles serum flecainide levels	Decrease flecainide dose by 50%
	Digoxin	Increases serum digoxin levels by small amount	Monitor serum digoxin level and indications of toxicity
	Alkalinizing agents, foods that increase urine pH to >7§, strict vegetarian diet	Promotes reabsorption increases blood levels, increases toxicity risk	Monitor serum levels
	Acidifying agents, foods that decrease urine pH to <5§ acidic juices	Increases renal elimination, decreases effectiveness	Monitor serum levels and clinical indicators of effectiveness
Mexiletine	Opioid analgesics, atropine, antacids	Slows absorption of mexiletine	Separate adminstration of antacids by at least 1 h

Table 16–15 ■ **Drug and Food Interactions: Selected Antiarrhythmics—cont'd**

Drug	Interacting Drug/Food	Possible Effect	Implications
	Metoclopramide	Speeds absorption	
	Phenytoin; phenobarbital, cigarette smoking	Increases metabolism and decreases effectiveness of mexiletine	Avoid concurrent use
	Alkalinizing and acidifying agents[§]	Same as with flecainide	Same as with flecainide
Procainamide[†]	Other antiarrhythmics	Additive effect (see amiodarone)	
	Antihypertensives, nitrates	Potentiates hypotensive effects	Monitor BP. Safety issues
	Drugs with anticholinergic properties	Additive anticholinergic effects	Monitor for dry mouth, wheezing, urinary retention orthostatic hypotension
	Ranitidine, quinidine, trimethoprim	Increases serum levels and effects of procainamide	Monitor for procainamide toxicity (tachycardia, confusion, drowsiness, nausea, and vomiting)
	Digoxin	Increases digoxin levels by 35%–85%	Dosage reduction required
	Metoprolol, propranolol	Increases serum levels and effects of these drugs	Dosage reduction may be required
	Quinidine	Inhibits propafenone metabolism	Avoid concurrent use
Quindinepercent[*,†,‡]	Digoxin	Increases serum levels and toxicity risk	Dosage reduction recommended
	Amiodarone	See amiodarone	See amiodarone
	Phenytain, phenobarbital	Increases metabolism and decreases effectiveness of quinidine	Monitor therapeutic effects
	Verapamil	Decreases metabolism and increases serum levels of quinidine	Monitor for toxicity
	Antihypertensives, nitrates, alcohol	Additive hypotension	
	Procainamide, propafenone, tricyclic antidepressants (TCAs)	Increases serum levels and risk for toxicity for each of these drugs	
	Drugs with anticholinergic properties	Additive anticholinergic effects	Monitor for dry mouth, wheezing, urinary retention, orthostatic hypotension
	Alkalinizing and acidifying foods and drugs[§]	See flecainide	
Sotalol	General anesthetics, IV phenytoin, CCBs	Additive myocardial depression	
	Digoxin	Additive bradycardia	
	Antihypertensives, nitrates, alcohol	Additive hypotension	

Continued

Table 16–15 ■ **Drug and Food Interactions: Selected Antiarrhythmics—cont'd**

Drug	Interacting Drug/Food	Possible Effect	Implications
	Amphetamines, ephedrine, epinephrine, norepinephrine, phenylephrine, pseudoephedrine	Unopposed alpha-adrenergic stimulation, leading to excessive HTN and bradycardia	Avoid concurrent use. Teach patient not to use OTCs without contacting health care provider
	Amiodarone, disopyramide, procainamide, quinidine	Increases proarrhythmia risk	Avoid concurrent use
	Clonidine	Potentiates rebound HTN when clonidine discontinued	Use caution and monitor BP closely when discontinuing clonidine
	Insulin, oral hypoglycemics	May alter effectivenss of diabetic drugs	Dosage adjustment of diabetic drugs may be requireds
	Monoamine oxidase inhibitors (MAOIs)	May result in increased HTN	Use cautiously within 14 d of MAOI

*Interacts with warfarin to increase anticoagulation. Monitor prothrombin time. Dosage of warfarin may need to be decreased. For amiodarone, the decrease may be 33%–50%.

†Interacts with cimetidine to increase serum levels of the antiarrhythmic. Choose different histamine$_2$ blocker. Monitor for toxicity if cimetidine must be used.

‡Interacts with rifampin to decrease serum levels and effectiveness of antiarrhythmic. If they must be used together, monitor for decreased therapeutic effect of antiarrhythmic, and adjust dosage as needed.

§Foods that alkalinize urine: all fruits except cranberries, prunes, plums; all vegetables; milk. Foods that acidify urine: cheeses, cranberries, eggs, fish, grains, meats, plums, poultry, prunes.

¶Drugs with anticholinergic properties: antihistamines, atropine, benztropine, haloperidol, phenothiazines, TCAs, trihexyphenidyl.

Clinical Use and Dosing

Atrial Arrhythmias (Atrial Fibrillation/Flutter, Atrioventricular Nodal Reentrant Tachycardia, Wolff-Parkinson-White Tachycardias)

All **antiarrhythmics** have some use in these disorders. Class IA drugs (**quinidine**, **procainamide**) are especially useful. **Quinidine** has a short-acting form that is given every 4 to 6 hours, a long-acting form for every 8-hour administration, and **Quinidex Extentabs**, which can be given bid (Table 16–16). It has been combined with **mexiletine** to enhance effectiveness and reduce adverse effects. **Procainamide** can be used in a hemodynamically stable patient for the acute treatment of focal atrial trachycardia and the acute management of stable atrial flutter (American College of Cardiology/American Heart Association/European Society of Cardiology [ACC/AHA/ESC], 2003; ACC/AHA/ESC, 2006). It can also be used in the long-term management of recurrent, well-tolerated atrial flutter if combined with an AV node blocking agent and no significant structural cardiac disease is present. **Procainamide's** half-life is only 3 to 4 hours, requiring frequent dosing. If around-the-clock **antiarrhythmic** activity is required, a sustained-release preparation must usually be given every 6 hours. Less frequent dosing is sometimes possible in renal disease, in which excretion is slowed. **Amirodarone** is very effective against supraventricular arrhythmias, especially in children, in whom it appears to be quite safe. The wide range of adverse reactions seen in adults and its many drug interactions make it a second-line drug choice. Reentrant supraventricular tachycardia is a major indication for **verapamil** (**Calan**, **Isoptin**). However, ICSI (2008a) states that it is ineffective and can increase the risk for ventricular fibrillation in patients with re-excitation. It can also be used to decrease the rate in atrial fibrillation/flutter with rapid ventricular response. The long-acting form has the advantage of once-daily administration. The high risk for clot formation associated with atrial fibrillation requires concurrent anticoagulation therapy with either **aspirin** or **warfarin**, depending on the risk profile of the patient.

Ventricular Arrhythmias (Ventricular Ectopic Beats, Ventricular Tachycardia, Ventricular Fibrillation)

Simple ventricular rhythm disturbances such as occasional PVCs are rarely treated in primary care. Complex ventricular irritability demonstrated with ventricular rhythm disturbances is associated with increased risk for MI and sudden death. Despite this fact, only symptomatic patients with underlying heart disease, malignant forms of arrhythmia such as recurrent ventricular tachycardia, and poor LV function seem to benefit from prophylactic antiarrhythmic therapy. Controlled trials of **antiarrhythmic** therapy in minimally symptomatic post-MI patients with reduced ejection fractions actually showed increased rates of arrhythmia-associated death in those treated. **Class IA** agents have moderate efficacy in treating

Table 16–16 ◉ **Dosage Schedule: Selected Antiarrhythmics**

Drug	Clinical Use	Starting Dose	Maintenance Dose	Maximum Dose (Adjusted Dose)	Plasma Concentration
Amiodarone	Ventricular arrhythmias (unlabeled use in PSVT, atrial fibrillation)	400–600 mg tid for 1–2 wk	400–600 mg/d 200 mg/d* † or PSVT, atrial fibrillation	1,000 mg	1–2 mcg/mL
Atenolol	Prevent primary arrhythmic event post-MI	100 mg daily or 50 mg bid	100 mg daily or 50 mg bid for at least 9 d: post-MI		
	Insufficient control of atrial fibrillation with digoxin	25–50 mg/d added to digoxin dose	100 mg/d; 50 mg/d if severe renal impairment		
Disopyramide	Ventricular arrhythmia (unlabeled use in PSVT)	150 mg q8h *Children:* mg/kg/d in 4 divided doses at q6h intervals: <1 yr = 10–30 1–4 = 10–20 4–12 = 10–15 12–18 = 6–15 *Adults:* <50 kg 400 mg/d *Adults:* >50 kg 400–800 mg/d in divided doses q6h for standard tablets; q12h for controlled release		For creatinine clearance <40 mL/min, dosage in adults is 100 mg q8h; further reductions as clearance decreases	2–4 mcg/mL
Flecainide*	Sustained ventricular tachycardia, PSVT	100 mg q12 h for ventricular tachycardia; 50 mg q12h for PSVT	100–150 mg q12h for ventricular tachycardia; 50–100 q12h for PSVT	Ventricular tachycardia: 400 mg/d; PSVT: 300 mg/d; adjust doses by 50-mg increments; minimum 4 d between adjustments	
Mexiletine	Ventricular arrhythmias	200 mg q8h (if rapid control of arrhythmia is essential, load with 400 mg)	200–300 mg q8h	1200 mg/d: adjust doses by 50–100-mg increments; minimum 2–3 d between adjustments	0.5–2 mcg/mL
Procainamide	Ventricular arrhythmias	750 mg q6h *Children:* 15–50 mg/kg/d in divided doses *Young adults:* 50 mg/kg/d in divided doses (q3–4h for tablets; q6h or q8h for sustained release) reduce dose if age >50 or with renal or hepatic impairment		4 g/d	3–10 mcg/mL (risk of cardiac and GI toxicity increases if >8 mcg/mL)

Continued

Table 16–16 ◉ **Dosage Schedule: Selected Antiarrhythmics—cont'd**

Drug	Clinical Use	Starting Dose	Maintenance Dose	Maximum Dose (Adjusted Dose)	Plasma Concentration
Propafenone*	Ventricular arrhythmias (unlabeled use in PSVT associated with WPW)	150 mg q8h	225–300 mg q8h	900 mg; increases doses at minimum of 3-d intervals	0.2–1.5 mcg/mL (nonlinear change in plasma level related to dose increase)
Propranolol	PSVT: atrial fibrillation; tachycardias associated with digitalis toxicity, excessive catecholamines, thyroid dysfunction	10–30 mg tid–qid given ac and hs; for atrial fibrillation uncontrolled by digoxin, add 40–80 mg of propranolol to digoxin dose		240 mg/d	
Quinidine	Premature atrial contraction, PSVT, atrial fibrillation, atrial flutter, atrioventricular nodal reentry; WPW, VC; ventricular tachycardia not associated with complete heart block	Single-dose 200-mg tablet to assess for idiosyncratic reaction	200–300 mg tid or qid for tablets; 300–600 mg q8h for sustained release†*	2–6 mcg/mL	
Sotalol	Ventricular arrhythmias	80 mg bid	240–320 mg/d in 2 divided doses; long half-life makes more than bid dosing unnecessary	640 mg; adjust doses at minimum 2 d interval	

PSVT = paroxysmal supraventricular tachycardia; MI = myocardial infarction; WPW = Wolff-Parkinson-White syndrome.
* Because of proarrhythmic effects, use with lesser arrhythmias is not recommended.
†Because the rate of absorption from various sustained-release formulations may be markedly different, they are not interchangeable.

ventricular arrhythmias and are sometimes prescribed. **Disopyramide** has a pronounced negative inotropic effect, however, which limits its usefulness. For patients with heart failure, discontinuation of most **antiarrythmics**, **CCBs**, and **NSAIDs** is recommended (American College of Cardiology/American Heart Association [ACC/AHA], 2009). Class IA agents in patients with reduced LVEF especially increase the risk of serious arrhythmias. This is also true for Class IC **flecainide** and **propafenone** and Class III **sotalol** (ACC/AHA, 2003). These drugs are both cardiodepressant and proarhythmic in heart failure patients. **Class IB** drugs are fairly weak **antiarrhythmics** for these problems and are either second-line drugs or used with **class IA** drugs. Their relatively long half-lives allow bid or tid dosing. They are well tolerated in HF, having little negative inotropic effect, with **mexiletine** more negatively inotropic than **tocainide**. **Class IC** drugs are moderately effective but are reserved for very refractory cases because of their proarrhythmic qualities. **Class II** drugs are useful in exercise-induced ventricular tachycardia but should be monitored with serial exercise testing to check efficacy. They are safe and especially useful in arrhythmias caused by ischemic heart disease because they are among the few drugs proven to reduce CAD mortality. Selection for $beta_1$ receptors reduces many of their adverse reactions. **Atenolol (Tenormin)**, has strong $beta_1$ selectivity, resulting in a low adverse effect profile, and is used for post-MI arrhythmia prophylaxis. **Propranolol (Inderal)**, a nonselective BB, is used with several arrhythmias. **Class III** drugs are the best choice for monomorphic ventricular tachycardia.

A common noncardiac cause of tachyarrhythmias is hyperthyroidism. **Propranolol**, a **class II** drug, slows the heart rate by its beta-blocking action, and has the added effect of preventing peripheral conversion of T4 to T3, thereby reducing the serum levels of the more active form of thyroid hormone.

Rational Drug Selection

Risk versus Benefit

The choice of **antiarrhythmic** drugs is usually based not only on benefit (correction or prevention of the rhythm) but also on risks (adverse effects and toxicity). Benefits may be assessed and drugs chosen by electrophysiological studies. When no agent meets electrophysiological study criteria for choice, empiric **amiodarone** may be prescribed because of its effects in all classes and because it has been shown to reduce mortality in cardiac arrest survivors from 50 to 20 percent at 2 years' post–cardiac arrest. The more potentially lethal the arrhythmia is, the more acceptable the risks become. In terms of prevention, only BBs have been definitively shown by research to reduce mortality in relatively asymptomatic patients. Risks related to adverse reactions are present in all **antiarrhythmics** and increase with higher doses and longer times of administration.

Concurrent Diseases

The presence of diseases in other organ systems may dictate the choice of drug, based on the effects of the **antiarrhythmic** on that system (bronchospasm in asthma, urinary retention in benign prostatic hyperplasia).

Cost

All **antiarrhythmics** are expensive. Cost data are provided in Table 16–17. Those requiring frequent monitoring by diagnostic tests need to have the cost of this monitoring factored into their cost. For example, **amiodarone** may require a chest x-ray every 3 to 6 months, pulmonary function tests, and ophthalmic examinations, as well as thyroid-stimulating hormone (TSH) and free thyroxine (T4) levels, dependent on the signs and symptoms found in the patient. This significantly raises the cost of this drug. Generic **procainamide** requires q6h to q8h dosing. Cost is increased significantly when generic is switched to the sustained-release form.

Table 16–17 ◆ **Available Dosage Forms: Selected Antiarrhythmics**

Drug	Dosage Form	How Supplied	Cost
Amiodarone (Cordarone) (Pacerone)	Tablets: 200 mg (G)	In bottles of 60, 100, 250, 500, and UD 100	$25
	200 mg (B) [Cordarone]	In bottles of 60 and UD 100	$218
	200 mg (B) [Pacerone]	In bottles of 60, 90, 500, and UD 100	$107
	400 mg (B) [Pacerone]	In bottles of 30, 100, 500, and UD 100	
Disopyramide (Norpace)	Capsules: 100 mg (G), 150 mg (G)	In bottles of 100 and 500	100 mg = $50; 150 mg = $53
	100 mg (B), 150 mg (B)	In bottles of 100 and 1,000	100 mg = $97; 150 mg = $114
	Capsules (CR): 100 mg (B), 150 mg (B)	In bottles of 100, 500, and UD 100	100 mg = $115; 150 mg = $137 $90
	150 mg (G)	In bottles of 100	
Flecainide (Tambocor)	Tablets: 50 mg (G), 100 mg (G), 150 mg (G)	In bottles of 100	50 mg = $60; 100 mg = $83; 150 mg = $127
	50 mg (B), 100 mg (B), 150 mg (B)	In bottles of 100 and UD 100	50 mg = $187; 100 mg = $292; 150 mg = $401
Mexiletine (Mexitil)	Capsules: 150 mg (G), 200 mg (G), 250 mg (G)	In bottles of 100 and UD 100 250 mg = $41	150 mg = $23; 200 mg = $27
Procainamide (Pronestyl) (Procanbid)	Tablets (extended release): 250 mg, 500 mg, 750 mg, 1,000 mg (all G) Procanbid tablets: 750 mg, 1,000 mg Capsules: 250 mg, 375 mg, 500 mg (G) Pronestyl capsules: 250 mg, 375 mg 500 mg (sustained release) (all B)	In bottles of 100 and 500 In bottles of 100 and 500 In bottles of 60 and UD 100 In bottles of 100, 250, and 1,000 In bottles of 100	500 mg = $33; 750 mg = $53; 1,000 mg = $67 250 mg = $13; 500 mg = $17 250 mg = $73; 375 mg = $77; 500 mg = $86

Continued

Table 16–17 ◆ **Available Dosage Forms: Selected Antiarrhythmics—cont'd**

Drug	Dosage Form	How Supplied	Cost
Propafenone (Rythmol)	Tablets: 150 mg (G), 225 mg (G), 300 mg (G) 150 mg (B), 225 mg (B), 300 mg (B) Capsules (SR): 225 mg (B), 325 mg (B), 425 mg(B)	In bottles of 100 and 500 In bottles of 100 and UD 100 In bottles of 100 In bottles of 100	150 mg = $53; 225 mg = $78; 300 mg = $167 225 mg = $445; 325 mg = $585 425 mg = $585
Quinidine sulfate	Tablets: 200 mg, 300 mg (G) Tablets (sustained release): 300 mg (G) Quinidex extendtabs: 300 mg	In bottles of 100 and 1,000 In bottles of 100 and 250 In bottles of 100, 250, and UD 100	200 mg = $22; 300 mg = $37 $30
Quinidine Gluconate	Tablets (sustained release): 324 mg	In bottles of 100, 250, and 500	$81
Sotalol (Betapace)	Tablets: 80 mg (G), 120 mg (G), 160 mg (G) 240 mg (G) 80 mg (B), 120 mg (B), 160 mg (B) 240 mg (B) Sotalol AF tablets: 80 mg, 120 mg, 160 mg Betapace AF tablets: 80 mg, 120 mg, 160 mg	In bottles of 100, 500, and 1,000 In bottles of 100, 500, and 1,000 In bottles of 100 and UD 100 In bottles of 100 and UD 100 In bottles of 60 and 100 In bottles of 60 and 100	120 mg = $28; 160 mg = $36 $49 80 mg = $274; 120 mg = $365 160 mg = $456; 240 mg = $592 80 mg = $94; 120 mg = $224; 160 mg = $155 80 mg = $151/60; 120 mg = $200/60; 160mg = $250/60

(G) = generic; (B) = brand.
Cost data are in 100 units unless otherwise noted.

Decision Steps

Because the margin between therapeutic efficacy and toxicity is narrow and the knowledge needed to prescribe these drugs is extensive, it is best to refer patients to a cardiologist for initiation of therapy. Phone consultation may also be required during therapy unless the provider has extensive experience with antiarrhythmic therapy. When this is not possible, Katsung (2004) recommends several important steps in deciding on therapy:

1. Any factor that might be precipitating the arrhythmia should be determined and eliminated. Especially relevant are adverse drug reactions, underlying disease states such as thyroid disorders, and potassium levels.
2. A firm arrhythmia diagnosis should be established. Use of inappropriate drugs because of a misdiagnosis of the arrhythmia can be catastrophic in some cases.
3. Establish a reliable baseline on which to judge the efficacy of any subsequent antiarrhythmic therapy. Methods include ambulatory monitoring, electrophysiological studies, and treadmill exercises.
4. The mere identification of an arrhythmia does not necessarily require its treatment. An excellent justification for conservative treatment was provided by the Cardiac Arrhythmia Suppression Trial (CAST).

Monitoring

Laboratory Data

Potassium concentration in the extracellular space is the major determinant of resting membrane potential and membrane stability. Potassium levels should always be checked and kept more than 4 mEq/L for patients with rhythm disturbances. Renal and hepatic functions (blood urea nitrogen [BUN], creatinine, transaminases) should be watched because they are the principal routes of excretion for **antiarrhythmic** drugs. Intervals for these tests depend on drug class. **Antiarrhythmics** tend to have narrow therapeutic ranges and are often given to patients who are taking other drugs with which they may interact, increasing the risk of toxicity or lack of efficacy. Serum drug levels should be monitored at regular intervals after steady state is achieved. Timing of the blood draw is critical. The sample is usually drawn 4 to 6 hours after the last oral dose so that a peak serum level is not mistaken for a steady-state level. Anticoagulation studies (prothrombin time [PT], international normalized ratio [INR], activated partial thromboplastin time [apt]) are discussed in Chapter 18. Laboratory studies related to the underlying disease that may be causing the arrhythmia are not discussed here.

Electrocardiogram

Monitoring 12-lead electrocardiograms (ECGs) for indications of efficacy and toxicity is essential, especially concerning drugs for which ECG changes are the primary indicators of such problems. The frequency of monitoring depends on the stability of the patient's drug regimen and the presence of symptoms.

Other Studies

Electrophysiological studies, echocardiography, and exercise stress testing are best done in consultation with a cardiologist. Monitoring for BBs is discussed in Chapter 14 and for CCBs earlier in this chapter. Monitoring parameters are further delineated in Table 16–18.

Patient Education

Cardiac rhythm disturbances tend to engender fear. A thin line exists between providing, on the one hand, enough information to have the patient appreciate the seriousness of the disorder (or the lack of seriousness in benign forms of arrhythmia) and, therefore, adhere to the treatment regimen and, on the other hand, so much information that fear or denial takes over and adherence suffers. Most patients and their families appreciate an honest discussion of the disorder and its treatment, accompanied by assurance of effective treatment for most forms of arrhythmia. Most **antiarrhythmics** have annoying adverse reactions, and patients are more likely to tolerate them when the importance of the drug is explained.

Administration

The patient should take the drug exactly as prescribed. For doses taken more than once daily, evenly space the

Table 16–18 **Monitoring Parameters for Selected Antiarrhythmics**

Drug	Parameters	Timing	Comments
Amiodarone	Chest x-ray, pulmonary function studies	Every 3–6 mo	High risk for pulmonary fibrosis. Risk of sudden cardiac death may outweigh risk associated with pulmonary dysfunction. Every effort should be made to rule out other treatable cause of pulmonary problem. Some providers schedule tests based on symptoms after 1 yr without problems
	Thyroid-stimulating hormone (TSH), Free T_4	Every 6 mo	Monitor closely for other indications of thyroid dysfunction as well
	Ophthalmic exam (slit lamp and fundoscopy)	Every 6 mo	Although rare, visual impairment may progress to permanent blindness. Any symptoms of impairment should result in prompt ophthalmic exam. Corneal microdeposits are reversible with reduction in dose and no reason to stop treatment
Flecainide*	ECG Liver function studies Serum drug levels		Watch for sinus node problems and AV block. Highly metabolized in liver. Liver disease may significantly increase free drug level. Keep trough <1 mcg/mL
Mexiletine*	Liver function studies		Aspartate aminotransferase (AST) elevations >3 times upper limit of normal (ULN) have been observed. Assess for other treatable causes such as CHF or acute MI before stopping drug
Procainamide†	Complete blood count (CBC) Antinuclear antibody (ANA) titer		At initiation of therapy to assess for blood dyscrasias At initiation of therapy and at any indication of lupuslike syndrome
Propafenone	Liver function studies		Highly metabolized by liver. Liver disease may increase bioavailability to 70%
Quinidine†	CBC, renal and liver function studies		Discontinue drug if blood dyscrasias or hepatic or renal dysfunction occurs
Sotalol	Fasting blood glucose		May affect insulin secretion and glucose metabolism. May mask indications of hypoglycemia in patients with diabetes

All require monitoring of potassium level and 12-lead ECG. Most require serum drug levels. Monitoring of renal function is prudent in all.
*Changes in urine pH can alter drug excretion. Monitor urinalysis on annual visits.
†ECG changes are the primary indicators of toxicity in these drugs. QRS >25% above normal or prolonged QT intervals suggest reduction in dose by as much as 50%.

doses. Abrupt withdrawal of these drugs may result in life-threatening arrhythmias, HTN, or myocardial ischemia. The patient should keep enough medication on hand for weekends, holidays, and vacations. For **amiodarone**, if a dose is missed at its usual time, it should not be taken at all that day; the patient should simply take the next day's dose. Its very long half-life maintains a stable dose. For **disopyramide**, **mexiletine**, **procainamide sustained-release**, **propafenone**, and **tocainide**, a dose that is missed should be taken as soon as it is remembered, unless the next dose is due in 4 hours or less. For **flecainide**, the missed dose should be taken unless the next dose is due in 6 hours, and for **sotalol**, 8 hours. For **quinidine** and standard formulations of **procainamide**, the separation is 2 hours.

Several drugs come in more than one formulation, from standard to sustained release (see Table 16–17). The patient should read the label carefully and follow the appropriate dosing schedule, especially if the drug is changed to a different form or a different drug. For sustained-release formulations, the tablets should not be crushed or chewed but must be swallowed whole. Patients who have difficulty in swallowing should be placed on standard formulations that can be crushed.

Food intake is a concern with some of the antiarrhythmics. **Sotalol** absorption is significantly decreased when it is taken with food. It should always be taken on an empty stomach. **Mexiletine**, **tocainide**, and **quinidine**, however, have uncomfortable GI adverse effects unless they are taken with food. Foods that alter urine pH affect the excretion of **flecainide**, **mexiletine**, and **quinidine** and should be avoided or taken in consistent amounts. (See Table 16–15 for a list of such foods.)

Drug interactions are frequent with both prescription and OTC drugs. The patient should consult the health-care provider before taking any other drugs, including OTC cold remedies.

Adverse Reactions

Dizziness is the most common adverse response. Changing position slowly, especially when arising from a lying position, decreases this reaction. Caution should be taken in driving or other activities that require alertness until the patient's response is known. Monitoring of pulse rate and rhythm and BP provides early indications of efficacy and toxicity. Patients should learn to take their own pulse and BP and check them whenever symptoms occur. Hypotension and slow, rapid, or irregular heart rates should be reported promptly. Bone marrow is affected in many classes. Patients should report fever, chills, sore throat, or unusual bruising to the health-care provider. Photosensitivity may occur through window glass, thin clothing, and sunscreens for patients who are taking **amiodarone**, **disopyramide**, or **quinidine**. Protective clothing and sunblock are recommended during therapy and for 4 months following it. Some find wearing dark glasses helpful. With **amiodarone**, a bluish discoloration of the skin in areas exposed to sunlight may occur. It is usually reversible and fades over several months. This drug is also associated with epididymitis. Patients should report pain or swelling in the scrotum. **Procainamide** occasionally is associated with a lupus-like syndrome. Joint swelling and rashes should be reported. Frequently using mouthwashes, practicing good oral hygiene, chewing sugarless gum, or sucking on hard candy may relieve the dry mouth commonly found with **disopyramide**. The patient should notify the health-care provider if dry mouth, constipation, difficulty in urinating, or blurred vision persists with this drug. Tremors are an early indication of excessive doses of **mexiletine** and should be reported promptly.

For all of these drugs, the importance of keeping follow-up appointments to monitor efficacy and adverse reactions cannot be overstated. Failure to discover problems early can result in permanent adverse changes for some drugs, and life-threatening events as well.

Because these drugs are Pregnancy Category C or D, female patients capable of childbearing should be made aware of the risks of these drugs, and contraception should be instituted before prescribing them.

Lifestyle Management

Lifestyle management is similar to that discussed for **ACEIs**. The patient should always wear a medical identification bracelet or necklace that states the name of the drug and the disorder for which it is being taken. Patient education related to **BBs** is discussed in Chapter 14.

NITRATES

Nitrates were first introduced for the treatment of angina in the 19th century. Their ability to affect both oxygen supply and demand and their effectiveness in rapid relief of acute angina have made them one important part to the treatment of this disorder.

Pharmacodynamics

Nitroglycerin (NTG) and its analogues act largely by providing more nitric oxide (NO) to vascular endothelium and arterial smooth muscle, resulting in vasodilation (Figure 16–5). All parts of the vascular system, from larger arteries to large veins, relax in response to **nitrates**. **Nitrates** affect the supply–demand equation on both sides. Dilation of venous capacitance vessels results decreased systemic vascular resistance (afterload), venous pooling, and decreased venous return to the heart, which leads to decreased preload. Arterial dilation, which occurs more commonly with higher doses, decreases systemic arterial pressure, resulting in decreased afterload. MOD is reduced by the reduced cardiac workload.

The decreased venous return decreases LV end-diastolic pressure (preload), resulting in decreased wall tension and an increased transmyocardial gradient. This increased gradient improves perfusion between the coronary arteries and the subendocardium and increases

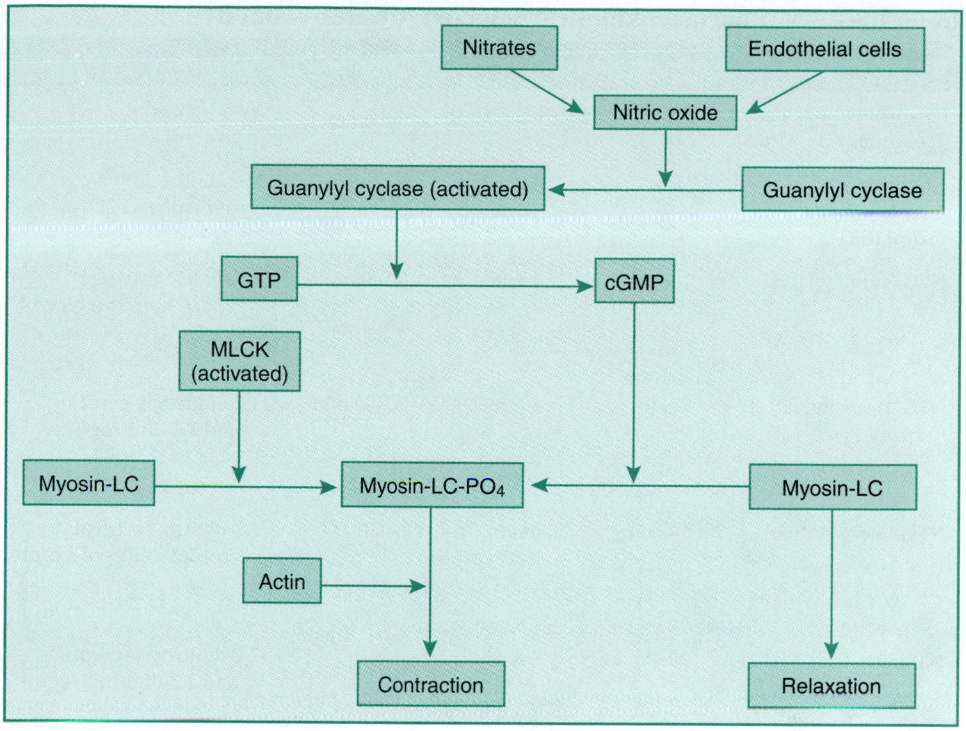

Figure 16–5. Action of substances that increase nitric oxide concentration in smooth muscle cells. Nitrates, nitrites, and other substances that increase nitric oxide concentration in smooth muscle cells potentiate the activation of guanylyl cyclase. Activated guanylyl cyclase then facilitates the production of cyclic guanosine monophosphate (cGMP). Through a series of not clearly known intermediate steps, the cGMP facilitates the dephosphorylation of the myosin light chain, resulting in muscle relaxation.

oxygen supply to the myocardium. Their coronary artery vasodilating effect—originally thought to be their primary role in improving MOD—is now thought to play a limited role because of atherosclerotic changes in the coronary arteries. They have little effect on angina associated with atherosclerotic CAD.

Indirect actions include reflex responses of baroreceptors and hormonal mechanisms to decreased arterial pressure. The primary mechanism is sympathetic discharge, resulting in tachycardia and increased myocardial contractility. Another action of clinical significance is on platelet aggregation. NO released from **NTG** increases cyclic guanosine monophosphate (cGMP), resulting in decreased platelet aggregation. This action is believed to play a role in reduction of infarct size and mortality post-MI for patients given IV **NTG** and may also exist for other forms of **NTG**.

Relaxation of smooth muscle of the bronchi, GI tract, and genitourinary tract also occurs but so briefly that this action is not considered clinically significant.

Pharmacokinetics

Absorption and Distribution

Nitrates are well absorbed by oral, buccal, sublingual, and transdermal routes (Table 16–19). Sublingual absorption is dependent on salivary secretion. Dry mouth (including drug induced) decreases absorption. **Amyl nitrite** is available in an inhaled form, providing for very rapid absorption.

Table 16–19 ▶ **Pharmacokinetics: Selected Nitrates**

Drug	Onset	Peak	Duration	Metabolite	Half-Life	Excretion
Amyl nitrate inhalant	0.5 min		3–5 min	None	UK	1/3 in urine
Isosorbide dinitrate, sublingual	2–5 min	6 min	1–3 h	Mononitrate	Drug 45 min Metabolite: 2–5 h	In urine
Isosorbide dinitrate, Oral	20–40 min	6 min	4–6 h	Isosorbide mononitrate	Drug: 45 min Metabolite: 2–5 h	In urine
Isosorbide dinitrate, oral (SR)	up to 4 h	6 min	6–8 h	Isosorbide mononitrate	Drug: 45 min Metabolite: 2–5 h	In urine

Continued

Table 16–19 ▶ **Pharmacokinetics: Selected Nitrates—cont'd**

Drug	Onset	Peak	Duration	Metabolite	Half-Life	Excretion
Isosorbide mononitrate, Oral	30–60 min	UK	7 h	Metabolized to glycerol and CO_2	UK	In urine and lung
Isosorbide mononitrate, oral (SR)	Slow	3–4 h	>12 h	Metabolized to glycerol and CO_2	UK	In urine and lung
NTG, sublingual	1–3 min	4 min	30–60 min	1,2-dinitrogly-cerol and 1,3-dinitroglycerol	Drug: 1–3 min Metabolites: approx. 40 min	In urine
NTG, translingual spray	2 min	4 min	30–69 min	1,2-dinitrogly-cerol and 1,3-dinitroglycerol	Drug: 1–3 min Metabolites: approx. 40 min	In urine
NTG buccal tablet	1–2 min	4 min	3–5 h	1,2-dinitrogly- cerol and 1,3-dinitroglycerol	Drug 1–3 min Metabolites: approx. 40 min	In urine
NTG oral (SR)	20–45 min	UK	3–8 h	1,2-dinitrogly- cerol and 1,3-dinitroglycerol	Drug: 1–3 min Metabolites: approx. 40 min	In urine
NTG topical ointment*	30–60 min	UK	2–12 h	1,2-dinitrogly- cerol and 1,3-dinitroglycerol	Drug: 1–3 min Metabolites: approx. 40 min	In urine
NTG transdermal patch	30–60 min	UK	Up to 24 h	1,2-dinitrogly-cerol and 1,3-dinitroglycerol	Drug: 1–3 min Metabolites: approx. 40 min	In urine

UK = unknown.
*Used almost exclusively in the hospital.
All have approximately 60% protein binding.
Half-life of NTG is 1–4 min; others have longer half-lives, with SR preparations up to 12 h.

Metabolism and Excretion

Oral **nitrates** have a significant hepatic first-pass effect. Hepatic organic nitrate reductase removes nitrate groups from the parent molecule, yielding less potent vasodilators than the parent drug and resulting in low bioavailability for most products. Oral **nitrates** must be given in sufficiently high doses to sustain blood levels despite the first-pass effect. **NTG** has a short half-life (1–4 min), but the two major metabolites (1,2 and 1,3 dinitrates) have longer half-lives and appear in substantial concentrations, making them responsible for some of the pharmacological activity. The dinitrates are further metabolized to mononitrates. **Isosorbide dinitrate** is metabolized to active metabolites that accumulate more than the parent drug with long-term therapy. Because **isosorbide mononitrate** is the major active metabolite of **isosorbide dinitrate** and most of the clinical activity is attributed to this metabolite, it is now available as a single-entity product with a bioavailability of nearly 100 percent.

The sublingual route avoids hepatic first-pass effect and is preferred for achieving a rapid blood level. The inhalation route has the same advantages. The buccal and transdermal routes also avoid the first-pass problems but have slower onsets of action. Total duration of effect by these routes is brief. When longer duration of action is needed, oral preparations are given.

Metabolism of **nitrates** leads to glucuronide derivatives and carbon dioxide excreted by the kidneys and the lungs. Table 16–19 depicts the pharmacokinetics of all formulations.

Pharmacotherapeutics

Precautions and Contraindications

Precautions and contraindications are largely related to the actions of these drugs. Vasodilation can result in increased intracranial pressure, so **nitrates** are contraindicated in head trauma or cerebral hemorrhage. Vasodilation can also result in postural hypotension. Patients with volume depletion and anemia should avoid using **nitrates.** *Drug Facts and Comparisons* (Wolters Kluwer Health, 2009) states that closed-angle glaucoma is also a contraindication because intraocular pressure (IOP) may be increased. Some individuals have hypersensitivity or idiosyncratic responses to **nitrates** and must avoid them. For the transdermal patches, allergy to their adhesive may limit their use.

Because the activity of these drugs may compromise maternal-to-fetal circulation, they are Pregnancy Category C. **Amyl nitrite** is Pregnancy Category X because it markedly reduces system BP and blood flow on the maternal side of the placenta.

It is not known if **nitrates** are excreted in breast milk. The importance of the drug for the mother and possible risks to the infant should be taken into consideration when deciding on nitrate use in nursing mothers.

Safety and efficacy in children have not been established.

Adverse Drug Reactions

The major adverse reactions are direct extensions of therapeutic vasodilation: orthostatic hypotension with potential for syncope, tachycardia, and throbbing headache. Hypotension may result in decreased diastolic filling pressure, and the tachycardia may result in decreased diastolic filling time, leading to myocardial ischemia, arrhythmias, and rebound HTN. Headache may be severe and persists in up to 50 percent of patients. For patients with severe, persistent headache, it may be necessary to use a different drug group to treat the disease process.

Less common adverse reactions include nausea, vomiting, incontinence of urine and feces, dysuria, impotence, and urinary frequency. Rash and cutaneous vasodilation with flushing may occur with transdermal applications and can be reduced by rotating the site of application.

Tolerance

With continuous exposure, smooth muscle develops clinically significant tolerance (tachyphylaxis). In well-controlled clinical trials, **nitrates** were no more effective than placebo after 18 to 24 hours of continuous therapy, particularly for long-acting/sustained-release preparations. The mechanisms by which this occurs are not fully understood. One mechanism proposed is that, over time, decreased substrate (sulfhydryl) results in decreased cGMP, leading to decreased vasodilation. Orally bioavailable compounds containing sulfhydryl groups, such as *N*-acetylcysteine, may diminish tolerance to the hemodynamic effects of **nitrates** in HF (Mehra et al, 1994), but additional research is needed for validation. Attempts to overcome **nitrate** tolerance by increasing dosage, even to doses far in excess of those commonly used, have failed. Only after **nitrates** have been absent from the body for 10 to 12 hours does their effectiveness return. See the section Clinical Use and Dosing for recommendations to overcome this problem.

Drug Interactions

Additive hypotension is possible with other drug classes that have actions or adverse effects of hypotension: **antihypertensives, BBs, CCBs, haloperidol (Haldol),** or **phenothiazines.** Drugs with anticholinergic effects may decrease absorption of sublingual or buccal NTG. **Aspirin** increases **nitrate** serum concentrations and may potentiate their action. **Nitrates** may decrease the pharmacological effects of **heparin.** Specific drug interactions and the appropriate actions to prevent them are given in Table 16–20.

Clinical Use and Dosing

Angina

Oxygen extracted from the coronary arteries is at maximum efficiency at all times, and there is no oxygen reserve during periods of increased oxygen demand. Ischemia occurs when demand exceeds supply. Increased oxygen supply is created by dilating the arteries to bring more blood flow to the myocardium. Unfortunately, CAD, usually associated with atherosclerosis and plaque formation, makes dilation of these arteries difficult, if not impossible. Although they have some ability to dilate the coronary arteries, **nitrates** are also able to facilitate movement of oxygen across the arterial–myocardial membrane and

Table 16–20 ■ **Drug Interactions: Nitrates**

Drug	Interacting Drug	Possible Effect	Implications
Isosorbide dinitrate	Antihypertensives, alcohol, BBs, phenothiazines	Additive hypotension	Monitor BP closely. isosorbide mononitrate Teach home BP monitoring
NTG	Antihypertensives, alcohol, BBs, CCBs, haloperidol, phenothiazines	Additive hypotension	Monitor BP closely. Teach home BP monitoring
	Agents with anticholinergic properties	May decrease absorption of SL and buccal formulations	Use other formulation if possible

their use in CAD relates as much to this action as it does to vasodilation. Ischemia caused by the imbalance between MOS and MOD produces pain (angina). There are three types of angina: chronic stable angina, unstable angina, and Prinzmetal's angina. Chronic stable angina (exertional angina) is caused by narrowing of the arterial lumen and hardening of the arterial walls, so that the affected vessels cannot dilate in response to the increased MOD associated with physical exertion or emotional stress.

For many patients with stable, predictable angina, **nitrates** are sufficient for control of symptoms. Dosage depends on formulation, with sublingual doses used to treat acute attacks and long-acting forms used for prevention (Table 16–21). Dosing for sublingual **NTG**, a short-acting form, is 0.4 to 0.6 mg every 5 minutes for up to three doses. If the angina is not relieved by the second dose, the recommendation is to take the third dose, call 911, and go to the hospital. Dosing for **isosorbide dinitrate**, a long-acting form, is 10 to 40 mg orally bid or tid; the sustained-release form is 40 to 80 mg daily. **Isosorbide mononitrate** dosing is 20 mg bid. For both long-acting forms, twice-daily dosing on an eccentric schedule, with doses separated by 7 hours, is preferred to reduce problems with tolerance. For variant (Prinzmetal's) angina, in which the mechanism may be largely related to vasospasm, long-acting **nitrates** are occasionally sufficient to control symptoms, although **CCBs** are often added to the treatment regimen. Dosing is similar. For unstable angina, the prophylactic value of long-acting **nitrates** is uncertain, but they may play a role, depending on the underlying pathology. In exertional angina, short-acting forms taken within 5 or 10 minutes of exercise may prevent the anginal episode. Dosing is usually 0.4 mg sublingually.

Patients with angina suggesting serious illness need immediate assessment in a monitored area of an emergency room. Early therapy for such patients includes **aspirin**, **nitroglycerine**, and **morphine**. Other **nitrates** may also be used. **Long-acting nitrates** appear to reduce mortality in trials that did not include thrombolysis (ICSI, 2008b). **Nitrate** therapy is appropriate for ischemic pain relief in these patients.

Optimal therapy for postinfarction angina is with **BBs** and **long-acting nitrates** (ICSI, 2008b). **Isosorbide dinitrate** is effective for this indication.

Table 16–21 ◉ **Dosage Schedule: Selected Nitrates**

Drug	Clinical Use	Starting Dose	Maintenance Dose	Maximum Dose
Isosorbide dinitrate SL, chewable	Treatment of angina	2.5–5 mg SL; 5 mg chewable	Titrate upward until angina relieved or adverse reactions limit	—
Isosorbide dinitrate, Oral	Treatment and prevention of angina; not for acute attack	5–20 mg q6h	10–40 mg bid (eccentric schedule 8 a.m. and 2 p.m.)	—
Isosorbide dinitrate oral SR	Same as oral	40 mg bid (eccentric schedule)	40–80 mg bid (eccentric schedule) or daily	—
Isosorbide mononitrate, Oral	Treatment and prevention of angina; not for acute attack	5–10 mg bid (eccentric schedule)	20 mg bid (eccentric schedule)	—
Isosorbide mononitrate, oral SR	Same as oral	30–60 mg qd	120 mg daily after several days on initial dose	240 mg/d
NTG SL	Prophylaxis	5–10 min prior to activities that might precipitate attack		3 tablets in 15 min
	Treatment of acute anginal attacks	0.4–0.6 mg tablet under tongue q 5 min times 3		3 tablets in 15 min
NTG, translingual spray	Prophylaxis	5–10 min prior to activities that might precipitate attack. Do not inhale spray	—	3 metered sprays in 15 min
	Treatment of acute anginal attacks	1–2 metered sprays onto or under tongue		3 metered sprays in 15 min

Table 16–21 ◉ **Dosage Schedule: Selected Nitrates—cont'd**

Drug	Clinical Use	Starting Dose	Maintenance Dose	Maximum Dose
NTG, oral SR	"Possibly effective" for prophylaxis or treatment of angina	2.5–2.6 mg tid or qid	Increase by 2.6/2.6 mg increments over a period of days or weeks until adverse reactions limit	2.6 mg qid
NTG, transdermal patch	Prevention of angina	0.2–0.4 mg/h on 12–14 h off 10–12 h	0.4–0.8 mg/h on 12–14 h; off 10–12 h	—

Heart Failure

Their role in reducing ventricular filling pressure and pulmonary and system vascular resistance gives **nitrates** a small place in the treatment of HF. **Isosorbide dinitrate** administered chronically has been shown to be effective in improving exercise capacity and in reducing symptoms. Its limited effect of systemic vascular resistance and the problem of tolerance mean that it is rarely single-drug therapy. Combining this drug with **hydralazine** has produced a more sustained improvement than either drug alone. With the advent of ACEIs and ARBs and the redefined role of BBs in HF, the newer guidelines no longer present a role for **nitrates** in the management of HF (see Chap. 36). No specific dosage schedule is provided for their use with HF.

Initiation of Therapy

Start low and go slow are the appropriate steps here. If the initial dose is too high, severe vascular headaches and the possibility of orthostatic hypotension may cause patients to stop taking the drug. Beginning low and advancing slowly over a period of 1 to 2 weeks usually results in the desired effects without the headaches.

Dosage increases should be made against the following parameters:

1. Reduced angina or lack of angina occurs with usual activity.
2. Heart rate at rest increases by no more than 15 bpm.
3. BP does not fall to the point of causing orthostatic hypotension.

Headache or its absence is not a reliable variable by which to judge therapy because tachyphylaxis for this adverse effect is common in a few weeks to 1 month.

Prevention of Tolerance

To prevent or reduce the development of tolerance, a **nitrate**-free interval of 10 to 12 h/d is required. Sustained-release preparations are more likely to lead to tolerance and should be avoided unless used daily. Short-acting products with bid/tid dosing are less likely to lead to tolerance. For bid dosing, use an eccentric dosing schedule separated by 7 hours (e.g., 7 a.m., 2 p.m.). Patients whose anginal symptoms occur at night may do best with a daytime **nitrate**-free interval, and the reverse holds for those whose symptoms occur during the daytime. If around-the-clock coverage is necessary for anginal symptoms, coverage with a BB or CCB during the **nitrate**-free interval may be needed.

CLINICAL PEARL

Patients with migraine headaches are especially at risk for **nitrate** headaches. Start them first on a **beta blocker** for migraine prophylaxis, and then add the **nitrate** to prevent the problem.

Class III drugs are **potassium channel blockers,** but they also have effects found in other classes. **Amiodarone, quinidine,** and **sotalol** all have potassium channel–blocking properties in addition to their effects on sodium channels or beta receptors. "Pure" **potassium channel–blocking drugs** are currently entering clinical trials. Potassium channel blockade would result in increased action potential duration, increased refractoriness, and reduced automaticity. They should be effective in treating reentry problems, in inhibiting ventricular fibrillation that is due to myocardial ischemia, and in improving contractility. An investigational D-isomer of the **class III drug sotalol** has no beta-blocking properties and thus no adverse reactions associated with beta blockade. It retains its effect on repolarization and would increase the instances in which it could be used.

Rational Drug Selection

Formulation and Cost

Sublingual NTG has rapid action, long-established efficacy, easy use, and low cost. A disadvantage is its short duration of action. It is also volatile and must be kept in a tightly capped, amber container and stored in a cool place. Once a bottle is opened, it is generally effective for only about 6 months. Onset and duration of action of a single metered dose of **translingual spray** is about the same as **sublingual NTG**. Each canister contains

200 doses and retains efficacy for up to 3 years. Some skill is required to use it. Cost per dose is substantially higher than for the sublingual form, but the prolonged shelf life helps reduce total cost. It is a good alternative for patients who wear dentures or have dry mucosa. **Oral NTG** has questionable efficacy and is available only in sustained release, a form associated with increased incidence of tolerance. **Transdermal** delivery systems offer easy use and release **NTG** at a constant rate to maintain steady-state plasma levels. They are also inexpensive, with cost at approximately $1 per day. Tolerance is an issue unless a **nitrate**-free interval is provided, and bioavailability varies significantly from patient to patient. Physical exercise and ambient temperatures may increase absorption.

Among the **oral nitrates, isosorbide dinitrate** provides sustained **nitrate** activity and better anginal prophylaxis. Single doses significantly improve hemodynamic parameters and exercise tolerance for up to 4 hours. Its action is not as rapid as **sublingual NTG** but does occur in 15 to 30 minutes, which is appropriate for prevention. Eccentric scheduling appears to balance the need for angina coverage and the avoidance of tolerance. In generic form, its cost is very low. Chewable and sublingual forms provide more rapid onset of action, but the duration of action falls to about 2 hours. Because there appears to be no clear benefit over **sublingual NTG**, the higher cost of these latter two forms does not seem to justify their use. **Isosorbide dinitrate** is also available in a sustained-release form that requires only bid or daily dosing, but it has highly variable intestinal absorption, and the risk of **nitrate** tolerance is higher unless it is used once daily.

Isosorbide mononitrate offers 100 percent bioavailability and the convenience of once-daily dosing but otherwise appears to have no significant clinical advantage over **isosorbide dinitrate. Nitrate** tolerance occurs less often for the regular formulation. The sustained-release form has the same problems with tolerance as other sustained-release formulations. Cost is significantly higher. Cost data for all **nitrates** is provided in Table 16–22.

Table 16–22 ◆ **Available Dosage Forms: Nitrates**

Drug	Dosage Form	How Supplied	Cost
Isosorbide dinitrate (Isordil, Sorbitrate)	Tablets: (sublingual) 2.5 mg (G)	In bottles of 100, 500, 1,000, and UD100	No data available on sublingual or chewable forms
	5 mg (G), 10 mg (G)	In bottles of 100, 1,000, and UD 100	
	2.5 mg (I), 5 mg (I)	In bottles of 100, 500, and Redipak 100	
	10 mg (I)	In bottles of 100	
	2.5 mg (S), 5 mg (S)	In bottles of 100	
	Tablets (chewable): 5 mg (S), 10 mg (S)	In bottles of 100 and 500	
	Tablets: (oral) 5 mg (G)	In bottles of 100, 1,000, and UD 100	
	10 mg (G)	In bottles of 100, 500, 1,000, and UD 100	$23
	20 mg (G)	In bottles of 90, 100, 120, 180, 240, 360, 500, 1,000, and UD 100	$32
	30 mg (G)	In bottles of 100, 500, 1,000, and UD 100	$23
	5 mg (I), 10 mg (I)	In bottles of 100, 500, 1,000, and Redipak 100	5 mg = $31; 10 mg = $37
	20 mg (I), 30 mg (I)	In bottles of 100, 500, and Redipak 100	20 mg = $60; 30 mg = $66
	40 mg (I)	In bottles of 100 and UD 100	$66
	5 mg (S), 10 mg (S)	In bottles of 100, 500, and UD 100	No data on Sorbitrate brand
	20 mg (S), 30 mg (S), 40 mg (S)	In bottles of 100 and UD 100	
	Tablets (sustained release): 40 mg (G)	In bottles of 90, 100, 250, 1,000, and UD 100	
	40 mg (I)	In bottles of 10, 500, and 1,000	
	Capsules (sustained release): 40 mg (I)	In bottles of 60 and 100	
	40 mg (Dilatrate-SR)	In bottles of 100 and 500	$68

Table 16–22 ◆ **Available Dosage Forms: Nitrates—cont'd**

Drug	Dosage Form	How Supplied	Cost
Isosorbide mononitrate (IMSO, Monoket, Imdur)	Tablets: 20 mg (G)	In bottles of 100 and 500	$34
	10 mg (Mo), 20 mg (Mo)	In bottles of 60, 100, 180, and UD 100	10 mg = $93; 20 mg = $135
	20 mg (M)	In bottles of 100 and UD 100	$170
	Tablets (extended release). 60 mg (G)	In bottles of 100	$33
	30 mg (Im), 60 mg (Im), 120 mg (Im)	In bottles of 30, 100, and UD 100	30 mg = $176; 60 mg = $184; 120 mg = $258
	60 mg (Isotrate ER)	In bottles of 100 and 500	
NTG (buccal) (Nitrogard)	Tablet, buccal, controlled release: 2 mg	In bottles of 100 and UD 100	No data on buccal tablets
	3 mg	In bottles of 100 and UD 100	
NTG (sublingual) (NitroQuick, Nitrostat)	Tablets: 0.3 mg (NQ), 0.4 mg (NQ)	In bottles of 100	0.4 mg = $14
	0.6 mg (NQ)	In bottles of 100	0.4 mg = $13
	0.3 mg (NS), 0.4 mg (NS), 0.6 mg (NS)	In bottles of 100	
NTG (Translingual)	Aerosol spray, translingual: 0.4 mg/metered dose	In 14.48 g (200 metered doses)	No data
NTG (Transdermal)	Patch: 0.2/16–62.5 (G), 0.4/32–125 (G)	In 30 patches	0.2 = $25; 0.4 = $23
	0.6/75–187.5 (G)	In 30 patches	0.6 = $34
	0.1/9 (M), 0.2/18 (M), 0.4/36 (M)	In 30 patches	0.2 = $67; 0.4 = $75
	0.6/54 (M)	In 30 patches	0.6 = $82
	0.1/20 (N), 0.2/40 (N), 0.3/60 (N)	In 30 and 100 patches and UD 30 and 100	0.2 = $67
	0.4/80 (N), 0.6/120 (N), 0.8/160 (N)	In 30 and 100 patches and UD 30 and 100	0.4 = $75; 0.6 = $83
	0.1/12.5 (T), 0.2/25 (T), 0.4/50 (T)	In 30 and 100 patches and UD 100	
	0.6/75 (T), 0.8/100 (T)	In 30 and UD 30	

(I) = Isordil brand; (S) = Sorbitrate brand. (M) = IMSO; (Mo) = Monoket; (Im) = Imdur. Patches: (M) = Minitran; (N) = NitroDur; (T) = Transderm-Nitro. Patch: First number is release rate in mg/h; second number is total NTG content in mg. If two total NTG content numbers are given, it is based on variable surface areas and NTG content in different patches by the same manufacturer.
Cost data are for 100 units except for patches, which are for 30 patches.

Monitoring

No specific monitoring parameters exist for **nitrates**.

Patient Education

Administration

Take the drug exactly as prescribed. For oral doses taken more than once daily, a **nitrate**-free interval of 10 to 12 hours is necessary to prevent **nitrate** intolerance. For bid dosing, an eccentric dosing schedule separated by 7 hours (e.g., 7 a.m., 2 p.m.) is best. If anginal symptoms occur at night, it may be best to have a daytime **nitrate**-free interval, with the reverse for symptoms occurring during the daytime. If round-the-clock coverage is necessary for anginal symptoms, coverage with a BB or CCB during the **nitrate**-free interval may be needed.

Several drugs come in more than one formulation, from standard to sustained release (see Table 16–22). The patient should read the label carefully and follow the appropriate dosing schedule. This is especially important if the drug is changed to a different form or a different drug. For sustained-release formulations, the tablets should not be crushed or chewed but must be swallowed whole. **Sublingual NTG** tablets may lose potency when stored. Store in tightly closed, amber glass containers. Tablets lose potency when exposed to air, heat, or moisture or when mixed with other tablets. Do not open the bottle frequently or keep bottles of tablets next to the body (e.g., in a shirt pocket) or in an automobile glove compartment. A burning sensation under the tongue is not a reliable method of testing potency. Adhere to the expiration date on the bottle, usually 6 months, and write the date the bottle was first opened on the bottle. If ordered for treatment of acute anginal attacks, **sublingual NTG** is the drug of choice. At the first sign of an attack, the patient should sit down and place one sublingual tablet under the tongue and allow it to dissolve. It should not be swallowed. If the pain is not relieved, repeat every 5 minutes for up to three doses. If the angina is not relieved by the second dose, the patient should take the third dose, call 911, and go directly to the hospital. Dry mouth may reduce the effectiveness of **sublingual NTG**. Dry-mouth problems should be discussed with the health-care provider. **Sublingual spray**, which is useful even with dry mouth, may be used in the same manner as the tablet. Lift the tongue and spray the dose under the tongue. **Transdermal patches** also require a **nitrate**-free interval of 10 to 12 hours. Follow the same instructions as for oral tablets related to this interval. The site of application should be changed each time, with the best sites being the anterior chest and the upper arms in areas not covered with hair. Remove the clear plastic cover over the medication side of the patch before applying. Apply firm pressure over the patch to ensure contact with the skin. Physical exercise and ambient temperatures may increase absorption by this route, resulting in more adverse effects.

For all forms, do not double doses and do not discontinue abruptly, which may result in rebound angina. Avoid concurrent use of **alcohol** with these drugs. Because some OTC drugs interact with **nitrates** or contain **alcohol**, do not take any new OTC drugs, including cold remedies, without first discussing this with the health-care provider.

Adverse Reactions

The major adverse reactions are throbbing headaches, rapid heart rates, and decreased BP when arising from a sitting or lying position, with the potential for fainting. Headache may be severe; although it should decrease with continued therapy, it persists in up to 50 percent of patients. It is less likely with lower doses and slow increases in doses. It is best treated with **acetaminophen (Tylenol)**. Report headaches to the health-care provider, who may alter the dose or change the drug. Rapid heart rates should also be reported right away. They may worsen the condition for which the **nitrate** is prescribed. Making position changes slowly minimizes the BP changes. When arising from lying down, the patient should sit on the edge of the bed for a few minutes before standing to allow the body to adjust to this different position.

The rashes, skin irritation, and flushing/blushing of the skin that may occur with **transdermal patches** can be reduced by rotating the site of application.

Incontinence of urine and bowel movements, pain on urination, frequent urination, and impotence are rare adverse responses. They should be reported so that a potential cause other than the **nitrate** can be ruled out or alterations in the drug regimen can be undertaken.

Because these drugs are Pregnancy Category C, female patients capable of childbearing should be made aware of the risks of these drugs, and contraception should be instituted before they are prescribed. **Amyl nitrite** is Pregnancy Category X and should not be prescribed in these circumstances.

Lifestyle Management

See the section **Angiotensin-Converting Enzyme Inhibitors and Angiotensin II Receptor Blockers**.

PERIPHERAL VASODILATORS

Peripheral vasodilators are used to treat HTN and PVD, although significant clinical improvement of PVD rarely occurs with these drugs alone. **Peripheral alpha$_1$ antagonists** and **central alpha$_2$ agonists** can be used for these purposes. They are discussed in Chapter 14. The focus of the discussion here is on two drugs, **hydralazine (Apresoline)** and **minoxidil (Loniten)**, and their use in treating HTN.

Pharmacodynamics

Peripheral vasodilators useful in the treatment of HTN act by direct relaxation and dilation of arteriolar smooth muscle, thereby decreasing PVR. They do not dilate the capacitance vessels (epicardial coronary arteries) and do not relax venous smooth muscle.

Pharmacokinetics

Absorption and Distribution

Hydralazine is well absorbed orally. Taking it with food increases absorption. It is widely distributed and crosses the placenta but enters breast milk in minimal amounts. It is compatible with breastfeeding, according to the American Academy of Pediatrics. **Minoxidil** is also well absorbed orally and widely distributed. It enters breast milk in larger amounts and should not be used while breastfeeding (Table 16–23).

Metabolism and Excretion

With **hydralazine**, bioavailability is low and variable among patients, based on their genetics. Rapid acetylators have greater hepatic first-pass metabolism, lower bioavailability, and less antihypertensive benefit than do slow acetylators. Although **hydralazine's** half-life is short, vascular effects persist longer than blood concentrations would suggest, based on the avid binding of this drug to vascular tissue. **Minoxidil** is not protein bound and has a higher bioavailability. Its half-life is also short, but it also has a longer antihypertensive effect because of the persistence of its active metabolite, minoxidil sulfate.

Pharmacotherapeutics

Precautions and Contraindications

Use cautiously in patients with cardiovascular disease. Myocardial ischemia may result from the increased oxygen demand associated with SNS stimulation. Because these drugs do not dilate the epicardial coronary arteries, the peripheral arterial vasodilation may "steal" blood flow

Table 16–23 ▶ **Pharmacokinetics: Selected Peripheral Vasodilators**

Drug	Onset	Peak	Duration	Protein Binding	Bioavailability	Half-Life	Elimination
Hydralazine PO	45 min	1–2 h	6–12 h	87%	30%–50%	3–7 h	12%–14% in urine
Minoxidil	30 min	2–3 h	24+ h	None	UK	4.2 h	20% in urine

UK = unknown.

from any ischemic region of the heart. If used alone, sodium and water retention may precipitate high-output CHF. Both problems are more likely to occur in older adults.

Cautious use is also recommended for patients with pulmonary HTN related to the potential for severe hypotension.

Both drugs are Pregnancy Category C and should be used only when benefits clearly outweigh risks. **Hydralazine** is excreted in breast milk but is compatible with breastfeeding, according to the American Academy of Pediatrics (Wolters Kluwer Health, 2009). **Minoxidil** is also excreted in breast milk, and nursing mothers should not use it. Safety and efficacy of both drugs have not been established by clinical trials with children, but children's doses are listed in the drug literature.

Adverse Drug Reactions

Decreased peripheral resistance secondary to peripheral vasodilation triggers compensatory responses in the SNS and in the RAA system. These responses prevent the orthostatic hypotension and sexual dysfunction caused by many other antihypertensives, but they precipitate added tachycardia, increased cardiac contractility and output, sodium and water retention, headache, and tachyphylaxis to the antihypertensive effects. **Hydralazine** sometimes induces a lupus-like syndrome. It appears to be dose related in that it occurs almost exclusively with doses above 50 mg/d. The incidence is highest in white women. A positive antinuclear antibody (ANA) test is found in these patients, but no renal impairment is seen. Discontinuing the drug reverses the syndrome, but the ANA does not return to normal until 6 to 8 months after the drug is stopped. **Minoxidil** has been associated with elongation, thickening, and enhanced pigmentation of fine body hair. This effect has resulted in its use in treating male pattern baldness.

Drug Interactions

Additive effects may occur with other **antihypertensives**. **NSAIDs** may decrease their antihypertensive effects. Interactions with **BBs** and **loop diuretics** are positive in that they prevent the adverse effects common to these drugs. Specific drug interactions and the appropriate actions to prevent them are given in Table 16–24.

Clinical Use and Dosing

Hypertension

The usual oral dose of **hydralazine** is 25 to 100 mg qid, which provides smooth control of BP regardless of acetylator type. The maximum dose recommended is 200 mg/d

Table 16–24 ■ **Drug Interactions: Peripheral Vasodilators**

Drug	Interacting Drug	Possible Effect	Implications
Hydralazine	Antihypertensives, alcohol, nitrates*	Additive hypotension	Avoid concurrent use or monitor BP closely
	MAOIs	Severe hypotension	Avoid concurrent use
	NSAIDs	Reduced antihypertensive effects	Choose different analgesic or anti-inflammatory
	Beta blockers	Increased blood levels of hydralazine	Used concurrently to treat adverse reactions. May require reduction of hydralazine dose.
Minoxidil	Antihypertensives, alcohol, nitrates, guanethidine	Additive hypotension	Avoid concurrent use or monitor BP closely
	NSAIDs	Reduced antihypertensive effects	Choose different analgesic or anti-inflammatory

*Hydralazine may be prescribed with isosorbide dinitrate to treat CHF.

to minimize the risk of the lupus-like syndrome. **Minoxidil** is usually started at 5 mg daily and increased at 3-day intervals to 10 mg/d, then 20 mg/d, and then 40 mg/d, each in two divided doses. Effective control of BP may occur at any of these doses. Adult's and children's doses are provided in Table 16–25.

The SNS stimulation and sodium and water retention problems associated with both of these drugs require the concurrent administration of a BB and a **loop diuretic**. BBs prevent the tachycardia, increased cardiac output, and increased renin release; **diuretics** prevent the salt and water retention caused by decreased renal sodium excretion.

Heart Failure

Hydralazine with concurrent administration of **isosorbide dinitrate** has been used to treat CHF. This combination has been demonstrated to reduce mortality in CHF, but is not a primary recommendation from current guidelines. The dosage is up to 800 mg tid to reduce afterload. This is not usually a long-term management solution unless the effects of an ACEI are desired in a patient with renal dysfunction. **ACEIs, ARBs, BBs, CGs (digoxin),** and **diuretics** are the drugs generally used to treat HF.

Rational Drug Selection

These drugs are third-line therapy for moderate to severe HTN.

Monitoring

These drugs have no specific monitoring requirements beyond those used for patients with HTN. HTN is discussed in Chapter 40 and HF in Chapter 36.

Patient Education

Administration

Patients should take the drug exactly as prescribed at the same time each day, even if they are feeling well. A missed dose should be taken as soon as it is remembered; doses should not be doubled. If more than two doses in a row are missed, the patient should consult the health-care provider. These drugs control but do not cure HTN. The patient should not stop or alter the dose without first contacting the health-care provider.

Hydralazine should be taken with meals to enhance absorption. **Minoxidil** may be taken without regard to meals or food.

Drug interactions occur with **NSAIDs** and some OTC drugs, especially cough, cold, and allergy remedies. The patient should not take any other drugs without first consulting the health-care provider.

Adverse Reactions

Hypotensive reactions are the most common. Changing position slowly and avoiding exercise in hot weather can decrease these reactions. The patient should learn home BP and pulse monitoring and report decreases in BP by more than 20 mm Hg or increases in pulse of more than 20 bpm above baseline. Dyspnea, pronounced dizziness, or nausea should be reported. Because fluid retention may occur, patients should weigh themselves daily and report weight gain of more than 5 lb in 1 week or more than 1 lb in 1 day, as well as swelling of hands, feet, or ankles or decreased urine output.

Because these drugs are Pregnancy Category C, female patients capable of childbearing should be made aware

Table 16–25 ◉ **Dosage Schedule and Available Dosage Forms: Peripheral Vasodilators**

Drug	Starting Dose	Maintenance Dose	Maximum Dose	Available Dosage Form
Hydralazine (Apresoline)	10 mg qid, After 2–4 d; may increase to 25 mg qid for the rest of the first week, then increase to 50 mg qid	25–100 mg qid. Once maintenance dose is achieved, may go to bid dosing	400 mg/d; To minimize risk of lupus-like syndrome, keep maximum dose <200 mg/d	Tablets: 10 mg, 25 mg, 50 mg, 100 mg
	Children: 0.75 mg/kg/d in four divided doses	Increase over next 3–4 wk to BP control. (see adult dose for protocol)	7.5 mg/kg or 200 mg/d	
Minoxidil (Loniten)	5 mg/d increased at 3-d intervals to 10 mg/d then 20 mg/d then 40 mg/d; each in two divided doses	5–40 mg/d in two divided doses	100 mg/d	Tablets: 2.5 mg, 10 mg
	Children <12 yr: 0.2 mg/kg/d in single dose	Increase dose in 50%–100% increments in 3-d intervals until BP control. Usual dose: 0.25–1 mg/kg/d	50 mg daily	

of the risks of these drugs, and contraception should be instituted before they are prescribed.

Lifestyle Management

Adherence with other interventions for HTN, such as weight reduction, low-sodium diet, smoking cessation, moderation of alcohol intake, regular exercise, and stress management, is as important as the drugs.

ANTILIPIDEMICS

Atherosclerosis is the major cause of CAD. It is characterized by deposits of cholesterol and other lipoproteins on the walls of arteries. Four major classes of lipoproteins are found in the serum of fasting individuals: low-density lipoproteins (LDLs), high-density lipoproteins (HDLs), very-low-density lipoproteins (VLDLs), and triglycerides. The risk for CAD is associated with serum cholesterol levels greater than 200 mg/dL, fasting triglyceride levels greater than 150 mg/dL, LDL levels greater than 100 mg/dL, and HDL levels less than 45 for men and 55 for women. Lifestyle and pharmacological therapies are directed toward bringing elevated levels of these lipoproteins down to specific levels associated with reduced cardiovascular disease risk. Raising HDL levels is also important but not yet a major part of the treatment protocol. Drugs differentially affect LDLs, HDLs, VLDLs, and triglyceride levels. The choice of drug is based on how that drug affects each of these.

This section focuses on the drugs used to lower plasma lipoprotein levels. The pathophysiology of atherosclerosis, the relationship of hyperlipidemia to atherosclerosis development, and the management of hyperlipidemia based on the National Cholesterol Education Program guidelines are discussed in Chapter 39.

Pharmacodynamics

Two pathways are involved in the metabolism of lipoproteins. The *exogenous pathway* is central to the lifestyle modifications that are the core of hyperlipidemia therapy. Drugs that affect absorption of fat and cholesterol in the intestine (**bile acid sequestrants**) and drugs that increase lipolysis of triglycerides via lipoprotein lipase (**fibric acid derivatives**) also have some of their mechanism of action through this pathway. VLDLs are synthesized and secreted by the liver into the circulation in the endogenous pathway. They are triglyceride rich, with some cholesterol present. VLDL interacts with lipoprotein lipase in the capillary endothelium to hydrolyze triglycerides into free fatty acids and glycerol, which are then absorbed by fat and muscle cells. About 50 percent of the VLDL remnants stay in the circulation and become intermediate-density lipoproteins (IDLs). IDLs are then enriched with cholesterol by hepatic triglyceride lipase to become LDLs, which carry about 75 percent of the circulating cholesterol.

LDL receptors in the liver are down-regulated by the presence of LDL; therefore, one mechanism for lowering LDL is drug therapy that increases the number of LDL receptors in the liver (**bile acid–binding resins, 3-hydroxy-3-methylglutaryl coenzyme A [HMG-CoA] reductase inhibitors**). Drugs that inhibit VLDL synthesis in the liver (**niacin, fibric acid derivatives**) also reduce LDL via the endogenous pathway.

Elevated lipoproteins, especially LDLs, have been associated with serious and potentially lethal cardiovascular disorders associated with atherosclerosis. HDLs, by contrast, exert antiatherogenic effects. Lowering LDL levels and raising HDL levels through diet, exercise, and drugs have been shown to decrease the progression of atherosclerosis. Drugs differentially affect LDL, HDL, and triglyceride levels. Their clinical application is based on how they affect each of these.

There are four general classes of lipid-lowering drugs: **niacin, fibric acid derivatives, bile acid sequestrants,** and competitive **inhibitors of HMG-CoA reductase** (Figure 16–6). Each is discussed separately.

Niacin decreases VLDL and LDL levels. The primary mechanism of action is probably inhibition of VLDL secretion, which, in turn, decreases production of LDL levels by 10 to 15 percent. Clearance of VLDL via the lipoprotein lipase pathway also results in lowering of triglyceride levels by 20 to 80 percent. HDL catabolism is concurrently decreased, resulting in elevations of HDL levels by 20 to 30 mg/dL. The drug has no effect on bile acid production. Reduction in circulating fibrinogen levels and increases

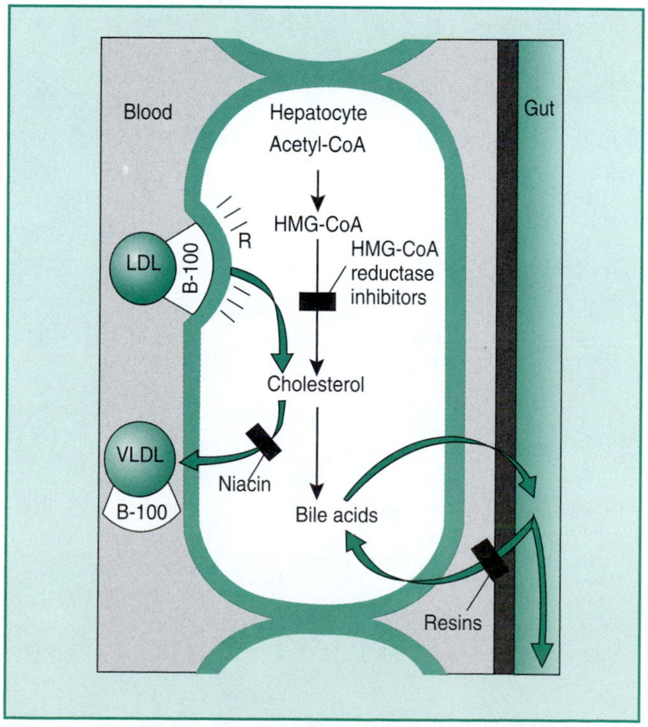

Figure 16–6. Sites of action of antihyperlipidemics.

in tissue plasminogen levels also decrease the risk for thrombogenesis.

Fibric acid derivatives (gemfibrozil [Lopid] and fenofibrate [Tricor]) increase lipolysis of triglycerides via lipoprotein lipase, resulting in a decrease of 50 percent or more in triglyceride levels. A decrease in VLDL is also related to decreased secretion by the liver. Only modest reductions in LDL levels (15%–20%) occur in most patients. Patients with combined hyperlipidemia may actually increase their LDL levels. HDL levels increase by 15 to 25 percent as a direct consequence of decreasing triglycerides.

Bile acid sequestrants (colestipol [Colestid] and cholestyramine [Questran]) exchange chloride ions for negatively charged bile acids, promoting a 10-fold increase in bile acid excretion. The increased clearance results in enhanced conversion of cholesterol to bile acids by the liver. Increased uptake of LDL from plasma results from up-regulation of high-affinity LDL receptors on cell membranes, especially in the liver. The net result is decreased LDL levels by 10 to 35 percent. HDL levels increase about 5 percent. Triglycerides may also rise initially, but they return to baseline within a few weeks.

Reductase inhibitors (atorvastatin [Lipitor], fluvastatin [Lescol], lovastatin [Mevacor], pravastatin [Pravachol], rosuvastatin [Crestor], and simvastatin [Zocor]) block synthesis of cholesterol in the liver by competitively inhibiting HMG-CoA reductase activity. They induce an increase in high-affinity LDL receptors, resulting in an increased catabolism of LDL and an increase in the liver's extraction of LDL precursors. The net result is decreased LDL levels by 25 to 63 percent. Modest decreases in triglycerides of 12 to 43 percent and increases in HDL of 8 to 17 percent also occur.

Pharmacokinetics

Absorption and Distribution

Absorption and distribution vary greatly among **antilipidemics** (Table 16–26). **Atorvastatin, niacin, fenofibrate, fluvastatin, gemfibrozil,** and **simvastatin** are all well absorbed. **Lovastatin, pravastatin,** and **rosuvastatin** are poorly absorbed. Food decreases the rate of absorption of most **reductase inhibitors.** Food intake increases the rate of absorption of **lovastatin** and **fenofibrate.** It does not affect absorption of the other **antilipidemics.**

Most are widely distributed and enter breast milk in variable amounts. **Cholestyramine** and **colestipol** are not absorbed at all and have no distribution. Their action is entirely related to binding bile acids in the gut.

Table 16–26 ▶ **Pharmacokinetics: Selected Antilipidemics**

Drug	Onset	Peak	Duration	Protein Binding	Bioavailability	Half-Life	Elimination
Atorvastatin	Rapid	1–2 h	20–30 h	>98%	14%. First pass (CYP3A4)	14 h	<2% in urine
Cholestyramine	24–48 h	1–3 wk	2–4 wk	NA	0%	UK	Insoluble complex in feces
Colestipol	24–48 h	1 mo	1 mo	NA	0%	UK	Insoluble complex in feces
Fluvastatin	1–2 wk*	4–6 wk*	UK	>98%	24% (IR); 29% (XR). Saturable first pass (CYP2C9)	<1 h	5% in urine, 90% in feces
Gemfibrozil	2–5 d*	4 wk*	Months	95%	UK	1.5 h	70% in urine, 6% in feces
Lovastatin	2 wk*	4–6 wk	6 wk	>95%	<5% (IR); 190% (XR). Extensive first pass (CYP3A4)	3–4 h	10% in urine, 83% in feces
Niacin		45 min	UK	UK	UK	45 min	88% unchanged in urine
Pravastatin	1–2 wk*	4–6 wk*	UK	50%	17%. Extensive first pass	1.8 h	20% in urine, 70% in feces
Rosuvastatin	UK	2–4 wk	UK	88%	20%. 10% metabolized by CYP2C9	19 h	90% in feces
Simvastatin	1–2 wk*	4–6 wk*	UK	95%	<5%. Extensive first pass (CYP3A4)	3 h	13% in urine, 60% in feces

NA = not applicable; UK = unknown.
*Effect on plasma lipids.

Metabolism and Excretion

Niacin, fenofibrate, and **gemfibrozil** have some metabolism by the liver but are excreted mostly unchanged in the urine. These drugs are affected by impaired renal function. The **reductase inhibitors** are extensively metabolized by the liver, often employing CYP 2C6 and 3A4 enzyme systems, and usually on first pass. This explains their universally low bioavailabilities, for they immediately release formulations from less than 5 percent for **simvastatin** to 24 percent for **fluvastatin.** The extended-release formulation of **lovastatin,** however, has a bioavailability of 190 percent. Because **reductase inhibitors** are largely excreted in bile and feces, with only small amounts excreted unchanged in the urine, plasma levels are not significantly affected by renal function but may increase markedly with hepatic failure and chronic alcoholic cirrhosis. Plasma half-lives are generally short (45 min to 3 h), with the exception of **atorvastatin,** whose half-life is 14 hours.

Bile-acid sequestrants bind with cholesterol in the intestine and are not metabolized by the liver. They are excreted in bound form in the feces.

Pharmacotherapeutics

Precautions and Contraindications

Active liver disease is a contraindication for all **antilipidemics** except the **bile acid sequestrants.** Marked persistent increases in serum transaminases and drug-induced hepatitis have occurred with **reductase inhibitors,** and they should be used with caution in any patient who consumes substantial quantities of alcohol or who has a history of liver disease. Cautious use of the **bile acid sequestrants** is suggested for patients with a history of constipation, and phenylketonuria (PKU) is a contraindication for **cholestyramine.** Severe renal impairment warrants cautious use of those drugs excreted largely unchanged in the urine (**niacin, fenofibrate,** and **gemfibrozil**). Some **niacin** products contain tartrazine (FDC yellow dye #5) and should be avoided for patients with an **aspirin** allergy. Because of its tendency to GI irritation, **niacin** should also be used cautiously for patients with a history of peptic ulcer disease.

Niacin, fenofibrate, and **gemfibrozil** are Pregnancy Category C. Risks and benefits should be weighed. All the **reductase inhibitors** are Pregnancy Category X and should not be given to women who have the potential to become pregnant. No Pregnancy Category has been assigned to the **bile acid sequestrants** because they are not absorbed systemically. All **antilipidemics** should be avoided during breastfeeding. Dosages of some **reductase inhibitors** (**atorvastatin, lovastatin, pravastatin,** and **simvastatin**) have been approved for children with heterozygous or homozygous familial hypercholesterolemias with some residual receptor activity. The safety of other **antilipidemics** has not been established for children under age 18.

Adverse Drug Reactions

Cutaneous flushing, especially of the face and upper body, has been associated with **niacin.** Gradually increasing initial low doses helps to reduce this adverse reaction. **Niaspan,** an extended-release form of **niacin,** can be administered at bedtime, with the smaller amount of cutaneous flushing occurring while the patient is sleeping to make the drug more easily tolerated.

Fenofibrate and **gemfibrozil** have a few GI symptoms, including dyspepsia, abdominal pain, and diarrhea. They may also produce cholelithiasis secondary to their increased cholesterol excretion into the bile. They are discontinued if gallstones are found. Both of these drugs have also been associated with mild to moderate decreases in hemoglobin, hematocrit, and WBCs. These levels tend to stabilize, however, with long-term management.

The **bile acid sequestrants'** major problems are GI effects, including constipation that may be severe and result in impaction. Constipation is more common in older adults. A laxative or stool softener may be helpful. Other GI symptoms include flatulence, nausea, vomiting, and abdominal pain. Headache is also common. Reduced folate levels have been reported with long-term use. Supplementation with folic acid is suggested. A fairly rare symptom is a burnt odor to the urine.

The **reductase inhibitors** all have headache as a common adverse reaction. **Atorvastatin** and **simvastatin** have the lowest adverse reaction profiles, with myalgia for the former and abdominal pain for the latter as the only adverse reactions besides headaches. **Fluvastatin, lovastatin,** and **pravastatin** all have GI-associated adverse reactions (dyspepsia, abdominal pain, flatulence, constipation, or diarrhea). Generally, these reactions are mild and transient.

Rhabdomyolysis with renal dysfunction secondary to myoglobinuria has occurred with **reductase inhibitors** and **fibric acid derivatives.** Although it occurs in only 0.1 to 0.5 percent of patients, when it does occur, it is serious. Myopathy should be considered in any patient with diffuse myalgias, muscle tenderness and weakness, and elevations in creatine kinase (CK) values more than 10 times the upper limit of normal. Consider temporarily withholding or discontinuing drug therapy in patients with a risk factor predisposing them to the development of renal failure secondary to rhabdomyolysis, including hypotension; major surgery or trauma; severe metabolic, endocrine, or electrolyte disorder; or uncontrolled seizures.

Drug Interactions

All **antilipidemics** except **niacin** affect **warfarin** activity: **Bile acid sequestrants** decrease its effect, and the other classes increase its effect. **Gemfibrozil** and **fenofibrate** have interactions with several other **antilipidemics.** All **reductase inhibitors—atorvastatin** most of all—increase **digoxin** levels. Systemic **imidazole** and **triazole** therapies increase **reductase inhibitor** levels by 20-fold. **Propranolol** decreases the antilipidemic activity of **reductase inhibitors**. **Niacin**, **erythromycin**, and **cyclosporine** all increase the risk of rhabdomyolysis when given with **reductase inhibitors**. Combining **reductase inhibitors** and **fibric acid derivatives** also increases the risk for rhabdomyolysis. Taking **lovastatin** with food enhances its blood levels. Specific drug interactions and the appropriate actions to prevent them are given in Table 16–27.

Table 16–27 ■ **Drug Interactions: Selected Antilipidemics**

Drug	Interacting Drug	Possible Effect	Implications
All reductase inhibitors	Digoxin	Slight elevation in digoxin levels. Concurrent administration with atorvastatin may increase steady-state levels by 20%	If unable to choose alternative drug, monitor for digoxin toxicity. Avoid concurrent use of atorvastatin
	Warfarin	Increased anticoagulant effect	Monitor PT/INR closely
	Itraconazole and other azole antifungals	Coadministration increases reductase inhibitor levels 20-fold	Temporarily interrupt reductase inhibitor if systemic azole antifungals needed
	Propranolol	Decreases antilipidemic activity	Choose alternative beta blocker
	Erythromycin, HIV protease inhibitors, nefazodone	Potent inhibitors of CYP3A4; may increase risk of myopathy	If must coadminister, monitor closely for myopathy
Atorvastatin	Maalox TC	Coadministration decreases atorvastatin level by 35%; LDL reduction is not altered	Separate doses by at least 1 h
	Norethindrone, ethinyl estradiol	Increases contraceptive levels by 30% and 20%, respectively	Choose alternative contraceptive or antilipidemic
	Colestipol	Coadministration decreases atorvastatin levels by 25%; LDL reduction > than either alone	May be therapeutic choice
	Erythromycin	Atorvastatin levels increased by 40%; increased myopathy risk	Choose alternative antibiotic
	Cyclosporine, gemfibrozil, niacin	Increased myopathy and rhabdomyolysis risk	Avoid concurrent use
Cholestyramine	Mycophenolate	Decreases area under curve (AUC) by 40%	Monitor for indications of rejection
	Piroxicam	Elimination enhanced	Choose alternative NSAID
	Thyroid hormones	Possible loss of efficacy with potential hypothyroidism	Choose alternative antilipidemic
	Vitamins A, D, E, K, and folic acid	May interfere with vitamin absorption, with resultant bleeding tendencies	With long-term therapy vitamins A and D may be given in water-miscible form; vitamin K can be supplemented parenterally or orally
	Warfarin	Decreased anticoagulant effect	Choose alternative antilipidemic, or monitor PT/INR more closely

Table 16–27 ■ **Drug Interactions: Selected Antilipidemics—cont'd**

Drug	Interacting Drug	Possible Effect	Implications
Fluvastatin	Alcohol	Daily intake of 20 g more than 2 h after evening meal or within 1 h of fluvastatin dose increases AUC by 30%	Avoid daily alcohol intake
	Niacin, propranolol, digoxin	Decreases fluvastatin bioavailability	Avoid concurrent administration
	Rifampin	May cause decrease in fluvastatin AUC and plasma clearance	Choose alternative antilipidemic
Gemfibrozil	Warfarin	Enhances anticoagulant effect	Choose alternative antilipidemic or monitor PT/INR closely
	Colestipol	Bioavailability of gemfibrozil reduced	Avoid concurrent use
	Lovastatin	Severe myopathy or rhabdomyolysis	Avoid concurrent use
	Pravastatin	Urinary excretion and protein binding reduced	Avoid concurrent use
Lovastatin	Isradipine	Increased lovastatin clearance with reduced effect	Choose alternative CCB
	Food	Taking on empty stomach decreases absorption by 30%	Take consistently with food
	Grapefruit	Large quantities may increase risk of myopathy	
Pravastatin	Cholestyramine, colestipol	Decreases pravastatin levels by 40%–50%	Take prevestatin 1 h before or 4 h after bile acid–binding resins
	Cyclosporine	Coadministration increases pravastatin level 7-fold	Separate doses as above

Clinical Use and Dosing

Increased Low-Density Lipoproteins

Niacin, **bile acid sequestrants**, and **reductase inhibitors** all reduce LDL.

Reductase inhibitors are first-line drugs in monotherapy and in combinations. Because of the diurnal pattern of cholesterol synthesis, **reductase inhibitors** are given in the evening in a single daily dose. **Rosuvastatin** is the newest drug in this class and the most potent with an adverse reactions profile similar to that of **atorvastatin.** The usual starting dose is 5 to 20 mg/d with a maximum of 40 mg/d. **Atorvastatin** is the next most potent and has the best adverse reaction profile. The usual dose is 10 mg/d initially increased at 2- to 4-week intervals up to 80 mg/d. Heterozygous familial hyperlipidemia (FH) in children 10 to 17 years of age has the same starting dose, but the maximum dose recommended is 20 mg/d. **Simvastatin** also has an excellent adverse reaction profile and is twice as potent on a weight basis as lovastatin and pravastatin. The initial dose is 20 to 40 mg/d, with a maximum of 40 mg/d. For adolescents (10–17 yr) with FH, the starting dose is 10 mg/d, with a maximum of 40 mg/d. **Lovastatin** has a midrange adverse reactions profile. Because it must be taken with food, it is given with the evening meal. Initial dose is 20 mg/d immediate release (IR) or 20 mg, 40 mg, or 60 mg daily of the extended release (XR), with dosage increases at 6- to 8-week intervals to a maximum dose of 80 mg/d. For adolescents with FH, the starting dose is 10 mg/d, with a maximum dose of 40 mg. **Pravastatin** is similar in potency and adverse effects profile to **lovastatin.** The initial dose is 40 mg/d, with a maximum of 80 mg. Pediatric doses for this drug are available for children as young as 8 years of age. For 8- to 13-year-olds, the dose is 20 mg/d, both initial and maximum doses. For 14- to 18-year-olds, the starting and maximum dose is 40 mg/d. **Fluvastatin** is about one-half as potent as **lovastatin** and has a midrange adverse reactions profile. The initial dose is 40 mg/d, with a maximum dose of 80 mg/d. Splitting the dose into bid doses slightly improves the LDL-lowering ability (Table 16–28). In general, children with high-risk lipid abnormalities should

Table 16–28 ● **Dosage Schedule: Selected Antilipidemics**

Drug	Indication	Starting Dose	Maintenance Dose	Maximum Dose
Atorvastatin	Hypercholesterolemia (Heterozygous familial and nonfamilial and mixed dyslipidemia)	10–20 mg daily. If >45% LDL reduction needed, 40 mg daily	10–80 mg daily. Dosage adjustments at 2–4 wk intervals	80 mg/d
	Heterozygous FH in children (10–17 yr)	10 mg/d	10–20 mg/d. Same dosage adjustments	20 mg/d
	Homozygous FH	10 mg/d	10–80 mg/d. Same dosage adjustments	80 mg/d
	Elevated TG (in combination with niacin or BAS)	10 mg/d	10–40 mg/d	40 mg/d
Cholestryamine	Hyperlipidemia	1 pkt (4 g) mixed in 6–8 oz juice as slurry; taken 30 min before, during, or 30 min after breakfast and dinner	2–4 pkt (8–16 g) mixed and taken as before	24 g/d
Colesevelam	Hyperlipidemia	3 tablets (1,875 mg) bid with meals or 6 tablets once daily with a meal	3,750–4,375 mg/d	4,375 mg/d
Colestipol	Hyperlipidemia	Granules: 5 g/d given once or in two divided doses. (Mix as cholestyramine above)	5–30 g/d. Dosage adjustments at 1–2 mo intervals	30 g/d
		Tablets: 2 g/d once or in two divided doses	2–16 g/d. Same dosage adjustments	16 g/d
Fenofibrate*	Hyperlipidemia, and adjunct for Hypertriglyceridemia	43–130 mg/d (Antara); 54–160 mg/d (Lofibra); 48–145 mg/d (Tricor) If renal impairment: 43 mg/d (Antara) If renal impairment: 48 mg/d (Tricor) If renal impairment: 67 mg/d (Lofibra)	Increase dose at 4–8 wk intervals to target lipid levels	130 mg/d 200 mg/d 145 mg/d
Fluvastain	Hyperlipidemia *Peds:* New indication for boys and girls 10–16 yrs of age and at least 1 yr post menarche.	40 mg/d	40 mg/d or 40 mg bid or 80 mg XR/d	80 mg/d
Gemfibrozil	Hypertriglyceridemia, adjunct	1,200 mg/d in two divided doses, 30 min before morning and evening meals	600–1200 mg bid	1,200 mg bid
Lovastatin	Hyperlipidemia and primary prevention of cardiac events from CHD	Adults: (IR) 20 mg/d with evening meal (XR) 20 mg, 40 mg, or 60 mg at bedtime	20–80 mg/d. 80 mg in two divided doses. Dosage adjustments at 4-wk intervals	80 mg/d 60 mg/d 40 mg/d
	Heterozygous FH in children (10–17 yr) (IR only) 10–20 mg/d	10 mg/d with evening meal	10–60 mg/d	
	Combination therapy with niacin or BAS		10–40 mg/d 20 mg/d	

Table 16–28 ● **Dosage Schedule: Selected Antilipidemics—cont'd**

Drug	Indication	Starting Dose	Maintenance Dose	Maximum Dose
Niacin (IR = Nicor; XR = Niaspan)	Hyperlipidemia, adjunct for high triglycerides or low HDL	(IR): 250 mg following the evening meal	1.5–2 g/d in two or three divided doses. Increase dose at 4–7 day intervals. If target lipid not met after 2 mo, may increase to 3 g/d	6 g/d
		(XR): 500 mg at bedtime for 1–4 wk	Increase to 1 g at bedtime during wks 5–8. If target not met, increase to 1,500 mg at bedtime	2 g/d
Pravastatin	Hyperlipidemia and primary prevention of cardiac events from CHD	40 mg once daily	40–80 mg once daily	80 mg/d
	Heterozygous FH in children	Children 8–13 yr: 20 mg once daily.	20 mg once daily	20 mg/d
		Children 14–18 yr: 40 mg once daily	40 mg once daily	40 mg/ d
Rosuvastatin	Hypercholesterolemia (Heterozygous familial and non-familial and mixed dyslipidemia)	5–10 mg once daily	5–40 mg once daily. Dosage adjustments at 2–4 wk intervals	40 mg/d
	Homozygous FH	20 mg once daily	20–40 mg once daily.	40 mg/d
	Combined BAS		Same dosage adjustments	10 mg/d
Simvastatin	Hypercholesterolemia (Heterozygous familial and nonfamilial and mixed dyslipidemia)	20–40 mg daily in the evening. 10 mg/d for older adults or renal impairment (Ccr <30 mL/min)	20–40 mg/d. 20 mg/d for older adults and renal impairment	80 mg/d (over 20 mg/d cautiously for older adults and renal impairment
	Homozygous FH	40 mg/d	40 mg once daily or 80 mg/d in three divided doses: 20 mg, 20 mg, and 40 mg at bedtime	80 mg/d
	Heterozygous FH in children (10–17 yr) Girls at least 1 yr post menarche.	10 mg/d	10–40 mg/d	40 mg/d

FH = familial hyperlipidemia; TG = triglycerides; BAS = bile acid sequestrants; (IR) immediate release; (XR) = extended release.
*Dosage recommendations for renal impairment are the same for older adults.

have drugs started at the lowest dose given once daily, usually at bedtime (McCrindle et al, 2007).

Chapter 39 presents further discussion on the use of **statins** for this indication. Recent clinical trials have shown that LDL lipid-lowering therapy can now be used in persons in categories (near but below the level required for the diagnosis of hyperlipidemia) in which Adult Treatment Panel III (ATP III) formerly could not make definitive recommendations. In general, these new trials strongly reinforce ATP III recommendations (Grundy et al, 2004).

Niacin is effective in lowering total cholesterol and triglyceride levels and raising HDL levels. As a B-complex vitamin, it is available OTC, but OTC doses are not sufficient to lower LDL. In prescription strength, **niacin** has been shown to reduce all-cause mortality for patients with CAD. Because of its many adverse reactions, it is most frequently given as adjunctive therapy with a **bile acid sequestrant** or a **reductase inhibitor** for patients with very high triglyceride and/or low HDL levels. For hyperlipidemia, a dose of 1.5 to 2 g/d is usually enough. The daily dose should be divided and given with meals, starting at 250 mg at bedtime and gradually increased at 4- to 7-day intervals (see Table 16–28).

Bile acid sequestrants are best for patients with a low CAD risk profile and moderately elevated LDL levels, but who are unable to reduce their LDL by diet alone. Their biggest drawback is their GI adverse effect profile. **Cholestyramine** and **colestipol** come in powdered form. The initial dose is 1 packet mixed with juice in a slurry. They are never swallowed in dry form. **Colestipol** and **colesevelam** come in tablet form. The dose is taken one half hour before, during, or one half hour after a meal for several days. Doses are increased gradually, based largely on GI adverse reactions. A common dose is 2 to 4 packets or 3 tablets at breakfast and supper.

Elevated Very-Low-Density Lipoproteins and Elevated Triglycerides

Fenofibrate and **gemfibrozil** are the most potent triglyceride-lowering agents because of their effect on VLDL, and they are generally used for this purpose. Doses vary not only by drug but also by brand of **fenofibrate**. Data from the Helsinki Heart Study resulted in the recommendation that this drug not be used for patients with combined hyperlipidemia who have CAD symptoms. In severe mixed hyperlipidemia, **niacin**, plus a **bile acid sequestrant** or a **reductase inhibitor**, often produces marked reduction in triglyceride levels. To prevent pancreatitis for patients with marked hypertriglyceridemia, **niacin** in large doses may be used for patients who do not respond to **fibric acid derivatives**.

Decreased High-Density Lipoproteins

Niacin is the most effective agent in increasing levels of HDL. **Gemfibrozil** and **fenofibrate** are the next best at increasing HDL, followed by the **reductase inhibitors. Rosuvastatin** and **simvastatin** match these other drugs in their ability to raise HDL. Although they are now recognized as a risk factor in heart disease, HDL levels are not usually treated alone. This factor is a bonus effect when choosing a drug to treat elevated LDL or VLDL levels.

Rational Drug Selection

In addition to the nature of the lipoprotein abnormality and the mechanism of action and adverse reaction profile of the drug, as discussed previously, factors taken into account in selecting the appropriate drug or drug combination include degree of CAD risk, age of the patient, and cost.

Degree of Coronary Artery Disease Risk

For all risk groups, dietary reduction in saturated fat and cholesterol is first-line therapy. When drug therapy is a necessary adjunct, the following pattern is helpful.

For high-risk CAD patients as defined by the National Cholesterol Education Program (NCEP, 2001), **reductase inhibitors** are the most cost-effective and should be tried first. When baseline LDL is greater than 130 mg/dL, relatively high doses or combining with other antiplipidemics may be needed (Cannon et al, 2004; Nissen et al, 2004). If patient response is inadequate after 4 months, switch to a different drug or try a combination of drugs. Combinations of **reductase inhibitors** with **bile acid sequestrants** or **niacin** have shown promise for the highest-risk patients who fail to respond to **reductase inhibitors** alone. The combination of a **reductase inhibitor** with **fibric acid derivatives** is to be avoided because of the increased risk for rhabdomyolysis. It is common that achievement of an LDL level less than or equal to 100 is difficult with only one drug class. Patients whose response is still inadequate should be referred to a lipid disorder specialist.

For moderate-risk CHD patients, drug therapy is based on 10-year CAD risk. If that risk is greater than 20 percent, **reductase inhibitors** are appropriate (NCEP, 2001). For lower levels of risk, drugs generally are not needed if dietary modifications are followed. For isolated low-HDL patients, aerobic exercise, smoking cessation, and weight loss if they are obese are added to the dietary therapy. There is to date no evidence that drug treatment to increase HDL levels reduces CHD risk. Further discussion occurs in Chapter 39.

Elevated triglycerides are not an independent risk factor for CAD, and no consensus exists about treating these elevations. **Fibric acid derivatives** are the drugs of choice when treatment is chosen. It is also the drug of choice for patients with very high triglyceride levels (greater than 800 mg/dL) who are at risk for pancreatitis because of this high level.

Age

The prevalence of hypercholesterolemia and CAD risk is greatest among people older than age 65 years. Because dietary therapy alone often fails to achieve the LDL goal in older adults, drug therapy is used as an adjunct. **Reductase inhibitors** are the first-line choice. These drugs are well tolerated in the older adult, with minor diarrhea and occasional sleep disturbances being the most common problems. Because these drugs may cause an elevation in liver enzymes, it is important to monitor LFTs in older patients. **Niacin** is effective, but it is not as well tolerated because its adverse reactions profile is more common in the older adult. It may also trigger hypotension and arrhythmias. Multiple daily dosing is required, which may increase the complexity of a drug regimen often already complex. **Niaspan** taken once daily at bedtime may address these problems. **Bile acid sequestrants** are safe for older adults, but their GI problems, especially the risk of constipation and impaction, and their effect on the absorption of many of the drugs that older adults are often also taking make them less desirable than **reductase inhibitors.**

Cost

Although it is usually not the first factor considered in choosing therapy, cost can be a factor, especially for older patients on fixed incomes. The generic formulation of **lovastatin** appears to be the cheapest among the **antilipidemics.** None of the **antilipidemics** are "cheap." Brand-name drugs are always more expensive than generic. Table 16–29 lists the costs for each of the drugs.

Monotherapy versus Multiple Drugs

According to the NCEP (2001), few patients can achieve lipid targets on one drug class alone. The high doses required to do so result in unacceptable adverse responses. Combinations of drugs are the rule to achieve the newer, lower target levels. The decision will shortly be made to lower the target LDL to less than 70 for high-risk patients. When this occurs, it will be practically impossible to achieve this level without drug combinations. Specific combinations have been discussed previously and are discussed in Chapter 39.

Table 16–29 ◆ **Available Dosage Forms: Selected Antilipidemics**

Drug	Dosage Form	How Supplied	Cost
Atorvastatin (Lipitor)	Tablets: 10 mg, 20 mg 40 mg, 80 mg	In bottles of 90, 5,000, and UD 100 In bottles of 90 and 500	10 mg = $210; 20 mg, 40 mg, and 80 mg = $303
Colestyramine (LoCholest, Questran)	Powder for suspension: 4 g (G)	In packets of 42 and 60 and 378 g cans	
	4 g (LCh)	In packets of 60 and 378 g cans	
	4 g (Q)	In packets of 60 and 378 g cans	$64/can and $145/60 pkt
	Powder for suspension, light: 4 g (G)	In packets of 60 and 21 g, 231 g, and 239 g cans	
	4 g (LCh)	In packets of 60 and 239 g cans	
	4 g (Q)	In packets of 60	$64/can and $145/60 pkt
Colestipol (Colestid)	Tablets: 1 g (B)	In bottles of 120 and 500	$69/120
	Granules: 5 g (B)	In packets of 30 and 90; in 300 g and 500 g bottles	$86/500 g bottle
Colesevelam (WelChol)	Tablets: 625 mg (B)	In bottles of 24 and 180	$153/180
Fenofibrate (Antara, Lofibra, Tricor)	Tablets: 48 mg, 145 mg (T)	In bottles of 90	48 mg = $271/90; 145 mg = $92/90
	Capsules: 43 mg, 87 mg, 130 mg (A)	In bottles of 30 and 100	43 mg = $32/30; 130 mg = $92/30
	Capsules: 67 mg, 134 mg, 200 mg (L)	In bottles of 100	67 mg = $35; 200 mg = $100
Fluvastatin (Lescol, Lescol XL)	Capsules: 20 mg, 40 mg (B)	In bottles of 30 and 100	20 mg = $54/30; 40 mg = $174
	Tablets XL: 80 mg (B)	In bottles of 30 and 100	$233
Gemfirbozil (Lopid)	Tablets: 600 mg (G)	In bottles of 60, 500, blister pack 25, and UD 100	$19/60
	600 mg (B)	In bottles of 60, 500, and UD 100	$99/60
Lovastatin (Mevacor)	Tablets: 10 mg (G)	In bottles of 30, 60, 100, 500, and 1,000	$25/60
	10 (B)	In UD 60	$75/60
	20 mg (G), 40 mg (G)	In bottles of 30, 60, 90, 100, 500, and 1,000	20 mg = $37/60; 40 mg = $62/60
	20 mg (B)	In bottles of 1,000, 10,000; UD 60, 90, 100	$136/60
	40 mg (B)	In bottles of 100, 10,000; UD 60 and 90	$244/60
(Altocor)	Tablets (XR): 10 mg, 20 mg, 40 mg, 60 mg (A)	In bottles of 30	No data No data
Niacin (Nicor, Niaspan)	Tablets: 500 mg (Nicor)	In bottles of 100	500 mg = $136;
	Tablets (XR): 500 mg, 750 mg, 1,000 mg (Niaspan)	In bottles of 100 In bottles of 100	750 mg = $193; 1,000 mg = $228

Continued

Table 16–29 ◆ **Available Dosage Forms: Selected Antilipidemics—cont'd**

Drug	Dosage Form	How Supplied	Cost
Pravastatin (Pravachol)	Tablets: 10 mg (B) 20 mg (B) 40 mg (B) 80 mg (B)	In bottles of 90 In bottles of 90, 1,000, and UD 100 In bottles of 90 and UD 100 In bottles of 90 and 500	$265/90 $269/90 $394/90 $394/90
Rosuvastatin (Crestor)	Tablets: 5 mg (B) 10 mg (B), 20 mg (B) 40 mg (B)	In bottles of 90 In bottles of 90 and UD 100 In bottles of 30 and UD 100	10 mg = $260; 20 mg = $260; 40 mg = $261
Simvastatin (Zocor)	Tablets: 5 mg (B) 10 mg (B) 20 mg (B), 40 mg (B), and 80 mg (B)	In bottles of 1,000 and UD 30, 60, 90, 100 In bottles of 1,000 and 10,000; UD 30, 90, 100 In bottles of 1,000 and 10,000; UD 30, 60, 90, and 100	$135/90 $180/90 20 mg and 40 mg = $313 80 mg = $316

(G) = generic; (B) = brand. Where there is more than one brand, the initials of the brand are used. Cost in 100 units unless otherwise stated (e.g., $135/90 tablets).

Monitoring

Measurement of the LDL cholesterol level is the top priority, although a lipid profile is usually done because it provides more data and is not more expensive. Lipid levels should be measured beginning about 4 to 6 weeks after initiation of therapy and then every 3 to 4 months until control is established. After that, every 6 to 12 months is usually enough.

Monitoring protocols for specific drugs in addition to the standard lipid levels are as follows. For **niacin**, LFTs, uric acid levels, and blood glucose levels are done initially at 4- to 6-week intervals until a stable dose is determined, and thereafter at 3- to 4-month intervals. For **reductase inhibitors**, LFTs are done prior to initiating therapy, every 4 to 6 weeks during the first 3 months of therapy, every 6 to 12 weeks for the rest of the first year, and then every 6 months. If aspartate aminotransferase (AST) or alanine aminotransferase (ALT) levels increase to three times that which is normal, reduce the dose or discontinue therapy. CK levels are monitored if muscle tenderness is exhibited. For **fibric acid derivatives**, LFTs should be assessed prior to initiating therapy and with the same protocol as **reductase inhibitors**.

Patient Education

The importance of patient education in the treatment of hyperlipidemia cannot be overemphasized because, in addition to appropriate drug therapy, lifestyle management is the key to success.

Administration

The patient should take the drug exactly as prescribed and not skip doses or double up on missed doses. **Bile acid sequestrants** are taken before meals, mixed and vigorously shaken with 4 to 6 oz water, milk, fruit juice, or other noncarbonated beverage. Rinsing the glass with a small amount of additional liquid ensures that the entire dose was taken. For patients who require thick liquids, these drugs can also be mixed with cereals or pulpy fruits such as applesauce. The powder cannot be taken dry. If other drugs are to be taken, administer them 1 hour before or 4 hours after the **bile acid sequestrant. Reductase inhibitors** are best taken in the evening because of their action on cholesterol synthesis. **Lovastatin** is the only **reductase inhibitor** that should be taken with food to improve its absorption; it is best taken with the evening meal. **Atorvastatin** can be taken at any time of the day and without regard to food.

Adverse Reactions

Cutaneous flushing, especially of the face and upper body, has been associated with **niacin. Aspirin** 325 mg taken 30 minutes prior to the dose can reduce or eliminate this response; hot fluids taken near the time of the dose make the flushing worse. Taking **niacin** with meals reduces the incidence of adverse reactions. A high-fiber diet or psyllium supplement just before a meal usually ameliorates the flatulence, constipation, or abdominal pain associated with bile acid sequestrants. Natural laxatives such as prunes or **stool softeners** can also be helpful. For these drugs and for **fibric acid derivatives**, the health-care provider should be notified of persistent constipation or flatulence. For all **reductase inhibitors**, muscle tenderness or pain may indicate a serious problem that may require discontinuance of the drug. It should be reported immediately to the health-care provider. **Fluvastatin, lovastatin**, and **pravastatin** all have GI-associated adverse reactions (dyspepsia, abdominal pain, flatulence, constipation, or diarrhea) and headache. Generally, these effects are mild and transient.

For all of these drugs, the importance of keeping follow-up appointments to monitor efficacy and adverse reactions cannot be overstated. Failure to discover problems early can result in increased risk for CAD and, for some drugs, life-threatening events.

Because the **reductase inhibitors** are Pregnancy Category D or X, female patients capable of childbearing should not take these drugs, or contraception should be instituted before prescribing them. The health-care provider should be notified if pregnancy is planned or suspected.

Lifestyle Management

For a cardiac-healthy lifestyle, it is important to stress the need for dietary restriction in fat, cholesterol, carbohydrates, and alcohol; regular aerobic exercise; and smoking cessation. Medication helps to control hyperlipidemia, but it does not cure it. Lifestyle management is discussed in more detail in Chapter 39.

DIURETICS

Diuretics are first-line therapy in the treatment of HF and HTN through their reduction in ECF volume. Of the several classes of **diuretics**, the ones most commonly used in primary care are the distal tubular (**thiazides** and **aldosterone antagonists**) and **loop diuretics**. These drugs are the focus of this discussion.

Pharmacodynamics

Disease processes that increase renal sodium and water retention result in increased ECF volume. This increased volume increases capillary hydrostatic pressure. Taken together, the result is increased afterload, which leads to HF. Increased ECF volume also contributes to HTN. **Diuretics** act to reduce this volume in different ways (Figure 16–7). The **loop diuretics** inhibit sodium reabsorption in the ascending loop of Henle. These drugs are short acting and cause a large natriuresis. The **thiazide-type diuretics** act on the distal renal tubule to inhibit sodium reabsorption. Their effect is generally longer lasting, and they cause less brisk diuresis. Both of these classes also result in increased potassium excretion. The **potassium-sparing diuretics** include **aldosterone antagonists** and agents that inhibit excretion of potassium distally. These agents are weak **diuretics**, often used in combination with **thiazides** to reduce potassium loss.

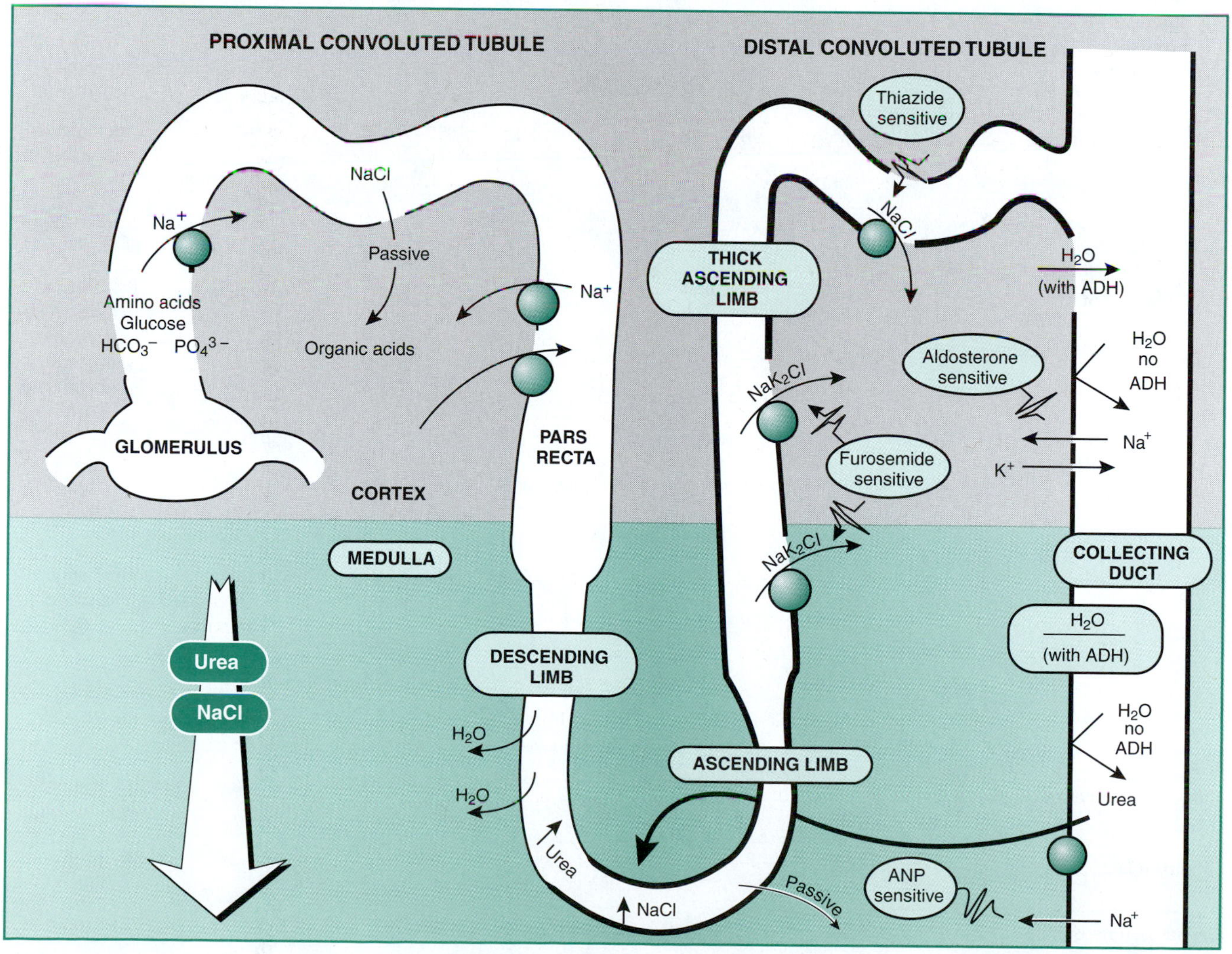

Figure 16–7. Sites of action of diuretics.

Initially, **diuretics** promote natriuresis, decrease plasma volume, and reduce cardiac output. With time, these effects return to baseline, but total peripheral resistance remains decreased. The mechanism behind this additional long-term effect of **diuretics** is not clearly known but may be related to the amount of sodium in the vessel walls themselves. Theoretically, sodium in vessel walls contributes to the ability of the vessels to constrict, and loss of sodium from the vessel walls may contribute to vasodilation, leading to decreased PVR. Decreased PVR reduces afterload to improve cardiac functioning and reduce BP.

Diuretics may also be used as adjunct therapy for disease processes in which the treatment itself may contribute to fluid retention—for example, use of **CCBs** and some **antiarrhythmics**.

There are many **diuretics** available. The focus of this section is on the most commonly seen drugs, with prototypical drugs from each class included.

Pharmacokinetics

Absorption and Distribution

Absorption and distribution vary among the **diuretics** (Table 16–30). **Thiazide** and **loop diuretics** are all well absorbed orally. Among the **potassium-sparing diuretics**, **spironolactone (Aldactone)** is well absorbed, **amiloride (Midamor)** is poorly absorbed, and **triamterene (Dyrenium)** has an absorption somewhere between the two. Food enhances the absorption of **metolazone (Zaroxolyn)**. All are widely distributed, cross the placenta, and enter breast milk. The **thiazides** enter intracellular spaces as well,

Table 16–30 ▶ **Pharmacokinetics: Selected Diuretics**

Drug	Onset (h)	Peak (h)	Duration (h)	Protein Binding	Bioavailability	Half-Life (h)	Elimination
Thiazide and Related Diuretics							
Chlorthalidone	2–3	2–6	24–72	UK	64%	35–50	Unchanged in urine
Hydrochlorothiazide	2	4–6	6–12	20%–80%	65%–75%	5.6–14.8	Unchanged in urine
Indapamide	1–2	2	up to 36	71%–79%	93%	14	~7% unchanged in urine
Metolazone	1	2	12–24	<20%	65%	No data	6%–15% in feces, partially excreted unchanged in urine
Loop Diuretics							
Bumetanide	0.5–1	1–2	4–6	94%–96%	72%–96%	1–1.5	50% in urine, 20% in feces
Furosemide	1	1–2	6–8	91%–97%	60%–64%	0.5–1 (increased in renal and hepatic impairment and in neonates)	Unchanged in urine
Potassium-Sparing Diuretics							
Amiloride	2	6–10	24	23%	15%–25%	6–9	50% in urine
Spironolactone	24–48	48–72	48–72	>98%	>90%	13–24	In urine and bile
Triamterene	2–4	6–8	12–16	50%–67%	30%–70%	3	21% in urine

UK = unknown.

which may explain their preferential use in refractory edema.

Metabolism and Excretion

The liver is the primary site of metabolism for all **diuretics**. **Furosemide (Lasix)** has nonhepatic and hepatic metabolism. All **diuretics** are excreted mostly unchanged in the urine. **Metolazone, bumetanide (Bumex)**, and **spironolactone** have some excretion in feces and bile. Plasma half-lives vary from 30 to 60 minutes for **furosemide** to 35 to 50 hours for **chlorthalidone**. Impaired renal or hepatic function increases the half-life of **furosemide**. Table 16–30 lists the pharmacokinetics for the selected drugs.

Pharmacotherapeutics

Precautions and Contradictions

All **diuretics** affect electrolytes. They should be carefully selected and used cautiously for patients with preexisting electrolyte abnormalities. **Potassium-sparing diuretics** have an absolute contraindication for patients with impaired renal function because of their tendency to produce hyperkalemia. Creatinine clearances less than 25 to 30 mL/min suggest careful monitoring of electrolytes and cautious use with all **diuretic** classes. Hepatic dysfunction suggests cautious use with all **diuretics**, especially those with some excretion in feces or bile.

For patients with a history of gout or renal calculi, cautious use of **thiazide** and **loop diuretics** and **spironolactone** is suggested because of the potential for hyperuricemia. **Diuretics** should be used cautiously for patients with diabetes, who may require alterations in their hypoglycemic regimen related to glucose intolerance.

Older adults are at increased risk for hypotension with these drugs and require careful BP monitoring and patient teaching about mobility. The use of **thiazide** and **loop diuretics** has been associated with increased fall risk in older adults.

Diuretics decrease plasma volume and may decrease placental perfusion. Several **thiazide** and **loop diuretics** are Pregnancy Category C and should be used only when benefits clearly outweigh risks. Jaundice and thrombocytopenia may be seen in neonates. **Spironolactone, hydrochlorothiazide**, and **chlorthalidone** are Pregnancy Category B. **Spironolactone** appears to be the best choice for pregnant women when a **diuretic** must be used. Safety has been established in children only for **furosemide, hydrochlorothiazide**, and **spironolactone**.

Adverse Drug Reactions

Electrolyte imbalances are common in all diuretic classes. **Thiazide** and **loop diuretics** cause hypokalemia and may cause hypercalcemia, hyponatremia, and hypomagnesemia. When it occurs, the hypomagnesemia must be corrected first to permit successful treatment of the hypokalemia. The average potassium loss is 0.6 mEq/L and is dose related. Increased sodium intake exacerbates the potassium loss. Metabolic alkalosis may be associated with the hypokalemia. **Potassium-sparing diuretics** cause hyperkalemia. Hyperuricemia may occur with all **diuretics; thiazide** and **loop diuretics** and **spironolactone** are the most likely to cause it, and **indapamide (Lozol)** is the least likely. The hyperuricemia itself is usually not treated unless gout or renal calculi develop.

Glucose intolerance is a problem with all **diuretic** groups; **thiazide** and **loop diuretics** cause the most difficulty, and **metolazone** and **indapamide** have the least effect. This intolerance is directly linked to the serum potassium level, and correcting hypokalemia often relieves the problem.

Hypotension secondary to fluid volume deficits can also occur with all **diuretics**. Starting with a low dose and increasing the dose gradually can reduce this problem.

Hyperlipidemia with increases in cholesterol, LDL, and triglycerides has been seen with **thiazide diuretics**. The elevations are transient and tend to return to baseline in about 6 months.

Gynecomastia occurs in 50 percent of patients receiving **spironolactone**, and impotence occurs in a smaller number. These can be distressing to men. **Loop diuretics** have a small risk for hearing loss and tinnitus.

Drug Interactions

All **diuretics** have potential additive hypotensive effects with other drugs that lower BP. Synergistic hypokalemia is probable between **thiazide** and **loop diuretics**, and additive hypokalemia may occur between these classes and **mezlocillin, piperacillin, ticarcillin, amphotericin B**, and **glucocorticoids**. Hypokalemia may increase the risk of **digitalis** toxicity. Concurrent administration of **potassium-sparing diuretics** and **ACEIs** may lead to significant hyperkalemia. Potassium preparations, including nonsodium salt substitutes, may also result in significant hyperkalemia.

Thiazide and **loop diuretics** decrease the renal excretion of **lithium** and may induce **lithium** toxicity. These two classes may decrease the action of **sulfonylureas** and **insulin. Thiazide diuretics** and **spironolactone** diminish the anticoagulant effects of **warfarin**, whereas **loop diuretics** enhance its anticoagulant effects. Additive ototoxicity occurs between **loop diuretics** and **aminoglycosides** and **cisplatin. NSAIDs** and **salicylates** may decrease the **diuretic** effectiveness of all classes.

Specific drug interactions and the appropriate actions to prevent them are given in Table 16–31.

Clinical Use and Dosing

Regardless of the clinical use, start with the lowest effective dose, increase the dose gradually to reduce the likelihood of adverse reactions, consider reducing doses where appropriate, and consider **potassium** supplementation or combination with a **potassium-sparing diuretic** when laboratory studies indicate it is appropriate.

Table 16–31 ■ **Drug Interactions: Selected Diuretics**

Drug	Interacting Drug	Possible Effect	Implications
Thiazide diuretics	Allopurinol	Concurrent use may increase incidence of hypersensitivity reactions	Avoid concurrent use
	Anticholinergics	Increased diuretic absorption	Monitor diuretic effect
	Anticoagulants	Diminished anticoagulant effect	Monitor PT/INR. Adjust anticoagulant dose prn.
	Antigout agents	Diuretic may increase uric acid levels	Choose different diuretic or adjust antigout agent dose
	Antineoplastics	Diuretic may prolong antineoplastic-induced leukopenia	Monitor WBC. Choose alternative diuretic.
	Bile acid–binding resins	Resins bind thiazides and reduce absorption by up to 85%	Give thiazide 2 h before or 4 h after bile acid–binding resin
	Calcium salts	Hypercalcemia may be worsened	Avoid concurrent use
	Diazoxide	Hyperglycemia, often with symptoms of frank diabetes	Choose alternative antihypertensive
	Digitalis glycosides	Digitalis toxicity and toxicity-induced arrhythmias	Monitor potassium level and administer supplement as needed
	Lithium	Decreased renal excretion of lithium, resulting in toxicity	Monitor lithium level closely, or choose alternative diuretic
	Loop diuretics	Synergistic diuresis and hypokalemic effects	Reduce doses of both or one of these unless planned for therapeutic reasons. Monitor electrolytes closely.
	NSAIDs	Some may reduce diuretic effect; concurrent administration of indomethacin has been associated with renal failure	Monitor diuresis. Avoid concurrent administration of indomethacin
	Sulfonylureas, insulin	Diuretics induce hyperglycemia and may decrease hypoglycemic effects	Monitor serum glucose. Adjust dose of hypoglycemic.
	Vitamin D	Biologic actions of vitamin D enhanced, resulting in hypercalcemia	Monitor serum calcium levels
Loop diuretics	Aminoglycosides, cisplatin	Increased risk for ototoxicity	Avoid concurrent use. If you must use aminoglycoside, use different diuretic during time it is administered.
	Anticoagulants	Enhanced anticoagulant activity	Monitor PT/INR. Adjust dose prn.
	Digitalis glycosides	Digitalis toxicity and toxicity-induced arrhythmias	Monitor potassium levels and administer potassium supplement prn
	Hydantoins	Reduces diuretic effect of furosemide	Monitor diuretic effect and adjust dose prn

Table 16–31 ■ **Drug Interactions: Selected Diuretics—cont'd**

Drug	Interacting Drug	Possible Effect	Implications
	Lithium	Decreased renal excretion of lithium, resulting in toxicity	Monitor lithium levels closely or choose different diuretic
	NSAIDs, salicylates	Reduces effects of diuretic	Monitor diuretic effect and adjust dose
	Sulfonylureas	Diuretic-induced hyperglycemia may reduce hypoglycemic effect	Monitor serum glucose and adjust dose of sulfonylurea, or choose different diuretic
	Theophylline	Actions of theophylline may be enhanced or inhibited	Monitor theophylline levels closely, or choose different bronchodilator
Potassium-sparing diuretics	ACE inhibitors, potassium preparations	Concurrent use may result in hyperkalemia	Avoid concurrent use. Choose differnt diuretic.
	Anticoagulants	Decreased anticoagulant effects	Monitor PT/INR and adjust dose prn
	Cimetidine	May increase bioavailability and decrease renal clearance of triamterene only	Choose alternative $histamine_2$ blocker
	Digitalis glycosides	Interaction complex and difficult to predict risk of toxicity	Monitor digitalis level closely or avoid concurrent use
	NSAIDs salicylates	Decreased diuretic effect; interaction with indomethacin has resulted in renal failure	Monitor diuretic effect. Avoid concurrent use with indomethacin.

Hypertension

Initial drug therapy for HTN is monotherapy, although rarely is one drug sufficient to achieve target BP. When the decision is made to begin drug therapy and there are no clear indications for another type of drug, a **thiazide-type diuretic** should be chosen because, in randomized controlled trials (RCTs) comparing **diuretics** with other classes of **antihypertensive drugs, diuretics** have been unsurpassed in preventing cardiovascular complications of HTN (ALLHAT Officers and Coordinators, 2002; Wright et al, 2009). The choice of **diuretic** should be based on level of kidney function. For estimated glomerular filtration rates (EGFR) higher than the mid–40 mL/min range, a **thiazide diuretic** should be used as **loop diuretics** are not as effective as **thiazides** in this setting. For EGFRs that are lower than the mid–40 mL/min range, **loop diuretics**, sometimes in combination with **metolazone**, are more appropriate and are most effective when dosed twice daily.

Diuretics are preferred as initial therapy for sodium-sensitive patients such as blacks, older adults, the obese, and those with renal insufficiency. **Thiazide diuretics** are generally not the first drugs of choice for patients with hyperlipidemia because of their potential for worsening the hyperlipidemia; however, lipid disorders do not contraindicate the use of **thiazide diuretics.**

All classes of **diuretics** have been used to treat HTN, but the best results are with thiazide-type diuretics. The dose-response curve of **diuretics** is fairly flat. Increasing the dose produces more adverse reactions with little change in therapeutic benefit. Dosage should be increased no sooner than 4 weeks, which is the length of time usually required to achieve optimal therapeutic effect. When a **thiazide diuretic** is added to an existing antihypertensive regimen, reduce the dosage of the other **antihypertensives** to prevent excessive hypotension and orthostasis.

Edema Associated With Congestive Heart Failure, Hepatic Cirrhosis, and Renal Disease

First-line therapy in treating CHF is with **ACEIs**, depending on the stage of the heart failure. Chapter 36 discusses the most appropriate drug for initiation of therapy based on stage. Drugs are often introduced in combinations. The role of **diuretics** is supplemental and part of a treatment regimen. The most effective class for this indication is the

loop diuretics. Torsemide is a very good long-acting **loop diuretic** that is especially useful in heart failure management. These drugs are effective in moderate to severe disease and can be used when Ccr is less than 25 mL/min. **Indapamide** is also indicated for edema associated with HF and is effective with these low Ccr levels. **Thiazide diuretics** may be used to treat the edema associated with mild HF, **corticosteroid** and **estrogen** therapy, premenstrual syndrome, and limited renal dysfunction. They are not useful if the Ccr is less than 25 mL/min. Among the **thiazides, hydrochlorothiazide** and **chlorthalidone** are the first choices for this indication. Intermittent dosing may be advantageous and reduce the incidence of adverse reactions. With premenstrual syndrome, the drug should be taken 3 to 5 days before menstruation and discontinued when menstruation begins. Frequent dosage adjustments may be necessary in edematous patients.

Dosages for both indications for each drug are indicated in Table 16–32.

Rational Drug Selection

Indications

When HTN is mild, **diuretic** therapy can be initiated with **hydrochlorothiazide** 50 mg. The ALLHAT trials (ALLHAT Officers and Coordinators, 2002; Wright et al, 2009) have consistently shown that **chlorthalidone (Thalitone)** initiated at 15 mg and increased as needed to a maximum of 50 mg, was superior to all other drugs in that trial in treating hypertension. For patients with renal impairment, the addition of **metolazone** 2.5 to 5 mg is helpful. When these conditions are moderate to severe, **furosemide** 20 to 40 mg is necessary. **Potassium-sparing diuretics** are relatively weak agents and are used mainly in conjunction with **thiazide** or **loop diuretics** to prevent hypokalemia (Table 16–33).

Concurrent Disease Processes

Increasing glucose levels can be a problem for patients with diabetes, and hyperuricemia can be a problem for

Table 16–32 ◉ **Dosage Schedule: Selected Diuretics**

Drug	Clinical Use	Starting Dose	Maintenance Dose	Maximum Dose
Amiloride	Adjunctive therapy for edema of CHF	5 mg daily	10 mg qd or 5 mg bid	20 mg/d
Bumetanide	Edema of CHF, hepatic cirrhosis, renal disease; useful as alternate for furosemide allergy	0.5 mg daily	2 mg/d; intermittent dosing every other day or 3–4 d with 1–2 d between is safest and most effective	10 mg/d
Chlorthalidone	Edema HTN	50–100 mg/d 25 mg/d	150–200 mg/d 25–50 mg/d	200 mg/d 100 mg/d
Furosemide	Refractory edema of CHF, hepatic cirrhosis, renal disease	20–80 mg daily or bid	Titrate in increments of 20–40 mg q6–8h; until desired diuresis; give bid 8 a.m. and 2 p.m.	600 mg/d; for CHF with chronic renal failure, doses of 2–2.5 g/d have been used
	HTN	40 mg bid	Titrate up or down to control HTN	
	Infants and children	2 mg/kg/d	Titrate in increments of 1 mg/kg q6–8h until desired diuresis	6 mg/kg/d
Hydrochlorothiazide	HTN Edema Infants <6 mo Infants 6 mo–2 yr Children 2–12 yr	12.5 mg/d 25–200 mg/d 3.3 mg/kg/d 12.5 mg/d 37.5 mg/d	25–50 mg qd or in two divided doses 25–100 mg/d 3.3 mg/kg/d Up to 37.5 mg/d Up to 100 mg/d; all infant and children doses given in two divided doses and based on body weight	50 mg/d 200 mg/d Rarely need more than 50 mg/d

Table 16–32 ● **Dosage Schedule: Selected Diuretics—cont'd**

Drug	Clinical Use	Starting Dose	Maintenance Dose	Maximum Dose
Indapamide	HTN	1.25 mg daily	2.5–5 mg daily; increase at 4-wk intervals if needed to control HTN	5 mg/d
	Edema of CHF	2.5 mg daily	If response not adequate in 1 wk, increase to 5 mg qd	5 mg/d
Metolazone (Zaroxolyn only)	Adjunct therapy for HTN Renal disease, CHF	2.5 mg daily 5 mg daily	5 mg daily 10 mg daily	20 mg daily 20 mg daily
Spironolactone	HTN	50 mg daily	50–100 mg daily or in two divided doses	100 mg/d
	Edema of CHF, hepatic cirrhosis, nephrotic syndrome	25–100 mg daily	25–200 mg/d in divided doses; if inadequate diuresis after 5 d add different diuretic or change diuretics	>100 mg/d; increased adverse reactions without improved therapy possible
	Children: edema	3.3 mg/kg/d as in single or divided doses	3.3 mg/kg/d	
	Children: HTN	1 mg/kg daily	1–2 mg/kg bid	
Triamterene	Edema of CHF, hepatic cirrhosis, steroid use	50 mg daily	50–100 mg bid	300 mg/d

CHF = congestive heart failure; HTN = hypertension.

Table 16–33 ◆ **Available Dosage Forms: Selected Diuretics (Replace)**

Drug	Dosage Form	How Supplied	Cost	Combinations
Amiloride (Midamor)	Tablets: 5 mg (B)	In bottles of 100	$51	With HCTZ (Moduretic)
Bumetanide (Bumex)	Tablet: 0.5 mg (B); 1 mg (B)	In bottles of 100, 500, and UD 100	0.5 mg = $48; 1 mg = $67	
	2 mg (B)	In bottles of 10 and UD 100	2 mg = = $112	
Chlorthalidone (Thalitone, Hygroton)	Tablets: 15 mg (T)	In bottles of 100	$150	
	25 mg (G)	In bottles of 100 and 1,000	$11.49	
	25 mg (T)	In bottles of 100		
	25 mg (H)	In bottles of 100		
	50 mg (G)	In bottles of 100, 250, and 1,000	$25.59	
	50 mg (H)	In bottles of 100		
	100 mg (G)	In bottles of 100, 500, and 1,000		
	100 mg (H)	In bottles of 100		

Continued

Table 16–33 ◆ **Available Dosage Forms: Selected Diuretics (Replace)—cont'd**

Drug	Dosage Form	How Supplied	Cost	Combinations
Hydroclorothiazide (Esidrix, Ezide, HydroDiuril, Oretic)	Tablets: 25 mg (G)	In bottles of 30, 100, 500, 1,000, 5,000, and UD 32 and 100	$5	With spironolactone (Aldactazide)
	25 mg (E)	In bottles of 100		
	25 mg (HD)	In bottles of 100 and 1,000	$16	With triamterene (Dyazide, Maxide)
	25 mg (O)	In bottles of 100, 1,000, and UD 100		
	50 mg (G)	In bottles of 30, 100, 500, 1,000, 5,000, and UD 100	$10	With hydralazine (Apresazide)
	50 mg (E)	In bottles of 100 and packs of 360 and 720		
	50 mg (Ez)	In bottles of 100 and 1,000		With captopril (Capozide)
	50 mg (HD)	In bottles of 100, 1,000, 5,000	$25	
	50 mg (O)	In bottles of 100, 1,000, and UD 100		With metoprolol (Lopressosor)
	100 mg (G)	In bottles of 30, 100, 250, 500, 1,000, and UD 100	$7	
	100 mg (HD)	In bottles of 100		With benazepril (Lotensin HCT)
	Micronized capsules: 12.5 mg	In bottles of 100		
	Solution: 50 mg/5 mL (G)	In 500 mL		
Indapamide (Lozol)	Tablets: 1.25 mg (B)	In bottles of 100	$59	
	2.5 mg (B)	In bottles of 100, 1,000, and UD 100	$109	
	2.5 mg (G)	In bottles of 100 and 1,000	$40	
Metolazone (Zaroxolyn, Mykrox)	Tablets: 2.5 mg (Z); 5 mg (Z); 10 mg (Z)	In bottles of 100, 1,000, and UD 100 (all doses)	2.5 mg = $71; 5 mg = $103; 10 mg = $127	
	0.5 mg (M)	In bottles of 100	0.5 mg = $107	
Spironolactone (Aldactone)	Tablets: 25 mg (G)	In bottles of 100, 250, 500, 1,000	$9	With HCTZ (Aldactazide)
	25 mg (A)	In bottles of 100, 500, 1,000, 2,500, and UD 100	$68	
	50 mg (A)	In bottles of 100 and UD 100	$118	
	100 mg (A)	In bottles of 100 and UD 100	$127	
Triamterene (Dyrenium)	Capsules: 50 mg (B)	In bottles of 100 and UD 100	$92	With HCTZ (Dyazide, Maxide)
	100 mg (B)	In bottles of 100, 1,000, and UD 100	$166	
Triamterene/HCTZ (G)	37.5 mg/25 mg (G)		Cost of generic combination: $5/30	

(G) = generic (note: HCTZ is the generic hydrochlorothiazide); (B) = brand. Where more than one brand exists, the initial of the brand is used to differentiate them.

patients with gout. In the order of most likely to least likely to have these adverse effects, the drugs are **thiazides, loop diuretics, potassium-sparing diuretics, metolazone,** and **indapamide.** Drug choices for patients with diabetes or gout are in the reverse order of this list. Low doses of **thiazide diuretics** can be used for patients with these disorders. Hypokalemia can be a significant problem for patients with cardiac disorders. Drugs likely to have this adverse reaction are the **loop** and **thiazide diuretics.** These drugs are still often chosen for their effects on the edema associated with HF. Careful monitoring of potassium levels must accompany their use with these patients. Hyperkalemia can be lethal for patients with renal failure and problematic for those with reduced renal function. **Potassium-sparing diuretics** are contraindicated in the former and rarely chosen in the latter. Both **potassium-sparing diuretics** and **thiazides** should be avoided for patients with Ccr less than 25 to 30 mL/min. **Loop diuretics, metolazone,** and **indapamide** are safe alternatives for these patients. Hyperlipidemia is usually a transient phenomenon, and there is no consensus on the restriction of a drug class because of it. **Indapamide** effectively controls mild to moderate HTN, with no adverse reaction of lipids and minimum impact on potassium, glucose, and uric acid. It appears to address most concerns.

Combinations

Metolazone by itself is not a strong **diuretic,** but as an adjunct to **loop diuretics** its synergistic effect frequently overcomes refractory cases or enables dosage reduction of the **loop diuretic,** resulting in fewer adverse reactions. Combining a potassium-wasting diuretic with a **potassium-sparing diuretic** can prevent hypokalemia. Some drugs come in this combination (**triamterene and hydrochlorothiazide [Maxzide], spironolactone and hydrochlorothiazide [Aldactazide]**), making it possible to take only one tablet.

Cost

Comparison of monthly cost for the average dosing of one of the selected **diuretics** in this section is listed in Table 16–33. The generic form of each of these drugs is less expensive than the brand name, and the value of generic **diuretics** is quite clear!

Monitoring

In addition to monitoring the clinical indicators (BP, heart rate, edema, weight gain, dyspnea, cough, urine output), it is also critical to monitor renal function, glucose level, and electrolytes. Prior to initiating therapy, BUN, creatinine, electrolytes (sodium, potassium, calcium, and magnesium), uric acid, and glucose levels should be drawn. The patient should return to the clinic 1 week after initial prescription for a follow-up visit to check the clinical indicators and their electrolytes. Potassium levels of 3.5 to 4 mEq/L are usually not an indication for supplementation in a noncardiac patient. Patients with cardiac disorders should have their potassium levels maintained at 4 to 4.5 mEq/L. Spacing of monitoring after the first visit depends on lability of symptoms and dosage adjustments. Specific indicators to monitor depend on the common adverse effects of the specific drug(s) being used. This topic is discussed further in Chapters 36 and 40.

Patient Education

Administration

Patients should take the drug exactly as prescribed, even if they are feeling well, and not skip or double doses. For drugs given twice daily, the morning dose should be taken at breakfast and the evening dose no later in the day than 4 p.m. These drugs increase urine output, and taking the drug later may make the patient get up at night to urinate. Some of these drugs come alone or in combination. Check with the pharmacist with each refill to make certain the drug is in the correct form.

Adverse Reactions

Hypotensive reactions are the most common. Changing position slowly, not using alcohol, not standing for long periods, and avoiding exercise in hot weather can decrease these reactions. These drugs are used to reduce fluid volume in the body. Weighing daily helps to monitor that fluid. The patient should notify the health-care provider if weight loss of more than 1 lb per day or 5 lb per week, excessive thirst, dry skin or mucous membranes, dizziness, muscle pain, weakness or cramps, nausea, vomiting, increased heart rate, or diarrhea occurs. These may indicate an abnormal potassium level.

Potassium-wasting **diuretics** may cause potassium loss from the body. The health-care provider monitors this loss with laboratory work. If instructed by the health-care provider, a diet high in potassium may be needed. Foods high in potassium include bananas, dates, figs, fish, citrus juices, melons, molasses, baked potatoes, prunes, soybeans, and tomatoes. If an oral potassium supplement is prescribed, powders or liquids can be diluted in at least 4 oz fruit juice to improve the taste. Tablets taken with meals reduce GI irritation.

Potassium-sparing diuretics cause the body to hold potassium. The health-care provider monitors this gain with laboratory work. Patients should not take potassium supplements or use salt substitutes that have potassium in them.

Occasionally, these drugs cause GI upset that may be reduced by taking them with meals. Use of a sunscreen prevents photosensitivity reactions, although these are rare.

Changes in blood sugar and other body chemicals may occur. Follow-up appointments that allow the health-care provider to assess levels of these chemicals and progression of the disease process are important.

Lifestyle Management

If these drugs are taken for HTN, it is important to continue with the other therapies for HTN, including weight loss, restricted sodium intake, stress reduction, regular aerobic exercise, not using tobacco products, and moderation in alcohol intake. These drugs help to control HTN but do not cure it. Patients should not use OTC preparations without first checking with the health-care provider. They may interact with these drugs or make the disease process worse.

Lifestyle management for the specific disorders managed in whole or part with **diuretics** is covered in Chapters 36 and 40.

REFERENCES

AACE Hypertension Task Force. (2006). American Association of Clinical Endocrinologists medical guidelines for clinical practice for the diagnosis and treatment of hypertension. *Endocrinology Practice, 12*(2), 193–222.

ALLHAT Officers and Coordinators for the ALLHAT Collaborative Research Group. (2002). Major outcomes in high-risk hypertensive patients randomized to angiotensin-converting enzyme inhibitor or calcium channel blocker vs diuretic: The Antihypertensive and Lipid-Lowering Treatment to Prevent Heart Attack (ALLHAT). *Journal of the American Medical Association, 288,* 2981–2997.

American College of Cardiology/American Heart Association (ACC/AHA). (2002). *ACC/AHA guideline update for the management of patients with chronic stable angina: A report to the American College of Cardiology/American Heart Association Task Force on Practice Guidelines.* Bethesda, MD: American College of Cardiology Foundation.

American College of Cardiology/American Heart Association (ACC/AHA). (2009). ACC/AHA guidelines for the diagnosis and management of heart failure in adults: A report of the American College of Cardiology Foundation/American Heart Association Task Force on Practice Guidelines developed in collaboration with the International Society for Heart and Lung Transplantation. *Journal of the American College of Cardiology, 53*(15), 1343–1382.

American College of Cardiology/American Heart Association/European Society of Cardiology (ACC/AHA/ESC). (2003). ACC/AHA/ESC guidelines for the management of patients with supraventricular arrhythmias—executive summary: A report of the American College of Cardiology/American Heart Association Task Force on Practice Guidelines and the European Society of Cardiology Committee for Practice Guidelines. *Journal of the American College of Cardiology, 42*(8), 1493–1531.

American College of Cardiology/American Heart Association/European Society of Cardiology (ACC/AHA/ESC). (2006). ACC/AHA/ESC 2006 guidelines for management of patients with atrial fibrillation—executive summary: A report of the American College of Cardiology/American Heart Association Task Force on Practice Guidelines and the European Society of Cardiology Committee for Practice Guidelines. *Journal of the American College of Cardiology, 4*(4), 854–906.

American Diabetes Association. (2009). Standards of medical care in diabetes. *Diabetes Care, 32*(Suppl. 1), 13–61.

Brenner, B., Cooper, M., DeZeeuw, D., Keane, W., Mitch, W., Parving, H., et al, RENAAL Study Investigators. (2001). Effects of losartan on renal and cardiovascular outcomes in patients with type 2 diabetes and nephropathy. *New England Journal of Medicine, 345*(12), 861–869.

Cannon, C., Braubwald, E., McCabe, C., Rader, D., Rouleau, J., Belder, R., et al. (2004). Intensive versus moderate lipid lowering with statins after acute coronary syndromes. *New England Journal of Medicine, 350*(15), 1495–1504.

Daniels, S., Greer, F., & Committee on Nutrition. (2008). Lipid screening and cardiovascular health in childhood. *Pediatrics, 122*(1), 198–208.

Digitalis Investigation Group. (1997). The effect of digoxin on mortality and morbidity in patients with heart failure. *New England Journal of Medicine, 336*(8), 525–533.

Elliot, W. (1996). Higher incidence of discontinuance of angiotensin converting enzyme inhibitors due to cough in black subjects. *Clinical Pharmacology and Therapy, 60,* 582–588.

Flather, M., Yusuf, S., Kober, L., Pffeffer, M., Hall, A., Murray, G., et al. (2000). Long-term ACE-inhibitor therapy in patients with heart failure or left-ventricular dysfunction: A systematic overview of data from individual patients. ACE-Inhibitor Myocardial Infarction Collaborative Group. *Lancet, 355,* 1575–1581.

Forclaz, A., Maillard, M., Nussberger, J., Brunner, H., & Burnier, M. (2003). Angiotensin II receptor blockade: Is there truly a benefit of adding an ACE inhibitor? *Hypertension, 41,* 31–36.

Grundy, S., Cleeman, J., Merz, C., Brewer, H., Jr., Clark, L., Hunninghake, D., et al. (2004). Implications of recent clinical trials for the National Cholesterol Education Program Adult Treatment Panel III guidelines. *Circulation, 110*(2), 227–239.

Gulati, M., Cooper-DeHoff, R., McClure, C., Jophnson, B., Shaw, L., Handberg, E., et al. (2009). Adverse cardiovascular outcomes in women with nonobstructive coronary artery disease. *Archives of Internal Medicine, 169*(9), 843–850.

Hecht, H., & Harman, M. (2003a). Comparison of effectiveness of statin monotherapy versus statin and niacin combination therapy in primary prevention and effects on calcified plaque burden. *American Journal of Cardiology, 91,* 348–350.

Hecht, H., & Harman, M. (2003b). Comparisons of the effects of atorvastatin versus simvastatin on subclnical atherosclerosis in primary prevention as determined by electron beam tomography. *American Journal of Cardiology, 91,* 42–45.

Hunt, S., Abraham, W., Chin, M., Feldman, A., Francis, G., Ganiats, T., et al. (2005, August). ACC/AHA guideline update for the diagnosis and management of chronic heart failure in the adults. A report of the American College of Cardiology/American Heart Association Task Force on Practice Guidelines. Bethesda, MD: American College of Cardiology Foundation (ACCF), 82 pp.

Institute for Clinical Systems Improvement (ICSI). (2004, February). Heart failure in adults. *Institute for Clinical Systems Improvement,* 83 pp. Retrieved May 25, 2004, from http://www.guideline.gov/summary/summary.aspx

Institute for Clinical Symptoms Improvement (ICSI). (2007, April). Stable coronary artery disease. *Institute for Clinical Symptoms Improvement,* 45 pp. Retrieved June 16, 2009 from http://www.guideline.gov/summary/summary/aspx (Note: This article has a 2009 update as an addendum.)

Institute for Clinical Symptoms Improvement (ICSI). (2008a, October). Atrial fibrillation. *Institute for Clinical Systems Improvement.* 62 pp. Retrieved June 5, 2009, from http://www.guideline.gov/summary/summary.aspx

Institute for Clinical Symptoms Improvement (ICSI). (2008b, October). Diagnosis and treatment of chest pain and acute coronary syndrome (ACS). *Institute for Clinical Symptoms Improvement.* 69 pp. Retrieved June 5, 2009, from http://www.guideline.gov/summary/summary.aspx

Kaiser Permanente Care Management Institute. (2006). Secondary prevention of coronary artery disease clinical practice guideline. *Kaiser Permanente Care Management Institute,* 117 pp. Retrieved June 16, 2009, from http://www.guideline.gov/summary/summary.aspx

Katsung, B. (2004). *Basic and clinical pharmacology* (12th ed.). Stamford, CT: Appleton and Lange.

Levine, A., Muller, C., & Levine, T. (1998). Effects of high-dose lisinopril-isosorbide dinitrate on severe mitral regurgitation and heart failure remodeling. *American Journal of Cardiology, 82*(6), 1299–1301.

Magee, L., Helewa, M., Moutquin, J., von Dadelszen, P., & Hypertension Guideline Committee, Society of Obstetricians and Gynaecologists of Canada. (2008, March). Treatment of the hypertensive disorders of pregnancy. In: Diagnosis, evaluation, and management of the hypertensive disorders of pregnancy. *Journal of Obstetrics and Gynaecology of Canada, 30*(3 Suppl. 1), 24–36.

McCrindle, B., Urbina, E., Dennison, B., Jacobson, M., Steinberger, J., Rocchini, A., et al, American Heart Association Atherosclerosis, Hypertension and Obesity in Youth Committee, American Heart Association Council of Cardiovascular Disease in the Young, American Heart Association Council on Cardiovascular Nursing. (2007). Drug therapy of high-risk lipid abnormalities in children and adolescents. *Circulation, 115*(14), 1948–1967.

Mehra, A., Shotan, A., Ostrzega, E., Hsueh, W., Vasquez-Johnson, J., & Elkeayam, U. (1994). Potentiation of isosorbide dinitrate effects with *N*-acetylcysteine in patients with chronic heart failure. *Circulation, 89,* 2595–2600.

Mente, A., deKoning, L., Shannon, H., & Anand, S. (2009). A systematic review of the evidence supporting a causal link between dietary factors and coronary heart disease. *Archives of Internal Medicine, 169*(7), 659–669.

Meyers, C., Carr, M., Park, S., & Brunzell, J. (2003). Varying cost and free nicotinic acid content in over-the-counter niacin preparations for dyslipidemia. *Annals of Internal Medicine, 139*(12), 996–1002.

National Cholesterol Education Program (NCEP). (2001). *Third report of the Expert Panel on Detection, Evaluation, and Treatment of High Blood Cholesterol in Adults (Adult Treatment Panel III).* Rockville, MD: National Institutes of Health, National Heart, Lung, and Blood Institute.

National Collaborating Centre for Chronic Conditions (NCCC). (2003). *Chronic heart failure: National clinical guideline for diagnosis and management in primary and secondary care.* Salisbury, Wiltshire, England: Sarum ColourView Group.

National High Blood Pressure Education Program (NHBPEP). (2003). *The seventh report of the Joint National Committee on Prevention, Detection, Evaluation, and Treatment of High Blood Pressure.* Rockville, MD: National Institutes of Health, National Heart, Lung, and Blood Institute.

Nissen, S., Tuzcu, E., Schoenhagen, P., Brown, B., Ganz, P., Vogel, R., et al. (2004). Effect of intensive compared to moderate lipid-lowering therapy on progression of coronary atherosclerosis: A randomized controlled trial. *Journal of the American Medical Association, 291*(9), 1071–1080.

Packer, M., Gheorghiade, M., Young, J., Constantini, P., Adams, K., Cody, R., et al. (1993). Withdrawal of digoxin from patients with chronic heart failure treated with angiotensin-converting enzyme inhibitors. RADIANCE Study. *New England Journal of Medicine, 329,* 1–7.

Pitt, B., Segal, R., Martinez, F., Meurers, G., Cowley, A., Thomas, I., et al. (1997). Randomized trials of losartan versus captopril in patients over 65 with heart failure (Evaluation of Losartan in the Elderly Study, ELITE). *Lancet, 349*(9054), 747–752.

Remuzzi, G., Schieppati, A., & Ruggenenti, P. (2003). Nephropathy in patients with type 2 diabetes. *New England Journal of Medicine, 346*(15), 1145–1151.

Schaefer, E., McNamara, J., Tayler, T., Daly, J., Gleason, J., Seman, L., et al. (2003). Comparison of effects of statins (atorvastatin, fluvastatin, lovastatin, pravastatin and simvastatin) on fasting and postprandial lipoproteins in patients with coronary heart disease versus control subjects. *American Journal of Cardiology, 93,* 31–39.

Schneck, D., Knapp, R., Ballantyne, C., McPherson, R., Chitra, R., & Simonson, S. (2003). Comparative effects of rosuvastatin and atorvastatin across their dose ranges in patients with hypercholesterolemia and without active arterial disease. *American Journal of Cardiology, 91,* 33–41.

Snow, V., Barry, P., Fihn, S., Gibbons, R., Owens, D., Williams, S., et al. (2004). Primary care management of chronic stable angina and asymptomatic suspected or known coronary artery disease: A clinical practice guideline from the American College of Physicians. *Annals of Internal Medicine, 141*(7), 562–567.

University of Michigan Health System. (2009, February). UMHS hypertension guideline. Retrieved June 5, 2009, from University of Michigan Health System: Guidelines for clinical care.

Uretsky, B., Young, J., Shahidi, F., Yellen, L., Harrision, M., & Joily, M. (1993). Randomized study assessing the effect of digoxin withdrawal in patients with mild to moderate chronic congestive heart failure: Results of the PROVED trial. *Journal of the American College of Cardiology, 22,* 955–962.

Veterans Health Administration, Department of Defense (VA/DoD). (2003). *VA/DoD clinical practice guidelines for the management of ischemic heart disease.* Washington, DC: Veterans Health Administration, Department of Defense.

Veverka, A. (2004, November). Angiotensin and aldosterone antagonists after acute myocardial infarction. *Drugs Facts and Comparisons NEWS,* 83–86.

Viscoli, C., Horwitz, R., & Singer, B. (1993). Beta-blockers after myocardial infarction: Influence of first-year clinical course on long-term effectiveness. *Annals of Internal Medicine, 118,* 99.

Wade, V., & Gleason, B. (2004). Dual blockade of the renin-angiotensin system in diabetic nephropathy. *Annals of Pharmacotherapy, 38*(7), 1278–1282.

Wolters Kluwer Health. (2009). *Drug facts and comparisons.* St. Louis, MO: Wolters Kluwer Health.

Wright, J., Probstfield, J., Cushman, W., Pressel, S., Cutler, J., Davis, B., et al, for the ALLHAT Collaborative Research Group. (2009). ALLHAT findings revisited in the context of subsequent analyses, other trials, and meta-analyses. *Archives of Internal Medicine, 169*(9), 832–842.

Yim, B., & Chong, P. (2003). Niacin-ER and lovastatin treatment of hypercholesterolemia and mixed dyslipidemia. *Annals of Pharmacotherapy, 37,* 106–115.

CHAPTER 17

DRUGS AFFECTING THE RESPIRATORY SYSTEM

Teri Moser Woo

Chapter Outline

Numerous medications are available to treat disorders of the respiratory system. Those discussed in this chapter include **bronchodilators**, which act on the bronchial smooth muscle to reverse bronchospasm, and **leukotriene receptor agents**, which act to decrease the inflammation in the lungs of patients with asthma. **Antihistamines**, **decongestants**, **expectorants**, and **antitussives** are over-the-counter (OTC) medications included in this chapter. **Inhaled anti-inflammatory medications** used for asthma and **intranasal steroids** used for the treatment of seasonal or perennial rhinitis are also discussed. Prescribing recommendations for the multiple medications used in the treatment of asthma or chronic obstructive pulmonary disease (COPD) are provided in Chapter 30. IV forms of respiratory medications, which are rarely used in primary care, are not discussed here.

BRONCHODILATORS

Beta$_2$ Receptor Agonists

Beta$_2$ receptor agonist bronchodilator agents are widely used in caring for all ages of patients to treat reversible bronchoconstriction caused by asthma or reactive airway disease (RAD). A variety of **beta-agonist bronchodilators** are available, and the medications come in a variety of forms and delivery systems. Albuterol (Ventolin, Proventil) is the most commonly prescribed drug in this class. Other sympathomimetic **bronchodilator** medications used in primary care are **metaproterenol** (Alupent), **terbutaline** (Brethine, Brethaire), **bitolterol** (Tornalate), **pirbuterol** (Maxair), **levalbuterol** (Xopenex), **formoterol** (Foradil), and **salmeterol** (Serevent).

Pharmacodynamics

Bronchodilators act on the smooth muscle of the bronchial tree to reverse bronchospasm, thereby decreasing airway resistance and residual volume and increasing vital capacity and airflow. **Beta agonists** stimulate beta$_2$ adrenergic receptors in the lung to increase production of cyclic adenosine monophosphate (cAMP) by activation of adenyl cyclase, the enzyme that catalyzes the conversion of adenosine triphosphate (ATP) to cAMP. Increased cAMP concentrations relax bronchial smooth muscle and inhibit release of mediators of immediate hypersensitivity from cells, especially from the mast cells.

The perfect **bronchodilator** would work only on the beta$_2$ receptors in the lungs and have no other actions or systemic effects. Unfortunately, all of the currently available preparations have some effects on other body systems, such as the cardiovascular system, skeletal muscles, and central nervous system (CNS).

Albuterol is a selective **beta$_2$ agonist** with some minor beta$_1$ activity. It can increase heart rate by directly stimulating beta$_2$ receptors in the heart and by stimulating beta$_2$ receptors in vascular smooth muscle. The effect on cardiac beta$_2$ receptors is of consequence only at high serum levels of **albuterol** because it has a low affinity for these receptors and there are fewer beta$_2$ receptors than beta$_1$ receptors in the heart. Stimulation of the beta$_2$ receptors in the vascular smooth muscle leads to vasodilation, a decrease in diastolic blood pressure, and therefore a reflex increase in heart rate. **Albuterol** causes beta$_2$ receptor stimulation of skeletal muscle that leads to tremors. **Albuterol** has fewer cardiac and CNS effects than some of the other **beta agonists** and is, therefore, often the drug of choice for first-line therapy. **Levalbuterol** is similar to **albuterol**, where the (S)-isomer from racemic **albuterol** is removed, leaving the (R)-isomer, which has less adverse effects. **Pirbuterol** is a selective **beta$_2$ agonist** that is structurally identical to **albuterol**, except for the substitution of a pyridine ring for the benzene ring in their chemical makeup.

Terbutaline has a pharmacodynamic profile similar to that of **albuterol**, in that it is a selective **beta$_2$ agonist** with minor beta$_1$ activity. **Terbutaline** is also noted to inhibit uterine contractions via its beta receptor–mediated action on uterine smooth muscle. **Metaproterenol** is also a selective **beta$_2$ agonist** with some beta$_1$ activity, although it is less selective than **albuterol** or **terbutaline**. **Bitolterol** is hydrolyzed by the esterases in the lung to colterol, or terbutylnorepinephrine, which is a selective **beta$_2$ agonist**.

Salmeterol and **formoterol** are unique in that they are long-acting inhaled **bronchodilators** with a 12-hour half-life. **Salmeterol** is more selective for beta$_2$ receptors than is **albuterol** and has minor beta$_1$ activity. **Salmeterol** and **formoterol** exert long-lasting bronchoprotection effects against allergen-, exercise-, histamine-, and **methacholine**-caused bronchospasm.

Pharmacokinetics

Absorption and Distribution

Albuterol is most commonly inhaled and gradually absorbed from the bronchi. The overall systemic concentration remains low following recommended doses. The low systemic concentration is because of the need to use only 5 percent of the dose required orally to achieve the desired effects. Oral forms of **albuterol** are well absorbed from the gastrointestinal (GI) tract, rapidly enter the bloodstream, and are widely distributed in the body fluids and tissues. Extended-release oral **albuterol** is formulated to be absorbed from the stomach more slowly. Breast milk excretion is not known.

Levalbuterol is minimally absorbed from the respiratory tract and its distribution is unknown.

Pirbuterol is minimally absorbed from the respiratory tract, with amounts below the limits of serum assay detected after administration via inhalation. Its distribution is unknown.

Terbutaline is available in inhaled, oral, and subcutaneous (SC) forms. The inhaled form of **terbutaline** is minimally absorbed from the respiratory tract. Approximately 33 to 50 percent of the oral form is absorbed from the GI tract and is widely distributed. If administered SC, **terbutaline** is almost completely absorbed and is widely distributed. It crosses the placenta and is excreted in breast milk.

Metaproterenol may be administered via the inhaled route or orally. Approximately 3 percent of the inhaled **metaproterenol** dose is absorbed intact through the lungs. Oral dosing results in approximately 10 percent of the dose being absorbed intact. Distribution of **metaproterenol** is unknown.

Bitolterol absorption is too low to be measured by serum assay; distribution is unknown.

Salmeterol administered via inhaler is absorbed via the lungs in small amounts; undetectable amounts are found in the serum with recommended doses. With chronic administration, **salmeterol** is detected in the serum at very low levels. **Salmeterol** is excreted in breast milk in small amounts, approximately equal to plasma levels.

Formoterol is an inhaled dry powder capsule administered via a unique Aerolizer Inhaler™. The powdered medication is quickly absorbed in the lungs, with an onset of 1 to 3 minutes. There are no human studies of distribution of **formoterol** into breast milk; in rat studies, the drug could be measured in milk.

Metabolism and Excretion

Most of the common **bronchodilators** are metabolized in the liver and excreted primarily in the urine.

Albuterol is metabolized into **albuterol** 49-O-sulfate, which has little or no beta adrenergic–stimulating effect and no beta adrenergic–blocking effect. Approximately 72 percent of inhaled **albuterol** is excreted in the urine within 24 hours of inhalation, 28 percent of this as unchanged drug and 44 percent as the metabolite. Another 10 percent of the inhaled **albuterol** is excreted in the feces. Oral administration of **albuterol** results in 65 to 90 percent of the dose being excreted in the urine over 3 days, the majority in the first 24 hours. About 4 percent of the oral **albuterol** dose is excreted in feces.

Levalbuterol is metabolized and excreted in the same fashion as **albuterol**.

Pirbuterol is not metabolized extensively, with 51 percent of the dose excreted in the urine as **pirbuterol** plus its sulfate conjugate. **Terbutaline** is partially metabolized in the liver, primarily to inactive sulfate conjugate, and is excreted in the urine. **Metaproterenol** is metabolized by the liver into its sulfate conjugate and excreted in the urine. **Bitolterol** is a prodrug that is hydrolyzed by esterases in tissue and blood to the active moiety colterol. Within 24 hours, 83 percent of the dose is excreted in the urine. After 72 hours, 85.6 percent of the dose has been excreted in the urine and 8 percent in the feces, as conjugated colterol.

Salmeterol xinafoate, as ionic salt, dissociates so that the **salmeterol** and 1-hydroxy-2-naphthoic acid (xinafoate) are metabolized and excreted independently. **Salmeterol** base is extensively metabolized by hydroxylation in the liver. Urinary elimination accounts for 25 percent of the drug, and 60 percent is eliminated in the feces over a period of 7 days. The xinafoate moiety has no apparent pharmacological activity, is extensively protein bound, and has a long elimination half-life of 11 days.

Formoterol fumarate is metabolized by glucuronidation in the liver. Renal elimination accounts for 59 to 62 percent of elimination; 32 to 34 percent is eliminated in the feces.

Table 17–1 shows the pharmacokinetic properties of selected **bronchodilators**.

Pharmacotherapeutics

Precautions and Contraindications

Sympathomimetic **bronchodilators** have relatively few contraindications to use. Cardiac arrhythmias associated with tachycardia, tachycardia, or heart block caused by digitalis intoxication, angina, narrow-angle glaucoma, organic brain damage (epinephrine only), and shock during general anesthesia with halogenated agents are all contraindications to **beta$_2$ agonists**. Because of these drugs' effects on the cardiovascular system, patients with hypertension, ischemic heart disease, coronary insufficiency, congestive heart failure, and a history of stroke and/or cardiac arrhythmias should be monitored closely for adverse effects during administration of any of the sympathomimetic **bronchodilators**. For patients with diabetes mellitus, there is a potential drug-induced hyperglycemia that may result in loss of diabetic control when using any of the **beta$_2$ agonists**, and their insulin dosage may need to be increased. For patients with hyperthyroidism, adverse reactions are more likely to occur with the use of **bronchodilators**. Patients taking **digoxin** require close monitoring when **albuterol** is started because **albuterol** increases the volume of distribution of **digoxin** and can cause up to a 30 percent decrease in blood

Table 17–1 ▶ **Pharmacokinetics: Selected Bronchodilators**

Drug	Onset	Peak	Duration	Half-Life	Metabolism	Elimination
Beta$_2$ Agonists						
Albuterol					Hepatic	Renal 90%; fecal
Inhalation	5–15 min	0.5–2 h	2–6 h	3.8 h		10%
Oral short-acting	15–30 min	2–3 h	4–6 h	2.7–5 h		
Oral extended-release			8–12 h			
Bitolterol				UK	Hydrolyzed by esterases in tissues and blood to colterol	Renal
Inhalation	3–4 min	0.5–1 h	5–8 h			
Formoterol	1–3 min	15 min	12 h	10-14 h	Hepatic	Renal
Levalbuterol	10–17 min	1.5 h	5–6 h	3.3–4.0 h	Hepatic	Renal
Metaproterenol				UK	Hepatic	Renal
Inhalation	1 min	1 h	1–2.5 h			
Nebulization	5–30 min	1 h	4 h			
Oral	15–30 min	1 h	4 h			
Pirbuterol	5 min	0.5–1 h	5 h	2 h	Hepatic	Renal
Inhalation	5 min	0.5–1 h	5 h			
Salmeterol	14 min	3–4 h	12 h	2.5 h	Hydroxylation	Feces
Inhalation						
Terbutaline				UK	Liver (partial)	Renal; small amount in bile, feces
Inhalation	5–30 min	—	3–6 h			
Oral	30 min	—	4–8 h			

Continued

Table 17–1 ▶ **Pharmacokinetics: Selected Bronchodilators—cont'd**

Drug	Onset	Peak	Duration	Half-Life	Metabolism	Elimination
Anticholinergic						
Ipratropium Inhalation	 15–30 min	 1–2 h	 4–5 h	2 h	Ester hydrolysis	Renal
Xanthine Derivatives						
Theophylline Immediate-release Extended-release Liquid		2h 4–7 h 1 h	—	*Children <6 mo:* >24 h; >6 mo: 1.1–3.7 h *Adult nonsmokers:* 8.7–2.2 h; *adult smokers:* 4–5 h; adults with COPD, congestive heart failure (CHF), cor pulmonale, or liver disease may exceed 24 h	Liver	Renal

UK = unknown.

digoxin levels. Patients with diagnosed or suspected pheochromocytoma should avoid the **beta-adrenergic antagonists** because severe hypertension may occur.

Lower doses of **bronchodilators** may be necessary in older adults because of increased sympathomimetic sensitivity.

In the **Salmeterol** Multicenter Asthma Research Trial (SMART), there was a small but statistically significant increase in respiratory-related and asthma-related deaths in the study population receiving **salmeterol** versus placebo (Nelson, et al, 2006). The study was terminated early owing to these findings. Further analysis indicates that the risk may be greater for African Americans than for white subjects (Nelson et al, 2006). The U.S. Food and Drug Administration (FDA) subsequently issued a black box warning for **salmeterol** and **formoterol** in 2005 and in December 2008 a follow-up FDA advisory was issued stating that the risks of **salmeterol (Serevent)** and **formoterol (Foradil)** outweighed the benefits and should not be used singly in asthma for all ages. The safety and risks of the **long-acting beta agonists (LABAs)** continued to be studied with an emphasis on examining the risk for intubation and death in patients who use **LABAs**. Salpeter, Wall, and Buckley (2010) conducted a meta-analysis of pooled data of randomized controlled trials (RCTs) totaling 36,588 patients and found a 2-fold increase in catastrophic events (asthma related intubations and death) in patients who were treated with **LABAs**. In February 2010 the FDA released a safety announcement regarding **LABAs**:

To ensure the safe use of these products:

- The use of **LABAs** is contraindicated without the use of an asthma controller medication such as an inhaled corticosteroid. Single-ingredient **LABAs** should only be used in combination with an asthma controller medication; they should not be used alone.
- **LABAs** should only be used long-term in patients whose asthma cannot be adequately controlled on asthma controller medications.
- **LABAs** should be used for the shortest duration of time required to achieve control of asthma symptoms and discontinued, if possible, once asthma control is achieved. Patients should then be maintained on an asthma controller medication.
- Pediatric and adolescent patients who require the addition of a **LABA** to an **inhaled corticosteroid** should use a combination product containing both an **inhaled corticosteroid** and a **LABA**, to ensure compliance with both medications. (http://www.fda.gov/Safety/MedWatch/SafetyInformation/SafetyAlertsforHumanMedicalProducts/ucm201003.htm)

Providers should use caution when prescribing **LABAs** and provide close follow-up to ensure patient safety.

Terbutaline is Pregnancy Category B; the rest of the **beta-agonist bronchodilators** are Pregnancy Category C. No reports linking the use of **albuterol** with human congenital anomalies have been published. **Terbutaline** is used during pregnancy to prevent contractions related to preterm labor. This is not an FDA-approved use; therefore, oral forms of the **beta agonists** should be used selectively in patients in labor. Inhaled forms of the **beta agonists** are less likely to affect uterine contractions.

Small amounts of **terbutaline** and **salmeterol** can be measured in breast milk. The other inhaled **beta-agonist bronchodilators** cannot be measured in breast milk, probably because of the small amount of drug that is used and absorbed. The use of inhaled **bronchodilators** during lactation is most likely safe, with careful monitoring of the infant.

Albuterol is used extensively in infants and children with minimal adverse effects. **Metaproterenol** may also be used in young children, although **albuterol** is generally the first-choice medication. Dosing guidelines are provided on the label by the manufacturer of **levalbuterol** for children down to age 6 years, although a study of safety and efficacy in 2- to 5-year-olds indicated that the drug was effective and well tolerated by younger children (Skoner et al, 2005). **Salmeterol** should not be prescribed to children younger than age 4 years. **Terbutaline** may be safely prescribed to children, although it is not a first-line **beta agonist** for asthma. The safety of **pirbuterol** and **bitolterol** for use in children aged 12 years and under has not been established.

Adverse Drug Reactions

Adverse reactions to the **beta-agonist bronchodilators** are usually transient and discontinuing the medication is not usually necessary, but a temporary reduction in the dose may alleviate some of the side effects. Slowly increase the dose after the reaction to the optimal dosing has subsided.

Supraventricular and ventricular ectopic beats have occurred with **beta-agonist** inhalation, but the incidence is low (**bitolterol** 0.5%, **terbutaline** about 4%, **pirbuterol** less than 1%). Tachycardia and palpitations are reported in 14 percent of patients who use these sympathomimetic **bronchodilators**.

The **beta-agonist bronchodilators** exhibit some CNS excitation effects, with tremors, dizziness, shakiness, nervousness, and restlessness reported in some patients. Headaches may occur with **bronchodilator** use in 2 to 28 percent of patients. Insomnia is rare, reported in 1 to 3 percent of patients.

Salmeterol has an increased risk of exacerbation of severe asthma symptoms if the patient is deteriorating. To avoid this risk, LABAs should not be started in patients with acutely deteriorating asthma.

Drug Interactions

Because of the cardiovascular effects of the **bronchodilators**, careful monitoring for drug interactions is necessary. If any of the **beta agonists** are prescribed with **digitalis glycosides**, caution and careful monitoring of the patient's electrocardiogram (ECG) is necessary because there is an increased risk of cardiac arrhythmia.

Beta agonists used with **beta-adrenergic blocking agents** (including ophthalmic preparations) may result in mutual inhibition of therapeutic effects. **Tricyclic antidepressants** and **monoamine oxidase inhibitors** (MAOIs) used with **albuterol, metaproterenol,** or **terbutaline** may potentiate the effects of the **bronchodilator** on the vascular system. Table 17–2 shows drug interaction information.

Table 17–2 ■ **Drug Interactions: Selected Bronchodilators**

Drug	Interacting Drug	Possible Effect	Implications
Beta$_2$ Agonists			
Albuterol	Digoxin	Digoxin serum levels may be decreased	Decreased dose of albuterol may be needed
	Other sympathomimetics	Additive effects	Serious adverse cardiac effects; do not use concurrently
	MAOIs	Potentiates albuterol	Severe hypertension, headache, hyperpyrexia, and possible hypertensive crisis; do not use concurrently
	Tricyclic antidepressants	Potentiates the pressor response of sympathomimetics	Arrhythmias if used concurrently
	Beta blockers (including ophthalmic agents)	Mutual inhibition of therapeutic effects	Should not be used together
	Cocaine	Increased CNS stimulation	Observe patients for cardiac and CNS effects
	Thyroid hormones	Cardiac effects of both drugs enhanced	Increased risk of coronary insufficiency from combined use of these drugs; avoid this combination in patients with preexisting cardiac disease
	Ritodrine	Increased CNS stimulation	Avoid concurrent use
Bitolterol	Other sympathomimetics	Additive effects	Serious adverse cardiac effects; avoid concurrent use of sympathomimetics
	MAOIs	Potentiates bitolterol	Severe hypertension, headache, hyperpyrexia, and possible hypertensive crisis; do not use together

Continued

Table 17–2 ▣ **Drug Interactions: Selected Bronchodilators—cont'd**

Drug	Interacting Drug	Possible Effect	Implications
	Tricyclic antidepressants	Potentiates the pressor response of sympathomimetics	May cause arrhythmias; do not use together
	Beta blockers (including ophthalmic agents)	Mutual inhibition of therapeutic effects	Should not be used together
Levalbuterol	Beta blockers	Mutual inhibition of therapeutic effects	Should not be used together
	MAOIs	Potentiates albuterol	Severe hypertension, headache, hyperpyrexia, and possible hypertensive crisis; do not use concurrently
	Tricyclic antidepressants	Potentiates the pressor response of sympathomimetics	Arrhythmias if used concurrently
	Digoxin	Digoxin serum levels may be decreased	Decreased dose of albuterol may be needed
	Other sympathomimetics	Additive effects	Serious adverse cardiac effects; do not use concurrently
Metaproterenol	Other sympathomimetics	Additive effects	Serious adverse cardiac effects; avoid concurrent use
	MAOIs	Potentiates metaproterenol	Severe hypertension, headache, hyperpyrexia, and possible hypertensive crisis; do not use together
	Tricyclic antidepressants	Potentiates the pressor response of sympathomimetics	May cause arrhythmias; do not use together
	Beta blockers (including ophthalmic agents)	Mutual inhibition of therapeutic effects	Should not be used together
	Inhalation anesthetics	Sensitizes the myocardium to the effects of metaproterenol	May cause arrhythmias; use with caution and, if possible, avoid concurrent use
	Theophylline or caffeine	Additive toxic effects	CNS stimulation or toxicity a concern; use with caution and close monitoring
	Thyroid hormones	Cardiac effects of both drugs enhanced	Increased risk of coronary insufficiency from the combined use of these drugs; use with caution in patients with preexisting cardiac disease
Pirbuterol	Other beta agonists	Additive effects	Increased adverse effects; avoid concurrent use
	MAOIs, tricyclic antidepressants	Potentiates pirbuterol	Severe hypertension, headache, hyperpyrexia, and possible hypertensive crisis; do not use within 14 d of each other
Salmeterol	Beta blockers (including ophthalmic agents)	Mutual inhibition	Avoid concurrent use
	MAOIs, tricyclic antidepressants	Potentiates vascular effects of salmeterol	Severe hypertension, headache, hyperpyrexia, and possible hypertensive crisis; do not use concurrently
Terbutaline	Halogenated anesthetics	Sensitizes the myocardium to the effects of terbutaline	Ventricular arrhythmias; do not use concurrently
	MAOIs, tricyclic antidepressants, maprotiline	Potentiates vascular effects of terbutaline	Severe hypertension, headache, hyperpyrexia, and possible hypertensive crisis; do not use concurrently
			Decreased antihypertensive effect; should not be used together

Table 17–2 ■ **Drug Interactions: Selected Bronchodilators—cont'd**

Drug	Interacting Drug	Possible Effect	Implications
	Beta blockers and other antihypertensive agents	Mutual inhibition	Do not use together
	Cocaine	Increased CNS and cardiac stimulation	Observe patients for arrhythmias
	Cardiac glycosides, levodopa	Increased potential for cardiac arrhythmias	Dosage of cardiac glycoside or levodopa should be decreased and the patient closely monitored
Anticholinergics			
Ipratropium	Cromolyn inhalation solution	Forms a precipitate when mixed together	Do not mix
Xanthine Derivatives			
Theophylline	Allopurinol, beta blockers, calcium channel blockers, cimetidine, ciprofloxacin oral contraceptives, corticosteroids, disulfiram, ephedrine, influenza virus vaccine, interferon, macrolides, mexiletine, quinolones, thiabendazole, thyroid hormones, carbamazepine, isoniazid, loop diuretics, fluvoxamine, ticlopidine, propafenone	Increased serum theophylline levels if taken concurrently	Lower doses of theophylline may be necessary; monitor theophylline level closely when starting, stopping, or changing the dose of these medications; doses of theophylline may need to be temporarily decreased after administration of influenza vaccine
	Aminoglutethimide, barbiturates, charcoal, hydantoins, ketoconazole, rifampin, smoking (cigarettes, marijuana), sulfinpyrazone, beta agonists, thioamines, carbamazepine, isoniazid, loop diuretics, lansoprazole, primidone, ritonavir	Decreased serum theophylline levels if taken concurrently	Increased doses of theophylline may be necessary; monitor theophylline level closely when starting, stopping, or changing the dose of these medications; theophylline toxicity may occur if these medications are stopped suddenly
	Inhalation anesthetics	Increased risk of cardiac arrhythmias	Avoid or use with caution
	Sympathomimetics	May cause excessive stimulation, nervousness, irritability, and insomnia	Avoid concurrent use or use with caution
	Lithium	Theophylline may increase renal clearance of lithium	Monitor lithium clinical effectiveness if theophylline is prescribed
	Zafirlukast	May increase theophylline levels if added to an existing theophylline regimen	Monitor theophylline levels closely after adding zafirlukast to the treatment regimen

Clinical Use and Dosing

Bronchospasm

The **bronchodilators** are used primarily in the treatment of bronchospasm associated with asthma, bronchitis (acute or chronic), and COPD.

The dose of **albuterol** metered-dose inhaler (MDI) in children over age 4 years and adults is two puffs every 4 to 6 hours. The dose of **albuterol (Ventolin, Proventil)** delivered via nebulizer for children over age 12 years as well as for adults is 2.5 mg (0.5 mL) in 2 mL normal saline; for younger children up to 15 kg, the dose is 0.1 to 0.15 mg/kg per dose. For children over 15 kg, the dose is the same as it is for adults, 2.5 mg/dose. Inhaled forms of **albuterol** may be repeated once after 5 to 10 minutes, up to two times (three doses total) during exacerbations. The oral **albuterol** dose in adults is 2 to 4 mg three or four times a day, up to a maximum of 32 mg/day. For children aged 6 to 12 years, 2 mg **albuterol** three or four times a day may be prescribed, although oral **albuterol** is rarely used in children. If prescribing to children under age 6 years **albuterol** syrup is dosed at 0.1 mg/kg three times a day. **Albuterol** syrup is rarely used because the inhaled form is more effective and has less adverse effects.

The recommended dose of **levalbuterol (Xopenex)** in adolescents over age 12 years and adults is 0.63 mg three times a day, every 6 to 8 hours. Dosing for children aged 6 to 11 years is 0.31 mg three times a day per the manufacturer's label, with routine dosing not to exceed 0.63 mg three times a day. In the Skoner and colleagues (2005) study, children aged 2 to 5 years were dosed at both 0.31 mg and 0.63 mg three times a day without regard to weight; both doses were tolerated by the children, although they had less variation in heart rate when dosed at 0.31 mg. The authors recommend dosing young children at 0.31 mg three times a day, but note that 0.63 mg may be indicated for some patients. *Expert Panel Report 3: Guidelines for the Diagnosis and Management of Asthma* (National Asthma Education and Prevention Program [NAEPP], 2007) recommend dosing **levalbuterol** via nebulizer, administering 0.31 to 1.25 mg in 3 mL of normal saline every 4 to 6 hours to children 4 years of age or younger, although the NAEPP notes that **levalbuterol** is not FDA approved for children younger than 6 years.

Metaproterenol (Alupent) comes in MDI, inhalation solution, and syrup forms. The dose of **metaproterenol** MDI in children over age 12 years and adults is two to three inhalations every 3 to 4 hours, not to exceed 12 inhalations per day. The dose of **metaproterenol** delivered via nebulizer in children age 12 years and older and adults is 0.1 to 0.2 mL of 5 percent solution diluted in 2.5 mL normal saline up to every 4 hours. **Metaproterenol** is also available in nebulizer solution. The dose for infants and children of **metaproterenol** nebulizer solution is 5 to 15 mg diluted in 2 to 3 mL of normal saline every 4 to 6 hours. For adolescents and adults, the dose of **metaproterenol** nebulizer solution is 10 to 15 mg every 4 to 6 hours. **Metaproterenol** MDI is not recommended for children under age 12 years; oral syrup or nebulizer solution is the suggested therapy in this age group. **Metaproterenol** syrup dose in children over age 9 years 20 mg (10 mL) three or four times a day. For children aged 6 to 9 years, the dose of **metaproterenol** syrup is 10 mg (5 mL) three or four times a day. The dose of **metaproterenol** in children aged 2 to 6 years is 1.3 to 2.6 mg/kg per day in doses divided to take three or four times a day. Children under age 2 years are dosed at 0.4 mg/kg per dose given three to four times a day; infants should be dosed every 8 to 12 hours.

Terbutaline is available in MDI (**Brethaire**), oral tablets (**Brethine**), or parenteral form for SC injection. The dose of **terbutaline** MDI in children age 12 and older and adults is two puffs every 4 to 6 hours. The dose of oral **terbutaline** for bronchospasm in adolescents age 15 or older and adults is 5 mg three times a day, with a maximum of 15 mg in 24 hours. For children aged 12 to 15 years, the dose of **terbutaline** is 2.5 mg three times a day, with a maximum dose of 7.5 mg in 24 hours. Children less than age 12 years are dosed at 0.5 mg/kg every 8 hours, which may be gradually increased up to 0.15 mg/kg per dose, with a maximum daily dose of 5 mg. The dose of parenteral **terbutaline** (**Brethine** injection) in adults is 0.25 mg SC in the lateral deltoid. The dose may be repeated in 15 to 30 minutes. The maximum dose is 0.75 mg in 4 hours.

Pirbuterol is available only in MDI form (**Maxair Autohaler**). The dose of **pirbuterol** in children over age 12 years and adults is one to two inhalations every 4 to 6 hours for a maximum of 12 inhalations in 24 hours. Younger children are dosed at 4 to 8 inhalations every 20 minutes for a total of three doses, then every 1 to 4 hours. Maintenance therapy for children and adults is two inhalations three to four times a day.

Bitolterol (Tornalate) is available in MDI form. The adult dose to treat acute bronchospasm is two puffs, 1 to 3 minutes apart, followed by a third puff if needed. For prevention of bronchospasm, the adult dose is two puffs every 8 hours. **Bitolterol** is not recommended for use in children younger than 12 years.

Salmeterol (Serevent DISKUS) is a long-acting **bronchodilator** available in powder for oral inhalation, packaged in a specially designed plastic delivery device that delivers 50 mcg per inhalation. The dose for children age 4 years and older and adults to control asthma and to prevent bronchospasm is one actuation/puff twice a day. **Salmeterol** is not to be used for short-term bronchospasm relief. If prescribing **salmeterol** for persistent asthma, the drug must be prescribed in conjunction with an inhaled **corticosteroid** or other asthma-controller medication. **LABAs** should be prescribed for as short a time as possible to get the asthma under control, and then patients are maintained on their controller medication. To prevent exercise-induced bronchospasm, the dose of one actuation/ puff (50 mcg) is inhaled 30 minutes before exercise. Patients who are using **salmeterol** twice a day for asthma control should not use an additional dose before exercise. Frequent use of **LABAs** for exercise-induced asthma is discouraged by the *Expert Panel 3* guidelines as they may be masking persistent asthma.

Patients also need to have a short-acting **bronchodilator** prescribed for them to use for short-term relief, and they need to be educated not to use **salmeterol** for acute exacerbations. **Salmeterol** is packaged in combination with **fluticasone (Advair DISKUS)** with differing dosages of **fluticasone** (100 mcg, 250 mcg, 500 mcg per actuation) combined with 50 mcg of **salmeterol (Advair DISKUS 100/50, Advair DISKUS 250/50, Advair DISKUS 500/50)**. The FDA recommends pediatric and adolescent patients who require the addition of a LABA to an inhaled corticosteroid be prescribed a combination product to increase compliance and ensure patient safety (U.S. Food and Drug Administration, 2010). Dosing is covered in the inhaled Corticosteroid section of this chapter.

Fomoterol is packaged as a 12-mcg, single-use dry powder capsule. Dosing for children older than age 5 years or adults is one capsule every 12 hours. Children younger than age 4 years cannot generate enough inspiratory flow to administer the dry powder capsules.

Ipratropium is an inhaled **anticholinergic** that may be used in combination with **albuterol** to treat asthma exacerbation in the emergency department (NAEPP, 2007). Hospital admission may be avoided by the addition of **ipratropium** to treatment regimen in cases of exacerbation seen in the clinic or emergency department. **Ipratropium** is the **bronchodilator** of choice in patients who are taking **beta blockers** or who do not tolerate **beta$_2$ agonists.**

Exercise-Induced Bronchospasm

Bronchodilators used just before exercise can prevent exercise-induced bronchospasm (EIB). The medications recommended by the *Expert Panel Report 3: Guidelines for the Diagnosis and Management of Asthma* (NAEPP, 2007) are inhaled **albuterol** or other **short-acting beta$_2$ agonist** and **salmeterol**. The dose of **albuterol** MDI to prevent exercise-induced bronchospasm is two puffs 15 minutes prior to exercise. **Albuterol** used this way should prevent exercise-induced bronchospasm for 2 to 3 hours. The dose of **salmeterol** is two puffs 30 to 60 minutes prior to exercise. **Salmeterol** should prevent exercise-induced bronchospasm for 10 to 12 hours. **Salmeterol** and other **long-acting beta$_2$ agonists** have shortened duration of action if used on a daily basis (NAEPP, 2007). **Cromolyn** or **nedocromyl** may be used before exercise, but they are not as effective as short-acting **beta$_2$ agonists. Leukotriene modifiers** may improve EIB in up to 50 percent of patients (NAEPP, 2007). Table 17–3 presents dosage recommendations.

Rational Drug Selection

The Expert Panel Report 3 does not differentiate or recommend a specific **short-acting beta$_2$ agonist** for use in asthma. Therefore, the practitioner who is prescribing for adults may choose any of the short-acting **bronchodilators.** Choosing an appropriate **bronchodilator** is a matter of the age of the patient and the cost.

Table 17–3 ◉ **Dosage Schedule: Selected Bronchodilators**

Drug	Indication	Dose	Comments
Beta$_2$ Agonists			
Albuterol	Bronchospasm associated with asthma or COPD	*Inhaled:* 2 puffs q4–6h *Nebulizer* (run over 10–15 min) *Adults:* dilute 0.5 mL of 0.5% solution in 3 mL normal saline OR give 1 unit dose *Children:* 0.01–0.05 mL/kg of 0.5% solution diluted in 2 mL normal saline *Oral* *Adults:* 2–4 mg tid or qid up to a max of 32 mg/day *Children 6–12 yr:* 2 mg tid or qid *Children <6 yr:* 0.1 mg/kg divided tid	May repeat dose in 20 min × 3 during exacerbations; check proper inhaler technique with every clinic visit min 0.25 mL max 1.0 mL
	Exercise-induced asthma	*Inhaled:* 2 puffs 5 min prior to exercise	
Bitolterol	Acute bronchospasm	*Inhaled* *Children >12 yr and adults:* 2 puffs 1–3 min apart, followed by a third puff if needed	Not recommended for children <12 yr
	Bronchospasm prevention	*Inhaled:* 2 puffs every 8 h	

Continued

Table 17–3 ◉ **Dosage Schedule: Selected Bronchodilators—cont'd**

Drug	Indication	Dose	Comments
Formoterol	Long-acting bronchodilator for preventing bronchospasm	*Children >5 yr and adults:* 12 mg (contents of one capsule) q12h	Should not be used as monotherapy for asthma
	Prevention of Exercise-induced asthma	*Children >5 yr and adults:* 12 mg (contents of one capsule) 15 min before exercise	Should not use a second dose within 12 h
Levalbuterol	Bronchospasm in patients with reversible obstructive airway disease	HFA MDI: ≥4 yr: 1–2 puffs every 4–6 h *Nebulizer* *Children ≥12 yr and adults:* 0.63 mg 3 times a day every 6–8 h; may be increased to 1.25 mg 3 times a day *Children 6–11 yr:* 0.31 mg 3 times a day every 6–8 h; not to exceed 0.63 mg 3 times a day *Children 2–6 yr:* Not labeled for use in this age. See comments	*Children 2–5 yr:* 0.31–0.63 mg every 6–8 h; 0.31 mg well tolerated (Skoner et al, 2005)
Metaproterenol	Bronchospasm associated with asthma or COPD	*Inhaler* *Children >12 yr and adults:* 2–3 inhalations every 3–4 h; do not exceed 12 inhalations/d *Nebulizer* *Children >6 yr and adults:* 0.1–0.2 mL of 5% solution diluted in 2.5 mL normal saline up to every 4 h *Hand bulb nebulizer* *Children >12 yr and adults:* 5–15 (usually 10) inhalations every 4 h or 3–4 times/d (chronic use) *Syrup* *Children >9 yr or who weigh >60 lb:* 20 mg (10 mL) tid or qid *Children 6–9 yr who weigh <60 lb:* 10 mg (5 mL) tid or qid *Children <6 yr:* 1.3–2.6 mg/kg/d in doses divided tid or qid	Metaproterenol MDI not recommended in children <12 yr: Nebulizer solution not recommended in children <6 yr; oral syrup is the suggested therapy in this age group
Pirbuterol	Bronchospasm associated with asthma	*Inhaled* *Children >4 yr and adults:* 2 puffs every 6–8 h (NIH guidelines)	Not recommended for children <4 yr
Salmeterol	Long-acting bronchodilator for preventing bronchospasm	*Inhaled DISKUS* *Children >4 yr and adults:* 1 actuation/puff bid, 12 h apart	Not to be used for short-term relief or acute exacerbations; patients need to have a short-acting bronchodilator also prescribed for them. If using salmeterol for asthma control, patients should not use another dose for exercise-induced asthma; a short-acting bronchodilator or cromolyn should be used
	Exercise-induced asthma	*Inhaled Diskus* 1 puff/actuation 30–60 min before exercise	
Terbutaline	Bronchospasm associated with asthma or COPD	*Inhaled* 2 puffs every 4–6 h; do not repeat more often than every 4–6 h	Not recommended in children <12 yr

Table 17–3 ◉ **Dosage Schedule: Selected Bronchodilators—cont'd**

Drug	Indication	Dose	Comments
		Oral *Children >15 yr and adults:* 5 mg tid; max 15 mg/24 h *Children 12–15 yr:* 2.5 mg tid; max 7.5 mg/24 h *Parenteral* *Adults:* 0.5 mg SC in the lateral deltoid; may repeat in 15–30 min; maximum dose is 0.5 mg in 4 h *Children <12 yr:* 0.05 mg/kg every 8 hr. May increase to 0.15 mg/kg dose. Maximum 5 mg/d	Terbutaline is used to control premature contractions in pregnant women, so use with care in the patient in the third trimester nearing due date because it may affect labor
Anticholinergics			
Ipratropium	Bronchospasm associated with asthma or COPD	*Acute Exacerbation of Asthma* (NIH guidelines) *Children:* Nebulization: 250 mcg of 20 min × 3 doses then every 2–4 h MDI: 4–8 puffs as needed *Children >12 yr and adults:* Nebulization 500 mcg of 30 min _ 3 then every 2–4 h MDI: 4–8 puffs as needed *Asthma Maintenance* (NIH Guidelines) *Children:* Nebulization: 250–500 mcg of 6 h MDI: 1–2 inhalations of 6 h; max 12 puffs/day *Children >12 yr and adults:* Nebulization: 250 mcg of 6 h MDI: 2–3 inhalations of 6 h; max 12 puffs/day *COPD* MDI: *Adults:* 2 puffs qid, may increase to 12 puffs/day Nebulizer: One unit-dose vial 500 mcg 3–4 times a day via nebulizer	Contraindicated in patients with soybean or peanut allergy. Ipratropium can be mixed with albuterol 0.5% solution for nebulizer use if used within 1 h
Combination Medications			
Albuterol/ ipratropium (Combivent)	Bronchospasm associated with COPD, not controlled with one bronchodilator alone	*Inhaled* *Adults:* 2 puffs qid *Children <12 yr:* 1–2 puffs qid *Nebulizer* *Adults:* 3 mL q4–6h *Children:* 1.5 to 3 mL q8h	Primarily used for COPD patients; simplifies medication regimen by combining two commonly prescribed medications
Xanthine Derivatives			
Theophylline	Bronchospasm associated with asthma, COPD, and bronchitis	The dose for asthma and COPD is variable with the patient's weight and serum theophylline levels *Adults* (>16): Initially: 6 mg/kg/24 h or 400 mg/24 h tid or qid; the dose is increased every 3 d in 25% increments until desired serum theophylline levels are achieved (ideally between 10 and 20 mcg/mL); max dose: 13 mg/kg/d	Dosing adjustments are made based on the serum theophylline level: If the level is 5–10 mcg/mL, the dose is increased by 25% every 3 days until desired serum concentrations of theophylline are reached; if the serum concentration is between 10 and 15 mcg/mL, maintain dosage if tolerated and

Continued

Table 17–3 ◉ **Dosage Schedule: Selected Bronchodilators—cont'd**

Drug	Indication	Dose	Comments
		Children 1–9 yr: Initially: 16 mg/kg/24 h; max 400 mg/d; dosage may be increased by 25% every 3 days to a maximum based on age (1–9 yr, max 24 mg/kg/day, 9–12 yr, max 20 mg/kg/day; 12–16 yr, max daily dose is 18 mg/kg Monitoring for serum theophylline levels is the same in children as for adults, with a steady state theophylline level of 5–15 mcg/mL the goal	recheck at 6- to 12-mo intervals; if level is 15–19.9 mcg/mL, consider decreasing dose by 10% to provide a greater margin of safety; if the level is 20–25 mcg/mL, then decrease dose by 10% and recheck level in 3 d; if serum level is 25–30 mcg/mL, then decrease subsequent doses by 25%, and redraw level in 3 d; if theophylline level is >30 mcg/mL, then skip next 2 doses, decrease dose by 50%, and recheck in 3 days
Caffeine citrate	Apnea of prematurity	Loading dose: 10–20 mg/kg Maintenance: 5 mg/kg/d	If theophylline has been given in last 3 d, decrease loading dose by 50%–75%

Patient Age

The only short-acting **bronchodilators** that can be prescribed for children under age 4 years are **albuterol** and **metaproterenol. Levalbuterol** is labeled to be used in children older than age 4 years, and the *Expert Panel 3* (NAEPP, 2007) guidelines indicate **levalbuterol** should not be used in children younger than age 4 years. **Albuterol** is by far the most often used medication in clinical practice and is safe to use even in infants.

Cost

Of the short-acting **bronchodilators, albuterol** is the least expensive, especially if a generic formula is prescribed.

Monitoring

There is no specific monitoring required for **bronchodilators.** As a part of overall asthma management, pulmonary function and response to **bronchodilators** should be monitored with a peak flowmeter. If a patient is on **digitalis,** an ECG should be done prior to starting a **beta agonist** and routinely during therapy to detect cardiac arrhythmias that may occur.

Patient Education

Administration

The **bronchodilator** should be used as prescribed. Overuse of **bronchodilators** will lead to increased adverse effects, and using the **bronchodilator** less than prescribed may lead to increased bronchospasm and decreased pulmonary function.

The administration of **bronchodilators** via MDI can be difficult for most adults and all children. Learning to coordinate the release of the medication from the inhaler with a deep breath is difficult. Written and pictorial instructions are available with the inhaler, but the provider must not assume that the patient understands the proper method of administering inhaled medications. It is recommended that a spacer device be used with MDIs (Aerochamber, InspirEase). Use verbal instructions as well as actual demonstration with a placebo inhaler to reinforce the written instructions. These instructions and demonstrations should be repeated at follow-up visits.

To use an inhaler properly, the patient should first exhale and then tilt the head slightly back and place the inhaler mouthpiece either about 2 inches from the open mouth or between the open lips. While inhaling, the patient should press down on the canister, breathe in slowly and deeply, and hold his or her breath for 10 seconds (count of 10) or as long as comfortable. If two puffs are prescribed, then the patient should wait at least 1 full minute between inhalations.

CLINICAL PEARL

Administering Medications Via A Nebulizer to Infants and Toddlers

Administering a medication via a nebulizer to an infant or toddler is, at times, a challenge. A pediatric mask may be used if the child tolerates it. One trick is to "blow" the nebulized medication into the patient's face near the nose and mouth. This is achieved by occluding the mouthpiece end of the unit and aiming the "tail" end toward the patient's nose and mouth. This is especially effective if the child is sleeping and needs the medication.

Another suggestion to parents of young children is to read a book to the child during the treatment or play an appropriate short video to make the time pass more quickly.

To assist with the delivery of inhaled medications, a spacer can be prescribed. The Aerochamber is a tube-like device that has pictures drawn on the outside to remind the patient of the proper technique for using the inhaler. For younger children and older adults, the InspirEase spacer gives a visual cue of the spacer bag deflating to help in taking a deep-enough breath, or an Aerochamber with the appropriate-size mask can be used. Both of these devices emit a whistling sound if the patient is taking too rapid a breath, giving a cue to breathe more slowly.

The use of a nebulizer should be demonstrated to the patient either in the clinic or by the home health agency that is providing the device. Specific instructions vary slightly with the manufacturer. The key points that should be covered with nebulizer use are accurate measurement of the medication (if using nebulizer solution) and appropriate cleaning of the equipment. Many nebulizer medications are available in unit-dose packaging, which, although more expensive, is helpful if patients have difficulty accurately measuring their medication.

Instructions for **salmeterol** dry powder DISKUS (**Serevent** DISKUS, **Advair** DISKUS) administration say that the patient should use the medication as prescribed and should not exceed the prescribed dose. Patients should not exhale or blow into the DISKUS. The DISKUS should not be washed or taken apart.

Formoterol (**Foradil** AEROLIZER) is a dry powder capsule administered via a patented aerolizer. The **Foradil** capsule is placed into the aerolizer, then the aerolizer is squeezed to break the capsule. The patient inhales the medication. Patients should receive clear instructions not to swallow the capsule.

Adverse Reactions

The patient should be instructed not to exceed the recommended dosage of the medication because excessive use may lead to increased adverse effects. Overuse of the **beta$_2$ agonist bronchodilators** can lead to seizures, hypokalemia, anginal pain, and hypertension. Patients should understand that they may have some **stimulant**-like effects (e.g., increased heart rate, tremors) when they initially begin the medication, but these effects should lessen if they use it correctly. Some patients may get a headache with the use of **bronchodilators.** Patients who experience GI upset when taking oral medications should take the medications with food. The patient should inform the provider if palpitations, tachycardia, chest pain, muscle tremors, dizziness, headache, or flushing occurs.

Lifestyle Management

Lifestyle management issues related to the disease process being treated should be discussed. They often include the following:

1. The patient needs to self-monitor respiratory status with a peak flowmeter to determine the effectiveness of the prescribed medication.
2. The patient should avoid or quit smoking.
3. The patient should avoid environmental triggers for asthma at home, work, and school.

Table 17–4 presents the available dosage forms of selected **bronchodilators.**

Xanthine Derivatives

Methylxanthines have declined in importance in the treatment of asthma, but some patients may still benefit from the use of **theophylline.** The other **methylxanthines** include **aminophylline** and **caffeine. Theophylline** and **caffeine** are closely related chemically in that **theophylline** is 1,3-dimethylxanthine and **caffeine** is 1,3,7-triethylxanthine, and they share many of the same effects on the body. Because many patients throughout the world consume **caffeine** in tea, coffee, and cola beverages

Table 17–4 ◆ **Available Dosage Forms: Selected Bronchodilators**

Drug	Dosage Form	How Suppied	Cost
		BETA$_2$ AGONISTS	
Albuterol			
Acuneb	0.63 mg/3 mL	3-mL vials	
	1.25 mg/3 mL	3-mL vials	
Ventolin HFA,	17 g (about 200 inhalations)	Metered-dose inhaler: 90 mcg/puff	$34.09
Ventolin syrup	480 mL	Syrup: 2 mg/5 mL	480 mL
	100, 500	Tablets: 2 mg, 4 mg	
	20 mL with dropper	Solution for nebulizer: 0.5% (5 mg/mL)	
	3-mL unit dose	Solution for nebulizer: 0.083% in unit-dose vial	
	24, 96	Rotacaps: 200 mcg	$37.92
		Ventolin HFA MDI	$38.99

Continued

Table 17–4 ◈ Available Dosage Forms: Selected Bronchodilators—cont'd

Drug	Dosage Form	How Suppied	Cost
		BETA$_2$ AGONISTS	
Proventil HFA	17 g (about 200 inhalations [ihn]) 100, 500 100 480 mL 20 mL with dropper 3-mL unit dose	Metered-dose inhaler: 90 mcg/puff Tablets: 2 mg, 4 mg Extended-release tabs: 4 mg Syrup: 2 mg/5 mL Solution for nebulizer: 0.5% (5 mg/mL) Solution for nebulizer: 0.083% in unit-dose vial Proventil HFA MDI	$55.09 $35.94
ProAir	200 inh	Inhaler: 90 mcg/puff	$45.99
Vospire	ER tabs	Extended-release tablets: 4 mg, 8 mg	
Generic	100, 500 480 mL 20 mL with dropper 3-mL unit dose	Tablets: 2 mg, 4 mg Syrup: 2 mg/5 mL Solution for nebulizer: 0.5% (5 mg/mL) 0.63 mg/3 mL neb soln Metered-dose inhaler 90 mcg/puff	2 mg =$ 17.77/100 4 mg = $24.98/100 $26.24/480 mL $20.60/20-mL bottle $39/25 unit dose containers $10.99
Bitolterol Tornalate	15 mL (about 300 inhalations)	Metered-dose inhaler: 0.37 mg/puff	$39
Formoterol Foradil Aerolizer Aerolizer Oxeze Turbohaler	12-mcg capsule	Powder for oral inhalation, 60 capsules	$170/60
Levalbuterol Xopenex HFA	HFA inhaler 45 mcg/inhalation Unit dose solution for nebulizer: 0.31 mg/3 mL 0.63 mg/3 mL 1.25 mg/3 mL Concentrated solution for inhalation: 1.25 mg/0.5 mL	15-mg inhaler 24 unit-dose vials 24 unit-dose vials 24 unit-dose vials 30	$48.99 $120.70/24 $123.91/24 $122.41/24 —
Metaproterenol Alupent	100, 1,000 480 mL 5-mL, 10-mL inhaler 2.5 mL 10-mL, 30-mL vials with dropper	Tablets: 10 mg, 20 mg Syrup: 10 mg/5 mL Metered-dose inhaler: 0.65 mg/puff Solution for inhalation: 0.4%, 0.6% Solution for inhalation: 5%	 $36.09
Metaprel	100 480 mL 10-mL inhaler 10 mL with dropper	Tablets: 10 mg, 20 mg Syrup: 10 mg/5 mL Metered-dose inhaler: 0.65 mg/puff Solution for inhalation: 5%	
Generic	100, 1,000 480 mL 2.5 mL 0.3-mL, 30-mL vials with dropper	Tablets: 10 mg, 20 mg Syrup: 10 mg/5 mL Solution for inhalation: 0.4%, 0.6% Solution for inhalation: 5%	$20.99/60 $12.00/240 mL $39.99/30 vials $18.99

Table 17–4 ◈ **Available Dosage Forms: Selected Bronchodilators—cont'd**

Drug	Dosage Form	How Suppied	Cost
		BETA$_2$ AGONISTS	
Pirbuterol			
Maxair Autoinhaler	14-g MDI (about 400 inhalations)	Inhaler: 0.2 mg/puff	$33.68
Salmeterol Inhaler			
Serevent Diskus	Diskus (60 inhalations)	Diskus Inhaler: 50 mcg/inhalation	$169
Terbutaline			
Generic	10.5-g MDI (about 300 inhalations) 100	Inhaler: 0.2 mg/puff Tablets: 2.5 mg, 5 mg	$10 2.5 mg = $49.99/100 5 mg = $51.10/100
Brethine	100, 1,000 2-mL ampule	Tablets: 2.5 mg, 5 mg Parenteral: 1 mg/mL	2.5 mg = $48.30/100
Bricanyl	100, 1,000 2-mL ampule Turbohaler: 0.5 mg/puff	Tablets: 2.5 mg, 5 mg Parenteral: 1 mg/mL	
		ANTICHOLINERGICS	
Ipratropium			
Atrovent HFA	12.9-g MDI (200 inhalations) 25 unit-dose vials (2.5 mL each) per foil pouch	Inhaler: 17 mcg/puff Solution for nebulizer: 500 mcg per unit-dose vial	$156.51/inhaler
		COMBINATION MEDICATIONS	
Albuterol-Ipratropium			
Combivent	14.7-g MDI (200 inhalations)	Inhaler: ipratropium 18 mcg/puff combined with albuterol 90 mcg/puff	$172.97
		XANTHINE DERIVATIVES	
Theophylline (immediate release)			
Slo-Phyllin	100 (dye-free) Pint	Tablets: 100 mg, 200 mg Syrup: 80 mg/5 mL	$15.99/60
Theolair	100 15 mL, 18.75 mL, 30 mL, 500 mL	Tablets: 125 mg, 250 mg Solution: 80 mg/15 mL	$31.99/60
Generic	100, 500, 1,000 15 mL, 30 mL, pint, gallon	Tablets: 100 mg, 200 mg, 300 mg Elixir: 80 mg/15 mL	$8.99/60
Theophylline (timed release)			
Generic Theophylline CR Slo-bid Gyrocaps	60, 180 100, 1,000	Timed-release 12-h capsule: 125 mg, 200 mg, 300 mg Timed-release capsules (8–12 h): 50 mg, 75 mg, 100 mg, 125 mg, 200 mg, 300 mg	125 mg = $43.57/60 200 mg = $29.99/60 300 mg = $49.99/60
Slo-Phyllin	100, 1,000	Timed-release capsules (8–12 h): 60 mg, 125 mg, 250 mg	$15.99/60
Theo-24	100, 500	Timed-release capsules (24 h): 100 mg, 200 mg, 300 mg	$27.81/60
Theo-Dur Sprinkles	100	Timed-release capsules (12 h): 50 mg, 75 mg, 125 mg, 200 mg	

Continued

Table 17–4 ◆ **Available Dosage Forms: Selected Bronchodilators—cont'd**

Drug	Dosage Form	How Suppied	Cost
XANTHINE DERIVATIVES			
Theo-Dur	100, 500, 1,000, 5,000	Timed-release tablets (8–24 h): 100 mg, 200 mg, 300 mg, 400 mg	
Uni-Dur	100	Timed-release scored tablets (24 h): 400 mg, 600 mg	
Uniphyl	100, 500	Timed-release tablets (24 h): 400 mg, 600 mg	$69.75/60 tablets
Generic	100	Timed-release tablets (24 h): 400 mg	$99.99/100 tablets

Soln=solution

and because many OTC preparations for analgesia contain **caffeine, caffeine** pharmacodynamics are discussed briefly here.

Pharmacodynamics

Theophylline and the other **methylxanthines** work directly by an unknown mechanism believed to be mediated by selective inhibition of specific phosphodiesterases (PDEs). This, in turn, produces an increase in cAMP, which then leads to bronchial smooth muscle and pulmonary vessel relaxation.

Theophylline and **caffeine** have an impact on most of the major body systems. They are powerful CNS stimulants, often causing insomnia and excitability. Although both drugs have cardiovascular effects, **theophylline** has a greater effect on the cardiovascular system. **Theophylline** directly stimulates the myocardium and increases myocardial contractility and heart rate. By relaxing vascular smooth muscle, **theophylline** dilates the coronary, pulmonary, and systemic blood vessels. Both **theophylline** and **caffeine** increase gastric acid secretion and may produce nausea and vomiting, although this reaction is probably due to CNS effects. Both **methylxanthines** stimulate skeletal muscle, causing tremors. **Theophylline** acts directly on the renal tubules to cause increased sodium and chloride excretion. By increasing renal blood flow (from increased heart rate) and the glomerular filtration rate, **theophylline** and **caffeine** also cause diuresis. Often, these effects occur even when **theophylline** is within the therapeutic range.

Pharmacokinetics

Absorption and Distribution

Methylxanthines, such as **theophylline**, are most commonly used in an oral form that is rapidly and completely absorbed from the GI tract. Delayed-release and extended-release tablets are also available, and their rate of absorption varies among the various formulations. The absorption of slow-release forms of **theophylline** can be significantly altered by gastric pH and food ingestion; therefore, patient education regarding the timing of these medications is important to the success of the medication. **Theophylline** distributes rapidly in nonadipose tissue and body water, including breast milk and cerebral spinal fluid. **Theophylline** crosses the placenta. The volume of distribution (Vd) for **theophylline** averages 0.45 L per kg of body weight (L/kg) and ranges from 0.3 to 0.7 L/kg from infants to adults. The volume of distribution may be altered in premature neonates, elderly patients, adults with cirrhosis, pregnant women during the third trimester, and critically ill patients, probably because of altered protein binding. Serum **theophylline** levels should be monitored closely in these patients. **Theophylline** distributes readily into breast milk with milk levels 70% of maternal serum levels.

Metabolism and Excretion

Theophylline is metabolized primarily in the liver, with very little or no first-pass effect. Metabolism is believed to occur over multiple parallel pathways, mediated by cytochrome P450 (CYP450) isoenzyme. Medications that induce CYP450 can significantly increase clearance of **theophylline.** In neonates, several of these pathways are undeveloped but mature slowly over the first year of life. **Caffeine** is a minor active metabolite of **theophylline** in older children and adults. In premature neonates and children younger than 6 months, **caffeine** has a long half-life because of their immature livers, which results in significant accumulation. As the liver matures, the half-life of **caffeine** shortens and, therefore, does not accumulate in older children and adults. Table 17–1 outlines the half-life of **theophylline** in various ages of patients with a variety of diseases. Patients with congestive heart failure, cor pulmonale, pulmonary edema, and prolonged fever can have decreased metabolism of **theophylline** and, therefore, need to be closely monitored. Smoking and high-protein diets can increase the **theophylline** excretion rate, and high-carbohydrate diets can decrease it.

Pharmacotherapeutics

Precautions and Contraindications

The only true contraindications to **theophylline** are hypersensitivity to any **xanthine**, peptic ulcer disease, and underlying seizure disorder. Contraindications to **caffeine** include hypersensitivity to **caffeine** and use of **caffeine** sodium benzoate formulation in neonates.

Because of its effects on the cardiovascular system, patients with hypertension, ischemic heart disease, coronary insufficiency, congestive heart failure, or a history of stroke and cardiac arrhythmias should be monitored closely for adverse effects while taking **theophylline**.

Excessive doses may lead to toxicity. Incidence of toxicity increases when serum **theophylline** levels are above 20 mcg/mL. Toxicity is found if serum **theophylline** levels reach 25 mcg/mL in 75 percent of patients. Toxicity should not occur at recommended dosages but may occur if **theophylline** clearance is decreased (hepatic impairment, chronic lung disease, cardiac failure, patients older than age 55, and infants under age 1 year).

Theophylline clearance may be decreased in patients over age 55.

Caffeine has a prolonged half-life of 72 to 96 hours in the neonate, whereas in infants over 9 months, children, and adults, the half-life is 5 hours.

Theophylline is Pregnancy Category C. There are no published reports linking **theophylline** with congenital defects. **Theophylline** crosses the placenta, and newborn infants may have therapeutic serum levels if maternal serum **theophylline** levels are in the high-normal range. Transient tachycardia, irritability, and vomiting can be found in newborns of women consuming **theophylline**.

With close monitoring, **theophylline** may be used in children. Infants younger than 1 year have decreased **theophylline** clearance and should have close monitoring of serum **theophylline** levels. **Theophylline** is used to treat apnea in preterm infants, with a therapeutic serum **theophylline** range of 5 to 10 mcg/mL. If levels are kept in this range, the neonate should not have signs of toxicity. **Caffeine** citrate is also commonly used to treat apnea of prematurity.

Adverse Drug Reactions

Adverse drug reactions are uncommon with serum **theophylline** levels below 20 mcg/mL, although some patients may show toxic effects between 15 and 20 mcg/mL, especially during initiation of therapy. The CNS adverse effects that may be seen include irritability, restlessness, seizures, and insomnia. Gastroesophageal reflux may occur. The cardiovascular adverse effects that may occur include palpitations, tachycardia, hypotension, and life-threatening arrhythmias. Other adverse effects include rash, diuresis, and tachypnea.

At serum **theophylline** levels above 20 mcg/mL, patients may experience nausea, vomiting, diarrhea, headache, insomnia, and irritability. At levels above 35 mcg/mL, the patient may have hyperglycemia, hypotension, cardiac arrhythmias, tachycardia, seizures, brain damage, and death.

Adverse effects of **caffeine** include cardiac arrhythmias, tachycardia, insomnia, agitation, irritability, headache, nausea, vomiting, and gastric irritation.

Drug and Food Interactions

Many medications act to either increase or decrease **theophylline** clearance due to metabolism via CYP450 isoenzyme CYP1A2, CYP2E1, and CYP3A3/4 substrate. These medications are shown in Table 17–2. Of significance is smoking tobacco, which increases **theophylline** clearance. **Theophylline** levels should be monitored closely if the patient begins or quits smoking while on **theophylline**. Nicotine replacement products (gum or patch) also affect **theophylline** clearance. **Theophylline** clearance may not return to normal for 3 months to 2 years after smoking cessation.

The sedative effects of **benzodiazepines** may be antagonized by **theophylline**. Concurrent use of **theophylline** with **beta$_2$ agonist bronchodilators** may result in additive toxicity. **Lithium** levels may be reduced by **theophylline**. The concurrent use of **tetracyclines** with **theophylline** may lead to an increased incidence of **theophylline** adverse reactions. See Table 17–2 for other drugs that affect **theophylline** levels or interact with **theophylline**.

Theophylline elimination may be influenced by the patient's diet. A diet that is low in carbohydrates and high in protein increases the elimination (shortens the half-life) of **theophylline**. A diet high in carbohydrates and low in protein decreases the elimination (lengthens the half-life) of **theophylline**. A diet that contains a lot of charcoal-broiled foods accelerates the hepatic metabolism of **theophylline** because of the high polycyclic hydrocarbon content.

Caffeine is metabolized via the CYP450 isoenzyme CYP1A2, CYP2E1, and CYP3A3/4 substrate; therefore, other drugs metabolized via these isoenzymes will possibly interact. **Cimetidine**, **ketoconazole**, **fluconazole**, **mexiletine**, and **phenylpropanolamine** may impair **caffeine** metabolism, leading to increased serum levels. **Caffeine** elimination may be increased by coadministration of **phenobarbital** and **phenytoin** (Takemoto et al, 2009).

Clinical Use and Dosing

Asthma and Chronic Obstructive Pulmonary Disease

The National Heart, Lung, and Blood Institute (NHLBI) *Expert Panel Report 3* (NAEPP, 2007), which provides guidelines for the management of asthma, recommends reserving **theophylline** for long-term control of asthma and an "alternative, not preferred" therapy in step 2 of asthma care. The *Expert Panel Report 3* recommends using **theophylline** as an alternative treatment in combination with inhaled **corticosteroids** (NAEPP, 2007). The guidelines recommend that **long-acting beta$_2$ agonists** (in combination with inhaled **corticosteroids**) be tried before **theophylline** because of toxicity issues with **theophylline. Theophylline** is not recommended for first-line therapy in the COPD patient, although if the patient has been stable on **theophylline**, there is no reason to discontinue the medication as long as serum **theophylline** levels are monitored.

The dose of **theophylline** for asthma and COPD varies with the patient's weight and serum **theophylline** levels. The adult patient (older than age 16 years) is started on a dose of 6 mg/kg per 24 hours or 400 mg/24 hours, whichever is less, divided at 6- to 8-hour intervals. The dose is increased every 3 days in 25 percent increments until the desired serum **theophylline** levels are achieved (ideally between 10 and 20 mcg/mL). The maximum dose for patients age 12 to 16 years is 13 mg/kg per day, and 10 mg/kg/day in healthy adolescents older than age 16 years and adults. Dosing adjustments are made based on the serum **theophylline** level. If the level is 5 to 10 mcg/mL, then the dose of **theophylline** is increased by 25 percent every 3 days until desired serum concentrations of **theophylline** are reached. If the serum concentration is between 10 and 15 mcg/mL, maintain dosage if tolerated and recheck at 6- to 12-month intervals. If the serum **theophylline** level is 15 to 19.9 mcg/mL, consider decreasing the dose by 10 percent to provide a greater margin of safety. If the serum **theophylline** level is 20 to 25 mcg/mL, then decrease the dose by 10 percent and recheck the level in 3 days. If the serum level is 25 to 30 mcg/mL, skip the next dose and decrease subsequent doses by 25 percent; redraw **theophylline** level in 3 days. If the **theophylline** level is above 30 mcg/mL, then skip the next two doses and decrease the dose by 50 percent; recheck in 3 days. If the patient has a serum **theophylline** level above 20 mcg/mL, consultation with a physician is indicated to determine if hospitalization for **theophylline** toxicity is warranted, based on clinical status.

The Expert Panel Report 3 (NAEPP, 2007) for the management of asthma in children indicates **theophylline** as alternative therapy in moderate persistent asthma, in combination with low-dose inhaled **corticosteroid** in children age 5 years or older. The initial dose of **theophylline** in children is 16 mg/kg per 24 hours up to a maximum of 400 mg per day. The dosage may be increased by 25 percent every 3 days to a maximum that is based on age. For children aged 1 to 9 years, the maximum is 24 mg/kg per day; for 9 to 12 years, the maximum dose is 20 mg/kg per day; for 12- to 16-year-old patients, the maximum daily dose is 18 mg/kg. If the patient is over age 16 years, then the dosing is the same as it is for adults, maximum 13 mg/kg per day. Monitoring for serum **theophylline** levels is the same in children as for adults, with a steady-state **theophylline** level of 5 to 15 mcg/mL the goal. **Theophylline** is not recommended for use in children with asthma younger than age 5 years because of altered metabolism during viral or febrile illnesses affecting serum concentration (NAEPP, 2007).

Apnea of Prematurity

A loading dose of **caffeine** citrate 10 to 20 mg/kg is given in the treatment apnea of prematurity, with a maintenance dose of 5 mg/kg per day. If **theophylline** has been given to the patient in the previous 3 days, the loading dose is decreased by 50 to 70 percent. Maintenance dose is adjusted based on clinical response and serum **caffeine** levels (8 to 20 mcg/mL). If **theophylline** is used to treat apnea of prematurity, the patient is given a loading dose of 4 mg/kg per dose, with a maintenance dose of 4 mg/kg per day in the premature infant or newborn up to age 6 weeks. The total daily dose is divided and administered every 12 hours. A recent RCT comparing **caffeine** and **theophylline** for the treatment of apnea of prematurity found both drugs are equally effective in decreasing apnea spells in infants less than 33 weeks' gestation, but caffeine is significantly more effective as prophylaxis against apnea in infants at risk (Skouroliakou, Bacopoulou, & Markantonis, 2009). The Skouroliakau and colleagues study found no sustained benefit of one drug over the other after the first week of therapy.

Rational Drug Selection

Because **theophylline** is the only **xanthine derivative** that is commonly used in asthma and COPD, the selection process basically involves choosing between the different forms of **theophylline** that are available on the basis of the cost and convenience of each of them. There are immediate-release, timed-release, and liquid formulas. Capsules that can be opened and sprinkled on soft foods are convenient for some patients.

Immediate Release

When therapy is initiated, the daily dose may be changing frequently based on serum **theophylline** levels, and immediate-release tablets or capsules should be prescribed. The variety of dosage tablets available (100 mg, 125 mg, 200 mg, 250 mg, 300 mg) makes titrating the dose easier if incremental increases or decreases are required. Immediate-release **theophylline** requires dosing every 6 to 8 hours. Children younger than age 12 years usually require every-6-hour dosing, whereas adolescents and adults usually require every-8-hour dosing, although this timing may vary by individual. The cost of immediate-release **theophylline** is slightly higher than that of most of the timed-release formulas because more doses are taken and, therefore, more tablets need to be dispensed in a month. Many patients are stabilized to a set dose per 24 hours and then switched to a timed-release formula.

Timed Release

The variety of available timed-release **theophylline** products are described in Table 17–4. The formulas range from

8- to 24-hour release. It is recommended that patients be stabilized on immediate-release formulas to determine the total 24-hour dose that is required and then switched to a timed-release formula of choice. With some timed-release **theophylline** formulas offering once-daily dosing, there is a definite improvement in convenience with the timed-release products. One caution for the patient is that the dose must be taken at the same time every day to have steady serum **theophylline** levels.

Liquid

The liquid forms of **theophylline** may be used for children or patients who have difficulty in swallowing pills or capsules. The liquid is available in 80 mg/15 mL.

Monitoring

The patient who is taking **theophylline** needs to be monitored closely for signs of toxicity. When therapy is initiated, **theophylline** levels should be drawn frequently as the dosage is titrated. If the patient is demonstrating any signs of toxicity, a serum **theophylline** level should be drawn. Once the patient is stabilized and has a steady **theophylline** level, then monitoring should be done every 6 to 12 months. More frequent levels may need to be done if a new medication is added to the patient's regimen (see Table 17–2) or if the patient has a change in overall health that may affect the ability to metabolize or excrete **theophylline. Theophylline** levels need to be timed to measure peak levels of the drug. A serum **theophylline** level should be drawn 1 to 2 hours after immediate-release formulas and 5 to 9 hours after the morning dose of sustained-release formulas. The patient should have a **theophylline** level drawn when changing brands of **theophylline** because the bioavailability varies among brands.

Patient Education

Administration

The patient should be instructed to take the medication exactly as prescribed. Missed doses or irregular timing of doses can cause wide variations in the serum **theophylline** level, resulting in either subtherapeutic or toxic levels. The patient may take the medication either with or without food, but consistency is important because food can alter the absorption of the medication. The patient should not chew or crush enteric-coated, sustained-release tablets or capsules.

Adverse Reactions

Toxicity should be discussed with any patient who is taking **theophylline.** Patients who are having signs of toxicity may mistakenly think they have a viral illness. Instead, patients with any unusual symptoms should contact their provider. The symptoms to report include nausea, vomiting, insomnia, jitteriness, headache, rash, severe GI pain, restlessness, convulsions, or irregular heartbeat.

The patient should avoid large amounts of **caffeine**-containing beverages, which can increase the adverse effects of **theophylline.** Explain that **theophylline** elimination may be influenced by the patient's diet. A diet that is low in carbohydrates and high in protein increases the elimination of **theophylline,** a diet that is high in carbohydrates and low in protein decreases the elimination of **theophylline,** and a diet that contains a lot of charcoal-broiled foods accelerates the hepatic metabolism of **theophylline.** Any drastic changes in patients' diets should be discussed with the provider, and a plan for monitoring developed.

The impact on serum **theophylline** levels that different drugs may have should be discussed with the patient. Any change in the patient's overall medication regimen should warrant a status review and possibly serum **theophylline** levels. The impact of smoking on **theophylline** levels should be discussed and patients advised to notify their provider if they start or stop smoking.

Lifestyle Management

Lifestyle management issues related to the disease process should be discussed. They often include the following:

1. The patient needs to self-monitor respiratory status with a peak flowmeter to determine the effectiveness of the medication prescribed.
2. The patient should avoid or quit smoking.
3. The patient should avoid environmental triggers for asthma at home, work, and school.

Anticholinergics

Inhaled **anticholinergics** are used primarily to treat COPD, although **ipratropium** may be used in combination with **albuterol** as the emergent treatment of an asthma exacerbation or when a patient is intolerant to **beta$_2$ agonists** (NAEPP, 2007). **Ipratropium bromide** (**Atrovent**) is a quaternary amine **anticholinergic** that is structurally similar to **atropine.** It is available as a single medication (**Atrovent**) or combined with **albuterol** (**Combivent**). **Tiotropium bromide** (**Spiriva**) is an inhaled **anticholinergic** available to treat COPD.

Pharmacodynamics

The action of each of the two inhaled **anticholinergics** is similar. **Ipratropium** acts to block the muscarinic cholinergic receptors by antagonizing the action of acetylcholine. Blocking the cholinergic receptors decreases the formation of cyclic guanosine monophosphate (cGMP), which leads to decreased contractility of the smooth muscle of the lungs, probably because of the actions of cGMP on intracellular calcium. The amount of bronchodilation caused by **ipratropium** inhalation is thought to reflect the level of parasympathetic tone. When inhaled, **ipratropium**'s actions are confined to the mouth and airways. **Tiotropium** exhibits its pharmacological action by inhibiting the muscarinic M_3 receptors in the lungs, causing smooth muscle bronchodilation.

Pharmacokinetics

Absorption and Distribution

Ipratropium, when inhaled, is poorly absorbed from both the lung and the GI tract. Only 1 to 2 percent of a dose is systemically absorbed. **Ipratropium** penetrates the CNS poorly. It is unknown whether **ipratropium** crosses the placenta. **Ipratropium** is excreted into breast milk in minimal amounts.

Tiotropium is administered via dry powder inhaler, has a bioavailability of 19.5 percent, and is 72 percent protein bound in human plasma. Similar to **ipratropium**, **tiotropium** demonstrates poor GI absorption when administered orally with an absolute bioavailability of 2 to 3 percent. **Tiotropium** does not cross the blood–brain barrier. **Tiotropium** is distributed in breast milk of rats; it is unknown whether it is excreted in human milk or whether it crosses the placenta.

Metabolism and Excretion

Most of the dose (90%) of **ipratropium** is swallowed and excreted in the feces unchanged. The portion of the dose that is absorbed is partially metabolized by ester hydrolysis to inactive metabolites. Approximately 50 percent of the absorbed drug is excreted unchanged in the urine. **Tiotropium** that is absorbed is eliminated unchanged in the urine.

Pharmacotherapeutics

Precautions and Contraindications

Ipratropium is contraindicated in patients with hypersensitivity to **atropine** or **atropine derivatives** and for those with **bromide** sensitivity.

Tiotropium is contraindicated in patients with hypersensitivity to **ipratropium** or **tiotropium.**

Ipratropium and **tiotropium** should not be used for the treatment of acute bronchospasm. The exception is if **ipratropium** is combined with **albuterol** emergency room treatment of acute bronchospasm (NAEPP, 2007).

Inhaled anticholinergics (ipratropium and **tiotropium)**, even though poorly absorbed systemically, should be avoided for patients with urinary retention, bladder neck obstruction, or prostatic hypertrophy because of the anticholinergic effects. Both drugs may increase intraocular pressure in patients with closed-angle glaucoma.

Ipratropium bromide is Pregnancy Category B and **tiotropium** is Pregnancy Category C. Their safety in pregnancy has had limited study; therefore, **inhaled anticholinergics** should be used in pregnancy only if clearly indicated. **Ipratropium** is excreted in breast milk in minimal amounts. **Atropine**, a chemically related drug, is considered safe during lactation. Because such small amounts of drug reach the breast milk, **ipratropium** is probably safe for use if needed during breastfeeding.

The safety and effectiveness of **ipratropium** have not been established in children under age 12 years. Providers may use **ipratropium** in younger children as an adjunct to **beta-agonist (albuterol)** therapy in acute exacerbations of asthma per the *NAEPP Expert Panel Report 3* (2007). **Tiotropium** is approved only for COPD, which does not normally occur in children. Safety and effectiveness of **tiotropium** in children have not been established.

Adverse Drug Reactions

The most common adverse drug reaction reported with ipratropium is cough. Also reported are the related symptoms of hoarseness, throat irritation, and dysgeusia. Nausea, vomiting, and dyspepsia are thought to be related to the local anticholinergic effects that **ipratropium** has on the GI system. Xerostomia (dry mouth) is reported in 2 percent of patients.

Dry mouth is the most commonly reported adverse reaction to inhaled **tiotropium (Spiriva HandiHaler)**, reported in 16 percent of patients in the manufacturer's clinical trials. Mouth irritation, pharyngitis, nasal congestion, sinusitis, headache, and upper respiratory infections occurred at slightly higher rates in patients using **Spiriva** than in those using a placebo in the initial clinical trials (Boehringer-Ingelheim, 2009).

Other anticholinergic effects that are reported (in less than 2% of patients) include urinary retention, dizziness, drowsiness, and constipation. Prostate disorders may also be noted (less than 2% reported) in patients using **ipratropium.** In a 4-year trial of **tiotropium (Spiriva HandiHaler)** constipation occurred at a slightly higher rate than it did in those using a placebo (5.1% vs. 3.7% in placebo patients). Patients with urinary retention were excluded from clinical trials, as there is an assumption that urinary retention will worsen with **anticholinergic** administration.

If **ipratropium** is accidentally sprayed in the eyes, the patient may experience temporary eye irritation, pain, mydriasis, blurred vision, cycloplegia (paralysis of the ciliary muscle), irritant conjunctivitis, and visual disturbances.

Rare allergic and anaphylactoid reactions may occur. Reactions include urticaria, maculopapular rash; bronchospasm; pruritus; laryngospasm; oropharyngeal edema; and angioedema of the tongue, lips, and face. The patient's history usually includes sensitivity to other drugs and foods. Allergy to soybeans, legumes, or soy lecithin appears to be correlated with hypersensitivity to **ipratropium bromide.**

Drug Interactions

Ipratropium and **tiotropium** are minimally absorbed into the systemic circulation after inhalation; therefore, there are no major drug interactions.

Patients who are concurrently using **cromolyn sodium** and **ipratropium bromide** via nebulizer should be cautioned not to mix the two, because a precipitate will form.

Clinical Use and Dosage

Chronic Obstructive Pulmonary Disease

The dose of **ipratropium** from an MDI is 18 mcg per spray. The dose of **ipratropium** for adults with COPD is two inhalations (36 mcg) four times a day, for a total of eight puffs per day. If needed, the patient may take up to 12 puffs per day (maximum of 216 mcg /24 h). If using a nebulizer, the dose of **ipratropium** is one unit-dose vial (500 mcg) three to four times a day via nebulizer, with doses 6 to 8 hours apart. Ipratropium may be mixed with **albuterol** if used within 1 hour.

Tiotropium (Spiriva) is a dry powder capsule administered via a patented HandiHaler device. The dosage for COPD is two inhalations of a single 18-μg capsule once daily.

The **ipratropium-albuterol** combination **(Combivent)** is indicated for second-line use for patients with COPD. It should be prescribed for patients already on a **bronchodilator** who continue to have bronchospasm that may benefit from a second **bronchodilator.** Each inhalation of **Combivent** administers 103 mcg of **albuterol** sulfate and 18 mcg of **ipratropium bromide.** The dose of **Combivent** is two inhalations four times a day. The patient may take additional inhalations but must not exceed 12 inhalations per 24 hours.

Asthma

The adult dose of **ipratropium** for asthma maintenance is two to three inhalations four times a day. It should not be used for exercise-induced asthma. For children under age 12 years, the dose is one or two inhalations every 6 hours. The dose of **ipratropium** solution in adults is 250 mcg administered via a nebulizer four times a day. The dose for children under age 12 years is 250 to 500 mcg every 8 hours. Infants are dosed at 125 to 250 mcg three times a day. Dosing for acute exacerbation of asthma per the National Institutes of Health (NIH) guidelines is found in Table 17–3. **Ipratropium** may be mixed with **albuterol** if the combination is used within 1 hour.

The **ipratropium-albuterol** combination **(Combivent)** is a second-line quick relief medication in the treatment of asthma. Each inhalation of **Combivent** administers 103 mcg of **albuterol** sulfate and 18 mcg of **ipratropium bromide.** The dose of **Combivent** in adults is two to three inhalations four times a day, and in children under age 12 years, one to two inhalations every 6 hours. The dose of nebulizer solution of **albuterol** (2.5 mg/3 mL) and **ipratropium** (0.5 mg/3 mL) is 3 mL every 4 to 6 hours for adults and 1.5 to 3 mL every 8 hours in children under age 12 years.

Tiotropium is not indicated for the treatment of asthma. The dosing for the treatment of COPD is one 18-μg capsule daily via HandiHaler.

Rational Drug Selection

Ipratropium is a second-line **bronchodilator** in the treatment of asthma and COPD. For the practitioner considering prescribing both **ipratropium** and **albuterol,** an appropriate choice would be the combination product **Combivent. Tiotropium (Spiriva)** is for use in COPD; cost and ease of use (dry powder vs. inhaler) may be the deciding factor.

Cost

The cost of a month's supply of **Atrovent HFA MDI** is $143.59 or more (http://www.drugstore.com). Generic **ipratropium** inhaler is not available. The cost of **Atrovent** inhalation solution is more than $200 for 150 unit-dose vials, and generic **ipratropium** inhalation solution is $57 (http://www.drugstore.com) for 150 unit-dose vials. The cost of the combination product **Combivent** is $158.69 (http://www.drugstore.com) or $76.56 for **Duoneb (ipratropium** and **albuterol nebulizer solution)** per month, a significant cost savings over prescribing the two products individually. The generic combination product is even less expensive at $13.97 for **ipratropium/albuterol nebulizer solution** (http://www.costco.com). The provider needs to be familiar with the cost to the patient for each medication when making decisions regarding prescribing. It may be less expensive to prescribe the combined medication for COPD, or, depending on the patient's prescription drug coverage, it may be less expensive to prescribe each product individually.

Tiotropium (Spriva) is available only as a dry powder capsule for use with the HandiHaler. The cost of 1 month's worth of capsules (30) is $223.07.

Monitoring

There is no specific laboratory monitoring necessary with the use of **ipratropium,** other than monitoring the disease process.

Patient Education

Administration

Ipratropium and **tiotropium** should be used as prescribed. Overuse of **bronchodilators** leads to increased adverse effects, and using the **bronchodilator** less than prescribed may lead to increased bronchospasm and decreased pulmonary function.

The administration of medication via an MDI can be difficult for most adults and all children. Learning to coordinate the release of the medication from the inhaler with a deep breath is difficult. Written and pictorial instructions are available with the inhaler, but the provider must not assume that the patient understands the proper method of administering inhaled medications. Use verbal instructions as well as actual demonstration with a placebo inhaler to reinforce the written instructions. These instructions and demonstrations should be repeated at follow-up visits.

CLINICAL PEARL

Spacers

Spacer devices usually require a prescription to be dispensed. The provider can often obtain samples of different spacers from manufacturers.

To use an inhaler properly, the patient should first exhale and then tilt the head slightly back and place the inhaler mouthpiece either about 2 inches from the open mouth or between the open lips. While inhaling, the patient should press down on the canister, breathe in slowly and deeply, and hold her or his breath for 10 seconds (count of 10) or as long as comfortable. If two puffs are prescribed, then the patient should wait at least 1 full minute between inhalations. If the patient is prescribed other inhalers, advise the patient to use the **ipratropium** first and wait 5 minutes before using the other inhalers as directed.

To assist with the delivery of inhaled medications, a spacer can be prescribed. The Aerochamber is a tube-like device that has pictures drawn on the outside to remind the patient of the proper technique to use in administering the inhaler. For younger children and older adults, the InspirEase spacer gives a visual cue of the spacer bag deflating to help in taking a deep enough breath. If the patient is taking too rapid a breath, both of these devices emit a whistling sound as a cue to breathe more slowly.

Administration of **ipratropium** via nebulizer is per the manufacturer's directions. One unit dose of **ipratropium** is administered every 6 to 8 hours. **Albuterol** can be added to the **ipratropium** if the mixture is used within 1 hour. **Cromolyn** will precipitate if added to **ipratropium** solution; the patient should be advised of this if both medications are prescribed. The nebulizer medication cup should be rinsed well between drugs if these two medications are to be used concurrently via nebulizer.

Regardless of administration method, patients should rinse their mouth with water after inhaling **ipratropium** or **tiotropium** to minimize dry mouth.

To prime the MDI, patients using **Combivent** are recommended to "test-spray" the oral inhalation aerosol three times into the air before using it the first time. The patient should also prime the MDI in this manner if the medication has not been used in more than 24 hours.

Spiriva should be administered via the patented HandiHaler device only. Capsules of **tiotropium (Spiriva)** dry powder are inserted into HandiHaler, and the medication is administered via breath actuation. The **Spiriva** package insert has step-by-step pictures and text explaining how to administer the medication.

Adverse Reactions

The patient should be advised that a cough may develop with either inhaled **anticholinergic** and that less common complaints of throat irritation, hoarseness, or dry mouth may occur. Using a spacer device and rinsing the mouth with water after administration will decrease the incidence of these adverse effects.

Other adverse effects occur less often, but patients should be aware of the possible adverse effects and be instructed to notify their provider if they begin to have adverse effects from the **ipratropium** or **tiotropium**.

Lifestyle Management

Lifestyle management issues related to the disease process should be discussed. They often include the following:

1. Patients need to self-monitor their respiratory status with a peak flowmeter to determine the effectiveness of the medication prescribed.
2. The patient should avoid or quit smoking.
3. The patient should avoid environmental triggers for asthma at home, work, and school.
4. Patients with COPD should avoid unnecessary exposure to viral respiratory infections.

Leukotriene Modifiers

Leukotriene receptor agonists (**LTRAs**) and **5-lipoxygenase pathway inhibitors** were developed with the theory that cysteinyl leukotrienes play a significant role in the chronic inflammation associated with asthma and allergy. Leukotrienes are substances that induce numerous effects that contribute to the inflammatory process, including smooth muscle contractility; neutrophil aggregation, degranulation, and chemotaxis; vascular permeability; and on lymphocytes. There are two **LTRAs** available for use in asthma, **zafirlukast (Accolate)** and **montelukast (Singulair)**, and one **5-lipoxygenase pathway inhibitor, zileuton (Zyflo)**.

Pharmacodynamics

Leukotriene-Receptor Agonists

Zafirlukast is a synthetic, selective, and competitive **LTRA** of leukotriene D4 and E4 (LTD4 and LTE4). These leukotrienes have been identified as components of slow-reacting substance of anaphylaxis. **Montelukast** is a selective **LTRA** that inhibits the cysteinyl leukotriene (CysLT1) receptor. It binds with high affinity and selectivity to the CysLT1 receptor. **Montelukast** inhibits the actions of LTD4 at the CysLT1 receptor. There is evidence that the cysteinyl leukotrienes contribute to the pathophysiology of asthma and allergy, including airway edema, smooth muscle constriction, and cellular changes associated with the inflammatory process. In vitro studies demonstrated that **zafirlukast** antagonized the contractile activity of three leukotrienes (LTC4, LTD4, and LTE4) in the conducting airway smooth muscle. **Montelukast** may also inhibit symptoms of allergic rhinitis, as leukotrienes are also released from the nasal mucosa during allergen exposure.

5-Lipoxygenase Pathway Inhibitors

Zileuton is an inhibitor of 5-lipoxygenase, the enzyme that catalyzes the formation of leukotrienes from arachidonic acid. By inhibiting 5-lipoxygenase, **zileuton** inhibits the formation of leukotrienes LTB_4, LTC_4, and LTE_4, identified as components of slow-reacting substance of anaphylaxis.

Pharmacokinetics

Absorption and Distribution

Zafirlukast is rapidly absorbed from the GI tract following oral administration. Peak plasma concentrations are reached in 3 hours. The bioavailability of **zafirlukast** may be decreased when taken with food, and it should be taken on an empty stomach. **Zafirlukast** is greater than 99 percent protein bound, primarily to albumin. **Zafirlukast** is excreted in breast milk in measurable amounts (50 ng/mL) compared with 255 ng/mL in plasma, when administered in healthy women in 40-mg/day dosages.

Montelukast is rapidly absorbed following oral administration, with peak plasma concentration achieved in 3 to 4 hours for the film-coated tablet and in 2 to 2.5 hours after administration of the chewable tablet. **Montelukast** is more than 99 percent protein bound. There is minimal distribution across the blood–brain barrier in rats; no human studies are available. **Montelukast** crosses the placenta in rats and is excreted in rat milk; there are no human studies available.

Zileuton is rapidly absorbed after oral administration, with a peak time of 1.7 hours. Food increases the maximum concentration (C_{max}) of **zileuton** up to 27 percent. **Zileuton** is 93 percent protein bound. **Zileuton** crosses the placental barrier in rats and is excreted in rat's milk. There are no controlled studies in pregnant women.

Metabolism and Excretion

Zafirlukast is extensively metabolized. In vitro studies using human liver microsomes showed that the hydroxylated metabolites of **zafirlukast** are formed through the CYP450 2C9 (CYP2C9) enzyme pathway. Additional studies using human liver microsomes show that **zafirlukast** inhibits CYP3A4 and CYP2C9 isoenzymes at concentrations close to the clinically achieved plasma concentrations. The metabolites of **zafirlukast** found in plasma are at least 90 times less potent LTD4 receptor antagonists than **zafirlukast**. Following oral administration of **zafirlukast**, urinary excretion accounts for approximately 10 percent of the dose, and the remainder is excreted in the feces. Unmetabolized **zafirlukast** is not found in the urine.

Montelukast is extensively metabolized by the liver, with no detectable amounts of metabolites found in the plasma. CYP3A4 and CYP2C9 are the liver enzymes involved with the metabolism of **montelukast**. **Montelukast** and its metabolites are excreted almost exclusively via the bile, with less than 0.2 percent excreted in the urine.

Zileuton is metabolized in the liver via CYP1A2, CYP2C9, and CYP3A4. Renal elimination is the primary method of elimination, with 94.5 percent eliminated in the urine.

Table 17–5 presents the pharmacokinetics of the **leukotriene modifiers**.

Pharmacotherapeutics

Precautions and Contraindications

The only true contraindication to the leukotriene modifiers **zafirlukast** and **montelukast** is hypersensitivity to any of the components of the medication. Chewable **montelukast** tablets are contraindicated in patients with phenylketonuria because the product contains phenylalanine. **Zileuton** is contraindicated in patients with active liver disease.

The **leukotriene modifiers** are not to be used for primary treatment of an acute asthma attack.

Zafirlukast should be used with caution in patients with hepatic dysfunction because it is extensively metabolized by the liver. If a patient has alcoholic cirrhosis, the clearance of **zafirlukast** is reduced about 50 to 60 percent. There is no need to adjust the dose of **montelukast** in the patient with mild to moderate hepatic insufficiency because the elimination is only slightly prolonged, although use should be avoided in patients with severe liver disease.

Leukotriene modifiers should not be abruptly substituted for inhaled or oral **steroids**. Caution is advised as systemic **corticosteroids** are reduced. There have been reports that the reduction of oral **steroid** dose in some patients on **zafirlukast** has been followed by eosinophilia, vasculitic rash, worsening pulmonary symptoms, cardiac complications, and/or neuropathy sometimes presenting as Churg-Strauss syndrome, a systemic eosinophilic rash.

Neuropsychiatric events have been reported in postmarketing surveillance of adult, adolescent, and pediatric patients taking **leukotriene modifiers**. The reported neuropsychiatric events include agitation, aggression, anxiousness, dream abnormalities and hallucinations, depression, insomnia, irritability, restlessness, suicidal

Table 17–5 ▶ **Pharmacokinetics: Leukotriene Modifiers**

Drug	Onset	Peak	Duration	Protein Binding	Bioavailability	Half-Life	Metabolism	Elimination
Montelukast	—	3–4 h	—	>99%	64%	2.7–5.5 h	Extensive hepatic	Bile
Zafirlukast	3–14 d	2–4 h	—	>99%	Unknown	About 10 h	Extensive hepatic	Feces: 90% Urine: 10%

thinking and behavior (including suicide), and tremor (FDA, 2009). Sleep disorders were more frequent in all three products than in placebo in the original clinical trials (FDA, 2009). The FDA (2009) recommends that patients be informed of the potential for neuropsychiatric events with these medications and should consider discontinuing **leukotriene modifiers** if the patient develops neuropsychiatric problems.

Zafirlukast and **montelukast** are Pregnancy Category B. **Zileuton** is Pregnancy Category C.

The safety and efficacy of **zafirlukast** has been established in children age 5 and older. **Montelukast** may be prescribed for children as young as age 12 months for chronic asthma. Safety and effectiveness of **Zileuton** in pediatric patients younger than age 12 years have not been established.

Caution should be used in prescribing any of the **leukotriene modifiers** to lactating women because the effects on infants are unknown.

Adverse Reactions

The most common adverse reaction reported with **zafirlukast** use is headache. GI upset, myalgias, and fever are reported in a small percentage of patients. There is a reported increase in respiratory infections in patients older than age 55 years who are taking **zafirlukast.** The respiratory infections were usually mild to moderate and associated with coadministration of inhaled **corticosteroids.**

The reported adverse reactions of those taking **montelukast** are similar to placebo.

Zileuton has similar effects to placebo in clinical trials, except for a significant increase in dyspepsia (8.2% vs. 2.9%) in patients treated with **zileuton.** Hepatic injury, including hepatitis and death, is reported, with 1.9 percent of patients exhibiting elevated ALT in the clinical trials.

Drug Interactions

Zafirlukast should be used with caution with any drug that is metabolized by CYP2C9 and CYP3A3/4 isoenzymes. Coadministration of **aspirin** with **zafirlukast** results in about a 45 percent increase in plasma **zafirlukast** level. **Erythromycin** coadministered with **zafirlukast** results in a 40 percent decrease in plasma **zafirlukast** level. Concurrent **terfenadine** use leads to decreased plasma **zafirlukast** levels, and **theophylline** use has a similar profile. When **warfarin** is prescribed to the patient taking **zafirlukast,** there is a clinically significant increase in prothrombin time (PT).

Monitor closely the patient who is taking drugs that are metabolized by CYP450 isoenzymes CYP2A6, CYP2C9, and CYP3A3/4 (**phenobarbital, rifampin**) concurrently with **montelukast.**

Coadministration with drugs metabolized by CYP3A4 and **zileuton** should be monitored closely as there is a theoretical interaction. Coadministration of **zileuton** and **theophylline** may elevate serum **theophylline** levels. A reduction of **theophylline** dose by 50 percent is recommended by the manufacturer of **Zyflo. Terfenadine** plasma levels are increased by up to 35 percent and clearance is reduced by 22 percent when administered with **zileuton.** Coadministration with **warfarin** may theoretically increase prothrombin time; monitoring closely is warranted.

Table 17–6 presents drug interactions.

Clinical Use and Dosing

Zafirlukast is indicated in the treatment of chronic asthma in children aged 5 years or older and adults. **Montelukast** is indicated for use in the treatment of persistent asthma for patients aged 12 months or older. **Montelukast** may be prescribed for the prevention of exercise-induced bronchoconstriction in adolescents age 15 years or older and adults. **Montelukast** may also be used to treat seasonal allergic rhinitis in patients 2 years or older and perennial allergic rhinitis in patients

Table 17–6 ■ **Drug Interactions: Leukotriene Modifiers**

Drug	Interacting Drug	Possible Effect	Implications
Montelukast	Phenobarbital	Decreases area under curve (AUC) of dose by about 40%	Monitor patient closely
	Rifampin	Decreased metabolism of montelukast	Monitor
Zafirlukast	Aspirin	Increased plasma levels of zafirlukast	Monitor
	Erythromycin	Decreased plasma levels of zafirlukast	Use together with caution
	Theophylline	Decreased plasma levels of zafirlukast	Use cautiously
	Warfarin	Increased PT	Closely monitor PT
	Drugs metabolized by CYP2C9: amitriptyline, diclofenac, ibuprofen, imipramine, phenytoin, tolbutamide	Possible interactions	Until more data known, zafirlukast should be used cautiously in patients stabilized on these medications

Table 17–6 ■ **Drug Interactions: Leukotriene Modifiers—cont'd**

Drug	Interacting Drug	Possible Effect	Implications
	Drugs metabolized by CYP3A4: alprazolam, astemizole, carbamazepine, cisapride, some corticosteroids, cyclosporine, diazepam, calcium channel blockers (felodipine, isradipine, nicardipine, nifedipine, nimodipine), diltiazem, erythromycin, lidocaine, lovastatin, midazolam, quinidine, simvastatin, triazolam, verapamil	Possible interactions	Until more data known, zafirlukast should be used cautiously in patients stabilized on these medications

6 months and older. **Zileuton** is indicated for the treatment of persistent asthma in children aged 12 years and older and adults.

The dose for **zafirlukast** is 20 mg twice daily in children aged 12 years or older and adults, and 10 mg twice a day for children aged 5 to 11 years. Because food reduces bioavailability of **zafirlukast**, it must be taken on an empty stomach.

The adult dosage (patients aged 15 years or older) of **montelukast** is 10 mg once a day in the evening. The dose of **montelukast** in children aged 6 to 14 years is 5 mg once a day in the evening. Children aged 2 to 5 years are dosed with 4 mg of **montelukast** before bed; children aged 12 to 24 months are prescribed 4 mg of oral granules. **Montelukast** may be taken without regard to meals. **Montelukast** is dosed the same for allergy as for asthma.

The dose of **zileuton** is 600 mg four times a day or two 600-mg extended-release tablets twice a day, 1 hour after meals. Table 17–7 shows the dosage schedule.

Rational Drug Selection

Drug selection is based on the age of the patient and convenience in dosing. Children under age 5 years may be prescribed only **montelukast**. **Montelukast** offers once-a-day dosing without regard to meals, which may make it more convenient than **zafirlukast**. **Zileuton** is dosed four times a day or extended-release twice a day. **Singulair (montelukast)** costs $134.96 for a 30-day supply (30 tablets) and **Accolate (zafirlukast)** costs $115.75 for 60 tablets, a 30-day supply (http://www.drugstore.com). A 30-day supply of **zileuton (Zyflo)** costs $687.66 (http://www.drugstore.com).

Monitoring

Monitoring of improving or worsening asthmatic symptoms, **bronchodilator** use, and pulmonary function is necessary to determine the efficacy of the **leukotriene modifiers**. Patients should be monitored for new onset of neuropsychiatric symptoms, including depression or behavior change.

Patient Education

Patient education focuses on proper dosing of the medication, adverse reactions, and the general asthma management plan. The incorporation of the **leukotriene** medications into the asthma treatment plan is covered in Chapter 30.

Administration

The patient must take the medication as prescribed, even if symptom free. These medications are not for acute episodes of asthma. Patients must continue to use the **bronchodilator** inhaler for acute episodes of bronchospasm. They are not to decrease or discontinue

Table 17–7 ● **Dosage Schedule: Leukotriene Modifiers**

Drug	Indication	Dose	Comments
Montelukast	Prophylaxis and chronic treatment of asthma	*Adults:* 10 mg once daily in p.m. *Children 6–14 yr:* 5 mg at bedtime *Children 2–5 yr:* 4 mg at bedtime *Children 12–24 mo:* 4 mg granules at bedtime	Not recommended for children <12 mo
Zafirlukast	Prophylaxis and chronic treatment of asthma	*Adults:* 20 mg bid *Children 5–11 yr:* 10 mg bid	Not recommended for children <5 yr; must be taken on an empty stomach

any of their other asthma medications unless instructed to do so by their health-care provider.

Zafirlukast must be taken on an empty stomach, whereas **montelukast** may be taken without regard to meals. **Zileuton** may be taken with or without food.

Pregnant or nursing women should not take these medications.

Patients should be aware of significant drug interactions with **leukotriene modifiers** because of the way these drugs are metabolized by the liver. Patients should be advised to discuss with their health-care provider any new medications that are prescribed or discontinued.

Adverse Reactions

Patients and parents of pediatric patients should be informed of the potential for neuropsychiatric events including agitation, aggression, anxiousness, dream abnormalities and hallucinations, depression, insomnia, irritability, restlessness, suicidal thinking and behavior (including suicide), and tremor. Any new neuropsychiatric symptoms should be reported to the provider.

Lifestyle Management

Lifestyle management issues related to the disease process should be discussed. They often include the following:

1. The patient needs to self-monitor respiratory status with a peak flowmeter to determine the effectiveness of the medication prescribed.
2. The patient should avoid or quit smoking.
3. The patient should avoid environmental triggers for asthma at home, work, and school.

Table 17–8 presents the available dosage forms.

RESPIRATORY INHALANTS

Corticosteroids

The *Expert Panel Report 3* states that **corticosteroids** are the "most potent and effective anti-inflammatory medication currently available" (NAEPP, 2007, p. 213). Their anti-inflammatory effects lead to reduction in the severity of asthma symptoms, increased peak flow readings, and decreased airway hyperresponsiveness. In general, inhaled **steroids** are safe and well tolerated at recommended dosages and can be used by both children and adults. **Corticosteroids** are also used intranasally for the treatment of allergic rhinitis.

The commonly prescribed inhaled **corticosteroids** for asthma are **beclomethasone dipropionate** (QVAR), **triamcinolone acetonide** (Azmacort), **budesonide** (Pulmicort), **flunisolide** (AeroBid), **mometasone furoate** (Asmanex Twisthaler), **fluticasone** (Flovent), and **ciclesonide** (Alvesco). There are significant differences between the different formulations in the amount of **steroid** delivered per inhalation, and they are not interchangeable without adjusting the inhalations per day.

The **corticosteroids** that are available for intranasal use are **beclomethasone** (Beconase), **triamcinolone** (Nasacort AQ), **budesonide** (Rhinocort Aqua), **flunisolide** (Nasalide, Nasarel), **mometasone** (Nasonex), **fluticasone** (Flonase), and **ciclesonide** (Omnaris).

Pharmacodynamics

In the treatment of asthma and allergic rhinitis, the primary actions of orally inhaled **corticosteroids** are anti-inflammatory. The inhaled **adrenocorticosteroids** inhibit the immunoglobulin E (IgE) and mast cell–mediated migration of inflammatory cells into the bronchial tissue (late-phase allergic reaction). The exact mechanism of action by which the inhaled **corticosteroids** inhibit bronchoconstrictor mechanisms and produce smooth muscle relaxation is unknown. The exact mechanism of action of **corticosteroids** on the nasal mucosa is unknown. Intranasal **corticosteroids** applied topically to the nasal tissues exert local anti-inflammatory effects without any systemic glucocorticoid effects.

Pharmacokinetics

Absorption and Distribution

Absorption of inhaled **corticosteroids** occurs from the lungs and from the GI tract. Approximately 10 to 30 percent of the dose from an MDI is delivered to the lungs. If a spacer device is not used, approximately 80 percent of the dose

Table 17–8 ◈ **Available Dosage Forms: Leukotriene Modifiers**

Drug	Dosage Form	How Supplied	Cost
Montelukast (Singulair)	Tablets: 10 mg Chewable tablets: 5 mg, 4 mg Granules: 4 mg/packet	80, 90, 100	$140 for 30 tablets 4 mg = $144/30 5 mg = $144/30 $145 for 30 packets
Zafirlukast (Accolate)	Tablets: 20 mg Tablets: 10 mg	60, 100	$116 for 60 tablets $111 for 60 tablets

from an MDI is swallowed, with the oral bioavailability differing from drug to drug.

Beclomethasone is rapidly absorbed from the nasal and pulmonary tissues and GI tract. Upon inhalation, 10 to 25 percent of the drug is deposited in the tissues of the mouth, trachea, and lungs, where it is completely absorbed. The remainder of the dose is swallowed. The oral bioavailability of inhaled **beclomethasone** is 20 percent. **Beclomethasone** is highly protein bound. **Beclomethasone** and its metabolites do not appear to distribute into the tissues, but **beclomethasone** does cross the placenta. With systemic administration, **steroids** are excreted in breast milk; it is unknown whether inhaled **beclomethasone** is found in breast milk.

Triamcinolone (Azmacort) MDI is packaged with a built-in spacer to enhance the delivery of the medication to the lungs. **Triamcinolone (Nasacort)** for intranasal use is delivered via intranasal metered-dose pump. **Triamcinolone** is rapidly and completely absorbed from lung tissues and nasal mucosa. It is distributed throughout the hilar areas of the lungs. The oral bioavailability of the swallowed portion of the dose is 10.6 percent. **Triamcinolone** is weakly protein bound and crosses the placenta. It is unknown whether inhaled **triamcinolone** is excreted in breast milk.

Approximately 20 percent of the inhaled dose of **budesonide** reaches the systemic circulation. Once absorbed from the nasal tissues or lungs, the distribution of **budesonide** is extensive. **Budesonide** is 88 percent protein bound. It is unknown if **budesonide** is excreted in breast milk, but it passes through the placenta.

Flunisolide is rapidly absorbed from the bronchial tree, with 10 to 20 percent of the inhaled dose distributing into the lungs. Fifty percent of an intranasal dose of **flunisolide** is absorbed into the systemic circulation. The oral bioavailability of the dose is 20 to 40 percent. **Flunisolide** crosses the placental barrier. Breast milk excretion is unknown.

Less than 1 percent of **mometasone** oral powder for inhalation is absorbed. With nasal administration the medication that is swallowed is absorbed, although plasma concentrations are near or below level of quantification. Breast milk excretion is unknown.

Fluticasone is primarily absorbed in the lung, resulting in systemic bioavailability of 30 percent of the dose. Intranasal **fluticasone** has a systemic bioavailability of less than 2 percent. It is highly lipid soluble and is rapidly distributed into the tissues. **Fluticasone** is 91 percent protein bound. **Fluticasone** crosses the placenta. Breast milk excretion is unknown.

Ciclesonide is minimally absorbed and what is absorbed is 99 percent protein bound in distribution.

Metabolism and Excretion

All inhaled **corticosteroids** have some portion of the dose that is swallowed. After GI absorption, they all undergo high first-pass liver metabolism.

In the lung, **beclomethasone** is rapidly metabolized to beclomethasone 17-monopropionate, and more slowly to free **beclomethasone**. Metabolites of **beclomethasone** are excreted mainly in the feces, with a small portion excreted in the urine.

Triamcinolone is metabolized into three less active ingredients: 6-β-hydroxy triamcinolone acetonide, 21-carboxytriamcinolone, and 21-carboxy-6-β-hydroxytriamcinolone acetonide. All of the metabolites of **triamcinolone** are eliminated in the feces.

Budesonide undergoes extensive first-pass metabolism into two main metabolites: 16-α-hydroxyprednisolone (24%) and 6-β-hydroxybudesonide (5%). The metabolites are excreted in the urine (66%) and the feces.

The part of the **flunisolide** dose that is swallowed is absorbed and metabolized by the liver into several metabolites. One of the metabolites has minor glucocorticoid activity. The drug is further metabolized into inactive metabolites. Excretion of inhaled **flunisolide** is not described, but oral doses are excreted equally in the feces and the urine.

Mometasone is extensively metabolized in the liver via CYP3A4 isoenzyme. It is excreted primarily via the bile; 74 percent of metabolites is excreted in feces.

Fluticasone is metabolized in the liver primarily by CYP3A4. The only detectable metabolite is a 1-β-carboxylic acid derivative. Excretion is primarily in the feces; less than 5 percent is excreted in the urine.

Ciclesonide is metabolized by CYP3A4 into an active metabolite, des-ciclesonide. Sixty-six percent of **ciclesonide** is excreted in the feces and approximately 20 percent in the urine.

Pharmacokinetics are presented in Table 17–9.

Pharmacotherapeutics

Precautions and Contraindications

All of the inhaled **corticosteroid** preparations are contraindicated in acute status asthmaticus or when intensive, acute therapy is warranted. They should not be used for relief of acute bronchospasm.

Care should be used when substituting any of the inhaled **corticosteroids** for oral **corticosteroid** therapy. There have been deaths due to adrenal insufficiency in asthmatic patients who were switched from oral to inhaled **corticosteroids**.

The risk for hypothalamic-pituitary-adrenal (HPA) suppression is low with inhaled **corticosteroids**, but the risk increases when inhaled **corticosteroids** are administered while the patient is taking oral **steroids**.

Inhaled **corticosteroids** should be avoided in patients with Cushing's syndrome. They should be used with caution in patients with ocular herpes simplex infections, tuberculosis, oral or nasal surgery or trauma, healing nasal septal ulcers, and untreated respiratory infection (viral, fungal, or bacterial).

All of the inhaled **corticosteroids** are Pregnancy Category C. There have been no well-controlled studies

Table 17–9 ▶ **Pharmacokinetics: Respiratory Inhalants**

Drug	Onset	Peak	Protein Binding	Bioavailability	Half-Life	Metabolism	Elimination
Corticosteroids							
Beclomethasone	Few days to 3 wk	—	—	<5%	15 h	Hepatic	Feces
Budesonide	—	—	88%	10%	2 h	Hepatic	Renal
Flunisolide	Few days to 4 wk	10–30 min	—	20%	1.8–2 h	Hepatic	Renal, feces
Fluticasone	—	—	91%	30%	—	Hepatic	Feces
Mometasone	11 h	1–2 wk	98%	—	5.8 h	Hepatic	Bile, renal
Triamcinolone	—	—	Weak	10%	0.5–1 h	Hepatic	Feces
Inhaled Antihistamine							
Azelastine	30 min–1 h	2–3 h	88%	40%	22 h	Hepatic	Feces
Anti-Inflammatory Agents							
Cromolyn sodium	—	—	—	<1%	—	Not metabolized	Bile, renal
Nedocromil	—	20 min	—	6–9%	1.5–2.3 h	Not metabolized	Renal: 64% Feces: 36%

of the effects of inhaled **corticosteroids** during pregnancy.

The use of high-dose inhaled **steroids** in children may inhibit growth, but so can poorly controlled asthma. There is a potential for slight growth delay (1 cm in height in the first year), but this is not sustained in subsequent years of treatment, is not progressive, and may be reversible (NAEPP, 2002). The long-term safety of **beclomethasone** in children under age 6 years has not been determined; doses higher than 400 mcg/day in younger children warrant close monitoring of growth. **Triamcinolone** inhalant therapy should not be prescribed to children under age 6 years, because the safety and efficacy have not been established. **Budesonide** safety has been determined for children as young as 6 months. Inhibition of growth has been noted in children on high-dose inhaled **fluticasone.** **Fluticasone** be prescribed with caution to children under age 4 years. **Mometasone** nasal spray may be prescribed for children as young as age 2 years, but the safety of **mometasone** oral inhalation powder for asthma management has not been established for children younger than age 12 years. The safety of inhaled **flunisolide** in children under age 6 years has not been established. Studies were conducted in children regarding safety of nasal **ciclesonide** in children aged 6 to 11 years; nasal **ciclesonide (Omnaris)** is considered safe and effective in children aged 6 years or older. During clinical trials the safety and efficacy of inhaled **ciclesonide (Alvesco)** was studied in children aged 4 to 11 years with asthma. To control asthma symptoms, **ciclesonide (Alvesco)** was determined to be safe, but not effective in children younger than 12 years.

Adverse Reactions

All of the inhaled **corticosteroids** have associated xerostomia, hoarseness (5% to 50% of patients), tongue and mouth irritation, flushing, and dysgeusia (altered taste sensation). Rash and urticaria have been reported with the use of **flunisolide, beclomethasone,** and **fluticasone.** Dysmenorrhea has been reported in 1 to 3 percent of patients using inhaled **fluticasone** and 4 to 9 percent using **mometasone** oral inhalation powder.

Local immunosuppression can lead to oral candidiasis with any of the inhaled **corticosteroids.** Cataracts can be induced with **corticosteroid** use, even with inhaled **corticosteroids.** Bronchospasm may occur with any of the inhaled **corticosteroids.**

With high-dose inhaled **corticosteroid** use, HPA suppression is theoretically possible. Concurrent use of systemic **corticosteroids** with inhaled **corticosteroids** increases the likelihood of HPA suppression, compared with the use of either one alone.

Pulmonary infiltrates with eosinophilia may occur with inhaled **flunisolide,** usually when inhalation

corticosteroid therapy replaces systemic **corticosteroid** therapy. The cause is unknown.

Intranasal **corticosteroid** use may cause nasal irritation, itching, sneezing, and nasal dryness. The patient may experience bloody nasal mucus or epistaxis.

Drug Interactions

There are no known drug interactions with inhaled **triamcinolone**, **flunisolide**, **mometasone**, **beclomethasone**, or **ciclesonide**.

Ritonavir significantly increases **fluticasone** serum concentrations and may lead to increased **corticosteroid** effects of **fluticasone. Ketoconazole** increases plasma concentration of **fluticasone** and **budesonide** when coadministered. The interaction is due to inhibition of CYP3A4 isoenzyme, the enzyme that metabolizes **fluticasone** and **budesonide.** There are no other known drug interactions, but close monitoring for **corticosteroid**-related side effects is advisable if coadministered with other drugs that are known to inhibit CYP3A4. Those drugs include **anastrozole** (Arimidex) in high doses, **delavirdine** (Rescriptor), **erythromycin, fluconazole** (Diflucan), **fluoxetine** (Prozac), **itraconazole** (Sporanox), **mibefradil** (Posicor), **nefazodone** (Serzone), **nelfinavir** (Viracept), **ritonavir** (Norvir), and **zileuton** (Zyflo). Drug interactions are presented in Table 17–10.

Clinical Use and Dosing

Asthma

The inhaled **corticosteroids** are the preferred long-term control medications for managing the inflammatory process associated with asthma (NAEPP, 2007). Dosages for the inhaled **corticosteroids** vary with the specific product and the delivery method. The patient with persistent asthma is started on inhaled **corticosteroids** according to the *Expert Panel Report 3* guidelines for the management of asthma discussed in detail in Chapter 30 (NAEPP, 2007). All patients with mild persistent asthma are started on a low dose of inhaled **corticosteroids.** Children older than age 12 years and adults may be treated with **cromolyn,**

Table 17–10 ■ **Drug Interactions: Respiratory Inhalants**

Drug	Interacting Drug	Possible Effect	Implications
Corticosteroids			
Beclomethasone	None known	—	—
Budesonide	Ketoconazole*	Increased budesonide concentrations and suppression of plasma cortisol levels	Observe the patient for increased corticosteroid-related side effects
Flunisolide	None known	—	—
Fluticasone	Ketoconazole* Ritonavir	Increased fluticasone concentrations and suppression of plasma cortisol levels	Observe the patient for increased corticosteroid-related side effects
Mometasone	None known	—	—
Triamcinolone	None known	—	—
Inhaled Antihistamines			
Azelastine	Cimetidine	The mean maximum concentration (C_{max}) and area under the curve (AUC) of azelastine is increased when coadministered with cimetidine	Monitor closely if coadministering
	Ethanol or other CNS depressants	Reduced mental alertness and impairment of CNS performance may occur	Use concurrently with caution
Anti-Inflammatory Agents			
Cromolyn	None known	—	—
Nedocromil	None known	—	—

*There are no other known drug interactions, but close monitoring is advisable if coadministered with other drugs that are known to inhibit CYP3A4. Those drugs include anastrozole in high doses, delavirdine, erythromycin, fluconazole, fluoxetine, itraconazole, mibefradil, nefazodone, nelfinavir, ritonavir, and zileuton.

nedocromil, **leukotriene modifiers**, or **theophylline** as alternative therapy. If the patient has moderate persistent asthma, then the patient is prescribed daily low- to medium-dose inhaled **corticosteroids** combined with a **long-acting beta agonist**. Alternatively, the patient can be prescribed medium-dose inhaled **corticosteroids** or a combination of low- to medium-dose inhaled **corticosteroids** and a **leukotriene modifier**. Severe persistent asthma requires daily high-dose inhaled **corticosteroids** and **long-acting beta agonists**. See Table 17–11 for dosing inhaled **corticosteroids** for children over age 5 years and adults. Chapter 30 should be referred to for comprehensive asthma management.

Table 17–11 ◉ **Dosage Schedule: Respiratory Inhalants**

Drug	Indication	Dose	Comments
Corticosteroids			
Beclomethasone	Asthma	*Children >5 yr and adults:* Low dose: 168–504 mcg daily in divided doses either bid, tid, or qid (4–12 puffs of 42 mcg) Medium dose: 504–840 mcg daily in divided doses (12–20 puffs of 42 mcg) High dose: >840 mcg daily in divided doses (>20 puffs of 42 mcg) *Children <5 yr:* Low dose: 80–160 mcg daily in divided doses (2–4 puffs 40 mcg/puff 1–2 puffs 80 mcg/puff) Medium dose: 160–320 mcg daily in divided doses (4–8 puffs 40 mcg/puff 2–4 puffs 80 mcg/puff) High dose: >320 mcg daily in divided doses (>8 puffs 40 mcg/puff >4 puffs 80 mcg/puff)	Patients should rinse their mouth with water after use; if needed, use inhaled bronchodilator first
	Allergic rhinitis	*Children >6 yr and adults:* 42 mcg/spray aqueous nasal spray: 1–2 sprays each nostril bid 42 mcg/spray nasal inhaler: 1 spray each nostril 2–4 times/d 84 mcg/spray aqueous nasal spray: 1–2 sprays each nostril once a day	Not recommended for use in children <6 yr
Budesonide	Asthma	*Adults:* Low dose: 200–400 mcg daily (1–2 inhalations daily) Medium dose: 400–600 mcg daily (2–3 inhalations daily) High dose: >600 mcg daily (>3 inhalations daily) *Children 12 mo–8 yr:* Pulmicort respules: Previously treated with bronchodilators alone: 0.25 mg twice daily or 0.5 mg daily, max 0.5 mg/d Previously treated with inhaled corticosteroids: 0.25 mg bid or 0.5 mg daily, max 2 mg/d Previously treated with oral corticosteroids: 0.5 mg or 1 mg daily, max 1 mg daily	Rinse mouth after use Has rapid onset for an inhaled steroid Improvement can occur within 24 h of beginning treatment, although maximum benefit may not be achieved for 1–2 wk Dose should be titrated to the lowest effective dose once asthma is controlled

Table 17–11 ◉ **Dosage Schedule: Respiratory Inhalants—cont'd**

Drug	Indication	Dose	Comments
		Children >6 yr: Low dose: 200 mcg daily (1 inhalation daily) Medium dose: 200–400 mcg daily (2–3 inhalations daily) High dose: >400 mcg/d (>2 inhalations daily)	
	Allergic rhinitis	*Children >6 yr and adults:* Initially 2 sprays in each nostril bid or 4 sprays once daily in the a.m. (max 4 sprays/nostril/d)	Blow nose prior to using For perennial rhinitis, gradually reduce over 2–4 wk to lowest effective dose
Flunisolide	Asthma	*Adults:* Low dose: 500–1,000 mcg daily (2–4 puffs daily divided in bid dose) Medium dose: 1,000–2,000 mcg daily (4–8 puffs divided bid) High dose: >2,000 mcg daily (>8 puffs divided bid) *Children >6 yr:* Low dose: 500–750 mcg (2–3 puffs daily) Medium dose: 1,000–1,250 mcg daily (4–5 puffs daily divided bid) High dose: >1,250 mcg daily (>5 puffs divided bid)	Rinse mouth after use If needed, use inhaled bronchodilator first Safety in children <6 yr has not been established
	Allergic rhinitis	*Adults:* Initially 2 sprays each nostril bid, maximum 8 sprays each nostril/d *Children 6–14 yr:* Initially 1 spray each nostril tid or 2 sprays each nostril bid; maximum 4 sprays/nostril/d	Blow nose prior to using Safety in children <6 yr has not been established
Fluticasone	Asthma	*Children >11 yr and adults:* Low dose: 88–264 mcg daily (2–6 puffs of 44 mcg/puff divided bid) Medium dose: 264–660 mcg daily (2–6 puffs of 110 mcg/puff daily divided bid) High dose: >660 mcg (>6 puffs 110 mcg/puff or >3 puffs 220 mcg/puff) *Children 4–11 yr:* Low dose: 88–176 mcg daily (2–4 puffs of 44 mcg/puff divided bid) Medium dose: 176–440 mcg daily (2–4 puffs 110 mcg/puff divided bid) High dose: >440 mcg (>4 puffs 110 mcg/puff or >2 puffs 220 mcg/puff)	Safety in children <4 yr has not been established
	Allergic rhinitis	*Children >11 yr and adults:* Initially 2 sprays each nostril once a day or 1 spray in each nostril bid; for maintenance, reduce dose to 1 spray each nostril daily	Safety in children <4 yr has not been established

Continued

Table 17–11 ◉ **Dosage Schedule: Respiratory Inhalants—cont'd**

Drug	Indication	Dose	Comments
		Children 4–11 yr: Initially 1 spray in each nostril once daily; may increase to 2 sprays in each nostril once daily if needed; for maintenance: 1 spray in each nostril once daily	
Fluticasone and Salmeterol (Advair)	Persistent asthma	*No prior inhaled corticosteroid:* *Children 4–11 yr:* Fluticasone 100 mcg/salmeterol 50 mcg 1 inhalation bid *Children ≥12 yr and adults:* Fluticasone 100 mcg/salmeterol 50 mcg 1 inhalation bid *Children and adults currently on inhaled corticosteroids:* Require dosing based on current steroid dose per manufacturer *COPD: Adults:* Fluticasone 250 mcg/salmeterol 50 mcg 1 inhalation bid	Titrate dose to lowest effective strength which maintains control of asthma
Mometasone	Allergic rhinitis	*Children 2–11 yr:* 1 spray each nostril once a day *Children ≥12 yr and adults:* 2 sprays each nostril twice a day.	
Asmanex Twisthaler	Asthma	*Children ≥12 yr and adults:* Previous Therapy — Recommended Starting Dose — Highest Recommended Daily Dose Bronchodilators alone — 220 mcg daily p.m. — 440 mcg Inhaled corticosteroids — 220 mcg daily p.m. — 440 mcg Oral corticosteroids — 440 mcg bid — 880 mcg	Contains lactose. If administered once a day, dose should be taken in the p.m. Safety not established in children <12 yr
Triamcinolone	Asthma	*Children >12 yr and adults:* Low dose: 400–1,000 mcg daily divided in bid, tid, or qid doses (4–10 puffs) Medium dose: 1,000–2,000 mcg daily in divided doses (10–20 puffs) High dose: >200 mcg daily in divided doses (>20 puffs) *Children 6–12 yr:* Low dose: 400–800 mcg per day in divided doses (4–8 puffs daily) Medium dose: 800–1,200 mcg daily in divided doses (8–12) High dose: >1,200 mcg daily in divided doses (>12 puffs)	Rinse mouth after use Safety in children <6 yr has not been established

Table 17–11 ◉ **Dosage Schedule: Respiratory Inhalants—cont'd**

Drug	Indication	Dose	Comments
	Allergic rhinitis	*Children >12 yr and adults:* 2 sprays in each nostril once daily; may increase if needed to a maximum of 8 sprays/d; reduce dose as condition improves *Children 6–12 yr:* 2 sprays each nostril once daily; may reduce as condition improves	Safety in children <6 yr has not been established
Inhaled Antihistamine			
Azelastine	Allergic rhinitis	*Children >12 yr and adults:* 2 sprays (137 mcg/spray) per nostril bid *Children 5–11 yr:* 1 spray per nostril bid	Safety in children <5 yr has not been established The unit must be primed before using for the first time by pumping the activator 4 times, until a fine mist occurs
Anti-Inflammatory Agents			
	Asthma	*Inhaled* *Children >5 yr and adults:* 4 puffs qid initially; wean down to 2 puffs bid to tid; may use 2 puffs prior to exercise or allergen exposure *Nebulizer* *Children >2 yr and adults:* 1 unit dose qid, weaning down to bid	Cromolyn must be used continuously 3–4 wk before maximum effect is achieved Cromolyn is very safe to use in children, with fewer side effects than inhaled steroids
	Allergic rhinitis	*Children >6 yr and adults:* 1 spray in each nostril 3–4 times a day; may increase dosage to 6/d if needed	Begin therapy 1 wk before known exposure; for allergic rhinitis, 2–4 wk of therapy may be needed to produce relief; blow nose prior to administering
Nedocromil	Asthma	*Inhaled* *Children >6 yr and adults:* 2 puffs qid *Nebulizer* *Children >2 yr and adults:* 1 ampule via nebulizer qid	Once control is established, the dose can be reduced to 3 times a day; after several weeks the dose can be further decreased to bid

Children with persistent asthma require daily anti-inflammatory therapy. Young children with mild persistent asthma are usually started on step 2 therapy, a low-dose inhaled **corticosteroids** (via nebulizer or MDI and mask), with an alternative therapy being **cromolyn** or **montelukast**. If the child has moderate persistent asthma, low-dose inhaled **corticosteroids** combined with **montelukast** or long-acting inhaled **beta agonist** are begun. Because **salmeterol** is not approved for children younger than age 4 years, an alternative treatment would be medium-dose inhaled **corticosteroids**, or low-dose inhaled **corticosteroids** combined with a leukotriene modifier (**montelukast**). High-dose inhaled **steroids** combined with a **long-acting inhaled beta agonist** or **montelukast** are prescribed for severe persistent asthma. The provider should be familiar with the differences in dosing young children and adults. The full *Expert Panel Report 3* guidelines for step-wise management of asthma are available in Chapter 30.

Allergic Rhinitis

Allergic rhinitis results when allergens come in contact with the nasal mucosa, causing a hypersensitivity reaction. Nasal **corticosteroids** are used to manage the inflammatory response associated with seasonal or perennial allergies. Intranasal **corticosteroids** may be used once or twice a day, depending on the drug chosen. Once clinical improvement occurs, usually in 3 to 7 days, the dose can be decreased. See Table 17–11 for dosing information.

Rational Drug Selection

The *Expert Panel Report 3* and update (NAEPP, 2007) do not recommend one inhaled **corticosteroid** over another; therefore, the choice is mostly based on ease of dosing and the adverse drug interactions and indications previously addressed. There are no generic equivalent formulas for the inhaled **corticosteroids** but there is generic **fluticasone** nasal spray, which may make cost a factor as more generic formulas are available.

Dosing

If a patient requires a high dose of inhaled steroid, the **beclomethasone** 42 mcg/puff dose would be more than 20 puffs per day, whereas the dose of **budesonide** would be eight or more puffs per day. High-dose **triamcinolone** would also be 20 puffs per day. **Fluticasone** and **flunisolide** have the highest steroid anti-inflammatory effect per puff, which makes dosing high-dose inhaled steroids more convenient (see Table 17–11 for dosing). If the patient requires a low dose or if trying to wean the dose, **beclomethasone** or **triamcinolone** would be the first choice.

Monitoring

The patient who is using inhaled **corticosteroids** needs to be monitored for adverse effects of the medication, effectiveness of the medication, and the asthma disease process. If high-dose inhaled **corticosteroids** are used for a long time, blood glucose and potassium should be monitored, as well as growth in young children.

Patient Education

Administration

Patients who are concurrently using an inhaled **bronchodilator** should administer the **bronchodilator** first and wait several minutes before using the inhaled **corticosteroid.** This procedure enhances the absorption of the **steroid** in the bronchial tree.

The administration of inhaled **corticosteroids** via an MDI can be difficult for most adults and all children. Learning to coordinate the release of the medication from the inhaler with a deep breath is difficult. Written and pictorial instructions are available with the inhaler, but the provider must not assume that the patient understands the proper method of administering inhaled medications. Use verbal instructions as well as actual demonstration with a placebo inhaler to reinforce the written instructions. These instructions and demonstrations should be repeated at follow-up visits.

To use an inhaler properly, the patient should first exhale and then tilt the head slightly back and place the inhaler mouthpiece either about 2 inches from the open mouth or between the open lips. While inhaling, the patient should press down on the canister, breathe in slowly and deeply, and hold his or her breath for 10 seconds (count of 10) or as long as comfortable. If multiple puffs are prescribed, then the patient should wait at least 1 full minute between inhalations.

To assist with the delivery of inhaled medications, spacers can be prescribed. The Aerochamber is a tube-like device that has pictures drawn on the outside to remind the patient of the proper techniques. For younger children and older adults, the InspirEase spacer gives a visual cue of the spacer bag deflating to help in taking a deep enough breath. Both of these devices cue the patient to breathe slowly by emitting a whistling sound if the patient is taking too rapid a breath.

Dry powder, breath-actuated inhalers require adequate inspiratory effort to deliver the medication into the bronchial tree. Patient self-administration should be observed to determine whether they are using the medication appropriately.

Patients should rinse their mouth with water after each use to help reduce dry mouth, hoarseness, and candidiasis infection.

The patient should clear the nasal passages of mucus prior to using intranasal **corticosteroids.** If the nasal passages are swollen and blocked, the patient should administer a topical decongestant prior to using intranasal **corticosteroids.** The medication is sprayed into the nasal passages. The patient does not need to inhale the medication. The patient should understand that the effects are not immediate and that clinical improvement may take 3 to 7 days. Rinsing the mouth with water after use will reduce the rare chance of candidiasis infection associated with intranasal **corticosteroid** use.

Inhaled **steroids** are not to be used as abortive asthma medications; they are for preventive therapy only. The provider should have patients bring in all their inhalers and review which are to be used for abortive therapy (**short-acting beta agonists**) and which are for preventive therapy. The patient should be advised to continue to use the inhaled **corticosteroid** even when not having asthma symptoms.

Adverse Reactions

The patient should be advised to notify the provider if sore mouth or throat occurs. Oral *Candida* infections are possible, and the patient should get prompt treatment. The patient should be aware of the possibility of dysphonia developing. Rinsing the mouth with water and using a spacer device will decrease its incidence.

Other adverse effects occur less often, but the patient should be aware of them and be instructed to notify the provider if adverse effects begin to develop from the inhaled medication.

Relatively few medications interact with the inhaled **corticosteroids. Ketoconazole** should be avoided for patients who are prescribed **fluticasone, ciclesonide,** and **budesonide**. Patients should be instructed to notify all providers that they are on inhaled **corticosteroids** to avoid possible interactions.

Lifestyle Management

Lifestyle management issues related to the disease process should be discussed. They often include the following:

1. Patients need to self-monitor their respiratory status with a peak flowmeter to determine the effectiveness of the medication prescribed.
2. The patient should avoid or quit smoking.
3. The patient should avoid environmental triggers for asthma at home, work, and school.

Available dosage forms are presented in Table 17–12.

Inhaled Anti-Inflammatory Agents

Cromolyn sodium and **nedocromil** are synthetic compounds that inhibit antigen-induced bronchospasm. **Cromolyn** was originally produced to be used as a **bronchodilator** but was found to have no **bronchodilator** activity. Nevertheless, **cromolyn** inhibits antigen-induced bronchospasm, blocks the release of histamine, and is a mast cell stabilizer. **Nedocromil** is similar to **cromolyn** in many ways, but there are distinct differences, which are discussed in this section.

Cromolyn (Intal) is used in the treatment of asthma; it (Nasalcrom) is also used in treating allergic rhinitis. **Nedocromil** (Tilade) is approved for use in patients with asthma who are not controlled with **beta agonists** alone.

Pharmacodynamics

Cromolyn and **nedocromil** both act to inhibit mast cell degranulation, which prevents the release of histamine and slow-reacting substance of anaphylaxis (SRS-A). Neither drug prevents the binding of IgE to the mast cell or the binding of antigen to IgE. **Cromolyn** and **nedocromil** also prevent the release of leukotrienes, which induce

Table 17–12 ◆ **Available Dosage Forms: Respiratory Inhalants**

Drug	Dosage Form	How Supplied	Cost
		CORTICOSTEROIDS	
Beclomethasone			
QVAR	40 mcg/puff 80 mcg/puff	7.3-g (100 inhalation) canister	$91.86 $109.99
Beconase AQ	Aqueous nasal inhaler: 42 mcg/spray	25-g canister (200 sprays)	$149.99
Budesonide			
Pulmicort Respules	0.25 mg/2 mL 0.5 mg/2 mL	2 mL ampules—30	$223/30 $259/30
Pulmicort Flexihaler	Flexihaler 90 mcg/dose Flexihaler: 180 mcg/dose	60 inh 120 inh	$114.46 $151.75
Rhinocort	Nasal spray: 32 mcg/spray	7 g (200 sprays)	$111.96
Flunisolide			
Aerobid	Inhaler: 250 mcg/puff	7-g canister (100 inhalation)	$96.44
Generic nasal spray	0.025% Solution Aqueous nasal spray: 25 mcg/spray	25-mL inhaler 29 mcg/act Solution 25 mL Bottle	$39.99 $45.99
Nasalide	Nasal solution: 25 mcg/spray	25-mL metered pump (200 sprays)	$51.59
Nasarel	Aqueous nasal spray: 25 mcg/spray	25-mL metered pump (200 sprays)	$48.99
Fluticasone			
Flovent HFA	Inhaler: 44 mcg/puff, 110 mcg/puff, 220 mcg/puff	44 mcg/puff in 7.9- (60 inh) and 13-g (120 inh) canisters; 110 mcg/puff in 13-g (120 inh) canister; 220 mcg/puff in 13-g (120 inh) canister	$71.47 44 mcg $90.47 110 mcg $141.37 220 mcg

Continued

Table 17–12 ◆ **Available Dosage Forms: Respiratory Inhalants—cont'd**

Drug	Dosage Form	How Supplied	Cost
		CORTICOSTEROIDS	
Flonase	50 mcg inhalation	120 sprays	$85.98
Generic	16 g bottle	50 mcg/actuation	$60/16-g bottle
Fluticasone/Salmeterol			
Advair 100/50 diskus	Fluticasone 100 mcg Salmeterol 50 mcg	60 doses/disk	$176
Advair 250/50	Fluticasone 250 mcg Salmeterol 50 mcg	60 doses/disk	$215.97
Advair 500/50	Fluticasone 500 mcg Salmeterol 50 mcg	14 doses/disk 60 doses/disk	$288 $274.97
Mometasone			
Nasonex	Nasal suspension 50 mcg/spray	17-g bottle	$116.82
Asmanex Twisthaler	Powder for oral inhalation 110 mcg/inh, 220 mcg/inh	110 mcg/inh: 30 inhalation 220 mcg/inh: 30 inhalation, 60 inhalation, or 120 inhalation	$97.99/30 inh $99.99/60 inh $218/120 inh
Triamcinolone			
Azmacort	Inhaler: 75 mcg/puff	20-g (240 inh) canisters	$91.29
Nasacort AQ	Aqueous nasal spray: 55 mcg/spray	10-g (100 sprays) canisters	$118
		INHALED ANTIHISTAMINE	
Azelastine			
Astelin	Aqueous nasal spray: 137 mcg/spray	30-mL bottles (100 sprays/bottle)	$117.27
		ANTI-INFLAMMATORY AGENTS	
Cromolyn Sodium			
Intal	Inhaler: 800 mcg/puff Solution for nebulizer: 20-mg/2-mL ampules	8.1-g (112 inh) canister 2-mL ampules (60, 120)	Temporarily not available
Nasalcrom OTC	Nasal solution: 5.2 mg/spray	13-mL (100 sprays) and 26-mL (200 sprays) metered pump	$16.29/26 mL $9.99/13 mL
Nedocromil			
Tilade	Inhaler: 1.75 mg per puff Solution for nebulizer: 11-mg/2.2-mL ampule	16.2-g (104 inh) canister 2-mL ampules (60, 120)	Temporarily not available

numerous effects that contribute to the inflammatory process in the lungs. **Nedocromil** additionally inhibits and prevents the release of platelet-activating factor (PAF). With continued use, **cromolyn** and **nedocromil** reduce bronchi hyperreactivity to stimuli such as cold air, allergens, and environmental irritants.

Neither drug has bronchodilator, antihistamine, or vasoconstrictor activity, and at therapeutic doses, neither has systemic activity.

Pharmacokinetics

Absorption and Distribution

Inhaled **cromolyn** is poorly absorbed systemically; only 8 percent of the dose is absorbed. Approximately 5 to 10 percent of the inhaled dose reaches the lungs, with the amount affected by the degree of bronchoconstriction present. Intranasal **cromolyn** is minimally absorbed. Distribution of the absorbed amount of the drug is unknown. Minimal amounts of **cromolyn** cross the placenta and distribute into breast milk.

Inhaled **nedocromil** is slowly absorbed from the lungs, with 6 to 9 percent of the dose having systemic bioavailability. Absorption of **nedocromil** is affected by exercise and decreased forced expiratory volume (FEV) measurements. Distribution is unknown. **Nedocromil** is thought to cross the placenta. It is unknown whether **nedocromil** is excreted in breast milk.

Metabolism and Excretion

The portion of the dose of **cromolyn** that is absorbed from the lung is rapidly excreted unchanged in the urine and bile. The remaining portion of the dose is exhaled or swallowed and excreted unchanged in the feces. **Nedocromil** is not metabolized and is excreted unchanged in the urine (64%) and feces (36%).

Pharmacotherapeutics

Precautions and Contraindications

Neither **cromolyn** nor **nedocromil** is a **bronchodilator**, and neither is contraindicated in the treatment of acute bronchospasm or status asthmaticus.

Hypersensitivity to **cromolyn** or **nedocromil** is a contraindication to their use.

Both **cromolyn** and **nedocromil** are Pregnancy Category B. These drugs should be used with caution in the lactating mother because their safety has not been established.

Cromolyn is safe for use in children as young as 2 years (nebulizer solution). Safety and efficacy of **nedocromil** in children under age 6 years have not been established.

Adverse Reactions

Cromolyn is generally well tolerated. Inhaled **cromolyn** may cause bronchospasm, which can be avoided by preadministering a **beta-agonist bronchodilator**. Throat irritation and cough are also reported. Intranasal **cromolyn** may produce nasal irritation and cause sneezing.

Nedocromil is well tolerated, with an unpleasant taste the most common (12.6%) reported adverse effect. Altered taste sensation (dysgeusia) has also been reported. Other reported adverse reactions are cough (7%), headache (6%), sore throat (5.7%), rhinitis (4.6%), and nausea (4%).

Drug Interactions

There are no clinically significant drug interactions with either **cromolyn** or **nedocromil**. **Cromolyn** solution for nebulizer use will form a precipitate if mixed with ipratropium solution.

Clinical Use and Dosing

Asthma

Cromolyn is considered an alternative long-term control drug for the treatment of mild persistent asthma. It is available in inhaled form and nebulizer solution. The dosage of **cromolyn** MDI for children older than 5 years and adults is two sprays (800 mcg/spray) inhaled four times a day at regular intervals. The dose of nebulizer solution of **cromolyn** is one ampule (20 mg) four times a day at regular intervals. The dose of **cromolyn** may be decreased after the patient is stabilized (usually after 4 wk) to two or three doses a day. If used concurrently with **bronchodilators**, the **bronchodilator** should be administered first. **Cromolyn** may be mixed with **albuterol** in a nebulizer cup to simplify dosing. The patient should understand that the effectiveness of **cromolyn** depends on using it regularly.

Oral **cromolyn** is also used for systemic mast cell disease (mastocytosis) and inflammatory bowel disease. Dosing for mastocytosis is 200 mg of **Gastrocrom** oral concentrate four times a day in adults and 100 mg four times a day in children aged 2 to 12 years. Initial adult dosing for inflammatory bowel disease is 200 mg four times a day of **Gastrocrom** oral concentrate, which may be doubled if not responding after 2 to 3 weeks to 400 mg four times a day. Children aged 2 to 12 years with inflammatory bowel disease are dosed at 100 mg four times a day. The dose may be doubled, but do not exceed 40 mg/kg/day (Takemoto et al, 2009).

The dose of **nedocromil** MDI in children age 6 years or older and adults is two inhalations four times a day at regular intervals. After good control is achieved, which usually takes several weeks, the patient's dose may be weaned to three times a day. After several weeks of good control, the patient may be further weaned to twice-a-day dosing, which is the minimal effective dose. Patients should understand that effective treatment depends on continued use, even if they are having no asthma symptoms.

Bronchospasm Prophylaxis

Cromolyn is indicated for patients with exercise-induced bronchospasm or individuals who have bronchospasm with known precipitating factors (e.g., pet exposure). The dose of **cromolyn** MDI for children aged 5 years or older and adults is two inhalations 10 to 15 minutes before exercise. If exercise is prolonged, the dose may be repeated. Nebulizer dosing in children aged 2 years or older and adults is 1 ampule administered via nebulized solution not more than 1 hour prior to exercise. For maximum effectiveness, the time between the use of inhaled **cromolyn** sodium and exercise should be as brief as possible.

Allergic Rhinitis

The dosage of **cromolyn** sodium nasal inhalation spray in children aged 6 years and older and adults is one spray in each nostril three to four times a day. The dose may be increased to six times a day if needed. The dose is administered while the patient is inhaling, and the nostrils should first be cleared of mucus. Two to 4 weeks of therapy may be needed to produce relief from perennial rhinitis.

Rational Drug Selection

The decision regarding which inhaled **anti-inflammatory** to use is often based on cost, availability, and patient variables such as age or ease of dosing. As of this writing, chlorofluorocarbon (CFC)-containing inhalers are being phased out, with **Intal** and **Tilade** scheduled for removal from the market on December 31, 2010. It is assumed manufacturers will develop CFC-free products, as seen in the inhaled **corticosteroids**.

Patient Variables

Cromolyn has dosage forms available for use in children as young as 2 years, whereas **nedocromil** is approved only for patients age 6 years and older.

Administration

Cromolyn comes in multiple formulations that allow the provider to match the patient's age and lifestyle with an administration form. **Cromolyn** MDI (**Intal**) has been discontinued in the United States, but inhalation solution for nebulizer use is available. **Nedocromil** is available only in MDI form, which is scheduled for removal in December 2010.

Cost

Cromolyn is available in generic nebulizer solution; the cost of 60 ampules is $94.99 (http://drugstore.com).

Monitoring

No specific monitoring is required other than monitoring associated with the disease process.

Patient Education

Administration

The administration of inhaled anti-inflammatory agents requires the patient to use the medication as prescribed. Neither **cromolyn** nor **nedocromil** is effective if not used at regular intervals. Clarification regarding the use of inhaled **bronchodilators** that can be used as needed and the inhaled **anti-inflammatory** agents will enable the patient to use the medication appropriately, as will a written plan.

The administration of **cromolyn** or **nedocromil** via an MDI can be difficult for adults and children alike. Learning to coordinate the release of the medication from the inhaler with a deep breath is difficult. Written and pictorial instructions are available with the inhaler, but the provider must not assume that the patient understands the proper method of administering inhaled medications. Use verbal instructions as well as actual demonstration with a placebo inhaler to reinforce the written instructions. These instructions and demonstrations should be repeated at follow-up visits. Do not assume that the patient who is already using another medication via MDI is using it correctly. These teaching steps should be used whenever a new medication is introduced.

To use an inhaler properly, the patient should first exhale, then tilt the head slightly back, and place the inhaler mouthpiece either about 2 inches from the open mouth or between the open lips. While inhaling, the patient should press down on the canister, breathe in slowly and deeply, and hold her or his breath for 10 seconds (count of 10) or as long as comfortable. If two puffs are prescribed, then the patient should wait at least 1 full minute between inhalations.

To assist with the delivery of inhaled medications, a spacer can be prescribed. The Aerochamber is a tube-like device that has pictures drawn on the outside to remind the patient of the proper technique to use in administering the inhaler. For younger children and older adults, the InspirEase spacer gives a visual cue of the spacer bag deflating to help them take a deep enough breath. If the patient takes a rapid breath, both devices emit a whistling sound to cue the patient to breathe more slowly.

The use of **cromolyn** via nebulizer must be demonstrated to the patient in the clinic or by the home health agency that is providing the nebulizer. Because the vials are premeasured, there is no concern about dosing error.

Adverse Reactions

At therapeutic dosages, minimal adverse reactions are reported. The patient should be instructed not to exceed the recommended dosage of the medication.

Lifestyle Management

Lifestyle management issues related to the disease process being treated should be discussed. They often include the following:

1. The patient needs to self-monitor respiratory status with a peak flowmeter to determine the effectiveness of the medication prescribed.
2. The patient should avoid or quit smoking.
3. The patient should avoid environmental triggers for the asthma at home, work, and school.

Inhaled Antihistamines

Azelastine (Astelin, Astepro) and **olopatadine (Patanase)** are the intranasal H_1 blockers currently available in the United States. They are used for the treatment of seasonal allergic rhinitis and vasomotor rhinitis.

Pharmacodynamics

Azelastine is an H_1 agonist and a potent inhibitor of histamine release from the mast cells. **Azelastine** and its metabolite desmethylazelastine inhibit the effects of histamine by competing with histamine for H_1 binding sites. **Azelastine** may also interfere with histamine- and leukotriene-induced bronchospasm. **Olopatadine** is a selective H_1 receptor antagonist.

Pharmacokinetics

Absorption and Distribution

Azelastine, administered intranasally, has a systemic oral bioavailability of 40 percent. Protein binding of azelastine is 88 percent and, for the active metabolite desmethylazelastine, is 97 percent. Peak serum concentrations are reached in 2 to 3 hours. Exact absorption information is unknown. Distribution is unknown, but because somnolence is a reported adverse effect, azelastine is assumed to enter the CNS. It is unknown whether azelastine crosses the placenta or is distributed in breast milk.

Olopatadine is absorbed from nasal mucosa and peaks in 15 minutes to 2 hours after administration. The portion of olopatadine absorbed is 55 percent protein bound.

Metabolism and Excretion

Azelastine is metabolized into the principal active metabolite, desmethylazelastine. Following intranasal dosing of azelastine to steady state, plasma concentration of desmethylazelastine is 20 to 30 percent of azelastine. Excretion of azelastine and desmethylazelastine is via the feces.

Olopatadine is not extensively metabolized and is eliminated in the urine.

Pharmacotherapeutics

Precautions and Contraindications

Some patients using intranasal azelastine may experience somnolence and should be cautioned not to drive or operate heavy equipment while using it. Patients should not use alcohol or other CNS depressants while using azelastine.

Olopatadine is contraindicated only in patients with nasal diseases other than allergies. Spraying into the eyes should be avoided.

It is unknown whether azelastine is excreted in breast milk. Use during lactation with caution. Olopatadine has been measured in the milk of nursing rats; no studies of use in lactating women have been done. Because seasonal allergic rhinitis is not generally a life-threatening disease, the benefits do not outweigh the unknown risks to the infant.

Azelastine and olopatadine are Pregnancy Category C. It should be used in pregnancy only if the potential benefits outweigh the risks to the fetus. There are no adequate studies in pregnant women. In animals receiving more than 240 times the normal dose, external and skeletal abnormalities have been noted.

Safety of azelastine in children under age 5 years and of olopatadine in children younger than age 12 years has not been established.

Adverse Reactions

The most commonly reported adverse reaction to azelastine is bitter taste (19%). Other reported adverse reactions are somnolence (11%), headache, weight gain (2%), and myalgia (1.5%). Local effects such as nasal irritation, epistaxis, sneezing, and rhinitis are also reported. Bitter taste (12.8%), headache (4.4%), and epitaxis (3.2%) are also reported in patients using intranasal olopatadine.

Drug Interactions

There is an additive impairment of CNS function when azelastine is used with ethanol or other CNS depressants. When azelastine is coadministered orally with cimetidine, the area under the curve (AUC) and C_{max} are increased by 65 percent. Data regarding interactions with intranasal azelastine and cimetidine are not available. Azelastine should be used cautiously with other antihistamines. There is theoretical additive CNS depression when olopatadine is administered with other CNS depressants or alcohol.

Clinical Use and Dosing

Allergic Rhinitis

Azelastine is approved for use in seasonal allergic rhinitis. It is used to treat the specific symptoms of rhinorrhea, sneezing, and nasal pruritus. The dose for children older than age 12 years and adults is two sprays (137 mcg/spray) per nostril twice a day. Children age 5 to 12 years should use one spray in each nostril twice a day.

Dosing for olopatadine is two sprays in each nostril twice a day in children older than age 12 years and in adults.

Rational Drug Selection

Oral Versus Intranasal Antihistamine

The provider may choose to use intranasal azelastine or olopatadine rather than a systemic antihistamine because of decreased adverse effects or fewer drug interactions noted with the intranasal product.

Cost

The cost of azelastine (Astelin) is $111.68 for a 30-mL bottle (http://drugstore.com). Olopatadine (Patanase) costs $114.17 for a 30.5-g bottle (http://drugstore.com).

Patient Variables

Azelastine should not be prescribed to children under age 5 years and olopatadine not prescribed to children younger than age 12 years. Both drugs should be used with caution in pregnant and lactating patients.

Monitoring

There is no specific monitoring required with the use of azelastine or olopatadine other than symptoms of allergic rhinitis to determine efficacy.

Patient Education

Administration

The patient should be instructed to prime the medication unit before use by pumping the activator four times, or until a fine mist appears. The patient should keep the sprayer pointed away from the face, other people, and pets when priming the medication. The patient should wipe the tip of the sprayer with a clean tissue after using and replace the cap between uses. To prevent the spread of infection, the sprayer should be used by only one person.

Adverse Reactions

The patient should be instructed about the most common adverse reactions. Caution regarding driving or operating heavy equipment while using **azelastine** should be stressed. The bitter taste that some patients experience may be decreased by drinking water or another fluid after administration. The patient should report any unusual adverse reactions to the provider.

The patient should be cautioned not to drink **alcohol** or take any other CNS depressants while using intranasal **azelastine.** The patient may not be aware that an intranasal medication can have an interaction with an orally administered medication, and therefore, the provider must give careful instructions before prescribing **azelastine.**

Lifestyle Management

Lifestyle management related to the disease process needs to be discussed with the patient. Points to discuss often include avoidance of known allergens and using environmental methods to control dust mites and other common allergens.

Oxygen

Oxygen is a basic element essential for human life; oxygen deprivation leads to rapid death. Therapy with **oxygen** is necessary for life in several diseases that interfere with normal oxygenation of blood and tissues. **Oxygen** as a therapeutic gas is delivered from steel containers and is 99 percent pure.

Pharmacodynamics

Oxygen is prescribed to treat hypoxia, or tissue deprivation of **oxygen.** Hypoxia can be caused by an inadequate supply of **oxygen** to the lungs, which can be due to poor ventilation or inadequate partial pressure of inspired **oxygen.** Inadequate pulmonary function can lead to hypoxia, as in a mismatch between ventilation and perfusion. Tissue hypoxia may occur with inadequate delivery of **oxygen** to the tissues, such as occurs in low cardiac output. Tissue hypoxia may also occur if the **oxygen** concentration of the blood is low, as occurs in anemia.

The effects of hypoxia can be observed in all major organ systems. The respiratory system increases the ventilatory rate and depth as a result of stimulation of carotid and aortic chemoreceptors. The heart increases cardiac output by increasing the heart rate. With severe hypoxia, bradycardia develops and ultimately leads to circulatory failure. The CNS is the most sensitive to hypoxia, with initial impaired judgment and psychomotor ability, leading to confusion; restlessness; and ultimately stupor, coma, and death.

Pharmacokinetics

The **oxygen** content of inhaled air is normally 20.9 percent, equivalent to a partial pressure of 159 mm Hg. As **oxygen** is inhaled, it enters the pulmonary airways and travels to the distal airways and alveoli. In the distal airways, the partial pressure of **oxygen** (Po_2) is decreased by dilution with carbon dioxide and water vapor and by uptake into the blood. The diffusion of **oxygen** into the pulmonary capillary blood is driven by the gradient between the Po_2 in mixed venous blood and that in the alveolar gas. The pressure gradient increases when 100 percent **oxygen** is administered, causing increased **oxygen** diffusion into the pulmonary capillary blood. **Oxygen** is delivered via the circulation to the tissue capillary beds, where **oxygen** is diffused by its higher partial pressure out of the blood and into the cells.

Oxygen in the blood is carried by the hemoglobin, with a small amount in physical solution in the plasma. The amount of **oxygen** carried by the hemoglobin depends on the partial pressure of carbon dioxide ($PaCo_2$) and is usually illustrated with the oxyhemoglobin dissociation curve.

Pharmacotherapeutics

Precautions and Contraindications

The only contraindication to **oxygen** use is concurrent smoking while the **oxygen** is running. **Oxygen** is a flammable gas that will ignite if a flame is too near. This has implications for chronic smokers, who should turn off their **oxygen** to smoke.

Oxygen should be prescribed to patients with chronic carbon dioxide retention with extreme caution and close monitoring. Because hypoxemia may be the primary stimulus for respiration in these patients, the lowest possible concentration of **oxygen** to avoid serious tissue hypoxia should be used. In patients with hypercapnia, the sudden increases in $PaCo_2$ produced by **oxygen** may result in cessation of respiration.

Adverse Drug Reactions

Dry Nasal Passages

The most common adverse drug reaction reported in patients who are administered **oxygen** is dry nasal passages from the flow of gas through the nasal cannula (NC). This can be prevented by administering humidified **oxygen** by mask or by keeping the flow rate low (less than 5 to 6 L/min).

Toxicity

Oxygen toxicity occurs when inspired concentrations of **oxygen** exceed those of air for prolonged periods of time.

Cell membrane damage and death are thought to be caused by increased production of reactive species such as superoxide anion, singlet **oxygen**, hydroxyl radical, and hydrogen peroxide. Some tissues, including the respiratory tract, the CNS, and the retina, are more sensitive to high **oxygen** concentration.

In the respiratory tract, inhalation of 100 percent **oxygen** for 6 to 8 hours can lead to decreased movement of tracheal mucus. In as little as 12 hours of 100 percent **oxygen**, the patient may experience tracheobronchial irritation and complain of chest tightness. After 17 hours, there is increased alveolar permeability and inflammation. Overall pulmonary function decreases after 18 to 24 hours of continuous 100 percent **oxygen.** After 24 hours of 100 percent **oxygen**, the patient usually has symptoms of nausea, vomiting, and anorexia. The patient may survive 1 week on toxic levels of **oxygen.** Death occurs from pulmonary edema.

Oxygen toxicity of the CNS does not occur until the partial pressure of inspired **oxygen** (PIo_2) is greater than 2 atm, which usually occurs in a hyperbaric chamber.

The retina of a premature neonate can be damaged by exposure to high levels of **oxygen** for prolonged periods. The development of retrolental fibroplasia is thought to be related to high levels of partial pressure of **oxygen** in arterial blood (Pao_2) administered to the neonate. Adults rarely have **oxygen**-induced retinopathy, even with hyperbaric levels.

Drug Interactions

There are no drug interactions with **oxygen**.

Clinical Use and Dosing

Oxygen is administered to treat hypoxia as determined by pulse oximetry or arterial or mixed venous blood gases. Hypoxia is usually a symptom or manifestation of an underlying disease, and therefore, **oxygen** therapy is not curative, but it does provide symptomatic and temporary improvement in the patient's status. The underlying cause of hypoxia needs to be treated.

Correction of Hypoxia

To correct hypoxia, **oxygen** is administered to the patient via a variety of **oxygen**-delivery systems. The provider chooses a delivery system based on the fraction or percentage of **oxygen** (FIo_2) that is desired for treatment. The goal of treatment is to maintain **oxygen** saturation above 90 percent.

An NC will deliver an FIo_2 of 0.24 to 0.35 if the flow of **oxygen** is at 5 to 6 L/min. Higher flow rates via NC dry out the nasal mucosa and will not achieve higher FIo_2 because the **oxygen** is mixed with ambient air. Humidified **oxygen** can be delivered to decrease nasal passage dryness. The percentage of **oxygen** that can be delivered via NC is 22 to 44 percent.

Masks cover the mouth and nose and allow for a higher concentration of **oxygen** to be delivered. **Oxygen** delivery via mask requires a flow rate above 5 L/min to avoid accumulation of exhaled air in the mask. A flow rate of 8 to 10 L/min is recommended. A simple face mask, which allows room air to dilute the **oxygen**, delivers 40 to 60 percent **oxygen** to the patient. A face mask with an **oxygen** reservoir provides a constant flow of **oxygen** at above 60 percent concentration. If the flow rate of **oxygen** is 6 L/min, then the **oxygen** concentration is 60 percent. The **oxygen** concentration increases by 10 percent for every liter per minute increase in flow. When 10 L/min of **oxygen** is delivered via a mask with an **oxygen** reservoir, the percentage of **oxygen** delivered reaches 100 percent. A Venturi mask allows for controlled percentages of **oxygen** to be delivered to patients. The mask can be adjusted to deliver 24, 28, 35, and 40 percent. This type of mask is used on patients with chronic hypercapnia (e.g., COPD patients) to tightly control the amount of **oxygen** delivered and avoid respiratory depression associated with high **oxygen** concentrations in these patients.

Oxygen may also be delivered by hood or tent to provide a known concentration to the patient, with little cooperation required from the patient. Flow rates must be high enough to prevent accumulation of carbon dioxide.

Monitoring

Monitoring the patient on **oxygen** is necessary to treat hypoxia and to avoid toxicity. The most accurate yet invasive method to monitor blood oxygenation is by arterial or mixed venous blood gas sampling. This procedure can be painful for the patient and requires rapid transport of the specimen to the laboratory. Blood gases have the advantage of providing additional information, besides oxygenation, regarding the patient's status that may assist in the treatment of the underlying cause of hypoxemia. Pulse oximetry is a noninvasive method of monitoring the patient receiving **oxygen** therapy. It measures the difference in absorption of light by oxyhemoglobin and deoxyhemoglobin in an accessible location, such as the finger, toe (in children), or ear. Pulse oximetry measures the hemoglobin saturation and not Po_2.

The need for continuing **oxygen** therapy should be monitored by drawing arterial blood gases after 1, 3, and 6 months of therapy.

Patient Education

Administration

The patient who is receiving home **oxygen** therapy requires knowledge of the appropriate use of **oxygen**, as well as education about safe administration.

The patient should use the **oxygen** as prescribed by the provider. Increasing or decreasing the flow rate of **oxygen** may have adverse effects. Using **oxygen** for fewer hours than prescribed will increase hypoxia and will have detrimental effects.

The patient should understand that **oxygen** is a flammable gas that should be kept away from open flame.

Patients who smoke should be cautioned not to smoke while their **oxygen** is running.

Adverse Reactions

There are minimal adverse reactions with the use of **oxygen**. The patient should be advised of the potential of developing dry nasal passages. Increasing hydration and increasing the humidity of the home will help somewhat.

Oxygen toxicity should be discussed and the patient advised to use the **oxygen** only as directed. Patients who begin to exhibit symptoms that may be related to toxicity should contact their health-care provider.

Lifestyle Management

Lifestyle management issues related to the disease process being treated should be discussed. They often include the following:

1. The patient should avoid or quit smoking.
2. COPD patients should avoid unnecessary exposure to viral respiratory infections.
3. Patients with COPD or other chronic respiratory diseases should avoid high altitudes.
4. Before traveling by air, the patient should contact the provider to formulate a plan of care.

ALLERGY MEDICATIONS

Antihistamines

Antihistamines are used in primary care to treat a variety of allergic conditions. This chapter addresses the **antihistamines** used to treat allergic symptoms specific to the respiratory tract. **Antihistamines** are also called **H_1 receptor antagonists**, which describes the action the medication has at the cellular level. This text uses **antihistamine**, the more commonly used name in clinical practice.

The first **antihistamines** became available in the 1940s, with the still widely used **diphenhydramine** first available in the 1950s. They are referred to as the first generation **antihistamines**. The 1980s brought a new generation of nonsedating **antihistamines** that provided relief to allergy sufferers without causing the drowsiness of the earlier medications. They are referred to as second generation **antihistamines**. New **antihistamines** that are longer acting and have better adverse effect profiles continue to be developed.

Pharmacodynamics

Antihistamines are H_1 receptor antagonists that reduce or prevent most of the physiological effects of histamine at the H_1 receptor site. **Antihistamines** compete with histamine for H_1 receptor sites on the effector cells. They do not prevent histamine release or bind with histamine that has already been released. They prevent, but do not reverse, responses mediated by histamine. The effects of **antihistamines** include inhibition of respiratory, vascular, and GI smooth muscle constriction by antagonism of the constrictor action on smooth muscle. **Antihistamines** strongly block the action of histamine that results in increased capillary permeability and formation of edema and wheal. They also decrease the flare and itch responses of histamine on peripheral nerve endings. Histamine-activated exocrine secretions (salivary, lacrimal) are decreased with the use of systemic **antihistamines**. **Antihistamines** with strong anticholinergic (**atropine**-like) properties may have an increased drying effect by decreasing secretions from cholinergically innervated glands.

The first generation **antihistamines** competitively antagonize the effects of histamine at the peripheral H_1 receptor sites in the GI tract, uterus, large blood vessels, and bronchial muscle. First generation **antihistamines** bind nonselectively to the central H_1 receptors and can cause both CNS stimulation and depression. CNS depression is found even with therapeutic doses of the first generation **antihistamines**. Some of the first generation **antihistamines** are more likely than others to depress the CNS, and patients vary in their sensitivity to the different preparations. Commonly prescribed first generation **antihistamines** include the ethanolamine drugs **diphenhydramine (Benadryl)** and **clemastine (Tavist)**, the alkylamines **brompheniramine (Dimetane)** and **chlorpheniramine (Chlor-Trimeton)**, the piperazine **hydroxyzine (Atarax, Vistaril)**, and the piperidine **cyproheptadine (Periactin)**.

Second generation **antihistamines** are selective for peripheral H_1 receptors and therefore as a group are less sedating. They do not cross the blood–brain barrier in appreciable amounts; consequently, very little of the second generation **antihistamines** gets into the brain. Their effects on performance and on objective measures of sedation vary little from those of a placebo. Second generation **antihistamines** that are commonly prescribed include the piperazine drug **cetirizine** (**Zyrtec**) and the piperidines **desloratadine (Clarinex)**, **fexofenadine (Allegra)**, and **loratadine (Claritin)**.

Antihistamines have other pharmacodynamic properties related to their central action rather than their histamine receptor blockade action. Several first generation **antihistamines** have significant antiemetic and antinausea properties owing to strong anticholinergic properties caused by the **antihistamine**'s binding to the muscarinic receptors. **Diphenhydramine** can be used to reverse the extrapyramidal adverse effects caused by **phenothiazines**. Probably because of their anticholinergic actions, some of the **antihistamines (diphenhydramine)** have effects on Parkinson's symptoms and may be effective in the early stages of treatment.

Pharmacokinetics

Absorption and Distribution

The first generation **antihistamines** are stable lipid-soluble amines that are well absorbed from the GI tract.

Diphenhydramine is widely distributed throughout the body tissues and fluids, including the CNS. It crosses the placenta and is found in breast milk. The distribution of **clemastine** is unknown, but the drug does cross the placenta and is distributed in breast milk. **Chlorpheniramine** is approximately 72 percent protein bound and is widely distributed in body tissue and fluids. **Chlorpheniramine** crosses the placenta and is found in breast milk. Distribution of **hydroxyzine** has not been fully described, and it is unknown whether it crosses the placenta or is distributed in breast milk. The distribution of **cyproheptadine, dimenhydrinate**, and **brompheniramine** is unknown.

The second generation **antihistamines** are rapidly absorbed from the GI tract, although concurrent food ingestion can decrease or delay absorption. **Fexofenadine** is rapidly absorbed, and absorption is not affected by food intake. Administration of **loratadine** with food decreases absorption up to 40 percent for the syrup or tablet and 48 percent for the rapid-disintegrating tablet. **Desloratadine** is well absorbed, and food intake dose not affect absorption. Absorption of **cetirizine** is slightly reduced by food intake. **Cetirizine** is widely distributed, except in the CNS, where concentrations are less than 10 percent of the peak serum concentration. It is unknown whether **cetirizine** crosses the placenta, but it has been measured in breast milk. **Fexofenadine** distribution is unknown. **Loratadine** is 97 percent protein bound and is excreted in breast milk. It is not known if **loratadine** crosses the placenta. **Desloratadine** is highly (82% to 87%) protein bound, it is not known whether it crosses the placenta, and only minimal amounts are excreted in breast milk.

Metabolism and Excretion

The first generation **antihistamines** are metabolized primarily in the liver. **Diphenhydramine** is metabolized in the liver, with the unchanged portion of the dose and metabolites excreted in the urine in 24 to 48 hours. **Clemastine** is extensively metabolized by an unknown mechanism. **Clemastine** and its metabolites are excreted primarily in the urine. Metabolism of **chlorpheniramine** is extensive, occurring first in the gastric mucosa and then on the first pass through the liver. Metabolites of **chlorpheniramine** are excreted in the urine, with the excretion rate dependent on the pH of the urine and urinary flow. **Cyproheptadine** is metabolized in the liver into several conjugated metabolites, with excretion in the urine and feces. **Hydroxyzine** is completely metabolized by the liver. Metabolism and excretion of **brompheniramine** and **dimenhydrinate** are unknown.

Most of the second generation **antihistamines** are metabolized by the liver to active metabolites by the hepatic microsomal P450 system. Consequently, metabolism of these drugs can be affected by competition for the P450 enzymes by other drugs. **Cetirizine** is minimally metabolized by the P450 enzymes and is primarily excreted unchanged in the urine. Approximately 5 percent of the dose of **fexofenadine** is metabolized, with 80 percent excreted in the feces and 11 percent excreted in the urine. **Loratadine** has a high first-pass effect and is metabolized in the liver to the active metabolite descarboethoxyloratadine. Patients with chronic liver disease have higher peak plasma concentrations (double the normal levels) of **loratadine** than do healthy patients. Elimination of **loratadine** is through the urine and feces.

See Table 17–13 for the pharmacokinetics.

Table 17–13 ▶ **Pharmacokinetics: Selected Antihistamines**

Drug	Onset	Peak	Duration	Protein Binding	Half-Life	Metabolism	Elimination
First Generation Antihistamines							
Brompheniramine	15–30 min	2–5 h	4–6 h	—	25 h	Hepatic	Renal
Clemastine	15–30 min	2–5 h	10–12 h (up to 24 h)	—	—	Probably hepatic	Renal
Chlorpheniramine	30–60 min	2–6 h	4–8 h	72%	*Adults:* 20–24 h *Children:* 10–13 h	Gastric mucosa and hepatic	Renal
Cyproheptadine	—	6–9 h	8 h	—	1–4 h	Hepatic	Primary renal; some in feces
Diphenhydramine	15–30 min	2–4 h	4–6 h	98%–99%	1–4 h	Hepatic	Renal
Hydroxyzine	15–60 min	—	4–6 h	—	3–20 h	Hepatic	Renal

Continued

Table 17–13 ▶ **Pharmacokinetics: Selected Antihistamines—cont'd**

Drug	Onset	Peak	Duration	Protein Binding	Half-Life	Metabolism	Elimination
Second Generation Antihistamines							
Cetirizine	Rapid	1 h	—	93%	8.3 h	Minimal 60% excreted unchanged	Renal, feces (10%)
Desloratadine	1 h	3 h	24 h	82–87%	27 h	Hepatic	Renal fecal
Fexofenadine	1 h	2.6 h	12 h	60–70%	14.4 h	95% excreted unchanged	Fecal (80%), renal (11%)
Loratadine	1–3 h	8–12 h	>24 h	97%	8.4 h	Hepatic CYP3A4 and CYP2D6	Fecal, renal

Pharmacotherapeutics

Precautions and Contraindications

The precautions and contraindications differ between the first generation and second generation antihistamines.

First Generation Antihistamines

Although first generation **antihistamines** are available without prescription and all **antihistamines** are widely prescribed, the provider must be aware of the precautions and absolute contraindications to the **antihistamines**.

The first generation **antihistamines** are generally safe and effective. **Antihistamines** are contraindicated in patients with narrow-angle glaucoma, lower respiratory tract symptoms (they thicken secretions and impair expectoration), stenosing peptic ulcer, symptomatic prostatic hypertrophy, bladder neck obstruction, pyloroduodenal obstruction, and MAOI use.

There are few but significant precautions to the first generation **antihistamines**. Because of the anticholinergic effects, caution is required for patients with a predisposition to urinary retention, history of bronchial asthma, increased intraocular pressure, hyperthyroidism, cardiovascular disease, or hypertension. **Antihistamines** cause varying degrees of sedation and drowsiness and reduce mental alertness; therefore, patients should not drive or perform other tasks requiring mental alertness while taking the first generation **antihistamines**. Children should be supervised when they are taking these medications and performing potentially unsafe activities such as swimming or bicycling.

The first generation **antihistamines—chlorpheniramine, brompheniramine, diphenhydramine, clemastine**, and **cyproheptadine**—are Pregnancy Category B. **Hydroxyzine** and **carbinoxamine** are the only first generation **antihistamines** classified as Pregnancy Category C.

First generation **antihistamines** are contraindicated in newborns and premature infants, who may have severe reactions (convulsions). Breastfeeding is also a contraindication for the use of first generation **antihistamines** because all of the medications are excreted in breast milk and they may decrease milk production.

Caution should be exercised with the use of first generation **antihistamines** in young children because a paradoxical CNS stimulation can occur. Do not exceed recommended dosages for each age group of children. **Chlorpheniramine, brompheniramine, cyproheptadine, dimenhydrinate**, and **diphenhydramine** are all labeled to be used in children over age 2 years. **Hydroxyzine** syrup may be prescribed for infants and children for pruritus.

Second Generation Antihistamines

The second generation **antihistamines** have only a few contraindications. The use of **astemizole** is contraindicated in patients with significant hepatic dysfunction and concomitant **erythromycin, clarithromycin, troleandomycin, quinine, ketoconazole**, or **itraconazole** therapy. Cases of torsade de pointes have been reported following **astemizole** use. Prolonged QT interval is a potential adverse effect of **astemizole**, which is contraindicated in patients with prolonged QT syndrome, hypokalemia, or hypomagnesemia (including patients on diuretics with a potential for causing these electrolyte imbalances). **Astemizole** is also contraindicated in patients on HIV **protease inhibitors, serotonin reuptake inhibitors, cisapride, sparfloxacin**, and **mibefradil. Astemizole (Hismanal)** and a previous second generation antihistamine **terfenadine** (Seldane) have been voluntarily removed from the market because of these potentially life-threatening drug interactions.

The second generation **antihistamines** are generally not recommended during pregnancy, especially during the third trimester, because of a seizure risk to the fetus. **Loratadine** and **cetirizine** are classified Pregnancy

Category B. The other second generation **antihistamines, loratadine, desloratadine**, and **fexofenadine**, are Pregnancy Category C, and their use should be avoided.

Fexofenadine are not recommended for children under age 6. **Loratadine** may be prescribed to children as young as age 2. **Cetirizine** syrup and **desloratadine** syrup may be used in children as young as 6 months.

Adverse Drug Reactions

As described previously, the major adverse reaction to first generation **antihistamines** is sedation, which can interfere with a patient's ability to function at work or school. Other central adverse effects include dizziness, tinnitus, lassitude, disturbed coordination, fatigue, headache, irritability, nervousness, blurred vision, diplopia, and tremors. The next most common adverse effects are GI and include increased or decreased appetite, nausea, epigastric distress, vomiting, constipation, and diarrhea. Dry mouth, urinary retention, and dysuria are also adverse effects reported in patients taking first generation **antihistamines**. The concurrent ingestion of **alcohol** or other CNS depressants produces an additive effect that further impairs function.

The second generation **antihistamines** have few central adverse effects. The major improvement in the second generation **antihistamines** is that the incidence of drowsiness is greatly reduced. They are well tolerated by the GI system and have a minimal incidence of dry mouth (less than or equal to 5%). Overall, when patients have adverse reactions to the first generation **antihistamines**, a change to a second generation drug often alleviates the problem.

Drug Interactions

The first generation **antihistamines** should be used with caution concurrently with any medication that has CNS depressant effects. All of the first generation **antihistamines** exhibit additive CNS sedation effects if coadministered with **ethanol, anxiolytics, sedatives, hypnotics**, and **barbiturates**. The anticholinergic effects of **antihistamines** may be enhanced if coadministered with **tricyclic antidepressants** and **phenothiazines**. It is recommended that H_1 agonists not be used within 2 weeks of **MAOIs** because of increased anticholinergic effects. **Cyproheptadine** may reverse the antidepressant effects of selective **serotonin reuptake inhibitors (SSRIs)**. Two **antihistamines** should not be prescribed at the same time to avoid additive anticholinergic and sedative effects.

The second generation **antihistamines**, although not sedating when used singly, may have additive CNS sedation effects if used with other CNS depressants (**barbiturates, anxiolytics, sedatives, hypnotics, ethanol**, and **benzodiazepines**). Concurrent use with another H_1 blocker may cause sedation.

Desloratadine and **loratadine** are extensively metabolized by the CYP450 enzymes, and coadministration of other medications that are also metabolized by these enzymes should be avoided, such as are **erythromycin, cimetidine**, and **ketoconazole**.

Table 17–14 presents drug interactions.

Table 17–14 ■ **Drug Interactions: Selected Antihistamines**

Drug	Interacting Drug	Possible Effect	Implications
First Generation Antihistamines			
Brompheniramine	MAOIs	MAOIs can prolong and intensify the effects of antihistamines	Avoid concurrent use
	Ethanol and other CNS depressants	Additive CNS depression	Use with caution
Clemastine	MAOIs	Additive anticholinergic effects	Concurrent use contraindicated
	Antimuscarinics: Tricyclic antidepressants, phenothiazines, ethanolamine-derivative H_1 blockers (clemastine, carbinoxamine, promethazine, trimeprazine) clozapine, cyclobenzaprine, disopyramide	Additive anticholinergic effects	Avoid concurrent use
	CNS depressants: Ethanol, antipsychotics, sedatives, hypnotics, opiate agonists, barbiturates	Enhanced CNS-depressant effect	Avoid concurrent use

Continued

Table 17–14 ■ Drug Interactions: Selected Antihistamines—cont'd

Drug	Interacting Drug	Possible Effect	Implications
Chlorpheniramine	MAOIs	Additive anticholinergic effects	Avoid concurrent use
	Antimuscarinics: Tricyclic antidepressants, phenothiazines, benztropine	Enhanced anticholinergic effects of chlorpheniramine	Chlorpheniramine has moderate anticholinergic effects and is preferable to other H_1 blockers when an H_1 blocker must be used
	CNS depressants	Enhanced CNS-depressant effect	Avoid concurrent use
Cyproheptadine	*Antimuscarinics:* Tricyclic antidepressants, phenothiazines, ethanolamine-derivative H_1 blockers (clemastine, diphenhydramine), benztropine	Increased anticholinergic effects of cyproheptadine	Avoid concurrent use
	CNS depressants: Barbiturates, ethanol, benzodiazepines, tricyclic antidepressants, opiate agonists	Enhanced CNS-depressant effect	Avoid concurrent use
	SSRIs	Reversal of antidepressant effects of SSRIs	Use cyproheptadine only if needed
Diphenhydramine	MAOIs	Additive anticholinergic effects	Do not use within 2 wk of each other
	Antimuscarinics: Tricyclic antidepressants, phenothiazines, ethanolamine-derivative H_1 blockers (clemastine, carbinoxamine, promethazine, trimeprazine) clozapine, cyclobenzaprine, disopyramide	Additive anticholinergic effects	Avoid or use with caution; monitor closely if coadministration is necessary
	CNS depressants: Ethanol, antipsychotics, sedatives, hypnotics, opiate agonists, barbiturates	Enhanced CNS-depressant effect	Avoid concurrent use
Hydroxyzine	MAOIs	May prolong and intensify the anticholinergic effects of antihistamines	Concurrent use contraindicated; avoid use within 2 wk of each other
	Antimuscarinics: Tricyclic antidepressants, phenothiazines, ethanolamine-derivative H_1 blockers (clemastine, carbinoxamine, promethazine, trimeprazine) atropine, benztropine	Additive anticholinergic effects	Avoid concurrent use
	CNS depressants: Ethanol, antipsychotics, sedatives, hypnotics, opiate agonists, barbiturates	Additive CNS-depressant effects	Avoid concurrent use

Table 17–14 ■ **Drug Interactions: Selected Antihistamines—cont'd**

Drug	Interacting Drug	Possible Effect	Implications
Second Generation Antihistamines			
Cetirizine	Theophylline:	May ↓ cetirizine clearance	Avoid concurrent use
	CNS depressants: Barbiturates, ethanol, benzodiazepines, tricyclic antidepressants, opiate agonists	Additive CNS-depressant effects and drowsiness	Use with caution
Desloratadine	Ketoconazole erythromycin	Increases plasma concentrations of desloratadine	Does not cause cardiac toxicity, but coadminister with caution
	CNS depressants	Additive CNS depression	Avoid or minimize concurrent use
Loratadine	Macrolide antibiotics (clarithromycin, erythromycin, troleandomycin)	Interferes with the metabolism of loratadine, resulting in increased serum concentrations of loratadine	Does not cause cardiac toxicity, but coadminister with caution
	CNS depressants: Barbiturates, ethanol, benzodiazepines, tricyclic antidepressants, opiate agonists	Additive CNS-depressant effects and drowsiness	Avoid or minimize concurrent use
Fexofenadine	Ketoconazole	↑ fexofenadine plasma levels	Avoid concurrent use
	Erythromycin	↑ fexofenadine levels	Avoid concurrent use
	Aluminum- and magnesium-containing antacids	↓ fexofenadine absorption	Administer fexofenadine 1 h before antacids
	Alcohol	CNS depression	Avoid concurrent use

Clinical Use and Dosing

Respiratory Allergies

Most of the **antihistamines** are effective in the treatment of seasonal allergic rhinitis and conjunctivitis. **Antihistamines** effectively treat the sneezing, rhinorrhea, watery eyes, and itching of eyes, nose, and throat associated with seasonal allergies or hay fever. The treatment decision is often made according to the adverse-effect profile and cost. Although the first generation drugs **diphenhydramine, chlorpheniramine, brompheniramine,** and **clemastine** are effective, inexpensive, and available without prescription, their adverse effect of drowsiness often prevents patients from being able to continue their daily activities. The usual adult dose of **diphenhydramine** for respiratory allergies is 25 to 50 mg every 4 to 6 hours. The adult dose of **chlorpheniramine** is 4 mg every 4 to 6 hours or 8 to 12 mg of the extended-release form every 8 to 12 hours. **Brompheniramine** is dosed at 4 mg every 4 to 6 hours in adults with respiratory allergies. Pediatric doses for these medications are given in Table 17–15.

If a patient cannot tolerate the first generation **antihistamines**, a second generation medication can be prescribed to treat respiratory allergies. The dose of **cetirizine** that should be prescribed for children over 12 years and adults is 5 to 10 mg/day given once a day. In children aged 6 to 11 years, the dose of **cetirizine** is 5 to 10 mg once daily. For **cetirizine** syrup prescribed to children aged 2 to 5 years, the dose is 2.5 mg (half tsp of 5 mg/5mL syrup) once daily. The dose of **cetirizine** may be increased to 5 mg/day, delivered as 5 mg once daily or 2.5 mg twice a day. Children aged 6 to 12 months are dosed at 2.5 mg once a day. Children aged 12 to 23 months are also prescribed 2.5 mg once a day, with an increase to 2.5 mg twice a day if needed. The dose of **fexofenadine** in healthy children aged 12 years or older and adults is 60 mg twice a day. Children aged 6 to 11 years should be prescribed 30 mg twice a day of **fexofenadine.** If a patient has renal impairment (creatinine clearance [CCr] less than 80 mL/min), the dose of **fexofenadine** is 60 mg once daily. The dose of **loratadine** in healthy children over age 6 years and adults is 10 mg once a day, with children aged 2 to 5 years prescribed 5 mg once a day. If an adult has renal or liver disease, the dose of **loratadine** is 10 mg every other day. **Desloratadine** is dosed at 5 mg once daily in children 12 years and older and adults. In patients with renal or hepatic impairment **desloratadine** is given

Table 17–15 ◉ **Dosage Schedule: Selected Antihistamines**

Drug	Indication	Dose	Comments
First Generation Antihistamines			
Brompheniramine	Allergic and vasomotor rhinitis, pruritus, conjunctivitis	*Adults:* 4 mg PO q4–6h ***or*** 8–12 mg of sustained-release form 2 to 3 times/d Maximum dose: 12 mg/24 h *Children 6–12 yr:* 2 mg q4–6h; max 12 mg/24 h *Children <6 yr:* 0.125 mg/kg/d in divided doses every 6–8 h	May be administered with or without food
Clemastine	Allergic rhinitis	*Children >12 yr and adults:* 1 mg bid *Children 6–12 yr:* 0.5 mg bid	May be administered without regard to meals
	Pruritus, mild urticaria, angioedema	*Children >12 and adults:* 2 mg bid *Children 6–12 yr:* 1 mg bid	May be administered without regard to meals
Chlorpheniramine	Allergic rhinitis, conjunctivitis, pruritus, urticaria	*Children >12 yr and adults:* 4 mg every 4–6 h; max 24 mg/d *Children 6–12 yr:* 2 mg every 4–6 hr; max 12 mg/d *Children 2–5 yr:* 1 mg every 4–6 h; max 4 mg/d *Extended-release form:* *Children >12 yr and adults:* 8–12 mg bid or tid; max 24 mg/d *Children 6–12 yr:* 8 mg once daily; max 12 mg/d *Children 2–5 yr:* use other forms	Administer with food or milk to minimize gastric irritation Do not crush or chew extended-release tablets
Cyproheptadine	Allergic rhinitis, conjunctivitis, pruritus, urticaria	*Children >14 yr and adults:* 4 mg q8–12h; usual range 12–16 mg/d; max dose 0.5 mg/kg/d *Children 7–14 yr:* 4 mg q8–12h; max 16 mg/d *Children 2–6 yr:* 2 mg q8–12h; max 12 mg/d	Administered without regard to meals
Diphenhydramine	Upper respiratory allergies	*Children >12 yr and adults:* 25–50 mg every 4–6 h; max 300 mg/d *Children 6–12 yr:* 12.5–25 mg q 4–6h; max 150 mg/24 h *Children 2–6 yr:* 6.25 mg; max 37.5 mg/24 h	May cause drowsiness; may cause excitability in young children
Hydroxyzine	Allergic and vasomotor rhinitis, pruritus	*Adults:* 25 mg 3–4 times/d *Children >6 yr:* 12.5–25 mg 3–4 times/d; max 50–100 mg/24 h *Children <6 yr:* 1–2 mg/kg every 6–8 h	May cause drowsiness
	Nausea/vomiting	*Adults:* 25–100 mg 3–4 times/d *Children 6–12 yr:* 12.5 mg every 6 h or 1–2 mg /kg/d/ in divided doses *Children <6 yr:* 12.5 mg every 6 h ***or*** 1–2 mg/kg/d in divided doses	May cause drowsiness
	Insomnia	*Adults:* 50–100 mg PO 30–60 min before bedtime	May cause drowsiness

Table 17–15 ◉ **Dosage Schedule: Selected Antihistamines—cont'd**

Drug	Indication	Dose	Comments
Second Generation Antihistamines			
Cetirizine	Seasonal or perennial rhinitis, chronic urticaria, pruritus	*Children >12 yr and adults:* 5–10 mg once a day *Children >6–11 yr:* 5–10 mg once a day *Children 2–5 yr:* 2.5 mg initially; can increase dose to 5 mg/d (either as one 5-mg dose or 2.5 mg q12h) *Children 6–12 mo:* 2.5 mg once daily *Children 12–23 mo:* 2.5 mg once daily; may be increased to 2.5 mg twice daily	May be administered without regard to food, but food may delay absorption by up to 1 h; patients with renal impairment (CCr <31 mL/min) decrease dose to 5 mg once daily
Desloratadine	Allergic rhinitis, chronic urticaria	*Children >12 yr and adults:* 5 mg once a day *Children 6–11 yr:* 2.5 mg once a day *Children 1–5 yr:* 1.25 mg once a day Children 6–12 mo: 1 mg once a day	
Fexofenadine	Allergic rhinitis	*Children >12 yr and adults:* 60 mg PO bid *Children 6–11 yr:* 30 mg PO bid	Dose without regard to meals; not recommended in children <12; patients with renal impairment (CCr <80 mL/min) reduce starting dose to 60 mg once daily
Loratadine	Allergic rhinitis, chronic urticaria	*Children >6 yr and adults:* 10 mg once daily *Children 2–5 yr:* 5 mg once daily	Dose without regard to meals; patients with renal impairment (CCr <30 mL/min) reduce starting dosage to 10 mg every other day

every other day. Pediatric dosing for the second generation **antihistamines** is found in Table 17–15.

Hypersensitivity Reactions

The first generation antihistamine **diphenhydramine** is usually the drug of choice for patients with acute hypersensitivity reactions. It is available in oral tablet, capsule, and liquid forms without prescription and in parenteral form for acute IM or IV use. The adult oral dose of **diphenhydramine** is 25 to 50 mg every 4 to 6 hours for hypersensitivity reactions. In children 6 to 12 years with hypersensitivity reactions, the dose of **diphenhydramine** is 12.5 to 25 mg every 4 hours. Children aged 2 to 6 years are prescribed **diphenhydramine** syrup, at a dose of 6.25 mg every 4 hours. In an acute hypersensitivity reaction, IM administration of **diphenhydramine** may be necessary. The adult dose of **diphenhydramine** is 10 to 50 mg deep IM or IV, with a maximum of 400 mg/day. In children, the dose is 1.25 mg/kg per dose or given deep IM every 4 hours, or 5 mg/kg/day divided every 6 to 8 hours, with a maximum daily **diphenhydramine** dose of 300 mg. **Cyproheptadine** is also indicated for use in hypersensitivity reactions. The adult dose of **cyproheptadine** is 4 mg three times a day. No second generation **antihistamines** are indicated for use in hypersensitivity reactions.

Urticaria and Angioedema

In urticaria, histamine is the primary mediator, and therefore, the **antihistamines** are the drugs of choice and quite effective. **Clemastine**, a very effective treatment for urticaria, is available in both tablet and liquid form for use with children (older than 6 years) and adults. **Hydroxyzine** is effective in the management of pruritus due to allergic conditions such as chronic urticaria and in histamine-mediated pruritus. It is also available in tablet and liquid form. **Hydroxyzine** may be used safely in children younger than age 6 years and, therefore, may be a better choice than **clemastine** in younger children with urticaria. **Cetirizine**, **desloratadine**, and **loratadine** may be prescribed for urticaria. See Table 17–15 for dosing information.

Nighttime Sleep Aid

Diphenhydramine is available without prescription as a sleep aid and is a safe treatment for occasional insomnia. The recommended dose for adults is 50 mg at bedtime. Table 17–15 presents dosing information.

Motion Sickness/Antiemetic

Dimenhydrinate (Dramamine) is used in the treatment and prevention of nausea, vertigo, and vomiting associated with motion sickness. Dosing for children aged 2 to 5 years is 12.4 to 25 mg every 6 to 8 hours, to a maximum of 75 mg/day. Children aged 6 to 12 years are given 25 to 50 mg of **dimenhydrinate** every 6 to 8 hours with a maximum of 150 mg/day. An alternative dose is 5 mg/kg per day divided into 4 doses. Children 12 years and older and adults are given 50 to 100 mg every 4 to 6 hours, not to exceed 400 mg/day. The onset of action of **dimenhydrinate** is 15 to 30 minutes, so predosing for motion sickness would require that the medication be taken with food or water at least 15 minutes before needed.

Rational Drug Selection

First Versus Second Generation Antihistamines

Although many of the first generation **antihistamines** are readily available without prescription, the common adverse effect of sedation prevents their use during the day by patients who need to be alert for work or school. The second generation **antihistamines** are well tolerated and do not impair daytime functioning. They are also longer acting, allowing for convenient once- or twice-a-day dosing.

Cost

The second generation **antihistamines** used to be more expensive than the first generation **antihistamines**, but with many second generation drugs now available in generic form, cost has less impact on decision making. Most insurance companies will not pay for the cost of the more expensive brand-name second generation **antihistamines**. For the patient, the cost is offset by the ability to perform daily functions more easily when taking the second generation medications.

Monitoring

No specific laboratory monitoring is necessary with **antihistamines**.

Patient Education

Patient education focuses on proper use of the medication, adverse reactions, and safety precautions while using the medications.

Administration

Patients should be instructed regarding the proper dosing of the drug. Especially if patients are switching from a shorter-acting first generation to a longer-acting second generation antihistamine, they need to be aware of the dosing schedule. Doses should not be doubled or increased unless prescribed by the health-care provider. The long-acting second generation **antihistamines** should not be taken closer together than prescribed, so missed doses need to be held until the time of the next dose (every 12 or 24 h).

Some **antihistamines** cause GI upset and need to be taken with food. **Loratadine** should be taken on an empty stomach because absorption may be decreased by as much as 60 percent.

Patients should be instructed not to crush or chew sustained-release tablets.

Adverse Reactions

Some **antihistamines** (first generation) may cause drowsiness, and patients should observe caution while driving or performing other tasks requiring alertness. Patients should avoid **alcohol** and other CNS depressants while taking **antihistamines.** Patients should be instructed to report excessive drowsiness to their health-care provider to determine whether another medication would provide therapeutic effects without sedation.

Patients taking **loratadine** should be aware of the serious interaction between the **antihistamines** and **macrolide antibiotics** and the oral **azol antifungals**. Written instructions regarding the specific medications to avoid are the most effective and safest method of ensuring that patients do not accidentally get placed on any new medication that would cause a serious adverse reaction. The additive CNS depression that occurs with the **antihistamine** and other **CNS depressants** (e.g., **alcohol**) should be addressed and the patient cautioned regarding driving or operating heavy machinery.

Lifestyle Management

Lifestyle management related to the disease process needs to be discussed with the patient. Points to discuss often include avoidance of known allergens and using environmental methods to control dust mites and other common allergens.

Available dosage forms are presented in Table 17–16.

COUGH AND COLD MEDICATIONS

Decongestants

Decongestants are widely used for congestion associated with the common cold and allergic rhinitis. Many preparations are available without a prescription, and they are available in many formulations. They come in liquid, tablet, capsule, nasal spray, or drops, providing a variety of methods of administration. Although patients may self-treat with **decongestants** and the health-care provider may rarely prescribe them, they are included here for the provider to learn about the proper dosing and potential adverse effects or drug interactions that may occur with these medications.

Pharmacodynamics

The **decongestants** are **alpha-adrenergic receptor agonists** (sympathomimetic) that produce vasoconstriction by stimulating alpha receptors within the mucosa of the respiratory tract, which temporarily reduces the swelling associated with inflammation of the mucous membranes. These sympathomimetic amines act on the alpha receptors of the vascular smooth muscle, causing vasoconstriction, pressor effects, and nasal

Table 17–16 ◈ **Available Dosage Forms: Selected Antihistamines**

Drug	Dosage Form	How Supplied	Cost
FIRST GENERATION ANTIHISTAMINES			
Brompheniramine			
Dimetapp Allergy	Capsules: 4 mg Scored tablets: 4 mg	24 24	$12.89/30 tablets
Bromfed	Brompheniramine 4 mg Pseudoephedrine 60 mg	30	$12.89/30 tabs
Children's Dimetapp Cold & Allergy	Brompheniramine 1 mg phenylephrine 2.5 mg	per 5 mL 12 oz	$10.99/12 oz
Clemastine			
Tavist	Scored tablets: 1.34 mg (1 mg clemastine) Scored tablets: 2.68 mg (2 mg clemastine)	8, 16 100	$8.79
Generic Syrup	Syrup: 0.67 mg (0.5 mg clemastine)/5 mL	4-oz bottles (5.5% alcohol)	$18.99/120 mL
Generic	Tablet: 1.34 mg (1 mg clemastine), 2.68 mg (2 mg clemastine)	100, 30, 60	1.34 mg = $26/100 2.68 mg = $18/30
Chlorpheniramine			
Chlor-Trimeton Allergy 4 hour	Tablets: 4 mg	24, 100	$6.29/24 tabs
Chlor-Trimeton Allergy 8 hour	Sustained-release tablets: 8 mg	15, 100	
Chlor-Trimeton Allergy 12 hour	Sustained-release tablets: 12 mg	10, 24, 100	$12.99
Chlor-Trimeton Syrup	Syrup: 2 mg/5 mL	4-oz bottles	
Generic	Tablets: 4 mg Syrup: 2 mg/5 mL	60, 100, 1,000 4-oz bottles	$10.99/60
Cyproheptadine			
Periactin	Tablets: 4 mg	100, 30	$16.99/30 tablets
Periactin Syrup	Syrup: 2 mg/5 mL	Pints (5% alcohol)	
Generic	Tablets: 4 mg Syrup: 2 mg/5 mL	30, 100, 250, 500, 1,000 Pints, gallons	$13.99/30 $18.99/120 mL
Diphenhydramine			
Benadryl Allergy	Capsules: 25 mg Tablets: 25 mg	24, 48, 100, 1,000 24, 48	 $14.29/100
Benadryl Dye-Free Allergy Softgels	Capsules: 25 mg	24	$4.99/24 capsules
Benadryl Allergy Liquid	Liquid: 12.5 mg/5 mL	4-oz, 8-oz bottles (no alcohol)	$9.49/8 oz $5.69/4 oz
Benadryl Dye-Free-Allergy Liquid	Liquid: 6.25 mg/5 mL	4-oz bottles (no alcohol)	$5.69/4 oz
Benadryl Allergy Chewables	Chewable tablets: 12.5 mg	24	$5.99/24 tabs
Generic	Capsules: 25 mg, 50 mg Tablets: 25 mg Syrup: 12.5 mg/5 mL Liquid: 6.25 mg/5 mL	30, 100, 1,000 24, 100, 48 4 oz (5% alcohol) 4 oz, 8 oz (0.5% alcohol)	$7.99/48.25 mg $4.99/48 tablets $2.39/4 oz
Hydroxyzine			
Atarax	Tablets: 10 mg, 25 mg, 50 mg, 100 mg Syrup: 10 mg/5 mL	100, 500 Pints (0.5% alcohol)	$44.99/30
Vistaril	Capsules: 25 mg, 50 mg, 100 mg Suspension: 25 mg/5 mL	100, 500 4 oz, pint bottles (no alcohol)	25 mg = $55/30 50 mg = $64/30 $103/240 mL

Continued

Table 17–16 ◆ **Available Dosage Forms: Selected Antihistamines—cont'd**

Drug	Dosage Form	How Supplied	Cost
	FIRST GENERATION ANTIHISTAMINES		
Generic	Tablets: 10 mg, 25 mg, 50 mg	100, 250, 500, 1,000	10 mg = $17.99 25 mg = $26.99 50 mg = $30.99
	Capsules: 25 mg, 50 mg, 100 mg Syrup: 10 mg/5 mL	100, 250, 500, 1,000 5-mL unit dose, 12.5 mL, 25 mL, pint	$7.99/240 mL
	SECOND GENERATION ANTIHISTAMINES		
Cetirizine			
Zyrtec	5 mg, 10 mg chewable tablets 1 mg/mL syrup 1 mg/mL prefilled single-use spoons 10 mg tablets	100 4 oz	$68.32 $12.99/120 mL $12.99/10 $39.99/70
Generic	10 mg tablets		$9.99/30
Fexofenadine			
Allegra	Tablets: 180 mg, 60 mg, 30 mg 30 mg/mL suspension	60, 100, 1,000 300 mL	180 mg = 80/30 60 mg = $99/60 $75.70/300 mL
Generic	Tablets: 180 mg, 60 mg, 30 mg	30, 90, 100	30 mg = $19.99/30 60 mg = $38.99/30 180 mg = $61.99/30
Loratadine			
Claritin	Tablets: 10 mg Syrup: 1 mg/mL Rapidly disintegrating tablets: 10 mg (Claritin Reditabs)	14, 30, 100, 500 Pints 30	$22.99/30 $10.99/4 oz
Alavert	Rapidly disintegrating tablets: 10 mg		$21.49/60
Generic	Tablets: 10 mg Syrup: 1 mg/mL		$8.99/30 $7.99/120 mL
Desloratadine			
Clarinex	Tablets: 5 mg Tablet rapidly disintegrating: 2.5 mg (Clarinex Reditabs) Syrup: 0.5 mg/mL	30 473 mL	$133/30 $147/30 $209.75/473 mL

decongestion. Other alpha effects include constriction of the GI and urinary sphincters, mydriasis, and decreased pancreatic beta cell secretion. **Pseudoephedrine (Sudafed)**, the most commonly used systemic **decongestant**, is noted to have mild CNS stimulant effects, especially in patients sensitive to sympathomimetic drugs. **Phenylpropanolamine**, which was often combined with an **antihistamine** in OTC cold medications, was removed from the market in 2005 after a public health advisory found an increased risk for hemorrhagic stroke in women. Other effects of the systemic **decongestants** are increased heart rate, force of contraction, and cardiac output. These effects are usually mild in healthy patients, and at appropriate dosages, decongestion occurs without dramatic blood pressure changes.

Pseudoephedrine is being replaced in some **decongestant** products with **phenylephrine** hydrochloride to deter the manufacture of methamphetamine, which uses **pseudoephedrine** as an ingredient. In 2006 the USA PATRIOT Act added the Combat Methamphetamine Epidemic Act that applies to all cough and cold products (including combination products) that contain the methamphetamine precursor chemicals **ephedrine, pseudoephedrine,** or **phenylpropanolamine.** The law includes a daily and 30-day limit on purchases of known methamphetamine precursors whether at a retail store or via the Internet. All potential precursors are to be stored behind the counter in retail stores and retailers are required ask for identification and keep a log of who is purchasing the drugs. Some states (Oregon) have made pseudoephedrine a Schedule III drug, requiring a prescription to be written by a provider who is licensed to prescribe controlled substances.

Topical decongestants are sympathomimetic amines that cause intense vasoconstriction when applied directly to swollen mucous membranes of the nasal passage. This shrinks the swollen membranes, causing almost immediate relief from nasal congestion. There are minimal systemic effects from topical use of nasal decongestants.

Pharmacokinetics

Absorption and Distribution

The oral decongestants are well absorbed from the GI tract and widely distributed. Pseudoephedrine is widely distributed and presumed to cross the blood–brain barrier and placenta. Small amounts of pseudoephedrine are excreted in breast milk.

Absorption and distribution of the topical decongestants have not been described.

Metabolism and Excretion

Pseudoephedrine is partially metabolized in the liver into norpseudoephedrine, an active metabolite. Pseudoephedrine and its metabolite are excreted in the urine, with 50 to 75 percent of the dose excreted as unchanged drug. Excretion of pseudoephedrine is highly dependent on the pH of the urine. If the urine is acidic (pH near 5), the rate of urinary excretion is increased. If the urine is alkaline (pH of 8), the rate of excretion is slowed, as some of the drug is reabsorbed into the renal tubule.

Metabolism of phenylephrine is via the enzyme monoamine oxidase in the liver. Excretion of phenylephrine or its metabolites has not been described.

Metabolism and excretion of the topical decongestants are not available.

Table 17–17 presents the pharmacokinetics of selected decongestant.

Pharmacotherapeutics

Precautions and Contraindications

There are only a few absolute contraindications to taking decongestants. The oral decongestants are absolutely contraindicated for patients on concurrent MAOI therapy. Concurrent use of these medications may result in severe headache, hypertension and hyperpyrexia, and possibly hypertensive crisis. Oral decongestants are also contraindicated for patients with severe hypertension or coronary artery disease.

Safety and efficacy of decongestant medications have been questioned after a number of reports of deaths of infants taking cold medications (Centers for Disease Control and Prevention, 2007). In October 2007 an FDA panel met and recommended all pediatric cough and cold medications be relabeled as not indicated for use in children under age 4 years. In October 2007 manufactures voluntarily removed all infant drop formulas of cough and cold medications from the market.

Topical imidazolines (oxymetazoline) are to be used with caution in children under age 6 years. Topical naphazoline is contraindicated for patients with glaucoma.

Adverse Drug Reactions

Adverse effects are minimal at recommended doses, unless a patient is sensitive to sympathomimetics. CNS effects may include anxiety, tenseness, restlessness, headache, light-headedness, dizziness, drowsiness, tremor, insomnia, hallucinations, psychological disturbances, CNS depression, and weakness. Of these CNS effects, the most common adverse effects are restlessness and tremors. Cardiovascular adverse effects include transient hypertension, arrhythmia, and cardiovascular collapse, with hypotension, palpitations, tachycardia, and bradycardia. These adverse reactions are rare at recommended doses in healthy individuals. Other adverse effects are nausea, vomiting, pallor, and, rarely, shortness of breath or respiratory difficulty (at higher doses).

Table 17–17 ▶ **Pharmacokinetics: Selected Decongestants**

Drug	Onset	Peak	Duration	Protein Binding	Half-Life	Metabolism	Elimination
Systemic							
Pseudoephedrine	30 min	—	4–8 h 12 h (extended release)	—	9–16 h	Hepatic	Renal 55%–75% as unchanged drug; affected urine by pH
Phenylephrine	15–20 min	—	2–4 h	—	2.5 h	—	—
Topical							
Phenylephrine	—	—	0.5–4 h	—	—	Hepatic, intestinal	Unknown
Oxymetazoline	—	—	—	—	—	—	—
Tetrahydrozoline			3 h	—	—	—	—

Topical **decongestants** have adverse reactions related to the intense vasoconstrictor effect of the nasal spray or sensitivity to additives such as sulfites. Transient stinging is the most common adverse effect reported with topical **decongestants.** Burning, sneezing, dryness, and local irritation are all reported with topical drugs. The most significant adverse reaction with topical **decongestants** is rebound congestion (rhinitis medicamentosa) with prolonged or chronic use. This does not occur with short-term (3- to 5-day) use.

Drug Interactions

The **MAOIs** and **beta-adrenergic blockers** increase the effects of **sympathomimetics**; therefore, patients taking these medications should avoid **decongestants. Phenothiazines** and **tricyclic antidepressants** potentiate the presser effects of **pseudoephedrine.** See Table 17–18 for further drug interactions.

Clinical Use and Dosing

Nasal Congestion

Oral **decongestants** are used for the temporary relief of nasal congestion due to the common cold, sinus infection, and allergic rhinitis. They may be used to promote nasal or sinus drainage and are also indicated in the relief of eustachian tube congestion. The adult dose of **pseudoephedrine** for nasal congestion is 60 mg every 4 to 6 hours. In children aged 6 to 12 years, the dose is

Table 17–18 ▣ **Drug Interactions: Selected Decongestants**

Drug	Interacting Drug	Possible Effect	Implications
Systemic			
Phenylephrine	MAOIs	Hypertensive crisis	Do not use within 14 d of each other
Pseudoephedrine	Caffeine, cocaine, and other sympathomimetic drugs	Additive sympathomimetic activity	Use concurrently with caution
	MAOIs, furazolidone, procarbazine	Concurrent use can prolong and intensify the cardiac stimulation and vasopressor effects, may lead to severe cardiovascular and cerebrovascular response	Avoid use within 14 d of each other
	Ergot alkaloids	Peripheral vasoconstriction, additive vasoconstriction	Avoid concurrent use
	Methyldopa, reserpine	Decreased antihypertensive effects	Monitor BP closely if using concurrently
	Thyroid hormones	Increased effects of both agents on the cardiovascular system	Use concurrently with caution
	Urinary alkalinizers: Sodium bicarbonate, sodium citrate, potassium citrate, sodium lactate, sodium acetate	Increased alkalinization of the urine leads to tubular reabsorption of pseudoephedrine	Observe for increased adverse effects; use together with caution
Topical			
Phenylephrine	MAOIs, tricyclic antidepressants	Hypertensive crisis	Do not use within 14 d of each other
	Beta blockers	May increase vasopressor effects of sympathomimetics	Monitor closely for adverse reaction
Oxymetazoline	MAOIs, tricyclic antidepressants	Hypertensive crisis	Do not use within 14 d of each other
	Beta blockers	May increase vasopressor effects of sympathomimetics	Monitor closely for adverse reaction
	Anesthetics: Cyclopropane, halothane	May sensitize the myocardium to sympathomimetics	Discontinue oxymetazoline prior to use
Tetrahydrozoline	None reported	—	—

30 mg every 4 to 6 hours, and in children aged 2 to 6 years, the dose of **pseudoephedrine** is 15 mg every 4 to 6 hours. **Pseudoephedrine** is no longer recommended for use in children younger than 4 years, but if prescribing, the dose of **pseudoephedrine** is 4 mg/kg per day divided in four-times-a-day doses. **Phenylephrine (Sudafed PE)** is dosed at 10 mg every 4 hours in children over age 12 years and adults (maximum 60 mg in 24 hours). Dosing of **phenylephrine** for children aged 6 to 12 years is 7.5 mg every 4 to 6 hours up to 30 mg per day. In children aged 2 to 6 years the dose of **phenylephrine** is 3.75 mg every 4 to 6 hours, up to 15 mg per day. **Phenylephrine** is not recommended for use in children younger than 2 years. Complete dosing of the different forms of the oral **decongestants** is found in Table 17–19.

Topical **decongestants** are indicated in the symptomatic relief of nasal congestion due to the common cold, sinus infection, and allergic rhinitis. As previously mentioned, topical **decongestants** are only for short-term (3- to 5-day) use because of the rebound congestion of long-term use. Nasal **decongestants** may also relieve ear block and pressure pain in air travel, especially if a patient is suffering from a common cold or sinus infection. The adult dose of **oxymetazoline** topical nasal spray is one or two drops or sprays of 0.05 percent solution in each nostril twice a day or up

Table 17–19 ◉ **Dosage Schedule: Selected Decongestants**

Drug	Indication	Dose	Comments
Systemic			
Phenylephrine	Nasal congestion	*Children >12 yr and adults:* 10 mg every 4 h	Maximum of 6 doses Not recommended for children <12 yr
Pseudoephedrine	Nasal congestion	*Children >12 yr and adults:* 60 mg every 4–6 hr (20 mL of 15 mg/5 mL liquid); max 240 mg/d *Children 6–12 yr:* 30 mg every 4–6 h (10 mL of 15 mg/5 mL liquid); max 120 mg/d *Children 2–6 yr:* 15 mg every 4–6 h (5 mL of 15 mg/5 mL liquid); max 60 mg/d *Children <2 yr:* 1 mg/kg/dose every 4–6 h, max 4 doses or *Extended-release (12-h formula):* *Children >12 yr and adults:* 120 mg every 12 h: max 240 mg/d *Children <12 yr:* not recommended *Extended release (24-h formula):* *Children >12 yr and adults:* 1 tablet; max 240 mg/d *Children <12 yr:* not recommended	Note: use of pseudoephedrine in children <2 yrs is not recommended as standard practice.
Topical			
Phenylephrine	Nasal congestion and eustachian tube congestion	*Children >12 yr and adults:* 1–2 sprays of 0.25% or 0.5% solution in each nostril every 4 h prn congestion; 1% solution can be used in adults with severe congestion *Children 6–12 yr:* 1–2 sprays of 0.25% solution in each nostril every 4 h prn congestion *Children 2–6 yr:* 2 drops or sprays of 0.125% or 0.16% solution to each nostril every 4 h as needed *Children 6 mo–2 yr:* 1–2 drops of 0.16% solution in each nostril every 3–4 h prn	Advise patients to use nasal decongestant spray for a maximum of 2–3 d in a row to avoid rebound congestion

Continued

Table 17–19 ◉ **Dosage Schedule: Selected Decongestants—cont'd**

Drug	Indication	Dose	Comments
Oxymetazoline	Nasal congestion	*Children >6 yr and adults:* use 1–2 drops or sprays of 0.05% solution in each nostril bid *Children 2–5 yr:* 1–2 drops of 0.025% solution in each nostril bid; do not use 0.05% solution in young children *Children <2 yr:* not recommended	Advise patients to use nasal decongestant spray for a maximum of 2–3 d in a row to avoid rebound congestion
Tetrahydrozoline	Nasal congestion	*Children >6 yr and adults:* 2–4 drops or 3–4 sprays of 0.1% solution in each nostril every 3–4 h prn Children <6 yr: 2–3 drops of 0.05% solution in each nostril every 3–4 h prn	Advise patients to use nasal decongestant spray for a maximum of 2–3 d in a row to avoid rebound congestion

to every 6 hours if needed. Children aged 2 to 5 years should use two to three drops of the 0.025 percent solution in each nostril. The use of 0.05 percent **oxymetazoline** should be avoided in children. The dose of topical **phenylephrine** nasal solution in adults is one to two sprays or drops of 0.25 or 0.5 percent solution every 4 hours as needed for congestion. Adults with severe congestion can use **phenylephrine** 1 percent solution. Children aged 6 to 12 years should use 0.25 percent solution, two sprays in each nostril every 4 hours. If the child is between age 6 months and 6 years, the 0.16 percent solution should be prescribed. The dose of **phenylephrine** in young children (younger than age 6 years) and infants is 1 to 2 drops or sprays every 4 hours. Use topical nasal **decongestants** sparingly in young children.

Table 17–19 presents dosing information.

Rational Drug Selection

Topical Versus Systemic

Topical **decongestants** are effective and have few adverse effects. Many health-care providers recommend them for short-term use for the common cold and sinusitis. A concern is the significant rebound congestion that occurs if the topical **decongestants** are used long term. It can occur in as little as a week of constant use. Therefore, topical **decongestants** for allergic rhinitis, although safe, must be accompanied with strict patient education to prevent rebound congestion. In patients who are sensitive to the drying effects of the topical **decongestants**, the oral form may be better tolerated. The reverse is also true; in patients sensitive to **sympathomimetics**, the topical **decongestants** are usually tolerated.

Short- Versus Long-Acting

There are short- and long-acting forms of both oral and topical **decongestants.** In general, the short-acting forms are better tolerated and have fewer adverse effects. The longer-acting forms are useful for patients who require all-day or all-night relief, if the patients can tolerate them.

Cost

Cost is usually not a major factor in prescribing **decongestants**, which are available OTC, and generic forms of all the medications are available.

Monitoring

There is no specific monitoring required with the **decongestants.**

Patient Education

Administration

The first concern that the health-care provider should address is self-prescribing and dosing of the nonprescription **decongestants.** Whether a drug interaction is a concern or a patient may be taking an inappropriate dose, it is important for the health-care provider to be aware that the patient may be taking a **decongestant**. A thorough history should include any self-prescribed medications and the amount and timing of these medications. Patient teaching should include proper dosing, especially in pediatric patients. Patients with cardiovascular disease, hyperthyroidism, diabetes mellitus, or prostatic hypertrophy should use these products sparingly and only on the advice of their health-care provider.

When topical **decongestants** are recommended, it is imperative that the patient be warned about rebound congestion and cautioned to use the medication for only 3 to 5 days or, for chronic allergic rhinitis use, only 2 of every 7 days.

Parents should be cautioned not to use adult-formula nasal sprays in children. There are children's strength **oxymetazoline** (0.025%) and **phenylephrine HCl** (0.125%) available.

Adverse Reactions

Patients should notify their health-care provider if insomnia, dizziness, weakness, tremor, or irregular heartbeat occurs with topical **decongestants.** Patients should be cautioned not to exceed the recommended dosage because higher doses cause nervousness, dizziness, or sleeplessness.

Lifestyle Management

Patients should maintain adequate hydration while taking decongestants to keep mucus mobile. They should also refrain from smoking when they are congested. Caffeine-containing products may cause tachycardia if ingested with **decongestants.**

Table 17–20 presents available dosage forms.

Antitussives

Antitussives are widely used by patients to self-treat coughs. It is essential for the health-care provider to

Table 17–20 ◆ **Available Dosage Forms: Selected Decongestants**

Drug	Dosage Form	How Supplied	Cost
	SYSTEMIC		
Pseudoephedrine Sulfate			
Afrin	Extended-release tablets: 120 mg (60 mg immediate release/60 mg extended release)	100	
Drixoral Non-Drowsy Formula	Extended-release tablets: 120 mg (60 mg immediate release/60 mg extended release)	20	$9.99/20 tablets
Pseudoephedrine HCl			
Sudafed	Tablets: 30 mg, 60 mg Extended release: 120 mg Liquid: 30 mg/5 mL	24, 48, 100, 1,000 10, 20 4 oz	$13.99/96 tablets
Generic	Tablets: 30 mg, 60 mg Liquid: 30 mg/5 mL	24, 100, 1,000 120 mL, 240 mL, pint, gallon	N/A
Phenylephrine			
Sudafed PE	10 mg tablet 2.5 mg/5 mL	18 tablets 36 tablets 48 tablets 4 oz	 $5.97 $10.49 $6.49.129 mL
	TOPICAL		
Phenylephrine			
Neo-Synephrine	Solution: 0.125%, 0.25%, 0.5%, 1%	30 mL, drops or spray bottle	$5.29/0.5 oz
Generic	Solution: 0.125%, 0.25%, 0.5%, 1%	30 mL, drops or spray bottle	$3.49/1.0 oz
Oxymetazoline			
Afrin Children's Nose Drops	Solution: 0.025%	20-mL bottle with dropper	
Afrin	Solution: 0.05%	15-mL spray bottle and 20-mL drops	$6.99/0.5 fl oz
4-Way Long Lasting Nasal	Solution: 0.05%	15-mL spray bottle	$4.99/0,5 oz
Dristan Long Lasting	Solution: 0.05%	15-mL, 30-mL spray bottle	
Neo-Synephrine 12 Hour	Solution: 0.05%	15-mL spray bottle	$6.19/0.5oz
Generic	Solution: 0.05%	15-mL, 30-mL spray bottle	$9.49/1.0 fl oz
Tetrahydrozoline			
Tyzine	Solution: 0.1%	15-mL spray, 30-mL drops	
Tyzine Pediatric Drops	Solution: 0.05%	15-mL drops	

educate the patient on the useful physiological mechanism a cough provides by clearing the airway of secretions and foreign material. Therefore, a cough should not be suppressed if it is protecting the airway. There are times when an **antitussive** is necessary to provide rest or sleep. The cough reflex is complicated, involving both the CNS and peripheral nervous system, as well as the smooth muscle of the bronchial tree. The drugs that can affect this complex mechanism are diverse, ranging from **bronchodilators** to drugs that act centrally or peripherally to suppress cough. This section discusses the nonprescription **antitussives dextromethorphan** and **benzonatate. Codeine,** which is also used as an **antitussive**, is covered in Chapter 15 with the other **opioids**. Dosing of **codeine** for **antitussive** use is included here.

Pharmacodynamics

Cough results when sensory stimuli or irritation in the bronchial tree stimulates cough receptors, probably located in the bronchial smooth muscle. A message is sent via the afferent nervous system to the cough centers in the medulla. **Antitussives** work either centrally or peripherally to affect the cough. The exact mechanism of action of antitussives is poorly understood. **Dextromethorphan,** the D isomer of the **codeine** analogue levorphanol, acts centrally in the cough center in the medulla to elevate the threshold for coughing. **Codeine** works as an antitussive through direct action on receptors in the cough center of the medulla, at lower doses than is required for analgesia. **Benzonatate (Tessalon)** is related to **tetracaine** and is thought to anesthetize the stretch receptors in the respiratory passages, thereby decreasing their activity and calming the cough peripherally at its source.

Pharmacokinetics

Absorption and Distribution

Dextromethorphan, codeine, and **benzonatate** are absorbed well from the GI tract. The distribution of **dextromethorphan** and **benzonatate** is unknown. **Codeine** is 7 percent protein bound and widely distributed, including in the CNS. **Codeine** freely crosses the placenta and is distributed into breast milk.

Metabolism and Excretion

Dextromethorphan is extensively metabolized by the liver and excreted in the urine, mostly as metabolites. **Codeine** is metabolized in the liver by glucuronidation into morphine and **norcodeine.** The metabolism of **codeine** into morphine is mediated by CYP450 2D6. **Codeine** is eliminated in the urine as unchanged drug, **norcodeine,** and free and conjugated **morphine.** The metabolism and excretion of **benzonatate** is unknown. See Table 17–21 for the pharmacokinetics of selected preparations.

Pharmacotherapeutics

Precautions and Contraindications

Antitussives are not to be used for persistent or chronic cough caused by smoking, asthma, or emphysema. In asthma, **antitussives** may impair expectoration and thus cause increased airway resistance. **Expectorants** must not be used by patients with excessive respiratory secretions for the same reason. Patients must be cautioned not to self-medicate their cough for long periods (more than 7 days) without seeking the care of their health-care provider. If high fever or rash accompanies a cough, patients must be seen by their health-care provider.

Benzonatate is contraindicated for patients allergic to **tetracaine, procaine,** or related compounds.

Dextromethorphan, codeine, and **benzonatate** can cause drowsiness, dizziness, nausea, and GI upset. In addition, patients taking **benzonatate** may experience headache, constipation, pruritus, skin eruptions, a sensation of burning eyes, a vague "chilly" sensation, chest numbness, and hypersensitivity.

Patients with hepatic function impairment should be monitored if **dextromethorphan** is prescribed because metabolism of the drug may be impaired. The metabolism of **codeine** can be affected by deficiency of CYP450D or by medications that may inhibit CYP2D6.

Table 17–21 ▶ Pharmacokinetics: Selected Cough Preparations

Drug	Onset	Peak	Duration	Protein Binding	Half-Life	Metabolism	Elimination
Antitussives							
Dextromethorphan	15–30 min	—	5–6 h	—	11 h	Extensive hepatic	Renal
Codeine (used as an antitussive)	30–60 min	1–2 h	4–6 h	7%	3–4 h	Primarily hepatic (CYP2D6)	Renal
Benzonatate	15–20 min	—	3–8 h	—	—	—	—
Expectorants							
Guaifenesin	Rapid	—	—	—	1 h	—	Renal

Codeine may cause dependence and should be used with caution in a patient with a history of substance abuse. Although dextromethorphan is not addictive, there have been reports of abuse of dextromethorphan-containing products, especially among teenagers. The FDA issued a Talk Paper in 2005 to warning the public, providers, and law enforcement of the potential for dextromethorphan abuse and as of 2010 has begun exploring whether dextromethorphan should become a scheduled drug.

Codeine causes decreased gastric motility and therefore should be used cautiously by patients with GI obstruction, ileus, or preexisting constipation. Patients with acute ulcerative colitis may be more sensitive to the constipating effects of codeine.

Dextromethorphan and codeine are Pregnancy Category C, but no teratogenic effects have been demonstrated. Codeine should be used with caution near term in pregnancy. Benzonatate is Pregnancy Category C and is to be given to pregnant women only if clearly needed. There are better-studied choices for antitussives in pregnancy, such as dextromethorphan or short-term codeine.

Drug Interactions

Use of antitussives with any CNS depressant may cause increased CNS depression. Concurrent use of dextromethorphan and MAOIs is contraindicated.

Codeine should be used with caution concurrently with medications that are metabolized by CYP2D6 isoenzymes. Quinidine has been shown to interfere with the metabolism of codeine. Other medications that inhibit CYP2D6 are amiodarone (Cordarone), tricyclic antidepressants, metoclopramide (Reglan), selective serotonin reuptake inhibitors (SSRIs), cimetidine (Tagamet), thioridazine (Mellaril), propafenone (Rythmol), and haloperidol (Haldol).

Drugs interactions are shown in Table 17–22.

Clinical Use and Dosing

Cough

Dextromethorphan, codeine, and benzonatate are used to control nonproductive cough. Antitussives should be used only for the nonproductive, irritant-like cough, after other pathology has been ruled out, specifically asthma or pneumonia. Antitussives are not to be used for asthmatic cough or for coughs accompanied by excessive respiratory secretions.

Dextromethorphan is available in many forms and either singly or in combination with expectorants. As it is available without prescription, it is widely used by patients to self-medicate their cough, not always appropriately. The adult dose of dextromethorphan is 10 to 30 mg every 4 to 8 hours. Children aged 6 to 12 years are given a dose of 5 to 10 mg every 4 hours or 15 mg every 6 to 8 hours. The dose of dextromethorphan in children aged 2 to 6 years is 2.5 to 7.5 mg every 4 to 8 hours, although current guidelines recommend not using cough medication in children with cough (Chang & Glomb, 2006).

Benzonatate is available only by prescription and is effective in controlling dry, irritant-like coughs. The dose for children aged 10 years and older and adults is 100 mg three times a day. Benzonatate does not cause CNS sedation and may be preferred over dextromethorphan or

Table 17–22 ■ Drug Interactions: Selected Cough Preparations

Drug	Interacting Drug	Possible Effect	Implications
Antitussives			
Dextromethorphan	MAOIs	Dextromethorphan can block neuronal uptake of serotonin and can increase concentrations of serotonin if combined with MAOIs; hypertensive or hyperpyretic crisis is possible	Use concurrently with caution, if at all; avoid use within 14 d
	SSRIs	SSRIs interfere with dextromethorphan metabolism, leading to toxicity	Use lower doses of dextromethorphan
	CNS depressants	Additive CNS depression	Use with caution
	Amiodarone, quinidine	These drugs inhibit CYP2D6; dextromethorphan toxicity may occur	Monitor for toxicity if prescribed concurrently
Codeine (used as an antitussive)	CNS depressants, alcohol	Additive CNS depression	Use cautiously and reduce dose to avoid additive effects
	Antihypertensive agents	Antagonizes antihypertensives	Monitor patients closely
	Antidiarrheals	Can lead to severe constipation	Use with caution; monitor the patient
Benzonatate	None known	—	—
Expectorants			
Guaifenesin	None known	—	—

codeine in patients who need to remain alert or who have a history of substance abuse and want to avoid opioids.

Codeine, a Schedule III, IV, or V medication (depending on combination with other medications), may be administered alone or in combination with another agent such as **guaifenesin** for cough suppression. The adult dose of **codeine** for cough suppression is 10 to 20 mg every 4 to 6 hours, with the maximum daily dose not exceeding 120 mg. Children aged 6 to 12 years can be prescribed 5 to 10 mg every 4 to 6 hours (maximum 60 mg/d). Current guidelines recommend against the use of **antitussives** in children (Chang & Glomb, 2006). Table 17–23 presents dosing information.

Rational Drug Selection

Patients may self-medicate their cough with a nonprescription form of **dextromethorphan**, and the health-care provider has little to do with the choice of the medication. (Advertising has the largest impact.) The health-care provider becomes involved when the patient asks for a recommended formula or if nonprescription products are not effective.

Cost

Although nonprescription **dextromethorphan** is less expensive than **benzonatate**- or **codeine**-containing preparations, patients with good prescriptive coverage may actually pay less out of pocket for the prescription product. Cost must therefore be evaluated on an individual basis.

Effectiveness

Patients might feel that a prescription medication is more effective than nonprescription, but **dextromethorphan** has been found to be as effective as **codeine** in the treatment of cough.

Monitoring

There is no specific monitoring required when prescribing **antitussive** medications.

Patient Education

Patient education centers on proper administration, adverse reactions, and drug interactions with the **antitussive** agents.

Administration

Patients should be aware of the proper dosing of **antitussive** medication. When they are self-medicating, they are often not following the recommended dosing schedule. The health-care provider needs to determine if the patient is taking the proper amount, measured with a calibrated measuring spoon (not a flatware teaspoon or tablespoon), and spacing the dosage appropriately. The medications may be taken without regard to food but may be better tolerated if taken with food or milk.

Table 17–23 ● **Dosage Schedule: Selected Cough Preparations**

Drug	Indication	Dose	Comments
Antitussives			
Dextromethorphan	Cough	*Children >12 yr and adults:* 10–30 mg every 4 h or 30 mg every 6–8 h	Do not exceed 120 mg in 24 h
		Children 6–12 yr: 5–10 mg every 4 h or 15 mg every 6–8 h	Do not exceed 60 mg in 24 h
		Children 2–6 yr: 2.5–5 mg every 4 h or 7.5 mg every 6–8 h	Do not exceed 30 mg in 24 h
		Children 7 mo–2 yr: 2–4 mg every 6–8 h	
Codeine (used as an antitussive)	Cough	*Adults:* 10–20 mg every 4 h	Do not exceed 120 mg in 24 h
		Children 6–12 yr: 5–10 mg every 4 h	Do not exceed 60 mg in 24 h
		Children 2–6 yr: 2.5–5 mg every 4 h	Do not exceed 30 mg in 24 h. Not recommended for acute or chronic cough in children.
Benzonatate	Cough	*Children >10 yr and adults:* 100 mg tid, up to 600 mg per day	Do not chew or crush capsules
Expectorants			
Guaifenesin	Cough	*Children >12 yr and adults:* 200–400 mg every 4 h	Maximum 2.4 g/24 h
		Children 6–11 yr: 100–200 mg every 4 h	Maximum 1.2 g/24 h
		Children 2–5 yr: 50–100 mg every 4 h	Maximum 600 mg/24 h

Adverse Reactions

CNS depression is the major concern. Some of the **antitussives** are in **alcohol**-containing syrup form, and others may cause sedation. Driving or operating hazardous machinery should be undertaken with caution, and not at all if the patient is sensitive to the sedating effects of the **antitussives.** Patients should also be aware that if they have long-term (occurring for more than 7 days) cough or cough accompanied by fever, they should be seen by their health-care provider.

Patients concurrently taking **MAOIs** should not take **antitussives. Antitussives** should be taken with caution if the patient is concurrently taking any other CNS sedating medications.

Lifestyle Management

The patient with a cough should be encouraged to increase fluid intake to improve the viscosity of the respiratory secretions. The patient should refrain from smoking and, if possible, stop smoking. Avoidance of respiratory irritants and people with respiratory infections will decrease the incidence of cough.

Table 17–24 presents available dosage forms.

Expectorants

Guaifenesin is the only expectorant ingredient listed by the FDA panel as having scientific evidence of safety and efficacy. **Guaifenesin** is indicated as an expectorant in the symptomatic treatment of cough due to the common cold and mild upper respiratory infections.

Pharmacodynamics

Guaifenesin's main mechanism of action is to increase the output of the respiratory tract by decreasing adhesiveness and surface tension. The increased flow of the thinned secretions promotes ciliary action and facilitates the removal of respiratory mucus. This changes a dry, nonproductive cough into a more productive cough.

Pharmacokinetics

Absorption and Distribution

Guaifenesin is rapidly absorbed from the GI tract after oral administration. Distribution is unknown. It is not known whether **guaifenesin** crosses the placenta or is distributed in breast milk.

Table 17–24 ◆ **Available Dosage Forms: Selected Cough Preparations**

Drug	Dosage Form	How Supplied	Cost
ANTITUSSIVES			
Dextromethorphan			
Scot-Tussen DM Cough Chasers	Lozenges: 2.5 mg	20	N/A
Hold DM	Lozenges: 5 mg	10	$2.99/10
Robitussin Cough Calmers	Lozenges: 5 mg	10	$10.49/12 oz
Supress Cough	Lozenges: 7.5 mg	1,000	$2.89/32
Robitussin Pediatric	Liquid: 7.5 mg/5 mL	120 mL, 240 mL	$10.49/12 fl oz
Vicks Formula 44	Liquid: 15 mg/5 mL	120 mL, 240 mL (contains 10% alcohol)	$7.99/8 oz
Vicks Formula 44 Pediatric	Liquid: 15 mg/15 mL (1 mg/mL)	120 mL (no alcohol)	N/A
Delsym	Sustained-action liquid: 30 mg/5 mL	89 mL	$11.89/5 oz
Codeine			
Codeine sulfate (used as an antitussive)	Tablets: 15 mg, 30 mg, 60 mg	100	$22.99/100
Benzonatate			
Tessalon Perles	Capsules: 100 mg	100, 1,000	$13.99/30 capsules
EXPECTORANTS			
Guaifenesin			
Robitussin	Syrup: 100 mg/5 mL	30 mL, 60 mL, 120 mL, 240 mL, pint, gallon (contains 3.5% alcohol)	$10.49/12 fl oz
Generic	Syrup: 100 mg/5 mL	120 mL, 240 mL, pint, gallon	$5.00/12 oz

Metabolism and Excretion

The exact mechanism of metabolism of **guaifenesin** is unknown. Its major metabolite, beta (2-methoxyphenoxy) lactic acid, is excreted in the urine.

Pharmacotherapeutics

Precautions and Contraindications

Guaifenesin is not to be used for persistent cough, such as that found with smoking, asthma, or emphysema. Cough related to heart failure or **angiotensin-converting enzyme (ACE) inhibitor** therapy should not be treated with **guaifenesin.** A cough accompanied by high fever or lasting longer than 7 days should be evaluated by a health-care provider.

Guaifenesin is Pregnancy Category C. There have been no problems documented in breastfeeding women taking this medication. Use in children as young as age 2 years is considered safe.

Adverse Drug Effects

GI upset, nausea, and vomiting are the most commonly reported adverse effects of **guaifenesin.** Drowsiness, diarrhea, dizziness, rash, and headache have also been reported. **Guaifenesin** is contraindicated only if the patient is hypersensitive to **guaifenesin.**

Drug Interactions

There are no drug interactions of significance with **guaifenesin;** however, **guaifenesin** may cause false readings in certain laboratory determinations of 5-hydroxyindoleacetic acid (5-HIAA) and vanillylmandelic acid (VMA).

Clinical Use and Dosing

Dry, Nonproductive Cough

Guaifenesin is indicated in the symptomatic relief of dry, nonproductive cough, with mucus in the respiratory tract. The dose of **guaifenesin** for children over age 12 years and adults is 200 to 400 mg every 4 hours. The **guaifenesin** dose in children aged 6 to 11 years is 100 to 200 mg every 4 hours. Children aged 2 to 5 years should be dosed with 50 to 100 mg of **guaifenesin** every 4 hours.

Monitoring

There is no specific laboratory monitoring required with the use of **guaifenesin.**

Patient Education

Administration

The patient should be aware of the proper dose of **guaifenesin.** The patient should be using a calibrated medication spoon and taking the appropriate dose per age.

Guaifenesin is an OTC product, and patients may self-medicate, often without proper understanding of the medication. The provider may assist the patient in making the proper choice of cough medication by explaining the difference between the OTC products **guaifenesin** and **dextromethorphan.** An explanation of the many combination products that are available and some guidance about appropriate use will assist the patient in making an informed choice.

Adverse Reactions

Although ADRs of **guaifenesin** are mild, patients should be instructed regarding the mild gastrointestinal upset that may occur.

Lifestyle Management

Patients should be instructed to remain well hydrated while taking **guaifenesin,** and they should refrain from smoking.

REFERENCES

Abramowicz, M. (2005). Drugs for asthma. *Treatment Guidelines from the Medical Letter, 3*(33), 33–38.

Apter, A. J., & Szefler, S. J. (2006). Advances and adult and pediatric asthma. *Journal of Allergy and Clinical Immunology, 117*(3), 512–518.

Berger, W. E. (2003). Levalbuterol: Pharmacologic properties and use in the treatment of pediatric and adult asthma. *Annals of Allergy, Asthma, and Immunology, 90*(6), 583–592.

Centers for Disease Control and Prevention. (2007). Infant deaths associated with cough and cold medications—two states, 2005. *Mortality and Morbidity Weekly Report, 56*(1), 104.

Chang, A. B., & Glomb, W. B. (2006). Guidelines for evaluating chronic cough in pediatrics: ACCP evidence-based clinical practice guidelines. *Chest, 129,* 260S–283S.

Drazen, J. M., Israel, E., Boushey, H. A., Chinchilli, V. M., Fahy, J. V., Fish, J. E., et al. (1996). Comparison of regularly scheduled with as-needed use of albuterol in mild asthma. *New England Journal of Medicine, 335*(12), 841–847.

Drombrowski, M., Thom, E., & McNellis, D. (1999). Maternal-fetal medicine units (MFMU) studies of inhaled corticosteroids during pregnancy. *Journal of Allergy and Clinical Immunology, 103*(2), S356–S359.

Hayden, M. L. (2004). Allergic rhinitis. *Nurse Practitioner, 29*(12), 26–37.

Ladebauche, P. (1997). Managing asthma: A growth and developmental approach. *Pediatric Nursing, 23*(1), 37–44.

Lieu, T. A., Quesenberry, C. P., Capra, A. M., Sorel, M. E., Martin, K. E., & Mendoza, G. R. (1997). Outpatient management practices associated with reduced risk of pediatric asthma hospitalization and emergency department visits. *Pediatrics, 100*(3, Pt. 1), 334–341.

Luskin, A. T. (1999). An overview of the recommendation of the working group on asthma and pregnancy. *Journal of Allergy and Clinical Immunology, 103*(2), S350–S353.

Man, S. E. P., & Sin, D. D. (2005) Inhaled corticosteroids in chronic obstructive pulmonary disease. *Drugs, 65*(5), 579–591.

National Asthma Education and Prevention Program (NAEPP). (2002). *The Expert Panel Report: Guidelines for the diagnosis and management of asthma. Updates on selected topics 2002* (NIH Publication No. 02–5074). Bethesda, MD: National Heart, Lung, and Blood Institute, National Institutes of Health.

National Asthma Education and Prevention Program (NAEPP). (2007). *The Expert Panel Report 3: Guidelines for the diagnosis and management of asthma.* Bethesda, MD: National Heart, Lung, and Blood Institute, National Institutes of Health. Retrieved from http://www.nhlbi.nih.gov/guidelines/asthma/

National Heart, Lung, and Blood Institute. (1995). *Global strategy for asthma management and prevention: NHLBI/WHO report* (NIH Publication No. 95–3659). Bethesda, MD: National Institutes of Health.

Nelson, H. S., Weiss, S. T., Bleecker, E. R., Yancey, S. W., Dorinsky, P. M., & the SMART Study Group. (2006). The Salmeterol Multicenter Asthma

Research Trial: A comparison of usual pharmacotherapy for asthma or usual pharmacotherapy plus salmeterol. *Chest, 129*(1), 15–26.

Parsons, J. P., & Mastronarde, J. G. (2005). Exercise-induced bronchoconstriction in athletes. *Chest, 128*(6), 3966–3974.

Salpeter, S. R., Wall, A. J., & Buckley, N. S. (2010). Long-acting beta-agonists with and without inhaled corticosteroids and catastrophic asthma events. *American Journal of Medicine, 123,* 322–328.

Simmons, M. S., Nides, M. A., Rand, C. S., Wise, R. A., & Tashkin, D. P. (1996). Trends in compliance with bronchodilator inhaler use between follow-up visits in a clinical trial. *Chest, 109*(4), 963–968.

Skoner, D. P., Greos, L. S., Kim, K. T., Roach, J. M., Parsey, M., & Baumgartner, R. A. (2005). Evaluation of the safety and efficacy of levalbuterol in 2- to 5-year-old patients with asthma. *Pediatric Pulmonology, 40*(6), 477–486.

Skouroliakou, M., Bacopoulou, F., & Markantonis, S. L. (2009). Caffeine versus theophylline of apnea of prematurity: A randomized controlled trial. *Journal of Paediatrics and Child Health, 45*(10), 587–592.

Takemoto, C. K., Hodding, J. H., & Kraus, D. M. (2009). *Pediatric dosage handbook* (16th ed.). Hudson, OH: Lexicomp.

Tashkin, D. P., Bleecker, E., Braun, S., Campbell, S., DeGraff, A. C., Hudgel, D.W., et al. (1996). Results of a multicenter study of nebulized inhalant bronchodilator solutions. *American Journal of Medicine, 100*(Suppl. IA), IA-62S–IA-68S.

U. S. Food and Drug Administration. (2010). FDA Drug Safety Communication: New safety requirements for long-acting inhaled asthma medications called long-acting beta-agonists (LABAs). Retrieved from http://www.fda.gov/Drugs/DrugSafety/PostmarketDrugSafetyInformationforPatientsandProviders/ucm200776.htm

U.S. Food and Drug Administration (2009). Updated information on leukotriene inhibitors: Montelukast (marketed as Singulair), zafirlukast (marketed as Accolate), and zileuton (marketed as Zyflo and Zyflo CR). Retrieved from http://www.fda.gov/Drugs/DrugSafety/PostmarketDrugSafetyInformationforPatientsandProviders/DrugSafetyInformationforHeathcareProfessionals/ucm165489.htm

VanAndel, A. E., Reisner, C., Menjoge, S. S., & Witek, T. J. (1999). Analysis of inhaled corticosteroid and oral theophylline use among patients with stable COPD from 1987 to 1995. *Chest, 115*(3), 703–707.

Wendel, P. J., Ramin, S. M., Barnett-Hamm, C., Rowe, T. F., & Cunningham, F. G. (1996). Asthma treatment in pregnancy: A randomized controlled study. *American Journal of Obstetrics and Gynecology, 175*(1), 150–154.

Zieger, R. S., Szefler, S. J., Phillips, B. R., Schatz, M., Martinez, F. D., Chinchilli, V. M., et al. (2006). Response to fluticasone and montelukast in mild-to-moderate persistent childhood asthma. *Journal of Allergy and Clinical Immunology, 117*(1), 45–52.

CHAPTER 18

DRUGS AFFECTING THE HEMATOPOIETIC SYSTEM

Teri Moser Woo

Chapter Outline

ANTICOAGULANTS AND ANTIPLATELETS

Thromboemboli are a common cause of morbidity and mortality. Venous thromboembolism occurs in approximately 100 of every 100,000 persons in the United States each year (American Heart Association Writing Group Members, 2010). Pulmonary embolism is a common complication of deep vein thrombosis (DVT), with silent pulmonary embolism occurring in up to one-third of patients with DVT (Stein, Matta, Musani, & Diaczok, 2010). The morbidity and mortality associated with these emboli could be significantly reduced by timely use of anticoagulation therapy. Oral anticoagulation therapy has been used in primary care for over 50 years, and the number of indications for its use has steadily increased. The introduction of **low-molecular-weight heparin** (LMWH) with less bleeding risk has allowed the outpatient use of injectable anticoagulation therapy as well. With more selective and reliable laboratory tests to monitor blood levels, the management of anticoagulation therapy has become a major tool in the prevention of thrombus formation in primary care.

Pharmacodynamics

Thrombi tend to develop whenever intravascular conditions promote activation of the clotting cascade. These conditions include injury to the intimal lining of the artery; roughing of this surface such as occurs in atherosclerosis; inflammation, which is a cardinal part of atherogenesis; traumatic injury; infection; alteration in the normal laminar blood flow; low blood pressure; or obstructions that cause blood stasis and pooling within the vessels. Although the exact details of the clotting mechanism are not fully understood, it is generally accepted that clotting occurs when several circulating proteins interact in a cascading series of limited proteolytic actions (Fig. 18–1). At each step, a precursor protein is converted to an active protease that activates the next clotting factor, and finally, a solid clot is formed. The key regulatory protein in this cascade that initiates blood coagulation is likely factor VII (McCance & Huether, 2010. The components involved at each stage are a protease from the preceding stage, a precursor protein, a protein activator, calcium, and an organizing surface provided by platelets.

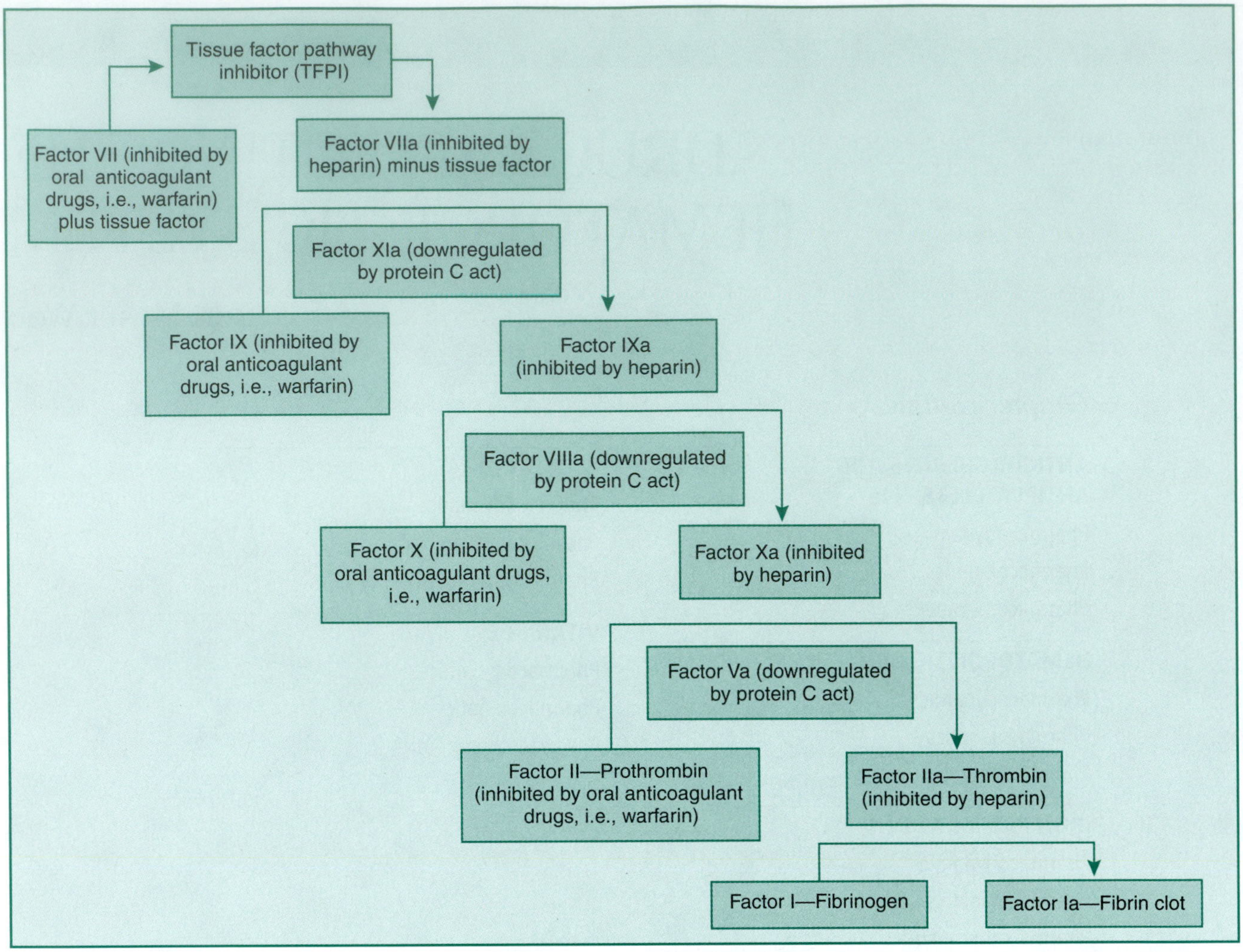

Figure 18–1. The clotting cascade.

Fibrinogen is the substrate for the enzyme thrombin (factor IIa). This protease is formed by activation of its precursor protein, prothrombin. Prothrombin is bound by calcium to a platelet surface, where activated factor X (Xa), in the presence of factor V (Va), converts it to circulating thrombin. Thrombin then converts fibrinogen to fibrin to form the clot. Venous thrombi are mainly fibrin and red blood cells (RBCs) and occur when the balance of the clotting pathway is altered by thrombophilic abnormalities, vessel wall damage, or stasis (Weitz, Hirsh, & Samama, 2004). Arterial thrombosis occurs when an atherosclerotic plaque is disrupted and a thrombus forms at the site of disruption (Weitz et al, 2004).

Oral anticoagulants such as **warfarin (Coumadin)** inhibit the hepatic synthesis of several clotting factors, including factor X. The decline in clotting factors is a function of the half-life of each factor, which varies from 5 hours for factor VII to 72 hours for factor II. Plasma also contains protease inhibitors that inactivate coagulation proteins. One of these factors is antithrombin III. **Heparin** inhibits the activity of several activated clotting factors by accelerating the activity of antithrombin III. LMWH **enoxaparin (Lovenox)** potentiates the activity of antithrombin III and inactivates factors Xa and IIa (thrombin). **Fondaparinux (Arixtra)** is a selective inhibitor of antithrombin III and a factor Xa inhibitor. An anticoagulant **rivaroxaban (Xarelto)**, approved in Europe, is currently in U.S. Food and Drug Administration (FDA) review and is a highly selective factor Xa inhibitor that inhibits thrombin formation and the development of thrombi. **Ximelagatran (Exanta)** is an oral anticoagulant that is awaiting further studies before it can gain FDA approval.

The formation of a clot also requires that platelets aggregate to form the organizing base for the clot. Platelets adhere to injured vessel walls, undergo granulate discharge, and aggregate into clumps, releasing biochemical mediators. Several factors affect platelet adherence, including sufficient concentrations of calcium in the platelet so that it can change shape, aggregate, degranulate, and activate arachidonic pathways. Adhesion occurs when the platelet receptor binds to von Willebrand factor, bridging the plate to injury site. Two of the mediators released by platelets are serotonin and histamine, which affect smooth muscle in the vascular endothelium causing an immediate temporary vasoconstriction. Vasoconstriction reduces blood flow and diminishes bleeding. Vasodilation follows to permit the inflammatory process to occur.

The arachidonic pathway uses cyclooxygenase to produce thromboxane A_2 (TXA_2), a prostaglandin, and prostacyclin I_2 (PGI_2). TXA_2 causes vasoconstriction and promotes degranulation of other platelets, which then release more adenosine diphosphate (ADP) to promote adherence. PGI_2 inhibits the effect of TXA_2 by promoting vasodilation and inhibiting platelet degranulation. The net effect is to permit platelet aggregation at the injury site but to prevent adherence to normal vascular endothelium. **Aspirin** antagonizes the cyclooxygenase pathway and interferes with platelet aggregation. **NSAIDs** have this same action. **NSAIDs** are not used as **antiplatelet drugs**, but this explains why concurrent use with **anticoagulants** is contraindicated (Kniff-Dutmer, Schut, & van der Laar, 2003). **Ticlopidine (Ticlid)** and **clopidogrel (Plavix)** reduce platelet aggregation by inhibiting the ADP pathway of platelets. Unlike **aspirin**, they have no effect on prostaglandin metabolism.

Aspirin and **ibuprofen** also have analgesic, antipyretic, and anti-inflammatory actions related to their cyclooxygenase (COX) activity. These actions are discussed in Chapter 25.

Pharmacokinetics

Absorption and Distribution

Heparin, including the low-molecular-weight drugs **dalteparin (Fragmin)**, **enoxaparin (Lovenox)**, **fondaparinux (Arixtra)**, and **tinzaparin (Innohep)** are not absorbed in the gastrointestinal (GI) tract and must be given IV or SC. The IV route is used in acute care. SC injection of **heparin** results in considerable individual variation in bioavailability. **LMWHs** have less variation, but bioavailability between drugs is not consistent, and these drugs are not interchangeable. Once absorbed, **heparin** is distributed in plasma and extensively protein bound. The LMWHs are distributed in plasma and have limited to no protein binding (Table 18–1). Volume of distribution (Vd) is different between the **LMWHs** and may factor into choosing among them for specific populations.

Table 18–1 ▶ **Pharmacokinetics: Selected Anticoagulants and Antiplatelets**

Drug	Onset	Peak	Duration	Protein Binding	Bioavailability/ Volume of Distribution	Half-Life	Elimination
Anticoagulants							
Dalteparin	—	4 h	Up to 24 h	—	87%/40–60 mL	3–5 h (increased in renal insufficiency)	In urine
Enoxaparin	—	3–5 h	12 h	—	100%/4.3 L	4.5 h	In urine
Heparin (SC only)	20–60 min	2–4 h	8–12 h	Extensive	—	1–3 h (nonlinear and dose dependent; 30 min for doses of 25 mcg/ kg vs. 150 min for doses of 400 mcg/kg); half-life shorter for patients with deep vein thrombosis (DVT) than those with pulmonary embolism; half-life may be prolonged in liver disease	50% unchanged in urine; some urine degradation products have anticoagulant activity; also eliminated by reticuloendothelial system (lymph nodes and spleen)
Fondaparinux	—	2 hr	—	None	100%/7–11 L	11–21 h	In urine
Tinzaparin	—	—	—	None	87%/3.1–5 L	3–4 h	In urine
Warfarin	—	3–5 d	2–5 d	99%	100%/0.14 L	40 h	92% in urine as metabolites

Continued

Table 18–1 ▶ **Pharmacokinetics: Selected Anticoagulants and Antiplatelets—cont'd**

Drug	Onset	Peak	Duration	Protein Binding	Bioavailability/ Volume of Distribution	Half-Life	Elimination
Antiplatelets							
Aspirin	5–30 min	1–3 h	3–6 h	Concentration-dependent low doses: (100 mcg/mL) = 90% high doses: (400 mcg/mL) = 76%	—	15–20 min	Renal excretion depends on urine pH; as pH increases from 5 to 8, renal clearance increases from 2%–3% to more than 80%
Clopidogrel	—	1 h	3–7 d	98%	50%	8 h	50% in urine; 46% in feces
Ticlopidine	2 h	8–11 d	2 wk	98%	—	12.6 h for single dose; 4–5 d with repeated dosing	60% in urine, 23% in feces; clearance decreases with age

The **coumarin derivative** most commonly used is **warfarin (Coumadin). Warfarin** is rapidly and completely absorbed orally. Although serum levels are found in 1 to 2 hours, the anticoagulation effect is dependent on depletion of clotting factors. Because factor II has a life of 72 hours, the full effect does not occur for 3 to 4 days. **Warfarin** is highly bound to plasma protein.

Rivaroxaban is rapidly absorbed when given orally and is 80 to 100 percent bioavailable and is highly protein bound. **Rivaroxaban** effects protime (PT) in 2 to 4 hours after the first tablet is ingested.

Aspirin is rapidly and completely absorbed after oral administration. Bioavailability is dependent on the dosage form, the presence of food, gastric emptying time, gastric pH, presence of antacids or buffering agents, and particle size. Bioavailability of enteric-coated forms is erratic. **Aspirin** is partially hydrolyzed during absorption and distributed to all body tissues and fluids, including fetal tissues and breast milk. Protein binding is highest with low plasma concentrations and lower with high concentrations.

Ticlopidine is rapidly absorbed after oral administration. Administration after meals increases the area under the curve (AUC) by 20 percent.

Clopidogrel is rapidly absorbed after oral administration. Bioavailability is not affected by food.

Metabolism and Excretion

Heparins are metabolized by the liver and the reticuloendothelial system. A secondary site of metabolism may be in the kidney. Clearance is nonlinear, and the half-life may be prolonged at higher doses and in liver disease.

In patients with severe renal insufficiency, **dalteparin** mean terminal half-life of anti-factor Xa may be considerably longer, with greater accumulation than in other patients. The AUC for anti-factor Xa is marginally increased with **enoxaparin** for mild to moderate renal insufficiency, but significantly increased with creatinine clearance (Ccr) less than 30 mL. **Tinzaparin** has a similar problem with a 24 percent reduction in clearance in severe renal insufficiency.

The risk of **fondaparinux**-associated major bleeding increases with age, from 1.8 percent for those under age 65 to 2.7 percent for those older than 75. This drug should be used cautiously in the elderly. It also has increased terminal half-life in renal impairment.

Warfarin is metabolized by hepatic microsomal enzymes cyproheptadine (CYP) 1A2 and 2C9 and is excreted primarily in the urine as inactive metabolites.

Rivaroxaban is metabolized by CYP 3A4 and 2J2 and is eliminated renally with a half -life of 7 to 11 hours.

Aspirin is extensively metabolized by the liver and excreted by the kidney. The amount excreted depends on urine pH. As pH increases, the amount excreted as unchanged drug increases from 2 or 3 percent to 80 percent.

Ticlopidine is extensively metabolized by the liver. Because of its nonlinear pharmacokinetics, clearance decreases markedly with repeated administration. In older adults, half-lives of 12.6 hours after the first dose increased to 4 to 5 days with repeated dosing. Steady-state levels occur in about 14 to 21 days. Trace amounts of intact drug are found in the urine, and one-third of the dose is excreted in feces and bile as intact drug. Clearance decreases with age. Renal impairment alters plasma levels but does not seem to affect platelet aggregation or bleeding times, except in moderately impaired patients.

Clopidogrel is a prodrug and the liver rapidly converts it to a metabolite that is the active **antiplatelet** compound. Plasma levels are significantly higher in the elderly but are not associated with differences in platelet aggregation and bleeding time, so no dosage adjustment is needed for this population. Steady state occurs in 3 to 7 days. It is excreted almost equally in urine and in feces, making it safer for patients with renal insufficiency.

Pharmacotherapeutics

Precautions and Contraindications

All **anticoagulants** are contraindicated for patients who are hypersensitive to the drug or actively bleeding or who have hemophilia, thrombocytopenia, severe hypertension (HTN), intracranial hemorrhage, infective endocarditis, active tuberculosis, or ulcerative lesions of the GI tract.

Heparins are contraindicated in advanced hepatic or renal disease. They may be used in patients who are actively bleeding to treat disseminated intravascular coagulation (DIC). **Heparin** is Pregnancy Category C. Although it does not cross the placenta, its use during pregnancy has been associated with unfavorable outcomes, including stillbirth and prematurity. It should be used only when clearly indicated. Safety has not been established in neonates. Some **heparin** preparations contain benzyl alcohol, which is known to cause "gasping syndrome," a fatal toxicity in neonates. Hyperkalemia may develop, and use for patients with diabetes or renal insufficiency requires care and frequent monitoring of activated partial thromboplastin time (aPTT). **Heparin** has been associated with fatal medication errors because of the different strengths of preparations available, including a highly concentrated 10,000 units in 1 mL. The Joint Commission has listed anticoagulant therapy as a National Patient Safety Goal requiring each facility have a plan in place to reduce patient harm.

LMWHs are contraindicated for patients with allergies to pork, sulfites, or benzyl alcohol; uncontrolled bleeding; and in patients who have antiplatelet antibodies. Renal impairment requires cautious use and is discussed in the metabolism and excretion section. Body weight less than 50 kg is also associated with markedly increased risk for bleeding; however, it is possible to adjust the dose of **enoxaparin** for patients with weights less than 45 kg. Cautious use is also indicated in untreated HTN, retinopathy (hypertensive or diabetic), severe liver disease, recent history of ulcer, or malignancy. **LMWH** should not be used for thromboprophylaxis in patients with mechanical prosthetic heart valves, especially pregnant women, as prosthetic heart valve thrombosis may occur. **Enoxaparin** is Pregnancy Category B. Teratogenicity and fetal death have been reported as well for **tinzaparin**, although a clear cause-and-effect relationship was not established. **Fondaparinux** is also listed as Pregnancy Category B without adequate or well-controlled studies in pregnancy. Institute for Clinical Systems Improvement (ICSI; 2005) states that **LMWHs** do not cross the placenta and do not cause teratogenicity or fetal bleeding, while acknowledging that use of **LMWHs** during pregnancy is controversial. The pharmacokinetics of **LMWHs** are altered during pregnancy. The American College of Chest Physicians (ACCP) recommends anti-factor Xa activity should be monitored if pregnant women are treated with **LMWH** (Hirsh, Guyatt, Albers, Harrington, & Schunemann, 2008). The use of **LMHW** during pregnancy requires consultation with a perinatologist regarding the benefit of treatment versus risk to the pregnant woman and fetus.

Hepatic dysfunction potentiates the response to **warfarin** through impaired synthesis of coagulation factors. Hypermetabolic states produced by fever or hyperthyroidism also increase responsiveness to **warfarin**, probably by increasing the catabolism of **vitamin K**–dependent coagulation factors. **Warfarin** should be used cautiously with these patients. Increased risk for bleeding is also an issue with older adults. Cautious use based on a balance between the potential for decreased risk of thromboembolism and the risk for bleeding is necessary for older adults with dementia or severe cognitive impairment; history of three falls within the previous year or recurrent, injurious falls; uncontrolled HTN; or who are nonadherent or unreliable (Sebastian & Tresch, 2000). **Warfarin** crosses the placenta and can cause hemorrhagic disorders in the fetus and serious birth defects. It is Pregnancy Category X and should not be administered during pregnancy. ICSI (2010) states that the amount of **warfarin** in breast milk is too small to affect the baby. **Warfarin** is considered safe during lactation, as minimal amount is excreted in breastmilk (LactMed, 2010).

Hypersensitivity to **aspirin** and cross-sensitivity with **NSAIDs** may occur, contraindicating the drug. **Aspirin** hypersensitivity is more prevalent in patients with asthma, nasal polyps, or chronic urticaria. Reye syndrome has been associated with its use in children and teenagers who have influenza or chickenpox. Reversible hepatotoxicity has occurred. Use **aspirin** cautiously in patients who have liver damage, preexisting hypoprothrombinemia, or vitamin K deficiency. **Aspirin** is Pregnancy Category C and Pregnancy Category D in the third trimester. **Aspirin** should be avoided during lactation, especially in young infants (LactMed, 2010). If a woman is on chronic high-dose **aspirin** therapy salicylates levels should be monitored in the infant (LactMed, 2010).

Patients with severe hepatic disease may have bleeding disorders; neither **clopidogrel** nor **ticlopidine** is recommended for these patients. They are also not recommended for patients with GI ulcers. Both drugs are Pregnancy Category B. Despite the lack of evidence of teratogenic potential with this drug, it should be used in pregnancy only when clearly indicated. Safety and efficacy in children under age 18 have not been established. Clearance of **ticlopidine** increases with age, and older adults' increased sensitivity to this drug requires close monitoring for adverse effects. Older adults have increased plasma levels of **clopidogrel**, but no dosage adjustments are needed. In older adults, **clopidogrel** is a safer drug. See discussion in Metabolism and Excretion section for more detail. **Ticlopidine** causes elevations in serum cholesterol (8% to 10%) and triglycerides within

1 month of therapy, and the higher levels persist. The ratios of subfractions of cholesterol remain unchanged. This may be a factor in choosing a drug for patients with dyslipidemias.

Adverse Drug Reactions

All **anticoagulants** can cause excessive bleeding. Several studies have shown that the incidence of bleeding severe enough to require hospitalization or transfusion is less than 5 percent. Risk of this complication is higher early in the initiation of therapy, with wide fluctuations in aPTT or international normalized ratio (INR) and in older adults, especially women above age 60. Patients with laboratory studies within the therapeutic range who exhibit this adverse reaction should be evaluated for underlying pathological processes that may be the source of the bleeding before implication of the **anticoagulant**.

Heparins can also cause thrombocytopenia and anemia. The incidence of thrombocytopenia is up to 30 percent and is more likely with bovine than with porcine heparin. Early thrombocytopenia occurs 2 to 3 days after initiating therapy, and a delayed form occurs 7 to 12 days after initiation. If the platelet count falls below 100,000/mm^3, the heparin should be discontinued. The antidote for **enoxaparin** overdose is **protamine sulfate** 1 mg for each mg of **enoxaparin**; for **dalteparin** and **tinzaparin**, it is 1 mg for each 100 anti-Xa international unit (IU) of **dalteparin**. Both are given by slow IV injection. There is no known antidote for **fondaparinux**. Because of **heparin's** short half-life, **heparin** overdose is usually treated by withdrawal of the drug. If treatment is required, **protamine sulfate** is also the antidote for **heparin** overdose.

Toxicity and overdose of **warfarin** are usually treated by withholding one or more doses. If it must be treated, **vitamin K** 1 to 10 mg is the antidote for **warfarin** overdose with minor bleeding; 5 to 50 mg may be used for frank bleeding.

Hemorrhagic skin necrosis in women and cyanotic toes in men have been observed in patients with therapeutic levels of **anticoagulants**. The mechanism appears to be related to a transient inhibition in proteins S and C in patients in whom these clotting factors are congenitally absent.

Although rare, allergic reactions do occur with **warfarin**. They are characterized by symmetrical, maculopapular, erythematous lesions. Some are isolated and some confluent. They tend to occur on the face, neck, and torso. Because of the length of time to therapeutic dose for **warfarin**, the drug reaction does not occur until the patient has been on the drug for 8 to 10 days.

Aspirin can produce gastric erosions that increase the risk of serious upper GI bleeding. This adverse effect is more likely when it is used in combination with other **anticoagulants** such as **warfarin**. Salicylism (tinnitus) associated with the use of **aspirin** occurs at serum levels above 200 mcg/mL. In addition to tinnitus, indications of **aspirin** toxicity are headache, hyperventilation, agitation, mental confusion, lethargy, diarrhea, and sweating. Severe toxic effects may occur at levels above 400 mcg/mL that occur with high doses. Such high doses are not used for **antiplatelet** therapy, so the management of severe toxicity is discussed in Chapter 25, which covers the use of **aspirin** for anti-inflammatory therapy.

> **CLINICAL PEARL**
>
> **Warfarin Allergic Patients**
>
> To maintain anticoagulation in patients with allergic reactions to **warfarin**, **enoxaparin or fondaparinux** can be given SC long term. The usual dose is 1 mg/kg.

Reversible neutropenia has occurred 3 weeks to 3 months after the initiation of therapy with **ticlopidine**. Severe neutropenia (less than 450 neutrophils/mm^3) or thrombocytopenia (less than 80,000 platelets/mm^3) is an indication to discontinue the drug.

Clopidogrel has been evaluated for safety in a very large number of patients and its tolerability is similar to that of **aspirin**, with approximately the same number of patients withdrawing from treatment because of adverse reactions.

Drug Interactions

Cephalosporins and **penicillins** given parenterally have both been associated with coagulopathies, increasing the risk of bleeding when given with **heparin**. Although not reported for these drugs when they are given orally, there is a theoretical increased risk for bleeding. Second and third generation **cephalosporins** and high doses of **penicillins**, regardless of route of administration, have also been associated with an increased bleeding risk with **warfarin** because they inhibit the cyclic interconversion of vitamin K.

Drugs that affect platelet functioning or cause hypoprothrombinemia, including **aspirin**, **NSAIDs**, **dipyridamole**, **quinidine**, and **valproic acid**, increase the risk of bleeding when used with any **anticoagulant**. Others are listed in Table 18–2.

Heparin and **LMWHs** have similar drug interactions, but also interact with **antiplatelets** (including **NSAIDs**) and **dextran**. Some natural products are also associated with increased risk for bleeding (see Table 18–2). Some of these are used as spices in cooking, and patients should be warned about their use. **Clopidogrel** has increased risk for bleeding from this same group of natural products.

Drugs potentiating and inhibiting **warfarin** are shown in Table 18–2. Drugs producing no effect were **antacids**, **atenolol**, **bumetanide**, **enoxacin**, **famotidine**, **fluoxetine**, **ketorolac**, **metoprolol**, **naproxen**, **nizatidine**, **psyllium**, and **ranitidine**. ICSI (2010) also does not include these drugs on a list of drugs interacting with **warfarin** with the exception of **antacids**, which they recommend be separated in administration. The ICSI website in the

Table 18–2 ■ **Drug Interactions: Selected Anticoagulants and Antiplatelets**

Drug	Interacting Drug	Possible Effect	Implications
Anticoagulants			
Dalteparin Enoxaparin	Salicylates, NSAIDs, dipyridamole sulfinpyrazone, ticlopidine	Increased risk of bleeding	
Fondaparinux, Tinzaparin	Thrombolytics, dextran, clopidogrel, some penicillins	Increased risk of bleeding	Avoid concurrent use
	Natural products: anise, arnica, chamomile, clove, feverfew, garlic, ginger, ginkgo, and panax ginseng	Increased risk of bleeding	Some are used as spices in cooking. Warn patients about this interaction and to avoid their concurrent use
Heparin	Cephalosporins and penicillins	Altered platelet aggregation and other coagulopathies with increased risk of bleeding	Mainly related to parenteral administration of these drugs; close monitoring required regardless of route of administration if used concurrently
	Nitroglycerin	Effect of heparin may be decreased	Reports are conflicting; monitor drug effects closely
	Platelet inhibitors: aspirin, salicylates, NSAIDs, dipyridamole, hydroxychloroquine, phenylbutazone, ticlopidine	Increased risk of bleeding	Avoid concurrent use
	Digitalis, tetracycline, nicotine, antihistamines	May partially counteract anticoagulant action	Avoid concurrent use
Warfarin	Alcohol (if concomitant liver disease), amiodarone, anabolic steroids, cimetidine, clofibrate, cotrimoxazole, erythromycin, fluconazole, isoniazid, metronidazole, omeprazole, phenylbutazone, piroxicam, propafenone, propranolol, sulfinpyrazone, citalopram, entacapone, sertraline, zileuton, Food/supplement: fish oil, mango	Evidence indicates it is highly probable that these drugs potentiate action with increased risk of bleeding	Avoid concurrent use; if necessary, dosage adjustment of warfarin may be required. Draw INR within 4 to 7 d of starting concerning drug.
	Acetaminophen, chloral hydrate, ciprofloxacin, celecoxib, disulfiram, itraconazole, quinidine, phenytoin, tamoxifen, pachitaxel, tolterodine, tetracycline, amoxicillin/clavulanate, azithromycin, levofloxacin, ritonavir, simvastatin, ropinirole, interferon, tramadol, Food: grapefruit ***Herbal supplements: dashen, dong quai, lycium barbarum, PC-SPES***	Evidence indicates these drugs probably potentiate action with increased risk of bleeding	Close monitoring of INR. Draw INR within 4 to 7 d of starting drug with possible interaction
	Aspirin	Increases risk of bleeding with higher doses; even low doses of aspirin (100 mg/d) have been associated with increased risk of minor bleeding	Avoid concurrent use
	Oral contraceptives	May decrease the anticoagulant effect	Use other birth control method
	Barbiturates, carbamazepine, chlordiazepoxide, cholestyramine, dicloxacillin, griseofulvin, nafcillin, rifampin, flu vaccine Foods: foods high in vitamin K,* large amounts of avocado, soy milk ***Herbs: ginseng***	Inhibits anticoagulant action	Avoid concurrent use of drugs. Maintain stable intake of foods high in vitamin K so that diet is balanced

Continued

Table 18–2 ■ **Drug Interactions: Selected Anticoagulants and Antiplatelets—cont'd**

Drug	Interacting Drug	Possible Effect	Implications
Antiplatelets			
Clopidogrel	Platelet inhibitors: aspirin, NSAIDs, dipyridamole, ticlopidine Anticoagulants: heparin and warfarin	Increased risk of bleeding	Avoid concurrent use except with aspirin in selected cases (see ACCP recommendations)
	Proton pump inhibitors Cimetidine, esomeprazole, fluoxetine, fluconazole, ketoconazole	Significant interaction that lowers antiplatelet effect of clopidogrel due to competitive inhibition of CYP2C19	The FDA recommends PPIs and other drugs that inhibit CYP2C19 be avoided in patients taking clopidogrel
	Phenytoin, tolbutamide, tamoxifen, torsemide, fluvastatin, and NSAIDs Natural products: see LMWHs above	May decrease metabolism and increase effects of interacting drugs	With high doses and based on data related to CYP450 2C9 inhibition.. No data to predict level of interaction. Use with caution
Ticlopidine	Platelet inhibitors: aspirin, NSAIDs, dipyridamole, clopidogrel Anticoagulants: heparin, LMWHs, and warfarin	Increased risk of bleeding	Avoid concurrent use
	Antacids	Concurrent administration results in 18% decrease in ticlopidine plasma levels	Separate drug administration; give ticlopidine first and antacids 1 h later
	Cimetidine	Chronic use of cimetidine reduced ticlopidine clearance by 50%	Use different histamine$_2$ blocker if reducing gastric acid is required
	Digoxin	Digoxin plasma levels decreased 15%	Avoid concurrent use
	Phenytoin	Elevated phenytoin plasma levels associated with somnolence and lethargy.	Use with caution and remeasure phenytoin levels
	Theophylline	Significantly increased theophylline elimination half-life with comparable reduction in total plasma clearance	Avoid concurrent use

*Foods high in vitamin K: asparagus, beans, broccoli, Brussels sprouts, cabbage, cauliflower, cheese, collards, fish, milk, mustard greens, pork, rice, spinach, turnips, yogurt.

Reference section has a large table of drugs that interact with **warfarin** and gives reasons for each interaction. The ICSI guidelines recommend measuring INR within 4 to 7 days when an interacting drug is added to the regimen (ICSI, 2010).

Clinical Use and Dosing

Prevention and Treatment of Thromboembolism

Warfarin is the drug of choice for the prevention of venous thrombosis, systemic thrombosis and pulmonary embolism. For prevention, **warfarin** should be given in a dose sufficient to maintain an INR between 2 and 3 (Hirsh et al, 2008). Loading doses are to be avoided. The average beginning dose is 5 mg daily (range 2.5 to 7.5 mg daily), with a recheck of INR in two to three doses. An initial dose of 7.5 mg may be given for patients who weigh more than 80 kg. Starting at doses higher than 10 mg does not result in a quicker therapeutic INR at day 4 or 5 (ICSI, 2010). Lower initiation doses should be considered for patients with any of the following (ICSI, 2010):

- Older than 75 years
- Multiple comorbid conditions
- Poor nutrition (low albumin)
- Elevated INR when off **warfarin**
- Elevated liver function tests
- Changing thyroid status

If the INR is greater than 2 after the first three doses, consider decreasing the dose by one-half. If INR rises rapidly, search for reasons such as drug interactions, poor nutritional status, infection or systemic disease process. Monitoring is discussed later.

Patients with acute pulmonary emboli (PE), DVT, or acute systemic embolization are admitted to the hospital for **heparin** therapy and then placed on oral anticoagulation. Alternative PE treatment is short-term treatment with **LMWH**, SC **fondaparinux**, then transitioning to oral **warfarin**. If PE is highly suspected, the ACCP recommends treatment with anticoagulants while awaiting diagnostic tests. In patients with acute PE, initial treatment is **heparin, LMWH**, or **fondaparinux** for at least 5 days and until INR is greater than or equal to 2.0 for at least 24 hours

(Hirsh et al, 2008). The ACCP recommends starting **warfarin** on the first day of treatment in conjunction with **heparin, LMWH,** or **fondaparinux.** Treatment for PE due to a transient (reversible) risk factor is **warfarin** for 3 months, after which the patient should be evaluated for risk/benefit ratio of long-term therapy (Hirsh et al, 2008). If at 3 months risk factors for bleeding are absent, the patient should receive long-term treatment, 6 to 12 months, maintaining an INR of 2.5 (range 2.0 to 3.0).

Deep Vein Thrombosis

The ACCP divides the treatment of acute DVT into acute treatment of DVT of the leg and treatment of upper extremity DVT. The initial treatment of acute DVT of the leg or upper extremity is short-term treatment with SC **LMWHs**, SC **fondaparinux**, or IV or SC **heparin** for at least 5 days and until the INR is 2.0 for at least 24 hours (Hirsh et al, 2008). **Warfarin** should be initiated on the first treatment day, as for PE. For a patient with an idiopathic DVT, the patient is maintained on **warfarin** with a target of 2.5 (range 2.0 to 3.0) for 6 to 12 months. If patients with idiopathic DVT request less frequent INR testing, they may be switched to "low-intensity" treatment (i.e., INR is kept between 1.5 and 1.9 with less frequent monitoring) after 3 months of conventional therapy (Hirsh et al, 2008).

Patients with an indwelling central line catheter are at risk for developing a DVT. In most patients with indwelling central venous catheter, the catheter is not removed if it is functional and is needed for therapy (i.e., chemotherapy). Treatment is the same as for leg DVT. If the catheter is removed, the patient should still receive at least 3 months of anticoagulant therapy (Hirsh et al, 2008).

All other patients requiring anticoagulant therapy can be safely started on **warfarin** as outpatients. Therapy is initiated with 5 mg daily unless the patient weighs less than 110 lb, is over age 75, or is at increased risk of bleeding. Patients with these weight, age, and risk parameters are started on 2.5 mg daily. Steady state is achieved in 5 to 7 days, at which time dosage adjustments are made, based on INR laboratory results. The goal of therapy is an INR of 2 to 3 for all treatment durations. Therapy is usually continued for 3 months for patients with a transient (reversible) DVT risk factor.

For patients with DVT or PE and cancer, the ACCP guideline recommends **LMWH** for the first 3 to 6 months of long-term **anticoagulant** therapy. Patients who have coagulopathies should be referred for management.

Air travel time longer than 8 hours places patients at risk of developing a DVT. The ACCP (Hirsh et al, 2008) recommends the following measures to prevent thrombus formation: wearing loose clothing, avoiding tight clothing around the waistline or lower extremities, achieving good hydration, and performing frequent calf muscle exercises. If patients have a high risk of developing a DVT, the ACCP recommends that they wear compression stockings providing 15 to 30 mm Hg of pressure during air travel. High-risk patients may also receive a single prophylactic dose of **LMWH** injected before travel (Hirsh et al, 2008).

For all patients, the ACCP stresses that immobility (bedrest) is counterproductive. They recommend ambulation as tolerated and the use of elastic compression stockings with a pressure of 30 to 40 mm Hg at the ankle for 2 years after an episode of DVT.

Dosage recommendations for anticoagulants are given in Table 18–3.

Table 18–3 ◉ **Dosage Schedule: Selected Anticoagulants and Antiplatelets**

Drug	Indication	Initial Dose	Maintenance Dose
Aspirin	MI and stroke prevention	300–325 mg daily	300–325 mg daily
Clopidogrel	Prevention of new ischemic event (CVA or MI) in patients with recent CVA, MI, or established PAD	75 mg once (may need 150 mg in some patients)	75 mg daily
	Acute coronary syndromes	300 mg once	75 mg daily. Aspirin 75–325 mg given concurrently
Dalteparin*	Prevention of DVT after abdominal surgery	2,500–5,000 IU on day of surgery	2,500–5,000 IU daily for 5–10 d postoperatively
	Hip replacement	2,500 2 h pre-op	2,500 IU evening post-op, then 5,000 IU daily for 5–9 d
Enoxaparin*	DVT and/or PE	1 mg/kg q12 h	Transition to warfarin
	Hip replacement and knee replacement	30 mg 12–24 h post-op or 40 mg 12 h pre-op	or 40 mg daily for 3 weeks
	Abdominal surgery	40 mg 2 h pre-op	40 mg daily for 7–10 d

Continued

Table 18–3 ◉ **Dosage Schedule: Selected Anticoagulants and Antiplatelets—cont'd**

Drug	Indication	Initial Dose	Maintenance Dose
Fondaparinux†	Hip-fracture surgery and hip or knee replacement	2.5 mg 6–8 h after surgery	2.5 mg for 24 d following hip-fracture surgery or 5–9 d for hip or knee replacement
	Therapy for DVT	Patients <50 kg: 5.0 mg daily Patients 50–100 kg: 7.5 mg daily Patients >100 kg: 10 mg daily	Continue same dose
Heparin	Preventive of postoperative thromboembolism	5,000 IU 2 h pre-op	5,000 U q8–12h for 7 d after surgery
Ticlopidine	Preventive of stroke in patients intolerant of aspirin	250 mg bid with food	250 mg bid with food
Tinzaparin*	DVT and/or PE	175 anti-Xa IU/kg	175 anti-Xa IU/kg daily for 6 d with transition to warfarin
Warfarin	Prevention and treatment of venous thrombosis, systemic embolism, and pulmonary embolism; prevention of embolic stroke in atrial fibrillation	5 mg daily; for patients < 50 kg; >age 75, or at increased risk of bleeding: 2.5 mg daily	Measure INR at 5–7 d and adjust to INR of 2–3
	Recurrent systemic embolism and mechanical heart valves		Measure INR at 5–7 d and adjust to INR of 3–4.5
	Total hip replacement or hip fracture surgery*	5 mg daily for patients <110 lb, >age 75, or at increased risk of bleeding: 2.5 mg daily	Measure INR at 5–7 d and adjust to INR of 2–3

*Doses reduced for severe renal impairment (Ccr <30 mL/min). Only outpatient indications are covered.

†Recommendation of American College of Chest Physicians. The ACCP also states that low-molecular-weight heparin may be used for hip fracture surgery, ischemic stroke with paralysis of lower extremities, and medical patients with clinical risk factors. Specific doses are not given for these indications, but fixed dose bid started postoperatively is recommended for surgical patients.

Prevention of Embolic Stroke in Atrial Fibrillation

Both **warfarin** and **aspirin** are effective for prevention of embolism in patients with nonvalvular atrial fibrillation (AF). **Warfarin** is more effective than **aspirin**, but is associated with a higher rate of bleeding (Hirsh et al, 2008) and requires monitoring that makes it more expensive. The ACCP (Hirsh et al, 2008) has given parameters to determine when to use each drug. For patients with persistent or paroxysmal AF at high risk for stroke, the recommendation is **warfarin** with a target INR between 2 and 3. High-risk patients are those with one of the following:

- Prior ischemic stroke, transient ischemic attack (TIA), or systemic embolism
- Age greater than 75 years
- Moderately or severely impaired left ventricular systolic function and/or congestive heart failure
- History of HTN
- History of diabetes mellitus

For patients with persistent AF, age 65 to 75 years, in the absence of other risk factors, antithrombotic therapy with either **warfarin** with the same INR target or **aspirin** 325 mg/day, are acceptable alternatives. In patients with persistent AF under age 65 and with no other risk factors, **aspirin** 75 to 325 mg/day is recommended. For patients with AF and mitral stenosis, the recommendations follow those for patients at high risk. If the valvular heart disease has resulted in valve replacement, the recommendations follow those for patients with heart valves, regardless of the presence or absence of AF.

For patients with mitral valve prolapse but no AF, TIAs, or ischemic stroke, the ACCP recommends against antithrombotic therapy (Hirsh et al, 2008). In patients with mitral valve prolapse with documented TIAs and ischemic stroke, the treatment is **antiplatelet** therapy, with **aspirin** 50 to 100 mg daily (Hirsh et al, 2008). If a patient continues to have TIAs or recurrent embolism while on **aspirin** therapy, **warfarin** with a target INR of 2 to 3 is recommended. Therapy is continued indefinitely in all these cases.

The ACCP guidelines are supported by the American Heart Association and American College of Cardiology Foundation (Hirsh et al, 2008). The American Academy of Family Physicians (AAFP) and the American College of Physicians (ACP) stress the importance of rate control with the chronic anticoagulation for the majority of patients (McNamara, Tamariz, Segal, & Bass, 2003; Snow et al, 2003). They recommend **atenolol, metoprolol, diltiazem,** or **verapamil** as the best drugs for rate control in this situation. **Digoxin** could be used as a second-line agent. These drugs are discussed in Chapter 16. The AAFP and ACP concur with the anticoagulation recommendations discussed previously, and suggest that most patients converted to sinus rhythm from AF should not be placed on rhythm maintenance therapy.

Cerebral ischemic event prevention in patients with noncardioembolic stroke or TIAs has a different set of recommendations. ACCP recommends three options for preventive therapy: **aspirin** 50 to 100 mg daily, the combination of **aspirin** (25 mg) and extended-release **dipyridamole** (200 mg bid), and **clopidogrel** 75 mg daily as acceptable options for therapy (Hirsh et al, 2008). For patients with moderate to high risk of bleeding, low doses of **aspirin** (50 to 100 mg daily) are recommended. Because **clopidogrel** is significantly more expensive than **aspirin,** it should be reserved for patients who cannot take **aspirin** for a variety of reasons.

Recurrent Embolism or Prosthetic Heart Valves

Warfarin is the drug of choice for patients with recurrent embolism or prosthetic heart valve. Therapy is initiated and maintained the same as for prevention of venous thrombosis, except that the target INR depends on the type of valve. The targets are shown in Table 18–4. Of note, patients who have mechanical valves and additional risk factors such as AF, myocardial infarction (MI), left atrial enlargement, endocardial damage, and low ejection fraction, 75 to 100 mg/day of **aspirin** should be added to their **warfarin** protocol. The same is true for patients with caged ball or caged disc valves. Long-term management of patients with bioprosthetic valves who are in sinus rhythm may be managed on 75 to 100 mg/day of **aspirin** alone (Hirsh et al, 2008). Therapy is continued indefinitely for mechanical heart valves. For systemic embolization that recurs after 6 months of therapy, therapy is usually continued for an additional 12 months.

The European Society of Cardiology recommends higher target INR (3.0 to 4.5) for mechanical prosthetic heart valves, with second generation valves being slightly lower at 2.5 to 3.0; however, the American Heart Association and the American College of Cardiology Foundation have recommendations consistent with ACCP guidelines (Hirsh et al, 2008).

Warfarin is contraindicated in pregnancy, and pregnant patients with prosthetic valves require management with **heparin** (ICSI, 2010). Of note, one study showed that two pregnant patients with mechanical heart valves had thrombotic complications when treated with **LMWH.** Because of this, the FDA and manufacturer have warned that **enoxaparin** is not indicated for prophylaxis for heart valve patients who are pregnant. Despite the ACCP presenting guidelines for the use of thrombotic agents during pregnancy, in general, pregnant patients with prosthetic heart valves should be managed by an anticoagulation specialist and perinatologist (Bates et al, 2008).

Table 18–4 **Recommended INR Values Based on Reason for Warfarin Use**

Reason for Use	INR range
Prevention of DVT, pulmonary embolism, or systemic embolism	2.0–3.0
Prevention of embolic stroke in patients with atrial fibrillation	2.0–3.0
Patients with St. Jude Medical bileaflet prosthetic heart valve	2.0–3.0
Patients with tilting disk valves and bileaflet prosthetic heart valves in aortic position	2.5–3.5
Patients with CarboMedics bileaflet valve or Medtronic Hall tilting disk prosthetic heart valve	2.0–3.0
Patients with mechanical valves and high risk (e.g., atrial thrombus, AF, hypercoagulable state, low ejection fraction)*	2.5–3.5
Patients with caged ball or caged disk prosthetic heart valves*	2.5–3.5
Patients with bioprosthetic valve in mitral position	2.0–3.0
Patients with bioprosthetic valve in aortic position	2.0–3.0

*In addition to **warfarin,** these patients should also receive **aspirin** 75–100 mg/d.

Prevention of Myocardial Infarction

Results of clinical trials have shown that several protocols are effective in prevention of MI in patients with chronic coronary artery disease. The ACCP presents a number of options for treatment in its guidelines (Hirsh et al, 2008). Patients with acute coronary syndrome with or without ST-segment elevation are treated with **aspirin** 75 to 162 mg daily initially, then long term at 75 to 100 mg daily. In patients who cannot tolerate **aspirin, clopidogrel** monotherapy at 75 mg/day is acceptable. Patients with symptomatic coronary artery disease may be treated with a combination of **aspirin** (75 to 100 mg/day) and **clopidogrel** (75 mg/day).

Patients who have already experienced an acute MI (AMI) also need to be maintained on anti-clot therapy. Patients who have AMI with ST-segment elevation (STEMI) are often treated acutely with **fibrinolytics,** then with ongoing therapy after hospital discharge. A number of options are available for post-AMI treatment. Patients with ST-elevation acute coronary syndrome are started on a loading dose of **clopidogrel** 300 mg for patients younger than 75 years of age and 75 mg for those older than 75 years, then maintained on 75 mg per day for 2 to 4 weeks. The ACCP recommends **clopidogrel** 75 mg daily for 12 months after hospital discharge (Hirsh et al, 2008). For patients who have access to an anticoagulant center that can closely monitor their therapy, the ACCP suggests high-intensity **warfarin** (INR 3–4) for up to 4 years (Hirsh et al, 2008). Another option is combining **aspirin** (75 to 100 mg/day) and moderate-intensity **warfarin** (INR 2 to 3) (Hirsh et al, 2008). Patients who have percutaneous coronary intervention are treated long term with **aspirin** 75 to 100 mg per day. Patients who have a bare metal stent placed are treated long term with a combination of **aspirin** (75 to 100 mg/d) and **clopidogrel** (Hirsh et al, 2008). For patients with congestive heart failure who do not have an ischemic etiology, neither **aspirin** nor **warfarin** is recommended by the ACCP (Hirsh et al, 2008).

The ACCP recommends patients with a moderate risk for a coronary event take a daily dose of **aspirin** (75 to 100 mg/d). Patients with a high risk of coronary event may be maintained on low-dose **warfarin** to a target INR of 1.5, and if INR can be easily monitored, the ACCP recommends the low-dose **warfarin** over **aspirin** (Hirsh et al, 2008). Patients with **aspirin** allergy and a moderate to high risk of cardiovascular event can be maintained on **clopidogrel.**

The appropriate dose of medication for prevention of cardiovascular disease in diabetic patients is not yet clearly determined by evidence. The increased prevalence of cardiovascular morbidity and mortality and disturbances in coagulation in diabetes patients leads to a recommendation of **aspirin** 75 to 162 mg/day by the American Heart Association (2010). **Aspirin's** possible role in **insulin** resistance (see On the Horizon: Aspirin) may also play a role in determining dose.

On The Horizon

ON THE HORIZON

Aspirin

Aspirin has a unique role in insulin resistance. Recent studies have implicated activation of the serine kinase IKK-beta, which plays a key role in inflammation, in the pathogenesis of insulin resistance. Chronic **aspirin** administration reverses glucose intolerance in rats (Renna, Vazquez, Lama, Gonzalez, & Maitello, 2009). High-dose **aspirin** short-term treatment in humans not only resulted in a reduction in fasting plasma glucose but also was associated with a 15 percent reduction in total cholesterol and C-reactive protein, a 50 percent reduction in triglycerides, and a 30 percent reduction in insulin clearance despite no change in body weight (Hundal et al, 2002). Chronic **aspirin** therapy in rats (equal to low dose for 6 weeks) partially reversed increased systolic blood pressure and the remodeling of renal and carotid arteries (Renna et al, 2009). This may provide a new target not only for treatment of type 2 diabetes but also for the formation of atherosclerosis, a prime culprit in thrombus generation.

Prevention of Postoperative Thromboembolism

All hospitals are required by the Joint Commission to have a formal, active strategy to prevent venous thrombosis. The ACCP recommends the use of **LMWH**, low-dose **heparin**, or **fondaparinux** as thromboprophylaxis in the following surgical procedures: moderate-risk major general surgery, higher risk patients who are having a major procedure for cancer, major vascular surgery, major gynecological surgery, major urological procedures, bariatric surgery, thoracic surgery, and many orthopedic surgeries (Hirsh et al, 2008). The length of treatment is determined by the type of surgery, ranging from a single dose with minor procedures to 10 days for most orthopedic procedures, to 28 days in high-risk patients, patients undergoing major gynecological surgery, and patients having major surgery for cancer (Hirsh et al, 2008).

Perioperative Therapy of Patients on Warfarin or Antiplatelet Therapy

Patients on **warfarin** therapy for prevention of thromboembolism who need an invasive procedure may require parenteral anticoagulation perioperatively. The decision to take a patient off **warfarin** and "bridge" with **heparin** is determined by balancing bleeding risk due to the surgical procedure and clotting risk due to the underlying disorder (ICSI, 2010). Patients who have procedures with a low bleeding risk (for example, skin biopsies, cataract eye surgery, and most dental procedures) can remain on **warfarin.** If a patient is at low thromboembolic risk (for example, atrial fibrillation without prior stroke or remote history of venous thrombosis), **warfarin** may be stopped 4 to 5 days prior to surgery and resumed the evening of surgery. If the patient is at high thromboembolic risk (for example, prosthetic heart valves), bridging with a therapeutic dose of **LMWH** or unfractionated **heparin** may be indicated (Hirsh et al, 2008).

In the hospital, patients can be placed on IV **heparin** that can be discontinued 3 hours before surgery, or the SC route can be continued and stopped 12 hours before surgery. Another approach is to continue **warfarin** but keep INR around 1.5 during the surgical procedure. This level has been shown to be safe in selected surgeries (Hirsh et al, 2008). In each case, **warfarin** therapy is restarted 12 to 24 hours postoperatively. For patients undergoing dental procedures, tranexamic acid mouthwash can be used without interrupting **anticoagulant** therapy. Because bridging therapy can be very complex, consultation with a hematologist or anticoagulation expert is suggested. ICSI (2010, p. 44) has a detailed table with a recommended bridging schedule.

The ACCP recommends that **antiplatelets** be discontinued before surgery (Hirsch et al, 2008). **Aspirin** should be stopped 7 to 10 days prior to surgery; **clopidogrel** should be stopped 7 days ahead; **ibuprofen** should be stopped 2 days ahead. Increased blood loss has occurred with patients on these drugs at the time of surgery. The drugs may be restarted 24 hours postoperatively.

Rational Drug Selection

Cost

Although SC administration of an **anticoagulant** (**heparin**) is usually a short-term measure, cost is still a significant factor. The difference in cost between **heparin** and the newer **LMWHs** is significant; the newer drugs are much more expensive. **Enoxaparin (Lovenox)** is $256.46 for ten 30-mg syringes and **fondaparinux (Arixtra)** is $593.04 for ten 2.5-mg syringes, whereas **heparin** is $29.99 for a 5-mL vial of 10,000 unit/mL solution, a 10-day supply at 5,000 units per dose (http://www.drugstore.com). When the cost of laboratory monitoring is factored into the equation, the difference in cost between the LMWHs and regular **heparin** is less dramatic. Of all the drugs used to prevent clotting, **aspirin** is by far the cheapest.

Routes of Administration

Oral anticoagulation is preferred because it does not require specialized equipment or skills to administer, and it is less expensive. For patients who cannot swallow or for other reasons cannot take an oral **anticoagulant**, SC injections of **heparin** in either standard or low-molecular-weight formulation can be used. Patients or their family members must be taught correct techniques for SC administration (Table 18–5).

Table 18–5 ◆ **Available Dosage Forms: Anticoagulants and Antiplatelets**

Drug	Dosage Form (Tablets/Capsules)	Other Forms	Cost
Aspirin	81-mg chewable (orange flavor)	–	
	165-mg enteric-coated		
	325-mg tablets		
	Also in film coated and caplets		
Clopidogrel (Plavix)	75-mg tablets (in 30, 90, and 500 tablets/bottle and 100-unit dose	–	$342/90 tabs.
Dalteparin (Fragmin)	–	2,500 U/0.2 mL; 5,000 U/0.2 mL; 7,500 U/0.3 mL; 10,000 U/mL. All doses are provided in single-dose prefilled syringe with 27 g × 0.5-in. needle 10,000 U/mL and 25,000 U/mL in multidose vials	No data
Enoxaparin (Lovenox)	–	30 mg/0.3 mL; 40 mg/0.4 mL; 60 mg/ 0.6 mL; 80 mg/0.8 mL; 100 mg/mL; 120 mg/0.8 mL; 150 mg/mL. All doses are provided in a single-dose prefilled syringe with 27 g × 0.5-in. needle. 300 mg/3 mL in multidose vial	30 mg = $183 40 mg = $244 60 mg = $367 80 mg = $489 100 mg = $612 Multidose vial = $174
Fondaparinux (Arixtra)	–	2.5 mg in 0.5-mL single-dose prefilled syringe with needle.	$594.04/10 single dose syringes
Heparin sodium	–	In multidose vials: 1,000 U/mL (1-, 10-, 30-mL vials) 2,000 U/mL (5-, 10-mL vials) 2,500 U/mL (5-, 10-mL vials) 5,000 U/mL (1-, 10-mL vials) 10,000 U/mL (0.5-, 1-, 4-, 5-, 10-mL vials) 20,000 U/mL (1-, 2-, 4-mL vials) 40,000 U/mL (1-, 2-, 5-mL vials)	10,000U/mL-5mL vial = $29.99
Ticlopidine (Ticlid)	250-mg tablets (In 30, 60, 100, 500, and 1,000 tablets/bottle)	–	$35/100 tabs
Tinzaparin (Innohep)		20,000 U/mL in 2-mL multidose vials	No data

Continued

Table 18–5 ◆ **Available Dosage Forms: Anticoagulants and Antiplatelets—cont'd**

Drug	Dosage Form (Tablets/Capsules)	Other Forms	Cost
Warfarin (Coumadin)	Scored tablets: 1-mg pink 2-mg lavender 2.5-mg green 3-mg tan 4-mg blue 5-mg peach 6-mg teal 7.5-mg yellow 10-mg white (In 100 and 1,000 tablets/bottle)	–	1 mg = \$27.00/100 2 mg = \$26.00/100 2.5 mg = \$28/100 3 mg = \$29/100 4 mg = \$27/100 5 mg = \$26/100 6 mg = \$33/100 7.5 mg = \$33/100 10 mg = \$33/100

Brand

Anticoagulant effects may vary slightly by brand. Because even small variances can cause significant differences in anticoagulation, brands should not be interchanged. **Warfarin** comes in a variety of tablet strengths, making it possible to be exact in dosing, and it is the preferred oral **anticoagulant**. The tablets are color coded by dose, which also makes it easier to be certain the patient takes the correct dose, especially if the dose is prescribed over the telephone. **LMWHs** are not interchangeable. There is only one brand name for each, but the patient cannot be changed from one drug to another, as their actions and indications vary. The same is true for the **antiplatelets**.

Monitoring

Monitoring for dosage adjustments of **warfarin** is by INR blood tests. Daily INRs are done initially to guard against excessive anticoagulation in unusually sensitive patients and are continued until the therapeutic range is achieved and maintained for at least 2 consecutive days. The testing interval is then lengthened to two or three times weekly for 1 or 2 weeks, then less often, depending on the stability of the INR results. If the INR results remain stable, testing is reduced to as seldom as every 6 weeks. Drawing the blood in the morning with the patient taking the drug in the evening provides more stable results and allows rapid dosage changes if necessary.

Point-of-care patient self-testing is now possible with a variety of machines. The feasibility and accuracy of patient self-testing at home has been evaluated in several small studies with promising results. Such self-testing with associated self-management provides increased freedom for the patient, especially if they travel. Hirsh, Fuster, Ansell, and Halperin (2003) discuss this option, including evaluations of various machines. They find that self-testing and self-management of anticoagulation therapy offer limited advantages. The outcomes of self-management versus clinic management in several studies were essentially the same (Hirsh et al, 2003; Menendez-Jandula et al, 2005).

Protocols for dosage adjustments vary, but to maximize safety and avoid wide swings in anticoagulation, 10 percent changes in weekly doses are best unless the INR is widely out of range. If the INR is too low, the total weekly dose is adjusted upward by 10 percent and the INR is rechecked in 2 weeks. If the INR is too high, the daily dose is held for 1 day and then the weekly dose is adjusted downward by 10 percent and the INR is rechecked in 2 weeks. If the INR is above therapeutic range but less than 5, the patient is not bleeding, and rapid reversal is not indicated for surgical intervention, then one dose can be omitted and daily INRs are drawn. **Warfarin** is then resumed at a lower dose when the INR is within therapeutic range. If the INR is greater than 5 but less than 9 and the patient is not bleeding, then two doses can be omitted and **warfarin** reinstated at a lower dose when the INR falls into the therapeutic range or the next dose may be omitted and **vitamin K** (1 to 2 mg) can be given orally. When more rapid reversal is required, **vitamin K** 2 to 5 mg orally can be given, anticipating the INR will return to a 2 to 3 range within 24 hours. When INR results are greater than 9 but with no serious bleeding, then **vitamin K** 3 to 5 mg may be given orally, anticipating that the INR will fall within 24 to 48 hours. For serious bleeding, **vitamin K** should be given by slow IV infusion in a dose of 10 mg, supplemented with transfusion of fresh plasma according to the urgency of the situation, and referral is suggested (Hirsh et al, 2003). If the INR has frequent variability, external reasons such as dietary changes, undisclosed drug use, poor adherence, and intermittent **alcohol** consumption are evaluated, and the INR is drawn daily or weekly until a stable INR is reached. Once a stable dose is reached, monitoring may be done every 3 months.

Computer-assisted **warfarin** dose regulation has been shown to be more effective than traditional dosing at maintaining therapeutic INR values (Hirsch et al, 2003). This is especially true when personnel are inexperienced. Many health systems have anticoagulant clinics that manage patients on anticoagulant therapy, leading to optimal outcomes for the patient.

Monitoring for dosage adjustment of **heparin** is by aPTT blood tests. The goal of therapy is 1.5 to 2.5 times the control. Platelet counts and hematocrit (Hct) are done every 2 or 3 days initially. Thrombocytopenia tends to occur about the fourth day and resolves despite continued **heparin** therapy. Thrombocytopenia severe enough to require discontinuing therapy may occur about the eighth day of therapy. After this time, periodic testing of platelet and Hct levels and testing for occult blood in the stool are done during the course of **heparin** therapy regardless of the route of administration. Low doses of SC **heparin** (5,000 U bid) do not require monitoring because this regimen does not prolong the aPTT.

For the **LMWHs**, the same periodic monitoring of platelet and Hct levels is required, but the likelihood of thrombocytopenia is much less. The recommended test for monitoring these drugs is anti-factor Xa assay. A standard curve is constructed for each different **LMWH** preparation. Although the aPTT may be prolonged in patients on **LMWH**, it does not reliably reflect their activity. In general, routine monitoring of factor Xa is not recommended, except in pregnant patients.

The dose of **aspirin** for **antiplatelet** therapy is low to moderate. The serum salicylate level is approximately 100 mcg/mL. At low doses, no specific monitoring is required, although **aspirin** will prolong bleeding time. **Clopidogrel** has a safety profile similar to that of **aspirin** and no routine monitoring is required.

Severe neutropenia and thrombocytopenia have occurred with the administration of **ticlopidine.** The onset of these problems occurred 3 weeks to 3 months after the start of therapy, with no documented cases beyond that time. It is essential that complete blood counts (CBCs) and white blood cell (WBC) differential counts be performed every 2 weeks, starting from the second week to the end of the third month of therapy. More frequent monitoring is necessary for patients whose absolute neutrophil counts consistently decline or are 30 percent lower than baseline counts. After the first 3 months of therapy, CBCs are needed only for patients with signs or symptoms suggesting an infection (*Drug Facts and Comparisons,* 2005).

Patient Education: Anticoagulants

Administration

Anticoagulants should be taken exactly as prescribed, at the same time each day, even if the patient is feeling well. Missed doses should be taken as soon as remembered the same day. Doses should not be doubled. The health-care provider should be informed of missed doses at the time of checkup or laboratory tests. Doses are highly individualized and are determined by the results of laboratory tests (INR for **oral anticoagulants** and aPTT, platelet counts, and Hct for **heparin** and anti-factor Xa assays for **LMWHs**). Patients should not change the dose unless directed to do so by the health-care provider and should have the laboratory tests drawn each time they are ordered.

Differences in anticoagulation effect can occur between brands. The drug is prescribed by brand name and should be consistently filled that way. **Warfarin** tablets are color coded by dose, and patients should learn the color code for the brand used. For the **heparins**, which are injectable, the patient or a family member must be taught correct SC injection technique.

Oral **anticoagulants** may be taken without regard to timing of food intake. The type of food, however, is important. Ingestion of large quantities of foods high in **vitamin K** may antagonize the **anticoagulant** effect. This does not mean that these foods must be avoided entirely. They are part of a well-balanced diet. They should be eaten in consistent amounts so that anticoagulation levels can be maintained at a consistent level. Patients should be given written information regarding **vitamin K** content of common foods. The U.S. Department of Agriculture (USDA) has an extensive handout on **vitamin K** content in many common foods available on the Internet (http://www.nal.usda.gov/fnic/foodcomp/Data/SR17/wtrank/sr17w430.pdf). Some patients may need a nutrition consultation to manage their diet. Drug interactions may also occur with some over-the-counter (OTC) drugs, particularly **aspirin, NSAIDs,** and cold remedies that contain these products, and with **alcohol.** Many drugs are also prepared in an **alcohol** base. Some **multivitamins** contain **vitamin K** and should not be taken. The patient should consult with the primary care provider or pharmacist before taking any OTC medications or new prescription medications.

Some natural products, including some used as spices in cooking, have interactions with **LMWHs** and **clopidogrel** (see Table 18–2). Patients should be taught to avoid use of these products or to use them in consistent amounts. They should also inform their health-care provider if they use them, as it may affect monitoring test results.

Clopidogrel should not be taken with **proton pump inhibitors (PPI)** such as OTC **omeprazole (Prilosec** OTC), as the **PPI** decreases the effectiveness of the **clopidogrel.**

Adverse Reactions

Unusual bleeding is the most common adverse effect for all **anticoagulants.** To prevent bleeding, the patient should use a soft toothbrush, avoid flossing, shave with an electric razor, and if cut, apply pressure for 5 to 10 minutes. If the bleeding does not stop, the patient should continue the pressure and contact the health-care provider. Whenever possible, IM injections should be avoided. If they must be given, apply pressure to the injection site for 2 to 5 minutes to prevent bleeding or hematoma formation. Applying ice to the site of an SC injection for about 30 seconds prior to injecting the heparin reduces the chances of bleeding and hematoma formation. The following should be reported to the health-care provider:

1. Any bleeding that does not stop within 5 minutes
2. Nosebleeds and bleeding gums
3. Red- or pink-tinged urine
4. Faintness or weakness
5. Headaches
6. Stomach pains
7. Skin rash or unusual bruising
8. Red, black, or tarry stools or diarrhea

Dermal necrosis occurs in a small percentage (0.01% to 0.1%) of patients taking **warfarin** and occurs on the third to eighth day of therapy. Skin necrosis is associated with protein C or protein S deficiency. Purple toe syndrome results from peripheral emboli that occur 3 to 10 weeks after therapy is started. Necrotic skin lesions and cyanotic or purple-appearing toes should be reported and **warfarin** stopped (ICSI, 2010).

Warfarin is contraindicated in pregnancy. Women who are capable of becoming pregnant should have this topic discussed with them, and contraception should be instituted before prescribing this drug.

To reduce the risk of adverse reactions, the patient should wear an identification bracelet that states the **anticoagulant** being taken. Inform all health-care providers about the anticoagulation therapy so that new prescriptions and any treatments can take it into account. The patient should consult the health-care provider before undergoing dental work or elective surgery.

Patient Education: Antiplatelets

Administration

Daily dosing is the usual way **aspirin** is taken for **antiplatelet** effects. Taking it with a full glass of water reduces the risk of lodging the drug in the esophagus. Because **aspirin** may cause GI upset, it should be taken with food or after meals. Enteric-coated forms are available but have slightly less reliable amounts of drug reaching the bloodstream. Enteric-coated tablets may not be crushed or chewed. For patients with difficulty in swallowing, liquid forms are available. **Aspirin** that has a strong vinegar-like odor should not be used.

Ticlopidine may also cause GI upset and ought to be taken with a full glass of water and with food or after meals.

Adverse Reactions

Toxicity to **aspirin** may occur even with small doses in some patients, who should immediately report to the health-care provider ringing in the ears (tinnitus), unusual headache, hyperventilation, agitation, mental confusion, lethargy, diarrhea, or sweating.

For **ticlopidine**, a decrease in the number of WBCs can occur, especially during the first 3 months of therapy. A severe decrease can increase risk for infection. Patients should obtain scheduled blood tests to detect reduced WBCs. Report to the health-care provider any indications of infection such as fever, chills, or sore throat. **Ticlopidine** can also affect liver function. Patients should promptly report severe or persistent diarrhea, skin rashes, yellow skin or sclerae, dark urine, or light-colored stools.

For both drugs and for **clopidogrel**, unusual bleeding is the most common adverse effect. To prevent bleeding, the patient should use a soft toothbrush, avoid flossing, shave with an electric razor, and if cut, apply pressure for 5 to 10 minutes. They should also inform health-care providers, including dentists, that they are taking these drugs before any surgery or procedure is scheduled or any new drug is prescribed.

HEMATOPOIETIC GROWTH FACTORS

Hematopoietic growth factors are glycoprotein hormones that regulate the proliferation and differentiation of hematopoietic progenitor cells in bone marrow. Produced by recombinant DNA technology, these factors include **erythropoietin, granulocyte colony–stimulating factor (G-CSF), granulocyte-macrophage colony–stimulating factor (GM-CSF)**, and **thrombopoietic growth factor**. Anemias due to deficiency in erythropoietin, such as those found in patients with end-stage renal disease or AIDS or patients undergoing chemotherapy; infections associated with myelosuppressive chemotherapy, myeloid cancers, and AIDS; and thrombocytopenia associated with all of these are among the most refractory to treatment. The introduction of these growth factors has made effective treatment possible. **Erythropoietin** is indicated for anemic patients (hemoglobin > 10 to ≤ 13 g/dL) with normal erythropoietin levels who wish to donate their own blood before high risk elective, noncardiac, nonvascular surgery for allogenic transfusions. **Granulocyte colony–stimulating factor** is used for neutropenic patients, particularly those with neutropenia caused by bone marrow transplant and some blood cancers (Brender, 2006).

Pharmacodynamics

Stem cells in the hematopoietic bone marrow respond to various colony-stimulating factors; megakaryocyte stimulators; and erythropoietin to produce mature WBCs, platelets, and erythrocytes. Erythrocyte differentiation proceeds from erythroblasts through normoblasts to reticulocytes and finally to mature erythrocytes, based on stimulation from erythropoietin, with additional support from GM-CSF and interleukin-3 (IL-3). Granulocytes (neutrophils, eosinophils, and basophils/mast cells) are fully matured in the bone marrow by stimulation from G-CSF, GM-CSF, and IL-3. The agranulocytes (monocytes and lymphocytes) are produced by the stimulation from GM-CSF, IL-3, and macrophage colony–stimulating factor (M-CSF) and are released into the bloodstream before they mature. Monocytes become mature macrophages within 1 or 2 days, and lymphocytes travel to the lymphoid tissues, where they are stimulated to differentiate into T cells or B cells. Platelets develop from megakaryocytes by a unique process of proliferations termed endomitosis. In this process, the megakaryocyte undergoes the nuclear phase of cellular division, but fails to undergo the cytoplasmic phase. Without cytokinesis, the cell does not divide into two daughter cells. Rather, the megakaryocyte expands to accommodate the doubling of its DNA content and breaks up into platelets. Optimal numbers of platelets and their precursors in the bone marrow is maintained by the actions of thrombopoietin, GM-CSF and IL-11 (McCance & Huether, 2010). The development of these blood cells is shown in Figure 18–2 with the controlling factor indicated.

Endogenous erythropoietin is produced by the normal kidney in response to tissue hypoxia. In anemia, more erythropoietin is produced, signaling the bone marrow to produce more erythrocytes. Unless a patient has an **iron** deficiency, a primary bone marrow disorder, or bone marrow suppression from drugs and chronic disease, this stimulation of erythrocyte production corrects the anemia. In addition to **iron**, erythropoiesis is dependent on sufficient amounts of **vitamin B_{12}** and **folic acid.** In end-stage renal disease, the kidney is unable to produce the erythropoietin necessary for the stimulation of erythrocyte growth. **Epoetin alfa (Epogen, Procrit)** and **darbepoetin alfa (Aranesp)** have the same biological effects as erythropoietin. Endogenous colony-stimulating factors respond to decreased leukocyte counts or the presence of infection to signal the production of leukocytes. G-CSF is lineage specific, supporting the proliferation and differentiation of neutrophils. GM-CSF is multipotential, stimulating proliferation and differentiation of early and late granulocyte progenitor cells, as well as erythroid and megakaryocyte progenitors. **Filgrastim (Neupogen)** and **pegfilgrastim (Neulasta)** have the same biological effects as G-CSF. **Sargramostim (Leukine)** has the same biological effect as GM-CSF.

Low platelet mass activates thrombopoietin (TPO), a human growth factor, increasing the number of megakaryocytes. IL-11 is a thrombopoietic growth factor that directly stimulates the maturation of megakaryocytes. The biological effects of **oprelvekin (Neumega)** are the same as those of thrombopoietin and IL-11.

Pharmacokinetics

Absorption and Distribution

All **hematopoietic growth factors** are well absorbed following SC injection. Some can be given IV. Their distribution is similar to that of their endogenous equivalents (Table 18–6).

Metabolism and Excretion

Darbepoetin alfa has a circulating half-life of about 49 hours post–SC injection. Following IV administration, the serum concentration is biphasic, with a distribution half-life of 1.4 hours and a mean terminal half-life of 21 hours. **Epoetin alfa** has a circulating half-life of 4 to 13 hours in patients with chronic renal failure (CRF). There is no apparent difference in half-life for patients on or not on dialysis. The half-life is about 20 percent shorter in healthy patients. **Filgrastim** has an elimination half-life of 3.5 hours in healthy patients and those with cancer. **Oprelvekin** has a half-life of 6.9 hours. **Pegfilgrastim** has a half-life of 15 to 80 hours. **Sargramostim** has a half-life after SC injection of 2.6 hours. All are eliminated by first-order kinetics. The exact method of metabolism and excretion is unknown in most these drugs, with some elimination thought to occur in the kidneys.

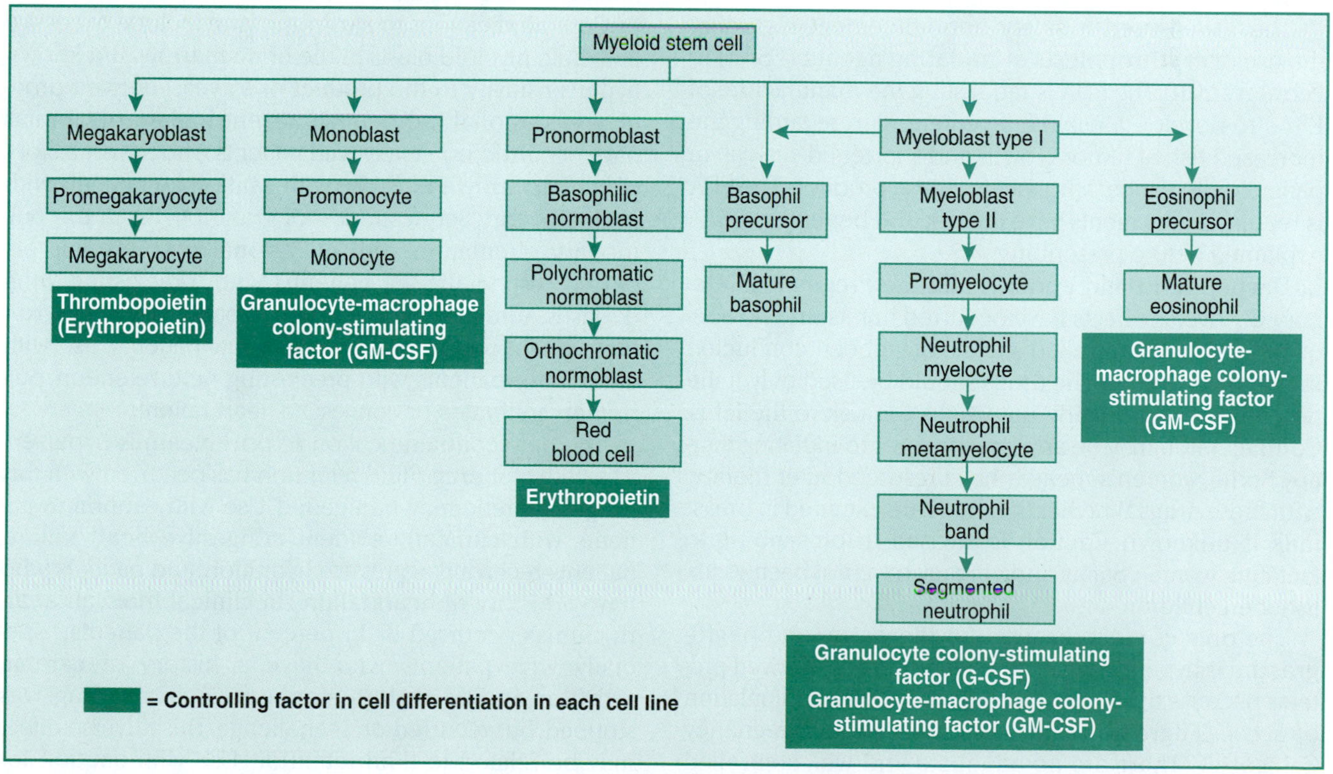

Figure 18–2. Development of blood cells.

Table 18–6 ▶ **Pharmacokinetics: Hematopoietic Growth Factors**

Drug	Onset	Peak	Duration	Half-life
Darbepoetin	2–6 wk (increase in reticulocytes)	34–90 h	UK	49 h (SC); 21 h (IV)
Epoetin alfa	7–10 d (increase in reticulocytes)	5–24 h	>24 h	4–13 h in chronic renal failure (about 20% shorter in healthy patients)
Filgrastim	–	2–8 h	–	3.5 h
Oprelvekin	5–9 d (increase in platelets)	3.2 h	7–14 d	6.9 h
Pegfilgrastim	–	2–8 h	–	15–80 h (SC)
Sargramostim	–	1–3 h	12 h	1.6–2.6 h

*Increase in reticulocytes.

Pharmacotherapeutics

Precautions and Contraindications

The only contraindication for **darbepoetin alfa** and **epoetin alfa** is uncontrolled HTN; increases in erythrocyte production may also be accompanied by increases in extracellular fluid (ECF) volume, which can increase blood pressure. Up to 80 percent of patients with CRF have HTN, which should be controlled before a patient starts therapy with these drugs and carefully monitored during such therapy. During early phases of therapy, when the Hct is increasing, about 25 percent of patients with CRF require initiation of or increases in **antihypertensive** therapy.

The FDA issued a safety announcement regarding the use of **erythropoiesis-stimulating agents (ESAs)** in February 2010. The FDA is requesting the manufacture of ESAs to develop a risk management plan regarding the increased risk of tumor growth and shortened survival in patients with cancer who receive these products. The FDA is requiring all patients have the risk and benefits of ESAs explained before prescribing.

Darbepoetin and **epoetin alfa** are Pregnancy Category C. Adverse effects have occurred in rats, and no adequate and well-controlled studies have been conducted in pregnant women. The drugs should be used only if the potential benefit clearly outweighs the risk to the fetus. Contraception may be appropriate prior to initiating therapy. Some women's menses have resumed after therapy with these drugs. Whether the drugs are excreted in breast milk is unknown. Caution is advised in prescribing to lactating women. Safety and efficacy have not been established in children.

The only contraindication for **filgrastim** and **pegfilgrastim** is hypersensitivity to *Escherichia coli*–derived proteins because this drug is derived from DNA manipulation of *E. coli*. **Filgrastim** and **pegfilgrastim** are Pregnancy Category C. There are no adequate and well-controlled studies in pregnant women. Adverse effects have been shown in pregnant animal studies. These drugs should be used only if the potential benefit clearly outweighs the risk to the fetus. Contraception may be appropriate prior to initiating therapy. Whether these drugs are excreted in breast milk is unknown. Caution is advised in prescribing to lactating women.

Serious long-term risks associated with daily **filgrastim** have not been identified in children aged 4 months to 17 years with severe chronic neutropenia. The safety and efficacy in neonates and patients with autoimmune neutropenia have not been established. Safety and efficacy have not been established in children for **pegfilgrastim.** Do not use the 6-mg fixed-dose syringe formulation in infants, children, and adolescents weighing less than 45 kg.

Contraindications to **sargramostim** include excessive leukemic myeloid blasts in the bone marrow and known hypersensitivity to the product or to yeast-derived products. Occasional transient supraventricular arrhythmias have occurred, especially with patients who have a history of cardiac arrhythmias. Use with caution for patients with such a history. Sequestration of granulocytes in the pulmonary circulation with occasional dyspnea has occurred, especially in patients with preexisting lung diseases. Administer with caution to patients with hypoxia. Fluid retention has occurred in a few patients. Use with caution for patients with preexisting fluid retention, pulmonary infiltrates, or congestive heart failure.

The only contraindication to **oprelvekin** is hypersensitivity to that drug. Fluid retention has occurred with this drug. A diuretic may be needed. Use with caution in patients with clinically evident congestive heart failure, patients receiving aggressive hydration, and patients who have a history of heart failure. In clinical trials, atrial arrhythmias occurred in 15 percent of the patients, especially with patients who have a history of cardiac arrhythmias. The rhythm stopped when the drug was stopped, but recurred on rechallenge. This adverse effect may be related to fluid retention. Use with caution for patients with such a history.

Oprelvekin is Pregnancy Category C. Adverse effects were noted in animal studies and there are no adequate, well-controlled studies in pregnant women. Use only if the potential benefit clearly outweighs the risk to the fetus. Contraception may be appropriate prior to initiating therapy. It is not known whether this drug is excreted in breast milk. Caution is advised in prescribing to lactating women.

There are no controlled trials that have established a safe and effective dose of **oprelvekin** in children. The administration of this drug to children, particularly under age 12, should be reserved for clinical trials with closely monitored safety assessments. Limited data are available from one clinical trial for pediatric patients receiving 50 mcg/kg per day. Adverse effects in this study were the same as for adults. No studies have been done to assess the long-term effects of its use on growth and development. Animal studies have shown bone and joint changes.

Sargramostim is Pregnancy Category C. There are no adequate and well-controlled studies in pregnant women. This drug should be used only if the potential benefit clearly outweighs the risk to the fetus. Contraception may be appropriate prior to initiating therapy. Whether this drug is excreted in breast milk is unknown. Caution is advised in prescribing to lactating women. Safety and efficacy in children have not been established.

Adverse Drug Reactions

Seizures have been observed in some patients being treated with **darbepoetin alfa** and **epoetin alfa** (2.5% of patients undergoing dialysis during the first 90 days of therapy). The relationship with seizure is uncertain, and the risk appears to lessen when the rate of increase in Hct is slower. Recommendations are that the dose be decreased if the hemoglobin (Hgb) increase exceeds 1 g/dL in any 2-week period.

The major adverse reaction is HTN. The risk is higher in patients with CRF, and the reaction is discussed in the Precautions and Contraindications section. Both of these drugs may increase the risk for cardiovascular events, especially thrombogenesis. The higher risk has, once again, been associated with rates of rise in Hgb and the target level of Hgb should be less than 12 g/dL.

As mentioned above, the FDA has issued a safety warning regarding the use of **ESAs** and decreased overall survival and/or increased risk of tumor progression has been reported in patients with breast, non-small cell lung, head and neck, lymphoid, and cervical cancers. The FDA is requiring that all patients have the risk and benefits of **ESAs** explained to them before the provider prescribes. Updates on the FDA warning can be found at the FDA website (www.fda.gov).

Allergic-type reactions have developed with **filgrastim** on initial and subsequent treatment in fewer than 1 in 4,000 patients. Skin, respiratory, and cardiovascular systems common to most hypersensitivity reactions are typical. Administration of **antihistamines, steroids, bronchodilators,** or **epinephrine** resulted in resolution. Symptoms recurred in more than 50 percent of the patients who were rechallenged with this drug. Such allergic reactions have not occurred in clinical trials of **pegfilgrastim.** Adult respiratory distress syndrome (ARDS) has been reported in neutropenic patients with sepsis receiving **filgrastim** and is postulated to be related to an influx of neutrophils to the sites of inflammation in the lungs. Patients receiving **pegfilgrastim** are also at risk. If ARDS develops, these drugs should be discontinued.

The adverse reactions with **oprelvekin** were mild to moderate in severity, reversible with discontinuance, and mainly similar to those of placebo groups when the dose was 50 mcg/kg. Tachycardia, edema, dizziness, conjunctival hemorrhage, and neutropenic fever were observed.

Adverse reactions to **sargramostim** include headache and transient pruritic rashes. Hypersensitivity reactions are rare. Cardiovascular, respiratory, and fluid retention problems are discussed in the Precautions and Contraindications section.

All of the **hematopoietic growth factors** can produce bone pain from the stimulation of the bone marrow. This may require analgesia.

Drug Interactions

Drug interactions for all the **hematopoietic growth factors** are minimum (Table 18–7). Only those drugs such as **lithium** that may potentiate myeloproliferative effects require avoidance of concurrent use or cautious use. There are no drug interactions reported with **darbepoetin alfa** or **oprelvekin**.

Table 18–7 ■ **Drug Interactions: Hematopoietic Growth Factors**

Drug	Interacting Drug	Possible Effect	Implications
Epoetin alfa	Heparin	May increase requirement for heparin anticoagulation during dialysis	Monitor aPTT carefully in dialysis patients
Filgrastim	Lithium	May potentiate the release of neutrophils	Drug interaction not fully studied; no recommendations at this time.
Pegfilgrastim	Antineoplastic agents	Simultaneous use may have adverse effect on rapidly proliferating neutrophils	Avoid use 24 h before or 24 h after chemotherapy
Sargramostim	Lithium	May potentiate myeloproliferative effects of sargramostim	Avoid concurrent use or use cautiously

Clinical Use and Dosing

Anemia Associated With Chronic Renal Failure

Darbepoetin alfa and **epoetin alfa** are the drugs of choice to elevate and maintain erythrocyte levels and decrease the need for transfusions. Patients both on dialysis and not on dialysis benefit equally. They not intended for immediate correction of severe anemia because it takes 7 to 10 days to see increases in reticulocyte counts. The starting dose for **epoetin alfa** is 50 to 100 U/kg given SC three times weekly. Maintenance doses are based on individual responses, and adjustments are based on Hct levels. The starting dose for **darbepoetin alfa** is 0.45 mcg/kg SC once weekly. Dosage adjustments are made no more frequently than once a month, because it takes that long to see increases in blood values. Table 18–8 shows guidelines for dosage adjustments for both drugs. Dosage adjustments are not to be made more than once monthly, based on the time it takes for erythroid progenitors to mature and red blood cell (RBC) survival time.

Table 18–8 ● Dosage Schedule: Hematopoietic Growth Factors

Drug	Indication	Initial Dose	Maintenance Dose
Darbepoetin alfa	Anemia in chronic renal failure	0.45 mcg/kg SC once weekly	Individualized: goal Hgb is 12 g/dL; as goal is approached the dose is reduced by 25%. If Hgb continues to increase, doses are withheld until it begins to drop. Then drug is restarted at a dose about 25% below previous dose. If Hgb increase is <1 g/dL over 4 weeks, and iron stores are adequate, dose may be increased by 25%. Further increases made at 4-wk intervals
	Cancer patients receiving chemotherapy	2.25 mcg/kg SC once weekly	Individualized to target Hgb. If <1 g/dL increase in Hgb after 6 wk of therapy, increase dose to 4.5 mcg/kg. If Hgb exceeds 12 g/dL, reduce dose by 25%. If Hgb exceeds 13 g/dL, withhold dose until Hgb ≤12 g/dL. Restart at dose 25% below previous dose
Epoetin alfa	Anemia in chronic renal failure	50–100 U/kg 3 times weekly	Individualized; reduced dose when hematocrit (Hct) approaches 36% or increases >4 points in any 2-wk period. Increase dose if Hct does not increase by 5–6 points after 8 wk of therapy and remains below target range of 30%–36%
	Zidovudine-treated HIV-infected patients	100 U/kg 3 times weekly for 8 wk	Individualized; when the desired response is attained, titrate to maintain it. If response is too low, increase by 50–100 U/kg 3 times weekly. Evaluate response every 4–8 wk and adjust by 50–100 U/kg increments. If response is too low at 300 U/kg, response is unlikely. If Hct exceeds 40%, stop dose until Hct is 36%, then resume treatment with a dose reduced by 25%
	Cancer patients on chemotherapy	150 U/kg 3 times weekly	If response is too low after 8 wk, increase dose up to 300 U/kg three times weekly; higher doses are not likely to produce a response. If Hct exceeds 40%, or increases >4% in any 2-wk period, stop dose until Hct is 36%, then resume treatment with a dose reduced by 25%
	Presurgery	300 U/kg/d *or*	Given 10 d prior to surgery, day of surgery, and for 4 d after surgery
		600 U/kg once weekly	Given 21, 14, and 7 d prior to surgery and then day of surgery
Filgrastim	Myelosuppressive chemotherapy	5 mcg/kg/d no earlier than 24 h after or 24 h before next dose of chemotherapy	Dose given daily for up to 2 wk. Discontinue therapy if ANC >10,000 mm^3 after expected nadir of chemotherapy
	Severe chronic neutropenia: Congenital cyclic/idiopathic	6 mcg/kg twice daily 5 mcg/kg daily	Individualized; reduce dose if ANC persistently >10,000 mm^3
Oprelvekin	Myelosuppressive chemotherapy	50 mcg/kg SC once daily; 6–24 hours after completion of chemotherapy	Continue dosing until the postnadir platelet count is ≥50,000 call/mcL. Dosing beyond 21 d is not recommended
Pegfilgrastim	Myelosuppressive chemotherapy	Single injection of 6 mg SC administered once per chemotherapy cycle	Do not give between 14 d before and 24 h after administration of cytotoxic chemotherapy

Anemia Related to Zidovudine Therapy

Epoetin alfa is the drug of choice to elevate and maintain erythrocyte levels and decrease the need for transfusions when the endogenous erythropoietin level is 500 mU/mL or less and the dose of **zidovudine** is 4,200 mg/week or less. The initial dose is 100 U/kg SC three times weekly for 8 weeks. Maintenance doses are based on individual responses, and adjustments are based on Hct levels. Table 18–8 shows the general guidelines for dosage adjustments. Dosage adjustments are timed as noted previously.

Anemia in Patients With Cancer on Chemotherapy

Darbepoetin alfa and **epoetin alfa** are drugs used to elevate and maintain erythrocyte levels and decrease the need for transfusions. The initial dose is 2.25 mcg/kg SC once weekly for **darbepoetin alfa** and 150 U/kg given SC three times weekly for **epoetin alfa.** Patients with lower baseline serum erythropoietin levels tend to respond more vigorously to this drug. Treatment is not recommended for patients with serum erythropoietin levels below 200 mU/mL. Dosage adjustments are made after 6 weeks for **darbepoetin alfa** and 8 weeks of therapy for **epoetin alfa.** Table 18–8 shows the general guidelines for dosage adjustments. Dosage adjustments are timed as noted previously.

Decreasing Blood Transfusions in Surgery Patients

Anemic patients scheduled to undergo elective, noncardiac, nonvascular surgery, with anticipated significant blood loss, benefit from **epoetin alfa** therapy to reduce the need for allogeneic blood transfusions. The recommended dose is 300 U/kg a day SC for 10 days prior to surgery, on the day of surgery, and for 4 days after surgery. An alternative dosing schedule is 600 U/kg once weekly at 21, 14, and 7 days before surgery, plus a fourth dose on the day of surgery. All patients on these regimens must receive adequate **iron** supplementation, beginning no later than the start of the **epoetin** therapy and continuing throughout the therapy.

Patients on Myelosuppressive Therapy

Filgrastim, pegfilgrastim, and **sargramostim** have been used for this indication. It is an off-labeled use in **sargramostim.** The recommended starting dose for **filgrastim** is 5 mcg/kg a day given as a single dose SC. Dosage adjustments are based on CBC and platelet data and are done in increments of 5 mcg/kg per day, according to the duration and severity of the absolute neutrophil count (ANC) nadir. It is given daily for up to 2 weeks until the ANC has reached 10,000 mm^3. Clinical trials have shown effective doses to be 4 to 8 mcg/kg a day. **Pegfilgrastim** is given as a once-only dose of 6 mg prior to the start of the chemotherapy cycle. Because it is an off-labeled use, the dosing schedule for **sargramostim** is not specified in the literature. Because of the specialty use of this drug and the need for IV administration, it is not discussed here.

Severe Chronic Neutropenia

Severe chronic neutropenia (SCN) can be congenital, cyclic, or idiopathic. Chronic administration of **filgrastim** reduces the incidence and duration of sequelae of neutropenia, such as fever, infection, and oropharyngeal ulcers. The initial dose for congenital SCN is 6 mcg/kg twice daily SC. For cyclic or idiopathic SCN, the initial dose is 5 mcg/kg every day. Dosage adjustments are based on the patient's clinical course and ANC.

Prevention of Severe Thrombocytopenia

Oprelvekin is used for prevention of severe thrombocytopenia and reduced need for platelet transfusion postmyelosuppressive therapy. It is given as one dose 6 to 24 hours after the completion of chemotherapy and continued on a daily basis until the postnadir platelet count is above 50,000. Dosing duration is between 14 and 21 days and dosing beyond 21 days is not recommended.

Other indications for the use of these drugs, including bone marrow transplant, are beyond the scope of this book.

Rational Drug Selection

The drug choice is based on its indication because each drug has very specific uses.

Monitoring

Monitoring parameters are different for each drug and are discussed specific to that drug.

Darbepoetin Alfa

Hgb levels are determined weekly until they have stabilized and the maintenance dose has been established. After dosage adjustments, weekly Hgb levels are also drawn for at least 4 weeks until it has been determined that the Hgb has stabilized in response to the new dose. Hgb is then monitored at regular intervals. Iron status should also be evaluated before and during treatment, since the majority of patients will require supplemental iron. Supplemental **iron** is recommended when the serum ferritin is less than 100 mcg/L or the serum transferrin is less than 20 percent.

Epoetin Alfa

Patients with CRF not on dialysis require monitoring of blood pressure and Hct no less frequently than patients maintained on dialysis. Hct is monitored twice weekly until it is stabilized in the target zone and the maintenance dose has been established and then for at least 2 to 6 weeks after each dosage adjustment. Maintenance monitoring is individualized, based on patient stability. In some patients, increases in blood urea nitrogen (BUN), creatinine, uric acid, phosphorus, and potassium have been noted. These values are routinely monitored in patients with CRF and require no additional monitoring.

Patients on **zidovudine** therapy for HIV infection require monitoring of Hct weekly until it is stabilized. Periodic monitoring thereafter is based on the progression of the disease.

During therapy with **epoetin alfa,** absolute and functional iron deficiency may develop. Functional iron deficiency is presumed to be based on inability to mobilize iron stores rapidly enough to support increased erythropoiesis. Transferrin saturation should be at least 20 percent, and ferritin should be at least 100 mcg/mL. Prior to initiating therapy and at regular intervals during therapy, determine transferrin and ferritin levels. Virtually all patients at some point require **supplemental iron.**

Delayed or diminished responses suggest referral to a hematologist. Possible common etiologies for patients who fail to respond or to maintain a response to doses within the recommended range for both **darbepoetin alfa** and **epoetin alfa** include the following:

1. Functional iron deficiency
2. Underlying infectious, inflammatory, or malignant disease
3. Occult blood loss
4. Underlying hematological diseases, such as thalassemia, refractory anemia, or myelodysplastic disorder
5. Vitamin B_{12} or folic acid deficiency
6. Hemolysis
7. Aluminum intoxication

Filgrastim

For patients on myelosuppressive chemotherapy, CBCs and platelet counts are done prior to initiating therapy and twice weekly during therapy. Following therapy, the same indicators are monitored around the time of the nadir of the chemotherapy. **Filgrastim** or **pegfilgrastim** therapy may be terminated when the ANC is 10,000 mm^3 or greater. For patients with SCN treated with **filgrastim,** CBCs with differential, platelet counts, and evaluation of bone marrow morphology and karyotype are done prior to initiating therapy. During the initial 4 weeks of therapy and for 2 weeks after any dosage adjustment, CBCs with differential and platelet counts are done. Once the patient is stable, monthly CBCs with differential and platelet counts are sufficient.

For **oprelvekin,** during dosing fluid balance needs to be monitored. If a **diuretic** is used, electrolyte balance may also need to be monitored. A CBC is drawn prior to chemotherapy and at regular intervals during therapy to monitor platelet counts. Monitoring continues during the time of expected nadir for the chemotherapy and until platelet counts are 50,000 or higher postnadir.

Patient Education

Administration

If the patient can safely and effectively self-administer these drugs, instruction is provided in correct SC injection technique and proper dosage (Table 18–9). Self-administration is common in patients with CRF. Detailed instructions on dilution and storage stability are included in the package insert.

Table 18–9 ◆ **Available Dosage Forms: Hematopoietic Growth Factors**

Drug	Dosage Form	Other Forms	Cost
Darbepoetin alfa (Aranesp)	Solution for SC injection: (in 1-mL single-dose vial) 25 mcg/mL; 40 mcg/mL; 60 mcg/mL; 100 mcg/mL; 150 mcg/mL; 200 mcg/mL; 300 mcg/mL and 500 mcg/mL		25 mcg = $124.69/vial; 40 mcg = $199.50/vial; 60 mcg = $299.25/vial; 100 mcg = $498.75/vial; 150 mcg = $748.13/vial; 200 mcg = $997.50/vial
Epoetin alfa (Epogen, Procrit)	Subcutaneous: (in 1-mL single-dose vials) 2,000 U/mL 3,000 U/mL 4,000 U/mL 10,000 U/mL 20,000 U/mL 40,000 U/mL	—	*Epogen* $125.20/vial, $269/vial, $527.73/vial *Procrit* $129.69/vial, $259/vial, $517/vial

Table 18–9 ◈ **Available Dosage Forms: Hematopoietic Growth Factors—cont'd**

Drug	Dosage Form	Other Forms	Cost
Filgrastim (Neupogen)	Subcutaneous: (in 1- and 1.6-mL single-dose vials; preservative-free) 300 mcg/mL	—	$202.50/1 mL vial $322.50/1.6 mL vial
Oprelvekin (Neumega)	Powder for injection: (in single-dose vial with diluent) 5 mg		No cost data
Pegfilgrastim (Neulasta)	Solution for injection (in single-dose syringe with needle) 10 mg/mL		$2,850.56 for 6 mg/ 0.6 mL
Sargramostim (Leukine)	Powder for injection (in vials) 250 mcg		No cost data
	Liquid: (in multidose vials) 500 mcg/mL		

Adverse Drug Reactions

HTN and allergic reactions are the two most common adverse reactions. Self-monitoring of blood pressure and signs and symptoms of an allergic reaction are taught.

IRON PREPARATIONS

Iron is an essential mineral in the production of Hgb, myoglobin, and a number of enzymes. Iron deficiency anemia results in problems with oxygen transport that affect the energy metabolism of every cell in the body. Iron deficiency anemia is commonly seen in infants, particularly premature infants; in children during rapid growth periods; and in pregnant and lactating women. It may also occur after gastrectomy and with malabsorption disorders, particularly those of the small bowel. The most common cause in adults is blood loss. Menstruation may cause the loss of more than 30 mg of iron with each period. Occult blood loss may occur from GI bleeding and from cancer. In an attempt to replace blood lost, erythropoiesis may occur at an increased rate and increased iron may be used and drawn from storage. Prevention and treatment of iron deficiency anemia are accomplished by administration of supplemental **iron**.

On The Horizon **ON THE HORIZON**

Interleukin-3, Stem Cell Factor, and Monocyte-Macrophage Colony–Stimulating Factor

IL-3, stem cell factor, and monocyte-macrophage colony–stimulating factor are currently in clinical trials. **IL-3** would provide broad-based therapy because it is involved in the generation and stimulation of all progenitor cells. Stem cell factor would provide therapy at an even earlier stage in blood cell development. Monocyte-macrophage colony–stimulating factor would provide a targeted approach to patients who do not require such a broad stimulation of blood cell growth.

Pharmacodynamics

Approximately 67 percent of total body **iron** is bound to heme in RBCs and muscle cells, and approximately 30 percent is stored bound to ferritin or hemosiderin mononuclear phagocytes and hepatic parenchymal cells. The remaining 3 percent is lost daily in urine, sweat, bile, and epithelial cells shed from the GI tract. Iron not lost is continuously recycled, as shown in Figure 18–3. Recycling is made possible by transferrin.

As iron deficiency develops, storage **iron** decreases and then disappears, followed by decreased serum ferritin and then serum **iron**. Finally, iron-binding capacity increases, resulting in a decrease in transferrin saturation. At this point, anemia develops. Administration of **iron** reverses the process so that eventually not only is serum iron improved but also iron storage is replenished. Management of anemia is discussed in Chapter 27.

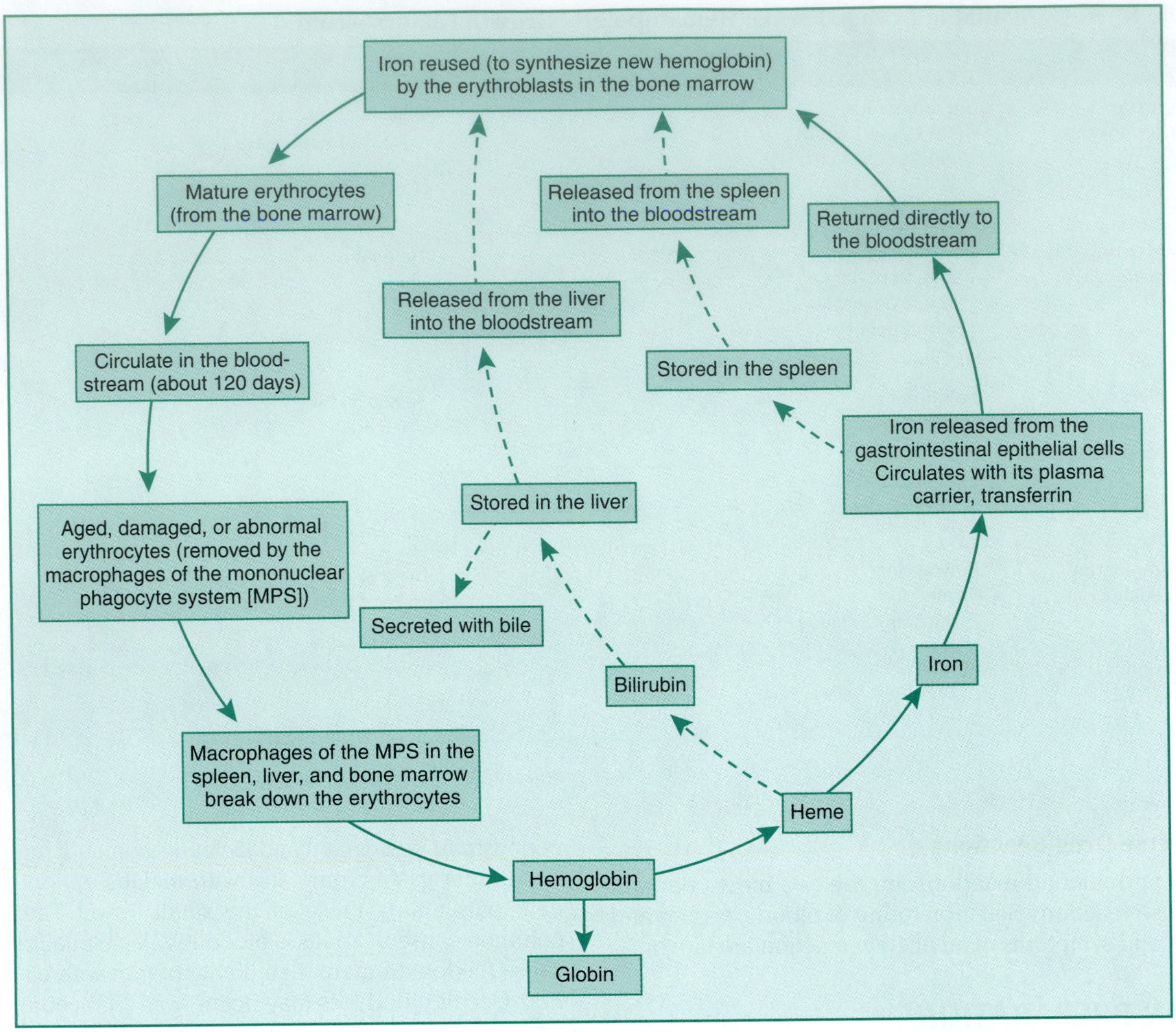

Figure 18–3. The iron cycle.

Pharmacokinetics

Absorption and Distribution

Only about 10 percent of the average daily dietary intake of **iron** is absorbed (1 to 2 mg/day) in patients with adequate **iron** stores. Absorption is enhanced in the presence of depleted **iron** stores and when erythropoiesis is increased. **Iron** is primarily absorbed in the duodenum and upper jejunum by an active transport mechanism. The ferrous form is absorbed three times more readily than the ferric form. The common ferrous forms (sulfate, gluconate, and fumarate) are absorbed almost on a milligram-for-milligram basis but differ in the amount of elemental **iron** each contains.

Factors that significantly affect absorption include sustained-release forms, dose, and the presence of food. Sustained-release or enteric-coated forms have less available **iron** because they transport the **iron** beyond the duodenum before it is released. As dose increases, the amount of **iron** absorbed increases, but the percentage of **iron** absorbed decreases. Food can decrease the absorption of **iron** by 40 to 66 percent, but gastric intolerance often requires administration with food. Concurrent administration of vitamin C may enhance absorption, but the literature is still controversial. Eggs and milk inhibit **iron** absorption.

Iron is transported via blood bound to transferrin. The transferrin–ferric iron complex is delivered to maturing erythroid cells, where transferrin receptors pick up and internalize the **iron** and release it within the cell.

Metabolism, Storage, and Excretion

Iron is stored as either ferritin or hemosiderin. Ferritin is more readily available and is water soluble. Hemosiderin is a particulate substance containing aggregates of ferric core crystals. Both are stored in macrophages in the liver, spleen, and bone marrow. Because the ferritin present in plasma is in equilibrium with stored ferritin, the plasma ferritin level can be used to estimate total-body iron stores.

There is no mechanism for excretion of iron. Iron is lost mainly through shedding of the GI mucosal cells, with small losses in urine, sweat, and bile. These losses total no more than 1 mg of **iron** per day. Because the body has no mechanism for excretion of **iron**, **iron** balance is achieved largely through control of the amount of **iron** absorbed in the gut.

Pharmacotherapeutics

Precautions and Contraindications

The only contraindications to the use of **iron** are hemochromatosis and hemolytic anemia. Tartrazine and sulfite are found in some **iron** formulations. Patients sensitive to them should not take these formulations.

Adverse Drug Reactions

GI symptoms are the most common adverse reactions and are usually mild. Irritation, anorexia, nausea and vomiting, constipation, or diarrhea may occur. Administering the **iron** with food reduces most of these problems. Stools may appear darker in color, which can present a problem in assessing GI bleeding. **Iron**-containing preparations may cause temporary staining of the teeth. Dilution of the drug reduces this problem.

Acute Toxicity

Acute **iron** toxicity is seen almost exclusively in children who have ingested many **iron** tablets. As few as 10 tablets of common oral **iron** preparations can be lethal in young children. Symptoms occur in four stages:

1. Within 1 to 6 hours, lethargy, nausea, vomiting, abdominal pain, tarry stools, weak and rapid pulse, hypotension, acidosis, and coma occur.
2. If not immediately fatal, symptoms may subside for about 24 hours.
3. Symptoms return in 12 to 48 hours and may also include diffuse vascular congestion, pulmonary edema, shock, acidosis, convulsions, anuria, hyperthermia, and death.
4. If the patient survives, in 2 to 6 weeks, pyloric stenosis, hepatic cirrhosis, and central nervous system (CNS) damage may be seen.

Treatment involves maintaining airway, respiration, and circulation. Perform gastric lavage with 1 to 5 percent **sodium bicarbonate** to convert the ferrous sulfate to ferrous carbonate, which is poorly absorbed and less irritating. Systemic chelation with **deferoxamine** IM is recommended for patients with serum **iron** levels above 350 mcg/dL.

Drug Interactions

Drug interactions involve chelation (**levodopa, penicillamine, quinolones**) or competition for absorption (**antacids, cimetidine, methyldopa, tetracyclines**). Food interactions occur with **vitamin C** (enhances absorption) and calcium (decreases absorption unless calcium carbonate is used). Drug interactions are shown in Table 18–10.

Clinical Use and Dosing

Oral **iron** therapy is used to prevent and treat iron deficiency anemia. Because they are more efficiently absorbed, ferrous salts should be used. Sustained-release and enteric forms should not be used because **iron** is best absorbed in the duodenum and jejunum. Different ferrous salts provide different amounts of **elemental iron**. In an iron-deficient patient, about 50 to 100 mg of **iron** can be incorporated into hemoglobin daily. The adult dose for **iron** replacement is 150 to 300 mg of elemental **iron** daily

Table 18–10 ■ **Drug Interactions: Iron**

Drug	Interacting Drug	Possible Effect	Implications
Iron	Antacids	Absorption reduced	Separate administration by at least 2 h
	Ascorbic acid	Absorption enhanced	Increase may not be significant; must be given concurrently
	Calcium	Coadministration decreases absorption of both; calcium carbonate does not decrease iron absorption	Separate administration by at least 2 h or use calcium carbonate for calcium supplementation and take between meals
	Chloramphenicol	Serum iron levels may be increased	—
	Cimetidine	Absorption reduced	Separate administration by at least 2 h
	Levodopa	Forms chelates with iron salts, decreasing levodopa levels by up to 90%	Avoid concurrent use

Continued

Table 18–10 ■ Drug Interactions: Iron—cont'd

Drug	Interacting Drug	Possible Effect	Implications
	Methyldopa	Methyldopa absorption decreased	Avoid concurrent use
	Penicillamine	Marked reduction in penicillamine absorption	Avoid concurrent use
	Quinolones	Decreased absorption of quinolones by up to 90%	Choose different antibiotic
	Tetracyclines	Coadministration decreases absorption and serum levels of both by up to 90%	Separate administration by at least 2 h
	Vitamin C	Absorption enhanced	May not be significant and requires concurrent administration

in two or three divided doses to correct **iron** deficiency rapidly. About 25 percent of ferrous salt given orally can be absorbed. Premature neonates require 2 to 4 mg of **elemental iron**/kg/day. Infants and young children require 4 to 6 mg/kg/day divided in 3 doses to treat severe iron deficiency and 3 mg/kg/day to treat mild to moderate iron deficiency. Doses for infants, children, and adults are provided in Table 18–11. If the patient cannot tolerate large doses, lower doses may be given, but resolving the deficiency takes longer. Treatment continues for 3 to 4 months after hemoglobin/hematocrit return to normal to correct the anemia and replenish **iron** stores.

Rational Drug Selection

Cost

Iron supplements are available in generic form and are not very expensive. The most expensive ferrous sulfate is **Fer-In-Sol**, a liquid form used mostly for infants and small children. Other liquid formulations were also expensive, but the least expensive was **ferrous sulfate elixir.** Costs of other forms are presented in Table 18–12. Generic **ferrous salts** are clearly less expensive, even though all of these compounds are OTC medications.

Formulation

Ferrous salts come in tablets, capsules, suspensions, drops, and chewable formulations (Table 18–12). Unless a patient's age or disease process makes swallowing difficult or impossible, the tablets are the cheapest, and they are easily digested and absorbed.

Monitoring

The reticulocyte count is measured 7 to 10 days after initiation of therapy because it is the first measurable response to **iron** therapy. A significant rise should be noted toward the normal 0.5 to 1.5 percent of the body's RBCs. Hemoglobin levels drawn at 2 weeks from initiation of therapy should indicate a rise in Hgb concentration of 0.1 to 0.2 g/100 mL per day of therapy. Normal Hgb levels of 14 to 18 g/dL in men and 12 to 16 g/dL in women should be reached in 1 to 3 months. Monitoring of RBC and Hgb levels thereafter is based on individual patient risk, response, and symptoms.

Patient Education

Prevention

Prevention of **iron** deficiency is the most important issue. The average American diet contains about 12 mg of **iron** daily. Twenty percent of this is absorbed in markedly deficient patients, but only 10 percent is absorbed in normal patients. This means that 0.6 to 1.2 mg of **elemental iron** is taken up under normal circumstances. This is an adequate requirement for men and postmenopausal women; however, menstruating women need 1.5 mg/day, and pregnant and lactating women need 2.5 mg/day. Eating **iron**-rich foods can prevent the need for **iron** supplements, especially in adults. Red meat is the best source of **iron**, but fish and **iron**-enriched breads and cereals are also good sources. The **iron** in eggs and green vegetables is not absorbed because it is bound to phosphates and phytates in these foods. Nutrition should be discussed, including **iron**-rich foods that are reasonable in cost. Most people who eat a balanced diet do not need **iron** supplements. Pregnant women, infants, and children during rapid growth periods usually need **iron** supplementation.

Administration

Patients should take **iron** as directed. If a dose is missed, they should take it as soon as it is remembered within 12 hours but not double doses. **Iron** should be taken on an empty stomach. If GI upset occurs, **iron** can be taken

Table 18–11 ◉ Dosage Schedule: Iron

Drug	Indication	Maintenance Dose
Iron	Replacement in iron-deficiency anemia	*Adults:* Ferrous sulfate 300–325 mg (60–65 mg of elemental iron) tid-qid Ferrous gluconate 300–325 mg (34–38 mg of elemental iron) qid Ferrous fumarate 200 mg (66 mg of elemental iron) tid-qid Ferrous fumarate 325 mg (106 mg elemental iron) bid-tid *Note:* Goal is 150–250 mg of elemental iron/d. RDA: Male >18 yr: 10 mg/d Female 11–50 yr: 15 mg/d Female >50 yr: 10 mg/d
		Children: 2–12 *yr:* goal is 4 to 6 mg/kg/d of elemental iron in 3 divided doses. 6 mo–2 yr: goal is up to 6 mg/kg/d of elemental iron in 3 divided doses. RDA: <5 months: 5 mg/d 5 mo to 10 yr: 10 mg/d Males: 11 to 18 yr: 12 mg/d Females: 11 to 18 yr: 15 mg/d
	Iron supplement in pregnancy and lactation	30 mg elemental iron daily (not taken with meals)

with food, but the amount absorbed will be less. Taking it with vitamin C or citrus juice may enhance absorption. Patients should avoid taking **iron** at the same time as milk, **antacids**, **tetracycline**, or **quinolones**, which decrease absorption, and drink liquid **iron** preparations in water or citrus juice or through a straw to prevent discoloration of teeth. Do not use sustained-release preparations.

Adverse Responses

Constipation is the most common problem. Increase fluids and fiber in the diet, especially **iron**-rich cereals. Stools may turn dark green or black. This color change is harmless. A stool softener may be used if needed to treat constipation.

Acute **iron** toxicity/poisoning can occur with an overdose. This is especially a problem with children, in whom as few as 10 of the commonly available **iron** tablets can be fatal. Keep **iron** preparations in childproof containers and in a locked medicine cabinet. Do not refer to vitamins or drugs as candy. Contact the local Poison Control Center immediately if overdose is suspected.

Detailed discussion of the management of **iron** deficiency anemia as well as other forms of anemia is presented in Chapter 27.

FOLIC ACID

Folic acid deficiency is most often related to inadequate dietary intake of green vegetables or excessive boiling of these vegetables in cooking. Other sources of

Table 18–12 ◆ Available Dosage Forms: Oral Iron

Drug	Dosage Form	How Supplied	Cost
Ferrous sulfate (20% elemental iron)	Ferrous sulfate: Tablets: 325 mg (65 mg elemental iron)	In bottles of 100, 1,000, and UD 100	$5.99/100 tablets
	Elixir: 220 mg/5mL (44 mg iron/5 mL)	In 473-mL bottle	
	Drops: 75 mg/0.6 mL (15 mg iron/0.6 mL)	In 50-mL bottle	
	Feosol: Capsules: 325 mg (65 mg iron)	In bottles of 100	$11.99/125 capsules
	FeroSul: Capsules: 325 mg (65 mg iron)	In bottles of 100 and 1,000	
	Fer-In-Sol: Drops: 75 mg/0.6mL (15 mg iron/0.6 mL)	In 50-mL bottle	$11.99/1.66 mL
	Fer-Gen-Sol: Drops: 75mg/0.6mL (15 mg iron/0.6 mL)	In 50-mL bottle	
Ferrous sulfate (Dried)	Feosol: Tablet: 200 mg (65 mg iron)	In bottles of 100	
	Feratab: Tablet: 300 mg (60 mg iron)	In UD 100	
	Ferrous sulfate: Slow-release tablet: 160 mg (50 mg iron)	In blister paks of 60	
	Slow Fe: Slow-release tablet: 160 mg (50 mg iron)	In bottles of 30	$24.39/90 tablets

Continued

Table 18–12 ◆ **Available Dosage Forms: Oral Iron—cont'd**

Drug	Dosage Form	How Supplied	Cost
Ferrous gluconate (12% elemental iron)	Ferrous gluconate: Tablet: 225 mg (28 mg iron)	In bottles of 100	$15.86/100 tablets
	Fergon: Tablet: 225 mg (27 mg iron)	In bottles of 100	$7.99/100 tablets
	Ferrous gluconate: Tablet: 300 mg (35 mg of iron); 324 mg (38 mg iron)	In bottles of 100	
	Tablet: 325 mg (36 mg iron)	In bottles of 1,000	
Ferrous fumarate (33% elemental iron)	Ferrous fumarate: Tablet: 90 mg (29.5 mg iron)	In bottles of 100	
	Ferrous fumarate: Tablet: 324 mg (106 mg iron)	In bottles of 100	
	Femiron: 63 mg (20 mg iron)		
	Hemocyte: Tablet: 324 mg (106 mg iron)	In bottles of 30 and 1,000	
	Ferrets: Tablet: 325 mg (106 mg iron)	In bottles of 60. Scored	
	Nephro-Fer: Tablet: 350 mg (115 mg iron)	In bottles of 30	
	Feostat: Chewable tablet: 100 mg (33 mg iron)	In UD 100	
	Ferro-Sequels: Timed-release tablet: 150 mg (50 mg iron)	In bottles of 30 and 90	
Carbonyl iron (pure iron microparticles)	Feosol: Tablet: 45 mg iron	In bottles of 30 and 60	$16.99/75 caplets
	Sundown tablet: 50 mg iron	In bottles of 200	
	Ircon: Tablet: 66 mg iron	In blister paks of 100	
	Icar: Chewable tablet: 15 mg iron	In bottles of 60 (grape flavor)	
	Suspension: 15 mg iron/1.25 mL	In 118 mL (grape and lemon flavors)	

Iron forms that come in combination with other minerals or vitamins are not included here.

folic acid deficiency include impaired absorption because of ileal disease or **phenytoin** use; increased demand during pregnancy, hyperthyroidism, hemolytic anemia, or malignancy; and impaired utilization for patients taking **methotrexate, triamterene,** and **trimethoprim.**

Pharmacodynamics

Exogenous **folate** is required for nucleoprotein synthesis and maintenance of normal erythropoiesis. **Folic acid** stimulates the production of erythrocytes, WBCs, and platelets. **Folic acid** undergoes a series of oxidative-reductive changes that result in the formation of tetrahydrofolic acid, a cofactor in transformation reactions in the biosynthesis of purines and thymidylates. Impaired thymidylate synthesis is thought to be the mechanism behind neural tube defects in the offspring of pregnant women with folic acid deficiency. Within 3 months of inadequate intake of **folates,** megaloblastic changes and anemia can develop. **Supplemental folic acid** is useful in preventing folic acid deficiency in high-risk patients with high folate requirements, such as pregnant women, and in alcoholics and patients with liver disease, who may have deficient storage of **folate.**

Pharmacokinetics

Absorption and Distribution

Only about 50 to 200 mcg of **folate** are absorbed from the daily intake of 500 to 700 mcg in the average diet. Pregnant women may absorb as much as 300 to 400 mcg of **folate** daily. Oral **folic acid supplements** are well absorbed from the proximal jejunum, and IM or SC administration also results in excellent absorption.

Metabolism, Storage, and Excretion

Folic acid is converted by the liver to its active metabolite (dihydrofolate reductase). Approximately 5 to 20 mg of **folate** are stored in the liver and other tissues extensively bound to plasma proteins. **Folates** are excreted in the urine and stool and destroyed by catabolism so that serum levels fall within days when intake is inadequate.

Pharmacotherapeutics

Precautions and Contraindications

The only contraindication is administration when vitamin B_{12} is deficient. **Folic acid** in doses greater than 0.1 mg/day may mask the indications of pernicious anemia in that the hematological symptoms are gone, but the neurological symptoms continue to progress. Except in pregnancy and lactation, daily doses of **folic acid** should not exceed 0.4 mg/day until pernicious anemia has been ruled out.

Folic acid is Pregnancy Category A. Pregnant women are more prone to develop folic acid deficiencies, and their diet should be supplemented. The recommended dietary allowance (RDA) for **folate** during pregnancy is 0.4 mg/day.

Adverse Drug Reactions

Rare transient rashes are the only adverse drug reaction.

Drug Interactions

Sulfonamides, methotrexate, and **triamterene** interfere with the activity of folate reductase and prevent the activation of **folic acid** (Table 18–13). Absorption is decreased if it is given concurrently with **sulfasalazine. Folic acid** requirements are increased in the presence of **estrogens, phenytoin,** and **glucocorticoids.**

Clinical Use and Dosing

Anemia Due to Folic Acid Deficiency

After pernicious anemia has been ruled out, the initial dose is up to 1 mg/day in adults and children. When clinical symptoms have subsided and the laboratory studies have normalized, maintenance doses range from 0.1 mg/day for infants to 0.8 mg/day for pregnant and lactating patients. Table 18–14 shows these dosages by age group. Chapter 27 discusses the management of pernicious anemia.

Prevention of Folic Acid Deficiency

Maintenance doses of **folic acid** may be sufficient to prevent folic acid deficiency in these patients if the upper limit for each age is used.

Doses of 0.4 mg prior to conception and throughout pregnancy have been associated with risk reductions of up to 50 percent for neural tube defects in the offspring. The U.S. Public Health Service recommends that all women of childbearing age who are capable of becoming pregnant consume 0.4 mg of **folic acid** daily. Because of the risks with higher doses of **folic acid** that B_{12} deficiency may be overlooked, total **folate** intake should not exceed 1 mg/day. Chapter 27 discusses the management of folic acid deficiency anemia with pregnancy considerations.

Folic Acid During Lactation

During lactation, **folic acid** requirements are markedly increased. Mothers who are breastfeeding and have folic acid deficiency require doses of 0.8 mg/day to prevent folic acid deficiency in their infants.

Rational Drug Selection

Folic acid is available OTC at less cost than in prescription form (Table 18–15).

Monitoring

The only specific monitoring parameters are those associated with managing the anemia that is being treated.

Table 18–13 ■ Drug Interactions: Folic Acid

Drug	Interacting Drug	Possible Effect	Implications
Folic acid	Aminosalicylic acid	Decreased serum folate levels	Avoid concurrent use
	Oral contraceptives	May impair folate metabolism and produce folate depletion, but the effect is mild and not likely to cause anemia	Monitor for clinical indications of anemia
	Sulfonamides	Prevent the activation of folic acid by causing a dihydrofolate reductase deficiency	Avoid concurrent use
	Methotrexate	Signs of folate deficiency have been reported	Monitor for indications of anemia
	Triamterene		
	Sulfasalazine		
	Hydantoins	An increase in seizure activity and a decrease in serum concentrations of the hydantoin to subtherapeutic levels Phenytoin may cause a decrease in serum folate levels, but clinically important anemia occurs in <1% of patients on long-term therapy	If folic acid is administered, a higher dose of phenytoin may be needed

Table 18–14 ◉ **Dosage Schedule: Folic Acid**

Drug	Indication	Initial Dose	Maintenance Dose
Folic acid	Treatment of megaloblastic anemia	Up to 1 mg/d until laboratory studies are normal	*Infants:* 0.1 mg/d *Children <4 yr:* 0.3 mg/d *Adults and children >4 yr:* 0.4 mg/d Pregnant and lactating women, patients who are alcoholic, and patients with liver disease: 0.8 mg/d
	Prevention of folic acid deficiency		*Infants:* 0.1 mg/d *Children <4 yr:* 0.3 mg/d *Adults and children >4 yr:* 0.4 mg/d Pregnant and lactating women, patients who are alcoholic, and patients with liver disease: 0.4 mg/d

Table 18–15 ◈ **Available Dosage Forms: Folic Acid**

Drug	Dosage Form	Other Forms	Cost
Folic acid (OTC)	Tablets: 0.4 mg, 0.8 mg		0.4 mg = $4.59/250 0.8 mg = $4.99/100
Folic acid (prescription)	Tablets: 1 mg	Multidose vial for injection (Folvite); 5 mg/mL	1 mg = $4.99/90 tablets

OTC = over the counter.

Patient Education

Although **folic acid** is part of a normal diet, **supplemental folic acid** should be taken only after consultation with a health-care provider. In particular, pregnant women and those who may become pregnant should discuss the need for **folic acid** with their provider. Foods high in **folate** include green vegetables (especially asparagus, lettuce, spinach, and broccoli), liver, yeast, and mushrooms, which should be included in a balanced diet.

VITAMIN B_{12}

Vitamin B_{12} deficiency can be caused by poor intake, impaired absorption, increased demand, or faculty utilization. Poor intake is rare, except in strict vegetarians who do not eat eggs or use dairy products. Impaired absorption is most often related to the lack of intrinsic factor found in pernicious anemia. Absorption can also be impaired by diseases of the ileum, by bacterial overgrowth from stasis such as occurs with severe constipation, and by altered digestive enzymes associated with gastrectomy. Faulty utilization is associated with rare genetic defects.

Pharmacodynamics

Vitamin B_{12} is critical to two essential enzyme systems. In one system, it is the cofactor in metabolism of methylmalonyl-CoA. When this metabolism does not take place, methylmalonyl-CoA accumulates, and abnormal fatty acids are synthesized. It is believed that these abnormal fatty acids in cell membranes of the CNS are responsible for the neurological manifestations of vitamin B_{12} deficiency. The other system involves **folate** metabolism. In the presence of vitamin B_{12} deficiency, the final steps in **folate** metabolism cannot occur, which explains why the megaloblastic anemia found in vitamin B_{12} deficiency can be partially corrected by **folic acid** administration. Management of anemia is discussed in Chapter 27.

Pharmacokinetics

Absorption and Distribution

Approximately 1 to 5 mcg of the daily dietary intake of 5 to 30 mcg is absorbed. In the stomach and duodenum, **vitamin B_{12}** complexes with intrinsic factor are secreted by the parietal cells of the gastric mucosa. This complex is then separated in the terminal ileum in the presence of calcium and absorbed by a highly specific receptor-mediated transport system. Patients with intrinsic factor deficits require parenteral administration of **vitamin B_{12}** to bypass this absorption problem. **Vitamin B_{12}** is well absorbed following IM and SC injection or intranasal administration. Plasma level peaks within 1 hour after injection.

Once absorbed, **vitamin B_{12}** is distributed throughout the body, bound to a plasma protein, transcobalamin II.

Metabolism, Storage, and Excretion

Excess **vitamin B_{12}** is stored mainly in the liver and released when needed to carry out normal cellular functions. Because the normal daily requirement of **vitamin B_{12}** is only about 2 mcg, it would take approximately 5 years for all the stored **vitamin B_{12}** to be exhausted and megaloblastic anemia to develop if **vitamin B_{12}** absorption stopped. After injection, **vitamin B_{12}** is stored in the liver for approximately 400 days.

Within 48 hours after injection, 50 to 98 percent of the dose appears in the urine. The major portion is excreted within the first 8 hours.

Pharmacotherapeutics

Precautions and Contraindications

The only contraindications to injectable **vitamin B_{12}** are hypersensitivity to cobalt, B_{12}, or any component of these and the presence of Leber's disease, a hereditary optic nerve atrophy. Severe and swift optic nerve atrophy occurs in patients with this disease who are treated with **cyanocobalamin.**

Pulmonary edema, peripheral vascular thrombosis, and congestive heart failure may occur early in treatment with **vitamin B_{12}**. Cautious use and careful monitoring are suggested. Blunted or impeded therapeutic response may occur in the presence of uremia, folic acid deficiency, concurrent infection, or iron deficiency.

Vitamin B_{12} (parenteral) is Pregnancy Category C. Adequate and well-controlled studies have not been done with pregnant women.

Adverse Drug Reactions

Hypokalemia and sudden death have occurred in severe megaloblastic anemia treated intensely. Serum potassium levels should be carefully monitored, and supplementation provided as needed.

Anaphylactic shock and death have occurred after parenteral administration. An interdermal test dose is given to patients sensitive to the cobalamins.

Transient diarrhea, urticaria, and pruritus may occur but are not common. Pain is common at the injection site.

Drug Interactions

Injectable **vitamin B_{12}** has few drug interactions. Several drugs, extended-release **potassium**, and excessive intake of **alcohol** or **vitamin C** may decrease absorption of oral **vitamin B_{12}**. Table 18–16 shows these drug interactions.

Clinical Use and Dosing

Prevention of Vitamin B_{12} Deficiency

Vitamin B_{12} is an essential vitamin, and needs increase during pregnancy. The National Academy of Sciences recommends oral doses of 2.2 mcg/day during pregnancy. **Vitamin B_{12}** is excreted in breast milk in concentrations that approximate the mother's vitamin B_{12} blood level. The Food and Nutrition Board of the National Academy of Sciences—National Research Council recommends 2.6 mcg/day during lactation, 0.3 to 0.5 mcg/day for infants under age 1, and 0.7 to 1.4 mcg/day for children aged 1 to 10 (Table 18–17).

Pernicious Anemia

Because the underlying problem in almost all cases of pernicious anemia is malabsorption, therapy with **vitamin B_{12}** is required for life. Oral, IM, and intranasal replacement is available. Oral **vitamin B_{12}** is useful only for patients who cannot take the parenteral form. Initial dosing is

Table 18–16 ■ **Drug Interactions: Vitamin B_{12}**

Drug	Interacting Drug	Possible Effect	Implications
Vitamin B_{12}	Aminosalicylic acid	Reduced biological and therapeutic action of B_{12} Abnormal Schilling test and symptoms of B_{12} deficiency	Avoid concomitant administration
	Chloramphenicol	Hematological effects of B_{12} may be decreased in patients with pernicious anemia	Choose a different antimicrobial
	Colchicine	May cause malabsorption of B_{12} (oral)	If unable to avoid concomitant use, administer B_{12} parenterally
	Aminoglycosides Extended-release potassium supplements Cimetidine Excessive intake of alcohol or vitamin C		

Table 18–17 ● **Dosage Schedule: Vitamin B_{12}**

Drug	Indication	Initial Dose	Maintenance Dose
Vitamin B_{12}	Pernicious anemia	1,000 mcg/d for 7 d IM or deep SC	If clinical improvement and reticulocyte response, give 100 to 1,000 mcg IM weekly for a month. Then give 1,000 mcg monthly for life of patient If neurological symptoms are present, a twice-monthly dose is recommended for 6 mo prior to beginning the monthly dose Nasal therapy would consist of 500 mcg cyanocobalamin weekly Oral therapy consists of 1,000 mcg daily for life
	Vitamin B_{12} deficiency without pernicious anemia	Cyanocobalamin: Parenteral *Adults:* 30 mcg/d for 5–10 d *Children:* For hematological signs: 10–50 mcg/d for 5–10 d For neurological signs: 100 mcg/d for 10–15 d Oral 1,000 mcg/d Hydroxocobalamin: *Adults:* 30 mcg/d for 5–10 d *Children:* 100 mcg doses to equal 1–5 mg over 2 wk	Parenteral *Adults:* 100–200 mcg monthly *Children:* For hematological signs: 100–250 mcg/d every 2–4 wk For neurological signs: 100 mcg once or twice weekly for several months, then taper to 250–1,000 mcg monthly by 1 y *Adults:* 100–200 mcg/mo *Children:* 30–50 mcg every 4 wk

1,000 mcg daily for 7 days by IM or deep SC injection. The hematological response to injected **vitamin B_{12}** is usually rapid. Reticulocytosis begins on the second or third day and is usually maximal by the fifth to tenth day. If there is clinical improvement and an appropriate reticulocyte response has occurred after 7 days of therapy, then 100 to 1,000 mcg IM are given weekly for a month. Doses of 1,000 mcg may be used, as excess **vitamin B_{12}** is excreted in the urine. By this time, the hematological values should be normal. Hgb and Hct levels should return to normal within 1 to 2 months. It may take up to 6 months to resolve neurological symptoms. If neurological symptoms are present, a twice-monthly dose is recommended for 6 months prior to beginning the monthly dose. Because pernicious anemia is not correctable, **vitamin B_{12}** must be taken once monthly for the life of the patient. Parental, nasal, or oral therapy may be used once a patient's B_{12} levels return to normal. Parenteral therapy consists of 1,000 mcg of **vitamin B_{12}** monthly. Nasal therapy would consist of 500 mcg of **cyanocobalamin** weekly. Oral therapy consists of 1,000 mcg daily for life. Oral therapy should be tried because of ease of administration and cost. Further discussion is found in Chapter 27.

Patients With Vitamin B_{12} Deficiency

For adults with vitamin B_{12} deficiency that is not pernicious anemia, 1,000 mcg of oral **cobalamin** are given until normal B_{12} levels are achieved—usually 6 to 12 weeks. In seriously ill patients, both **vitamin B_{12}** and **folic acid** may need to be administered. Dosages for children vary, based on the presence of hematological versus neurological signs. Oral doses up to 1,000 mcg have been used; however, oral therapy is not usually recommended for deficiency states in children.

Unnecessary Vitamin B_{12} Therapy

Some well-meaning health-care providers have given parenteral **vitamin B_{12}** to patients with fatigue or other vague symptoms. Sometimes these patients report feeling better, in all probability related to a placebo effect. There is no indication that **vitamin B_{12}** is useful for patients who do not have a deficiency state. Although the risk in giving this drug is low, a better approach is to determine the patient's underlying problem, such as depression, anxiety, or the presence of an inflammatory disease or other disorder that may inhibit erythropoiesis.

Rational Drug Selection

Of the two main parenteral forms of **vitamin B_{12}**, **cyanocobalamin (Crystamine, Cyanoject, Cyomin)** is less protein bound and has a shorter duration of action than **hydroxocobalamin (Hydrobexan, Hydro-Cobex, Hydro-Crysti-12)** (Table 18–18). The latter form may mean less frequent injections, but antibody reactions are more common with this form. Either one works as well.

For patients with pernicious anemia, dietary deficiency, or inadequate secretion of intrinsic factor, **intranasal cyanocobalamin (Nascobal)** has been approved by the FDA for maintenance therapy of patients with hematological remission after initial treatment. Once-weekly dosing of **cyanocobalamin** gives a 500-mcg dose.

Oral replacement may be used once the patient has reached normal vitamin B_{12} levels via parenteral administration. Oral **cyanocobalamin** offers ease of administration and is inexpensive ($5.99 for 60 tablets at http://www.drugstore.com).

Monitoring

Sudden drops in serum potassium levels have been reported with **vitamin B_{12}** therapy. Serum potassium levels should be monitored closely for the first 48 hours and **supplemental oral potassium** given if needed. Reticulocyte counts, Hct, iron, folic acid, and vitamin B_{12} serum levels are obtained prior to treatment, between the fifth and the seventh day of therapy, at one month, then every 3 to 6 months. If folate levels are also low, **folic acid** may need to be administered. Monitoring for **folic acid** is discussed in the section on that drug. Relapse of symptoms is not uncommon in the presence of continuing therapy. Hematological evaluations should continue at regular intervals throughout the patient's lifetime, based on the individual's response to therapy.

Patient Education

Administration

Orally administered **vitamin B_{12}** should be taken with meals to increase absorption. It may be taken with fruit juices, but ascorbic acid alters the stability of the drug. Expensive vitamin preparations are no more efficacious than are less costly ones. Vitamins are not a substitute for a well-balanced diet.

Treating pernicious anemia requires administrating **vitamin B_{12}** for the rest of the patient's life. Failure to do so leads to the return of anemia and the development of incapacitating and irreversible damage to spinal cord nerves. IM injections should be given in large muscles such as the buttock or thigh, and SC injections should be given deeply in these same areas.

Adverse Drug Reactions

Diarrhea, itching, and urticaria may sometimes temporarily occur. Hypokalemia has occurred early in the treatment of severe anemia. Health-care providers should monitor for this problem. Diets high in potassium may help. Rare cardiac and pulmonary symptoms have occurred. Patients should report shortness of breath, swelling in the lower legs or ankles, and pain or redness in the calves.

Table 18–18 ◆ **Available Dosage Forms: Vitamin B_{12}**

Drug	Dosage Form	How Supplied	Cost
Vitamin B_{12}	Tablet: 100-mcg, 500-mcg and 1,000-mcg	In bottles of 100	500 mcg = $5.99/100 tablets 1000 mcg = $10.79/100 tablets
Big-Shot B_{12}	Tablet: 5,000 mcg	In bottles of 30 and 60	5000 mcg = $34.99/120 tablets
Vitamin B_{12}	Lozenges: 100-mcg 250-mcg and 500-mcg	In bottles of 100 In bottles of 100 and 250	2500 mcg = $6.49/50 lozenges 5000 mcg = $6.49/30 lozenges
Nascobal	Intranasal: 500 mcg/0.1 mL (500 mcg in each activation)	In 2.3 mL-bottle In 5 mL-bottle	$277.97/2.3 mL
Hydroxocobalamin, crystalline (Hydro Cobex, Hydro-Crysti 12, LA-12)	Injection: 1,000 mcg/mL	In 30-mL multidose vial	
Cyanocobalamin, crystalline (vitamin B_{12})	Tablet: 500 mcg and 1,000 mcg	In bottle of 100	
Cyanocobalamin, crystalline (vitamin B_{12}, Crystamine, Crysti 1000 Cyanojet, Cyomin, Rubesol-1000)	Injection: 1,000 mcg/mL	In 1 mL vial In 10- and 30-mL multidose vials	1 mL vial = $35.99/25 vials $19.99/30 mL $13.99/10mL

REFERENCES

Albers, G., Amarenco, P., Easton, J., Sacco, R., & Teal, P. (2004). Antithrombotic and thrombolytic therapy for ischemic stroke: The Seventh ACCP Conference on Antithrombotic and Thrombolytic Therapy. *Chest, 126*(Suppl. 3), 483S–512S.

American Heart Association. (2010). Diabetes and aspirin. Retrieved from http://www.americanheart.org/presenter.jhtml?identifier=3044772

American Heart Association Writing Group Members, Lloyd-Jones, D., et al. (2010). Heart disease and stroke statistics 2010 update: A report from the American Heart Association. *Circulation, 121,* e46–e215.

Bates, SM, Greer, IA, Pabinger, I, Sofaer, S, Hirsh, J. (2008). Venous thromboembolism, thrombophilia, antithrombotic therapy, and pregnancy: American College of Chest Physicians Evidence-Based Clinical Practice Guidelines (8th Edition). Chest 133(6 Suppl):844S-86S

Boden, W. (2003). Practical approach to incorporating new studies and guidelines for antiplatelet therapy in the management of patients with non–ST-segment elevation acute coronary syndrome. *American Journal of Cardiology, 93*(1), 69–72.

Brender, E. (2006). Granulocyte-stimulating factor. *JAMA, 295,* 1088.

Coomarasamy, A., Honest, H., Papaioannou, S., Gee, H., & Khan, K. (2003). Aspirin for prevention of preeclampsia in women with historical risk factors: A systematic review. *Obstetrics and Gynecology, 101,* 1319–1332.

Diner, B. (2003). Anticoagulation or antiplatelet therapy for non-rheumatic atrial fibrillation and flutter. *Annals of Emergency Medicine, 41*(1), 141–143.

Hirsh, J., Fuster, V., Ansell, J., & Halperin, J. (2003). American Heart Association/American College of Cardiology Foundation guide to warfarin therapy. *Circulation, 107*(12), 1692–1711.

Hirsh, J., Guyatt, G., Albers, G. W., Harrington, R., & Schunemann, H. J. (2008). Antithrombotic and thrombolytic therapy. Executive summary: *American College of Chest Physicians evidence-based clinical practice guidelines* (8th edition). *Chest, 133,* 71S–109S.

Hundal, R., Petersen, K., Mayerson, A., Randhawa, P., Inzucchi, S., Shoelson, S., et al. (2002). Mechanism by which high-dose aspirin improves glucose metabolism in type 2 diabetes. *Journal of Clinical Investigation, 109*(10), 1321–1326.

Hurlen, M., Abdelnoor, M., Smith, P., Erikssen, J., & Arnesan, H. (2002). Warfarin, aspirin or both after myocardial infarction. *New England Journal of Medicine, 347,* 969–974.

Institute for Clinical Systems Improvement (ICSI). (2010). *Antithrombolic therapy supplement* (8th ed.). Bloomington, MN: ICSI Health Care Guideline. Retrieved from http://www.icsi.org.

Kniff-Dutmer, E., Schut, G., & van der Laar, M. (2003). Concomitant coumarin-NSAID therapy and risk for bleeding. *Annals of Pharmacotherapy, 37*(1), 12–16.

LactMed (2010). Warfarin. LactMed. National Library of Medicine: Bethesda, MD. Retrieved from http://toxnet.nlm.nih.gov/cgi-bin/sis/search/f?./temp/~HQpIfb:1

Lee, A., Levine, M., Baker, R., Bowden, C., Kakkar, A., Prins, M., & Gent, M. (2003). Low-molecular-weight heparin versus a coumarin for the prevention of recurrent venous thrombosis in patients with cancer. *New England Journal of Medicine, 349,* 146–153.

McCance, K., & Huether, S. (2010). *Pathophysiology: The biological basis for disease in adults and children* (6th ed.). St. Louis, MO: Mosby.

McNamara, R., Tamariz, L., Segal, J., & Bass, E. (2003). Management of atrial fibrillation: A review of the evidence for the role of pharmacologic therapy, electrical cardioversion and echocardiography. *Annals of Internal Medicine, 139,* 1018–1033.

Menendez-Jandula, B., Sosuto, J., Oliver, A., Montserrat, I., Quintana, M., Gich, I., et al. (2005). Comparing self-management of oral anticoagulant therapy with clinic management. *Annals of Internal Medicine, 142*(1), 1–10.

Nowak, S., & Jaber, L. (2003). Aspirin dose for prevention of cardiovascular disease in diabetics. *Annals of Pharmacotherapy, 37*(1), 116–121.

Renna, N. F., Vazquez, M. A., Lama, M. C., Gonzalez, E. S., & Maitello, R. M. (2009). Effect of chronic aspirin administration on an experimental model of metabolic syndrome. *Clinical and Experimental Pharmacology and Physiology, 36,* 162–168.

Salem, D., Stein, P., Al-Ahmad, A., Bussey, H., Horstkotte, D., Miller, N., et al. (2004). Antithrombotic therapy in valvular heart disease—native and prosthetic: The Seventh ACCP Conference on Antithrombotic and Thrombolytic Therapy. *Chest, 126*(Suppl. 3), 457S–482S.

Sebastian, J., & Tresch, D. (2000). Use of oral anticoagulants in older patients. *Drugs and Aging, 16,* 409–435.

Singer, D., Albers, G., Dalen, J., Go, A., Halperin, J., & Manning, W. (2004). Antithrombotic therapy in atrial fibrillation: The Seventh ACCP Conference on Antithrombotic and Thrombolytic Therapy. *Chest, 126*(Suppl. 3), 429S–456S.

Snow, V., Weiss, K., LeFevre, M., McNamara, R., Bass, E., Green, L., et al, for the AAFP/ACP Panel on Atrial Fibrillation. (2003). Management of newly detected atrial fibrillation: A clinical practice guideline from the American Academy of Family Physicians and the American College of Physicians. *Annals of Internal Medicine, 139*(12), 1009–1017.

Stein, P. D., Matta, F., Masani, M. H., & Diaczok, B. (2010). Silent pulmonary embolism in patients with deep venous thrombosis: A systemic review. *American Journal of Medicine, 123,* 426–431.

Tang, E., Lai, C., Lee, K., Wong, R., Cheng, G., & Chan, T. (2003). Relationship between patients' warfarin knowledge and anticoagulation control. *Annals of Pharmacotherapy, 37*(1), 34–39.

Weitz, J. I., Hirsh, J., & Samama, M. M. (2004). New anticoagulant drugs: The Seventh ACCP Conference on Antithrombotic and Thrombolytic Therapy. *Chest, 126,* 265S–286S.

Wells, P., Holbrook, A., & Crowther, N. (1994). The interaction of warfarin with drugs and food: A critical review of the literature. *Annals of Internal Medicine, 121,* 676–683.

CHAPTER 19

DRUGS AFFECTING THE IMMUNE SYSTEM

Teri Moser Woo

Chapter Outline

Primary care providers prescribe **immunizations** frequently, with pediatric providers prescribing many **vaccines** daily. Although vaccination is typically associated with children, the Centers for Disease Control and Prevention (CDC) recommends a number of **vaccines** for adolescents and adults. A dramatic decrease is seen in **vaccine**-preventable diseases when mass campaigns are implemented, with cases of invasive *Haemophilus influenzae* decreasing 99 percent, pertussis decreasing 93 percent, and hepatitis A dropping 91 percent (CDC, 2010g; Immunization Action Coalition, 2010).

The immunization schedules may change, but the underlying premise of preventing the spread of infectious disease through mass immunization of susceptible populations does not change. The success of mass vaccination is measured not only in decreased numbers of vaccine-preventable illnesses but also in the resurgence of diseases such as polio and measles when programs are halted (Katz, 2005; Roush, Murphy, & the Vaccine-Preventable Disease Table Working Group, 2007; World Health Organization [WHO], 2006). This chapter discusses **immunizations**, **immune globulin serums**, and the diagnostic drugs used in primary care, such as **purified protein derivative (PPD)** for tuberculosis (TB) screening. The immunomodulators **cyclosporine** and **azathioprine** are addressed. The use of **interferon** is not discussed here because it is usually prescribed by specialty care providers.

IMMUNIZATIONS

Vaccination is the single best technique for preventing infectious disease. Vaccines exist for many diseases that affect adults and children. This section of the chapter discusses active immunization with either attenuated or inactivated infective agents, the recommended schedule of immunizations for adults and children, and the true precautions and contraindications to immunization. Issues surrounding immunization such as barriers to immunization are discussed, as well as immunization of special populations and travel immunizations.

Vaccines are divided into two different types: those that are made from attenuated ("modified-live") or inactivated ("killed") infective agents. Attenuated vaccines include measles, mumps, and rubella (MMR); oral polio (OPV); varicella virus (Varivax, ProQuad); yellow fever (YF-Vax); live, attenuated virus influenza vaccine (Flumist); rotavirus (Rotarix, RotaTeq); varicella zoster (Zostavax); and bacilli Calmette-Guérin (BCG). Inactivated vaccines include diphtheria, tetanus, and pertussis (DTP, DTaP, DT, Td, Tdap), *H. influenzae* type B (HIB), hepatitis A and B, influenza (Fluzone), meningococcal (Menactra, Menomune), inactivated polio vaccine (IPV), human papillomavirus vaccine (Gardasil, Cervarix), pneumococcal polysaccharide (PPV23), and pneumococcal conjugate vaccine (PCV13). Cholera, Japanese encephalitis virus, and plague vaccine are other inactivated vaccines. Typhoid vaccine is available in an inactivated form and an oral live, attenuated form. The pharmacodynamics of each vaccine is discussed according to its category. Note that the information is included in this chapter.

ATTENUATED VACCINES

Influenza Live, Attenuated Influenza Vaccine

Pharmacodynamics

Influenza reaches epidemic levels in the winter months in temperate areas and was responsible for 36,000 deaths per year in the United States between 1990 and 1999 (Fiore et al, 2009). Influenza live, attenuated influenza vaccine (LAIV) (Flumist) is a trivalent vaccine containing two strains of influenza A and one of influenza B, the strains depending on the predicted circulating influenza virus strains. The vaccine is cold adapted, meaning the virus replicates easily in the mucosa of the nasopharynx, and temperature sensitive so it does not replicate effectively at core body temperature (38°C to 39°C).

Pharmacokinetics

The LAIV (Flumist) vaccine is administered intranasally with half of the dose administered in each nostril. The 50 percent mean clearance time is 50 minutes (range 40 to 60). Mucosal immunoglobulin A (IgA) antibodies peak in 2 to 11 weeks following vaccination (McCarthy & Kockler, 2004). Viral shed in nasopharyngeal secretions has been noted for an average of 7.6 days in a sample of children in day care (Vesikari et al, 2006). In 5- to 49-year-olds, 30 percent had viral shedding after receiving LAIV, with maximal shedding at 2 days' post-vaccine (Fiore et al, 2009).

Pharmacotherapeutics

Precautions and Contraindications

LAIV is contraindicated in patients with egg or egg product hypersensitivity.

LAIV is contraindicated in persons with asthma, reactive airways disease, or other chronic disorders of the pulmonary or cardiovascular systems; persons with other underlying medical conditions, including such metabolic diseases as diabetes, renal dysfunction, and hemoglobinopathies; and persons with known or suspected immunodeficiency diseases or who are receiving immunosuppressive therapies (Fiore et al, 2009).

Patients who are immunocompromised or who have HIV should not be vaccinated with LAIV.

LAIV should not be administered to patients who have had Guillain-Barré syndrome.

LAIV is Pregnancy Category C, and pregnant women should not be vaccinated with influenza LAIV. Caution should be used with administration to nursing mothers, as there is a possibility of viral shed in breast milk.

Use of live influenza vaccine is contraindicated in children under age 2 years owing to significant increased incidence of reactive airway disease and asthma. The vaccine is also contraindicated in children or adolescents receiving aspirin or other salicylates because of the association of Reye syndrome with wild-type influenza infection.

Adverse Drug Reactions

LAIV is usually well tolerated with generally mild and transient adverse effects. Among healthy adults, vaccine recipients reported 3 to 10 percent more cough, runny nose, nasal congestion, sore throat, and chills than placebo recipients, which was considered significant (Fiore, 2009). No serious adverse reactions have been reported in either children (older than age 2 years) or adult vaccine recipients.

Drug Interactions

The administration of LAIV and concurrent use of antivirals active against influenza A and/or B viruses has not been studied. The manufacturer recommends waiting 48 hours after discontinuing antivirals before administering LAIV.

LAIV should not be administered to children under age 17 years on aspirin therapy owing to the theoretical increased risk for Reye syndrome.

LAIV may be concurrently administered with measles, mumps, rubella (MMR) and varicella with no problems noted in developing an immune response. LAIV may be simultaneously administered with any of the inactivated **vaccines.** Inactivated or live **vaccines** may be administered the same day as LAIV, but if not administered the same day, the two live vaccines need to be separated by 4 weeks.

Clinical Use and Dosing

Children and adults aged 9 years through 49 years should receive 0.2 mL of LAIV as soon as it becomes available in the fall. Children aged 5 to 8 who have not had previous **influenza vaccination** should receive two doses (0.2 mL each) separated by 4 weeks (CDC, 2010i). Children who have previously received **influenza vaccine** need only one dose (0.2 mL).

LAIV (Flumist) comes prepackaged in prefilled single-use sprayers. The **vaccine** is thawed by holding the sprayer in the palm of the hand. It may also be thawed in the refrigerator and stored for up to 24 hours before use. Half of the dose is administered in one nostril while the patient is in an upright position; then the second half is administered in the second nostril.

Monitoring

Laboratory monitoring is not necessary after LAIV administration.

Patient Education

Because LAIV is a live virus **vaccine,** recipients should be advised to stay away from close contact with immunocompromised persons for 7 days after administration, although the risk is theoretical. Patients should report serious or moderate reactions, such as difficulty breathing, wheezing, hives, swelling, unusual weakness, and temperature 38.9°C or higher to their health-care provider.

Measles, Mumps, and Rubella Vaccine

Pharmacodynamics

Immunization with MMR or **measles vaccine** alone stimulates the immune system to produce disease-specific antibodies by inducing a subclinical infection with attenuated virus particles. This subclinical infection is not contagious. The vaccine-induced antibodies are capable of virus neutralization by complement activation, induction of cell-mediated immunity, and opsonization. The available single-agent and other combination vaccines include **measles virus vaccine (Attenuvax), mumps virus vaccine live (Mumpsvax), rubella (Meruvax II), rubella and mumps (Biavax II), and measles and rubella virus vaccine live (M-R-Vax II).** In 2005, a vaccine that added **varicella** to MMR (MMRV) received licensing (ProQuad) and is discussed in the next section.

Pharmacokinetics

The MMR vaccine is administered SC. Following SC injection, antibodies are detectable in 2 weeks (rubella may take 2 to 6 wk) in 95 percent of patients vaccinated, and immunity occurs in about 10 days. Immunity persists for 15 years or more, with permanent immunity developing in most patients. More than 99 percent of people who receive two doses of MMR separated by at least 1 month develop evidence of immunity to measles, which is why the current recommendation is for two doses. Mumps outbreaks in New York in 2005 and Iowa in late 2005 and early 2006 indicate that effectiveness of MMR against mumps is 80 percent after one dose and 90 percent after two doses, based on limited data (CDC, 2006a). Immunity to mumps persists for at least 20 years.

Pharmacotherapeutics

Precautions and Contraindications

MMR contains live, attenuated virus, and virus has been detected for 1 to 4 weeks after vaccination in the pharynx or nose of most patients who receive the vaccine; however, this does not appear to cause virus transmission.

According to the CDC, there are relatively few true contraindications to administering **MMR vaccine.** They include previous anaphylactic reaction to the MMR vaccine or any component of the **vaccine,** including **neomycin** (topically or systemically administered) or gelatin. A history of contact dermatitis to **neomycin** is not a contraindication to MMR. Anaphylactic reaction or hypersensitivity to eggs is no longer a contraindication to MMR.

Immunosuppression can potentiate virus production, and therefore, MMR vaccination is not recommended for immunocompromised patients. In patients with HIV infection, MMR vaccine can be administered if the patient is asymptomatic or without evidence of severe immunosuppression (CDC, 2006c). MMR should not be given to patients who are severely immunocompromised because of cancer, leukemia, or lymphoma or who are on immunosuppressive drug therapy, including high-dose **steroids** (Prednisone greater than 2 mg/kg/day or 20 mg/day in patients weighing more than 10 kg) or radiation therapy (CDC, 2006c). MMR may be given to close contacts of immunosuppressed patients, including health-care workers.

MMR vaccination is generally deferred if a patient has a moderate or severe febrile illness and is given when the patient recovers from the acute phase of the illness. Minor illnesses, with or without fever (diarrhea, upper respiratory infection, or otitis media), are not contraindications to MMR vaccination, and vaccination should not be postponed.

On The Horizon — **QUADRIVALENT INFLUENZA VACCINE**

Historically influenza vaccine has been a trivalent vaccine with two strains of influenza A and one of B. There is a quadrivalent nasal influenza vaccine developed by MedImmune in clinical trials that contains two strains of influenza A (influenza A/H1N1, A/H3N2) and two of influenza B (B/Yamagata and B/Victoria). Early trials are promising. It is likely that in the next 5 years there will be quadrivalent nasal and injectable influenza vaccine.

Patients who receive blood products should wait 3 months before administration of MMR (CDC, 2006a; Merck, 2010). Patients who receive **immune globulin** should wait 3 to 11 months before administering MMR (American Academy of Pediatrics [AAP], 2009b).

MMR vaccine should not be given to pregnant women or women who may become pregnant within 3 months after administration. There is a theoretical possibility of congenital rubella syndrome in the infant if the mother is given **rubella vaccine** when pregnant. Women should be asked if they are pregnant before administration of MMR and advised to avoid pregnancy for 3 months after administration of the vaccine. Pregnancy in the mother of a patient receiving MMR is not a contraindication.

MMR may be administered to breastfeeding women.

The MMR vaccine may be safely administered to children of all ages, although it may not be immunogenic in infants under age 12 months. If MMR or monovalent **measles vaccine** is administered to a child under age 12 months, then the child should be revaccinated with MMR at 12 to 15 months of age and receive a third dose of MMR at age 4 to 6 years.

Adverse Drug Reactions

Approximately 5 to 15 percent of children develop a fever of at least 103°F (39.5°C) after vaccination with MMR. The fever usually occurs 7 to 12 days after MMR vaccination. The fever usually lasts 1 to 2 days, and the patient is otherwise asymptomatic. MMR may cause a transient maculopapular rash 7 to 10 days after vaccination in 5 percent of patients.

Thrombocytopenia is a rare adverse reaction that may occur within 2 months of administration of MMR **vaccine**. The incidence of thrombocytopenia is 1 case per 1 million doses upon passive surveillance in the United States and 1 case per 30,000 to 40,000 doses in prospective studies. The clinical course of thrombocytopenia is generally benign and transient.

Drug Interactions

MMR should not be administered to patients receiving **immunosuppressants**, including high-dose **corticosteroids**, **interferon**, and **antineoplastic drugs**, because they may have insufficient response to immunization. Patients may remain susceptible despite immunization. The AAP states, "Children receiving <2 mg/kg per day of **prednisone** or its equivalent, or <20 mg/day if they weigh more than 10 kg, can receive **attenuated live-virus vaccines** during **corticosteroid** treatment" (AAP, 2009a).

The **MMR vaccine** may be inactivated by IG. To avoid inactivation of the attenuated virus, administer the MMR **vaccine** at least 14 to 30 days before or 3 months after the IG. If IG is being given in preparation for international travel, the MMR vaccine should be administered at least 2 weeks before IG.

MMR is not contraindicated if a PPD was done recently. PPD should be delayed for 4 to 6 weeks after an MMR has been given because it may interfere with the tuberculin skin test.

Administration of the MMR and **varicella vaccines** is compatible if done on the same day, with different needles, and at separate sites. If the two live **vaccines** are not given at the same time, an interval of 1 month between MMR and **varicella vaccine** is indicated. MMRV (ProQuad) is indicated for simultaneous vaccination against measles, mumps, rubella, and varicella in children 12 months to 12 years of age.

Clinical Use and Dosing

MMR is routinely given SC at 12 to 15 months of age with a repeat dose at age 4 to 6 years. The second dose of MMR may be given as soon as 4 weeks after the first dose, which is indicated during an epidemic or before international travel. Those children who have not received their second dose of MMR by age 12 should have it at that time. Adults born in 1957 or later who are at least age 18 (including those born outside the United States) should receive at least one dose of MMR if there is no serological proof of immunity or documentation of a dose given on or after the patient's first birthday. Health-care workers and other adults in high-risk groups, such as students entering college, military recruits, and international travelers, should receive a total of two doses of MMR. Adults born before 1957 are considered immune, but proof of immunity may be desirable for health-care workers. See Tables 19–1 and 19–2 for further information on routine dosing. The catch-up schedule for dosing children who are behind in the routine vaccine schedule is found in Table 19–3.

If administering a single-agent vaccine, the dosing is as follows: **Measles vaccine** is recommended in times of outbreak if exposure is considered likely. If **measles vaccine** is given before age 12 months, then reimmunization with MMR is recommended at age 12 to 15 months and again at school entry (age 4 to 6 years). **Mumps** vaccination is usually given in the form of MMR. If indicated in time of outbreak, the patient may receive one SC dose of **mumps vaccine**. **Rubella virus vaccine** is given as a single SC injection. **Rubella vaccine** is routinely given to nonimmune postpartum women before hospital discharge.

Monitoring

Laboratory monitoring is not necessary after MMR administration. Rubella titer may be drawn to determine if a patient is immune.

Patient Education

All patients or the parents or guardians of the patients are required by law to receive Vaccine Information Statements (VISs) that are developed by the CDC. They are available in a variety of languages, and every effort to provide

Table 19–1 **Recommended Immunization Schedule for Persons Aged 0 Through 6 Years—United States, 2011**

Recommended Immunization Schedule for Persons Aged 0 Through 6 Years—United States • 2011

For those who fall behind or start late, see the catch-up schedule

Vaccine ▼ Age ▶	Birth	1 month	2 months	4 months	6 months	12 months	15 months	18 months	19–23 months	2–3 years	4–6 years
Hepatitis B[1]	HepB	HepB			HepB						
Rotavirus[2]			RV	RV	RV[2]						
Diphtheria, Tetanus, Pertussis[3]			DTaP	DTaP	DTaP	see footnote[3]	DTaP				DTaP
Haemophilus influenzae type b[4]			Hib	Hib	Hib[4]	Hib					
Pneumococcal[5]			PCV	PCV	PCV	PCV				PPSV	
Inactivated Poliovirus[6]			IPV	IPV	IPV						IPV
Influenza[7]					Influenza (Yearly)						
Measles, Mumps, Rubella[8]						MMR		see footnote[8]			MMR
Varicella[9]						Varicella		see footnote[9]			Varicella
Hepatitis A[10]						HepA (2 doses)				HepA Series	
Meningococcal[11]										MCV4	

Range of recommended ages for all children

Range of recommended ages for certain high-risk groups

This schedule includes recommendations in effect as of December 21, 2010. Any dose not administered at the recommended age should be administered at a subsequent visit, when indicated and feasible. The use of a combination vaccine generally is preferred over separate injections of its equivalent component vaccines. Considerations should include provider assessment, patient preference, and the potential for adverse events. Providers should consult the relevant Advisory Committee on Immunization Practices statement for detailed recommendations: **http://www.cdc.gov/vaccines/pubs/acip-list.htm.** Clinically significant adverse events that follow immunization should be reported to the Vaccine Adverse Event Reporting System (VAERS) at **http://www.vaers.hhs.gov** or by telephone, **800-822-7967**.

1. **Hepatitis B vaccine (HepB).** (Minimum age: birth)
   At birth:
   - Administer monovalent HepB to all newborns before hospital discharge.
   - If mother is hepatitis B surface antigen (HBsAg)-positive, administer HepB and 0.5 mL of hepatitis B immune globulin (HBIG) within 12 hours of birth.
   - If mother's HBsAg status is unknown, administer HepB within 12 hours of birth. Determine mother's HBsAg status as soon as possible and, if HBsAg-positive, administer HBIG (no later than age 1 week).

   Doses following the birth dose:
   - The second dose should be administered at age 1 or 2 months. Monovalent HepB should be used for doses administered before age 6 weeks.
   - Infants born to HBsAg-positive mothers should be tested for HBsAg and antibody to HBsAg 1 to 2 months after completion of at least 3 doses of the HepB series, at age 9 through 18 months (generally at the next well-child visit).
   - Administration of 4 doses of HepB to infants is permissible when a combination vaccine containing HepB is administered after the birth dose.
   - Infants who did not receive a birth dose should receive 3 doses of HepB on a schedule of 0, 1, and 6 months.
   - The final (3rd or 4th) dose in the HepB series should be administered no earlier than age 24 weeks.
2. **Rotavirus vaccine (RV).** (Minimum age: 6 weeks)
   - Administer the first dose at age 6 through 14 weeks (maximum age: 14 weeks 6 days). Vaccination should not be initiated for infants aged 15 weeks 0 days or older.
   - The maximum age for the final dose in the series is 8 months 0 days
   - If Rotarix is administered at ages 2 and 4 months, a dose at 6 months is not indicated.
3. **Diphtheria and tetanus toxoids and acellular pertussis vaccine (DTaP).** (Minimum age: 6 weeks)
   - The fourth dose may be administered as early as age 12 months, provided at least 6 months have elapsed since the third dose.
4. ***Haemophilus influenzae* type b conjugate vaccine (Hib).** (Minimum age: 6 weeks)
   - If PRP-OMP (PedvaxHIB or Comvax [HepB-Hib]) is administered at ages 2 and 4 months, a dose at age 6 months is not indicated.
   - Hiberix should not be used for doses at ages 2, 4, or 6 months for the primary series but can be used as the final dose in children aged 12 months through 4 years.
5. **Pneumococcal vaccine.** (Minimum age: 6 weeks for pneumococcal conjugate vaccine [PCV]; 2 years for pneumococcal polysaccharide vaccine [PPSV])
   - PCV is recommended for all children aged younger than 5 years. Administer 1 dose of PCV to all healthy children aged 24 through 59 months who are not completely vaccinated for their age.
   - A PCV series begun with 7-valent PCV (PCV7) should be completed with 13-valent PCV (PCV13).
   - A single supplemental dose of PCV13 is recommended for all children aged 14 through 59 months who have received an age-appropriate series of PCV7.
   - A single supplemental dose of PCV13 is recommended for all children aged 60 through 71 months with underlying medical conditions who have received an age-appropriate series of PCV7.
   - The supplemental dose of PCV13 should be administered at least 8 weeks after the previous dose of PCV7. See *MMWR* 2010:59(No. RR-11).
   - Administer PPSV at least 8 weeks after last dose of PCV to children aged 2 years or older with certain underlying medical conditions, including a cochlear implant.
6. **Inactivated poliovirus vaccine (IPV).** (Minimum age: 6 weeks)
   - If 4 or more doses are administered prior to age 4 years an additional dose should be administered at age 4 through 6 years.
   - The final dose in the series should be administered on or after the fourth birthday and at least 6 months following the previous dose.
7. **Influenza vaccine (seasonal).** (Minimum age: 6 months for trivalent inactivated influenza vaccine [TIV]; 2 years for live, attenuated influenza vaccine [LAIV])
   - For healthy children aged 2 years and older (i.e., those who do not have underlying medical conditions that predispose them to influenza complications), either LAIV or TIV may be used, except LAIV should not be given to children aged 2 through 4 years who have had wheezing in the past 12 months.
   - Administer 2 doses (separated by at least 4 weeks) to children aged 6 months through 8 years who are receiving seasonal influenza vaccine for the first time or who were vaccinated for the first time during the previous influenza season but only received 1 dose.
   - Children aged 6 months through 8 years who received no doses of monovalent 2009 H1N1 vaccine should receive 2 doses of 2010–2011 seasonal influenza vaccine. See *MMWR* 2010;59(No. RR-8):33–34.
8. **Measles, mumps, and rubella vaccine (MMR).** (Minimum age: 12 months)
   - The second dose may be administered before age 4 years, provided at least 4 weeks have elapsed since the first dose.
9. **Varicella vaccine.** (Minimum age: 12 months)
   - The second dose may be administered before age 4 years, provided at least 3 months have elapsed since the first dose.
   - For children aged 12 months through 12 years the recommended minimum interval between doses is 3 months. However, if the second dose was administered at least 4 weeks after the first dose, it can be accepted as valid.
10. **Hepatitis A vaccine (HepA).** (Minimum age: 12 months)
    - Administer 2 doses at least 6 months apart.
    - HepA is recommended for children aged older than 23 months who live in areas where vaccination programs target older children, who are at increased risk for infection, or for whom immunity against hepatitis A is desired.
11. **Meningococcal conjugate vaccine, quadrivalent (MCV4).** (Minimum age: 2 years)
    - Administer 2 doses of MCV4 at least 8 weeks apart to children aged 2 through 10 years with persistent complement component deficiency and anatomic or functional asplenia, and 1 dose every 5 years thereafter.
    - Persons with human immunodeficiency virus (HIV) infection who are vaccinated with MCV4 should receive 2 doses at least 8 weeks apart.
    - Administer 1 dose of MCV4 to children aged 2 through 10 years who travel to countries with highly endemic or epidemic disease and during outbreaks caused by a vaccine serogroup.
    - Administer MCV4 to children at continued risk for meningococcal disease who were previously vaccinated with MCV4 or meningococcal polysaccharide vaccine after 3 years if the first dose was administered at age 2 through 6 years.

The Recommended Immunization Schedules for Persons Aged 0 Through 18 Years are approved by the Advisory Committee on Immunization Practices (**http://www.cdc.gov/vaccines/recs/acip**), the American Academy of Pediatrics (**http://www.aap.org**), and the American Academy of Family Physicians (**http://www.aafp.org**).

Department of Health and Human Services • Centers for Disease Control and Prevention

Table 19–2 **Recommended Immunization Schedule for Persons Aged 7 Through 18 Years—United States, 2011**

Recommended Immunization Schedule for Persons Aged 7 Through 18 Years—United States • 2011

For those who fall behind or start late, see the schedule below and the catch-up schedule

Vaccine ▼ Age ▶	7–10 years	11–12 years	13–18 years
Tetanus, Diphtheria, Pertussis[1]		Tdap	Tdap
Human Papillomavirus[2]	see footnote [2]	HPV (3 doses)(females)	HPV series
Meningococcal[3]	MCV4	MCV4	MCV4
Influenza[4]	Influenza (Yearly)		
Pneumococcal[5]	Pneumococcal		
Hepatitis A[6]	HepA Series		
Hepatitis B[7]	Hep B Series		
Inactivated Poliovirus[8]	IPV Series		
Measles, Mumps, Rubella[9]	MMR Series		
Varicella[10]	Varicella Series		

Range of recommended ages for all children

Range of recommended ages for catch-up immunization

Range of recommended ages for certain high-risk groups

This schedule includes recommendations in effect as of December 21, 2010. Any dose not administered at the recommended age should be administered at a subsequent visit, when indicated and feasible. The use of a combination vaccine generally is preferred over separate injections of its equivalent component vaccines. Considerations should include provider assessment, patient preference, and the potential for adverse events. Providers should consult the relevant Advisory Committee on Immunization Practices statement for detailed recommendations: **http://www.cdc.gov/vaccines/pubs/acip-list.htm**. Clinically significant adverse events that follow immunization should be reported to the Vaccine Adverse Event Reporting System (VAERS) at **http://www.vaers.hhs.gov** or by telephone, **800-822-7967.**

1. **Tetanus and diphtheria toxoids and acellular pertussis vaccine (Tdap).** (Minimum age: 10 years for Boostrix and 11 years for Adacel))
   - Persons aged 11 through 18 years who have not received Tdap should receive a dose followed by Td booster doses every 10 years thereafter.
   - Persons aged 7 through 10 years who are not fully immunized against pertussis (including those never vaccinated or with unknown pertussis vaccination status) should receive a single dose of Tdap. Refer to the catch-up schedule if additional doses of tetanus and diphtheria toxoid–containing vaccine are needed.
   - Tdap can be administered regardless of the interval since the last tetanus and diphtheria toxoid–containing vaccine.
2. **Human papillomavirus vaccine (HPV).** (Minimum age: 9 years)
   - Quadrivalent HPV vaccine (HPV4) or bivalent HPV vaccine (HPV2) is recommended for the prevention of cervical precancers and cancers in females.
   - HPV4 is recommended for prevention of cervical precancers, cancers, and genital warts in females.
   - HPV4 may be administered in a 3-dose series to males aged 9 through 18 years to reduce their likelihood of genital warts.
   - Administer the second dose 1 to 2 months after the first dose and the third dose 6 months after the first dose (at least 24 weeks after the first dose).
3. **Meningococcal conjugate vaccine, quadrivalent (MCV4).** (Minimum age: 2 years)
   - Administer MCV4 at age 11 through 12 years with a booster dose at age 16 years.
   - Administer 1 dose at age 13 through 18 years if not previously vaccinated.
   - Persons who received their first dose at age 13 through 15 years should receive a booster dose at age 16 through 18 years.
   - Administer 1 dose to previously unvaccinated college freshmen living in a dormitory.
   - Administer 2 doses at least 8 weeks apart to children aged 2 through 10 years with persistent complement component deficiency and anatomic or functional asplenia, and 1 dose every 5 years thereafter.
   - Persons with HIV infection who are vaccinated with MCV4 should receive 2 doses at least 8 weeks apart.
   - Administer 1 dose of MCV4 to children aged 2 through 10 years who travel to countries with highly endemic or epidemic disease and during outbreaks caused by a vaccine serogroup.
   - Administer MCV4 to children at continued risk for meningococcal disease who were previously vaccinated with MCV4 or meningococcal polysaccharide vaccine after 3 years (if first dose administered at age 2 through 6 years) or after 5 years (if first dose administered at age 7 years or older).
4. **Influenza vaccine (seasonal).**
   - For healthy nonpregnant persons aged 7 through 18 years (i.e., those who do not have underlying medical conditions that predispose them to influenza complications), either LAIV or TIV may be used.
   - Administer 2 doses (separated by at least 4 weeks) to children aged 6 months through 8 years who are receiving seasonal influenza vaccine for the first time or who were vaccinated for the first time during the previous influenza season but only received 1 dose.
   - Children 6 months through 8 years of age who received no doses of monovalent 2009 H1N1 vaccine should receive 2 doses of 2010-2011 seasonal influenza vaccine. See *MMWR* 2010;59(No. RR-8):33–34.
5. **Pneumococcal vaccines.**
   - A single dose of 13-valent pneumococcal conjugate vaccine (PCV13) may be administered to children aged 6 through 18 years who have functional or anatomic asplenia, HIV infection or other immunocompromising condition, cochlear implant or CSF leak. See *MMWR* 2010;59(No. RR-11).
   - The dose of PCV13 should be administered at least 8 weeks after the previous dose of PCV7.
   - Administer pneumococcal polysaccharide vaccine at least 8 weeks after the last dose of PCV to children aged 2 years or older with certain underlying medical conditions, including a cochlear implant. A single revaccination should be administered after 5 years to children with functional or anatomic asplenia or an immunocompromising condition.
6. **Hepatitis A vaccine (HepA).**
   - Administer 2 doses at least 6 months apart.
   - HepA is recommended for children aged older than 23 months who live in areas where vaccination programs target older children, or who are at increased risk for infection, or for whom immunity against hepatitis A is desired.
7. **Hepatitis B vaccine (HepB).**
   - Administer the 3-dose series to those not previously vaccinated. For those with incomplete vaccination, follow the catch-up schedule.
   - A 2-dose series (separated by at least 4 months) of adult formulation Recombivax HB is licensed for children aged 11 through 15 years.
8. **Inactivated poliovirus vaccine (IPV).**
   - The final dose in the series should be administered on or after the fourth birthday and at least 6 months following the previous dose.
   - If both OPV and IPV were administered as part of a series, a total of 4 doses should be administered, regardless of the child's current age.
9. **Measles, mumps, and rubella vaccine (MMR).**
   - The minimum interval between the 2 doses of MMR is 4 weeks.
10. **Varicella vaccine.**
    - For persons aged 7 through 18 years without evidence of immunity (see *MMWR* 2007;56[No. RR-4]), administer 2 doses if not previously vaccinated or the second dose if only 1 dose has been administered.
    - For persons aged 7 through 12 years, the recommended minimum interval between doses is 3 months. However, if the second dose was administered at least 4 weeks after the first dose, it can be accepted as valid.
    - For persons aged 13 years and older, the minimum interval between doses is 4 weeks.

The Recommended Immunization Schedules for Persons Aged 0 Through 18 Years are approved by the Advisory Committee on Immunization Practices (**http://www.cdc.gov/vaccines/recs/acip**), the American Academy of Pediatrics (**http://www.aap.org**), and the American Academy of Family Physicians (**http://www.aafp.org**).

Department of Health and Human Services • Centers for Disease Control and Prevention

Table 19–3 Catch-Up Immunization Schedule for Persons Aged 4 Months Through 18 Years Who Start Late or Who Are More Than 1 Month Behind

Catch-up Immunization Schedule for Persons Aged 4 Months Through 18 Years Who Start Late or Who Are More Than 1 Month Behind—United States • 2011

The table below provides catch-up schedules and minimum intervals between doses for children whose vaccinations have been delayed. A vaccine series does not need to be restarted, regardless of the time that has elapsed between doses. Use the section appropriate for the child's age

Vaccine	Minimum Age for Dose 1	Minimum Interval Between Doses: Dose 1 to Dose 2	Dose 2 to Dose 3	Dose 3 to Dose 4	Dose 4 to Dose 5
PERSONS AGED 4 MONTHS THROUGH 6 YEARS					
Hepatitis B[1]	Birth	**4 weeks**	**8 weeks** (and at least 16 weeks after first dose)		
Rotavirus[2]	6 wks	**4 weeks**	**4 weeks**[2]		
Diphtheria, Tetanus, Pertussis[3]	6 wks	**4 weeks**	**4 weeks**	**6 months**	**6 months**[3]
Haemophilus influenzae type b[4]	6 wks	**4 weeks** if first dose administered at younger than age 12 months **8 weeks (as final dose)** if first dose administered at age 12–14 months **No further doses needed** if first dose administered at age 15 months or older	**4 weeks**[4] if current age is younger than 12 months **8 weeks (as final dose)**[4] if current age is 12 months or older and first dose administered at younger than age 12 months and second dose administered at younger than 15 months **No further doses needed** if previous dose administered at age 15 months or older	**8 weeks (as final dose)** This dose only necessary for children aged 12 months through 59 months who received 3 doses before age 12 months	
Pneumococcal[5]	6 wks	**4 weeks** if first dose administered at younger than age 12 months **8 weeks (as final dose for healthy children)** if first dose administered at age 12 months or older or current age 24 through 59 months **No further doses needed** for healthy children if first dose administered at age 24 months or older	**4 weeks** if current age is younger than 12 months **8 weeks (as final dose for healthy children)** if current age is 12 months or older **No further doses needed** for healthy children if previous dose administered at age 24 months or older	**8 weeks (as final dose)** This dose only necessary for children aged 12 months through 59 months who received 3 doses before age 12 months or for children at high risk who received 3 doses at any age	
Inactivated Poliovirus[6]	6 wks	**4 weeks**	**4 weeks**	**6 months**[6]	
Measles, Mumps, Rubella[7]	12 mos	**4 weeks**			
Varicella[8]	12 mos	**3 months**			
Hepatitis A[9]	12 mos	**6 months**			
PERSONS AGED 7 THROUGH 18 YEARS					
Tetanus, Diphtheria/ Tetanus, Diphtheria, Pertussis[10]	7 yrs[10]	**4 weeks**	**4 weeks** if first dose administered at younger than age 12 months **6 months** if first dose administered at 12 months or older	**6 months** if first dose administered at younger than age 12 months	
Human Papillomavirus[11]	9 yrs	**Routine dosing intervals are recommended (females)**[11]			
Hepatitis A[9]	12 mos	**6 months**			
Hepatitis B[1]	Birth	**4 weeks**	**8 weeks** (and at least 16 weeks after first dose)		
Inactivated Poliovirus[6]	6 wks	**4 weeks**	**4 weeks**[6]	**6 months**[6]	
Measles, Mumps, Rubella[7]	12 mos	**4 weeks**			
Varicella[8]	12 mos	**3 months** if person is younger than age 13 years **4 weeks** if person is aged 13 years or older			

1. **Hepatitis B vaccine (HepB).**
   - Administer the 3-dose series to those not previously vaccinated.
   - The minimum age for the third dose of HepB is 24 weeks.
   - A 2-dose series (separated by at least 4 months) of adult formulation Recombivax HB is licensed for children aged 11 through 15 years.
2. **Rotavirus vaccine (RV).**
   - The maximum age for the first dose is 14 weeks 6 days. Vaccination should not be initiated for infants aged 15 weeks 0 days or older.
   - The maximum age for the final dose in the series is 8 months 0 days.
   - If Rotarix was administered for the first and second doses, a third dose is not indicated.
3. **Diphtheria and tetanus toxoids and acellular pertussis vaccine (DTaP).**
   - The fifth dose is not necessary if the fourth dose was administered at age 4 years or older.
4. ***Haemophilus influenzae* type b conjugate vaccine (Hib).**
   - 1 dose of Hib vaccine should be considered for unvaccinated persons aged 5 years or older who have sickle cell disease, leukemia, or HIV infection, or who have had a splenectomy.
   - If the first 2 doses were PRP-OMP (PedvaxHIB or Comvax), and administered at age 11 months or younger, the third (and final) dose should be administered at age 12 through 15 months and at least 8 weeks after the second dose.
   - If the first dose was administered at age 7 through 11 months, administer the second dose at least 4 weeks later and a final dose at age 12 through 15 months.
5. **Pneumococcal vaccine.**
   - Administer 1 dose of 13-valent pneumococcal conjugate vaccine (PCV13) to all healthy children aged 24 through 59 months with any incomplete PCV schedule (PCV7 or PCV13).
   - For children aged 24 through 71 months with underlying medical conditions, administer 1 dose of PCV13 if 3 doses of PCV were received previously or administer 2 doses of PCV13 at least 8 weeks apart if fewer than 3 doses of PCV were received previously.
   - A single dose of PCV13 is recommended for certain children with underlying medical conditions through 18 years of age. See age-specific schedules for details.
   - Administer pneumococcal polysaccharide vaccine (PPSV) to children aged 2 years or older with certain underlying medical conditions, including a cochlear implant, at least 8 weeks after the last dose of PCV. A single revaccination should be administered after 5 years to children with functional or anatomic asplenia or an immunocompromising condition. See *MMWR* 2010;59(No. RR-11).
6. **Inactivated poliovirus vaccine (IPV).**
   - The final dose in the series should be administered on or after the fourth birthday and at least 6 months following the previous dose.
   - A fourth dose is not necessary if the third dose was administered at age 4 years or older and at least 6 months following the previous dose.
   - In the first 6 months of life, minimum age and minimum intervals are only recommended if the person is at risk for imminent exposure to circulating poliovirus (i.e., travel to a polio-endemic region or during an outbreak).
7. **Measles, mumps, and rubella vaccine (MMR).**
   - Administer the second dose routinely at age 4 through 6 years. The minimum interval between the 2 doses of MMR is 4 weeks.
8. **Varicella vaccine.**
   - Administer the second dose routinely at age 4 through 6 years.
   - If the second dose was administered at least 4 weeks after the first dose, it can be accepted as valid.
9. **Hepatitis A vaccine (HepA).**
   - HepA is recommended for children aged older than age 23 months who live in areas where vaccination programs target older children, or who are at increased risk for infection, or for whom immunity against hepatitis A is desired.
10. **Tetanus and diphtheria toxoids (Td) and tetanus and diphtheria toxoids and acellular pertussis vaccine (Tdap).**
    - Doses of DTaP are counted as part of the Td/Tdap series.
    - Tdap should be substituted for a single dose of Td in the catch-up series for children aged 7 through 10 years or as a booster for children aged 11 through 18 years; use Td for other doses.
11. **Human papillomavirus vaccine (HPV).**
    - Administer the series to females at age 13 through 18 years if not previously vaccinated or have not completed the vaccine series.
    - Quadrivalent HPV vaccine (HPV4) may be administered in a 3-dose series to males aged 9 through 18 years to reduce their likelihood of genital warts.
    - Use recommended routine dosing intervals for series catch-up (i.e., the second and third doses should be administered at 1 to 2 and 6 months after the first dose). The minimum interval between the first and second doses is 4 weeks. The minimum interval between the second and third doses is 12 weeks, and the third dose should be administered at least 24 weeks after the first dose.

Information about reporting reactions after immunization is available online at **http://www.vaers.hhs.gov** or by telephone, **800-822-7967**. Suspected cases of vaccine-preventable diseases should be reported to the state or local health department. Additional information, including precautions and contraindications for immunization, is available from the National Center for Immunization and Respiratory Diseases at **http://www.cdc.gov/vaccines** or telephone, **800-CDC-INFO** (800-232-4636).

Department of Health and Human Services • Centers for Disease Control and Prevention

adequate information to the patient or parent before immunization should be made. These statements are available at the CDC Web site or at http://www.immunize.org in multiple languages (Table 19–4).

The SC injection of MMR may sting the patient, who may have post-injection discomfort.

The VIS states that 5 to 15 percent of patients may experience a fever of up to 103°F (39.5°C) approximately 7 to 12 days after administration of MMR. The patient may also experience rash, malaise, or sore throat.

Table 19–4 Vaccine Information Statements

Vaccine Information Statements (VISs) are available from the Centers for Disease Control and Prevention (CDC) or your local health department for the following vaccines. They have also been translated into the languages listed below. A PDF version of these VISs (English and other languages) can be found at http://www.immunize.org.

VACCINES	
Anthrax	Meningococcal
Chickenpox	Measles, mumps, and rubella
Diphtheria, tetanus, and pertussis	Pneumococcus
HIB	Polio (oral and inactivated)
Hepatitis A	Rabies
Hepatitis B	Rotavirus
Influenza	Smallpox
Japanese encephalitis	Td, Tdap
Lyme disease	Typhoid
	Yellow fever

LANGUAGES	
Arabic	Korean
Armenian	Laotian
Bosnian	Marshallese
Burmese	Portuguese
Cambodian	Polish
Chinese	Punjabi
Croatian	Romanian
Farsi	Russian
French	Samoan
German	Serbo-Croatian
Haitian	Somali
Hindi	Spanish
Hmong	Tagalog
Ilokano	Thai
Italian	Turkish
Japanese	Vietnamese

Measles, Mumps, Rubella and Varicella Vaccine

Pharmacodynamics

Similar to MMR, the MMRV (ProQuad) vaccine is a live, attenuated virus vaccine that produces a subclinical infection, creating active immunity to measles, mumps, rubella, and varicella viruses.

Pharmacokinetics

The MMRV vaccine is administered SC. Following SC injection of the first dose, the response rate at 6 weeks for patients is 91.2 percent for varicella, 97.4 percent for measles, 98.8 percent for mumps, and 98.5 percent for rubella (Merck, 2010). More than 99 percent of people who receive two doses of MMRV separated by at least 3 months develop evidence of immunity to all four covered viruses; for that reason the current recommendation is for two doses.

Pharmacotherapeutics

Precautions and Contraindications

The contraindications for MMRV are the same as for MMR.

A history of anaphylactic reaction to **neomycin** or gelatin or any other component of the **vaccine**. Immediate treatment for anaphylaxis reaction should be available when administering MMRV.

MMRV is contraindicated in patients with primary or acquired immunodeficiency, including patients with immunosuppression associated with HIV/AIDS and patients with blood dyscrasias, leukemia, lymphomas of any type, or other malignant neoplasms affecting the bone marrow or lymphatic system. Immunosuppressive therapy, including high-dose **steroids**, may result in a more extensive vaccine-associated rash or disseminated disease. Low-dose, replacement, or short-burst therapy for asthma are not contraindications for MMRV administration.

MMRV should not be administered to a pregnant patient and the manufacturer recommends pregnancy should be avoided for at least 3 months following vaccination (Merck, 2010). MMRV (ProQuad) is Pregnancy Category C.

If a patient has untreated tuberculosis or a febrile illness with temperature greater than 101.3°F (38.5°C), then vaccination with MMRV should be deferred until the patient is well.

Because of the increased risk of fever and febrile seizures with MMRV, it should be used with caution in patients with a history of cerebral injury, seizures, or other conditions in which physiological stress due to fever should be avoided.

No data is available on the development of thrombocytopenia in patients vaccinated with MMRV (ProQuad). Because of the known risk for thrombocytopenia with MMR, use caution when administering MMRV.

Vaccination with MMRV should be avoided for 3 months after a blood transfusion or **immune globulin** administration.

Adverse Drug Reactions

The adverse drug reactions seen in MMRV are similar to MMR, except patients are more likely to develop fever and rash. There is a risk for developing a fever 7 to 12 days after MMR administration. In pre-licensure studies MMRV fever (equal to or greater than 102°F; equal to or greater than 39°C) was seen in 21.5 percent of patients, compared to 14.9 percent of patients receiving MMR (CDC, 2010h). Post-licensure studies of febrile seizures post-MMRV vaccination indicate one additional febrile seizure occurred 5 to 12 days after vaccination per 2,300 to 2,600 children aged 12 to 23 months, who had received the first dose of **MMRV vaccine** compared with children who had received the first dose of **MMR vaccine** and **varicella vaccine** administered as separate injections at the same visit (CDC, 2010h). This increased risk of febrile seizure is not seen after the second dose of MMRV administered at the 4- to 6-year visit.

There is a slightly increased risk of developing a measles-like rash from 2.1 percent with MMR alone to 3 percent with MMRV.

Additional adverse reactions include pain at injection site (22%), erythema (14.4%), and swelling (8.4%), similar to what is seen in patients receiving MMR (Merck, 2010).

Drug Interactions

Drug interactions with MMRV are the same as for MMR: immunosuppressants, **immune globulin**, **tuberculin skin tests**, and **salicylates**.

Clinical Use and Dosing

MMRV is also given SC at 12 to 15 months of age. The first dose may be given any time before age 12 years. Use of MMRV for the repeat dose at 4 to 6 years is well tolerated and results in higher levels of varicella antibodies (Reisinger et al, 2006). Three months should elapse before a second dose of MMRV is administered. MMRV may be administered one month after a dose of MMR.

Patient Education

The CDC recommends providers administering MMRV to children have a conversation with parents regarding the increased risk of fever and febrile seizures with the combination vaccine (CDC, 2010h). Parents of children should be informed about the slightly increased risk of febrile seizures 5 to 12 days after receiving the MMRV combination (Marin, Broder, Temte, Snider, & Seward, 2010). This risk will need to be weighed against the discomfort of two injections.

Oral Poliovirus Vaccine

Although **oral polio vaccine** (OPV) is no longer used in the United States, it is still used in other countries because of administration ease and low cost.

Pharmacodynamics

OPV stimulates the immune system to produce antipoliovirus antibodies against Sabin poliovirus types 1, 2, and 3. After oral administration, the live, attenuated virus enters the small intestine, where it replicates in the villous epithelial cells. These specialized epithelial cells transport the viral antigens to the B cells and macrophages, which process and produce antipoliovirus antibodies. In 1 to 2 weeks after a dose of OPV, antibodies are present. The live, attenuated poliovirus lingers in the gastrointestinal (GI) tract for 4 to 6 weeks, inducing both mucosal and serum antipoliovirus antibodies. The local secretory (intestinal) immune responses to OPV are greater than those induced by IPV. OPV induces intestinal immunity against wild strains of poliovirus; IPV does not. At least two doses of OPV are necessary for intestinal immunity. OPV may induce a herd type of immunity because of the spread of live, attenuated viruses to susceptible contacts during the viral shedding period of 4 to 6 weeks after dosing. Three doses of OPV result in sustained, lifelong immunity.

Pharmacokinetics

After oral administration of OPV, antibody stimulation occurs within 7 to 10 days. Poliovirus antibodies have been found in serum, nasal secretions, saliva, duodenal fluids, urine, and feces. Poliovirus antibodies are distributed into breast milk.

Pharmacotherapeutics

Precautions and Contraindications

An anaphylactic reaction to any previous dose of OPV is a contraindication to its use. Patients with neomycin or streptomycin hypersensitivity also should not receive OPV because these agents are contained in OPV in small quantities.

OPV should be delayed if a patient has a moderate or severe febrile illness or severe respiratory infection. Administration of OPV with current viral GI infection, ongoing diarrhea, or vomiting is contraindicated. Vomiting may prevent the vaccine from reaching the stomach and small intestine. Diarrhea may increase transit time, preventing proper contact of the vaccine viruses with villous intestinal cells, and lead to decreased immune response. Vaccine administration should be delayed until the vomiting and diarrhea have been resolved.

There is a risk that immunocompromised individuals may develop poliomyelitis from use of live poliovirus, which is in OPV. Cancer, leukemia, lymphoma, radiation therapy, and immunodeficiency, including HIV or AIDS, are contraindications to OPV use. Drugs that affect the immune system, including high-dose **steroids**, are also a contraindication to OPV use. There is a chance that immunosuppressed individuals may contract OPV-associated poliomyelitis from coming in contact with a patient who is shedding the virus. IPV is the drug of choice in immunocompromised patients. IPV should also be used if household members are immunocompromised.

Vaccination of pregnant women should be avoided. OPV is Pregnancy Category C. If exposure to poliomyelitis is imminent and immediate protection is needed, vaccinate with OPV or IPV according to the adult dosing schedule.

OPV is safe during breastfeeding and is routinely given during infancy.

Adverse Drug Reactions

The administration of OPV is associated with a low incidence (1 case/2.6 million doses) of paralytic poliomyelitis in patients who receive the vaccine and in household contacts. Vaccine-associated paralytic poliomyelitis (VAPP) is most likely to occur after the first dose of OPV. Household contacts are put at risk of developing VAPP because poliovirus is shed in the feces for 6 to 8 weeks after a dose of OPV. There is no risk of VAPP with the use of IPV, which is why, as of January 2000, IPV is the drug of choice for routine childhood immunization against polio in the United States.

Drug Interactions

OPV should not be administered to patients receiving **immunosuppressants**, including **corticosteroids**, **interferon**, and **antineoplastic drugs**, because there may be insufficient response to immunization. Patients may remain susceptible despite immunization. IPV is the recommended drug to use in these patients.

The CDC recommends that administration of live-virus **vaccines** be separated by intervals of at least 1 month, unless data are available regarding simultaneous vaccination (**MMR**, **hepatitis B vaccine** [**HBV**], **DTP**, **DTaP**, **influenza**, and **HIB** may be given with OPV). Concurrent administration of OPV and **cholera vaccine**, **parenteral typhoid vaccine**, or **plague vaccine** should generally be avoided because of increased adverse effects. Concurrent administration of **oral typhoid vaccine** live may result in decreased immune responses to OPV. IG may be given with OPV.

Clinical Use and Dosing

To eliminate the risk of VAPP, the CDC recommended in January 2000 an all-IPV schedule for childhood immunizations. OPV may be used only for special circumstances, such as mass vaccination campaigns to control outbreaks of paralytic polio and in unvaccinated children who will be traveling in less than 4 weeks to areas where polio is endemic or epidemic. OPV may be used in children who have received at least two doses of IPV and whose parents do not accept the recommended number of vaccine injections. VAPP should be discussed with these parents before administering OPV. See Tables 19–1, 19–2, and 19–3 for dosing schedules.

Patient Education

All patients or their parents or guardians are required by law to receive CDC VISs, which are available in a variety of languages. Every effort should be made to provide adequate information to patients and parents before immunization.

If a patient receives OPV, the patient and family should be instructed that virus is shed in the stools for 6 to 8 weeks and that good hand washing is crucial to preventing the small chance of contracting VAPP from the infected feces.

As previously mentioned, VAPP should be discussed with the parent or, if applicable, the patient before administering OPV.

Rotavirus Vaccine

Pharmacodynamics

Rotavirus is the leading cause of gastroenteritis in infants and young children worldwide. Almost every child in the United States will become infected with rotavirus by age 5 years, causing 400,000 doctor visits, and 55,000 to 70,000 hospital admissions (CDC, 2006b). **RotaTeq** is a live oral vaccine that contains five strains of rotavirus (G1, G2, G3, or G4, P7). **Rotarix** is indicated for the prevention of rotavirus gastroenteritis caused by G1, G3, G4, and G9. Both vaccines are live vaccines that replicate in the small intestine and induce active immunity against rotavirus.

Pharmacokinetics

Pharmacokinetic information regarding **rotavirus vaccine** is not available.

Pharmacotherapeutics

Precautions and Contraindications

Because **rotavirus vaccine** is a live virus vaccine, it should not be administered to infants who are or may be potentially immunocompromised including infants with blood dyscrasias, leukemia, lymphomas, or other malignant neoplasms; infants on immunosuppressive therapy; infants with primary and acquired immunodeficiency states including HIV/AIDS; and infants who have received blood transfusions or blood products in the past 42 days.

Infants who have a febrile illness should have the **vaccine** delayed, except when withholding the vaccine creates greater risk to the patient. A minor upper respiratory infection with low-grade fever (under 100.5°F) is not a reason for withholding **rotavirus vaccine**. The virus should not be administered to infants with acute gastroenteritis until it improves.

Rotavirus may be shed in the stools of patients receiving the **vaccine** (8.9% of patients in clinical trials); therefore, it is prudent to use caution if the infant will have close contact with persons with malignancies or who are otherwise immunocompromised, and contacts who are receiving immunosuppressive therapy.

Adverse Drug Reactions

A previous live rhesus rotavirus–based **vaccine** (**RotaShield**) was withdrawn from the market after it was found to be associated with intussusception. The risk for intussusception was evaluated in a large clinical trial of more than 70,000 infants, which found no association with intussusception and administration of **RotaTeq** or **Rotarix** (CDC, 2006b, 2009). The CDC has conducted a large ($N = 69{,}625$) study and determined there was no increased risk of developing intussusception from either currently available **rotavirus vaccine** (CDC, 2009). The CDC continues to monitor this.

GI symptoms are the major reported adverse effects in the clinical trials of **RotaTeq**. There was a slight increase incidence of vomiting in the **RotaTeq** patients (6.7% vs. 5.4% for placebo after dose 1, 5.0% vs. 4.4% for placebo after dose 2, and 3.6% vs. 3.2% for placebo after dose 3), as well as a slight increase in reports of diarrhea in the **RotaTeq** group (10.4% vs. 9.1% in placebo after dose 1, 8.6% vs. 6.4% in placebo group after dose 2, and 6.1% vs. 5.4% in placebo after dose 3). Symptoms of irritability did not differ between **RotaTeq** and placebo infants in all three doses.

Rotarix clinical trials found no increase in fever, diarrhea, or fussiness in patients who received **Rotarix** over placebo. Patients who received **Rotirix** had a slightly increased (13% versus 11%) incidence of vomiting in the week after administration.

Drug Interactions

During clinical trials, **RotaTeq** and **Rotarix** were routinely administered concurrently with DTaP, IPV, HIB, HBV, and **pneumococcal conjugate vaccine**. There was no evidence of reduced antibody response to these vaccines when administered with **RotaTeq** or **Rotarix** (CDC, 2009).

Clinical Use and Dosing

RotaTeq vaccination consists of a series of three ready-to-use oral liquid doses. The **vaccine** is administered orally beginning at 6 to 12 weeks of age with the second and third doses delivered in 4- to 10-week intervals. All doses of the **vaccine** should be delivered by age 32 weeks. **RotaTeq** was administered to preterm (25 to 36 wk gestation) infants according to their age in weeks, and there was no difference in adverse effects between the **vaccine** and the placebo. There are insufficient data on safety and efficacy outside of these age ranges.

Rotarix is a two-dose schedule of 1 mL per dose given at 2 to 4 months of age. The two doses may be administered between 6 and 24 weeks of age. The two doses should be administered at least 4 weeks apart.

The CDC has recommendations for both **rotavirus vaccines**, including the maximum age for the first dose, which is 14 weeks 6 days (CDC, 2009). If a child inadvertently given the first dose after 15 weeks and 0 days, then the series should be continued and completed by 8 months 0 days (CDC, 2009). **Rotavirus vaccine** may be administered before, after or concurrently with any blood product or antibody-containing product (IG). Ideally the series should all be the same **rotavirus** product, but if it is unknown whether the patient received **RotaTeq** or **Rotarix**, then the series should be completed with the product available to the clinic (CDC, 2009).

If the patient regurgitates, spits out or vomits the **rotavirus** vaccine, it should not be readministered.

Children who have had rotavirus gastroenteritis before completing the series should start or complete the series according to the standard schedule.

Patient Education

All patients or their parents or guardians are required by law to receive CDC VISs, which are available in a variety of languages. Every effort should be made to provide adequate information to patients and their parents before immunization.

Because **rotavirus vaccine** is a live vaccine shed in the stool, caregivers should encourage strict hand washing practices.

Parents should be instructed to report any adverse reactions to their health-care provider. Providers should fill out a Vaccine Adverse Event Reporting System (VAERS) form, available at http://www.vaers.hhs.gov/

Varicella Virus Vaccine

Pharmacodynamics

Varicella virus vaccine (**Varivax**) is a live **vaccine** that produces IgG antibody humoral immune response to varicella zoster virus (VZV). Vaccinated patients also have cell-mediated immune response, with activation of both CD41 helper T cells and CD81 T lymphocytes. Efficacy of **varicella vaccine** is measured by protection against disease and by protection against severe disease. Efficacy of one dose of **varicella vaccine** is 94.4 percent over a 10-year period, with protection against household exposure 90.2 percent (CDC, 2007b). The two-dose regimen is 98.3 percent effective against any disease and 96.4 percent effective against household exposure (CDC, 2007b). Vaccination appears to prevent serious disease even in patients who do not seroconvert. Post-vaccination cases of varicella are mild (less than 50 lesions, frequently not vesicular, mild or no fever) and patients recover quicker than when infected with wild virus (CDC, 2007b).

Pharmacokinetics

A single SC dose of **varicella virus vaccine** given to children aged 12 months to 12 years stimulates IgG antibody production and results in seroconversion rates of 85.7 percent 6 weeks after the first dose (CDC, 2007b). According to the CDC (2007b), in children aged 12 months to 12 years who are administered a second dose with 3 months between doses, there is a 99.6 percent response seroconversion rate. When the second dose is given at age 4 to 6 years, the response is 99.4 percent seroconversion rate. In patients, aged 13 and older, seroconversion rates are 78 to 82 percent; a second dose results in 99 percent seroconversion in adolescents and adults. Waning immunity has not been demonstrated, with high antibody levels measured for at least 10 years after vaccination.

Post-exposure prophylaxis with **varicella vaccine** is effective in preventing varicella disease. Administration to unvaccinated children within 3 days of exposure to varicella rash is 90 percent effective in preventing varicella and 70 percent effective if administered within 5 days of exposure (CDC, 2007b). Post-exposure prophylaxis is 100 percent effective in decreasing the severity of disease.

Pharmacotherapeutics

Precautions and Contraindications

Patients with **neomycin** or gelatin hypersensitivity should not receive **varicella vaccine** because there are small quantities of each in the **vaccine**.

Varicella vaccine should be delayed if a patient has a moderate or severe illness, with or without fever.

There is a risk that immunocompromised individuals will develop varicella from use of live virus for vaccination. Cancer, leukemia, lymphoma, radiation therapy, and immunodeficiency are contraindications to **varicella vaccine** use. Patients with symptomatic HIV infection should not receive **varicella vaccine.** Regarding asymptomatic HIV infected children, the CDC states, "HIV-infected children with CD4+ T-lymphocyte percentage >15 percent should be considered for vaccination with the single antigen **varicella vaccine**" (CDC, 2007b, p. 24).

Drugs that affect the immune system, including high-dose **steroids**, also contraindicate **varicella vaccine** use. Patients who are on systemic **steroids** (e.g., for asthma) may be vaccinated if they are receiving less than 2 mg/kg or less than 20 mg per day of **prednisone** and are not otherwise immunocompromised (CDC, 2007b).

Varicella vaccine may be given to a patient if an immunocompromised person is in the household. The patient who develops a rash after vaccination should avoid contact with the immunocompromised person for the duration of the rash, although there has been no evidence of transmission of virus to an immunocompromised person in post-licensure monitoring of more than 55 million doses (CDC, 2007b).

Vaccination of pregnant women should be avoided. **Varicella vaccine** is Pregnancy Category C. Pregnancy should be avoided for 1 to 3 months after vaccination. The manufacturer of **Varivax** has established a pregnancy registry to monitor maternal–fetal outcomes of pregnant women inadvertently administered the **varicella virus vaccine** live 3 months before or during pregnancy. For information about the registry, call 1-800-986-8999. In 10 years of monitoring via the pregnancy registry, no cases of congenital varicella syndrome or congenital varicella birth defects have been documented (CDC, 2007b). **Varicella vaccine** may be given if there is a pregnant household contact, such as the patient's mother. **Varicella vaccine** may be given to a nursing mother if the risk of exposure to natural VZV is high. It is not known if it is excreted in breast milk.

Adverse Drug Reactions

The reactions reported most frequently in children and adults that can be attributed to **varicella vaccine** include fever, injection site reaction, and a vesicular rash. In healthy children, fever of 102°F or higher is reported in 14.7 percent of vaccine recipients. Pain or discomfort at the injection site is reported in 19.3 percent, with 3.4 percent of patients developing a vesicular rash at the injection site. A generalized vesicular rash developed in 3.8 percent of patients, with the median number of five or fewer lesions in healthy children. The vesicular rash occurs within 26 days of injection with **varicella vaccine**.

Adult and adolescent patients require two injections and have similar adverse reactions. Fever in vaccine recipients aged 12 years and older was defined as a temperature of 100°F or higher. After the first dose of **varicella vaccine**, 10.2 percent reported fever, and 9.5 percent reported fever after the second dose. Localized reaction at the injection site was reported in 3 percent of adolescent and adult patients after the first dose and in 1 percent after the second dose. A generalized vesicular rash was reported by 5.5 percent after the first dose and 0.9 percent after the second dose.

Drug Interactions

Varicella vaccine should not be administered to patients receiving **immunosuppressants**, including high-dose **corticosteroids**, **interferon**, and **antineoplastic drugs**, because response to immunization may be insufficient. Patients may remain susceptible despite immunization. Patients receiving **prednisone** up to 20 mg per day or less than 2 mg/kg per day for less than 2 weeks may receive **varicella vaccine** (CDC, 2007b).

Whether **varicella vaccine** may be inactivated by **IG** is unknown, although other live-virus vaccines may be inactivated. **Varicella vaccine** should not be given for 3 to 11 months after **IG** is administered depending on the **IG** produced (CDC, 2007b). The CDC recommends that **IG** preparations should not be administered for 2 weeks after **varicella vaccine** is given; the manufacturer recommends waiting 2 months. If **IG** is given in the interval after vaccination, the recipient should be either revaccinated in 5 months or tested for varicella immunity 6 months later and revaccinated if indicated.

The **MMR** and **varicella vaccines** are compatible if they are administered on the same day, with different needles, and at separate sites, or in the form of **MMRV**. If the two live vaccines are not given at the same time, an interval of 1 month between **MMR** and **varicella vaccine** is indicated. **Varicella vaccine** may be given simultaneously with **DTaP**, **DT**, **Td**, **HIB**, **IPV**, **OPV**, **PCV13**, or **HBV**, using separate sites of injection.

Although no adverse effects from the use of **salicylates** or **aspirin** (**ASA**) have been reported, the manufacturer recommends avoidance of **ASA** for 6 weeks after vaccination.

Reye syndrome, which affects children younger than age 15 exclusively, has been associated with **aspirin** use following active varicella infection. Children who are on therapeutic ASA therapy may be vaccinated with the **varicella vaccine,** with close clinical monitoring. According to the CDC, vaccination is thought to present less risk than natural **varicella vaccine** in these children (2007b).

Clinical Use and Dosing

The CDC and the American Academy of Pediatrics (AAP) recommend that all healthy children who lack a reliable history of varicella infection be routinely vaccinated at age 12 to 15 months. A second dose of **varicella vaccine** is recommended at age 4 to 6 years (before entering kindergarten). The second dose may be administered earlier, as long as the interval between the two doses is more than 3 months.

Healthy adolescents age 13 and older, who have no history of varicella infection and who have not previously received **varicella vaccine,** should be administered two doses 4 to 8 weeks apart.

The Advisory Committee on Immunization Practices (ACIP) of the CDC recommends that all healthy adults be screened for varicella immunity and adults without immunity should receive **varicella vaccine.** Attention should be given to those adults at high risk of exposure or transmission of varicella disease. They include adults who live in households with children, live or work in an environment in which varicella transmission is likely (teachers, health-care workers, day-care workers) or could occur (college dorm, correctional institution, military), or have household contact with an immunocompromised person; nonpregnant childbearing women; and international travelers. Performing serological testing of adults before administering is optional and may be cost effective. The **varicella vaccine** dose for adults is two doses, separated by 4 to 8 weeks.

Administration error: If a child is accidentally administered **zoster vaccine (Zostavax)** instead of **varicella vaccine (Varivax),** then it should be counted as a valid vaccine and reported to the VAERS whether or not an adverse reaction occurs. The child will still require two doses of **varicella vaccine.**

Monitoring

There is no need to do post-vaccination titers after patients receive the **varicella vaccine.** At this time there is no commercially available test to determine immunity from **varicella** vaccine, just disease-induced immunity; therefore, the test may detect a false-positive outcome (CDC, 2007b).

Patient Education

All patients or their parents or guardians are required by law to receive CDC VISs, which are available in a variety of languages. Every effort should be made to provide adequate information to patients and their parents before immunization.

There may be transient burning or stinging at administration.

Patients should be informed that there is a small chance that they may develop a fever, reaction at the injection site, or vesicular rash after administration of **varicella vaccine.**

Zoster Vaccine

Pharmacodynamics

Shingles is a localized and painful cutaneous eruption caused by the reactivation of varicella zoster virus, the same virus that causes chickenpox in children. The varicella virus becomes latent in the neuronal cell bodies and becomes reactivated to cause shingles. The triggers for reactivation are not well understood, but it is known that cell-mediated immunity may prevent reactivation. The lifetime incidence of shingles is 1 in 3 and it affects approximately 1 million patients in the United States annually (CDC, 2008).

Zoster vaccine (Zostavax) is a live, attenuated varicella zoster vaccine from the same strain used to develop the **varicella vaccine (Varivax, ProQuad).** The **zoster vaccine** reduced the risk of developing zoster by 51.3 percent in pre-licensure trials and 66.5 percent effective in preventing post-herpetic neuralgia in the study group that was followed for 3 years. The vaccine also reduces severity of zoster by 57 percent in the vaccine recipients who developed post-herpetic neuralgia.

The **zoster vaccine** has been studied and approved by the U.S. Food and Drug Administration (FDA) for adults aged 60 years and older. The vaccine is most effective in patients aged 60 to 69 years and least effective in patients over age 80 years (CDC, 2008). The **zoster vaccine** is currently being studied for use in patients aged 50 years and older (Tyring et al, 2007).

CLINICAL PEARL

Administering Multiple Vaccines

Currently a child from age 12 to 18 months should receive six possible injections. This can be traumatic for patient and parent. Most public health officials recommend giving all the recommended vaccines at one visit; therefore, the child who is 15 months old could be getting as many as all six injections at that visit. Using combined vaccines is best **(Pediarix, Pentacel)** to decrease the number of injections or spread the administration of the vaccines over two or three visits. If it is necessary to give all the vaccines in one visit, as in the case of upcoming international travel or a history of unreliable attendance at well-child examinations, two people can administer the vaccines simultaneously. Giving the vaccines simultaneously makes the process faster and simpler for the patient and the person administering the **vaccine.** The CDC has guidelines for administering multiple injections to infants located in Appendix D of the *Pink Book* at http://www.cdc.gov/vaccines/pubs/pinkbook/downloads/appendices/D/site-map.pdf.

Pharmacokinetics

A single SC 0.65-mL dose of **zoster vaccine** produces a peak in cell-mediated response to varicella zoster in 1 to 3 weeks. Patients in the 60-to-69 age group demonstrated a better immune response to the vaccine than patients over age 70 years.

Pharmacotherapeutics

Precautions and Contraindications

Zoster vaccine should not be administered to patients with a history of anaphylactic reaction to **neomycin**, gelatin, or any other component of the **vaccine**.

Patients with primary immunodeficiency states should not be administered **zoster vaccine**. As **zoster vaccine** is a live, attenuated virus, patients with leukemia, lymphoma, cancer of the bone marrow or lymphatic system, or AIDS should not be given the vaccine, as they may develop disseminated disease. Patients receiving high-dose **corticosteroids** (greater than 20 mg/d of **prednisone**) for more than 2 weeks should wait at least a month after **prednisone** is stopped to get the **zoster vaccine**.

Zoster vaccine (Zostavax) is not approved for women of childbearing age and should not be administered to pregnant women.

Zoster vaccine should not be administered to patients with active tuberculosis or acute illness, or with fever.

Adverse Drug Reactions

The most common adverse drug reactions to **zoster vaccine** reported during the clinical trials were related to the injection site. Pain/tenderness (33.4%), erythema (33.7%), swelling (24.9%), and pruritus (6.6%) are all reported by patients receiving **zoster vaccine**. Headache was reported by 1.4 percent of patients who received the **zoster vaccine** versus 0.8 percent of patients who received a placebo.

Drug Interactions

Antiviral drugs (acyclovir, famciclovir, and **valacyclovir)** should be stopped at least 24 hours before **zoster vaccine** is administered. **Antivirals** should not be used for at least 14 days after vaccination (CDC, 2008).

Zoster vaccine can be administered before, after or at the same time as blood product or antibody-containing products.

Patients who are taking high-dose **corticosteroids** (greater than 20 mg/d **prednisone**) should not be vaccinated and need to be off **prednisone** for a month before vaccination. Short-term **corticosteroids** (less than 14 d) or low-dose (less than 20 mg/d) **prednisone** may be vaccinated with **zoster virus**.

Patients taking low-doses of **methotrexate** (less than or equal to 0.4 mg/kg/wk), **azathioprine** (less than or equal to 3.0 mg/kg/d), or **6-mercaptopurine** (less than or equal to 1.5 mg/kg/d) for treatment of rheumatoid arthritis, psoriasis, polymyositis, sarcoidosis, or inflammatory bowel disease may be vaccinated with **zoster vaccine** (CDC, 2008).

Clinical Use and Dosing

A single dose of **zoster vaccine** is recommended for all adults ages 60 years or older. The dose is 0.65 mL administered in the SC tissue of the deltoid region. The vaccine is given even if a patient has a history of herpes zoster (CDC, 2008). It is not necessary to screen for history of varicella disease or **vaccine**, nor is it necessary to test for varicella immunity prior to immunization. Studies are currently under way to lower the age for administration to 50 years.

Zoster vaccine is not recommended for patients who have received the **varicella vaccine**, although patients in the approved age range have most likely had wild varicella infection.

Patients with chronic medical conditions (e.g., chronic renal failure, diabetes mellitus, rheumatoid arthritis, and chronic pulmonary disease) may be vaccinated (CDC, 2008). **Zoster vaccine** should be deferred in patients with severe illness or with fever. It may be administered if the patient has a minor acute illness without fever (that is, an upper respiratory infection).

Zoster vaccine may be administered with other common vaccines in this age group, **Td, Tdap**, and **pneumococcal**. Administration of **zoster vaccine** and other live virus vaccines should be separated by 4 weeks.

Patients who are immunosuppressed have greater morbidity and mortality from herpes zoster. If patients will be initiating immunosuppressive therapy or have diseases that might lead to immunodeficiency, **zoster vaccine** should be administered as soon as possible while their immunity is still intact. **Zoster vaccine** should be administered at least 14 days before immunosuppressive therapy is started. **Zoster vaccine** should be avoided for at least 24 months after stem cell transplant (CDC, 2008).

Antiviral medications should be avoided for 14 days after **zoster vaccine**.

Administration error: If a child is accidentally administered **zoster vaccine (Zostavax)** instead of **varicella vaccine (Varivax)**, then it should be counted as a valid vaccine and reported to the VAERS whether or not an adverse reaction occurs. If an adult over age 60 is administered the **varicella vaccine (Varivax)**, it is not considered a valid dose and the patient is administered **zoster vaccine (Zostavax)** the same day (CDC, 2008). If the **zoster vaccine** is not administered the same day, then a dose of **zoster vaccine** should be administered at least 28 days later.

Monitoring

There is no specific monitoring of patients after receiving the **zoster vaccine**.

Patient Education

All patients who receive vaccines are required by law to receive a Vaccine Information Statement in the appropriate language.

Patients should be informed they may have discomfort at the injection site, including pain, swelling, erythema, and pruritus. See Table 19–5.

Recommended Adult Immunization Schedule

UNITED STATES · 2011

Note: These recommendations *must* be read with the footnotes that follow containing number of doses, intervals between doses, and other important information.

Figure 1. Recommended adult immunization schedule, by vaccine and age group

<table>
<tr><th>VACCINE ▼ / AGE GROUP ▶</th><th>19–26 years</th><th>27–49 years</th><th>50–59 years</th><th>60–64 years</th><th>≥65 years</th></tr>
<tr><td>Influenza[1,*]</td><td colspan="5">1 dose annually</td></tr>
<tr><td>Tetanus, diphtheria, pertussis (Td/Tdap)[2,*]</td><td colspan="4">Substitute 1-time dose of Tdap for Td booster; then boost with Td every 10 yrs</td><td>Td booster every 10 yrs</td></tr>
<tr><td>Varicella[3,*]</td><td colspan="5">2 doses</td></tr>
<tr><td>Human papillomavirus (HPV)[4,*]</td><td>3 doses (females)</td><td></td><td></td><td></td><td></td></tr>
<tr><td>Zoster[5]</td><td></td><td></td><td></td><td colspan="2">1 dose</td></tr>
<tr><td>Measles, mumps, rubella (MMR)[6,*]</td><td colspan="2">1 or 2 doses</td><td colspan="3">1 dose</td></tr>
<tr><td>Pneumococcal (polysaccharide)[7,8]</td><td colspan="4">1 or 2 doses</td><td>1 dose</td></tr>
<tr><td>Meningococcal[9,*]</td><td colspan="5">1 or more doses</td></tr>
<tr><td>Hepatitis A[10,*]</td><td colspan="5">2 doses</td></tr>
<tr><td>Hepatitis B[11,*]</td><td colspan="5">3 doses</td></tr>
</table>

*Covered by the Vaccine Injury Compensation Program.

For all persons in this category who meet the age requirements and who lack evidence of immunity (e.g., lack documentation of vaccination or have no evidence of previous infection)

Recommended if some other risk factor is present (e.g., based on medical, occupational, lifestyle, or other indications)

No recommendation

Report all clinically significant postvaccination reactions to the Vaccine Adverse Event Reporting System (VAERS). Reporting forms and instructions on filing a VAERS report are available at http://www.vaers.hhs.gov or by telephone, 800-822-7967.

Information on how to file a Vaccine Injury Compensation Program claim is available at http://www.hrsa.gov/vaccinecompensation or by telephone, 800-338-2382. Information about filing a claim for vaccine injury is available through the U.S. Court of Federal Claims, 717 Madison Place, N.W., Washington, D.C. 20005; telephone, 202-357-6400.

Additional information about the vaccines in this schedule, extent of available data, and contraindications for vaccination also is available at http://www.cdc.gov/vaccines or from the CDC-INFO Contact Center at 800-CDC-INFO (800-232-4636) in English and Spanish, 24 hours a day, 7 days a week.

Figure 2. Vaccines that might be indicated for adults based on medical and other indications

<table>
<tr><th rowspan="2">INDICATION ▶
VACCINE ▼</th><th rowspan="2">Pregnancy</th><th rowspan="2">Immuno-compromising conditions (excluding human immunodeficiency virus [HIV])[3,5,6,13]</th><th colspan="2">HIV infection[3,6,12,13] CD4+ T lymphocyte count</th><th rowspan="2">Diabetes, heart disease, chronic lung disease, chronic alcoholism</th><th rowspan="2">Asplenia[12] (including elective splenectomy) and persistent complement component deficiencies</th><th rowspan="2">Chronic liver disease</th><th rowspan="2">Kidney failure, end-stage renal disease, receipt of hemodialysis</th><th rowspan="2">Healthcare personnel</th></tr>
<tr><th><200 cells/μL</th><th>≥200 cells/μL</th></tr>
<tr><td>Influenza[1,*]</td><td colspan="8">1 dose TIV annually</td><td>1 dose TIV or LAIV annually</td></tr>
<tr><td>Tetanus, diphtheria, pertussis (Td/Tdap)[2,*]</td><td>Td</td><td colspan="8">Substitute 1-time dose of Tdap for Td booster; then boost with Td every 10 yrs</td></tr>
<tr><td>Varicella[3,*]</td><td colspan="3">Contraindicated</td><td colspan="6">2 doses</td></tr>
<tr><td>Human papillomavirus (HPV)[4,*]</td><td></td><td colspan="8">3 doses through age 26 yrs</td></tr>
<tr><td>Zoster[5]</td><td colspan="3">Contraindicated</td><td></td><td colspan="5">1 dose</td></tr>
<tr><td>Measles, mumps, rubella (MMR)[6,*]</td><td colspan="3">Contraindicated</td><td colspan="6">1 or 2 doses</td></tr>
<tr><td>Pneumococcal (polysaccharide)[7,8]</td><td></td><td colspan="7">1 or 2 doses</td><td></td></tr>
<tr><td>Meningococcal[9,*]</td><td colspan="5">1 or more doses</td><td></td><td colspan="3"></td></tr>
<tr><td>Hepatitis A[10,*]</td><td colspan="6">2 doses</td><td></td><td colspan="2"></td></tr>
<tr><td>Hepatitis B[11,*]</td><td colspan="2"></td><td colspan="2"></td><td colspan="2">3 doses</td><td colspan="3"></td></tr>
</table>

*Covered by the Vaccine Injury Compensation Program.

For all persons in this category who meet the age requirements and who lack evidence of immunity (e.g., lack documentation of vaccination or have no evidence of previous infection)

Recommended if some other risk factor is present (e.g., on the basis of medical, occupational, lifestyle, or other indications)

No recommendation

These schedules indicate the recommended age groups and medical indications for which administration of currently licensed vaccines is commonly indicated for adults ages 19 years and older, as of February 4, 2011. For all vaccines being recommended on the adult immunization schedule, a vaccine series does not need to be restarted, regardless of the time that has elapsed between doses. Licensed combination vaccines may be used whenever any components of the combination are indicated and when the vaccine's other components are not contraindicated. For detailed recommendations on all vaccines, including those used primarily for travelers or that are issued during the year, consult the manufacturers' package inserts and the complete statements from the Advisory Committee on Immunization Practices (http:// www.cdc.gov/vaccines/pubs/acip-list.htm).

The recommendations in this schedule were approved by the Centers for Disease Control and Prevention's (CDC) Advisory Committee on Immunization Practices (ACIP), the American Academy of Family Physicians (AAFP), the American College of Obstetricians and Gynecologists (ACOG), and the American College of Physicians (ACP).

U.S. DEPARTMENT OF HEALTH AND HUMAN SERVICES
CENTERS FOR DISEASE CONTROL AND PREVENTION

Continued

Table 19–5 **Recommended Adult Immunization Schedule—cont'd**

Footnotes

Recommended Adult Immunization Schedule—UNITED STATES · 2011

For complete statements by the Advisory Committee on Immunization Practices (ACIP), visit www.cdc.gov/vaccines/pubs/ACIP-list.htm.

1. Influenza vaccination

Annual vaccination against influenza is recommended for all persons aged 6 months and older, including all adults. Healthy, nonpregnant adults aged less than 50 years without high-risk medical conditions can receive either intranasally administered live, attenuated influenza vaccine (FluMist), or inactivated vaccine. Other persons should receive the inactivated vaccine. Adults aged 65 years and older can receive the standard influenza vaccine or the high-dose (Fluzone) influenza vaccine. Additional information about influenza vaccination is available at http://www.cdc.gov/vaccines/vpd-vac/flu/default.htm.

2. Tetanus, diphtheria, and acellular pertussis (Td/Tdap) vaccination

Administer a one-time dose of Tdap to adults aged less than 65 years who have not received Tdap previously or for whom vaccine status is unknown to replace one of the 10-year Td boosters, and as soon as feasible to all 1) postpartum women, 2) close contacts of infants younger than age 12 months (e.g., grandparents and child-care providers), and 3) healthcare personnel with direct patient contact. Adults aged 65 years and older who have not previously received Tdap and who have close contact with an infant aged less than 12 months also should be vaccinated. Other adults aged 65 years and older may receive Tdap. Tdap can be administered regardless of interval since the most recent tetanus or diphtheria-containing vaccine.

Adults with uncertain or incomplete history of completing a 3-dose primary vaccination series with Td-containing vaccines should begin or complete a primary vaccination series. For unvaccinated adults, administer the first 2 doses at least 4 weeks apart and the third dose 6–12 months after the second. If incompletely vaccinated (i.e., less than 3 doses), administer remaining doses. Substitute a one-time dose of Tdap for one of the doses of Td, either in the primary series or for the routine booster, whichever comes first.

If a woman is pregnant and received the most recent Td vaccination 10 or more years previously, administer Td during the second or third trimester. If the woman received the most recent Td vaccination less than 10 years previously, administer Tdap during the immediate postpartum period. At the clinician's discretion, Td may be deferred during pregnancy and Tdap substituted in the immediate postpartum period, or Tdap may be administered instead of Td to a pregnant woman after an informed discussion with the woman.

The ACIP statement for recommendations for administering Td as prophylaxis in wound management is available at http://www.cdc.gov/vaccines/pubs/acip-list.htm.

3. Varicella vaccination

All adults without evidence of immunity to varicella should receive 2 doses of single-antigen varicella vaccine if not previously vaccinated or a second dose if they have received only 1 dose, unless they have a medical contraindication. Special consideration should be given to those who 1) have close contact with persons at high risk for severe disease (e.g., healthcare personnel and family contacts of persons with immunocompromising conditions) or 2) are at high risk for exposure or transmission (e.g., teachers; child-care employees; residents and staff members of institutional settings, including correctional institutions; college students; military personnel; adolescents and adults living in households with children; nonpregnant women of childbearing age; and international travelers).

Evidence of immunity to varicella in adults includes any of the following: 1) documentation of 2 doses of varicella vaccine at least 4 weeks apart; 2) U.S.-born before 1980 (although for healthcare personnel and pregnant women, birth before 1980 should not be considered evidence of immunity); 3) history of varicella based on diagnosis or verification of varicella by a healthcare provider (for a patient reporting a history of or having an atypical case, a mild case, or both, healthcare providers should seek either an epidemiologic link with a typical varicella case or to a laboratory-confirmed case or evidence of laboratory confirmation, if it was performed at the time of acute disease); 4) history of herpes zoster based on diagnosis or verification of herpes zoster by a healthcare provider; or 5) laboratory evidence of immunity or laboratory confirmation of disease.

Pregnant women should be assessed for evidence of varicella immunity. Women who do not have evidence of immunity should receive the first dose of varicella vaccine upon completion or termination of pregnancy and before discharge from the healthcare facility. The second dose should be administered 4–8 weeks after the first dose.

4. Human papillomavirus (HPV) vaccination

HPV vaccination with either quadrivalent (HPV4) vaccine or bivalent vaccine (HPV2) is recommended for females at age 11 or 12 years and catch-up vaccination for females aged 13 through 26 years.

Ideally, vaccine should be administered before potential exposure to HPV through sexual activity; however, females who are sexually active should still be vaccinated consistent with age-based recommendations. Sexually active females who have not been infected with any of the four HPV vaccine types (types 6, 11, 16, and 18, all of which HPV4 prevents) or any of the two HPV vaccine types (types 16 and 18, both of which HPV2 prevents) receive the full benefit of the vaccination. Vaccination is less beneficial for females who have already been infected with one or more of the HPV vaccine types. HPV4 or HPV2 can be administered to persons with a history of genital warts, abnormal Papanicolaou test, or positive HPV DNA test, because these conditions are not evidence of previous infection with all vaccine HPV types.

HPV4 may be administered to males aged 9 through 26 years to reduce their likelihood of genital warts. HPV4 would be most effective when administered before exposure to HPV through sexual contact.

A complete series for either HPV4 or HPV2 consists of 3 doses. The second dose should be administered 1–2 months after the first dose; the third dose should be administered 6 months after the first dose.

Although HPV vaccination is not specifically recommended for persons with the medical indications described in Figure 2, "Vaccines that might be indicated for adults based on medical and other indications," it may be administered to these persons because the HPV vaccine is not a live-virus vaccine. However, the immune response and vaccine efficacy might be less for persons with the medical indications described in Figure 2 than in persons who do not have the medical indications described or who are immunocompetent.

5. Herpes zoster vaccination

A single dose of zoster vaccine is recommended for adults aged 60 years and older regardless of whether they report a previous episode of herpes zoster. Persons with chronic medical conditions may be vaccinated unless their condition constitutes a contraindication.

6. Measles, mumps, rubella (MMR) vaccination

Adults born before 1957 generally are considered immune to measles and mumps. All adults born in 1957 or later should have documentation of 1 or more doses of MMR vaccine unless they have a medical contraindication to the vaccine, laboratory evidence of immunity to each of the three diseases, or documentation of provider-diagnosed measles or mumps disease. For rubella, documentation of provider-diagnosed disease is not considered acceptable evidence of immunity.

Measles component: A second dose of MMR vaccine, administered a minimum of 28 days after the first dose, is recommended for adults who 1) have been recently exposed to measles or are in an outbreak setting; 2) are students in postsecondary educational institutions; 3) work in a healthcare facility; or 4) plan to travel internationally. Persons who received inactivated (killed) measles vaccine or measles vaccine of unknown type during 1963–1967 should be revaccinated with 2 doses of MMR vaccine.

Mumps component: A second dose of MMR vaccine, administered a minimum of 28 days after the first dose, is recommended for adults who 1) live in a community experiencing a mumps outbreak and are in an affected age group; 2) are students in postsecondary educational institutions; 3) work in a healthcare facility; or 4) plan to travel internationally. Persons vaccinated before 1979 with either killed mumps vaccine or mumps vaccine of unknown type who are at high risk for mumps infection (e.g. persons who are working in a healthcare facility) should be revaccinated with 2 doses of MMR vaccine.

Rubella component: For women of childbearing age, regardless of birth year, rubella immunity should be determined. If there is no evidence of immunity, women who are not pregnant should be vaccinated. Pregnant women who do not have evidence of immunity should receive MMR vaccine upon completion or termination of pregnancy and before discharge from the healthcare facility.

Healthcare personnel born before 1957: For unvaccinated healthcare personnel born before 1957 who lack laboratory evidence of measles, mumps, and/or rubella immunity or laboratory confirmation of disease, healthcare facilities should 1) consider routinely vaccinating personnel with 2 doses of MMR vaccine at the appropriate interval (for measles and mumps) and 1 dose of MMR vaccine (for rubella), and 2) recommend 2 doses of MMR vaccine at the appropriate interval during an outbreak of measles or mumps, and 1 dose during an outbreak of rubella. Complete information about evidence of immunity is available at http://www.cdc.gov/vaccines/recs/provisional/default.htm.

7. Pneumococcal polysaccharide (PPSV) vaccination

Vaccinate all persons with the following indications:

Medical: Chronic lung disease (including asthma); chronic cardiovascular diseases; diabetes mellitus; chronic liver diseases; cirrhosis; chronic alcoholism; functional or anatomic asplenia (e.g., sickle cell disease or splenectomy [if elective splenectomy is planned, vaccinate at least 2 weeks before surgery]); immunocompromising conditions (including chronic renal failure or nephrotic syndrome); and cochlear implants and cerebrospinal fluid leaks. Vaccinate as close to HIV diagnosis as possible.

Other: Residents of nursing homes or long-term care facilities and persons who smoke cigarettes. Routine use of PPSV is not recommended for American Indians/Alaska Natives or persons aged less than 65 years unless they have underlying medical conditions that are PPSV indications. However, public health authorities may consider recommending PPSV for American Indians/Alaska Natives and persons aged 50 through 64 years who are living in areas where the risk for invasive pneumococcal disease is increased

8. Revaccination with PPSV

One-time revaccination after 5 years is recommended for persons aged 19 through 64 years with chronic renal failure or nephrotic syndrome; functional or anatomic asplenia (e.g., sickle cell disease or splenectomy); and for persons with immunocompromising conditions. For persons aged 65 years and older, one-time revaccination is recommended if they were vaccinated 5 or more years previously and were aged less than 65 years at the time of primary vaccination.

9. Meningococcal vaccination

Meningococcal vaccine should be administered to persons with the following indications:

Medical: A 2-dose series of meningococcal conjugate vaccine is recommended for adults with anatomic or functional asplenia, or persistent complement component deficiencies. Adults with HIV infection who are vaccinated should also receive a routine 2-dose series. The 2 doses should be administered at 0 and 2 months.

Other: A single dose of meningococcal vaccine is recommended for unvaccinated first-year college students living in dormitories; microbiologists routinely exposed to isolates of *Neisseria meningitidis*; military recruits; and persons who travel to or live in countries in which meningococcal disease is hyperendemic or epidemic (e.g., the "meningitis belt" of sub-Saharan Africa during the dry season [December through June]), particularly if their contact with local populations will be prolonged. Vaccination is required by the government of Saudi Arabia for all travelers to Mecca during the annual Hajj.

Meningococcal conjugate vaccine, quadrivalent (MCV4) is preferred for adults with any of the preceding indications who are aged 55 years and younger; meningococcal polysaccharide vaccine (MPSV4) is preferred for adults aged 56 years and older. Revaccination with MCV4 every 5 years is recommended for adults previously vaccinated with MCV4 or MPSV4 who remain at increased risk for infection (e.g., adults with anatomic or functional asplenia, or persistent complement component deficiencies).

Table 19–5 Recommended Adult Immunization Schedule—cont'd

10. Hepatitis A vaccination

Vaccinate persons with any of the following indications and any person seeking protection from hepatitis A virus (HAV) infection:

Behavioral: Men who have sex with men and persons who use injection drugs.

Occupational: Persons working with HAV-infected primates or with HAV in a research laboratory setting.

Medical: Persons with chronic liver disease and persons who receive clotting factor concentrates.

Other: Persons traveling to or working in countries that have high or intermediate endemicity of hepatitis A (a list of countries is available at http://wwwn.cdc.gov/travel/contentdiseases.aspx).

Unvaccinated persons who anticipate close personal contact (e.g., household or regular babysitting) with an international adoptee during the first 60 days after arrival in the United States from a country with high or intermediate endemicity should be vaccinated. The first dose of the 2-dose hepatitis A vaccine series should be administered as soon as adoption is planned, ideally 2 or more weeks before the arrival of the adoptee.

Single antigen vaccine formulations should be administered in a 2-dose schedule at either 0 and 6–12 months (Havrix), or 0 and 6–18 months (Vaqta). If the combined hepatitis A and hepatitis B vaccine (Twinrix) is used, administer 3 doses at 0, 1, and 6 months; alternatively, a 4-dose schedule may be used, administered on days 0, 7, and 21–30, followed by a booster dose at month 12.

11. Hepatitis B vaccination

Vaccinate persons with any of the following indications and any person seeking protection from hepatitis B virus (HBV) infection:

Behavioral: Sexually active persons who are not in a long-term, mutually monogamous relationship (e.g., persons with more than one sex partner during the previous 6 months); persons seeking evaluation or treatment for a sexually transmitted disease (STD); current or recent injection-drug users; and men who have sex with men.

Occupational: Healthcare personnel and public-safety workers who are exposed to blood or other potentially infectious body fluids.

Medical: Persons with end-stage renal disease, including patients receiving hemodialysis; persons with HIV infection; and persons with chronic liver disease.

Other: Household contacts and sex partners of persons with chronic HBV infection; clients and staff members of institutions for persons with developmental disabilities; and international travelers to countries with high or intermediate prevalence of chronic HBV infection (a list of countries is available at http://wwwn.cdc.gov/travel/contentdiseases.aspx).

Hepatitis B vaccination is recommended for all adults in the following settings: STD treatment facilities; HIV testing and treatment facilities; facilities providing drug-abuse treatment and prevention services; healthcare settings targeting services to injection-drug users or men who have sex with men; correctional facilities; end-stage renal disease programs and facilities for chronic hemodialysis patients; and institutions and nonresidential day-care facilities for persons with developmental disabilities.

Administer missing doses to complete a 3-dose series of hepatitis B vaccine to those persons not vaccinated or not completely vaccinated. The second dose should be administered 1 month after the first dose; the third dose should be given at least 2 months after the second dose (and at least 4 months after the first dose). If the combined hepatitis A and hepatitis B vaccine (Twinrix) is used, administer 3 doses at 0, 1, and 6 months; alternatively, a 4-dose Twinrix schedule, administered on days 0, 7, and 21 to 30, followed by a booster dose at month 12 may be used.

Adult patients receiving hemodialysis or with other immunocompromising conditions should receive 1 dose of 40 μg/mL (Recombivax HB) administered on a 3-dose schedule or 2 doses of 20 μg/mL (Engerix-B) administered simultaneously on a 4-dose schedule at 0, 1, 2, and 6 months.

12. Selected conditions for which Haemophilus influenzae type b (Hib) vaccine may be used

1 dose of Hib vaccine should be considered for persons who have sickle cell disease, leukemia, or HIV infection, or who have had a splenectomy, if they have not previously received Hib vaccine.

13. Immunocompromising conditions

Inactivated vaccines generally are acceptable (e.g., pneumococcal, meningococcal, influenza [inactivated influenza vaccine]) and live vaccines generally are avoided in persons with immune deficiencies or immunocompromising conditions. Information on specific conditions is available at http://www.cdc.gov/vaccines/pubs/acip-list.htm.

Oral Typhoid Vaccine

Pharmacodynamics

Typhoid vaccines are used to increase resistance to enteric fever caused by *Salmonella typhi.* Typhoid fever is spread by ingesting water contaminated by feces from infected persons. Worldwide, an estimated 22 million cases of typhoid fever occur annually (Brunette, Kozarsky, Magill, & Shtim, 2010). The risk is greatest in travelers to South Asia, although the disease can be seen in East and Southeast Asia, Africa, the Caribbean, and Central and South America (Brunette et al, 2010). **Oral typhoid vaccine (Vivotif Berna)** is a live, attenuated vaccine, Ty21a. The **oral vaccine** is ingested and works in the small intestine to synthesize a lipopolysaccharide that evokes a protective immune response. The vaccine is estimated to be 50 to 80 percent effective in preventing typhoid fever. Efficacy of protective immunity depends on the size of the bacterial inoculum consumed.

Pharmacokinetics

The absorption, distribution, and metabolism of **oral typhoid vaccine** are unknown.

Pharmacotherapeutics

Precautions and Contraindications

Hypersensitivity to **typhoid vaccine** is a contraindication to its use.

Because **oral typhoid vaccine** is a live, attenuated virus, it should not be administered to immunocompromised patients, including those who are HIV infected.

Do not administer it to a patient with acute febrile illness or an acute GI illness (diarrhea).

Oral typhoid vaccine is Pregnancy Category C. It is not known if the vaccine is harmful to the fetus. If it is necessary to vaccinate a pregnant patient, inactivated vaccine is recommended.

Oral typhoid vaccine is not recommended for use in children younger than age 6 years. Use inactivated vaccine in young children.

Adverse Drug Reactions

Adverse effects of **oral typhoid vaccine** are infrequent and transient and resolve with intervention. Abdominal pain, diarrhea, vomiting, fever, headache, and rash have been reported.

Drug Interactions

The antimalarial drug **mefloquine (Lariam)** can inhibit the growth of the live Ty21a strain in vitro. It is recommended that **oral typhoid vaccine** be given either 24 hours before or 24 hours after **mefloquine.**

Immunosuppressants may cause insufficient response to the vaccine.

The manufacturer recommends that **oral typhoid vaccine** not be administered to individuals receiving **sulfonamides** and **antibiotics,** which may be active against the vaccine strains and prevent a sufficient degree of multiplication to induce a protective immune response.

Clinical Use and Dosing

Oral typhoid vaccine is used for primary immunization against *S. typhi* infection in the following:

1. Travelers to areas where a risk of exposure to *S. typhi* is recognized.

2. People who have household contact with a documented typhoid fever carrier.
3. Laboratory workers who have frequent contact with *S. typhi*.

For primary immunization of patients over age 6 years, the dose is 1 capsule on alternate days (days 1, 3, 5, 7) for a total of 4 doses. The capsule needs to be taken 1 hour before meals with a glass of cold water (not warmer than body temperature). The vaccine capsule should be swallowed whole. Ideally, the patient should finish the four doses at least 1 week prior to exposure or travel.

A booster dose of four capsules, given every other day, is recommended every 5 years under conditions of repeated exposure.

Monitoring

There is no specific monitoring of patients after receiving **oral typhoid vaccine**.

Patient Education

The **oral typhoid vaccine** should be taken exactly as prescribed. It must be taken on an empty stomach with cold water. Every-other-day dosing should be explained. The patient must understand that all four doses must be taken, at least 1 week prior to travel, to provide the best protection.

Although the possible adverse effects of the **vaccine** are mild and usually transient, the patient should be informed about them.

The best protection against typhoid fever is food and water precautions to prevent contracting *S. typhi*.

Yellow Fever Vaccine

Pharmacodynamics

Yellow fever is a viral illness spread by some species of mosquitoes in Central and South America and in tropical regions of Africa. Yellow fever is endemic in sub-Saharan Africa and tropical South America (Brunette et al, 2010). The CDC estimates the risk of an unvaccinated traveler contracting yellow fever during a 2-week visit to West Africa as 10 cases per 100,000 and 1 case per 100,000 travelers to South America (Brunette et al, 2010). All travelers should use personal protective measures to avoid mosquito bites to prevent yellow fever transmission.

Vaccination is recommended for travel to endemic areas. Certification of **yellow fever vaccine** may be required for all persons aged 9 months or older to enter certain countries in endemic areas. Current recommendations are listed at the CDC Travel Web site: *Yellow Book*, Chapter 2: Pre-Travel Consultation (http://www.cdc.gov/travel). **Yellow fever vaccine (YF-Vax)** is a live, attenuated virus that is prepared by culturing the 17D strain virus in a living chick embryo.

Pharmacokinetics

After SC administration of the **vaccine**, active immunity to yellow fever occurs in 7 to 10 days and lasts for 10 years or more. The World Health Organization publishes international health regulations requiring revaccination at 10-year intervals for those at high risk.

Pharmacotherapeutics

Precautions and Contraindications

Yellow fever vaccine should be avoided in any patient with a history of egg hypersensitivity or sensitivity to chicken protein.

Because **yellow fever vaccine** is a live, attenuated virus, it is contraindicated in immunocompromised patients, including those who are HIV infected with a CD4 T-lymphocyte less than 15 percent, patients with primary immunodeficiencies, malignant neoplasms, transplant patients or other patients on immunosuppressive therapies (CDC, 2009). The vaccine should be used with caution in HIV infected patients with CD4 counts 15 to 24 percent. **Yellow fever vaccine** is contraindicated in patients with a thymus disorder.

Defer vaccination with **yellow fever vaccine** for 8 weeks following blood or plasma transfusion.

Yellow fever vaccine is Pregnancy Category C. It is not known if the **vaccine** is harmful to the fetus. Vaccinate only those pregnant women who are at high risk of contracting the disease. Use with caution in breastfeeding women.

Yellow fever vaccine is contraindicated in infants younger than 6 months. Use with caution in infants aged 6 to 8 months. Rare cases of encephalitis have occurred in infants of this age who have received **yellow fever vaccine.**

Yellow fever vaccine should be used with caution in patients who are aged 60 years or older. VAERS reports indicate an increase in serious adverse events after vaccination of patients aged 60 and older. If patients are traveling to endemic areas, **vaccination** risks need to be weighed against the risk of exposure to the yellow fever virus.

Adverse Drug Reactions

Up to 10 percent of patients experience fever or malaise, usually 7 to 14 days after administration of **yellow fever vaccine**. Myalgia or headache is reported in 2 to 5 percent of **vaccine** recipients. Incidence of mild adverse events has been 25 percent or less in clinical trials (CDC, 2002). Anaphylaxis may occur and **epinephrine** should be on hand when administering the vaccine.

A very rare reaction is **yellow fever vaccine**–associated viscerotropic disease, with symptoms of fever and multiple organ failure (CDC, 2002). The rate is higher among persons 60 years or older, 1/100,000 in 60- to 69-year-olds and 2.3/100,000 in persons aged 70 or older (Brunette et al, 2010. The case-fatality ratio for **yellow fever vaccine**–associated viscerotropic disease is 53 percent. The onset of illness is an average of 3.5 days after vaccination.

Yellow fever vaccine–associated neurological disease is a conglomerate of clinical syndromes including meningoencephalitis, Guillain-Barré syndrome, encephalomyelitis, bulbar palsy, and Bell's palsy. Adverse neurological outcomes are usually seen among infants as encephalitis, but may occur at any age.

Drug Interactions

Concurrent vaccination with **yellow fever vaccine** and **hepatitis A vaccine** (HAV) and HBV, **meningococcal vaccine** (Menomune), **typhoid fever vaccine** (Typhim Vi), and **measles vaccine** does not appear to affect response to **yellow fever vaccine** (CDC, 2002).

Immunosuppressants may cause insufficient response to the **yellow fever vaccine.**

Preservatives in diluent may kill the live virus in the vaccine. **Yellow fever vaccine** should be reconstituted with the diluent supplied with the vaccine.

Clinical Use and Dosing

Immunization against yellow fever is recommended for all people over age 9 months who are living in or traveling to endemic areas. Vaccination is required by international regulations for travel to certain countries. The dose is a single 0.5-mL dose given SC. The vaccine should be repeated every 10 years.

Monitoring

There is no specific monitoring of patients needed after receiving **yellow fever vaccine** other than for the rare adverse drug reactions (ADRs) listed previously.

Patient Education

Patients should be educated about the mild transient adverse effects that can occur from **vaccine** administration.

Patients should be instructed about protecting themselves against mosquitoes. Insect repellant and proper protective clothing and netting provide the best defense against insect-borne diseases.

Bacillus Calmette-Guérin Vaccine

Pharmacodynamics

Immunization with **bacillus Calmette-Guérin** (BCG) **vaccine** lowers the risk of serious complications of primary TB in children. It is not widely used in the United States, but is given to infants and young children in countries where TB is endemic. BCG is an immune stimulant used to produce immunity against TB. Vaccination with BCG stimulates natural infection with *Mycobacterium tuberculosis* and results in a cell-mediated immune reaction and immunity against TB. Vaccination with BCG causes variable degrees of protection against TB. The protective effect of BCG use in children against miliary and meningeal TB is about 80 percent. It is less effective in adults.

Pharmacokinetics

BCG is administered percutaneously. Specific pharmacokinetic information is not available. Duration of protection against TB varies according to the potency of the strain of BCG used. TB sensitivity may last up to 10 years.

Pharmacotherapeutics

Precautions and Contraindications

Patients with active TB should not receive BCG. PPD skin testing should be performed on all patients over 2 months of age who are receiving BCG.

Cancer, leukemia, lymphoma, radiation therapy, and immunodeficiency are contraindications to BCG use. Patients with symptomatic or asymptomatic HIV infection should not receive BCG. Drugs that affect the immune system, including high-dose **steroids**, are also a contraindication to BCG use.

Precautions should be taken to avoid accidental exposure to BCG solutions during preparation and administration because these solutions contain live, attenuated *M. tuberculosis.*

BCG is Pregnancy Category C. The CDC does not recommend the use of BCG in pregnant women.

The World Health Organization recommends that HIV-infected infants not receive BCG even in areas of high TB activity because of the risk of disseminated BCG disease (WHO, 2007).

Adverse Drug Reactions

A normal reaction to the **BCG vaccine** are skin lesions that appear within 10 to 14 days after the multiple-puncture disc application of BCG. The lesions consist of small red papules at the site of administration. The papules reach maximum diameter (3 mm) after 4 to 6 weeks and then scale away and slowly subside. Six months after vaccination, there is usually no visible sign of vaccination, although faint disc marks may be noted.

Lymphadenopathy may occur in a regional lymph node that resolves spontaneously.

Osteomyelitis is a rare occurrence (1/1 million doses). BCG-induced osteomyelitis affects the epiphyses of the long bones and can occur from 4 months to 2 years after administration.

Rarely, lupoid-like skin reactions have occurred. It has been recommended that patients who experience lupus-like symptoms after BCG administration be treated with isoniazid (INH) for 3 months.

Disseminated BCG infection and death are very rare (about 1/5 million doses) and usually occur in children with impaired immune systems.

Drug Interactions

Antituberculosis agents (**rifampin**, **INH**, **streptomycin**) and **immunosuppressives** may interfere with the development of an appropriate immune response to BCG administration.

BCG administration will cause PPD skin tests to give false-positive readings for up to 10 years after administration.

After 10 years, a positive PPD usually indicates infection with *M. tuberculosis*.

Clinical Use and Dosing

In the United States, BCG is administered only in very special circumstances, such as unavoidable risk of exposure to *M. tuberculosis* and failure of other methods of prevention and control of TB. With the reemergence of drug-resistant TB, the use of BCG is being reevaluated.

The ACIP has set clear criteria for the use of BCG in the United States: "BCG vaccination should be considered for infants and children who reside in settings in which the likelihood of *M. tuberculosis* transmission and subsequent infection is high provided no other measures can be implemented (e.g., removing child from the source of infection). In addition, BCG vaccination may be considered for health-care workers who are employed in settings in which the likelihood of transmission and subsequent infection with *M. tuberculosis* strains resistant to INH and rifampin is high" (CDC, 1996b).

BCG is given to healthy infants from birth to 2 months without TB skin testing. After that, BCG is given only to children with negative Mantoux skin tests.

The administration of BCG must be exactly as the manufacturer directs. The vaccine is dropped onto clean, dry skin over the deltoid muscle and spread over the area to be punctured, using the edge of the multipuncture disc. The prongs of the disc are coated with the virus by lightly dipping them into the spread vaccine. The prongs of the disc are pressed into the skin and held for 5 to 10 seconds. After the disc is removed, the vaccine is respread to fill all the puncture areas. Additional **vaccine** may be applied to ensure a "wet" vaccine site. The vaccinated area needs to be kept dry for 24 hours. No dressing is required.

The dose for infants 1 month or younger is diluted to 50 percent by adding 2 mL of sterile water to the vaccine.

The person administering the **vaccine** should take precautions against coming in contact with the live virus.

Monitoring

There is no specific monitoring of patients who receive BCG, although providers are reminded it may affect TB test results.

Patient Education

The patient or parent should be instructed that the **vaccine** contains live virus and that the site should not be touched. The **vaccine** site should be kept clean until the local reaction has resolved.

Clear instructions regarding the normal skin reaction should be given to the patient or parent prior to administration.

INACTIVATED VACCINES

Diphtheria, Tetanus, and Pertussis Vaccine

Pharmacodynamics

Various combinations of **diphtheria, tetanus,** and **pertussis vaccines** are available on the market. Regardless of the combination of **vaccines,** the basic pharmacodynamic principles are the same.

Diphtheria toxoid induces the production of antibodies against the exotoxin excreted by *Corynebacterium diphtheriae.* Complete immunization (four doses, then boosters every 10 yr) induces specific antibodies and reduces the incidence of diphtheria by more than 95 percent. Immunized persons who develop diphtheria have milder illness. Infection with *C. diphtheriae* does not confer immunity, and previously infected persons should still receive **toxoid.**

Adsorbed **tetanus toxoid** contains antigens that induce the production of antibodies against the exotoxin excreted by *Clostridium tetani.* The duration of immunity against *C. tetani* is about 10 years. Natural immunity to *C. tetani* does not occur in the United States, and even patients with previous *C. tetani* infection should receive the **tetanus toxoid.**

Pertussis vaccine contains inactivated pertussis antigens. **Acellular pertussis vaccine** contains one or more immunogens derived from *Bordetella pertussis* and, unlike whole-cell vaccine, contains little or no endotoxin. Immunization with **pertussis vaccine** produces antibodies against *B. pertussis.* The efficacy of **whole-cell pertussis vaccine** for children exposed to pertussis who received at least three doses of DPT is estimated at 59 to 90 percent. **Whole-cell pertussis vaccine, DPT** is no longer available in the United States. **Acellular pertussis vaccine** has a clinical efficacy of 79 to 93 percent in protecting against clinical pertussis after household exposure. Vaccinated patients who do contract pertussis usually have a milder case. **Pertussis vaccine** is always given in combination with diphtheria and tetanus vaccines (DTaP, Tdap, Tdap).

Pharmacokinetics

The DTaP vaccine is given IM. Ninety percent of patients who receive three doses develop protective immunity against diphtheria and tetanus. Patients who receive four doses of DTaP have immunity that persists for 10 years or more. In patients who receive four doses of DTaP, immunity to pertussis begins to wane after 4 to 6 years. Ten years after immunization, fewer than 50 percent of **vaccine** recipients have protective antibodies against *B. pertussis,* which is why a booster dose of **Tdap** is recommended in adolescents, who make up 34 percent of active pertussis cases (CDC, 2006d). Vaccination is also recommended for all adults, including health-care workers and caregivers of infants younger than 12 months of age (CDC, 2006e).

Pharmacotherapeutics

Precautions and Contraindications

In the United States, it is currently recommended that DTaP be used for primary immunization of infants and children. Therefore, the precautions and contraindications to DTaP are discussed here, and DTP is not discussed, although the contraindications are the same for each vaccine. Tdap is discussed later in this section.

The true contraindication to DTaP vaccination is a patient who experienced an immediate anaphylactic reaction with a previous dose. Encephalopathy that occurred within 7 days of a previous dose, unexplained by another cause, is a possible contraindication to further pertussis vaccine use (CDC, 2006c). In this case, DT should be substituted for DTaP.

Patients with unstable, progressive neurological problems may have the vaccine deferred until the neurologic status is clarified.

Precautions associated with DTaP include a previous temperature of 105°F (40.5°C) or higher within 48 hours after a dose, history of continuous crying (more than 3 h) within 48 hours of a dose, convulsions within 3 days of a previous dose, and collapse or shock-like state (hypotonic-hyporesponsive episode) within 48 hours of a previous dose. Although these precautions were once considered contraindications, they are now considered precautions because they have not been proved to cause permanent sequelae.

Additional precautions include seizures 3 days or less after a previous dose of DTaP, persistent or inconsolable crying lasting more than 3 hours within 48 hours of a previous dose, Guillain-Barré syndrome (GBS) less than 6 weeks after a previous dose of tetanus toxoid–containing vaccine, or moderate or severe acute illness with or without fever (CDC, 2006c).

DTaP may be given to immunocompromised patients or patients on immunosuppressive therapy, although the immune response to the vaccine may be less than optimal. Patients with HIV infection may be immunized.

Temperature less than 104°F (less than 40.5°C), fussiness, or mild drowsiness after a previous dose of DTaP, family history of seizures, family history of an adverse event after a DTP vaccine, or stable neurological condition are not contraindications to vaccinating with DTaP.

Infants born prematurely should begin the vaccine series based on their date of birth, with the first vaccine given routinely at age 2 months.

The ACIP has recommended that pregnant women receive a booster of Td if it has been 10 or more years since their last tetanus vaccine. Pregnant adolescents may be vaccinated with Tdap (CDC, 2006c). Td is Pregnancy Category C, but it has been used extensively worldwide in pregnant women with no adverse effects reported.

Patients with a minor acute or febrile illness, including otitis media, may be immunized. Immunization should be delayed in cases of moderate or severe illnesses, with or without fever.

The contraindications to DT include patients older than age 7 years; give Td. The contraindications to DT or Td include hypersensitivity to any component of the vaccine and moderate-to-severe illness, with or without fever. Do not postpone for minor illness, including otitis media.

The contraindications to Tdap include Guillain-Barré syndrome 6 weeks or sooner after previous use of tetanus toxoid–containing vaccine, previous arthus reaction after receiving tetanus or diphtheria vaccine, or a progressive neurological disorder (CDC, 2006e).

Tdap or Td should be deferred in a patient with moderate or severe illness, with or without fever. Fever with previous DTaP vaccine is not a reason to withhold Tdap vaccine (CDC, 2006e).

Adverse Drug Reactions

Injection site reactions of mild to moderate pain, erythema, swelling, and induration may last for a few days after injection. Transient low-grade fever, chills, malaise, generalized aches and pains, and headache may occur. Fever was common after DPT and less common after DTaP. Drowsiness, fretfulness, and GI upset may occur. Pain at injection site is the most frequent adverse event reported for Tdap (CDC, 2006d, 2006e).

Seizures may occur and are more likely in children with a history of seizures, although less common now that DPT is no longer used in the United States. Seizures may be related to fever, and antipyretic prophylaxis is recommended every 4 to 6 hours in children with a history of febrile seizures after DTaP administration to decrease the incidence of febrile seizure after vaccination.

Drug Interactions

Coadministration of radiation therapy, antineoplastic agents, or immunosuppressives can decrease the immunological response to the DTaP vaccine.

DTaP, DT, and Td should not be administered concurrently with cholera vaccine, typhoid vaccine, or plague vaccine; there may be accentuated adverse effects. DTaP, DT, Tdap, or Td may be coadministered with HBV, HIB, meningococcal, influenza, hepatitis A, and pneumococcal vaccines.

Clinical Use and Dosing

DTaP is routinely given at age 2 months, 4 months, 6 months, 15 to 18 months, and 4 to 6 years. DT, if used, is given on the same schedule.

As a booster, Tdap is recommended at age 11 to 12 years. Tdap (ADACEL) is labeled for use in persons aged 11 to 64 years. Tdap (BOOSTRIX) is labeled for persons 10 to 64 years. Patients should receive a booster dose of Td or Tdap every 10 years. If a patient older than age 7 years has never been immunized, the primary series of Td is 3 doses. The first dose is followed by the second dose 4 weeks later. The third dose is given 6 to 12 months after the second dose. Every adult needs a booster every 10 years after completion of the primary series of 3 doses.

Monitoring

There is no laboratory monitoring needed with DTaP, DT, Tdap, or Td vaccine.

Patient Education

The parent or patient should receive a VIS prior to administration of vaccine. Any questions or concerns regarding the vaccine should be addressed.

The most common adverse reaction after DTaP, Tdap, or Td injection is pain and erythema at the injection site. Advise the patient to take acetaminophen for discomfort for the first 24 hours after injection.

Post-vaccination fever, myalgia, and headache can be treated with acetaminophen or ibuprofen prophylaxis. Pre-medicating with **antipyretics** before vaccination is not routinely recommended.

Haemophilus B Conjugate Vaccine

Pharmacodynamics

HIB conjugate vaccine consists of the HIB capsular polysaccharide covalently linked to another antigen to increase immunogenicity. **HIB conjugate vaccine** exposure stimulates the immune system to produce HIB capsule–specific antibodies that destroy the capsule. This makes the organism vulnerable to antibody- and cell-mediated immunity. Unconjugated capsule polysaccharide vaccines cause B-cell stimulation only. By conjugating the capsule polysaccharide, T-cell stimulation occurs as well. **HIB conjugate vaccine** comes singly and in combination with other vaccines (HBV/HIB [Comvax], DTaP/HIB [TriHibit], DTaP/IPV/HIB [Pentacel]).

Pharmacokinetics

HIB is administered IM. Antibodies are detected approximately 1 to 2 weeks after administration. The HIB is more immunogenic in older children; therefore, only one dose is needed for children receiving their first dose at age 15 months or older.

Ideally, the patient should receive the same conjugate vaccine product for all of the primary series of immunizations. However, when different products are given for the series, serum antibodies are similar to those of patients who received all the same formula.

The anticapsular antibodies may cross the placenta and are distributed in breast milk.

Pharmacotherapeutics

Precautions and Contraindications

Anaphylactic reaction to the vaccine or any component is a contraindication to HIB.

Moderate to severe illness, with or without fever, may be a reason to delay vaccine. Minor illness, including otitis media, is not a reason to delay administration.

HIB vaccine should be administered only to children under age 6 years.

Adverse Drug Reactions

The most common adverse reaction following HIB is pain, redness, and swelling at the injection site. These symptoms are mild and usually last less than 24 hours. Systemic reactions are infrequent, and when HIB is given with DTaP, there is no increased incidence of systemic reaction over DTaP given alone.

Drug Interactions

There are no known interactions.

Clinical Use and Dosing

Dosing of HIB depends on the vaccine used. **HibTITER** (HbOC) and **ActHib** (PRP-T) are given at 2 months, 4 months, 6 months, and a booster at 12 to 15 months. **PedvaxHIB** (PRP-OMP) is given at 2 months, 4 months, and a booster at 12 to 15 months. HIB/HBV (Combax) is given and 2, 4 and 12 to 15 months. **Pentacel** (DTaP/OPV/HIB) can be administered at 2, 4, 5 and 15 to 18 months. **TriHIBit** (DTaP/HIB) can be administered as the booster DTaP dose at 12 to 18 months if the primary HIB series was completed at least 6 months before. The first dose of HIB can be given at age 6 weeks but no earlier. Any HIB vaccine can be used for the booster dose at age 12 to 15 months.

If a child is receives the first dose at age 15 months or older but younger than 5 years, only one dose of HIB is needed.

Monitoring

No laboratory monitoring is necessary.

Patient Education

Parents should receive a VIS prior to administration of the **vaccine**. Any questions or concerns regarding the **vaccine** should be addressed.

The most common adverse reaction after HIB injection is pain and erythema at the injection site. Advise the parent to give acetaminophen for discomfort for the first 24 hours after injection.

Inactivated Poliovirus Vaccine

Pharmacodynamics

IPV is a parenteral noninfectious suspension of three types of inactivated poliovirus. The IPV available in the United States since the late 1980s is of enhanced potency and is highly immunogenic. IPV inhibits pharyngeal acquisition of poliovirus and, to a lesser extent, provides gut immunity. IPV is available in combination with **diphtheria, tetanus, pertussis,** and **hepatitis B** (Pediarix) or in combination with DTaP and HIB (Pentacel).

Pharmacokinetics

After IM administration of two doses, approximately 95 percent of patients have antibodies to polio. After three doses, 99 to 100 percent of patients have high antibody titers.

Pharmacotherapeutics

Precautions and Contraindications

A history of immediate hypersensitivity reaction after receiving IPV is a contraindication. Patients with **neomycin**, **streptomycin**, or **polymyxin B** hypersensitivity should not receive the vaccine because there are small amounts of these substances in the vaccine.

IPV is the preferred drug (over OPV) in immunosuppressed patients, although a protective immune response cannot be guaranteed. IPV can be administered to patients with HIV disease.

If it is needed to protect the patient, IPV may be administered during pregnancy. IPV is Pregnancy Category C.

IPV can be used in infants as young as 6 weeks of age.

Adverse Drug Reactions

Injection site reaction is reported in 13 percent of patients. Systemic reactions are infrequent, and when IPV is given with DTaP, there is no increased incidence of systemic reaction over DTaP given alone.

Drug Interactions

The immune response to IPV may be diminished if the patient is taking **immunosuppressant** medication. Revaccinate 3 months after discontinuing **immunosuppressants**.

IPV can be coadministered with all other childhood vaccines.

Monitoring

There is no need for laboratory monitoring after administration of IPV.

Patient Education

Parents should receive a VIS prior to administration of the **vaccine**. Any questions or concerns regarding the vaccine should be addressed.

The most common adverse reaction after IPV injection is pain and erythema at the injection site. Advise the parent to give **acetaminophen** for discomfort.

Hepatitis B Virus Vaccine

Pharmacodynamics

HBV is produced by recombinant DNA technology from common baker's yeast that is genetically modified to synthesize HbsAg. Active immunization with HBV stimulates the immune system to produce antihepatitis B surface antigen antibodies (anti-HBs). HBV is available in combination with **diphtheria, tetanus, acellular pertussis,** and **inactivated polio vaccine** (Pediarix), in combination with HAV (Twinrix), and in combination with HIB (Comvax).

Pharmacokinetics

Three doses of HBV induce protective antibody response in more than 95 percent of infants, children, and adolescents and in more than 90 percent of adults. Anti-HBs appear in the serum 2 weeks after IM administration. The minimum anti-HB titer needed to provide protection against hepatitis B is 10 milli-international units (mIU)/mL.

Pharmacotherapeutics

Precautions and Contraindications

The only true contraindication to HBV is hypersensitivity to yeast or other components of the vaccine.

Moderate or severe illness, with or without fever, is a contraindication to HBV.

Patients with renal disease requiring hemodialysis or patients with immunosuppression may require larger doses to achieve adequate serum levels of anti-HBs.

HBV is Pregnancy Category C. The CDC (2006i) has stated that HBV may be given in pregnancy if indicated.

Adverse Drug Reactions

Localized reaction at the injection site is reported by 17 percent of HBV vaccine recipients. Approximately 15 percent of patients report systemic complaints, including fatigue, weakness, malaise, fever, headache, nausea or vomiting, diarrhea, and pharyngitis. Serum sickness has occurred days to weeks after administration of HBV. A very rare side effect is alopecia (occurs 5/1 billion doses).

Drug Interactions

Patients who are taking **immunosuppressants** or **antineoplastic agents** may require larger doses or additional doses of HBV to achieve adequate anti-HB titers.

Clinical Use and Dosing

Vaccination with HBV is recommended for all ages, particularly patients at high risk of contracting hepatitis B. Those at high risk include IV drug users, infants born to mothers who are HbsAg-positive, hemodialysis patients, sexually active people with multiple partners, incarcerated people, international travelers, household contacts of hepatitis B carriers, and sexual contacts of hepatitis B carriers. Patients who are getting tattoos or who share razors,

> **CLINICAL PEARL**
>
> **Administering Injections**
>
> A technique to help older children, adolescents, or adults who are anxious about receiving injections is to encourage them to take slow, deep breaths. Younger children (5-year-olds) can be told to pretend they are blowing up a balloon. Have the patient inhale and exhale two or three times, and then, on the third or fourth exhalation, administer the injection.

toothbrushes, or body-piercing jewelry are also at risk of contracting hepatitis B. Health-care workers, day-care staff, and other people who may have exposure to body fluids also have a greater risk of contracting hepatitis B.

The ACIP and the AAP recommend universal vaccination of all infants as a comprehensive strategy to control hepatitis B. The current recommendations for childhood immunizations include administering the three-dose HBV series to newborns or at age 11 to 12 years to children not previously vaccinated. The series can be started at any age, although it is recommended that preterm infants be at least 1 month of age before starting HPV series (CDC, 2005a). Some states are requiring proof of HBV series completion for entry to the 7th grade.

Vaccination with HBV is recommended for all adults who are at high risk of contracting hepatitis B infection. The ACIP has issued a recommendation that HBV be offered to unvaccinated adults assumed to be at risk, including patients of sexually transmitted disease treatment clinics, HIV treatment facilities, drug abuse treatment programs, correctional facilities, chronic hemodialysis treatment centers, and services providing care to developmentally delayed adults (CDC, 2005a).

CLINICAL PEARL

Patients With Shot Phobia

In older children and adults who have a true phobia of injections, use **EMLA** cream to anesthetize the injection area. Have the patient apply the disk or cream 1 hour prior to the scheduled administration time, or the cream can be applied in the clinic and the injection administered after 1 hour.

The recommended schedule for vaccinating infants with HBV is to give the first dose at birth or before age 2 months. The second dose is given at age 1 to 4 months. Dose 3 is given at age 6 to 18 months. The rules regarding minimum HBV dose spacing in older children and adults are that there must be 4 weeks between doses 1 and 2, 2 months between doses 2 and 3, and 4 months between doses 1 and 3, allowing the series to be completed in as little as 4 months. The series is never restarted, no matter how long it has been since the previous dose.

The recommended dosing of HBV is provided in Table 19–6.

Table 19–6 ● Recommended Doses of Currently Licensed Formulations of Hepatitis B Vaccine by Age Group and Vaccine Type

	Single-Antigen Vaccine			Combination Vaccine						
	Recombivax HB	*Engerix-B*		*†Comvax**	*x§*		*Pediarix*			*Twinri*
Age group	Dose (mcg)	Volume (mL)	Dose (mcg)	Volume (mL)	Dose (mcg)	Volume (mL)	Dose (mcg)	Volume (mL)	Dose (mcg)	Volume (mL)
>6 wk to 4 yr* or 6 yr†	NA	NA	NA	NA	5	0.5	0	0.5	NA**	NA
Children (0–19 yr)	5	0.5	10	0.5	5*	0.5	10†	0.5	NA	NA
Adolescents 11–15 yr	10‡	1.0‡	10	0.5	NA	NA	NA	NA	NA	NA
11–19 yr	5	0.5	10	0.5	NA	NA	NA	NA	NA	NA
Adults (= 20 yr)	10	1.0	20	1.0	NA	NA	NA	NA	20§	1.0
Hemodialysis Patients and Other Immunocompromised Persons										
<20 yr§§	5	0.5	10	0.5	NA	NA	NA	NA	NA	NA
= 20 yr	40¶¶	1.0	40***	2.0	NA	NA	NA	NA	NA	NA

*_Combined hepatitis B–*Haemophilus influenzae* type b conjugate vaccine. This vaccine cannot be administered at birth, before age 6 wk, or after age 71 mo.
†_Combined hepatitis B–diphtheria, tetanus, and acellular pertussis-inactivated poliovirus vaccine. This vaccine cannot be administered at birth, before age 6 wk, or at age = 7 yr.
§_Combined hepatitis A and hepatitis B vaccines. This vaccine is recommended for persons aged =18 yr who are at increased risk for both hepatitis B virus and hepatitis A virus infections.
¶_Recombinant hepatitis B surface antigen protein dose.
**_Not applicable.
‡_Adult formulation administered on a two-dose schedule.
§§_Higher doses might be more immunogenic, but no specific recommendations have been made.
¶¶_Dialysis formulation administered on a three-dose schedule at age 0, 1, and 6 mo.
***_Two 1.0-mL doses administered at one site, on a four-dose schedule at ages 0, 1, 2, and 6 mo.
(Centers for Disease Control, 2005a).

HBV is generally given IM but may be given SC if IM injections are contraindicated (as in hemophiliacs). HBV should be given IM in the deltoid or anterolateral thigh. The immunogenicity of HBV is decreased when given in the buttock. HBV should not be given with the same syringe or at the same site as **hepatitis B immune globulin (H-BIG)**.

Patients who do not develop a serum anti-HB antibody response (greater than or equal to 10 mIU/mL) after three doses of HBV should be revaccinated with one to three doses. If the patient does not respond after three additional doses, he or she is unlikely to respond to any additional doses.

Monitoring

Susceptibility testing before HBV vaccination is not routinely indicated for children or adolescents. Testing for previous infection may be considered in adults in high-risk groups with high rates of hepatitis B infection, such as users of IV drugs, gay men, and household contacts of hepatitis B carriers.

Routine post-vaccination testing for anti-HBs is not necessary. Post-vaccination testing is advised 1 to 2 months after the third dose of HBV for those whose subsequent management is determined by their anti-HB status: (1) those at risk for occupational exposure risk from sharp injuries, (2) those with HIV infection, (3) hemodialysis patients, (4) immunocompromised patients at risk of contracting hepatitis B, (5) regular sexual contact of hepatitis carriers, and (6) infants born to HbsAg-positive mothers.

Patient Education

Parents should receive a VIS prior to administration of the vaccine. Any questions or concerns regarding the vaccine should be addressed.

The most common adverse reaction after HBV injection is pain and erythema at the injection site. Advise the parent to give **acetaminophen** for discomfort for the first 24 hours after injection.

Hepatitis A Virus Vaccine

Pharmacodynamics

HAV vaccine is used to confer immunity to hepatitis A in people at risk of contracting the disease. With HAV administration, stimulation of specific antibodies takes place without producing disease symptoms. Serum antibody titers after HAV are lower than those resulting from hepatitis A infection. Serum antibody titer of 20 mIU/mL is considered protective. There are two HAV products available. Both provide immunity with a two-dose schedule.

Pharmacokinetics

HAV is administered IM. One dose of HAV can induce seroconversion in 88 percent of patients by 15 days and 99 percent of patients by 1 month. This rapid seroconversion from a single dose can provide protection for at least 12 months. Administration of a second dose at 6 to 12 months after the first dose provides 100 percent protection. The duration of the **vaccine** protection has not been determined yet, as long-term efficacy has not been established. Theoretically, antibody levels should last 20 years or more. The CDC does not recommend any post-vaccination monitoring of serological response because of the high vaccine response in children and adults (CDC, 2006f).

Pharmacotherapeutics

Precautions and Contraindications

HAV should not be administered to patients with a previous history of severe reaction to HAV.

Moderate or severe illness, with or without fever, is a contraindication to HAV.

Patients with immunosuppression may be given HAV, but they may have lower antibody titers than immunocompetent people.

HAV is Pregnancy Category C. The CDC (2007a) has stated HAV may be given in pregnancy if indicated and that it poses no risk to the fetus.

The safety and effectiveness of HAV in children under age 12 months has not been established.

Adverse Drug Reactions

The most frequently reported adverse reaction to HAV is soreness at the injection site (56% in adults and 15% in children). Headache and malaise are other minor adverse reactions that have been reported.

Drug Interactions

Patients who are taking **immunosuppressants** or **antineoplastic agents** may have a decreased immunological response to HAV.

Clinical Use and Dosing

HAV vaccine provides pre-exposure protection from hepatitis A infection in adults and children. HAV is recommended for people who are at increased risk for infection and for any person wishing to obtain immunity.

The CDC previously recommended vaccination for children living in states in which the 1987 to1997 annual hepatitis A rate was 20 or more cases per 100,000 population. These states, listed by occurrence rate, are Arizona (48 cases/100,000), Alaska, Oregon, New Mexico, Utah, Washington, Oklahoma, South Dakota, Idaho, Nevada, and California (20 cases/100,000). In the 2006 Recommended Childhood Immunization Schedule, the ACIP, AAP, and American Academy of Family Physicians (AAFP) recommend that all children begin HAV at age 1, regardless of location. Providers can visit the CDC hepatitis A Web site at http://www.cdc.gov/hepatitis/index.htm for the latest information on hepatitis A.

People at increased risk for hepatitis A infection who should be routinely vaccinated include the following:

1. People over age 1 year who are traveling or working in countries that have high or intermediate endemic

infection. All of South America, Africa, Greenland, and Asia have a high incidence of hepatitis A infection. Russia and eastern Europe are areas of intermediate prevalence. IG is recommended for children under age 1 who are traveling to these areas.
2. Men who have sex with men.
3. Illegal drug users.
4. People who have an occupational risk for infection, including those who work with hepatitis A–infected primates or with hepatitis A in a research laboratory setting.
5. People with clotting factor disorders.
6. People with chronic liver disease.

Two different HAV products are currently available, **HAVrix** and **VAQTA**, as well as a combination product that combines HAV and HBV, **Twinrix**. **HAVrix** is available in two strengths: 1,440 enzyme-linked immunoassay units (EL.U) and 720 EL.U. The adult (age 19 years and older) dose is 1,440 EL.U administered in a two-dose schedule, 6 to 12 months apart. The pediatric (age 1 to 18 years) dose of **HAVrix** is 720 EL.U, administered in a two-dose schedule 6 to 12 months apart. **VAQTA** is available in two strengths: adult, which has 50 antigen U/1-mL dose, and pediatric-adolescent strength, which has 25 U/0.5-mL dose. The dose for adults is 50 U administered 6 months apart. The dose for children aged 1 to 18 years is 25 U administered 6 to 18 months apart. **Twinrix** is **HAVrix** (720 EL.U) combined with **Engerix-B** (20 mcg) and is approved for persons 18 years and older. The dosing schedule of **Twinrix** is 1.0 mL in 3 doses, at 0, 1, and 6 months.

HAV is injected IM into the deltoid muscle. Injection in the gluteal region results in suboptimal response. Patients with impaired an immune system may require additional doses to obtain an adequate anti–hepatitis A response.

Monitoring

Pre-immunization testing of children for hepatitis A antibodies is generally not recommended. Pretesting may be cost effective in adults who have a high likelihood of immunity from prior infection, such as those who have lived in areas of high hepatitis incidence, those older than 40, and those with a history of jaundice that potentially may have been hepatitis A infection (CDC, 2006f).

Post-immunization testing is not indicated in immunocompetent persons because of the high seroconversion rates in children and adults who receive HAV. Post-immunization testing is warranted in immunocompromised patients who may have suboptimal response to the **vaccine**.

Patient Education

Parents should receive a VIS prior to administration of the vaccine. Any questions or concerns regarding the **vaccine** should be addressed.

The most common adverse reaction after HAV injection is pain and erythema at the injection site. Advise the patient to take acetaminophen for discomfort for the first 24 hours after injection.

> **CLINICAL PEARL**
>
> **Bioterrorism**
>
> Providers need to have a basic understanding of vaccines available against possible biological weapons. The CDC Web site has an area dedicated to bioterrorism located at www.bt.cdc.gov/bioterrorism/. There are vaccines available for anthrax and smallpox, although this chapter does not discuss them because they are not currently recommended. Full prescribing information for both the anthrax and the smallpox vaccines are also available at the CDC National Immunization Web site at http://www.cdc.gov/nip/publications/acip-list.htm.

Human Papillomavirus Vaccine

Pharmacodynamics

Human papillomavirus (HPV) causes cervical cancer, the second-biggest cause of female cancer mortality worldwide, with an estimated 288,000 deaths yearly (WHO, 2011). "Genital HPV infection is extremely common and most often remains subclinical, but a proportion of the infected individuals with low-risk HPV types such as HPV-6 or HPV-11 will develop genital warts, whereas a subset of women with high-risk HPVs such as HPV-16 or HPV-18 will develop preneoplastic lesions of cervical intraepithelial neoplasia (CIN)" (WHO, 2005, p. 85). Approximately 500,000 cases of genital warts occur in men and women in the United States annually (CDC, 2010b). Two vaccines to treat HPV are currently available: **Gardisil** is a quadrivalent human papillomavirus recombinant vaccine that provides immunity against types 6, 11, 16, 18, and **Cervarix** a bivalent vaccine against HPV strains 16 and 18.

Pharmacokinetics

Cervarix (HPV2) is well tolerated after IM injection at 0, 1, and 6 months with a 99.8 percent antibody response, providing 100 percent efficacy against HPV 16 cervical infections and 89.6 percent efficacy against HPV 16 plus HPV 18 cervical infections (Pagliusi & Aguado, 2004). **Gardasil** (HPV4) has also demonstrated 100 percent efficacy in women against HPV 16 infection (median follow-up 17.4 months) using a 0-, 2-, and 6-month schedule of vaccination (Koutsky et al, 2002). **Gardasil** (HPV4) is 89.4 percent effective in preventing genital warts in males caused by HPV 6, 11, 16, and/or 18 strains (CDC, 2010b).

Pharmacotherapeutics

Precautions and Contraindications

The only true contraindication to HPV **vaccine** is severe allergic reactions to any component of the **vaccine**.

Gardasil should not be administered to patients allergic to yeast.

Both **vaccines** have a reported adverse effect of syncope. Patients should be observed for 15 minutes after administration and put in supine or Trendelenburg position if they become symptomatic.

Both **HPV vaccines** are rated Pregnancy Category B. They are not recommended for use in pregnancy. No causally associated adverse pregnancy outcome has been reported in preclinical or post-licensure studies. If a patient is administered **HPV vaccine** during pregnancy a registry has been set up by both manufacturers to report exposure (telephone: **Gardasil**, Merck & Co. at 800-986-8999; **Cervarix**, GlaxoSmithKline at 888-452-9622). Pregnancy testing is not needed before vaccination.

Adverse Drug Reactions

Pain, redness, and swelling at the injection site were the most commonly reported local adverse reaction, reported in over 20 percent of subjects receiving the **vaccines**.

The most common general adverse events were fatigue, headache, myalgias, and arthalgias.

The most common serious reaction to **HPV vaccine** is syncopal episodes. Reports of falling with injury due to syncope after receiving HPV have been reported; recommendations are that all patients who receive the **HPV vaccine** be observed for 15 minutes after administration.

Drug Interactions

No known drug interactions occur with **HPV vaccine**. **Immunosuppressants** may reduce the immune response to the vaccine.

Clinical Use and Dosing

Dosing of the **HPV vaccines** vary with drug and gender of the patient.

HPV4 (Gardasil) is approved for use in girls and women age 9 to 26 years of age to prevent cervical, vulvar, and vaginal cancer caused by HPV types 16 and 18 and genital warts (condyloma acuminata) caused by HPV types 6 and 11. HPV4 is recommended for all girls starting at age 11 to 12 years, but may be started as young as age 9 years. The dosing schedule is three doses of 0.5 mL given IM at 0, 2, and 6 months.

HPV4 (Gardasil) is approved for the prevention of genital warts caused by HPV types 6 and 11 in males. The **HPV4** vaccine may be given to males ages 9 to 26 years to prevent genital warts (CDC, 2010b). The dosing schedule for **HPV4** in males is 0.5 mL given IM at 0, 2, and 6 months.

HPV2 (Cervarix) is approved to prevent cervical cancer caused by HPV types 16 and 18 in females aged 10 to 25 years. **HPV2** is recommended by the ACIP as one of the two **HPV vaccines** for routine vaccination of females beginning at age 11 to 12 years (CDC, 2010a). The dose of **HPV2 (Cervarix)** is three 0.5 mL doses, at 0, 1 and 6 months.

After patients receive **HPV vaccine**, they should be monitored for 15 minutes because of the risk for syncope after the vaccine.

Monitoring

No ongoing monitoring of patients is needed after vaccination with **HPV vaccine**.

Patient Education

Parents should receive a VIS prior to administration of the vaccine. Any questions or concerns regarding the **vaccine** should be addressed.

Patients should be informed of the risk for syncope and why they need to be monitored after administration of HPV.

The most common adverse reactions after **HPV** injection are pain, erythema, and swelling at the injection site. Advise the patient to take acetaminophen for discomfort for the first 24 hours after injection.

Influenza Vaccine

Pharmacodynamics

Influenza vaccine (Agriflu, Fluogen, FluShield, Fluzone) is multivalent **vaccine** that contains three different viral subtypes. Each year, the World Health Organization recommends to the FDA's Vaccines and Related Biologic Products Advisory Committee what strains will be included in the following year's **vaccine**. Data from the WHO Influenza Surveillance Network are used to determine the composition of the Northern and Southern Hemisphere influenza **vaccine** for the following season. Because influenza viruses are constantly changing and immunity wanes over time, annual immunization is required. The previous year's **vaccine** cannot be used for the current year.

Influenza virus vaccine imparts immunity by stimulating production of antibodies that are specific to the disease strain. Patients who receive the **vaccine** are immune only to the strains included in the **vaccine** for that year.

Pharmacokinetics

The **influenza vaccine** is administered IM. The **vaccine** produces protective antibodies within 10 to 14 days. The duration of immunity generally lasts from 6 months to 1 year.

Pharmacotherapeutics

Precautions and Contraindications

Anaphylactic reaction to the **influenza vaccine**, eggs, or egg products is a contraindication to the use of **influenza vaccine**. If the patient's status is unclear, skin testing for egg allergy can clarify whether the vaccine can be given. Thimerosal is used as a preservative in the vaccine; therefore, patients with hypersensitivity to thimerosal should not receive the **influenza vaccine**. Some of the **influenza vaccines** contain sulfites; care should be taken to check the ingredients listed on the packaging prior to administering vaccine to a patient with sulfite hypersensitivity.

Patients with an active neurological disorder should defer the **vaccine** until the condition stabilizes. Any patient with a history of Guillain-Barré syndrome (GBS) less than 6 weeks after a previous dose of **influenza vaccine** should not receive the vaccine.

Patients with HIV disease may be immunized with **influenza vaccine**, but they may have lower vaccine-induced antibody levels.

Patients with an acute febrile illness should defer the **vaccine** until their symptoms subside. **Influenza vaccine** is Pregnancy Category C, but according to the CDC (2010i) **influenza vaccine** may be safely administered to pregnant women. **Influenza vaccine** may be administered to lactating women with no effect on the infant.

The safety of **influenza vaccine** has not been established in children younger than 6 months of age.

Administration error: The dosing schedules for children and adults for injectable **influenza vaccine** are different. If an adult is accidentally administered a pediatric dose (0.25 mL), the adult should receive and additional pediatric dose (0.25 mL) the same day. If the mistake is not discovered until later, a full adult dose is administered. If a child is administered an adult dose, no action needs to be taken.

Adverse Drug Reactions

Adverse reactions to the **influenza vaccine** are usually mild and more common in children than in adults.

Local injection site reaction occurs in about 23 percent of patients.

In addition, 5 to 10 percent of patients experience mild systemic adverse effects, including low-grade fever, malaise, and myalgia.

Rarely, a patient has an immediate hypersensitivity reaction to the **vaccine**, including urticaria, angioedema, bronchospasm, and/or anaphylactic shock. These reactions are most likely the result of hypersensitivity to residual egg protein.

Drug Interactions

Patients who are taking **immunosuppressants** or **antineoplastic** agents may have a decreased immunological response to **influenza vaccine.**

Medications that may have inhibited clearance after administration of **influenza vaccine** include **theophylline, phenytoin,** and **warfarin.** Reports concerning impaired drug clearance are conflicting, and the concurrent administration of **influenza vaccine** to patients taking these medications is not contraindicated.

Clinical Use and Dosing

The **influenza vaccine** should be administered annually to all persons aged 6 months and older, including pregnant women. The optimal time for organized vaccination programs is October through mid-November.

Travelers to areas in which influenza is endemic should be vaccinated 2 to 4 weeks prior to travel.

The dose of **influenza vaccine** is as follows:

1. Patients aged 9 years or older are given one 0.5-mL dose of **influenza vaccine** annually.
2. Adults aged 65 years or older may receive high-dose **influenza vaccine (Fluzone High-Dose).**
3. Previously vaccinated children aged 3 to 8 are given one 0.5-mL dose.
4. Children aged 3 to 8 who have never been vaccinated receive 0.5 mL, with a repeat dose in 4 weeks.
5. Children aged 6 to 35 months who have been previously vaccinated receive 0.25 mL of vaccine.
6. Children aged 6 to 35 months who have not been previously vaccinated with **influenza vaccine** receive 0.25 mL, with a second dose in 4 weeks.

Monitoring

There is no laboratory monitoring needed after patients receive the **influenza vaccine.**

Patient Education

Parents should receive a VIS prior to administration of vaccine. Any questions or concerns regarding the vaccine should be addressed.

The most common adverse reaction after **influenza vaccine** injection is pain and erythema at the injection site. Some patients may also experience low-grade fever and malaise. Advise the patient to take acetaminophen for discomfort for the first 24 hours after injection.

Pneumococcal Vaccine

Pharmacodynamics

There are two types of **pneumococcal vaccine (Pneumovax 23, Prevnar)** currently available. **Polyvalent pneumococcal polysaccharide vaccine (PPV)** contains 23 highly purified capsular polysaccharides from *Streptococcus pneumoniae.* These are the 23 most prevalent or invasive pneumococcal types, accounting for at least 90 percent of all blood isolates associated with clinical infection. PPV stimulates the immune system to produce pneumococcus capsule–specific antibodies. These antibodies presumably destroy the capsule, making the pneumococcus vulnerable to antibody- and cell-mediated immunity. Clinical trials suggest a protective efficacy of 60 to 90 percent. The 23-valent **PPV** has limited immunogenicity in children younger than 2 years. The 23-valent vaccine was approved by the FDA in 1977.

In February 2000, the FDA approved the first **vaccine** to prevent invasive pneumococcal disease in infants and children, **pneumococcal 7-valent conjugate vaccine (Prevnar).** The vaccine targeted the seven most common strains of pneumococcus, which accounted for 80 percent of invasive disease in infants. With universal vaccination of children under the age of 5 years with **PCV7**, invasive pneumococcol disease decreased by 76 percent over

10 years of use (CDC, 2010c). In spite of this reduction, there were still cases of invasive pneumococcal disease in children caused by strains not in the PCV7 vaccine.

In 2010 the FDA approved a **13-valent conjugate vaccine (Prevnar13; PCV13)**, which is active against six additional strains of pneumococcus, responsible for 64 percent of invasive pneumococcal disease in children vaccinated with PCV7 (CDC, 2010c). The vaccine is approved for use in patients up to age 5 years (high-risk patients up to age 71 months), but it is not meant to replace the 23-valent vaccine, which is approved for high-risk children over age 2 years.

Pharmacokinetics

PPV is administered either SC or IM. Immunity after SC or IM injection occurs in 2 to 3 weeks. Serotype-specific antibodies decline after 5 to 10 years. Children may decline to pre-vaccination levels in 3 to 5 years, especially asplenic children and children with sickle cell disease.

PCV13 is administered IM, with measurable titers present 1 month after the fourth dose.

Pharmacotherapeutics

Precautions and Contraindications

Previous anaphylactic reaction to the vaccine or any component is a contraindication to its use.

Moderate to severe illness, with or without fever, is a reason to defer the vaccine until the patient has improved.

Pneumococcal vaccine should be given at least 10 to 14 days before elective splenectomy, organ transplant, immunosuppressive therapy, or chemotherapy. Patients with Hodgkin's disease and immunosuppressed patients have suboptimal antibody response to vaccination.

Use PPV cautiously in patients with idiopathic thrombocytopenic purpura (ITP), as PPV has been associated with relapse of ITP.

PPV is Pregnancy Category C. Use of the vaccine during the first trimester should be avoided. It is not known if the vaccine is excreted in breast milk.

PPV 23-valent vaccine is not recommended in children under 2 years.

PCV13 is not for use in adults.

Adverse Drug Reactions

Seventy-two percent of PPV recipients report local injection site reactions of erythema, induration, and soreness that last up to 48 hours. Occasionally, low-grade fever and arthralgia have been reported. High fever is rare.

During clinical trials of Prevnar, adverse effects were generally mild and included local injection site reaction, irritability, drowsiness, and decreased appetite. Approximately 21 percent of children in the vaccine group had a fever of 100.8°F or higher, compared with 14 percent of the control group. During clinical trials of PCV13 (Prevnar 13) infants had redness (24.3%), swelling (20.1%) and tenderness (62.5%) at the injection site, and experienced fever (24.3%), irritability (85.6%) and increased sleep (71.5%) after the first dose at approximately the same rate as infants who received PCV7 (CDC, 2010f).

Drug Interactions

No known drug interactions have occurred.

Clinical Use and Dosing

Dosing of PPV is based on the age and medical condition of the patient:

1. PPV is recommended for all adults aged 65 or older. The dose is 0.5 mL IM or SC. Revaccinate (a second dose) if the original vaccination was 5 years or more ago *and* the patient was under age 65 when the dose was given.
2. People aged 2 years to 65 years who have chronic illness and who are at increased risk of morbidity or mortality from pneumococcal disease should receive PPV. These risk factors include chronic cardiac or pulmonary disease, chronic liver disease or alcoholism, diabetes mellitus, and cerebrospinal fluid leaks. The dose of PPV is 0.5 mL given IM or SC once. Revaccination is not recommended in these populations.
3. Immunocompetent patients aged 2 years to 65 years with functional or anatomic asplenia (including sickle cell anemia) should receive 0.5 mL IM or SC. Revaccination is recommended 5 years or more after the first dose; if the patient is under 10 years old, revaccination should be considered 5 years after the first dose.
4. Immunocompromised patients (including HIV infection); those with chronic renal failure, hematological malignancy, Hodgkin's disease, lymphoma, or multiple myeloma; patients receiving immunosuppressive therapy; and patients who have received an organ or bone marrow transplant should receive a dose of 0.5 mL IM or SC. Revaccination should be considered if the first vaccine was 5 years or more ago; in children under age 10, revaccination is considered 5 years after the first dose.
5. Adult smokers between the ages of 19 and 64 years should be given one dose of PPV.
6. Patients with asthma between the ages of 19 and 64 years should receive one dose of PPV.
7. One dose of PPV at 12 and 24 months following bone marrow transplant.
8. A dose of PPV is administered 2 or more months after last dose of PCV13 to children age 2 years or older.

The suggested dosing schedule for PCV13 is four doses given at 2, 4, 6, and 12 to 15 months of age. Children who are not vaccinated with PCV 13 at the routine infant vaccine times, should be dosed following the Catch Up schedule (see Table 19–3).

Monitoring

No laboratory monitoring is necessary.

Patient Education

Parents should receive a VIS prior to administration of the **vaccine**. Any questions or concerns regarding the vaccine should be addressed.

The most common adverse reaction after **pneumococcal vaccine** injection is pain and erythema at the injection site. Advise the patient to take **acetaminophen** for discomfort for the first 24 hours after injection.

Meningococcal Vaccine

Pharmacodynamics

Two **meningococcal vaccines** are currently approved in the United States. **Meningococcal polysaccharide vaccine (MPSV) groups A, C, Y, and W-135 (Menomune A/C/Y/W-135).** MPSV is for use against meningococcemia and meningitis caused by *Neisseria meningitidis* serogroups A, C, Y, and W-135. **MCV4 (Menactra, Menveo)** is a tetravalent **meningococcal conjugate vaccine** that also provides protection against serogroups A, C, Y, and W-135.

Based on multistate surveillance data from July 1994 to June 2002, *N. meningitidis* serogroup C accounted for 63 percent of meningococcal disease, serogroup B for 25 percent, and serogroups Y and W-135 for most of the remaining cases (CDC, 2005c). Serogroup A is rare in the United States but the most common cause of epidemics in Africa and Asia.

Both **meningococcal vaccines** induce the formation of bactericidal antibodies to meningococcal antigens. Post-immunization seroconversion rates for **Menomune A/C/Y/W-135** reported by the manufacturer in children aged 2 years to 12 years were group A, 72 percent; group C, 58 percent; group Y, 90 percent; and group W-135, 82 percent. Among 20,000 military recruits under epidemic conditions, the **vaccine** demonstrated 90 percent efficacy against serogroup C. **MCV4 (Menactra, Menveo)** demonstrated similar efficacy in patients age 11 to 55 years in clinical trials (CDC, 2005c, 2010e).

Limitations of the **meningococcal polysaccharide vaccine (Menomune)** include the following: Serogroup C polysaccharide is poorly immunogenic among children aged less than 2 years, it does not confer long-lasting immunity, and it does not cause a sustainable reduction of nasopharyngeal carriage of *N. meningitidis* (CDC, 2005c). Conjugation of polysaccharide (as in **MCV4**) to a protein carrier changes the immune response from T cell independent to T cell dependent, leading to stronger response to the vaccine and reduction of asymptomatic carrier state (CDC, 2006d).

Pharmacokinetics

Protective antibody levels may be achieved within 7 to 10 days after vaccination. The measurable levels of antibodies to serogroups A and C decrease during the first 3 years following vaccination. This decrease occurs more rapidly in infants and young children than it does in adults.

Pharmacotherapeutics

Precautions and Contraindications

Previous anaphylactic reaction to any component of the vaccine is a contraindication to its use.

Moderate to severe illness, with or without fever, is a reason to defer the **vaccine** until the patient has improved.

The expected immune response may not be obtained if the **vaccine** is used in patients on immunosuppressive therapy.

Menomune A/C/Y/W-135 should not be given to pregnant women. It is not recommended for children under age 2 years. **MCV4 (Menactra)** is approved for use in children age 2 years or older and adults; it is not recommended in adults older than 55 years. **MCV4 (Menveo)** is not recommended for children younger than 11 or adults older than 55 years.

MPSV (Menomune) is the only vaccine approved for adults older than age 55 years.

Adverse Drug Reactions

Adverse reactions to either **vaccine** are mild and consist of pain and tenderness at the injection site for 1 to 2 days.

Drug Interactions

There are no known drug interactions to this **vaccine**.

Clinical Use and Dosing

The ACIP (CDC, 2005c) recommends routine vaccination of young adolescents (defined as aged 11 to 12 years) with **MCV4** at the preadolescent health-care visit or on entering high school (age 15). The ACIP also recommends that the following high-risk groups receive meningococcal vaccine:

1. Patients with deficiencies in late complement components (C3, C5, to C9).
2. Persons with functional or actual asplenia.
3. Research, industrial, and clinical laboratory personnel who routinely are exposed to *N. meningitidis* in solution that may be aerosolized.
4. Travelers to, and residents of, hyperendemic areas such as sub-Saharan Africa. Epidemics have occurred recently in Saudi Arabia, Kenya, Tanzania, Burundi, and Mongolia.
5. College freshmen living in dorms.
6. Military recruits.

MCV4 is administered IM as a single 0.5-mL dose. The dose of **Menomune** for all ages is a single SC 0.5-mL dose.

In patients age 2 years to 10 years, **MCV4 (Menactra)** is the preferred vaccine. Adults over age 55 years should receive **MPSV**.

Revaccination may be indicated for persons at high risk for infection (travel to or living in epidemic areas) who were previously vaccinated with **MPSV** or **MCV4**. Children who were vaccinated between age 2 and 6 years old should be considered for revaccination with **Menactra** in 3 years if they remain at high risk. If previous dose was given at age 7 years or older, either brand of MCV4 may be given after 5 years. Revaccination with MCV4 of high-risk older children and adults may be considered in 5 years after the first dose of MPSV or MCV4.

The ACIP recommendations for booster vaccination of adolescents with MCV4 will change with the 2011 immunization schedule due to waning antibody levels within 5 years of vaccination (Brady, 2011). A booster dose of MCV4 is recommended at age 16 years in children who received their first dose of MCV4 at age 11 to 12 years. Adolescents who receive their first dose of MCV4 at age 13 to 15 years should receive a booster dose at age 16 to 18 years, or up to 5 years after the first dose (Brady, 2011).

Monitoring

Laboratory monitoring is not necessary with this vaccine.

Patient Education

Parents should receive information regarding the benefits and risks of the vaccine prior to administration. Any questions or concerns regarding the vaccine should be addressed.

The most common adverse reaction after vaccine injection is pain and erythema at the injection site. Advise the patient to take acetaminophen for discomfort for the first 24 hours after injection.

Lyme Disease Vaccine

Pharmacodynamics

Lyme disease is a vector-borne illness caused by ticks infested with *Borrelia burgdorferi*. Recombinant Lyme disease vaccine (LYMErix, Immulyme) imparts immunity against *B. burgdorferi* by stimulating production of antibodies to the lipoprotein OspA. OspA is a lipoprotein of the *B. burgdorferi* spirochete. The mechanism by which Lyme disease vaccine works is thought to be by antibody killing of the spirochete in the tick. Transmission of the OspA antibody occurs while the tick is feeding on the blood of an immunized host, and the antibodies kill the spirochete even before transmission occurs. In February 2002, SmithKline Beecham, the maker of the only approved Lyme disease vaccine, LYMErix, discontinued its production after there were concerns about the side effects of the vaccine, although an FDA investigation did not find the vaccine to be dangerous. The long-term immunity for patients who previously received the vaccine is unknown.

Typhoid Vaccine

Pharmacodynamics

Typhoid vaccines (Typhoid Vaccine, Typhim Vi) are used to increase resistance to enteric fever caused by *S. typhi*. The efficacy of protective immunity depends on the size of the bacterial inoculum consumed.

There are two parenteral typhoid vaccines available, a heat- and phenol-inactivated vaccine (Typhoid Vaccine) and a purified Vi polysaccharide (Typhim Vi). Efficacy of Typhoid Vaccine is 71 to 77 percent. The efficacy of Typhim Vi is 49 to 87 percent in reducing disease incidence. Typhim Vi is used in the United States, and a second brand of Vi polysaccharide, Typherix, is used in Canada.

Pharmacokinetics

Absorption, distribution, and metabolism of typhoid vaccine are unknown.

Pharmacotherapeutics

Precautions and Contraindications

Hypersensitivity to typhoid vaccine is a contraindication to its use.

Do not administer to a patient with acute febrile illness.

Typhoid vaccine is Pregnancy Category C. It is not known if the vaccine is harmful to the fetus. If vaccinating a pregnant patient is necessary, inactivated vaccine is recommended.

Typhim Vi and Typherix are not recommended for children under age 2.

Adverse Drug Reactions

Vaccine recipients report local injection site reactions of erythema, induration, and soreness that begin within 24 hours and last 1 to 2 days. Systemic symptoms including low-grade fever, headache, and myalgias have been reported. High fever is rare.

Drug Interactions

If possible, plague vaccine should not be given at the same time as typhoid vaccine to avoid the possibility of accentuated adverse effects.

Immunosuppressants may cause insufficient response to the vaccine.

Clinical Use and Dosing

Typhoid vaccine is used for primary immunization against *S. typhi* infection in the following:

1. Travelers to areas where a risk of exposure to *S. typhi* is recognized.
2. Persons with household contact with a documented typhoid fever carrier.
3. Laboratory workers with frequent contact with *S. typhi*.

The dose of Typhim Vi and Typherix in children older than age 2 years and adults is 0.5 mL SC. A booster dose should be administered every 2 years to patients at continued risk of contracting typhoid.

Monitoring

There is no laboratory monitoring needed after typhoid vaccine.

Patient Education

Parents should receive information regarding the benefits and risks of the **vaccine** prior to administration. Any questions or concerns regarding the vaccine should be addressed.

The most common adverse reaction after **typhoid** vaccination injection is pain and erythema at the injection site. Advise the patient to take **acetaminophen** for discomfort for the first 24 hours after injection.

The best protection against typhoid fever is food and water precautions to prevent contracting *S. typhi*.

Cholera Vaccine

Pharmacodynamics

Cholera vaccine is a suspension of equal parts inactivated Ogawa and Inuba serotypes of killed *Vibrio cholerae*. **Cholera vaccine** provides active immunity against cholera. The vaccine is 50 percent effective in reducing disease in endemic areas. The manufacture and sale of the only licensed **cholera vaccine** in the United States (Wyeth-Ayerst) has been discontinued. It has not been recommended for travelers because of the brief and incomplete immunity if offers. No cholera vaccination requirements exist for entry or exit in any country" (CDC, 2005b).

Japanese Encephalitis Virus Vaccine

Pharmacodynamics

Japanese encephalitis (JE) is the most common form of viral encephalitis in Asia and is spread by mosquitoes. An estimated 35,000 to 50,000 cases occur annually. JE is usually severe, resulting in death in 20 to 30 percent of cases, miscarriage in pregnant women, and serious neurological outcomes in 30 to 50 percent of infected patients (CDC, 2010d). Two vaccines are available. Inactivated mouse brain **JE virus vaccine (JE-VAX)** is an inactivated vaccine derived from infected mouse brain. Production of **JE-VAX** ceased in 2010. Currently the only vaccine in production in the United States for JE is an **inactivated Vero cell culture-derived vaccine (IXIARO)**.

Pharmacokinetics

JE-VAX is administered in a three-dose schedule, administered at 0, 7, and 30 days, provides the highest level of immunity against JE. Length of full protection against JE is unknown, although immunity is known to last for 12 months after a 3-dose initial series.

IXIARO is administered via a two-dose schedule, at 0 and 28 days; 96 percent of **vaccine** recipients demonstrated an adequate level of immunity against JE. Length of full protection against JE is unknown

Pharmacotherapeutics

Precautions and Contraindications

Previous anaphylactic reaction to any component of the **vaccine**, including thimerosal, is a contraindication to its use.

Pregnancy is a contraindication to **JE-VAX** and **IXIARO** use.

IXIARO is not approved for children younger than age 17 years (CDC, 2010d). Until safety data are available on **IXIARO**, all currently available doses of **JE-VAX** are reserved for children.

Adverse Drug Reactions

Overall, 20 percent of recipients experience adverse effects from the **JE-VAX** vaccine. **Vaccine** recipients report local injection site reactions of erythema, induration, and soreness. Systemic symptoms including low-grade fever, headache, rash, chills, dizziness, and malaise. Adverse reactions occur usually within 48 hours but may occur as long as 10 days after vaccination.

Generalized urticaria and angioedema of the face, lips, and oropharynx may occur in about 1 to 104 per 10,000 doses of **JE-VAX**. Most patients are successfully treated with **antihistamines** or **corticosteroids**. Patients with a history of allergies are more likely to develop this reaction. Patients should be advised to remain in areas in which medical intervention is available for 10 days after administration, as delayed allergic response may occur.

IXIARO appears to have the same reported adverse reactions as placebo. As only 5,000 doses had been administered prior to approval, post-licensure surveillance is ongoing. Report any significant adverse effects to the VAERS.

Drug Interactions

There are no known drug interactions.

Clinical Use and Dosing

The ACIP recommends that **JE-VAX** be administered to those who plan on residing in areas in which JE is endemic or epidemic. The probability of JE viral infection and illness increases with the duration of the stay in rural endemic areas. Current information on locations of JE virus transmission can be obtained from the CDC *Yellow Book* or Travel Web site (http://www.cdc.gov/travel).

JE-VAX or **IXIARO** is not recommended for all travelers to Asia. The **vaccine** should be offered to people spending a month or longer in endemic areas during the transmission season, especially if they are traveling to rural areas. It should also be offered to those who will be spending extensive time outdoors during their travel.

The dose of **JE-VAX** for children aged 3 years and older is a series of three SC doses of 1 mL each, given on days 0, 7, and 30. An abbreviated dosing schedule may be used if necessary, with dosing at 0, 7, and 14 days (only in special circumstances and not recommended routinely). The dose in children aged 1 to 3 years is identical except that the dose is 0.5 mL SC. Safety in infants under age 1 is not known. A booster dose of 1.0 mL (0.5 mL in children younger than 3 years) may be administered 2 years after the primary series.

The dose of IXIARO is two 0.5-mL doses administered IM 28 days apart. The series should be completed at least 1 week before potential exposure to Japanese encephalitis virus. Need for a booster is not known, as the vaccine is newly approved. Providers are referred to the CDC Travel Web site for dosing information (http://www.cdc.gov/travel). IXIARO is not licensed for use in children younger than 17 years as of this date (CDC, 2010d).

Monitoring

There is no monitoring needed after the vaccine.

Patient Education

Patients should receive information regarding the benefits and risks of the **vaccine** prior to administration. Any questions or concerns regarding the vaccine should be addressed.

The most common adverse reactions after vaccination are pain and erythema at the injection site and low-grade systemic symptoms. Adverse reactions may occur up to 10 days after immunization. Patients are advised not to travel outside the United States for 10 days after administration in case of adverse reaction.

Personal protection against mosquitoes is essential for all travelers to endemic areas. Patients should be advised to protect themselves by wearing long-sleeved shirts and long pants. Use of insect repellant should be encouraged. **Permethrin** should be applied to clothing.

Plague Vaccine

Pharmacodynamics

Plague vaccine is a whole-cell vaccine consisting of a suspension of inactivated plague bacilli (*Yersinia pestis*) is no longer available in the United States. Vaccination against plague is not required by any country as a condition for entry. Travelers who may be exposed to plague should carry prophylactic antibiotics (**doxycycline**, or **trimethoprim-sulfamethoxazole** for children less than 8 years of age) and use them according to the CDC guidelines for plague, which can be found at the CDC Traveler's Health Web site, http://www.cdc.gov/travel

Rabies Vaccine

Pharmacodynamics

Rabies vaccine (Imovax, RabAvert) is a preparation of inactivated rabies virus, which induces active immunity. The two products available differ only in the cell culture used to develop the vaccine. **Imovax** uses human diploid cell (HDC) culture, and **RabAvert** uses purified chick embryo cell culture.

Pharmacokinetics

An antibody response to **rabies vaccine** can be measured in 7 to 10 days after administration. Antibodies persist for 2 years.

Pharmacotherapeutics

Precautions and Contraindications

Previous anaphylactic reaction to any component of the vaccine, including neomycin, is a contraindication to its use.

Moderate to severe illness, with or without fever, is a reason to defer the **vaccine** until the patient has improved.

The expected immune response may not be obtained if the **vaccine** is used in patients on immunosuppressive therapy.

Rabies vaccine is Pregnancy Category C. Pregnancy is not a contraindication to post-exposure vaccination of pregnant women. Safety in children under age 6 has not been established.

Adverse Drug Reactions

Local reactions, including pain, erythema, and swelling of the injection site, have been reported by 30 to 70 percent of **vaccine** recipients. Systemic reactions have been reported by 5 to 40 percent of recipients. Systemic reactions include headache, nausea, abdominal pain, muscle aches, and dizziness. Three cases of a neurological illness resembling Guillain-Barré syndrome have been reported.

A serum sickness–like reaction has been reported among about 6 percent of patients who received booster doses of **Imovax**.

Drug Interactions

Long-term therapy with **chloroquine (Aralen)** can interfere with the active antibody response to rabies vaccine.

Patients who are taking **immunosuppressants** or **antineoplastic agents** may have a decreased immunological response to rabies vaccine.

Rabies IG (RIG) can partially suppress the antibody response to **rabies vaccine**. Follow the CDC recommendations for simultaneous administration exactly, and give no more than recommended dose of **RIG**.

Clinical Use and Dosing

Rabies vaccine can be given for primary or pre-exposure vaccination or as part of post-exposure prophylaxis. Pre-exposure vaccination is recommended to high-risk groups, such as veterinarians, animal handlers, and certain laboratory workers. Post-exposure prophylaxis is recommended if the patient has a bite from a rabid animal that penetrates the skin. Post-exposure vaccine administration should always be accompanied by the use of **RIG**.

Pre-exposure vaccine dosing consists of three 1-mL IM injections of **vaccine** in the deltoid muscle. The doses are given on day 0, day 7, and either day 21 or day 28. A booster dose of 1 mL is given every 2 years to those considered at frequent risk if their serum antibody titer is less than 1:5. Persons considered at frequent risk include veterinarians, animal control officers, wildlife officers, and staff where rabies is enzootic. In very high-risk patients, those who work in research laboratories or vaccine production facilities, a serum rabies antibody test should be done every 6 months and vaccine administered if levels are less than 1:5.

Post-exposure prophylaxis always includes administration of both **passive antibody** and **vaccine**, with the exception of those who have previously received complete vaccination (pre-exposure or post-exposure). For post-exposure vaccination, the ACIP recommends four doses of **rabies vaccine**. The dose is 1 mL given IM on days 0, 3, 7, and 14, with RIG given on day 0 (Rupprecht et al, 2010). For those who have previously been vaccinated, two doses of **rabies vaccine** are given on days 0 and 3, with no RIG needed.

Monitoring

Patients who receive a four-dose schedule of **rabies vaccine** do not need post-vaccination serological testing (Rupprecht et al, 2010).

Patient Education

Patients should receive information regarding the benefits and risks of the **vaccine** prior to administration. Any questions or concerns regarding the vaccine should be addressed. The need for repeated doses should be discussed.

The most common adverse reactions after rabies vaccination injection are pain and erythema at the injection site and systemic symptoms including headache, nausea, abdominal pain, muscle aches, and dizziness. Advise the patient to take **acetaminophen** for discomfort.

Table 19–7 presents issues concerning immunizations.

IMMUNE GLOBULIN SERUMS

IG serums provide passive immunity to infectious diseases. The choice of IG is determined by the types of products available, the type of antibody desired, route of

Table 19–7 **Issues in Immunization**

Childhood Immunization Ideally, immunizations should be given as a part of comprehensive child health care. It is widely recognized that childhood immunizations are the most cost-effective way of preventing infectious diseases in children. Identified barriers to childhood immunization include the following: 1. Financial, with low socioeconomic status placing a child at risk of underimmunization 2. Family structure issues, such as single or teen parenthood (Bates & Wolinsky, 1998) 3. Perceived attitudes regarding the benefit of immunization 4. Provider policies and practices that lead to missed vaccine opportunities during clinic visits
Standards for Child and Adolescent Immunization Practices (National Vaccine Advisory Committee, 2009) **AVAILABILITY OF VACCINES** 1. Vaccination services are readily available. 2. Vaccinations are coordinated with other health-care services and provided in a medical home when possible. 3. Barriers to vaccination are identified and minimized. 4. Patient costs are minimized.
ASSESSMENT OF VACCINATION STATUS 5. Health-care professionals review the vaccination and health status of patients at every encounter to determine which vaccines are indicated. 6. Health-care professionals assess for and follow only medically indicated contraindications.
EFFECTIVE COMMUNICATION ABOUT VACCINE BENEFITS AND RISKS 7. Parents/guardians and patients are educated about the benefits and risks of vaccination in a culturally appropriate manner and in easy-to-understand language.
PROPER STORAGE AND ADMINISTRATION OF VACCINES AND DOCUMENTATION OF VACCINATIONS 8. Health-care professionals follow appropriate procedures for vaccine storage and handling. 9. Up-to-date, written vaccination protocols are accessible at all locations where vaccines are administered. 10. Persons who administer vaccines and staff who manage or support vaccine administration are knowledgeable and receive ongoing education. 11. Health-care professionals simultaneously administer as many indicated vaccine doses as possible. 12. Vaccination records for patients are accurate, complete, and easily accessible. 13. Health-care professionals report adverse events following vaccination promptly and accurately to the Vaccine Adverse Events Reporting System (VAERS) and are aware of a separate program, the National Vaccine Injury Compensation Program (NVICP). 14. All personnel who have contact with patients are appropriately vaccinated.
IMPLEMENTATION OF STRATEGIES TO IMPROVE VACCINATION COVERAGE 15. Systems are used to remind parents/guardians, patients, and health-care professionals when vaccinations are due and to recall those who are overdue. 16. Office- or clinic-based patient record reviews and vaccination coverage assessments are performed annually. 17. Health-care professionals practice community-based approaches.

Table 19–7 Issues in Immunization—cont'd

Standards for Adult Immunization Practices (National Vaccine Advisory Committee, 2009)

MAKE VACCINATIONS AVAILABLE.

1. Adult vaccination services are readily available.
2. Barriers to receiving vaccines are identified and minimized.
3. Patient "out-of-pocket" vaccination costs are minimized.

ASSESS PATIENTS' VACCINATION STANDARDS.

4. Health-care professionals routinely review the vaccination status of patients.
5. Health-care professionals assess for valid contraindications.

COMMUNICATE EFFECTIVELY WITH PATIENTS.

6. Patients are educated about risks and benefits of vaccination in easy-to-understand language.

ADMINISTER AND DOCUMENT VACCINATIONS PROPERLY.

7. Written vaccination protocols are available at all locations where vaccines are administered.
8. Persons who administer vaccines are properly trained.
9. Health-care professionals recommend simultaneous administration of indicated vaccine doses.
10. Vaccination records for patients are accurate and easily accessible.
11. All personnel who have contact with patients are appropriately vaccinated.

IMPLEMENT STRATEGIES TO IMPROVE VACCINATION RATES.

12. Systems are developed and used to remind patients and health-care professionals when vaccinations are due and to recall patients who are overdue.
13. Standing orders for vaccinations are employed.
14. Regular assessments of vaccination coverage levels are conducted in a provider's practice.

PARTNER WITH THE COMMUNITY.

15. Patient-oriented and community-based approaches are used to reach the target.

Immunization in Special Populations

Pregnant Patients

The ACIP has published guidelines for vaccinating pregnant women (CDC, 1998 updated, 2007a): "The risk from vaccination during pregnancy is largely theoretical. The benefit of vaccination among pregnant women usually outweighs the potential risk for disease when (a) the risk for disease exposure is high, (b) infections would pose a special risk for the mother or fetus, and (c) the vaccine is unlikely to cause harm" (CDC, 1998, updated, 2007).

Generally, live-virus vaccines are contraindicated in pregnant women because of the possible risk of transmission to the fetus. If a woman is inadvertently given live-virus vaccine while pregnant, she should be counseled about the potential effects on the fetus. It is not normally an indication to terminate pregnancy.

Recommendations for Vaccination During Pregnancy Include the Following:

Vaccine	May Be Given if Indicated	Contraindicated During Pregnancy	Comments
Routine			
Hepatitis B	X		The theoretical risk to the fetus is low from the inactivated vaccine
MMR		X	
Meningococcal			Safety has not been evaluated in pregnant women
Td	X		
Tdap			Pregnancy is not a contraindication for Tdap administration. ACIP recommends Td when tetanus and diphtheria protection is required during pregnancy. In some situations (pregnant adolescent, health-care worker or child-care provider), health-care providers can choose to administer Tdap instead of Td to add protection against pertussis.
Varicella		X	

Continued

Table 19–7 **Issues in Immunization—cont'd**

Vaccine	May Be Given if Indicated	Contraindicated During Pregnancy	Comments
Human papillomavirus (HPV)			Not recommended during pregnancy
Influenza (inactivated)	X		Recommend for all women pregnant during flu season
Influenza (LAIV)		X	
Pneumococcal			The safety of the pneumococcal vaccine in the first trimester of pregnancy has not been determined
IPV			Vaccination of pregnant women should be avoided, although no adverse effects have been documented. If the woman is at risk, IPV may be administered.
Travel and Others Anthrax			Vaccinate only if benefits outweigh risks to fetus
BCG		X	
Japanese encephalitis (JE)			The vaccine should not be routinely administered during pregnancy. If a pregnant woman will be moving to an area of high risk of JE, then vaccination should be considered.
Meningococcal (MPSV)	X		
Rabies	X		
Typhoid (parenteral and oral)			It is not known if the vaccine is harmful to the fetus. If necessary to vaccinate a pregnant patient, inactivated vaccine is recommended.
Vaccinia (smallpox)			Vaccinia vaccine should not be administered to pregnant women for routine nonemergency indications. Pregnant women who have had a definite exposure to smallpox virus (i.e., face-to-face, household, or close-proximity contact with a smallpox patient) and are, therefore, at high risk for contracting the disease, should be vaccinated.
Yellow fever			It is not known if the vaccine is harmful to the fetus. Only vaccinate pregnant women who are at high risk of contracting disease.
Zoster		X	
Immunocompromised Patients For practical considerations, persons with immunocompromising conditions may be divided into three groups:			
1. Persons who are severely immunocompromised not as a result of HIV infection 2. Persons with HIV infection 3. Persons with conditions that cause limited immune deficits (e.g., asplenia, renal failure) that may require use of special vaccines or higher doses of vaccines but that do not contraindicate use of any particular vaccine ACIP recommendation for vaccinations is based on where the patient falls within these three groups.			
1. Persons who are severely immunocompromised not as a result of HIV infection: In general, these patients should not be administered live vaccines. Measles, mumps, and rubella (MMR) vaccine is not contraindicated for the close contacts. Passive immunization with immune globulin should be considered for immunocompromised persons instead of or in addition to vaccination. 2. In general, persons known to be HIV infected should not receive live-virus or live-bacteria vaccines. MMR vaccination is recommended for all children and for adults when otherwise indicated, regardless of their HIV status. Enhanced inactivated polio vaccine (eIPV) is the preferred polio vaccine for persons known to have HIV infection. Pneumococcal vaccine is indicated for all HIV-infected persons ≥2 yr of age. 3. Persons with conditions that cause limited immune deficits (e.g., asplenia, renal failure) that may require use of special vaccines or higher doses of vaccines but that do not contraindicate use of any particular vaccine. Persons with these conditions are generally not considered immunosuppressed for the purposes of vaccination and should receive routine vaccinations with both live and inactivated vaccines according to the usual schedules.			

Table 19–7 **Issues in Immunization—cont'd**

Travel Immunization International travel is becoming more common, with jet travel allowing people to travel great distances in a few hours. With international travel comes exposure to infectious diseases not common in the United States. Patients should be advised to begin to prepare for their trip at least 8 wk prior to departure. To determine what vaccines the traveling patient will need, the provider can consult with a local travel clinic or the CDC. The CDC Web site has a travel information section, maintained by the National Center for Infectious Disease (http://www.cdc.gov/travel/). The Web site allows the provider or patient to inquire into recommendations based on the region the patient will be traveling to. Information on traveling with children, outbreaks, and special needs travelers is also located at this site. The CDC also publishes an annual guide, *The Yellow Book: Health Information for International Travel.* In addition to special immunizations required by travel, patients should also have all of the recommended routine immunizations for their age, including influenza vaccine. Patients should have a copy of their current immunizations included with their travel documents.

administration, timing, and other considerations. IG products that may be used in primary care include **immune globulin IM (IGIM, BayGam; GamaSTAN S/D), hepatitis B immune globulin (H-BIG, HepaGam B), tetanus immune globulin (TIG, HyperTET S/D), respiratory syncytial virus immune globulin (RSV-IGIV, RespiGam), varicella-zoster immune globulin (VZIG), rabies immune globulin (RIG, HyperRab S/D, Imogam), Rh_0(D) immune globulin (RhoGAM, HyperRHO-S/D), and vaccinia immune globulin (VIG).**

Pharmacodynamics

IGs are derived from the pooled plasma of adults, processed by cold ethanol fractionation. It consists primarily of immunoglobulin fraction (95% IgG) and is not known to transmit hepatitis, HIV, or other infectious diseases. The concentrated protein solution contains specific antibodies in proportion to the infectious and immunization experience of the donor population from which the plasma was derived. **IG serums** undergo processing to remove and inactivate viruses, including hepatitis A, B, and C; parvovirus B-19; and HIV. Specific **IGs** differ from **IGIM**, which is sometimes referred to as gamma globulin, in that they have high levels of a specific IG.

IGIM (BayGam; GamaSTAN S/D) is a sterile preparation of concentrated antibodies. **IGIM** provides protection against hepatitis A and measles through passive transfer of antibody. It may be used for pre-exposure prophylaxis or post-exposure prevention in the treatment of hepatitis A; it is used post-exposure in measles.

Hepatitis B immune globulin (HBIG, HepaGam B) is a sterile solution of **IGs** (10% to 18%) against HbsAg. Anti-HBsAg antibodies are collected from donors with high titers of anti-HBsAg. **HBIG** is used to provide passive immunity to patients following exposure to blood infected with hepatitis B, sexual and household contacts of hepatitis B virus–infected people, and infants born to HbsAg-positive mothers.

Tetanus immune globulin (TIG, HyperTET S/D) is prepared from the plasma of adults who are hyperimmunized with tetanus toxoid. TIG contains antibodies that neutralize the exotoxin produced by *Clostridium tetani.* The passive immunity bestowed by **TIG** is capable of attenuating or preventing tetanus infection by binding free exotoxin.

Respiratory syncytial virus immune globulin (RSV-IGIV) is a polyclonal human hyperimmune globulin. The product is prepared by extracting IgG antibodies from the plasma of humans who have high titers of antibodies against respiratory syncytial virus (RSV). Resistance to RSV disease is via cellular and humoral immunity. RSV-IGIV does not protect the nasal mucosa from RSV and thus does not prevent acquired immunity to RSV.

Varicella-zoster immune globulin (VZIG) is derived from human plasma and consists of IgG, with trace amounts of IgA and IgM. **VZIG** is used primarily for passive immunization of high-risk susceptible patients after exposure to chickenpox or herpes zoster. The administration of **VZIG** has shown to significantly reduce the mortality in untreated patients.

Rabies immune globulin (RIG, HyperRab S/D, Imogam) is primarily **gamma globulin. RIG** is used to provide passive immunity to rabies in patients exposed to the virus. Rabies antibodies neutralize the rabies virus to retard its spread and to inhibit its effectiveness.

Rh_0(D) immune globulin (RhoGAM, HyperRHO S/D) is used to prevent isoimmunization in Rh_0(D)-negative women exposed to Rh_0(D)-positive blood. **Rh_0(D) immune globulin** is a solution containing IgG antibodies against erythrocyte antigen Rh_0(D), collected from the plasma of human donors. It is believed that the anti-Rh_0(D) antibodies in **Rh_0(D) immune globulin** interact directly with the Rh_0(D) antigens, preventing interaction between the antigens and the maternal immune system. **Rh_0(D) immune globulin** prevents the development of erythroblastosis fetalis in current or subsequent pregnancies.

Vaccinia immune globulin intravenous (VIGIV) provides passive immunity for smallpox associated eczema vaccinatum, severe or progressive vaccinia, and vaccinia infections in patients with skin conditions (impetigo, poison ivy, eczema, varicella zoster) that would lead to severe rash with smallpox infection.

Pharmacokinetics

IGIM, when used for pre-exposure prophylaxis for hepatitis A, confers protection for less than 3 months. It is greater than 85 percent effective in preventing hepatitis A if given within 2 weeks after exposure. IGIM can be given to prevent or modify measles in susceptible persons if used within 6 days of exposure.

HBIG is slowly absorbed, with antibodies appearing in 1 to 6 days and peak levels reached in 3 to 9 days. The antibodies remain in the serum for up to 2 months. HBIG probably crosses the placenta and may be distributed in breast milk.

TIG is given IM, with peak levels of IgG noted 2 days after administration. The half-life of IgG in circulation is 3.5 to 4.5 weeks.

RSV-IGIV is administered IV on a monthly basis. The serum half-life of RSV-IGIV is 22 to 28 days.

VZIG is administered IM, with peak IgG levels obtained in 2 days after administration. It is the most effective if administered within 4 days of exposure to VZV. Antibody protection lasts 3 weeks.

RIG is administered by infiltrating the wound with half of the dose and giving the other half of the dose IM in a separate limb from the injury.

Rh_o(D) immune globulin pharmacokinetics is not well described. Peak antibody levels are reached in 5 to 10 days after IM administration. Anti-Rh_o(D) antibodies are not detectable 6 months after administration of **Rh_o(D) immune globulin.**

VIGIV peaks in 2 hours and has a half-life of 30 days.

Pharmacotherapeutics

Precautions and Contraindications

An allergic response to IGIM or anti-IGA antibodies is a contraindication to IG serum use, as is thimerosal allergy.

Patients with IgA deficiency often develop antibodies against IgA and are more likely to have anaphylactic or immune-mediated adverse reaction to pooled IG products.

RSV-IGIV is contraindicated in patients with cyanotic congenital heart disease.

Live-virus vaccines should not be administered within 3 months of an IG serum.

Pregnancy is not a contraindication to most IG serums.

VIGIV is contraindicated in patients with vaccinia keratitis.

VIGIV may cause falsely high blood glucose readings on some test systems due to the maltose in the preparation. Blood glucose testing should be done with a glucose-specific method.

Adverse Drug Reactions

Local reactions include tenderness and pain in the injection site that may last for several hours.

Systemic reactions include urticaria and angioedema. Less frequently reported adverse reactions include emesis, chills, fever, myalgia, lethargy, and nausea.

Drug Interactions

IG serums interfere with the immune response to live-virus vaccines.

Clinical Use and Dosing

IG serums are used to prevent disease by either pre-exposure or post-exposure administration. The clinical use and dosing of the IG serums are detailed in Table 19–8.

Monitoring

Laboratory monitoring is not necessary. The patient's Rh status should be determined prior to administering **Rh_o(D) immune globulin.**

Patient Education

Patients should receive information regarding the benefits and risks of the IG prior to administration. Any

Table 19–8 ◉ **Dosage Schedule: Immune Globulins**

Drug	Indication	Dose	Comments
I/gamma globulin	Hepatitis A prophylaxis	Length of stay: <3 mo, give 0.02 mL/kg IM. Prolonged (>3 mo), give 0.06 mL/kg and repeat every 4 to 6 mo	Effective if given before exposure or within 2 wk of exposure
	Measles	Give 0.25 mL/kg IM. If child is also immunocompromised, give 0.5 mL/kg IM	Must be given within 6 d of exposure to measles
	Immunoglobulin	Deficiency 0.66 mL/kg every 3–4 wk	
Hepatitis B immune globulin (HBIG)	After exposure to blood infected with hepatitis B (HBV)	Children ≥12 mo and adults: Administer 0.06 mL/kg IM within 24 h; repeat in 28–30 d Children <12 mo: 0.5 mL x 1	Give hepatitis B vaccine within 7 d and repeat at 1 and 6 mo
	Sexual contacts of HBV-infected people	Administer 0.06 mL/kg IM within 14 d of sexual contact	Give hepatitis B vaccine within 7 d and repeat at 1 and 6 mo
	Infants born to HbsAg-positive mothers	Administer 0.5 mL IM within 12 h of birth	Give hepatitis B vaccine within 12 h of birth and repeat at 1 or 2 and at 6 mo

Table 19–8 ◉ **Dosage Schedule: Immune Globulins—cont'd**

Drug	Indication	Dose	Comments
Tetanus immune globulin (TIG)	Passive immunization against tetanus	Clean minor wounds: No TIG necessary. Give Td/DTaP if indicated All other wounds (may be contaminated with dirt, feces, soil, saliva, and puncture wounds). Unknown or <3 doses of DTaP/Td: Give adults 250 U TIG, children 4 U/kg of TIG, give a booster dose of TD/DTaP History of >3 doses of tetanus toxoid: No TIG, no Td/DTaP booster	
Respiratory syncytial virus immune globulin (RSV-IGIV)	RSV prophylaxis in high-risk children	*Children <24 mo with bronchopulmonary dysplasia or chronic lung disease:* Give 750 mg/kg IV once monthly throughout RSV season *Infants <6 mo born at 32 wk gestation or earlier or infants <12 mo of age if less than 28 wk gestation:* Give 750 mg/kg IV once monthly throughout RSV season	Medication should be infused at a rate of 1.5 mL/kg/h for the first 15 min, then increase to 3 mL/kg/h for 15 min, maximum rate of 6 mL/kg/h
Varicella-zoster immune globulin (VZIG)	Passive immunization for high-risk patients exposed to varicella	Administer VZIG within 96 h of exposure *Adults and adolescents:* 125 U/10 kg, up to 625 U maximum	VZIG administration is recommended in the following groups: Immunocompromised patients (patients with HIV, cancer, or receiving immunosuppressive therapy), neonates of women who have symptoms of varicella at delivery, premature neonates exposed postnatally, pregnant women
		Children and infants: 125 U/10 kg, rounded to nearest 125 U >40 kg: 625 U IM 30.1–40 kg: 500 U 20.1–30 kg: 375 U 10.1–20 kg: 250 U <10 kg: 125 U	Patients should meet the additional requirements: 1. Not immune to varicella 2. Significant exposure <96 h prior to VZIG administration; significant exposure defined as household contact, playmate contact (>1 h contact), hospital contact (in same room)
Rabies immune globulin (RIG)	Provides passive immunity to rabies	Previously unvaccinated against rabies: Administer 20 IU/kg up to 7 d after the first dose of rabies vaccine	Post-exposure prophylaxis always includes administration of both passive antibody and vaccine, with the exception of those who have previously received complete vaccination. For postexposure vaccination, the ACIP recommends that 4 doses of rabies vaccine be given, with RIG given at the same time as the first vaccine dose
Rh_o (D) immune globulin (RhoGAM)	Rh isoimmunization prophylaxis	Administer 300 mcg IM at 28 wk gestation and/or within 72 h of an Rh-incompatible delivery, miscarriage, abortion, or transfusion accident Administer 50 mcg IM if pregnancy terminated prior to 13 weeks gestation	Each vial or syringe (~300 mcg) prevents sensitization to a volume of up to 15 mL of Rh-positive red blood cells

questions or concerns regarding the vaccine should be addressed.

The most common adverse reactions after IG administration are pain and erythema at the injection site.

DIAGNOSTIC BIOLOGICALS

Tuberculin Purified Protein Derivative

The diagnostic biological agent that is commonly used in primary care is **tuberculin PPD**. PPD is used to screen asymptomatic individuals for infection with *M. tuberculosis*.

Pharmacodynamics

PPD is administered intradermally to asymptomatic individuals. Once a person has become sensitized to mycobacterial antigens, a hypersensitivity reaction occurs to the administration of the intradermal PPD. In sensitive people, the reaction includes induration and erythema at the site of administration. A positive reaction to PPD indicates that the person at some time has had a TB infection. A positive test does not indicate an active infection but rather that further testing is indicated. See Chapter 45 for more information regarding TB evaluation.

Pharmacotherapeutics

Precautions and Contraindications

Do not administer PPD to known tuberculin-positive reactors because they may have a severe reaction, including ulceration and necrosis at the site of administration.

SC administration should be avoided, as a general febrile reaction or acute inflammation may occur.

Skin testing of immunodeficient people may not be accurate because skin-test responsiveness may be suppressed.

Skin test responsiveness may be delayed in the older adult patient.

PPD testing is safe in pregnancy, during lactation, and in children of all ages, including infants.

Adverse Drug Reactions

In highly sensitive people, vesiculation, ulceration, and necrosis can occur at the administration site. A normal adverse reaction is a minimal amount of bleeding at the administration site.

Drug Interactions

Live-virus vaccines (MMR, **varicella**) can suppress the reaction to PPD if given within 4 to 6 weeks prior to the PPD. PPD can be administered at the time that MMR and **varicella vaccines** are administered.

Patients who have been vaccinated with BCG generally are sensitive to PPD.

Immunosuppressant medications can suppress the reaction to PPD testing.

Clinical Use and Dosing

The Mantoux PPD test containing 5 tuberculin units (TU) is the preferred test because the interpretation of the reaction has been standardized. Previously, multiple puncture tests were used, and there were many problems with interpretation.

The test consists of injecting 5 TU of PPD intradermally. A small white bleb should appear at the injection site if it is done correctly. Reactions are read in 48 to 72 hours after administration. For patients who may be highly sensitized, a test dose of 1 TU is used.

Determining the results of the skin test is based on the likelihood of infection and the risk of active TB if infection has occurred. If the patient is HIV-positive or has fibrotic lesions on chest x-ray, a reaction of 5-mm or more induration is considered positive. A reaction of 10-mm or more induration is considered positive in other at-risk patients, including infants and children. In patients who are not in any high-risk category or high-risk environment, a result of 15-mm or more induration is considered positive.

Patients are considered high risk if they have any of the following: (1) diabetes mellitus; (2) prolonged therapy with adrenocorticosteroids; (3) immunosuppressive therapy; (4) hematological and/or reticuloendothelial diseases, such as leukemia or Hodgkin's disease; (5) injection drug users known to be HIV-seronegative; (6) end-stage renal disease; or (6) any clinical presentation that includes substantial rapid weight loss or chronic malnutrition.

People who are in a high-incidence group with a skin test reaction of 10-mm or more induration are candidates for preventive therapy, even if they do not have any of the risk factors. High-incidence groups include the following: (1) foreign-born persons from high-prevalence countries, (2) medically underserved low-income populations, and (3) residents of facilities for long-term care.

Monitoring

The PPD should be read by an experienced health-care professional who has been trained in the proper method of interpreting the results.

Patient Education

Patients must have an understanding of the reason for PPD testing and why the test must be read in 48 to 72 hours.

Adverse reactions are rare in patients who are not already sensitized to TB.

IMMUNOMODULATORS

Although not generally prescribed by primary care providers, two immunomodulator medications commonly prescribed to patients by specialty providers are covered in this chapter. **Cyclosporine (Sandimmune)** is prescribed to organ transplant patients and is used for severe rheumatoid arthritis. **Azathioprine (Imuran)** is also prescribed for transplant patients and patients with severe rheumatoid arthritis. The topical immunomodulators **pimecrolimus (Elidel)** and **tacrolimus (Protopic)** are discussed in the integumentary medications (Chapter 23).

Pharmacodynamics

Cyclosporine is an oral and parenteral immunosuppressive agent. It is believed to act by inhibiting the production or release of various lymphokines. The actions of the T-helper cell, the mediators of cellular immunity and tissue rejection, are impaired. **Cyclosporine** may inhibit T-suppressor cells. **Cyclosporine** also inhibits the synthesis of gamma-interferon. **Cyclosporine** does not cause myelosuppression.

Azathioprine is an oral and parenteral immunosuppressive that decreases the metabolism of purines and may inhibit DNA and RNA synthesis. It may interfere with coenzyme functioning, decreasing cellular metabolism. **Azathioprine** has the ability to inhibit the delayed hypersensitivity reaction and cellular cytotoxic activity that occur during renal transplantation.

Pharmacokinetics

Absorption and Distribution

After oral administration, approximately 20 to 50 percent of **cyclosporine** is absorbed. Absorption from the GI tract is highly variable. It is widely distributed throughout the body, crosses the placenta, and is excreted in breast milk.

Azathioprine is well absorbed following oral administration. It is widely distributed and crosses the placenta.

Metabolism and Excretion

Cyclosporine undergoes extensive first-pass metabolism. It is metabolized extensively by the liver cytochrome P450 3A (CYP450 3A) enzyme system. Elimination of **cyclosporine** and its metabolites is primarily through the bile and feces, with only 6 percent excreted renally.

Azathioprine is metabolized in the liver to its active metabolite, mercaptopurine. The metabolites and some unchanged **azathioprine** are excreted in the urine.

Pharmacotherapeutics

Precautions and Contraindications

Hypersensitivity to the medication or components of the product is a contraindication to its use. **Cyclosporine** has a black box warning regarding anaphylaxis with IV administration. Oral **cyclosporine** preparations contain corn, castor oil, and/or olive oil, and patients with hypersensitivity to these food products should avoid its use.

Patients with renal dysfunction should be monitored for worsening renal function while taking **cyclosporine**. **Azathioprine** can accumulate in patients with renal impairment, possibly causing toxicity.

Hepatic dysfunction can affect the metabolism of both drugs.

Both **cyclosporine** and **azathioprine** are contraindicated in pregnancy and breastfeeding.

Cyclosporine has a black box warning regarding increased susceptibility for severe, even fatal infections.

Azathioprine has a black box warning regarding increased risk of developing neoplasms.

Adverse Drug Reactions

Nephrotoxicity is the most common adverse effect of **cyclosporine** therapy. **Cyclosporine** may also cause hypertension; headaches; GI upset; hirsutism (50% of patients); gingival hyperplasia (4% to 16%); hypercholesterolemia; and neurological effects such as seizures, tremor, paresthesias, and mood changes.

Hepatic failure can occur with **azathioprine** use. Nausea and vomiting occurred in 12 percent of patients. Patients taking **azathioprine** should be monitored for bone marrow suppression. Other adverse effects reported are fever, rash, pancreatitis, alopecia, and retinopathy.

Drug Interactions

Cyclosporine interacts with many drugs, especially those metabolized by the hepatic enzymes

Azathioprine suppresses the immune system; therefore, live or inactivated vaccines should not be given to patients receiving this drug. OPV should not be administered to household contacts of patients taking **azathioprine.** It may take the immune system 3 to 12 months to return to normal after administration of **azathioprine.** Other drug interactions are shown in Table 19–9.

Clinical Use and Dosing

Cyclosporine and **azathioprine** are usually prescribed by specialty providers. If in consultation with a specialist, the primary care provider is prescribing these products for rheumatoid arthritis, the dosing is as follows: **Cyclosporine** is started at 1.25 mg/kg twice daily and may increase by 0.5 to 0.75 mg/kg/day at 8 weeks and at 12 weeks, if indicated. Maximum dose is 4 mg/kg/day. Decrease dose by 25 to 50 percent if adverse effects occur. **Azathioprine** is begun at 1 mg/kg/day in one to two divided doses. The dose can be increased in 6 to 8 weeks, by 0.5 mg/ kg/day. The dose can be increased every 4 weeks to a maximum of 2.5 mg/kg/day.

Monitoring

Patients prescribed these medications need monitoring of their blood pressure, renal function, and hepatic function. Patients taking **cyclosporine** also need to have serum **cyclosporine** levels checked periodically. Patients taking **azathioprine** need a complete blood count (CBC) and serum amylase drawn periodically.

Patient Education

Patients should be instructed to take the medication exactly as prescribed.

Table 19–9 ■ **Drug Interactions: Immunomodulators**

Drug	Interacting Drug	Possible Effect	Implications
Azathioprine	Live vaccines (MMR, varicella)	Decreased antibody response to vaccine	Wait 3 mo to 1 yr after stopping azathioprine before administering live vaccines
	Allopurinol	Increased pharmacological and toxic effects of azathioprine	Avoid concurrent use, or reduce dose of azathioprine by one-third to one-half
	Angiotensin-converting enzyme (ACE) inhibitors	May induce severe leukopenia or anemia	
	Methotrexate	May increase plasma levels of azathioprine metabolite 6-MP	Avoid concurrent use
	Anticoagulants	Decreased effectiveness of anticoagulants	Avoid concurrent use
	Alkylating agents/antineoplastic agents	Prior treatment with alkylating agents puts patient at higher risk of developing neoplasms or infection	
	Cyclosporine	Cyclosporine plasma levels might be decreased	
Cyclosporine	*Nephrotoxic drugs:* amphotericin B, acyclovir, aminoglycosides, foscarnet, NSAIDs, vancomycin, ganciclovir	Additive nephrotoxicity	
	Immunosuppressants	Increased risk of lymphoma and infection	
	Potassium-sparing diuretics: amiloride, spironolactone, triamterene	Hyperkalemia	Monitor potassium levels
	Drug metabolized by CYP450 3A isoenzyme inhibitors: calcium channel blockers, androgens, clarithromycin, azole antifungals, methylprednisolone, allopurinol, bromocriptine, danazol, erythromycin, dalfopristin, metoclopramide	Increased cyclosporine levels, leading to cyclosporine toxicity	Monitor cyclosporine levels
	Drugs metabolized by CYP450 3A isoenzyme inducers: nafcillin, moda?nil, troglitazone, rifampin, carbamazepine, pentobarbital, phenytoin, octreotide, ticlopidine, primidone	Decreased cyclosporine levels	Monitor cyclosporine levels if any of these drugs are added or deleted from medication regimen
	Vaccines	Decreased effectiveness of vaccines	Wait at least 3 mo after therapy with cyclosporine is completed to administer live vaccines
	Digoxin	Increased digoxin levels	Monitor digoxin levels
	Prednisolone	Increased prednisolone levels	
	Lovastatin	Increased lovastatin levels	
	Grapefruit juice	Increased cyclosporine levels	
	Protease inhibitors	Cyclosporine toxicity	
	SMX/TMP	Decreased blood levels of cyclosporine	
	Clonidine	Interferes with clonidine pharmacokinetics	
	Metoclopramide (oral)	Increases oral bioavailability of cyclosporine by 30%	Monitor cyclosporine concentrations
	Colchicine	Nephrotoxicity and azotemia	Avoid concurrent use
	Orlistat	Altered bioavailability of cyclosporine	Monitor if using concurrently

Any symptoms of adverse reactions should be reported to the provider immediately. The patient should be cautioned to report any flu-like symptoms, which may be a sign of hepatic or renal dysfunction.

REFERENCES

American Academy of Pediatrics. (2009a). Immunocompromised children. In L. K. Pickering (Ed.), *Red book: 2009 Report of the Committee on Infectious Diseases* (28th ed., pp. 72–86). Elk Grove Village, IL: American Academy of Pediatrics. Retrieved June 3, 2010, from http://aapredbook.aappublications.org/cgi/content/full/2009/1/1.7.3

American Academy of Pediatrics. Measles. (2009b) In L. K. Pickering (Ed.), *Red book: 2009 Report of the Committee on Infectious Diseases* (28th ed., pp. 444–455). Elk Grove Village, IL: American Academy of Pediatrics. Retrieved June 3, 2010, from http://aapredbook.aappublications.org/cgi/content/full/2009/1/3.77

American College Health Association (ACHA). (2000). *Recommendations for institutional prematriculation guidelines.* Baltimore: ACHA. Retrieved from http://www.acha.org

Bates, A. S., & Wolinsky, F. D. (1998). Personal, financial, and structural barriers to immunization in socioeconomically disadvantaged urban children. *Pediatrics, 101*(4), 591–596.

Brady, M. T. (2011). Changes in MCV4 use include booster dose for adolescents. *AAP News, 32*(1), 1.

Brunette, G. W., Kozarsky, P. E., Magill, A. J., & Shtim, D. R. (2010). The pre-travel consultation, travel-related vaccine-preventable diseases. *CDC health information for international travel 2010: The yellow book.* Centers for Disease Control: Atlanta, GA.

Centers for Disease Control and Prevention (CDC). (1996a). Prevention of plague: Recommendations of the ACIP. *Morbidity and Mortality Weekly Report, 45*(RR-14), 1.

Centers for Disease Control and Prevention (CDC). (1996b). The role of BCG vaccine in the prevention and control of tuberculosis in the United States: A joint statement by the advisory council of the elimination of tuberculosis and the ACIP. *Morbidity and Mortality Weekly Report, 45*(RR-4), 1–18.

Centers for Disease Control and Prevention (CDC). (1997a). Control and prevention of meningococcal disease and control and prevention of serogroup C meningococcal disease: Evaluation and management of suspected outbreaks. Recommendations of the ACIP. *Morbidity and Mortality Weekly Report, 46*(RR-5), 1–21.

Centers for Disease Control and Prevention (CDC). (1997b). Pertussis vaccination: Use of acellular pertussis vaccines among infants and young children: Recommendations of the ACIP. *Morbidity and Mortality Weekly Report, 46*(RR-7), 1–25.

Centers for Disease Control and Prevention (CDC). (1997c). Poliomyelitis prevention in the United States: Introduction of a sequential vaccination schedule of inactivated poliovirus vaccine followed by oral poliovirus vaccine. Recommendations of the ACIP. *Morbidity and Mortality Weekly Report, 46*(RR-3), 1–25.

Centers for Disease Control and Prevention (CDC). (1999). Human rabies prevention—United States, 1999: Recommendations of the ACIP. *Morbidity and Mortality Weekly Report, 48*(RR-1), 1–33.

Centers for Disease Control and Prevention (CDC). (2002). Yellow fever vaccine: Recommendations of the Advisory Committee on Immunization Practices (ACIP). *Morbidity and Mortality Weekly Report, 51* (RR-17), 1–11.

Centers for Disease Control and Prevention (CDC). (2005a). A comprehensive immunization strategy to eliminate transmission of hepatitis B virus infection in the United States. *Morbidity and Mortality Weekly Report, 54*(RR-16), 1–23.

Centers for Disease Control and Prevention (CDC). (2005b). Cholera. *Centers for Disease Control Division of Bacterial and Mycotic Diseases.* Retrieved April 15, 2006, from http://www.cdc.gov/ncidod/dbmd/diseaseinfo/cholera_g.htm#Is%20a%20vaccine%20available%20to%20prevent%20cholera

Centers for Disease Control and Prevention (CDC). (2005c). Prevention and control of meningococcal disease. Recommendations of the Advisory Committee on Immunization Practices (ACIP). *Morbidity and Mortality Weekly Report, 54*(RR07), 1–21.

Centers for Disease Control and Prevention (CDC). (2006a). CDC Health Advisory: Multi-state mumps outbreak. *Centers for Disease Control Health Alert Network.* Retrieved April 15, 2006, from http://www.phppo.cdc.gov/HAN/ArchiveSys/ViewMsgV.asp?AlertNum=00243

Centers for Disease Control and Prevention (CDC). (2006b). CDC's Advisory Committee recommends new vaccine to prevent rotavirus. *Centers for Disease Control National Immunization Program* [Press release, February 21, 2006]. Retrieved from http://www.cdc.gov/nip/pr/pr_rotavirus_feb2006.pdf

Centers for Disease Control and Prevention (CDC). (2006c). General recommendations on immunization: Recommendations of the Advisory Committee on Immunization Practices (ACIP). *Morbidity and Mortality Weekly Report, 55*(RR-15), 1–48.

Centers for Disease Control and Prevention (CDC). (2006d). Preventing tetanus, diphtheria, and pertussis among adolescents: Use of tetanus toxoid, reduced diphtheria toxoid and acellular pertussis vaccines: Recommendations of the Advisory Committee on Immunization Practices (ACIP). *Morbidity and Mortality Weekly Report, 55*(RR-3), 1–43.

Centers for Disease Control and Prevention (CDC). (2006e). Preventing tetanus, diphtheria, and pertussis among adults: Use of tetanus toxoid, reduced diphtheria toxoid and acellular pertussis vaccines: Recommendations of the Advisory Committee on Immunization Practices (ACIP). *Morbidity and Mortality Weekly Report, 55*(RR-17).

Centers for Disease Control and Prevention (CDC). (2006f). Prevention of hepatitis A through active or passive immunization: Recommendations of the Advisory Committee on Immunization Practices (ACIP). *Morbidity and Mortality Weekly Report, 55*(RR07), 1–23.

Centers for Disease Control and Prevention (CDC). (2006g). Rotavirus. *Centers for Disease Control National Immunization Program.* Retrieved from http://www.cdc.gov/nip/diseases/rota/rota-faqs.htm

Centers for Disease Control and Prevention (CDC). (2006h). Smallpox Supplemental Fact Sheet: Investigational vaccinia immune globulin (VIG) information. *Centers for Disease Control* Emergency Preparedness & Response. Retrieved April 15, 2006, from http://www.bt.cdc.gov/agent/smallpox/vaccination/vig.asp

Centers for Disease Control and Prevention (CDC). (2006i). A comprehensive immunization strategy to eliminate transmission of hepatitis B virus infection in the United States. *Morbidity and Mortality Weekly Report, 55*(R16), 1–25.

Centers for Disease Control and Prevention (CDC). (2007a). *Guidelines for vaccinating pregnant women.* Retrieved from http://www.cdc.gov/vaccines/pubs/downloads/b_preg_guide.pdf

Centers for Disease Control and Prevention (CDC). (2007b). Prevention of varicella: Recommendations of the Advisory Committee on Immunization Practices. *Morbidity and Mortality Weekly Report, 56*(RR-4).

Centers for Disease Control and Prevention (CDC). (2008). Prevention of herpes zoster: Recommendations of the Advisory Committee on Immunization Practices. *Morbidity and Mortality Weekly Report, 57*(RR-5).

Centers for Disease Control and Prevention (CDC). (2009). ACIP provisional recommendations for the use of yellow fever vaccine. Retrieved from www.cdc.gov/vaccines.

Centers for Disease Control and Prevention (CDC). (2010a). FDA licensure of bivalent human papillomavirus vaccine (HPV2, Cervarix) for use in females an updated HPV vaccination recommendations from the Advisory Committee on Immunization Practices (ACIP). *Morbidity and Mortality Weekly Report, 59*(20), 626–629.

Centers for Disease Control and Prevention (CDC). (2010b). FDA licensure of quadrivalent human papillomavirus vaccine (HPV4, Gardasil) for use in males and guidance from the Advisory Committee on Immunization Practices (ACIP). *Morbidity and Mortality Weekly Report, 59(20), 630–632.*

Centers for Disease Control and Prevention (CDC). (2010c). Invasive pneumococcal disease in young children before licensure of 13-valent pneumococcal conjugate vaccine—United States, 2007. *Morbidity and Mortality Weekly Report, 59*(09), 253–257.

Centers for Disease Control and Prevention (CDC). (2010d). Japanese encephalitis vaccines: Recommendations of the Advisory Committee on Immunization Practices (ACIP). *Morbidity and Mortality Weekly Report, 59*(RR-1).

Centers for Disease Control and Prevention (CDC). (2010e). Licensure of a meningococcal conjugate vaccine (Menveo) and guidance for use—Advisory Committee on Immunization Practices (ACIP). *Morbidity and Mortality Weekly Report, 59*(09), 273.

Centers for Disease Control and Prevention (CDC). (2010f). Licensure of a 13-valent pneumococcal conjugate vaccine (PCV13) and recommendations for use among children—Advisory Committee on Immunization Practices (ACIP). *Morbidity and Mortality Weekly Report, 59*(09), 258–261.

Centers for Disease Control and Prevention (CDC). (2010g). Notifiable diseases/deaths in selected cities weekly information. *Morbidity and Mortality Weekly Report, 58*(51 & 52), 1458–1469.

Centers for Disease Control and Prevention (CDC). (2010h). Use of combination measles, mumps, rubella, and varicella vaccine: Recommendations of the Advisory Committee on Immunization Practices. *Morbidity and Mortality Weekly Report, 59*(RR-3). Retrieved from http://www.cdc.gov/mmwr/pdf/rr/rr5903.pdf

Centers for Disease Control and Prevention (CDC). (2010i). Prevention and control of influenza with vaccines: Recommendation of the Advisory Committee on Immunization Practices (ACIP). *Morbidity and Mortality Weekly Report, 59*(RR08), 1–62.

Fiore, A. E., Shay, D. K., Broder, K., Isakander, J. K., Uyeki, T. M., Mootrey, G., et al. (2009). Prevention and control of seasonal influenza with vaccines: Recommendations of the Advisory Committee on Immunization Practices (ACIP). *Morbidity and Mortality Weekly Report, 58*(RR08), 1–52.

Franco, E. L., & Harper, D. M. (2005). Vaccination against human papillomavirus infection: A new paradigm in cervical cancer control. *Vaccine, 23,* 2388–2394.

Harrison, L. H., Dwyer, D. M., Maples, C. T., & Billman, L. (1999). Risk of meningococcal infection in college students. *Journal of the American Medical Association, 281*(20), 1906–1910.

Immunization Action Coalition. (2010). Vaccines work! CDC statistics demonstrate dramatic declines in vaccine-preventable diseases when compared with pre-vaccine era. Immunization Action Coalition. Retrieved from http://www.immunize.org/catg.d/p4037.pdf

Katz, S. L. (2005). A vaccine-preventable infectious disease kills half a million children annually. *Journal of Infectious Diseases, 192,* 1679–1680.

Koutsky, L. A., Ault, K. A., Wheeler, C. M., Brown, D. R., Barr, E., Alvarez, F. B., et al. (2002). A controlled trial of a human papillomavirus type 16 vaccine. *New England Journal of Medicine, 347*(21), 1645–1651.

Marin, M., Broder, K. R., Ternte, J. L., Snider, D. E., & Seward, J. F. (2010). Use of combination measles, mumps, rubella, and varicella vaccine: Recommendations of the Advisory Committee on Immunization Practices (ACIP). *Morbidity and Mortality Weekly Report, 59*(RR-3), 1–11.

McCarthy, M. W., & Kockler, D. R. (2004). Trivalent intranasal influenza vaccine, live. *The Annals of Pharmacotherapy, 38*(12), 2086–2093.

Merck & Co. (2010). M-M-R II (Measles, mumps and rubella virus vaccine live). Whitehouse Station, NJ: Merck. Retrieved from http://www.merck.com/product/usa/pi_circulars/m/mmr_ii/mmr_ii_pi.pdf

Pagliusi, S. R., & Aguado, M. T. (2004). Efficacy and other milestones for human papillomavirus vaccine introduction. *Vaccine, 23,* 569–578.

Reisinger, K. S., Brown, M. L., Xu, J., Sullivan, B. J., Marshall, G. S., Nauert, B., et al. (2006). A combination measles, mumps, rubella, and varicella vaccine (ProQuad) given to 4- to 6-year-old healthy children vaccinated previously with M-M-RII and Varivax. *Pediatrics, 117*(2), 265–272.

Roush, S. W., Murphy, T. V., & the Vaccine-Preventable Disease Table Working Group. (2007). Historical Comparisons of Morbidity and Mortality for Vaccine-Preventable Diseases in the United States. *Journal of the American Medical Association, 298*(18), 2155–2163.

Rupprecht, C. E., Briggs, D., Brown, C. M., Franka, R., Katz, S. L., Kerr, H. D., & Cieslak, P. R. (2010). Use of a reduced (4-dose) vaccine schedule for postexposure prophylaxis to prevent human rabies. *Morbidity and Mortality Weekly Report, 59*(RR-02), 1–9.

Shinefield, H., Black, S., Digilio, L., Reisinger, K., Blatter, M., Gress, J. O., et al. (2005). Evaluation of a quadrivalent measles, mumps, rubella and varicella vaccine in healthy children. *Pediatric Infectious Disease Journal, 24*(8), 665–669.

Tyring, S. K., Diaz-Mitoma, F., Padget, L. G., Nunez, M., Poland, G., Cassidy, W. M., & the Protocol 009 Study Group. (2007). Safety and tolerability of a high-potency zoster vaccine in adults >/= 50 years of age. *Vaccine, 25*(10), 1877–1883.

Vesikari, T., Karvonen, A., Korhonen, T., Edelman, K., Vainionpaa, R., & Salmi, A. (2006). A randomized, double-blind study of the safety, transmissibility and phenotypic and genotypic stability of cold-adapted influenza virus vaccine. *Pediatric Infectious Diseases Journal, 25*(7), 590–595.

World Health Organization (WHO). (1998). District guidelines for yellow fever surveillance (Publication No. [WHO/EPI/GEN] 98.09). Geneva, Switzerland: World Health Organization.

World Health Organization (WHO). (2005). Viral Cancers. *In State of the Art of Vaccine Research and Development.* (Publication No. WHO/IVB/05). Geneva, Switzerland: World Health Organization.

World Health Organization (WHO). (2006). Global case count (Polio cases from 01 March 2005 to 28 February 2006). *Global Polio Eradication Initiative.* Retrieved from http://www.polioeradication.org/casecount.asp

World Health Organization (WHO). (2011). Human papillomavirus infection and cervical cancer. Retrieved from http://www.who.int/vaccine_research/diseases/hpv/en/

CHAPTER 20

DRUGS AFFECTING THE GASTROINTESTINAL SYSTEM

Teri Moser Woo

Chapter Outline

There is a wide variety of drugs that are used to treat disorders affecting the gastrointestinal (GI) tract. **Cholinergic drugs** increase gastric acid secretion and increase peristalsis; **anticholinergic drugs** inhibit gastric acid secretion and decrease peristalsis. These drugs are discussed in Chapter 14. **Phenothiazines** have antiemetic properties and some **narcotic analgesics** or their derivatives are used to treat diarrhea and are discussed in Chapter 15. Several groups of drugs are used almost exclusively to treat GI disorders, such as **antacids, antidiarrheals, antiemetics, laxatives,** and drugs used to decrease gastric acid production. These drugs are discussed in this chapter. IV forms of GI drugs not used in primary care are not discussed in this chapter.

ANTACIDS

Antacids are weak bases that react with hydrochloric acid (HCl) to form a salt and water. They are used to reduce gastric acidity in the treatment of gastroesophageal reflux and peptic ulcer disease. Various combinations of metallic cation (aluminum, calcium, magnesium, and sodium) and basic anion (hydroxide, bicarbonate, carbonate, citrate, and trisilicate) can be used. Most **antacids** in current use have as their cation aluminum, calcium, or magnesium, and their anion is usually hydroxide (OH), bicarbonate (HCO_3), or carbonate (CO_3). The buffering capacity of the other two anions is too limited to be clinically effective.

Pharmacodynamics

Antacids neutralize gastric acidity, which causes an increase in the pH of the stomach and duodenal bulb. They also inhibit the proteolytic activity of pepsin and increase lower esophageal sphincter tone. **Aluminum-based** products inhibit smooth muscle contraction and thus slow gastric emptying. **Calcium-based** antacids are also used to treat calcium-deficiency states, such as those that occur postmenopause and in chronic renal failure. They are also used to bind phosphates in chronic renal failure, as are **aluminum-based antacids. Magnesium-based antacids** are used to treat magnesium deficiencies from malnutrition, alcoholism, or magnesium-depleting drugs. The use of drugs as nutrient therapy is discussed in Chapter 9.

Acid-neutralizing capacity (ANC) varies between products and is expressed in milliequivalents (mEq) of HCl required to keep an **antacid** suspension at pH 3.5 for 10 minutes in vitro. **Antacids** must neutralize at least 5 mEq per dose. Those with higher ANC values are more likely to be effective in vivo. **Sodium bicarbonate** and **calcium carbonate** have the highest ANC but are not used for chronic therapy because of their systemic effects. Suspensions have greater ANC than do powders or tablets.

Pharmacokinetics

Absorption and Distribution

Aluminum- and magnesium-based antacids are not absorbable with routine use. With chronic use, 5 to 20 percent of magnesium and smaller amounts of aluminum may be absorbed. These small amounts that are absorbed are widely distributed, cross the placenta, and appear in breast milk. Aluminum concentrates in the central nervous system. **Calcium-based antacids** require **vitamin D** for absorption from the GI tract. The small amount that is absorbed enters the extracellular fluid, crosses the placenta, and enters breast milk.

If ingested in a fasting state, **antacids** reduce acidity for approximately 20 to 40 minutes. If taken 1 hour after a meal, acidity is reduced for 2 to 3 hours. A second dose given 3 hours after a meal maintains the reduced acidity for more than 4 hours after the meal.

Metabolism and Excretion

The action of **antacids** occurs locally in the GI tract with minimal absorption, and so there is minimal metabolism. **Magnesium-based antacids** are excreted in the urine. **Aluminum-based antacids** bind with phosphate ions in the intestine to form insoluble aluminum phosphate, which is excreted in the feces. **Calcium-based antacids** are excreted mainly in feces, with 20 percent eliminated in urine.

Table 20–1 shows the pharmacokinetic properties of selected **antacids**.

Pharmacotherapeutics

Precautions and Contraindications

All **antacids** are contraindicated in the presence of severe abdominal pain of unknown cause, especially if accompanied by fever. **Calcium-based antacids** are contraindicated in the presence of hypercalcemia and renal calculi.

Renal impairment presents several issues for patients who take **antacids. Magnesium-based antacids** are contraindicated in patients with renal failure and used with caution for patients with any degree of renal insufficiency because the malfunctioning kidney is unable to excrete magnesium, and hypermagnesemia may result. Prolonged use of **aluminum-based antacids** for patients with renal failure may result in or worsen dialysis osteomalacia. Aluminum is not easily removed by dialysis because it is bound to albumin and transferrin, which do not cross the

Table 20–1 ▶ **Pharmacokinetics: Selected Antacids**

Drug	Onset	Peak	Duration	Acid-Neutralizing Capacity (ANC)	Half-Life	Elimination
Aluminum hydroxide	Slightly delayed	30 min	30 min–1 h on empty stomach; 3 h after meals	3.2 (AlternaGEL) 2.0 (Amphojel) 10.6	Unknown	As aluminum phosphate in feces
Magnesium hydroxide	Immediate	30 min	30 min–1 h on empty stomach; 3 h after meals	11.4	Unknown	In urine
Aluminum hydroxide-magnesium hydroxide combinations	Immediate	30 min	30 min–1 h on empty stomach; 3 h after meals	2.7 (Maalox) 5.7 (Maalox HRF) 5.1 (Mylanta)	Unknown	In urine and feces
Calcium carbonate	Slightly delayed	30 min	30 min–1 h on empty stomach; 3 h after meals	10	Unknown	Mostly in feces; 20% in urine

dialysis membrane. As a result, aluminum is deposited in bone, and osteomalacia occurs. Elevated tissue aluminum levels also contribute to the development of dialysis encephalopathy.

Many **antacids** have high sodium content. Patients with hypertension (HTN), congestive heart failure (CHF), marked renal failure, or those on low-sodium diets should use a low-sodium preparation.

Adverse Drug Reactions

Aluminum- and **calcium-based antacids** cause constipation; **magnesium-based antacids** cause diarrhea. Alkalosis may occur but tends to be a clinically significant problem only for patients with renal impairment.

Drug Interactions

All **antacids** have drug interactions with orally administered weakly acidic and weakly basic drugs, decreasing or increasing their absorption and, therefore, their effects. Enteric coating on drugs is used to protect them from the acid of the stomach, and the coating dissolves in the more basic medium of the duodenum. Concurrent administration of **antacids** with enteric-coated drugs destroys the coating, alters their absorption, and increases the risk for adverse reactions. Some **antacids** adsorb or bind to the surface of other drugs, resulting in decreased bioavailability. **Magnesium hydroxide (Milk of Magnesia, Maalox, Mylanta)** has the greatest ability to adsorb and **calcium carbonate** and **aluminum hydroxide (AlternaGEL, Amphojel)** have intermediate ability to adsorb certain drugs.

Increasing urinary pH affects the rate of elimination by inhibiting the excretion of weakly basic drugs and increasing the elimination of weakly acidic ones. Separating the administration of the **antacid** and the interacting drug by at least 2 hours and giving the interacting drug first in this sequence often can avoid these problems. Table 20–2 provides specific information on drug interactions with selected **antacids**.

Clinical Use and Dosing

Hyperacidity

Antacids are used for symptomatic relief of stomach upset associated with the hyperacidity of heartburn, acid indigestion, and "sour stomach." Because they are sold over the counter (OTC), doses may vary, as patients choose the amount they think they need to relieve symptoms. Generally, dosing is 1 to 2 tablets or 1 to 2 tablespoons of suspension taken intermittently. Dosing of common **antacids** is found in Table 20–3.

Peptic Ulcer Disease

Although the main factor in most duodenal ulcers and many gastric ulcers is infection with *Helicobacter pylori,* hyperacidity is also a factor in peptic ulcer disease (PUD). **Antacids** were formerly considered step 1 in PUD management, but the current guidelines follow a stepped-down approach and treatment is begun with a **proton pump inhibitor.** Patients with uncomplicated PUD can benefit from 15 to 30 mL of **antacid** suspension 1 to 3 hours after meals and at bedtime and often select to do this before consulting a

Table 20–2 ■ Drug Interactions: Selected Antacids

Drug	Interacting Drug	Possible Effect	Implications
All antacids	Weakly acidic drugs (e.g., digoxin, phenytoin, chlorpromazine, isoniazid, ketoconazole)	Decreased absorption with possible decreased drug effects	Separate administration by at least 2 h, giving the antacid after the drug
	Weakly basic drugs (e.g., pseudoephedrine, levodopa)	Increased absorption with possible toxicity or adverse reactions	Separate administration by at least 2 h, giving the antacid after the drug
	Drugs acidic at the time of excretion (e.g., salicylates)	Enhanced excretion	May be used therapeutically to treat salicylate toxicity. Otherwise, avoid concurrent use or alter dosage of drug
	Drugs basic at the time of excretion (e.g., quinidine, amphetamines)	Decreased excretion	Avoid concurrent use or alter dosage of drug
	Drugs with enteric coating	Antacids may destroy the coating, resulting in altered absorption or adverse reactions	Avoid concurrent use or separate administration by at least 2 h, giving the antacid after the drug
	Buffered aspirin products	Alkalinization of urine accelerates aspirin excretion, and systemic alkalosis and increased sodium load may occur	Caution against use of these antacid-analgesic combinations in chronic pain syndromes. Not an issue if used only intermittently

Continued

Table 20–2 ■ **Drug Interactions: Selected Antacids—cont'd**

Drug	Interacting Drug	Possible Effect	Implications
Aluminum-based antacids	Allopurinol, chloroquine, corticosteroids, ethambutol, histamine$_2$ blockers, iron salts, phenothiazines, tetracyclines, thyroid hormones, ticlopidine	Decreased pharmacological effect of the drug	Avoid concurrent use or separate administration by at least 2 h, giving the antacid after the drug
	Benzodiazepines	Increased pharmacological effect of the drug	Avoid concurrent use
Calcium-based antacids	Fluoroquinolones, hydantoins, iron salts, salicylates, tetracyclines	Decreased pharmacological effect of the drug	Avoid concurrent administration
	Quinidine	Increased pharmacological effect of the drug	Avoid concurrent administration
Magnesium-based antacids	Benzodiazepines, corticosteroids, histamine$_2$ blockers, hydantoins, iron salts, nitrofurantoin, phenothiazines, tetracyclines, ticlopidine	Decreased pharmacological effect of the drug	Avoid concurrent administration
	Quinidine, sulfonylureas	Increased pharmacological effect of the drug	Avoid concurrent administration

Table 20–3 ◉ **Dosage Schedule: Selected Antacids**

Drug	Indication	Dosage Schedule
Aluminum hydroxide	Hyperphosphatemia	Tablets or capsules: 500–1,500 mg with meals Suspension: 30 mL with meals
	Hyperacidity	*Adults:* Tablets or capsules: 500–1,500 mg 3–6 times daily between meals and at bedtime Suspension: 5–30 mL prn between meals and at bedtime Children: 300 to 900 mg per dose between meals and at bedtime
Calcium carbonate	Calcium deficiency in chronic renal failure	*Adults:* Tablets 1,000 mg/d
	Postmenopause or osteoporosis	*Adults:* Tablets 1,200–1,500 mg/d
	Hyperacidity	*Children >11 yr and adults:* TUMS (500 mg calcium carbonate) chew 2–4 tablets for symptoms, not to exceed 15 tablets/d *Children 5 yr to 11 yr:* 800 mg calcium carbonate for symptoms, do not exceed 4800 mg per day *Children 2–5 yr:* 400 mg as needed, do not exceed 1,200 mg/d
Magnesium hydroxide	Hyperacidity	*Children >12 yr and adults:* Tablets: 622–1,244 mg up to qid Liquid: 5–15 mL up to qid with water Liquid concentrate: 2.5–7.5 mL up to qid with water
	Laxative	*Adults:* 30–60 mL at bedtime with water *Children:* 2–5 yr: 5–15 ml/d at bedtime 6–11 yr: 15–30 ml/d at bedtime
Aluminum hydroxide-magnesium hydroxide combinations	Hyperacidity	Tablets: 1 or 2 prn
	Peptic ulcer disease	Suspension: 15–30 mL prn Suspension: 15–30 mL 1 h and 3 h after meals and at bedtime
	Gastroesophageal reflux disease	*Children >12 yr and adults:* Suspension: 5–30 mL every 30–60 min for acute management; 5–30 mL 1 h and 3 h after meals and at bedtime for maintenance *Infants and children <12 yr:* Suspension: 0.5 mL/kg (average dose 2–15 mL) 1–2 h after meals or feedings

health-care provider. Additional doses may be used for recurring symptoms. Because ANC is higher in patients with uncomplicated PUD, combined **antacids** with both **aluminum hydroxide** and **magnesium hydroxide** are best unless the patient also has renal insufficiency or failure. Further discussion of PUD occurs in Chapter 34.

Gastroesophageal Reflux Disease

Lifestyle management and drugs to increase lower esophageal sphincter tone are central to the management of gastroesophageal reflux disease (GERD), but there is a role for **antacids** in mild disease. The current guidelines recommend the step-up approach, in which **antacids** and **histamine$_2$ receptor antagonists (H_2RAs)** are used with lifestyle modifications initially, or a step-down approach in which **proton pump inhibitors (PPIs)** are the first step. In either approach, when **antacids** are used, they are given with **H_2RAs** and suspensions are generally used. For acute management, **antacid** doses may be given every 30 to 60 minutes until symptoms are relieved; for maintenance, doses are given 1 and 3 hours after meals and at bedtime. Additional doses may be given for recurring symptoms. Dosing of **antacids** is found in Table 20–3. Further discussion of GERD occurs in Chapter 34.

Hyperphosphatemia

Aluminum carbonate (Basalgel) and **aluminum hydroxide** have been used, along with a low-phosphate diet, to treat hyperphosphatemia in patients with chronic renal failure. They have also been used to prevent the formation of phosphate urinary stones. The dose is 30 mL of suspension with each meal.

Calcium Deficiency

Calcium carbonate (Tums) is routinely used to treat calcium deficiency states associated with chronic renal failure, postmenopause, and osteoporosis. Tablets, often in chewable form, are commonly used. A dose of 1,000 mg/day of **calcium carbonate** is sufficient to provide adequate **calcium** for patients with chronic renal failure. Higher doses are needed for osteoporosis prevention, 1,000 mg daily for men and for premenopausal women and 1,500 mg/day of **calcium** for postmenopausal women. Doses higher than 2,000 mg/day are not advised because of increased adverse effects. Patients with osteoporosis require a combination of **calcium**, **Vitamin D**, and another bone density–building medication such as a **bisphosphonate**.

Rational Drug Selection

In addition to consideration of adverse drug reactions and the indications discussed previously, other major factors used to choose among antacids are ANC, sodium content, and cost.

Acid-Neutralizing Capacity

Combination products that contain **aluminum hydroxide** and **magnesium hydroxide** have the highest ANC (see Table 20–1). When moderate to severe hyperacidity is a factor in the disease process under treatment, these drugs are chosen over other **antacids**.

Sodium Content

Sodium content of **antacids** may be significant. Patients who must restrict sodium intake (e.g., those with HTN, CHF, or marked renal failure) should use a low-sodium **antacid**. The sodium content is listed on the product label.

Cost

Antacids are sold OTC. In general, they are inexpensive, but the cost of a high-dose regimen varies significantly. Because these drugs are OTC, costs may vary and "shopping" different stores and using generic forms of the drug may yield cost savings.

Monitoring

No specific monitoring is required beyond that related to the disease process for which the patient is being treated. Serum phosphate, potassium, and calcium levels may be monitored periodically during chronic use. These drugs may cause increased serum calcium and decreased serum phosphate. Chronic **magnesium hydroxide** use may cause elevated magnesium levels in patients with renal failure or the elderly with decreased renal function.

Patient Education

Administration

Antacids should be taken as prescribed, especially related to mealtimes. For best effects, take 1 to 3 hours after meals and at bedtime. To prevent chewable tablets from entering the small intestine in undissolved form, they must be chewed thoroughly before they are swallowed and followed with half a glass of water. Suspensions should be shaken before administration (Table 20–4).

Antacids have many drug interactions when taken concurrently with other drugs because the altered acidity of the stomach affects acid labile drugs. **Antacids** may bind with many drugs affecting their absorption. The dose of **antacid** may need to be separated from the dose of another drug by as much as 2 hours. Health-care providers should instruct the patient in timing the administration of such drugs. Patients should be told not to begin taking OTC **antacids** on their own without first consulting their health-care provider or the pharmacist to discuss any potential drug interactions.

Calcium-based antacids should not be administered with food containing large amounts of oxalic acid (e.g., spinach, rhubarb) or phytic acid (e.g., bran, cereals). These foods decrease the absorption of **calcium**. Taking these **antacids** with food that contains phosphorus (milk or other dairy products) may lead to milk-alkali syndrome (nausea,

Table 20–4 ◆ **Available Dosage Forms: Selected Antacids**

Drug	Dosage Form	How Supplied
Aluminum hydroxide (AlternaGEL)	Liquid: 600 mg/5 mL	In 150-mL and 360-mL bottles
(Amphojel)	Tablets: 300 mg, 600 mg	In bottles of 100 tablets
(Alu-Tab)	Tablets: 500 mg	In bottles of 250 tablets
(Alu-Cap)	Capsules: 400 mg	In bottles of 100 capsules
(Dialume)	Capsules: 500 mg (sodium content <1.2 mg)	In bottles of 500 capsules
(Generic)	Suspension: 320 mg/5 mL Concentrated suspension: 450 mg/5 mL Concentrated suspension: 675 mg/5 mL Concentrated liquid: 600 mg/5 mL	In bottles of 360 and 480 mL In bottles of 500 mL (peppermint flavor) In bottles of 180, 500 mL (creamsicle flavor) In bottles of 30, 180, 480 mL
Calcium Carbonate (Amitone) (Mallamint) (Alka-Mints)	Tablets, chewable: 350 mg (sodium content <2 mg) Tablets, chewable: 420 mg (sodium content <0.1 mg) Tablets, chewable: 850 mg (sodium content <5 mg)	In bottle of 100 (peppermint flavor) In bottles of 1000 (mint flavor) In bottles of 75 (spearmint flavor)
Calcium carbonate (Tums)	Tablets, chewable: 500 mg (sodium content <2 mg) Extra-strength, chewable: 750 mg (sodium content <4 mg) Ultra, chewable: 1,000 mg (sodium content <4 mg)	In bottles of 36, 75, 150, 400 tablets In bottles of 24, 48, 96 tablets (assorted flavors) In bottles of 36, 72 tablets (assorted flavors)
(Generic)	Tablets: 500 mg, 600 mg, 650 mg, 1,250 mg	In bottles of varying number 60–1,000
	Suspension: 1,250 mg/5 mL	In bottles of 500 mL (mint flavor)
Magnesium hydroxide (Phillips' Chewables)	Tablets: 311 mg	In bottles of 100, 200 tablets (mint flavor)
(Phillips' Milk of Magnesia)	Liquid: 400 mg/5 mL Concentrated liquid: 800 mg/5 mL	In bottles of 120, 360, 780 mL In bottles of 240 mL
(Generic)	Liquid: 400 mg/5 mL	In bottles of 360 mL, pint, gallon
Aluminum hydroxide–magnesium hydroxide combinations (Maalox)	Tablets/chewable: 200 mg aluminum, 200 mg magnesium Extra-strength: 350 mg aluminum, 350 mg magnesium Suspension: 200 mg aluminum, 225 mg magnesium/5 mL; and 300 mg aluminum, 600 mg magnesium/5 mL	In bottles of 100 tablets (mint flavor) In bottles of 38, 75 tablets (mint cream flavor) In bottles of 148, 355, and 769 mL (mint cream and cherry cream flavors)
(Mylanta)	Tablets/chewable: 200 mg aluminum, 200 mg magnesium, 20 mg simethicone Double-strength: 400 mg aluminum, 400 mg magnesium (For all tablets: Sodium content is 0.77 mg) Suspension: 200 mg aluminum, 225 mg magnesium/5 mL; and 300 mg aluminum, 600 mg magnesium/5 mL (For all liquids: Sodium content is 0.58 mg)	In bottles of 12, 40, 48, 100, 180 tablets In bottles of 24, 60 tablets (mint and cherry) In bottles of 150, 360, and 720 mL

vomiting, confusion, and headache). Taking these **antacids** with an acidic fruit juice may improve absorption.

Adverse Reactions

Patients should be told to consult their health-care provider before taking **antacids** for more than 2 weeks if a problem recurs, if relief is not obtained, or if symptoms of GI bleeding (black, tarry stools; coffee-ground emesis) occur.

Aluminum- and calcium-based antacids may cause constipation. Methods of preventing constipation such as increased bulk in the diet, greater fluid intake, and more mobility should be recommended. A **stool softener** may be needed to treat constipation related to **antacid** use. **Magnesium-based antacids** may cause diarrhea. Increased fiber in the diet may help this problem.

Lifestyle Management

Lifestyle management issues related to the disease process should be discussed. They often include smoking avoidance or cessation, inappropriate body positions while sleeping, foods that irritate the gastric mucosa (e.g., spicy foods) or stimulate acid production (e.g., **alcohol**), and foods that decrease lower esophageal sphincter tone (e.g., fatty food, chocolate, and caffeine).

ANTIDIARRHEALS

Diarrhea is a common reason for self-treatment and for patients to seek treatment from a health-care provider. Much of the diarrhea seen in a primary care setting has an infectious etiology, is food or drug induced, or is the result of inflammatory bowel disease. Diarrhea that lasts for less than 2 weeks is considered acute; if it lasts more than 2 weeks, it is considered chronic. Most episodes are acute and self-limiting, with few serious consequences. The exception is diarrhea in children, for whom dehydration can occur rather quickly, even with short-term diarrhea. Chronic diarrhea can result in weight loss, dehydration, perianal skin breakdown, and nutritional deficits.

Diarrhea that is drug induced may be treated simply by removal of the offending drug. Food-induced diarrhea related to food poisoning and other diarrheas of an infectious etiology may require **antimicrobial** therapy depending on the pathogen. Drugs used to treat infectious diseases are the subjects of Chapter 24. The focus of this chapter is drugs used for symptomatic relief. Some drugs used to treat diarrhea are chemically related to **opioids. Opioids** are discussed further in Chapter 15.

Anticholinergic agents are also sometimes used to treat diarrhea and are discussed in Chapter 14. This chapter does not discuss the diagnosis of diarrhea.

Pharmacodynamics

Three main classes of drugs are used to treat diarrhea: **absorbent preparations (kaolin and pectin** [Kapectolin] and **bismuth subsalicylate** [Pepto-Bismol, Kaopectate Liquid]), **opiates (diphenoxylate with atropine** [Lomotil], **diphenoxin with atropine** [Motofen], and **loperamide** [Imodium]), and **anticholinergics. Anticholinergics** are useful only for inflammatory bowel disease.

Kaolin is a clay-like powder that attracts and holds onto bacteria, and **pectin** thickens the stool by absorbing moisture in the stool. They do not affect total water loss, however. Commonly used to treat simple diarrhea, the combination was rated by the U.S. Food and Drug Administration (FDA) in 1986 as "safe and effective"; however, there are no specific trials to demonstrate this.

Bismuth subsalicylate appears to have **antisecretory** and **antimicrobial** effects in vitro and may have some **anti-inflammatory** effects. The **salicylate** moiety provides the **antisecretory** effect, and the **bismuth** moiety may exert direct **antimicrobial** effects against bacterial and viral enteropathogens. Because of these effects, it is also used as part of a multidrug regimen for the eradication of *H. pylori.*

Diphenoxylate with **atropine** is a constipating **meperidine** congener that lacks **analgesic** activity. High doses (4–60 mg), however, can cause **opioid** activity, including euphoria, and physical dependence with chronic use. The addition of **atropine** provides **anticholinergic** effects that decrease secretion in the bowel and slow peristalsis.

Loperamide binds to the opiate receptors of the intestinal wall leading to slowed gastric motility. It also reduces fecal volume, increases viscosity and bulk, and diminishes the loss of fluid and electrolytes.

Pharmacokinetics

Absorption and Distribution

Kaolin and pectin act locally in the bowel and are not systemically absorbed (Table 20–5). **Bismuth subsalicylate** undergoes chemical dissociation in the GI tract; the **salicylate** moiety is absorbed, with plasma levels similar to those of **aspirin.** There is only negligible absorption of the bismuth moiety. **Diphenoxylate with atropine** and **difenoxin with atropine** are both well absorbed from the GI tract. Their distribution is unknown, but they do enter breast milk. The **atropine** in the drug readily crosses the blood–brain barrier and the placenta and enters breast milk. It also produces mild to moderate **anticholinergic** effects. Forty percent of **loperamide** is absorbed after oral administration, but it does not cross the blood–brain

Table 20–5 ▶ **Pharmacokinetics: Selected Antidiarrheals**

Drug	Onset	Peak	Duration	Half-Life	Elimination
Bismuth subsalicylate	—	—	—	2–3 h for low doses: 15–30 h for larger doses	>90% of salicylate in urine
Difenoxin with atropine		20–40 min	3–4 h	24–72 h	Excreted as conjugates in urine and feces
Diphenoxylate with atropine	45–60 m	2 h	3–4 h	2.5 h (12–14 h for the metabolite)	14% of drug and metabolites in urine; 49% in feces
Loperamide	1 h	2.5–5 h	10 h	10.8 h (range 9.1–14.4 h)	25% unchanged in feces; 1.3% in urine as free drug and glucuronic acid conjugate

barrier well, so there are limited central nervous system (CNS) effects.

Metabolism and Excretion

The **salicylate** portion of **bismuth subsalicylate** is metabolized in the liver and more than 90 percent is excreted in urine. **Diphenoxylate with atropine** is rapidly and extensively metabolized to diphenoxylic acid, which is biologically active and its main metabolite. It is excreted in urine and feces. **Difenoxin with atropine** is rapidly metabolized to an inactive hydroxylated metabolite. Both the drug and its metabolite are excreted, mainly as conjugates, in the urine and feces. **Loperamide** is partially metabolized by the liver and undergoes enterohepatic recirculation to be completely metabolized. Most is eliminated in feces, with a minimal amount excreted in urine.

Pharmacotherapeutics

Precautions and Contraindications

Drugs that reduce intestinal motility or delay intestinal transit time have induced toxic megacolon, especially in patients with inflammatory bowel disease. **Diphenoxylate with atropine, difenoxin with atropine,** and **loperamide** should be used cautiously for these patients and promptly discontinued if abdominal distention occurs. Because of their hepatic metabolism and renal excretion, these drugs should also be used with extreme caution in patients with advanced hepatorenal disease and in all patients with abnormal liver function studies because hepatic coma may be precipitated.

The **atropine** component of **diphenoxylate** and **difenoxin** contraindicates their use in narrow-angle glaucoma and requires cautious use in prostatic hyperplasia. Children, especially those with Down syndrome, have increased sensitivity to **atropine**. This drug should be avoided or used with extreme caution in children. It is not recommended for use in children younger than 12 years. This drug may prolong or aggravate diarrhea associated with organisms that penetrate the intestinal mucosa, such as *Escherichia coli, Salmonella,* and *Shigella* or in pseudomembranous colitis associated with broad-spectrum **antimicrobial** therapy. It should not be used in these conditions.

The **salicylate** component of **bismuth subsalicylate** contraindicates its use in children or teenagers during or after recovery from chickenpox or flu-like illness. It is also contraindicated for patients with **aspirin** hypersensitivity.

All **antidiarrheals** require cautious use in older adults and others in whom impaction is a high risk. Older adults are especially sensitive to **diphenoxylate** or **difenoxin** because of the **atropine** content and **anticholinergic** properties.

Pregnancy categories vary among the antidiarrheal drugs. **Kaolin** and **pectin** are Pregnancy Category B. All others are Pregnancy Category C except **loperamide**, which is Pregnancy Category B. However, there are no adequate and well-controlled studies in pregnant women for any of these drugs, and safety during pregnancy has not been established.

Some of the drugs are excreted in breast milk, and the safety of any of the **antidiarrheals** has not been established in lactating women. They should be avoided or used with caution.

None of the **antidiarrheals** has established safety for children younger than age 2 years. All have published children's doses. It is important to keep in mind that dehydration may influence younger children's response to these drugs. **Antidiarrheals** are contraindicated in the treatment of diarrhea in most children; the standard of care is oral rehydration therapy (ORT) to treat electrolyte and fluids loss of diarrhea.

Adverse Drug Reactions

The main adverse drug reaction for all **antidiarrheals** is rebound constipation. For **bismuth subsalicylate**, additional reactions that all patients should be warned about are gray black stools and black tongue, results of the **bismuth**. Patients should be told to expect this reaction and that it does not indicate GI bleeding.

The adverse reactions associated with the other two drugs are related to their **anticholinergic** and **opioid**-like effects. **Diphenoxylate** and **difenoxin** (both with **atropine**) may exhibit **anticholinergic** adverse reactions such as dry mouth and mucous membranes, flushing, tachycardia, and urinary retention, especially in children. **Loperamide** also exhibits these reactions, but to a lesser degree. Both drugs have CNS reactions of dizziness and drowsiness, **loperamide** less so than **diphenoxylate** or **difenoxin** (both with **atropine**). Because they cross the blood–brain barrier better, **diphenoxylate** and **difenoxin** (both with **atropine**) also exhibit sedation, headache, and, in higher doses or with chronic use, euphoria or depression, although **difenoxin** exhibits these slightly less so than **diphenoxylate**.

Drug Interactions

Bismuth subsalicylate may potentiate the risk for toxicity if taken with **aspirin** and the risk for hypoglycemia if given in large doses with **insulin** or **oral hypoglycemics. Diphenoxylate with atropine, difenoxin with atropine** and **loperamide** all have additive or potentiating CNS effects with other CNS depressants and additive **anticholinergic** effects with other drugs that share these effects. There are few other drug interactions (Table 20–6).

Clinical Use and Dosing

Simple, Acute Diarrhea

After the cause of the diarrhea has been determined and, if possible, eliminated, absorbent preparations are commonly used for relief of symptoms in adults. **Kaolin-pectin** or **bismuth subsalicylate** taken after each loose stool may be effective. The majority of acute diarrheal illnesses are self-limiting, and the main concern is to maintain hydration.

Table 20–6 ■ **Drug Interactions: Selected Antidiarrheals**

Drug	Interacting Drug	Possible Effect	Implications
Bismuth subsalicylate	Aspirin	May potentiate salicylate toxicity	Avoid concurrent use
	Tetracycline	May decrease GI absorption	Separate administration by 2 h
	Thrombolytics, warfarin, heparin	Large doses may increase risk for bleeding	Avoid concurrent use or use small doses; monitor clotting studies closely
	Insulin, oral hypoglycemics	Large doses increase risk of hypoglycemia	Avoid concurrent use or use small doses
Diphenoxylate with atropine	CNS depressants, including alcohol, antihistamines, opioids, sedative hypnotics	Additive/potentiating CNS depression	Monitor patient closely if these drugs must be given concurrently
	Monoamine oxidase inhibitors (MAOIs)	Because chemical structure is similar, concurrent use may precipitate hypertensive crisis	Avoid concurrent use or within 14 d of use of MAOIs
	Drugs that have anticholinergic properties	Additive anticholinergic effect	Monitor for toxicity; treat symptoms with good oral hygiene, hard candy, sugarless gum
Kaolin-pectin	Digoxin, chloroquine	Decreases GI absorption	Avoid concurrent use or separate doses by at least 2 h, giving kaolin-pectin last
Loperamide	CNS depressants, including alcohol, antihistamines, opioids, sedative hypnotics	Additive/potentiating CNS depression	Monitor patient closely if these drugs must be given concurrently
	Drugs that have anticholinergic properties	Additive anticholinergic effect	Monitor for toxicity; treat symptoms with good oral hygiene, hard candy, sugarless gum

Hydration can usually be maintained in adults, even with profuse diarrhea, by the use of oral fluids. Commercial hydrating fluids (**Pedialyte**, **Rehydralyte**) or powdered salts are available; adding a pinch of table salt and a half-teaspoon of honey to an 8-oz glass of fruit juice also makes a hydrating solution for older children and adults. Nondiet colas that have been allowed to lose their carbonation may also be used in older children and adults. Alternate these solutions with 8-oz glasses of water to which has been added one-quarter teaspoon of baking soda to replenish the electrolytes commonly lost in acute, infectious diarrhea (sodium, potassium, bicarbonate, and chloride).

Children with severe diarrhea need **oral rehydrating solutions (ORS)** to prevent dehydration. Examples include **Infalyte**, **Kao-Lectrolyte**, and **Pedialyte**. These OTC products are available in pharmacies or supermarkets. If the child does not like the flavor, one-quarter teaspoon of sugar-free Kool-Aid powder may be added. Jell-O, water, or sports drinks should be avoided because they do not contain enough sodium. For infants, a homemade recipe includes one-half cup infant rice cereal mixed with 16 oz of water and one-quarter teaspoon of salt. Children should be given **ORS** to satisfy their thirst for at least 6 hours and often for 24 hours. Infants and young children need electrolyte replacement with their fluids, whereas older children and adults may be able to be rehydrated with fluids alone. Full management of acute diarrhea is not within the scope of this chapter.

If the absorbents do not resolve the diarrhea, **diphenoxylate** or **difenoxin** (both with **atropine**) or **loperamide** may be added. **Diphenoxylate with atropine** is given three to four times daily rather than after each loose stool. **Difenoxin with atropine** is dosed both after each stool or every 3 to 4 hours as needed to avoid exceeding the maximum 24-hour dose. Antidiarrheals are generally not recommended in children.

Unlike acute diarrhea, chronic diarrhea requires etiological diagnosis and specific therapy for that diagnosis. Simply suppressing symptoms is not sufficient.

> **CLINICAL PEARL**
>
> **Oral Rehydration Therapy**
>
> Evaluation of the effectiveness of oral rehydration is based on at least three wet diapers per 24 hours in infants. For children older than 1 year, avoid all fruit juices and other drinks that contain fructose because they usually make the diarrhea worse. If the infant or child is drinking milk or lactose-based formula, try withholding milk or lactose products. Resolution of the diarrhea strongly suggests lactose intolerance.

Chronic Diarrhea Associated With Inflammatory Bowel Disease

Steroids and **sulfasalazine** are needed to control diarrhea in exacerbation of inflammatory bowel disease. **Loperamide** 4 mg initially, followed by doses of 2 to 4 mg four times a day, may be used as adjunct therapy, and it may lead to substantial clinical improvement, especially if combined with added fiber in the diet and **anticholinergics**. If clinical improvement is not observed with doses of 16 mg/day for at least 10 days, symptoms are unlikely to be controlled by further use of this drug.

Chronic Diarrhea Associated With Pancreatic Insufficiency

Malabsorption due to pancreatic insufficiency requires use of enzyme supplements. **Antidiarrheal** medications are not generally used for this indication.

Chronic Infantile Diarrhea

Bismuth subsalicylate has been used to treat chronic infantile diarrhea. The dose is 2.5 mL every 4 hours for children 2 to 24 months; 5 mL for children 24 to 48 months; and 10 mL for children 48 to 70 months (Taketomo, Hodding, & Kraus, 2009).

Traveler's Diarrhea

Bismuth subsalicylate appears to have antibacterial and antisecretory properties and is used to treat traveler's diarrhea in doses of two tablets or 2 fluid oz before each meal and at bedtime (4 times/d) for up to 3 weeks during brief periods of high risk (Centers for Disease Control and Prevention [CDC], 2009). The management of traveler's diarrhea can be divided into prevention and treatment. The most important risk factor for acquiring this disorder is the patient's destination. High-risk areas include Latin America, Africa, parts of the Middle East, the Dominican Republic, Haiti, and Asia. Intermittent-risk areas include southern Europe, Israel, South Africa, and a number of the Caribbean islands. Numerous studies performed around the world have shown that enterotoxigenic *E. coli* is the most common causative organism. Oral **antimicrobials** are also used for both prevention and treatment of this disorder; the provider should refer to the CDC Travel Web site for current antimicrobial recommendations. **Bismuth subsalicylate** has been effective in decreasing the duration and severity of diarrhea associated with Norwalk virus (CDC, 2009). Symptomatic management in adults includes **bismuth subsalicylate** two tablets or 30 mL of liquid every 30 minutes for no more than eight doses per day for no longer than 48 hours. **Loperamide** 4 mg initially, followed by 2 mg after each loose stool with no more than 8 mg/day for no longer than 48 hours, may also be used. Doses are smaller for children.

Table 20–7 provides adults' and children's doses of selected antidiarrheals.

Rational Drug Selection

Indication

For acute diarrhea, any of the **antidiarrheals** is appropriate. The more severe the diarrhea is, the less likely it will be that absorbent agents will help. **Bismuth subsalicylate**

Table 20–7 ● Dosage Schedule: Selected Antidiarrheals

Drug	Indication	Initial Dose	Additional Doses
Bismuth subsalicylate*†	Acute diarrhea	*Adults:* 524 mg every 30 min or 1,048–1,200 mg every 60 min as needed	Not to exceed 4.2 g/24 h
		Children 9–12 yr: 262–300 mg every 30–60 min as needed	Not to exceed 2.4 g/24 h
		Children 6–9 yr: 176 mg every 30–60 min as needed	Not to exceed 1.4 g/24 h
		Children 3–6 yr: 88 mg every 30–60 min as needed	Not to exceed 704 mg/24 h
		Children <3 yr weighing >13 kg: 88 mg *Children <3 yr weighing 6.4–8 kg:* 44 mg May repeat q4h; not to exceed 6 doses/24 h	May repeat q4h; not to exceed 6 doses/24 h
	Traveler's diarrhea	524 mg (2 tablets or 30 mL of 262 mg/15 mL liquid) every 30 min for up to 8 doses	Not to be used for more than 48 h
Difenoxin with atropine	Acute diarrhea	*Adults: 2 mg*	1 mg after each loose stool or 1 mg every 3–4 h as needed. Total 24 hours dose not to exceed 8 mg
Diphenoxylate with atropine	Acute diarrhea	*Adults:* 5 mg tid to qid initially	5 mg daily as needed; not to exceed 20 mg/d
		Children 2–12 yr: all doses qid and in liquid form *2 yr/11–14 kg:* 1.5–3 mL *3 yr/12–16 kg:* 2–3 mL *4 yr/14–20 kg:* 2–4 mL *5 yr/16–23 kg:* 2.5–4.5 mL *6–8 yr/17–32 kg:* 2.5–5.5 mL *9–12 yr/23–55 kg:* 3.5–5 mL	Reduce dosage as soon as control of symptoms is achieved; maintenance dosage may be as low as one-fourth of initial daily dose; maximum daily dose 20 mg

Table 20–7 ● **Dosage Schedule: Selected Antidiarrheals—cont'd**

Drug	Indication	Initial Dose	Additional Doses
Kaolin-pectin	Acute diarrhea	*Adults:* 60–120 mL after each loose stool *Children >12 yr:* 40–60 mL after each loose stool *Children 6–12 yr:* 30–60 mL after each loose stool *Children 3–6 yr:* 15–30 mL after each loose stool	
Loperamide	Acute diarrhea, traveler's diarrhea	*Adults:* 4 mg initially	2 mg after each loose stool; not to exceed 8 mg/d for OTC use or 16 mg/d for prescription use
		Children 9–11 yr or 30–47 kg: 2 mg initially	1 mg after each loose stool; not to exceed 6 mg/24 h; OTC use not to exceed 48 h
		Children 6–8 yr or 24–30 kg: 1 mg initially	1 mg after each loose stool; not to exceed 4 mg/24 h; OTC use not to exceed 48 h
	Chronic diarrhea associated with inflammatory bowel disease	*Adults only:* 4 mg initially	2 mg after each loose stool until symptoms resolved; maintenance dose is usually 4–8 mg/d in divided doses; not to exceed 16 mg/d

*The dosage schedule for eradication of *Helicobacter pylori* is discussed in Chapter 34.

†Avoid bismuth subsalicylate in pediatric patients with influenza or chicken pox because of the risk of Reye syndrome.

and **loperamide** are the only drugs indicated for traveler's diarrhea. **Loperamide** is the only drug with an indication for use with inflammatory bowel disease.

Cost

Brand names are more expensive than generic formulations, and there is no significant clinical difference between the two. **Diphenoxylate with atropine** generic is $13.99 for 30 tablets, whereas the brand **Lomotil** is $41.99 (http://drugstore.com). **Loperamide (Imodium)** is available OTC and is $9.99 for 24 tablets, or the generic **loperamide** at $5.99 (http://drugstore.com).

Monitoring

There is no specific monitoring beyond that required for the disease process being treated. Patients with chronic diarrhea may benefit from monitoring of hydration status and electrolyte studies.

Patient Education

Administration

Despite the fact that many of these drugs are available OTC, they are not innocuous drugs. Patients need to be informed that they should take the **antidiarrheal** exactly as directed; do not make up missed doses or double doses, and do not exceed the maximum number of doses recommended for 24 hours. The health-care provider should be notified if the diarrhea continues beyond 48 hours, or if abdominal pain, fever, or distention occurs.

Tablets may be administered with food if GI irritation occurs (Table 20–8). They may also be crushed and taken with fluid. Chewable tablets may be chewed or allowed to

Table 20–8 ◆ **Available Dosage Forms: Selected Antidiarrheals**

Drug	Dosage Form	How Supplied
Bismuth subsalicylate (Pepto-Bismol, Kaopectate)	Tablets/chewable: 262 mg	In bottles of 30, 42 (cherry flavor); 24, 42 (original flavor); <2 mg sodium
	Liquid: 262 mg/15 mL	In bottles of 120, 240, 360, 480 mL; 5 mg sodium/15 mL
	Liquid: 524 mg/15 mL	In bottles of 120, 240, 360 mL; <5 mg sodium/15 mL
Difenoxin with atropine (Motofen)	Tablets: 1 mg difenoxin and 0.025 mg atropine sulfate	In bottles of 50 and 100. White, scored.
Diphenoxylate with atropine (Lomotil)	Tablets: 2.5 mg diphenoxylate, 0.025 mg atropine sulfate	In bottles of 100, 500, 1,000, 2,500
	Liquid: 2.5 mg diphenoxylate, 0.025 mg atropine sulfate/5 mL	In bottles of 60 mL (cherry flavor) 15% alcohol; with dropper

Continued

Table 20–8 ◈ **Available Dosage Forms: Selected Antidiarrheals—cont'd**

Drug	Dosage Form	How Supplied
(Generic)	Tablets: 2.5 mg diphenoxylate, 0.025 mg atropine sulfate Liquid: 2.5 mg diphenoxylate, 0.025 mg atropine sulfate/5 mL	In bottles of 100, 500, 1,000, 2,500 In bottles of 10, 60 mL
Kaolin-pectin (Kapectolin, Kao-Spen)	Suspension: 5.2 g kaolin plus 260 mg pectin/30 mL; 5.85 mg kaolin plus 130 mg pectin/30 mL Also comes in combinations with paregoric, bismuth, carboxy-methylcellulose, and others	
Loperamide (Imodium A-D)	Tablets: 2 mg Liquid: 1 mg/5 mL	In packets of 6, 12 In bottles of 60, 90, 120 mL (cherry/licorice flavor)
(Imodium)	Capsule: 2 mg	In bottles of 100, 500
(Generic)	Capsule: 2 mg Liquid: 1 mg/5 mL	In bottles of 100, 500, 1,000 In bottles of 60, 118 mL

dissolve. Calibrated measuring devices should be used for liquid preparations. Suspensions should be shaken before they are measured and administered.

Drug interactions may occur, especially with **diphenoxylate with atropine** and **loperamide**. Patients should be told not to take any OTC **antidiarrheal** if they are taking other drugs, especially **digoxin**, **cephalosporin antimicrobials**, **warfarin**, or **heparin**, or CNS depressants (including **alcohol**) without first contacting their healthcare provider.

Adverse Reactions

All **antidiarrheals** have the potential for rebound constipation. As soon as symptoms of diarrhea are reduced, the dosage of the **antidiarrheal** drug should be reduced; it should be stopped as soon as symptoms resolve.

Bismuth subsalicylate can turn the tongue and stools gray black. Patients should be told that this reaction can be expected and that it does not indicate GI bleeding.

Diphenoxylate and **difenoxin** (both with **atropine**) can cause dry mouth and mucous membranes. These symptoms can be improved by good oral hygiene, sucking hard candy, or chewing sugarless gum. Flushing, tachycardia, and urinary retention may also occur. These symptoms are especially notable in children and in older men. They may necessitate stopping the drug. **Loperamide** also exhibits these reactions but to a lesser degree. Both drugs can produce CNS reactions of dizziness and drowsiness, **loperamide** less so than **diphenoxylate** or **difenoxin** (both with **atropine**). Driving or other activities requiring mental alertness should be avoided until the patient's response to the drug is known.

Lifestyle Management

Adding fiber to the diet and using **oral rehydrating solutions** were discussed previously. The importance of washing one's hands after each bowel movement should be stressed. Education about maintaining nutritional intake is also important. Sometimes patients think that they can stop their diarrhea by stopping their food intake. Resting the GI tract briefly (e.g., for 24 hr) may be appropriate, but reducing fluid intake is never appropriate, and food intake should be restarted after the GI rest.

A bland food diet can assist in maintaining nutrition and is also helpful in reducing the diarrhea. Stopping milk or other lactose-based food products for a few days may give an indication whether the diarrhea is associated with lactose intolerance.

CYTOPROTECTIVE AGENTS

Peptic ulceration can be caused by a variety of conditions, some of which are iatrogenic. The administration of **NSAIDs**, for example, has been associated with gastric mucosal damage and ulcer formation. Ulcer formation and GI bleeding related to **NSAID** use often occur without warning. Patients at high risk are those with previous history of ulcers, also on steroids, on high doses of **NSAIDS**, concurrently taking anticoagulants, or older than 75 years. Among the agents used to treat or prevent ulcer formation are two **cytoprotective agents**, **sucralfate** (**Carafate**) and **misoprostol** (**Cytotec**). These drugs are the focus of this section.

Pharmacodynamics

Sucralfate is a basic aluminum salt of a sulfated disaccharide, which is believed to act by polymerization and selective binding to necrotic ulcer tissue, where it covers the ulcer site and acts as a barrier to acid, pepsin, and bile salts. It has no acid-neutralizing activity, and little is absorbed, although some aluminum salts are released. In addition, the drug may directly absorb bile salts and stimulate endogenous prostaglandin synthesis. **Prostaglandins** are central to the formation and maintenance of the protective mucosa of the GI tract.

Misoprostol is a methyl analogue of prostaglandin E_1. The principal mechanism of action of this drug appears to be inhibition of gastric secretion through inhibition of histamine-stimulated cyclic adenosine monophosphate (AMP) production. Over a dosage range of 50 to 200 mcg, it inhibits basal and nocturnal gastric acid secretion and acid secretion in response to a variety of stimuli, including meals, histamine, and coffee by binding to prostaglandin E receptors. It has no significant effect on fasting or postprandial gastrin or on intrinsic factor output; however, it produces a moderate decrease in pepsin concentration during basal conditions.

Misoprostol also has mucosal protective qualities. Prostaglandin E receptors have a high affinity for **misoprostol** and for its acid metabolite. These receptors facilitate the production of mucus and bicarbonate. They also allow the drug taken with food to be effective, despite the lower serum concentration.

Misoprostol also produces uterine contractions that may endanger pregnancy. See discussion below.

Pharmacokinetics

Absorption and Distribution

Sucralfate is minimally absorbed (Table 20–9). Its action is largely topical. **Misoprostol** is rapidly and extensively absorbed after oral administration. Distribution of this drug is unknown.

Metabolism and Excretion

Because it is essentially not absorbed, more than 90 percent of **sucralfate** is excreted in feces. **Misoprostol** is rapidly converted to its free acid, which is responsible for its clinical activity. It does not affect the cytochrome P450 (CYP450) enzyme systems. The half-life of this drug is 20 to 40 minutes, but renal impairment results in a doubling of this half-life. The metabolite is excreted in urine.

Pharmacotherapeutics

Precautions and Contraindications

Because its action is topical, there are no specific precautions or contraindications for **sucralfate**. It is Pregnancy Category B. Its safety and efficacy have not been established in children.

Misoprostol must be used with caution in renal impairment. Its half-life, maximum concentration and the area under the curve (AUC) double with renal insufficiency. No routine dosage adjustments have been recommended, but dosage may need to be reduced if the usual dose is not tolerated. In older adults (older than 64 years), the AUC for the acid metabolite of **misoprostol** is increased. The cause may be decreased renal functioning associated with aging, and recommendations are the same as for renal impairment.

Misoprostol is Pregnancy Category X. It may cause abortion, premature birth, or birth defects. Uterine rupture has been reported in women who were administered **misoprostol** to induce labor. It should not be administered to pregnant women to treat NSAID-induced ulcers. Patients should be warned of the abortifacient properties of the drug and be advised not to give it to others (http://www.drugs.com).

Misoprostol is metabolized in the mother to misoprostol acid that is excreted in breast milk. Caution is advised when administered to a nursing woman.

Safety and efficacy in children younger than 18 years have not been established.

Adverse Drug Reactions

Adverse reactions in clinical trials with **sucralfate** were minor and rarely led to discontinuance of the drug. Constipation, the most frequent complaint, occurs in only 2 percent of patients. Other adverse reactions, including dizziness and gastric discomfort, occurred in less than 0.5 percent of patients.

Adverse reactions with **misoprostol** were largely GI or gynecological. Diarrhea is the most common complaint (13% to 40% of patients). Abdominal pain, nausea, and flatulence occur in small numbers of patients and are difficult to separate from the symptoms of the disorder for which the drug was prescribed. Postmenopausal bleeding, spotting (0.7%), cramps (0.6%), hypermenorrhea (0.5%), menstrual disorder (0.3%), and dysmenorrhea (0.1%) occur in women. Reactions related to pregnancy were discussed previously.

Drug Interactions

Sucralfate may decrease the absorption of several drugs when given concurrently or prior to their administration

Table 20–9 ▶ **Pharmacokinetics: Cytoprotective Agents**

Drug	Onset	Peak	Duration	Protein Binding	Half-Life	Elimination
Misoprostol	Minutes	12–15 min	3–6 h	<90%	20–40 min (doubles in renal impairment)	80% in urine
Sucralfate	30 min	UK	5 h	UK	6–20 h	90% in feces

UK = unknown.

(Table 20–10). Separating the administration of the interacting drug by at least 2 hours and giving the interacting drug first can often solve the problem.

The only drug of concern with **misoprostol** is the potential for increased diarrhea risk with **magnesium-based antacids.** Food can decrease maximum plasma concentrations, but this has little clinical significance.

Clinical Use and Dosing

Prophylaxis and Treatment of Duodenal Ulcers Associated With NSAID Use

NSAIDs inhibit prostaglandin synthesis and damage the mucosal lining of the stomach, which may result in ulcer formation. The first choice is to discontinue the NSAID. **Misoprostol** is approved by the FDA for prophylaxis or treatment of duodenal ulcers that are due to use of NSAIDs for those patients who must continue NSAID use. Dosage is 200 mcg four times a day with food (Table 20–11). If this dose cannot be tolerated, 100 mcg can be used. **Misoprostol** should be taken with meals and at bedtime. The drug is taken for the duration of NSAID therapy.

Because **misoprostol** commonly causes a dose-dependent diarrhea and other GI symptoms, and because its stimulant effect on the uterus contraindicates its use for women with childbearing potential, its use as prophylaxis is reserved for those with high risk for and little tolerance of the GI hazards of **NSAIDs.**

In a *Cochrane Review* of the literature regarding prevention of NSAID-induced gastroduodenal ulcers, **misoprostol** significantly reduced the risk of endoscopic ulcers. **Misoprostol** 800 mg/day was more effective than 400 mg/day in gastric ulcers, but not duodenal ulcers (Rostom et al, 2002).

Treatment of Duodenal Ulcers From Other Causes

Sucralfate can be used for short-term (up to 8 wk) treatment of active duodenal ulcer. Dosage is 1 g four times a day on an empty stomach, 1 hour before meals and at bedtime. Healing usually occurs within 2 weeks. Maintenance therapy after the ulcer has healed is 1 g twice a day. **Sucralfate** has off-labeled uses in treating gastric and esophageal ulcers, with the same dosing schedule. It appears to have some advantage over **antacids** and **H_2RAs** in stress ulcer prophylaxis.

Although more effective than placebo, **misoprostol** is less effective than **H_2RAs** or **PPIs** for treatment of duodenal ulcers from other causes. In doses greater than 400 mcg/day, it has an off-labeled use for treatment of duodenal ulcers not responsive to **H_2RAs.**

Rational Drug Selection

Drug selection is based on indications cited previously (Table 20–12). **Sucralfate** is preferred over **misoprostol**

Table 20–10 ■ Drug Interactions: Cytoprotective Agents

Drug	Interacting Drug	Possible Effect	Implications
Misoprostol	Magnesium-based antacids	Increased risk for diarrhea	Choose different antacid
	Food	Maximum plasma concentrations of acid metabolite are diminished when taken with food	Little clinical significance, but best taken on empty stomach
Sucralfate	Aluminum-based antacids	Increased constipation risk; increase in total body burden of aluminum	Choose different antacid
	Anticoagulants	Decrease in effect of warfarin	Avoid concurrent use
	Digoxin	Reduced serum levels of digoxin; reduced effects	Avoid concurrent use
	Hydantoins	Absorption may be decreased	Separate administration by 2 h and give hydantoin first
	Ketoconazole, quinolones	Bioavailability decreased	Separate administration by 2 h and give drugs first
	Quinidine	Reduced serum levels of quinidine; reduced effects	Separate administration by 2 h and give quinidine first

Table 20–11 ● Dosage Schedule: Cytoprotective Agents

Drug	Indication	Dosage Schedule
Misoprostol	Prophylaxis and treatment of duodenal ulcers due to NSAID use	200 mcg qid with food. Last dose usually at bedtime. Taken for duration of NSAID therapy. If this dose is not tolerated, 100 mcg qid may be used
Sucralfate	Active duodenal ulcer	1 g qid taken 1 h before meals and at bedtime.
	Maintenance after healing of duodenal ulcer	1 g bid taken on empty stomach

Table 20–12 ◆ **Available Dosage Forms: Cytoprotective Agents**

Drug	Dosage Form	How Supplied
Misoprostol (Cytotec)	Tablets: 100 mcg	In bottles of 60, 100 tablets
	Tablets: 200 mcg	In bottles of 60, 100 scored tablets
Sucralfate (Carafate	Tablets: 1 g	In bottles of 100, 120, 500 tablets
	Suspension: 1 g/ 10 mL	In bottles of 420 mL

for treatment of active duodenal ulcers not caused by NSAIDs. **Sucralfate** is also the drug of choice for women of childbearing age.

Monitoring

No specific monitoring parameters exist for these drugs. Monitoring should relate to the disease process being treated. Women of childbearing age should have a negative pregnancy test before misoprostol is prescribed to them.

Patient Education

Administration

Patients should be taught to take the drug exactly as prescribed. **Sucralfate** is taken on an empty stomach, **misoprostol** with food. Advise the patient to continue the therapy even if feeling better. **Sucralfate** is given for 4 to 8 weeks to ensure ulcer healing; **misoprostol** is given for the duration of NSAID therapy. Missed doses should be taken as soon as remembered unless it is almost time for the next dose. Doses should not be doubled. Women of childbearing age should have a negative pregnancy test and start **misoprostol** on day 2 or 3 of their menstrual period.

Adverse Reactions

Increased fluid intake, dietary bulk, and exercise may reduce the incidence of constipation associated with **sucralfate**. Diarrhea may occur with **misoprostol**. If it continues for more than 1 week, the health-care provider should be notified. The patient should also report onset of black, tarry stools or severe abdominal pain, which may indicate treatment failure and the onset of GI bleeding.

Women of childbearing age should be informed that **misoprostol** will cause spontaneous abortion. The drug should not be prescribed until contraceptive therapy is established and the patient has a negative serum pregnancy test within 2 weeks of starting therapy. If pregnancy is suspected, the drug should be immediately stopped and the health-care provider notified so that pregnancy testing can be performed.

Lifestyle Management

Lifestyle management related to peptic ulcers is discussed in Chapter 34.

ANTIEMETICS

Nausea and vomiting are common complaints in primary care and have a multitude of causes. Treatment is often nonpharmacological, but **antiemetics** may also be used to provide symptom relief and prevent fluid and electrolyte disturbances. This section discusses drugs used for these purposes.

Drug classes with **antiemetic** properties commonly used include **antihistamines, phenothiazines, sedative hypnotics, cannabinoids,** and **5-HT$_3$ receptor antagonists.** The **antihistamines** most commonly used for these **antiemetic** properties are **dimenhydrinate** (Dramamine), **diphenhydramine** (Benadryl), **hydroxyzine** (Vistaril), and **meclizine** (Antivert). The **phenothiazines** include **prochlorperazine** (Compazine) and **promethazine** (Phenergan). The **cannabinoid dronabinol** (Marinol) is used for nausea and vomiting associated with cancer. The **5-HT$_3$ receptor antagonists** include **palonosetron** (Aloxi), **dolasetron mesylate** (Anzemet), **granisetron** (Kytril, Sancuso), and **ondansetron** (Zofran). A miscellaneous **antiemetic** not from the previous classes of drugs is **trimethobenzamide** (Tigan). Each of these drugs is discussed in this section.

Pharmacodynamics

Antihistamines that possess significant **antiemetic** activity have strong **anticholinergic** effects as well as histamine$_1$-blocking effects. Blockade of histamine$_1$ receptors results in decreased exocrine gland secretion (e.g., salivary and lacrimal). First generation **antihistamines** with strong **anticholinergic** properties bind to central cholinergic receptors and produce **antiemetic** effects, decreasing nausea, and vomiting. They are especially helpful in the nausea associated with motion sickness because of their depression of conduction in the vestibulocerebellar pathway. The **antiemetic** drugs in this class are **dimenhydrinate, diphenhydramine, hydroxyzine,** and **meclizine.**

Phenothiazines block dopamine receptors in the chemoreceptor trigger zone (CTZ). They also bind to and block cholinergic, alpha$_1$-adrenergic, and histamine$_1$ receptors.

Although all **phenothiazines** have these actions to some degree, their use as **antiemetics** is limited by their sedating and extrapyramidal effects. The **antiemetic** drugs in this class are **prochlorperazine** and **promethazine.** They are less sedating and have **antiemetic** effects at lower doses than some other **phenothiazines. Metoclopramide** also blocks dopamine receptors and has been used as an **antiemetic**. Its main use, however, is as a **prokinetic**, and it is discussed in that section of this chapter.

Cannabinoids work in the CNS similar to cannabis (marijuana) to prevent nausea and vomiting associated with cancer chemotherapy and as an appetite stimulant, especially in HIV patients.

The 5-HT_3 **receptor antagonists** block serotonin both peripherally on vagal nerve terminals and centrally in the chemoreceptor trigger zone. Chemotherapy causes the release of serotonin from the enterochromaffin cells; pretreatment with a 5-HT_3 **receptor antagonist** decreases emesis.

Trimethobenzamide is a miscellaneous **antiemetic** agent that inhibits emetic stimulation of the CTZ.

Pharmacokinetics

Absorption and Distribution

All of these drugs are well absorbed after oral administration (Table 20–13). Oral liquid formulations provide the most reliable absorption. The **antihistamines, phenothiazines,** and 5-HT_3 **receptor antagonists** come in IV form.

Table 20–13 ▶ **Pharmacokinetics: Selected Antiemetics**

Drug	Onset	Peak	Duration	Protein Binding	Half-Life	Elimination
Dimenhydrinate						
PO	15–60 min	1–2 h	3–6 h	UK	UK	In feces via biliary excretion
PO ER	UK	UK	12 h	UK	UK	
IM	20–30 min	1–2 h	3–6 h	UK	UK	
PR	30–45 min	UK	6–12 h	UK	UK	
Diphenhydramine						
PO	15–60 min	1–4 h	4–8 h	98%–99%	2.4–7 h	In feces via biliary excretion
IM	20–30 min	1–4 h	4–8 h	98%–99%	2.4–7 h	
Hydroxyzine						
PO, IM	15–30 min	2–4 h	4–6 h	UK	3 h	In feces via biliary excretion
Meclizine	30–60 min	UK	4–24 h (dose dependent)	UK	6 h	UK
Prochlorperazine						
PO	30–40 min	UK	10–12 h	>90%	UK	Half in urine; half by enterohepatic circulation
PR	60 min	UK	3–4 h	>90%	UK	
IM	10–20 min	10–30 min	3–4 h	>90%	UK	
Promethazine						
PO	10 min	UK	4–12 h	65%–90%	UK	Half in urine; half by enterohepatic circulation
PR	20 min	UK	12 h	65%–90%	UK	
IM	20 min	UK	12 h	65%–90%	UK	
Trimethobenzamide						
PO	10–40 m	UK	3–4 h	UK	UK	In urine
PR	10–40 m	UK	3–4 h	UK	UK	
IM	15–35 m	UK	2–3 h	UK	UK	
Dronabinol						
PO	0.5-1 hr	2-4 hr	4-6 hr	97%	4 hr	Feces and urine
Dolasetron						
PO		1 hr			8 hr	Urine and feces
IV		0.6 hr			10 min	Urine and feces
Ondansetron		2 hr			3 hr	Urine and feces

ER = extended release; PR = per rectum; UK = unknown.

Prochlorperazine, promethazine, and **trimethobenzamide** have formulations for administration by the rectal route. The IM and rectal routes are commonly used when vomiting is present.

Distribution of **antihistamines** is not clearly known, but **phenothiazines** are widely distributed, cross the blood–brain barrier and placenta, and enter breast milk. As a result, they are associated with more adverse reactions.

Metabolism and Excretion

Dimenhydrinate, diphenhydramine, and **hydroxyzine** are extensively metabolized by the liver and eliminated in feces by biliary excretion. The **cannabinoid dronabinol** undergoes extensive first-pass hepatic metabolism and is eliminated as active and inactive metabolite in the feces and urine. The **5-HT$_3$ receptor antagonists** undergo extensive first-pass metabolism and are eliminated in the urine and feces. **Trimethobenzamide** is metabolized by the liver and is excreted in urine. The **phenothiazines** are metabolized by the liver into active compounds that persist for prolonged periods. They are eliminated half by the kidney in urine and half through enterohepatic circulation. The fetus, infants, and older adults have diminished capacity to metabolize and excrete **phenothiazines.**

Pharmacotherapeutics

Precautions and Contraindications

The drug class determines the precautions and contraindications. **Antihistamines** have **anticholinergic** properties and have precautions and contraindications similar to **anticholinergics.** Cautious use in narrow-angle glaucoma, seizure disorders, pyloric obstruction, hyperthyroidism, cardiovascular disease, and prostatic hypertrophy is in order. Because they are metabolized so extensively by the liver, they are contraindicated in severe liver disease. Cautious use is also suggested for older adults, and dosage reductions may be required.

Dimenhydrinate and **diphenhydramine** are Pregnancy Category B, and they are safe for use in children. **Meclizine** is also Pregnancy Category B. Safety and efficacy of **meclizine** has not been established in children less than 12 years or during lactation. **Hydroxyzine** is Pregnancy Category C, but has been used safely during labor. Safety in lactation and in children has not been established, but it has been used for both, and children's doses are published.

Phenothiazines produce extrapyramidal reactions and are contraindicated in Parkinson's disease. They are also contraindicated in narrow-angle glaucoma, bone marrow depression, and severe cardiovascular or hepatic disease because of their serious adverse reactions. Cautious use is suggested in respiratory impairment caused by acute pulmonary infection or chronic respiratory disorders, such as severe asthma or emphysema. "Silent pneumonia" may develop in these patients when they are treated with **phenothiazines.** Because these drugs suppress the cough reflex, aspiration of vomitus is possible, and they should be used cautiously where aspiration is a risk. Although all of these points are important to consider, they are less likely to be a problem in very short-term use as an **antiemetic.**

The **phenothiazines** are Pregnancy Category C. They have dosing schedules for children.

Dronabinol contains cannabinoid and sesame oil and should not be used by anyone sensitive to these ingredients. **Dronabinol** should be used with caution in patients with a history of seizure disorder because it may lower the seizure threshold. Patients with cardiac disorders should be monitored for hypotension, possible hypertension, syncope, or tachycardia.

The **5-HT$_3$ receptor antagonists** may mask progressive ileus. **Zofran ODT** disintegrating tablets contain aspartame and should be used with caution in patients with phenylketonuria.

Adverse Drug Reactions

The most common adverse reactions for **antihistamines** are drowsiness and the common **anticholinergic** effects of dry mouth, blurred vision, and urinary retention. Paradoxical excitation may occur in children. Pain at the injection site occurs in IM injections.

Phenothiazines produce drowsiness as well, but they also produce serious adverse reactions that sometimes occur even with short-term use and low doses. These reactions include extrapyramidal reactions such as dystonia, akathisia, and tardive dyskinesia. Other serious concerns are their ability to mask acute symptoms of surgical and neurological conditions and the potential for agranulocytosis 4 to 10 weeks after initiation of therapy.

Promethazine has been known to cause fatal respiratory depression in children younger than 2 years of age and has a black box warning regarding its use in children. In children older than age 2 years, the lowest effective dose should be used and coadministration of respiratory depressants should be avoided.

Other adverse reactions are associated with the **anticholinergic** effects of phenothiazines drugs and include dry mouth, dry eyes, blurred vision, constipation, and urinary retention. They also discolor urine pink to reddish brown, and patients should be told that this reaction does not indicate hematuria.

The **cannabinoid dronabinol** may cause euphoria, depression, dizziness, paranoid thoughts, somnolence, and abnormal thoughts. Cardiac effects include palpitations, tachycardia, and hypotension. Seizure and seizure-like activity have been reported in patients receiving **Marinol** capsules in postmarketing surveillance.

The **5-HT$_3$ receptor antagonists** have the common side effects of constipation, headache, fatigue, dizziness, and diarrhea. Less common but concerning are rare cases of tachycardia, bradycardia, hypotension, and QT prolongation.

Drug Interactions

Antihistamines and **phenothiazines** have additive CNS depression with other drugs that produce CNS depression and additive **anticholinergic** effects with other drugs that have **anticholinergic** effects or adverse reactions.

Phenothiazines also have additive hypotensive effects with **antihypertensive** agents or acute ingestion of **alcohol**. Concurrent administration of **lithium** increases the risk for extrapyramidal reactions, and **phenothiazines** may mask the signs of **lithium** toxicity. **Antithyroid agents** increase the risk for agranulocytosis.

The **cannabinoid dronabinol** interacts with other CNS depressants, causing additive CNS depression with **benzodiazepines, barbiturates, alcohol opioids, antihistamines, muscle relaxants,** and other **CNS depressants.** Dronabinol has been studied and administered with **cytotoxic agents, anti-infective agents, sedatives,** or **opioid analgesics** without significant adverse effects.

These and additional drug interactions are listed in Table 20–14.

Table 20–14 ■ **Drug Interactions: Selected Antiemetics**

Drug	Interacting Drug	Possible Effect	Implications
Dimenhydrinate, diphenhydramine, hydroxyzine, meclizine	Alcohol, other antihistamines, opioids, sedative hypnotics, other CNS depressants	Additive CNS depression	Avoid concurrent use or warn patient of drowsiness and its consequences
	Aminoglycosides, ethacrynic acid, other ototoxic drugs	May mask indications of ototoxicity of these drugs	Avoid concurrent use
	Tricyclic antidepressants (TCAs), monoamine oxidase inhibitors, quinidine, and other drugs with anticholinergic properties	Additive anticholinergic effects	Avoid concurrent use or provide patient education about ways to reduce or treat anticholinergic effects
	Azole antifungals	Plasma levels (including metabolites) may be increased	Choose different antiemetic
	Macrolide antibiotics	Plasma levels (including metabolites) may be increased	Choose different antiemetic
	Serotonin reuptake inhibitors	Plasma levels (including metabolites) may be increased	Choose different antiemetic
Prochlorperazine, promethazine	Antihypertensives, nitrates, and acute ingestion of alcohol	Additive hypotensive effects	Avoid concurrent administration or monitor blood pressure closely
	Alcohol, antihistamines, antidepressants, opioids, sedative hypnotics, and other CNS depressants	Additive CNS depression May increase TCA serum levels	Avoid concurrent administration or warn about drowsiness and its risks; select different antiemetic or antidepressant other than TCA
	Antihistamines, antidepressants, atropine, haloperidol, other phenothiazines, and other drugs with anticholinergic properties	Additive anticholinergic effects	Avoid concurrent use or provide patient education about ways to reduce or treat anticholinergic effects
	Lithium	Lithium increases risk of extrapyramidal symptom (EPS) reactions; prochlorperazine may mask indications of lithium toxicity	Avoid concurrent use

Table 20–14 ■ **Drug Interactions: Selected Antiemetics—cont'd**

Drug	Interacting Drug	Possible Effect	Implications
	Antithyroid agents	Increased risk for agranulocytosis	Choose different antiemetic
	Antacids	Concurrent administration may decrease absorption	Separate administration or give antiemetic by IM or rectal route
Trimethobenzamide	Alcohol, antihistamines, antidepressants, opioids, sedative hypnotics, and other CNS depressants	Additive CNS depression	Avoid concurrent use or warn patient of drowsiness and its consequences
Dronabinol	Alcohol, benzodiazepines, barbiturates, CNS depressants	Additive CNS depression	Write for smallest practical amount of dronabinol
	Tricyclic antidepressants (Amitriptyline, amoxapine, desipramine,)	Additive tachycardia, hypertension, drowsiness	Avoid concurrent administration if possible
	Theophylline	antagonizes	
Dolasetron	Drugs that prolong QT interval		
Ondansetron	Potent inducers of CYP3A4 (i.e., phenytoin, carbamazepine, and rifampicin)	Clearance of ondansetron was significantly increased and ondansetron blood concentrations were decreased	No dosage adjustment necessary
	Apomorphine	Increased apomorphine levels	Avoid concomitant use
	P-glycoprotein inhibitors	ondansetron levels increased	

Clinical Use and Dosing

The only clinical use presented here is to treat nausea and vomiting. Table 20–15 shows the dosing schedules for each of the drugs for this purpose. Other uses for these drugs are discussed in Chapter 15.

Rational Drug Selection

Treatment of Nausea and Vomiting Due to Drugs or Gastroenteritis

Nausea and vomiting as an adverse effect of medication or gastroenteritis often improve with treatment using an antiemetic. Because of their low side effect profile and tolerance, the **5-HT$_3$ receptor antagonists** are being used extensively to treat nausea and vomiting. The **phenothiazines** are also a good choice for initial and short-term treatment of nausea, except in children. **Trimethobenzamide** is also effective. The **antihistamines** can also be used and, because they have less serious adverse reactions, are better for longer-term applications. All are available in a variety of dosage forms so that they need not be taken orally by a patient who is nauseated. **Dronabinol** is approved only for use in **chemotherapy**-associated nausea and vomiting, and appetite stimulation.

Motion Sickness

Antihistamines are useful for this indication because they act on the vestibular system and the CTZ to help control the nausea and vomiting associated with vestibular dysfunction. They also provide rapid onset of action and have a prolonged effect. **Dimenhydrinate** and **meclizine** are the most commonly used. **Meclizine** is also used to treat vertigo. The **phenothiazines** are not effective for motion sickness or vestibular disease because their site of action does not involve the vestibular system.

Vomiting Due to Gastroparesis

For this indication, **prokinetic** drugs are best. They are discussed later in this chapter.

Monitoring

When **antiemetic** drugs are used for a single dose or very short term, no specific monitoring is required beyond that associated with the disease process and the potential fluid and electrolyte shifts that may result from vomiting. If treatment is needed for longer than a few days, the following monitoring parameters are suggested. **Promethazine** has been associated with bone marrow depression. A complete blood count (CBC) prior to initiation of therapy is

Table 20–15 ◉ **Dosage Schedule: Selected Antiemetics**

Drug	Indications	Dosage Schedule	Notes
Dimenhydrinate	Antiemetic	*Children >12 yr and adults:* 50 mg PO/IM or 25 mg ER capsules q4h; not to exceed 400 mg/d PR = 50–100 mg q6–8h	For motion sickness, give dose 1–2 h prior to departure or ER dose 12 h prior to departure
		Children 6–12 yr: 25–50 mg (PO/IM) q6–8h; not to exceed 150 mg/d	Use calibrated measuring device when giving liquid doses
		Children 8–12 yr: PR = 25–50 mg q8–12h	
		Children 6–8 yr: 12.5–25 PR q8–12h	
		Children 2–6 yr: Up to 12.5–25 mg q6–8 h; not to exceed 75 mg/d	
Diphenhydramine	Antiemetic	*Adults:* 25–50 mg q6h PO; 10–50 mg q2–3h IM; not to exceed 300 mg/d	For motion sickness, give dose 1–2 h prior to departure or ER dose 12 h prior to departure
		Children: >20 lb (9.1 kg): 12.5–25 mg 3–4 times daily (5 mg/kg) not to exceed 300 mg/d	
		Children: 1–1.5 mg/kg q4–6h PO; not to exceed 300 mg/d	Use calibrated measuring device when giving liquid doses.
		IM = 1.25 mg/kg qid; not to exceed 300 mg/d	Capsules may be emptied and contents taken with food or water
			Give IM into deep, well-developed muscle; avoid SC administration
Hydroxyzine	Antiemetic	*Children >12 yr and adults:* 25–100 mg PO/IM tid or qid	Tablets may be crushed and capsules opened and administered with food or fluid for patients with difficulty in swallowing
		Children 6–12 yr: 12.5–25 mg q6h *Children <6 yr:* 12.5 mg q6h (General calculation for children: 0.5 mg/kg q6h)	Give IM into deep, well-developed muscle using Z track. Do not use deltoid. Injection is painful. Rotate sites frequently. Avoid SC or IV administration
Meclizine	Motion sickness	Tablet: 25–50 mg	Take 1 h prior to travel. May repeat dose every 24 h for duration of journey
	Vertigo	Tablet: 25–100 mg daily in divided doses	
	Nausea and vomiting in pregnancy	Lowest dose that relieves nausea	Based on lowest risk of teratogenicity (see text)
Prochlorperazine	Antiemetic	*Children >12 yr and adults:* 5–10 mg PO/IM tid or qid; may also give 30 mg once daily or 10 mg bid of ER PR = 25 mg bid; not to exceed 40 mg/d *Children 18–39 kg:* 2.5 mg PO/PR tid or 5 mg bid; not to exceed 15 mg/d *Children 14–17 kg:* 2.5 mg PO/PR bid or tid; not to exceed 10 mg/d *Children 9–13 kg:* 2.5 mg PO/PR qd or bid; not to exceed 7.5 mg/d *Children 2–12 kg:* 132 mcg/kg IM in single dose	Do not crush or chew ER capsules. Administer with food or milk or a full glass of water to minimize GI distress. Dilute syrup in citrus or chocolate-flavored drinks Give IM into deep, well-developed muscle. Keep patient recumbent for at least 30 min following injection to avoid hypotensive effects

Table 20–15 ● **Dosage Schedule: Selected Antiemetics—cont'd**

Drug	Indications	Dosage Schedule	Notes
Promethazine	Antiemetic	*Adults:* 25 mg PO/IM/PR q4h *Children >2 yr:* 0.25–0.5 mg/kg q4–6h PO/IM/PR	For motion sickness, give dose 1–2 h prior to departure Administer with food, water, or milk to minimize GI distress. Tablets may be crushed and mixed with food or fluids for patients with difficulty in swallowing Use calibrated measuring device when giving liquid doses Give IM into deep, well-developed muscle; SC administration may cause tissue necrosis Do not administer to children <age 2 yr
Trimethobenzamide	Antiemetic	*Adults:* 250 mg PO tid/qid; IM/PR = 200 mg tid/qid *Children 15–45 kg:* 100–200 mg PO/PR tid/qid or 15 mg/kg/d in 3–4 divided doses *Children <15 kg:* 100 mg PR tid/qid	Capsules can be opened and contents mixed with food or fluid for patients with difficulty in swallowing. Inject deep into well-developed muscle to minimize tissue irritation.
Dronabinol	Refractory nausea and vomiting associated with cancer chemotherapy	*Adults and children:* 5 mg/m^2 1–3 h before chemotherapy. Then every 2–4 h after chemo. May increase as needed by increments of 2.5 mg/m^2 to a max of 15 mg/m^2	Individualize the dosing
Dolasetron	Prevention of nausea and vomiting after chemotherapy or surgery	*Children ≥16 yr and adults:* 100 mg within 1 hr before chemotherapy or 2 hr before surgery *Children 2 yr–16 yr:* 1.8 mg within 1 hr of chemotherapy or 1.2 mg within 2 hr before surgery	
Ondansetron	Prevention of nausea and vomiting associated with chemotherapy.	*Adults:* 24 mg administered 30 min before the start chemotherapy or 8 mg tid *Children 4–11 yr:* 4 mg tid	

ER = extended release; PR = per rectum.

appropriate. **Phenothiazines** have also been associated with blood dyscrasias that tend to occur between week 4 and week 10 of therapy. A CBC may be done prior to initiation and after 4 weeks of therapy.

Patient Education

Administration

These drugs should be taken as prescribed (Table 20–16). Each of them has special considerations related to administration, which are presented in Table 20–15. For all of the drugs used to treat motion sickness, take 1 to 2 hours prior to departure, except for extended-release **dimenhydrinate**, which is taken 12 hours before departure. For all liquid formulations, use a calibrated measuring device to attain an accurate dose. For all injections, administer deep into well-developed muscle, and avoid the deltoid and subcutaneous (SC) injections. For **hydroxyzine** also use a Z-track method of injection. All tablets except extended-release ones can be crushed or mixed with food, water, or milk to minimize GI distress and for patients who have difficulty with swallowing. Capsules can be opened and emptied to allow mixing for the same reasons.

Adverse Reactions

Single-dose or short-term use has relatively few adverse reactions. All are associated with drowsiness, dry mouth, dry eyes, constipation, and urinary retention. **Phenothiazines** turn the urine pink to reddish brown. Patients need to be told that this effect does not constitute hematuria.

Table 20–16 ◈ **Available Dosage Forms: Selected Antiemetics**

Drug	Dosage Form	How Supplied
Dimenhydrinate (Dramamine)	Tablets: 50 mg	In bottles of 12, 36, 100 scored tablets
	Chewable tablets: 50 mg	In bottles of 8, 24 scored tablets
	Injection: 50 mg/mL	In 1-mL ampules and 5-mL vials
	Liquid: 12.5 mg/4 mL	In 90 mL (cherry flavor); 5% alcohol
	Liquid: 15.62 mg/5 mL	In 480 mL
(Generic)	Tablets: 50 mg	In bottles of 12, 100, 300, 500, 1,000 tablets
	Injection: 50 mg/mL	In 1-mL ampules and 1-, 10-mL vials
	Liquid: 12.5/4 mL	In pint and gallon
Diphenhydramine (Benadryl)	Soft gels: 25 mg	In 24 capsules
	Tablets: 25 mg	In 24, 100 tablets
	Chewable tablets: 12.5 mg	In 24 tablets (grape-flavor); have phenylalanine
	Liquid: 6.25 mg	In 236 mL (dye-free); 118 mL (cherry flavor)
	Injection: 50 mg/mL	In 1-mL ampules, 10-mL vials, and 1-mL syringe
(Generic)	Soft gels: 25 mg	In 30, 100, 1000 capsules
	Capsules: 50 mg	In bottles of 100, 1,000 capsules
	Syrup: 12.5 mg/5 mL	In 118 mL
	Injection: 50 mg/mL	In 1-mL ampules and 10-mL vials
Hydroxyzine (Atarax)	Tablets: 10 mg, 25 mg, 50 mg	In bottles of 100, 500 tablets
	Tablets: 100 mg	In bottles of 100 tablets
	Syrup: 10 mg/5 mL	In pints
(Vistaril)	Capsules: 25 mg, 50 mg, 100 mg	In bottles of 100, 500 capsules
	Oral suspension: 25 mg/5 mL	In 120 mL and 473 mL (lemon-flavored)
	Injection: 25 mg/mL	In 10-mL vials
	Injection: 50 mg/mL	In 1-, 2-, 10-mL vials
(Generic)	Tablets: 10 mg, 25 mg, 50 mg	In bottles of 100, 250, 500, 1,000 tablets
	Capsules: 25 mg, 50 mg, 100 mg	In bottles of 100, 500, 1,000 capsules
	Syrup: 10 mg/5 mL	In 12.5 mL, 25 mL, and pints
	Injection: 25 mg/mL	In 1-mL and 10-mL vials
	Injection: 50 mg/mL	In 2-mL ampules, 1- and 2-mL syringes, and 1-, 2-, 10-mL vials
Meclizine (Antivert)	Tablets: 12.5 mg	In bottles of 30, 60, 100, 500, 1,000, and UD 100
	25 mg	In bottles of 12, 20, 30, 60, 100, 500, 1,000, and UD 32 and 100
	25 mg, chewable	In bottle of 20, 30, 60, 100, 1,000, and UD 100
	50 mg	In bottles of 100

Table 20–16 ◆ **Available Dosage Forms: Selected Antiemetics—cont'd**

Drug	Dosage Form	How Supplied
	Capsules: 25 mg	In bottles of 100
Prochlorperazine (Compazine)	Tablets: 5 mg, 10 mg, 25 mg	In bottles of 100, 1,000 tablets
	Spansules (SR): 10 mg, 15 mg, 30 mg	In bottles of 50, 500 SR capsules
	Syrup: 5 mg/5 mL	In 120 mL; fruit flavor
	Injection: 5 mg/mL	In 2-mL ampules, 10-mL vials, and 2-mL syringes
	Suppositories: 2.5 mg, 5 mg, 25 mg	In 12s; individually foil wrapped
(Generic)	Tablets: 5 mg, 10 mg, 25 mg	In bottles of 12, 30, 100, 1,000 tablets
	Injection: 5 mg/mL	In 2-mL ampules and 2-mL and 10-mL vials
Promethazine (Phenergan)	Tablets: 12.5 mg, 25 mg	In bottles of 100 scored tablets
	Tablets: 50 mg	In bottles of 100 tablets
	Syrup: 6.25 mg/5 mL	In 118 and 473 mL
	25 mg/5 ml	In 473 mL
	Suppositories: 12.5 mg, 25 mg, 50 mg	In 12s; individually foil wrapped
	Injection: 25 mg/mL, 50 mg/mL	In 1-mL ampules
(Generic)	Tablets: 12.5 mg	In bottles of 100 tablets
	Tablets: 25 mg, 50 mg	In bottles of 100, 1,000 tablets
	Syrup: 6.25 mg/5 mL	In 118 mL
	Suppositories: 50 mg	In 12s; individually foil wrapped
	Injection: 25 mg/mL, 50 mg/mL	In 1-mL ampules and 10-mL vials
Trimethobenzamide (Tigan)	Capsules: 100 mg	In bottles of 100 capsules
	Capsules: 250 mg	In bottles of 100, 500 capsules
	Pediatric suppositories: 100 mg	In 10 individually foil wrapped
	Suppositories: 200 mg	In 10, 50 individually foil wrapped
	Injection: 100 mg/mL	In 2-mL ampules, 20-mL vials, and 2-mL syringe
(Generic)	Capsules: 250 mg	In bottles of 100, 500 tablets
	Pediatric suppositories: 100 mg	In 10 individually foil wrapped
	Suppositories: 200 mg	In 10, 50 individually foil wrapped
	Injection: 100 mg/mL	In 2-mL ampules and 20-mL vials
Dronabinol	Capsules: 2.5 mg, 5 mg, 10 mg	60
Dolasetron	Tablets: 50 mg, 100 mg	5
Ondansetron	Tablets: 4 mg, 8 mg ODT (disintegrating tab): 4 mg ODT: 8 mg Oral solution 4 mg/5 ml	30 30 10, 30 50 ml

Longer-term administration of **phenothiazines** is not recommended because of potentially serious adverse reactions. Patients should be told the indications of dystonia, akathisia, and tardive dyskinesia and to stop the drug and report these immediately.

Phenergan should not be administered with other respiratory depressants in children.

Dronabinol (Marinol) may cause euphoria and behavior changes. Patients should not drive until they know how they will respond to the medication.

Lifestyle Management

Nausea and vomiting are often self-limiting disorders. Before drug therapy begins, unless there is clear indication of fluid or electrolyte disturbances, nonpharmacological interventions can be tried. Resting the GI tract for a brief time (8 hr) by taking only clear liquids in small amounts is often helpful. Clear liquids are those that can be held up to light and seen through. For infants, ORS (discussed in the **Antidiarrheals** section) such as **Pedialyte** may be used instead of other clear liquids. Formula and milk should be withheld for these 8 hours. For breastfed babies, continue breastfeeding, but nurse on only one side at each feeding during the first 8 hours. Older children and adults can take any clear liquid and require ORS only if they appear dehydrated. Remember, this treatment does not mean as much clear liquid as the patient can hold. Start with small amounts and gradually increase the intake.

After 8 hours without vomiting, start with bland food such as saltine crackers, honey on white bread, bland soup, rice, or mashed potatoes. For babies, start with applesauce, strained bananas, and rice cereal. If the baby takes only formula, give 1 or 2 oz less than usual with each feeding. Breast-fed babies can return to regular breastfeeding after 1 hour without vomiting. Most patients will be back on a regular diet within 24 hours.

EMETICS

Poisoning is a serious problem in the United States, despite extensive prevention programs. According to the American Association of Poison Control Centers, nearly 2 million poisoning cases are documented each year, and many more go unreported. In the past, vomiting to remove a poison was advised in some circumstances. However, problems occurred with use of **emetics** so that they are no longer recommended. Poisoning is now treated with antidotes or gastric lavage. For this reason, emetics are not discussed in this book.

HISTAMINE$_2$ RECEPTOR ANTAGONISTS

Histamine$_2$ blockers (also known as **histamine$_2$ antagonists** [H_2RAs]) inhibit acid secretion by gastric parietal cells through a reversible blockade of histamine at histamine$_2$ receptors. They are used to reduce gastric acid in patients who are temporarily not taking anything by mouth and for prophylaxis and management of duodenal and gastric ulcers and GERD. They are also used to treat heartburn, acid indigestion, and "sour stomach."

Pharmacodynamics

Gastric parietal cells have three receptors that can be stimulated to cause the parietal cell to produce H+: acetylcholine, gastrin, and histamine$_2$. H_2RAs are reversible competitive blockers of histamine at histamine$_2$ receptors. They are highly selective, do not affect histamine$_1$ receptors, and are not **anticholinergic** agents. They are potent inhibitors of all phases of gastric acid secretion, including that caused by **muscarinic agonists** and gastrin. Fasting and nocturnal secretions and those stimulated by food, **insulin**, **caffeine**, pentagastrin, and betazole are all inhibited. Because they do not inhibit **acetylcholine**, they reduce gastric acid secretion by only 35 to 50 percent.

The volume and hydrogen ion concentration of gastric juice, gastric emptying, and the lower esophageal sphincter pressure are all affected to varying degrees by different drugs in this class. **Cimetidine (Tagamet)**, **ranitidine (Zantac)**, and **famotidine (Pepcid)** have no effect on gastric emptying. **Cimetidine** and **famotidine** have no effect on lower esophageal sphincter pressure. **Ranitidine**, **nizatidine (Axid)**, and **famotidine** have little or no effect on fasting or postprandial serum gastrin. **Ranitidine** does not affect pepsin secretion or pentagastrin-stimulated intrinsic factor secretion.

Ranitidine is 5 to 12 times more potent and **famotidine** is 30 to 60 times more potent than **cimetidine** in controlling gastric acid secretion, but there is no clear evidence that greater potency has any clinical advantage. Treatment failures have occurred with each of these drugs, and it is doubtful that treatment failure with one drug in the class can be corrected by changing drugs within the class.

Pharmacokinetics

Absorption and Distribution

All drugs in the class are well absorbed following oral administration (Table 20–17). The absorption of **cimetidine**, **famotidine**, and **ranitidine** may be decreased by **antacids** but is unaffected by food. The absorption of **nizatidine** is decreased by 10 percent by **aluminum and magnesium hydroxides.** With food, AUC and maximum concentration of **nizatidine** increases by 10 percent. **Cimetidine** and **ranitidine** also have IM routes of absorption. All agents enter breast milk and cerebrospinal fluid.

Metabolism and Excretion

All agents are metabolized to differing degrees by the CYP450 enzyme system of the liver and excreted in differing percentages as unchanged drug in the urine.

Table 20–17 ▶ **Pharmacokinetics: Histamine$_2$ Blockers**

Drug	Onset	Peak	Duration	Protein Binding	Bio- availability	Half-Life	Metabolized	Elimination
Cimetidine	30 min	45–90 min	4–5 h	13%–25%	60%–70%	2 h	30%–40%	48% unchanged in urine
Famotidine	60 min	1–4 h	1–4 h	15%–20%	40%–45%	2.5–3.5 h	30%–35%	25%–30% unchanged in urine
Nizatidine	60 min	0.5–3 h	UK	35%	>90%	1–2 h	<18%	60% unchanged in urine, <6% in feces
Ranitidine	60 min	1–3 h	1–3 h	15%	50%–60%	2–3 h	<10%	30%–35% unchanged in urine

UK = unknown.

Nizatidine has at least one metabolite that has histamine-blocking activity. All others are metabolized to inactive compounds.

Pharmacotherapeutics

Precautions and Contraindications

Renal impairment requires cautious use of the H$_2$RAs and dosage adjustments. Patients with renal impairment are more subject to the CNS adverse reactions. Older adults may have reduced renal function, and these drugs should be used cautiously with this age group. **Cimetidine** seems to have the most problems with decreased renal clearance, and **ranitidine** the fewest.

Hepatocellular injury may occur with **nizatidine**, as evidenced by elevated liver enzymes (Alanine transaminase [ALT], aspartate aminotransferase [AST], or alkaline phosphatase). These abnormalities are reversible with discontinuation of the drug. Because of this risk, it should not be used for patients with a history of liver disease.

Occasional reversible hepatitis or hepatocellular disorders have occurred with **ranitidine.** It is contraindicated for patients with a history of liver disease.

H$_2$RAs are Pregnancy Category B; however, there are no adequate and well-controlled studies of these agents in pregnant women. They should be used only when the potential benefits outweigh the potential risks to the fetus.

These drugs vary in their excretion in breast milk. **Cimetidine** is excreted in breast milk in milk:plasma ratios of 5:1 to 12:1. Potential daily dose to the infant is 6 mg. Do not nurse. **Famotidine** is excreted in the breast milk of rats. It is not known whether it is excreted in human breast milk. The decision to discontinue the drug is made based on the need of the mother for the drug. **Nizatidine** is excreted in breast milk in a concentration of 0.1 percent of the oral dose in proportion to plasma concentrations. Once again, the decision to discontinue the drug is made based on the need of the mother for the drug. **Ranitidine** is excreted in breast milk with milk:plasma ratios of 1:1 to 6.7:1. Exercise caution when giving to nursing mother.

There has been extensive study of the H$_2$RAs in the past few years as a part of the Best Pharmaceuticals for Children Act. Safety and efficacy of **ranitidine** have been established in children age 1 month to 16 years. **Famotidine** is labeled safe for infants and children as young as neonates, although children younger than one year have experienced agitation that stopped when **famotidine** was stopped (U.S. Food and Drug Administration, 2010).

Adverse Drug Reactions

All of these drugs have similar adverse reaction profiles. **Cimetidine** appears to have the greatest degree of antiandrogenic reactions (e.g., gynecomastia and impotence). Reversible CNS (e.g., mental confusion, agitation, psychosis, depression, and disorientation) adverse reactions have also occurred with this drug.

Hematological adverse reactions include agranulocytosis, granulocytopenia, thrombocytopenia, and aplastic anemia. These reactions are rare but should be monitored. Other less common adverse drug reactions include drowsiness, dizziness, constipation or diarrhea, and nausea. Adverse drug reactions related to liver function are discussed in the Precautions and Contraindications section.

Drug Interactions

Many of the drug interactions with this class of drugs are related to their metabolism by the CYPP450 enzyme system of the liver. **Cimetidine** is the most problematic because it uses several isoenzymes (CYP1A2, CYP2C9, and CYP2D6). Any drug metabolized extensively by these isoenzymes will have its metabolism inhibited by **cimetidine**, with a risk for increased plasma levels and toxicity for that drug. **Famotidine, nizatidine,** and **ranitidine** have less effect on the CYP system and use a narrower number of isoenzymes in their metabolism. Although they still have drug interactions, they are fewer than with **cimetidine.** Table 20–18 provides

Table 20–18 ▣ **Drug Interactions: Histamine$_2$ Blockers**

Drug	Interacting Drug	Possible Effect	Implications
Cimetidine	Benzodiazepines, caffeine, calcium channel blockers, carbamazepine, labetalol, metoprolol, metronidazole, pentoxifylline, propafenone, propranolol, quinidine, quinine, sulfonylureas, tacrine, theophylline, triamterene, tricyclic antidepressants, valproic acid, warfarin*	Decreased hepatic metabolism of these drugs	Select different histamine$_2$ blocker Monitor drug levels of those with narrow therapeutic range or potential for cardiac rhythm disturbances
	Ferrous salts, indomethacin, ketoconazole, tetracyclines	Action of these drugs decreased because of decreased absorption	Avoid concurrent administration; separate doses or select different histamine$_2$ blocker
	Digoxin	Decreased serum digoxin concentrations during co-administration	Select different histamine$_2$ blocker
	Flecainide	Increased drug effects of flecainide	Select different histamine$_2$ blocker
	Narcotic analgesics	Toxic effects (e.g., respiratory depression) may be increased	Select different histamine$_2$ blocker
	Procainamide	Increased plasma levels of procainamide and its cardioactive metabolite by decreasing renal tubular secretion	Select different histamine$_2$ blocker; ranitidine was shown to have similar action in only one study, so best not to choose that drug
	Tocainide	Decreased drug effects of tocainide	Select different histamine$_2$ blocker
	Cigarette smoking	Smoking reverses cimetidine-induced inhibition of nocturnal gastric secretion, hindering ulcer healing	Avoid cigarette smoking
Famotidine	Ketoconazole	Action of drug decreased by reduced absorption	Separate administration by at least 1 h and give ketoconazole first
	Food	May increase bioavailability of famotidine	No clinical significance
Nizatidine	Salicylates	Increased serum salicylate levels when given to patients receiving high doses (3.9 g/d) of salicylate	Monitor salicylate levels or select different histamine$_2$ blocker
	Food	May increase bioavailability of nizatidine	No clinical significance
Ranitidine	Diazepam	Decreased drug effects of diazepam due to decreased drug absorption	Separate doses by at least 1 h and give diazepam first
	Sulfonylureas	Increased hypoglycemic effects of glipizide or glyburide	Dosage adjustments may be needed
	Warfarin	May interfere with warfarin clearance; data conflicting	Monitor PT/INR more closely; may need dosage adjustment
All histamine$_2$ blockers	Alcohol	May increase blood alcohol levels	Avoid use of alcohol
	Antacids, anticholinergics, metoclopramide	May decrease absorption of cimetidine, ranitidine; less effect on nizatidine and famotidine	Separate dose by at least 1 h for cimetidine and ranitidine; no special precautions needed for nizatidine and famotidine

INR = international normalized ratio; PT = prothrombin time.
*Although interactions with these drugs are not listed for other histamine$_2$ blockers, some effect is probable, even though it is not to the same extent.

a list of drug interactions for the various **histamine$_2$ blockers**.

Clinical Use and Dosing

Gastroesophageal Reflux Disease

GERD in adults is treated with stepped therapy. Current guidelines recommend choosing between two different approaches to treatment (Institute for Clinical Systems Improvement [ICSI], 2006). In both approaches, lifestyle modifications occur throughout the treatment. In step-up guidelines, **histamine$_2$ blockers** are added to **antacid** therapy or used to replace high-dose **antacid** therapy, providing better symptom relief and increasing esophageal healing to about 50 percent. Standard dosing is shown in Table 20–19. If no esophageal erosive disease is present, twice-daily dosing is effective. Once-daily dosing of H_2RAs is not effective in treating GERD.

In the step-down approach, patients are started on PPIs and once the patient is symptom free for 4 weeks, he or she steps down to a lower PPI dose or switches to a H_2RA. Chapter 34 discusses management of GERD by both approaches and provides an algorithm for each. Because these drugs are now available OTC, many patients may have used these drugs as self-tried therapy before seeking care. It is important to seek this information in the initial history.

Table 20–19 ● **Dosage Schedule: Histamine$_2$ Blockers**

Drug	Indication	Initial Dose	Maintenance Dose
Cimetidine	Short-term treatment of active duodenal ulcer	*Adults:* 800 mg at bedtime or 300 mg qid with meals and at bedtime or 400 mg bid	*Adults:* 400 mg at bedtime; dosage not to exceed 2.4 g/d. In severe renal impairment, use 300 mg every 8–12 h
		Children: 20–40 mg/kg/d in 4 divided doses	*Children:* 20 mg/kg/d; 10–15 mg/kg/d in renal impairment
	Duodenal ulcer prophylaxis	*Adults:* 300 mg bid or 400 mg at bedtime	Same
	Treatment of active benign gastric ulcer	*Adults:* 800 mg at bedtime or 300 mg qid with meals and at bedtime	800 mg at bedtime. In severe renal impairment, use 300 mg every 8–12 h. No information concerning usefulness of treatment periods >8 wk
	GERD	*Adults:* 800 mg bid in morning and at bedtime or 400 mg qid with meals and at bedtime	*Adults:* Same dose for up to 12 wk. Use >12 wk has not been established. May go as high as 600 mg qid if needed. In severe renal impairment, use 300 mg every 8–12 h
		Children: 20–40 mg/kg/d in 4 divided doses	
	Pathological hypersecretory conditions	*Adults:* 300 mg qid with meals and at bedtime	*Children:* 20 mg/kg/d; 10–15 mg/kg/d if renal impairment Individualize dose. Do not exceed 2,400 mg/d. Continue as long as clinically indicated
	Heartburn, indigestion, sour stomach	*Adults:* 200 mg (OTC) with water as symptoms occur	Take up to 400 mg bid. Do not take maximum dose for more than 2 wk without consulting health care provider
Famotidine	Short-term treatment of active duodenal ulcer	*Adults:* 40 mg/d at bedtime or ≤20 mg bid (in morning and at bedtime)	*Adults:* 20 mg at bedtime for up to 8 wk. Most heal in 4 wk. If CCr <10 mL/min, give 20 mg at bedtime or increase dosing interval to 36–48 h
		Children: 1–2 mg/kg/d in 1 or 2 divided doses	*Children:* Same dose for up to 8 wk Most heal in 4 wk
	Duodenal ulcer prophylaxis	*Adults:* 20 mg at bedtime	Same
	Treatment of benign active gastric ulcer	*Adults:* 40 mg at bedtime	Same dose. If CCr < 10 mL/min, give 20 mg at bedtime or increase dosing interval to 36–48 h. No data to support treatment beyond 8 wk
	GERD	*Adults:* 20 mg bid (in morning and at bedtime)	*Adults:* 20 mg for up to 6 wk. If erosive disease, 20–40 mg bid for up to 12 wk
		Children: 1–2 mg/kg/d in 1 or 2 divided doses	*Children:* Same dose. Treatment trial for 2–4 wk
	Heartburn, acid indigestion, and sour stomach	*Adults:* Relief: 10 mg (1 tablet) with water Prophylaxis: 10 mg 1 h prior to meal that is expected to cause symptoms	Can be used up to bid for <2 wk

Continued

Table 20–19 ● **Dosage Schedule: Histamine$_2$ Blockers—cont'd**

Drug	Indication	Initial Dose	Maintenance Dose
Nizatidine	Short-term treatment of active duodenal ulcer	*Adults:* 300 mg at bedtime or 150 mg bid (in morning and at bedtime)	300 mg at bedtime. If CCr 20–50 mL/min, give 150 mg at bedtime. If CCr < 20 mL/min, give 150 mg every 2 or 3 d
	Maintenance of healed duodenal ulcer	*Adults:* 150 mg at bedtime	150 mg at bedtime
	GERD	*Adults:* 150 mg bid (in morning and at bedtime)	150 mg bid
Ranitidine	Short-term treatment of active duodenal ulcer	*Adults:* 100–150 mg bid (in morning and at bedtime) or 300 mg at bedtime	150 mg at bedtime. If CCr <50 mL/min, give 150 mg at bedtime
	Duodenal ulcer prophylaxis	*Adults:* 150 mg at bedtime	150 mg at bedtime
	Treatment of benign active gastric ulcer	*Adults:* 150 mg bid (in morning and at bedtime)	150 mg at bedtime
	GERD	*Adults:* 150 mg bid (in morning and at bedtime); if erosive disease, give 150 mg qid	*Adults:* 150 mg bid. If CCr <50 mL/min, give 150 mg at bedtime. If erosive disease, give 150 mg bid.
		Children: 2–4 mg/kg/d in two divided doses	*Children:* 2 mg/kg/d in 2 divided doses
	Pathologic hypersecretory conditions	*Adults:* 150 mg bid (in morning and at bedtime)	Individualize dose; doses up to 6 g/d have been used
	Heartburn, acid indigestion, and sour stomach	*Adults:* Relief: 75 mg up to bid	Can be used up to bid for <2 wk

GERD = gastroesophageal reflux disease.
For all children <12 years of age, consultation with pediatric specialist is advised.

Infants and children with GERD have also been successfully treated with **histamine$_2$ blockers** for several years with good response and few adverse reactions (Stansbury, 2004). The North American Society for Pediatric Gastroenterology, Hepatology, and Nutrition (NASPGHAN) and European Society for Pediatric Gastroenterology, Hepatology, and Nutrition (ESPGHAN) international consensus on the diagnosis and management of gastroesophageal reflux (GER) and GERD no longer recommends empiric treatment with **H$_2$RAs** in infants (Vandenplas et al, 2009).

Dosing of **histamine$_2$ blockers** for infants and children is shown in Table 20–19. Once again, twice-daily dosing is required.

A more detailed discussion of the management of GERD is found in Chapter 34.

Peptic Ulcer Disease

With the advent of the discovery that the cause of PUD is usually an infection rather than excessive acid due to stress, diet, smoking, **alcohol** consumption, and **NSAIDs**, the treatment pattern has changed. Most patients will have tried an OTC H$_2$RA before they present with peptic ulcer symptoms. There is no treatment protocol that includes **histamine$_2$ blockers** when eradication of *H. pylori* as the source of the ulcer is required. Continued acid suppression may be accomplished with H$_2$RAs after the peptic ulcer has healed. A more detailed discussion of the management of PUD is found in Chapter 34.

Heartburn, Acid Indigestion, and "Sour Stomach"

Relief of symptoms may be provided by OTC use of **H$_2$RAs**. However, it is important for patients to be informed about the potential for drug interactions.

All Uses

Regardless of the reason for which the H$_2$RA is prescribed, consideration of renal function is important in determining dosage. In the presence of renal impairment, dosage intervals need to be increased. For **cimetidine**, the interval is increased if the renal impairment is severe; for **famotidine**, if creatinine clearance (CCr) is less than 10 mL/min; and for **nizatidine** and **ranitidine**, if CCr is less than 50 mL/min.

Rational Drug Selection

No specific H$_2$RA is preferred over another for effectiveness. Choice is based on cost and whether the patient is taking other drugs that might have interactions with the specific H$_2$RA.

Cost

Generic formulations are always less expensive than brand names. OTC drugs are usually less expensive than prescriptions, but because their dose is lower, the cost difference is lost in the increased number of pills required.

Other Drugs

Cimetidine has the most drug interaction potential. Other **histamine$_2$ blockers** have fewer listed drug interactions.

Monitoring

Because of the potential for hepatocellular damage, patients who require higher doses or more than short-term use of this class of drugs should have laboratory testing of liver function prior to initiation of therapy and at regular intervals throughout therapy.

Renal impairment influences drug dosing for all drugs in this class. Patients who require higher doses or more than short-term therapy or for whom renal impairment is a likely risk (e.g., older adults) should have renal function assessment done prior to initiation of therapy.

Patient Education

Administration

Instruct patients to take the drug as prescribed for the full course of therapy, even if they are feeling better. If a dose is missed, it should be taken as soon as remembered but not if it is almost time for the next dose. Do not double doses.

H_2RA should be taken with meals or immediately afterward and at bedtime to achieve the best effects. Doses taken once daily are best taken at bedtime. Oral suspensions are shaken prior to administration, and unused portions are discarded after 30 days. The foil is removed from **ranitidine** effervescent tablets or granules, and they are dissolved in 6 to 8 oz of water before they are taken. The available dosage forms of H_2RAs are found in Table 20–20.

If the patient is also taking antacids or other drugs whose interaction with H_2RA produces interference with absorption, the drugs' administration should be separated by at least 30 minutes to 1 hour. **Sucralfate** should be taken 2 hours after the H_2RA.

Patients taking OTC preparations are not to take the maximum doses continuously for more than 2 weeks without consulting their health-care provider. A diagnostic work-up is in order under these circumstances.

Adverse Reactions

H_2RA may cause drowsiness or dizziness. Caution patients to avoid driving or other activities requiring alertness until their response to the drug is known.

For male patients taking **cimetidine**, warn about the potential for gynecomastia and impotence. Because other

Table 20–20 ◆ **Available Dosage Forms: Histamine$_2$ Receptor Antagonists**

Drug	Dosage Form	How Supplied
Cimetidine (Tagamet)	Tablets: 100 mg Tablets: 200 mg, 300 mg Tablets: 400 mg Tablets: 800 mg Liquid: 300 mg/5 mL Injection: 300 mg/2 mL	In bottles of 16, 32, 64 tablets In bottles of 100 tablets In bottles of 60 tablets In bottles of 30 tablets In 240 mL (mint-peach flavor) In single-dose vials, disposable syringes, and 8-mL multiple-dose vials
(Generic)	Tablets: 200 mg, 300 mg, 400 mg, 800 mg Liquid: 300 mg/5 mL Injection: 300 mg/2 mL	In bottles of 100, 500, 1,000 tablets In 240 mL and 470 mL (mint-peach flavor) In 2-mL and 8-mL vials
Famotidine (Pepcid)	Tablets: 10 mg Tablets: 20 mg, 40 mg Powder for oral suspension: 40 mg/5 mL when reconstituted Injection: 10 mg/mL	In packets of 12 tablets In bottles of 30, 90, 100 tablets In bottles of 400 mg (cherry-banana-mint flavor) In 2-mL single-dose and 4-mL multidose vials
Nizatidine (Axid)	Capsule: 150 mg Capsule: 300 mg	In bottles of 60 capsules In bottles of 30 capsules
Ranitidine (Zantac)	Tablets: 150 mg Tablets: 300 mg Effervescent tablets: 150 mg Geldose: capsules: 150 mg Syrup: 15 mg/mL Efferdose: granules: 150 mg Injection: 25 mg/mL	In bottles of 60, 500 tablets In bottles of 30, 250 tablets In bottles of 30, 60 tablets In bottles of 30 capsules In 480 mL In 1.44-g packets In 2-mL, 10-mL, and 40-mL vials and 2-mL syringes
(Generic)	Syrup: 15 mg/mL	In 10 mL

drugs in the class are less likely to cause these problems, a different drug may be selected.

Advise patients to report the onset of black, tarry stools. They are not adverse reactions to the drug but may indicate GI bleeding. Sore throat, diarrhea, rash, confusion, or hallucinations should also be reported promptly. These adverse reactions may require dosage alteration or discontinuation of the drug. Increasing the fluid and fiber in the diet may minimize constipation.

Lifestyle Management

Smoking interferes with the absorption of H_2RA and increases gastric acid secretion. Advise the patient to stop smoking. **Alcohol** and products containing **aspirin** or **NSAIDs** and some foods may also increase gastric acid secretion; they should be avoided. Other lifestyle modifications are discussed in Chapter 34.

PROKINETICS

Prokinetic drugs, also known as gastrointestinal stimulants, stimulate the motility of the GI tract without stimulating gastric, biliary, or pancreatic secretions. These drugs are used in the management of a wide range of disorders in which reduced GI motility is a problem, including gastroparesis associated with diabetes mellitus, GERD, and emesis associated with cancer chemotherapy. Only one drug remains in this class since the removal of **cisapride (Propulsid)** from the market in 2004, **metoclopramide** (Reglan), which will be discussed in this section.

Pharmacodynamics

Metoclopramide stimulates motility in the upper GI tract. Its mode of action is unclear but appears to be related to sensitizing tissues to the action of acetylcholine. The action does not depend on an intact vagal innervation system, but **anticholinergic** drugs can reverse the action. This drug increases the tone and amplitude of gastric contractions, relaxes the pyloric sphincter and duodenal bulb, and increases peristalsis of the duodenum and jejunum, resulting in accelerated gastric emptying and increased speed of gastric transit. It has almost no effect on the colon or gallbladder. For patients with GERD secondary to decreased lower esophageal sphincter pressure (LESP), **metoclopramide** produces dose-related increases in LESP. These effects begin at doses as low as 5 mg and continue through 20-mg doses.

This drug also has some actions similar to the **phenothiazines** and **dopamine antagonists** and produces sedation and, rarely, extrapyramidal symptoms (EPS). It also induces release of prolactin and transiently increases circulating aldosterone levels. As mentioned in the **Antiemetics** section, it also has **antiemetic** properties as a result of its antagonism of central and peripheral dopamine receptors. Dopamine produces vomiting by stimulation of the CTZ, and **metoclopramide** blocks this stimulation.

Pharmacokinetics

Absorption and Distribution

Metoclopramide is well absorbed after oral administration (Table 20–21) and has an injectable formulation. It has low protein binding and high bioavailability.

Metoclopramide is widely distributed throughout body tissues, crosses the blood–brain barrier and the placenta and enters breast milk in concentrations greater than in plasma.

Metabolism and Excretion

Metoclopramide is partially metabolized by the liver. Because it is excreted in urine, clearance is affected by renal function. In patients whose creatinine clearance is less than 40 mL/min, the recommended dose is cut in half.

Pharmacotherapeutics

Precautions and Contraindications

Metoclopramide has a black box warning because of the risk of developing tardive dyskinesia. The risk for tardive dyskinesia increases with longer length of treatment. **Metoclopramide** should be discontinued if patients develop signs of movement disorder. Treatment should not exceed 12 weeks, except in rare cases.

Metoclopramide is contraindicated in the presence of disorders in which stimulation of GI motility might be dangerous (GI hemorrhage, mechanical obstruction, new surgery on the GI tract, or perforation). Its dopamine-associated activity affects the CNS, and the drug is used cautiously with patients who have a history of depression. Depression with symptoms ranging from mild to severe, including suicide ideation, have been reported. Patients

Table 20–21 ▶ **Pharmacokinetics: Prokinetic Agents**

	Onset	Peak	Duration	Protein Binding	Bioavailability	Half-Life	Elimination
Metoclopramide PO IM	30–60 m 10–15 m	1–2 h 1–2 h	1–2 h 1–2 h	30% 30%	65%–95% 65%–95%	2.5–5 h 2.5–5 h	85% in urine after 72 h (25% as unchanged drug); clearance affected by renal function

who are at risk for EPS also require cautious use of this drug.

Because **metoclopramide** is excreted primarily through the kidneys, it should be used with caution for patients with renal impairment. Dosage adjustments are mentioned above. It undergoes minimal hepatic metabolism and is safe to administer to patients with impaired hepatic function as long as their renal function is normal.

Metoclopramide is Pregnancy Category B; however, there are no adequate and well-controlled studies in pregnant women. Case reports to date have not been associated with fetal harm, but the drug should be prescribed only when the benefits clearly outweigh the risks to the fetus.

Metoclopramide is excreted in breast milk and concentrates at about twice the plasma level at 2 hours after taking the dose. However, in a mother taking 30 mg/day, the infant would receive less than 45 mg/day, which is still much less than the recommended maximum dose for infants. Exercise caution when giving to a nursing mother, but recognize that there appears to be little, if any, risk to the infant.

Infants and children aged 21 days to 3.3 years with symptomatic GERD have been treated with **metoclopramide** at a daily dosage of 0.5 mg/kg without difficulty. Stansbury (2004) recommends a dose of 0.3 mg/kg/day. She also recommends that the drug not be given to children with a seizure disorder, based on its activity in the CNS.

Adverse Drug Reactions

The most serious adverse reaction, the development of tardive dyskinesia, is discussed above. Other adverse reactions associated with **metoclopramide** include depression, dizziness, diarrhea, and hypoglycemia in patients with diabetes. Less common adverse reactions include galactorrhea, amenorrhea, gynecomastia, impotence secondary to hyperprolactinemia, and fluid retention secondary to transient elevations in **aldosterone.** Approximately 20 to 30 percent of all patients taking this drug experience some adverse reaction. The incidence correlates with the dose and duration of therapy.

Drug Interactions

Drug interactions with **metoclopramide** are largely related to its cholinergic and dopaminergic activities. Additive CNS depression occurs with other **CNS depressants,** and increased risk of EPS occurs with other drugs that have the potential for EPS. Drugs with **anticholinergic** effects reverse the action of metoclopramide, and the reverse is also true. There is a potential for hypertensive crisis if administered with **MAOIs.**

Table 20–22 provides a more detailed list of these drug interactions.

Clinical Use and Dosing

Gastroesophageal Reflux Disease

The principal effect of **metoclopramide** in the management of GERD is on symptoms of postprandial and daytime heartburn. For adults, if symptoms occur throughout the day, 10 mg taken 30 minutes prior to each meal and at bedtime is recommended (Table 20–23). When symptoms are confined to specific situations such as after

Table 20–22 ■ **Drug Interactions: Prokinetic Agents**

Drug	Interacting Drug	Possible Effect	Implications
Metoclopramide	Alcohol, antidepressants, antihistamines, opioids, and sedative hypnotics	Additive CNS depression; increases rate of absorption of alcohol	Avoid concurrent use or warn of potential CNS depression
	Haloperidol, phenothiazines, other drugs with EPS effects	Increased risk of extrapyramidal reactions	Avoid concurrent use; select different prokinetic
	Anticholinergics and opioids	Effects of metoclopramide on GI motility may antagonize these drugs	If not used therapeutically, avoid concurrent use
	Cimetidine	Reduced bioavailability of cimetidine	Select different histamine$_2$ blocker
	Digoxin	Decreased absorption, plasma levels, and therapeutic effects	Capsules, elixir, and tablets with high dissolution rate are least affected; use these formulations if both drugs must be given
	Levodopa	These drugs have opposite effects on dopamine receptors: bioavailability of levodopa increased; effects of metoclopramide decreased	Avoid concurrent use; metoclopramide is relatively contraindicated for patients with Parkinson's disease
	Monoamine oxidase inhibitors (MAOIs)	Metoclopramide releases catecholamines that may produce hypertension in patients taking MAOIs	Use cautiously concurrently, if at all; monitor blood pressure closely

Table 20–23 ◉ **Dosage Schedule: Prokinetic Agents**

Drug	Indication	Dosage Schedule	Notes
Metoclopramide	GERD	*Adults:* Treatment: 10–15 mg qid (30 min before meals and at bedtime) Prophylaxis: 20 mg at bedtime	Some patients respond to doses as low as 5 mg. Dose not to exceed 0.5 mg/kg/d. Therapy not to exceed 8 wk. Patients with CCr <40 mL/min, initiate therapy with half the recommended dose.
	Diabetic gastroparesis	*Adults:* 10 mg qid (30 min before meals and at bedtime) *Children:* 0.4–0.8 mg/kg/d in 4 divided doses (30 min before meals and at bedtime)	

GERD = gastroesophageal reflux disease.

the evening meal, a single 10- to 20-mg dose 30 minutes prior to that meal or at bedtime is effective in preventing the symptoms.

Occasionally, patients who are more sensitive to the therapeutic dose (e.g., older adults) require only 5 mg per dose. Children require daily doses at 0.3 mg/kg in three divided doses (30 min prior to each meal). For patients whose CCr is less than 40 mL/min, doses are reduced (see above).

Diabetic Gastroparesis

Metoclopramide has an indication for treatment of diabetic gastroparesis. Dosage is 10 mg 30 minutes before meals and at bedtime for 2 to 8 weeks. The route of administration is based on the severity of symptoms. If only the earliest manifestation of gastroparesis is present, oral administration is adequate. If the symptoms are more severe, parenteral therapy with 10 mg IV over 1 to 2 minutes for up to 10 days may be needed before oral therapy can be initiated. Rectal formulations can be made by a pharmacist to avoid the IV route. The suppositories each contain 25 mg of **metoclopramide** in polyethylene glycol. One suppository is administered 30 to 60 minutes before each meal and at bedtime. After symptoms are resolved (no more than 8 wk of therapy), the drug is stopped and reinstituted at the earliest indications of symptom return.

Diabetics often experience renal impairment. Because **metoclopramide** is excreted principally by the kidney, those patients with CCr below 40 mL/min should have their therapy initiated at approximately half the recommended dosage. Depending on clinical efficacy and safety considerations, the dosage may be increased or decreased as appropriate.

Rational Drug Selection

Efficacy

Metoclopramide has demonstrated limited symptomatic improvement and endoscopically demonstrated esophageal healing for patients with GERD. Given its significantly higher cost, however, it is difficult to justify its use in place of H_2RAs or PPIs.

Length of Therapy

Metoclopramide is not used for management of GERD if treatment must be long term. With longer than 8 weeks of therapy, there is a much higher risk for adverse reactions, including EPS.

Concomitant Diseases

Metoclopramide should be used cautiously for patients with diseases that place them at risk for EPS disorders or for patients taking drugs that place them at risk for these disorders. Other considerations based on concomitant disorders are discussed in the Precautions and Contraindications section.

Monitoring

Because of the need to adjust dosage in the presence of renal impairment, renal function should be assessed before therapy with **metoclopramide** is begun. No other monitoring is required except that for the disease process being treated.

Patient Education

Administration

Advise the patient to take the drug exactly as prescribed (Table 20–24). **Metoclopramide** is taken 30 minutes before each meal and at bedtime. If a dose is missed, it should be taken as soon as the patient remembers unless it is almost time for the next dose. Do not double doses or exceed the recommended dose.

Adverse Reactions

Metoclopramide may cause drowsiness. Caution patients to avoid driving or other activities that require alertness until their response to the drug is known. Concurrent use of other **CNS depressants**, including **alcohol**, makes this problem worse and causes additive CNS depression.

Warn patients taking **metoclopramide** to notify their health-care provider immediately if involuntary movement of the eyes, face, or limbs occurs, which may be EPS related.

Table 20–24 ◆ **Available Dosage Forms: Prokinetic Agents**

Drug	Dosage Form	How Supplied
Metoclopramide (Reglan)	Tablets: 5 mg Tablets: 10 mg Syrup: 5 mg/5 mL Injection: 5 mg/mL	In bottles of 100 tablets In bottles of 100 scored tablets In 480 mL and unit dose 10 mL In 2-, 10-mL ampules and 2-, 10-, 30-mL vials
(Generic)	Tablets: 5 mg Tablets: 10 mg Syrup: 5 mg/5 mL Injections: 5 mg/mL	In bottles of 100, 500, 1,000 tablets In bottles of 100, 500, 1,000, 2,500 tablets In 480 mL and unit dose 10 mL In 2-mL ampules and 2-, 10-, 20-, 30-mL vials

Lifestyle Management

Lifestyle modifications are tried before any drug in the management of both GERD and diabetic gastroparesis. First, patients should try to avoid **alcohol**, **NSAIDs**, large meals, fatty foods, chocolate, **caffeine**, citrus, and food or fluid intake within 3 hours of going to bed at night. They should also attempt smoking cessation, weight loss, and sleeping with the head of the bed elevated. These modifications are discussed in more detail in Chapter 34.

PROTON PUMP INHIBITORS

PPIs are **antisecretory** drugs used to treat gastric conditions characterized by hyperacidity. They are used for erosive gastritis, GERD, and Zollinger-Ellison syndrome and as part of a multidrug regimen for short-term treatment of active PUD, especially duodenal ulcers caused by *H. pylori*.

Pharmacodynamics

PPIs do not exhibit **anticholinergic** or **histamine$_2$-blockade** properties but suppress gastric acid secretion These drugs reduce H+ secretion by inhibition of the H+/K+/ATPase enzyme system at the secretory surface of the parietal cell itself to block the final step in H+ secretion. The effect is dose related and inhibits basal and stimulated acid secretion regardless of the stimulus. They reduce gastric acid by more than 90 percent and frequently produce achlorhydria. Serum gastrin levels increase parallel with inhibition of the acid secretion. The decrease in acid secretion lasts for up to 72 hours after each dose. Gastric acid secretion begins within 3 to 5 days after the drug is discontinued and returns to pretreatment levels within 1 to 2 weeks with **omeprazole (Prilosec)**, 4 weeks with **esomeprazole** (**Nexium**) and **lansoprazole** (**Prevacid**), or 3 months with **pantoprazole** (**Protonix**). When **PPIs** were first introduced, there was concern about this degree of acid reduction and its potential effects on digestion and intrinsic factor production.

Normal physiological effects related to suppression of gastric acid secretion result in decreased blood flow to the antrum, pylorus, and duodenal bulb. Increased serum pepsinogen levels and decreased pepsin activity also occur. As with other drugs that increase gastric pH, related increases in nitrate-reducing bacteria and elevation of nitrate concentration in gastric juice occur in patients with gastric ulcer. Compensatory increases in serum gastrin levels develop initially, but no further increase occurs with continued treatment, and there are no apparent ill effects from this increase.

Pharmacokinetics

Absorption and Distribution

All of these drugs are acid labile and so most are formulated as enteric-coated granules (Table 20–25). Absorption is rapid and begins after the granules leave the stomach and reach the less acidic duodenum. Peak plasma concentrations are approximately proportional, but because of a saturable first-pass effect, **omeprazole** has a greater than linear response when given in doses above 40 mg. **Esomeprazole** peak increases proportionally when the dose is increased, and there is a 3-fold increase in the AUC from 20 to 40 mg. The AUC is decreased by 43 to 53 percent after food intake compared to fasting conditions for this drug. **Esomeprazole** should be taken at least 1 hour before meals.

Peak and AUC of **lansoprazole** are diminished by 50 to 70 percent if the drug is given after food as opposed to the fasting state. It should be given on an empty stomach.

When **pantoprazole** is given with food, absorption may be delayed by 2 hours or longer. Taking **rabeprazole** (**Aciphex**) with a high-fat meal may delay its absorption by up to 4 hours. In each case, the peak and AUC are not altered.

All drugs are distributed to the parietal cells of the stomach. They all cross the placenta. **Omeprazole** has been measured in breast milk of women. The other PPIs have been found in breast milk in animal studies.

Metabolism and Excretion

These drugs are extensively metabolized by CYP450 2C19 and CYP450 3A4, and several metabolites have been identified. These metabolites appear to have little or no antisecretory activity. **Omeprazole** is metabolized by

Table 20–25 ▶ **Pharmacokinetics: Proton Pump Inhibitors**

Drug	Onset	Peak	Duration	Protein Binding	Bioavailability	Half-Life	Elimination
Esomeprazole	UK	1.5 h	UK	97%	64% (single dose); 90% (multiple doses)	1–1.5 h	80% in urine as metabolite; <1% unchanged drug
Lansoprazole	1 h	1.7 h	>24 h	97%	>80%	1.5 h; increases to 3.2–7.2 h in hepatic impairment	33% in urine; remainder in feces
Omeprazole	1 h	0.5–3.5 h	>72 h	95%	30%–40%; increases to 100% in hepatic impairment	30–60 min; increases to 3 h in hepatic impairment	77% in urine; remainder in feces
Pantoprazole	UK	2.5 h	>24 h	98%	77%	1 h	71% in urine as metabolite; 18% in feces
Rabeprazole	<1 h	2–5 h	UK	96.3%	52%	1–2 h	90% in urine as metabolites; 10% in feces
Dexlansoprazole		4–5 h		96.1%		1–2 h	50.7% is excreted in the urine and 47.6% in the feces

the CYP450 system and may interact with other drugs also metabolized by this system. **Lansoprazole** and **dexlansoprazole** are metabolized by the CYP450 3A4 and CYP450 2C19 isoenzyme systems; however, they do not have clinically significant drug interactions related to this metabolic site.

In patients with varying degrees of hepatic disease, the mean plasma half-life of each of these drugs increases from a low of 3 hours with **omeprazole** to a high of 9 hours for **pantoprazole.** The plasma elimination half-life of these drugs does not reflect the duration of suppression of gastric acid secretion, apparently because of prolonged binding to the parietal H+/K+/ATPase enzyme.

Little unchanged drug is excreted in the urine, but 33 to 90 percent of the metabolites is excreted in the urine. The rest is excreted in feces. A significant biliary excretion route is implied, especially for **omeprazole** and **lansoprazole.** Older adults have somewhat decreased elimination rates of all of these drugs, perhaps related to the decreased renal function associated with aging.

Pharmacotherapeutics

Precautions and Contraindications

The only true contraindication to the PPIs are hypersensitivity to the ingredients.

The **PPIs** are extensively metabolized in the liver; therefore, they should be used cautiously in patients with hepatic dysfunction and the elderly. No dosage adjustments are recommended for these patients, however.

Omeprazole is Pregnancy Category C. In animal studies, doses far in excess of those given to humans produced increased fetal lethality. Sporadic reports have been received of congenital anomalies in infants born to women receiving **omeprazole** during pregnancy. An expert review of published data on experiences of **omeprazole** use during pregnancy by the Teratogen Information System (TERIS) concluded that therapeutic doses during pregnancy are unlikely to post a substantial teratogenic risk. There have been no adequate and well-controlled studies in pregnant women. Use in pregnancy only if the potential benefits outweigh the potential risks to the fetus.

Lansoprazole, esomeprazole, pantoprazole, and **rabeprazole** are Pregnancy Category B, but there have been no adequate and well-controlled studies in pregnant women for these drugs, either. Use in pregnancy only if the potential benefits outweigh the potential risks to the fetus.

Omeprazole has been measured in human breast milk and the other drugs in this class have exhibited drug in the breast milk in animal studies. The decision to discontinue the drug or discontinue nursing should take into account the importance of the drug to the mother.

The safety and efficacy of **pantoprazole** and **rabeprazole** have not been established in children younger than age 12 years. **Esomeprazole, omeprazole,** and **lansoprazole** have been found safe and efficacious for short-term treatment of GERD and erosive esophagitis in pediatric patients and are FDA approved for use in children as young as 1 year of age.

Adverse Drug Reactions

These drugs are generally well tolerated when used for short-term treatment, and the adverse reactions that did occur in more than 1 percent of patients in clinical trials included dizziness, drowsiness, abdominal pain, constipation, diarrhea, and flatulence. It is difficult to determine if the GI-related symptoms were associated with the disease or the drug.

PPIs have now been on the market long enough to have a large body of long-term safety data. Ali, Roberts, and Tierney (2009) conducted an extensive review of the literature to determine the long-term safety of **PPIs** and the authors suggest the combined body of knowledge raises concerns. There is evidence for significant nutrient deficiencies in patients taking **PPIs** long term. **Iron, vitamin** B_{12}, and **calcium** all need an acid environment for optimal absorption. The **PPIs** are so effective in reducing acid production that patients are at risk for iron deficiency anemia, vitamin B_{12} deficiency, and calcium deficiency (Ali et al, 2009; Lodato et al, 2010). Patients on long-term **PPIs** may be at risk for osteoporosis and increased hip fractures, especially when combined with other risk factors for fracture such as age and female gender (Ali et al, 2009; Corley, Kubo, Zhao, & Quesenberry, 2010; Lodato et al, 2010; Thomson, Sauve, Kassam, & Kamitakahara, 2010).

Stomach acid provides a natural defense against microbial pathogens. Patients on long-term PPI therapy have an increased risk of *Clostridium difficile*, salmonella, and camphylobacter infections (Ali et al, 2009). Patients on **PPIs** also have an increased risk of pneumonia.

There are cellular level changes that occur with long-term **PPI therapy,** including hyperplasia of enterochromaffin-like cells, leading to a concern about the development of gastric cancers (Ali et al, 2009; Lodato et al, 2010; Vandenplas et al, 2009). Atrophic gastritis has been noted in patients taking **omeprazole** long term, and chronic atrophic gastritis is a risk factor for developing gastric carcinoid tumors (Lodato et al, 2010). In spite of these cellular changes, at this time there is not strong evidence for the development of gastric cancers from long-term PPI use (Lodato et al 2010; Thomson et al, 2010).

Drug Interactions

Drug interactions with **PPIs** relate to their use of the CYP450 enzyme system for metabolism and the change in bioavailability of concurrently administered drugs requiring an acid environment for absorption. **PPIs** may decrease the effects of **atazanavir, indinavir,** and **nelfinavir** and coadministration is not recommended. All **PPIs** may interfere with absorption of drugs given orally that depend on an acidic gastric pH to be effective. These drugs include **ketoconazole, esters of ampicillin, digoxin,** and **iron** salts. Increased monitoring of INR is required if **warfarin** is administered with **PPIs.**

Clopidogrel (**Plavix**) has a black box warning regarding concerns for poor metabolizers of CYP2C19 and concurrent administration of medications that interfere with CYP2C19. Coadministration of **clopidogrel** and **omeprazole** has been shown to decrease the active metabolite of **clopidogrel** by 46 percent, leading to decreased effectiveness. Clinically, a decrease in the antiplatelet effect of **clopidogrel** may lead to increased clot formation. The FDA issued a warning in November 2009 to avoid concurrent use of **PPIs** and **clopidogrel**, followed by an update in February 2010 that states the following:

Until further information is available FDA recommends the following:

- Healthcare providers should continue to prescribe and patients should continue to take **clopidogrel** as directed, because **clopidogrel** has demonstrated benefits in preventing blood clots that could lead to a heart attack or stroke.
- Healthcare providers should re-evaluate the need for starting or continuing treatment with a **PPI**, including **Prilosec OTC**, in patients taking **clopidogrel**.

These and other interactions are shown in Table 20–26.

Clinical Use and Dosing

Duodenal and Gastric Ulcers

Treatment for patients with uncomplicated gastric ulcers includes testing and treating for *H. pylori* and acid suppressive therapy with **PPIs. Lansoprazole, omeprazole, esomeprazole,** and **rabeprazole** are used for treatment of active duodenal ulcer and active benign gastric ulcer. The once-daily dose is taken before a meal, preferably in the morning (Table 20–27). Treatment is for 12 weeks.

Table 20–26 ■ **Drug Interactions: Proton Pump Inhibitors**

Drug	Interacting Drug	Possible Effect	Implications
Esomeprazole	Benzodiazepines	Oxidative metabolism of BDZ decreased. Reduced clearance and increased half-life	Reduce dose of BDZ or increased dose interval
	Clarithromycin	Increased concentrations of both drugs	No action required
Lansoprazole	Theophylline	10% increase in theophylline clearance	Additional titration of theophylline dosage may be required

Continued

Table 20–26 ■ **Drug Interactions: Proton Pump Inhibitors—cont'd**

Drug	Interacting Drug	Possible Effect	Implications
Omeprazole	Clarithromycin	Coadministration may result in increased plasma levels of both drugs	This combination is among the FDA-approved treatment options for *Helicobacter pylori* eradication
	Benzodiazepines, phenytoin	103% increase in diazepam half-life; 15% reduced clearance of phenytoin	Use lansoprazole or select a treatment regimen that does not require a proton pump inhibitor if the interacting drugs must be given
	Sulfonylureas	Concurrent use may increase serum sulfonylurea concentration, increasing hypoglycemic effects	No specific action beyond monitoring blood glucose
Rabeprazole	Clarithromycin	Increased concentrations of both drugs	No action required; may be part of *H. pylori* protocol
All PPIs	Sucralfate	Decreased absorption of proton pump inhibitor	Take proton pump inhibitor 30 min prior to sucralfate
	Ketoconazole, esters of ampicillin, digoxin, iron salts	Proton pump inhibitors decrease absorption of these drugs	Avoid concurrent administration; for digoxin, monitor serum levels closely
	Azole antifungals (itraconazole, ketoconazole, etc.)	Bioavailability of azole decreased due to high gastric pH interference with table dissolving	Avoid concomitant administration
	Digoxin	Increased serum digoxin levels	Magnitude of change may not be clinically significant, but need to monitor
	Salicylates	Enteric-coated salicylates may dissolve more rapidly, increasing gastric adverse response	Separate administration by at least one hr and give salicylate first
	Warfarin	Prolonged elimination of warfarin; increased INR	Increase monitoring frequency

Table 20–27 ◉ **Dosage Schedule: Proton Pump Inhibitors**

Drug	Indication	Initial Dose	Maintenance Dose
Esomeprazole	GERD with erosive esophagitis	20 or 40 mg daily for 4–8 wk 20 mg daily for 4 wk	20 mg/d
	Symptomatic GERD *Helicobacter pylori* eradication/prevent duodenal ulcer	Triple therapy: Esomperazole 40 mg daily + amoxicillin 1g bid + clarithromycin 500 mg bid for 7–10 d	
Lansoprazole	Duodenal ulcer	15 mg qd for 4 wk *H. pylori:* Triple therapy: Lansoprazole 30 mg bid + amoxicillin 1 g bid + clarithromycin 500 mg tid for 10 d Double therapy: Lansoprazole 30 mg tid + amoxicillin 1 g tid for 14 d	15 mg qd
	Benign gastric ulcer	30 mg daily for <8 wk	
	Erosive esophagitis	30 mg daily for <8 wk	15 mg qd
	Hypersecretory disorders	60 mg daily	Up to 90 mg bid; doses >120 mg/d must be divided

Table 20–27 ◉ Dosage Schedule: Proton Pump Inhibitors—cont'd

Drug	Indication	Initial Dose	Maintenance Dose
	Erosive esophagitis	*Children 12–17 yr and adults:* 30 mg once daily for up to 8 wk *Children 1–11 yr:* ≤30 kg: 15 mg daily for up to 12 wk >30 kg: 30 mg daily for up to 12 wk	If not healed, repeat dose for additional 8 wk Increase to 30 mg bid in patients who remain symptomatic after 2 wk of therapy
	Gastric ulcer associated with NSAID therapy	30 mg daily for up to 8 wk	15 mg/d for up to 12 wk
	GERD	*Children 12–17 yr and adults:* 15 mg daily for up to 8 wk *Children 1–11 yr:* ≤ 30 kg: 15 mg daily for up to 12 wk > 30 kg: 30 mg daily for up to 12 wk	
Omeprazole	Duodenal ulcer	20 mg daily for 4–8 wk *H. pylori:* Triple therapy: Omeprazole 20 mg bid + clarithromycin 500 mg bid + amoxicillin 1 g bid for 10 d Double therapy: Omeprazole 40 daily + clarithromycin 500 mg tid for 14 d; then omeprazole 20 mg daily for 14 additional days	
	Benign gastric ulcer	40 mg daily for 4–8 wk	
	Erosive esophagitis	20 mg daily for 4–8 wk	20 mg qid
	GERD	*Children 2–18 yr:* ≤20 kg: 10 mg daily for 4–8 wk >20 kg: 20 mg daily for 4–8 wk	Note: On a per-kg basis doses are higher for children than adults.
	Hypersecretory disorders	60 mg daily	Up to 120 mg tid; doses >80 mg/d must be divided
Pantoprazole	Symptomatic GERD	20–40 mg daily for 7–10 d	20 mg/d
	GERD with erosive esophagitis	40 mg daily for up to 8 wk	40 mg/d If not healed, repeat same dose for additional 8 wk
	Hypersecretory disorders	Individualized. 40 mg bid; may treat for up to 2 yr	Doses up to 240 mg/d have been used
Rabeprazole	Duodenal ulcers	20 mg daily after the morning meal for up to 4 wk	If not healed, repeat dose for 4 wk
	GERD	20 mg daily for 4 wk	If symptoms, repeat dose for 4 wk
	Erosive esophagitis	20 mg daily for 4–8 wk	If not healed, repeat dose for 4 wk
	H. pylori eradication/ prevent duodenal ulcer	Triple therapy: Rabeprazole 20 mg bid + amoxicillin 1 g bid + clarithromycin 500 mg bid for 7 d	
	Hypersecretory disorders	Individualized: 60 mg daily; may treat for up to 1 yr	Dose up to 100 mg/d or 60 mg bid have been used
Dexlansoprazole	Erosive esophagitis	Treatment: 60 mg daily for 8 wk Maintenance for healed EE: 30 mg daily for up to 6 mo	Moderate hepatic dysfunction: 30 mg/d Not recommended for children <18 yr
	GERD	30 mg daily for 4 wk	

Further discussion of multidrug treatment for *H. pylori* is found in Chapter 34.

More than 90 percent of duodenal ulcers and 80 percent of gastric ulcers are thought to be related to infection with *H. pylori.* Multiple treatment regimens are available for *H. pylori* eradication; triple regimens combine a **PPI** with two antibiotics for 14 days and the quadruple regimen combines a **PPI** with two antibiotics and bismuth subsalicylate (Lew, 2009). Acid suppression by the **PPI** in conjunction with the **antimicrobial** helps alleviate the ulcer-related symptoms, heals gastric mucosal inflammation, and may enhance the efficacy of the **antimicrobial** agent against *H. pylori* at the mucosal surface. Eradication of *H. pylori* significantly affects healing and recurrence rates. The recurrence rate of peptic ulcers is 6 to 15 percent for patients taking **antimicrobial** therapy versus 80 percent recurrence for those on conventional **antisecretory** therapy. Chapter 34 discusses the treatment of peptic ulcer disease in depth and Table 34–6 discusses triple and quadruple therapy for gastric ulcers. Any of the **PPIs** can be used in these protocols. See Table 20–28.

Gastroesophageal Reflux Disease

For most patients, GERD is treated with stepped therapy. The steps are based on symptom relief and degree of esophageal damage. Either the step-up approach or the step-down approach may be used. There is evidence supporting both and the provider may select either. Regardless of the approach chosen, lifestyle modifications occur throughout therapy. They are discussed in detail in Chapter 34.

The step-up approach begins with lifestyle modifications and OTC **antacids** followed by **H_2RAs** and **PPIs** in later steps. If symptoms are refractory after 4 to 8 weeks of therapy or if endoscopy shows evidence of erosive disease, **PPIs** become central to management. They replace

Table 20–28 ◆ Available Dosage Forms: Proton Pump Inhibitors

Drug	Dosage Form	How Supplied	Cost
Esomeprazole (Nexium)	Capsules: delayed-release: 20 mg, 40 mg	In bottles of 90, 1,000 capsules and UD 30 and 100	$124/30
Lansoprazole (Prevacid)	Capsules, delayed-release: 15 mg, 30 mg	In bottles of 100, 1,000 capsules	15 mg: $169.99/30 30 mg: $597.99/100
	Prevacid OTC: Capsules, delayed-release: 15 mg	In 14, 28, 42 packets	$11.99/14 $20.99/28 $25.99/42
	Tablets: orally disintegrating, delayed-release: 15 mg, 30 mg	In UD 30s (strawberry flavor)	$126/30 $427/100
	Granules for oral suspension, delayed-release: 15 mg	In UD 30s (strawberry flavor)	
Lanprazole (generic)	Capsules, delayed-release: 15 mg	In 30s	$99.99/30
Omeprazole (Prilosec)	Capsules, delayed-release: 10 mg, 20 mg	In bottles of 30, 90, 1,000 capsules	10 mg: $34.36/30 20 mg: $98.99/90
	Prilosec OTC: Tablets, delayed-release: 20 mg	In 14, 28, 42 packets	$12.99/14 $16.40/28 $27.99/42
	Capsules: 40 mg	In bottles of 100, 1,000 capsules and UD 30	$190/30
Omeprazole (generic)	Tablets: 20 mg	In 14, 28, 42 packets	$9.99/14 $17.99/28 $20.99/42
Pantoprazole (Protonix)	Tablets: delayed-release: 20 mg 40 mg	In bottles of 90 tablets	$282/90
		In bottles of 90, 100, 1,000 tablets and blister pak of 10	$282/90
Rabeprazole (Aciphex)	Tablets, delayed-release: 20 mg	In bottles of 30, 90 tablets and UD 100	$117/30
Dexlansoprazole (Kapidex) Dexilant	Delayed-release capsules: 30 mg, 60 mg 60 mg capsule	In bottles of 30, 90, 100 30	30 mg $127.98/30 60 mg $127.98/30 60 mg $95.99/30

the H2RAs. This is the last phase that is appropriately managed by the primary care provider, after which referral to a gastroenterologist is appropriate. The step-up approach is best for patients with mild disease and/or only occasional symptoms.

The step-down approach begins with a standard dose of a PPI every morning for 8 weeks (ICSI, 2006). If symptoms are not resolved, the dose of PPI is doubled (twice-a-day dosing) for another 4- to 8-week trial period (American Gastroenterological Association [AGA] Institute Medical Position Panel, 2008). After 4 weeks, a lower PPI dose is tried. If there is no relief after 8 weeks of twice-a-day PPI, then the patient warrants a referral to a gastroenterologist. The goal is to step down to the lowest PPI dose or transition to a H_2RA if symptoms are relieved. The step-down approach is more appropriate for those with moderate to severe disease and/or daily symptoms.

Whether the step-up or the step-down approach is chosen, failure to achieve symptom relief after 3 months or the presence of symptoms that suggest complications move the recommendations of all groups to referral to gastroenterology. PPIs may mask the symptoms of gastric cancers, and the provider should keep this in mind. The presence of alarm symptoms (dysphagia, painful swallowing, noncardiac chest pain, weight loss, hematemesis, and choking) suggests endoscopy as part of the initial evaluation.

All PPIs are approved for the treatment of GERD. The once-daily dosing is taken before breakfast. The length of therapy is 4 to 8 weeks. In the rare patient whose healing does not occur by then, an additional 4 weeks may be needed. Nonresponsive patients require referral to a gastroenterology specialist. Patients may need long-term intermittent therapy for GERD. Dosage schedules for GERD are found in Table 20–27.

Hypersecretory Conditions (Including Zollinger-Ellison Syndrome)

All PPIs can be used to treat hypersecretory conditions such as Zollinger-Ellison syndrome. These disorders usually require higher dosing than does GERD or PUD and vary depending on the drug used. Some patients with Zollinger-Ellison syndrome have been treated continuously for more than 5 years.

Rational Drug Selection

Drug Interactions

For patients taking drugs metabolized by the CYP450 system, **lansoprazole** is the best choice. Although all **PPIs** are metabolized by CYP450 enzymes, **lansoprazole** appears to have no clinically significant drug interactions with **warfarin** or other drugs metabolized by CYP450. All the **PPIs** interact with **atazanavir** equally.

Difficulty in Swallowing

For patients with difficulty in swallowing, **omeprazole**, **esomeprazole**, and **lansoprazole** capsules can be opened and the intact granules sprinkled on 1 tablespoon of applesauce and swallowed immediately. Do not chew or crush the granules. **Lansoprazole** comes as a quick-dissolve tablet (**Prevacid SoluTab**) or as granules for suspension (**Prevacid for Oral Suspension**) that are mixed in 30 ml of water. **Omeprazole (Prilosec for Delayed-Release Oral Suspension)** comes as granules for suspension that are mixed with water and left to thicken for 2 to 3 minutes before administration. **Pantoprazole (Protonix)** comes as granules for delayed-release suspension that are mixed in applesauce or apple juice. The instructions with **rabeprazole** specifically state not to crush the tablet. All the **PPIs** have an enteric coating, even the granules; therefore, none of them should be crushed or chewed.

Patients with tube feedings require a formulation that will not clog the tube. **Omeprazole** capsules or granules may be used in patients on tube feedings. An **omeprazole** capsule may be opened and mixed with an acidic juice or **omeprazole** granules may be mixed with water in a catheter-tip syringe and administered after waiting 2 to 3 minutes for the mixture to thicken. **Pantoprazole** granules are emptied into the barrel of a syringe and 10 ml of apple juice is added; additional apple juice may be needed to rinse the syringe of granules. **Lansoprazole** granules for suspension or quick-dissolve tablets should not be used for nasogastric feedings. A **lansoprazole** capsule may be opened and mixed with 40 ml of apple, cranberry, grape, orange, tomato, or V-8 juice and administered via nasogastric tube.

Helicobacter Pylori Treatment

To increase adherence, choose the least complex regimen with the fewest adverse reactions that still has a high eradication rate. Chapter 34 has more discussion of this treatment.

Monitoring

The only monitoring relates to the disease process being treated. However, patients taking **proton pump inhibitors** to treat ulcers should be tested for *H. pylori* infection. Patients taking **PPIs** should stop therapy for 2 weeks before undergoing urea breath testing to diagnose this infection or be tested via stool antigen testing. **PPIs** alone rarely eradicate *H. pylori* infection, but they can suppress it so that testing during **antisecretory** therapy may lead to false-negative results.

Patient Education

Administration

Patients should take the drug exactly as prescribed, even if they are feeling better. If a dose is missed, it should be taken as soon as the patient remembers it, unless it is almost time for the next dose. Do not double up on doses.

All of these drugs are taken before a meal. Drugs taken once daily are preferably taken in the morning. These drugs may safely be taken with antacids.

Patients who have difficulty swallowing should be instructed not to chew or crush tablets or granules. Patients or caregivers should have clear instructions on how to administer **PPIs** to those with swallowing problems or tube feedings.

Adverse Reactions

PPIs may occasionally cause drowsiness or dizziness. Patients should avoid activities that require mental alertness until their response to the drug is known. Advise patients to promptly report to their health-care provider the onset of black, tarry stool; diarrhea; abdominal pain; or persistent headache, which may indicate progression of the disease or adverse drug effects.

Lifestyle Management

Lifestyle modifications are always attempted before drugs are used to treat GERD. They are also often used prior to treatment of the other indications for **PPIs.** These modifications are discussed more detail in Chapter 34.

LAXATIVES

Constipation is a common affliction caused by everything from lack of sufficient fluids, fiber, and exercise to serious GI diseases to iatrogenic causes secondary to adverse reactions to drugs. It is among the most frequent reasons for self-medication and is particularly troublesome to older adults.

Treatment often takes the form of **laxative** use. More than $500 million is spent annually in the United States on **laxatives.** The pathophysiology of constipation varies with its cause, and the action of the drug chosen to treat the constipation must also vary to match the cause. In light of these differences, six main classes of drugs are used to promote evacuation of the bowel: stimulants, osmotics, **bulk-producing laxatives**, lubricants, surfactants, and **hyperosmolar laxatives.** Each class is discussed in this section. Because each **laxative** has several brand names, only the generic name is used.

Pharmacodynamics

Stimulants

The stimulant **laxatives** have a direct action on intestinal mucosa by stimulating the myenteric plexus. Stimulants facilitate the release of prostaglandins and increase cyclic adenosine monophosphate (cAMP) concentration. This increase in cAMP increases the secretion of electrolytes and stimulates peristalsis. Drugs in the stimulant class include **cascara, senna, bisacodyl,** and **castor oil.**

The **stimulants** are used most often for treatment of constipation associated with reduced mobility, constipating drugs, reduced motility, neurogenic bowel secondary to spinal cord injury, and irritable bowel syndrome. They are also used to prepare the bowel for radiological or surgical procedures.

Osmotics

The class of **osmotics** exerts its effects mainly by drawing water into the intestinal lumen to increase intraluminal pressure. These drugs are hypertonic salt-based solutions that cause the diffusion of fluid from the plasma into the intestine to dilute the solution to an isotonic state. The magnesium salts also cause an increase in the release of cholecystokinin by the duodenum. Sulfate salts are considered the most powerful. Drugs in this class include **magnesium hydroxide, magnesium citrate, sodium phosphate, polyethylene glycol electrolyte solution,** and **polyethylene glycol (PEG) 3350.**

Polyethylene glycol electrolyte solution is used to cleanse the entire GI tract for diagnostic purposes, to flush poisons from the system, and to remove parasites. PEG 3350 powder is used for constipation.

Bulk-Producing Laxatives

The **bulk-producing laxatives** are the safest and most physiological because their action is similar to that achieved by increasing fiber in the diet. They do not hinder absorption of nutrients and are less likely to be habit forming. The **bulk-producing laxatives** consist of natural and semisynthetic polysaccharides and cellulose. When combined with water in the intestine, they produce mechanical distention resulting in an increase in peristalsis. Drugs in this class include **psyllium, methylcellulose,** and **polycarbophil.**

The **bulk-producing laxatives** may be used for long-term management of simple, chronic constipation, especially if it is related to low fiber intake in the diet. They are also useful in situations in which straining at stool is to be avoided and in the management of chronic, watery diarrhea.

Lubricants

Mineral oil is the main ingredient in lubricant laxatives. Its action is to retard colonic absorption of fecal water and soften the stool. It does not stimulate peristalsis. It is used to soften stool associated with fecal impaction. **Mineral oil** also lubricates the intestine to facilitate the passage of stool. Major concerns with the use of **mineral oil** are that it may decrease absorption of fat-soluble vitamins, and there is concern for aspiration in children younger than 4 years of age.

Surfactants

Surfactants are often referred to as "stool softeners" because they reduce the surface tension of the oil–water interface on the stool and facilitate admixture of fat and water into the stool, producing an emollient action. Drugs in this class are the **docusate compounds: docusate sodium, docusate calcium,** and **docusate potassium.**

Surfactants are most beneficial when feces are hard or dry, in anorectal conditions in which passage for firm stool is painful, and in situations when straining at stool is to be avoided. **Docusate sodium** can be safely administered to all ages from infants to the elderly.

Hyperosmolar Laxatives

Hyperosmolar laxatives are often listed as "miscellaneous," but they share a similar mechanism of action.

Glycerin produces local irritation and, as a hyperosmotic compound, draws water from the extravascular spaces into the lumen of the intestine, resulting in more liquid stool. **Lactulose** is a hyperosmotic disaccharide. In the colon, resident bacteria transform the drug into lactic acid and acetic and formic acids. These acids exert an osmotic effect by drawing water from the extravascular spaces into the intestinal lumen.

Glycerin is used to treat fecal impaction and patients with neurogenic bowel, in which the bowel is filled with feces that cannot be evacuated. **Lactulose** is used to treat chronic constipation in older adults, but it also is the only laxative used to treat hepatic encephalopathy. It lowers the pH of the colon, which in turn inhibits the diffusion of ammonia across colonic membranes.

Pharmacokinetics

Absorption and Distribution

Absorption is highly variable between classes from no absorption for the **bulk-forming laxatives** to 3 percent or less for all other classes except the **magnesium salts**, of which up to 30 percent may be absorbed (Table 20–29). **Magnesium salts** are widely distributed, cross the placenta, and enter breast milk. Small amounts of metabolites of **bisacodyl** have been found in breast milk. The remaining drugs in each class have no distribution, with their action being localized in the intestine.

Metabolism and Excretion

Locally acting drugs have no specific metabolism and are excreted in feces. The liver metabolizes small amounts of **bisacodyl**. **Glycerin** is 80 percent metabolized by the liver and 10 to 20 percent by the kidney. **Magnesium salts** are metabolized by the liver and excreted primarily by the kidney.

Pharmacotherapeutics

Precautions and Contraindications

Precautions and contraindications vary by class of **laxative**, but all share the contraindication of use in the presence of nausea, vomiting, or undiagnosed abdominal pain or if bowel obstruction is suspected or diagnosed. Other precautions and contraindications are specific to a class or a drug.

Stimulants

Bisacodyl is to be used with caution in the presence of severe cardiovascular disease. The extract of **cascara sagrada** contains **alcohol** and should be avoided by people with **alcohol** intolerance.

Castor oil is contraindicated in pregnancy because it has been associated with induction of uterine contractions. **Cascara derivatives** are Pregnancy Category C. **Bisacodyl** is safe to use in pregnancy and is listed as Pregnancy Category B.

Cascara sagrada is excreted in breast milk and may increase the incidence of diarrhea in the nursing infant.

Osmotics

Magnesium hydroxide is contraindicated in the presence of any degree of renal insufficiency because the kidney may be unable to excrete excessive magnesium ions. Hypermagnesemia, hypocalcemia, and heart block also contraindicate their use. Because large quantities of **polyethylene glycol electrolyte solution** must be taken,

Table 20–29 ▶ **Pharmacokinetics: Selected Laxatives**

Drug Class	Onset	Peak	Site of Action	Elimination
Stimulants	6–10 h 0.25–1 h bisacodyl PR 2–6 h castor oil	UK	Colon Colon Small intestine	Mostly in feces
Osmotics (magnesium salts)	0.5–3 h	UK	Small and large intestine	Primarily in urine
Bulk-forming	12–24 h	2–3 d	Small and large intestine	In feces
Lubricants	6–8 h PO 2–15 min PR	UK	Colon Colon	In feces
Surfactants	24–48 h PO 2–15 min PR	UK	Small and large intestine	Small amount absorbed is eliminated in bile
Hyperosmolar	0.25–0.5 h glycerin 24–48 h lactulose	UK UK	Colon Colon	UK Small amount absorbed is excreted unchanged in urine

PR = per rectum; UK = unknown.

these salts are used cautiously for patients with diminished gag reflex unless it is being administered by nasogastric tube. **Osmotics** should be avoided in patients with bowel obstruction or ileus.

Magnesium hydroxide is Pregnancy Category B. **Polyethylene glycol electrolyte solution** is Pregnancy Category C, as is **PEG 3350**.

PEG 3350 (Miralax) should not be used in children younger than 4 years of age. The use of **polyethylene glycol electrolyte solution** to treat constipation in children is contraindicated because of concerns about electrolyte disturbance.

Bulk-Forming Laxatives

Bulk-forming laxatives are used with caution for patients with a narrowed esophageal or intestinal lumen. Some dosage forms contain sugar or salt and should be avoided by patients who must restrict these substances. **Bulk-forming laxatives** should be avoided in patients who are impacted.

Bulk-forming agents are not given a specific pregnancy category but have been safely used during pregnancy.

Lubricants

Lipid pneumonia has occurred in patients who aspirated **mineral oil**. The very young, older adults, people with dysphagia, and debilitated patients are at highest risk.

Although no specific pregnancy category is listed for **mineral oil**, it should be avoided during pregnancy because chronic use decreases the absorption of fat-soluble vitamins and causes hypoprothrombinemia in the newborn.

Surfactants

Docusate compounds have no specific contraindications or precautions. They have not been given a specific pregnancy category but have been safely used during pregnancy.

Hyperosmolar

Hyperosmolar agents are used with caution in the presence of volume depletion. Older adults are especially at risk for dehydration. Hyperglycemia has been noted in some patients taking **lactulose**, and it is used with caution in the presence of diabetes mellitus.

Glycerin is Pregnancy Category C; **lactulose** is Pregnancy Category B. It is not known if **lactulose** is excreted in breast milk.

Other general **laxative** precautions include the following:

1. Abuse and dependency: Chronic use of **laxatives**, particularly **stimulants**, may lead to **laxative** dependency, which in turn may result in fluid and electrolyte imbalances, steatorrhea, osteomalacia, and vitamin and mineral deficiencies. The "laxative abuse syndrome" is most commonly seen in women with depression, personality disorders, or anorexia nervosa. Cathartic colon can also result. The pathology resembles ulcerative colitis.
2. Tartrazine sensitivity: Some of these products contain tartrazine, which may cause allergic types of reactions, including bronchial asthma, in susceptible individuals. Although the incidence of this sensitivity in the general population is low, it is frequently seen in patients who also have aspirin sensitivity.

Adverse Drug Reactions

Adverse drug reactions are most commonly extensions of the drug's action and include excessive bowel activity, cramping, flatulence, and bloating. Perianal irritation may also develop.

Allergic reactions such as urticaria, dermatitis, rhinitis, and bronchospasm have occurred when patients accidentally inhaled **bulk-forming laxatives**. **Phenolphthalein** may cause a skin hypersensitivity characterized by a fixed drug eruption. Discontinue the drug if this occurs.

Drug Interactions

Because most **laxatives** have local activity and limited absorption, few drug interactions occur. Table 20–30 lists those drug interactions.

Clinical Use and Dosing

All **laxatives** are used to treat constipation or to prepare the bowel for a procedure. Specific uses for each class are discussed in the Pharmacodynamics section. Table 20–31 lists the dosing schedules for each indication.

Rational Drug Selection

The choice of drug to treat constipation depends on the severity of the constipation, the reason for it, and the speed with which resolution is needed. Drugs are used only after the reason for the constipation has been corrected if possible (stop or decrease the dose of the drug that induced the constipation). Indications for the use of each class of drug are presented in the Pharmacodynamics section.

Rapid Response and Short Term

Stimulants are the drug of choice when rapid response is needed. All are equally effective. They should be used only for the short term, however. Safer drugs can be used for long-term management when speed is not the main issue. The choice of drug depends largely on cost.

Osmotic laxatives work quickly as well. **Magnesium hydroxide** produces evacuation in 6 to 8 hours and is generally administered before bedtime. **PEG 3350** produces a bowel movement in 1 to 3 days. **Docusate sodium** is the preferred **surfactant**.

Slower Response and Long Term

Bulk-forming laxatives are the drug of choice when rapid response is not needed and long-term management with the least adverse reactions is desired. They are especially

Table 20–30 ■ Drug Interactions: Selected Laxatives

Drug	Interacting Drug	Possible Effect	Implications
All laxatives	Other orally administered drugs	May decrease absorption of other orally administered drugs because of increased motility and decreased transit time	Separate administration by at least 1 h
Bisacodyl	Antacids, histamine$_2$ blockers, proton pump inhibitors	May remove enteric coating of tablets	Separate administration or select different laxative
Lactulose	Antimicrobials	Concurrent use may decrease effectiveness of lactulose used in hepatic encephalopathy	If concurrent use cannot be avoided, dosage adjustments of lactulose may be required
	Antacids	May decrease the effect of lactulose on colon pH	Separate doses by at least 1 h
Magnesium salts	Fluoroquinolones, nitrofurantoin, tetracycline	May decrease absorption of these drugs	Avoid concurrent administration
Mineral oil	Docusate compounds	Concurrent use may increase mineral oil absorption	Avoid concurrent use
	Foods	May decrease absorption of vitamins A, D, E, K	
Psyllium	Digoxin, salicylates, warfarin	May decrease absorption of these drugs	Separate administration by at least 1 h and give drug before psyllium

Table 20–31 ◉ Dosage Schedule: Selected Laxatives

Drug	Indication	Dose	Notes
Bisacodyl	Constipation	*Children >12 yr and adults:* Tablets: 10–15 mg once daily PR: 10 mg once daily *Children 2–11 yr:* Tablets: 5 mg (0.3 mg/kg) once daily PR: 5 mg once daily *Children <2 yr:* PR: 5 mg single dose	Up to 30 mg have been used as preparation for bowel procedure
Cascara sagrada	Constipation	*Children >12 yr and adults:* Tablets: 300 mg–1 g once daily Extract tablet: 200–400 mg daily Fluid extract: 0.5–1.5 mL daily Aromatic fluid extract: 2–6 mL daily *Children 2–11 yr:* Tablets: 150–500 mg once daily Extract tablet: 100–200 mg once daily Fluid extract: 0.25–0.75 mL once daily Aromatic fluid extract: 1–3 mL once daily *Children <2 yr:* Fluid extract: 0.12–0.38 mL once daily Aromatic fluid extract: 0.5–1.5 mL once daily	Tablets and liquids come in combinations with docusate and milk of magnesia
Castor oil	Constipation	*Children >12 yr and adults:* 15–60 mL in a single dose *Children 2–11 yr:* 5–15 mL in a single dose	

Continued

Table 20–31 ◉ Dosage Schedule: Selected Laxatives—cont'd

Drug	Indication	Dose	Notes
Docusate	Constipation	*Calcium* *Adults:* 240 mg once daily *Children >6 yr:* 50–150 mg once daily *Potassium* *Adults:* 100–300 mg once daily *Children >6 yr:* 100 mg once daily at bedtime *Sodium* *Children >12 yr and adults:* 50–500 mg once daily *Children 6–11 yr:* 40–120 mg once daily *Children 3–6 yr:* 20–60 mg once daily *Children <3 yr:* 10–40 mg Suppository: *Adults:* 50–100 mg or 1 suppository	
Glycerin PR	Constipation	*Children >6 yr and adults:* 2–3 g as suppository or 5–15 mg as enema *Children <6 yr:* 1–1.7 g as a suppository or 2–5 mL as enema	
Lactulose	Constipation	*Adults:* 15–30 mL once daily *Children:* 7.5 mL once daily	May use up to 60 mg/d; unlabeled use
	Hepatic encephalopathy	*Adults:* 30–45 mL tid–qid *Children and adolescents:* 40–90 mL daily in divided doses *Infants:* 2.5–10 mL daily in divided doses	May be given q1–2h initially; goal is 2–3 soft stools/d; discontinue if diarrhea develops
Magnesium salts	Constipation	*Hydroxide (milk of magnesia)* *Children >12 yr and adults:* 30–60 mL once daily (in concentrate: 10–20 mL once daily) *Children 6–11 yr:* 15–30 mL in single or divided doses *Children 2–5 yr:* 5–15 mg in divided doses	
	Bowel prep or bowel cleanout if impacted	*Citrate* *Children >12 yr and adults:* 240 mL *Children 6–11 yr:* 100 mL	
Polyethylene glycol/electrolyte solution	Bowel prep	*Adults:* 240 mL every 10 min (up to 4 L) until fecal discharge is clear with no solid material *Children:* 25–40 mg/kg/h until fecal discharge is clear with no solid material	Tastes salty, making it difficult to take. Ice it. May suck on hard candy or breath mints to make more palatable
PEG 3350 (Miralax)	Constipation	*Adults:* oral 17 g daily *Children >4 yr:* 0.7–1.5 g/kg daily, do not exceed 17 g	Mix with 4 to 8 oz of beverage
Psyllium	Constipation	*Adults:* 1–2 tsp/packet/wafer (3–6 g psyllium) in or with a full glass of liquid bid–tid *Children >6 yr:* 1 tsp/packet/wafer (1.5–3 g psyllium) in or with ½–1 glass of liquid bid–tid	Up to 30 g/d in divided doses Up to 15 g/d in divided doses
Senna	Constipation	*Children >12 yr and adults:* 360 mg–2 g at bedtime *Children 6–11 yr:* 50% of adult dose *Children 1–5 yr:* 33% of adult dose Rectal: *Children >12 yr and adults:* 30 mg qid–bid	Fletcher's Castoria lists a children's dose of 10–15 mL (6–15 yr) and 5–10 mL (2–5 yr)

PR = per rectum.

suited to older adults. The choice of product depends upon the patient's acceptance of texture and taste. **Lactulose** can be used if the **bulk-forming laxatives** do not work or are not well tolerated. It works well in older adults and children.

Special Indications

Polyethylene glycol electrolyte solution is the best drug for cleansing the bowel in preparation for radiological or surgical procedures. It is very effective and does not produce electrolyte disturbances.

Lactulose is effective in reducing ammonia levels in the blood and brain with patients who have hepatic encephalopathy. It prevents absorption of ammonia from the intestine and produces diarrhea that flushes the ammonia out. Dietary adjustments to reduce ammonia production are simultaneously implemented.

Pregnancy

For pregnant women, **bulk-forming laxatives** and **surfactants** are safe and effective for regular use throughout pregnancy. **Magnesium hydroxide** is Pregnancy Category B and can be used intermittently.

> **CLINICAL PEARL**
>
> **Polyethylene Glycol/Electrolyte Solution**
>
> The taste of polyethylene glycol/electrolyte solution is quite salty, and many patients find it difficult to consume the required volume in the required amount of time. Place the container of solution in ice in a basin. Do not pour it over ice, which will melt and increase the volume the patient must consume. Have the patient drink 240 mL of fluid each 10 minutes and give a Tic-Tac or similar small mint-flavored hard candy to suck on between glasses of the drug. This reduces the salty taste in the mouth and makes the drug more palatable.

The Precautions and Contraindications section lists the pregnancy categories for other drugs, including those that should not be used during pregnancy.

Monitoring

In general, the monitoring for patients taking **laxatives** for more than 6 months includes laboratory assessment of fluid and electrolyte status, especially potassium and in the case of **magnesium hydroxide** use, magnesium level. For patients taking **lactulose** for hepatic encephalopathy, the overall management of this disorder requires careful monitoring because it is a serious disease with a high potential for complications. Monitoring includes serum electrolytes for hypokalemia and hypernatremia. For older adults taking **lactulose** for more than 6 months to manage their constipation, laboratory assessment of potassium, chloride, and carbon dioxide should be done periodically or with any indication of fluid or electrolyte disturbance.

Patient Education

Laxatives should not be taken in the presence of nausea, vomiting, or abdominal pain. These symptoms may indicate serious disorders that may be the cause of the constipation and that require a work-up. Patients should not take a **laxative** but instead contact their health-care provider.

Administration

Rapid-acting **laxatives** are best taken in the morning; slower-acting ones are best taken at bedtime. Taking a **laxative** on an empty stomach and with a full glass of water will produce more rapid results. Do not crush or chew enteric-coated tablets. Liquids can be given with fruit juice. For infants, taking liquids with fruit juice may mask any unpleasant taste. Suspensions are shaken before they are taken. Effervescent tablets are dissolved in a full glass of water before they are taken.

Table 20–32 ◆ **Available Dosage Forms: Selected Laxatives**

Drug	Dosage Form	How Supplied
Bisacodyl (Dulcagen)	Tablets: 5 mg	In bottles of 100 tablets
	Suppositories: 10 mg	In 12 individually foil wrapped
(Dulcolax)	Tablets: 5 mg	In bottles of 10, 25, 50, 100, 1,000 tablets
	Suppositories: 10 mg	In 2, 4, 8, 16, 50 individually foil wrapped
(Fleet)	Tablets: 5 mg	In bottles of 24 tablets
	Suppositories: 10 mg	In 4 individually foil wrapped
Cascara sagrada	Tablets: 325 mg	In bottles of 100 tablets
	Aromatic fluid extract	In 120 mL and in pints
Docusate calcium (Surfak)	Capsules: 50 mg	In bottles of 30, 100 capsules
	Capsules: 240 mg	In bottles of 7, 30, 100, 500 capsules

Continued

Table 20–32 ◈ **Available Dosage Forms: Selected Laxatives—cont'd**

Drug	Dosage Form	How Supplied
Docusate potassium (Diocto-K, Dialose, Kasof)	Capsules: 100 mg	In bottles of 36, 100 capsules (Dialose), 100 capsules (Diocto-K)
	Capsules: 240 mg	In bottles of 30, 60 capsules (Kasof)
Docusate sodium (Colace)	Capsules: 50 mg, 100 mg	In bottles of 30, 60, 250, 1,000 tablets
	Syrup: 60 mg/15 mL	In 240 and 480 mL
	Liquid: 150 mg/15 mL	In 30 and 480 mL (with calibrated dropper)
(Generic)	Capsules: 50 mg	In bottles of 100 capsules
	Capsules: 100 mg and 250 mg	In bottles of 100, 1000 capsules
	Syrup: 50 mg/15 mL	In 15 and 30 mL
	Syrup: 60 mg/15 mL	In pints and gallons
Glycerin (Sani-Supp)	Adult suppositories	In 10, 25, 50 individually foil wrapped
	Pediatric suppositories	In 10, 25 individually foil wrapped
(Generic)	Adult suppositories	In 10, 12, 25, 50, 100 individually foil wrapped
	Pediatric suppositories	In 10, 12, 25 individually foil wrapped
Lactulose (Cephulac, Chronulac, Enulose)	Syrup: 10 g lactulose/15 mL	In 480 mL and 1.9 L (Cephulac) In 240 and 960 mL (Chronulac) In pint and 1.89 L (Enulose)
(Generic)	Syrup: 10 g lactulose/15 mL	In 240 and 960 mL
Magnesium sulfate (Epsom salts)	Granules: 40 mEq Mg^{2+} per 5g	In 150- and 240-g packets and 4 lb
Magnesium hydroxide (Milk of Magnesia)	Chewable tablets: 300 mg and 600 mg	In bottles of 100 and 200 tablets
	Liquid: 80 mEq Mg^{2+} per 30 mL	In 180, 360, 480, 960 mL
	Concentrate:	In 100, 400, 480 mL (lemon flavor); 240 mL (strawberry and orange cream flavors)
Magnesium citrate	Liquid: 77 mEq Mg^{2+}per 100 mL	In 240, 296, 300 mL
Phenolphthalein (Ex-Lax)	Tablets: 90 mg	In 8, 30, 60 tablets
	Chocolate tablets: 90 mg	In 6, 18, 48, 72 chewable tablets
(Feen-a-Mint)	Tablets: 97.2 mg	In 12, 30, 60 regular tablets; 20 chewable tablets
	Chocolate tablets: 65 mg	In 4, 18, 36 chocolate-mint flavor chewable tablets
	Gum: 97.2 mg/piece	In 5, 16, 40 peppermint-flavored pieces of gum
Polyethylene glycol/electrolyte solution (Colyte, GoLYTEly)	In oral solution or powder for oral solution	In gallon containers
Psyllium (Fiberall, Konsyl, Metamucil)	Powder: 3.4 g psyllium/5 mL	In 284 and 426 g (Fiberall) In 210, 420, 630, 960 g and 30, 100 unit-dose packets (Metamucil) In 325, 500 g (Konsyl)
	Powder: 6 g psyllium/5 mL	In 300, 450 g and 25 unit-dose 6 g packets
	Wafers: 1.7 g psyllium	In 24 wafers (Metamucil)

Table 20–32 ◆ **Available Dosage Forms: Selected Laxatives—cont'd**

Drug	Dosage Form	How Supplied
	Wafers: 3.4 g psyllium	In 14 wafers (Fiberall)
	Effervescent powder: 3.4 g/5 mL	In 30, 100 single-dose packets (Metamucil)
Senna (Senokot, Fletcher's Castoria)	Tablets: 187 mg	In 20, 50, 100, 1,000 tablets (Senokot)
	Granules: 326 mg	In 60, 170, 340 g (Senokot)
	Syrup: 218 mg/5 mL	In 60, 240 mL (Senokot)
	Liquid: 33.3 mg/mL	In 75, 150 mL
PEG 3350 (Miralax)	Powder for oral solution: 17 g	In 17 g/packet, 255 g, 527 g

Suppositories are usually given close to the time that a bowel movement is desired. Lubricate them with a water-soluble lubricant and insert far enough into the rectum to pass the internal rectal sphincter. Encourage the patient to retain the suppository for 15 to 30 minutes before expelling.

Some liquid **laxatives** have special storage requirements and manufactures recommendations should be followed.

Adverse Reactions

The most common adverse drug reactions are excessive bowel activity, cramping, flatulence, and bloating. Perianal irritation may also occur.

Allergic reactions such as a rash, rhinitis, and bronchospasm have occurred when patients accidentally inhaled **bulk-forming laxatives**. Be careful when pouring the powder to avoid this possibility. **Phenolphthalein** may cause a skin hypersensitivity rash. Advise the patient to notify the health-care provider if this occurs. The drug is discontinued and a different **laxative** chosen if the need for a laxative continues.

Teach patients the indications of a fluid or electrolyte disturbance and have them report these symptoms promptly.

Lifestyle Management

Prevention is the key with regard to constipation. Lifestyle management should be a major focus. Stress the need for adequate fluids, fiber, and exercise. **Laxatives** are last-resort and temporary measures. They are not intended for long-term management in most cases.

Misconceptions about bowel function should be corrected. Different people have different bowel patterns, all of which may be normal and not signal pathology. Stressing this point is especially important for older adults, who were often taught in their youth that maintenance of health depended on having one bowel movement every day.

Constipation in children may be a control issue or signal pathology. Discuss this topic with the parents. A trial of a **laxative** concurrently with behavior modification is appropriate, but the child needs to be monitored for the need for referral for a GI work-up.

REFERENCES

Ali, T., Roberts, D. N., & Tierney, W. M. (2009). Long-term safety concerns with proton pump inhibitors. *American Journal of Medicine, 122,* 896–903.

American Gastroenterological Association (AGA) Institute Medical Position Panel. (2008). American Gastroenterological Association medical position statement on the management of gastroesophageal reflux disease. *Gastroenterology, 135,* 1383–1391.

Centers for Disease Control and Prevention (CDC). (2005). Foodborne illness. Retrieved May 21, 2010, from http://www.cdc.gov/ncidod/dbmd/diseaseinfo/foodborneinfections_g.htm

Centers for Disease Control and Prevention (CDC). (2006). Traveler's diarrhea. Retrieved May 21, 2010, from http://www.cdc.gov/ncidod/dbmd/diseaseinfo/travelersdiarrhea_g.htm#prevent

Centers for Disease Control and Prevention (CDC). (2010). Traveler's diarrhea. CDC Health Information for International Travel 2010: The Yellow Book. Retrieved from http://wwwnc.cdc.gov/travel/yellowbook/2010/chapter-2/travelers-diarrhea.aspx

Corley, D. A., Kubo, A., Zhao, W., & Quesenberry, C. (2010). Proton pump inhibitors and histamine-2 receptor antagonists are associated with hip fractures among at-risk patients. *Gastroenterology,* March 27, 2010, Epub ahead of print.

Gold, B., Colletti, R., Abbot, M., Czinn, S., Elitsur, Y., Hassall, E., et al. (2000). *Helicobacter pylori* infection in children: Recommendations for diagnosis and treatment. *Journal of Pediatric Gastroenterology, 31*(5), 490–497.

Institute for Clinical Systems Improvement (ICSI). (2006). *Initial management of dyspepsia and GERD.* Institute for Clinical Systems Improvement, July 2006. Retrieved from http://www.icsi.org

Laine, L., Franz, J., Baker, A., & Neil, G. (1997). A United States multicenter trial of dual and proton pump inhibitor-based triple therapies for *Helicobacter pylori. Alimentary Pharmacologic Therapy, 11,* 913–917.

Lew, E. (2009). Peptic ulcer disease. In N. J. Greenberger (Ed.), *Current diagnosis & treatment gastroenterology, hepatology, & endoscopy* (3rd ed.). New York: McGraw Hill.

Lodato, F., Azzaroli, F., Turco, L., Mazzella, N., Buonfiglioli, F., Zoli, M., et al. (2010). Adverse effects of proton pump inhibitors. *Best Practices in Research and Clinical Gastroenterology, 24*(2), 193–201.

Rostom, A., Dube, C., Wells, G. A., Tugwell, P., Welch, V., Jolicoeur, E., et al. (2002). Prevention of NSAID-induced gastroduodenal ulcers. *Cochrane Database of Systematic Reviews 4,* Art. No. CD002296. This version first published online July 24. 2000. Last assessed as up to date May 12, 2009.

Stansbury, A. (2004). GER and GERD in children. *American Journal for Nurse Practitioners, 8*(3), 37–44.

Takemoto, C.K., Hodding, J.H., & Kraus, D.M. (2009). Pediatric Dosage Handbook 16th Edition. Hudson, Ohio:LexiComp.

Thjodleifsson, B. (2003). Treatment of acid-related disease in the elderly with emphasis on the use of proton pump inhibitors. *Drugs and Aging, 19*(12), 911–927.

Thomson, A. B. R., Sauve, M. D., Kassam, N., & Kamitakahara, H. (2010). Safety of the long-term use of proton pump inhibitors. *World Journal of Gastroenterology, 16*(19), 2323–2330.

U.S. Food and Drug Administration (2010). Pediatric labeling changes through December 21, 2010. Retrieved from http://www.fda.gov/downloads/ScienceResearch/SpecialTopics/PediatricTherapeuticsResearch/UCM163159.pdf

Vandenplas, Y., Rudolph, C. D., DiLorenzo, C., Hassall, E., Liptak, G., Mazur, L., et al. (2009). Pediatric gastroesophageal reflux clinical practice guidelines: Joint recommendations of the North American Society for Pediatric Gastroenterology, Hepatology, and Nutrition (NASPGHAN) and the European Society for Pediatric Gastroenterology, Hepatology, and Nutrition (ESPGHAN). *Journal of Pediatric Gastroenterology and Nutrition, 49,* 498–547.

CHAPTER 21

DRUGS AFFECTING THE ENDOCRINE SYSTEM

Marylou Robinson and Anita Lee Wynne

Chapter Outline

BISPHOSPHONATES

Bone is dynamic tissue that undergoes a continuous process of resorption (osteoclastic activity) and formation (osteoblastic activity) throughout life. Under normal physiological states, the two processes are about equal. Skeletal mass is usually maximal at about age 35, and declines in women after age 40 and men after age 50. The rate of decline becomes most rapid in women within 2 years of menopause, with one-third to one-half of all bone that will be lost going during the first 5 years after menopause. The cycle of bone remodeling takes longer to complete and the rate of mineralization slows with aging. As the life expectancy of women reaches the mid-80s, osteopenia in perimenopausal women takes on epidemic proportions (50%), especially among white and Asian women in industrial societies (International Osteoporosis Foundation [IOF], 2009). Men experience bone loss as well, but at later ages and slower rates than women. Initial bone mass is also about 30 percent higher in men than it is in women, so the loss is less disabling (McCance & Huether, 2006). The femoral neck and lumbar vertebrae lose the most. Cortical (compact) bone, which is 80 percent of the skeleton, is lost less rapidly than is cancellous (spongy) bone. Bone loss is related to smoking, calcium deficiency, magnesium deficiency, vitamin D deficiency, high-protein intake, excess phosphorus intake, overly vigorous exercise, certain prescription and over-the-counter (OTC) drugs, **alcohol** intake, and reduced physical activity. It is estimated that 24 million Americans have osteoporosis, of which 80 percent are women. Chapters 48 and 51 discuss this concern as it relates to women's health.

In addition to normal aging, pathophysiological conditions can also alter the balance between resorption and formation. Even a minor imbalance can have devastating effects. For example, if bone resorption exceeds formation by only 2 percent per year, in 20 years 40 percent of skeletal mass will be lost. Malignancy, syndromes of ectopic calcification, and Paget's disease are examples of pathological conditions associated with altered bone remodeling.

Pharmacodynamics

The remodeling cycle is initiated by osteoclastic activity. In response to microfractures and other damage associated with normal wear and tear, osteoclasts are drawn to the damaged area of the trabecula, attach to its surface, and resorb the damaged and surrounding bone, creating a resorption pit (Fig. 21–1). Resorption is accomplished by pseudopodia, which attach tightly to the bone surface and secrete acids and enzymes that dissolve bone. The osteoclasts then leave the area and osteoblasts move in, line up to cover the surface of the pit, and form new bone. **Bisphosphonates** adhere tightly to bone and, by

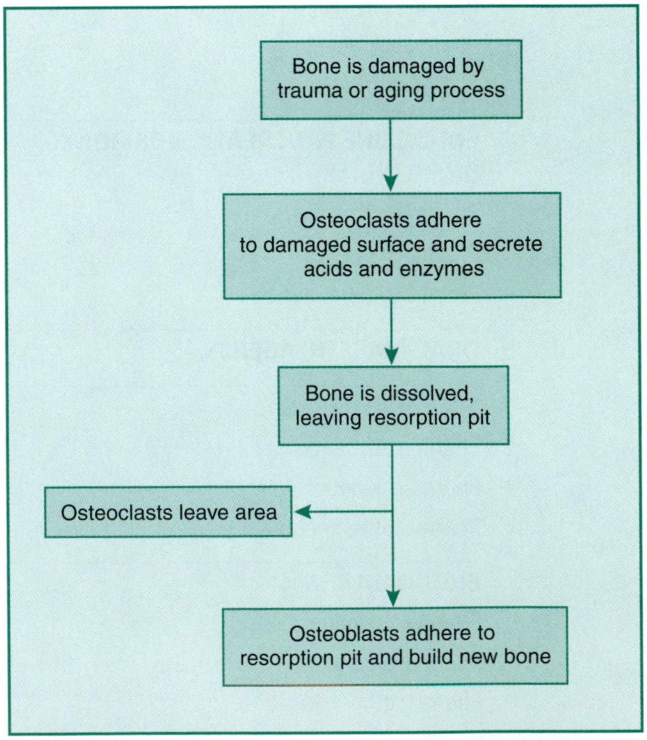

Figure 21–1. Bone remodeling. Damaged bone sections are removed by osteoclasts that use pseudopods to attach to bone surface. Bone is dissolved, leaving a resorption pit. The osteoclasts then leave the site of damage. Osteoblasts enter the resorption pit and build new bone. The process takes 4 to 5 months.

inhibiting osteoclastic activity, are potent inhibitors of both normal and abnormal bone resorption. Among this group of drugs, **etidronate (Didronel)** reduces both bone resorption and bone formation because formation is coupled with resorption. **Pamidronate (Aredia)** and **risedronate (Actonel)** inhibit bone resorption without inhibiting bone formation and mineralization. **Alendronate (Fosamax)** is a highly selective inhibitor of bone resorption and is 100 to 500 times more potent than the other drugs. It does not interfere with osteoclast recruitment or attachment, but it does inhibit osteoclastic activity. **Tiludronate (Skelid)** inhibits osteoclastic activity through two different mechanisms. It inhibits protein-tyrosine-phosphatase, resulting in detachment of osteoclasts from the bone surface, and it inhibits the osteoclastic proton pump. **Zoledronic acid (Zometa)** inhibits osteoclastic activity and induces osteoclast apoptosis. It also inhibits the increased osteoclastic activity and skeletal calcium release induced by various stimulatory factors released by tumors. **Ibandronate (Boniva)** inhibits osteoclast activity and reduces bone resorption and turnover based on its affinity for hydroxyapatite, which is part of the mineral matrix of the bone. All reduce vertebral fractures, only **aldendronate, risedronate,** and **zoledronic acid** have demonstrated nonvertebral fracture reductions; it cannot be assumed the others can achieve the same end point (*Drug Facts and Comparisons*, 2009). **Aledronate** and **risedronate** have been studied in men, but transferability of results with other medications is considered a safe assumption. Because **pamidronate** is available only in parenteral form, and **zoledronic acid** is available only for IV use, they are not discussed here in detail except to alert the primary care provider about monitoring the drug and its place in the total treatment regimen of the patient.

Pharmacokinetics

Absorption and Distribution

All oral **bisphosphonates** potentially cause gastric irritation; therefore, they must be taken with the patient upright and fasting. Absorption and bioavailability of oral doses are significantly reduced by the presence in the gut of food or other preparations containing divalent cations. To enhance gastric emptying, the patient takes the drug with 8 oz of water. No other food or drink should be ingested, and the patient must remain upright for at least half an hour (1 hour with **ibandronate**). Table 21–1 shows the effect of food, coffee, and juice on bioavailability.

Table 21–1 ▶ **Pharmacokinetics: Bisphosphonates**

Drug	Onset of Effect	Peak	Duration	Bioavailability (With/Without Food)	Steady-State V_d Exclusive of Bone	Half-Life (Normal Renal Function)	Elimination
Alendronate	1 mo	3–6 mo	7 mo (following after discontinuation of the drug)	0.7% in females 0.59% in males Reduced 40% when taken with food; 60% with coffee or juice	28 L/kg or more	10 yr (in bone)	50% in urine
Etidronate	1 mo	Unknown	1 yr (following after discontinuation of the drug)	1% Reduced when taken with food or juice	1.37 L/kg	More than 90 d (in bone	Absorbed dose: 50% in urine Unabsorbed dose: in feces
Ibandronate	UK	0.5–2 hr	Up to 1 mo	0.6% absorbed; less with food	90 L	10–60 hr	50%–60% urine; unabsorbed in feces
Risedronate	Days	1 h	16 mo (following after discontinuance of drug	0.63% Reduced by 55% when taken with food	6.3 L/kg	Terminal half-life 480 h	50% of absorbed drug in urine; rest in feces
Tiludronate	UK	2 h	UK	6% Reduced when taken with food	1 to 4.6 mg/L	150 h	60% in urine

UK = unknown; V_d = volume/density.

These drugs are all mainly distributed to bone. Their terminal half-life in bone is exceedingly long, varying from more than 10 years for **alendronate** to more than 90 days for **etidronate**. The half-life of **risedronate** is much shorter at 480 hours; **ibandronate** is 220 hours; **zoledronic acid** is 167 hours; and **tiludronate** is 150 hours, but these times are thought to represent the dissociation of the drug from the bone surface, rather than its time within the bone. Their volumes of distribution exclusive of bone vary significantly from 90 L/kg for **ibandronate** to 1.3 L/kg for **etidronate**.

Most **bisphosphonates** are Pregnancy Category C. **Pamidronate** is category D. *Drug Facts and Comparisons* (2009) states that fetal anomalies have occurred in animal studies and there are no adequate and well-controlled studies in pregnant women and recommends use of all **bisphosphonates** only when they are clearly needed and the benefits to the mother outweigh the potential hazards to the fetus. Excretion in breast milk is minimal if at all; however, all **bisphosphonates** are used with extreme caution during breastfeeding.

Safety and efficacy in children have not been established, but children have been treated with **etidronate** (Pregnancy Category B) at doses recommended for adults to prevent heterotopic ossifications or soft tissue calcifications. The epiphyseal changes that occurred were reversible with discontinuation of the drug.

Metabolism and Excretion

There is no evidence that any of the **bisphosphonates** are systemically metabolized. Drug that is not distributed to bone is largely excreted in the urine. Because of the fairly exclusive renal excretion and the high volumes of distribution exclusive of bone, these drugs are not recommended for patients with moderate to severe renal impairment (serum creatinine greater than 4.9; creatinine clearance [CCr] less than 30 to 35 mL/min), and dosage adjustments may be necessary if the drug must be given.

Pharmacotherapeutics

Precautions and Contraindications

There are no absolute contraindications except uncorrected hypocalcemia and documented Barrett's esophagus (American Society of Health-System Pharmacists [AHFS], 2009). Cautious use is recommended for patients with gastrointestinal (GI) disorders. The risk for severe esophageal adverse reactions is greater in patients who lie down after taking these drugs or who fail to swallow them with a full glass (8 oz) of water. **Etidronate** has been withheld from patients with enterocolitis because diarrhea has occurred in some patients, particularly at high doses.

Etidronate has also been associated with fractures in patients with Paget's disease when they are given high doses or when therapy lasts longer than 6 months. These patients must be carefully monitored with x-rays and laboratory work to assess for these lesions.

Adverse Drug Reactions

All oral **bisphosphonates** have GI adverse drug reactions including abdominal pain, nausea, flatulence, constipation/diarrhea, acid regurgitation, and taste perversion. Other GI reactions include esophageal ulcer formation and gastritis. These reactions are seen more often in patients with Paget's disease. Rarely were any of these drugs discontinued because of these adverse reactions.

Another common adverse drug reaction for all **bisphosphonates** is musculoskeletal pain. Once again, it was more common for patients with Paget's disease and more common with **risedronate**. In higher doses, pain incidence also increased in about 20 percent for patients taking **etidronate**. Musculoskeletal pain occurred in about 6 percent of patients taking **alendronate** and **ibandronate**.

Rare reports of osteonecrosis of the jaw have been reported associated with active dental disease or invasive procedures, especially in cancer patients. Most cases are associated with the IV forms of **bisphophonates**, but oral medications also carry the risk after 3 years of use. If elective dental procedures are planned, drug cessation for 3 months pre- and postprocedure may decrease the risk (Ruggiero et al, 2009).

Recent concerns have arisen about increased risk of atrial fibrillation. Conflicting data exist on whether IV and oral **bisphophonates** are linked to this cardiac rhythm. Recommendations to halt use have not been made in those with atrial fib or for those at risk for other reasons (Institute for Clinical Systems Improvement [ICSI], 2008; U.S. Food and Drug Administration, 2009a).

IV formulations are associated with higher renal toxicity risk, especially with rapid infusion. Checking serum creatinine prior to every dose is recommended.

Drug Interactions

Because of these drugs' adverse reactions on the GI tract, drug interactions are most common with other drugs that affect the GI tract. **Histamine$_2$ blocking agents** double **alendronate** bioavailability, but the impact is unknown (*Drug Facts and Comparisons,* 2009). **Calcium supplements** and **antacids** interfere with **bisphosphonate** absorption when taken within 1 hour of each other. The risk of GI bleeding is increased when **aspirin** and **NSAIDs** are concomitantly taken. **Aspirin** may decrease the bioavailability of **tiludronate** by up to 50 percent when taken 2 hours after the **tiludronate**. Although **indomethacin** increases the bioavailability of **tiludronate** by 2- to 4-fold, the bioavailability is not significantly altered by **diclofenac**; therefore, each **NSAID** must be considered individually. Table 21–2 presents these and other drug interactions.

Concurrent use of **bisphosphonates** and other drugs known to build bone density, such as **estrogens** and **SERMs**, prove to have additive bone density, but fracture reduction potential is unknown. Use of multiple drugs should be reserved for those patients with

Table 21–2 ■ **Drug and Food Interactions: Bisphosphonates**

Drug	Interacting Drugs and Food	Possible Effect	Implications
Alendronate	Ranitidine, aspirin, NSAIDs	Bioavailability doubled Increases risk of GI bleeding with doses more than 10 mg/d	Clinical significance unknown Avoid concurrent use
	Any food	Bioavailability decreased by 40%	Take 30 min or more before any food intake
	Coffee, orange juice	Bioavailability decreased by 60%	Take 30 min or more before intake
Etidronate	Warfarin	INR may increase when added to regimen that includes warfarin.	Increase INR monitoring
Ibandronate	Ca++, aluminum, Mg++ and iron products Food & milk products	Decreased absorption	Take 60 min prior to food or mineral products
Risedronate	Any food	Bioavailability decreased	Take 30 min or more before any food intake
Tiludronate	Aspirin	Tiludronate bioavailability decreased by up to 50% when aspirin taken 2 h after the tiludronate	Avoid concurrent use or give aspirin more than 2 h after tiludronate
	Indomethacin	Increases tiludronate bioavailability 2- to 4-fold	Clinical significance unknown
	Any food	Bioavailability decreased by 90%	Take after overnight fast and 4 h before standard breakfast
Zoledronic acid	Concurrent use loop diuretics or aminoglycosides	Increases hypocalcemia risk	Check Ca++ levels before
All bisphosphonates	Calcium supplements, antacids	Interferes with bisphosphonate absorption Bioavailability may be decreased by 60% when given within 1 h	Take most bisphosphonates at least 30 min before; ibandronate requires 1 hour before

suspected lower response rates or significant risk profiles (ICSI, 2008).

Clinical Use and Dosing

Osteoporosis

Expert clinical trial data support the use of **bisphosphonates** for prevention and treatment of osteoporosis and its risk for fractures in men and postmenopausal women, especially vertebral fractures. The best trials have been done with **alendronate, ibandronate,** and **risedronate** (ICSI, 2008) and have received U.S. Food and Drug Administration (FDA) approval for this indication. **Ibandronate** and **zoledronic acid** come in an IV form and **alendronate** has an oral solution for those patients unable to take tablets. **Raloxifene (Evista),** a **selective estrogen receptor modulator,** is also approved for osteoporosis prevention and is discussed in Chapter 22.

Practitioners should consider prophylactic use of **bisphosphonates** in patients with early osteopenia related to long-term use of medications that contribute to bone loss such as **thyroid hormone, aromatase inhibitors,** and **glucocorticoids** (AHFS, 2009). It is recommend that all adults taking more than 7.5 mg of **prednisone** or its equivalent for more than 3 weeks be given **alendronate** or **risedronate** AACE (Hodgson et al, 2003; *Drug Facts and Comparisons,* 2009). In very high-risk patients, a maximum 2-year use of **teriparatide (Forteo),** a parathyroid hormone, may be more efficacious (ICSI, 2008). The bone mass benefit disappears after **teriparatide** discontinuance, a decline not seen with the **bisphosphonates** for 5 years.

Initial doses for prevention of bone loss for **alendronate and risedronate** are 5 mg/day or 35 mg/week. For treatment of existing osteoporosis, the dose of **alendronate** doubles to 10 mg/day or 70 mg/week, and the dose of **risedronate** increases to 75 mg for two consecutive days or 150 mg once a month. The Scottish Intercollegiate Guidelines Network (SIGN, 2004) is less conservative and recommends the same doses for both prevention and treatment as are listed above for treatment. Therapy with 10 mg daily can increase bone density by up to 10 percent after 3 years and can decrease vertebral and hip fractures by 50 percent (Table 21–3). Use for more than 4 years is currently under review concerning its efficacy or safety.

The initial and maintenance dosage of **ibandronate** for both prevention and treatment is one 2.5-mg tablet taken daily or one 150-mg tablet taken once monthly on the same date of each month. The IV dose is 3 mg given over 30 seconds and repeated every 3 months, a schedule that must be closely maintained for best results.

Table 21–3 ● **Dosage Schedule: Bisphosphonates**

Drug	Indication	Initial Dose	Maintenance Dose	Renal Use Parameter
Alendronate	Osteoporosis: men, post-menopausal women, glucocorticoid-induced	Prevention: 5 mg/d or 35 mg/wk Treatment: 10 mg/d or 70 mg/wk	5 mg/d or 35 mg/wk 10 mg/d or 70 mg/wk	CCr 35–60: no dosage adjustment CCr 35: use not recommended
	Paget's disease	40 mg/d	40 mg/d for 6 mo; re-treat if needed with same dose only after 6 mo post-treatment evaluation	As above
Etidronate	Paget's disease	5 mg/kg/d	5–10 mg/kg/d not to exceed 6 mo or 11–20* mg/kg/d not to exceed 3 mo; re-treat if needed with same dose only after 3–6 mo post-treatment evaluation	Serum creatinine 2.5–4.9, reduce dose Creatinine more than 5: use not recommended
	Heterotropic ossification: hip replacement	20 mg/kg/d for 1 mo preoperatively	20* mg/kg/d for 3 mo postoperatively	As above
	Spinal cord injury	20 mg/kg/d for 2 wk	10 mg/kg/d for 10 wk	As above
Ibandronate	Osteoporosis	Prevention and treatment	2.5 mg daily or 150 mg monthly; IV 3 mg over 30 second bolus	CCr <30 contraindicated
Risedronate	Osteoporosis: men, postmenopausal women, glucocorticoids-induced	Prevention and treatment	5 mg/d or 35 mg/wk or 75 mg on two consecutive dates monthly or 150 mg/month. Not to exceed 10 mg/kg/d for 6 mo or 11–20 mg/kg/d for 3 mo.	
	Paget's disease	30 mg/d	30 mg/d for 2 mo; re-treat if needed with same dose only after 2 mo post-treatment evaluation	CCr less than 30: use not recommended
Tiludronate	Paget's disease	30 mg/d	400 mg/d for 3 mo; re-treat if needed with same dose only after 3 mo post-treatment evaluation	CCr less than 30: use not recommended
Zoledronic acid (Reclast)	Osteoporosis	Treatment and prevention	5 mg IV infusion yearly	If serum Cr greater than 4.5 consider risks
	Paget's disease	Treatment	5 mg IV infusion yearly	

*Doses in excess of 20 mg/kg/d or for longer than 6 mo have been associated with increased risk for fracture.

Another IV osteoporosis treatment and fracture prevention medication is **zoledronic acid** (5 mg), which is taken only yearly.

Although its labeled use is for treatment of Paget's disease, **etidronate** has been prescribed, as an off-labeled use, to treat postmenopausal osteoporosis and prevent further bone loss in early postmenopausal women. Dosage is 400 mg daily for 14 days, followed by 76 days of **elemental calcium**, 500 mg daily. This drug also has an off-labeled use in the treatment of **glucocorticoid-induced** bone loss in postmenopausal women. Dosage is 400 mg daily for 1 month and then 400 mg daily for 2 weeks every third month, plus **calcium** and **ergocalciferol.** None of the major guidelines mention **etidronate** for this indication.

Although the focus of this chapter section is **bisphosphonates, intranasal calcitonin** (Hodgson et al, 2003; SIGN, 2004), **calcium**, and **vitamin D** (Hodgson et al, 2003; ICSI, 2008; SIGN, 2004) have been recommended as complementary agents. **Calcitonin** is less effective than are the **bisphosphonates**, but it is useful for those who cannot take them. Use is limited to those patients who are more than 5 years postmenopause, those who cannot remain upright, and those who are not allergic to salmon. Alternative agents such as **phytoestrogens, synthetic isoflavones, natural progesterone cream, magnesium, vitamin K,** and **eicosapentaenoic acid** have also been subjected to limited randomized clinical trials. Findings from these trials have been inconsistent in their support of these alternative agents (ICSI, 2008; Whelen, Jurgens, Bowles, & Doyle, 2009).

Paget's Disease

All **bisphosphonates** are used to treat Paget's disease when the alkaline phosphatase is at least twice the upper limit of normal. They may also be used for those who are asymptomatic or at risk for future complications from their disease. Symptomatic Paget's disease is best treated with **etidronate. Editronate** slows accelerated bone turnover in pagetic lesions and, to a lesser extent, in normal bone. This reduced turnover is accompanied by symptomatic improvement, including less bone pain and decreased bone fractures. Initial dose is 5 to 10 mg/kg daily for up to but not exceeding 6 months or 11 to 20 mg/kg daily, not to exceed 3 months. The higher doses are reserved for times when lower doses are ineffective, when there is an overriding need for suppression of increased bone turnover, or when prompt reduction of elevated cardiac output is required. Doses greater than 20 mg/kg daily are not recommended. Retreatment for relapse is acceptable only after more than 90 drug-free days and when there is evidence of active disease. Dosage is the same as for initial treatment.

Treatment with **alendronate** using doses of 40 mg daily for 6 months, has produced highly significant decreases in serum alkaline phosphatase as well as in urinary markers of bone collagen degradation (*Drug Facts and Comparisons,* 2009). Retreatment may be considered after a 6-month post-treatment evaluation period. **Risedronate** treatment is 30 mg daily for 2 months. In patients with this treatment protocol, bone turnover returned to normal in a majority of the patients and no evidence of new fractures was found (*Drug Facts and Comparisons,* 2009). Retreatment requires a post-treatment evaluation time of 2 months. **Tiludronate** treatment is 400 mg daily for 3 months. Patients on this protocol had a reduction toward normal in the rate of bone turnover and a reduced number of osteoclasts. Retreatment occurs only after a 3-month post-treatment evaluation. **Pamidronate** IV is useful in patients with moderate to severe Paget's disease. For all of these drugs, indications for retreatment are evidence of active disease or failure to normalize alkaline phosphatase levels.

Patients with Paget's disease benefit from **supplemental calcium** and **vitamin D** if their dietary intake is not adequate. Consideration must be given to spacing the administration of the **calcium supplement** and the **bisphosphonate** to prevent reduction in bioavailability.

Heterotopic Ossification

When heterotopic ossification is a complication of total hip replacement, **etidronate** may be used at 20 mg/kg daily for 1 month preoperatively and 20 mg/kg daily for 3 months postoperatively. **Etidronate** is also used when this problem occurs secondary to spinal cord injury. The dosage then is 20 mg/kg daily for 2 weeks, followed by 10 mg/kg daily for 10 weeks, begun as soon as possible after the injury and prior to evidence of heterotopic ossification.

Other uses of **bisphosphonates** to treat the hypercalcemia of malignancy are with parenteral dosage forms and are usually reserved for use by specialists. These uses are not discussed here.

Rational Drug Selection

Alendronate, ibandronate, risedonrate, and **zoledronic acid** are approved by the FDA for prevention and treatment of osteoporosis in postmenopausal women, but some health-care providers have used **etidronate.** There have been no randomized, controlled studies comparing the FDA-approved drugs with **etidronate,** but the same bone mineral density has not been achieved by cyclic use of **etidronate** as has been achieved by the use of the other drugs. In addition, 3- to 4-year studies of **etidronate** are inconclusive with regard to fracture prevention.

For the treatment of Paget's disease, **bisphosphonates** may be used, but **ibandronate** does not have approval for this indication. **Etidronate** has been used longer for this indication and has midrange adverse drug reactions. Clinical trials reported in *Drug Facts and Comparisons* (2009), however, showed increased efficacy of **alendronate** over **etidronate** in suppression of alkaline phosphatase, with a response rate of 85 percent for **alendronate** as compared with 30 percent for etidronate and 0 percent for placebo. In addition, **alendronate** produced mild, transient, and asymptomatic decreases in serum calcium and phosphate as compared with **etidronate.** *Drug Facts and Comparisons* also reported a positive-controlled study conducted in Europe, with treatment groups taking 400 mg/day of **tiludronate** versus 400 mg/day of etidronate for 6 months. **Tiludronate** was more efficacious than etidronate in that trial. **Risedronate** has the highest adverse drug reaction profile. With consideration of all these factors, the drugs of choice appear to be **alendronate** and **tiludronate** (Table 21–4).

Monitoring

Before beginning treatment, rule out common treatable disorders that can also cause low bone density. These include hyperparathyroidism, vitamin D deficiency, hyperthyroidism, and renal disease. Tests for these disorders are serum calcium and albumin, 25-hydroxy vitamin D, thyroid-stimulating hormone (TSH), and serum creatinine levels, respectively. Serum creatinine levels are drawn prior to initiating therapy. Dosage alterations or contraindications to using specific **bisphosphonates** occur with serum creatinine levels above 2.5 mg/dL. Because **bisphosphonates** inhibit intestinal calcium transport, careful monitoring of serum calcium should be done during therapy. Phosphate, magnesium, and potassium should also be monitored because these electrolytes may be altered by **bisphosphonate** administration.

Elevation of alkaline phosphatase is a major indicator of Paget's disease and its reduction is an indicator of the efficacy of treatment. Alkaline phosphatase should be monitored prior to initiating therapy, at the end of each cycle of therapy, and prior to initiating any retreatment.

Measurement of bone mineral density is the most accurate predictor of fracture risk and efficacy of these drugs. Each 10 percent change below peak bone mass is associated with a doubling of the fracture risk for patients

Table 21–4 ◈ **Available Dosage Forms: Bisphosphonates**

Drug	Dosage Form	How Supplied	Cost Generic
Alendronate (Fosamax)	Tablets: 5 mg	Bottles 30 & 100	$88/30; $293/100
	10 mg	Bottles 30 & 100	$88/30; $293/100;
	35 mg	In UD 4 and 20	$82/4; $61/4;* $410/20
	40 mg	Bottle 30	$198/30
	70 mg	In UD 4 and 20	$82/4; $61/4;* $410/20
	Oral solution: 70 mg	In 75 mL UD4	$96/4 brand only
Etidronate (Didronel) Generic available	Tablets: 200 mg	In bottles of 60	$210/60
	400 mg	In bottles of 60	$420/60
Ibandronate (Boniva) brand only	Tablets: 150 mg	In UD of 3	$329/3
	1 mg/mL IV	UD	$494/dose
Risedronate (Actonel) brand only	Tablets: 5 mg	In bottles of 30	$108/30
	30 mg	In bottles of 30	$759/30
	35 mg	UD of 4	$101/4
	75 mg	Dose pack of 2	$110/2
	150 mg	In UD of 3	$329/3
Tiludronate (Skelid) brand only	Tablet: 240 mg	In foil strips of 56	$642/56
Zoledronic acid (Reclast) brand only	5 mg/100 mL IV dose	UD	$1,275/dose

Prices from *Red Book 2009* (113th ed.) AWP unless noted.
*Medicaid Federal Upper Price Limit. **On 2009 major store $4 price list.

with osteoporosis. Dual energy x-ray absorptiometry (DEXA) is the gold standard by which bone mineral density and therapy are monitored. Initial evaluation with DEXA can also suggest when a disease process other than aging is the probable cause of the bone loss. Once therapy has been established, DEXA is repeated 1 year later to determine progress. Whether to repeat DEXA at later dates is controversial. According to the American Association of Clinical Endocrinologists (AACE) (Hodgson et al, 2003), DEXA should be used for:

1. Women who are estrogen-deficient, to make decisions about therapy.
2. Women who have vertebral abnormalities or osteopenia detected on x-ray, to confirm the diagnosis.
3. Patients being treated for osteoporosis, to monitor for treatment efficacy.
4. Patients receiving long-term glucocorticoid therapy to guide therapy to preserve bone mass.
5. Patients with asymptomatic primary hyperthyroidism or other diseases associated with high risk for osteoporosis, to make therapy decisions.
6. All women older than 40 years who have sustained a fracture.
7. All women older than 65 years.

The ICSI (2008) adds the following risk factors:

1. Body weight of less than 127 lb or body mass index (BMI) less than or equal to 20.
2. Smoking and/or alcohol intake of more than 2 drinks per day.
3. Surgical menopause at younger than 40 years.
4. On hormone replacement for more than 10 to 15 years.
5. Premenopausal women with amenorrhea for more than 1 year.
6. Anyone with severe loss of mobility (unable to ambulate outside one's dwelling without a wheelchair) for more than 1 year.
7. Significant kyphosis or height loss of more than 4 cm (1.6 in.).
8. Solid organ or allogenic bone marrow transplant recipients.
9. Bariatric surgery patients.
10. Patients with chronic disease, such as rheumatoid arthritis, ankylosing spondylitis, inflammatory bowel disease, prolonged hyperthyroidism (or exuberant thyroid hormone replacement), and hyperparathyroidism.

Patient Education

Administration

Take the oral drugs first thing in the morning, at least 30 minutes prior to other medications, beverages, or food (60 min for **ibandronate**). **Etidronate** and **tiludronate** should be taken 2 hours before any food. **Alendronate**, **ibandronate**, **risedronate**, and **tiludronate** should be taken with 8 oz of plain water. Mineral water, coffee, orange juice, and other beverages greatly reduce absorption. If **supplemental calcium** or **antacids** are taken, the **bisphosphonate** must be administered at least 1 hour before these other drugs. If a daily dose is missed, skip that dose and resume taking the drug the next morning. For **ibandronate,** if the once-monthly dose is missed, and the next scheduled dose is more than 7 days away, the patient should take one 150-mg tablet in the morning following the date that it is remembered and then return to the every month schedule on the original schedule. Do not double doses or take later in the day. Remaining upright for at least 30 minutes after taking the oral medications (60 min for **ibandronate**) facilitates passage to the stomach and minimizes the risk for esophageal irritation. The IV forms of **zoledronic acid** and **ibandronate** can be taken without regard for food, but must be given by health-care professionals.

Adverse Reactions

GI distress is the most common adverse reaction. If needed, aluminum- or magnesium-containing antacids may be taken more than 2 hours after the **bisphosphonate.** If diarrhea occurs with etidronate, notify the health-care provider, who may divide the dose throughout the day to control the diarrhea. Female patients should advise their health-care provider if pregnancy is planned or suspected or if they are breastfeeding. The drug may have to be changed or stopped.

Lifestyle Management

Eat a balanced diet with adequate amounts of **calcium** and **vitamin D**. Supplemental **calcium** and **vitamin D** are typically needed. Participate in regular exercise; it is beneficial for cardiovascular fitness as well as preserving bone mass. Reduce or stop behaviors such as smoking and **alcohol** intake that increase the risk of osteoporosis. Because relapse is not uncommon, keeping follow-up appointments to monitor progress, even after the drug is discontinued, is important.

HYPOTHALAMIC AND PITUITARY HORMONES

A combination of neural and endocrine systems located in the hypothalamus and the pituitary gland mediates control of metabolism, growth, and certain aspects of reproduction. The hormones involved in these hypothalamus-pituitary-hormone axes are adrenocorticotropic hormone, corticotropin-releasing hormone, follicle-stimulating hormone, growth hormone, growth hormone–binding protein, growth hormone–releasing hormone, gonadotropin-releasing hormone, insulin-like growth factor 1, luteinizing hormone, luteinizing hormone–releasing factor, prolactin-releasing factor, prolactin, somatotropin-releasing factor, thyrotropin-releasing hormone, and thyroid-stimulating hormone. The reproductive hormones are covered in Chapter 22, the corticosteroid-related hormones are covered in Chapter 25, and the thyroid-related hormones are discussed later in this chapter. This section discusses the growth hormone axis. Drugs affecting this axis are often prescribed by specialists, and the role of the primary care provider is largely to monitor the drug and its place in the total treatment regimen of the patient.

On The Horizon — CLODRONATE (BONEFOS)

Research on using bisphosphonate adjuvant therapy to decrease the risk of bone metastasis in breast cancer is active, but the results are uncertain.

Pharmacodynamics

The hypothalamus-pituitary–growth hormone axis (Fig. 21–2) begins with growth hormone–releasing hormone (GHRH), which is secreted by the hypothalamus in response to decreased serum glucose levels in the body (hypoglycemia stimulates secretion, and hyperglycemia inhibits it). GHRH then binds to receptors in the anterior pituitary, resulting in the secretion by that gland of growth hormone (GH) (also called somatotropin). GH is a single peptide that attaches to receptors that allow it to pass through the cell membrane. Once inside cells, GH fosters protein synthesis, fat breakdown, and tissue growth. GH also causes hyperglycemia by decreasing glucose utilization by cells and increasing the rate by which glycogen is broken down into glucose. Both GHRH and GH have now been synthesized by recombinant DNA technology and

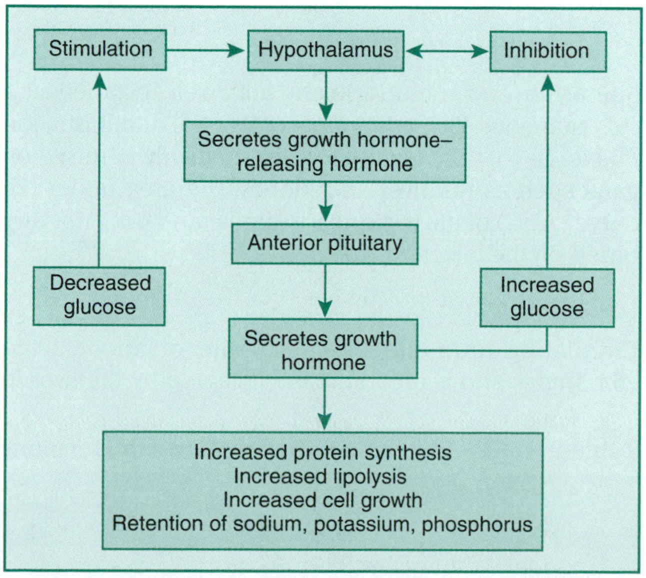

Figure 21–2. Hypothalamus-pituitary–growth hormone axis.

are available in drug form. They produce the same actions as the natural hormones.

The primary role of GHRH at this time is as a diagnostic tool for evaluation of children of short stature with subnormal GH responses to conventional stimuli in order to assess for dysfunction of the hypothalamus or the pituitary. It will not be discussed further.

Administration of **somatrem** and **somatropin**, results in an initial **insulin**-like effect, with increased tissue uptake of both glucose and amino acids and decreased lipolysis. Within a few hours, there is a peripheral **insulin** antagonistic effect, with impaired glucose uptake and increased lipolysis. These drugs also stimulate synthesis of somatomedins in the growth plate cartilage and the liver, resulting in increased linear, organ, and skeletal growth and increased cellular protein synthesis. Children with GH deficiency sometimes also experience hypoglycemia that is improved by administration of these drugs. Patients receiving these drugs may also experience reduction in fat stores and decreased mean cholesterol levels, but they are not used specifically for these reasons clinically. The retention of sodium, potassium, and phosphorus that occurs is also not a part of the treatment goal. Reduction of wasting and cachexia are desired effects when used in AIDS patients **(Serostim only)** (U.S. Food and Drug Administration, 2003).

In cases of overabundance of growth axis hormones (acromegaly), pituitary surgical interventions are primary interventions, but the recurrence rate sometimes requires the use of **somatostatin analogues** such as **octreotide (Sandostatin)** (Cozzi et al, 2006). These **GH** suppressant agents are also used in GI bleeds and cases of severe diarrhea in AIDS patients. The benefit of using **GH** for AIDS wasting is reversed if the analogues are also used. These high cost parenteral medications are not further discussed in this chapter.

Pharmacokinetics

Absorption and Distribution

Somatrem and **somatropin** are both well absorbed after subcutaneous (SC) or intramuscular (IM) administration (Table 21–5). They tend to localize to highly perfused organs, such as the liver and kidney. The area under the curve (AUC) of the two drugs is similar and does not vary based on the injection type or site.

Metabolism and Excretion

Circulating hormone has a half-life of about 20 to 25 minutes and is predominantly cleared by the liver. In the kidney, both drugs are filtered by the glomerulus, reabsorbed in the proximal tubule, and broken down within the renal cells into amino acids that return to the circulation. The total mean half-life of both drugs from administration to elimination is 3.8 to 4.9 hours. Active blood levels persist for up to 36 hours. Consistent with the role of the liver and the kidney in the elimination of these drugs, there is a reduction in hormone clearance in patients with hepatic or renal dysfunction.

Pharmacotherapeutics

Precautions and Contraindications

Somatrem and **somatropin** are contraindicated in patients with closed epiphyses and those with evidence of active tumor growth. They are used cautiously in growth hormone deficiency due to intracranial tumor because they increase the tumor growth. Patients with coexisting adrenocorticotropic hormone deficiency may experience increased symptoms of this disorder, therefore, **somatrem** or **somatropin** should be used cautiously with these patients. Serum levels of inorganic phosphorus, alkaline phosphatase, and parathyroid hormone may increase with **somatropin** therapy. Changes in thyroid hormone laboratory measurements have also occurred. This makes management of thyroid disorders more difficult. In addition, untreated hypothyroidism prevents optimal response to GH therapy. If GH must be used for patients with thyroid dysfunction, frequent monitoring of thyroid function and adequate treatment with thyroid hormone is necessary (*Drug Facts and Comparisons,* 2009).

Insulin resistance may be induced by **somatrem** or **somatropin** therapy. The drugs are used cautiously with diabetic patients and those with glucose intolerance or risk of metabolic syndrome. Close monitoring of glucose levels is critical.

The safety and efficacy of synthetic **growth hormones** have not been established in pregnancy and lactation. They are Pregnancy Category C and should be used only if clearly needed.

Adverse Drug Reactions

Approximately 30 to 40 percent of patients on **somatrem** and 2 to 4.7 percent of patients on **somatropin** developed persistent antibodies, making them less likely to respond to the drug. Other adverse reactions were rare and included pain at the injection site, hyperglycemia, hypothyroidism, and edema secondary to retained sodium.

Table 21–5 ▶ **Pharmacokinetics: Growth Hormones**

Drug	Onset (of Effect)	Peak (Drug in Plasma)	Duration (Drug in Plasma)	Bioavailability	Half-Life (Normal Renal Function)	Elimination
Somatrem, somatropin	Within 3 mo	7.5 h	36 h	75% (SC) 63% (IM)	3.8 h (SC) 4.9 h (IM)	By liver and kidney

Drug Interactions

Glucocorticoid therapy and **estrogens** may inhibit the growth-promoting effect of the synthetic **growth hormones. Anticonvulsants** may have more severe side effects. **Insulin** may lose its effectiveness.

Clinical Use and Dosing

Growth Failure Associated With Chronic Renal Insufficiency

Somatropin is used to treat children with growth failure up to the time of renal transplantation (National Institute for Health and Clinical Excellence [NICE], 2002). The weekly dosage is 0.35 mg/kg given SC. No studies have been done to date on its use after transplantation. GH is known to increase the side effects of **cyclosporine**, so it is typical 1 year after transplant for endocrinologists to evaluate continued need for GH. To optimize therapy for patients receiving hemodialysis, these patients should receive their injections at night, just prior to going to sleep, or at least 3 to 4 hours after dialysis to prevent hematoma formation caused by the **heparin**. Patients undergoing chronic cycling peritoneal dialysis (CCPD) receive their injections in the morning after they have completed dialysis. Patients undergoing chronic ambulatory peritoneal dialysis (CAPD) receive their injections in the evening at the time of the overnight exchange.

Long-Term Treatment of Growth Failure in Children

Who Lack Adequate Endogenous GH

Somatrem and all forms of **somatropin** (except **Serostim**) have been used for this indication. Dosage of **somatrem** is up to 0.1 mg/kg three times weekly, titrated to individual patient response. Doses in excess of 0.3 mg/kg have resulted in risks of known effects of excess human GH. Dosage of the various forms of **somatropin** varies by drug, with selected forms shown in Table 21–6.

Turner's Syndrome

Somatropin is approved for long-term treatment of short stature associated with Turner's syndrome. The weekly dose of **Nutropin** is 0.375 mg/kg or less, divided into equal doses three to seven times per week and given SC. Specific dosing scheduling is individualized based on patient and drug manufacturer. Introduction of **estrogen** to stimulate puberty should be delayed as long as possible for best terminal height achievement (Chernausek, Attie, Cara, Rosenfeld, & Frane, 2000).

Somatropin Deficiency

Patients must meet strict criteria before **somatropin** is prescribed, and tests related to these criteria are usually done by the endocrinology team. For children, the recommended weekly dose of **Humatrope** is 0.18 mg/kg, divided into equal doses and given either on 3 alternate days or six times per week SC. For adults, the recommended SC dose is started at 0.006 mg/kg given daily and increased to a maximum of 0.0125 mg/kg daily, based on patient response. Again, practitioners are cautioned to reference the dosing schedules of each individual brand, as they all vary.

Rational Drug Selection

Choice of drug is based on indication and other variables considered by the endocrinology team. Costs are significant and coordination with patient assistance and prior authorization of insurance programs is typically needed.

Table 21–6 ● **Dosage Schedule: Selected Growth Hormones**

Indication	Drug*	Initial Dose	Maintenance Dose
Growth failure related to chronic renal failure	Nutropin	0.35 mg/kg	0.35 mg/kg/wk (see note in text regarding hemodialysis)
Growth failure due to inadequate endogenous growth hormone	Protropin	0.1 mg/kg	0.1–0.3 mg/kg 3 times/wk; not to exceed 0.3 mg/kg
	Genotropin	0.16 mg/kg	0.16–0.24 mg/kg/wk in equal doses divided into 6–7 injections
	Humatrope	*Children:* 0.18 mg/kg	0.18–0.3 mg/kg/wk divided into equal doses, given on 3 alternate days or 6 d/wk
		Adults: 0.006 mg/kg	0.006 mg/kg/d
	Norditropin	0.024 mg/kg	0.024–0.034 mg/kg, given 6–7 times weekly
	Nutropin	0.3 mg/kg	0.3 mg/kg/wk
Turner's syndrome	Nutropin	0.375 mg/kg	0.375 mg/kg/wk divided into equal doses, given 3–7 times/wk
Somatropin deficiency	Humatrope	*Children:* 0.18 mg/kg	0.18–0.3 mg/kg/wk divided into equal doses, given on 3 alternate days or 6 d/wk
		Adults: 0.006 mg/kg	0.006 mg/kg/d

Many additional formulations available with unique dosing patterns.

Monitoring

Prior to initiating and throughout therapy, hepatic and renal function studies are done. Patients with thyroid dysfunction, diabetes mellitus, or glucose intolerance have their disease processes more carefully monitored, as discussed in the Precautions and Contraindications section.

Monitoring of bone age by x-ray is done to evaluate growth and to determine epiphyseal closure (typically age 14 or 15 in girls, 15 or 16 in boys). The schedule for this assessment is determined by the endocrinology team. Dosing is typically halted when growth is less than 2 cm over the previous year (NICE, 2002). Monitoring for increasing alkaline phosphates, hypertension, and acromegalic changes (in adults) is indicative of excessive dosing. Abuse of all of these drug formulations exists for illegal athletic performance enhancement and touted antiaging properties. Excessive requests for refills should be monitored.

Patient Education

These drugs are usually given at home by a family member or self-administered. Education is directed to both the patient and the person who will administer the drug. These are injected drugs. Information about proper use and disposal of needles and syringes and cautions against reuse of needles is important.

Administration

These drugs have specific reconstitution and storage requirements (Table 21–7). Storage for all of them is at temperatures from 2°C to 8°C (36°F to 46°F). They are not to be frozen. Each brand has a specific reconstitution formula, and the patient or family member should be taught that formula. Reconstituted vials are stable in refrigeration for 14 to 28 days, depending on the brand (except for **Serostim**, which is stable for only 24 hours).

The techniques for SC injection and site selection must be taught. The dosage schedule must be reviewed. **Somatropin** injections should be at least 48 hours apart. Because these drugs are given in weekly schedules, a calendar marked with the days of the week when the drug is to be given may be helpful.

Adverse Reactions

Adverse reactions are minimal. Patients and their parents, if appropriate, should be taught to report persistent pain at the injection site and edema. Because of the potential for hyperglycemia, patients should also be taught the signs and symptoms of this disorder and what to do, should it occur.

Lifestyle Management

Emphasize the need for regular follow-up visits with the endocrinology team to ensure appropriate growth rate, evaluate laboratory work, and determine bone age by x-ray.

EXOCRINE PANCREATIC ENZYMES

The pancreas is both an exocrine gland and an endocrine gland. The exocrine functions of the gland are related to secretion of enzymes into the gut for digestion. Disorders that decrease pancreatic function impair the production and secretion of these enzymes and, therefore, impair

Table 21–7 ◆ **Available Dosage Forms: Selected Growth Hormones**

Drug	Dosage Form	How Supplied
Somatrem (Protropin)	Powder for injection: 5 mg per vial 10 mg per vial	In carton of 2 vials and 10-mL multidose vials In carton of 2 vials and two 10-mL multidose vials
Somatropin (Genotropin) miniquick)	Powder for injection: 0.2-mg vial; 0.4-mg vial; 0.6-mg vial; 0.8-mg vial; 1-mg vial; 1.2-mg vial; 1.4-mg vial; 1.6-mg vial; 1.8-mg vial; 2-mg vial	Preservative free. In single-use syringe with 2-chamber cartridge. In 7s
(Gentropin)	Powder for injection: 1.5-mg vial 5.8-mg vial; 13.8-mg vial	In 1.5 mg Intra-mix 2-chamber cartridge with needle In Intra-mix 2-chamber cartridges with needle or without needle. In 1s and 5s
(Humatrope)	Powder for injection: 5 mg 6 mg 24 mg	In vial with 5 mL of diluents In vials with diluents In cartridge with prefilled syringe and diluent
(Norditropin)	Powder for injection: 4 mg and 8 mg Injection: 5 mg/1.5 ml; 10 mg/1.5 ml; and 15 mg/1.5 ml	In vials with diluents In cartridges
(Nutropin)	Powder for injection: 5-mg vial and 10-mg vial Depot: 13.5 mg, 18 mg, and 22.5 mg AQ: 10-mg vial	In cartons of 2 vials with 10-mL multidose vial of diluent In single-use vials with 1.5-mL diluent and needles In-2-mL multidose vials. In 6s

digestion. Two major disorders that are characterized by decreased pancreatic functioning are cystic fibrosis and pancreatitis. Bariatric procedures may also induce need for enzymatic supplementation.

Cystic fibrosis (CF) affects approximately 30,000 people in the United States. Once a disease of childhood, improved and aggressive management has resulted in a mean survival age of almost 25 years; 25 percent of patients survive into their 30s and 40s. Initially, this disorder is an obstructive lung disease, but plugging of the pancreatic ducts eventually results in pancreatic insufficiency, with resultant malabsorption of protein, fat, and carbohydrates.

Acute pancreatitis and chronic pancreatitis are both characterized by inflammation of the pancreas that results in swelling and obstruction of the pancreatic ducts. This obstruction leads not only to activated enzymes digesting the pancreas itself, but also to failure of the enzymes to reach the duodenum and thus the same malabsorption problems as occur in CF. Only bariatric surgery patients exhibiting malabsorption issues need enzyme supplementation.

Pharmacodynamics

The enzymes secreted by the exocrine pancreas are trypsinogen (protein digestion), chymotrypsin (protein digestion), amylase (carbohydrate digestion), and lipase (fat digestion). These enzymes are secreted into the bowel distal to the stomach because some of them are irreversibly inactivated by pH values of 4 or less. **Pancreatin (Ku-Zyme)** contains primarily amylase, lipase, and protease and **pancrelipase (Pancrease)** contains principally lipase and also some amylase and protease. These two drugs substitute for pancreatic enzymes and hydrolyze fats to glycerol and fatty acids, change proteins into peptides and amino acids, and convert starch into dextrins and sugars.

Pharmacokinetics

Absorption and Distribution

These agents exert most of their effects in the duodenum and upper jejunum with limited if any systemic distribution. Because they are permanently inactivated by gastric acid and pepsin secretion, problems in drug delivery by the oral route may occur. Enteric coating may prevent destruction or inactivation by gastric acid but inhibit enzyme delivery to the duodenum. For this reason, it is important to synchronize the delivery of the drug with gastric emptying, and the drug must be taken immediately before or with a meal.

Metabolism and Excretion

Because these drugs are simply enzyme delivery systems and there is limited if any systemic distribution, there is no metabolism or excretion beyond that which would normally occur in the body with the secretion of these enzymes.

Pharmacotherapeutics

Precautions and Contraindications

Pancrelipase is derived from a porcine source. Patients with hypersensitivity to pork proteins should not use this drug. They increase uric acid levels and may be an issue for those with gout or renal impairment. **Pancreatin** is derived from porcine, bovine, or vegetable sources, depending on the brand. Patients with cultural concerns or hypersensitivity to hog or beef protein may benefit from those products derived from vegetable sources.

These drugs are contraindicated during acute exacerbations of chronic pancreatitis. During this time, patients receive nothing by mouth to rest the GI tract and have no need for these enzymes. The presence of these enzymes during that time would only exacerbate the pancreatic disorder.

It is not known whether these drugs can cause fetal harm when administered to a pregnant woman. **Pancrease** and **Pancrease MT** are Pregnancy Category B; all others are Pregnancy Category C. Because there are no well-controlled studies on pregnant women, they should be given only if the benefit to the mother outweighs any risk to the fetus. It is also not known whether these drugs are excreted in breast milk and so should be used cautiously by nursing mothers.

Adverse Drug Reactions

High doses have been associated with GI symptoms such as nausea, cramping, abdominal pain, diarrhea, and colonic strictures. Extremely high doses may cause hyperuricosuria and hyperuricemia.

Irritation of the skin and mucous membranes occurs less commonly. Powder spilled on the hands may cause local irritation. The dust of finely powdered concentrates irritates the nasal mucosa and respiratory tract. Inhalation of airborne powder can precipitate an asthma attack.

Drug and Food Interactions

Calcium- and **magnesium-based antacids** may decrease the effectiveness of the enzymes (Table 21–8). The ability of **oral iron** to increase serum iron levels may be reduced by concomitant administration of **pancreatin** or **pancrelipase.** Alkaline foods destroy the coating of enteric-coated products, resulting in destruction of the enzymes by gastric acids.

Clinical Use and Dosing

Enzyme Replacement in Patients With Deficient Exocrine Pancreatic Secretions, Cystic Fibrosis, Chronic Pancreatitis, Pancreatic Insufficiency and Steatorrhea of Malabsorption Syndromes, and Postgastrectomy

The dosing and schedule are the same for each of these conditions. Although each drug is specified in lipase, protease, and amylase units, the drugs are prescribed in units of lipase. Children 6 months to 1 year initiate therapy with 2,000 U of lipase per meal (Table 21–9). Because the

Table 21–8 ■ **Drug and Food Interactions: Pancreatic Enzymes**

Drug	Interacting Drug	Possible Effect	Implications
Pancreatin, pancrelipase	Calcium carbonate, magnesium hydroxide	Decreases effectiveness of pancreatin and pancrelipase	Avoid concurrent administration
	Oral iron	Decreases the serum iron response	Avoid concurrent administration
	Alkaline foods	Destroys coating on enteric-coated products	Give enzymes first and separate administration by at least 1 h

only the two brands of **pancreatin** are available in doses less than 4,000 U and capsules cannot be divided, these two brands, or a tablet or powdered form of **pancrelipase (Viokase powder)** (0.7 g), are typically used for this age group. **Pancrelipase (Zenpop)** was approved in 2009 for children less than 12 months at doses of 2,000 to 4,000 per 120 mL of formula or incidence of breastfeeding. Capsules must be opened and sprinkled directly into the infant's mouth or on applesauce; the medication cannot be dissolved in milk or formula. Children 1 to 6 years initiate therapy with 4,000 to 8,000 U of lipase sprinkled on acidic foods such as applesauce or commercially prepared bananas or pears. Several brands of both drugs have dosage forms that can deliver this dose. Initial doses for children 7 to 12 years are 4,000 to 12,000 U of lipase. Initial therapy for adults is 4,000 U of lipase with each meal or snack (300 mg for every 17 g of dietary fat). Dosages may be increased as needed, based on patient response.

Postpancreatectomy and Ductal Obstructions Caused by Cancer of the Pancreas or Common Bile Duct

The dosing and schedule for these indications is 8,000 to 16,000 U of lipase at 2-hour intervals. In severe deficiencies, the dose may be increased to 64,000 to 88,000 U of lipase with meals, or the frequency of administration may be increased to hourly intervals unless nausea, cramps, or diarrhea occurs.

Rational Drug Selection

Cost

There are many available dosages and brands of these drugs (Table 21–10). **Pancrealipase** drugs with higher lipase units are more expensive, but are about as expensive as it would be to take enough of the lower-dose tablets to gain the higher dose. Given this fact, the dose per unit of lipase is about the same across brands. There are OTC tablets for **pancreatin.** With this drug, it is sometimes less expensive to purchase the higher-dosage brands when these doses are required than it is to double or triple the lower-dose brand.

Brand

It is important to remember that the various brands are not bioequivalent. Each drug varies in the number of units of lipase, protease, and amylase present. Despite cost variables, it is not possible to change brands solely because the dosage has changed. When it is necessary to change brands, the health-care provider should monitor the effect

Table 21–9 ◉ **Dosage Schedule: Pancreatic Enzymes**

Drug	Indication	Initial Dose	Maintenance Dose
Pancreatin, pancrelipase	Enzyme replacement in patients with deficient exocrine pancreatic secretions, cystic fibrosis, chronic pancreatitis, pancreatic insufficiency and steatorrhea of malabsorption syndromes, and post-gastrectomy	*Children <12 mo:* 2,000 to 4,000 units of lipase per 120 mL of formula or breastfeeding episode *Children 1–6 yr:* 4,000–8,000 units of lipase *Children 7–12 yr:* 4,000–12,000 Units of lipase Adults: 4,000–48,000 units of lipase with each meal or snack	Maintenance dose is within dosage range stated for initial therapy, based on end points of growth curves and minimized symptoms
Pancrelipase powder	Cystic fibrosis	0.7 g with meals	0.7 g with meals
Pancrelipase	Postpancreatectomy and ductal obstructions caused by cancer of the pancreas or common bile duct	8,000–16,000 units of lipase at 2-h intervals	Dose may remain same or be increased to 64,000–88,000 Units of lipase with meals, or frequency may be increased to hourly intervals unless nausea, cramps, or diarrhea occurs

Table 21–10 ◆ **Available Dosage Forms: Pancreatic Enzymes in Units**

Drug	Lipase	Protease	Amylase	How Supplied
Pancreatin				
Ku-Zyme	1,200	15,000	15,000	In bottles of 100
Kutrase	2,400	30,000	30,000	In bottles of 100
Pancrelipase				
Pancrease MT 4	4,000	12,000	12,000	In bottles of 100
Pancrecarb MS 4 Delay Release	4,000	25,000	25,000	In bottles of 100
Pancrelipase	4,500	25,000	20,000	In bottles of 100 & 250
Pangestyme EC Delay Release	4,500	25,000	20,000	In bottles of 100 & 250
Panocaps Delay Release	4,500	25,000	20,000	In bottles of 100 & 250
Lipram 4500 Delay Release	4,500	25,000	20,000	In bottles of 100 & 250
Ultrase	4,500	25,000	20,000	In bottles of 100
Creon 5 Delay Release	5,000	18,750	16,660	In bottles of 100 & 250
Zenpep Delay Release	5,000	17,000	27,000	In bottles of 12 & 100
Pancrelipase tab	8,000	30,000	30,000	In bottles of 100 & 500
KU-Zyme HP	8,000	30,000	30,000	In bottles of 100
Panokase tab	8,000	30,000	30,000	In bottles of 100 & 500
Plaretase 8000 tab	8,000	30,000	30,000	In bottles of 100 & 500
Viokase 8 Tab	8,000	30,000	30,000	In bottles of 100 & 500
Pancrecarb MS-8 Delay Release	8,000	45,000	40,000	In bottles of 100 & 250
PAN-2400	9,816	60,214	75,900	In bottles of 100
Lipram-PN10 Delay Release	10,000	30,000	30,000	In bottles of 100
Pancrease MT 10	10,000	30,000	30,000	In bottles of 100
Zenpep Delay Release	10,000	34,000	55,000	In bottles of 12 & 100
Creon 10 Delay Release	10,000	37,500	33,200	In bottles of 100 & 250
Palcaps 10 Delay Release	10,000	37,500	33,200	In bottles of 100 & 250
Pangestyme CN-10 Delay Release	10,000	37,500	33,200	In bottles of 100
Lipram-UL 12 Delay Release	12,000	39,000	39,000	In bottles of 100
Pangestyme UL12 Delay Release	12,000	39,000	39,000	In bottles of 100
Ultrase MT 12	12,000	39,000	39,000	In bottles of 100
Zenpep delayed release	15,000	51,000	82,000	In bottles of 12 & 100
Pancrelipase	16,000	48,000	48,000	In bottles of 100 & 250
Pangestyme MT16 Delay Release	16,000	48,000	48,000	In bottles of 100
Panocaps MT16 Delay Release	16,000	48,000	48,000	In bottles of 100
Lipram-P16 Delayed Release	16,000	48,000	48,000	In bottles of 100
Pancrease MT 16	16,000	48,000	48,000	In bottles of 100
Pancrecarb MS-16 Delay Release	16,000	52,000	52,000	In bottles of 100 & 250
Pancrelipase tab	16,000	60,000	60,000	In bottles of 100 & 500
Viokase 16 tab	16,000	60,000	60,000	In bottles of 100 & 500

Continued

Table 21–10 ◆ **Available Dosage Forms: Pancreatic Enzymes in Units—cont'd**

Drug	Lipase	Protease	Amylase	How Supplied
Viokase Powder	16,800	70,000	70,000	In 227 g
Lipram-UL 18 Delay Release	18,000	58,500	58,500	In bottles of 100
Pangestyme UL 18 Delay Release	18,000	58,500	58,500	In bottles of 100
Ultrase MT 18	18,000	58,500	58,500	In bottles of 100
Liprase-PN20 Delayed release	20,000	44,000	56,000	In bottles of 100
Pancrease MT 20	20,000	44,000	56,000	In bottles of 100
Panocaps MT20 Delay Release	20,000	44,000	56,000	In bottles of 100
Lipram-UL20 Delay Release	20,000	65,000	65,000	In bottles of 100 & 500
Pangestyme UL 20 Delay Release	20,000	65,000	65,000	In bottles of 100
Ultrase MT 20	20,000	65,000	65,000	In bottles of 100 & 500
Zenpep Delay Release	20,000	68,000	109,000	In bottles of 12, 100 & 500
Creon 20 Delay Release	20,000	75,000	66,400	In bottles of 100 & 250
Liproam-CR20 Delay Release	20,000	75,000	66,400	In bottles of 100 & 250
Palcaps 20 Delay Release	20,000	75,000	66,400	In bottles of 100 & 250
Pangestyme CN-20 Delay Release	20,000	75,000	66,400	In bottles of 100

*All drugs, including delayed release, are capsules unless noted otherwise.

of the new drug on end points. Treatment failures have been reported in cystic fibrosis patients when brand-name products were replaced by a generic or when one product was switched for another (*Drug Facts and Comparisons*, 2009).

Monitoring

Assessment of the efficacy of pancreatic enzyme replacement and the dosage of drug required is accomplished by determining which dose minimizes steatorrhea and maintains good nutritional status. The assessment of the end points in children is aided by charting growth curves. Other data include skinfold thickness, arm muscle circumference, and laboratory values such as albumin, cholesterol, glucose, hemoglobin, hematocrit, transferrin, and electrolytes. Because these drugs may produce elevated uric acid levels, serum and urine are tested for uric acid at regular intervals. Stools are monitored for fat content (steatorrhea), and the patient is told to report foul-smelling and frothy stools.

Patient Education

Administration

All doses are taken immediately before or with meals or snacks. Capsules may be opened and sprinkled on food. Capsules with enteric-coated beads should not be chewed. They may be sprinkled on soft food that is not hot and that can be swallowed without chewing, such as applesauce or gelatin. Swallow immediately because the proteolytic enzymes may irritate the mucosa. Following with a glass of water or juice or eating immediately after taking the drug helps to ensure that the medication is swallowed and does not remain in contact with the mouth and esophagus for long periods. **Pancrelipase** is destroyed by acid. **Sodium bicarbonate** or **aluminum-based antacids** may be used with preparations without enteric coating to neutralize gastric pH. **Calcium- and magnesium-based antacids** should not be used for this purpose because they interfere with drug action. Enteric-coated beads are designed to withstand the acid pH of the stomach. Enteric-coated formulations should not be mixed with alkaline food prior to ingestion, or the coating will be destroyed.

The various brands of these drugs are not bioequivalent or interchangeable. Use the same brand consistently unless told to change by the health-care provider. This is especially important for OTC brands. Variability in manufacturing standards and bioavailability has prompted the FDA to require all pancreatic enzymes to obtain approval from the FDA as of April 2010 or they will be removed from the market (U.S. Food and Drug Administration, 2009b).

Adverse Reactions

Adverse reactions are usually GI in nature. The lowest effective dose should be used. Report to the health-care provider nausea, stomach cramps, abdominal pain, or diarrhea. Dosages or brands may need to be changed if symptoms persist. Irritation of the skin and mucous membranes can also occur. Powder spilled on the hands may cause local irritation. Wash it off immediately. There is no other treatment required. The dust of finely powdered concentrates may irritate the nasal mucosa and respiratory tract. Inhalation of airborne powder can precipitate an asthma attack. The patient should tell the health-care provider whether he or she has asthma or any other chronic lung condition.

Lifestyle Management

Pancreatic enzyme replacement is only part of the treatment regimen. It will not be successful without adherence to the rest of the treatment regimen. Dietary recommendations depend on the reason enzyme replacement is needed, but generally the diet is high calorie, high protein, and low fat. For children with cystic fibrosis, the diet is high calorie, high protein, and high fat. The dosage of the enzyme replacement is based on fat content of the diet, so the amount of fat in each meal should be fairly consistent. Small, frequent meals are often better tolerated than three large meals, especially when the reason for the enzyme replacement is cystic fibrosis, postoperative gastrectomy, or bariatric procedure.

ENDOCRINE PANCREATIC HORMONES (INSULIN)

Insulin is a small protein molecule secreted by the beta cells of the pancreas. It is essential to the utilization of glucose by all body cells. Disorders of **insulin** secretion and utilization are found in diabetes mellitus, and the primary use of insulin as a drug is the treatment for this disorder. Type 1 diabetes, which accounts for 10 percent of total diabetes, results from an autoimmune destruction of the beta cells of the islet of Langerhans of the pancreas, which leads to **insulin** deficiency. Before hyperglycemia occurs, 80 to 90 percent of the function of **insulin**-secreting beta cells must be lost. Beta cell abnormalities are present long before the acute clinical onset of type 1 diabetes.

Regardless of the cause, the pathology is probably disequilibrium between the relative excess production of glucagon by the pancreatic A cells and the lack of **insulin** produced by the B cells. This ratio of **insulin** to glucagon in the portal vein—not the concentration of each hormone—controls hepatic glucose and fat metabolism, two major problems in type 1 diabetes. The recognition that the totality of the metabolic pathology is a factor of both of these hormones may eventually lead to a different approach to diabetes management.

Because there is a lack of **insulin** production by the beta cells of the islet of Langerhans, successful treatment requires **insulin** replacement. If the disease progresses without treatment, diabetic ketoacidosis (DKA), weight loss, and muscle wasting may develop. Chapter 33 discusses the treatment of both type 1 and type 2 diabetes, including the use of insulin. Figure 33–1 depicts the pathological cause of the various symptoms of type 1 diabetes. This chapter discusses **insulin** the drug.

Pharmacodynamics

Insulin is normally released from pancreatic beta cells at a constant low basal rate with intermittent bursts in response to a variety of stimuli, including stress, vagal activity, and high blood glucose levels. Figure 21–3 shows one mechanism for the stimulation of **insulin** release from beta cells. Once the **insulin** has arrived at an **insulin**-sensitive cell, it is bound to specialized receptors that are found on the cell membrane. These receptors foster changes within the cell membrane that result in translocation of certain proteins, such as glucose transporters, from sequestered sites within the cell to the cell surface. Once on the cell surface, the transporter facilitates the intake of glucose by the cell. Several hormonal agents such as **corticosteroids** lower the affinity of the **insulin** receptor, and others such as GH increase this affinity. **Insulin** promotes the storage of fat as well as glucose and influences cell growth and metabolic functions in a wide variety of tissues.

Action on Glucose Transporters

The GLUT 1 **insulin** transporter is found in all tissue, especially in red blood cells and in the brain. It is associated with basal uptake of glucose and transport of glucose across the blood–brain barrier. The GLUT 2 transporter is found in the beta cells of the pancreas and in the liver, kidney, and gut. It regulates **insulin** release and glucose homeostasis. Defects in this receptor are thought to contribute to the reduced **insulin** secretion seen in type 2 diabetes. The GLUT 3 transporter is located in the brain, kidney, and placenta and is related to uptake of glucose in neurons and some other tissues. The GLUT 4 transporter is located in muscle and adipose tissue. It is the transporter most associated with lowering blood glucose (BG) levels and is the primary influence in glucose uptake, especially during exercise. It is also the one most associated with **insulin** resistance in type 2 diabetes. GLUT 5 transporters are found in the gut and the kidney. They are associated with intestinal absorption of fructose.

The total number of **insulin** receptors can be down-regulated by such factors as obesity and long-standing hyperglycemia. This may explain why weight loss can be a significant factor in diabetes management.

Action on the Liver

Insulin acts on the liver to increase storage of glucose as glycogen and resets the liver after food intake by reversing the amount of catabolic activity. **Insulin** also decreases urea production, protein catabolism, and cyclic adenosine monophosphate (cAMP) in the liver; promotes triglyceride synthesis; and increases potassium and phosphate uptake by the liver.

Action on Muscle Cells

Insulin promotes protein synthesis by increasing amino acid transport and by stimulating ribosomal activity. It also promotes glycogen synthesis to replace glycogen stores used during muscle activity.

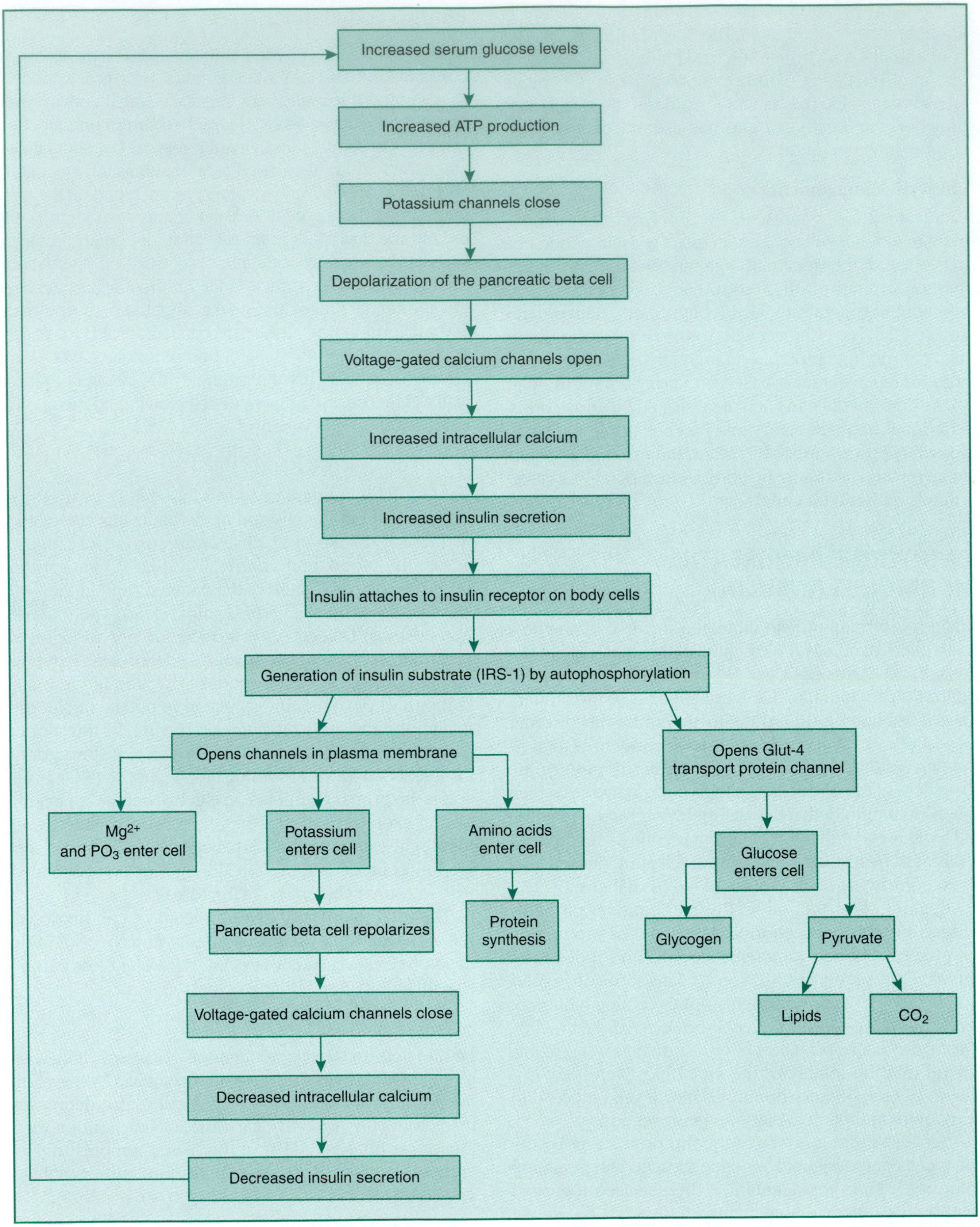

Figure 21–3. Mechanism of insulin release from beta cells.

Action on Adipose Tissue

Finally, **insulin** reduces the circulation of free fatty acids and promotes the storage of triglycerides in adipose tissue. This process is accomplished, in part, by suppression of cAMP production and dephosphorylation of the lipases in fat cells.

Administration of **insulin** acts on each of these receptors to produce the same effect as the naturally occurring hormone. Although it is given largely to control BG in patients with diabetes, that is not its only effect on the body.

Pharmacokinetics

Absorption and Distribution

Insulin is absorbed from SC or IM injection sites because it would be destroyed by proteolytic enzymes in the stomach if given orally. Absorption rate is determined by type of insulin, injection site, and volume injected. It may also be given via IV; the drug is placed directly into circulation without the need for absorption. **Insulin** preparations are divided into three types, based on onset, duration, and peak intensity of action. Table 21–11 presents each of these types. Because **human insulin** has a more rapid onset and shorter duration of action that pork or beef **insulin**, and because it is less antigenic, it has replaced animal **insulin.** Injection sites in the abdomen have as much as 50 percent more absorption than the arm, followed by the thighs and buttocks.

Insulin can also be absorbed via the nasal mucosa. Because **insulin** is a large peptide molecule, nasal absorption requires transport assistance and finding the best transporter has delayed the formulation of a drug for some time. Powdered forms of **human insulin** for inhalation are in trials (Cefalu, 2007; Rosenstock, Hollander, Chevalier, & Iranmanes for the SERENADE Group, 2008) and a gel form remains under study (D'Souza, Mutalik, Venkatesh, Vidyasagar, & Udupa, 2005). Pulmonary inhalation of insulin is not the sole answer to the problem of adherence by patients who do not want to inject themselves, but it has been demonstrated to be an effective mode of delivery and "the new insulin inhalers can be considered as a 'brick in the wall'" (Cefalu, 2007, p. 440).

Types of Insulin

Lispro is an **insulin** analogue produced by recombinant DNA technology. It is created by reversing two amino acids on the insulin B chain. This ultrashort-acting **insulin** has the same method of binding to **insulin** receptors, the same circulating half-life, and the same immunogenicity as **regular insulin.** Its onset of action, however, is much shorter—15 minutes—and it reaches its peak within 1 hour. Clinical trials have demonstrated that optimal time for preprandial injection of this **insulin** is 15 minutes rather than the 30-minute interval used for **regular insulin.** The duration of action of this **insulin** is not increased with a larger dose. It is compatible with **neutral protamine Hagedorn (NPH). Insulin aspart**, homologous with **regular human insulin** except for one amino

Table 21–11 ▶ **Pharmacokinetics: Insulins**

Drug	Onset (h)	Peak (h)	Duration (h)*	Elimination	Compatibility
Rapid-Acting					
Insulin aspart	0.25	1–3	3–5	In urine	No other insulin
Insulin glulisine	0.25	0.5–1.5	1–2.5	In urine	NPH
Lispro	0.25	0.5–1.5	2–5	Ultralente; NPH	
Short-Acting					
Regular	0.5–1	2–4	8–12	Very little unchanged insulin is excreted in the urine	
Intermediate-Acting					
NPH	1–1.5	4–12	24	Very little unchanged insulin is excreted in the urine	Regular, Glulisine, Lipro
Long-Acting					
Insulin glargine	1.1	5	24	In urine	No other insulin
Insulin detemir	1.3	3–8	15.5–23.2	In urine	No other insulin
PZI	4–8	14–24	36	Very little unchanged insulin is excreted in the urine	Regular

*Clinically significant duration of action is shorter than the pharmacokinetic duration of action. The clinically significant duration of action for short-acting insulins is approximately 4 h; for intermediate-acting insulins, it is approximately 6–8 h; and for long-acting insulins, it is approximately 12 h.

acid, has a rapid onset of action similar to **insulin lispro. Insulin glulisine** is created by replacing lysine and glutamic acid on the **insulin** B chain. Its profile is similar to that of **lispro.**

Regular insulin is a short-acting form whose effect appears within 30 minutes of injection and generally lasts for 8 to 12 hours. The clinically significant duration of action is slightly less, at 4 to 6 hours.

Neutral protamine Hagedorn (NPH) or **isophane** is an **intermediate-acting insulin.** The onset of action is delayed by combining the **insulin** with protamine. After SC injection, proteolytic enzymes degrade the protamine in **NPH** to permit absorption of the **insulin.** Its onset of action is 1 to 1.5 hours, and its duration is 12 to 24 hours, although the duration is usually no longer than 16 hours in actual clinical effect.

Insulin glargine is created by substituting glycine and arginine for other amino acids in **human insulin.** It has a unique AUC profile that has no pronounced peak, as small amounts of **insulin** are released slowly resulting in a constant concentration/time profile over 24 hours. This profile has resulted in improved glycemic control in large, diverse populations with long-standing type 2 diabetes. One large study (Davies, Storms, Shutler, Bianchi-Biscay, & Gomis for the AT.LANTUS Study Group, 2005) showed a low incidence of severe hypoglycemia even in a simple subject-administered titration algorithm. Another study (White, Chase, Arslanian, & Tamborland for the 4030 Study Group, 2009) found greater reductions in glucose variability for **insulin glargine** when compared with **NPH insulin.** Because variability in blood glucose has been associated with an increased incidence of diabetic complications, this is an important finding (Kilpatrick, Rigby, & Atkin, 2008; Marfella et al, 2009). **Insulin detemir** is an **insulin** analogue that differs from **human insulin** by a single amino acid deletion and the acylation of myristic acid to the B terminus of the molecule. These changes prolong absorption from the subcutaneous depot, resulting in a more prolonged, less peaked absorption compared to that of **NPH insulin.** It has a pharmacokinetic profile similar to **insulin glargine** (Porcellati et al, 2007). **Insulin** is widely distributed to most body tissues.

Metabolism and Excretion

Insulin is metabolized by the liver, the kidney, and muscle cells. Almost all of it is metabolized, and a very small amount is excreted unchanged in the urine.

Pharmacotherapeutics

Precautions and Contraindications

The only contraindications to **insulin** are hypoglycemia and hypersensitivity to any of the ingredients in the product. **Human insulin** derived by recombinant DNA technology from *Escherichia coli* bacteria or yeast rarely poses hypersensitivity problems.

Some studies with **human insulin** have shown increased circulating levels of insulin in patients with renal failure (*Drug Facts and Comparisons,* 2009). Because renal insufficiency and failure are common complications of diabetes, careful glucose monitoring and dose adjustments are needed for patients with renal dysfunction.

Studies have also shown increased circulating levels of **insulin** in patients with hepatic function impairment. Hepatic failure is uncommon in diabetes, but careful glucose monitoring and dose adjustments are needed for these patients as well.

Pregnancy requires careful diabetes management. **Human insulin** does not cross the placenta and is the drug of choice for pregnant women and those considering pregnancy. Most **insulin** is Pregnancy Category B; however, **insulin aspart, insulin glargine, insulin glulisine,** and **insulin determir** formulations have not been studied in pregnant women and use during pregnancy is on a risk/benefit basis. They are listed as Pregnancy Category C. Although human **insulin** is excreted in breast milk, because it is given by injection, it is not absorbed intact by the breastfeeding infant. Inadequate or excessive **insulin** treatment of mothers with diabetes, however, reduces milk production. It is not known if **insulin aspart, insulin glargine, insulin glulisine,** and **insulin detemir** are excreted in breast milk and so caution should be exercised in administering these drugs to nursing mothers. **Insulin** can be used safely in infants and children.

Hypothyroidism may delay **insulin** turnover, requiring less **insulin** to treat diabetes.

Hyperthyroidism may cause an increase in the renal clearance of **insulin.** Patients with either of these concurrent diseases require more frequent monitoring of glucose levels than other patients with diabetes when **insulin** management is required.

Insulin resistance, a suboptimal response of **insulin**-sensitive tissues (especially in the liver, muscle, and adipose tissue) to **insulin** occurs more commonly in patients with type 2 diabetes, but may occur in patients with either type of diabetes. The result is an increased rate of endogenous glucose production secondary to increased glucagon levels because liver cells do not receive feedback messages about the amount of insulin being secreted or the amount of glucose already in the bloodstream. Type 2 diabetes is also associated with down-regulation of **insulin** receptors in skeletal muscle resulting in insulin resistance. Patients who have this problem may require more than 1.5 U of **insulin** per kilogram of body weight each day in the absence of ketoacidosis or acute infection. Patients who may exhibit this resistance include obese patients; patients with acanthosis nigricans, ketoacidosis, or endocrinopathies; and patients with **insulin** receptor defects who may need to have their diabetes managed by an endocrinologist.

Adverse Drug Reactions

Two life-threatening adverse reactions are central to patient management with **insulin**: hypoglycemia and diabetic ketoacidosis. One is associated with too much **insulin** or not enough food and the other with too little **insulin**.

Hypoglycemia

Hypoglycemia may result from an excessive **insulin** dose, excessive work or exercise without eating, food that is not absorbed in the usual manner because of a postponed or omitted meal, or an illness that results in vomiting or diarrhea. It may also be associated with concurrent administration of another drug that increases the hypoglycemic effects of **insulin**. **Alcohol** is especially risky in this regard because it not only induces hypoglycemia but also masks the signs and symptoms of the disorder. Table 21–12 shows these drug interactions. Signs and symptoms of hypoglycemia include decreased levels of consciousness, hunger, diaphoresis, weakness, dizziness, and tachycardia. The peak of action for each type of **insulin** is the most likely time for a hypoglycemic reaction. This is especially important when more than one type of **insulin** is being used and the peaks of the different types of **insulin** coincide. Mild episodes of hypoglycemia can be treated with oral **glucose**. Adjustments in **insulin** dosage, meal patterns, or exercise may be needed. More severe episodes, with coma, seizure activity, or neurological impairment, require treatment with IM or SC **glucagon** or concentrated IV **glucose**. Additional carbohydrate intake and observation are necessary because hypoglycemia may recur after apparent clinical recovery.

Diabetic Ketoacidosis (DKA)

Diabetic ketoacidosis (DKA) may result from stress, illness, infection, or **insulin** omission. It may also develop slowly after a long period of adequate control of BG. Children with undiagnosed type 1 diabetes may present with DKA at the time of diagnosis. Signs and symptoms of DKA include drowsiness, dim vision, and Kussmaul's respiration. Indications of hyperglycemia that may precede DKA and give warning of its impending occurrence include polyuria, polydipsia, polyphagia, weight loss and fatigue, vomiting, dehydration, ketone odor to the breath, and abdominal pain. Treatment requires hospitalization and is directed at the acid–base and fluid imbalances that result, as well as the elevated BG. IV fluids, correction of the acidosis and hypotension, and low-dose regular **insulin** given SC or by IV infusion are required.

Drug Interactions

Many drugs either decrease or increase the effects of **insulin** because of their effects on BG. Table 21–12 shows these interactions. **Beta blockers** are especially problematic because they can increase **insulin** resistance, producing hyperglycemia, but can also mask most of the signs and symptoms of hypoglycemia. The one indication of hypoglycemia that **beta blockers** do not mask is diaphoresis, and people with diabetes who must take **beta blockers** for a concurrent disease or condition should be taught to test their blood sugar level whenever they experience diaphoresis.

Clinical Use and Dosing

Type 1

Because patients with type 1 diabetes mellitus (formerly called **insulin**-dependent) do not produce **insulin**, they must receive **insulin** replacement. A wide variety of regimens are used in this treatment, including **regular insulin** only delivered via **insulin** pump and mixtures of short-acting and intermediate-acting or short-acting and long-acting **insulin** given in multiple doses from two to four times daily (Table 21–13). Chapter 33 discusses the management of type 1 diabetes mellitus in more detail.

Table 21–12 ■ **Drug Interactions With Insulin**

Interacting Drug	Possible Effects	Implications
Acetazolamide, AIDS antivirals, asparaginase, calcitonin, corticosteroids, cyclophosphamide, dextrothyroxine, diazoxide, diltiazem, dobutamide, epinephrine, estrogens, ethacrynic acid, isoniazid, lithium carbonate, morphine sulfate, niacin, phenothiazines, phenytoin, nicotine, thiazide diuretics, thyroid hormones	Decreases hypoglycemic effect of insulin	Close monitoring of blood glucose levels is required if concurrent administration
Alcohol, anabolic steroids, beta-adrenergic blockers*, chloroquine, guanethidine, lithium carbonate, monoamine oxidase inhibitors, mebendazole, octreotide, pentamidine, phenylbutazone, pyridoxine, salicylates, sulfinpyrazone, sulfonamides, tetracyclines	Increases hypoglycemic effect of insulin	Close monitoring of blood glucose levels is required if concurrent administration

*Cardioselective beta-adrenergic blockers (those affecting only or mainly $beta_1$ receptors) are less likely to affect insulin's hypoglycemic effect and may be acceptable alternatives for patients who must take beta-adrenergic blockers.

Table 21–13 ● Dosage Schedule: Insulin

Drug	Indication	Schedule	Initial Dose	Comments
Insulin aspart* and Insulin glulisine	Type 1	Use in combination with IA or LA due to its rapid onset and short duration. *Start meal within 5–10 min of injection.*	50%–70% of total daily insulin requirement as aspart. Remainder as IA or LA insulin	May need increased basal insulin or more total daily insulin to prevent premeal hyperglycemia
		May also be used in insulin pumps	50% of total daily dose as meal related and remainder on pump	
Insulin glargine	Type 1	Use as single dose (once daily) at bedtime. Given with RA at meals	Glargine to = 50% of daily insulin dose at bedtime, then split rest of insulin dose with short-acting insulin at meal times	Calculate total daily insulin requirement at 0.3 U/kg/d
		As single dose at bedtime given with 70/30 mixed insulin	Glargine to = 50% of daily insulin dose at bedtime; 70/30 mixed insulin at bedtime and morning for rest of daily dose	
	Type 2	As single dose with oral agent	As single dose in morning with oral agent	See text for notes on use
Insulin detemir	Type 1	Use as single dose (once daily) at bedtime. Given with RA at meals.	Detemir to = 50% of daily insulin dose at bedtime, then split rest of insulin dose with short-acting insulin at meal times 0.1–0.2 units/kg in the evening	Calculate total daily insulin requirement at 0.3 U/kg/d
	Type 2	As a single dose with oral agent Twice daily	0.1–0.2 units/kg or 10 units	Dosage adjusted to achieve glycemic goals
Insulin lispro*	Type 1	Use in combination with IA or LA insulin due to its rapid onset and short duration of action	50%–70% of total daily insulin dose as lispro given 15–30 min before meals. Remainder as IA given 2/3 in morning and 1/3 in evening or as LA given in morning	Draw lispro into the syringe first if mixing with IA or LA insulin Inject immediately after mixing. Concentrations higher, duration shorter if given in abdomen
Regular	Type 1	Used in combination with IA or LA insulin due to its rapid onset and short duration of action	50%–70% of total daily insulin dose as regular given 30–60 min before meals. Remainder as IA given 2/3 in morning and 1/3 in evening or as LA given in morning	Also comes in U 500 for patients who need high doses (e.g., insulin resistance)
NPH	Type 1	Often used in combination with RA insulin. Comes in 70% IA and 30% RA mixed insulin and 50/50 mixed	Give bid with 2/3 of daily dose in morning and 1/3 in evening. Same protocol with 70/30 or 50/50.	See text related to mixing
	Type 2	With oral agent for type 2 patients who cannot control with oral agent and lifestyle modifications alone	10 U of NPH or Lente at bedtime with oral agent in morning	Individualized

RA = rapid acting; IA = intermediate acting; LA = long acting.
NOTE: Usual daily insulin requirement is 0.6–0.8 U/kg/d for adults and 0.8–1.2 U/kg/d for children during rapid growth. For drugs with*, daily insulin requirement is 0.05–1 U/kg/d.
These do not represent all possible combinations or scheduling protocols.

Type 2

Patients with type 2 diabetes (formerly called non–insulin-dependent) produce **insulin**, but they may not produce enough to meet the body's needs. They also have **insulin** receptor defects, **insulin** resistance, and altered hepatic glucose metabolism. **Insulin** is prescribed when their disease process cannot be adequately controlled by diet, exercise, weight reduction, and oral agents. Chapter 33 discusses the pharmacological management of type 2 diabetes mellitus.

Dosing

Average **insulin** doses are 0.6 to 0.8 U/kg of body weight per day. Obese patients may require more than 100 units per day. How the doses are dispersed throughout the day depends on the pharmacokinetics of the type of **insulin** used. For example, for bid dosing, two-thirds of the total daily dose is given in the morning and one-third in the evening in most cases. One way to give **insulin glargine** is to calculate the daily dose of **insulin** at 0.3 U/kg and start bedtime **glargine** at 50 percent of the total dose and split the remaining 50 percent with **short-acting insulin** before meals. For type 2 diabetics, **insulin glargine** can be initiated at a dose of approximately 0.1 U/kg while simultaneously starting an oral agent. A third possibility is to calculate the daily dose of **insulin** at 0.3U/kg and use **premixed 70/30 insulin** with two-thirds of the total daily dose in the morning and one-third of the dose in the evening. Table 33–7 lists the commonly used **insulin** regimens.

Mixing

Mixing **insulins** is common practice in diabetic regimens, but not all **insulins** are compatible with each other or make good combinations. Table 21–11 has a column that lists compatibilities. *Drug Facts and Comparisons* (2009) recommends that when mixing two different types of **insulin**, always draw clear **insulin** into the syringe first. Patients will have a consistent response if the method of mixing is standardized. All premixed formulations of **insulin** (**70/30 Novolin**, **70/30 Humulin**, and **50/50 Humulin**) contain NPH (percentage is first number) and **regular** (percentage is second number) **insulin**. These **premixed insulins** remain stable at room temperature for 1 month or for 3 months under refrigeration. NPH and **regular insulin** mixed in plastic or glass syringes may be stored for 1 week at room temperature and 14 days if refrigerated. With the increasing use of **lispro**, **an ultrashort-acting insulin**, it has been mixed with a longer-acting **insulin** to provide sustained insulin activity. It can be mixed with NPH immediately before injection without affecting its rapid absorption. **Lispro** is now available in premixed formulations Regardless of the **insulin** mixture used, the patient should standardize the interval between mixing the **insulins** and injecting them.

Switching Insulins

Each **insulin** has unique characteristics and neither brand of **insulin** nor type of syringe nor needle should be changed without monitoring by the health-care provider. The provider may want, however, to switch from an **insulin** formulation that has peaks in its action to one that does not (**insulin glargine**). If changing from a treatment regimen with an **intermediate- or long-acting insulin** to a regimen with **insulin glargine**, the amount and timing of the **short-acting insulin**, **insulin analogue (lispro)**, or **oral antidiabetic** may need to be adjusted. This is especially true for patients who have developed **insulin** antibodies and require high doses of **insulin**. In one clinical study with **insulin**-naïve patients with type 2 diabetes and already being treated with **oral antidiabetic** agents, **insulin glargine** was started at 10 U once daily and subsequently adjusted based on the patient's response to a total daily dose between 2 U and 100 U. In other clinical studies, when patients were switched from once-daily NPH to once-daily **insulin glargine**, the initial dose was usually not changed. If the change was from bid NPH to **insulin glargine**, to avoid hypoglycemia the initial dose of **insulin glargine** was reduced by 20 percent and then adjusted based on patient response (*Drug Facts and Comparisons*, 2009). Regardless of the drugs involved in the switch, careful monitoring of BG is required during the transition period.

Hyperkalemia

IV infusions of **glucose** and **insulin** produce a shift of potassium into cells and lower serum potassium levels. This treatment is usually reserved for hospitalized patients with very high potassium levels or those at risk for cardiac arrhythmias.

Severe Ketoacidosis or Diabetic Coma

Regular insulin given IV is used for rapid effect in severe ketoacidosis or diabetic coma. Because there is a high risk for inducing hyperosmolar coma with this therapy, these patients are also hospitalized.

Pregnancy

For treatment of gestational diabetes and for management of patients with diabetes who become pregnant, **insulin** is the drug of choice. **Oral hypoglycemic agents** are contraindicated in pregnancy. Any of the **insulin** treatment regimens used for people with diabetes may be used. Special care must be taken to avoid hypoglycemic episodes.

Rational Drug Selection

Method of Delivery

Concerning method of delivery, most patients with diabetes inject their **insulin** based on a specific regimen. Any **insulin** shown in Table 21–14 is appropriate for this use. Several rapid-acting formulations are now being used in

Table 21–14 ◈ **Available Dosage Forms: Insulin**

Drug	Dosage Form and How Supplied
Ultra-Short-Acting Insulin	
Lispro/Humalog	100 U/mL in 10-mL vials and 3-mL cartridges and 3-mL disposable pen insulin delivery devices
Aspart/NovoLog	100 U/mL in 3-mL PenFill cartridges and 10-mL vials
Glulisine/Apidra	100 U/mL in 3-mL OptiClik cartridge and 10-mL vials
Short-Acting Insulin	
Regular/Novolin R (human)	100 U/mL in 10-mL vials
Regular/Novolin R PenFill (human)	100 U/mL in 3-mL cartridge (for NovoPen)
Regular/Novolin R PenFill (human)	100 U/mL in 3-mL prefilled syringes
Regular Humulin-R (human)	100 U/mL in 10-mL vials
Regular/Humulin-R (Concentrated)	500 U/mL in 20-mL vials
Intermediate-Acting Insulin	
NPH/Humulin-N (human)	100 U/mL in 10-mL vials and 3-mL cartridges
NPH/Novolin-N (human)	100 U/mL in 10-mL vials
NPH/Novolin PenFill (human)	100 U/mL in 3-mL cartridge (for NovoPen)
NPH/Novolin Prefilled (human)	100 U/mL in 3-mL prefilled syringes
Mixed Insulin	
NPH and Regular/Humulin 70/30 (human)	100 U/mL in 10-mL vials and 3-mL cartridges
NPH and Regular/Novolin 70/30 (human)	100 U/mL in 10-mL vials
NPH and Regular/Novolin 70/30 PenFill (human)	100 U/mL in 3-mL cartridge (for NovoPen)
NPH and Regular/Novolin 70/30 Prefilled (human)	100 U/mL in 3-mL prefilled syringes
NPH and Regular/Humulin 50/50 (human)	100 U/mL in 10-mL vials
Aspart /NovoLog Mix 70/30	100 U/mL in 3-mL PenFill cartridges and 10-mL vials
Lispro/protamine sulfate 50/50 mix	100 U/mL in 3-mL disposable pen and KwikPen delivery device and in 10-mL vials
Lispro/protamine sulfate 75/25 mix	100 U/mL in 3-mL disposable pens and in 10-mL vials
Long-Acting Insulin	
Glargine (Lantus)	100 U/mL in 3-mL Opticlik and 3-mL SoloStar cartridges and 10-mL vials
Detemir (Levemir)	100 U/mL in 10-mL vials

insulin pumps. Specially formulated insulins can also be administered via inhalation. This latter form may address some of the issues of nonadherence associated with having to inject the medicine.

Response to Intermediate-Acting Insulin

Approximately one-third of patients have either a delayed or early response to intermediate-acting insulin. Although these patients may be placed on any insulin regimen that includes intermediate-acting insulin, in the design of the regimen, this response should be considered.

Half of these patients with altered responses are early responders who experience their peak insulin effect at the early time in the range for that insulin (e.g., 4 hours for NPH; 7 hours for Lente). They are at high risk to become hypoglycemic, often in the early afternoon after a morning dose. They should have their intermediate-acting insulin dose split into two-thirds in the morning and one-third before dinner. The half that are delayed responders experience their peak effect in the late time in the range for that insulin and may experience hypoglycemia in the late evening to early night hours. These patients require a reduction in intermediate-acting insulin dose and the addition of a short-acting insulin in the morning. These regimens are among those discussed in Chapter 33.

Level of Intensity of Control

Results of the Diabetes Control and Complications Trial (DCCT, 1993) indicate that tighter controls to lower BG levels significantly reduced the risk of complications associated with diabetes. This trial conclusively demonstrated, in patients with type 1 diabetes, that the risk for development or progression of retinopathy was reduced by 76 percent, for nephropathy by 50 percent, for neuropathy by 60 percent, and for cardiovascular disease by 35 percent. These benefits were observed with an average glycosylated hemoglobin (HbA_{1c}) of less than 7 percent. This has been further supported in other studies (Kilpatrick, Rigby, & Atkin, 2008; Marfella et al, 2009). The American Diabetic Association, Canadian Diabetic

Association, and the European Association for the Study of Diabetes now recommend that HbA_{1c} levels of less than 7 percent are desirable for most diabetic patients. The reduction in risk in the DCCT correlated continuously with reduction in HbA_{1c}. This relationship implies that complete normalization of glycemic levels may prevent complications. These benefits have also been demonstrated for patients with type 2 diabetes. DCCT patients on tight control used combinations of **short-acting and intermediate-acting insulin** given three to four times per day. Those on very tight control used **long-acting insulin** at night, and **short-acting insulin** before each meal or more frequently, based on self-monitored glucose measurements. A third group used an **insulin** pump. Patients who are intelligent, well motivated, and reliable can be taught to regulate their blood sugar with this degree of control. Less capable patients risk hypoglycemic reactions on this regimen and might not be appropriate candidates or may need higher fasting blood glucose targets than the more capable patients.

Presence of Complications Such as Retinopathy and Neuropathy

Patients with complications such as retinopathy and neuropathy may find it difficult to draw up their own **insulin. Premixed insulin** may assist with this problem. Choice of **insulin** is based on the commercial availability of **premixed insulin** or those that can be safely stored for some time after mixing. These complications are discussed in Chapter 33.

Type 2 Diabetes Mellitus Unable to Control

About 28 percent of patients with type 2 diabetes use some form of **insulin** to control blood glucose levels and limit complication risks (Agency for Healthcare Research and Quality [AHRQ], 2008). Patients with type 2 diabetes who are not controlled on oral agents and have postprandial hyperglycemia can have a **rapid-acting insulin** added immediately prior to meals. Patients who have fasting hyperglycemia can have bedtime **NPH** added. If they have overall poor control, intensive **insulin** therapy is used.

A systematic review of 45 research studies comparing the newer premixed **insulins** and the newer **insulin analogues** with other diabetic medicines for type 2 diabetes (AHRQ, 2008) have indicated risks and benefits for each choice.

- The premixed **insulin analogues** are better at lowering HbA_{1c} and preprandial blood glucose than are the oral **antidiabetic agents**; however, they have more risk for hypoglycemia.
- The premixed **insulin analogues** and the newer premixed **insulins** are associated with less weight gain than all of the oral **antidiabetic agents** except **metformin** and the **gliptins**.
- Long-acting **insulin analogues** appear to be more effective than premixed **insulin analogues** in lowering fasting blood glucose levels, but the reverse is true for lowering blood glucose levels after a meal with high sugar content.
- The newer premixed **insulins** are better at lowering HbA_{1c} and postprandial glucose than **long-acting insulin**; however, they carry a higher risk for hypoglycemia.
- Cost is a major factor with all the newer **insulin analogues**, regardless of formulation; they are significantly more expensive than either **regular** or **NPH insulins**.

The number of times the drug must be administered (complexity) was not discussed in this article, but the more complex the regimen, the greater is the risk for nonadherence. These data are further supported by studies conducted in 2009 (Buse et al, 2009; Heise et al, 2009; Umpierrez et al, 2009). Table 21–13 and Chapter 33 provide more information on dosing.

Monitoring

Two categories of monitoring are needed for diabetics: (1) control of BG and (2) signs of complications.

Control of Blood Glucose

For patients with type 1 and 2 diabetes, the goals of therapy are preprandial BG levels of 90 to 130 mg/dL, postprandial BG levels less than 180 mg/dL; bedtime glucose levels of 100 to 140 mg/dL, and HbA_{1c} levels of less than 7 percent (American Diabetes Association, 2009). Patients with comorbid diseases, the very young, older adults, and others with unusual conditions or circumstances may warrant different treatment goals. HbA_{1c} levels of 7 correspond roughly to a BG level of 150 mg/dL when it is referenced to a nondiabetic value of 6. HbA_{1c} values can be increased by iron-deficiency anemia, **alcohol** use, and lead toxicity and can be decreased by chronic blood loss, chronic renal failure, and pregnancy when performed by some techniques. These potential confounding variables should be considered in assessing changes in HbA_{1c} levels.

Preprandial BG can be assessed by self-monitoring as often as before every meal and at bedtime. Preprandial BG level assessment should be augmented by monitoring HbA_{1c}, because this value reflects the average BG level over a period of 120 days. Assessment intervals by healthcare providers are based on the degree of control, medication regimen, and other variables, such as financial resources and insurance coverage. For patients with type 1 diabetes, assessment of HbA_{1c} is usually done quarterly. It is done at least every 6 months for patients with type 2 diabetes. Intervals between testing are based on clinical variables, including the long-term degree of glycemic control. Chapter 33 includes more discussion of this monitoring.

Signs of Complications

The most common complications of diabetes are nephropathy, retinopathy, peripheral and GI neuropathies, hypertension, cardiovascular disease, dyslipidemia, and skin breakdown, especially on the feet. Monitoring guidelines and goals for lipid levels were added to the American Diabetes Association Clinical Practice Guidelines in 2005 and were updated in 2009. DKA may occur in patients with type 1 diabetes, and hyperosmolar hyperglycemic nonketotic syndrome may occur in patients with type 2 diabetes. All patients with diabetes may experience hypoglycemic episodes. Tight glycemic control with the use of **insulin** is one way to prevent or reduce these complications. All patients with diabetes should be taught how to monitor for and manage these complications. Providers need to be aware of the physical examination and laboratory evaluations that are appropriate to determine the degree of glycemic control and define associated complications and risk factors. Prevention, evaluation, and management of these complications as they relate to pharmacological therapies are discussed in the American Diabetes Association clinical practice recommendations. These updated recommendations were published in the January 2009 issue of *Diabetes Care.*

Patient Education

Administration

The number, type, and amount of daily **insulin** administrations depend on BG levels, diet, and exercise. The primary care provider must work with the patient to establish the diet-exercise-**insulin**-glucose monitoring regimen with active patient participation.

Each type of **insulin** has a specific pattern of onset, peak, and duration. **Lispro, Aspart,** and **glulisine** are injected within 15 minutes before a meal. **Regular insulin** is injected 30 to 60 minutes before a meal. **Insulin glargine** and **insulin detemir** are given once daily in the morning 15 to 30 minutes before the first meal. For **insulin suspensions** (NPH, NPL), ensure uniform dispersion of **insulin** by rolling the vial gently between the hands until the color is even. Avoid vigorous shaking, which produces air bubbles or foam. **Lispro** and **regular insulins** are clear solutions and do not require dispersion of suspended particles. Do not use them if they are cloudy, discolored, or unusually viscous, which may indicate loss of potency.

Vials of **insulin** not in use should be refrigerated in temperatures from 36°F–46°F. Extreme temperatures (greater than 86°F or less than 28°F) and excessive agitation should be avoided to prevent loss of potency, clumping, frosting, or precipitation. **Insulin** in use may be kept at room temperature < 86°F.

Insulin is also available in syringe pens. They come in 3-mL syringes, with each milliliter containing 100 U of **insulin**. Both single type and premixed **insulins** come in this formulation. Table 21–14 depicts these formulations.

Maintenance doses of **insulin** are administered SC. The patient must be taught the technique for drawing up the correct dose and for SC injection. Only **insulin** syringes should be used to draw up **insulin** dosages. Sites should be rotated, but because the abdomen, arm, and leg have different absorption rates, rotation should occur within one general area (e.g., the abdomen). As a general rule, do not administer within 1 inch of the same site for 1 month. **Regular insulin** given IV is reserved for severe DKA and diabetic coma.

Exercise increases the rate of absorption from injection sites and increases glucose recycling, both of which may result in increased risk for hypoglycemia if the dose of **insulin** is unchanged. Exercise should be planned and consistent within a treatment regimen.

When different types of **insulin** are mixed, always draw clear **insulin** into the syringe first. The order of mixing and the procedure used, including the model or brand of syringe and needle, should not be changed from dose to dose. Patients stabilized on a mixture of **insulins** should have a consistent response if the procedure is the same each time. **Premixed insulin** is available commercially and may be used if the type and concentration mix fit the patient. Some formulations cannot be mixed and patients should be so informed.

Most **insulin**, including premixed types, is stable at room temperature for 1 month and for 3 months if refrigerated between 2°C and 8°C (36°F to 46°F). Mixtures involving **lispro** that patients mix themselves must be given immediately after they are mixed. Other mixtures (e.g., **regular and NPH**) are stable for 7 days at room temperature and 14 days if refrigerated. Patients should be taught storage requirements for their specific **insulin**.

Different brands of **insulin** are not bioequivalent. The patient should not change brands without first consulting the health-care provider, who will arrange for close monitoring if the change is appropriate.

Adverse Reactions

The most common adverse drug reactions are actually an extension of the action of the **insulin**. Hypoglycemia can be life threatening and has a higher risk of occurrence as the intensity of therapy increases. The patient should be taught the signs and symptoms of hypoglycemia and the appropriate treatment for it, based on whether it is mild, moderate, or severe. Diet and exercise affect **insulin** dosage. Decreased food intake, increased time between the injection of **insulin** (especially short-acting formulations) and food intake, or increased activity may decrease **insulin** requirements and increase the risk for hypoglycemia.

Alcohol intake is especially dangerous for patients with diabetes. The effect of **alcohol** on BG is dependent on the amount ingested and the relationship to food intake.

Alcohol is not metabolized to glucose and inhibits gluconeogenesis. If it is ingested without food, hypoglycemia can result, even at levels that do not exceed mild intoxication. Not only can it cause hypoglycemia but also it can mask the signs and symptoms of the disorder. For patients using insulin, the Clinical Practice Recommendations (American Diabetes Association, 2009) recommend no more than two alcoholic beverages (one alcoholic beverage equals 12 oz beer, 5 oz wine, or 1.5 oz distilled spirits) with and in addition to the regular meal plan. The calories from this alcohol must be calculated as part of the total caloric intake and substituted as one alcoholic beverage that equals two fat exchanges. Reduction of or abstinence from alcohol is preferable.

Hyperglycemia is less immediately life threatening than hypoglycemia but still is an indication of poor control of BG, and it may be life threatening if it is high enough to produce ketosis. Patients should be taught to recognize early indications of hyperglycemia and the treatment for it.

Accurate monitoring of BG levels is central to managing dosages of insulin and to monitoring for adverse drug reactions. The patient should be taught fingerstick BG self-monitoring.

Lifestyle Management

Management of type 1 or type 2 diabetes involves diet, exercise, weight control, and self-monitoring of BG, as well as administration of insulin. Studies across age groups and ethnicities (Amati et al, 2009; Lawerence et al, 2009; Mayer-Davis et al, 2009; Mozaffarian et al, 2009) have shown that lifestyle management of risk factors makes a significant difference in the new-onset of diabetes and in its successful management. Patient teaching related to management of diabetes is discussed in Chapter 33.

ORAL DIABETIC AGENTS

Ninety percent of patients with diabetes mellitus have type 2 diabetes. The pathogenesis of type 2 diabetes is complex, and manifestations vary greatly across patients. Plasma insulin levels in type 2 diabetes may by low, normal, or high. The main physiological alteration in type 2 diabetes is insulin resistance, a suboptimal response of insulin-sensitive tissues (especially in the liver, muscle, and adipose tissue) to insulin. The result is four primary alterations in glucose metabolism: (1) insufficient production of endogenous insulin by the beta cells of the pancreas, (2) tissue insensitivity to insulin, (3) impaired response of the beta cells to BG levels, and (4) excessive production of glucose by the liver secondary to increased glucagon levels. Glucagon-like peptide 1 (GLP-1), an incretin hormone released by the intestine throughout the day and increased in response to a meal, stimulates insulin secretion by the beta cells and suppresses glucagon secretion by the liver. GLP-1 levels are decreased in type 2 diabetes.

These patients do not have an absence of insulin secretion, although some may eventually develop absence of insulin. If the pancreas is the major organ involved in type 1 diabetes, the liver and the incretin hormone system are the major organs in type 2. Type 2 diabetics have few and nonspecific pancreatic changes. Many years of compensatory hyperinsulinemia may occur before the onset of clinical symptoms of diabetes. Eventually the beta cell responsiveness to glucose stimulus diminishes and hyperglycemia prevails.

Adipose tissue also does not take up glucose in response to insulin, resulting in obesity. Increased visceral fat shows an inverse relationship with insulin sensitivity (Bloomgarden, 2003). Because the link between obesity and type 2 diabetes is firmly established, oral hypoglycemic agents and other oral antidiabetic agents should be considered in relation to their tendency to contribute to weight gain, to their being weight neutral, or contribute to weight loss.

Finally, type 2 diabetes is associated with down-regulation of insulin receptors in skeletal muscle. The gradual onset and progression of type 2 diabetes allows patients to adapt to the symptoms without realizing that the disease process is producing them. The complications noted in the discussion of type 1 diabetes are also present in type 2 diabetes and may occur more commonly in the latter.

Because there is sufficient endogenous insulin supply to inhibit the development of DKA, insulin is not mandatory, although it may be used later in the disease process or during acute illness or stress. Patients can, however, develop hyperglycemic, hyperosmolar nonketosis (HHNK). Oral hypoglycemic agents and other oral antidiabetic agents are effective in addressing one or more of the metabolic defects in type 2 diabetes; insulin is added during episodes when glycemic control is not possible with oral agents alone, as discussed earlier.

On The Horizon **INHALED INSULIN**

Inhaled insulin formulations continue to be developed. **Technosphere Inhaled Insulin** has been shown to be well tolerated and have excellent glycemic control with clinically meaningful reductions in HbA_{1c} levels. Postprandial blood glucose levels are also reduced (Rosenstock et al, 2008). This drug is in clinical trials.

SULFONYLUREAS

The first class of oral drugs developed to manage patients with type 2 diabetes mellitus was the sulfonylureas. They are true **oral hypoglycemics** and are useful only for patients with some endogenous **insulin** secretion. Although they are still important for that indication, their risk for hypoglycemia and their limited action on **insulin** resistance has resulted in their movement from first-line status to second line.

Pharmacodynamics

Sulfonylureas cause an increase in endogenous **insulin** secretion by the beta cells of the pancreas related to increased cAMP generation. They may improve the binding between **insulin** and **insulin** receptors or increase the number of receptors, thereby having a limited ability to improve **insulin** utilization by the tissues. Hypoglycemic effects appear to be due to increased endogenous **insulin** production and to improved beta cell sensitivity to BG levels or suppression of glucose release by the liver. **Sulfonylureas** also potentiate the effect of antidiuretic hormone and may produce a mild diuresis. They are useful for patients with type 2 diabetes who are not controlled with lifestyle modifications alone. They are efficacious in about 50 percent of patients with type 2 diabetes for total control of BG and in about 30 percent of patients for improved glucose levels without total control, but their use fails to continue to manage BG levels for the long term in about 36 percent of patients. They appear to be similar to **metformin** in lowering HbA_{1c} levels by about 1.5 percent (Nathan et al, 2009). The glucose-lowering effect of these drugs is rapid compared to some other **antidiabetic agents**, but the maintenance of glycemic targets over time is not as good as monotherapy with **metformin** (Nathan et al, 2009).

Pharmacokinetics

Absorption and Distribution

All **sulfonylureas** are well absorbed after oral administration and all except **glipizide (Glucotrol)** can be taken with food (Table 21–15). Absorption of **glipizide** is delayed by the presence of food in the gut. **Tolbutamide, glyburide,** and **glipizide** are more effective when taken 30 minutes prior to a meal. **Tolazamide (Tolinase)** is absorbed more slowly than the other **sulfonylureas**.

Although the mechanisms of action are similar for all **sulfonylureas**, the **first** and **second generations** differ

Table 21–15 ▶ **Pharmacokinetics: Sulfonylureas**

Drug	Onset (h)	Peak (h)	Duration (h)	Protein Binding	Half-Life (h)	Metabolism	Elimination
First Generation							
Chlorpropamide	1	3–6	25–60	99%	36 (prolonged by renal disease)	80% metabolized in liver; activity unknown	Excreted 100% in urine, renal elimination may be hastened by increased urine pH
Tolazamide	4–6	1–6	12–24	99%	7	Metabolized in liver to several mildly active metabolites	Excreted 100% in urine
Tolbutamide	1	4–6	6–12	99%	4.5–6.5	Oxidized in liver to inactive metabolites	Excreted 100% in urine
Second Generation							
Glipizide	1–1.5	1–2	10–16	99%	2–4	Metabolized in liver to inactive metabolites	Excreted 80%–85% in urine
Glyburide				99%		Metabolized in liver to weakly active metabolites	Excreted as metabolites in bile and urine, approximately 50% by each route
Nonmicronized	2–4		24		10		
Micronized	1	1.5–3	24		4		
Glimepiride	2	2–3	24	99.5%	5	Completely metabolized by liver	Excreted 60% in urine and 40% in feces

UK = unknown.

in absorption. **Second generation** compounds are more nonpolar and lipophilic. Therapeutically effective doses and serum concentrations are lower because of their intrinsic potency and ability to cross plasma membranes. All **sulfonylureas** are highly bound to plasma proteins, especially albumin, but the **first generation** binding is ionic whereas the **second generation** binding is not. Because they have ionic bonds, **first generation** drugs are more likely to be displaced from their binding sites by drugs that competitively bind to proteins (e.g., **warfarin, phenylbutazone).** Displacement would result in a greater hypoglycemic effect and may account for the increased risk for hypoglycemia found with **first generation** drugs.

Chlorpropamide and **tolbutamide** enter breast milk. **Glyburide (DiaBeta)** reaches high concentrations in bile and crosses the placenta.

Metabolism and Excretion

All **sulfonylureas** are metabolized in the liver to active or inactive metabolites. The hypoglycemic effects of these drugs may be prolonged by severe liver disease because of reduced metabolism. Differences exist among the **sulfonylureas** in the duration of hypoglycemic effects, in part because of their metabolism. **Tolbutamide** is short acting because it is rapidly metabolized to an inactive metabolite by the liver. **Tolazamide** has two active metabolites that are less potent than the parent compound.

All **sulfonylureas** are excreted primarily in the urine; **first generation** are excreted 100 percent and **second generation** has both urine and feces elimination routes. **Glyburide** is excreted as metabolites in bile and urine, approximately 50 percent by each route. The renal elimination of **chlorpropamide** may be sensitive to changes in urine pH, with urinary alkalinization hastening its excretion. The half-life of this drug is prolonged in renal disease.

Pharmacotherapeutics

Precautions and Contraindications

All **sulfonylureas** are contraindicated for patients with hypersensitivity to the drugs or the compounds in which they are mixed. Cross-sensitivity may occur with other **sulfonamides**, including **thiazide diuretics**.

Although the **sulfonylureas** are listed as Pregnancy Category C (**glyburide** is Pregnancy Category B), because abnormal blood glucose levels during pregnancy may be associated with a higher incidence of congenital abnormalities, **insulin** is the drug of choice for management of diabetes during pregnancy, and **oral hypoglycemic agents** should not be used. All **sulfonylureas** except **glyburide** are teratogenic in animals. There are no adequate studies in pregnant women. Prolonged severe hypoglycemia has occurred in neonates born to mothers on a **sulfonylurea** at the time of delivery. If these drugs must be used during pregnancy, discontinue use 2 to 4 weeks before the expected delivery date.

Chlorpropamide and **tolbutamide** are known to enter breast milk; it is not known if other **sulfonylureas** are also excreted in breast milk. Because of the potential for hypoglycemic reactions in nursing infants, **sulfonylureas** are contraindicated in nursing mothers. Safety and efficacy of these drugs in children have not been established; however, with the increased incidence of type 2 diabetes in children, studies may be conducted to address the possible use of these drugs in children.

Other conditions in which **sulfonylureas** should not be used include type 1 diabetes; DKA or diabetic coma; and uncontrolled infection, burns, or trauma. Patients with adrenal or pituitary insufficiency are especially susceptible to hypoglycemia, and **sulfonylureas** should be used cautiously and patients monitored more frequently if they have these comorbid conditions. Severe hepatic impairment may cause inadequate hepatic release of glucose in response to hypoglycemia. Renal impairment may cause decreased elimination, leading to accumulation of these drugs and resulting in hypoglycemia. All **sulfonylureas** should be used with extreme caution for patients with hepatic or renal impairment, and liver and renal function should be monitored frequently if they must be used.

Older adults and debilitated patients are particularly susceptible to the hypoglycemic action of **sulfonylureas** (Nathan et al, 2009), and the signs and symptoms of hypoglycemia may be difficult to recognize. **Long-acting agents** should be avoided, and **short-acting agents** should be used with caution with these patients.

A boldfaced warning in all **sulfonylurea** material states that the administration of **oral hypoglycemic** drugs has been reported to be associated with increased cardiovascular mortality as compared to treatment with diet alone or diet plus **insulin**. This warning is based on the study conducted by the University Group Diabetes Program. Patients who were treated for 5 to 8 years with diet plus **tolbutamide** had a rate of cardiovascular mortality approximately 2.5 times that of patients treated with diet alone. A significant increase in total mortality was not observed. Although only one drug in the **sulfonylurea** class was shown to produce this problem, this warning was extended to the entire class because of their close similarities in mode of action and chemical structure. These concerns were not substantiated by the UK Prospective Diabetes Study (UKPDS), or Action in Diabetes and Vascular Disease: Preterax and Diamicron MR Controlled Evaluation (ADVANCE) studies (Nathan et al, 2009) but the warning has remained.

Adverse Drug Reactions

All **sulfonylureas** may produce severe hypoglycemia. **Second generation drugs** are less likely than **first generation drugs** to have this adverse reaction. Others at high risk have been discussed in the Precautions and

Contraindications section. Hypoglycemia may be difficult to recognize in patients who are concurrently taking **beta blockers** because these drugs mask the signs and symptoms of hypoglycemia, with the exception of diaphoresis. Hypoglycemia is also more likely when caloric intake is reduced, after severe or prolonged exercise, when **alcohol** is consumed, or when more than one glucose-lowering agent is used.

Weight gain of approximately 2 kg is common following the initiation of **sulfonylurea** therapy (Nathan et al, 2009). The relationship of poor weight control to less than optimal diabetes management has been discussed in other sections.

Gastrointestinal disturbances (nausea, epigastric fullness, and heartburn) are the most common adverse reactions. They tend to be dose related and disappear when the dose is reduced. Diarrhea has been associated with **glipizide** use; taste alteration has been associated with **tolbutamide** use. Cholestatic jaundice is rare but requires discontinuation of the drug.

Dermatological reactions include rashes, pruritus, erythema, and urticaria. These tend to be transient and may disappear despite continued use of the drug. Photosensitivity can also occur, and patients should use sunblock and wear covering clothing when exposed to sunlight.

Syndrome of inappropriate secretion of antidiuretic hormone (SIADH) has occurred after administration of **sulfonylureas**, especially with patients who also have congestive heart failure or hepatic cirrhosis. These drugs stimulate ADH release, augmenting hypothalamic-pituitary release of ADH. The result is excessive water retention and dilutional hyponatremia. **Glipizide**, **tolazamide**, and **glyburide** are mildly diuretic.

Hemolytic anemia, agranulocytosis, leukopenia, and thrombocytopenia have occurred but are rare. Patients should have initial and annual complete blood counts done.

The increased **insulin** secretion generated by **sulfonylureas** has been associated with weight gain and hyperinsulinemia. Combination with **metformin** (**Glucophage**) reduces these adverse effects.

Drug Interactions

Sulfonylureas interact with a large number of drugs that either increase or decrease their hypoglycemic effect (Table 21–16). **Alcohol** interacts with these drugs to produce a disulfiram-like syndrome, characterized by facial flushing and occasional breathlessness but without the nausea, vomiting, and hypotension seen in a true alcohol–disulfiram reaction. This reaction occurs in about 33 percent of patients concurrently ingesting **alcohol** and **chlorpropamide**. It is uncertain whether this reaction occurs with **glyburide** and **glipizide**. No cases have been reported with **glimepiride** (**Amaryl**).

Clinical Use and Dosing

Type 2 Diabetes Mellitus

Both **first and second generation sulfonylureas** are used to treat type 2 diabetes. They are effective as add-on therapy with patients who have previously used diet, exercise, weight control, and **metformin**. Equivalent therapeutic doses vary from 1 mg to 1,000 mg, depending on the drug (Table 21–17). **Micronized glyburide** 3-mg tablets provide serum concentrations that are not bioequivalent to those from the conventional formulation group. When transferring patients from any **sulfonylurea** to **micronized glyburide**, the dose must be retitrated. Although all the drugs are listed as once-daily doses, many of the drugs work equally well when the daily dose is divided and given bid, especially when higher doses are required. The dose is highly individualized, based on BG

Table 21–16 ■ Drug Interactions: Sulfonylureas

Drug	Interacting Drug	Possible Effect	Implications
All sulfonylureas	Androgens, anticoagulants,* chloramphenicol, fluconazole, gemfibrozil, histamine$_2$ blockers, magnesium salts, methyldopa, MAO inhibitors, NSAIDs (except diclofenac), phenylbutazone, probenecid, salicylates, sulfonamides, tricyclic antidepressants, urinary acidifiers	Enhance the hypoglycemic effect of the sulfonylurea	Avoid concurrent administration or monitor blood glucose levels closely if drug must be given
All sulfonylureas	Beta-adrenergic blockers, cholestyramine, diazoxide, hydantoins, rifampin, thiazide diuretics, urinary alkalinizers	Decrease the hypoglycemic effect of the sulfonylurea	Avoid concurrent administration or monitor blood glucose levels closely
Glimepiride*	In addition to drugs with all sulfonylureas: corticosteroids, phenothiazines, thyroid products, estrogens, oral contraceptives, nicotinic acid, sympathomimetics, and isoniazid	May cause loss of glucose control because these drugs can cause hyperglycemia	If concurrently administered, monitor closely for loss of glucose control; when they are withdrawn, monitor closely for hypoglycemia

The changes in prothrombin time/international normalized ratio (PT/INR) were so small that they are unlikely to be clinically significant.
*Concurrent administration of glimepiride and warfarin did not alter the pharmacokinetic properties of warfarin.

Table 21–17 ● **Dosage Schedule: Sulfonylureas**

Drug	Initial Dose	Maintenance Dose	Maximum Dose
First Generation			
Chlorpropamide	Moderately severe, middle-aged stable adults: 250 mg Older adults: 100–125 mg Severe disease: 250 mg	250 mg/d before morning meal 100–250 mg/d before morning meal 500 mg/d before morning meal	750 mg/d
Tolazamide	100 mg	If fasting blood glucose (FBS) less than 200 mg/dL give 100 mg/d before morning meal If FBS more than 200 mg/dL give 250 mg/d before morning meal If patient malnourished, underweight, or elderly, give 100 mg/d before morning meal If more than 500 mg/d, divide dose and give bid before morning and evening meal	1,000 mg/d
Tolbutamide	1,000 mg	500–2,000 mg/d, divide dose and give bid before morning and evening meal	2,000 mg/d
Second Generation			
Glipizide			
Glipizide (G)	5 mg	5–15 mg/d 30 min before morning meal	40 mg/d
Glucotrol (B)	Older adults, liver disease: 2.5 mg	15–40 mg/d. Doses more than 15 mg/day: divide and give bid before morning and evening meal; adjust doses in 2.5–5 mg increments several days apart	
Glipizide XL (G) Glucotrol XL (B)	5 mg	10–20 mg/d 30 min before morning meal; adjust doses in 2.5–5 mg increments several days apart	40 mg/d
Glyburide			
Glyburide (G) DiaBeta (B)(Generic available in both micronized and non-micronized formulations)	2.5 mg	1.25–20 mg/d before morning meal. Dose more than 10 mg/d: divide and give bid; adjust dose in increments of 2.5 mg at weekly intervals	12 mg/d for micronized; 20 mg/d for non-micronized
Glynase (B) (Micronized formulation)	1.5 mg	0.75–6 mg/d before morning meal. Dose more than 10 mg/d: divide and give bid before morning and evening meal; adjust dose in increments of 1.5 mg at weekly intervals	12 mg/d
Glimepiride			
Glimepiride (G) Amaryl (B)	1 mg	1–4 mg/d before morning meal. After reaching 2-mg dose, increase in increments of no more than 2 mg at 1–2 wk intervals	8 mg/d

readings. Start with the lowest dose and increase every 4 to 7 days, based on glucose control. In general, one-half the maximum dose is usually the maximally efficient dose for glucose control. If the blood glucose level goal is not achieved on one-half the maximum dose, consider adding a drug from a different class.

Neurogenic Diabetes Insipidus

For neurogenic diabetes insipidus, **chlorpropamide** in doses of 200 mg to 500 mg has been used. This is an off-labeled use.

Rational Drug Selection

Age

Chlorpropamide and **glyburide** should be avoided in older adults. They are associated with more severe hypoglycemia in this age group (Nathan et al, 2009). Use a shorter-acting agent such as **glipizide. Chlorpropamide** should be suitable for a young adult patient with no renal dysfunction, on no other medication, and not using alcohol.

Sulfonylureas are not currently approved for use in children, although studies in the pediatric population with **second generation agents** are ongoing. Pediatric endocrinologists have used them with **metformin**, when monotherapy with **metformin** has been unsuccessful. Referral to a pediatric endocrinologist may be necessary.

Cost

The most expensive drug is **chlorpropamide**, the remaining **sulfonylureas** are all less expensive, with generic brands less expensive and brand names more expensive. Among the brand names, **Amaryl (glimepiride)** is the least expensive and compares favorably with generic forms of the other drugs in terms of cost. Table 21–18 includes available dosage forms with the cost index for each of these drugs. Cost in retail dollars is presented for **second generation** brand-name drugs.

Concurrent Disease

In the presence of renal impairment, **glipizide** and **tolbutamide** are reasonable choices because they are oxidized in the liver to inactive metabolites. **Glyburide** is also a reasonable choice because 50 percent of it is excreted in bile, which gives an alternative route for excretion. **Tolazamide** is also safe to use, with creatinine clearance (CCr) less than 30 mL/min.

Taking Multiple Medications

Second generation sulfonylureas are best for patients who are taking multiple medications to minimize potential drug interactions. **Second generation sulfonylureas** also have the advantage of once-daily administration, thereby reducing the complexity of the drug regimen and improving adherence. Among this group of drugs, **glimepiride** binds to different **insulin** receptors than do other **sulfonylureas** and may be effective when others are not. It is also associated with a lower incidence of hypoglycemic reactions.

Concurrent Administration With Insulin

Sulfonylureas have been concurrently administered with **insulin** with some success for patients who are not

Table 21–18 ◆ Available Dosage Forms: Sulfonylureas

Drug	Dosage Form	Cost Index	Cost
Chlorpropamide (G) (100-mg tablet * and **)	100 mg in 100-, 250-, 500-, and 1,000-tablet bottles	1	
	250 mg in 100-, 500-, and 1,000-tablet bottles	2	
Glimepiride (G)* and **	1 mg in 30-, 100-, 500-, and 1,000-tablet bottles	0.2	$10/100 (G) $61/100 (B)
	2 mg in 30-, 100-, 500-, and 1,000-tablet bottles	0.4	$10/100 (G)/100 $96/100 (B)
	4 mg in 30-, 100-, 250-, 500-, and 1,000-tablet bottles	0.7	$10/100 (G) $175/100 (B)
Amaryl (B) (glimepiride)	1 mg in 100-tablet bottle		$61.22/100
	2 mg in 100-tablet bottle		$95.54/100
	4 mg in 100-tablet bottle		$174.78/100
Glipizide (G) * and **	5 mg in 100-, 500-, and 1,000-tablet bottles	0.3	$19.98/100 (G)
	10 mg in 100-, 500-, and 1,000-tablet bottles	0.6	$21.66/100 (G)
Glucotrol (B)	5 mg (scored) in 100- and 500-tablet bottles	0.3	$74/100 (B)
	10 mg (scored) in 100- and 500-tablet bottles	0.6	$120/100 (B)
Glipizide XL	2.5 mg in bottles of 30		$35/90
	5 mg in 100- and 500-tablet bottles	0.3	$35/90
	10 mg in 100- and 500-tablet bottles	0.5	$60/90
Glucotrol XL (B)	2.5 mg in 30-tablet bottles		$63/90 (B)
	5 mg in 100- and 500-tablet bottles		$63/90 (B)
	10 mg in 100- and 500-tablet bottles		$105/90 (B)
Glipizide/ Metformin	2.5 mg/250 mg in 100-tablet bottles		UK
	2.5 mg/500 mg in 100-tablet bottles		$125/100
	5 mg/500 mg in 100-tablet bottles		$106.65/100
Metaglip (B)	2.5 mg/250 mg in 100-tablet bottles		$108/100 (B)
	2.5 mg/500 mg in 100-tablet bottles		UK
	5 mg/500 mg in 100-tablet bottles		$111/100 (B)

Table 21–18 ◈ **Available Dosage Forms: Sulfonylureas—cont'd**

Drug	Dosage Form	Cost Index	Cost
Glyburide (G) (2.5 mg and 5 mg * and **)	1.25 mg in 50-, 100-, and 500-tablet bottles	0.6	$27.17/100
	1.5 mg (micronized) in 100-, 500-, and 1,000-tablet bottles		
	2.5 mg in 90-, 100-, 500-, and 1,000-tablet bottles	0.3	$24.41/100
	3 mg (micronized) in 100-, 500-, and 1,000-tablet bottles		
	4.5 mg (micronized) in 100-, 500-, and 1,000-tablet bottles		
	5 mg in 90-, 100-, 500-, and 1,000-tablet bottles and blister packs of 25, 100, and 600 tablets	0.4	$22.12/100
	6 mg (micronized) in 100-, 500-, and 1,000-tablet bottles		
DiaBeta	1.25 mg (scored) in 50-tablet bottles	0.4	$47/100
	2.5 mg (scored) in 100-, and 500-tablet bottles	0.3	$79/100
	5 mg (scored) in 500- and 1,000-tablet bottles	0.5	$121/100
Glynase (micronized) (3 mg and 6 mg * and **)	1.5 mg (scored) in 100-tablet bottles	1.5	$83/100
	3 mg (scored) in 100-, 500-, and 1,000-tablet bottles	0.4	$117/100
	6 mg in 100- and 500-tablet bottles	0.7	$185/100
Glyburide/ Metformin (G)	1.25 mg/250 mg in 100-tablet bottles		$67/100
	2.5 mg/500 mg in 100-tablet bottles		$77/100
	5 mg/500 mg in 100-tablet bottles		$84/100
Glucovance (B) (glyburide/ metformin)	1.25 mg/250 mg in 100-tablet bottles		$127/100
	2.5 mg/500 mg in 100-tablet bottles		$143/100
	5 mg/500 mg in 100-tablet bottles		$153/100
Tolazamide (G)	100 mg in 100- and 250-tablet bottles	0.1	$40/100
	250 mg in 100-, 200-, 500-, and 1,000-tablet bottles	0.2	$59/100
	500 mg in 100-, 250-, and 500-tablet bottles	0.4	$102/100
Tolbutamide (G)	500 mg in 100-, 500-tablet bottles	0.2	$44/100
Orinase (B)	500 mg (scored) in 200-tablet bottles	0.2	

Cost index based on cost per 100 mg of chlorpropamide.
Drugs at Walmart $4 for 30-day supply and $10 for 90-day supply are marked with *. Those at Target $4 for 30-day supply are marked with **.

CLINICAL PEARL

Tolazamide has the added advantage that it may be crushed and put down a nasogastric tube or sprinkled on applesauce or other soft food for patients who have difficulty in swallowing tablets.

controlled on diet, exercise, weight control, and **metformin**. The drugs most commonly used are **second generation sulfonylureas**. The only drug that has had the research necessary to obtain formal FDA approval for this indication is **glimepiride**. There is further discussion in the **insulin** section related to type 2 diabetes in this chapter and in Chapter 33.

Monitoring

HbA_{1c} is the preferred tool for monitoring long-term BG control. As discussed in the **insulin** monitoring section, it provides an indication of the average BG level over the past 120 days. Standards vary from laboratory to laboratory, but in general, each 1 percent change in HbA_{1c} equals a change in BG of about 30 mg/dL. The goal for patients with type 2 diabetes is the same as the goal for type 1. (HbA_{1c} less than 7%). Glycated albumin (fructosamine) is also sometimes used for monitoring, although it is not recommended as a substitute for HbA_{1c} except in situations such as hemolytic anemia in which HbA_{1c} cannot be used. It indicates the average BG for the past 1 to 3 weeks and is used to assess short-term control. The minimum goal for fructosamine levels is 325 mmol or less, with a goal for intensive therapy of 287 mmol or less. All decreases in these monitoring parameters are beneficial, even if the goal is not met.

The American Diabetes Association (2009) recommends that patients with type 2 diabetes be tested by HbA_{1c} every 6 months if they are meeting glycemic goals and at least every 3 months if their therapy has changed or they are not meeting glycemic goals. Patients who have gestational diabetes should be encouraged to do self-monitoring of capillary BG. Patients who do not want to do self-monitoring should be monitored with HbA_{1c} testing, following the same schedule as patients with type 2 diabetes.

The goal for patients with type 2 diabetes who do not desire intensive therapy in terms of preprandial and fasting blood glucose (FBS) levels is 90 to 130 mg/dL, and bedtime glucose levels should be 100 to 140 mg/dL. Fair control is considered to be 120 to 180 mg/dL, and anything higher is unacceptable control. Those who desire and are willing to undertake the requirements of intensive therapy have a FBG goal of 110 mg/dL. For both of these the HgA_{1c} goal is less than 7 percent. Self-monitoring of preprandial BG by fingerstick is usually done less often than for patients on **insulin** because the drugs have different pharmacokinetic profiles. Patients are taught to keep a diet, drug, and BG level diary, and these diaries are reviewed at each health-care provider visit.

Patient Education

Administration

Patients are taught to take the medication exactly as prescribed, at the same time each day, preferably before or with the morning meal. All **sulfonylureas** except **glipizide** may be taken with food. **Glipizide** must be taken 30 minutes before a meal to prevent a reduction in absorption. If a dose is missed, instruct the patient to take it as soon as remembered unless the timing of the dose will produce a risk for hypoglycemia. Doses should not be taken if the patient is unable to eat.

Adverse Reactions

The most common adverse reactions are gastrointestinal. If GI upset is a problem, notify the health-care provider. The dose may be divided and given twice daily to reduce this adverse effect. The most serious potential adverse reaction is hypoglycemia. Teach the patient the signs and symptoms of hypoglycemia and how to treat it. The treatment is the same as that discussed in the **Endocrine Pancreatic Hormones (Insulin)**, Patient Education section. Caution the patient to avoid concurrent administration of other drugs without first discussing them with the health-care provider. Many drugs increase or decrease the effectiveness of **sulfonylureas** and can produce hypoglycemia or hyperglycemia. This is especially a problem with **alcohol** because it both produces hypoglycemia and masks the indications of this adverse reaction. **Alcohol** may also produce a disulfiram-like reaction when combined with some **sulfonylureas**.

Because these drugs may produce alterations in red and white blood cell and platelet formation, patients should notify their health-care provider promptly if they experience sore throat, rash, or unusual bruising or bleeding. **Sulfonylureas** may also produce an antidiuretic effect, and patients should promptly report unusual weight gain, swelling of the ankles, drowsiness, or shortness of breath.

Lifestyle Management

Management of type 2 diabetes involves diet, exercise, weight control, and self-monitoring of BG, as well as administration of **oral hypoglycemics**. Further patient teaching related to management of diabetes is discussed in Chapter 33.

BIGUANIDES

The **biguanides** are **oral antihyperglycemic drugs** used in the treatment of type 2 diabetes mellitus. Their pharmacology and chemistry are different from the **oral hypoglycemics** so that they form a different class. To date **metformin (Glucophage)** is the only drug in this class used clinically. Because its actions directly address the major pathological defects in type 2 diabetes, it has moved to first-line therapy in adults and children older than 10 years of age.

Monotherapy with **metformin (Glucophage)** has proved effective as initial drug therapy. If monotherapy with **metformin** is not effective, it has proved very successful as combination therapy with a variety of drugs from other **antidiabetic agent** classes or **insulin**. This section discusses **metformin**. Information provided is also true for the long-acting form, **Fortamet**, and for **Glumetza** unless specifically addressed.

On The Horizon **DAPAGLIFLOZIN**

The kidney filters 160 mg of glucose daily, with 90 percent being reabsorbed by sodium-glucose cotransporter 2 (SGLT2) and 10 percent by SGLT1 in the renal tubules. **Dapagliflozin**, a novel inhibitor of renal SGLT2, allows an insulin-dependent approach to type 2 diabetes treatment. One study (List, Woo, Morales, Tang, & Fiedorek, 2009) found improved hyperglycemia with a reduction in HbA_{1c} of 0.9 percent and mild weight loss in study subjects. This drug is in clinical trials.

Pharmacodynamics

Metformin increases peripheral glucose uptake and utilization (**insulin** sensitivity), decreases hepatic glucose production, and decreases intestinal absorption of glucose. Together, these actions address the primary pathological defects of type 2 diabetes to improve glucose tolerance and lower both basal and postprandial plasma glucose levels. Unlike the **sulfonylureas, metformin** does not stimulate **insulin** release from the pancreatic beta cells, and so does not produce hypoglycemia in diabetic or nondiabetic patients except in specific circumstances (see the Adverse Effects section). **Metformin** also does not cause hyperinsulinemia.

The magnitude of decline in fasting BG concentrations with **metformin** therapy is directly proportional to the level of fasting hyperglycemia. Patients with higher BG levels experience a greater percentage of decrease in BG and HbA_{1c} levels than those with lower BG levels.

Metformin also has a modestly favorable impact on lipids because of its actions in the liver. In clinical studies, **metformin** alone lowered mean fasting serum triglycerides (16%), total cholesterol (5%), and low-density lipids (LDL) (8%), and increased high-density lipids (HDL) (2%). The same was true when **metformin** was combined with a **sulfonylurea** or other **antidiabetic**, but the magnitude of the changes was less for the combination (*Drug Facts and Comparisons*, 2009).

In contrast to patients taking **sulfonylureas**, patients taking **metformin** do not gain weight. In fact, they often lose weight. Because obesity is a major factor in the pathogenesis of type 2 diabetes, this is an important drug action.

Metformin also inhibits platelet aggregation and reduces blood viscosity. This property is a factor in its use in metabolic syndrome, which is discussed below.

Pharmacokinetics

Absorption and Distribution

Metformin is 50 to 60 percent absorbed after oral administration under fasting conditions. The extended-release form of the drug has a different absorption profile from the immediate-release form (Table 21–19). Food decreases the extent and slightly delays the absorption in the immediate-release form, with an approximately 40 percent decrease in C_{max} and a 25 percent decrease in AUC. It is not known if these are clinically relevant. The extent of absorption from the extended-release form (**Fortamet**) was

Table 21–19 ▶ **Pharmacokinetics: Antihyperglycemic Drugs**

Drug	Onset*	Peak*	Duration*	Protein Binding	Bioavail-ability	Half-Life	Excretion
Metformin IR and solution	Days	1–8 h	UK	Minimal	50%–60% if taken fasting; nonlinear; reduced by food intake	6.2 h (plasma) 17.6 h (blood)	100% excreted unchanged in urine
Metformin ER, Fortamet, and Glumetza	Days	3–10 h (mean of 6–7) h	UK	Minimal	Increased by 60% with food for Fortamet and Glumetza	UK	In urine
Acarbose	0.5–1 h	1 h	2–3 h		Less than 2% in plasma	2 h	51% in feces as unabsorbed drug; 34% in urine
Miglitol	0.5–1 h	2 h	3h		100% in extracellular fluids at 25 mg; 50%–70% at higher doses	Normal renal function: 2 h Renal impairment: CCr < 25: 4 h	95% in urine as unchanged drug
Nateglinide	20 min	1 h	4h	98%	73%	1.5 h	83% in urine; 10% in feces
Pioglitazone	UA	2–4 h	UA		99%	3–7 h	15%–30% in urine
Repaglinide	0.5 h	1 h	1.4 h		100%	1–1.4 h	90% in feces; 8% in urine
Rosiglitazone	UA	1–3 h	UA		99%	3–4 h	64% in urine; 23% in feces

UA = data unavailable; UK = unknown.
*Of antihyperglycemic effect.

increased by approximately 60 percent when given with food. **Glumetza** must be administered immediate after a meal to maximize absorption. The rate and extent of absorption with **metformin** solution is comparable with that of the tablets under fasting or fed conditions (*Drug Facts and Comparisons,* 2009). Absorption is also not linearly related to dose. The higher the dose the patient takes, the lower the percentage that is absorbed. Increased doses do not result in proportionally increased amounts of drug in the body.

Metformin is negligibly bound to plasma proteins. Plasma half-life is 6.2 hours, but the half-life in the blood is 17.6 hours, suggesting that RBCs may be a compartment of distribution. The apparent volume of distribution is very high and averages 654 L following single doses of 850 mg.

Metabolism and Excretion

There is no hepatic metabolism for metformin, and it is excreted unchanged in the urine. There is no biliary excretion. Renal clearance is 3.5 times that of CCr, indicating that renal tubular secretion is the major route of elimination.

Data suggest a trend toward higher C_{max} and AUC values for **Glumetza** in Asian subjects when compared with white, Hispanic, and African American subjects. This difference does not appear to be clinically significant.

Pharmacotherapeutics

Precautions and Contraindications

There are two major contraindications to **metformin** use: (1) renal disease or dysfunction and (2) metabolic acidosis. Males with serum creatinine levels 1.5 or higher, females with levels 1.4 or higher, and patients of either gender with abnormal CCr rates should not receive **metformin** because of its heavy dependence on renal function for elimination (ICSI, 2004). Patients with acute or chronic metabolic acidosis and patients at high risk for lactic acidosis because of tissue hypoperfusion or hypoxia (e.g., severe dehydration, heart failure, respiratory failure, and chronic alcoholism with severe liver damage) also should not receive this drug (ICSI, 2004). Lactic acidosis is a rare, but serious complication that can occur with **metformin** because of its accumulation during treatment. When it occurs, it is fatal 50 percent of the time. The risk for lactic acidosis increases in the presence of renal dysfunction, making the interaction of these two contraindications more serious than either one alone.

Although there is no specific contraindication for hepatic dysfunction, it has been associated with some cases of lactic acidosis. **Metformin** should not be used for patients with clinical and laboratory evidence of hepatic disease.

Cautious use is suggested with patients over age 80 because of the probability of decreased renal function. Limited data suggest that total plasma clearance is decreased and half-life is prolonged in healthy older adults as compared with healthy young subjects (*Drug Facts and Comparisons,* 2009). These data suggest that the change in pharmacokinetics is primarily accounted for by change in renal function. For older adults, CCr should be tested before beginning therapy and at least annually during therapy.

Metformin should also be temporarily withheld (48 hours before to 48 hours after the procedure) from patients undergoing radiological studies that involve an iodine-based contrast medium because such materials may result in altered renal function and have been associated with lactic acidosis in patients receiving **metformin**. **Metformin** should be reinstituted only after renal function has been reevaluated and found to be normal. It should also be temporarily withheld from patients undergoing surgical procedures in which fluid will be withheld because of the risk for dehydration and hypoperfusion that may result in lactic acidosis. The time frame for withholding the drug is the same.

A decrease in vitamin B_{12} levels to subnormal without clinical manifestations has been observed in about 7 percent of patients receiving **metformin**. This decrease is probably due to interference with **vitamin B_{12}** absorption from the intrinsic factor–**vitamin B_{12}** complex. Patients with or at risk for anemia associated with altered **vitamin B_{12}** utilization should have the disorder treated and under control before beginning metformin therapy.

Metformin is listed as Pregnancy Category B, but it is not recommended for use during pregnancy. The consensus among experts is that **insulin** should be used to control BG during pregnancy (see the **Sulfonylureas Precautions and Contraindications** section, related to pregnancy). Studies in rats indicate that **metformin** is excreted in breast milk in levels approximately the same as in the plasma. Similar studies have not been conducted in nursing mothers. Because the potential for hypoglycemia in nursing infants may exist, decide whether the patient should discontinue nursing or discontinue **metformin** based on the importance of the drug to the mother.

Use of **metformin** in 10- to 16-year-old children is supported by evidence from adequate and well-controlled clinical trials with children of this age with type 2 diabetes; the trials demonstrated a similar response in glycemic control and adverse reactions to those seen in adults. Studies in children younger than 10 years have not been conducted. **Glumetza** has not been studied in children younger than 18 years of age and is not recommended for children.

The safety and efficacy of **metformin ER** have not been established in children.

Adverse Drug Reactions

The most common adverse reaction involves GI disturbances (e.g., abdominal bloating, diarrhea, nausea, vomiting, and an unpleasant metallic taste). These adverse reactions are usually transient and resolve in about

2 weeks without a change in dose. They may be reduced by initiating therapy with a low dose and titrating the dose up slowly.

Lactic acidosis is rare and was discussed in the Precautions and Contraindications section. Hypoglycemia is also rare unless there is a concurrent reduction in caloric intake, an increase in strenuous exercise not compensated for with increased caloric intake, or concurrent use of another glucose-lowering drug or **alcohol** (ICSI, 2004). Older adults, debilitated and malnourished patients, and those with adrenal or pituitary insufficiency are also at increased risk for hypoglycemia.

Drug Interactions

Cationic drugs that are eliminated by renal secretion (e.g., **amiloride, digoxin, morphine, procainamide, quinidine, ranitidine, triamterene, trimethoprim**, and **vancomycin**) may compete with **metformin** for its elimination pathway (Table 21–20). Dosage adjustments may be needed in **metformin** or the interacting drugs.

Cimetidine increases the peak **metformin** plasma level by 60 percent, with an increase of 40 percent in its AUC. **Furosemide** increases these levels by 15 percent without any significant change in renal clearance. Both of these drugs may increase the effects of **metformin** because of these alterations. Dosage adjustment for **metformin** may be necessary.

Nifedipine increases absorption and may increase the effects of **metformin**. It concurrently increases the amount excreted in the urine, however, so that the total effect may be small.

Clinical Use and Dosing

Type 2 Diabetes Mellitus

Metformin is indicated as monotherapy and as added therapy for patients with type 2 diabetes who cannot achieve adequate BG control on diet, exercise, weight control, and a **sulfonylurea** alone. The HgA_{1c} lowering commonly achieved with this drug alone is 1.5 to 2 percent (ICSI, 2004). It is especially useful for obese patients because it is not associated with weight gain and may produce some weight loss. Its positive effect on lipids creates a clear advantage for patients with hyperlipidemia. The pharmacodynamics of **metformin** are different from those of **sulfonylureas** so that the two drugs taken together potentiate each other's actions. In clinical trials, both the fasting and the postprandial BG levels of patients decreased by 20 to 30 percent. Because this drop is so dramatic, it is important to monitor BG levels closely when **metformin** is added to the treatment regimen of a drug that can produce hypoglycemia.

Metformin is available in 500-mg, 850-mg, and 1-g tablets in IR and ER formulations and in an oral solution of 500 mg/5 mL. Begin therapy with 500 mg bid with the morning and evening meal or 850 mg bid with the morning and evening meal for adults (Table 21–21). For children the starting dose is 500 mg bid with the morning and evening meals. The dose is increased in increments of 500 mg at weekly intervals for both adults and children or 850 mg every other week for adults. The most common adverse reactions are GI disturbances. If they occur, the starting dose can be lower or the current dose can be held at that level and not increased. The symptoms will most likely resolve in about 2 weeks, at which time the dosage can be increased again until target BG levels are reached. The maximum dose recommended is 2,550 mg/day for adults or 2,000 mg/day for children. The maximum dose should be divided and given tid to reduce GI reactions.

Conversion of IR Formulation to ER Formulation

Clinical trials have shown that patients treated with the IR formulation of **metformin** who were switched to the ER

Table 21–20 ■ **Drug Interactions With Metformin**

Interacting Drug	Possible Effect	Implications
Alcohol	Potentiates the effect of metformin on lactate metabolism	Warn patients against excessive alcohol intake while taking metformin.
Amiloride, digoxin, morphine, procainamide, quinidine, ranitidine, triamterene, trimethoprim, vancomycin	May compete for elimination pathway	Dosage adjustments may be needed for metformin or interacting drug.
Beta-adrenergic blockers	May mask signs and symptoms of hypoglycemia	Does not affect diaphoresis as indicator of hypoglycemia; teach patient to check blood glucose level if experiencing diaphoresis.
Cimetidine, furosemide	Increases plasma levels of metformin without concurrent increase in renal excretion	Dosage adjustments of metformin may be needed.
Iodine-based contrast media	May affect renal function and increase the risk for lactic acidosis	Withhold metformin for 48 h before and after procedure in which contrast is used.
Nifedipine	Enhances absorption of metformin and may increase effects	Dosage adjustments of metformin may be needed.

Table 21–21 ◉ **Dosage Schedule: Metformin**

Drug	Dosage Schedule
Immediate Release	
Metformin IR 500-mg (generic) and Glucophage IR 500-mg tablets and Riomet 500-mg/5-mL solution	*Adults and children >17 yr:* Week 1: 500 mg bid at morning and evening meal. Maximum dose 2,550 mg Week 2: 1,000 mg q AM and 500 mg at evening meal Week 3: 1,000 mg q AM and 1,000 mg at evening meal Week 4: 1,500 mg q AM and 1,000 mg at evening meal *Children 10–16 yr:* (Same as adult). Maximum dose 2,000 mg
Metformin IR 850-mg (generic) and Glucophage IR 850-mg tablets	*Adults and children > 17 yr:* Weeks 1 & 2: 850 mg daily at morning meal. Maximum dose: 2,550 mg Weeks 3 and 4: 850 mg q am and 850 mg at evening meal Week 5: 850 mg at breakfast, 850 mg at lunch, and 850 mg at evening meal
Extended Release	
Metformin ER 500-mg (generic), Glucophage XR 500-mg tablets (B), Fortamet (B) and Glumetza (B)	*Adults and Children >17 yr:* Week 1: 500 mg daily at evening meal. Week 2: 1,000 mg daily at evening meal Week 3: 1,500 mg daily at evening meal Week 4: 2,000 mg daily at evening meal
Metformin ER 750-mg (generic) and Glucophage ER 750-mg tablets	*Adult and Children >17 yr:* Weeks 1 & 2: 750 mg daily at evening meal Weeks 3 and 4: 1,500 mg daily at evening meal Week 5: 2,250 mg daily at evening meal

formulation could safely be transferred with the same total daily dose. Close monitoring of glucose levels is recommended during the transition.

Concomitant Metformin and Sulfonylurea Therapy in Adults

If a patient is not responsive to 4 weeks of the maximum dose of **metformin** monotherapy, gradual addition of a **sulfonylurea** may be considered. With concomitant therapy, the desired BG level may be obtained by adjusting the dose of either drug. However, if the patient experiences a hypoglycemic episode, reduce the **sulfonylurea** dose rather than the **metformin** dose, because the former drug is more likely to be the source of the problem. There are combination formulations that include **metformin** plus **glipizide (Metaglip)**, and **metformin** plus **glyburide (Glucovance)**. These combination drugs are administered similarly to **metformin IR** and carry the precautions/contraindication, adverse effects and drug interactions of both drugs.

If a patient has not met BG and HgA_{1c} targets by 3 months of combination therapy, consider adding **insulin** to the regimen. This patient may benefit from referral to an endocrinologist.

Concomitant Metformin and Thiazolidinediones

Thiazolidinediones can also be added to a treatment regimen when the patient has not achieved blood glucose targets on **metformin** alone or in combination with other drugs. The starting dose is based on the patient's current regimen of each of the drugs. The starting doses of these drugs are discussed in their section below. There are combination formulations that include **metformin** plus **pioglitazone (ActoPlus Met** and **ActoPlus Met XR)** and **metformin** plus **rosiglitazone (Avandamet)**. The same issues related to administration and combining that are stated with **sulfonylureas** apply, as does the information about achieving target HbA_{1c} goals.

Concomitant Metformin and Meglitinides

These drugs can be added to a treatment regimen when the patient has not achieved blood glucose targets on **metformin** alone or in combination with other drugs. The starting dose is based on the patient's current regimen of each of the drugs. The starting doses of these drugs are discussed in their section below. There is a combination formulation of **metformin** plus **repaglinde (PrandiMet)**. The same data apply to the combination as stated above.

Concomitant Metformin and Gliptins

All of the **gliptins** have been approved for this combination. The starting doses of these drugs are discussed in their section below. There is a combination formulation of **sitagliptin plus metformin (Janumet)**. It is given twice daily with meals with a gradual dose escalation to reduce the adverse GI reaction caused by **metformin** (Reynolds, 2009; *Drug Facts and Comparisons*, 2009).

Concomitant Metformin and Insulin Therapy

Initiate **metformin IR or ER** at 500 mg once daily in patients on **insulin** therapy. For patients who do not respond adequately, increase the dose of **metformin** by 500 mg daily after 1 week and by 500 mg daily every week thereafter until adequate glycemic control is achieved. The maximum daily dose is the same as for **metformin** alone for both adults and children. The **insulin** dose should then be decreased by 10 to 25 percent when the FBG decreases to less than 120 mg/dL.

Metabolic Syndrome

Metformin inhibits platelet aggregation and decreases blood viscosity. It is recommended in a treatment protocol that includes **angiotensin converting enzyme** (ACE) **inhibitors** or **angiotensin II receptor blockers** (ARBs), **statins**, and **aspirin** in the treatment of **insulin** resistance syndromes including metabolic syndrome (Bloomgarden, 2003). Chapter 33 has more discussion of this syndrome, which includes obesity, hypertension, hyperlipidemia, and **insulin** resistance.

Prevention of Conversion of Prediabetes to Diabetes

The Diabetes Prevention Program Research Group (2002) tested **metformin** and lifestyle modifications as methods for preventing the conversion of prediabetes to type 2 diabetes. This group also looked at the cost effectiveness of this intervention (2003) and found that both of these interventions were cost effective across subjects, regardless of age, ethnicity, or gender, and affordable in routine clinical practice. Because prevention of movement from prediabetes to diabetes is a primary goal of treatment directed at children who may develop type 2 diabetes, **metformin** has become first-line therapy for this indication. This is discussed further in Chapter 33. Table 21–22 lists the available dosage forms of **metformin**, including the ER and oral solution formulations.

Monitoring

Before initiating therapy and at least annually thereafter, assess renal function. Assessment is by serum creatinine and CCr initially and then by serum creatinine annually.

For patients with increased risk for developing altered renal function, the assessment should be made more

Table 21–22 ◈ Available Dosage Forms: Metformin

	Dosage Form	How Supplied	Cost
Metformin IR (generic)	Tablets: 500 mg;	In bottles of 100, 1,000, 2,000, and UD 100	$22.00
	850 mg;	In bottles of 100, 500, 1,000, and UD 100	$87.00
	1,000 mg	In bottles of 100, 500, 1,000, and UD 100	$50.00
Metformin ER	Tablets: 500 mg;	In bottles of 100, 500, and 1,000	$19 per 90 tablets
	750 mg	In bottles of 100, 500, and 1,000	$90 per 90 tablets
Glucophage IR (brand name)	Tablets: 500 mg	In bottles of 100 and 500	$117.00
	850 mg	In bottles of 100	$87.00
	1,000 mg	In bottles of 100	$235.00
Glucophage ER (brand name)	Tablets: 500 mg	In bottles of 100	$70.00 per 60 tablets
	750 mg	In bottles of 100	$140.00 per 90 tablets
Glipizied/metformin (generic)	Tablets: 2.5 mg/500 mg	In bottles of 100	$125.0
	5 mg/500 mg	In bottles of 100	$107.00
Glyburide/metformin (generic)	Tablets: 1.25 mg/250 mg	In bottles of 100	$67.00
	2.5 mg/500 mg		
	5 mg/500 mg	In bottles of 100	$77.00
		In bottles of 100	$84.00
Glucovance (glyburide/metformin) (brandname)	Tablets: 1.25 mg /250 mg	In bottles of 100	$127.00
	2.5 mg/500 mg		
	5 mg/500 mg	In bottles of 100	$143.00
		In bottles of 100	$153.00
Glumetza ER (brand name)	Tablets: 500 mg	In bottles of 100	$190
	1,000 mg	In bottles of 100	NA
Fortamet ER (brand name)	Tablets: 500 mg	In bottles of 180	$417.00 per 180 tablets
	1,000 mg	In bottles of 180	$939.00 per 180 tablets
Riomet (brand name)	Oral solution: 500 mg per 5 mL	In bottles of 118 mL and 473 mL	$130.00 for 473 mL

Cost is per 100 tablets unless otherwise noted.
IR = immediate release; ER = extended release.

> **CLINICAL PEARL**
>
> When **metformin** is added to a **sulfonylurea** in a diabetic regimen, the increased sensitivity to **insulin** caused by **metformin** results in less need for the insulin secretion generated by the **sulfonylurea.** If the BG level drops too much, the dose of the **sulfonylurea** should be reduced.

often. Patients who have been previously well controlled on **metformin** who are no longer controlled or who develop illnesses that place them at risk for metabolic acidosis should be assessed for evidence of ketoacidosis or lactic acidosis. Assessment includes serum electrolytes and ketones, BG, and, if indicated, blood pH and lactate levels. Lactic acidosis is characterized by elevated blood lactate levels (greater than 5 mmol/L), decreased blood pH, and electrolyte disturbances with an increased anion gap. Because impaired hepatic function may significantly decrease the ability to clear lactate, liver function studies should be done before therapy is initiated.

Response to **metformin** therapy is assessed by daily to weekly monitoring of fasting and postprandial BG and by monitoring HbA_{1c} every 3 months or monitoring fructosamine every 2 months. During initial therapy and with each incremental increase, fasting BG is used to evaluate response. After the patient is stabilized on a specific dose, monitoring with fasting BG and HbA_{1c} levels every 6 months is sufficient.

Some patients with inadequate **vitamin B_{12}** or **calcium** intake or absorption may be predisposed to developing subnormal **vitamin B_{12}** levels. Assessment for this problem is done by red blood cell indices drawn at initiation of therapy and every 2 to 3 years thereafter.

Patient Education

Administration

Patients are taught to take the drug at the same time each day exactly as prescribed. **Metformin** and **Foramet** are taken once daily, usually in the morning. **Glumetza** is taken once daily in the evening with food. The tablets should be swallowed whole and not cut, crushed, or chewed. Because the titrating doses will change weekly or every other week, a card or calendar is helpful to remind patients of the schedule. If a dose of **metformin** is missed, it is taken as soon as it is remembered unless it is about time for the next dose. Do not double doses. If a dose of the long-acting drugs **(Fortamet and Glumetza)** is missed, patients resume taking the drug according to schedule. Unlike **metformin** monotherapy, the combination drug **PrandiMet** is taken 15 minutes prior to a meal instead of with food.

Explain to the patient that **metformin** helps to control hyperglycemia, but it does not cure diabetes. The therapy will be long term.

Adverse Reactions

The most common adverse reactions are GI disturbances. If they occur, they may be reduced by taking the drug with food rather than before the meal. The health-care provider should be notified of GI disturbances so that the dose may be kept at the current level until they resolve. Even with the same dose, GI disturbances will usually resolve in about 2 weeks. If the GI disturbances include vomiting or diarrhea or the patient develops a fever, the drug is stopped and the health-care provider notified. Dehydration may result and presents a risk for the patient to develop lactic acidosis and decreased renal function. Patients are taught the signs and symptoms of lactic acidosis (e.g., chills, dizziness, low blood pressure, muscle pain, sleepiness, trouble breathing, slow heart rate, and weakness) and to report them immediately.

Lactic acidosis may also develop from any incident that results in hypoperfusion or hypoxia. A patient who is to undergo a procedure with an **iodine-based contrast medium** or surgery in which fluid will be withheld will be temporarily taken off **metformin;** the health-care provider should be notified if one of these procedures is anticipated.

Hypoglycemia is less common than with other glucose-lowering drugs but may occur when **metformin** is given with one of these drugs. Patient instruction for hypoglycemia has been discussed in the **Endocrine Pancreatic Hormones (Insulin)** and **Sulfonylureas** sections. Adverse reactions for the combination drugs include those of both drugs.

Metformin may cause an unpleasant or metallic taste. This reaction usually resolves spontaneously in a few weeks.

Lifestyle Management

Type 2 diabetes is a chronic illness managed with diet, exercise, weight control, and self-monitoring of BG, as well as drug therapy. Further patient teaching related to management of diabetes is discussed in Chapter 33.

ALPHA-GLUCOSIDASE INHIBITORS

The **alpha-glucosidase inhibitors** are **oral antihyperglycemic drugs** used in the treatment of type 2 diabetes mellitus. Their pharmacodynamics are different from those of the **sulfonylureas** and the **biguanides.** The action of this class has proved to reduce blood glucose both as added therapy for patients who cannot achieve control on diet alone and as added therapy for patients whose blood glucose cannot be controlled by lifestyle modifications and other **oral antidiabetic** agents. These drugs are not given as monotherapy; they are adjunct to other therapy for type 2 diabetes.

Pharmacodynamics

Alpha-glucosidase inhibitors do not act directly on any of the defects in metabolism seen in type 2 diabetes mellitus. They competitively inhibit the absorption of complex carbohydrates (CHO) from the small bowel. Their chemical structure is a pseudo-tetrasaccharide that binds to alpha glucosidase. Because this structure is so similar to the CHO molecule, digestive enzyme activity is partially diverted from CHO digestion while it is trying to digest the **alpha-glucosidase inhibitor.** This effectively delays the digestion of CHO and permits CHOs that would normally have been digested in the upper small bowel to move farther down in the bowel. The lower parts of the bowel have the necessary enzymes to digest this CHO, but, because they are not normally active in this process, enzyme induction is required. The process of induction takes weeks to months, and during this time patients may experience intestinal flatus and abdominal distention. **Alpha-glucosidase inhibitors** have no inhibitory activity against lactase and do not induce lactose intolerance.

Alpha-glucosidase inhibitors lower BG levels after meals. The higher that the postprandial BG level is, the larger the reduction will be that this drug can provide. As a consequence of plasma glucose reduction, they also reduce glycosylated hemoglobin levels. The mean reduction in HbA_{1c} is 0.77 percent, postprandial BG reduction is approximately 50 mg/dL, and fasting BG reduction is 20 mg/dL (*Drug Facts and Comparisons,* 2009).

Unlike the many other classes of **antidiabetic agents,** they do not enhance pancreatic beta cell secretion of **insulin** and so do not produce hypoglycemia in diabetic or nondiabetic patients, except in special situations. Like **metformin,** they are not associated with weight gain and diminish the weight-increasing effects of **sulfonylureas** when given in combination with them. Their activity is effective on any CHO food intake, including liquid diets taken via nasogastric tube.

Pharmacokinetics

Absorption and Distribution

Less than 2 percent of **acarbose** is systemically absorbed as active drug. The remainder is active in the GI tract with no systemic distribution. **Miglitol** is completely absorbed in the GI tract at 25-mg doses, and 50 to 70 percent is absorbed at higher doses. Its volume of distribution of 0.18 is consistent with distribution primarily into extracellular fluids.

Metabolism and Excretion

Acarbose and **miglitol** are metabolized exclusively by intestinal bacteria and digestive enzymes. The minimal amount of drug absorbed is excreted by the kidneys. The plasma elimination half-life of both drugs is about 2 hours, so drug accumulation does not occur with tid dosing. The mean steady-state AUC and maximum concentration of this drug were 1.5 times higher in older adults taking **acarbose,** but this was neither statistically nor clinically significant. This change was not seen with **miglitol.**

Pharmacotherapeutics

Precautions and Contraindications

Alpha-glucosidase inhibitors should not be used for patients with bowel diseases such as inflammatory bowel disease, bowel obstruction or risk factors for it, chronic intestinal disease associated with marked digestive disorders, or conditions that may deteriorate as a result of increased gas in the intestine.

Plasma concentrations of **alpha-glucosidase inhibitors** were 5 times higher in patients with severe renal impairment (CCr less than 25 mL/min); however, dosage adjustments to compensate for this are not possible because the drugs act locally (*Drug Facts and Comparisons,* 2009). Long-term studies with diabetic patients with renal impairment have not been conducted. Therefore, treatment with these drugs is not recommended for these patients.

The safety of **alpha-glucosidase inhibitors** in pregnant women has not been established. Although they are listed as Pregnancy Category B, they should not be used in pregnancy unless clearly needed. As previously discussed with other oral agents, **insulin** is the drug of choice for pregnant diabetics. In a study, a small amount of **acarbose** was excreted in the breast milk of rats. It is not known if it is excreted in human breast milk, and it should not be used in lactating women. **Miglitol** is excreted in human breast milk to a small degree. Total excretion in breast milk accounts for 0.02 percent of a 100-mg maternal dose. Although the levels in breast milk are exceedingly low, it also should not be used for lactating women.

Safety and efficacy in children have not been established for either drug.

Adverse Drug Reactions

GI symptoms are the most common adverse reactions. Approximately 77 percent of patients taking **acarbose** and 41 percent of patients taking **miglitol** experience flatulence, the leading reason for discontinuance of the drug. Approximately 33 percent of patients taking **acarbose** and 29 percent of patients taking **miglitol** experience diarrhea, whereas 21 percent report abdominal pain while taking **acarbose** and 12 percent while taking **miglitol.** These adverse effects can be reduced by slow titration to maximal dose.

Because of their mechanism of action, **alpha-glucosidase inhibitors** alone do not cause hypoglycemia but may do so in combination with other drugs which lower blood glucose, such as **sulfonylureas.** Treatment

CLINICAL PEARL

Starting the **alpha-glucosidase inhibitor** at 25 mg daily for 1 week and increasing the dose to 25 mg bid for 1 week and then to 25 mg tid for 1 week decreases the incidence of GI-adverse responses.

Table 21–23 ▣ **Drug Interactions: Alpha-Glucosidase Inhibitors**

Drug	Interacting Drug	Possible Effect	Implications
Acarbose, miglitol	Digoxin	Serum digoxin concentrations may be reduced with reduced therapeutic effect	Choose another antihyperglycemic drug
	Digestive enzymes and intestinal absorbents	Reduced effect of alpha-glucosidase inhibitor	Do not take concomitantly
Miglitol	Propranolol	Reduces bioavailability of propranolol by 40%	Avoid current use
	Ranitidine	Reduces bioavailability of ranitidine by 60%	Avoid current use

of this hypoglycemia cannot be accomplished with the usual ingestion of sucrose (hard candy or soft drinks), fructose, or starches because **alpha-glucosidase inhibitors** delay the absorption of these disaccharides. Because there is no inhibitory activity against lactase or monosaccharides, milk, lactose, and glucose can be used to treat the hypoglycemia.

Reversible increases in serum transaminases (alanine aminotransferase [ALT] and aspartate aminotranspeptidase [AST]) have occurred with doses greater than 200 mg tid of **acarbose.** Hepatic abnormalities improved or resolved with discontinuance of the drug. This laboratory change has not been reported with **miglitol.**

Drug Interactions

The literature on drug interactions related to **acarbose** is contradictory. The package insert reports no interference with the pharmacokinetics or pharmacodynamics of **digoxin, nifedipine, propranolol,** or **ranitidine.** *Drug Facts and Comparisons* (2009), however, states that **acarbose** interferes with **digoxin** absorption, resulting in decreased serum concentration that may diminish the therapeutic effects of the **digoxin.**

Miglitol has drug interactions with several drugs, including **digoxin, propranolol,** and **ranitidine.** Both **acarbose** and **miglitol** may have their therapeutic effects reduced by concurrent administration with digestive enzymes or intestinal absorbents. Table 21–23 shows drug interactions for these two drugs as reported in *Drug Facts and Comparisons* (2009).

Clinical Use and Dosing

Management of type 2 diabetes mellitus is the only indication for these drugs. They are useful for patients with high postprandial BG levels. The initial dose of both drugs is 25 mg tid taken with the first bite of each meal (Table 21–24). Taking the dose with the first bite is critical; a space between administration of the drug and ingestion of food decreases its effect, and no effect occurs if it is taken after a meal. The dose is increased in increments of 25 mg with each meal (75 mg/day) at 4- to 8-week intervals. The maintenance dose is usually 50 mg tid, although some patients may benefit from increasing the dose to 100 mg tid. If no further reduction in postprandial BG is achieved at the higher dose, consider reducing the dose to 50 mg tid.

Because patients with low body weight are at higher risk for elevations in serum transaminase, the dose should be not be higher than 50 mg tid for patients weighing less than 60 kg, and the 100-mg tid dose should be reserved for patients weighing more than 60 kg. The maximum dose is 100 mg tid.

When given in combination with a **sulfonylurea** or **metformin**, the drop in postprandial BG may be significant. It is important to monitor BG levels closely when

Table 21–24 ◉ **Dosage Schedule: Alpha-Glucosidase Inhibitors**

Patient Population	Initial Dose	Incremental Dosage Increases
Weight more than 60 kg (most patients)	25 mg tid with the first bite of each meal for 4 wk	Weeks 5–8: 50 mg tid with first bite of each meal Weeks 9–12: 100 mg tid with first bite of each meal
Weight less than 60 kg	25 mg tid with the first bite of each meal for 4 wk	Weeks 5–8: 50 mg tid with first bite of each meal; then maintain this dose
Patients with poor GI tolerance	25 mg daily with first bite of evening meal for 2 wk	Weeks 3–4: 25 mg tid with first bite of morning and evening meal Weeks 5–12: 25 mg tid with first bite of each meal Week 13: Begin 50 mg tid with first bite of each meal; then maintain this dose

alpha-glucosidase inhibitors are added to the treatment regimen to avoid hypoglycemia.

Rational Drug Selection

Adverse Reactions

Elevated serum transaminase levels have been reported in long-term studies of **acarbose**, usually with doses up to 300 mg tid. These elevations appear to be dose related and disappeared with maximum doses at 100 mg tid. There have been no reported hepatic adverse reactions and no reported changes in liver function tests with miglitol.

The percentage of patients experiencing GI adverse effects in clinical trials is slightly lower with **miglitol**. Patients at risk for this adverse effect might be tried first on **miglitol**.

Drug Interactions

Miglitol has reported drug interactions with **propranolol** and **ranitidine**. Patients who must take these medications might benefit from choosing **acarbose**.

Monitoring

Before initiating therapy and at least annually thereafter, assess renal function. For patients with increased risk beyond their diabetes for developing altered renal function, the assessment timing should be related to the disease process that produces the added risk. **Alpha-glucosidase inhibitors** are not recommended for patients with renal impairment. Assessment of renal function includes serum electrolytes, blood urea nitrogen (BUN), and serum creatinine. A similar assessment is required related to hepatic function for patients taking **acarbose**. Because **acarbose** has been associated with reversible elevations in serum transaminase, these values should be assessed every 3 months for the first year.

Response to **alpha-glucosidase inhibitor** therapy is assessed by regular monitoring of fasting and postprandial BG. During initial therapy and with each incremental increase, fasting BG is used to evaluate response. After the patient is stabilized on a specific dose, monitoring with fasting BG and HbA_{1c} levels every 3 to 6 months is sufficient.

Patient Education

Administration

Patients are taught to take these drugs with the first bite of each meal. The need for this timing of administration must be stressed because taking it too soon reduces its effect and taking it after a meal means no effect. Because the titrating doses may change at 4- to 8-week intervals, a card or calendar is helpful to remind them of the schedule. Explain to the patient that **alpha-glucosidase inhibitors** help to control hyperglycemia, but they do not cure diabetes. The therapy is long term.

Adverse Reactions

The most common adverse reactions are GI disturbances. If they occur, the health-care provider should be notified so that the dose may be adjusted. These effects can be reduced or prevented by slow titration of the dose. Even without changing the dose, GI disturbances usually resolve in about 2 weeks.

Hypoglycemia is less common than with other glucose-lowering drugs but may occur when **alpha-glucosidase inhibitors** are given with **insulin, sulfonylureas,** or **repaglinide (Prandin).** The usual treatment for hypoglycemia with sucrose, fructose, or starches does not resolve the problem for patients on **alpha-glucosidase inhibitors** because it interferes with the absorption of these carbohydrates. An 8-oz glass of milk or lactose tablets can be used to treat the hypoglycemia because **alpha-glucosidase inhibitors** do not affect lactose metabolism. Severe hypoglycemia may need to be treated with IV glucose or glucagon. Patients should wear identification that states they are taking an **alpha-glucosidase inhibitor** and the source of simple carbohydrate that should be used in case of hypoglycemia.

Lifestyle Management

Type 2 diabetes is a chronic illness managed with diet, exercise, weight control, and self-monitoring of BG, as well as drug therapy. Further patient teaching related to management of diabetes is discussed in Chapter 33. Table 21–25 shows the available dosage forms of the alpha-glucosidase inhibitors.

CLINICAL PEARL

The delayed absorption of carbohydrates caused by **alpha-glucosidase inhibitors** results in less need for the insulin secretion generated by a **sulfonylurea.** If the BG level drops too much, the dose of the **sulfonylurea** should be reduced.

On The Horizon — MONOTHERAPY WITH RIMONANANT

The endocannabinoid system regulates energy homeostasis and lipid and glucose metabolism through G protein-coupled cannabinoid (CB1) receptors located in the brain, adipose tissue, liver, skeletal muscle, and pancreas. CB1 antagonism in these tissues directly modulates fat disposition in liver and adipose tissues, fatty acid synthesis, and glucoses disposal. (Rosenstock et al, 2009) studied the effects of monotherapy with **rimonanant,** a CB1 receptor antagonist. Therapy with this drug resulted in improved glycemic control (HbA_{1c} reduced 0.5%), weight loss (–3.8 kg), and improved lipid profiles in drug-naïve patient with type 2 diabetes. At this time the drug is not FDA approved and the company is not actively pursuing its development.

Table 21–25 ◆ **Available Dosage Forms: Alpha-Glucosidase Inhibitors**

Drug	Dosage Form and How Supplied	Cost
Acarbose (Precose)	25 mg in 100-tablet bottles	$82
	50 mg (scored) in 100-tablet bottles & UD 100	$88
	100 mg in 100-tablet bottles and UD 100	$90
Miglitol (Glyset)	25 mg in 100-tablet bottles	UK
	50 mg in 100-tablet bottles	
	100 mg in 100-tablet bottles	

THIAZOLIDINEDIONES

The **thiazolidinediones** (TDZs) are **oral antihyperglycemic drugs** used in the treatment of type 2 diabetes mellitus. Their actions have lowered BG levels as monotherapy for patients who cannot achieve BG control with diet alone, and they have proved very successful as added therapy for patients who cannot be controlled by lifestyle modifications or other **antidiabetic agents. Troglitazone (Rezulin)**, the first **TDZ**, was approved in March 1997. It was removed from the market in 1999 because of the adverse reactions associated with liver damage. **Pioglitazone (Actos)** and **rosiglitazone (Avandia)** are newer drugs in this class. They have been associated with less risk of liver damage, but the potential for increased cardiovascular risk has been postulated, and in 2009 the American Diabetes Association and the European Association for the Study of Diabetes recommended that **rosiglitazone** no longer be used to treat type 2 diabetes. This recommendation is discussed in the Precautions and Contraindications section. The Canadian Diabetes Association, however, disagrees with this recommendation and states that there is insufficient cause to exclude **rosiglitazone** (Woo for the Canadian Diabetic Association 2008 Clinical Practice Guidelines Steering Committee, 2009). Because this drug remains on the market and there is controversy about its cardiac risk, it is included in this section.

Pharmacodynamics

TDZs improve glycemic control by improving **insulin** sensitivity, a major pathological problem with type 2 diabetes. They are effective only in type 2 diabetes because they depend on the presence of **insulin** for their action. They are highly selective activators of the peroxisome proliferator-activated receptor gamma, a nuclear receptor that regulates gene transcription, resulting in expression of proteins that improve **insulin** action in the cell. This action leads to increased utilization of available **insulin** by the liver and muscle cells and also in adipose tissue. In addition, these drugs reduce hepatic glucose production. Taken together, these actions improve glucose tolerance and lower both basal and postprandial plasma glucose levels. Unlike the **sulfonylureas, TDZs** do not produce hypoglycemia in diabetic or nondiabetic patients, except in special situations, and do not cause hyperinsulinemia because they do not stimulate **insulin** release from the pancreatic beta cells. Like **metformin**, they have a modest impact on lipids because of their actions in the liver. In clinical studies, **pioglitazone** lowered serum triglyceride levels and increased HDL levels. Although total cholesterol and LDL levels increased slightly, the LDL fractions became larger and less dense. The end result, however, was no change in the serum HDL to total cholesterol ratio, so this risk factor for cardiovascular disease did not improve and there appears to be an increased risk for cardiovascular events with **rosiglitazone** (Nathan et al, 2009; *Drug Facts and Comparisons,* 2009).

Pharmacokinetics

Absorption and Distribution

Pioglitazone and **rosiglitazone** are rapidly absorbed after oral administration. Food does not alter the extent of absorption, but it does delay the time until peak concentration is reached. Both drugs are extensively bound to plasma proteins, with a mean volume of distribution (V_d) ranging from 0.63 L/kg for **pioglitazone** to 17.6 L/kg for **rosiglitazone.** This difference in V_d might be a factor in drug choice for patients with high extracellular fluid levels.

Metabolism and Excretion

Both drugs are highly metabolized by the liver into metabolites and **pioglitazone** has at least two active metabolites. Hepatic function impairment increased C_{max} for both drugs and AUC levels for **rosiglitazone.** The **pioglitazone** site of metabolism in the liver results in inhibition of the CYP450 2C8, 3A4, and 1A1 isoenzymes. Drugs using these isoenzymes are likely to have drug interactions. In vitro drug studies suggest that **rosiglitazone** does not inhibit any of the major CPY450 enzyme systems. It is predominantly metabolized by CYP450 2C8 and, to a lesser extent, 2C9.

Mean plasma elimination half-life ranges from 3 to 7 hours, with 23 percent of **rosiglitazone** and its metabolites recovered in the feces and 64 percent in the urine. **Pioglitazone** is excreted 15 to 30 percent in the urine.

CLINICAL PEARL

When **thiazolidinediones** are added to a **sulfonylurea** in a diabetic regimen, the increased sensitivity to insulin caused by the **thiazolidinedione** results in less need for the **insulin** secretion generated by the **sulfonylurea**. If the BG level drops too much, the dose of the **sulfonylurea** should be reduced.

The mean **pioglitazone** C_{max} and AUC values are increased 20 percent and 60 percent in women. The mean oral clearance of **rosiglitazone** in women is 6 percent lower compared to men (*Drug Facts and Comparisons*, 2009).

Pharmacotherapeutics

Precautions and Contraindications

The metabolites of these drugs have been found in increased concentrations in patients with chronic liver disease. Although available clinical data to date show no evidence of hepatotoxicity induced by **pioglitazone** or **rosiglitazone**, it is prudent to remember that these drugs are structurally similar to **troglitazone** and may demonstrate similar problems with time. Serum transaminase levels must be checked at the start of therapy and frequently during therapy. Specific monitoring times are discussed in the Monitoring section. These drugs should not be initiated in patients with ALT levels greater than 2.5 times the upper limit of normal. They should be discontinued if the patient develops jaundice or has laboratory measurements suggesting liver injury (e.g., ALT greater than 3 times the upper limit of normal).

An increase in plasma volume (fluid retention) with a resultant increase in body weight and decrease in hemoglobin of less than or equal to 1 percent with **rosiglitazone** and 2 to 4 percent with **pioglitazone** has been noted in some patients. This may not present a problem for patients with New York Heart Association class I or II heart disease, but these drugs should be used with caution if administered to class III or IV heart disease patients. They may exacerbate or lead to heart failure. This is more likely if the patient is on a combination of a **TDZ** and **insulin**.

Recent studies (Nissen & Wolski, 2007; Richter et al, 2007; Selvin et al, 2008; Singh, Loke, & Furberg, 2007) have found an increase in cardiovascular morbidity and mortality for **rosiglitazone**. In 2009, the American Diabetes Association and the European Association for the Study of Diabetes produced a consensus algorithm that included the recommendation that **rosiglitazone** not be used in the treatment of type 2 diabetes based on accumulating data questioning the safety of this drug. Although **rosiglitazone** is still available, it now has a black box warning regarding its cardiotoxicity. Nathan (2009), writing for the American Diabetes Association and the European Association for the Study of Diabetes Consensus Committee, states that "given the other options available, the consensus group agreed unanimously to withdraw our previous recommendation of **rosiglitazone**" (p. e59). The Canadian Diabetes Association disagrees with this recommendation. They base this in part on recent studies (ACCORD and RECORD), which have not clearly shown increased cardiac risk (Woo et al, 2009). In premenopausal anovulatory patients with **insulin** resistance, **TDZ** treatment may result in resumption of ovulation. If pregnancy is not desired, a birth control method should be instituted prior to beginning therapy.

There are no adequate and well-controlled studies of the use of **pioglitazone** or **rosiglitazone** in pregnant women. Some animal studies have shown fetal death and growth retardation. These drugs are listed as Pregnancy Category C; **TDZs** should not be used during pregnancy unless the potential benefit clearly outweighs the risk. **Insulin** is the drug of choice for treatment of diabetes during pregnancy.

It is not known whether these drugs are excreted in human breast milk. They are secreted in the milk of lactating rats. Do not administer these drugs to lactating women. Safety and efficacy in children younger than 18 years have not been established.

Adverse Drug Reactions

TDZs are generally well tolerated, and all reported adverse reactions (except those associated with hepatic injury discussed in the Precautions and Contraindications section) have been no more common than those seen with placebo.

Drug Interactions

Administration of **pioglitazone** with an **oral contraceptive** that contains **ethinyl estradiol** and **norethindrone** reduces the plasma concentrations of both components by 30 percent. These changes, added to the resumption of ovulation that occurs in some anovulatory women, could result in loss of contraception. A higher dose of **oral contraceptive** or an alternative birth control method may be needed.

Pioglitazone is metabolized by the CPY450 3A4 isoenzyme system. Specific formal pharmacokinetic interaction studies have not been conducted with other drugs also metabolized by this system (e.g., **erythromycin, calcium channel blockers, corticosteroids, cyclosporine, HMG-CoA reductase inhibitors**). One anecdotal report by Slim, Salem, Zani, and Biour (2009) found a case of **pioglitazone**-induced rhabdomyolysis in a 52-year-old man when this drug was added to a treatment regimen with **gliclazide** and **acarbose**. The rhabdomyolysis resolved when the **pioglitazone** was discontinued. In vitro, **ketoconazole** appears to significantly inhibit **pioglitazone** metabolism. Until data are available, it is prudent to avoid these drug combinations or to carefully monitor patients concurrently taking **pioglitazone** and any of the drugs also metabolized by the CYP450 3A4 isoenzyme system. Table 21–26 presents drug interactions with **thiazolidinediones**.

Clinical Use and Dosing

The only approved indication for these drugs is as therapy for type 2 diabetes mellitus patients not controlled by diet alone or diet and an **oral antidiabetic agent** or **insulin**.

Monotherapy

Clinical trials have been conducted to study the use of both **pioglitazone** and **rosiglitazone** as monotherapy for

Table 21–26 ▣ **Drug Interactions With Thiazolidinediones**

Drug	Interacting Drug	Possible Effect	Implications
Pioglitazone	Oral contraceptives	Oral contraceptives with ethinyl estradiol and norethindrone show reduced plasma contraceptive components	May result in loss of contraception; consider higher dose of contraceptive or alternative method
	Atorvastatin	Concurrent use for 7 d shows in increase in serum concentrations of both drugs	Monitor BG closely
	Ketoconazole	Coadministration shows in increase in pioglitazone AUC and C_{max}. Ketoconazole significantly inhibits pioglitazone metabolism.	Avoid concurrent use. Select different antifungal agent. If both must be given, monitor glycemic control closely.
	Nifedipine	Concurrent use shows in increase in nifedipine-ER concentrations	Unknown clinical significance
Pioglitazone and rosiglitazone	Bile acid sequestrants	Pharmacological effects of thiazolidinedione may be decreased; bile acid sequestrant reduces absorption	Avoid concurrent use; separate doses by 4 h, giving thiazolidinedione first

patients previously treated only with diet. The current Standards of Medical Care in Diabetes of the American Diabetes Association (2009), however, recommend that these drugs be used as add-on therapy when blood glucose targets are not achieved by lifestyle modifications and **metformin.** Doses of 15 to 30 mg/day of **pioglitazone** were associated with decreased fasting BG by 39 mg/dL for the 15-mg dose and 58 mg/dL for the 30-mg dose. Glycosylated hemoglobin (HgA_{1c}) was reduced by 0.9 percent for the 15-mg dose and 1.3 percent for the 30-mg dose.

The initial dose of **pioglitazone** may be either 15 mg or 30 mg and the dose may be increased in 15-mg increments to a maximum dose of 45 mg/day (Table 21–27). Because effectiveness of therapy is best evaluated by HgA_{1c} values, it is recommended that the adequate time

Table 21–27 ◉ **Dosage Schedule: Thiazolidinediones**

Drug	Indication	Initial Dose	Maintenance Dose
Pioglitazone	Monotherapy (see text for more discussion)	15–30 mg daily	May increase in increments up to maximum dose of 45 mg/d
	Combined with sulfonylurea	15–30 mg daily	Continue current sulfonylurea dose; decrease dose of sulfonylurea if hypoglycemia results. Maximum dose of pioglitazone 45 mg/d
	Combined with metformin	15–30 mg daily	Continue metformin dose. Maximum dose is 45 mg/d
	Combination with insulin	15–30 mg once daily	15–30 mg/d. Decrease insulin dose by 10%–25% if hypoglycemia or FBG <100 mg/dL
Rosiglitazone	Monotherapy	4 mg/d in single dose or in divided doses twice daily	If inadequate response in 12 wk, increase to 8 mg/d in single or divided doses. Maximum dose is 8 mg/d
	Combined with metformin	4 mg/d in single dose or in divided doses twice daily	May be increased to 8 mg if inadequate control after 12 wk. Maximum dose is 8 mg/d
	Combination with insulin	4 mg once daily	Do not exceed 4 mg/d. Decrease insulin dose by 10%–25% if hypoglycemia or FBG <100 mg/dL

period for evaluation of drug effectiveness is 3 months unless glycemic control deteriorates.

Rosiglitazone in doses of 8 mg/day reduced fasting BG by 40.8 mg/dL and HgA_{1c} by 0.53 percent. Four-milligram doses reduced fasting BG by 25.4 percent and HgA_{1c} by 0.27 percent. **Rosiglitazone** is usually initiated at 4 mg/day as a single dose. If single-dose therapy is not effective, the dose may be divided into twice-daily dosing or increased incrementally to a maximum dose of 8 mg/day (see Tables 21–26 and 21–27). As with **pioglitazone**, evaluation of adequacy of response requires 12 weeks of therapy.

Combination Therapy With Sulfonylureas

When used as added therapy to management with a **sulfonylurea**, initiate **pioglitazone** with either the 15- or 30-mg dose. For **rosiglitazone**, initiate therapy at 4 mg/day in single or divided doses. Continue the current dose of the **sulfonylurea**. If the response in terms of glycemic control is inadequate, increase the dose of the TDZ at 8 to 12 weeks, not to exceed the maximum mg/day (see Table 21–27).

The pharmacodynamics of **TDZs** are different from that of **sulfonylureas** so that the two drugs taken together potentiate each other's actions. Both fasting and postprandial BG levels of patients decrease. It is important to monitor BG levels closely when **TDZs** are added to the treatment regimen to avoid hypoglycemia.

Combination Therapy With Metformin

TDZs have been approved for combination therapy with **metformin**. This combination is discussed in the **Biguanides** section.

Combination Therapy With Insulin

For patients stabilized on **insulin**, continue the **insulin** dose while initiating the TDZ. For **pioglitazone**, initiate the dose at 15 to 30 mg once daily. For **rosiglitazone**, initiate the dose at 4 mg once daily and do not increase this dose. For both drugs, decrease the **insulin** dose by 10 to 25 percent if the patient reports hypoglycemia or if the FBG decreases to less than 100 mg/dL. Further adjustments are individualized based on glucose-lowering response (see Table 21–27).

Monitoring

Serum transaminase (ALT) levels must be checked at the start of therapy. **TDZs** are not started if the pretreatment serum ALT level is more than 2.5 times the upper limit of normal (ULN). Once therapy is started, ALT is checked every 2 months for the first 12 months and periodically thereafter. If the ALT increases to more than 1.5 to 2 times the ULN, liver function tests are done every week until levels return to normal. The drug is discontinued if the ALT level is more than 3 times the ULN. The cost of this amount of monitoring must be considered in the total cost of therapy with these drugs.

If any patient develops symptoms suggesting hepatic dysfunction, the decision whether to continue the therapy with **pioglitazone** or **rosiglitazone** is guided by clinical judgment pending laboratory evaluation. If jaundice is observed, therapy is discontinued.

Due to contradictory evidence on the cardiotoxicity of **rosiglitazone**, patients taking this drug should have their cardiac function evaluated on a regular basis. This evaluation should look for indications of myocardial ischemia and heart failure.

Response to TDZ therapy is assessed by regular monitoring of fasting BG and HgA_{1c}. During initial therapy and with each incremental increase, fasting BG is used to evaluate response. After the patient is stabilized on a specific dose, monitoring with fasting BG and HgA_{1c} levels every 3 to 6 months is sufficient.

Patient Education

Administration

Pioglitazone is to be taken once daily in the morning. If it is missed, it can be taken as soon as remembered. If the dose is missed for the entire day, the dose should not be doubled the next day. Explain to the patient that **pioglitazone** helps to control hyperglycemia, but it does not cure diabetes. The therapy is long term.

Rosiglitazone may be taken once daily or twice daily in divided doses. The dosing schedule should not be changed without consultation with the health-care provider. If the dose is missed for the entire day, the dose should not be doubled the next day. Explain to the patient that **rosiglitazone** helps to control hyperglycemia, but it does not cure diabetes. The therapy is long term.

Adverse Reactions

TDZs are generally well tolerated and adverse reactions are rare. The one adverse reaction of concern is hepatocellular injury. Advise the patient to report immediately any signs of hepatic dysfunction such as nausea, vomiting, abdominal pain, fatigue, anorexia, jaundice, or dark urine. Explain to the patient that hepatic function must be carefully monitored and that it is essential to keep follow-up appointments for laboratory work.

Hypoglycemia is not a risk with monotherapy, but may occur when **TDZs** are given with another glucose-lowering drug. The usual treatment for hypoglycemia with sucrose, fructose, or starches will resolve the problem. Management of hypoglycemia is discussed in the Patient Education sections of the **Endocrine Pancreatic Hormones (Insulins)** and **Sulfonylureas** sections.

Cardiac risk has been discussed above. Patients should report immediately any chest pain, shortness of breath, peripheral edema, or indications of impending stroke.

Female patients using **oral contraceptives** for birth control and premenopausal anovulatory patients should be informed about the possible need to increase the dose of **oral contraceptive** or choose an alternative birth control method.

Lifestyle Management

Type 2 diabetes is a chronic illness managed with diet, exercise, weight control, and self-monitoring of BG, as well as drug therapy. Further patient teaching related to management of diabetes is discussed in Chapter 33. Table 21–28 depicts the available dosage forms of **thiazolidinediones**.

MEGLITINIDES

The **meglitinides** have a different mechanism of action than any of the other drugs used to treat type 2 diabetes. They are **short-acting insulin secretagogues**. Their action has proved helpful in lowering BG levels as monotherapy for patients who cannot achieve BG control with diet alone, and they have proved successful in combination with **metformin** for patients who cannot be controlled by lifestyle modifications or either agent taken alone. Current guidelines suggest these drugs be used as add-on therapy. **Repaglinide (Prandin)** can also be used in combination with **TDZs**. **Repaglinide** was approved in April 1998, and **nateglinide (Starlix)** was approved in December 2000. This section discusses these two drugs.

Pharmacodynamics

Meglitinides close ATP-dependent potassium channels in the beta cell membrane by binding at specific receptor sites. This potassium channel blockade depolarizes the beta cell and leads to an opening of calcium channels. The resultant influx of calcium increases the secretion of **insulin**. Because its time in the plasma is less than 2 hours, the effect is very short. The ion channel mechanism is highly tissue selective, with low affinity for heart and skeletal muscle, which reduces the potential adverse effects of these tissues.

The end result of **meglitinide** stimulation of **insulin** secretion is lower postprandial BG levels. They do not directly affect fasting BG levels or any of the other defects in metabolism seen in type 2 diabetes mellitus. They are most useful in patients whose primary glucose alteration is postprandial hyperglycemia.

Pharmacokinetics

Absorption and Distribution

After oral administration, **meglitinides** are rapidly and completely absorbed from the GI tract. They are highly bound to albumin for distribution, primarily to beta cell membranes. Peak plasma levels occur within 1 hour. The presence of food in the gut does not affect AUC, but there is a delay in C_{max} and time to peak plasma concentration (T_{max}). Both drugs are taken 20 minutes before a meal.

Metabolism and Excretion

Both drugs are completely metabolized by oxidative biotransformation and direct conjugation with glucuronic acid. The CYP450 enzyme system, particularly 2C9 for **nateglinide** and 3A4 for **repaglinide**, is involved in their metabolism. The metabolites of **nateglinide** are less potent **antidiabetic agents**, but the metabolites of **repaglinide** do not contribute to any glucose-lowering effect.

This drug is rapidly eliminated from the plasma, with a half-life of 1 to 1.5 hours. Within 96 hours after administration of **repaglinide** and 6 hours of **nateglinide**, the drugs and their metabolites are recovered in the feces and in the urine. Table 21–19 depicts the pharmacokinetics of these drugs.

Table 21–28 ◆ **Available Dosage Forms: Thiazolidinediones**

Drug	Dosage Form	Cost
Pioglitazone (Actos)	15 mg in 30-, 90-, and 500-tablet bottles 30 mg in 30-, 90-, and 500-tablet bottles 45 mg in 30-, 90-, and 500-tablet bottles	$469/100 $691/100 $753/100
ActoPlus Met (Piogliazone and Metformin)	15 mg/500 mg in 60- and 180-tablet bottles 15 mg/850 mg in 60- and 180-tablet bottles	$358/100 $358/100
ActoPlus Met XR (Piogliazone and Metformin)	15 mg/ER 1,000 mg in 30-, 60-, and 90-tablet bottles 30 mg/ER 1,000 mg in 30-, 60-, and 90-tablet bottles	
Rosiglitazone (Avandia)	2 mg in 30-, 60-, 100-, and 500-tablet bottles 4 mg in 30-, 60-, 100-, and 500-tablet bottles 8 mg in 30-, 60-, 100-, and 500-tablet bottles	$272/100 $421/100 $715/100
Avandamet (Rosiglitzaone and Metformin)	1 mg/500 mg in bottles of 60 tablets 2 mg/500 mg in bottles of 60 tablets 2 mg/1,000 mg in bottles of 60 tablets 4 mg/500 mg in bottles of 60 tablets 4 mg/1,000 mg in bottles of 60 tablets	$113/100 $261 $242 $421 $421

Pharmacotherapeutics

Precautions and Contraindications

In clinical trials, patients with moderate to severe hepatic impairment had higher and more prolonged serum concentrations of both total and unbound **meglitinides** than did healthy subjects. This drug should be used cautiously with patients who have hepatic impairment, and longer intervals between dosage adjustments should be used.

Repaglinide and **nateglinide** are Pregnancy Category C. Nonteratogenic skeletal deformities occurred in test animals. There are no adequate and well-controlled trials in pregnant women. **Insulin** is the drug of choice for treating diabetes in pregnant women. **Meglitinides** should not be used during pregnancy.

Both drugs are excreted in the breast milk of test animals. It is not known if it is excreted in human breast milk. Because the potential exists for hypoglycemia in nursing infants, they should not be used with lactating women.

No studies have been done to test these drugs' safety and efficacy in children.

Adverse Drug Reactions

The risk for hypoglycemia with **meglitinides** is about the same as with **glyburide** and **glipizide.** Patients with hepatic insufficiency, older adults, and debilitated and malnourished patients are at higher risk for hypoglycemia. The frequency of hypoglycemia is also greater for patients who have not been previously treated with oral hypoglycemic agents or whose HbA_{1c} is less than 8 percent. Careful timing of administration with regard to meals lessens the likelihood of this adverse reaction.

The risk for weight gain is similar to the **sulfonylureas.** Poor weight control is an issue in the management of type 2 diabetes in relation to complication development.

Drug Interactions

Because the CYP450 3A4 enzyme system is involved in the metabolism of **repaglinide** and both 2C9 (70%) and 3A4 (30%) in the metabolism of **nateglinide**, drugs that induce these isoenzymes (e.g., **rifampin, barbiturates, carbamazepine)** may increase **meglitinide** metabolism (Table 21–29). These isoenzymes are among the most used widely by drugs for metabolism; other drug reactions may be found as this drug is used.

Antifungal agents such as **ketoconazole** and **miconazole**, and **antimicrobial agents** such as **erythromycin** inhibit **repaglinide** metabolism and may increase the risk for hypoglycemia by raising blood levels of the drug.

Any drug that alters BG levels has the potential to alter the glycemic control effects of **meglitinides.** Drugs that alter BG levels are shown in Table 21–12. **Meglitinides** can potentiate the action of drugs that are highly protein bound by competing for their binding sites (e.g., **NSAIDs, salicylates, sulfonamides, warfarin, beta-adrenergic blockers,** and **monoamine oxidase inhibitors**). Table 21–29 shows drug interactions for the **meglitinides.**

Clinical Use and Dosing

Monotherapy

Of the two drugs currently available in the United States, **repaglinide** is almost as effective as **metformin**, decreasing HbA_{1c} levels by about 1.5 percent. **Nateglinide** is somewhat less effective in lowering HbA_{1c}. For monotherapy, if the patient has not previously been treated with oral agents or if the HbA_{1c} is less than 8 percent, the initial dose is 0.5 mg tid 30 minutes or less before each meal for **repaglinide** and 120 mg following the same schedule for **nateglinide.** If the HbA_{1c} is 8 percent or more or the patient is being switched from another oral agent, the initial dose is 1 to 2 mg tid for **repaglinide.** The dose does not change for **nateglinide** for HgA_{1c} less than 8 percent, but

Table 21–29 ■ Drug Interactions With Meglitinides and Repaglinide

Interacting Drug	Possible Efect	Implications
Drugs that induce CYP450 3A4	Increases metabolism and decreases effect of repaglinide and nateglinide	Closely monitor blood glucose levels and patient response
Drugs that induce CYP450 2C9	Increases metabolism and decreases the effect of nateglinide	Closely monitor blood glucose levels and patient response
Ketoconazole, miconazole, and potentially other "azoles"	Inhibits meglitinide metabolism and may increase risk for hypoglycemia	Closely monitor blood glucose levels and patient response Choose a different antifungal
Erythromycin and potentially other macrolides	Inhibits meglitinide metabolism and may increase risk for hypoglycemia	Closely monitor blood glucose levels and patient response Choose a different class of antimicrobial
Any drug that increases or decreases BG levels	May alter glycemic effects of meglitinide and increases risk for lack of control or hypoglycemia	Closely monitor blood glucose levels and patient response

it may be reduced to 60 mg tid 30 minutes before each meal if the patient is near goal HgA_{1c} (less than 7%) when treatment is initiated.

Combination With Metformin

Initial **repaglinide** dosing in combination with **metformin** is the same as with monotherapy if there is inadequate control with **metformin** and **repaglinide** is being added. **Metformin** can also be added to **repaglinide** therapy if there is inadequate control with **repaglinide** alone. Follow the initial dosing regimen for **metformin**.

Initial dosing for **nateglinide** with **metformin** is also the same as with monotherapy and for the same reasons and with the same protocol. Additional data on this combination are found in the **Biguanides** section.

For Both Uses

Doses are always administered 0 to 30 minutes prior to each meal (Table 21–30). The patient who does not eat does not use the drug. If extra meals are eaten, extra doses are taken. Dosage changes are based on fasting BG and HbA_{1c} levels. With **repaglinide**, the preprandial dose should be doubled, up to 4 mg, until satisfactory BG response is achieved. The initial dose and the maintenance dose are the same for **nateglinide**. Allow at least 1 week to assess patient response before adjusting a dose. The maximum daily dose is 16 mg for **repaglinide** and 720 mg for **nateglinide**. No dosage adjustments are required based on age, race, or gender. Table 21–30 shows the dosage schedules for these drugs.

Monitoring

The only monitoring required with this drug is periodic monitoring of fasting BG and HbA_{1c}. These values should be determined prior to initiation of therapy to determine baseline values and contribute to the decision about initial dose. Thereafter, they are used to monitor patient response.

Patient Education

Administration

Timing of the drug in relation to food is critical. The drug may be taken 30 minutes or less before a meal. If a meal is omitted, the drug should not be taken. If a meal is added to the patient's usual eating pattern, an additional dose should be taken. The total daily dose, however, should not exceed 16 mg for **repaglinide** or 720 mg for **nateglinide**. The preprandial dose should not be altered without first consulting the health-care provider.

Adverse Reactions

The only adverse effect associated with this drug is hypoglycemia. The risk is about the same as for patients taking **glipizide** or **glyburide**. Patients should be taught how to recognize and manage hypoglycemia, should it occur, as was discussed earlier in the Patient Teaching sections on **insulin** and **oral hypoglycemics**.

Table 21–30 ● **Dosage Schedule: Meglitinides Repaglinide**

Drug	Indication	Initial Dose	Maintenance Dose
Nateglinide	Monotherapy or combination with metformin for patient not previously managed with other agent and HgA_{1c} <8%	120 mg taken 20–30 min before each meal	Same as initial dose. Maximum dose 720 mg/d.
	Monotherapy or combination with metformin when target HgA1c is near <7% at initiation of therapy	60 mg taken 20–30 min before each meal	Same as initial dose. Maximum dose 720 mg/d.
Repaglinide	Monotherapy for patient not previously managed with oral agent and HbA_{1c} less than 8%	0.5 mg taken 30 min or less before each meal	Double preprandial dose, up to 4 mg, until blood glucose reaches target level. Dose increases at 1-wk intervals. Maximum dose 16 mg/d.
	Monotherapy for patient switching from other oral agent and HbA_{1c} 8% or more	1–2 mg taken 30 min or less before each meal	Double preprandial dose, up to 4 mg, until blood glucose reaches target level. Dose increases at 1-wk intervals. Maximum dose 16 mg/d.
	Combination therapy adding metformin	If HbA_{1c} less than 8%, dose is 0.5 mg. If HbA_{1c} is 8% or more, dose is 1–2 mg. Dose taken 30 min or less before a meal.	Double preprandial dose, up to 4 mg, until blood glucose reaches target level. Dose increases at 1-wk intervals. Maximum dose 16 mg/d.

Lifestyle Management

Type 2 diabetes is a chronic illness managed with diet, exercise, weight control, and self-monitoring of BG, as well as drug therapy. Further patient teaching related to management of diabetes is discussed in Chapter 33.

Table 21–31 shows available dosage forms and how they are supplied.

DIPEPTIDYL PEPTIDASE-4 INHIBITORS

The **dipeptidyl peptidase-4 inhibitors** (**gliptins**) are the newest class of **antidiabetic agents** with the first drug in the class, **sitagliptin**, approved in 2006 and **saxagliptin** approved in August 2009. **Vildagliptin** is not yet approved in the United States, but is being used in other parts of the world. Newer insights into the pathogenesis of type 2 diabetes have postulated a role for the incretin hormones. The action of **gliptins** is different from other **antidiabetic agents** because they act on the incretin hormone system to have an indirect effect to increase **insulin** production. Although the improvement in glycemic control is moderate and no more than with **metformin**, they are well tolerated, have a low risk for hypoglycemia, do not cause weight gain, and can be given orally once a day. These are in contrast to the common adverse effects of existing **antidiabetic agents**. Although they have been approved for monotherapy, they are best used as add-on therapy in combination with **metformin** as second-line therapy.

Pharmacodynamics

Pathophysiological defects in type 2 diabetes mellitus include an increased hepatic glucose output associated in part with increased secretion of glucagon by pancreatic alpha cells and decreased amount and functioning of the insulin secreted by the pancreatic beta cells. Glucagon-like peptide (GLP-1) is an incretin hormone derived from the gut that stimulates glucose-dependent insulin secretion, enhances insulin gene transcription and insulin biosynthesis, enhances cellular transformation from pancreatic ductal tissues to beta cell tissue, increases beta cell mass by cellular neogenesis and proliferation, inhibits beta cell apoptosis, suppresses glucagon secretion, inhibits gastric emptying, and reduces appetite and food intake (Drucker & Nauck, 2006; Pande, 2009). The actions of this peptide address several defects found in type 2 diabetes. Circulating levels of GLP-1 are significantly reduced in type 2 diabetes. GLP-1 receptors have been found in the stomach, intestine, central nervous system, kidney, heart and lungs (Pande, 2009). Dipeptidyl peptidase-4 (DPP-4) rapidly inactivates GLP-1, contributing to the defects seen in type 2 diabetes. Therapeutic approaches to enhance the actions of GLP-1 and thereby prolong the beneficial effects of this incretin hormone include GLP-1 receptor agonists and inhibitors of DPP-4. This section will focus on the latter. Because they are commonly referred to as **gliptins**, this name will be used to denote DPP-2 inhibitors. These drugs have demonstrated efficacy in reducing pre- and postprandial glucose levels, reducing HbA_{1c} levels and promoting weight loss in obese diabetics. Although **gliptins** enhance the activity of GLP-1, they reduce postprandial glucose concentration by stimulating insulin secretion and suppressing glucagon secretion, but have no direct effect on insulin action to increase glucose utilization and so do not address cellular insulin resistance (Man et al, 2009).

Pharmacokinetics

Absorption and Distribution

After oral administration, these drugs are rapidly absorbed from the GI tract with 87 percent bioavailability for **sitagliptin (Januvia)**, 85 percent for **vildagliptin (Glavus)**, and 75 percent for **saxagliptin (Onglyza)**. They can be taken with or without food. The volume of distribution of **sitagliptin** is approximately 198 L. Older adults have a greater volume of distribution of **saxagliptin** than do younger patients.

Metabolism and Excretion

Sitagliptin undergoes minimal metabolism, primarily involving CYP3A4 and CYP2C8. No active metabolites are produced. Mild hepatic insufficiency appears to have no clinically significant effect on its metabolism (Migoya et al, 2009). **Vildagliptin** also undergoes minimal metabolism, but there is a primary metabolite. **Saxagliptin** is metabolized by CYP 3A4. There is one active metabolite.

The major route of excretion is renal and involves active tubular secretion for all of these drugs. A large portion

Table 21–31 ◈ **Available Dosage Forms: Meglitinides**

Drug	Dosage Form	How Supplied	Cost
Nateglinide (Starlix)	Tablets: 60 mg 120 mg	In bottles of 100 In bottles of 100	$164/100 tablets $166/100 tablets
Repaglinide (Prandin)	Tablets: 0.5 mg, 1 mg, and 2 mg	In bottles of 100, 500, and 1,000	$214/100 tablets for all
PrandiMet (Repaglinide and Metformin)	Tablets: 1 mg/500 mg Tablets: 2 mg/ 500 mg	In bottles of 20 and 100 In bottles of 20 and 100	$190/100 tablets for all

is eliminated unchanged in the urine. Decreased renal function results in reduced renal clearance, but not to a degree that is clinically significant.

Table 21–32 shows the pharmacokinetics of these drugs.

Pharmacotherapeutics

Precautions and Contraindications

Because of their high dependence on the renal system for elimination, these drugs should be used cautiously with those with impaired renal function. A risk for toxicity exists for patients with end-stage renal disease and for those with moderate to severe renal impairment. Dosage adjustments for renal impairment for patients taking **sitagliptin** are given in Table 21–34. No dosage adjustments are given for the other drugs in this class. Older adults are more likely to have renal impairment, so kidney function should be considered for initial dosing and periodically monitored when these drugs are used in this population.

Gliptins are Pregnancy Category B; however, no well-controlled trials have been performed in humans related to pregnancy. These are relatively new drugs without long-term exposure to the pregnant diabetic population. Some other drug classes have historically shown adverse effects only after long-term use has provided a larger number of patient exposures. **Gliptins** should be used in pregnant women only if the benefits outweigh potential teratogenic effects.

It is unknown if **gliptins** pass into breast milk and infant risk has not been determined. Caution should be used when these drugs are given to nursing mothers.

Safety and efficacy in children (under 18 years of age) have not been established and these drugs are not used in type 1 diabetes.

Adverse Drug Reactions

The risk for hypoglycemia is low when **gliptins** are given as monotherapy or in combination with **metformin** (Pande, 2009; Tahrani, Piya, & Barnett, 2009; *Drug Facts and Comparisons,* 2009). The most common adverse effects are GI symptoms, headache, and increased upper respiratory infections, but the incidences for all of these are less than 5 percent.

Drug Interactions

Coadministration of **gliptins** with **ACE inhibitors** has been associated with increased risk of angioedema (Brown, Bylers, Carr, Maldonado, & Warner, 2009); however, the absolute risk is small. **Digoxin** had an increase of 11 to 18 percent in its AUC when coadministered with **sitagliptin.** This small increase in **digoxin** exposure is unlikely to be clinically important (*Drug Facts and Comparisons,* 2009). No drug interaction has been observed between **digoxin** and **saxagliptin.**

Gliptins have limited hepatic metabolism with CYP 3A4 and CYP 2C8. Until there is more long-term experience with these drugs, other drugs that use these same isoenzyme systems should be monitored for potential interactions. One anecdotal incident involving a 75-year-old woman (DiGregorio & Pasikhova, 2009) suggested a possible drug interaction between **sitagliptin** and **lovastatin** (a drug metabolized by the CYP 3A4 isoenzyme) that resulted in rhabdomyolisis. Table 21–33 shows the drug interactions with these drugs.

Clinical Use and Dosing

Gliptins are indicated as monotherapy and in combinations with or added to other antihyperglycemic drugs for the treatment of patients with type 2 diabetes who cannot

Table 21–32 ▶ Pharmacokinetics: Dipeptidyl Peptidase-4 Inhibitors (Gliptins)

Drug	Onset*	Peak*	Duration*	Protein Binding	Bioavailability	Half-Life	Excretion
Sitagliptin (Januvia) (B)	UK	1–4 h	24 h	38%	87%	12.4 h	87% in urine, 13% in feces
Vildagliptin (Glavus) (B)	UK	1–2 h	12–24 h	UK	85%	1.7–3.3 h	33% in urine Renal clearance 22% lower in older adults
Saxagliptin (Onglyza) (B)	UK	2 h	12–24 h	UK	75%	2.2–3.8 h	70% in urine

Table 21–33 ■ Drug Interactions With Dipeptidyl Peptidase-4 Inhibitors (Gliptins)

Drug	Interacting Drug	Possible Outcomes	Implications
Sitagliptin	Digoxin	AUC of digoxin increased 11%	Monitor patients receiving digoxin.
	Warfarin	No interactions found	No dosage adjustments required.
	Drug metabolized by CYP 450 system	No interactions found	Clinical studies have shown a very low propensity for causing drug interaction with substrates of CYP 3A4, 2C8, or 2C9.

achieve adequate blood glucose control with diet, exercise, weight control, **metformin**, and other drugs. They are especially useful for obese patients because they are not associated with weight gain and have been associated with weight loss in some patients. They could be especially beneficial in patients whose weight significantly increases cardiovascular risk (Kendall, Cuddihy, & Bergenstal, 2009). They are generally not appropriate as first-line therapy except for selected patients due to cost and lack of long-term safety data.

Monotherapy

All of the **gliptins** have been approved for monotherapy. **Sitagliptin** is administered in a once daily dose of 100 mg (*Drugs Facts and Comparisons,* 2009). Dosages are reduced for decreased creatinine clearance. One study reported by Chahal and Chowdhury (2007) found that drug-naïve patients taking 50-mg doses reduced their HbA_{1c} by 0.8 percent over a 12-week study period. Another 24-week study found reduction of 0.8 percent for patients taking 100 mg and 0.9 percent for patients taking 200 mg. A third study (Raz et al, 2006) found no benefit of treatment over 200 mg compared to 100 mg.

Vildagliptin is administered in bid dose of 50 mg for a total daily dose of 100 mg. Studies done with 25 mg bid doses have yielded HbA_{1c} reductions of 0.6 percent, 50 mg bid yielded reductions of 0.7 to 0.8 percent, and 100 mg once daily yielded reductions of 0.9 percent (Chahal & Chowdhury, 2007). This drug has been submitted for approval by the FDA, but has not yet received it.

Saxagliptin was approved in August 2009 for monotherapy and in combination with **metformin.** It is administered once daily with dose ranges between 2.5 and 10 mg.

Combination With Metformin

All of the **gliptins** have been approved for use in combination with **metformin.** A 54-week study of the efficacy and safety of combined therapy with **sitagliptin** and **metformin** in patients with type 2 diabetes found that initial treatment with either drug alone or in combination provided substantial and durable glycemic control and improved markers of beta cell function, and was generally well tolerated. Changes in HbA_{1c} levels were essentially the same for each arm of the study. Mean body weight decreased the most in the drug combination group (Williams-Herman et al, 2009). The dosages used in this study were **sitagliptin** 100 mg, **metformin** either 1,000 mg or 2,000 mg, and **sitagliptin** 100 mg combined with each of the two doses of **metformin.** In other studies (Chahal & Chowdhury, 2007), the addition of **sitagliptin** 100 mg daily to the treatment regimen for patients who were not well controlled on **metformin** greater than 1,500 mg daily resulted in increased reductions in HbA_{1c} levels of 0.7 percent.

Vildagliptin has also been studied in combination with **metformin** mainly as add-on therapy. The addition of **vildagliptin** 50 mg in patients already taking **metformin** 1,500 to 3,000 mg resulted in additional reduction of HbA_{1c} of 0.6 percent and for those given 100 mg (50 mg bid) the reduction was 1.1 percent (Chahal & Chowdhury, 2007). The pharmacokinetic interaction of the two drugs is not clinically significant so that no dosage adjustment is required for either drug (He et al, 2009).

Combination With Thiazolidinediones

Both **sitagliptin** and **vildagliptin** have been approved for use in combination with **TDZs**. The **TDZs** are associated with more adverse effects than the **gliptins**, and the combination of the two carries this concern. This is especially related to the weight gain and potential increased cardiovascular risk associated with **TDZs**.

When **sitagliptin** 100 mg was added to a treatment regimen for patients not well controlled on **pioglitazone** 30 and 45 mg in one study, the HbA_{1c} reductions were 0.7 percent and 0.9 percent, respectively (Chahal & Chowdhury, 2007). In a 24-week trial of patients inadequately controlled on **pioglitazone** 45 mg, **vildagliptin** 50 mg and 100 mg were used as add-on therapy, resulting in HbA_{1c} reductions of 0.8 percent and 1.0 percent, respectively. In another trial, drug-naïve patients were placed directly on the combination of **vildagliptin** 100 mg and **pioglitazone** 30 mg, which resulted in a HbA_{1c} reduction of 1.9 percent compared with 1.1 percent for the **vildagliptin** alone and 1.4 percent for **pioglitazone** monotherapy (Chahal & Chowdhury, 2007).

Combination With Sulphonylureas

No specific studies were found that used combinations of **gliptins** and **sulfonylureas**; however, such a combination is possible when patients are inadequately controlled with a **sulfonylurea.** If a **gliptin** is used in combination with a **sulfonylurea**, the dose of the **sulfonylurea** should be lowered to reduce the risk of **sulfonylurea**-induced hypoglycemia.

Table 21–34 gives the dosage schedule for these drugs.

Table 21–34 ● **Dosage Schedule for Dipeptidyl Peptidase-4 Inhibitors (Gliptins)**

Drug	Initial Dose	Maintenance Dose	Maximum Dose
Sitagliptin	100 mg once daily	100 mg once daily	200 mg total daily dose
Vildagliptin	50 mg bed	50 mg bid or 100 mg once daily	100 mg daily
Saxaglitpin	2.5 mg once daily	2.5–10 mg once daily	10 mg once daily

Rational Drug Selection

Age

Gliptins have been studied in the elderly population. Despite the concerns raised above about renal function, **gliptins** are effective and well-tolerated treatment options in elderly patients with type 2 diabetes. They demonstrate similar improvement in glycemic control as **metformin**, for example, with similar improvements in glycemic control and better GI tolerability (Schweizer, Dejager, & Bosi, 2009). Dosage adjustments may be made as needed for renal function, but are published only for **sitagliptin**.

Daily Glucose Fluctuations

There is increasing evidence that rapid glucose fluctuations over a daily period might play an important role in diabetic complications. One study did a side-by-side comparison of **sitagliptin** 100 mg taken once daily and **vildagliptin** 50 mg taken bid, looking at the variation of glucose fluctuations (Marfella et al, 2009). There were smaller fluctuations in interprandial glucose levels in the **vildagliptin** group treated bid versus the **sitagliptin** group treated once daily. In choosing between these drugs, flattening acute glucose fluctuations may be a decision factor.

Weight/Obesity

In two separate studies comparing a **gliptin** with a **TDZ**, body weight decreased for the patients on the **gliptin** and increased for patients on the **TDZ** (Blonde et al, 2009; Bolli, Dotta, Colin, Minic, & Goddman, 2009). **Sulphonylureas** have also been associated with weight gain. Both **gliptins** and **metformin** are weight neutral or associated with weight loss. These drugs are especially appropriate for overweight diabetic patients. Because all **gliptins** are weight neutral or promote weight loss, this is not a variable to choose among the various **gliptins**.

Cost

As is usually true for new classes of drugs that have required significant research and development costs, the **gliptins** are expensive. To date there is not much variability among the drugs in terms of cost. Drug cost may be a factor in choosing to use another drug class rather than a **gliptin**; it is not a factor in choosing among the drugs in this class.

Monitoring

Before initiating therapy and at least annually thereafter, assess renal function. Assessment is by serum creatinine and CCr initially and then by serum creatinine annually. Dosage adjustments are required based on creatinine clearance. For patients with increased risk for developing altered renal function, the assessment should be made more often.

Response to **gliptin** therapy is assessed by daily to weekly monitoring of fasting and postprandial BG and by monitoring HbA_{1c} every 3 months or monitoring fructosamine every 2 months. During initial therapy and with each incremental increase, fasting BG is used to evaluate response. After the patient is stabilized on a specific dose, monitoring with fasting BG and HbA_{1c} levels every 6 months is sufficient.

Patient Education

Administration

Sitagliptin is taken once daily in the morning. If the dose is missed it should be taken as soon as remembered. If the dose is missed for the entire day, it should not be doubled the next day. **Vildagliptin** is taken twice daily in divided doses. The dosage schedule should not be changed without consultation with the health-care provider. If the dose is missed it should be taken as soon as remembered. If one of the twice-daily doses is missed and the missed dose is near the time of the second dose, the missed dose may be skipped and the second dose taken on schedule. **Saxagliptin** is taken once daily in the morning. If the dose is missed, it should be taken as soon as remembered. If the dose is missed for the entire day, it should not be doubled the next day. With all three drugs, it is important to do a fingerstick blood glucose reading as soon as the missed dose is discovered and this reading should be discussed with the health-care provider regarding any dosage adjustments that may be needed.

Adverse Reactions

Gliptins are generally well-tolerated and adverse reactions occur in only a small percentage of those taking the drugs. Hypoglycemia is not anticipated with monotherapy, but may occur when these drugs are combined with another glucose-lowering agent. The usual treatment for hypoglycemia with sucrose, fructose or starches will resolve the problem. Management of hypoglycemia is discussed in the Patient Education sections under **Endocrine Pancreatic Hormones (Insulin)** and **Sulphonylureas**.

Lifestyle Management

Type 2 diabetes is a chronic illness managed with diet, exercise, weight control, and self-monitoring of BG, as well as drug therapy. Further patient teaching related to management of diabetes is discussed in Chapter 33. Available dosage forms are shown in Table 21–35.

GLUCAGON-LIKE PEPTIDE-1 AGONISTS

Another new class of drugs that acts on the incretin sytem are the **glucagon-like peptide-1 agonists (GLP-1)**. The first drug in this class, **exenatide (Byetta)**, was approved in April 2005, and a second drug, **liraglutide**, has been submitted for FDA approval. Glucagon-like peptide 1 is a naturally occurring peptide produced in the small intestine that potentiates glucose-stimulated **insulin** secretion. Although the **gliptins** stimulate this secretion indirectly, **GLP-1 agonists** directly bind to the GLP-1 receptor in the pancreatic beta cell and acts as an incretin mimetic. Improvement in glycemic control with a reduction in HbA_{1c}

Table 21–35 ◆ **Available Dosage Forms: Dipeptidyl Peptidase-4 Inhibitors (Gliptins)**

Drug	Dosage Form	How Supplied	Cost
Sitagliptin (Januvia) (B)	Tablets: 25 mg and 50 mg 100 mg	In 30- and 90-tablet bottles and UD blister pack 100 In 30-, 90-, 500-, and 1,000-tablet bottles and UD blister pack 100	Not yet available
Sitagliptin/metformin (Janumet) (B)	Tablets: 50 mg/500 mg 50 mg/1,000 mg	In 60-, 180-, and 1,000-tablet bottles and UD 50 for both strengths	Not yet available
Saxagliptin (Onglyza) (B)	Tablets: 2.5 mg 5 mg	In 30- and 90-tablet bottles In 30-, 90-, and 500-tablet bottles and blister packs of 100	Not yet available

of 0.5 to 1 percent has been demonstrated when added to other **antidiabetic agents.** These drugs have a low risk for hypoglycemia but are given by injection, and **exenatide** must be given twice daily. **Exenatide** has been approved as add-on therapy for patients who are taking **metformin**, a **sulfonylurea**, a TDZ, a combination of **metformin** and a **sulfonylurea**, or a combination of **metformin** and a TDZ.

Pharmacodynamics

The role of GLP-1 in the incretin system was discussed in the previous section. **Exenatide** is a homologue of the human GLP-1 sequence but it has a longer circulating half-life. It binds avidly with the GLP-1 receptor on the pancreatic beta cell to augment glucose-mediated **insulin** release. It also enhances other antihyperglycemic actions of the incretins, such as moderating **glucagon** secretion and lowering **glucagon** concentrations during periods of hyperglycemia. This latter effect leads to decreased hepatic glucose output and decreased **insulin** demand. Each of these effects occurs only in the presence of increased glucose and these effects subside as blood glucose concentrations decrease and approach euglycemia. **GLP-1 agonists** improve glycemic control by reducing fasting and postprandial glucose concentrations. They also slow gastric emptying and reduce appetite, making them either weight neutral or promoting weight loss, a significant factor in type 2 diabetes. In published studies, **exenatide** was associated with weight loss of 2 to 3 kg over 6 months (Nathan et al, 2009).

Pharmacokinetics

Absorption and Distribution

Exenatide is slowly absorbed following subcutaneous injection, reaching median peak plasma concentrations in 2.1 hours. **Liraglutide** reaches peak concentration later at 9 to 12 hours. Absorption is similar for both drugs, whether given in the upper arm, abdomen, or thigh. The mean volume of distribution for **exenatide** is 28.3 L.

Metabolism and Excretion

The metabolic fate of **exenatide** is not clear, but it is excreted predominantly by glomerular filtration with subsequent proteolytic degradation. **Liraglutide** is metabolized to a number of minor metabolites, which are excreted in both urine and feces. Table 21–36 presents pharmacokinetic information on these two drugs.

Pharmacotherapeutics

Precautions and Contraindications

Patients with severe GI disease (e.g., ulcerative colitis, Crohn's disease) should not use these drugs because of their effects on gastric emptying. Anecdotal postmarketing cases of acute pancreatitis have been reported in patients treated with **exenatide**. The number of pancreatitis cases is small, and whether the relationship is causal or coincidental is not clear at this time. Patients should report persistent, severe abdominal pain, which may be accompanied by vomiting; these are hallmark symptoms of pancreatitis.

Table 21–36 ▶ **Pharmacokinetics: Glucagon-Like Peptide-1 and Amylin Agonists**

Drug	Onset*	Peak*	Duration*	Protein Binding	Bioavailability	Half-Life	Excretion
Exenatide	UK	2.1 h	10 h	UK	UK	2.4 h	Mainly in urine
Liraglutide	UK	9–12 h	UK	UK	51%	11–15 h	As metabolites in urine and feces
Pramlintide	UK	19–21 min	UK	40%	30%–40%	48 min	As metabolites in urine

The drug should be used cautiously in older adults and those with mild to moderate renal impairment, although the manufacturer suggests that age does not influence the pharmacokinetics of **exenatide**. End-stage renal disease patients did show a decrease in **exenatide** clearance; therefore, **exenatide** is not recommended for patients with end-stage renal disease. No dosage adjustments are required for older adults or those with mild to moderate renal impairment for either **exenatide** or **liraglutide**.

Both drugs are listed as Pregnancy Category C based on studies in pregnant laboratory animals. No studies have been conducted on pregnant women. It is not known if these drugs are excreted in breast milk. The decision whether to discontinue either breastfeeding or the drug should take into account the drug's importance to the mother.

Adverse Drug Reactions

Exenatide has been associated with a relatively high frequency of GI disturbances, with 30 to 45 percent of treated patients experiencing one or more episodes of nausea, vomiting, or diarrhea (Nathan et al, 2009). These adverse reactions tend to abate over time. The same adverse reactions were seen in clinical trials with **liraglutide**.

Drug Interactions

The major drug interactions for both drugs relate to their action in slowing gastric emptying. Separating the administration of the interacting drug and **exenatide** or **liraglutide** will usually resolve the problem. The International Normalized Ratio (INR) increases and the risk of bleeding also increases when **exenatide** is coadministered with **warfarin**; these two drugs should not be used concurrently. **Digoxin** pharmacokinetics is also altered by **exenatide** and **liraglutide** and these drugs should also not be used concurrently. Table 21–37 lists the drug interactions for these drugs.

Clinical Use and Dosing

Neither of these drugs has been approved for monotherapy to treat type 2 diabetes. They are add-on therapies for patients already taking other diabetic drugs. Manufacturers of **liraglutide** are seeking approval for monotherapy as well as add-on therapy. Regardless of the other diabetic drug being taken, the initial dose of **exenatide** is 5 mcg subcutaneously twice daily 60 minutes before morning and evening meals (or the two main meals of the day, approximately 6 or more hours apart). Based on clinical

Table 21–37 ■ **Drug Interactions With GLP-1 and Amylin Agonists**

Drug	Interacting Drug	Possible Outcomes	Implications
Exenatide and liraglutide	Acetaminophen	Acetaminophen AUC and C_{max} decreased and T_{max} increased when coadministered	Give acetaminophen at least 1 h before or 4 h after exenatide.
Exenatide and liraglutide	Digoxin	Coadministration of repeated doses of exenatide decreased digoxin C_{max} 17% and delayed T_{max} by about 2.5 h	Avoid concurrent use unless both are specifically needed. If so, monitor digoxin level and cardiac rhythm closely.
Exenatide	Lovastatin	Lovastatin AUC decreased by 40% and C_{max} by 28% and T_{max} delayed by 4 h when drugs coadministered	Give lovastatin at least 1 h before or 4 h after exenatide.
Exenatide and liraglutide	Oral antibiotics and oral contraceptives	Slowed gastric emptying may reduce extent and rate of oral medications that require rapid GI absorption	Take these drugs at least 1 h before exenatide.
Exenatide	Warfarin	Exenatide may lead to increased INR and increased bleeing when coadministered with warfarin	Avoid concurrent use unless both are specifically needed. If so, monitor INR closely.
Pramlintide	Drugs that alter GI motility (e.g., anticholinergics	Pramlintide may increase the effects of drugs that slow gastric emptying	Patients using these drugs have not been studied. Avoid concurrent use at this time.
Pramlintide	Orally administered drugs (e.g., analgesics, antibiotics, contraceptives)	Pramlintide has potential to delay absorption if coadministered	Administer interacting drug at least 1 h prior to or 2 h after pramlintide injection.

Table 21–37 ■ **Drug Interactions With GLP-1 and Amylin Agonists—cont'd**

Drug	Interacting Drug	Possible Outcomes	Implications
Pramlintide	Acetaminophen	Acetaminophen C_{max} decreased 29% and T_{max} increased 48–72 min when coadministered or given within 2 h of pramlintide injection	Separate dosing by more than 2 h. Give acetaminophen prior to pramlintide.
Pramlintide	Sulfonylureas, ACE inhibitors, fibrates, fluoxetine, pentoxifylline, propoxyphene, salicylates and sulfonamide antibiotics)	Increase the blood glucose lowering effect and susceptibility to hypoglycemia	If must be given, monitor blood glucose levels closely, which may mean frequent fingerstick blood glucose testing and teach patient signs and symptoms of hypoglycemia.

response, the dose of **exenatide** can be increased to 10 mcg twice daily after 1 month of therapy. **Liraglutide** is administered once daily.

Combination With Metformin, or a TDZ

When **exenatide** is added to **metformin** or TDZ therapy, the current dose **metformin** or TDZ can be continued, as it is unlikely that the dose of either **metformin** or the TDZ will require adjustment because of hypoglycemia.

Combination With Sulfonylurea

When **exenatide** is added to **sulfonylurea** therapy, a reduction in the **sulfonylurea** dose may be considered to reduce the risk of hypoglycemia.

Rational Drug Selection

To date there is only one drug in this class that has FDA approval. However, if **liraglutide** is approved, it will have the advantage as **exenatide** of once daily dosing. There is no other significant difference between **exenatide** and **liragulutide** in terms of precautions or contraindications, adverse effects, or drug interactions.

Monitoring

Glycemic control is monitored based on diabetic guideline protocol. If the patient must also take **warfarin**, INR is monitored closely and if the patient is on **digoxin**, the levels of this drug and cardiac response to it are monitored closely. Renal function studies are monitored based on diabetic guideline protocols.

Patient Education

Administration

Each dose of **exenatide** should be administered as a subcutaneous injection in the thigh, abdomen, or upper arm about 60 minutes before morning and evening meals. Doses should be at least 6 hours apart. **Exenatide** should not be taken after a meal. If a dose is missed, the patient should resume the treatment regimen as prescribed with the next scheduled dose.

Exenatide is dispensed for injection in prefilled pens, which are available in 5-mcg and 10-mcg doses. Explain to the patient that the pen must match the prescribed dosage. Each pen contains 60 doses to provide 30 days of twice-daily injections. The drug comes with a pen-user manual, which the patient should read along with the patient-information insert before starting drug therapy and each time the prescription is refilled. The manual includes information on setting up a new pen and using the pen for subsequent injections, storing and disposing of the pen and needles, and cleaning the outside of the pen. Needles are not included and must be purchased separately.

Adverse Reactions

The most common adverse reactions are GI disturbances that tend to subside with time. **Exenatide** may reduce appetite, the amount of food eaten, and patient weight. No changes in dose are needed, as the reactions actually have a positive effect on diabetes.

When taking **exenatide**, patient blood glucose levels should be checked before and after every meal and at bedtime. Hypoglycemia should not occur unless the patient is also taking a **sulfonylurea.** Hypoglycemic reactions should be reported to the health-care provider so that dosage may be adjusted if needed. Explain the signs and symptoms of hypoglycemia to the patient regardless of the drug combination, and teach the patient how to treat low blood glucose, which is discussed in Chapter 33.

Lifestyle Management

Type 2 diabetes is a chronic illness managed with diet, exercise, weight control, self-monitoring of BG, and drug therapy. Further patient teaching related to management of diabetes is discussed in Chapter 33. Available dosage forms are shown in Table 21–38.

AMYLIN AGONISTS

Amylin agonists are a synthetic analogue of the beta cell hormone amylin. To date there is only one drug in this class, **pramlintide (Symlin)**, an adjunct therapy for both

Table 21–38 ◆ **Available Dosage Forms: GLP-1 and Amylin Agonists**

Drug	Dosage Form	How Supplied	Cost
Exenatide (Byetta) (B)	Injection solution: 250 mcg/mL	In 1.2-mL (5 mcg) and 2.4-mL (10-mcg) prefilled pens. (60 doses)	1.2-mL pen: Each $245 2.4-mL pen: Each $272
Pramlintide (Symlin) (B)	Injection solution: 0.6 mg/mL and 1 mg/mL	In 5-mL vials (0.6 mg/mL) In 1.5- and 2.7-mL multidose pen-injectors (1 mg/mL)	5-mL vial: Each $190 2.7-mL pen: $294 for 2 syringes per box

type 1 and type 2 diabetes. In type 1 diabetes, **pramlintide's** use is for patients who use mealtime **insulin** therapy and have failed to achieve their glycemic target despite optimal **insulin** therapy. In type 2 diabetes, **pramlintide's** use is for patients who use mealtime **insulin** therapy, with or without a concurrent **sulfonylurea** or **metformin** and still have not achieved their glycemic target. Like the **GLP-1 agonists**, **pramlintide** lowers glucose by acting on glucagon secretion and slowing gastric emptying. Its adverse effects and administration via injection are also like the **GLP-1 agonists**. Currently, it is approved for use in the United States only as an add-on therapy with **regular insulin** or **rapid-acting insulin analogues**.

Pharmacodynamics

Amylin is colocated with **insulin** in secretory granules and cosecreted with **insulin** by pancreatic beta cells in response to food intake. Both amylin and **insulin** show similar fasting and postprandial patterns in healthy individuals. Amylin affects the rate of postprandial glucose by slowing gastric emptying; by suppressing glucagon secretion, which leads to decreased endogenous glucose output by the liver; and by centrally mediated modulation of appetite. Patients with type 1 and type 2 diabetes have dysfunctional beta cells resulting in reduced secretion of both **insulin** and amylin in response to food.

Pramlintide acts as an amylin mimetic to modulate gastric emptying, prevent postprandial risk in plasma glucagons, and improve satiety leading to decreased caloric intake and potential weight loss. In clinical studies, HbA_{1c} has decreased 0.5 to 0.7 percent (Nathan et al, 2009), and weight loss associated with this drug is about 1 to 1.5 kg over 6 months.

Pharmacokinetics

Absorption and Distribution

Pramlintide is slowly absorbed from injection sites in the upper arm, abdomen, or thigh. Injection into the arm results in higher exposure to the drug with greater variability compared with injection into the abdomen or thigh.

The drug does not bind extensively to plasma cells or albumin, so pharmacokinetics are relatively insensitive to changes in binding sites.

Metabolism and Excretion

Pramlintide is metabolized primarily by the kidneys, and its primary metabolite (2-37 pramlintide) has a similar half-life and is biologically active. AUC values are relatively constant with repeat dosing, indicating lack of bioaccumulation. Table 21–36 shows the pharmacokinetics of this drug.

Pharmacotherapeutics

Precautions and Contraindications

No consistent age-related differences in drug activity have been shown in clinical studies with older adults, but, given its real metabolism, it seems prudent to use caution or closely monitor older adults on this drug. Studies of patients with moderate or severe renal impairment did not show increased exposure or decreased clearance of the drug, but caution seems prudent given its renal metabolism.

Although **pramlintide** alone does not cause hypoglycemia, it is coadministered with **insulin**; therefore, the risk for hypoglycemia increases. **Pramlintide** is not the best choice for patients who have recurrent episodes of severe hypoglycemia or hypoglycemic unawareness. Older adults are prone to hypoglycemic unawareness, a reason to use the drug with caution in that population.

Confirmed diagnosis of gastroparesis or the required use of drugs to stimulate GI motility also contraindicates using this drug.

Pramlintide is Pregnancy Category C. No adequate and well-controlled studies have been conducted on pregnant women. Increases in congenital anomalies were observed in fetuses of rats treated with this drug, but no such changes were noted in rabbits. The potential risks to the fetus must be balanced with the needs of the mother for the drug when deciding to prescribe it.

Whether this drug is excreted in human milk is unknown. Administer to nursing women only if it is determined that the potential benefit outweighs the potential risk to the infant.

Adverse Drug Reactions

Most adverse effects are GI disturbances. The incidence of nausea was higher at the beginning of treatment and decreased with time in most patients. The incidence and severity of nausea were reduced by gradual titration to the recommended dose. The risk for hypoglycemia is discussed in the Precautions and Contraindications section.

Pramlintide has a **black box warning** about the increased risk for severe hypoglycemia when this drug is used in conjunction with **insulin**.

Drug Interactions

Drug interactions are based largely on other drugs that increase or decrease the actions of **pramlintide.** Drugs that alter GI motility and orally administered drugs that depend on gastric emptying time for absorption interact because of **pramlintide's** slowing of gastric emptying. Drugs that affect blood glucose levels and those with an adverse effect of hypoglycemia interact because of **pramlintide's** blood glucose lowering effects.

Acetaminophen has the only drug interaction not based directly on the actions of **pramlintide. Pramlintide** alters the pharmacokinetics of **acetaminophen**; therefore, their administration times must be separated.

Table 21–37 shows these interactions.

Clinical Use and Dosing

Pramlintide is used in treating type 1 and type 2 diabetes, and dosage differs depending on the type of diabetes.

Type 1 Diabetes

Initiate **pramlintide** at a dose of 15 mcg and titrate the dosage up in 15-mcg increments as tolerated to a 30- or 60-mcg maintenance dose. When the dose is initiated, the dosage of the preprandial **rapid-acting** or **short-acting insulin** (including fixed-mix **insulin**) is reduced by 50 percent. Pre- and postprandial blood glucose and bedtime glucose levels are monitored frequently. The dose of the **pramlintide** is then increased to the next increment when no clinically significant nausea has occurred for at least 3 days. If significant nausea persists at the 46- or 60-mcg dosage, reduce the dose back to 30 mcg. If the 30-mcg dosage is not tolerated, consider discontinuing the drug. Dosage increases are based on achieving the glycemic target. After a maintenance dose of **pramlintide** is achieved, **insulin** doses may be adjusted to optimize glycemic control.

Type 2 Diabetes

Initiate **pramlintide** at 60 mcg. Reduce the dose of preprandial **rapid-acting** or **short-acting insulin** (including fixed-mix **insulin**) by 50 percent. Monitor pre- and postprandial blood glucose and bedtime glucose levels frequently. Then increase the dose of the **pramlintide** to 120 mcg when no clinically significant nausea has occurred for 3 to 7 days. If significant nausea continues at the 120-mcg dose, decrease the dose to 60 mcg. Adjust the **insulin** dose to optimize glycemic control once the target dose of **pramlintide** is achieved and nausea has subsided.

Monitoring

The only monitoring required for this drug is that associated with the management of diabetes.

Patient Education

Administration

Pramlintide is administered by subcutaneous injection in the thigh or abdomen, but not in the upper arm because of variability of absorption. It is given immediately before each major meal containing at least 250 kcal or at least 30 g of carbohydrate. Because **pramlintide** cannot be mixed with any form of **insulin,** it is administered in a separate syringe from **insulin.** The injection site for **pramlintide** should be at least 2 inches away from the injection site for the **insulin.**

Pramlintide is available in 5-mL vials and in a multidose, prefilled pen for injection. Pen-injectors are available in these doses: a 60 pen-injector for 15-, 30-, 45-, and 60-mcg dosing, and a 60 pen-injector for 60-mcg and 120-mcg dosing. Patients should confirm they are using the correct pen-injector to deliver their prescribed dose. A package insert provides instructions for using the pen-injector. Needles are not included with the pen and must be purchased separately.

The table below gives the amount of **pramlintide** to draw up from a multidose vial.

Pramlintide Dose in Micrograms	Amount to Draw Up in a U-100 Insulin Syringe
15	2.5
30	5
45	7.5
60	10
120	20

Inform patients that if a dose is missed, they should wait until the next meal and take the usual dose of **pramlintide** at that meal.

Adverse Reactions

Most of the adverse reactions are GI disturbances and most patients experience nausea that subsides over time. The presence or absence of nausea is used to adjust doses and needs to be reported to providers. **Pramlintide** may reduce appetite, the amount of food eaten, and patient weight. These reactions have a positive effect on diabetes and no changes in treatment regimen are required based on them.

Patients on the drug should check blood glucose levels before and after every meal and at bedtime. Because this drug is taken with **insulin,** patients have an increased risk for severe hypoglycemic reactions. Hypoglycemic reactions should be reported to the health-care provider so that dosage adjustments can be made if needed. Explain the signs and symptoms of hypoglycemia and how to treat low blood glucose, which is discussed in Chapter 33, to the patient.

Lifestyle Management

Type 2 diabetes is a chronic illness managed with diet, exercise, weight control, self-monitoring of BG, and drug therapy. Further patient teaching related to management of diabetes is discussed in Chapter 33. Table 21–38 shows available dosage forms.

GLUCAGON

Glucagon is a hormone secreted by the pancreas. It has several actions, but its primary use clinically is in elevating BG levels for diabetic patients who have hypoglycemia, or as an oral diabetic agent for insulin overdose. It is also used to reverse the hypoglycemia induced by **insulin** shock therapy in psychiatric patients and has an off-labeled use in cardiovascular emergencies such as shock. Gastroenterologists use it to relax the GI musculature to facilitate radiographic examinations and scoping procedures. The increase in BG in patients who have been NPO for hours prior to a scheduled GI procedure can also be considered beneficial.

This drug is administered SC, IM, or IV. Most of the drugs in this book are oral preparations because that is the route most used in primary care. **Glucagon,** however, is used in urgent care and primary care settings in its IM or IV form, so it is included.

Pharmacodynamics

Glucagon is a polypeptide hormone produced by the alpha cells of the islets of Langerhans in the pancreas. It accelerates liver glucogenolysis by stimulating cAMP synthesis and increasing phosphorylase kinase activity. This results in increased breakdown of glycogen to glucose and inhibition of glycogen synthesis. The end result is an elevation in BG levels. **Glucagon** also stimulates hepatic gluconeogenesis by promoting the uptake of amino acids and converting them to glucose precursors. When administered parenterally, **glucagon** also produces relaxation of the smooth muscle of the GI tract, decreases gastric and pancreatic secretions, and increases myocardial contractility. These latter actions are not the primary reason for its clinical use, however.

Pharmacokinetics

Absorption and Distribution

Glucagon is well absorbed after parenteral administration. Its distribution is unknown.

Metabolism and Excretion

It is extensively metabolized by the liver and kidney and degraded in the plasma.

Plasma half-life is about 8 to 18 minutes.

Pharmacotherapeutics

Precautions and Contraindications

The only contraindication to **glucagon** is hypersensitivity to it. It should be given with caution to patients with insulinoma or pheochromocytoma. It may produce an initial increase in BG in these patients, but because of its **insulin**-releasing effect, it may subsequently cause hypoglycemia. It also stimulates catecholamine release, causing a marked increase in blood pressure in patients with pheochromocytoma. It has positive inotropic and chronotropic effects in all patients.

Glucagon is Pregnancy Category B, but there are no adequate and well-controlled studies in pregnant women. It should be used in pregnancy only if clearly indicated. Because **insulin** is the drug of choice in managing gestational diabetes and other diabetic patients during their pregnancy, the potential for a hypoglycemic reaction exists. The rapid resolution of any moderate to severe hypoglycemia is clearly in the best interests of the fetus and would override any concerns about potential risk from exposure to **glucagon.** It is not known whether this drug is excreted in breast milk. Caution should be used in giving it to a nursing mother.

Adverse Drug Reactions

The most frequent adverse reactions are nausea and vomiting. These may occur because of a possible reactive hypoglycemia after the initial BG rise. Rare allergic reactions resulting in urticaria, respiratory distress, and hypotension have been reported, possibly related to the phenol and glycerin in some products.

Drug Interactions

The **anticoagulant** effects of **oral anticoagulants** may be increased, with the possibility of bleeding. This interaction may occur after several days of therapy and appears to be dose related. This interaction is not associated with single-dose therapy to resolve a hypoglycemic reaction. The hyperglycemic response is prolonged with **epinephrine.** The response is blunted with **phenytoin.**

Clinical Use and Dosing

Reversal of hypoglycemia is the main use for this drug (Table 21–39). **Glucagon** counteracts severe hypoglycemic reactions in diabetic patients and in psychiatric patients recovering from **insulin** shock. BG levels of patients with type 1 diabetes do not respond as well as those of patients with type 2, and patients with type 1 diabetes often require concurrent administration of carbohydrates. Because all of its actions depend on the presence of glycogen in the liver, **glucagon** is of little or no help in states of starvation, adrenal insufficiency, or chronic hypoglycemia. Supplemental glucose is typically used to help reverse severe hypoglycemia.

An off-labeled use for **glucagon** is in the treatment of **propranolol and calcium channel blocker** overdose. Its

Table 21–39 ◉ **Dosage Schedule: Glucagon**

Indication	Initial Dose	Additional Doses
Hypoglycemia	Children, weight <20 kg: 0.5 mg SC, IM, or IV Adult and children, weight > 20 mg: 1 mg SC, IM, or IV	If response not adequate in 5–15 min, administer 1–2 additional doses; accompany with IV glucose if patient fails to respond.
Hypoglycemia in infants	0.3 mg/kg	0.3 mg/kg may be repeated q4h as needed
Insulin shock	After 1 h of coma: inject 0.5–1 mg SC, IM, or IV	If no response in 10–25 min, repeat dose. On awakening, feed patient orally as soon as possible.

use in these situations is based on its effects on smooth muscle and myocardial contractility and resultant increase in heart rate and blood pressure.

Monitoring

Monitoring of BG immediately prior to and after the injection is the only requirement.

Patient Education

Patients with diabetes who are at high risk for hypoglycemia may keep this drug on hand to be mixed and injected by a family member if oral **glucose supplements** are contraindicated with loss of consciousness or swallowing impairment. Education of the family member would include recognition of and testing for hypoglycemia and the procedure for mixing and administering **glucagon** parenterally (Table 21–39). Table 21–40 lists the available dosage forms of **glucagon**.

THYROID AGENTS

Thyroid hormones include both natural and synthetic compounds. The natural hormones are derived from beef and pork thyroid glands. Because their content and bioavailability are not consistent from dose to dose, they have largely been replaced with the synthetic compounds. This section discusses the synthetic thyroid hormones.

Pharmacodynamics

The hypothalamus-pituitary-thyroid hormone axis begins with the secretion of thyrotropin-releasing hormone (TRH) by the hypothalamus in response to cold, stress, and decreased levels of thyroxine (T4). TRH stimulates the synthesis and release of thyroid-stimulating hormone (TSH) by the anterior pituitary. TSH, in turn, stimulates an adenylyl cyclase mechanism in the thyroid cells to (1) immediately increase the release of stored thyroid hormones; (2) increase iodine uptake and utilization; (3) increase the synthesis of the two thyroid hormones, tri-iodothyronine (T3) and T4; and (4) increase the synthesis and secretion of prostaglandins by the thyroid gland. When thyroid hormones are secreted, they create a negative feedback loop, inhibit TRH and TSH secretion, and decrease further thyroid hormone synthesis and secretion. Figure 21–4 depicts the hypothalamus-pituitary-thyroid hormone axis.

As shown in Figure 21–4, **thyroid hormones** increase all the metabolic processes of the body and are central to the growth and differentiation of body tissues. The mechanism by which **thyroid hormones** exert their effect is not well understood, but it is believed that most of their effects are exerted through control of DNA transcription and protein synthesis. Administration of **synthetic thyroid hormones—levothyroxine** (T4), **liothyronine** (T3), and **liotrix** (a 4:1 mixture of T4 and T3)—produces the same effects on body tissues as the body's own **thyroid hormones** and produces the negative feedback loop to reduce further secretion of TSH and thyroid hormones.

Table 21–40 ◆ **Available Dosage Forms: Glucagon**

Drug	Dosage Form
Glucagon	1 mg powder for injection in vial with 1 mL of diluent, $84 dose
	Emergency kit prefilled syringe 1 mg, $113 dose
	(Use immediately after reconstitution; may be kept at 5°C for 48 h)

Pharmacokinetics

Absorption and Distribution

Levothyroxine (T4) is variably absorbed, with 48 to 79 percent of the dose absorbed after oral administration (Table 21–41). Fasting increases its absorption, and malabsorption syndromes cause excessive fecal loss of this drug. **Liothyronine** (T3) is 95 percent absorbed within 4 hours after administration. More than 99 percent of both circulating hormones are bound to serum proteins, including thyroid-binding globulin (TBg), thyroid-binding prealbumin (TBPA), and albumin (TBa). The higher affinity of T4 for TBg and TBPA as compared with T3 partially explains the higher serum levels and longer half-life of T4. T4 and T3 exist in the body in equilibrium between bound and free drug, but only the free drug produces the hormone's effects.

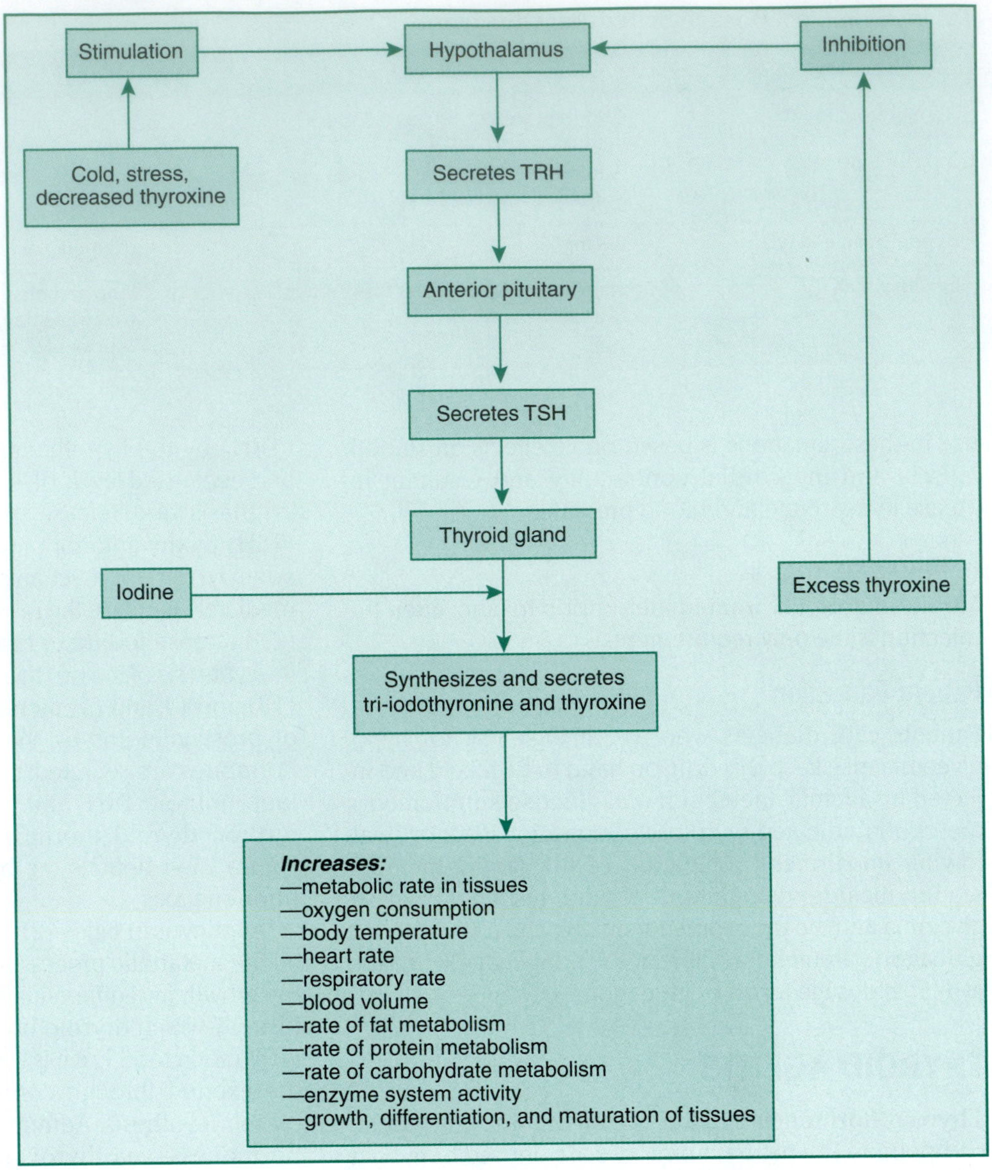

Figure 21–4. Hypothalamus-pituitary-thyroid hormone axis.

Metabolism and Excretion

Thyroid hormones are distributed to most body tissues. They do not readily cross the placenta, and minimal amounts are excreted in breast milk.

Under normal body functioning, the ratio of T4 to T3 released from the thyroid gland is 20:1. Approximately 35 percent of T4 is converted in peripheral tissues to T3 so that 80 percent of T3 comes from monodeiodination of T4. This process of deiodination of T4 occurs in the liver, kidney, and other body tissues, especially the skeletal muscles. The conjugated hormones then reenter the hepatic circulation, where they are excreted in the feces via bile.

Pharmacotherapeutics

Precautions and Contraindications

Thyroid hormone replacement is contraindicated after recent myocardial infarction (MI) or in thyrotoxicosis

Table 21–41 ▶ **Pharmacokinetics: Oral Thyroid Hormones**

Drug	Onset*	Peak*	Duration*	Biological Potency	Half-Life	Excretion
Levothyroxine (T4)	48 h	1–3 wk	1–3 wk	1	6–7 d**	In feces via bile
Liothyronine (T3)	48 h	24–72 h	72 h	4	1–2 d	In feces via bile

*Effects on thyroid function tests.
**3–4 d in hyperthyroidism; 9–10 d in myxedema.

uncomplicated by hypothyroidism. When hypothyroidism is a complicating or causative factor in MI or heart disease, judicious use of small doses of **thyroid hormone** may be called for. Cardiovascular disease, particularly coronary artery disease, may worsen when **thyroid hormones** are given. The increased heart rate associated with **thyroid hormone** administration increases oxygen demand by the heart muscle and decreases oxygen supply by reducing diastolic filling time. If **thyroid hormone** is required for patients who have cardiovascular disease, the lowest dose possible is used and with careful monitoring of signs and symptoms of worsening cardiovascular disease.

Long-term **levothyroxine** therapy has been associated with decreased bone density in the hip and spine in both premenopausal and postmenopausal women. To avoid this problem, the drug should be used only after appropriate clinical evaluation. When the drug is necessary, use only the lowest dose possible to achieve the desired effects, and periodically monitor the patient for osteoporosis.

Thyroid hormone therapy for patients with concomitant diabetes insipidus or adrenal insufficiency exacerbates the intensity of their symptoms. Dosage adjustments downward in **thyroid hormone** may be required. Severe or prolonged hypothyroidism can lead to decreased adrenocortical function. When thyroid replacement therapy is begun, the metabolism increases at a greater rate than adrenocortical activity and can precipitate adrenocortical insufficiency. Supplemental **adrenocorticosteroid** may be needed.

Adverse Drug Reactions

Adverse reactions other than those associated with hyperthyroidism due to overdose are rare. If the patient experiences indications of hyperthyroidism (increased heart rate, cardiac arrhythmias, chest pain, tremors, nervousness, insomnia, irritability, diarrhea, vomiting, weight loss, menstrual irregularities, or heat intolerance), the TSH level should be assessed and appropriate dosage adjustments made.

Drug Interactions

Bile-acid sequestrants, iron salts and **antacids** decrease the absorption of orally administered **thyroid preparations. Estrogens** increase TBg and may therefore decrease the response to **thyroid hormone. Thyroid hormones** may decrease the effectiveness of **warfarin, digoxin,** and **beta blockers.** Table 21–42 mentions these and other drug interactions.

Many drugs affect thyroid function tests and may interfere with correct assessment of thyroid status. These

Table 21–42 ■ **Drug Interactions With Thyroid Hormones**

Interacting Drug	Possible Outcomes	Implications
Beta-adrenergic blockers	Actions of beta-adrenergic blocker may be impaired when patient is converted to euthyroid state	Monitor response to beta-adrenergic blockers; assess for continued need for drug or for dosage adjustment.
Carbamazepine, hydantoins, Phenobarbital, rifamycins	Increased hepatic degradation of T4 Increased levothyroxine requirements	Monitor thyroid function closely
Cholestyramine, colestipol	Interferes with thyroid hormone absorption with loss of efficacy	Administer at least 4 h apart
Digoxin	Serum levels of digoxin reduced when hypothyroid patient is converted to euthyroid state	Monitor response to digoxin and serum levels; assess for need for dosage adjustment
Estrogens	Increases TBg and may decrease response to thyroid hormone	Monitor therapeutic response
Glucorticoids	Concurrent use may decrease peripheral conversion of T4 to T3	Monitor thyroid function and symptoms of hypothyroidism
Metformin, meglitinides, sulfonylureas, TDZs and insulin	Initiating thyroid hormones may cause increases in insulin or oral hypoglycemic requirements	Monitor BG closely
Sertraline (an SSRI)	Increased levothyroxine requirements	Monitor thyroid function closely or select different SRI
Tricyclic antidepressants	Concurrent use may increase toxic effects of both drugs. Toxic effects may include increased risk of dysrhythmias and CNS stimulation.	Avoid concurrent use
Warfarin	Increased anticoagulant action	May need to decrease dose of warfarin; monitor PT/INR carefully

INR = international normalized ratio; PT = prothrombin time.

drugs are discussed in Chapter 41. High-fat meals and those with high fiber may decrease absorption up to 40 percent.

Clinical Use and Dosing

Hypothyroidism

Treatment of hypothyroidism follows the "start low and go slow" principle to avoid excessive increase in metabolism before the body has a chance to adapt to the increase. For adults, **levothyroxine** is started at 50 mcg daily and is increased in increments of 25 mcg/day at 2- to 4-week intervals to 100 to 150 mcg/day. The target dose is based on TSH levels and is approximately 1.7 mcg/kg/day. Older adults may require less than 1 mcg/kg/day. An initial dose of 25 to 50 mcg/day is recommended with gradual dosage increases of 12.5 to 25 mcg/day at 6- to 8-week intervals. Lower doses and longer intervals for changing doses are required for patients with cardiovascular impairment or long-standing hypothyroidism. In these cases or in severe hypothyroidism, the initial dose is 12.5 to 25 mcg/day, increased by 25 mcg/day at 4-week intervals. The target dose is also based on TSH levels. Most patients require no more than 200 mcg/day. Failure to respond adequately to doses of 300 mcg/day suggests lack of adherence or malabsorption; however, reduction in sensitivity to thyroid hormone is possible.

Liothyronine (T3) is started at 25 mcg/day. Dosage is increased by 12.5 to 25 mcg/day at 1- to 2-week intervals until a maintenance dose of 25 to 50 mcg is reached.

Liotrix is started with 50 mcg of **levothyroxine/** 12.5 mcg of **liothyronine** per day. Doses are increased by 50/12.5 mcg at 4-week intervals until a maintenance dose of 50 to 100/12.5 to 25 is reached. For patients with myxedema or hypothyroidism with cardiovascular disease, the doses are reduced. This formulation is claimed to follow a more natural hormone secretion pattern; however, a meta-analysis demonstrated no benefits with combination medications including improved mental health and quality of life measures (Grozinski-Glasberg et al, 2006). The subset of post–total thyroidectomy patients may be the exception (Cooper, 2003).

For all of these drugs, dosages are different for infants, children, and geriatric patients. Table 21–43 presents the dosing schedules for all of these age groups.

Table 21–43 ● **Dosage Schedule: Thyroid Hormones**

Drug	Indication	Initial Dose	Maintenance Dose
Levothyroxine	Hypothyroidism and congenital hypothyroidism	*Adults:* 50 mcg daily	Increase dose by 25 mcg at 4- to 6-wk intervals to maintenance dose of 100–150 mcg daily
		Older adults: 12.5–25 mcg daily	Increase dose by 25 mcg daily at 6-wk intervals to maintenance dose of 100–150 mcg daily
		Children >12 yr: 2–3 mcg/kg daily	Increase in increments of 2 mcg/kg/d at 4- to 6-wk intervals to maintenance dose of 150–200 mcg daily
		Children 6–12 yr: 4–5 mcg/kg daily	Increase in increments of 4 mcg/kg/d at 4- to 6-wk intervals to maintenance dose of 100–150 mcg daily
		Children 1–5 yr: 5–6 mcg/kg daily	Increase in increments of 3 mcg/ kg/d at 2- to 4-wk intervals to maintenance dose of 75–100 mcg daily
		Children 6–12 mo: 6–8 mcg/kg daily	Increase in increments of 5 mcg /kg/d at 2- to 4-wk intervals to maintenance dose of 50–75 mcg daily
		Infants 3–6 mo: 8–10 mcg/kg daily	Increase in increments of 5 mcg/kg/d at 4- to 6-wk intervals to maintenance dose of 25–50 mcg daily
		Infants 0–3 mo: 10–15 mcg/kg	Dosage may be increased after 4–6 wk to 50 mcg daily
		Infants less than 2,000 g or at risk for cardiac failure: 25 mcg daily	For infants with congenital hypothyroidism, initiate therapy with full dose as soon as diagnosis is made
Liothyronine	Mild hypothyroidism	*Adults:* 25 mcg daily	Increase in increments of 12.5–25 mcg daily at 1- to 2-wk intervals to maintenance dose of 25–75 mcg daily
		Older adults or patients with cardiovascular disease: 5 mcg daily	Increase in increments of no more than 5 mcg daily at 2-wk intervals

Table 21–43 ● **Dosage Schedule: Thyroid Hormones—cont'd**

Drug	Indication	Initial Dose	Maintenance Dose
	Congenital hypothyroidism	5 mcg daily	Increase in increments of 5 mcg every 3–4 d until desired response Maintenance dose for infants a few months old is 20 mcg daily; for children age 1 yr, dose is 50 mcg daily; above 3 yr, use adult dose
	Simple nontoxic goiter	5 mcg daily	Increase in increments of 5 mcg every 1–2 wk When dose of 25 mcg daily is reached increase by 12.5–25 mcg daily every 1–2 wk Usual maintenance dose is 75 mcg daily
	Myxedema	5 mcg daily	Increase in increments of 5 mcg every 1–2 wk When dose of 25 mcg daily is reached, increase by 12.5–25 mcg daily every 1–2 wk Usual maintenance dose is 50–100 mcg daily
Liotrix	Hypothyroidism	*Adults:* 30 mg daily	Increase in increments of 15 mg every 2–3 wk to maintenance dose of 60–120 mg daily
		Children and infants with congenital hypothyroidism	Follow dosage recommendations for levothyroxine (see available dosage forms table for T4 equivalents for liotrix)

Hashimoto's Thyroiditis

Approximately 70 percent or more of patients with Hashimoto's thyroiditis go on to develop permanent hypothyroidism. If hypothyroidism develops, the treatment regimen is the same as for other causes of hypothyroidism, as discussed previously.

TSH Suppression in Thyroid Cancer, Nodules, and Euthyroid Goiter

The required maintenance dosage for this indication is larger than that for hypothyroidism. The initial dose of **levothyroxine** is 50 to 100 mcg/day, and the dose is increased until the TSH level declines to 0.05 to 0.3 mU/L. This therapy is relatively contraindicated in older adults and in patients with cardiovascular disease.

Thyroid Suppression Therapy

The dose is 2.5 mcg/kg daily for 7 to 10 days for this indication. These doses usually yield normal serum T4 and T3 levels without a response to TSH.

CLINICAL PEARL

Increasing the dose by 25 percent usually results in adequate coverage during pregnancy. Recheck TSH levels in 4 weeks to determine any dosage adjustment.

Pregnancy

Untreated hypothyroidism during pregnancy may increase the incidence of maternal complications, spontaneous abortion, fetal death or stillbirth, low birth weight, and abnormal fetal brain development (American Association of Clinical Endocrinologists [AACE], 2006). These outcomes can be avoided by thyroid hormone replacement (AACE, 2006; American College of Obstetricians and Gynecologists [ACOG], 2008). Because **thyroid hormones** are Pregnancy Category A, replacement is advised for all symptomatic pregnant women. Therapy begun before pregnancy should not be stopped. The increased metabolic rate common to pregnancy often requires higher doses. Increasing a patient's maintenance dose by 25 percent usually provides adequate coverage, but may require a 45 percent increase. T4 requirements increase by the eighth week and typically plateau at 16 weeks. TSH levels should then be checked every trimester to determine the need for any further dosage adjustment. Both the AACE and ACOG recommend **levothyroxine.**

Hormones are excreted in breast milk, but have not been associated with adverse effects. Infants must be monitored after birth for issues related to maternal levels. Infants born with thyroid deficiency are at high risk for adverse results.

Postpartum thyroiditis (5% to 10% of deliveries and miscarriage, abortion, and ectopics) can result in either hypo- or hyperthyroid states. Current ACOG (2007) recommendations do not suggest screening before or after deliveries unless patients are symptomatic. AACE (2006) guidelines support routine screening. Women with symptoms may or may not be treated within the first 8 to 12 weeks postpartum, as hormonal levels typically return to normal. **Propanolol** may be used for symptom control of hyperthyroid symptoms. Interestingly, elevated TSH is not strongly associated with postpartum depression. Those who have rebalanced levels within a few months are at risk for future thyroid imbalances within the next 5 to 10 years (Abalovich, Amino, & Barbour, 2007).

Congenital Hypothyroidism

Congenital hypothyroidism occurs in 1:3,000 to 4,000 newborns. Of all the causes of mental retardation, it is the easiest to screen for and treat. Most impacted infants have no signs or symptoms. **Levothyroxine** is the drug of choice. The recommended doses for this indication are based on the infant's weight. Full doses are started immediately on diagnosis of the condition. Tablets may be crushed and added to infant formula. Congenital hypothyroidism requires referral to an endocrinologist. There is some evidence that soy may impair **thyroxine** absorption from the gut, so special attention is given to monitoring in infants requiring soy-based formula (Messina & Redmond, 2006); this precaution does not pertain to adults.

Inappropriate Use of Thyroid Hormones

Obesity

In euthyroid patients, hormone replacement doses are ineffective for weight reduction. Larger doses may produce serious or even life-threatening toxicity, particularly when given with anorexiants. Use of **thyroid hormones** for this indication is not justified.

Infertility

Thyroid hormone therapy is *not* justified for the treatment of infertility in male or female patients unless the condition is accompanied by hypothyroidism.

Depression

Use of thyroid supplementation for chronic depressive states has long-term advocates, but blinded, placebo-controlled research does not support its use. Quality of life, perceived energy levels and complaints of hypothyroid symptoms are not altered with other than standard doses of thyroid medications (Walsh et al, 2006). Therefore, practitioners are cautioned not to up dosages "to feel better" due to the chronic bone issues.

Lithium preparations are antithyroid and can cause goiter. The goiter size will eventually increase TSH levels toward normal. Patients can develop overt hypothyroidism. Treated patients should be monitored using T4 levels.

CLINICAL PEARL

Levothyroxine tablets can be crushed and suspended in a small amount of formula or water for infants who cannot swallow whole tablets. For children who cannot swallow the intact tablet, it may be crushed and sprinkled over a small amount of food such as cooked cereal or applesauce. The suspension cannot be stored for any period of time. The tablet should be crushed, mixed to form a suspension, and given immediately.

Rational Drug Selection

Pharmacokinetics

Levothyroxine (T4) is the drug of choice for thyroid replacement and suppression therapy because of its longer half-life. This means that it can safely be withheld for up to 2 weeks, if necessary, without altering the patient's thyroid status. Because **T4** is converted to **T3** in the body, use of this drug produces both hormones. Both **levothyroxine** and **liothyronine** (T3) have content stability, but **liothyronine** is 3 to 4 times more active than **levothyroxine**, and this greater potency increases the risk for cardiotoxicity. **Levothyroxine** should be used with patients who have cardiovascular disease.

Cost

Generic forms of **levothyroxine** and the brands **Levoxyl** and **Levothroid** typically have similar low costs. The generic form of **levothyroxine sodium** has recently received FDA bioequivalence with the brand **Synthroid**. Cost varies between **Synthroid** and the other brands and the generic form of **levothyroxine** and also between strengths of the same drug. Cost data are included in Table 21–44, including available dosage forms of **levothyroxine** and **liothyronine**.

Ease of monitoring

Levothyroxine is the easiest to monitor via TSH and free T4 laboratory measurements of thyroid function. The monitoring of therapy with these laboratory tests is more difficult with **liothyronine**. Its best use is for TSH suppression. **Liotrix** offers no clear benefit over either of the other drugs on any of these parameters.

Monitoring

Thyroid function is monitored with TSH and free **T4** levels. Because of the negative feedback loop between TSH and **thyroid hormones**, elevations in TSH indicate insufficient **thyroid hormone**, and TSH levels below desired levels indicate excessive **thyroid hormone**. TSH and free **T4** levels are checked initially and at 6 weeks after the first adjustment. Recheck the levels 4 months after achieving target dose, and adjust the dose to keep TSH within normal limits. Remember steady state must be present to have reliable values; steady state takes 4 to 6 weeks to be achieved. Once the adult primary hypothyroid patient is stable on an appropriate dose, TSH can be checked only

Table 21–44 ◆ **Available Dosage Forms: Selected Thyroid Hormones**

Drug	Dosage Form	How Supplied	Cost per 100 Only
Levothyroxine, Levothroid, and Levoxyl			
Generic**	Tablets: 25 mcg, 50 mcg, 75 mcg, 88 mcg, 100 mcg, 112 mcg, 125 mcg, 150 mcg, 175 mcg, 200 mcg, 300 mcg	All doses in bottles of 100 tablets	25 mcg = $23*; 50 mcg = $26*; 75 mcg = $29*; 88 mcg = $30*; 100 mcg = $30*; 112 mcg = $34*; 125 mcg = $35*; 137 mcg = $35; 150 mcg = $36*; 175 mcg = $43*; 200 mcg = $44*; 300 mcg = $60*
Levothroid	Tablets: 25 mcg, 50 mcg, 75 mcg, 88 mcg, 100 mcg, 112 mcg, 125 mcg, 137 mcg, 150 mg, 200 mcg, 300 mcg	All doses in bottles of 100 tablets	25 mcg = $13; 50 mcg = $15; 75 mcg = $16; 88 mcg = $16; 100 mcg = $17; 112 mcg = $18; 125 mcg = $19; 137 mcg = $20; 150 mcg = $20; 175 mcg = $22; 200 mcg = $25; 300 mcg = $34
Levoxyl	Tablets: 25 mcg, 50 mcg, 75 mcg, 88 mcg, 100 mcg, 112 mcg, 125 mcg, 137 mcg, 150 mg, 175 mcg, 200 mcg, 300 mcg	All doses in bottles of 100 tablets	25 mcg = $36; 50 mcg = $40; 75 mcg = $55; 175 mcg = $65; 200 mcg = $66; 300 mcg = $235
Synthroid brand	Tablets: 25 mcg, 50 mcg, 75 mcg, 88 mcg, 100 mcg, 112 mcg, 125 mcg, 137 mcg, 150 mg, 200 mcg, 300 mcg	All doses in bottles of 100 tablets	25 mcg = $45; 50 mcg = $51; 75 mcg = $57; 88 mcg = $58; 100 mcg = $58; 112 mcg = $67; 125 mcg = $68; 137 mcg = $70; 150 mcg = $70; 175 mcg = $83; 200 mcg = $83; 300 mcg = $114
Liothyronine			
Cytomel Generic available	Tablets: 5 mcg, 25 mcg, and 50 mcg	All doses in bottles of 100 tablets	5 mcg = $86; 25 mcg = $113; 50 mcg = $170
Levothyroxine & Liothyronine (Thyrolar)	Tablets: 12.5 mcg/3.1 mcg; 25 mcg/6.25 mcg; 50 mcg/12.5 mcg; 100 mcg/25 mcg; 150 mcg/37.5 mcg	All doses in bottles of 100 tablets	Tablets: 12.5 mcg/3.1 mcg = $55; 25 mcg/6.25 mcg = $61; 50 mcg/12.5 mcg = $76; 100 mcg/25 mcg = $89; 150 mcg/37.5 mcg = $109

This table does not include all available forms. Selected dosage forms are given for levothyroxine and liothyronine only. All cost data are for 100 tablets. Prices from *Red Book 2009* (113th ed.) AWP unless noted.
*Medicaid Federal Upper Price Limit. **On 2009 major store $4 price list.

annually; serum T4 measurements are unreliable for monitoring **levothyroxine** dosing. The exception is for secondary hypothyroidism. In that case, TSH is typically suppressed and the T4 is used to regulate dosing. See Chapter 41 on additional thyroid disease care.

Infants must be checked every 1 to 2 months. Children should be monitored every 3 to 6 months, especially during growth spurts. Age-based normal values from a consistently used ordering laboratory should be used for dose adjustments.

Diagnostic TSH levels (0.5 to 5.0 mU/L) are not the same as therapeutic levels. Newest TSH levels for maintaining dosing have been revised to be 0.3 to 3.0 mU/L. Laboratory workups plus patient symptomology are used to find the right dosing with most patients best maintained between 1.0 and 2.5 mU/L. Hormone overreplacement (low TSH with normal T4 and T3) results in a subclinical hyperthyroidism. Dangers include bone thinning and cardiac irregularities.

Patient Education

Administration

Thyroid hormones are taken as a single daily dose in the morning before breakfast to prevent insomnia. Taking **levothyroxine** on an empty stomach enhances absorption. Other types may be taken without regard to food. If a dose is missed, it may be taken that same day as soon as it is remembered. If more than three doses are missed, the health-care provider should be informed

Caution patients not to change brands of thyroid preparation. Though generics are bioequivalent, major medical groups (American Thyroid Association, Endocrine Society, and American Association of Clinical Endocrinologists) believe they are not bioidentical therapeutically (2006). If brands are switched to generics, retitrating of doses over several months may be required. The additional costs of laboratory tests may offset any cost savings from selecting another manufacturer.

Although some health food stores may sell **dessicated thyroid** preparations OTC at a lower cost, these formulations do not have consistent amounts of **thyroid hormone** in them and should not be substituted for the prescribed drug. The serum fluctuations are more likely to cause cardiac symptoms than are the synthetic versions. They are primarily pork derivations.

Brand-name manufacturers have color-coded the tablets to assist in identification of dosing that does not follow most other medications. Unusual dosing levels (i.e., 88 or 112 mcg) require careful attention. Shortened dosing intervals facilitate intermediate dosing levels that can eliminate the need for pill splitting. The colorations are not standardized across manufacturers.

The potential confusion with unusual dosing formulations is compounded by most doses coming in micrograms, not milligrams. Care must be taken in writing prescriptions to avoid dosing errors, for example, 100 mcg = 0.1 mg and 75 mcg = 0.075 mg.

Adverse Drug Reactions

Teach the patient how to measure pulse rate. If the pulse rate is greater than 100 beats per minute, the dose should be withheld and the health-care provider notified. This may indicate excessive amounts of hormone. Other signs or symptoms that require notification include nervousness, chest pain, HTN, and unexplained weight loss of more than 2 lb in 1 week. Extreme fatigue may indicate inadequate dosing.

Some children on thyroid hormone therapy may experience partial hair loss. This is usually temporary, but parents and children should be informed that it may happen.

Lifestyle Management

Thyroid disorders are usually chronic illnesses managed with self-monitoring of symptoms as well as drug therapy. Emphasize the importance of keeping follow-up appointments for evaluation of thyroid function. For children, evaluation of physical and psychomotor growth and development is also central to their management. Explain to the patient that replacement therapy must be taken for life (except in cases of transient hypothyroidism). The drug will treat the disorder but not cure it. Further patient teaching related to management of thyroid disorders is discussed in Chapter 41.

ANTITHYROID AGENTS

Antithyroid agents function by either inhibiting the synthesis of thyroid hormones or destroying thyroid gland tissue. They are used to treat hyperthyroidism. Hyperthyroidism, also known as *thyrotoxicosis,* occurs when there is a breakdown in the feedback loop and the body's tissues are exposed to excessive levels of thyroid hormone. The cause of this excessive secretion varies, with the most common cause an autoimmune disorder called Graves' disease, which accounts for 60 to 90 percent of all hyperthyroidism (AACE, 2006). The hyperfunction of the thyroid gland leads to suppression of TSH and TRH, because the immune system is not controlled by feedback from the elevated levels of thyroid hormone.

Hyperfunction of the thyroid gland results in a dramatic increase in iodine uptake and thyroid gland metabolism. A disproportionate increase in T3 production is combined with a decreased concentration of thyroid-binding globulin so that increased circulating levels of **thyroid hormone** are seen. These hormones are responsible for many thyrotoxic symptoms. Severe levels may lead to thyroid storm, a life-threatening situation not covered in this chapter.

Regardless of the etiology of hyperthyroidism, the clinical features are attributable to metabolic effects of increased circulating levels of **thyroid hormone**. These effects include heat intolerance and increased sensitivity to stimulation by the sympathetic division of the autonomic nervous system. Table 41–3 (Chapter 41) shows the most common systemic effects of hyperthyroidism and discusses the management of hyperthyroidism.

The two drugs used in the outpatient setting to treat hyperthyroidism are **propylthiouracil** (PTU) and **methimazole** (**Tapazole**), referenced in the literature as the **thionamides** or **thioureas**. Because **radioactive iodine 131** is prescribed and administered by specialists in hospital environments, it will not be discussed here in detail. Nonradioactive **iodine** solutions can also be used.

Pharmacodynamics

Propylthiouracil (PTU) and **methimazole** (**Tapazole**) inhibit the synthesis of **thyroid hormones**. They do not inactivate existing thyroxine and tri-iodothyronine that are stored in the thyroid gland or that are circulating in the blood, nor do they interfere with the effectiveness of exogenous **thyroid hormones**. PTU partially inhibits the peripheral conversion of T4 to T3. Both drugs are concentrated in the thyroid gland; however, neither of these drugs treats the underlying pathology in hyperthyroidism, **Iodine tablets and solutions** (SSKI or **Lugol's**) are no longer first-line medications; however, they have a role in preoperative thyroid cancer care, in thyroid storm, and in individuals requiring persistent thyroid suppression if first line care does not achieve desired outcomes. A bolus increase in iodine intake can have a suppressive effect on normal hormone synthesis for up to 10 days (longer in those previously receiving I^{131}. This suppression is the basis for **iodine** use in cases of radiation bomb or reactor accidents, a topic beyond the scope of this text. The reader is referred to http://www.fda.gov or a major pharmaceutical reference text for dosing recommendations at the time of the incident.

1^{131}, like other **iodine** substances, is preferentially taken up by the thyroid gland via the sodium/iodine symptorter. Agents that affect any **iodine** uptake include cigarette smoking and perchlorate, a possible water contaminant.

1^{131} can be used to help diagnose whether thyroid masses localize uptake of **iodine** before or after ablation therapy. It is also given to cancer patients post-thyroidectomy to continue eradication of abnormal tissue. The radiation destroys local tissue. Because thyroid cells preferentially take up **iodine** molecules, the impact is mostly limited to thyroid tissue. Controversy exists whether long-term outcomes of survival or recurrence are altered for patients with low-risk masses.

Pharmacokinetics

Absorption and Distribution

PTU is rapidly absorbed after oral administration, reaching a peak serum level within 1 hour (Table 21–45). This drug is highly protein bound (75% to 80%) and concentrates in the thyroid gland. Concentrations in breast milk are low, and it crosses the placenta in low concentrations. Currently it is used only in adults (U.S. Food and Drug Administration, 2009c).

Methimazole is completely absorbed after oral administration but at variable rates. This drug is not protein bound and also concentrates in the thyroid gland. Concentrations in breast milk are high, and it readily crosses the placenta in high concentrations. It is associated with birth defects in early pregnancy (U.S. Food and Drug Administration, 2010).

I^{131} comes in capsules and solutions that must be prepared in special nuclear isotope pharmacies. It is rapidly absorbed by the thyroid, even faster under autoimmune conditions. I^{131} uptake by thyroid tissues is facilitated by following a low iodine diet for a week prior to scanning. Controversy exists about appropriate dosing. Research has not established optimal doses, but higher levels have been associated with phenomena wherein thyroid tissues are "stunned" and do not absorb as much isotope. This is being investigated, as is a lesser "stun" factor with different iodine isotopes (Norden, Larsson, & Tedelind, 2007). The higher doses, however, have better longer-term results.

I^{131} can be the initial therapy, but frequently is administered after the **thionamides** have returned the patient to a near euthyroid state. Pretreatment may increase success of sustained good outcomes and decreases the possible transient spike in hyperthyroid symptoms at the onset of therapy. Elders and those with cardiovascular (CV) disease are more vulnerable to these spike effects (ACCE, 2006). Pretreatment is stopped 6 days prior to the isotope dosing. Ablation of thyroid tissue is achieved with one dose 80 percent of the time.

Metabolism and Excretion

PTU is completely metabolized by the liver with a significant first-pass effect. **Methimazole** is mostly metabolized by the liver, but some drug (10%) is excreted unchanged in the urine. Both drugs have a short half-life, but this has little influence on the duration of **antithyroid** action or the dosing intervals because they are concentrated in the thyroid gland. Most states no longer require I^{131} patients to remain hospitalized to monitor excretion. Body or blood dosimetry is not done except for those with distant metastasis.

Pharmacotherapeutics

Precautions and Contraindications

Pregnancy creates a serious cautionary condition for the use of **antithyroid** drugs. I^{131} is contraindicated (Category X) due to infant impact when it crosses the placenta and into breast milk (AACE, 2006). **Methimazole** is associated with birth defects, leaving PTU as the option for early pregnancy when it is clinically necessary to administer an **antithyroid** drug. PTU and **methimazole** cross the placenta and can induce goiter and even cretinism in the fetus. Pregnancy typically reduces Graves' disease symptoms, so dosing is lower than normal and drops as the pregnancy advances (ACCE, 2006). The newborn should be tested at birth.

Adverse Drug Reactions

The most common serious adverse reaction to therapy with PTU and **methimazole** is agranulocytosis and possible aplastic anemia. This risk is higher for patients who already have decreased bone marrow reserve, for those

Table 21–45 ▶ **Pharmacokinetics: Antithyroid Drugs**

Drug	Onset*	Peak*	Duration*	Bioavailability	Protein Binding	Placental Transport and Breast Milk Levels	Half-Life	Excretion
Methimazole	1 wk	4–10 wk	Weeks	80%–95%	0%	High	6–13 h	Less than 10% in urine
Propylthiouracil	10–21 d	6–10 wk	Weeks	80%–95%	75%–80%	Low	1–2 h	35% in urine

*Effect on thyroid function.

older than 40 years, and for those receiving more than 40 mg/day. The patient's bone marrow function must be monitored, and the patient taught to report symptoms of this disorder. These drugs must be discontinued, should this adverse reaction occur. It is important to remember that about 10 percent of patients with untreated hyperthyroidism have leukopenia (WBC count less than 4,000/mm^3), often with related granulocytopenia.

Drug-induced hepatitis and abnormal hair loss may occur with either drug. The FDA (U.S. Food and Drug Administration, 2010) issued a black box warning concerning PTU and liver failure. PTU should be reserved for those patients where surgery or **methimazole** is not appropriate. Use in pediatric patients is restricted unless there is a **methimazole** allergy (U.S. Food and Drug Administration, 2009c). Less serious and less frequent adverse reactions to PTU and **methimazole** include drowsiness, headache, paresthesias, vertigo, diarrhea, nausea, arthralgia, and a pruritic skin rash. The nausea and skin rash are more common with PTU, but there is an element of cross-sensitivity with **metimazole.**

I^{131} is considered safe for outpatient therapy. There can be localized pain and edema for 2 to 3 weeks if **thionamides** were not used prior to treatment. Short-dose **corticosteroids** help alleviate it. Household contacts can be contaminated via saliva, urine, or direct radiation exposure. Not sharing eating utensils, avoiding sexual and other close contact, like sleeping alone, is recommended for 2 days to 3 weeks depending on dosing, even though studies have demonstrated exposures well below levels of concern. Dosing for thyroid cancer is higher than it is for hyperthyroidism therapy. Controversies exist over long-term (40-yr) minimal increases in post-therapy malignancies.

Many patients complain of dry mouth. Use of lemon candies within the first 24 hours remains contentious, but is considered appropriate thereafter. **Iodine-free laxatives** can be used to purge residual radioactive activity from the colon if normal bowel movements do not occur within the first day.

Drug Interactions

Any drugs that produce bone marrow depression have an additive effect with **antithyroid** drugs (Table 21–46). Additive **antithyroid** effects occur with **lithium, potassium iodide**, or **sodium iodide** given with PTU. **Potassium iodide** and **amiodarone** decrease **antithyroid** effects when given with **methimazole.** The risk of agranulocytosis is increased with concurrent administration of phenothiazines with **methimazole** and PTU. The anticoagulant activity of **warfarin** may be potentiated by the anti–**vitamin K** activity attributed to PTU.

Patient treated with I^{131} and later treated with **amiodarone** may develop hypothyroidism, sometimes acutely This is in contrast to the **amiodarone**-induced hyperthyroid effects found in most other circumstances.

Clinical Use and Dosing

Hyperthyroidism/Graves' Disease

Any of the **antithyroid** drugs may be used in adults. PTU is available in 50-mg tablets. The dose varies from 150 to 300 mg daily. Because of its short half-life, the dose is divided and taken three times daily. **Methimazole** comes in 5- and 10-mg tablets, and dosing is usually started at 10 to 15 mg daily. **Methimazole** works faster than PTU with fewer side effects. Ross's report in *UpToDate* (Ross, 2008) states low doses are as efficacious as higher doses except when treating severe cases and very enlarged goiters. For moderate disease the dose is 30 to 40 mg/day and for severe disease the dose is 60 mg/day. All doses divided equally and given every 8 hours.

PTU is initiated with 300 mg/day in three equally divided doses given 8 hours apart. Patients with severe hyperthyroidism may have initial doses of 400 to 900 mg/day depending on the severity of the disease. Maintenance doses are 100 to 150 mg/day. Treatment is for 6 to 18 months, with most patients being treated for 1 year.

Toxic Goiter

Patients with toxic goiter require higher doses of **antithyroid** drugs. **Methimazole** is initiated at dose of 60 mg/day

Table 21–46 ■ **Drug Interactions With Antithyroid Drugs**

Drug	Interacting Drug	Possible Effect	Implications
Methimazole, propylthiouracil	Any drug that produces bone marrow depression	Additive bone marrow depression	Monitor white blood cell counts with differential; dosage adjustments or discontinuance of one of the drugs may be needed.
Propylthiouracil	Lithium, potassium iodide, Warfarin	Additive antithyroid effects Anticoagulant effects potentiated	Avoid concurrent administration. Monitor PT/INR closely.
Methimazole	Potassium iodide, amiodarone	Decreased antithyroid effects	Avoid concurrent administration.
Methimazole, propylthiouracil	Phenothiazines	Increased risk for agranulocytosis	Avoid concurrent administration.

INR = international normalized ratio; PT = prothrombin time.

divided into three equal doses given 8 hours apart. PTU is initiated with 600 to 900 mg/day in three equally divided doses given 8 hours apart. Maintenance doses are the same as for hypothyroidism. Some treatment regimens give **methimazole** or PTU for 1 month to "calm" the thyroid and then administer a dose of **radioactive iodine**.

Rational Drug Selection

Pregnancy and Lactation

Because the amount of drug that crosses the placenta is lower with PTU, the lowest effective dose of this drug is selected if one must be used. In many pregnant women, the thyroid dysfunction diminishes as the pregnancy continues, so that the drug's dose can be reduced. In some cases, the drug can be withdrawn 2 to 3 weeks prior to delivery. Postpartum patients receiving **antithyroid** drugs should not nurse their infants. If it is necessary, however, PTU is the preferred drug.

Cost

There is a significant difference in cost between **methimazole** and **propylthiouracil.** Unless the provider is willing to try once-daily dosing and sees this as an advantage, PTU is about 10 percent of the cost of **methimazole.** A cost index is included in Table 21–47 that shows available dosage forms of these two drugs. Cost of I^{131} runs thousands of dollars, with additional charges for hospital services, scanning requirements, and special handling. Costs for simple **iodine** (SKKI or **Lugol's**) are extremely low.

Monitoring

TSH and free T4 levels are evaluated prior to beginning therapy and whenever symptoms recur, whenever dosages are adjusted, and every 2 to 3 months throughout therapy. Overt symptoms typically resolve weeks before laboratory values stabilize. TSH levels may be misleading, especially early in therapy. If the hyperthyroid state has been prolonged, the pituitary axis may not become rebalanced for months (Ross, 2008). T4 and T3 levels are monitored with the thionamides because the T3 may stay high even though the T4 returns to a normal baseline. Once TSH is back to normal, monitoring of T3 is no longer necessary. In addition to laboratory assessment, both the provider and the patient should regularly assess for signs and symptoms of hyperthyroidism (too low a dose) or hypothyroidism (too high a dose).

It should be understood that the majority of patients receiving antithyroid medication will develop hypothyroidism either immediately or over time. Recurrent hyperthyroidism is more likely in smokers and those who do not remain euthyroid for more than 6 months. Therefore, monitoring TSH levels after therapy is completed becomes a long-term primary care responsibility.

To monitor for the risk for agranulocytosis, a complete blood count, including white blood cell count and differential, is done prior to initiating therapy, if symptoms suggestive of this disorder occur, and periodically throughout therapy. This adverse reaction may develop rapidly, usually within the first 2 months of therapy. During that time, both the provider and the patient should be especially vigilant. It is more common in persons older than 40 years and those who are receiving more than 40 mg/day. Monitoring may be more frequent for these patients.

Drug-induced hepatitis has become a concern, especially with PTU. Liver function tests should be done prior to any thioamide therapy, especially if there are any indications of hepatic issues, with monitoring during and six months after treatment (U.S. Food and Drug Administration, 2009c).

Table 21–47 ◆ Available Dosage Forms: Antithyroid Drugs

Drug	Dosage Form	Cost
Methimazole (Tapazole)	5-mg (scored) tablet	$42*/100
	10-mg (scored) tablet	$72/100
Propylthiouracil (PTU)	50-mg tablet	$21/100

*Medicaid Federal Upper Limit.

Patient Education

Administration

If the drug is to be taken every 8 hours, it is not necessary to awaken at night to take the drug at exactly 8-hour intervals because the drug is concentrated in thyroid tissue. If a dose is missed, the patient should take it as soon as remembered. If it is almost time for the next dose, the two doses may be taken together. The health-care provider should be notified if more than one dose is missed so that an assessment of thyroid function can be made.

Dietary sources of **iodine** should be discussed and reduced or eliminated. They interfere with the action of the **antithyroid** drugs. Many OTC drugs, especially those used to treat colds, also have **iodine** in them. Teach the patient to read the labels.

Adverse Reactions

The most common potential adverse reaction related to PTU and **methimazole** is agranulocytosis. Patients are taught to report sore throat, fever, chills, rash, and unusual bleeding or bruising, as well as the reason for it.

Another potential adverse reaction is drug-induced hepatitis. Patients are also taught to report headache, malaise, weakness, and yellowing of the eyes or skin and the reasons for it. The patient should be told that any abnormal hair loss is probably temporary.

I^{131} may have a slight overall mortality from cardiovascular deaths in patient cohorts followed for over 40 years. The increased risk of cerebrovascular accident (CVA) is probably due to the effects of hyperthyroidism, not the radiation itself. Any suppressed testicular function returns to normal quickly. Any link to an increased risk of ophthalmopathy already associated with Graves' disease is controversial, but probably unfounded.

Lifestyle Management

Hyperthyroidism and goiter are often chronic illnesses managed with self-monitoring of symptoms as well as drug therapy. Emphasize the importance of keeping follow-up appointments for evaluation of thyroid function. For children, evaluation of physical and psychomotor growth and development is also central to their management. Explain to the patient that **antithyroid** drug therapy will be required for 6 to 18 months and perhaps longer, because recurrence of hyperthyroidism happens in 70 percent of patients. The drug will treat the disorder but may not cure it. Further patient teaching related to management of thyroid disorders is discussed in Chapter 41.

REFERENCES

Abalovich, M., Amino, N., & Barbour, L. (2007). Management of thyroid dysfunction during pregnancy and postpartum: An Endocrine Society clinical practice guideline. *Journal of Clinical Endocrinology and Metabolism, 92,* S1–S47.

ADVANCE Collaborative Group. (2008). Intensive blood glucose control and vascular outcomes in patients with type 2 diabetes. *New England Journal of Medicine, 358*(24), 2560–2572.

Agency for Healthcare Research and Quality (AHRQ). (2008). Comparative effectiveness, safety and indications of pre-mixed insulin analogues for adults with type 2 diabetes. Retrieved August 28, 2009, from http://effectivehealthcare.ahrq.org

Amati, F., Dube, J., Coen, P., Stefanovic-Racic, M., Toledo, F., & Goodpastor, B. (2009). Physical inactivity and obesity underlie the insulin resistance of aging. *Diabetes Care, 32*(8), 1550–1552.

American Association of Clinical Endocrinologists (AACE). (2006). American Association of Clinical Endocrinologists medical guidelines for clinical practice for the evaluation and treatment of hyperthyroidism and hypothyroidism. (Amended version from original *Endocrine Practice 2002, 8*[6], 457–469.) Retrieved August 10, 2009, from http://www.aace.com/pub/pdf/guidelines

American College of Obstetricians and Gynecologists (ACOG). (2007, October 1). *Routine thyroid screening not recommended for pregnant women* [Press release]. Retrieved August 10, 2009, from http://www.acog.org

American College of Obstetricians and Gynecologists (ACOG). (2008). *Thyroid disease in pregnancy* (ACOG Practice Bulletin No. 37. Bulletin originally published 2002; reaffirmed 2008). Retrieved August 10, 2009, from http://www.acog.org

American Diabetes Association. (2009, January). Standards of medical care in diabetes-2009. *Diabetes Care, 32*(Suppl. 1), 13-61

Anand, S., Yusuf, S., Vuksan, V., Devanesen, S., Teo, K., Montague, P., et al. (2000). Differences in risk factors, atherosclerosis, and cardiovascular disease between ethnic groups in Canada: The Study of Health Assessment and Risk in Ethnic Groups (SHARE). *Lancet, 356,* 279–284.

Andukuri, R., Drincic, A., & Rendell, M. (2009). Alogliptin: A new addition to the class of DPP-4 inhibitors. *Diabetes, Metabolic Syndrome and Obesity: Targets and Therapy, 2,* 117–126.

Bartels, D. (2004). Adherence to oral therapy for type 2 diabetes: Opportunities for enhancing glycemic control. *Journal of the American Academy of Nurse Practitioners, 16*(1), 8–16.

Bash, L., Selvin, E., Steffes, M., Coresh, J., & Astor, B. (2008). Poor glycemic control in diabetes and the risk of incident chronic kidney disease even in the absence of albuminuria and retinopathy: Atherosclerosis Risk in Communities (ARIC) study. *Archives of Internal Medicine, 168*(22), 2440–2447.

Blonde, N., Dagogo-Jack, S., Banerji, M., Pratley, R., Marcellari, A., Braceras, R., et al. (2009, October). Comparison of vildagliptin and thiazolidinedione as add-on therapy in patients inadequately controlled with metformin: Results of the GALIANT trial—a primary care, type 2 diabetes study. *Diabetes, Obesity and Metabolism, 11*(10), 978–986.. Retrieved August 20, 2009, from http://www.ncbi.nlm.nih.gov/sites/entrez

Bloomgarden, Z. (2003). American Association of Clinical Endocrinologists (AACE) consensus conference on insulin resistance syndrome. *Diabetes Care, 26*(4), 1297–1303.

Bolli, G., Dotta, F., Colin, L., Minic, B., & Goodman, M. (2009). Comparison of vildagliptin and pioglitzaone in patients with type 2 diabetes inadequately controlled with metformin. *Diabetes, Obesity and Metabolism, 11*(6), 589–595.

Brown, N., Bylers, S., Carr, D., Maldonado, M., & Warner, B. (2009). Dipeptidyl peptidase-IV inhibitor use associated with increased risk of ACE inhibitor-associated angioedema. *Hypertension, 54*(3), 516–523.

Buse, J., Wolffenbuttel, B., Herman, W., Shermonsky, N., Jiang, H., Fahrbach, J., et al. (2009). Durability of basal versus lispro mix 75/25 insulin efficacy (DURABLE) trial 24 week results. *Diabetes Care, 32*(6), 1007–1013.

Cefalu, W. (2007, February). Point: Pulmonary inhalation of insulin: Another "brick in the wall". *Diabetes Care, 30,* 439–441.

Chahal, H., & Chowdhury, T. (2007). Gliptins: A new class of oral hypoglycaemic agent. Retrieved August 19, 2009 from http://qjmed.oxfordjournals.org/cgi/content/full/hcm081v1

Cheng, J. (2009). The benefit and risk of antidiabetic agents used in patients with heart disease. *Journal of Pharmacy Practice, 22*(2), 179–193.

Chernausek, S., Attie, K., Cara, J., Rosenfeld, R., & Frane, J. (2000). Growth hormone therapy of Turner syndrome: The impact of age of estrogen replacement on final height. *Journal of Clinical Endocrinology and Metabolism, 85*(7), 2439–2445.

Cooper, D. (2003). Combined T4 and T3 therapy—back to the drawing board. *Journal of the American Medical Association, 290*(22), 3002–3004.

Cozzi, R., Montini, M., Attanasio, R., Albizzi, M., Lasio, G., Lodrini, S., et al (2006). Primary treatment of acromegaly with octreotide LAR. *Journal of Clinical Endocrinology and Metabolism, 91*(4), 1397–1403.

Craig, K., Donovam, K., Munnery, M., Owens, D., Williams, J., & Phillips, A. (2003). Identification and management of diabetic nephropathy in the diabetes clinic. *Diabetes Care, 26*(6), 1806–1811.

Daly, A., Warshaw, H., Pastors, J., Franz, M., & Arnold, M. (2003). Diabetes medical nutrition therapy: Practical tips to improve outcomes. *Journal of the American Academy of Nurse Practitioners, 15*(5), 206–211.

Davies, M., Storms, F., Shutler, S., Bianchi-Biscay, M., & Gomis, R., for the AT.LANTUS Study Group. (2005). Improvement of glycemic control in subjects with poorly controlled type 2 diabetes. *Diabetes Care, 28*(6), 1282–1288.

DeFronzo, R., Fleck, P., Wilson, C., & Mekki, Q., on behalf of the Alogliptin Study 010 Group. (2008). Efficacy and safety of the dipeptidyl peptidase-4 inhibitor alogliptin in patients with type 2 diabetes and inadequate glycemic control: A randomized, double-blind placebo-controlled study. *Diabetes Care, 31*(12), 2315–2317.

Diabetes Control and Complications Trial Research Group. (1993). The effect of intensive treatment of diabetes on the development and progression of long-term complications in insulin-dependent diabetes mellitus. *New England Journal of Medicine, 329,* 997.

Diabetes Prevention Program Research Group. (2002). Reduction in the incidence of type 2 diabetes with lifestyle intervention or metformin. *New England Journal of Medicine, 346*(6), 393–403.

Diabetes Prevention Program Research Group. (2003). Within-trial cost-effectiveness of lifestyle intervention or metformin for the primary prevention of type 2 diabetes. *Diabetes Care, 26*(9), 2518–2523.

DiGregorio, R., & Pasikhova, Y. (2009). Rhabdomyolisis caused by a potential sitagliptin-lovastatin interaction. *Pharmacotherapy, 29*(3), 352–356.

Drucker, D., & Nauck, M. (2006). The incretin system: Glucagon-like peptide-1 receptor agonists and dipeptidyl peptidase-4 inhibitors in type 2 diabetes. *Lancet, 368*(9548), 1696–1705.

Drug facts and comparisons. (2009). St. Louis, MO: Wolters Kluwer Health.

D'Souza, R., Mutalik, S., Venkatesh, M., Vidyasagar, S., & Udupa, N. (2005). Nasal insulin gel as an alternate to parenteral insulin: Formulation, preclinical, and clinical studies. *AAPS PharmSciTech, 6*(2), 3184–3189.

Grozinski-Glasberg, S., Fraser, A., Nashshoni, E., Weizman, A., & Leibovici, L.. (2006). Thyroine-triiodothyronine combination therapy versus thyroxine monotherapy for clinical hypothyroidism: Meta-analysis of randomized controlled trails. *Journal of Clinical Endocrinology and Metabolism, 91*(7), 2592–2599.

He, Y., Sabo, R., Picard, F., Wang, Y., Herron, J., Ligueros-Saylan, M., et al. (2009). Study of the pharmacokinetic interaction of vildagliptin and metformin in patients with type 2 diabetes. *Current Medical Research and Opinion, 25*(5), 1265–1272.

Heise, T., Heinemann, L., Hovelmann, U., Brauns, B., Nosek, L., Haahr, H., et al. (2009). Biphasic insulin aspart 30/70: Pharmacokinetics and pharmacodynamics compared with once-daily biphasic human insulin and basal-bolus therapy. *Diabetes Care, 32*(8), 1431–1433.

Hodgson, S., Watts, N., Bilezikian, J., Clarke, B., Gray, T., Harris, D., et al. (2003). American Association of Clinical Endocrinologists medical guidelines for clinical practice for the prevention and treatment of postmenopausal osteoporosis: 2001 edition with selected updates for 2003. *Endocrinology Practice, 9*(6), 544–564.

Howard, A., Arnsten, J., & Gourevitch, M. (2004). Effect of alcohol consumption on diabetes mellitus: A systematic review. *Annals of Internal Medicine, 140*(3), 211–219.

Institute for Clinical Systems Improvement (ICSI). (2004). *Management of type 2 diabetes.* Bloomington, MN: Author. Retrieved June 15, 2005, from http://www.guideline.gov/summary/summary.aspx

Institute for Clinical Systems Improvement (ICSI). (2008). *Diagnosis and treatment of osteoporosis.* Bloomington, MN: Author. Retrieved August 3, 2009, from http://www.ICSI.org/osteoporosis

International Osteoporosis Foundation (IOF). (2009). Facts and statistics about osteoporosis and its impact. Retrieved August 3, 2009, from http://www.iofbonehealth.org

Joint statement of the U.S Food and Drug Administration's decision regarding bioequivalence of levothyroxine sodium. (2004). *Thyroid 2004, 14,* 486.

Kahn, S., Haffner, S., Heise, M., Herman, W., Holman, R., Jones, N., et al, for the ADOPT Study Group. (2007). Glycemic durability of rosiglitazone, metformin, or glyburide monotherapy. *New England Journal of Medicine, 355*(23), 2427–2443.

Kendall, D., Cuddihy, R., & Bergenstal, R. (2009). Clinical application of incretin-based therapy: Therapeutic potential, patient selection and clinical use. *European Journal of Internal Medicine, 20*(Suppl. 2), 329–339.

Kilpatrick, E., Rigby, A., & Atkin, S. (2008). A1C variability and the risk of microvascular complications in type 1 diabetes: Data from the Diabetes Control and Complications Trial. *Diabetes Care, 31*(11), 2198–2202.

Lawerence, J., Mayer-Davis, E., Reynolds, K., Beyer, J., Pettit, D., D'Agostino, R., et al, for the SEARCH for Diabetes in Youth Study Group. (2009). Diabetes in Hispanic American youth: Prevalence, incidence, demographics, and clinical characteristics: The SEARCH for diabetes in youth study. *Diabetes Care, 32*(3), S123–S132.

List, J., Woo, V., Morales, E., Tang, W., & Fiedorek, F. (2009). Sodium-glucose cotransport inhibition with dapagliflozin in type 2 diabetes. *Diabetes Care, 32*(4), 650–657.

Man, C., Bocj, G., Giesler, P., Serra, D., Saylan, M., Foley, J., et al. (2009). Dipeptidyl peptidase-4 inhibition by vildagliptin and the effect on insulin secretion and action in response to meal ingestion in type 2 diabetes. *Diabetes Care, 32,* 14–18.

Marfella, R., Barbieri, M., Grella, R., Rizzo, M., Nicoletti, G., & Paolisso, G. (2009, March 5). Effects of vildagliptin twice daily vs. sitagliptin once daily on 24-hour acute glucose fluctuation. *Journal of Diabetes and its Complications, 24*(2), 79–83.. Retrieved August 20, 2009, from http://www.ncbi.nlm.nih.gov/sites/entrez

Mayer-Davis, E., Beyer, J., Bell, R., Dabelea, D., D'Agostino, R., Imperatore, G., et al, and the SEARCH for Diabetes in Youth Study Group. (2009). Diabetes in African American youth: Prevalence, incidence, demographics, and clinical characteristics: The SEARCH for diabetes in youth study. *Diabetes Care, 32*(3), S112–S122.

McCance, K., & Huether, S. (2006). *Pathophysiology: The biological basis for disease in adults and children* (5th ed.). St. Louis, MO: Mosby.

Messina, M., & Redmond, G. (2006). Effects of soy protein and soybean isoflavones on thyroid function in healthy adults and thyroid patients: A review of the relevant literature. *Thyroid, 16*(3), 249–258.

Migoya, E., Stevens, C., Bergman, A., Luo, W., Lasseter, K., Dilzer, S., et al. (2009). Effect of moderate hepatic insufficience on the pharmacokinetics of sitagliptin. *Canadian Journal of Clinical Pharmacology, 16*(1), e165–170.

Mozaffarian, D., Kamineni, A., Carnethon, M., Djousse, L., Mukamal, K., & Siscovick, D. (2009). Lifestyle risk factors and new-onset diabetes mellitus in older adults: The Cardiovascular Health Study. *Archives of Internal Medicine, 169*(8), 798–807.

Nathan, D., Buse, J., Davidson, M., Ferrannini, E., Holman, R., Sherwin, R., et al. (2009). Medical management of hyperglycemia in type 2 diabetes: A consensus algorithm for the initiation and adjustment of therapy: A consensus statement of the American Diabetes Association and the European Association for the Study of Diabetes. *Diabetes Care, 32*(1), 193–203.

Nathan, D., for the American Diabetes Association and European Association for the Study of Diabetes Consensus Committee. (2009). Medical management of hyperglycemia in type 2 diabetes: A consensus algorithm for the initiation and adjustment of therapy: A consensus statement of the American Diabetes Association and the European Association for the Study of Diabetes [Response letter]. *Diabetes Care, 32*(5), e59.

National Institute for Health and Clinical Excellence (NICE). (2002). TA42 growth hormone deficiency (children)—human growth hormone: Guidance. Retrieved August 6, 2009, from http://guidance.nice.org.uk/TA42/Guidance/pdf/English

Nissen, S., & Wolski, K. (2007). Effect of rosiglitazone on the risk of myocardial infarction and death from cardiovascular disease. *New England Journal of Medicine, 356*(24), 2457–2471.

Norden, M., Larsson, F., & Tedelind, S. (2007). Down-regulation of the sodium/iodide symporter explains I^{131}-induced thyroid stunning. *Cancer Research (Baltimore), 67*(15), 7512–7517.

Porcellati, F., Rossetti, P., Busciantella, N., Marzotti, S., Lucidi, P., Luzio, S., et al. (2007). Comparison of pharmacolinetics and dynamics of the long-acting insulin analogs glargine and detemir at steady state in type 1 diabetes. *Diabetes Care, 30*(10), 2447–2452.

Raz, I., Hanefeld, M., Xu, L., Caria, C., Williams-Herman, D., & Khatami, H. (2006). Efficacy and safety of the dipeptidyl peptidase-4 inhibitor sitagliptin as monotherapy in patients with type 2 diabetes mellitus. *Diabetologia, 49*(11), 2564–2571.

Remuzzi, G., Schieppati, A., & Ruggenenti, P. (2003). Nephropathy in patients with type 2 diabetes. *New England Journal of Medicine, 346*(15), 1145–1151.

Reynolds, J. (2009). Fixed-dose combination of sitagliptin and metformin for the treatment of type 2 diabetes. *Diabetes, Metabolic Syndrome and Obesity: Targets and Therapy, 2,* 127–134.

Richter, B., Bandeira-Echtler, E., Bergerhoff, K., Clar, C., & Ebrahim, S. (2007, July 18). Rosiglitazone for type 2 diabetes mellitus. *Cochrane Database Systematic Review, 3,* CD006063. Retrieved August 10, 2009, from http://ncbi.nlm.nih.gov/pubmed/17636824

Rosenstock, J., Bergenstal, R., DeFronzo, R., Hirsch, I., Klonoff, D., Boss, A., et al, for the 0008 Study Group. (2008). Efficacy and safety of technosphere inhaled insulin compared with technosphere powder placebo in insulin-naïve type 2 diabetes suboptimally controlled with oral agents. *Diabetes Care, 31*(11), 2177–2182.

Rosenstock, J., Hollander, P., Chevalier, S., & Iranmanesh, A., for the SERENADE Group. (2008). SERENADE: The study evaluating rimonabant efficacy in drug-naïve diabetic patients. Effects of monotherapy with rimonabant, the first CB1 receptor antagonist, on glycemic control, body weight, and lipid profile in drug-naïve type 2 diabetes. *Diabetes Care, 31*(11), 2169–2176.

Ross, D. (2008, November 12). Thiomamides in the treatment of Graves' disease. *UpToDate*. Retrieved June 3, 2009, from http://www.uptodate.com

Ruggiero, S., Dodson, T., Assall, L., Landesberg, R., Mari, R., & Mehrotra, B. (2009). American Association of Oral & Maxillofacial Surgeons position paper on bisphosphonate-related osteonecrosis of the jaws. *Journal of Oral and Maxillofacial Surgery, 67*(Supp. 1), 2–12.

Schmidt, M., Duncan, B., Vigo, A., Pankow, J., Ballantyne, C., Couper, D., et al, for the ARIC Investigators. (2003). Detection of undiagnosed diabetes and other hyperglycemic states: The Atherosclerosis Risk in Communities Study. *Diabetes Care, 26*(5), 1338–1343.

Schweizer, A., Dejager, S., & Bosi, E. (2009). Comparison of vildagliptin and metformin monotherapy in elderly patients with type 2 diabetes: A 24-week, double-blind, randomized trial. *Diabetes, Obesity and Metabolism, 11*(8), 804–812.

Scottish Intercollegiate Guidelines Network (SIGN). (2004). *Management of osteoporosis: A national guideline.* Edinburgh, Scotland: Author. Retrieved August 3, 2009, from http://www.sing.ac.uk/guidelines

Selvin, E., Bolen, S., Yeh, H., Wiley, C., Wilson, L., Marinopoulos, S., et al. (2008). Cardiovascular outcomes in trials of oral diabetes medications: A systematic review. *Archives of Internal Medicine, 168*(19), 2070–2080.

Singh, S., Loke, Y., & Furberg, C. (2007). Long-term risk of cardiovascular events with rosiglitazone. *Journal of the American Medical Association, 298*(10), 1189–1195.

Slim, R., Salem, C., Zani, M., & Biour, M. (2009). Pioglitazone-induced rhabdomyolysis. *Diabetes Care, 32,* e84.

Tahrani, A., Piya, M., & Barnett, A. (2009). Saxagliptin: A new DPP-4 inhibitor for the treatment of type 2 diabetes mellitus. *Advanced Therapies, 26*(3), 249–262.

Umpierrez, G., Jones, S., Smiley, D., Mulligan, P., Keyler, T., Temponi, A., et al. (2009). Insulin analogs versus human insulin in the treatment of patients with diabetic ketoacidosis: A randomized controlled trial. *Diabetes Care, 32*(7), 1164–1169.

U.S. Food and Drug Administration. (2003). Approval letter (for Serostim). Retrieved August 6, 2009, from http;//www.accessdata.fda.gov/scripts/cder/drugsatfda/index.cfm

U.S. Food and Drug Administration. (2009a). *Early communication of an ongoing safety review on bisphosphonates.* Retrieved August 3, 2009, from http://www.fda.gov/Drugs/DrugSafety/PostmarketDrugSafetyInformationfor PatientsandProviders/ucm070303

U.S. Food and Drug Administration. (2009b). *FDA approves pancreatic enzyme replacement product for marketing in the United States.* Retrieved September 1, 2009, from http://www.fda.gov/NewsEvents/Newsroom.PressAnnouncements/ucm149579.htm

U.S. Food and Drug Administration. (2009c). *Propylthiouracil-induced liver failure.* Retrieved June 5, 2009, from http://www.fda.gov/Drugs/DrugSafety/PostmarketDrugSafetyInformationforPatientsandProviders/ucm162701

U.S. Food and Drug Administration. (2010). *FDA drug safety communication: New boxed warning on severe liver injury with propylthiouracil.* Retrieved April 21, 2010, from http://www.fda.gov/Drugs/DrugSafety/PostmarketDrugSafetyInformationfor PatientsandProviders/ucm209023.htm

Walsh, J., Ward, L., Burke, V., Bhagat, C., Shiels, L., Henley, D., et al. (2006). Small changes in thyroxine dosage do not produce measurable changes in hypothyroid symptoms, well-being, or quality of life: Results of a double-blind, randomized clinical trial. *Journal of Clinical Endocrinology & Metabolism, 91*(7), 2624–2630.

Welschen, L., Bloemenday, E., Ipels, G., Decker, J., Heine, R., Stalman, W., et al. (2005). Self-monitoring of blood glucose in patients with type 2 diabetes who are not using insulin. *Diabetes Care, 28*(6), 1510–1517.

Whelen, A., Jurgens, T., Bowles, S., & Doyle, H. (2009). Efficacy of natural health products in treating osteoporosis: What is the quality of internet patient advice? *Annals of Pharmacotherapeutics, 43*(5), 899–907.

White, N., Chase, P., Arslanian, S., Tamborlane, W. and for the 4030 Study Group. (2009, March). Comparison of glycemic variability associated with insulin glargine and intermediate-acting insulin when used as the basal component of multiple daily injections for adolescents with type 1 diabetes. *Diabetes Care, 32,* 387–393.

Williams-Herman, D., Johnson, J., Teng, R., Luo, E., Davies, M., Kaufman, K., et al. (2009). Efficacy and safety of initial combination therapy with sitagliptin and metformin in patients with type 2 diabetes: A 54-week study. *Current Medical Research and Opinion, 25*(3), 569–583.

Woo, V., for the Canadian Diabetic Association 2008 Clinical Practice Guidelines Steering Committee. (2009). Medical management of hyperglycemia: A consensus algorithm for the initiation and adjustment of therapy: A response to Nathan et al. *Diabetes Care, 32,* e34.

CHAPTER 22

DRUGS AFFECTING THE REPRODUCTIVE SYSTEM

Taynin Kopanos

Chapter Outline

There are many medications that are prescribed for reproductive problems in both men and women. This chapter discusses **androgens** and **antiandrogens**, commonly prescribed for men, as well as appropriate prescribing of these medications for women. Prescribing of **estrogens** and **progesterone**, as well as their antagonists, is reviewed, as well as drugs for lactation and erectile dysfunction. Medications discussed in this chapter are limited to medications prescribed in primary care and gynecology and do not include medications prescribed in specialty endocrine or reproductive health care.

ANDROGENS AND ANTIANDROGENS

Testosterone is the primary male **androgen**. In many tissues, its activity depends on reduction to dihydrotestosterone, which binds to cytosol-receptor proteins. The androgen-receptor complex is then transported to the nucleus of the cell, where it initiates transcription events and cellular changes. Endogenous androgens are responsible for the following:

- Normal growth, maturation, and maintenance of the male sex organs and secondary sexual characteristics
- The skeletal growth spurt in adolescence and for the termination of linear growth by fusion of the epiphyseal growth plate
- Activation of sebaceous gland, accounting for some cases of acne during puberty
- Enhancing production of erythropoietic stimulating factor, resulting in increased red blood cell production
- Playing a role in libido

A more detailed discussion of the roles of **androgens** is seen in the Pharmacodynamics section.

The **androgens** (**testosterone propionate** [in oil, Depo-Testerone], **testosterone enanthate** [in oil, Delatestryl], **testosterone cypionate** [in oil, Depo-Testosterone], **methyltestosterone** [Android, Methitest, Testred, Virilon], **testosterone gel** [AndroGel 1%,

Testim], fluoxymesterone, transdermal testosterone [Testoderm, Androderm], and buccal testosterone [Striant]) have been used to treat disorders in both the male and female reproductive systems. **Androgens** are indicated for the symptomatic treatment of (1) deficiency states in males associated with hypogonadism and, (2) in both sexes for disorders such as cancer and HIV. **Androgen** therapy has also been used to treat libido, endometriosis, and postmenopausal symptoms in women. However, there is limited evidence supporting the correlation of testosterone levels and symptom reduction in women. **Androgens** have also been used illicitly to enhance athletic performance and increase muscle mass.

Antiandrogens fall into several different categories. **Androgen hormone inhibitors** in this section are also known as **5-alpha-reductase inhibitors.** These enzyme inhibitors block the conversion of testosterone to dihydrotesterone. Key agents in this class include **finasteride** (Propecia, Proscar) and **dutasteride** (Avodart). This class of drugs is used to treat benign prostatic hyperplasia, and **finasteride** (Propecia) has been approved to treat male-pattern baldness. **Leuprolide acetate** (Lupron) is a **gonadotropin-releasing hormone analogue**, also known as a **luteinizing hormone-releasing hormone antagonist.** These agents create a reversible chemical orchiectomy state in males and an oophorectomy state in females. Through this mechanism of action, these agents are effective in the treatment of advanced prostatic cancer and for the management of endometriosis and uterine leiomyomata (fibroids). **Flutamide** (Eulexin), **bicalutamide** (Casodex), and **nilutamide** (Nilandron) are **direct antiandrogens**; these agents inhibit androgen uptake or nuclear binding of androgen at target tissues. These agents are used as part of a combination therapy treatment of prostatic carcinoma. **Spironolactone** (Aldactone) is an aldosterone antagonist and inhibitor of 5-alpha-reductase that is indicated for use as a potassium-sparing diuretic (see Chapters 36 and 40 for further discussion regarding cardiovascular use). Additionally, it has an off-labeled use in the treatment of female hirsutism and acne due to its **antiandrogenic** properties. Symptoms of premenstrual syndrome/premenstrual dysphoric disorder (PMS/PMDD) have also been relieved by spironolactone doses of 25 mg four times a day beginning on day 14 of the menstrual cycle. Box 22–1 provides information on **antiandrogens.** Note the discussion in this chapter focuses on utilization and monitoring of androgen therapy in the primary care setting rather than in specialized practice.

Pharmacodynamics

Testosterone is the most important **androgen** in humans. It is highly protein bound, and only a small portion (2%) is found free in plasma and converted to dihydrotestosterone in the skin, prostate, seminal vesicles, and epididymis. In men, testosterone is produced primarily within the testes in interstitial or Leydig cells, located in the spaces between the seminiferous tubules. The testis, like the ovary, has both reproductive and endocrine functions. Women produce small amounts of testosterone

BOX 22–1 COMPOUNDS WITH ANTIANDROGENIC PROPERTIES

The problems of reduced potency in the oral form and the virilizing side effects of **androgens** led investigators to develop drugs that inhibit synthesis and block sex hormone production receptors. This approach of countering the effects of undesirable **androgen** excess has enabled therapy at higher dosages. Dihydrotestosterone is the essential androgen in the prostate. The effect of **androgens** can be reduced by inhibiting 5-alpha-reductase in its target tissues. PSA levels and digital prostate examination are required monitoring for men on these agents. Users of $alpha_1$-˜adrenergic antagonists may experience hypotension, syncopy, impotence, and decreased libido. Caution is advised with concurrent use of agents that potentiate the $alpha_1$-adrenergic blocking, and agents that increase the risk of hypotension.

Finasteride (Propecia, Proscar)

Finasteride, a steroid-like drug, inhibits 5-alpha-reductase, an intracellular enzyme that converts testosterone to 5-alpha-dihydrotestosterone (DHT). It has a 100-fold selectivity for 5-alpha-reductase type 2, the isoenzyme found primarily in the prostate, seminal vesicles, epididymides, and hair follicles. It is well absorbed orally, and the reduction in DHT begins within 8 hours of administration and lasts for about 24 hours. **Finasteride** undergoes extensive hepatic metabolism, with 39 percent being excreted in the urine and 57 percent in feces.

Approximately 90 percent is bound to plasma proteins. The FDA approved doses of 5 mg per day to treat benign prostatic hyperplasia (BPH). Although early improvement may be seen, 6 to 12 months of therapy may be needed to determine if a beneficial response has been achieved. Most patients experience a rapid regression in prostate gland size and about 50 percent experience an increase in urinary flow and improvement in BPH symptoms (*Drug Facts and Comparisons,* 2005). In 1998, the FDA approved a 1-mg dose for treating male pattern baldness. Three months of therapy are usually required to demonstrate benefits. Stopping the drugs reverses the effect within 12 months. The main undesirable adverse effects are decreased libido and impotence, which occur with both doses.

BOX 22–1 **COMPOUNDS WITH ANTIANDROGENIC PROPERTIES—cont'd**

Dutasteride (Avodart)

Like **finasteride, dutasteride** inhibits 5-alpha-reductase, an intracellular enzyme that converts testosterone to 5-alpha-dihydrotesterone (DHT). It inhibits both type 1 and type 2 forms of the isoenzyme. It does not bind to the human androgen receptor. It is absorbed well after oral administration and reaches peak serum concentration within 2 to 3 hours; however, peak clinical effect does not occur until 6 to 12 months of therapy have been completed. Heavily bound to plasma protein (99%), it is extensively metabolized by the liver, utilizing the CYP450 3A4/5 substrate. The drug and its metabolites are excreted mainly in feces (45%). Only trace amounts are found in the urine. This drug is approved for the treatment of BPH. BPH patients treated with this drug had a decrease of 94 percent of DHT after 1 year. Because of its long half-life, serum concentrations remain detectable for up to 6 months after discontinuance of treatment. **Dutasteride** is absorbed through the skin, so women who are pregnant or may become pregnant should not handle **dutasteride** capsules due to the potential risk of fetal anomaly to a male fetus. The main undesirable adverse effects are decreased libido and impotence.

Leuprolide Acetate (Lupron)

Leuprolide is a luteinizing hormone–releasing agonist. This drug produces gonadal suppression when blood levels are continuous in the treatment of prostate cancer. It may be given in a dose of 1 mg SC daily or IM every 3 months in the depot formulation. Mean plasma levels are achieved in 4 hours and are maintained after an initial drop in concentration. It has even greater suppression when used with **flutamide.** In pediatric patients, its use is to treat central precocious puberty. In gynecology, its use is in reducing uterine fibroids, endometriosis, and polycystic ovary syndrome. Approximately 90 percent of women with unstaged endometriosis have relief of pain, and 50 percent regain fertility with **leuprolide.**

Flutamide (Eulexin, Euflex)

Flutamide behaves like a competitive antagonist at the **androgen** receptor site, although it is truly a nonsteroidal agent. It has been used with **leuprolide** for the treatment of advanced prostate cancer and with female **androgen** excess syndrome. The adverse effects in men are gynecomastia and reversible liver toxicity. **Flutamide** is rapidly absorbed orally. It is metabolized into six compounds and bound 97 percent to plasma proteins, reaching a steady state by the fourth dose. **Flutamide** is excreted in the urine but has not required changes in dose unless renal function is less than 29 mL/min. There is a black box warning regarding hepatic failure, hepatic encephalopathy, and death with this agent. Most of these events have occurred within the first 3 months of therapy. Baseline and every month liver function testing is necessary for the first 4 months of therapy, and then periodically. Medication should be discontinued if any symptoms of hepatic injury or jaundice develop.

Spironolactone (Aldactone)

Spironolactone is another competitive inhibitor of dihydrotestosterone, **aldosterone,** interferes with the **androgen** receptors in the prostate. It also reduces 17-alpha-hydroxylase activity, lowering plasma levels of **testosterone** and androstenedione. Refer to Chapter 16 for its uses as a diuretic. **Spironolactone** is absorbed orally, reaches peak levels in 2 hours, and is metabolized by the liver and excreted through the portal system. **Spironolactone** has short-term use for primary hyperaldosteronism in patients preoperatively. It is used long term for those patients who are not good candidates for surgery or those with idiopathic hyperaldosteronism. There are also edematous conditions that require potassium conservation, such as congestive heart failure and cirrhosis of the liver associated with ascites. An off-labeled use is in females with androgen excess for the treatment of hirsutism and acne in dosages of 50 to 200 mg/day. Adverse reactions are usually dose related and reversible when the drug is discontinued. The commonest adverse reactions are GI upset, drowsiness, gynecomastia, impotence, cutaneous eruptions, and urticaria. Early animal chronic toxicity studies demonstrated tumorigenicity; therefore, use should be balanced against risk (there is a black box warning regarding this concern). This drug is contraindicated in pregnancy, yet the American Academy of Physicians has stated that it is compatible with breastfeeding. Although this drug is classified as a diuretic, its use in premenstrual syndrome is probably effective because of its antiandrogen effect, even at low doses (25 to 50 mg daily).

in the menstruating ovary and the adrenals, and both sexes produce testosterone peripherally from androstenedione, dehydroepiandrosterone (DHEA), and dehydroepiandrosterone sulfate (DHEAS).

At puberty, the normal male produces testosterone that stimulates maturation of the male reproductive tract and causes penile and scrotal growth. Secondary sexual characteristics associated with androgens also become noticeable. Skin changes occur, resulting in pubic, axillary, and facial hair growth, along with stimulation of sebaceous glands, making the skin thicker and oilier. Even the vocal cords become thicker, resulting in a lower-pitched voice.

Lean body mass increases and more growth occurs in all bones, with epiphyseal closure occurring at around 21 years of age. Androgens continue to play a crucial in the maintenance of sexual function across the male lifespan. Androgen levels remain stable until age 55 years, when a gradual decline begins. At 70 years, a more rapid decline in hormone levels occurs, and men experience decreased muscle mass, strength, and libido. Androgens have metabolic effects in protein metabolism, liver synthesis of clotting factors, and renal production of erythropoietin. Androgens affect lipoprotein metabolism, resulting in lower high-density lipoprotein (HDL). For example, men have HDLs of 20 to 40 mg/dL, and women have HDLs in the range of 40 to 60 mg/dL.

The use of synthetic **androgens** is intended to supplement or replace endogenous hormones. The mechanism of action and effects of synthetic **androgens** are similar to those described above. When men attempt to improve athletic prowess by taking large doses of exogenous **testosterone,** the normal feedback mechanisms in the male reproductive process is altered and spermatogenesis is reduced through suppression of follicle-stimulating hormone (FSH).

Pharmacokinetics

Absorption and Distribution

Several delivery modes for **testosterone replacement** are available. Oral **testosterone** is rapidly metabolized by the gut as methyltestosterone and fluoxymesterone and is converted in its target tissues by the enzyme 5-alpha-reductase. The further conversion of **testosterone** to estradiol by cytochrome P450 (CYP450) aromatase occurs in adipose tissue, the liver, and the hypothalamus. Buccal administration lengthens the half-life. IM administration (esters) in depot preparations can last 2 to 4 weeks. **Depo-Testosterone** is slowly absorbed into the bloodstream between dosing intervals. Varying rates of absorption from IM administration are associated with this method, and significant fluctuation in serum testosterone levels and effects are reported. For this reason, the selection of transdermal or implanted **testosterone** therapy may be preferred. Transdermal application is available in either a topically applied gel or through patch delivery systems. Both gel and patch delivery methods require once-daily application to intact, nonscrotal skin. These agents **(Androderm, AndroGel,** and **Testim)** are well absorbed through the skin and result in rises in serum **testosterone** levels within 2 to 4 hours of application. **Testoderm** is associated with a rapid return to baseline within 2 hours after removal. Other transdermal formulations have continuous absorption during a 24-hour dosing period. Specific precautions with the use of transdermal applications will be discussed later in this section. **Testopel** is a subcutaneous pellet that produces sustained **testosterone** effects for 3 to 6 months. The use of this subcutaneous version requires specific provider training in appropriate technique for in-office administration.

Testosterone in plasma is 98 percent bound to a specific testosterone-estradiol-binding globulin known as sex hormone–binding globulin (SHBG). SHBG is increased in plasma by **estrogen, thyroid hormone,** and cirrhosis of the liver. It is decreased by **androgens, growth hormone,** and obesity. The final 2 percent remains free to enter the cell (*Drug Facts and Comparisons,* 2010).

Metabolism and Excretion

Testosterone uses the CYP450 3A4 substrate for metabolism. Forty-four percent of **testosterone** degradation occurs in the liver, where it is inactivated to androsterone and etiocholanolone, and then conjugated and excreted in the urine. The majority (90%) is excreted in the urine and 6 percent is excreted in the feces. There is considerable variation in the reported half-life of **testosterone:** from 10 to 100 minutes. The amount of bound **testosterone** will determine the percentage of free drug and the free drug concentration determines half life.

Onset, Peak, and Duration

Oral administration of **testosterone** reaches peak levels in 2 hours, buccal in 1 hour, and IM in 8 days to 2 weeks. Onset, peak, and duration of action of transdermal forms vary. Table 22–1 depicts the pharmacokinetics of the various formulations of **androgens** and **antiandrogens,** including the variable half-lives of transdermal formulations.

Pharmacotherapeutics

Precautions and Contraindications

Contraindications for the use of **testosterone** include male breast cancer, prostate cancer, pregnancy (Category X due to fetal harm/virilization of the female fetus), and lactation.

Transdermal systems and **testosterone gel** are not indicated for women and must not be used by them. Safety and efficacy of **Testoderm** and **AndroGel** products in pediatric patients have not been established. Men who use topical gels must not have skin contact with pregnant women or with children, as skin-to-skin transfer of **testosterone** may occur. Men should wash their hands after application and allow skin to dry before it touches clothing to decrease risk of inadvertent transfer of medication.

Edema, with or without congestive heart failure, may be a serious complication. These drugs should be used cautiously in patients with preexisting cardiac, renal, or hepatic disease and frequent monitoring is required (see the Monitoring section). In addition to discontinuing the drug, **diuretic** therapy may be needed.

Men, especially elderly men, treated with **androgens** are at increased risk for developing prostatic hypertrophy, prostatic hyperplasia, and prostatic carcinoma. The treatment of hypogonadal men with **testosterone** may potentiate

Table 22–1 ▶ **Pharmacokinetics: Androgens and Antiandrogens**

Drug	Onset	Peak	Duration	Protein Binding (in %)	Half-Life	Elimination
Androgens						
Testosterone cypionate (in oil) (Depo-Testerone)	UK	UK	2–4 wk	98%	8 d	90% in urine as conjugates and metabolites; 6% in feces
Testosterone enanthate (in oil) (Delatestryl)	UK	UK	2–4 wk	98%	8 d	90% in urine as conjugates and metabolites; 6% in feces
Testosterone propionate (in oil) (Testex)	UK	UK	2–4 wk	98%	8 d	90% in urine as conjugates and metabolites; 6% in feces
Testosterone, buccal (Striant)	UK	10–12 h	12 h	UK	10–100 min	90% in urine. Avoids first pass effects of liver. Metabolized in liver and reproductive tissue
Methyltestosterone (Methitest, Testred, Virilon)	UK	UK	1–3 d	98%	10–100 min	90% in urine as conjugates and metabolites; 6% in feces
Fluoxymesterone	UK	UK	UK	98%	9.2 h	90% in urine as conjugates and metabolites; 6% in feces
Testosterone (Testoderm); Must apply to scrotal skin	UK	2–4 h	*		*	90% in urine as conjugates and metabolites; 6% in feces
Testosterone (Testoderm TTS); Apply to nonscrotal skin	UK	2–4 h	*		*	90% in urine as conjugates and metabolites; 6% in feces
Testosterone (Androderm); Apply to nonscrotal skin	UK	4–6 h	24 h		24 h	90% in urine as conjugates and metabolites; 6% in feces
Testosterone gel (AndroGel 1%, Testim)	30 min	4 h	48 h		5 d	90% in urine as conjugates and metabolites; 6% in feces
Antiandrogens						
Finasteride	NA	1–2 h	24 h	None	Normal renal function: 4.8–6 h Men >70 yr: 7 h	39% urine, 57% feces.
Leuprolide (11.25 mg Depo)	NA	Depot: 4 h	4 wk	45%–49%	NA	NA
Flutamide	NA	2 h	6 h	94%–96%	Normal renal function: 8 h Impaired renal function: slightly more than 8 h	Total: mainly in urine Unchanged: 4.2% in feces
Spironolactone (off-labeled use)	24–28 h	48–72 h	48–72 h	90%	1.3–2 h	Total: renal Unchanged: NA

NA = not available; UK = unknown.
*Serum levels return to normal within 2 h of removal. Serum levels plateau after 3–4 wk of use.

sleep apnea. This risk increases in men with obesity or chronic lung disease.

The areas of clinical usage of **androgens** that are more controversial include stimulating growth in boys with delayed puberty, in aging men to increase strength and muscle mass, and in athletes to improve competitive performance. In this last area, there has been abuse by coaches and athletes alike. The adverse effects far outweigh the potential benefits. It is advisable for primary care providers to refer these patients for consultation with endocrine specialists regarding initiating therapies for these populations.

Because of the abuse potential of **anabolic steroids**, providers must supply their federal narcotic identification number (Drug Enforcement Administration [DEA] number) on all prescriptions written for hormone combinations with **androgens**. Patients receiving steroid therapy require periodic laboratory and clinical evaluation. Prescribers may wish to limit prescription quantities and refills to match monitoring time frames to aid in adherence to follow-up evaluations and to reduce the potential for misuse.

Adverse Drug Reactions

The **androgens** as a class are potent agents, and can have serious or even fatal reactions if used improperly. When properly used **androgens** mimic the bodies endogenous processes. However, prolonged use of high doses of **androgens** has been associated with the development of potentially life-threatening hepatitis, hepatic neoplasms, cholestatic hepatitis, jaundice, and hepatocellular carcinoma. Cholestatic hepatitis and jaundice occur at relatively low doses of **fluoxymesterone** and **methyltestosterone**. It is reversible with drug discontinuance.

Sex specific side effects have been reported with the use of **androgen therapy**. Men may develop gynecomastia and reduced sperm levels that threaten fertility. Acne and baldness may occur, even with short-term therapy. Men can paradoxically have decreased libido, depression, and headache with exogenous administration of **androgens**. Scrotal pain, groin pain, or changes in urination may be associated with stimulation and changes of the prostate gland and need further evaluation. Men may develop priapism (a sustained erection) and will require education to seek emergent evaluation if this occurs. In women, menstrual irregularities may occur with these drugs through suppression of gonadotropin secretion, and hypercalcemia and virilization are reported.

All patients on **androgen therapy** may experience gastrointestinal (GI) symptoms, including nausea, vomiting, change in liver function, edema, and cholestatic jaundice. Suppression of clotting factors, as well as increased red blood cell production, can contribute to hemorrhage and thrombus formation simultaneously.

Both **testosterone** and **anabolic steroids** have the potential for abuse. The **anabolic steroids** have a high anabolic, low androgenic ratio of activity. The U.S. Food and Drug Administration (FDA) warns that **androgens** may cause peliosis hepatis. Peliosis is the replacement of normal liver tissue with bloody cysts. This vascularity may cause a silent, fatal abdominal hemorrhage. Liver tumors that are benign or malignant may develop. The lipoprotein changes with these steroids may hasten coronary artery disease. Drugs classified as **anabolic steroids** are **oxymetholone**, **stanozolol**, **oxandrolone**, **nandrolone phenylpropionate**, and **nandrolone decanoate**.

Drug Interactions

Various drug interactions have been reported with **androgens**. The main classes of associated drug interactions with **androgens** include **anticoagulants**, **diabetic agents**, and **corticosteroids**. The interaction of **anticoagulants** such as **warfarin (Coumadin)** with the **17-alkyl testosterone** derivatives has the most significant potential problem. The **17-alkyl testosterone** drugs are the **methyl-** and **fluoxy-forms** used for hypogonadism and male climacteric.

Although **testosterone** has been used for breast tenderness in the past, its use is discouraged because of lack of proven efficacy and the masculinizing effect that it has on women. Laboratory values of decreasing protein-bound T_4 and increased T_3 uptake need to be mentioned, but because the free T_4 levels are not affected, no deficiency state occurs. Table 22–2 presents drug interactions.

Table 22–2 ■ **Common Drug Interactions: Androgens and Antiandrogens**

Drug	Interacting Drug	Possible Effect	Implications
Androgens			
Testosterone	Anticoagulants	Increased anticoagulant effect	More frequent monitoring of prothrombin time
	Imipramine	Paranoid response	Consider switching to another class of antidepressants
	Diabetic agents	Decrease blood sugar	Frequent blood sugar monitoring. Dose adjustment of diabetic agents
	Cyclosporine	Impaired hepatic metabolism	Consider switching to another agent
Antiandrogens			
	Nevirapine	Combination induces hepatic metabolism of finasteride	Monitor for effectiveness of finasteride
Leuprolide	Pituitary, gonadotropic, and gonadal function Lab tests	Misleading results	Consider if lab test reports show unexpected values

Table 22–2 ■ **Common Drug Interactions: Androgens and Antiandrogens–cont'd**

Drug	Interacting Drug	Possible Effect	Implications
Flutamide	Warfarin	Increased INR and risk of bleeding	Monitor INR closely. As lutamide is indicated for advanced prostate cancer, the option to select an alternative treatment may be limited.
Spironolactone	Renal impairment and agents that affect renal function	Alteration in renal function and electrolytes	Monitor potassium levels in young patients with reduced renal function and in patients >65 yr
	Digitalis	May increase or decrease digitalis half-life	Monitor closely for signs of digitalis toxicity and electrolyte and digitalis levels. Consider alternative treatments.
	Potassium	Additive effect—increases risk of hyperkalemia	Recommend alternative
	Eplerenone (aldosterone receptor antagonist used for CHF)	Severe hyperkalemia	Combination is contraindicated. Do NOT use together; select an alternative agent.

Clinical Use and Dosing

The primary clinical use of these agents is for the replacement or augmentation of endogenous **androgen** for primary hypogonadal males or hypogonadotropic hypogonadism and for male climacteric. **Testosterone enanthate** demonstrated 30 years of clinical use, and the World Health Organization (WHO) selected it as the prototype hormone in its contraceptive efficacy studies. In rare situations, **androgens** are used in endometriosis, in refractory anemia, and with **estrogen** for osteoporosis and loss of libido. **Androgens** have anabolic effects with food and exercise for postoperative trauma patients and with some types of metastatic breast cancer. The masculinizing effect on women detracts from wider usage. **Testosterone** is controversial in pediatrics as a height stimulator and in sports as a performance enhancer. Primary care providers prescribe **androgens** largely for replacement therapy, and for that reason this discussion is limited. The use of **testosterone** with **estrogen** for osteoporosis and symptomatic treatment of hot flashes and decreased libido can be found in Chapter 38. Table 22–3 presents the dosage schedule for **androgens** and **antiandrogens**.

Table 22–3 ◉ **Dosage Schedule: Androgens and Antiandrogens**

Drug	Indication	Dose
Transdermal Androgens		
Testoderm	Replacement therapy for primary or hypogonadotropic hypogonadism	6 mg/d applied to scrotal area. (TTS can be applied to nonscrotal skin.) System should be worn for 22–24 h. If product comes off after it has been worn >12 h, do not reapply; wait until the next routine application time.
Androderm	Replacement therapy for primary or hypogonadotropic hypogonadism	5 mg/d. Apply to a clean, dry area of skin on back, abdomen, upper arms, or thighs. Avoid applying over bony prominences. System is worn 24 h.
AndroGel 1% or Testim	Replacement therapy for primary or hypogonadotropic hypogonadism	5–10 g applied once daily (preferably in the morning) to clean, dry, intact skin of the shoulders and/or upper arms or abdomen. Open packet and squeeze entire contents into the palm of the hand and apply immediately to the application site. Allow site to dry for a few minutes prior to dressing. Wash hands with soap and water after application. Do not apply gel to the genitals. Do not apply Testim to the abdomen. Wait 5–6 h before showering or swimming.

Continued

Table 22–3 ● **Dosage Schedule: Androgens and Antiandrogens—cont'd**

Drug	Indication	Dose
Antiandrogens		
Finasteride	Benign prostatic hyperplasia Androgenic alopecia	Oral: 5 mg daily, with or without meals Oral: 1 mg daily, with or without meals
Leuprolide	Prostatic carcinoma	SC: 1 mg daily IM: 3.75 mg q 1 month or 11.25 mg q 3 months or 30 mg q 4 months
Flutamide	Prostatic carcinoma	Oral: 250 mg 3 times/d at 8-h intervals for a total daily dosage of 750 mg
Spironolactone (off-labeled use)	Hirsutism	Oral: 50–200 mg/d; 50 mg bid on days 4–21 of the menstrual cycle may help reduce risk of menorrhagia that occurs with higher doses

Rational Drug Selection

Slow-Acting Versus Long-Acting Form

As discussed previously, there are various formulations of **androgen supplementation** from which a provider may select. There are various advantages and concerns to each formulation that should be considered. Providers should include patient preference, adherence concerns, and lifestyle as factors in agent selection.

IM forms have longer half-lives than do oral and transdermal agents, but less uniform absorption and steady serum drug levels. IM aqueous preparations need to be administered two to three times per week. The patient or a family member can be taught to administer these long-term medications to simplify daily routines. Preparations in oil can be administered at 2- to 4-week intervals. Oral preparations cause less discomfort to administer, but may cause gastric irritation and require twice-daily administration. Transdermal agents have demonstrated improved steady-state hormone levels; however, concerns with transfer to partners and children need to be considered. Subcutaneous pellets offer a long-acting option with infrequent administration (q 3 to 6 months). However, this formulation does not afford for easy dose titration and requires specialty skill in administration.

Cost

Oral testosterone products are less expensive those administered via other routes, in part because equipment and technical skills are not required for administration. **Buccal preparations** avoid the 44 percent metabolism in the liver, but the tablets are more costly. **Transdermal patches** are the most recent addition to **hormone replacement therapy** for men and women, and the convenience is associated with increased cost. Transdermal is the preferred route of administration for children because there are no taste issues or painful injections, and older adults with poor eyesight or swallowing problems have less difficulty with patch application.

In addition to the health-care needs and delivery preference, agent selection may also be influenced by a third-party payer source. Frequently, the patient's third-party payer (insurance) limits available formulations. Table 22–4 presents the available dosage forms.

Monitoring

Clients using supplemental and replacement **androgen therapy** will require monitoring for serum testosterone levels as well as therapeutic effect. Considerable and more frequent monitoring is necessary when higher doses are administered.

Table 22–4 ◆ **Available Dosage Forms: Androgens and Antiandrogens**

Drug	Dosage Form	How Supplied	Cost
Androgens			
Testosterone, Buccal (Striant)	Buccal: 30 mg testosterone	In blister packs of 10 systems	$247.03 (60 tabs)
Testosterone cypionate (in oil) (Depo-Testerone)	IM: 100 mg/mL 200 mg/mL	In 10-mL vials In 1- and 10-mL vials	34.99 for 200/ml (1 ml vial); $74.99 100 mg/ml (10 ml vial); $125.98 200 mg/ml (10 ml vial)

Table 22–4 ◆ **Available Dosage Forms: Androgens and Antiandrogens—cont'd**

Drug	Dosage Form	How Supplied	Cost
Testosterone enanthate (in oil) (Delatestryl)	IM: 200 mg/mL	In 5-mL multidose vials and 1-mL single-dose syringe with needle	5 mL = $79.99/units of 5
Testoderm	Topical: 10 mg, 15 mg	In packs of 30	NA
Androderm	Topical: 2.5 mg/24 h, 5 mg/24 h	2.5 mg/24 h in packs of 60 5 mg/24 h in packs of 30	$225.31 $232.04
AndroGel 1%	Topical: 1% testosterone	In 30 packets containing 2.5 to 5 g or in metered-dose pumps to deliver a total of 75 g	$163.75/75 units of 2.5 g $189.26/150 units of 5 mg $189.26/150 pump units
Testim	Topical: 1% testosterone	In 30 packets/tubes of 5 g	$267.48
Methyltestosterone (Methitest [M]; Testred [T];	Tablets: 10 mg (G), 10 mg (M)	In bottles of 100	$172.94/100 [M]
	25 mg (G), 25 mg (M)	In bottles of 100 and for (M) also in bottles of 1000	$279.99/100 [T]
Virilon [V])	Capsules: 10 mg (T); 10 mg (V)	In bottles of 100 and for (V) also in bottles of 1000	[V] NA
Fluoxymesterone	Tablets: 10 mg	In bottles of 100	$84.89 for 30 tabs
Antiandrogens			
Finasteride	Oral tablet	1 mg, 5 mg	$52.99 for 30 5-mg tabs $179.97 for 100 1-mg tabs
Leuprolide	Injection Lyophilized for injection	5 mg/mL in 2.8-mL multidose vial 7.5 mg, 11.25 mg, 15 mg, 22.5 mg, 30 mg in single-use kit	$497.84 IM: $590.39 for 1–3.75 mg q 1 month; $1,735.09 for 1–11.25 mg q 3 months; $2,745.09 for 1–30 mg q 4 months
Flutamide	Capsule Tablet	125 mg 250 mg	$263.99 for 180 capsules
Spironolactone (off-labeled use)	Tablet	25 mg, 50 mg, 100 mg	$15.99, $21.00, $35.00 by respective strength

In general, all patients on **androgen therapy** will require serum testosterone level monitoring, lipid tracking, liver function tests, and complete blood count evaluation. The goal of therapy is to maintain normal range serum testosterone levels. These laboratory evaluations should be performed at baseline and at 6-month intervals while on therapy. Closer monitoring of serum testosterone is needed at initiation and during dose titration. Male patients will additionally require prostate-specific antigen (PSA) and digital prostate evaluation prior to initiation of therapy and throughout the duration of treatment due to the increased risk of prostate hypertrophy and cancer associated with androgens. Abnormalities of liver function and elevation of lipids can be seen with these agents, as well as polycythemia.

Calcium levels in serum and urine may become abnormal in patients with metastatic breast cancer. **Methyltestosterone** and **fluoxymesterone** are apt to cause hepatic toxicity, and liver function tests should be drawn every 6 months. Individuals with renal or cardiovascular comorbidities will also require monitoring of electrolytes and for symptoms of edema and congestive heart failure (CHF). Blood glucose levels and antidiabetic medication may be affected by **androgen** therapy, and closer monitoring will be required. When using **testosterone** in prepubertal males, perform an x-ray every 6 months for bone maturation to avoid early closure of epiphyseal centers.

Patient Education

Administration

Avoid coadministering with other medications that cause gastric irritation. With buccal forms, food or liquids reduce absorption. Do not swallow buccal tablets; instead, park the tablet between gums and teeth. If the skin is sensitive to the patch adhesive, a small application of **aerosolized cortisone (e.g., Asthmacort or Nasacort)** to the skin will reduce irritation without loss of efficacy. Specific descriptions of how to apply transdermal systems is given in Table 22–3.

Adverse Reactions

Common adverse drug reactions and site effects of **androgens** have been discussed previously in this section. Some adverse effects are reversible if the drug is reduced or temporarily stopped. Significant adverse events with the use of **androgens** include hepatic injury, worsening of cardiovascular comorbidities, prostatic hypertrophy, and female virilization.

Hepatic injury has been associated with the use of orally administered synthetic **androgen** agents. Additional use of agents that are associated with risk of hepatic injury should be avoided to prevent additive hepatic risk. Patient education should include a discussion regarding the need to report abdominal pain, jaundice, anorexia, muscle pain, and weakness as these may be symptoms of hepatic injury. Patients with underlying dyslipidemia or angina may experience a worsening of symptoms, and should be further evaluated. Caution women to report signs of virilization such as hoarseness, hair thinning, and menstrual disruption. Older men should be routinely screened with questions regarding changes in urine stream and nighttime voiding patterns, as they may develop prostatic hypertrophy with secondary urinary retention while on **androgen** therapy.

Lifestyle Management

Children and young adults with hypogonadism need to treat their chronic problem cautiously because long-term use of **androgens** can precipitate adverse reactions. If managed early and carefully, males with hypogonadism may be able to conceive a child. Adolescents requiring therapy need to know that **testosterone** replacement is a far different matter from **anabolic steroid** use by the athlete looking for a competitive edge in an upcoming sports event. Older patients need to reduce sodium in their diet to avoid CHF while on **androgen** therapy.

ESTROGENS AND ANTIESTROGENS

Estrogen, like **testosterone**, is an endogenous hormone with multiple actions. The primary role of **estrogen** is the maturation and function of the female reproductive system. However, because there are estrogen receptor sites in the bone, cardiovascular system, central nervous system, and gastrointestinal tract, estrogen exerts significant nonreproductive health effects.

The first supplemental **estrogens** were prescribed for replacement therapy more than 50 years ago. The first marketed **estrogens** were **conjugated equine estrogens (Premarin)**. Later, **estrogens** were **esterified (80% estrone sulfate; 15% sodium equilin sulfate)**, and other synthetic and bioidentical formulations have been introduced to the market. **Estradiol** was synthesized into oral and IM preparations, vaginal creams, transdermal patches, and vaginal rings for 3-month administration. **Ethinyl forms** of **estradiol** became the primary forms of **estrogen** used in combination (preparations containing both **estrogen** and **progesterone**) **oral contraception. Ethinyl estradiol** has approximately 10 times the potency of **estradiol. Phytoestrogens** and **estrogen**-like herbal preparations have shown symptomatic improvement with perimenopausal symptoms. Studies have yet to demonstrate if **phytoestrogens** and **estrogen**-like herbal preparations convey the same cardioprotective and osteoporosis prevention benefits of traditional **estrogen** therapy. Extensive discussion of the use of **estrogens, phytoestrogens**, and related herbal therapies both for hormonal replacement and for prevention of osteoporosis is found in Chapter 38. Whereas the following section focuses the discussion on **estrogen** and its related pharmacodynamic/pharmacokinetic principles for prescribing, it should be noted that the use of **estrogen**-only products is contraindicated in women with an intact uterus. For women with an intact uterus, combination **estrogen** and **progesterone** products should be used. An extended discussion regarding the use of **estrogen** in the treatment of menopause and contraception is presented in Chapters 31 and 38. Information about **antiestrogens** is presented in Box 22–2.

Pharmacodynamics

Estrogens occur naturally in several forms. The primary sources of estrogen in the normally cycling adult woman is the ovarian follicle, which secretes 70 to 500 mcg of estradiol daily, depending on the phase of the menstrual cycle (*Drug Facts and Comparisons*, 2010). This estradiol is converted to estrone, which circulates in about equal amounts to the estradiol and to small amounts of estriol. After menopause, most endogenous estrogen is generated from conversion by peripheral tissues of androstenedione, secreted by the adrenal cortex, to estrone.

Effects of estrogen on the reproductive system include maturation of reproductive organs; development of secondary sexual characteristics; regulation of the menstrual cycle; and endometrial regeneration postmenstruation. Estrogen also effects closure of long bones after the pubertal growth spurt; maintains bone density by decreasing rate of bone resorption through antagonizing the effects of parathyroid hormone (PTH); maintains normal structure of skin and blood vessels through its actions on the endothelial cells in the arterial walls, including the induction of nitric oxide to facilitate vasodilation and oxygen uptake by cells; alters plasma lipids (increased HDL, slight reduction in low-density lipoprotein [LDL], reduced total cholesterol, increased triglycerides) through its action in the liver; reduces motility of the bowel through its modulation of sympathetic nervous system control over smooth muscle; alters production and activity of selected proteins,

BOX 22–2 ANTIESTROGENS

Although naturally occurring hormones such as **progesterone** and **testosterone** may modify the action of **estrogen,** the following discussion focuses on the synthetic **estrogen antagonists.** Drugs in this class may have limited use by most practitioners in primary care. **Clomiphene** is used for ovulation stimulation by infertility clinics. **Danazol** is primarily used for endometriosis by gynecologists, and **tamoxifen** is used for female cancers by oncologists.

Clomiphene (Clomid)

Clomiphene was the first chemical used to initiate ovulation in normogonadotropic, normoprolactinemic, and anovulatory patients. It has also been used as a component in the management of luteal-phase dysfunction, oligo-ovulation, artificial insemination, unexplained infertility, and in vitro fertilization. Although **clomiphene** has been used for 30 years, it is still a drug that remains in a specialized practice setting. The list of adverse side effects are hot flashes, multiple gestation, visual symptoms, cervical mucus abnormalities, luteal-phase defect, luteinized unruptured follicle syndrome, ovarian cancer, teratogenicity, enlargement of ovarian cysts, and liver disease.

The agonist–antagonist characteristics of **clomiphene** depend on the hormone climate. **Clomiphene** initiates ovulation in the presence of high **estrogen** levels in anovulatory females. It does this as long as other endogenous mechanisms trigger an LH surge and follicle rupture. **Clomiphene** blocks endogenous estrogen-negative feedback at the level of the hypothalamus. It also elevates **estrogen** and **progesterone** levels higher than normal. Its function may even affect the ovary and pituitary glands. **Clomiphene** also decreases serum insulin-like growth factors and increases SHBG, which assists those infertile women with polycystic ovary (PCO) disease. It has direct antiestrogenic effects on the endometrium and cervical mucus-producing glands. Elevated estrogen levels of women in the reproductive years can override the direct antiestrogen effects on the endometrium and cervical mucus.

This compound is active when taken orally, but little is known about its metabolism. Half of the compound is excreted in the feces within 5 days of administration. The hypothesis is that it is excreted through a slow enterohepatic pathway.

Danazol (Danocrine)

Although the major use of **danazol** has been to treat endometriosis, it has been employed in severe fibrocystic breast changes, hematological disorders, and idiopathic thrombocytopenic purpura. **Danazol** must be used with great caution in hepatic dysfunction, and carries a black box warning for this and for the risk of thromboembolism. The list of adverse effects is long, which is, in part, why this drug is not indicated for most primary care settings.

Danazol suppresses the pituitary-ovarian axis; inhibiting the midcycle surge of LH and FSH to suppress ovarian function. It has weak progestational and androgenic properties, as does its major metabolite, ethisterone. **Danazol** binds to **androgen, progesterone,** and **glucocorticoid** receptors and alters androgen metabolism. It does not inhibit aromatase, the enzyme required for **estrogen** synthesis. It also increases the clearance rate of **progesterone** by competing with the hormone for binding proteins. **Danazol** is taken orally and is slowly metabolized by the liver (CYP450 3A4 inhibitor), being excreted primarily in the urine after a 24-hour half-life.

Tamoxifen (Nolvadex)

Tamoxifen is the first agent in the **selective estrogen receptor modulator (SERM)** class of medications used to treat conditions that respond to adding or withdrawing **estrogens.** As the class name implies, these agents target selective estrogen receptors, while not stimulating others. It is used primarily as part of adjuvant therapy for breast cancer in patients with estrogen receptor (ER)–positive tumors. Recent studies have demonstrated a reduction in breast cancer in those individuals at high risk for developing the disease within 5 years. In the Gail model, age, family history, medical history of premalignant biopsies, and age at first live birth calculate the patient's absolute risk.

An antiestrogen in mammary tissue, **tamoxifen** blunts the effect of estrogen and has direct antigrowth activity of its own in the absence of **estrogen.** The mechanism may be that it blocks estradiol-induced cancer cell growth by altering the local production of growth factors and/or inhibiting the development of the tumor's blood supply. **Tamoxifen** continues to stimulate estrogen receptors in the endometrial tissue, and causes hyperplasia in the postmenopausal woman's endometrium and vagina. Several large-scale, longitudinal trials are under way to evaluate its effectiveness in preventing disease in high-risk women. The results will try to address its potential benefits on bone and lipids while reducing the risk on breast tissue.

This is a nonsteroidal agent that is given orally. Peak plasma levels are reached in a few hours with an initial half-life of 7 to 14 hours. The liver extensively metabolizes **tamoxifen,** and 65 percent of the drug is excreted through the gut within 2 weeks.

Raloxifene (Evista)

Raloxifene is also a **SERM.** Indications initially were for osteoporosis prevention in women who cannot or will not take **hormone replacement therapy.** Postmarketing studies have shown a positive lipid effect, which may improve cardiovascular disease risk. Results from the recent MORE randomized trial demonstrated a 76 percent reduced risk of invasive

Continued

BOX 22–2 **ANTIESTROGENS—cont'd**

breast cancer among the women taking **raloxifene** for osteoporosis. This was attributed to the effect of the drug on ER-positive tumors. This drug can be used only in women past menopause who have never had thromboembolic problems.

Raloxifene is a **selective estrogen receptor modulator** similar to **tamoxifen** with different degrees of **estrogen agonist or antagonist** activity in different tissues. It is an **estrogen agonist** on bone and an **antagonist** on breast and uterus. Unlike **tamoxifen,** it appears to be neutral on the vaginal tissues. A comparison of the beneficial effect on bone mineral density is slightly less than that of **estrogen.** Whether this bone effect will decrease the incidence of fractures has yet to be proved.

Raloxifene is taken orally without regard to meals, with a 60 percent absorption rate, but is extensively glucuronidated, and only 2 percent is bioavailable. It is excreted though the GI tract with a half-life of 32.5 hours.

Raloxifene is not indicated for pediatric patients or for premenopausal women. Concomitant **hormone replacement therapy** is not recommended.

The primary reasons sited by patients for discontinuing therapy were hot flashes and leg cramps. One reported that these symptoms may have lasted up to 6 months.

Raloxifene is highly bound (95%) to plasma proteins. Close monitoring or alternative treatments should be considered for patients using bile acid **sequestrants, thyroid hormones,** and **warfarin.**

One short-term trial indicated that it might be effective for prevention of postmenopausal bone loss without the risk for breast or uterine cancer. It may also have a beneficial effect on lipid metabolism. More studies are needed to validate that the effect on lipids actually confers a cardioprotective effect. This drug may be useful for nurse practitioners in primary care practices, but at this time, the long-term safety effects are not known. Like **estrogens,** there is some increase in thromboembolic disease, and it is teratogenic for women at risk of pregnancy.

Patients on concurrent anticoagulant therapy will require frequent INR levels initially during therapy, and dose adjustments of anticoagulants may be needed. Women should also be advised to continue with supplemental **calcium** and **vitamin D** for bone health.

Raloxifene can be administered orally without regard to food. Patients need to know that hot flashes can sometimes occur at the beginning of therapy, even in postmenopausal women.

The risk of thromboembolic disease (1%) is the same as it is for **estrogen** users. Individuals on **raloxifene** should discontinue use 72 hours prior to surgery to decrease risk of thrombosis and embolism. When traveling, patients should get up and move around every hour to avoid long periods of inactivity.

resulting in higher levels of thyroxine-binding globulin, sex-hormone binding globulin, transferrin, and renin substrate; enhances coagulability of blood by increasing the production of fibrinogen; and facilitates loss of intravascular fluid into extracellular space by its action on the renin-angiotensin-aldosterone cycle (retention of sodium and water by the kidney) resulting in edema and decreased extracellular fluid (ECF) volume. In the brain, estrogen maintains stability of the thermoregulatory center.

Control of estrogen secretion is by the hypothalamus through the pituitary gland. Gonadotropin-releasing hormone (GnRH) from the hypothalamus controls FSH and luteinizing hormone (LH) from the anterior pituitary. FSH and LH stimulate follicular development in the ovary. In the presence of adequate estrogen, LH surge is responsible for ovulation. Primary hormone pathways in the reproductive system are modulated by both negative and positive feedback loops.

Pharmacokinetics

Absorption and Distribution

Estrogens used as therapy are well absorbed in oral, transdermal, and parenteral administration routes. Orally administered **estrogen**, whether tablet or the newer chewable form is well absorbed given its lipophilic nature. However, oral **estrogens** are subject to extensive hepatic first-pass metabolism and require larger doses in order to achieve significant bioavailability. Substitution of an ethinyl group along with the **estrogen** or **estrogen** stabilized with piperazine has inhibited the first-pass effect, and allows for lower dosing amounts. The current dosing scheme has accounted for bioavailability, and prescribing clinicians are not required to make dosing adjustments. **Conjugated estrogens** are well absorbed from the GI tract. The tablet releases the drug slowly over several hours.

Compared to **oral estradiol**, transdermal formulations are metabolized in the skin to a small extent and are not subject to hepatic first-pass. This results in a therapeutic serum level of **estradiol** with lower circulating levels of **estrone** and its metabolites so that smaller total doses are required. An additional benefit of transdermal patches is that they release a constant stream of hormone, providing a steady serum hormone level. Topical applications given vaginally for local action are still usually sufficient to cause systemic effects. Topical delivery formulations include creams, hormone-impregnated rings, and tablets.

Vaginal absorption varies among women and treatment will require titration to achieve symptom control and limit unnecessary **estrogen** exposure. More of the hormone is absorbed if the degree of atrophy is great in the surrounding tissues.

Parenteral formulations that have an oil-based preparation have slow absorption with a prolonged duration of action. A single dose of IM **estradiol valerate** or **estradiol cypionate** is absorbed over several weeks.

The majority of **estradiol estrogen** (69% to 80%) binds strongly to the SHBG, and another 18 to 30 percent binds to albumin with less affinity. The remaining 1 to 2 percent free and unbound fraction is physiologically active and is responsible for the observed effects of estrogen. The distribution of exogenous forms of **estrogen** is similar to that of endogenous forms.

Metabolism and Excretion

The liver converts **estradiol** into less potent metabolites, **estrone** and **estriol**, which are excreted in the bile. A significant portion undergoes enterohepatic recirculation in the liver, resulting in undesirable side effects such as increased clotting factors and plasma renin substrate. The water-soluble forms that result from this recirculation are acidic, favoring renal excretion. **Estrogen** formulations that are administered by nonoral routes are not subject to first-pass metabolism, but they still undergo significant hepatic uptake, metabolism, and enterohepatic recycling.

Onset, Peak, and Duration

Naturally occurring estradiol levels vary during the menstrual cycle. Supplemental **estrogen** has a rapid onset of action ranging from less than an hour to 3 hours, depending on route of administration. Peak concentrations occur within the first days of use, and patients generally report symptoms improvement within the first few days of therapy. Duration of action depends on the route of delivery, and can range from several hours to a few days. The majority of patients report symptoms of **estrogen** deficiency after missing several days of therapy. Table 22–5 presents the pharmacokinetics of **estrogens**.

Pharmacotherapeutics

Estrogens have been synthesized for several decades and used in the primary care setting for replacement after oophorectomy and in natural menopause for treatment of hot flashes, vaginal atrophy, and irregular menstrual bleeding. The first **oral contraceptive** pills contained only **progesterone**. However, these early **progesterone**-only pills were associated with significant breakthrough bleeding. To combat that problem, **estrogen** was added to contraceptive pills in the 1960s. These early combined **progesterone/estrogen** pills used much higher doses of **estrogen** than is currently used in combined contraceptive pills. The dose of **estrogen** needed for contraception is higher than the dosage needed for replacement therapy. The potency ratio of replacement **estrogens** to

Table 22–5 ▶ **Pharmacokinetics: Estrogens and Antiestrogens**

Drug	Site of Metabolism	Active Metabolism	Half-Life (in hours by formulation and metabolites in individuals with normal renal function)	Elimination
Estrogens				
Ethinyl estradiol	Liver	Estradiol Estrone	1–2 4–18	Urine Feces
Conjugated estrogens	Liver	Estradiol Estrone	1–2 4–18	Urine
Estradiol transdermal system	Skin/Liver	Estrone	1–4 4–18 estrone	Urine
Estradiol vaginal ring	Vagina/Liver	Estrone	1–2	Unchanged: NA
Antiestrogens				
Clomiphene	NA	NA	5–7 d	42.4% feces; 7.8% in urine
Danazol	Liver	NA	24	NA
Tamoxifen	Liver	*N*-desmethyl-tamoxifen	5–7 d 14 d (metabolite)	Primarily in feces
Raloxifene	Liver		32.5	Primarily in feces

NA = not available.

contraception **estrogens** is approximately 1:10. Chapter 38 goes into greater detail about replacement **estrogens**, and Chapter 31 deals with **estrogen** use as a contraceptive. Many nurse practitioners commonly prescribe **oral contraceptives** for a noncontraceptive use in the treatment of dysmenorrhea, cycle control, and acne management, and for other secondary benefits. **Oral contraceptives** may be also prescribed to treat amenorrhea and hirsutism associated with polycystic ovary disease.

Precautions and Contraindications

There are absolute and relative contraindications that clinicians must consider when initiating **estrogen** therapy. Absolute contraindications include: current or prior history of an estrogen dependant cancer, current pregnancy, undiagnosed dysfunctional uterine bleeding, deep vein thromboembolism, arterial thromboemboli within the prior year, clotting disorders, and severe hepatic disease. Relative contraindications require added discussion with patients regarding the risk of **estrogen** therapy and its perceived benefits. Relative contraindications include cardiovascular disease, uncontrolled hypertension, diabetes mellitus, gallbladder disease, obesity, endometriosis, seizure disorder, and migraine. Women who experience migraine with aura are at increased risk for stoke and should not be prescribed **estrogen.** Women with an intact uterus should not be prescribed unopposed **estrogen** because of the risk of endometrial hyperplasia and endometrial cancer.

Estrogens have been implicated in the risk of endometrial cancer. The rates have increased dramatically since 1969 as the dose of **estrogen** for both contraception and replacement has significantly decreased. At the same time, the survival rate of woman with endometrial cancers has been higher in **estrogen** users than in those who do not use **estrogen**—perhaps in part due to early detection, as women on **estrogen** are required to have routine follow-up care. "Natural" and synthetic **estrogens** have the same risks for users. The absolute and relative contraindications for **estrogen** use are looked at in more detail in Chapters 31 and 38, with special emphasis on the most current clinical trials such as the Women's Health Initiative (WHI). The WHI findings have had a considerable impact on the prescribing patterns of clinicians and the perception of hormone therapy by the public. It is critical that prescribers understand the current state of the literature and can adequately evaluate the risks versus the benefits of **estrogen**-containing therapies, and partner with patients to determine the best course of treatment.

Although it was thought that **estrogen replacement therapy** (ERT) and **estrogen plus progestin therapy** (HRT) would provide some protection against coronary heart disease (CHD), the results of several trials from the PEPI trials (Writing Group of the PEPI Trial, 1996) to the WHI (Writing Group for the Women's Health Initiative Investigators, 2002) have shown that not only does **HRT** not provide protection, it actually may cause some increase in morbidity and mortality related to CHD. Women in the ERT-only arm of the trials tended to show no change in CHD. The WHI study revealed a higher incidence of CHD, stoke, and thromboemboli in women taking **HRT** therapy. The **estrogen**-only arm of the WHI was halted early due to increased stroke risk in women on estrogen alone.

Increased risk for thromboembolic events has been a long-standing concern related to **hormone replacement**, whether **estrogen** alone or in combination with **progestins.** The WHI found significantly increased risk for stroke in postmenopausal women on both **ERT** and **HRT.** For **HRT**, the risk was apparent in each decade of age, but for **ERT** the risk appeared to emerge after age 60 years (Langer, 2005). The risk for venous thromboembolic disease, including pulmonary embolism, was doubled in women in the **HRT** arm, with no difference based on age. There was a nonsignificant increase by about one-third with **ERT** alone (Anderson et al, 2004). There is some evidence to suggest that the timing of initiation of **ERT** and **HRT** may play a role in the CHD and atherosclerosis. The highest risk for cardiovascular events occurs within the first year of therapy.

Several design limitations have been identified in the WHI trial that deserve consideration when prescribing **ERT** and **HRT.** The majority of women in the WHI study were older (mean age of 63 yr) and had been menopausal for almost a decade, were not experiencing menopausal symptoms, and many of the participants had comorbidities of obesity and cardiovascular disease. Findings from the Women's HOPE (Health, Osteoporosis, Progestin, Estrogen) study, along with age-adjusted meta-analysis, suggest that lower doses of **estrogen** and **progesterone** may not raise the risk of CVD, and that women who initiate treatment at the time of menopause may not be at as great a risk for heart disease–related complications as women who started HRT at an older age (greater than age 65 years) and more distant from menopause (greater than 10 years) (Warren, 2010).

Estrogens are Pregnancy Category X. Use of **estrogens** during pregnancy is contraindicated because of the high rate of teratogenicity in male and female offspring. In the past, **estrogens** were used empirically to treat women who habitually aborted. However, research has shown there is no benefit in using **estrogens** for preventing miscarriages and there are risks to the developing fetus.

These precautions for any therapy that contains **estrogen** are the same regardless of the indication. The exception is that **ethinyl estradiol** is contraindicated in patients who smoke and are older than 35 years, but smoking patients may use postmenopausal **hormone replacement therapy** (ERT/HRT). The interaction of **estrogens** and smoking showing dose-related morbidity and mortality has been well documented. However, all women on **estrogen** products should be counseled on smoking cessation.

Adverse Drug Reactions

Most of the adverse reactions to **estrogens** are dose related. As a result, the majority of adverse effects are seen in patients using **oral contraceptives.** Some of the most concerning adverse reactions with **estrogen** are cardiovascular and hematological—myocardial infarction, hypertension, alteration in clotting factors, and thromboembolism. Unopposed **estrogen** use in women with an intact uterus increases the risk of abnormal uterine bleeding, endometrial hyperplasia, and gynecological cancers, and should not be prescribed. Women using **estrogen** therapy need adequate screening for risks that may predispose them to greater risk of adverse events, and should receive education on the risks and possible warning symptoms associated with these events. Additional adverse reactions are discussed in further detail in subsequent chapters. See Chapter 31 for managing migraine headaches, mood changes, eye discomfort, skin pigmentation, breast changes, weight gain, change in vaginal secretion, and leg discomforts. The adverse reactions more common with menopausal **estrogens** are elevation of systemic blood pressure, gall bladder disease, and irregular bleeding. See Chapter 38 for managing the undesirable adverse effects of menopausal **estrogens.** Women who have estrogen-dependent tumors may have worsening of their cancer while on any form of **estrogen** therapy; therefore, it is not advised for women with a current cancer or a history of estrogen-dependent cancer to use **estrogen** therapies.

Drug Interactions

Estrogens interfere with laboratory measurements of endocrine and liver function tests and thyroid-binding globulin. In addition, the prothrombin time and factors VII, VIII, IX, and X show increased levels in patients taking **estrogens** at the time of testing. Women may experience impaired glucose tolerance and increased triglycerides when oral **estrogens** are administered. The most common drug interactions are with **anticoagulants, tricyclic antidepressants, barbiturates, antituberculosis drugs, corticosteroids, seizure control medication,** and drugs for spasticity. Table 22–6 presents drug interactions.

Clinical Use and Dosing

Relief of Perimenopausal and Postmenopausal Symptoms

Relief of menopausal vasomotor symptoms can be dramatic after the initiation of hormonal therapy. The lowest effective dose of **estrogen** should be used for the shortest duration possible. **Estrogen** is available in various

Table 22–6 ■ **Common Drug Interactions: Estrogens and Antiestrogens**

Drug	Interacting Drug	Possible Effect	Implications
Estrogens			
Estrogens	Oral anticoagulants	Estrogens increase the risk of thromboembolitic events	The use of estrogen-containing products is contraindicated in individuals at high risk for coagulopathy
	Fosamprenavir	Alter efficacy of both agents; alter hepatic metabolism	Combination is contraindicated. Use nonhormonal contraception
	Benzodiazepines, rifampin	Barbiturates, rifampin, and other agents that induce hepatic microsomal enzymes with concomitant estrogens may produce lower estrogen levels than expected	Use a backup birth control method
	Corticosteroids	Estrogen coadministration may reduce the clearance and increase the elimination half-life of corticosteroids	It may be necessary to lower steroid dosage if there is an increase in adverse effects
	Dantrolene	Hepatotoxicity occurred more often in women >35 yr receiving dantrolene and estrogen	Check liver function tests after first 4 wk of therapy in women >35 yr
	Anticonvulsants	Breakthrough bleeding, spotting, and pregnancy have resulted when these medications were used concurrently. A loss of seizure control has also been suggested and may be due to fluid retention	Check blood levels of seizure medications after first 2 wk of therapy. Use a backup birth control method or switch to an IUD is preferred.

Continued

Table 22–6 ■ **Common Drug Interactions: Estrogens and Antiestrogens—cont'd**

Drug	Interacting Drug	Possible Effect	Implications
Antiestrogens			
Clomiphene	Bromsulphalein (BSP) lab studies	BSP retention of >5% reported in 10%–20% of patients; retention is usually minimal but elevated during prolonged clomiphene administration or with apparently unrelated liver disease. In some, preexisting BSP retention decreased even though clomiphene was continued. Other liver function tests usually normal	Use other liver function tests when patient is taking clomiphene
Danazol	Insulin and diabetic agents	Insulin requirements may increase in patients with diabetes; abnormal glucose tolerance tests may be seen	More frequent glucose monitoring; possible decreased dosing of anti-diabetic agents
	Warfarin	Prolongation of PT reported with concomitant use	Measure PT more frequently
	Amiodarone, clarithromycins, erythromycins	QT prolongation, cardiac arrhythmias	Avoid combination/select alternative agents
	Statin agents	Inhibits metabolism of statin agent, increases risk rhabdomyolysis	Avoid combination/select alternative agents
Tamoxifen	Anticoagulants	Hypoprothrombinemic effect may be increased by concurrent tamoxifen administration	Monitor PT more frequently. Consider a nonhormonal, non-SERM alternative
	Medications that utilize the CYPP450 3A4, 2C9, 2D6 pathways	Altered metabolism	Evaluate each agent individually
	Lab studies	T_4 elevations occurred in a few postmenopausal patients but not accompanied by clinical hyperthyroidism	Measure TSH instead of T_4
Raloxifene	Bile acid sequestrants (Cholestyramine)	Raloxifene absorption and enterohepatic cycling reduced 60%;	Avoid combination. Consider statins to decrease cholesterol
	Warfarin	In single-dose studies, 10% decreases in PT have been observed	Monitor PT closely, or consider alternative agent to raloxifene
	Thyroid agents	Combination may cause hypothyroidism	Separate dosing by at least 12 hours; closely monitor TSH at initiation of therapy—may require increased dose of thyroid hormones while using raloxifene

formulations, including estrogens derived from animal, plant, and synthetic sources. For women who have no objections to **estrogens** from animal sources, **conjugated equine estrogen (Premarin)** is available in doses from 0.3 mg to 2.5 mg. Suppression of hot flashes has been shown to be best at 0.625 mg, followed by 0.45 mg and 0.3 mg/day (Liu, 2004). Studies reported by Liu indicate that vasomotor symptoms begin to decrease by the second week of therapy and reach maximal effect by the eighth week of therapy. Dosage increases should not occur, however, until at least a 6- to 8-week interval to give the drug time to reach maximal effect at that dose.

Micronized estradiol (Estrace, Gynodiol) is the only bioidentical **estrogen**-alone product that is available in pill form. It is available in 0.5 mg to 2 mg doses. Suppression is found at 1-mg and 2-mg doses. The typical regimen is 1 mg taken daily. The lower dose (0.5 mg) has been used for osteoporosis prevention and is less useful for vasomotor symptom relief. Other agents, primarily **bisphosphonates**, should be considered if treatment of osteoporosis is the primary goal of therapy.

For women who prefer **estrogens** derived from plant sources, **estrone**-based drugs are available. **Synthetic conjugated estrogen-A (Cenestin)** is available in doses from 0.3 mg to 1.25 mg. Studies reported by Liu (2004) found that the majority (77%) of women randomized to **Cenestin** required a total daily dose of 1.25 mg to relieve vasomotor symptoms, whereas the remaining 23 percent required 0.625 mg or less. By week 8, the vasomotor symptoms were significantly decreased. **Synthetic conjugated estrogen-B (Enjuvia)** is available in doses of 0.3 mg to 1.25 mg, with the lower dose producing relief in many women. **Estropipate (Ogen, Ortho-EST)** is also derived from plant sources and available in 0.75-mg to 6-mg tablets. Following the rule to use the lowest dose to control symptoms, the dosing regimen should start at 0.75 mg.

Findings from the WHI, Women's HOPE study, and multiple meta-analyses suggest that therapy to treat the vasomotor symptoms associated with menopause at the onset of menopause should be done in an effort to reduce adverse cardiovascular events (Warren, 2010). When initiating therapy, begin with lowest starting dose of the selected **estrogen** product. Clinicians may wish to initiate an even slower taper or defer to a specialist for those women who have relative contraindications or precautions to **estrogen** therapy and who still elect to proceed with **estrogen** therapy. One proposed example is to use small doses (0.3 mg) of **conjugated estrogens** every other day for 2 months. Then, gradually increase the **estrogens** to daily use for another 2 months. If symptoms such as bleeding or breast pain do not occur, increase the **estrogen** up to 0.625 mg daily. Some women may need only the lower **estrogen** dosages to adequately control their symptoms as long as they have an adequate diet. Remember, **estrogen** must be partnered with **progesterone** to prevent endometrial hyperplasia and cancer in women with an intact uterus. ERT and HRT should be reevaluated on an annual basis, with the goal of utilizing therapy for 5 or less years.

Many of these drugs are available in transdermal systems. Most of them are indicated for the dual management of vasomotor and urogenital symptoms.

Complementary and alternative therapies include **phytoestrogens**, botanicals, and herbs. These alternatives have varying degrees of effectiveness and research support. They are discussed in some depth in Chapter 38.

Prevention and Management of Vulvovaginal Atrophy and Dryness

Decline in estrogen causes the vaginal mucosa and vulvar skin to become thin and atrophic. The result is discomfort, itching, dyspareunia, and increased cases of vaginitis. Low-dose oral ERT with **estrogen** from both plant and animal sources has been shown to decrease vaginal pH, thus reducing vaginal infections. It also thickens and revascularizes the vaginal epithelium, increases the number of superficial cells, and reverses vaginal atrophy (Liu, 2004). **Vaginal estrogen** also produces these positive effects and the changes begin in as short a time frame as 2 weeks. Topical creams and intravaginal delivery of **estrogen** are equally as efficacious as oral agents in the management of vulvovaginal symptoms.

Reduced Risk for Colon Cancer

Colorectal cancer is the third most common cancer in women in the United States and the third most common cause of cancer death in women (Thorneycroft, 2004). Because this cancer is also associated with aging, it clearly is a cancer to be considered concurrently with menopause. ERT and HRT have shown to reduce the risk of colon cancer. A thorough discussion regarding the risks and benefits of ERT and HRT is needed for patients to make informed decisions about ERT and HRT. Currently, the use of **estrogen**-containing products for colon cancer risk reduction alone is not indicated.

Prevention and Treatment of Osteoporosis

Estrogen is associated with bone formation and has osteoprotective benefits. Until recently, **estrogen** had been the gold standard for both prevention and treatment of osteoporosis. **Estrogens** prevent osteoporosis by reducing the bone-resorbing action of PTH. Estrogen receptors have been found in bone, which validates the hypothesis that estrogen may have direct effects on bone remodeling. Studies have shown that there is a direct correlation between rate of bone loss in menopausal women and estradiol levels (Fitzpatrick, 2004). Bone resorption has also been shown to be highest in the first postmenopausal year. Bone density declines between 1 and 4 percent in the first several years after menopause, and then stabilizes to about 1 percent per year. Women in the immediate postmenopausal years are the ones who are most in need of protection from osteoporosis.

Chapter 38 looks at the use of **estrogen** alone and in combination with other drugs in the treatment of osteoporosis. ERT and HRT use can significantly slow the natural progression of bone loss in postmenopausal women. Numerous studies have shown significant improvement in bond mineral density (BMD) and the reduction of hip and vertebral fractures in women using ERT and HRT. However, current practice trends are leaning away from selecting ERT and HRT exclusively for the prevention of osteoporosis. The WHI findings that ERT and HRT raised the risk for coronary events, stroke, pulmonary emboli, and breast cancer in women who took a combination of **estrogen** and **progesterone** have led leading national women's health organizations, including the FDA and U.S. Preventative Services Task Force, to encourage clinicians to consider alternative options for osteoporosis prevention and treatment when women are not experiencing moderate to severe menopausal symptoms. Balancing the risks and benefits of **estrogen** therapy and the availability of other drugs to prevent and treat osteoporosis should be discussed with women, who can then make an intelligent decision about whether to use **estrogen.** Dosing is the same for osteoporosis as recommendations for HRT and ERT dosing for menopausal symptoms. Long-term efficacy of taking **estrogen** in lower doses for prevention of osteoporosis remains unknown at this time.

Contraception

There are currently two formulations of **estrogen** available in combination **contraceptive** preparations, **ethinyl estradiol** (EE) and **mestranol. Mestranol** is the weaker of the two preparations, and must be metabolized into EE before it is able to bind with **estrogen** receptors. Fifty mcg of **mestranol** is equivalent to 35 mcg of EE. EE is the **estrogen** used in the vast majority of hormonal **contraceptive** formulations in wide use today. Most preparations used today contain between 20 and 35 mcg of EE. The **estrogen** component of **hormonal contraception** improves efficacy by suppressing FSH release, and therefore development of a dominant follicle. **Estrogen** also adds to cycle control, decreasing irregular bleeding patterns commonly found with **progestin**-only methods.

Combined oral contraceptives come in three main formulations. The most common formulation is a monophasic **combined oral contraceptive** (COC) that contains the same dose of hormone in each active pill. Biphasic pills alter the hormone dose in the middle of the cycle, and triphasic pills alter the **estrogen** dose, the **progesterone** dose, or both each week during a 28-day-dose pack. Additionally, there are **progesterone**-only contraceptives available that are discussed later in this chapter. Table 31–2 in Chapter 31 summarizes the brand-name and synthetic hormone formulas currently available. Rather than repeat this extensive list, the reader is referred to that table.

The theoretical effectiveness of prevention of pregnancy with COCs is 99 percent or greater. Patients who receive education on the proper use of COCs have lower discontinuation rates, and therefore fewer unwanted pregnancies. Additionally, clinicians should provide patients with information on **emergency hormonal contraception** and use a backup method such as **spermicide** and condoms. Commonly used OCs are presented in Chapter 31.

As the different COCs have similar effectiveness and are well tolerated, choosing among them may seem difficult. Although there are some advantages to selecting one type of **progesterone** option over another, for the majority of patients it is generally best to use a drug that has the lowest **estrogen** dose while still offering cycle control. Prescribers need to be familiar with the prescribing details of at least one preparation that does not contain **estrogen:** an "ultralow dose" or 20-mcg EE pill (e.g., for women over 35 yr or those who smoke more than 15 cigarettes/d), a **monophasic** COC, a **multiphasic** COC, and a nondaily administration method for women who have difficulty with daily regimens. Details on selecting among these options and a discussion of drug and patient variables to consider are presented in detail in Chapter 31.

Off-Labeled Uses

COCs have been used to treat conditions for which a formal FDA approval has not been awarded. Many of these off-labeled uses have considerable literature and research to support clinical use, and some pharmaceutical companies have sought FDA approval for specific agents for marketing purposes (such as acne management). Prescribers must disclose to patients when agents are being used for off-labeled purposes, and a thorough review of the risks and benefits and informed consent obtained. Table 22–7 presents the dosage schedule of **estrogens** other than those used for **contraception.**

Rational Drug Selection

Short Acting Versus Long Acting

Most women receive oral daily doses of **estrogen.** In this manner, a consistent and expected level is maintained. Some women may have problems remembering or difficulty in swallowing the oral form, and transdermal or parenteral administration is possible. Giving injections every 3 to 4 weeks is uncomfortable, and the daily levels may vary, depending on the circulation in the muscle into which the dose is injected.

Table 22–7 ◉ **Dosage Schedule: Estrogens and Antiestrogens**

Drug	Indication	Dosage
Estrogens		
Ethinyl estradiol	Moderate to severe vasomotor symptoms associated with menopause	0.02–0.1 mg/d
	Female hypogonadism	0.05 mg 1–3 times/d for first 2 wk of theoretical menstrual cycle; follow with progestin during last half of cycle
	Breast cancer (female)	1 mg 3 times/d chronically (palliation—BY SPECIALIST ONLY)
	Prostate cancer	0.15–2 mg/d chronically (palliation—BY SPECIALIST ONLY)

Table 22–7 ◉ **Dosage Schedule: Estrogens and Antiestrogens—cont'd**

Drug	Indication	Dosage
Conjugated estrogens	Moderate to severe vasomotor symptoms associated with menopause	0.3–1.25 mg/d cyclically
	Atrophic conditions caused by deficient endogenous estrogen production such as atrophic vaginitis and kraurosis vulvae	0.3–1.25 mg or more daily cyclically
	Female hypogonadism	2.5–7.5 mg daily, in divided doses for 20 d, followed by rest period of 10 d
	Female castration; primary ovarian failure	1.25 mg/d
	Osteoporosis	0.625 mg/d cyclically
	Mammary carcinoma (palliation)	10 mg 3 times/d for at least 3 mo
Estradiol transdermal system	Moderate to severe vasomotor symptoms associated with menopause; female hypogonadism; female castration; primary ovarian failure; atrophic conditions caused by deficient endogenous estrogen production such as atrophic vaginitis and kraurosis vulvae; prevention of osteoporosis/loss of bone mass	Menopause: start 0.025 or 0.05 mg applied twice weekly; adjust dose as necessary to control symptoms; attempt to taper or discontinue at 3- to 6-mo intervals; apply on clean, dry area on trunk of body but not breasts
Estradiol vaginal ring	Atrophic vaginitis	Insert ring as deeply as possible in upper third of vaginal vault; remains in place for 3 mo
Estradiol	Moderate to severe vasomotor symptoms associated with menopause; female hypogonadism; female castration; primary ovarian failure; atrophic conditions caused by deficient endogenous estrogen production, such as atrophic vaginitis and kraurosis vulvae; prevention of osteoporosis/loss of bone mass	Menopause symptoms: 0.05–2 mg/d Osteoporosis prevention: 0.5 mg/d cyclically
	Prostate cancer (specialty management)	1–2 mg 3 times/d
	Breast cancer (inoperable) (specialty management)	10 mg 3 times/d for at least 3 mo
Antiestrogens		
Clomiphene	Treatment of ovulary failure in patients desiring pregnancy whose partners are potent and fertile	First course: 50 mg/d for 5 d
	Off-labeled uses: Treatment of male infertility; however, use is controversial and further study is needed	50–400 mg/d for 2–12 mo
Danazol	Endometriosis	100–200 mg/d bid; consider downward titration
	Fibrotic breast disease	50–200 mg/d bid
	Hereditary angioedema	Starting dose: 200 mg 2–3 times/d; after favorable response, decrease dose by 50% or less at 1- to 3-mo intervals
	Off-labeled uses: precocious puberty, gynecomastia, menorrhagia	
Tamoxifen	Breast cancer (adjuvant therapy; advanced disease therapy) Off-labeled use: mastalgia, preventive therapy in high-risk breast cancer.	20–40 mg twice daily (a.m. and p.m.) or 20 mg daily; some studies have used dosages of 10 mg 2–3 times/d for 2 yr and 10 mg twice daily for 5 yr; the reduction in recurrence and mortality was greater in those studies that used the drug for 2 yr than in those that used it for <2 yr; there was no indication that doses >20 mg/d were more effective; optimal duration of adjuvant therapy unknown
Raloxifene	Prevention of osteoporosis in postmenopausal women	60 mg daily, which may be administered any time of the day without regard to meals

Formulation

Oral formulations of **estrogen** are the most commonly selected formulation by patients and prescribers, but there may be reasons for selecting another formulation. Most **estrogens** are available in transdermal formulation. The major advantage of transdermal formulations is their once- or twice-weekly application. A disadvantage is the incidence of skin irritation that occurs in 20 to 40 percent of users (Wysocki & Alexander, 2005). Vaginal instillation is possible for patients unable to tolerate oral formulations or for severe urethral and urogenital atrophy, as in vulvar dystrophies and dyspareunia. Low-dose **vaginal estrogens** (with the ring or cream) are not associated with as much risk of endometrial hyperplasia as are the oral forms. In addition, use of the **estradiol**-releasing vaginal ring has a positive effect on urethral and vaginal atrophy symptoms. **Estrace** has a bioidentical vaginal cream approved for the treatment of vaginal and urinary symptoms. The usual doses for all the creams include nightly application. Topical application with vaginal rings and vaginal tablets may be preferred by patients, as these may be perceived as easier to administer and less "messy" than the creams. The differences between the oral versus topical formulations are 2-fold: (1) The oral formulations retain the positive effects of ERT that accrue because of liver metabolism and the topical formulations lose this benefit; and (2) the total amount of **estrogen** to which the body is exposed is less with the topical formulations, which may be a consideration for women who have risk factor concerns with ERT. A dose of 25 mcg per day of **estradiol** administered vaginally in contrast to estrogen creams does not significantly raise blood levels of **estrogen**, especially if vaginal cornification has already taken place. Studies reported by Thorneycroft (2004) found no evidence of increased risk of CHD, breast cancer, or endometrial cancer with the use of vaginal ERT. There was a slight increase in endometrial hyperplasia and it might be prudent to withdraw patients periodically from vaginal ERT treatment.

Cost

Pricing on oral **estrogen** and **estrogen**-combination products can vary significantly. As oral preparations have been around the longest, several generic versions are available and are the least expensive. Several vaginal creams now have generic versions available. The latest products and brand-name products tend to be the most expensive. Transdermal preparations, the vaginal ring, and prepackaged punch-out cards or dial packs for convenience are generally priced higher. Cost is may be a determining factor in product selection for women on Medicare, those who have fixed incomes, or those who have multiple medications to purchase.

Route of Administration

As previously discussed, route of administration affects hepatic metabolism of **estrogen** and can reduce potential side effects and risks. Beyond these considerations, patient preference and affordability determine route selection. Oral formulations are typically preferred by patients and are easy for most patients to administer at mealtime or bedtime. A small percentage of women experience elevated triglycerides with oral **estrogens**, and these patients can avoid liver metabolism of the medication through transdermal absorption. Transdermal patches allow patients the freedom of less frequent dosing, and may be preferred by caregivers who assist patients with limited dexterity and an inability to swallow. Vaginal application reduces liver metabolism but is absorbed less after severe vaginal atrophy is treated. Estrogen levels are not as high after the first 6 months of therapy. As some older women lack the finger dexterity to fill an applicator and instill the cream, clinicians should assess the ability of patients to use this route of administration. Table 22–8 presents the available dosage forms of **estrogen**.

Monitoring

Oral contraception, ERT and HRT are chronic medications that are taken for months or years. If the patient has a coexisting medical condition, such as one of those listed in Chapters 31 and 38, monitoring of adverse effects is necessary. Schedule 1-month, 3-month, 6-month, or annual evaluation appointments, depending on the degree of illness or the severity of symptoms. Patient education regarding the symptoms and reporting of potentially worrisome adverse effects are necessary at the institution of therapy. Drawing baseline blood tests including a lipid panel and ordering mammograms prior to prescribing ERT or HRT are recommended. Additionally, women

Table 22–8 ◆ **Available Dosage Forms: Estrogen and Antiestrogens**

Drug	Dosage Form	How Supplied (Note: clinicians can prescribe smaller quantities)	Cost
Estrogens, Oral			
CONJUGATED ESTROGENS			
(Premarin)	Tablets: 0.3 mg	In bottles of 100, 1,000 tablets	$56.99/30
	0.45 mg	In bottles of 100 and UD 100 tablets	$51.99/30
	0.625 mg	In bottles of 1,000 and UD 100 tablets	$50.97/30
	0.9 mg	In bottle of 100 tablets	$49.99/30
	1.25 mg	In bottles of 100, 1,000 tablets	$50.00/30

Table 22–8 ◆ **Available Dosage Forms: Estrogen and Antiestrogens—cont'd**

Drug	Dosage Form	How Supplied (Note: clinicians can prescribe smaller quantities)	Cost
(Cenestin)	Tablets: 0.3 mg, 0.45 mg	In bottles of 30, 100, 1,000 tablets	Flat priced across all strengths $58.17/30
	0.625 mg	In bottles of 30, 100, 1,000 tablets	
	0.9 mg	In bottles of 30, 100, 1,000 tablets	
	1.25 mg	In bottles of 30, 100, 1,000 tablets	
Enjuvia	Tablets: 0.3 mg, 0.45 mg, 0.625 mg, 1.25 mg	In bottles of 30 tablets	$54.02 for 30 tabs of 0.3 mg Flat prices for other doses at $160.91 for 100 tabs
Esterified Estrogens			
(Menest)	Tablets: 0.3 mg	In bottles of 100 tablets	$27.99/30
	0.625 mg	In bottles of 100 tablets	$35.99/30
	1.25 mg	In bottles of 100 tablets	$41.15/30
	2.5 mg	In bottles of 50 tablets	$61.72/30
Estropipate (Piperazine Estrone Sulfate)			
(Ogen)	Tablets:	In bottles of 30, 100, 500 tablets	
	0.7 mg		$39.99/30
	1.5 mg		$52.99/30
	3 mg		$82.99/30
Estradiol			
(Femtrace [F] is estradiol acetate)	Tablets:	In bottles of 100 tablets	
	0.45 mg		$165.59/100
	0.9 mg		$160.99/100
	1.8 mg		$201.41/100
(Estrace [E], Gynodiol [Gyn], and the generic form are micronized estradiol)	Tablets: 0.5 mg (G)	In bottles of 100 tablets	$9.99/100
	0.5 mg (E)	In bottles of 100 tablets	$57.49/100
	0.5 mg (Gyn)	In bottles of 30, 100 tablets	
	0.9 (F)	In bottles of 100 tablets	
	1 mg (G)	In bottles of 100, 500 tablets	$18.99/100
	1 mg (E)	In bottles of 100, 500 tablets	$59.66/100
	1 mg (Gyn)	In bottles of 30, 100 tablets	
	1.5 mg (Gyn)	In bottles of 30, 100 tablets	$22.99/100
	1.8 mg (F)	In bottles of 100 tablets	
	2 mg (G)	In bottles of 100, 500 tablets	$15.99/100
	2 mg (E)	In bottles of 100, 500 tablets	$68.99/100
	2 mg (Gyn)	In bottles of 30, 100 tablets	
Estrogens, Topical			
Estradiol Transdermal (Release Rate in mg/24 h)			
(Menostar)	0.014	In 4	$60.99/4
(Alora)	0.025	In calendar packs (8 systems)	
	0.05	In calendar packs (8 systems)	$49.67/8
	0.075	In calendar packs (8 systems)	$44.15/8
	0.1	In calendar packs (8 systems)	$49.68/8

Continued

Table 22–8 ◆ **Available Dosage Forms: Estrogen and Antiestrogens—cont'd**

Drug	Dosage Form	How Supplied (Note: clinicians can prescribe smaller quantities)	Cost
(Climara)	0.025	In 4	Flat pricing for all strengths $57.55/ box of 4
	0.0375	In 4	
	0.05	In 4	
	0.6	In 4	
	0.075	In 4	
	0.1	In 4	
(Esclim)	0.025	In patient packs (8 systems)	
	0.0375	In patient packs (8 systems)	
	0.05	In patient packs (8 systems)	
	0.075	In patient packs (8 systems)	
	0.1	In patient packs (8 systems)	
(Vivelle and Vivelle-Dot)	0.025	In calendar packs (8 systems)	$51.99/8 patches
	0.0375	In calendar packs (8 systems)	$51.99/8 patches
	0.05	In calendar packs (8 systems)	$54.94/8 patches
	0.075	In calendar packs (8 systems)	$54.94/8 patches
	0.1	In calendar packs (8 systems)	$54.94/8 patches
(Estradiol transdermal system)	0.05	In 4	
	0.1	In 4	
(Estraderm)	0.05	In calendar packs (8 and 24 systems)	$54.99/8 patches
	0.1	In calendar packs (8 and 24 systems)	$54.99/8 patches
Emulsion (Estrasorb)	2.5 mg	In 1.74-g pouches	$16.95/6 packets
Gel (Estrogel)	0.75 mg estradiol	In 1.25-g UD; 80-g tubes, 93-g pumps	$68.94/50 grams
Estrogens, Injectable			
Estradiol Valerate In Oil			
(Delestrogen)	10 mg/mL;	In 5-mL multidose vials	$79.99/vial
	20 mg/mL;		$111.99/vial
	40 mg/mL		$177.99/vial
Estradiol Cypionate In Oil			
(Depo-Estradiol)	5 mg/mL	In 5-mL vials	$45.99/vial
Estrogens, Vaginal			
(Vagifem [V]; Estrace [E]; Premarin [P]; Ogen [O]; Estring [ES]; Femring [FE])	Tablets, vaginal: 2.5 mcg estradiol (V)	In bottles of 8, 18 tablets	$44.92/8; $90.46 per 18
	Cream: 0.1 mg estradiol (E) 0.625 mg conjugated estrogen (P) 1.5 mg estropipate (O)		$108.49/42.5 g
	Ring: 2 mg estradiol (ES)		$154.06/unit
	0.05 mg/d estradiol acetate (FE)		$156.19/unit
	0.1 mg/d estradiol acetate0 (FE)		$108.56/unit
Antiestrogens			
Clomiphene (Clomid [C], Milophene [M], Serophene [S])	Tablets: 50 mg (G)	In bottles of 10, 30 tablets	$84.99/30
	(C), (M), (S)	In bottles of 30 tablets	$75.94 [C]/5 $55.38 [S]/5
Danazol	Tablets: 50 mg,	In bottles of 100 tablets	$52.99/30
	100 mg		$68.60/30
	200 mg		$110.76/30

Table 22–8 ◆ **Available Dosage Forms: Estrogen and Antiestrogens—cont'd**

Drug	Dosage Form	How Supplied (Note: clinicians can prescribe smaller quantities)	Cost
Raloxifene (Evista)	Tablets: 60 mg	In UD30, 100, 2,000 tablets	$107.89/30
Tamoxifen (Nolvadex)	Tablets: 10 mg (G),	In bottles of 60, 180, 500, 1,000, and UD 100 tablets	
	10 mg (N)	In bottles of 60	
	20 mg (G),	In bottles of 30, 90, 100, 500, 1,000, and UD 100 tablets	$21.99/30
	20 mg (N)	In bottles of 30 tablets	

G = generic.

should have annual mammograms, pelvic evaluations, and cardiovascular assessments while on ERT or HRT. Patients with diabetes need to perform daily blood glucose measurements until stable on ERT or HRT, as adjustment to diabetes agents may be needed. Patients with hypertension need monthly blood pressure readings. Patients with seizure disorders will need initial increased frequency of laboratory monitoring of seizure medications and then every 6 months, as **estrogen** therapy may alter drug metabolism, affecting therapeutic levels of **antiepileptic** medications.

Patient Education

Administration

Patients taking **oral hormonal contraceptives** and HRT need to take the drug daily at about the same time to avoid breakthrough bleeding. Specific patient education regarding anticipated transient and nuisance side effects at the time of initiating therapy will improve adherence to therapy. Women may experience transient adverse effects such as mild nausea and breast tenderness or midcycle spotting during the first 2 months of therapy. Sometimes taking the medication at bedtime solves the nausea problem. Advise the patient to seek follow-up to discuss alternatives to oral therapy if nausea or vomiting or other issues make oral therapy unsuccessful. Also advise the patient to rotate the application sites for transdermal patches and to avoid applying patches to breast tissue.

Devices to improve adherence to a daily regimen include Mediset boxes and ways of making the drug part of the daily routine. For example, some women find it easier to put the **birth control** packet by their toothbrush or alarm clock to avoid forgetting the medication.

Adverse Reactions

The breasts, uterus, and vagina are more obvious organs dependent on **estrogen**. Although adverse drug reactions were discussed earlier in this section, clinicians need to communicate the following information to patients who are initiating or renewing **estrogen**-containing prescriptions. Leg pain, visual disturbances, and severe headache could herald thromboembolic phenomena that could be life threatening. Patients who smoke and those who are diabetic are at increased risk for this type of complication. Abnormal bleeding patterns or genital pain needs to be reported in all age groups. In younger women who experience irregular bleeding, infection or pregnancy is suspected, but bleeding in a postmenopausal woman may be the first symptom of uterine or ovarian cancer. Dysfunctional uterine bleeding in any perimenopausal or postmenopausal woman should be considered to be cancer until proved otherwise, and the appropriate steps should be taken to determine the presence or absence of cancer.

Lifestyle Management

Smoking increases the risk of thrombolytic events in patients taking **estrogen**. The use of **estrogen**-containing **contraception** in women who smoke and are over the age of 35 is contraindicated, and all patients who smoke should be counseled on the added risks associated with concurrent tobacco use and **estrogen** products. Patients who quit smoking for at least 1 year are considered nonsmokers.

Routine exercise and dietary changes have been associated with a reduction in vasomotor symptoms of menopause and reduced symptoms of dysmenorrhea.

The use of condoms and barrier devises to reduce the risk of sexually transmitted infections is also an important component of contraceptive management, and should be assessed and encouraged at prescription initiation and refill.

PROGESTERONES AND PROGESTERONE ANTAGONISTS

The **progesterones** include **progesterone** (Prometrium, Progesterone in Oil, Crinone, Prochieve), **medroxyprogesterone acetate** (Provera), **norethindrone** (Aygestin), and **megestrol acetate** (Megace). Most are used in **oral contraceptives** and for HRT. Many formulations (sometimes referred to as "generations") of **progesterone** have been developed to address issues of mood change, breakthrough bleeding, and sensitivity to progesterone agents.

Currently there are several different **androgen**-derived **progestins** available in **oral contraceptive** preparations: **norethindrone**, **norethindrone acetate**, **ethynodiol diacetate**, **norgestrel**, **desogestrel**, **levonorgestrel**, and **norgestimate**. **Norethindrone acetate** and **ethynodiol diacetate** are converted to **norethindrone** in the body. **Levonorgestrel** is the levorotatory form of **norgestrel** and its active metabolite.

Desogestrel and **norgestimate** offer a decrease in androgenicity when compared to other progesterones. **Desogestrel** undergoes conversion to its active metabolite **etonogestrel**. **Etonogestrel** is the **progestin** used in the vaginal ring. **Norelgestromin** is the primary metabolite of **norgestimate**, and is available as a contraceptive patch. Decreased androgenicity theoretically reduces adverse effects on carbohydrate and lipid metabolism found in previous formulations, as well as improves acne and hirsutism. **Medroxyprogesterone acetate** is available for injectable contraception.

Drospirenone is a **progestin** developed as a derivative of **spironolactone**. As a derivative of **spironolactone**, it has a mild diuretic effect as well as antimineralocorticoid effects. The drug has been granted FDA approval for the treatment of premenstrual syndrome and contraception when it is a component of a COC pill. **Drospirenone** may cause hyperkalemia and should be used cautiously with women who are using drugs that cause a potassium-sparing effect, such as **ACE-inhibitors**, or have underlying renal disease. Box 22–3 presents information on **progesterone antagonists**.

BOX 22–3 PROGESTERONE ANTAGONISTS

Mifepristone (Mifeprex)

Mifepristone was approved by the FDA on September 28, 2000, for termination of intrauterine pregnancy. It has a long half-life (18 h) and may prolong the follicular phase of the subsequent cycle. It is strongly bound to plasma proteins (98%). This binding is saturable and the drug has nonlinear pharmacokinetics with relation to plasma concentration and clearance. The antiprogestational activity results from competitive interaction with **progesterone** at **progesterone** receptor sites. The drug inhibits the activity of both endogenous and exogenous **progesterone.** When there is no **progesterone** to maintain a pregnancy, termination results. In 85 percent of women, **mifepristone** will act as an abortifacient when used in conjunction with **misoprostol** during the first 7 weeks of pregnancy. Women should expect to experience bleeding or spotting for an average of 9 to 16 days. Persistent heavy or moderate bleeding for more than 30 days could indicate an incomplete abortion. There are very specific requirements associated with administration of this drug, and it is best done in clinics that can meet these requirements. The drug is available only from the manufacturer and not through licensed pharmacies.

Mifepristone also exhibits antiglucocorticoid and weak antiandrogenic activity. Off-labeled uses in the treatment of endometriosis, Cushing's syndrome, and uterine leiomyomata are under study.

Pharmacodynamics

Effects of progestin on the reproductive organs include thickening of the endometrium and increasing its complexity in preparation for pregnancy; thickening of cervical mucus; thinning the vaginal mucosa; and relaxation of smooth muscles of the uterus and fallopian tube. During pregnancy, progestin maintains the thickened endometrium, relaxes myometrial muscles, thickens the myometrium for labor, is responsible for placental development, and prevents lactation until the fetus is born. In the absence of pregnancy, the reduced production of estrogen and progestin by the corpus luteum results in the shedding of endometrium to produce menstruation. Progestin is also responsible for alveolobular development of the secretory apparatus of the breast. Progestin also has actions outside the reproductive system. It stimulates lipoprotein activity and seems to favor fat deposition; increases basal insulin levels and insulin response to glucose; promotes glycogen storage in the liver; promotes ketogenesis; competes with aldosterone in the renal tubule to decrease Na+ resorption; increases body temperature; and increases ventilatory response to CO_2 resulting in a measurable decrease in $PaCO_2$. The latter occurs only during pregnancy.

Thickening of the endometrium related to estrogen stimulation is thought to increase the risk for endometrial cancer and studies have supported a direct correlation between ERT use and an increased incidence of endometrial cancer (Thorneycroft, 2004). To prevent this occurrence, **progestins** have been added to **HRT**. Concerns about HRT raised by the WHI are presented earlier in this chapter and are discussed in Chapter 38.

Pharmacokinetics

Absorption and Distribution

Progesterone is rapidly absorbed following any route of administration. Oral **progestins** are rapidly absorbed from the GI tract and quickly undergo hepatic degradation. Following IM administration, **progesterone in oil** is rapidly absorbed and undergoes hepatic metabolism. Long-acting forms can be maintained for 3 to 6 months. Gel formulation has sustained-release properties, so absorption can be lengthened to 50 hours. Subdermal implants of **progesterone** are also available. In the United States, **Implanon** is available to providers who have completed specific training on insertion. Subdermal implant **progesterone** is well absorbed through the dermis at a continuous rate. **Progesterone** binds to plasma albumin and corticosteroid-binding globulin.

Metabolism and Excretion

Oral progesterone is rapidly metabolized in the first pass through the liver. In the liver, **progesterone** is metabolized to **pregnanediol** and with the glucuronide metabolites conjugated with glucuronic acid. It is excreted in the urine. IM and implantable **progesterone** is extensively bound to serum proteins, and its metabolites are excreted 60 percent by the kidney and 10 percent through the bile and feces. The gel formulation is also eliminated through the renal route.

Onset, Peak, and Duration

Onset, peak, and duration vary based on the form of **progesterone.** After oral administration, the peak concentrations for oral **progesterone** occur after 1 to 2 hours. Half-life also varies by form of **progesterone** and can be from 4 to 40 hours. IM preparations reach peak levels by 24 hours and have a half-life of approximately 10 weeks. The liver quickly metabolizes the gel formulation, but the long absorption half-life provides the steady serum concentrations. The absorption half-life of the vaginal gel can be from 25 to 50 hours. Table 22–9 presents the pharmacokinetics of **progestins.**

Pharmacotherapeutics

Precautions and Contraindications

Patients with thromboembolic disease or a history of it should not use **progestins.** Breast cancer may be worsened under hormone influence. Patients with impaired liver function would have trouble metabolizing exogenous hormones.

Mental depression has been associated with both short-acting and long-acting **progestins.** The drug may need to be discontinued if depression recurs or occurs to a serious degree.

Fluid retention may occur. Patients with disorders that may be affected negatively by excess fluid (e.g., epilepsy, migraine, asthma, congestive heart failure, or renal dysfunction) require careful observation.

A decrease in glucose tolerance has been observed in a small percentage of patients on **estrogen-progestin** combination drugs. Diabetic patients should increase their glucose monitoring when receiving **progestin** therapy.

Progesterone is Pregnancy Category D and **norethindrone acetate** is Pregnancy Category X. **Progesterone gel** is used to support embryo implantation and maintain pregnancies as part of assisted reproductive technology (ART) treatments. Lactation may be enhanced by **medroxyprogesterone,** although the effects on the infant have not been determined.

Adverse Drug Reactions

The most common adverse reaction associated with **progestins** is irregular, breakthrough vaginal bleeding. Some patients may experience amenorrhea. Acne and chloasma have occurred with several of the more **androgenic progestin** products. Patients report increased breast tenderness and galactorrhea. Nausea, depression, and weight gain have also been reported.

Injectable and implanted **progesterone** for contraception use is associated with increased incidence of weight change and irregular menstrual bleeding. Because of low

Table 22–9 ▶ **Pharmacokinetics: Progesterones and Progesterone Antagonists**

Drug	Peak	Active Metabolite	Half-Life	Elimination
Progesterones				
Progesterone	1–2 h	5β-pregnan-3A, 20A-diol glucuronide	8–9 h	50%–60% in urine, 10% in bile and feces; small amount unchanged in bile
Progesterone gel	3.5 h (on daily dosing) 5.4 h (for bid dosing)	5β-pregnan-3A, 20A-diol glucuronide	45 h (for daily dosing) 25.9 h (for bid dosing)	50%–60% in urine, 10% in bile and feces; small amount unchanged in bile
Medroxyprogesterone acetate		5β-pregnan-3A, 20A-diol glucuronide	IM: 10 wk	15%–22% in feces; small amount unchanged in bile
Megestrol acetate	2.2 h	5β-pregnan-3A, 20A-diol glucuronide	34.2 h (mean)	50%–60% in urine, 10% in bile and feces; small amount unchanged in bile
Progesterone Antagonists				
Mifepristone (Mifeprex)	1–3 h	3 active metabolites	20–54 h	NA

NA = not available.

estrogen levels associated with IM **progestin (Depo-Provera)**, patients on this therapy are at increased risk for osteoporosis. In 2004, the FDA issued a black box warning for **Depo-Provera**. In the warning, the FDA cautions about using this form of contraception for longer than 2 years unless other forms of contraception are not viable options. The bone density loss may extend beyond the duration of treatment. Clinicians need to perform a risk assessment and have a thorough discussion of this information with patients prior to the initiation of therapy. Delays to return to fertility may also occur with IM **progestin** use.

Drug Interactions

The two drugs known to have specific interactions are **aminoglutethimide** and **rifampin**. The primary result is to decrease effectiveness of **progestin** therapy, and the result can be unplanned pregnancy. In addition to drug–drug interactions, **progesterone** can cause erroneous laboratory results in testing hepatic function, coagulation, thyroid, metyrapone, and other endocrine functions. Table 22–10 presents drug interactions.

Clinical Use and Dosing

Progestins are used for their effect on endometrial tissue. The major uses of **progestational hormones** are for perimenopausal and postmenopausal **hormonal therapy**, and as a **contraceptive** alone and in combination with **estrogen**.

Perimenopausal and Postmenopausal Hormone Replacement

Combinations of **estrogen** and **progestin** are used when the uterus is intact. The risk for endometrial cancer secondary to endometrial hyperplasia has been consistently demonstrated in research studies of ERT. The risk exists for all dose levels of ERT. To prevent this increased incidence, **progestins**, which reduce the buildup of endometrial tissue, are added to the treatment regimen. There are several combination therapies for use in menopause. These are discussed in more detail in the Rational Drug Selection section.

Progestin-Only Contraception

Progestins exhibit a negative effect in the hypothalamic-pituitary-ovarian axis, essentially suppressing the LH surge necessary for ovulation. They also cause thickening of cervical mucous, making penetration by sperm difficult. Tubal motility is slowed, delaying transport of the ovum and sperm. In addition, **progestins** cause atrophy of the endometrium, preventing implantation.

There are several brand-name **progestin-only pills** available that each contain 0.35-mg **norethindrone**. These pills contain no **estrogen** and are primarily used with special populations in which **estrogen** is contraindicated because of medical conditions or breastfeeding.

Because **progestin-only pills** contain very low levels of hormone, users need to be particularly diligent to take their medications correctly.

The FDA approved the use of **medroxyprogesterone acetate (Depo-Provera)** for contraception in 1993. When administered IM at the recommended 150-mg dose every 3 months (12 wk), it inhibits secretion of gonadotropins, which prevents follicular maturation and results in endometrial thinning. Most women using **Depo-Provera** experience disruption in menstrual bleeding patterns. These disruptions include irregular or unpredictable bleeding, spotting, or, rarely, heavy or continuous bleeding. Over half of all women on IM therapy will experience amenorrhea or some form of irregular menstrual bleeding. If abnormal bleeding persists or is severe, it should be investigated to

Table 22–10 ■ **Common Drug Interactions: Progesterones and Progesterone Antagonists**

Drug	Interacting Drug	Possible Effect	Implications
Progesterones			
Progesterone	Lab studies	Results of hepatic function, coagulation tests (increase in prothrombin; factors VII, VIII, IX, and X), thyroid, metyrapone test, and endocrine functions may be affected by progestins	Anticipate that laboratory levels of liver function and hormonal assays may not be accurate while the patient is taking these drugs
Medroxyprogesterone acetate (DMPA)	Aminoglutethimide	Aminoglutethimide may increase the hepatic metabolism of DMPA	Chemotherapy drug used for metastatic cancer. If spotting occurs, give DMPA earlier than 12 wk
Progesterone Antagonists			
Mifepristone (Mifeprex)	Agents that utilize the CYP450 3A4 pathway	Multiple interactions regarding changes in agent metabolism	Seek alternative options or close monitoring based on agents

rule out an underlying pathology. **Depo-Provera** has been associated with reduced bone density after chronic administration. Women using this form of **contraception** need to be made aware of the potential for osteoporosis, and this risk should be considered in choosing this form of **contraception.** Adolescents and young adults are of special concern, because growth in bone mineral density is largest during this age group and loss at this time reduces the total bone mass available later in life. As with all **progestin** products, there is a risk for thromboembolic events.

Off-Labeled Use of Progestins

Other off-labeled uses for **progestins** in the treatment of dysmenorrhea, endometriosis, hirsutism, and menstrual bleeding disorders are implemented when **estrogen** is contraindicated. The gel form of **progesterone** is used to assist in fertility programs for women with **progesterone** deficits. Refer to Chapter 31 for a more detailed discussion of **progesterone** as **contraception** and to Chapter 38 for its use in conjunction with **estrogen** for postmenopausal **hormone therapy.** Table 22–11 presents the dosage schedule of **progestins** and **progesterone antagonists.**

Rational Drug Selection

Short Acting Versus Long Acting

Oral contraceptive products are dosed in a convenient dial pack. These products are short acting, and the patient chooses when to stop and become fertile again. **Progesterone** is available for **contraception** in two parenteral forms which are long acting, and both have greater than 99 percent theoretical efficacy. Patient preference is a primary concern when selecting the route for contraceptive delivery with **progesterone** agents. For patients who have

Table 22–11 ● Dosage Schedule: Progesterones and Progesterone Antagonists

Drug	Indication	Dose
Progesterones		
Progesterone	Amenorrhea (primary and secondary)	400 mg q d × 10 d 5–10 mg IM daily for 6–8 consecutive d
	Abnormal uterine bleeding caused by hormonal imbalance in the absence of organic pathology	5–10 mg IM daily for 6 doses
	Infertility (gel only)	90 mg vaginally once daily (twice daily if complete ovarian failure)
	Off-labeled uses: premature labor, premenstrual syndrome (PMS) (suppositories)	
Medroxyprogesterone acetate	Secondary amenorrhea	5–10 mg daily for 5–10 d
	Contraception	150 mg IM q 3 months
	Abnormal uterine bleeding caused by hormonal imbalance in the absence of organic pathology	5–10 mg daily for 5–10 d, beginning on the 16th or 21st day of menstrual cycle
Megestrol acetate	Appetite enhancement in patients with AIDS (suspension only); treatment of anorexia, cachexia, or an unexplained significant weight loss in patients with AIDS; tumors (tablets only); palliative treatment of advanced carcinoma of the breast or endometrium	Initial dose is 800 mg/d (20 mL/d); shake the suspension well before using; in clinical trials evaluating different dose schedules, daily doses of 400 and 800 mg/d were clinically effective
Norethindrone acetate (Aygestin)	Secondary amenorrhea, and abnormal uterine bleeding caused by hormonal imbalance in the absence of organic pathology	2.5–10 mg/d for 5–10 d during the second half of the theoretical menstrual cycle. Withdrawal bleeding usually occurs within 3–7 d
	Endometriosis	Initial dose: 5 mg/d for 2 wk. Increase in 2.5 mg/d increments every two wk until 15 mg/d. Hold at this level for 6–9 mo or until breakthrough bleeding requires temporary termination
Progesterone Antagonists		
Mifepristone (Mifeprex)(Restricted access in the US)	Termination of intrauterine pregnancy through 49 d of pregnancy	Day 1: 600 mg as single oral dose Day 3: If termination has not occurred, 400 mcg of misoprostol are taken
	Cushing's syndrome	200 mg/d
	Tamoxifen-resistant breast cancer with progesterone receptors	

Continued

Table 22–11 ◉ **Dosage Schedule: Progesterones and Progesterone Antagonists—cont'd**

Drug	Indication	Dose
Combinations of Estrogen and Progestins	Prevention of endometrial hyperplasia in perimenopausal and postmenopausal women (HRT)	Estrogen (0.625 mg) plus medroxyprogesterone acetate (MPA) 2.5 mg/d (Prempro) Estrogen (0.625 mg) plus micronized progesterone 100 mg d Estrogen (0.625 mg)/d plus MPA 10 mg for 10–12 d Estrogen (0.625 mg)/d plus MPA 5 mg for 14 d (Premphase) Estrogen (0.625 mg)/d plus micronized progesterone 200 mg for 12 d Estrogen (0.625 mg) for d 1–25 plus MPA (5 mg)10 d 16–25 Estrogen (0.625 mg) plus progestin Monday through Friday

difficulty remembering to take the medication daily, the use of a long-acting method may be preferred. Table 22–12 presents available dosage forms.

Prevention of Endometrial Cancer

Endometrial cancer is a risk associated with estrogen therapy. In an attempt to decrease this risk, combinations of **estrogen** and a **progestin** have been prescribed to perimenopausal and postmenopausal women who have an intact uterus. The following is a partial list of available products and dosing patterns of HRT:

1. **Estrogen** (0.625 mg) plus **medroxyprogesterone acetate** (MPA) 2.5 mg daily **(Prempro)**. Of note, this is the medication used in the WHI study in which concern was raised about increased CHD risk.
2. **Estrogen** (0.625 mg) plus **micronized progesterone** 100 mg daily
3. **Estrogen** (0.625 mg) daily plus **MPA** 10 mg for 10 to 12 days
4. **Estrogen** (0.625 mg) daily plus **MPA** 5 mg for 14 days **(Premphase)**
5. **Estrogen** (0.625 mg) daily plus **micronized progesterone** 200 mg for 12 days (Writing Group from PEPI trial)
6. **Estrogen** (0.625 mg) days 1 to 25 plus **MPA** days 16 to 25 (the first regimen used, which has the disadvantage of more hot flashes)
7. **Estrogen** (0.625 mg) plus **progestin** Monday through Friday (may experience more hot flashes)

When initiating therapy in older women, begin with low doses (0.3 mg) of **conjugated estrogens** every other day for 2 months. Next, increase the **estrogens** to daily doses. Use for another 2 months. Add a **progestin** from the treatment regimens above if patient has a uterus. If symptoms such as bleeding or breast pain do not occur,

Table 22–12 ◆ **Available Dosage Forms: Progesterone and Progesterone Antagonists**

Drug	Dosage Form	How Supplied	Cost
Progesterones			
(Prometrium)	Capsules: 100 mg; 200 mg	In bottles of 100 capsules	$52.91/30 $92.87/30
Progesterone in oil	Injection: 50 mg/mL	In 10-mL multidose vials	
(Crinone)	Vaginal gel: 4% (45 mg) 8% (90 mg)	1.25-g gel in 6s	
		1.25-g gel in 6s and 18s	$79.94/8.7 g
(Prochieve)	Vaginal gel: 4% (45 mg) 8% (90 mg)	1.25-g gel in 6s	$152.42/1.45 g
		1.25-g gel in 6s and 18s	$220.99/1.45 g
Medroxyprogesterone acetate (MPA)	Tablets: 2.5 mg (G)	In bottles of 30, 90, 100, 500, 1,000 tablets	
	2.5 mg (P)	In bottles of 30, 100 tablets	$35.99/30
(Provera)	Tablets: 5 mg (G)	In bottles of 30, 100, 500, 1000 tablets	
	5 mg (P)	In bottles of 30, 100 tablets	$44.99/30
	Tablets: 10 mg (G)	In bottles of 30, 40, 50, 100, 250, 500 tablets	
	10 mg (P)	In bottles of 30, 100, 500 and UD 10 tablets	$54.99/30

Table 22–12 ◆ **Available Dosage Forms: Progesterone and Progesterone Antagonists—cont'd**

Drug	Dosage Form	How Supplied	Cost
Megestrol acetate (Megace)	Tablets: 20 mg (G)	In bottles of 100 and UD 100 tablets	$37.99/30
	20 mg (M)	In bottles of 100 tablets	
	Tablets: 40 mg (G)	In bottles of 100, 500, UD 100 tablets and blister packs of 25	$52.99/30
	40 mg (M)	In bottles of 100, 250, 500	
	Suspension: 40 mg/mL (G) and (M)	In 240 mL (lemon-lime flavor)	$131.33 (G); $167.52 (M)/240 ml
Norethindrone acetate (Aygestin)	Tablets: 5 mg (G) and	In bottles of 50 tablets	
	5 mg (A)	In bottles of 50 tablets	$85.31/30
Mifepristone (Mifeprex)	Not available in licensed pharmacies Must obtain from drug manufacturer		
Combinations of estrogen and progestins	Tablets: 0.625 mg conjugated estrogen + 2.5 mg MPA (PP)	In dial pack 28s	$62.33/pack
(PremPro [PP])	Tablets: 0.625 mg conjugated estrogens + 5 mg MPA (PP)	In dial pack 28s	$60.25/pack
(Premphase [PPh])	Tablets 0.3 mg conjugated estrogen + 1.5 mg MPA	In dial pack 28s	$117.08/84
(Femhrt [F])			
(Activella [A])	Tablets: 0.5 mg conjugated estrogen + 1.5 mg MPA	In dial pack 28s	$64.19/pack
(Ortho-Prefest [OP])			
Combipatch [CP]	Tablets: 0.625 mg conjugated estrogens + 5 mg MPA (PPh)	In dial pack 28s (14 of each drug)	$117.08/84
	Tablets: 5 mcg ethinyl estradiol + 1 mg norethindrone (F)	In bottles of 90 and blister pack 28s	$123.05/90
	Tablets: 1 mg estradiol + 0.5 mg norethindrone (A)	In dial pack 28s	$198.83/140
	Tablets: 1 mg estradiol + 0.09 mg norgestimate (OP)	In blister pack 30 (15 of each drug)	
	Transdermal patch: 0.05 mg estradiol + 0.14 mg norethindrone (CP)	9 cm². In 8s	$39.20/8
	Transdermal patch: 0.05 mg estradiol + 0.25 mg norethindrone (CP)	16 cm². In 8s	$55.99/8 patches

G = generic.

increase the **estrogen** up to 0.625 mg daily. Some women may need only the lower **estrogen** dosages as long as they have an adequate diet. Use of formulations other than oral may reduce the need for the addition of **progestin** because of reduced cancer risk. This reduced risk for different **estrogen** formulations is discussed in the **estrogen** therapy Rational Drug Selection section.

Vaginal Bleeding

The most common reason women give for discontinuing HRT is unacceptable vaginal bleeding. Continuous regimens (1 and 2 in the list above) eliminate monthly withdrawal bleeding, but they are associated with a higher rate of breakthrough bleeding, especially in the first 6 months and this is most likely in women who are more recently postmenopausal because endogenous production of **estrogen** is more labile from cycle to cycle in these women. Currently available data suggest the most positive risk/benefit profiles for all indications for HRT may accrue when the therapy is started near the time of menopause onset. The use of cyclical or sequential therapy (3 to 7 above) reduces the risk for breakthrough bleeding and is preferred until endogenous hormone production stabilizes, typically 2 to 3 years after menopause. Differences in potency of various progestins may result in differences in rates of bleeding. The PEPI study found **micronized progestin** was associated with less bleeding during the first 6 months than either continuous or cyclical MPA (Lindenfeld & Langer, 2002).

Effects on Lipids

Different types of **progestin** not only have differing effects on the endometrium, they also have differing effects on **estrogen**-associated benefits to lipids. **Norethindrone acetate** has been shown to reverse these benefits on HDL cholesterol while still offering effective endometrial protection. MPA and **micronized progestin** do not attenuate the effects of **estrogen** on lipid levels. **Norgestimate** improves HDL to a level intermediate between MPA and **micronized progestin,** also while providing good endometrial protection (Langer, 2005).

Monitoring

Pretreatment physical examination to assess health and possible contraindications to **progestins** is mandatory. Examination should be age specific. Patients with seizure disorders need monitoring of their symptoms because increased fluid retention may lower the seizure threshold. Women with migraines are vulnerable to any changes in physiological states, and fluid retention may give them cyclic migraines. Depression should be assessed early in therapy for those women with a history of previous affective disorders. Patients with diabetes may see changes in blood glucose levels, indicating more frequent measurement. Patients with a history of or risk for thromboembolic events or who use tobacco products should not use these products or should have careful monitoring for early indications of this problem. Additionally, women on injectable **progesterone** will require education and possible screening for osteoporosis based on age and risk factors.

Women on **HRT** require careful monitoring for cardiovascular, thromboembolic, and cancer risks. Monitoring for these risks is discussed in Chapter 38.

Patient Education

Administration

Most hormone regimens require daily dosing for efficacy, especially for the **progestin-only oral contraceptive.** The most common adverse effect is breakthrough bleeding, especially if doses are missed. The injectable form requires administration every 12 weeks, so a follow-up appointment should be scheduled for the time the injection is due to avoid loss of pregnancy protection. The use of injectable **progesterone** for contraception requires added screening at initial administration. Patients must present for initial administration of an injectable **progesterone** therapy while they are actively menstruating and have a negative pregnancy test. The use of injectable **progesterone** is associated with significant teratogenic effects. Patient-specific education regarding the need to maintain the specific redosing schedule should also be provided.

Estrogen/progestin combinations used for **HRT** require daily dosing. No specific instructions are required beyond those usually given for oral drugs.

Adverse Reactions

Progestins should not be used in the first 12 weeks of gestation because of masculinization of the female fetus. Depression and mood swings are common and represent a significant factor in postmenopausal **HRT** cessation. Irregular menstrual patterns and unpredictable spotting contribute to a proportion of women stopping **progestin-only** oral contraceptives. Breast tenderness and galactorrhea are the third most common reason women switch from a **progesterone contraceptive** and another reason that postmenopausal women stop HRT altogether.

Lifestyle Management

Progesterone therapy may be associated with hyperpigmentation and weight gain. To help reduce these complications, clinicians should encourage patients to use sunscreen to prevent skin changes, such as blotchy pigmentation, while using **progestins,** and promote routine physical exercise to combat the increase in body weight sometimes seen with **Depo-Provera.**

Smoking cessation is encouraged in all patients, but especially in young women using **hormonal contraception.** The association of both **estrogen** and **progesterone** with morbidity and mortality in patients older than 35 years who smoke may be a powerful motivator to quit smoking.

OTHER DRUGS AFFECTING THE REPRODUCTIVE SYSTEM

Other drugs affecting the reproductive system include those that are commonly used to treat infertility (**GnRH, FSH, LH,** and **human chorionic gonadotropin** [**hCG**]), those used as **lactation inhibitors** (**bromocriptine**), and those used in erectile dysfunction.

Drugs Commonly Used in Fertility Clinics

Gonadotropin-Releasing Hormone

GnRH is produced in the arcuate nucleus of the hypothalamus and controls the release of FSH and LH for both males and females. GnRH is used as a stimulant in pulsatile doses if the patient has a functional pituitary gland and an ovary to produce the LH surge initiating ovulation. **GnRH agents** may be used in pulsate form to stimulate ovulation, treat endometriosis and uterine fibroids, and as continuous therapy to suppress prostate cancer. **Leuprolide acetate (Lupron, Lupron Depot)** may be administered subcutaneously (SC) or IM. **Zoladex** is an SC implant that is used to treat prostate cancer, breast cancer, and severe endometriosis. It is administered every 28 days.

The use of **GnRH** is contraindicated in conjunction with medications that stimulate ovarian function. The use of **GnRH** for infertility treatments may result in multiple gestations. Long-term use of **GnRH** agents may result in bone demineralization, and DEXA (Dual Energy X-ray Absorptiometry) scans should be considered for patients who require ongoing treatment. Patients may report hot flashes, headache, and menstrual irregularities during treatment.

Follicle-Stimulating Hormone/Gonadotropins

FSH has an analogue, **human menopausal gonadotropin** (**hMG**) (**follitropin** [**Fertinex**], **menotropins** [**Pergonal,**

Humegon]). The drug is used in fertility treatments for both men and women. In men, the use of **gonadotropins** stimulates spermatogenesis and in women stimulates the maturation of follicles and ovulation. These agents are administered IM. Onset, peak, and duration are not established for all agents. These agents are used in specialty practices. As these agents are used to stimulate ovarian function, there is a risk of hyperstimulation syndrome that can cause ovarian enlargement, ascites, hydrothorax, hypovolemia, hemoperitoneum, fever, or arterial thromboembolism.

Luteinizing Hormone and Human Chorionic Gonadotropin

Luteinizing hormone (LH) has the analogue **hCG (A.P.L., Chorex-5, Profasi)**. Like FSH, LH is produced in the anterior pituitary and used in conjunction with FSH to stimulate ovulation. It also stimulates the corpus luteum to produce progesterone and androgens. No LH preparation is available for use clinically. Instead, a similar preparation, **hCG**, is substituted successfully.

Lactation Inhibitors

Bromocriptine

Although not a true hormone, **bromocriptine (Parlodel)** has an inhibitory effect on the pituitary gland that produces prolactin. It is widely used for shrinking pituitary prolactin-secreting tumors, reducing the prolactin levels of idiopathic prolactinemia, galactorrhea, and infertility. **Bromocriptine** is similar to dopamine in structure and binds to dopamine receptors within the pituitary gland to inhibit prolactin secretion. It is well absorbed from the GI tract and can begin to exert an effect within 2 hours of administration. **Bromocriptine** is metabolized through the CYP450 3A4 substrate, and excreted primarily in bile. When used for hyperprolactinemic indications, the initial dosage is 0.5 to 2.5 mg daily with meals; 2.5 mg may be added as tolerated every 3 to 7 days or until optimal therapeutic response is achieved. Therapeutic dosage is usually 5 to 7.5 mg, with a range of 2.5 to 15 mg/day.

For acromegaly, the initial dose is 1.25 to 2.5 mg for 3 days on retiring. An additional 1.25 to 2.5 mg is added as tolerated every 3 to 7 days. Therapeutic dosage is usually 5 to 7.5 mg, with a range of 20 to 30 mg/day.

Multiple drugs interact with **bromocriptine**. Some of the most notable interactions include **acetaminophen, erythromycin, phenothiazines, sympathomimetics, isometheptene**, and **phenylpropanolamine**.

Drugs Used for Erectile Dysfunction

Phosphodiesterase Type 5 Inhibitors

Erectile dysfunction (ED) is a common health condition that is associated with increased age and various comorbidities, such as diabetes and hypertension. The causes of erectile dysfunction are beyond the scope of this text. However, clinicians should complete a full history and physical to confirm proper diagnosis prior to initiating medication therapy. This section focuses on ED treatment with the use of **phosphodiesterase type 5 inhibitors (PDE5 inhibitors)**.

Sildenafil citrate (Viagra), the first **PDE5 inhibitor** indicated for the treatment of impotence in men with ED, was originally studied as a selective **vasodilator** for use in angina. Although not effective in the coronary arteries, it was effective as a selective inhibitor of cyclic guanosine monophosphate (cGMP), specific **PDE5**. This **PDE5** has a 10-fold selectivity for the enzyme that produces smooth muscle relaxation in the corpus cavernosum of the penis. As smooth muscles in the corpus cavernosum relax, blood flow into the penis is increased, resulting in an erection. There is no drug effect without sexual stimulation. It is rapidly absorbed after oral administration and eliminated by hepatic metabolism (mainly CYP450 3A4). Ingestion of food reduces its rate of absorption. The peak onset occurs 60 minutes after dosing, with duration up to 4 hours. About 80 percent is eliminated in the feces, with most of the remaining eliminated in the urine.

For erectile dysfunction, the dosage of **sildenafil** is 50 mg (25 to 100 mg, based on effectiveness) taken as needed approximately 1 hour before sexual activity. The maximum recommended frequency is once a day. Studies in healthy elderly volunteers (over 65 years) showed a reduced clearance with free plasma concentrations 40 percent higher than in younger volunteers (18 to 45 years). An initial starting dose of 25 mg is recommended for men over age 65 years.

There is an absolute contraindication for concomitant use with any form of **nitrates** because of the risk of severe hypotension, cardiovascular collapse, and death. Other potential drug interactions are many, including **antifungals, macrolide antibiotics** (such as **erythromycin**), **cimetidine, rifampin, alpha blockers, nonspecific beta blockers**, and **diuretics**. Do not use these drugs concomitantly or adjust doses of the **phosphodiesterase inhibitor** downward. Common adverse effects include headaches, flushing, dyspepsia, and blue-hue vision change.

All **PDE5 inhibitors** have been shown to have equal efficacy in treating ED. The main difference between the agents is longer duration of action. **Vardenafil (Levitra)** shares a pharmacokinetic profile similar to that of **sildenafil**, but is purported to have a shorter time to onset of action and is ten times more potent than **sildenafil**. The starting dose is 10 mg taken approximately 60 minutes before sexual activity. The dose may be increased to 20 mg or decreased to 5 mg based on efficacy and adverse effects. As with **sildenafil**, there is reduced clearance in elderly patients, with plasma concentrations up to 52 percent higher. A lower starting dose of 5 mg is recommended with this population. No adjustments are required for renal impairment, but the same recommendations are made as above related to drug interactions. **Tadalafil (Cialis)** has a different chemical structure that the other two PDE5

inhibitors. This allows for greater binding affinity in skeletal smooth muscle, the testes, and prostate, and less affinity in the retina. This may account for the low back pain and decreased incidence of visual disturbances with **tadalafil** that some users report. The recommended starting dose is 10 mg taken 30 minutes prior to anticipated sexual activity. The dose may be increased to 20 mg or decreased to 5 mg based on individual efficacy and tolerability. For patients with renal impairment (Creatinine clearance 31 to 50 mL/min), a starting dose of 5 mg not more than once daily is recommended. Use caution in patients taking other drugs that are potent inhibitors of CYP450 3A4 (see **sildenafil** drug interactions above). In patients using other CYP450 3A4 medications, dosage adjustment is a maximum recommended dose of **tadalafil** 10 mg, not to exceed one dose every 72 hours.

All **PDE5 inhibitors** share the same contraindication in patients who are using nitrates because of a risk of severe hypotension. Concurrent use with alpha blockers is also not recommended because of additive hypotensive effects. Patients with underlying cardiovascular disease require additional pretreatment evaluation. The American College of Cardiology (ACC) and the American Heart Association (AHA) have suggested that patients with unstable coronary artery disease, active ischemia, heart failure, and low blood pressure, and patients on multiple antihypertensive agents or medications that inhibit the CYP 450 3A4 pathway should not take **PDE5 inhibitors. Vardenafil** can cause QT prolongation and should not be used in patients with underlying arrhythmias, on dysrhythmic medications, or with hepatic insufficiency.

Patient education regarding the anticipated effectiveness of therapy and potential side effects should be given at the initiation of therapy and at each refill. Patients who experience chest pain or dizziness with sexual activity should refrain from additional use of these agents and sexual activity until these individuals have been reevaluated. Priapism is a rare but emergent adverse event that can occur with **PDE5 inhibitors.** Patients who experience an erection that lasts for longer than 4 hours need to be evaluated in the emergency department. While patients are on this therapy, periodic medication and health evaluation of them are encouraged to identify any new potential cardiovascular or health risks that may alter the ability to continue ED therapy.

The effects of **PDE5 inhibitors** for treating women with sexual dysfunction have been evaluated in small clinical trials. The results are mixed, with many studies unable to demonstrate efficacy. **PDE5 inhibitors** have been used to treat NICU (neonatal intensive care unit) infants with persistent pulmonary hypertension (Baquero, Soliz, Neira, Venegas, & Sola, 2006).

REFERENCES

Agency for Healthcare Research and Quality. (2005). Hormone therapy for the prevention of chronic conditions in postmenopausal women. Retrieved October 21, 2009, from http://www.ahrq.gov/clinic/uspstf05/ht/htpostmenrs.htm

Agency for Healthcare Research and Quality. (2005). Management of menopausal related symptoms. Retrieved October 21, 2009, from http://www.ahrq.gov/clinic/tp/menopstp.htm.

American College of Rheumatology. (2004). Concomitant teriparatide plus raloxifene for the treatment of postmenopausal osteoporosis: Results from a randomized placebo-controlled trial. Retrieved October 28, 2005, from http://www.rheumatology.org/press/2004

Anderson, G., Judd, H., Kaunitz, A., Barad, D., Beresford, S., Pettinger, M., et al. (2003). Effects of estrogen plus progestin on gynecologic cancers and associated diagnostic procedures: The Women's Health Initiative Randomized Trial. *Journal of the American Medical Association, 290*(13), 1739–1748.

Anderson, G., Limacher, M., et al. and The Women's Health Initiative Steering Committee. (2004). Effects of conjugated equine estrogen in postmenopausal women with hysterectomy: The Women's Health Initiative randomized trial. *Journal of the American Medical Association, 291,* 1701–1712.

Archer, D. (2004). Hormonal therapy and the postmenopausal woman: Current clinical challenges. *Portraits and Passages: Women's Health Through the Prime of Life.* CE # 04-17.

Baquero, H., Soliz, A., Neira, F., Venegas, M. E., & Sola, A. (2006). Oral sildenafil in infants with persistent pulmonary hypertension of the newborn: A pilot randomized blinded study. *Pediatrics, 117*(4), 1077–1083.

Barrett-Conner, E., Grady, D., & Stefanick, M. (2005). The rise and fall of menopausal hormone therapy. *Annual Review of Public Health, 26,* 115–140.

Boyack, M., Lookinland, S., & Chasson, S. (2002). Efficacy of raloxifene for treatment of menopause: A systematic review. *Journal of the American Academy of Nurse Practitioners, 14*(4), 150–165.

Brucker, M. (2002). What's a woman to do? *Association of Women's Health, Obstetric and Neonatal Nurses Lifelines, 6*(5), 408–417.

Cummings, S., Eckert, K., Grady, D., Powles, T., Cauley, L., Norton, L., et al. (1999). The effect of raloxifene on risk of breast cancer in postmenopausal women. *Journal of the American Medical Association, 281*(23), 2189–2197.

Drug facts and comparisons. (2010). St. Louis, MO: Wolters Kluwer Health.

Epocrates. (2009). Epocrates Rx pharmaceutical reference. Retrieved between October 21, 2009, and November 23, 2009. www.epocrates.com

Fitzpatrick, L. (2004). Estrogen and bone health. *The Female Patient, 29*(Suppl.), 4–9.

Garnero, P., Stevens, R., Ayres, S., & Phelps, K. (2002). Short-term effects of new synthetic conjugated estrogens on biochemical markers of bone turnover. *Journal of Clinical Pharmacology, 42,* 290–296.

Greenspan, S., Emkey, R., Bone, H., Weiss, S., Bell, N., Downs, R., et al. (2002). Significant differential effects of alendronate, estrogen or combination therapy on the rate of bone loss after discontinuation of treatment of postmenopausal osteoporosis: A randomized, double-blind, placebo-controlled trial. *Archives of Internal Medicine, 137*(11), 875–883.

Hatcher, R., Trussell, J., Stewart, F., Nelson, A., Cates, W., Guest, F., et al. (2004). *Contraceptive technology* (18th ed.). New York: Ardent Media.

Hatcher, R., Trussell, J., Nelson, A., Cates, W., & Stewart, F. (2007). *Contraceptive technology* (19th ed.). New York: Ardent Media.

Institute for Clinical Systems Improvement (ICSI). (2004). *Diagnosis and treatment of osteoporosis.* Bloomington, MN: Author. Retrieved July 11, 2005, from http://www.guideline.gov/summary/summary.aspx

Jamal, S., Leiter, R., Bayoumi, A., Bauer, D., & Cummings, S. (2004). Clinical utility of laboratory testing in women with osteoporosis. *Osteoporosis International, August 31.* Retrieved October 25, 2005, from http://www.osteoporosis.ca/english/For%20Health%20Professionals/Research

Kern, L., Powe, N., Levine, M., Fitzpatrick, A., Harris, T., Robbins, J., et al. (2005). Association between screening for osteoporosis and the incidence of hip fracture. *Annals of Internal Medicine, 142*(3), 173–181.

Kong, Y., & Penninger, J. (2004). Molecular control of bone remodeling and osteoporosis. *Experimental Gerontology, 35*(8), 947.

Kritz-Silverstein, D., & Barrett-Connor, E. (1996). Long-term postmenopausal hormone use, obesity, and fat distribution in older women. *Journal of the American Medical Association, 275*(1), 46–49.

Langer, R. (2005). Postmenopausal hormone therapy. *CME Bulletin of the American Academy of Family Physicians, 4*(1), 1–10.

Lindenfeld, E., & Langer, R. (2002). Bleeding patterns of hormone replacement therapies in the postmenopausal estrogen and progestin interventions trial. *Obstetrics and Gynecology, 100,* 853–863.

Liu, J. (2004). Use of conjugated estrogens after the Women's Health Initiative. *The Female Patient, 29,* 8–13.

Liu, J., Burdette, J., Xu, H., Gu, C., van Breeman, R., Bhat, K., et al. (2001). Evaluation of estrogenic activity of plant extracts for the potential treatment of menopausal symptoms. *Journal of Agricultural and Food Chemistry, 49,* 2472–2479.

Marx, P., Schade, G., Wilbourn, S., Blank, S., Moyer, D., & Nett, R. (2004). Low dose (0.3 mg) synthetic conjugated estrogen A is effective for managing atrophic vaginitis. *Maturitas, 47*(1), 47–55.

National Osteoporosis Foundation. (2005, September). Physician's guide to prevention and treatment of osteoporosis. Retrieved October 25, 2005, from http://www.nof/org/physguide/inside

North American Menopause Society. (2004). Treatment of associated vasomotor symptoms: Position statement of the North American Menopause Society. *Menopause, 11,* 11–33.

North American Menopause Society. (2005). The role of testosterone therapy in postmenopausal women: Position statement of the North American Menopause Society. Retrieved October 21, 2009, from http://www.menopause.org/Portals/0/Content/PDF/PStestosterone05.pdf

North American Menopause Society. (2006). Management of osteoporosis in postmenopausal women: 2006 position statement of the North American Menopause Society. Retrieved October 21, 2009, from http://www.menopause.org/Portals/0/Content/PDF/psosteo06.pdf

North American Menopause Society. (2007). The role of local vaginal estrogen for treatment of vaginal atrophy in postmenopausal women: 2007 position statement of the North American Menopause Society. Retrieved October 21, 2009, from http://www.menopause.org/Portals/0/Content/PDF/PSvagestrogen07.pdf.

North American Menopause Society. (2008). Estrogen and progestogen use in postmenopausal women: July 2008 position statement of the North American Menopause Society. Retrieved October 21, 2009, from http://www.menopause.org/PSHT08.pdf

Prentice, R. L., Manson, J. E., Langer, R. D., Anderson, G. L., Pettinger, M., Jackson, R. D., et al. (2009). Benefits and risks of postmenopausal hormone therapy when it is initiated soon after menopause. *American Journal of Epidemiology, 170,* 12–23.

Rossouw, J., Anderson, G., Prentice, R., Lacroix, A., Kooperberg, C., Stefanick, M., et al. (2002). Risks and benefits of estrogen plus progestin in healthy postmenopausal women: Principal results from the Women's Health Initiative Randomized Controlled Trial. *Journal of the American Medical Association, 288*(3), 321–333.

Sarrel, P. (2004). Vasomotor and vascular consideration. *The Female Patient* (Suppl. February), 10–18.

Scottish Intercollegiate Guidelines Network (SIGN). (2003). *Management of osteoporosis: A national guideline.* Edinburgh, Scotland: Author. Retrieved July 11, 2005, from http://www.guideline.gov/summary/summary.asp

Siminoski, K., Leslie, W., Frame, H., Hodsman, A., Josse, R., Khan, A., et al. (2005). Recommendations for bone mineral density reporting in Canada. *Canadian Association of Radiologists Journal, 56*(3), 178–188. Retrieved October 25, 2005, from http://www.osteoporosis.ca/english/For%20Health%20Professionals/Research

Stevens, R., Roy, P., & Phelps, K. (2002). Evaluation of single- and multiple-dose pharmacokinetics of synthetic conjugated estrogens, A (Cenestin) tablets: A slow-release estrogen replacement product. *Journal of Clinical Pharmacology, 42,* 332–341.

Thorneycroft, I. (2004). Unopposed estrogen and cancer. *The Female Patient,* (Suppl. to February), 19–26.

UpToDate. (2009a). *Overview of Contraception.* Waltham, MA. Retrieved October 21, 2009, from http://www.uptodate.com/online/content/topic.do?topicKey=gen_gyne/3029&selectedTitle=2~150&source=search_result

UpToDate. (2009b). *Treatment of menopausal symptoms with hormone therapy.* Waltham, MA. Retrieved October 21, 2009, from http://www.uptodate.com/online/content/topic.do?topicKey=r_endo_f/9609&selectedTitle=2~150&source=search_result

UpToDate. (2009c). *Treatment of male sexual dysfunction.* Waltham, MA. Retrieved October 21, 2009, from http://www.uptodate.com/online/content/topic.do?topicKey=r_endo_m/6961&selectedTitle=1~150&source=search_result

U.S. Department of Health and Human Services. (2004). *Bone health and osteoporosis: A report of the Surgeon General.* Rockville, MD: U.S. Department of Health and Human Services, Office of the Surgeon General. Retrieved from http://www.surgeongeneral.gov/library

U.S. Food and Drug Administration (FDA). (2004). *Safety Alerts: Depo-Provera (medroxyprogesterone acetate injectable suspension.* Retrieved from http://www.fda.gov/Safety/MedWatch/SafetyInformation/SafetyAlertsforHumanMedicalProducts/ucm154784.htm

Warren, M. P. (2010). Hormone therapy for menopausal symptoms: Putting benefits and risks into perspective. *The Journal of Family Practice, 59*(12), E1–E7.

Writing Group for the Women's Health Initiative Investigators. (2002). Risks and benefits of estrogen plus progestin in healthy postmenopausal women. *Journal of the American Medical Association, 288*(3), 321–323.

Writing Group of the PEPI Trial. (1996). Effects of hormonal therapy on bone mineral density: Results from the post-menopausal estrogen/progestin interventions (PEPI). *Journal of the American Medical Association, 276*(17), 1398–1396.

Wysocki, S., & Alexander, I. (2005). Bioidentical hormones for menopause therapy: An overview. *Women's Health Care: A Practical Journal for Nurse Practitioners, 4*(2), 9–17.

CHAPTER 23

DRUGS AFFECTING THE INTEGUMENTARY SYSTEM

Teri Moser Woo

Chapter Outline

This chapter discusses a wide variety of medications used to treat disorders of the skin or integumentary system, including topical anti-infective medications used to treat bacterial, fungal, and viral infections of the skin; topical **corticosteroids** and **immunomodulators** used for a variety of inflammatory diseases; and topical **antipsoriasis** and acne medications. Systemic medications used for skin disorders are discussed here only if not covered in another chapter. Systemic **antibiotics** and **antifungal** medications used to treat more serious skin infections, with the exception of **griseofulvin** and **terbinafine**, are discussed in Chapter 24. Systemic medications used for acne are discussed in this chapter, with the exception of systemic **antibiotics**, which are also covered in Chapter 24.

ANTI-INFECTIVES

Topical Antibacterials

Bacterial infections of the skin are common with patients of all ages. **Antibacterial** medications commonly used in primary care include topical agents and oral **antibiotics**. The most common pathogens seen in bacterial skin infections are *Staphylococcus aureus* and *Streptococcus pyogenes*. Skin infections with gram-negative bacilli are rare, but they may occur in patients who are immunocompromised or patients with diabetes. These patients usually require IV **antibiotic** therapy for their infections. Impetigo is usually treated topically unless it is a moderate to severe case. Commonly used drugs for impetigo are **mupirocin (Bactroban, Centany)**, **retapamulin (Altabax)**, **neomycin**, **bacitracin**, and **polymyxin B**. A combination product that is available over the counter (OTC) combines **neomycin**, **bacitracin**, and **polymyxin B (Neosporin, Triple Antibiotic Ointment)** or just **bacitracin** and **polymyxin B (Polysporin, Double Antibiotic Ointment)**. Moderate to severe impetigo, a boil or abscess, perianal streptococcal infections, and cellulitis all require prompt treatment with appropriate systemic **antibiotics**. Methicillin resistant *Staphylococcus aureus* (MRSA) is increasing in prevalence and providers need to have a suspicion for MRSA in the differential of any skin infection. If MRSA is suspected, appropriate systemic antibiotics should be used (TMP/SMZ, **clindamycin** or **doxycycline**).

Pharmacodynamics

Topical or systemic antibacterial agents may be either bacteriostatic or bactericidal. **Mupirocin** is bacteriostatic at low concentrations and bactericidal at high concentrations. **Mupirocin** is structurally unrelated to other topical antibiotic agents. It acts by binding to bacterial isoleucyl-tRNA synthetase. It thus inhibits bacterial protein synthesis. **Retapamulin** is bacteriostatic against *S. aureus* and *S. pyogenes* by inhibiting bacterial protein synthesis. **Bacitracin** is bacteriostatic but may also be bactericidal, depending on the antibiotic concentration and the susceptibility of the organism. **Bacitracin** inhibits the cell wall synthesis of the organism. **Erythromycin** binds to the 50 S ribosomal subunit, inhibiting bacterial protein synthesis. It is effective against a wide range of microorganisms. Information regarding the pharmacodynamics of the topical agents **neomycin** and **polymyxin B** is unavailable.

Pharmacokinetics

Absorption and Distribution

The topical agents commonly used to treat bacterial skin infections are minimally absorbed through normal skin. **Mupirocin** has minimal absorption of 0.3 percent when administered topically. If it is applied to large areas of abraded skin, it may allow for deeper penetration into the epidermal layers. **Mupirocin** may be applied intranasally, and there is no evidence of systemic absorption if used this way. Distribution of **mupirocin** is unknown.

Retapamulin ointment is minimally absorbed via intact or abraded skin. Three percent of patients had measurable **retapamulin** levels (0.5 mg/mL) after 1 day of administration to intact skin. Distribution is unknown.

Bacitracin, when used topically, is minimally absorbed. However, **bacitracin** is readily absorbed through large areas of denuded or burned skin. Topical preparations of **bacitracin** that include **neomycin** and polymyxin B are minimally absorbed through normal skin. Distribution of **bacitracin**, **neomycin**, and **polymyxin B** is unknown. Absorption and distribution of the oral **antibiotics** used to treat skin infections are discussed in Chapter 24.

Metabolism and Excretion

Metabolism and excretion of the topical antibacterial agents **mupirocin**, **bacitracin**, **neomycin**, and **polymyxin B** are unknown. **Retapamulin** is metabolized by liver enzymes in vitro; excretion is not known because of the low systemic absorption with topical administration. Information regarding the metabolism and excretion of topical **erythromycin** is also unavailable.

Pharmacotherapeutics

Clinical Use and Dosing

Impetigo

Impetigo is a superficial skin infection caused by *S. aureus*, *S. pyogenes*, or both. Treatment with an **antibiotic** that is effective against both organisms, either topical or oral, ensures successful treatment. Bullous impetigo is usually pure *S. aureus* and should be treated with an **antibiotic** that has good staph coverage.

If only one or two lesions are present, the patient may be treated with topical OTC **antibiotic** ointments such as **bacitracin** or a combination product that combines **bacitracin**, polymyxin B, with or without **neomycin** (**Polysporin, Neosporin, Double Antibiotic Ointment, Triple Antibiotic Ointment**). Either **bacitracin** alone or the combination **antibiotic** product is applied to affected area two to five times per day until the lesions clear. If the patient has up to five singular lesions, topical **mupirocin** ointment may be applied tid until the lesions are healed (5 to 14 days). Topical **retapamulin** is applied twice a day for 5 days. **Mupirocin** and **retapamulin** are available only by prescription. There are no reported drug interactions with the topical antibiotics (Table 23–1).

Oral **antibiotics** are indicated if the patient has more than five lesions or if the lesions continue to worsen after 2 or 3 days of topical **antibiotic** treatment. **Antibiotics** that are effective against *S. aureus* or *S. pyogenes* include **cephalexin (Keflex), amoxicillin/potassium clavulanate**

Table 23–1 ■ **Drug Interactions: Selected Anti-Infectives Used for Skin Disorders**

Drug	Interacting Drug	Possible Effect	Implications
Antibacterial			
Bacitracin	None reported		
Mupirocin	None reported with topical use		
	Other nasal products	Decreased effectiveness of intranasal mupirocin	Avoid use of other nasal products concurrently with intranasal mupirocin
Neomycin	None reported		
Polymyxin B	None reported		
Retapamulin	None reported		
Antifungal			
Butenafine	None reported		
Ciclopirox olamine	None reported		
Clotrimazole	Nystatin and amphotericin B	The azole antifungals could interfere with the action of either amphotericin B or nystatin by depleting polyene binding sites; this appears to be the most significant when the azole antifungal is given prior to amphotericin B	Do not use concurrently
	Spermicides (nonoxynol-9 and octoxynol)	Clotrimazole intravaginal preparations should not be administered concurrently with nonoxynol-9 and octoxynol; clotrimazole may inactivate the spermicides, leading to contraceptive failure	Do not use concurrently
Econazole	Topical corticosteroids	Corticosteroids may inhibit the antifungal activity of econazole against *Candida albicans* in a concentration-dependent manner	Avoid the use of topical steroids with econazole. Choose another topical anti fungal
Gentian violet	None reported		
Ketoconazole	None reported		

Continued

Table 23–1 ■ **Drug Interactions: Selected Anti-Infectives Used for Skin Disorders—cont'd**

Drug	Interacting Drug	Possible Effect	Implications
Miconazole	None reported		
Naftifine	None reported		
Nystatin	Topical clotrimazole (theoretically, all azoles)	Topical azoles compete for binding sites with nystatin	Do not use concurrently
Oxiconazole	None reported		
Sertaconazole	None reported		
Sulconazole	None reported		
Terbinafine	None reported		
Tolnaftate	None reported		
Antivirals			
Acyclovir	None reported		
Docosanol	None reported		
Penciclovir	None reported		

(Augmentin), and **dicloxacillin.** If MRSA is suspected **clindamycin, TMP/SMZ,** or **doxycycline** should be prescribed depending on local resistance patterns. A macrolide **antibiotic** such as **erythromycin** or **azithromycin (Zithromax)** can be used if the patient is penicillin allergic and MRSA is not suspected. There is some resistance of *S. aureus* to **erythromycin,** so the patient needs to be monitored closely. The patient treated with systemic **antibiotics** should be treated for 10 days (5 days with **azithromycin**).

Furuncle

Furuncle, commonly known as a boil or abscess, is usually caused by *S. aureus.* Treatment of a small abscess may include warm packs and systemic **antibiotics** that are effective against *S. aureus.* A larger abscess usually requires incision and drainage, as well as systemic **antibiotics** that provide coverage for *S. aureus.* Gram's stain and culture of the drainage from the abscess can determine if the organism will be sensitive to the **antibiotic** of choice. Prior to Gram's stain results, an appropriate first-line antibiotic would be **cephalexin, amoxicillin-clavulanic acid,** or **dicloxacillin.** Length of treatment should be 10 days, unless longer treatment is indicated by clinical progress.

Cellulitis

Cellulitis is a painful bacterial infection involving the soft tissue. The patient may become septic if left untreated. The causative organisms are most commonly *Streptococcus pneumoniae, S. aureus,* MRSA, or, in children, *Haemophilus influenzae.* Treatment with systemic **antibiotics** that are effective against these organisms is essential. If the clinical picture warrants it, an initial dose of an intramuscular (IM)-administered **antibiotic** such as **ceftriaxone** may be given, followed by oral **antibiotic** treatment. Oral **antibiotic** therapy with a broad-spectrum **antibiotic** such as **amoxicillin-clavulanate** or a broad-spectrum **cephalosporin** is indicated. MRSA patients may require parenteral **antibiotics** initially before oral **antibiotics** are started. Tissue aspirate cultures can guide the practitioner in determining if the organism is sensitive to the **antibiotic** of choice.

Nasal MRSA Carrier

Eradication of nasal MRSA colonization in adult patients and health-care workers may be achieved with intranasal **mupirocin.** Intranasal **mupirocin** is supplied in 1-g, single-use tubes and should be used twice a day. The patient applies approximately half the ointment from a single-use tube of nasal ointment into one nostril and the other half into the other nostril in the morning and evening for 5 days. Children may require smaller amounts of ointment.

Rational Drug Selection

Antibacterial Activity

The choice of a topical antibiotic is based on susceptibility. **Mupirocin** and **retapamulin** are considered a broad-spectrum topical **antibiotic. Bacitracin** and the combination of **bacitracin, neomycin,** and **polymyxin B** are OTC products that combine different antimicrobial spectrums to provide a single broad-spectrum product. **Mupirocin** is considered a broader spectrum **antibiotic** than the **double-** or **triple-antibiotic** formula. If resistance to the topical product is suspected or if the infection is not responding to topical **antibiotics,** then systemic **antibiotics** are warranted.

Cost

The OTC topical **antibiotic** products are relatively inexpensive. **Bacitracin** is usually sold as a generic product and is quite inexpensive. The combination product of **neomycin**, polymyxin B, and **bacitracin** is available in brand names (**Neosporin**), which are slightly more expensive than the generic product (**triple-antibiotic ointment**). Likewise the **double-antibiotic** brand-name products (**Polysporin**) are more expensive than generic **double-antibiotic** ointment. The brand-name products are usually less than $10 per 30-g tube, and the generic product approximately $5 for a 30-g tube. **Mupirocin** is more expensive: A 30-g tube of **Bactroban** cream is $92 and a 22-g tube of **Bactroban** ointment is $62; **generic mupirocin** is $35 for a 22-g tube (http://www.drugstore.com). A 15-g tube of **retapamulin** (**Altabax**) is $95 (http://www.drugstore.com).

Combination Products

Due to the possibility of developing **neomycin** sensitivity, most providers are recommending that patients use **double-antibiotic** (**Polysporin**) rather than **triple-antibiotic** (**Neomycin**) products.

Monitoring

No specific monitoring is required beyond that related to the disease process for which the patient is being treated.

Patient Education

Administration

Patients should be taught how to appropriately apply the **topical antibiotic ointment**. They should be instructed to wash their hands before applying the ointment or to use a gloved hand. The **antibiotic** ointment should be applied sparingly only to the affected infection area. Overapplication of the **antibiotic** ointment can increase adverse effects. Patients should not use the **antibiotic** ointment for longer than 1 week unless instructed to do so by their provider. To avoid contamination of the **antibiotic** ointment, care must be taken not to touch the tip of the **antibiotic** ointment container to the infected area or to any other surface.

Adverse Reactions

The patient should be instructed that adverse reactions to topical **antibiotics** are rare but that skin irritation is possible with any topical ointment. Any adverse reactions should be reported to the provider as soon as possible, and the **antibiotic** ointment should then not be used until the patient is instructed otherwise. The patient should not use the **antibiotic** ointment over large surface areas (more than 20% of body surface) without prior instruction from the provider.

Lifestyle Management

Patients need to be instructed on general infection control measures, especially if the patient has impetigo or MRSA is suspected; both are highly contagious diseases. Patients should wash their hands after any contact with the infected area. Within the family, the patient infected with impetigo should use care not to share towels or other utensils with other family members to prevent the spread of infection to other family members. The patient should be instructed to wash the impetigo lesions twice a day with antibacterial soap.

Antifungals

Fungal infections of the skin are common in all age groups. Infants and immunocompromised patients may have thrush and *Candida* infections in the diaper area. Tinea corporis, also known as ringworm, can be found in patients of all ages. Tinea capitis is most common in children. Tinea pedis, also known as athlete's foot, can be found at any age but generally in postpubertal patients. Fungal overgrowth occurs in immunocompromised patients or patients on antibiotics.

Antifungal medications are used to treat superficial fungal infections caused by dermatophytic fungi and yeast. The topical **antifungal** medications can be roughly divided into three major categories and two medications that are not classified. The four major categories are **polyene antibiotic antifungals**, the **topical azoles**, the **benzylamines**, and the **allylamine antifungals**. **Ciclopirox olamine** and **tolnaftate** do not fit into these categories. **Gentian violet**, an older **antifungal**, is also not classified.

The topical **azoles**, which include **clotrimazole** (**Lotrimin**), **ketoconazole** (**Nizoral, Extina**), **miconazole** (**Monistat**), **econazole** (**Spectazole**), **sertaconazole** (**Ertaczo**), **oxiconazole** (**Oxistat**), and **sulconazole** (**Exelderm**), are active against common dermatophytes and yeasts. **Terbinafine** (**Lamisil**) is a topical **allylamine antifungal** indicated for the treatment of tinea versicolor, tinea pedis, and tinea corporis. Another topical **allylamine antifungal**, **naftifine** (**Naftin, Naftine-MP**), is indicated in the treatment of tinea curis, tinea corporis, and interdigital tinea pedis. **Butenafine** (**Mentax**) is a **benzylamine antifungal** indicated for the topical treatment of tinea versicolor due to *Malassezia furfur* (formerly *Pityrosporum orbiculare*); interdigital tinea pedis; tinea corporis; and tinea cruris due to *Epidermophyton floccosum*, *Trichophyton mentagrophytes*, *Trichophyton rubrum*, and *Trichophyton tonsurans*. **Ciclopirox olamine** (**Loprox**) is a broad-spectrum **N-hydroxypyridinone antifungal**. **Tolnaftate** (**Tinactin**) is an OTC product used to treat superficial fungal infections. **Nystatin** is an **antifungal antibiotic** that is both fungistatic and fungicidal and is active against a wide variety of yeasts and yeast-like fungi. Systemic **antifungals** are used to treat tinea capitis and onychomycosis. **Griseofulvin** (**Grifulvin V, Grisactin**) is the first-line drug choice in the treatment of tinea capitis. Onychomycosis may be treated with topical **ciclopirox** (**Penlac**) or systemic **griseofulvin**, **ketoconazole** (**Nizoral**), **itraconazole** (**Sporanox**), or **terbinafine** (**Lamisil**). The pharmacological management of systemic fungal infections is discussed in Chapter 24.

Pharmacodynamics

Topical Antifungals

Nystatin is a **topical antifungal antibiotic** that is nearly identical to **amphotericin B** in structure. **Nystatin** is a **polyene antifungal.** It is effective only against *Candida.* **Nystatin** binds to sterols in the cell membranes of both fungal and human cells. When the **nystatin** binds to the sterols in the cell membrane of the fungus, it causes a change in membrane permeability that allows leakage of intracellular components.

Gentian violet is bactericidal to gram-positive organisms in very high concentration. It inhibits the growth of *Candida* and *Candida albicans.*

The **topical azole antifungals** all act in a similar fashion. They appear to alter the fungal cell membrane by inhibiting ergosterol synthesis through interacting with 14-alpha-demethylase, an essential component of the membrane. This causes leakage of cellular contents, such as potassium- and phosphorus-containing compounds. **Clotrimazole** is active against a wide variety of fungi, yeasts, and dermatophytes. Organisms that are susceptible to **clotrimazole** include *Aspergillus fumigatus, C. albicans, Cephalosporium, M. furfur, T. rubrum,* and some strains of *S. aureus* and *S. pyogenes.* **Miconazole** inhibits the growth of common dermatophytes *T. rubrum, T. mentagrophytes, C. albicans,* and the active organism in tinea versicolor, *M. furfur.* **Ketoconazole** is a broad-spectrum antifungal agent that is active against the dermatophytes *T. rubrum; T. mentagrophytes; T. tonsurans; Microsporum canis; E. floccosum;* and the yeast organisms *C. albicans, Candida tropicalis, Pityrosporum ovale,* and *P. orbiculare,* also known as *M. furfur,* the organism responsible for tinea versicolor. **Econazole** and **oxiconazole** have activity similar to that of **ketoconazole. Sertaconazole** is only indicated for use in the treatment of interdigit tinea pedis and is active against *T. rubrum, T. mentagrophytes,* and *E. floccosum.*

Terbinafine and **naftifine** are allylamine **antifungals** that probably exert their antifungal effectiveness by inhibiting squalene epoxidase, a key enzyme in sterol biosynthesis in fungi. This results in the accumulation of squalene within the fungal cell and causes fungal cell death. **Terbinafine** has fungicidal activity against dermatophytes. It is less active, however, against *Candida.*

Tolnaftate distorts hyphae and stunts mycelial growth in susceptible fungi.

Butenafine is the first of a newer class of topical **antifungal** agents, the **benzylamines. Butenafine** is effective against *C. albicans.* It acts to inhibit fungal ergosterol biosynthesis by interfering with the conversion of squalene into 2,3-oxidosqualene. At higher concentrations, **butenafine** may exert a direct membrane-damaging effect on fungal cell membranes. It is also active against *T. rubrum* and *T. mentagrophytes.*

Ciclopirox olamine is a broad-spectrum **antifungal** agent. It acts on the cell membrane to block transmembrane transport of amino acids into the fungal cell. At higher concentrations, the fungal cell membrane integrity is altered, allowing leakage of intracellular material. It inhibits the growth of pathogenic dermatophytes, yeasts, and *M. furfur.* **Ciclopirox nail lacquer** penetrates the nail to achieve minimum inhibitory concentrations (MIC) levels high enough to be fungicidal to most organisms responsible for onychomycosis.

Systemic Antifungals

The systemic **antifungal** agents used in the treatment of fungal infections of the skin include **griseofulvin**; the **azoles ketoconazole, itraconazole,** and **fluconazole**; and the oral allylamine **terbinafine.**

Griseofulvin is an **antifungal antibiotic** produced by certain species of *Penicillium.* **Griseofulvin** exerts its fungistatic activity by disrupting the mitotic spindle structure of the fungal cell. This arrests metaphase cell division. **Griseofulvin** may also produce defective DNA. **Griseofulvin** has an affinity to keratin precursor cells. It is deposited in the keratin precursor cells, which are gradually exfoliated and replaced by uninfected tissue. **Griseofulvin** has a greater affinity for diseased tissue than for healthy tissue. It is tightly bound to the new keratin, which becomes highly resistant to fungal infections.

Fluconazole is a synthetic, broad-spectrum **triazole antifungal** agent of the imidazole class. **Fluconazole** has a broader spectrum than the other **imidazole antifungals. Fluconazole** exerts its effect by altering the fungal cell membrane. It is a highly selective inhibitor of fungal CYP450 and sterol 14-alpha-demethylase. This inhibition results in increased cellular permeability, causing leakage of cellular contents.

Ketoconazole alters the permeability of the cell membrane and inhibits fungal synthesis of phospholipids. **Itraconazole** is a synthetic **triazole antifungal** medication that is closely related to **ketoconazole.** Similar to **ketoconazole,** it exerts its effect by altering the fungal cell membrane. **Itraconazole** inhibits the CYP450-dependent synthesis of ergosterol, which increases cellular permeability and causes leakage of cellular contents.

Terbinafine is an **allylamine antifungal** that exerts its antifungal effect through interfering with fungal sterol biosynthesis by inhibiting the enzyme squalene monooxygenase. This causes accumulation of squalene, which weakens the cell membrane in sensitive fungi. The accumulation of squalene within the fungal cell causes fungal cell death. **Terbinafine** has fungicidal activity against dermatophytes. It is less active against *Candida.* **Naftifine**'s mechanism of action is not known, but it probably works similarly to **terbinafine.**

Pharmacokinetics

Absorption and Distribution

Topical Antifungals

Topical **antifungals** are poorly absorbed from intact skin. **Nystatin** is not absorbed from intact skin or mucous membranes. Absorption information on **gentian violet** is unavailable. The topical **azoles** have little or no systemic absorption following topical application. When applied topically, **ciclopirox olamine** is minimally absorbed (average of 1.3%). **Butenafine**, when applied topically, is absorbed through the skin into the systemic circulation in amounts that have not been quantified. Absorption and distribution of **tolnaftate** have not been described. **Terbinafine** may be systemically absorbed when applied topically. **Naftifine** is minimally absorbed when applied topically, with 4.2 percent of the dose absorbed. Systemic absorption of topically administered **terbinafine** is much lower than that of orally administered **terbinafine**.

Systemic Antifungals

Griseofulvin and **terbinafine** are the two systemic **antifungals** discussed in this chapter, as they are primarily used in dermatological diseases. See Chapter 24 for further information on systemic **antifungal** medications.

Griseofulvin is poorly absorbed, and therefore oral formulations have been developed in an attempt to increase bioavailability. Microsize **griseofulvin** has a variable and unpredictable oral absorption. Ultramicrosize **griseofulvin** has almost complete absorption. Oral **griseofulvin** is absorbed mainly from the duodenum. Absorption of oral microsize **griseofulvin** may be increased by intake of high-fat food. **Griseofulvin** is widely distributed and concentrates in the skin, hair, nails, fat, and skeletal muscles. **Griseofulvin** does cross the placenta. Distribution in breast milk is unknown but should be assumed because of **griseofulvin**'s affinity for fat.

Terbinafine, when administered orally, is well absorbed from the gut. Bioavailability is approximately 40 percent. Administration with food increases the serum area under the curve (AUC) of **terbinafine** by 20 percent. **Terbinafine** is widely distributed, including the central nervous system (CNS), hair, and nailbeds. Following 2 weeks of therapy at recommended doses, **terbinafine** remains in the skin for up to 3 months. The drug may be detected in the nails for up to 90 days following treatment. It is unknown whether **terbinafine** crosses the placenta, but **terbinafine** is excreted in the breast milk of nursing mothers with a milk/plasma ratio of 7:1.

Metabolism and Excretion

Topical Antifungals

Topical **antifungals** are either not absorbed or absorbed minimally. Therefore, metabolism information regarding nystatin, **tolnaftate, oxiconazole, sulconazole, butenafine, sertaconazole, ciclopirox olamine**, and topical **ketoconazole** is not available. Topically administered **miconazole** is minimally absorbed following application to intact skin, with 1 percent of a dose applied six times daily for 14 days recovered in urine and feces. Metabolism of oral **miconazole** occurs mainly in the liver, and the small amount of topical medication that is absorbed is assumed to be also metabolized in this manner. Topical application of **econazole** results in lower systemic absorption. Less than 1 percent of an applied dose is recovered in urine and feces. Metabolism of **econazole** is unknown. There is little systemic absorption of **clotrimazole** following topical application. The small amounts absorbed are metabolized in the liver and excreted in the bile.

Systemic Antifungals

Griseofulvin is metabolized in the liver, mainly through oxidative demethylation and conjugation with glucuronic acid. The major metabolite is inactive. **Griseofulvin** is excreted through the urine, feces, and perspiration.

Terbinafine is metabolized in the liver through oxidation and hydrolysis to five inactive metabolites. Seventy percent of the oral **terbinafine** dose is excreted in the urine as conjugated and unconjugated metabolites. Clearance of **terbinafine** is decreased by approximately 50 percent in patients with renal impairment or hepatic cirrhosis.

Pharmacotherapeutics

Precautions and Contraindications

Topical Antifungals

There are few contraindications to the topical **antifungal** medications. Hypersensitivity to the antifungal agent or any of the components of the formulation is a contraindication. Patients with **azole** hypersensitivity are often sensitive to all **azole** derivatives. The **antifungal** agent should be discontinued if sensitization occurs. The use of **antifungals** around the eyes should be avoided. Gentian violet is contraindicated in ulcerated areas and in patients with porphyria. **Ketoconazole** cream contains sulfites that may cause allergic types of reactions, including anaphylactic symptoms and life-threatening or less severe asthmatic episodes in susceptible persons. **Ciclopirox topical nail lacquer (Penlac)** should not be used in immunocompromised or diabetic patients with onychomycosis.

The topical **antifungals** that are classified Pregnancy Category B are **clotrimazole, oxiconazole, ciclopirox olamine, naftifine,** and **butenafine.** The topical **antifungals** classified as Pregnancy Category C are **nystatin, ketoconazole, gentian violet, sulconazole, tolnaftate, miconazole, sertaconazole,** and **econazole.** Of these, only **ketoconazole** and **econazole** have demonstrated teratogenic effects in animal tests with doses 10 times the maximum recommended human dose. Therefore, **ketoconazole** and **econazole** should be used in pregnant women only when potential benefits to the mother outweigh the potential risk to the fetus. Although systemic absorption following topical application is extremely low, caution is advised in prescribing **econazole** or **ketoconazole** to breastfeeding women. The use of topical antifungals on the breast during lactation is not advised. If antifungal medication is needed to treat such a topical infection in a lactating woman, application of oral nystatin suspension to the affected area on the breast is suggested for safety.

The safety of topical antifungals for infants and children varies from product to product. Nystatin, gentian violet, and miconazole are all safe for use in infants and children. Econazole is safe for topical use in children as young as 3 months. Tolnaftate, topical ketoconazole, and topical clotrimazole are contraindicated in children younger than 2 years, although topical clotrimazole is used for short periods in children younger than 2 without adverse effects. The safety of ciclopirox olamine for use in children younger than 10 years has not been established. Butenafine, oxiconazole, sertaconazole, terbinafine, and naftifine have not had safety and effectiveness established for children younger than 12 years.

Systemic Antifungals

Griseofulvin should be used cautiously in patients with hepatic disease. It may be hepatotoxic on rare occasions. Patients with systemic lupus erythematosus (SLE) or lupus-like syndromes should use griseofulvin with caution because it has been known to exacerbate lupus. Griseofulvin is contraindicated in patients with porphyria or hypersensitivity to griseofulvin. There is a possibility of cross-sensitivity to griseofulvin in patients with penicillin hypersensitivity because griseofulvin is produced by a species of *Penicillium*. This cross-sensitivity is theoretical, and patients have been treated with griseofulvin without adverse effects.

Griseofulvin is Pregnancy Category C. Its use should be avoided in pregnant women because some women who received the drug during pregnancy reportedly have had spontaneous abortions or delivered infants with congenital abnormalities. Griseofulvin may be used safely in children as young as 2 years.

Terbinafine is contraindicated in patients who have known hypersensitivity to terbinafine or any of its components. Terbinafine should be used with caution in patients with hepatic disease or renal impairment (creatinine clearance 50 mL/min). Dosage adjustment may be needed in these patients. Terbinafine is rated Pregnancy Category B. Terbinafine should be used in pregnancy only if the potential benefit to the mother outweighs the potential risk to the fetus; treatment of onychomycosis can be postponed until after pregnancy is completed. It is recommended that terbinafine not be used during pregnancy. Oral terbinafine treatment is not recommended during lactation. After oral administration, terbinafine is excreted into the breast milk and can be found in the breast milk in a milk/plasma ratio of 7:1. A decision should be made whether to discontinue breastfeeding or to discontinue terbinafine. Terbinafine may be prescribed for children 4 years of age or older to treat tinea capitis.

Adverse Drug Reactions

Topical Antifungals

Adverse reactions are minimal with topical antifungal medications. Nystatin may cause mild skin irritation when applied topically to some patients, usually related to the preservative (parabens) in the formulation. The main adverse reaction seen in gentian violet is staining of the skin and clothing, which can be significant. It may also cause local burning and skin reactions when used on the oral mucosa or other mucous membranes. The topical azoles may all cause itching, stinging, burning, or general skin irritation. Note that cross-sensitization among the topical azoles has been reported. Adverse reactions to topical azoles occur in approximately 1 to 3 percent of patients treated. The only adverse reaction reported with tolnaftate is mild skin irritation. The allylamine antifungals butenafine and naftifine may cause burning, stinging, dryness, erythema, pruritus, local irritation, and rash. Ciclopirox olamine may cause skin irritation, pruritus at the application site, redness, pain, burning, and worsening of clinical symptoms. Ciclopirox nail lacquer may cause change in shape or discoloration of nail.

Systemic Antifungals

The most common adverse reaction with griseofulvin is hypersensitivity, such as skin rashes, urticaria, and rarely angioedema. Less commonly reported adverse reactions are oral thrush, nausea, vomiting, epigastric distress, and diarrhea. Several CNS effects have been reported. Headache occurs frequently in the beginning of therapy but often disappears with continued therapy. Other CNS adverse effects include fatigue, dizziness, insomnia, confusion, and impaired performance of routine activities. Hepatitis and elevated hepatic enzymes have been reported in a few patients after prolonged use or high doses of griseofulvin. A rare adverse effect of granulocytopenia or leukopenia has been reported from prolonged use of high doses of griseofulvin. Griseofulvin should be discontinued if the patient exhibits these conditions. When rare serious reactions occur with griseofulvin, they are usually associated with high doses or long periods of therapy.

Approximately 17 percent of patients taking oral terbinafine experience adverse reactions. The most common adverse reactions with oral terbinafine are gastrointestinal (GI) symptoms such as diarrhea (5.6%), dyspepsia (4.3%), abdominal pain (2.4%), nausea (2.6%), and flatulence. Two to three percent of patients taking oral terbinafine reported headache, dizziness, rash (unspecified), urticaria, and pruritus. Elevated liver enzymes occurred in 2 to 3 percent of patients taking terbinafine. Dysgeusia occurs in 2 percent of patients. Rare but serious adverse reactions observed with oral terbinafine include serious skin reactions (Stevens-Johnson syndrome and toxic epidermal neurolysis). Rare cases of blood dyscrasia have been reported with **terbinafine** use. Severe neutropenia, lymphopenia, thrombocytopenia, and agranulocytosis have all been reported with oral **terbinafine** use. In clinical trials, 1 to 2 percent of patients treated with oral **terbinafine** developed decreased absolute lymphocyte cells (less than 1,000/mm^3). These hematological adverse reactions are reversible with discontinuation of oral **terbinafine.**

Drug Interactions

Topical Antifungals

There are few drug interactions found with topical antifungal medications. The only significant interactions noted for topical **antifungals** are with **clotrimazole** and **econazole. Clotrimazole** and theoretically the other azole **antifungals** inhibit the synthesis of the fungal sterol ergosterol; the polyene **antifungals**, such as amphotericin B and **nystatin**, act by binding to ergosterol. Therefore, the azole **antifungals** could interfere with the action of either **amphotericin B** or **nystatin** by depleting polyene-binding sites. This appears to be the most significant when the **azole antifungal** is given prior to **amphotericin B. Clotrimazole** intravaginal preparations should not be administered concurrently with **nonoxynol-9** and **octoxynol. Clotrimazole** may inactivate the **spermicides**, leading to contraceptive failure. **Corticosteroids** may inhibit the antifungal activity of **econazole** against *C. albicans* in a concentration-dependent manner. When the concentration of **corticosteroid** is equal to the concentration of **econazole**, the antifungal activity of **econazole** is inhibited. When the **corticosteroid** concentration is 10 percent of that of **econazole**, there is no inhibition of antifungal activity.

Systemic Antifungals

Systemic antifungal medications have a number of drug interactions. **Griseofulvin** can increase some of the effects of **ethanol**, causing the patient to experience tachycardia, diaphoresis, and flushing. **Griseofulvin** can accelerate the hepatic metabolism of some medications. **Griseofulvin** may also decrease the hypoprothrombinemic activity of **warfarin**, which decreases its anticoagulant effect. Prothrombin time should be monitored closely if **griseofulvin** is either added or discontinued from **warfarin** therapy. **Estrogens** or **estrogen-containing oral contraceptives** can be affected by coadministration of **griseofulvin.** Patients may experience breakthrough bleeding, amenorrhea, or unintended pregnancy. They should use an alternative or second form of contraception while they are taking **griseofulvin** and for 1 month after **griseofulvin** is discontinued. **Griseofulvin** may reduce **cyclosporine** levels, resulting in decreased pharmacological effects. An increase in **cyclosporine** dose may be necessary if **griseofulvin** is added. A second dosage adjustment may be necessary if **griseofulvin** is discontinued. Serum **salicylate** concentrations may be decreased with **griseofulvin** use. Certain medications, including **barbiturates** and **primidone**, may impair the absorption of **griseofulvin**, resulting in decreased serum concentrations. Food can also affect the absorption of **griseofulvin.** Eating a high-fat meal at the time of dosing may increase microsize **griseofulvin** absorption.

Terbinafine clearance is affected by a number of medications. It is decreased by **cimetidine** and **terfenadine** and increased by **rifampin. Caffeine** clearance is decreased by **terbinafine. Cyclosporine** clearance is increased by **terbinafine. Theophylline** clearance is decreased by **terbinafine.** Patients taking **theophylline, aminophylline,** or **cyclosporine** concurrently with **terbinafine** should be monitored closely for increased or decreased effects of these medications with a narrow therapeutic window. **Terbinafine** may affect the metabolism of **warfarin,** leading to bleeding and coagulopathy.

Clinical Use and Dosing

Candidiasis

There are more than 150 recognized species of *Candida* that can cause a variety of clinical syndromes that are termed candidiasis and usually categorized by the site of involvement. The most common sites for mucocutaneous candidiasis are the mouth, where it causes stomatitis or thrush; the esophagus, where it causes esophagitis; and the vagina, where it causes yeast vaginitis. *Candida* can also be invasive or systemic, aspects that are not discussed in this chapter. In most patients, candidiasis is an opportunistic disease. *C. albicans* is the most common pathogen in humans; another common pathogen in humans is *C. tropicalis. C. albicans* is part of the normal human flora of the mouth, GI tract, and vagina. It normally lives in balance with other microorganisms within the body. When drugs or conditions, such as broad-spectrum **antibiotics, corticosteroids,** diabetes mellitus, or HIV infection, offset this balance, *C. albicans* may become a pathogen and cause mucocutaneous disease. *Candida* species may be transmitted from person to person, by direct contact either by hands or sexual contact, or during birth from colonized vagina to neonatal oropharynx. Candidiasis has emerged as the most common opportunistic fungal disease.

The first-line treatment for cutaneous *Candida* infections are the OTC **azoles, miconazole** and **clotrimazole,** which are applied twice daily to the affected skin area until clear (Table 23–2). For thrush in patients older than 3 years, a 10-mg **clotrimazole troche** is slowly and completely dissolved in the mouth five times a day for 14 days. Longer therapy may be needed in immunosuppressed patients.

For the patient who does not tolerate the azole **antifungals, nystatin** can be prescribed. **Nystatin** in cream, ointment, or powder formulation can be applied to the affected area two to three times per day until

Table 23–2 ◉ **Dosage Schedule: Selected Anti-Infectives Used to Treat Skin Disorders**

Drug	Indication	Dosage
Antibacterial		
Bacitracin	Minor cuts, wound, impetigo (1 or 2 lesions only)	Apply a small amount to the affected area once or twice daily; do not use >1 wk
Mupirocin	Impetigo	Apply a small amount to the lesions tid; may cover with gauze
	Nasal colonization with MRSA	Half the ointment from a single-use tube of nasal ointment into one nostril, and the other half into the other nostril bid for 5 d; children may require smaller amounts of ointment
Retapamulin	Impetigo	Age ≥9 mo: apply thin layer twice daily for 5 days. Reevaluate if no improvement in 3 to 4 d
Neomycin	Minor cuts, wounds, impetigo (1 or 2 lesions only)	Apply a small amount to the affected area 1–2 times daily; do not use >1 wk
Polymyxin B	Minor cuts, wounds, impetigo (1 or 2 lesions only)	Apply a small amount to the affected area 1–2 times daily; do not use >1 wk
Double antibiotic (polymyxin B, bacitracin)	Minor cuts, wounds, impetigo	Apply small amount 1–3 times daily to affected area
Triple-antibiotic ointment (polymyxin B, neomycin, bacitracin)	Minor cuts, wounds, impetigo (1 or 2 lesions only)	Apply a small amount to the affected area 1–3 times daily; do not use >1 wk
Antifungals		
Butenafine	Tinea corporis, tinea cruris	Apply to affected and immediately surrounding area once daily for 2 wk
Ciclopirox olamine	Tinea corporis, tinea cruris	Massage into affected skin bid for at least 2 wk Treat tinea pedis for 4 wk
Clotrimazole	Oral candidiasis	Adults and children >3 yr: 1 troche 5 times daily for 14 consecutive d; dissolve slowly in mouth Children <3 yr: Not recommended
	Fungal skin infections, including candidiasis	Apply to affected area bid for 2 wk
	Tinea pedis	Treat tinea pedis for 4 wk
Econazole	Tinea corporis, tinea cruris Tinea pedis	Apply to affected area once daily for 2 wk minimum Apply once daily; treat for 4 wk minimum
Gentian violet	Oral candidiasis	All ages: apply with cotton swab to entire inner surface of the mouth twice daily until clear
Ketoconazole	Tinea corporis, tinea cruris Tinea pedis	Apply once daily to affected area for 2 wk Apply once daily; treat for 6 wk
Miconazole	Fungal skin infections, including candidiasis Tinea pedis	Apply to affected area 2–3 times daily for 2 wk Treat tinea pedis for 4 wk minimum
Naftifine	Tinea corporis, tinea cruris, tinea pedis	Apply cream once daily until clear, up to 4 wk; gel is applied bid until clear
Nystatin oral suspension	Oral candidiasis	Adults and children: 2–3 mL in each inner cheek (total dose 4–6 mL) qid; have patient hold medication in mouth as long as possible before swallowing; treat for 48 h after clinical cure to prevent relapse Infants: 1 mL each cheek qid (2 mL/dose total), until 48 h after clinical cure; may apply medication to inner cheeks and tongue with cotton swab prior to administering the 1-mL dose via dropper

Table 23–2 ◉ **Dosage Schedule: Selected Anti-Infectives Used to Treat Skin Disorders—cont'd**

Drug	Indication	Dosage
Nystatin cream or ointment	Cutaneous ***Candida*** infections	All ages: apply to affected areas 2 or 3 times/d until clear
Oxiconazole	Tinea corporis, tinea capitis, tinea pedis	Apply to affected area once or twice/d for 2 wk Apply 1 or 2 times daily; treat for 4 wk
Sertaconazole	Interdigital tinea pedis in immunocompetent patients	Dry area Apply to affected and adjacent areas bid for 4 wk
Sulconazole	Tinea corporis, tinea cruris Tinea pedis	Massage medication into affected area once or twice a day for 3 wk Apply bid for 4 wk
Terbinafine	Tinea corporis, tinea cruris Tinea pedis	Apply to affected and immediate surrounding areas bid until clinical symptoms are significantly improved, usually 1 wk Apply to affected and immediately surrounding area bid until symptoms are significantly improved, usually 2 wk
Tolnaftate	Tinea pedis	Apply to affected area bid for 2–3 wk; if skin is thickened, treatment may take 4–6 wk; apply sparingly and massage in well; for maintenance or prophylaxis, apply powder once daily
Antivirals		
Acyclovir	Initial herpes genitalis Mucocutaneous herpes simplex virus (HSV) infections in immunocompromised patients	Apply to lesion every 3 h, 6 times daily for 7 d
Docosanol	Recurrent oral-facial herpes simplex episodes	Gently rub into affected area 5 times daily until healed. Begin treatment at earliest sign or symptom
Penciclovir	Recurrent herpes labialis (cold sores) on lips and face	Apply q2h while awake for 4 d; begin treatment at earliest sign or symptom

MRSA = methicillin-resistant *staphylococcus aureus.*

clear (Table 23–3). Cream is preferred to ointment in intertriginous areas. Treatment should continue for at least 2 weeks. For thrush, the dose in adults and children is 4 to 6 mL of **nystatin** suspension, which is swished around the mouth and swallowed four times per day. The dose in infants is 2 mL, with 1 mL applied on each side of the mouth four times per day. The dose of **nystatin** for neonates is 0.5 mL applied to each side of the mouth four times per day. Adults and older children can use **nystatin** troches, which are slowly dissolved in the mouth. Treatment should continue until symptoms have been resolved for 48 hours.

For refractory oral candidiasis, **gentian violet** may be used. The dose in infants is 3 to 4 drops of a 0.5 percent solution on the tongue or on the inner cheeks after feeding twice per day. Alternatively, a cotton-tipped swab can be dipped into the **gentian violet** and swabbed onto the inner cheeks and tongue. In adults and older children, a 1 or 2 percent solution may be applied to the affected area twice daily. The patient is to avoid swallowing the solution. Care should be used when applying **gentian violet**, which will stain any skin or clothing that it touches.

Second-line treatment for cutaneous *Candida* infections includes other prescription **azole antifungal** medications. **Econazole** is applied to the affected area twice daily for at least 2 weeks. **Ketoconazole** is applied once daily for at least 2 weeks. **Oxiconazole** is applied to the affected and immediately surrounding areas once or twice daily until clear. **Sulconazole** may be gently massaged into the affected areas and surrounding skin once daily until clear.

Other **antifungals** effective against *Candida* species include **ciclopirox olamine, naftifine,** and **butenafine. Ciclopirox olamine** is gently massaged into the affected skin and surrounding area twice daily until clinical improvement occurs. **Naftifine** is gently massaged into the affected area once a day for the cream formulation and twice a day for the gel formulation, until clinical clearing is observed. Topical **butenafine** is used in adults and children older than 12 years, and it is applied to the

Table 23–3 ■ **Available Dosage Forms: Selected Anti-Infectives Used to Treat Skin Infections**

Drug	Dosage Form	How Supplied	Cost
Antibacterials			
Bacitracin (OTC)			
• Baciguent	500 U/g ointment	In 15- and 30-g tubes	
• Generic	500 U/g ointment	In 1-, 15-, and 30-g tubes, 1-lb tubs	$4.29
Mupirocin (Rx)			
• Bactroban	2% ointment	In 22-g tubes	$73.50
	2% cream	In 15-g tubes	$62.17
	2% cream	In 30-g tubes	$92.21
	2% nasal ointment	In 10 × 1-g tubes	$45.99
Retapamulin (Rx) Altabax	1% ointment	In 5-g tubes	$49
		In 10-g tubes	$75
		In 15-g tubes	$95
Neomycin (OTC)			
• Myciguent	3.5 mg/g ointment or cream	In 15-g and 30-g tubes	
• Generic	3.5 mg/g ointment	In 15-g tubes	
		In 30-g tubes	
Triple-antibiotic ointment (polymyxin B, neomycin, and bacitracin) (OTC)			
• Neosporin Maximum Strength	Polysporin 10,000 U/g, neomycin 3.5 mg/g, bacitracin 400 U/g	In 15-g tubes	$10
• Generic	Polysporin 5,000 U/g, neomycin 3.5 mg/g, bacitracin 400 U/g	In 2.4-g tubes	$6.74
		In 9.6-g tubes	
		In 15-g tubes	
		In 30-g tubes	
Antifungals			
Butenafine (Rx)		In 15 g tube	$50.99
• Mentax	1% cream	In 30 g tube	$119.78
Lotrimin ultra (OTC)	1% cream	In 24-g tubes	$10.99 (12 g)
Ciclopirox olamine (Rx)			
• Loprox	0.77% cream	In 15 g tube	$24.99
		In 30 g tube	$44.99
		In 90 g tube	$109.99
Generic	0.77% lotion	In 30 mL	$107.88 (30 g)
		In 60 mL	$147
		In 90 g-tubes	$254.40
Clotrimazole			
• Lotrimin (Rx)	1% cream	In 15 g	
	1% lotion	In 30 g	
	1% solution	In 90 g	
		In 30 mL	
		In 10 mL	$8.49
		30 mL	
• Lotrimin AF (OTC)	1% cream	In 12 g	$9.49
		In 24 g	$12.99
	1% lotion	In 10 mL	
• Generic	1% cream	In 30 g	$8.99
Econazole (Rx)			
• Spectazole	1% cream	In 15 g	$27
		In 30 g	$46
		In 85 g	$90

Table 23–3 ■ **Available Dosage Forms: Selected Anti-Infectives Used to Treat Skin Infections—cont'd**

Drug	Dosage Form	How Supplied	Cost
Generic	1% cream	In 15-g tubes	$15.99
	1% cream	In 30-g tubes	$24.05
	1% cream	In 85-g tubes	$49.99
Gentian violet (OTC)	1% solution	In 30 mL	$4.99
	2% solution		$10.99
Ketoconazole			
• Nizoral	2% cream	In 15 g	
		In 30 g	
		In 60 g	
	2% shampoo	In 4 oz	
		In 120 mL	$31.57
• Nizoral A-D Shampoo (OTC)	1% shampoo	In 4 oz	
		In 7 oz	$15.49
• Generic	2% cream	In 15-g tubes	$19.99
	2% cream	In 30-g tubes	$27.28
	2% cream	In 60-g tubes	$35.99
	2% shampoo	In 120-mL bottles	$27.53
Miconazole			
• Monistat Derm (Rx)			
	2% cream	In 15 g	$32
	2% cream	In 28 g	$41.99
• Micatin (OTC)	2% powder	In 3 oz	$7.29
• Desenex OTC	2% spray	In 3 oz	$7.49 (28 g)
• Generic	2% cream	In 3 oz	$12.99 (28 g)
Naftifine (Rx)			
• Naftin	1% cream	In 15 g tubes	$31.69
		In 30 g tubes	$101.62
		In 60 g tubes	$183.77
	1% gel	In 20 g tubes	
		In 40 g tubes	$147
		In 60 g tubes	$208.50
Nystatin (Rx)			
• Nilstat	100,000 U/g cream (topical)	In 15 g	
		In 30 g	
	100,000 U/g ointment (topical)	In 15 g	
		In 30 g	
• Mycostatin	100,000 U/mL suspension (PO)	In 60 mL with dropper, 16 oz	
	Pastilles 200,000 U each (PO)	In 30s	$28.99
		In 15 g	
	100,000 U/g cream	In 15 g	
		In 30 g	$35.19
		In 30 g	
	100,000 U/g powder (topical)	In 15 g	
		In 30 g	$83.69
• Generic	100,000 U/g cream (topical)	In 15 g	$12.99/2 tubes
		In 30 g	
	100,000 U/g ointment (topical)	In 30 g	$12.99 (15 g)
	100,000 U/g cream (topical)		
	100,000 U/g ointment (topical)		
• Generic	100,000 U/mL suspension	In 180 mL	$42.98
	100,000 U/mL suspension	In 60 mL	$22.59

Continued

Table 23–3 ■ **Available Dosage Forms: Selected Anti-Infectives Used to Treat Skin Infections—cont'd**

Drug	Dosage Form	How Supplied	Cost
Oxiconazole (Rx)			
• Oxistat	1% cream	In 15 g	$48.99
		In 30 g	$83.58
		In 60 g	$157.99
	1% lotion	In 30 mL	$93.13
Sertaconazole			
• Ertaczo	2% cream	In 30 g tubes	$57.05
Sulconazole (Rx)			
• Exelderm	1% cream	In 15 g	$58.25
		In 30 g	$95.06
		In 60 g	$121.42
	1% solution	In 30 mL	$76.46
Terbinafine			
• Lamisil AT (OTC)	1% cream	In 12 g	$15.79 (30 g)
		In 24 g	
• Lamisil Solution	1% solution	In 30 mL	$10.99
Tolnaftate (OTC)			
• Tinactin	1% cream	In 15 g	
		In 30 g	$11.99
	1% solution	In 10 mL	
	1% powder	In 45 g	
		In 108 g	$7.99
	1% spray powder	In 100 g	$7.59
		In 150 g	$7.99
		In 133 g	$7.99
	1% spray liquid	In 120 mL	
• Aftate	1% gel	In 15 g	
• Generic	1% cream	In 15 g	
	1% solution	In 10 mL	
	1% powder	In 45 g	
	1% spray powder	In 105 g	
Antivirals			
Acyclovir (Rx)	5% cream	In 5-g tubes	$152.90
		In 2-g tubes	$69.44
• Zovirax	5% ointment	In 3-g tubes	
		In 15-g tubes	$171.35
Penciclovir (Rx)			
• Denavir	1% cream	In 1.5 g	$53.80
Docosanol			
• Abreva (OTC)	10% cream	In 2 g	$18.99

affected areas once daily until clear. Safety in children younger than 12 years has not been established.

An optional second-line treatment for oropharyngeal candidiasis (thrush) is systemic **fluconazole**. The dosage in adults is 200 mg orally (PO) on the first day, then 100 mg PO once daily for 14 days. Dosing in children, infants, and neonates older than 14 days is 6 mg/kg PO on the first day, followed by 3 mg/kg PO once daily for 14 days. Neonates younger than 14 days have the same dose as infants, except it should be given every 72 hours instead of once daily until age 2 weeks. Clinical improvement is rapid with **fluconazole**, with lesions on the inner cheeks often clearing within the first 1 or 2 days of treatment, but treatment should continue for the full 14 days. This point should be stressed to patients.

Tinea Capitis

Tinea capitis is commonly called ringworm of the scalp. The causative organisms are *Microsporum* species and *T. tonsurans*. *Microsporum* presents usually with broken hairs and a fine gray scale. *Trichophyton* causes "black dot" tinea, which presents with tiny black dots that are the remains of broken hair shafts. Definitive diagnosis is obtained by fungal culture. As fungal cultures may take 2 to 4 weeks for results, treatment is begun while awaiting results.

Treatment of tinea capitis consists of oral **antifungal** therapy with **griseofulvin** and biweekly shampooing with **sporicidal shampoo.** Tinea capitis should always be treated with a systemic **antifungal.** The treatment of choice is **griseofulvin,** with treatment to continue for 6 to 8 weeks or until 2 weeks after potassium hydroxide (KOH) or culture is negative. The dosing for **griseofulvin microsize** for adults is 500 mg daily in one or two doses. For children, the dose of **griseofulvin microsize** is 11 mg/kg/day in a single dose. For **ultramicrosize griseofulvin,** the adult dose is 330 to 375 mg/day, and the pediatric dose is 7.3 mg/kg/day in a single dose. **Griseofulvin** is absorbed more easily with a high-fat meal (whole milk, cheese, or ice cream), and the patient should be instructed about this point when beginning treatment.

The patient should also be treated with a **sporicidal shampoo** such as **selenium sulfide** or **ketoconazole.** The patient should shampoo with either the **selenium sulfide** 2.5 percent shampoo or **ketoconazole** 2 percent shampoo twice weekly until clear. Close contacts should be empirically treated with **sporicidal shampoo** twice per week. Six weeks of **griseofulvin** combined with **selenium sulfide** shampoo for 6 weeks results in an 89 percent clinical cure (Lorch Dauk, Conroy, Blumer, O'Riordan, & Furman, 2010).

If the patient is not responding to therapy, a culture should be obtained if it has not already been started. Cases resistant to **griseofulvin** may be treated with systemic **terbinafine, fluconazole,** or **itraconazole,** based on the sensitivity of the organism as determined by culture. Resistance to **griseofulvin** is not common, but by culturing the patient at the beginning of therapy, the provider will have sensitivity studies on which to base the treatment decision if there is no response after 4 weeks of treatment. Dosing information regarding systemic **terbinafine, fluconazole,** and **itraconazole** can be found in Chapter 24.

Tinea Corporis

Tinea corporis is a superficial fungal infection of the skin, also known as ringworm. The causative organism is *M. canis, T. tonsurans, or E. floccosum.* Tinea corporis presents as an annular lesion with raised borders and a clear center. There may be scaling and usually some erythema. It is spread by direct contact with an infected person or animal. Diagnosis is made by KOH scrapings, Wood's lamp, or fungal culture. Treatment is topical **antifungal** cream, with **miconazole, tolnaftate,** or **clotrimazole** the most common medications used. Other topical **antifungals** may be used, including **terbinafine, butenafine, sulconazole, naftifine, ciclopirox olamine, ketoconazole,** and **econazole.**

Tinea Cruris

Tinea cruris is also known as jock itch. It is a superficial fungal infection of the groin, upper thighs, and intertriginous folds. It is more common in males and rarely occurs before adolescence. The causative fungal organisms are *E. floccosum, T. rubrum,* and *T. mentagrophytes. C. albicans* may also be a causative organism. The lesions are scaly with a raised border, erythematous, and slightly brown in color. The treatment for tinea cruris is the same topical **antifungal** medications that are used for tinea corporis, with the same dosing schedule.

Tinea Pedis

Tinea pedis is a superficial fungal infection of the skin of the feet, commonly called athlete's foot. It is caused by the dermatophytes *E. floccosum, T. rubrum,* and T. *mentagrophytes. C. albicans* may also be a causative organism. Tinea pedis is more common in males and rarely occurs before puberty. Diagnosis is made by the classic clinical presentation of scaling, maceration, fissuring, and inflammation on the feet, especially in the inner digital areas. Treatment for tinea pedis is the same topical agents used for tinea corporis. Length of treatment is extended with tinea pedis, often with 4 weeks of treatment needed.

Tinea Versicolor

Tinea versicolor is a superficial fungal infection of the skin caused by *P. orbiculare.* Clinically, tinea versicolor appears as multiple scaling, oval maculae that may be hypopigmented or hyperpigmented. The treatment for tinea versicolor consists of topical application of **selenium sulfide shampoo** or a topical **antifungal. Selenium sulfide shampoo** is applied to the tinea versicolor patch and left on for 10 to 15 minutes every day for 1 week. **Selenium sulfide** can be used prophylactically once a month. The topical **azoles miconazole, clotrimazole,** and **econazole** may be used twice a day for 2 to 4 weeks in the treatment of tinea versicolor.

Onychomycosis

Onychomycosis, also known as tinea unguium, is a fungal infection of the nail, either fingernail or toenail. Treatment of onychomycosis usually involves months of a treatment with a systemic antifungal medication. Topical treatment is usually not effective with the exception of **ciclopirox nail lacquer (Penlac).** The most commonly prescribed systemic medications for onychomycosis are **griseofulvin, ketoconazole, itraconazole,** and **terbinafine.** Recent studies have demonstrated added effectiveness when topical **ciclopirox** and systemic **antifungals** are combined. Clearing of onychomycosis takes months of treatment regardless of treatment modality.

Griseofulvin has been used extensively in the treatment of onychomycosis and has a proven safety profile in adults and children. The medication should be administered for at least 4 months for onychomycosis of the fingernail. Treatment of the toenail should last at least 6 months. Renal, liver, and hematopoietic functions should be measured at least every 8 weeks during therapy. The adult dose of **griseofulvin microsize** for onychomycosis is 750 mg to 1 g/day in divided doses; the dose for **ultramicrosize** is 660 mg to 750 mg/day. The dose for children is 11 mg/kg/day of **microsize griseofulvin** and 7.3 mg/kg/day of **ultramicrosize griseofulvin**. The medication should be taken with a high-fat meal.

Ketoconazole may be used to treat onychomycosis but is usually not a first-line choice because of the associated possibility of hepatotoxicity. The dose of **ketoconazole** in adults is 200 mg daily for 4 to 6 months. The dose for children is 3.3 to 6.6 mg/kg/day in a single dose. Liver function tests should be done prior to beginning therapy and monthly for the whole course of therapy.

Itraconazole may be used for first-line therapy in adult patients with onychomycosis if a patient cannot tolerate **griseofulvin**. **Itraconazole** may be dosed in one of two methods, either daily dosing or pulse dosing. The daily dosing regimen for adults with toenail onychomycosis is 200 mg daily for 12 weeks. The pulse regimen for adults with toenail involvement is 400 mg/day for 1 week per month for 3 to 4 consecutive months. If only the fingernail area is involved, the adult dose is 200 mg bid for 7 days, then 3 weeks without treatment, and then 200 mg bid for 1 additional week. Safety in children has not been established, but multiple studies in children older than 3 years have reported no serious adverse affects (Suarez & Friedlander, 1998). For onychomycosis, the pediatric pulse dose is 5 mg/kg/day for 1 week per month for 3 to 4 consecutive months. For any patient who takes **itraconazole** for more than 8 consecutive weeks, liver enzymes and electrolytes should be drawn prior to and every 8 weeks during treatment. **Itraconazole** should not be administered to pregnant women or women considering pregnancy.

Systemic **terbinafine** has shown to be useful in the treatment of onychomycosis in both pediatric and adult trials. **Terbinafine** has an extremely long half-life, with persistence due to binding to lipophilic keratinocytes, and it can be found in toenails for 6 months after the start of a 3-month period of therapy. The dose for treating onychomycosis of the fingernail is 250 mg daily for 6 weeks. To treat an infected toenail, the dose is 250 mg daily for 12 weeks. Liver enzymes and complete blood count (CBC) should be monitored every 6 weeks if treatment lasts longer than 6 weeks. Because onychomycosis is not a serious or life-threatening disease, therapy in pregnant women should be deferred until the pregnancy is over.

Topical **ciclopirox nail lacquer (Penlac)** is applied once daily to the infected nail, preferably at bedtime. The solution is applied to the entire nailbed and surrounding 5 mm of skin. The solution must remain on the nail 8 hours before bathing. Once a week (every 7 days) previous coats of lacquer are removed with alcohol and excess nail is trimmed and filed. This routine is repeated for 48 weeks. Once a month the health-care provider should remove any unattached infected nail, and trim and file the horny material. The patient should not use nail polish during treatment.

Combining an oral **antifungal** with topical **ciclopirox** has been found in multiple studies to be more effective than either treatment alone. The combination of **terbinafine** and **ciclopirox** has the most published studies (Avner, Nir, & Henri, 2005; Baran & Kaoukhov, 2005; Gupta, Onychomycosis Combination Therapy Study Group, 2005). Dosing **ciclopirox** daily for 48 weeks combined with **terbinafine** 250 mg/day for 12 weeks or **terbinafine** 250 mg/day for 4 weeks, then 4 weeks of rest and an additional 4 weeks of **terbinafine** produced similar cure rates (70.4% vs. 66.7%) (Gupta et al, 2005). A slightly higher cure rate (88.2%) is achieved when **terbinafine** 250 mg/day for 16 weeks is combined with 9 months of topical **ciclopirox** (Avner et al, 2005). Although further studies are needed, it is reasonable to consider combining therapies in patients with onychomycosis.

Rational Drug Selection

Indication

For the treatment of thrush or oral candidiasis, the drug of choice is generally **nystatin**, with its low adverse effect profile and high efficacy. For treating topical dermatophyte infections, generally the OTC **azoles** are the first-line therapy because they are easily available without prescription and are low cost. If OTC products are not effective, then a broader spectrum **antifungal** can be prescribed, with little difference found in efficacy in treating common organisms that cause tinea infections. If treating tinea capitis or onychomycosis, **griseofulvin** is generally the drug of choice on account of its proven safety profile in both adults and children. If the patient is unable to tolerate **griseofulvin** and a culture-confirmed dermatophyte has been identified, then **itraconazole** and **ketoconazole** are appropriate second-line medications.

Cost

The cost of medication varies greatly among the **antifungals**. Generally, OTC products are less expensive than prescriptions. In the treatment of thrush, **nystatin** is a low-cost, effective therapy for topical fungal infections and is usually covered by insurance plans. When treating cutaneous fungal infections, the OTC products **clotrimazole** and **miconazole** should be the first medications used because of their low cost and their safety profile. If they are ineffective, then a prescription product with a broader spectrum may be used, but it is generally more expensive. In the treatment of tinea pedis, **tolnaftate** is available OTC in a variety of formulations; the generic products are generally the least expensive. **Griseofulvin** is the least expensive systemic antifungal. The cost of onychomycosis treatment is significant, with oral **terbinafine (Lamisil)** costing $325 for 30 tablets (http://www.costco.com). Topical **ciclopirox (Penlac)** is significantly less expensive at $143 for a 6.6-mL bottle.

Patient Variables

Many patients cannot tolerate systemic **antifungals** due to liver toxicity. Topical **ciclopirox** nail lacquer provides an alternative treatment for patients with onychomycosis who cannot tolerate systemic **antifungals**.

Monitoring

The patient being treated for oral candidiasis should be monitored for efficacy of treatment, with no laboratory monitoring necessary. The patient being treated for tinea capitis will need monitoring for adverse effects from the systemic **antifungals.** All of the systemic **antifungal** agents can possibly cause some alteration in hepatic function. If the patient is to be on continuous therapy, then baseline and ongoing monitoring of liver function is necessary. If liver enzymes become elevated, the medication should be discontinued. The patient being prescribed **griseofulvin** will require renal, liver, and hematopoietic function measurements every 8 weeks during therapy. Patients receiving **ketoconazole** require liver function tests prior to beginning therapy and monthly for the whole course of their treatment. Patients on **itraconazole** need liver enzyme and electrolyte studies if the medication is prescribed for longer than 8 consecutive weeks. In that case, liver function and electrolytes should be monitored prior to beginning therapy and every 8 weeks during treatment. Liver enzymes and CBC should be monitored every 6 weeks in the patient receiving **terbinafine** who is treated for longer than 6 weeks.

Patient Education

Administration

Instruct patients to take the drug as prescribed for the full course of their treatment, even if they note clinical improvement. In the treatment of oral candidiasis, the patient should be instructed to continue therapy until 2 days after symptoms have disappeared. When treating infants with thrush, all pacifiers and bottle nipples should be washed in warm, soapy water and soaked in hot or boiling water for 20 minutes between each use. This step is important to prevent reinfection of the infant with candidiasis. If treated with **gentian violet,** the patient should be warned that **gentian violet** will stain skin and clothing. If oral candidiasis is treated with **clotrimazole** troche, patients should be instructed to slowly dissolve the troche in their mouth, not chew.

Patients using topical **antifungals** for dermatophyte infections of the skin should be instructed to apply the medication to the infected area and the immediate surrounding area for the full length of treatment. Treatment is often continued beyond the point of clinical clearing to prevent recurrence of the infection. Generally, avoid occlusive dressings, which provide favorable conditions for yeast growth.

The treatment of tinea capitis or onychomycosis involves long-term therapy with oral **antifungal** medications. The patient should be encouraged to continue the medication for the full length of treatment and take the medication as prescribed. **Griseofulvin** must be taken with a high-fat meal to ensure adequate absorption of the medication. **Itraconazole** should be taken with food. **Ketoconazole** and **terbinafine** may both be taken without regard to meals.

In treating topical dermatophyte infections such as tinea corporis or ringworm, family members and pets should be checked for signs of infection and be treated also.

Adverse Reactions

The patient should be given written and oral instructions regarding the adverse drug reactions that may be expected with the medication that is being prescribed. If the patient is prescribed systemic **antifungal** medication, then an explanation of the possible adverse effects and the necessity for laboratory monitoring should be discussed. Patients should be instructed to immediately report to their provider any flu-like symptoms, which may be a sign of hepatic toxicity.

Topical Antivirals

Topical **antivirals** are used to treat herpes simplex virus (HSV) and herpes zoster. The **oral antiviral medications** used to treat these conditions and varicella are discussed in Chapter 24. The two herpes simplex virus infections that are treated with topical medications are HSV-1 and HSV-2, with HSV-1 generally associated with nongenital infection and HSV-2 with genital infection. There are three topical **antiviral** medications: **acyclovir (Zovirax), penciclovir** (Denavir), and the OTC product **docosanol** (Abreva).

Pharmacodynamics

Both **acyclovir** and **penciclovir** must be phosphorylated to be active against herpes simplex virus. Intracellularly, both medications are converted to monophosphate forms by viral thymidine kinases, then further converted to diphosphate and finally to triphosphate by various cellular enzymes. **Acyclovir** triphosphate competes with deoxyguanosine triphosphate for a position in the DNA chain of the herpes virus. Once incorporated in the DNA chain, it terminates DNA synthesis. **Penciclovir** triphosphate selectively inhibits viral DNA polymerase by competing with deoxyguanosine triphosphate. This inhibits viral replication. In vitro, **penciclovir** triphosphate is retained inside the HSV-infected cells for 10 to 20 hours, compared with 0.7 to 1 hour for **acyclovir.**

Pharmacokinetics

Absorption and Distribution

After topical application of **acyclovir, penciclovir,** or **docosanol** there is minimal absorption, and no drug is detected in the blood or urine after application.

Pharmacotherapeutics

Precautions and Contraindications

The only true contraindication to **acyclovir, penciclovir,** or **docosanol** is hypersensitivity to the product or any of its components. **Acyclovir** should be used with caution in patients with **ganciclovir** hypersensitivity in that these two drugs have similar chemical structures, and there may be cross-sensitivity.

Acyclovir ointment is classified as Pregnancy Category B, although no complete or well-controlled pregnancy studies have been performed in humans. **Penciclovir** is classified as Pregnancy Category B. No adverse effects on pregnancy outcomes or fetal development are found in animal studies. However, there have been no adequate or well-controlled studies in pregnant women.

Orally administered **acyclovir** is excreted in breast milk. It is unknown whether topical **acyclovir** is excreted in breast milk. Because topical **acyclovir** cannot be measured in the serum, it is assumed that it is not excreted in breast milk. It is not known if **penciclovir** is excreted in human milk after topical administration. Both medications should be used with caution in a nursing mother until further studies clarify their safety.

Safety and effectiveness in pediatric patients have not been established for **penciclovir** or **docosanol**. **Acyclovir** is approved for use in children and adults.

Adverse Drug Reactions

Although **systemic acyclovir** has extensive adverse reactions, topical **acyclovir** has only transient local adverse reactions. The most common reaction to topical **acyclovir** use is mild pain with transient burning or stinging in 28.3 percent of patients. Pruritus is reported by 4.1 percent of patients, with rash and local edema found in less than 1 percent.

Double-blind, placebo-controlled trials of **penciclovir** cream found no difference in the frequency of adverse events for both treatment groups. When 5 percent **penciclovir** cream (not currently available in the United States) was used, mild erythema was reported in 50 percent of subjects.

The only adverse reactions reported for **docosanol** is irritation at the site of application.

Drug Interactions

There are no known drug interactions identified with topical **acyclovir, penciclovir,** or **docosanol.**

Clinical Use and Dosing

Herpes Simplex

Acyclovir is indicated in the management of initial episodes of herpes genitalis and in limited, non–life-threatening, mucocutaneous HSV infections in immunocompromised patients. There is no clinical evidence for the benefit of using **acyclovir** in the immunocompetent patient, although decreased viral shedding may be noted. Topical **acyclovir** is applied to cover all lesions every 3 hours six times a day for 7 days. The dose size per application should be approximately a 0.5- to 1-inch ribbon of ointment per 4 square inches of surface area. A glove or finger cot should be used to apply the medication to prevent autoinoculation of other body sites and transmission of infection to other people.

Penciclovir is indicated in the treatment of recurrent herpes labialis (cold sores) on the lips and face. Application to mucous membrane is not recommended. In adults, **penciclovir** 1 percent cream is applied every 2 hours while awake, with treatment started as early as possible (during the prodrome or when lesions appear).

Docosanol (Abreva) is the only OTC product available for the treatment of herpes labialis. It is applied to the cold sore five times a day until healed. Treatment should begin at first sign of outbreak.

Herpes Zoster

Neither topical **acyclovir** nor topical **penciclovir** is indicated in the treatment of herpes zoster.

Varicella

Although oral **acyclovir** is used in the treatment of varicella, topical **acyclovir** does not have this indication. **Penciclovir** is not used in the treatment of varicella.

Rational Drug Selection

Efficacy

Penciclovir is the first topical antiviral medication that has been clinically proved to be effective in the treatment of herpes labialis (cold sores). **Docosanol** is effective in decreasing duration of cold sore outbreak, but must be started early in course of outbreak to be effective, whereas **penciclovir** may be started anytime in the disease course. Although **acyclovir** may be used for herpes labialis, it has not been clinically proved to be effective in the treatment of HSV infections in immunocompetent patients. In genital herpes, **acyclovir** is the drug of choice for primary lesions in immunocompromised patients.

Cost

Because topical **acyclovir** and **penciclovir** are both unique antiviral agents, their cost is not generally used as part of the decision of whether to prescribe the drug in treatment. **Denavir (penciclovir)** costs $54 for a 1.5-g tube and **Zovirax (acyclovir)** costs $69 for a 2-g tube. A 2-g tube of the OTC product **docosanol (Abreva)** is available for $15 (http://www.drugstore.com).

Monitoring

There is no laboratory monitoring necessary for patients treated with topical **acyclovir** or **penciclovir.** Monitoring for the adverse reactions noted previously is the only monitoring needed.

Patient Education

Administration

Patients should be instructed to start therapy with **acyclovir** as early as possible after the onset of the signs and symptoms of HSV infection. When applying **acyclovir,** patients should first wash their hands thoroughly and use a finger cot or rubber glove to apply the ointment to prevent the spread of infection. They should apply enough ointment to thoroughly cover all lesions. Patients should be instructed that **acyclovir** might cause transient burning, stinging, itching, and rash. They should notify their primary care provider if these symptoms become pronounced or persist.

Patients should be instructed to begin therapy with **penciclovir** as soon as symptoms begin, during the prodrome or when lesions appear. They should wash their hands thoroughly after applying **penciclovir** to prevent the spread of infection. Patients should avoid application on or near the eyes or mucous membranes. Although adverse reactions are rare, patients should be instructed to report any skin irritation to their provider.

Treatment with **docosanol** should begin at the earliest sign or symptom. Patients should wash hands before and after application. The medication should be rubbed in completely. Patients are to use the medication five times a day until cold sores are healed.

AGENTS USED TO TREAT ACNE

Acne is the most common skin condition in the United States, affecting approximately 40 to 50 million Americans (American Academy of Dermatology, 2009). Close to 100 percent of adolescents have at least an occasional comedone or pustule (American Academy of Dermatology, 2009). Acne can occur at any age, with up to 25 percent of adults having some degree of acne. Acne is classified as mild, moderate, or severe, and pharmacological intervention is based on the severity of acne. The bacterium commonly found in acne is *Propionibacterium acnes (P. acnes)*; thus, treatment often includes antibiotics active against *P. acnes* (Strauss et al, 2007).

The medications used in the treatment of acne may be either topical agents or systemic. The topical agents used for acne can be divided into two categories: **retinoids** and **antibiotics.** Oral medications for systemic use are divided into three categories: oral **antibiotics** (discussed in Chap. 24), hormonal therapy (discussed in Chap. 31), and **isotretinoin**, an oral **retinoid.** Oral **antibiotics** are prescribed for moderate to severe acne, and **isotretinoin** is prescribed for severe nodulocystic acne.

The pharmacological management of acne is discussed in Chapter 32.

Pharmacodynamics

Topical Retinoids

Tretinoin is a naturally occurring derivative of vitamin A that is structurally related to **isotretinoin.** After topical administration, **tretinoin** appears to prevent horny cell cohesion and to increase epidermal cell turnover. It effects mitotic activity through irritation of the follicular epithelium. This decreases microcomedo formation. The increased turnover of follicular epithelial cells causes extrusion of comedones that have already formed. Formation of new comedones is prevented through sloughing and expulsion of horny cells from the follicle. **Tretinoin** reduces the cell layers of the stratum corneum from 14 to 5 layers. **Tretinoin** does not affect the bacteria found in *P. acnes.* Topical **tretinoin** is also used in the treatment of fine wrinkling, mottled hyperpigmentation, roughness, and laxity of the skin associated with sun damage.

Adapalene is a topical retinoid-like drug used for the treatment of mild to moderate acne vulgaris. **Adapalene** binds to specific retinoic acid nuclear receptors but does not bind to the cytosolic receptor protein. Although the exact mode of action of **adapalene** is not known, it is suggested that topical **adapalene** may normalize the differentiation of follicular epithelial cells, resulting in decreased microcomedo formation. It is also a modulator of cellular differentiation, keratinization, and inflammatory processes, all of which represent important features in the pathology of acne vulgaris.

Tazarotene is a retinoid prodrug that is converted to its active form, AGN 190299, which is the cognate carboxylic acid of tazarotene. The exact mechanism of action of **tazarotene** in the treatment of acne is not well defined, but it is believed that the drug works by normalizing epidermal differentiation and by reducing the influx of inflammatory cells into the skin.

Topical Antibiotics

Benzoyl peroxide has antibacterial activity against *P. acnes,* the predominant organism in sebaceous follicles and comedones of acne vulgaris. This antibacterial activity is presumably due to the release of active or free-radical oxygen capable of oxidizing bacterial proteins. **Benzoyl peroxide** also has a drying effect, removes excess sebum, causes mild desquamation, and has a sebostatic effect.

Erythromycin is a bacteriostatic **macrolide antibiotic** but may be bactericidal in high concentrations. The mechanism by which topical **erythromycin** acts in reducing inflammatory lesions of acne vulgaris is unknown, but it is presumably due to its antibiotic actions.

Topical **clindamycin** demonstrates in vitro activity against isolates of *P. acnes,* the common bacteria found in acne vulgaris. **Clindamycin** also inhibits lipase-producing organisms, reducing the concentration of free fatty acids in sebum from approximately 14 percent to 2 percent after application. These free fatty acids are possibly a cause of the inflammatory lesions associated with acne.

The mechanism of action by which **tetracycline** improves acne is unknown. Systemic **tetracycline** seems to decrease the amount of free fatty acids present in acne lesions. It appears that topical **tetracycline** has a localized effect in which the medication is delivered to the pilosebaceous apparatus and adjacent tissues. **Tetracycline** is active against *P. acnes,* but there are reports of resistance developing.

Metronidazole is classified as an antiprotozoal and antibacterial agent. The mechanism by which topical **metronidazole** acts in reducing the inflammatory lesions in acne rosacea is unknown.

The mechanism of action for **azelaic acid** in acne vulgaris is its antimicrobial effect against *P. acnes* and

Staphylococcus epidermidis. The mechanism of action may be due to inhibition of microbial cellular protein synthesis. **Azelaic acid** decreases the inflammation associated with acne lesions by reducing the concentration of bacteria present in the skin. **Azelaic acid** may also cause normalization of keratinization, leading to an anticomedonal effect. It may also decrease microcomedone formation by reducing the number and size by of keratohyalin granules and the amount and distribution of filaggrin in epidermal layers. **Azelaic acid** does not effect sebum excretion.

The mechanism of action of **dapsone (Aczone)** in the treatment of acne is unknown.

Systemic Retinoids

Isotretinoin is an isomer of *all-trans* retinoic acid, a metabolite of retinol (vitamin A). Its actions include normalization of the keratinizing process of the follicular epithelium and reduction of sebocyte number with decreased sebum synthesis. Sebum lipid production and composition are altered during **isotretinoin** therapy, with sebum production reversibly reduced to 10 percent of pretreatment levels. **Isotretinoin**, if given in high doses, can reduce the concentration of *P. acnes* bacteria through decreased sebum production.

Pharmacokinetics

Absorption and Distribution

Topical Retinoids

Tretinoin, administered topically, is minimally absorbed systemically. Prolonged treatment or administration to large body surface areas can increase systemic absorption. **Adapalene**, when applied topically to the skin, has minimal absorption. Trace amounts of **adapalene** have been found in the plasma of acne patients after chronic topical application. **Tazarotene**, when administered topically to the skin, has minimal systemic absorption because of its rapid metabolism in the skin to the active metabolite. In clinical trials, topical use of **tazarotene** determined that systemic absorption of the total dose was less than 1 percent without occlusion. Even treating psoriasis by applying **tazarotene** to 20 percent of the total body surface area led to systemic absorption of less than 1 percent after 7 days of treatment.

Topical Antibiotics

Benzoyl peroxide is absorbed by the skin in unknown amounts. Absorption of topical **erythromycin** is unknown. **Clindamycin**, when applied topically, does exhibit some systemic absorption, depending on the surface area covered. Following multiple topical applications at a concentration equivalent to 10 mg, very low levels of **clindamycin** are present in the serum. Topically applied **tetracycline** does not appear to be absorbed through the skin in sufficient quantities to be detected systemically. **Metronidazole** is absorbed when applied topically but in very small amounts. When 1 mg is applied to the face, the resulting serum concentration is approximately 100 times less than one 250-mg tablet taken orally. Approximately 4 percent of topically applied **azelaic acid** is absorbed systemically.

Systemic Retinoids

The oral bioavailability from oil-filled capsules of **isotretinoin** is approximately 23 to 25 percent. Increased plasma levels may be found if the drug is taken with food. **Isotretinoin** is 99.9 percent plasma protein bound. Although severe fetal abnormalities have been noted, it is not known whether **isotretinoin** crosses the placenta. Distribution of **isotretinoin** is unknown.

Metabolism and Excretion

Topical Retinoids

A minimal amount of **tretinoin** is absorbed systemically. This trace amount is metabolized by the CYP450 hepatic enzyme system. Approximately 1 to 5 percent of a topically applied dose is excreted in the urine within 24 hours. The metabolism of topically applied **adapalene** is unknown. Excretion appears to be primarily by the biliary route. **Tazarotene** is rapidly metabolized in the skin to the active metabolite, tazarotenic acid, which is systemically absorbed and further metabolized by the liver to sulfoxides, sulfones, and other metabolites. Elimination of the metabolites is via fecal and renal pathways.

Topical Antibiotics

Benzoyl peroxide metabolism and excretion are unknown. Although topical **erythromycin** absorption is minimal, oral administration demonstrates that **erythromycin** is metabolized in the liver to several inactive metabolites. Excretion of **erythromycin** is mainly via the bile. Topical **clindamycin** is absorbed and metabolized into two active metabolites, clindamycin sulfoxide and N-desmethyl **clindamycin**, as well as other inactive metabolites. Following oral dosage, only about 10 percent is excreted in the urine as active drug and metabolites and 3.6 percent in the feces; the remainder is excreted as inactive metabolites. Approximately 80 percent of a dose of oral **metronidazole** is metabolized by side-chain oxidation and glucuronide conjugation into inactive metabolites. The major route of elimination of **metronidazole** and its metabolites is through the urine. Topically applied **azelaic acid** is minimally absorbed and is mainly excreted unchanged in the urine.

Systemic Retinoids

Isotretinoin is metabolized in the liver primarily via oxidation. It is unknown whether its metabolite is pharmacologically active. The metabolites are eliminated renally, and unchanged drug and metabolites are excreted in the feces.

Pharmacotherapeutics

Precautions and Contraindications

Topical Retinoids and Topical Antibiotics

Topical retinoids should be avoided in patients with eczema, sunburn, or skin abrasions at the site of application. **Topical retinoids** are contraindicated in lactating women. Safety and efficacy in children younger than 12 years have not been established. All three topical retinoids—**tretinoin, adapalene,** and **tazarotene**—are classified as Pregnancy Category C.

Topical **antibiotics** used in acne treatment have few true contraindications. **Benzoyl peroxide** may exhibit cross-sensitivity with benzoic acid derivatives. **Erythromycin**, when applied topically, is contraindicated only when the patient is hypersensitive to **erythromycin** or to any component of the preparation. Topical **clindamycin** is contraindicated in any patient who is hypersensitive to **clindamycin** or **lincomycin.** It is also contraindicated in patients with a history of regional enteritis, ulcerative colitis, or antibiotic-associated colitis. Topical **tetracycline** preparations contain sodium sulfites and are contraindicated in patients sensitive to sulfites or **tetracycline. Azelaic acid** has not been well studied in patients with dark skin and should be used cautiously in these patients to avoid hypopigmentation. **Metronidazole** for topical use contains parabens, and therefore any patient who is sensitive to parabens or **metronidazole** should not use it. **Azelaic acid** is classified as Pregnancy Category B. Because small amounts of **azelaic acid** are absorbed systemically and may be excreted in breast milk, caution should be exercised in administering it to lactating women. Safety and efficacy of **azelaic acid** in children younger than 12 years have not been established.

Systemic Retinoids

Isotretinoin should be avoided in patients with retinoid hypersensitivity, including **vitamin A, tretinoin,** and **etretinate.** Patients with parabens hypersensitivity should avoid **isotretinoin** because the drug is prepared with parabens, a preservative. Patients with a risk for osteoporosis (osteomalacia and anorexia nervosa) should avoid taking **isotretinoin** due to decreased bone mineral density seen during treatment. In a study of pediatric patients reported on the **Accutane** label, 7.9 percent had decreases in lumbar spine bone mineral density (BMD) of more than 4 percent (adjusted for body mass index); 10.6% patients had decreases in total hip BMD of more than 5 percent. Adolescents who participate in impact sports while taking **isotretinoin** are at risk for bone injuries. **Isotretinoin** is classified Pregnancy Category X and is absolutely contraindicated in pregnancy. It may cause severe malformations of the craniofacial, cardiac, thymic, and CNS structures. Many such infants have several malformations. Spontaneous abortions and premature births have also been reported. The drug should not be administered to any woman of childbearing age until after pregnancy has been excluded and appropriate birth control measures are used for at least 1 month. Patients should also avoid pregnancy for at least 1 month after discontinuation of **isotretinoin.** Breastfeeding is not recommended during **isotretinoin** treatment because of the potential adverse affects to the nursing infant. **Isotretinoin** was relabeled to include safety and efficacy information for 12- to 17-year-olds. Caution should be exercised in administering **isotretinoin** to patients with hyperlipidemia, as patients may have increased lipids during therapy. **Isotretinoin** should be prescribed cautiously to patients with psychotic disorders; it may cause major depression, psychosis, and, rarely, suicidal ideation.

Adverse Drug Reactions

Topical Retinoids

Topical retinoids all cause some degree of skin irritation. Burning or pruritus immediately after applying a topical retinoid is common. All three retinoid products cause erythema, scaling, xerosis, and peeling. These symptoms occur frequently and appear to be necessary for the therapeutic effect. Because photosensitivity may occur with topical retinoid use, patients should use sunscreen to prevent severe sunburn. Both **tretinoin** and **tazarotene** may cause skin discoloration, hyperpigmentation, or hypopigmentation, which will resolve after discontinuation of the medication.

Topical Antibiotics

Topical **antibiotics** used in the treatment of acne all cause some dryness, erythema, burning, peeling, and itching. **Benzoyl peroxide** may also cause marked peeling and desquamation, which appears to be a necessary component of the therapeutic effect. **Benzoyl peroxide** may also cause photosensitivity. Allergic contact sensitization may occur with any of the topical antibiotics used in the treatment of acne vulgaris. In patients with dark complexions, skin hypopigmentation may occur with the use of topical **azelaic acid.**

Systemic Retinoids

Isotretinoin has multiple reported significant adverse reactions. The most commonly reported adverse reactions involve mucocutaneous effects. Cheilitis (inflammation of the lips) occurs in more than 90 percent of patients. Dry skin, pruritus, and skin fragility occur in approximately 80 percent of patients. Conjunctivitis is reported by 40 percent of patients, with facial skin desquamation and drying of mucous membranes reported by approximately 30 percent of patients treated with **isotretinoin.** Patients also report xerosis, xerostomia, and epistaxis. These mucocutaneous drying effects of **isotretinoin** are dose related and are usually reversible after discontinuation of therapy.

Isotretinoin administration has resulted in alteration of lipid profiles in 25 percent of patients treated, including elevated triglyceride concentrations, a decrease in high-density lipoproteins (HDL) in 15 percent of patients, and hypercholesterolemia in 7 percent of patients. **Alcohol** consumption may potentiate serum triglyceride elevations. Lipid alterations occur most frequently at dosages greater than 1 mg/kg/day and are reversible upon discontinuation of **isotretinoin.**

Elevation of serum glucose and fasting serum blood glucose has been reported. Exacerbation of diabetes mellitus can occur. Decreases in hemoglobin and hematocrit concentrations have been reported in 10 to 20 percent of patients. Forty percent of patients prescribed **isotretinoin** may have increased sedimentation rates. Patients may also experience anemia and thrombocytopenia.

CNS effects include headache (5%), lethargy, and fatigue. **Isotretinoin** has also been associated with pseudotumor cerebri (benign increased intracranial pressure). Symptoms include headache, visual disturbances, and papilledema. In the postmarketing period, depression has been reported, as have psychosis and, rarely, suicidal ideation. If patients report depression, immediate discontinuation of therapy is indicated. Depression appears to subside with discontinuation of therapy and to recur upon reinstitution of therapy.

Adverse GI reactions include anorexia, nausea and vomiting, increased appetite, and thirst. Eighty percent of patients report dry mouth when taking **isotretinoin.** Inflammatory bowel disease, including regional enteritis, may occur.

Musculoskeletal adverse effects such as arthralgia and myalgia are reported in approximately 16 percent of patients taking **isotretinoin.** Skeletal abnormalities have been reported in adults and children receiving excessive doses (more than 2 mg/kg/d for prolonged periods, 6 mo–2 yr). BMD decreases have seen in pediatric patients when administered a single course of **isotretinoin** at normal dosages. Adolescent or adult athletes who participate in sports with a repetitive impact may be at increased risk for bone-related injuries due to the decreased BMD seen with **isotretinoin** use.

Isotretinoin has been associated with rare cases of hepatitis. Transient increases in alkaline phosphates, lactate dehydrogenase, AST, ALT, GGTP, and LDH have been reported in 10 to 20 percent of patients. If elevated hepatic enzymes persist or if symptoms of hepatitis develop, **isotretinoin** should be discontinued.

Ophthalmic adverse effects including corneal opacification have been reported in patients receiving **isotretinoin** for acne. This ocular effect is reversible with complete resolution or continuing resolution at 6 to 7 weeks following discontinuation of therapy. Of patients taking **isotretinoin,** 25 percent report visual disturbances, including blurred vision, decreased visual acuity, tunnel vision, photophobia, and diplopia.

Isotretinoin may cause transient changes in urinalysis findings, with increased white cells in urine (10% to 20%), proteinuria, microscopic or gross hematuria (less than 10%), and nonspecific urogenital findings in 5 percent of patients. Less than 1 percent of patients have abnormal menses.

Drug Interactions

Topical Retinoids and Topical Antibiotics

Topical retinoids should not be used concomitantly with other topical medications that have strong drying effects, such as **benzoyl peroxide, salicylic acid,** or **lactic acid** (Table 23–4). Medicated or abrasive soaps or cleaners should also be avoided because they can potentiate the skin irritation caused by **topical retinoids.** Products that contain **alcohol,** lime, menthol, spices, or perfumes can further dry and irritate the skin and should not be used with **topical retinoids.** Before **topical retinoids** are begun, the effects of strong topical drying agents need to subside to prevent significant skin irritation. Patients using **tazarotene** should exercise caution with other medications causing photosensitization (**tetracycline**) because severe sunburn may occur. **Topical retinoids** should not be used in the same areas of skin at the same time as **benzoyl peroxide** or **topical antibiotics.** A physical incompatibility between the medications or a change in pH may reduce the efficacy of **topical retinoids** if used simultaneously. When used together for clinical effect, these medications should be used at different times of the day,

Table 23–4 ■ Drug Interactions: Selected Acne Medications

Drug	Interacting Drug	Possible Effect	Implications
Topical Acne Medications			
Retinoids			
• Adapalene	Benzoyl peroxide Salicylic acid Lactic acid Medicated or abrasive soaps or cleaners	Increased skin irritation Potentiate the skin irritation caused by topical retinoids	Avoid concurrent use of topical medications that have strong drying effects, such as benzoyl peroxide, salicylic acid, or lactic acid
	Products that contain alcohol, lime, menthol, spices, or perfumes	Dry and irritate the skin	Concurrent use should be avoided Should not be used with topical retinoids Before beginning adapalene, the effects of strong topical drying agents need to subside to prevent significant skin irritation

Table 23–4 ■ **Drug Interactions: Selected Acne Medications—cont'd**

Drug	Interacting Drug	Possible Effect	Implications
Tazarotene	Photosensitizers (tetracycline)	Increased photosensitivity	Avoid concurrent use because severe sunburn may result
	Skin irritants (products that contain alcohol, lime, menthol, spices, or perfumes; medicated or abrasive soaps or cleaners)	Potentiate the skin irritation caused by topical retinoids	Concurrent use should also be avoided Before beginning tazarotene, the effects of strong topical drying agents need to subside to prevent significant skin irritation
Tretinoin	Benzoyl peroxide and topical antibiotics Topical sulfur, resorcinol, benzoyl peroxide, or salicylic acid Abrasive soaps and cleansers	A physical incompatibility between the medications or a change in pH may reduce the efficacy of topical retinoids if used simultaneously	Tretinoin should not be used in the same areas of skin at the same time as benzoyl peroxide or topical antibiotics; separate use in the same areas by many hours (a.m.–p.m. dosing)
	Products that contain alcohol, lime, menthol, spices, or perfumes	Potentiate the skin irritation caused by topical retinoids Increased skin irritation	Concurrent use should be avoided
Topical antibiotics			
• Azelaic acid	No known interactions		
• Benzoyl peroxide	Topical retinoids PABA-containing sunscreens Other topical acne agents	A physical incompatibility between the medications or a change in pH may reduce the efficacy of topical retinoids if used simultaneously May transiently discolor skin Additive irritant effects	Avoid use in the same area of skin at the same time Avoid concurrent use If using concurrently, observe for severe skin irritation
• Clindamycin	Erythromycin	Antagonize each other	Do not use concurrently
• Erythromycin	Clindamycin	Antagonize each other	Do not use concurrently
	Other topical acne agents (especially abrasives and keratolytics)	Additive irritant effects	Avoid concurrent use
Metronidazole	Oral anticoagulants	May potentiate effects of anticoagulant	Drug interaction less likely with topical metronidazole use but should be kept in mind in concurrent use
Dapsone	TMP/SMX	Levels of dapsone and its metabolites increased in the presence of TMP/SMX	Exposure from the proposed topical dose is about 1% of that from the 100 mg oral dose, even when coadministered with TMP/SMX
Systemic Acne Medication			
Isotretinoin	Vitamin A	Potentiate the toxic effects of isotretinoin	Do not take concurrently
	Alcohol	Potentiate the toxic effects of isotretinoin	Avoid concurrent use
	Tetracycline	May increase incidents of pseudotumor cerebri	Avoid concurrent use
	Drying agents, such as benzoyl peroxide, or other medicated or abrasive soaps or alcohol-containing products	Can potentiate the drying effects of isotretinoin	Observe for skin irritation if using concurrently
	Ethanol	Can increase the hypertriglyceridemic effects of isotretinoin	Postpone lipid determinations for at least 36 h following ethanol consumption, if patients are taking isotretinoin
	Carbamazepine	Reduced carbamazepine levels with concurrent use	Monitor closely if using concurrently

PABA = para-aminobenzoic acid.
TMP/SMX – trimethoprim/sulfamethoxazole

such as morning and night, to minimize possible skin irritation. **Topical antibiotics** have fewer significant drug interactions than systemic antibiotics. **Benzoyl peroxide** can interact with **topical retinoids**, as noted previously. **PABA sunscreens** may transiently discolor the skin if used concurrently with **benzoyl peroxide**. All of the **topical antibiotics** may have possible additive irritation when used with other topical acne agents (especially abrasives or keratolytics). **Azelaic acid** has no known drug interactions.

Systemic Retinoids

Concomitant use of **isotretinoin** and other sources of **vitamin A** can potentiate the toxic effects of **isotretinoin**. **Alcohol** may also potentiate the toxic effects of **isotretinoin**. **Tetracycline** may increase the incidence of pseudotumor cerebri. Simultaneous use of **isotretinoin** and other drying agents, such as **benzoyl peroxide** or other medicated or abrasive soaps or **alcohol**-containing products, can potentiate the drying effects of **isotretinoin**. **Ethanol** can increase the hypertriglyceridemic effects of **isotretinoin**. Lipid determinations should be postponed for at least 36 hours after **ethanol** consumption.

Clinical Use and Dosing

Acne Vulgaris

Topical retinoids are applied to the skin once daily (Table 23–5). In the evening before retiring, the patient applies a thin film of medication after washing with a gentle cleaner. Care should be taken to avoid the eyes, lips, and mucous membranes. It is recommended that the patient wait 20 to 30 minutes after cleaning before applying **tretinoin**. Patients should wash their hands immediately after applying **topical retinoids**.

Table 23–5 ● **Dosage Schedule: Selected Acne Medications**

Drug	Indication	Dosage	Notes
Topical Acne Medications			
Retinoids			
• Adapalene	Acne vulgaris	Apply to affected acne areas once daily at bedtime after washing with gentle cleanser	
• Tazarotene (0.1%)	Mild to moderate facial acne vulgaris	Apply a thin film of tazarotene in the evening after washing with a gentle cleaner	Avoid eyes, lips, and mucous membranes; patients should wash their hands immediately after applying medication; women of childbearing age should begin the medication during their normal menses
• Tretinoin	Acne vulgaris	Apply sparingly to affected acne areas once daily at bedtime; adjust frequency or strength as tolerated	Wait 20–30 min after cleaning with a gentle cleanser before applying tretinoin; patients should wash their hands immediately after applying medication
Topical Antibiotics			
• Azelaic acid	Mild to moderate inflammatory acne vulgaris	Massage thin film into affected areas bid	Apply to clean, dry skin; wash hands after application; if persistent irritation occurs, may decrease dose to once daily
• Benzoyl peroxide	Mild to moderate acne vulgaris	Cleansers: wash affected areas once or twice daily Other forms: apply to affected acne areas once daily; may increase to 2–3 times daily if tolerated	Wet areas to be washed with benzoyl peroxide cleanser, cleanse, rinse well, then pat dry If excessive dryness or peeling occurs, patient should reduce the number of applications per day
• Benzoyl peroxide and erythromycin gel (Benzamycin)	Acne vulgaris	Apply to affected acne areas bid	Apply to clean, dry skin; may decrease application to once daily if excessive irritation occurs
• Benzoyl peroxide and clindamycin gel (Benzaclin, Duac)	Acne vulgaris	Apply bid (Benzaclin) Apply once daily (Duac)	Apply to clean dry skin. Wash hands after applying medication
• Clindamycin	Acne vulgaris	Apply thin film bid to affected acne areas Pledget: apply to all affected areas bid	Wash hands after applying medication More than one pledget may be used; remove the pledget from the foil just before use and discard after single use

Table 23–5 ◉ **Dosage Schedule: Selected Acne Medications—cont'd**

Drug	Indication	Dosage	Notes
• Erythromycin	Acne vulgaris	Apply a thin layer to affected acne areas bid	Wash hands after applying medication
• Metronidazole	Acne rosacea	Apply to affected areas bid	Wash hands after applying; improvement should be noted in 3 wk
Dapsone (Aczone)	Acne vulgaris	Children >12 yr and adults: Apply pea-size amount to skin that has been washed and patted dry. Apply twice a day in the a.m. and p.m.	Wash hands after use. Reevaluate if no improvement after 12 wk
Systemic Acne Medication			
Isotretinoin • Accutane	Severe, recalcitrant nodulocystic acne, unresponsive to conventional therapy including systemic antibiotics	Initially: 0.5–1 mg/kg/d divided bid; severe acne may require 2 mg/kg/d; treatment continues for 15–20 wk; may discontinue if nodule count decreases by 70% before end of treatment	Isotretinoin is rarely prescribed by primary care providers; its use is usually reserved for specialty dermatology practice because of multiple adverse effects; because of the extremely high risk of adverse outcomes in the fetus, including deformities and fetal death, written consent should be obtained from the childbearing-age female patient before prescribing isotretinoin; two reliable forms of contraception should be used by childbearing-age patients; monthly pregnancy testing before, during, and 1 mo after therapy is discontinued is required in female patients; patient must register with iPledge

Topical antibiotics are applied to affected acne areas twice daily in a thin film. Patients should wash their skin with a gentle cleanser and pat dry before applying. **Benzoyl peroxide** cleanser may be used for cleaning once or twice daily. Patients should wet the skin areas to be treated prior to administration, rinse thoroughly after cleaning, and pat dry. With other dosage forms of **benzoyl peroxide,** patients may gradually increase application to two or three times daily if tolerated. If bothersome or excessive dryness or peeling occurs, patients should reduce the number of applications per day. **Clindamycin** should be applied to all of the affected areas twice daily. If using the pledget formulation, more than one pledget may be used. Patients should remove the pledget from the foil just before use and discard after a single use. Patients should be instructed to wash their hands thoroughly after the use of any **topical antibiotic.**

There are combination products available that combine a **topical antibiotic** with **benzoyl peroxide** (Benzamycin, Benzaclin, Duac). **Benzamycin,** a product that combines **benzoyl peroxide** and **erythromycin** gel, is unique in that the medication is supplied in a package in which the two medications are separate and are then mixed immediately prior to dispensing. This combination product forms a gel and should be stirred prior to application. **Benzamycin** should be stored in the refrigerator and expires 3 months after reconstitution. The product should not be allowed to freeze. **Benzamycin Pak** is also a combination of **benzoyl peroxide** and **erythromycin** packaged in single-use foil pouch that the patient opens and then mixes the two ingredients in the palm before applying to acne-affected areas. **Benzamycin Pak** does not require refrigeration. Products that combine **benzoyl peroxide** with **clindamycin** (**Benzaclin, Duac**) are also effective in acne treatment. Patients should apply these products to clean, dry skin twice daily for **Benzamycin** or **Benzaclin** and once daily before bed for **Duac.** If irritation occurs, patients may decrease application to once daily. It must be pointed out that all **benzoyl peroxide–containing** products bleach fabrics and hair, and care should be taken when handling such products.

Dapsone gel should be applied twice a day to skin that has been washed and patted dry. A pea-size amount of **dapsone** gel is spread into a thin layer over all acne-affected areas. Patients should wash their hands after application.

Because of its severe adverse effects, **isotretinoin** is usually prescribed only by dermatologists. It must be stressed that, because of the safety issues, primary care providers usually do not prescribe this medication. All female patients who are prescribed **isotretinoin,** as well as the prescriber, are registered with iPledge (http://www.iPledgeprogram.com), a program committed to preventing pregnancy while patients are taking **isotretinoin.**

Acne Rosacea

The topical treatment of rosacea consists of application of topical **antibiotics** or **benzoyl peroxide. Metronidazole** is often used as the initial therapy. **Metronidazole** 0.75 percent cream or gel (**MetroGel**) or 1 percent emollient cream (**Noritate**) is applied in a thin film twice a day after washing with a gentle cleanser. There may be some mild skin irritation associated with topical **metronidazole** use. Significant therapeutic results should be noticed within 3 weeks. Clinical studies have demonstrated continuing improvement through 9 weeks of therapy. Patients may use cosmetics after application of topical **metronidazole.** If irritation occurs, patients should reduce frequency, interrupt therapy, or discontinue use. Avoid getting **metronidazole** in the eyes.

Rosacea may also be treated with combination products that combine an **antibacterial** with a **keratolytic.** Formulas that combine **sulfacetamide** 10 percent and **sulfur** 5 percent (**Clenia, Rosula, Sulfacet-R**) are applied one to three times a day to clean skin. **Sulfacetamide** and **sulfur washes** (**Clenia, Rosula Cleanser**) are used once or twice a day. Another product available is **azelaic acid** 15 percent gel (**Finacea**), which is an antibacterial/antikeratinizing agent. It is applied to clean, dry skin twice a day. Patients should avoid getting any of these products in their eyes and wash their hands after applying.

Rational Drug Selection

Severity

The choice of acne medications is generally dependent on the severity of the acne on presentation. Mild acne is generally treated with **benzoyl peroxide**, which is available by prescription and in OTC preparations. **Benzoyl peroxide** alone often treats mild acne. Mild to moderate acne may be treated with the combination of **benzoyl peroxide** and another topical antibiotic such as **Benzamycin**, which contains **benzoyl peroxide** and **erythromycin** or a combination of **benzoyl peroxide** and **clindamycin** (**Benzaclin, Duac**). A combination retinoid product such as **Epiduo Gel** (**adapalene** and **benzoyl peroxide**) may be used. **Topical retinoids** are used for moderate to severe acne. In the treatment of moderate acne, a combination of **oral antibiotics** and either **topical antibiotics** or **topical retinoids** may be used. Hormonal therapy is indicated in mild to moderate acne in women (**Ortho-Tri-Cyclen, Estrostep Fe, Tri-Sprintec**). **Isotretinoin** is used in the treatment of recalcitrant nodulocystic acne, with its use reserved for the most severe patients. Dosage for selected acne medications are found in Table 23–6.

Cost

The least expensive topical acne medications are **benzoyl peroxide**, which is available OTC, and topical

Table 23–6 ◆ Available Dosage Forms: Selected Acne Medications

Drug	Dosage Form	How Supplied	Cost
TOPICAL ACNE MEDICATIONS			
Retinoids			
Adapalene (Rx)	0.1% cream	In 45 g	$259.33
Differin	0.1% gel	In 45 g	$259.98
	0.1% solution	In 30 mL	$83.69
Tazarotene (0.1%) (Rx)			
Tazorac	0.1% aqueous gel	In 30 and 100 g	$567.63 (100g)
	0.05% cream	In 60 g	$344.48
	0.05% cream	In 30 g	$170.29
	0.1% cream	In 60 g	$361.52
	0.1% cream	In 30 g	$177.88
	0.05% gel	In 100 g	$538.66
	0.1% gel	In 100 g	$567.63
	0.05% gel	In 30 g	$168.89
	0.1% gel	In 30 g	$177.88
Tretinoin (Rx)			
• Avita	0.025% cream	In 20 g	$69.21
		In 45 g	$79.99
	0.025% gel	In 45 g	$141.07
• Retin-A	0.25%, 0.05%, 0.1% cream	In 20, 40 g	
	0.25%, 0.01% gel	In 15, 45 g	
	0.05% liquid	In 28 mL	
	0.025% cream	In 20 g	$85.59
	0.05% cream	In 20 g	$97.85
	0.1% cream	In 20 g	$112.51

Table 23–6 ◆ **Available Dosage Forms: Selected Acne Medications—cont'd**

Drug	Dosage Form	How Supplied	Cost
	0.025% cream	In 45 g	$152.46
	0.05% cream	In 45 g	$162.17
	0.1% cream	In 45 g	$188.18
	0.01% gel	In 15 g	$75.83
	0.025% gel	In 15 g	$64.81
	0.01% gel	In 45 g	$149.46
	0.025% gel	In 45 g	$150.50
• Generic	0.25% cream	In 20 g	$39.99
	0.05% cream	In 20 g	$45.99
	0.1% cream	In 20 g	$46.19
	0.025% cream	In 45 g	$59.19
	0.05% cream	In 45 g	$73.49
	0.1% cream	In 45 g	$105.99
	0.01% gel	In 15 g	$35.99
	0.025% gel	In 15 g	$35.99
	0.01% gel	In 45 g	$79.50
	0.025% gel	In 45 g	$75.85
• Retin-A Micro	0.1% aqueous gelatin microspheres	In 20, 40 g	
	0.04% gel	In 20 g	$123.70
	0.1% gel	In 20 g	$117.51
	0.04% gel	In 45 g	$202.59
	0.1% gel	In 45 g	$199.75
Topical Antibiotics			
Azelaic acid (Rx)			
Azelex	20% cream	In 30 g	$181.32
		In 50 g	$262.74
Dapsone (Rx) (Aczone)	5% gel	In 30 g	$176
		In 60 g	$318
Benzoyl peroxide			
• Benzac AC	2.5% gel	In 60 g	$28.99
• Benzac AC 5	5% gel	In 60 g	$96.95
• Benzac AC 10	10% gel	In 60 mg	$92.87
• Benzac AC	2.5% gel	In 90 g	$22.99
• Benzac AC Wash	5% liquid	In 226 mL	$139.37
• Benzac AC Wash	10% liquid	In 226 mL	$135.67
• Benzac AC Wash	2.5%	In 240 mL	$36
• Benzac W	2.5% gel	In 60 g	$26.99
• Benzac W	5% gel	In 60 g	$27.99
• Benzac W	10% gel	In 60 g	$28.99
• Benzac W	10% gel	In 90 g	$24.99
• Benzac W Wash	5% liquid	In 226 mL	$135.67
• Benzac W Wash	10% liquid	In 226 mL	$139.85
• Desquam-X	5% gel	In 42.5 g	$14.99
• Desquam-X	10% gel	In 42.5 g	$15.99
• Desquam-X	5% gel	In 85 g	$25.99
• Desquam-X	10% gel	In 85 g	$26.99
• Desquam-X	5% liquid	In 140 mL	$20.99
• Desquam-X	10% liquid	In 140 mL	$20.98
• Desquam-E	2.5% gel	In 42.5 g	$21.99
• Desquam-E 5	5% gel	In 42.5 g	$22.99
• Desquam-E 10	10% gel	In 42.5 g	$21.99
• Dryox Wash 5 (OTC)	5% cleansing solution	In 240 mL	
• Dryox Wash 10 (OTC)	10% cleansing solution	In 240 mL	
• Dryox 2.5 (OTC)	2.5% gel	In 30 g	
		In 60 g	

Continued

Table 23–6 ◈ **Available Dosage Forms: Selected Acne Medications—cont'd**

Drug	Dosage Form	How Supplied	Cost
• Dryox 5 (OTC)	5% gel	In 30 g In 60 g	
• Dryox 10 (OTC)	10% gel	In 30 g In 60 g	
• Dryox 20 (OTC)	20% gel	In 30 g In 60 g	
• Oxy 10 Wash (OTC)	10% cleansing solution	In 120 mL	$5.59
• Oxy 5 Advanced Formula for Sensitive Skin (OTC)	5% gel	In 30 g	$5.59
• Oxy 10 Maximum Strength Advanced Formula (OTC)	10% gel	In 30 mg	$5.39
• Fostex 10% Wash (OTC)	10% cleansing solution		
• Fostex Bar	10% bar	In 106 g	
Benzoyl peroxide			
Generic (OTC and Rx)	5% mask	In 30 mL	
	10% lotion	In 30 mL	
	5% gel	In 45 g	
	10% gel	In 45, 90g	
	2.5% gel	In 60 g	$23.99
	5% gel	In 45 g	$12.99
	10% gel	In 45 mg	$13.99
	5% gel	In 90 g	$21.99
	5% gel	In 60 g	$24.99
	10% gel	In 60 g	$25.99
	10% gel	In 90 g	$29.99
Benzoyl peroxide-erythromycin gel (Benzamycin) (Rx)	Erythromycin 3% and benzoyl peroxide 5% gel	In 60 packets In 46.6 g	$142.45 $217.57
Benzoyl peroxide/clindamycin (Rx)			
• Benzaclin	50 g/jar		$195.42
• Duac	45 g/tube		$186.67 (1 kit)
Adapalene and benzoyl peroxide (Rx) Epiduo Gel Adapalene 1% and benzoyl peroxide 2.5% gel 45 g gel $219.56			
Clindamycin (Rx)			
• Cleocin T	1% gel	In 30 g In 60 g	$62.98 $104.98
	1% lotion	In 60 mL	$86.09
	10 mg/mL topical solution	In 30 mL with applicator In 60 mL with applicator	$27.65 $69.29
	1 mL solution/pad	In 60s (pledgets)	$76
• C/T/S	10 mg/mL solution	In 30 mL with applicator In 60 mL with applicator	
• Generic	10 mg/mL gel	In 30 g In 60 g	$17.99 $34.99
	10 mg/mL lotion	In 60 mL	$39.99
	10 mg/mL topical solution	In 30 mL In 60 mL	$14.99 $16.99
	10% swab	In 60 swabs	$39.99
Erythromycin (Rx)			
• A/T/S	2% solution	In 60 mL	
	2% gel	In 30 g	

Table 23–6 ◆ **Available Dosage Forms: Selected Acne Medications—cont'd**

Drug	Dosage Form	How Supplied	Cost
• Emgel	2% gel	In 27 g	
		In 50 g	
• Erygel	2% gel	In 5 g	
		In 30 g	$30.50
		In 60 g	$57.99
• Erycette	2% saturated swabs	In 60 pads	$30.99
• T-Stat	2% saturated swabs	In 60 swabs	$28.99
	2% solution	In 60 mL, applicator optional	$25.99
• Akne-Mycin	2% ointment	In 25 g	No cost
• Generic	2 % solution		
	2% gel	In 30 g	$18.65
	2% gel	In 60 g	$38.65
	2% pad	In 60	$48.89
	2% solution	In 59 mL	$26.13 (60 mL)
Metronidazole (Rx)	0.75% gel	In 28.4 g, 45 g	$64.79
MetroGel	1% gel	60 g	$200
		60g kit with Cetaphil	$196
• Noritate	1% cream	In 60 g	$149
SYSTEMIC ACNE MEDICATIONS			
Isotretinoin (Rx)			
• Accutane	10-, 20-, 40-mg capsules	In 100s	

erythromycin and **clindamycin.** Of the retinoids, the least expensive is **tretinoin,** at a cost of $31 for a 15-g tube of the generic formula and $40 (**Ativa**) to $50 (**Retin-A**) for the brand-name products. **Tazarotene (Tazorac)** is quite expensive, with the cost of a 30-g tube $107. **Adapalene (Differin)** costs approximately $109 for a 45-g tube. The cost of **isotretinoin** ranges from $100 to $500 per month, based on the dose prescribed.

Metronidazole treatment for acne rosacea is quite expensive; **Noritate** costs $149 per 60-g tube and **Metrogel** $200 for a 60-g tube (http://www.drugstore.com).

Monitoring

There is no special laboratory monitoring required with the use of **topical antibiotics** or **topical retinoids.** The primary care provider may be involved in the monitoring of the patient who is started on **isotretinoin** by the dermatologist. Monitoring required for this patient includes baseline CBC, both baseline and monthly liver function tests throughout treatment, baseline and monthly pregnancy testing throughout treatment, and serum lipid profile. Serum electrolytes should be drawn as baseline and after 4 to 6 weeks of treatment. An ophthalmological examination is also required for prescribing **isotretinoin.** If visual difficulties occur, an ophthalmological examination is required, with a second examination 6 to 7 weeks after discontinuation of the medication.

Patient Education

Administration

When **retinoids** are applied topically, it should be explained that the increased turnover of follicular epithelial cells causes extrusion of comedones, even comedones that may not be seen on the skin surface. Clinically, this causes an initial worsening of acne, as comedones that were previously under the skin are extruded. This "worsening" of acne is not a reason for discontinuation of treatment, and the patient should be reassured that the face will clear after approximately 6 to 8 weeks of treatment. The patient should also be instructed to use the medication as prescribed; there is no improved response to topical **retinoids** if they are used more often than recommended, but there is a dramatic increase in skin irritation.

The manufacturer has developed an extensive patient education curriculum for the prescriber of **isotretinoin** to use with patients. This kit includes written and video information, as well as the consent forms that are required when treating patients with **isotretinoin.** It is recommended that any provider who is prescribing **isotretinoin** use this extensive curriculum prior to and during treatment.

Adverse Reactions

It is important to instruct patients that all **topical antibiotics** used in the treatment of acne may cause skin irritation to some degree. **Benzoyl peroxide** may cause excessive drying, photosensitivity, and allergic contact sensitization. **Tetracycline** may cause discoloration of the skin; patients should inform their provider immediately and discontinue the medication. **Azelaic acid** may cause skin hypopigmentation in patients with dark complexions. Patients should be instructed to notify their provider if this problem develops.

Isotretinoin has many significant adverse reactions, as previously described. Patients should be fully informed about these adverse reactions prior to beginning therapy and should have written information to refer to at home if any adverse effects occur.

Lifestyle Management

The nonpharmacological management of acne includes gentle facial cleansers such as mild soaps or facial washes. Scrubbing, picking, and squeezing of comedones should be avoided. Patients should be advised to use skin products that will not aggravate their acne. That includes oil-based cosmetics, hair spray, mousse, and facial creams and moisturizers. **Sunscreens** that are oil free should be used at all times because of the increased photosensitivity due to acne preparations.

TOPICAL CORTICOSTEROIDS

Topical corticosteroids are adrenocorticosteroid derivatives incorporated into a vehicle suitable for application to the skin. The chemical structure is often modified to make them more lipid soluble and to increase potency. Structural changes also decrease mineralocorticoids' effects.

Pharmacodynamics

The therapeutic effects of topical **corticosteroids** are due to their nonspecific anti-inflammatory effects. They act against most causes of inflammation, including mechanical, chemical, microbiological, and immunological. At the cellular level, they appear to inhibit the formation, release, and activity of endogenous mediators of inflammation, such as prostaglandins, kinins, histamines, liposomal enzymes, and the complement system. When applied to inflamed skin, **steroids** inhibit the migration of macrophages and leukocytes into the area by reversing vascular dilatation and permeability. This results in decreasing edema, erythema, and pruritus by suppressing DNA synthesis. **Corticosteroids** applied topically have an antimitotic effect on epidermal cells. This is their primary action in proliferative disorders such as psoriasis.

At the molecular level, unbound **corticosteroids** readily cross the cell membrane and bind with high affinity to specific cytoplasmic receptors. Inflammation is reduced by diminishing the release of leukocytic acid hydrolyses. **Corticosteroids** also prevent macrophage accumulation at inflamed sites. Interference with leukocyte adhesion to the capillary wall and reduction of capillary membrane permeability and subsequent edema also reduce inflammation.

Pharmacokinetics

Absorption and Distribution

Absorption of **topical corticosteroids** varies, depending on the drug used, the vehicle used, the amount of skin surface area the medication is applied to, and the condition of the skin. Absorption is enhanced by increased skin temperature, hydration, and application to denuded areas, intertriginous areas, or skin surfaces with a thin stratum corneum layer (face or scrotum). Occlusive dressings enhance skin penetration and therefore increase drug absorption. Infants and children have more body surface area compared to body weight, and therefore proportionally more medication is absorbed into their system.

The penetration of **topical steroid** through the skin varies with the vehicle the medication is in. Ointments are more occlusive and therefore more potent. Creams are less occlusive and usually less potent. Lotions are usually the least potent. Gels, aerosols, lotions, and solutions are useful in hairy areas.

Occlusive dressings such as plastic wrap increase skin penetration approximately 10-fold by increasing the moisture content of the stratum corneum. This may be beneficial in resistant cases but may also lead to increased adverse effects because increased absorption of the **corticosteroid** may produce systemic side effects.

The relative potency of a product depends on several factors, including the characteristics and concentration of the drug, the vehicle used, and the vasoconstrictor assay. The vasoconstrictor assay is developed by applying an agent to the skin under occlusion and assessing the area of skin blanching. Other assays of **steroid** potency involve suppression of erythema and edema following experimentally induced inflammation. **Corticosteroids** distribute into breast milk and cross the placenta.

Metabolism and Excretion

Following topical administration, **corticosteroids** enter the bloodstream and are metabolized and excreted via the same pathways as systemic **steroids. Corticosteroids** are metabolized in the liver, although some topical preparations are partially metabolized in the skin. Inactive metabolites, as well as a small portion of unchanged drug, are excreted in the urine.

Pharmacotherapeutics

Precautions and Contraindications

Corticosteroids are contraindicated in any patient with a history of hypersensitivity to other **corticosteroids** or any ingredient in the preparation.

Corticosteroids are contraindicated as monotherapy in primary bacterial infections, treatment of rosacea, or acne vulgaris. Use of high-potency or very-high-potency agents on the face, groin, or axilla is contraindicated. Ophthalmic use should be reserved for specialty practice only, because prolonged ocular exposure may cause steroid-induced glaucoma and cataracts. When applied to the eyelids or the skin near the eyes, the drug may enter the eyes.

Corticosteroids are Pregnancy Category C. **Corticosteroids** are teratogenic in animals when administered systemically at relatively low dosages. There are no adequate and well-controlled studies of **topical steroid** use in pregnant women. Therefore, use during pregnancy is advised only if the potential benefits outweigh the potential hazards to the fetus. In pregnant patients, do not use extensively.

Systemic **corticosteroids** are excreted into breast milk in quantities not likely to have an adverse effect on the infant. Nevertheless, exercise caution when administering **topical steroids** to a nursing mother.

Children may be more susceptible to topical **corticosteroids'** effects because of their larger body surface area compared to weight. Therefore, in infants and young children, the lowest effective strength of **topical steroid** should be used to prevent systemic **corticosteroid** effects. Use of high-potency or very-high-potency agents should be avoided. Hypothalamic-pituitary-adrenal (HPA) axis suppression, Cushing's syndrome, and intracranial hypertension have been reported in children receiving topical **corticosteroids**. Many of the topical **corticosteroids** have been relabeled recently and are not to be used in children due to HPA suppression. Chronic **corticosteroid** therapy in children may interfere with growth and development.

The normal inflammatory response to local infections may be masked by topical **corticosteroids**.

Adverse Drug Reactions

Topical corticosteroid preparations may all cause localized skin irritation (pruritus, dryness, burning, and dermatitis). Use of **topical corticosteroids** also increases the risk for secondary infection due to immunosuppression. Other localized effects include acneiform rash, allergic contact dermatitis, folliculitis, hypertrichosis, miliaria, and maceration of the skin. Skin atrophy, hypopigmentation, striae, and xerosis may occur. Tolerance may occur with prolonged use of **topical corticosteroids**. Tolerance is reversible and may be prevented by interrupted or cyclic schedules of application for chronic dermatological conditions.

Systemic absorption may produce reversible HPA axis suppression, Cushing's syndrome, hyperglycemia, and glycosuria. They are more likely to occur with occlusive dressings and with more potent steroid preparations. Patients with liver failure or children may be at higher risk for systemic **steroid** effects.

Following prolonged application of **topical corticosteroid** around the eyes, cataracts and glaucoma may develop.

Changing to a less potent **topical corticosteroid** preparation may minimize the risk of adverse reactions.

Drug Interactions

There are no significant drug interactions noted with topical **corticosteroid** use.

Clinical Use and Dosing

Inflammatory Skin Diseases

Topical **corticosteroids** are used for numerous inflammatory or pruritic dermatoses. Some of the conditions for which **topical corticosteroids** have been proved effective are contact dermatitis, atopic dermatitis, nummular eczema, lichen planus, lichen simplex chronicus, insect bite reactions, discoid lupus erythematosus, and seborrheic dermatitis. Low-dose **topical corticosteroid** may also be used in the treatment of first- and second-degree localized burns and sunburns. The usual dose of a **topical corticosteroid** is to apply it sparingly to affected areas two to four times per day (see Table 23–7). **Topical corticosteroids** have a repository effect; with continuous use, one or two applications per day may be as effective as three or more. One dosing schedule that may be used is to apply the medication twice daily until clinical response is achieved, and then only as frequently as needed to control symptoms.

Table 23–7 ● **Dosage Schedule: Selected Topical Corticosteroids**

Drug	Dosage	Comments
Low Potency		
Hydrocortisone 1% or 2.5%	Apply a thin layer 2–4 times daily	May be used in children
Triamcinolone acetonide 0.025%	Apply a thin layer 3–4 times daily	May be used in children
Intermediate Potency		
Hydrocortisone valerate 0.2%	Apply a thin layer 2–3 times daily	Should be used with caution on face; use lower potency on face
Triamcinolone acetonide 0.1%	Apply a thin layer 3–4 times daily	Should be used with caution on the face; choose lower potency for face
Betamethasone valerate 0.12%	Apply a small amount of foam bid; massage into affected areas until foam disappears	Dispense a small amount of foam onto a clean plate or other cool surface (not on the hand)
Desoximetasone 0.05%	Apply thin film and massage in bid	Not recommended for use in children <10 yr
Mometaxone furoate 0.1%	Apply thin film once daily	Do not occlude

Continued

Table 23–7 ● **Dosage Schedule: Selected Topical Corticosteroids—cont'd**

Drug	Dosage	Comments
High Potency		
Betamethasone dipropionate augmented 0.05% (cream or lotion)	Apply thin film 1–2 times/d until clear; maximum of 45 g of cream or 50 mL of lotion/wk	Avoid abrupt cessation if used for chronic conditions; not recommended in children
Triamcinolone acetonide 0.5% (Aristocort, Kenalog)	Apply sparingly to affected area 2–3 times daily until clear	Avoid abrupt cessation if used for chronic condition; use with caution and sparingly in children
Halcinonide 0.1%	Apply sparingly 2–3 times/d	Avoid abrupt cessation if used for chronic condition; use with caution and sparingly in children
Super-High Potency		
Betamethasone dipropionate, augmented 0.05% (ointment or gel)	Apply thin film 1–2 times daily	Maximum of 45 g/wk; do not occlude
Clobetasol propionate 0.05%	Apply thin layer and rub in gently bid	Maximum of 50 g/wk and maximum therapy length 2 wk; doses as low as 2 g/d may cause HPA axis suppression
Flurandrenolide 4-mcg/cm^2 tape	Apply tape to clean, dry skin every 12 h	Do not use tape with intertrigo or serum-exuding lesions

Another dosing schedule that may be used to achieve therapeutic response with fewer adverse effects is short-term or intermittent therapy with high-potency agents for a short period (3 or 4 consecutive days per week or once per week). This may be more effective and cause fewer adverse effects than continuous use of lower-potency products.

It must be stressed that **topical corticosteroids** should not be abruptly discontinued. After long-term use or after using a high-potency agent, a rebound effect may occur. To prevent a rebound effect, switch to a less potent agent, alternate **topical corticosteroids** and emollient products, or gradually reduce the frequency of application (similar to tapering oral corticosteroids).

In children, low- to mid-potency agents should be used. Low-potency **topical corticosteroids** should also be used on body sites with a thinner stratum corneum layer (face, scrotum, axilla, and skinfolds). If treating large surface areas, a lower-potency agent should be used. Higher-potency agents should be used for areas such as the palms and soles, which are more resistant to treatment. Higher-potency agents are also used for crusting and thickened conditions, which are also more resistant to treatment.

Treatment with very-high-potency topical **corticosteroids** should not exceed 2 consecutive weeks. The total dosage should not exceed 50 g/week because of potential HPA axis suppression.

To increase absorption of **corticosteroids,** occlusive dressings may be used. The technique for properly using occlusive dressings is as follows: First, the area must be soaked in water and gently washed. While the skin is still moist, the medication is gently rubbed into the affected area. The area is then covered with plastic wrap. For hands, a plastic glove may be used; for feet, a plastic bag may be used; and a shower cap may be used for the scalp. After the plastic is applied, the edges should be sealed with tape to ensure that the wrap adheres closely to the skin. Do not use for more than 12 hours in a 24-hour period. This technique should not be used with very-high-potency **topical corticosteroids.**

Psoriasis

Topical corticosteroids are used to treat psoriasis because of their anti-inflammatory effects on the plaques. Moderate- to high-potency **steroids** are used because the psoriasis lesions are generally steroid resistant. Occlusion with plastic may be necessary for best results. The **steroid** cream or ointment is applied two to three times per day. Intermittent or "pulse" therapy minimizes some of the adverse effects and has the best long-term outcome. If using topical **corticosteroids** in the intertriginous areas or on the face, a low-dose medication should be chosen. Regardless of the **topical corticosteroid** preparation, 3 weeks of continuous use is the limit, and patients should be discouraged from using **steroids** for longer periods. **Topical corticosteroids** should be reserved for psoriasis flare, with other medications used for ongoing therapy.

Rational Drug Selection

Potency

The choice of **steroid** based on potency is determined by the area of skin to be treated, the condition of the area, and the patient's condition (Table 23–8). In general, low- to mid-potency **topical corticosteroids** are used on children. On the face or other areas with thin skin, low-potency agents should be used. High-potency agents may be used for brief periods, up to 2 weeks, in areas that are resistant to lower-potency treatment. There are many available **topical steroid** preparations, and it is impossible for

Table 23–8 ◈ **Available Dosage Forms: Topical Corticosteroids**

Drug	Potency	Dosage Form	How Supplied	Cost
Alclometasone dipropionate				
Aclovate	Low	0.05% ointment and cream	In 15, 45, 60 g	$71.77
		0.05% cream (gsk)	15, 45 g	$29.39, $59.79
Amcinonide				
• Cyclocort	High	0.1% ointment, cream	In 15, 30, 60 g	
		0.1% lotion	In 20, 60 mL	
		0.1% cream (fuj)	15-, 30-, 60-g tubes	$25.49, $36.09, $57.19
		0.1% ointment (fuj)	15-, 30-, 60-g tubes	$25.49, $36.09, $56.59
Augmented betamethasone		0.05% emollient cream	In 15, 45 g	
dipropionate	High	0.05% lotion	In 30, 60 mL	
• Diprolene	Super high	0.05% ointment and gel	In 15, 45 g	
• Diprolene AF	High	0.05% cream (sch)	In 15-, 50-g tubes	$47.69, $104.39
		0.05% lotion	In 30-, 60-mL bottles	$60.59, $113.86
	Super high	0.05% gel	In 15-, 50-g tubes	$49.58, $104.12
		0.05% ointment	In 15-, 50-g tubes	$53.40, $112.44
Betamethasone dipropionate	High	0.05% cream and ointment	In 15, 45 g	$12.99, $16.99
• Diprosone	Intermediate	0.05% lotion	In 60 mL	$21.99
	High	0.05% cream and ointment	In 15, 45 g	$13.51, $19.67
• Generic	Intermediate	0.05% lotion	In 20, 60 mL	
		0.05% cream	In 15-, 45-g tubes	$9.99, $11.99
		0.05% lotion	In 60-mL bottles	$21.99
		0.05% ointment	In 15-, 45-g tubes	$9.99, $11.99
Betamethasone valerate				
• Luxiq	Intermediate	0.12% foam	In 50 g, 100 g	$159.84, $291.59
• Valisone	Intermediate	0.1% cream	In 15, 45 g	
	High	0.1% ointment	In 15, 45 g	
• Generic	Intermediate	0.1% cream	In 15, 45 g	
		0.1% ointment	In 15-, 45-g tube	$ 7.99, $15.87
Clobetasol propionate		0.05% ointment, gel	In 15, 30, 45 g	
• Temovate	Super high	0.05% scalp application	In 25, 50 mL	
		0.05% cream	In 15-, 30-, 45-g tubes	$39.83, $54.33, $74.35
			In 60-g tubes	$104.84
		0.05% gel	In 15-, 30-, 60-g tubes	$39.83, $54.33, $90.33
		0.05% ointment	In 15-, 30-, 45-g tubes	$39.83, $54.33, $74.35
			In 60-g tubes	$90.33
		0.05% solution	In 25-, 50-mL bottles	$49.09, $80.95
Clocortolone pivalate				
• Cloderm	Intermediate	0.1% cream	In 15, 45 g	
		0.1% cream	15-, 45-g tubes	$33.73, $73.61
Desonide				
• DesOwen	Intermediate	0.05% cream, ointment	In 15, 60 g	
		0.05% lotion	In 60, 120 mL	
		0.05% cream	In 15-, 60-g tubes	$12.99, $24.99 (generic)
		0.05% lotion	In 118-, 59-mL bottles	$183.17, $123.38
		0.05% ointment	In 15-, 60-g tubes	$16.09, $40.76 (generic)
• Tridesilon	Intermediate	0.05% cream, ointment	In 15, 60 g	
		0.05% ointment	In 15-, 60-g tubes	$16.09, $40.76 (generic)

Continued

Table 23–8 ◈ **Available Dosage Forms: Topical Corticosteroids—cont'd**

Drug	Potency	Dosage Form	How Supplied	Cost
Desoximetasone				
• Topicort	High	0.05% gel	In 15, 60 g	
		0.25% cream, ointment	In 15, 60 g	
Generic	Intermediate	0.05% cream	In 15, 60 g	
		0.25% cream	In 15-, 60-g tube	$64.99, $229.99
		0.5% gel	In 15-g tubes	$66.69
		0.25% ointment	In 15-, 60-g tubes	$87.31, $259.99
Dexamethasone				
• Decaspray	Low	0.04% spray	In 25 g	
Diflorasone diacetate				
Generic	High	0.05% cream	15 g	$27.99
			30 g	$52.81
			60 g	$101.11
		0.05% ointment	15 g	$37.05
			30 g	$42.29
			60 g	$100.50
• Psorcon	Super high	0.05% gel	15 g	
			30 g	
			60 g	
Fluocinolone acetonide				
• Generic	Intermediate	0.025% cream	15 g	$46.10
			60 g	$38.99
		0.025% ointment	15 g	$33.47
			60 g	$38.99
		0.1% solution	20 ml	$53.29
			60 ml	$20.45
Fluocinonide				
• Lidex	High	0.05% cream	15 g	$48.69
			30 g	$69.49
			60 g	$110.19
		0.05% ointment	15 g	$48.69
			30 g	$69.49
			60 g	$110.19
		0.05% gel	15 g	$48.69
			30 g	$69.49
			60 g	$110.19
	0.05% solution		20 ml	$41.49
			60 ml	$104.49
• Generic	High	0.05% cream	15 g	$11.99
			30 g	$12.99
			60 g	$22.71
		0.05% ointment	15 g	$19.99
			30 g	$28.61
			60 g	$50.96
		0.05% gel	60 g	$50.71
		0.05% solution	60 ml	$27.23
• Lidex E	High	0.05% emollient cream	15 g	$48.69
			30 g	$69.49
			60 g	$110.19
• Fluocinonide E (generic)	High	0.05% emollient cream	15 g	$20.18
			30 g	$28.60
			60 g	$47.84
Flurandrenolide				
• Cordran	Super high	4 mcg/cm² tape	24" × 3" roll	$53.63
			80" × 3" roll	$105.02
Cordran Tape		4 mcg/sq cm	Rolls: 24 m × 3 in	$53.63
			Rolls: 80" × 3"	$105.02

Table 23–8 ◆ **Available Dosage Forms: Topical Corticosteroids—cont'd**

Drug	Potency	Dosage Form	How Supplied	Cost
Fluticasone propionate				
Cutivate	Intermediate	0.05% cream	In 15, 30, 60 g	
	0.005% ointment	In 15 and 60 g		
		0.05% cream	In 15-, 30-, 60-g tubes	$32.99, $62.99, $217.11
		0.05% lotion	In 60-mL bottles	$454.60 (120-mL bottle)
		0.005% ointment	In 15-, 30-, 60-g tubes	$32.99, $44.99, $128.28
Halcinonide				
• Halog	High	0.1% emollient cream	In 15, 30, 60 g	
• Halog	High	0.1% cream, ointment	In 15, 30, 60 g	
		0.1% solution	In 20, 60 mL	$33.99, $68.99
		0.1% cream	In 15-, 30-, 60-, 240-g tubes	$28.99, $74.86, $183.06
• Halog-E		0.1% cream	In 30-, 60-g tubes	$74.86, $183.06
Halobetasol propionate				
• Ultravate	Super high	0.05% cream, ointment	In 15, 45 g	
		0.05% ointment	In 15-, 50-g tubes	$64.78, $180.27
		0.05% cream	In 15-, 50-g tubes	$63.16, $152.54
Hydrocortisone				
• Hytone	Low	1% cream, ointment	In 30, 120 g	
		1% lotion	In 120 mL	
		2.5% cream, ointment	In 30, 60 g	
		2.5% lotion	In 60 mL	
		2.5% cream	In 28.4-, 56.8-g tubes	$42.99, $68.59
		2.5% cream	In 30-g tubes	$8.19
		2.5% ointment	In 28.4-g tubes	$42.99
		2.5% lotion	In 59-mL bottle	$63.99
• Cortisone 10 (OTC)	Low	1% cream, ointment	In 30 g	
• Cortisone 5 (OTC)		0.5% cream	In 60 g	
• Generic	Low	1% cream, ointment	In 20, 30, 120 g, 1 lb	$11.99 (15g), $11.99 (28g)
		2.5% cream, ointment	In 20, 30, 120 g, 1 lb	$13.67 (30g)
Hydrocortisone acetate				
• Maximum Strength Cortaid (OTC)	Low	1% cream, ointment	In 15, 30 g	$8.49
Hydrocortisone butyrate				
• Locoid	Intermediate	0.1% ointment, cream	In 15, 45 g	
		0.1% solution	In 20, 60 mL	
		0.1% cream	In 15-g tubes	$67.49
		0.1% lipocream	In 15-, 45-g tubes	$85.41, $174.86
		0.1% cream	In 45-g tubes	$183.83
		0.1% ointment	In 15-, 45-g tubes	$15.89, $29.59
		0.1% solution	In 20-, 60-mL bottles	$79.28, $219.43
Hydrocortisone valerate				
• Westcort	Intermediate	0.2% cream or ointment	In 15, 45, 60 g	
		0.2% ointment	In 15-, 45-, 60-g tubes	$22.39, $40.79, $48.39
		0.2% cream	In 15-, 45-, 60-g tubes	$22.39, $40.79, $48.39
Mometasone furoate				
• Elocon	Intermediate	0.1% ointment, cream	In 15, 45 g	
		0.1% lotion	In 27.5, 55 mL	
		0.1% cream	In 15-, 45-g tubes	$47.68, $79.13
		0.1% ointment	In 15-, 45-g tubes	$49.85, $76.45
		0.1% lotion	In 30-, 60-mL bottles	$49.85, $86.71

Continued

Table 23–8 ◆ **Available Dosage Forms: Topical Corticosteroids—cont'd**

Drug	Potency	Dosage Form	How Supplied	Cost
Triamcinolone acetonide				
• Aristocort	Low	0.025% cream, ointment	In 15, 60 g, 1 lb	
	Intermediate	0.1% cream, ointment	In 15, 60, 240 g	
	High	0.5% cream	In 15, 240 g	
• Aristocort A		0.025% cream	In 15-, 60-g tubes	$11.99, $40.99
		0.5% cream	In 15-g tubes	$12.99
		0.1% ointment	In 15-, 60-g tubes	$11.99 (15 g)
• Kenalog	Low	0.025% cream, ointment	In 15, 80, 240 g	
		0.025% lotion	In 60 mL	
	Intermediate	0.1% cream	In 15, 60, 80, 240 g	
		0.1% lotion	In 60 mL	
		0.2% aerosol	In 23, 63 g	
	High	0.5% cream	In 20 g	
		aerosol spray	In 63-g units	$118.99
		0.025% ointment	In 80-g tubes	$21.69
		0.1% cream	In 15-, 60-, 80-g tubes	$18.99 (15 g)
• Kenalog		0.1% ointment	In 15-, 60-g tubes	$19.59, $40.29
• Kenalog		0.5% cream	In 20-g tubes	$54.99
• Kenalog		0.025% lotion	In 60-, 60-mL bottles	$46.99
		0.1% lotion	In 60-mL bottles	$51.99
• Triamcinolone		0.1% cream	In 454-g jars	$15.69
		0.1% cream	In 15-g tubes	$11.99
		0.1% cream	In 80-g tubes	$12.99
• Triamcinolone		0.1% ointment	In 15-g tubes	$11.99
		0.1% ointment	In 80-, 454-g tubes	$18.99 (80 g)
• Triamcinolone		0.5% cream (generic)	In 15-g tubes	$12.99

any practitioner to be familiar with all of them. It is reasonable for the practitioner to be familiar with one or two agents in each potency category. Each provider needs to be familiar with what medications are allowed from each category in the formulary he or she is using.

Vehicle

The vehicle used may increase or decrease the potency of the **corticosteroid.** As previously mentioned, ointments are more occlusive and are effective for dry or scaly lesions. Creams may be used more frequently on oozing lesions on intertriginous areas, where the occlusive effects of ointments may cause increased adverse effects. Gels, aerosols, lotions, and solutions are used on hairy areas. The urea that is added to some products may enhance the penetration of **hydrocortisone** and other **steroids** by hydrating the skin. **Steroid-impregnated tape (Cordran)** is useful for occlusive therapy in small areas.

Cost

In general, lower-potency and generic products are less expensive than higher-potency and brand-name products, although this difference may be offset by increased efficacy in short-term burst therapy with some dermatoses. Therefore, cost must be evaluated, and the practitioner must determine whether it will be a part of the drug-selection process. Cost must also come into effect when prescribing off-formulary. If possible, prescribe medications that will be covered by the patient's insurance.

Monitoring

Adrenal function should be monitored in children if a high-potency **steroid** or occlusion is used. Adrenal function should also be assessed in adults who are applying more than 50 g weekly of a high-potency **steroid** preparation. Growth should be monitored in children who are using mid- or high-potency **topical corticosteroids.** The patient should also be monitored for adverse effects, as noted previously. Laboratory studies that should be obtained for patients on high-dose **steroids** are blood glucose and serum potassium levels.

Patient Education

Administration

The patient should be instructed to use the **topical corticosteroid** *exactly* as prescribed. Demonstration of the amount of medication that should be applied will be helpful for most patients. The provider can use a sample-size dose in the area to be treated to show the amount of medication to use. Demonstrate applying a pea-size amount of **topical corticosteroids** and spreading it thinly over the affected area. The patient should also understand the serious adverse effects that may occur with overuse of **topical corticosteroids.** If mid- or high-potency **topical steroids** are prescribed, the patient must understand that these medications are much stronger than, for example, **hydrocortisone** 1 percent cream, and that these medications therefore have more significant adverse effects associated with them if they are not used appropriately. If occlusion is to be used, clear directions regarding it need to be provided to the patient, preferably in writing.

Adverse Reactions

The patient should have written information regarding the adverse effects that may occur with overuse of **corticosteroids.** Patients should report any adverse effects, including worsening of their condition. When prescribing **topical corticosteroids** to children, the provider must clearly outline the course of treatment for the parent. If mid-potency **steroids** are used in children, the parent should understand the concern about growth in children. Patients should also be instructed not to abruptly discontinue their **topical steroid** medications, which also may cause adverse effects.

Lifestyle Management

Patients who are using **topical corticosteroids** often can benefit from nonpharmacological management. Many conditions require the use of moisturizers or emollients to provide optimal outcome in the disease process. Patients should be encouraged to use these nonpharmacological measures, in addition to the prescribed **topical corticosteroid**, to have the most optimal management of their skin condition. Bathing may improve the outcome with some skin conditions, but this must be individualized based on the patient and the condition.

TOPICAL IMMUNOMODULATORS

The **immunomodulators** are a class of topical medications used in the short-term or intermittent long-term treatment of atopic dermatitis. **Pimecrolimus (Elidel)** and **tacrolimus (Protopic)** are a second-line therapy after **topical corticosteroid** treatment failure for atopic dermatitis.

Pharmacodynamics

The therapeutic effects of the topical **immunomodulators** are related to their ability to inhibit calcineurin. The topical **immunomodulators** work through inhibition of phosphorylase activity of the calcium-dependent serine/threonine phosphatase calcineurin and the dephosphorylase activity of the nuclear factor of activated T-cell protein (NF-ATp). NF-ATp is a factor necessary for the cytokines IL-2, IL-4, and IL-5. They might also inhibit the transcription and release of other T-cell proteins which can contribute to allergic inflammation. **Tacrolimus** has been found to inhibit T cells, Langerhans cells, mast cells, and keratinocytes, with skin biopsy after topical tacrolimus treatment finding markedly diminished T-cell and eosinophilic activity in the epidermal cells. **Pimecrolimus** was specifically developed to treat inflammatory skin conditions and is active by binding to FKBP/macrophilin 12 and interfering with calcineurin action. It inhibits the release of inflammatory cytokines and mediators from mast cells.

Pharmacokinetics

Absorption and Distribution

Topical **tacrolimus** and **pimecrolimus** are minimally absorbed. **Pimecrolimus** is 74 to 87 percent protein bound and **tacrolimus** is 99 percent bound to alpha-acid glycoprotein. Distribution into breast milk is not known. It is not known if these drugs cross the placenta.

Metabolism and Excretion

Both **tacrolimus** and **pimecrolimus** are metabolized in the liver via the CYP3A4 system. **Pimecrolimus** is excreted primarily in the feces as metabolites. **Tacrolimus** is eliminated primarily in the bile.

Pharmacotherapeutics

Precautions and Contraindications

The only contraindication to either **tacrolimus** or **pimecrolimus** is hypersensitivity to the product or any component of the cream. The products should not be applied to a site with active cutaneous viral infection. Both products have received an U.S. Food and Drug Administration (FDA) black box warning regarding the long-term safety of **topical immunosuppressant calcineurin inhibitors** due to rare cases of malignancy (skin and lymphoma) that have been reported in patients using the topical forms of these medications. The FDA advisory stated, "Animal studies have shown that three different species of animals developed cancer following exposure to these drugs applied topically or given by mouth, including mice, rats and a recent study of monkeys" (FDA, 2006). Both **tacrolimus** and **pimecrolimus** should be avoided in children younger than 2 years and in immunosuppressed patients. Consider discontinuing the medication if lymphadenopathy of unknown etiology or infectious mononucleosis occurs. Use of these products should be avoided in malignant or premalignant skin conditions. Any bacterial or viral skin infections should be cleared before starting either product.

Both **tacrolimus** and **pimecrolimus** are Pregnancy Category C and should be avoided in the pregnant patient. Neither product is recommended in the breastfeeding mother, as breast milk excretion is unknown. Both products are not to be used in children younger than 2 years. If prescribing **tacrolimus** to children 2 to 15 years, the 0.03 percent ointment is recommended.

Adverse Drug Reactions

Tacrolimus and **pimecrolimus** both may have a local reaction at the site of application, consisting of burning, pruritus, and tingling. Headache is a reported adverse effect of both medications.

Drug Interactions

There are drug interactions reported with topical application of **tacrolimus** or **pimecrolimus**. There is a theoretical interaction between CYP3A4 inhibitors in widespread erythrodermic diseases due to increased absorption and patients should be observed for toxicity.

Clinical Use and Dosing

Pimecrolimus is to be used as a second-line drug in the short-term or intermittent long-term treatment of mild to moderate atopic dermatitis in immunocompetent patients older than 2 years. **Pimecrolimus (Elidel)** is applied to affected areas twice daily. The area where the medication is applied should not be occluded. **Tacrolimus (Protopic)** is used for short-term or intermittent long-term treatment of moderate to severe atopic dermatitis in children older than 2 years and adults. Children aged 2 to 15 years should use 0.03 percent strength, and patients 16 years or older can use either 0.03 or 0.1 percent strength. The **tacrolimus** ointment is applied twice a day and should not be occluded or applied to wet skin. **Tacrolimus** ointment should be continued for 1 week after the resolution of symptoms. The patient should be reevaluated 6 weeks after therapy is started.

Rational Drug Selection

Drug selection is based on the severity of atopic dermatitis, as **tacrolimus** is approved for moderate to severe disease and **pimecrolimus** is approved for mild to moderate disease. The cost of **Elidel** for a 30-g tube is $101 and a 30-g tube of **Protopic** 0.03 percent is $133 (http://www.drugstore.com).

Monitoring

Monitor patients' skin for worsening conditions such as pruritus, erythema, excoriation, and lichenification.

Patient Education

Administration

Patients should use the medication exactly as prescribed. When applying the medication the patient should be instructed to avoid contact with eyes, nose, mouth, and cut or scraped skin. The patient should be instructed not to occlude the area that the medication is applied to. Hands should be washed with soap and water before and after application of the medication. It may take 2 to 3 weeks for improvement and patients need to be advised of this.

Adverse Reactions

Patients should contact their provider if any signs of infection occur. Patients should also report lymphadenopathy or other adverse effects they experience.

Lifestyle Management

Patients using either **tacrolimus** or **pimecrolimus** should avoid exposure to sunlight, and artificial light sources such as tanning beds. Patients should use sunscreen and lip sunscreen (SPF [sun protection factor] 15 or higher) and wear protective clothing such as wide-brimmed hats. Patients can continue to use emollients for their atopic dermatitis.

TOPICAL ANTIPSORIASIS AGENTS

The management of psoriasis consists of topical medication and phototherapy for mild to moderate psoriasis (less than 20% of the body involved) and for severe psoriasis (more than 20% of the body involved) the addition of systemic medications. Patients with severe disease are usually referred to a dermatologist, and therefore systemic treatments with **immunosuppressants (Amevive, Raptiva, methotrexate)**, **retinoids (Soriatane)**, and **tumor necrosis factor blocker (Enbrel)** are not covered in this chapter. Providers need to be mindful of the negative emotional impact of psoriasis and refer patients for more intensive therapy and/or mental health therapy if needed (Skevington, Bradshaw, Hepplewhite, Dawkes, & Lovell, 2006.)

Topical therapy recommended by the American Academy of Dermatology evidence-based guidelines (Menter et al, 2009) for psoriasis consists of **topical steroids, tar,** or **keratolytic shampoos** for scalp involvement, and **keratolytic** agents **(anthralin** and **calcipotriene)** for thick plaques, applied topically. **Topical immunomodulators (tacrolimus, pimecrolimus)** may also be used. The combination of **topical steroids** and the **vitamin D derivative anthralin (Dovonex)** works better than either agent alone. Management of psoriasis is discussed in Chapter 32.

Pharmacodynamics

Calcipotriene, a vitamin D_3 derivative, regulates cell differentiation and proliferation and suppresses lymphocyte activity. In humans, the natural supply of vitamin D depends mainly on exposure to the ultraviolet rays of the sun for conversion of 7-dehydrocholesterol to vitamin D_3 in the skin. After entering the bloodstream, it is metabolized in the liver and kidneys to its active vitamin D form. Vitamin D_3 receptors occur in many parts of the body, including the skin cells known as keratinocytes. **Calcipotriene** has a similar affinity for the vitamin D receptor in the keratinocyte.

Anthralin is an antimitotic agent that is used for chronic psoriasis. It has an antiproliferative effect. The mechanism for the antipsoriasis effect of **anthralin** is unknown, but it inhibits cellular respiration by inactivation of mitochondria.

Coal tar affects psoriasis by enzyme inhibition and antimitotic action. It is manufactured as a by-product of the processing of coke and gas from bituminous coal and is extremely complex, rich in polycyclic hydrocarbons, and variable in composition. Little is known about its mechanism of action. It is used mainly in combination with ultraviolet B (UVB) for this indication.

Tazarotene is a topical retinoid prodrug that is used in the treatment of psoriasis. The exact mechanism of action is unclear at this time. Following topical application, **tazarotene** undergoes esterase hydrolysis to the active form, AGN 190299, which is the cognate carboxylic acid of **tazarotene.** It is believed that the drug works by normalizing epidermal differentiation, reducing hyperproliferation, and reducing the influx of inflammatory cells into the skin.

Pharmacokinetics

Absorption and Distribution.

Approximately 6 percent of **calcipotriene** is absorbed systemically when it is applied topically to psoriasis plaques. Distribution of **calcipotriene** is unknown. There is evidence that **calcipotriene** does cross the placenta. It is not known whether **calcipotriene** is excreted in breast milk.

Absorption and distribution of **anthralin** are unknown, as is the absorption of **coal tar.**

When administered topically to the skin, **tazarotene** has minimal systemic absorption because of its rapid metabolism in the skin to the active metabolite, tazarotenic acid, which is systemically absorbed and further metabolized. There is no apparent accumulation of **tazarotene** within body tissues. Retinoids may cross the placenta, and therefore it is assumed that **tazarotene** is also harmful to the fetus. It is not known if **tazarotene** is distributed into human breast milk; however, animal studies show that single topical doses of radiolabeled **tazarotene** are detected in maternal milk.

Metabolism and Excretion

Approximately 6 percent of a topical dose of **calcipotriene** is systemically absorbed when it is applied to psoriatic skin. Once absorbed, **calcipotriene** is rapidly and extensively metabolized in the liver into inactive metabolites. **Calcipotriene** is excreted in the bile.

Tazarotene is rapidly metabolized in the skin to the active metabolite, tazarotenic acid, which is absorbed and further metabolized. Tazarotenic acid is hydrophilic and quickly metabolized systemically. It is more than 99 percent plasma protein bound. Metabolism of **tazarotene** to tazarotenic acid occurs via esterase hydrolysis in the skin. After systemic absorption, it is hepatically metabolized to sulfoxides, sulfones, and other metabolites. Elimination is via the fecal and renal routes.

The metabolism and excretion are unknown for **anthralin** and **coal tar.**

Pharmacotherapeutics

Precautions and Contraindications

Calcipotriene should not be prescribed to any patients with preexisting hypercalcemia or evidence of vitamin D toxicity. It should also not be used in any patient with hypercalciuria, as this may increase renal calculi formation. **Calcipotriene** should not be applied to the face, as there have been several reports of facial dermatitis following application of this drug to the face. **Calcipotriene** is contraindicated in any patient with known hypersensitivity to any components of the preparation.

The safety and efficacy of **calcipotriene** in children have not been established. Children are at a greater risk of developing systemic adverse effects. **Calcipotriene** should be used cautiously in the elderly because patients older than 65 years have significantly more severe skin-related reactions than do younger patients treated with topical medication.

Calcipotriene is classified as Pregnancy Category C. **Calcipotriene** should be avoided during breastfeeding because adverse effects on the nursing infant may occur.

Anthralin is contraindicated in any patient with known hypersensitivity to **anthralin** or any component of the product. It should not be used on the face. Use of **anthralin** on acutely or actively inflamed psoriasis eruptions is contraindicated.

Coal tar preparations should not be applied to abraded skin. They should also be avoided on skin that is inflamed, broken, or infected because exacerbation of the condition can occur and systemic absorption of the drug can be increased. Sunlight (UV) exposure should be avoided for at least 24 hours after application of **coal tar** products unless patients are otherwise directed by their care provider. Exposure to sunlight causes a photosensitivity reaction. **Coal tar** is classified as Pregnancy Category C. It is not known what effects **coal tar** may have on the fetus. Whether **coal tar** is distributed into breast milk is unknown, although it is advised that **coal tar** should be used by lactating women only when clearly needed.

Tazarotene should not be used on eczematous skin because it may cause severe irritation and worsen eczema.

Tazarotene should be used cautiously in patients with known retinoid hypersensitivity reactions. Exposure to sunlight should be avoided, as well as UV exposure (including sun lamps). Patients must be warned of their increased photosensitivity and their increased potential for sunburn while using **tazarotene. Tazarotene** is classified as Pregnancy Category X and is contraindicated in women who are pregnant or may be considering pregnancy. Adequate pregnancy prevention is essential when childbearing-age women are prescribed **tazarotene.** It is not known if **tazarotene** is distributed into human breast milk; however, it should be used cautiously for breastfeeding women. The safety and efficacy of **tazarotene** in children younger than 12 years have not been established.

Adverse Drug Reactions

The most common reactions reported by patients using topical **calcipotriene** are skin irritation, burning, and pruritus, which affect up to 20 percent of patients during therapy. One to 10 percent of patients report erythema, xerosis, and exfoliative dermatitis. There are also rare reports of allergic contact dermatitis. Hypercalcemia and hypercalciuria occur almost exclusively when the recommended dosage of 100 g/week is exceeded. A significant increase in urine calcium is seen when **calcipotriene** is administered at the maximum weekly dose (100 g/wk) for 4 weeks.

The most significant adverse reaction noted in the use of **anthralin** is staining and discoloration of the uninvolved skin. Skin irritation is also noted. Permanent staining of clothes and bathroom fixtures may occur.

Coal tar may stain hair or fabrics. Excessive or long-term use may cause folliculitis, sensitization, and photosensitivity.

The most commonly reported adverse reactions from **tazarotene** topical use are burning, stinging, xerosis, and erythema. Worsening of psoriasis may occur. Skin irritation and skin pain may also develop. Reactions reported in less than 10 percent of patients include rash, desquamation, irritant contact dermatitis, and skin inflammation. Photosensitivity may occur with **tazarotene**.

Drug Interactions

No drug interactions with **calcipotriene** have been reported (Table 23–9). However, concurrent administration of high-dose **calcipotriene** with other agents may produce hypercalcemia. Those agents include **vitamin D** or **vitamin D analogues** or **calcium supplements**. Avoid prescribing large doses of **calcipotriene** to patients taking **vitamin D analogues** or **calcium supplements**.

Anthralin may not be used concurrently with **topical corticosteroid**. A withdrawal period of 1 week from **topical corticosteroid** is necessary before beginning therapy with **anthralin**.

Coal tar preparations may interact with **tetracycline**, **psoralens**, and **topical retinoids**, and concomitant use should be avoided.

Concomitant use of **tazarotene** and other topical medications that have strong drying effects, such as **benzoyl peroxide**, **salicylic acid**, or **sulfur** preparations, should be avoided. The manufacturer suggests that a patient's skin "rest" until the effects of such preparations subside before using **tazarotene**.

Clinical Use and Dosing

Psoriasis

Calcipotriene is applied in a thin film to the affected psoriasis plaques and rubbed into the skin gently and completely (Table 23–10). In adults, the ointment is applied twice daily in the morning and evening. The patient does not exceed 100 g/week of **calcipotriene** applied to the skin because of increased adverse drug reactions (ADRs) of hypercalcemia or parathyroid hormone suppression (Menter et al, 2009). Safety and efficacy in children have not been established. For the treatment of mild to moderate scalp psoriasis, the patient applies the topical solution twice daily. Improvement will be noted as soon as 1 to 2 weeks after treatment has begun. The patient should be reevaluated after 6 to 8 weeks. **Calcipotriene** may be used in combination with topical **steroids**. A combination of **calcipotriene** and **betamethasone propionate (Dovobet)** ointment is available for use.

Coal tar preparations have been used for over 100 years for the treatment of psoriasis. With newer psoriasis products available, the American Academy of Dermatology ranks **coal tar** as having Level II evidence for efficacy; more effective products such as topical **corticosteroids** or

Table 23–9 ■ Drug Interactions: Selected Psoriasis Medications

Drug	Interacting Drug	Possible Effect	Implications
Anthralin	Topical corticosteroids	Long-term use of corticosteroids may destabilize psoriasis, and withdrawal may cause rebound phenomenon	A withdrawal period of 1 wk from topical corticosteroid is necessary before beginning therapy with anthralin
Calcipotriene	Agent that may cause hypercalcemia: vitamin D, vitamin D analogues, calcium supplements	Concurrent administration of *high-dose* calcipotriene may produce hypercalcemia	Avoid using large doses of calcipotriene in patients taking vitamin D analogues or calcium supplements
Coal tar products	Tetracycline	Increased photosensitivity	Avoid concurrent use
	Psoralens	Increased photosensitivity, severe sunburn	Avoid concurrent use
	Topical retinoids	Increased photosensitivity	Avoid concurrent use
Tazarotene	Photosensitizers (tetracycline)	Increased photosensitivity	Avoid concurrent use; severe sunburn may result
	Skin irritants (products that contain alcohol, lime, menthol, spices, or perfumes; medicated or abrasive soaps or cleaners)	Potentiates the skin irritation caused by topical retinoids	Concurrent use should also be avoided

Table 23–10 ◉ **Dosage Schedule: Topical Psoriasis Medications**

Drug	Dosage	Notes
Anthralin	Begin with 0.1% strength. Apply a small amount to psoriasis lesions and rub in gently, avoiding healthy surrounding skin. Leave on for 10 min and wash off thoroughly. After 1 wk, contact time can be increased to 15–20 min. Increase strength of medication in incremental steps Scalp cream should be applied to scalp after combing hair to remove scale. Leave on for 10–20 min and rinse well. Begin with 0.25% strength and use daily for at least 1 wk. Increase strength if needed	Anthralin may stain skin and clothes. May alternate anthralin with other therapies (retinoids, topical steroids, UV light). Discontinue when lesions are healed and skin looks and feels normal
Calcipotriene	Apply bid to affected area; rub in gently and completely. Treat for 6–8 wk	Improvement is usually noted after 1 to 2 wk
Coal tar products	Cream or ointment preparations: Apply enough to cover the affected area and rub in gently, once or twice daily Shampoo: Apply to wet hair, massage in, and rinse; repeat application and leave on for 5 min. Rinse thoroughly after application Cleansing bar or gel formulas: Apply to the affected area, rub in gently, leave on for 5 min, and then remove excess Coal tar solution: May be used full strength or diluted in 3 parts water and applied to a cotton or gauze pad, then massaged gently into the affected area Baths: The solution may also be used as a bath by adding 4 to 6 tbsp coal tar solution to a tub of lukewarm water. The patient should be immersed into the bath to soak for 10–20 min. Bathing should be performed once daily to once every 3 d; the usual duration of therapy is 30–45 d. The patient must rinse skin thoroughly after a coal tar bath if exposure to UV or sunlight is to follow	All products are staining
Tazarotene	The 0.05% or 0.1% gel is applied in a thin film once daily, in the evening, to psoriatic lesions	Apply to clean, dry skin. No more than 20% of body surface area should be covered

vitamin D derivatives are available (Menter et al, 2009). Regardless, a variety of **tar** preparations, including creams, shampoos, ointments, lotions, gels, and oils are available. The **tar** preparation is applied to the affected psoriatic lesions once or twice daily. For cream or ointment preparations, the patient should apply enough to cover the affected area and rub in gently. Shampoo should be applied to wet hair, massaged in, and then rinsed. The application is then repeated and left on for 5 minutes. The shampoo should be rinsed out thoroughly after application. The cleansing bar or gel formulas should be applied to the affected area, rubbed in gently, and left on for 5 minutes; then the excess is removed. **Coal tar** solution may be used full strength or diluted in three parts water, applied to a cotton or gauze pad, and then massaged gently into the affected area. The solution may also be used as a bath by adding 4 to 6 tablespoons of **coal tar** solution to a tub of lukewarm water. The patient should be immersed into the bath to soak for 10 to 20 minutes. Bathing should be performed once daily to once every 3 days; the usual duration of therapy is 30 to 45 days. Patients must rinse their skin thoroughly after a **coal tar** bath if exposure to UV or sunlight is to follow.

The American Academy of Dermatology (AAD) ranks **tazarotene** as having Level I evidence for efficacy in treating psoriasis, with 50 percent or more improvement seen in the majority of patients (Menter et al, 2009). **Tazarotene** should be applied to clean, dry skin. The 0.05 percent or 0.1 percent gel is applied once daily in the evening to psoriatic lesions for 12 weeks. The patient should use enough to cover only the lesions with a thin film. No more than 20 percent of body surface area should be covered. Because unaffected skin may be more susceptible to irritation, avoid application of **tazarotene** to these areas. **Tazarotene** was investigated for up to 12 months during clinical trials for psoriasis. The AAD notes **tazarotene** is best used in combination with topical **corticosteroids** (Menter et al, 2009).

Anthralin is an older treatment for psoriasis that used to be the mainstay of therapy. The AAD currently rates the evidence regarding **anthralin** use for psoriasis as Level III evidence; better treatment choices are available. However, **anthralin** may still be an appropriate therapy for some patients.

When prescribing **anthralin** to a patient who has never used the medication, use a low-concentration product (0.1%). The medication is applied to the psoriatic lesions and rubbed gently until the medication has been absorbed. Take care not to get the **anthralin** on the healthy surrounding skin. The patient should take care not to apply excessive medication, which increases staining of skin and clothes. After the medication has been rubbed in, it is left on 10 to 20 minutes, then washed off in the shower. After 1 week, the length of time the medication is in contact with the skin can be increased to 15 to 20 minutes. The strength of **anthralin** can be increased in increments (0.25%, 0.5%, 1%) as tolerated. Some patients require the medication to be applied and left on for 60 minutes for improvement in their psoriatic lesions. Treatment should be continued until the lesions are completely healed (when nothing is felt with the fingers and the texture of the skin is completely normal).

Rational Drug Selection

Potency

With multiple medications available for treatment of psoriasis, the provider must decide which medication provides the most improvement to psoriatic lesions without severe adverse effects (Table 23–11). Response to **antipsoriasis medications** is highly individualized; therefore, different medications may be needed for similar presentation of psoriasis.

Vehicle

The patient's clinical presentation often determines which antipsoriasis medication should be used first. Large surface areas may respond to bath emulsions of **coal tar** solutions, where large surface areas can be treated. For scalp psoriasis, **coal tar** shampoo may be used or **anthralin** cream applied to the scalp. **Anthralin** can be irritating to the skin at higher strengths; therefore, lower-strength products should be begun, and the strength increased in increments.

Cost

Of the psoriasis medications, **coal tar** and **topical corticosteroids** are the least expensive. **Anthralin** cream (Zithranol-RR) is expensive ($156 for a 45-g tube), as is **calcipotriene (Dovonex)** ($284 for a 60-g tube), **calcitriol (Vectical)** ($485 for a 100-g tube) and **tazarotene** (Avage) ($182 for a 30-g tube of cream) (http://www.drugstore.com).

Monitoring

The patient who is being treated for psoriasis should be monitored for the effectiveness of therapy and for adverse effects of the medication. There is no laboratory monitoring required unless treatment levels of **calcipotriene** approach 100 g/week. At that point, serum and urine

Table 23–11 ◆ **Available Dosage Forms: Selected Psoriasis Medications**

Drug	Dosage Form	How Supplied	Cost
Anthralin (Rx)			
• Drithocreme	0.1%, 0.25%, 0.5%, 1% cream	In 50-g tubes	
• Dritho-Scalp	0.25%, 0.5% scalp cream	In 50-g tubes	
• Lasan	0.4% ointment	In 60-g tubes	
	0.1%, 0.2%, 0.4%, 1% cream	In 65-g tubes	
• Psoriatec cream	1%	In 50-g tubes	$93.99
Calcipotriene (Rx)			
Dovonex	0.005% ointment	In 60-g tubes	$145.29
	0.005% cream	In 60-g tubes	$303.51
	0.005% solution	In 60-mL bottles	$323.98
Coal tar products (OTC)			
• Ionil Shampoo	5% shampoo	In 946 mL	$29.99
• Zetar	30% coal tar emulsion	In 177 mL and 6 oz	
	1% shampoo	In 6 oz	
• Medotar	1% coal tar ointment	In 480 g	
• MG217 Medicated	2% coal tar ointment	In 108, 480 g	
• Fototar	2% cream	In 85, 480 g	
• MG217 Dual Treatment	5% coal tar lotion	In 120 mL	
• Tegrin for Psoriasis	5% coal tar lotion	In 177 mL	
• Oxipor VHC	48.5% coal tar lotion	In 57, 118 mL	
• Various generic	20% coal tar	In 120 mL, pint, and gal	
Tazarotene			
Tazorac	0.05% gel	In 30-g tubes	$180.39
		In 100-g tubes	$601.14
	0.1% gel	In 30-g tubes	$191.64
		In 100-g tubes	$638.75

calcium should be measured to determine the patient's risk for hypercalcemia or hypercalciuria.

Patient Education

Administration

Patients should be instructed to use their psoriasis medications exactly as prescribed. **Vitamin D derivatives** need to be applied as directed, as more than 100 g/week may cause hypercalcemia. Medications such as **coal tar** or **anthralin** may cause staining or discoloration of the skin, especially if not used correctly. Use of **tazarotene** on healthy skin increases adverse reaction. The patient should be advised not to increase the number of doses per day; doing so increases adverse effects.

Adverse Reactions

The patient should be instructed that **anthralin** might stain skin, bathroom fixtures, and clothes. Proper application of topical medications will not only optimize treatment but also decrease the adverse effects of the medication. The provider should review the use of medication prior to any change in therapy. Some psoriasis medications cause photosensitivity; therefore, the patient should be instructed to apply sunscreen or avoid sun exposure during therapy.

TOPICAL ANTISEBORRHEIC MEDICATIONS

Topical **antifungals** are the treatment mainstay for seborrheic dermatitis (Naldi & Rebora, 2009). In addition, **antiseborrheic shampoos** and **topical steroid** preparations may be use used. **Selenium sulfide** and **pyrithione zinc** are commonly used seborrhea shampoos. **Tar shampoo** is another therapy choice. **Sulfacetamide sodium** is another option and is available in lotion form and in combination with other **antiseborrheic medications** in many formulations.

Pharmacodynamics

Seborrhea is an inflammatory dermatitis that produces erythematous patches and scales. **Selenium sulfide (Selsun)** appears to have a cytostatic effect on the cells of the epidermis and follicular epithelium, leading to reduced corneocyte production. **Pyrithione zinc (Head & Shoulders)** is a cytostatic agent that reduces the cell turnover rate. Its mechanism of action is thought to be a nonspecific toxic effect on the epidermal cells. **Tar** derivatives treat seborrhea by correcting abnormal keratinization and by decreasing epidermal proliferation and dermal infiltration. **Tar** derivatives also decrease pruritus. The antifungals **ketoconazole (Nizoral)** and **ciclopirox** work against dandruff and seborrheic dermatitis because of activity against *Pityrosporum ovale*, a pathogen implicated in seborrhea. **Sulfacetamide sodium (Sebizon)** is an antibacterial agent that exerts a bacteriostatic effect against gram-positive and gram-negative microorganisms, the common organisms isolated from secondary cutaneous infections.

Pharmacokinetics

Absorption and Distribution

Absorption and distribution of **topical selenium sulfide, pyrithione zinc, ketoconazole,** and **sulfacetamide sodium** are unknown.

Metabolism and Excretion

Metabolism and excretion of topical **selenium sulfide, pyrithione zinc, ketoconazole,** and **sulfacetamide sodium** are unknown.

Pharmacotherapeutics

Precautions and Contraindications

Selenium sulfide is contraindicated in patients with acute inflammation and exudate, as absorption can be increased. It is also contraindicated in patients who are sensitive to any ingredients. There are no contraindications to the use of **pyrithione zinc. Tar** preparations should not be used on open or infected lesions or on areas of acute inflammation. **Ketoconazole** is contraindicated only for patients who are hypersensitive to any component of the product. It also contains sulfites, and patients who are sensitive to sulfites should be advised not to use **ketoconazole** shampoo. **Sulfacetamide sodium** should not be prescribed if sensitivity to **sulfonamides** is present, because cross-reactions to topical **sulfa** preparations may occur.

Selenium sulfide is Pregnancy Category C, as is **sulfacetamide sodium.** Some **tar** preparations **(Zetar)** are Pregnancy Category C, and others have no pregnancy warnings listed. **Tar** preparations should not be used in children younger than 2 years. **Ketoconazole shampoo** is Pregnancy Category C.

Adverse Drug Reactions

Skin irritation can occur with any of the **topical antiseborrheic** products. They may also cause greater-than-normal hair loss, hair discoloration, and scalp and hair oiliness or dryness. **Ketoconazole shampoo** may interfere with permanent wave solution.

Drug Interactions

There are no identified drug interactions with any of the **topical antiseborrheic** products.

Clinical Use and Dosing

Seborrhea and Dandruff

Selenium sulfide shampoo is available as an OTC product, which is 1 percent **selenium sulfide** (Selsun Blue,

Head & Shoulders Intensive), or by prescription, which contains 2.5 percent **selenium sulfide (Excel, Selsun)**. **Selenium sulfide shampoo** is massaged into wet hair and left on for 2 to 3 minutes before rinsing thoroughly. It should be applied twice a week until the dandruff is under control, usually within 2 weeks, and then weekly to maintain control. **Ketoconazole shampoo** is applied to wet hair, lathered, rinsed, and then repeated. It should be used every 3 to 4 days for up to 8 weeks. **Ciclopirox shampoo (Loprox)** is applied to wet hair and worked into a lather, then left on for 3 minutes and the hair then rinsed well. **Ciclopirox** shampoo is used twice a week for 4 weeks. **Pyrithione zinc** is the active ingredient in OTC dandruff shampoos such as **Head & Shoulders**. A bar soap containing **pyrithione zinc** (ZNP Bar) is available for use on body areas with seborrheic dermatitis. **Pyrithione zinc** is applied to wet skin or hair, lathered, rinsed, and repeated; the treatment is repeated once or twice weekly to maintain control of dandruff or seborrhea. **Tar shampoos** are available OTC and range in strength from 0.5 percent (DHS Tar) to 12 percent (**Extra Strength Denorex) coal tar**. The different products vary in their application instructions from daily to weekly, and the patient should be advised to follow the label instructions (Table 23–12). The variety of **antiseborrheic medications** and their dosage forms are found in Table 23–13.

Cradle Cap

Cradle cap in infants that is resistant to nonpharmacological treatment is treated with low-strength **selenium sulfide shampoo** (1%), which is applied in small amounts to the infant's scalp, massaged in, and rinsed well. The shampoo

Table 23–12 ● **Dosage Schedule: Topical Antiseborrheic Medications**

Drug	Indication	Dosage	Notes
Ketoconazole shampoo	Dandruff	Apply to wet hair. Apply and massage into scalp for 1 min, rinse, and repeat, leaving on scalp for 3 min. Use twice weekly for 4–8 wk, with at least 3 d between shampooing	Ketoconazole shampoo is available in 1% (OTC) or 2% (Rx) formulas. There is no information regarding efficacy of choosing one over the other
Pyrithione zinc	Dandruff	Shampoo is applied to wet hair, lathered, rinsed, and repeated. Repeat once or twice weekly to maintain control of dandruff.	Keep out of eyes
	Seborrheic dermatitis	Use pyrithione zinc bar or shampoo. Wet skin, lather, rinse, and repeat. Repeat once or twice weekly to maintain control of seborrhea	
Selenium sulfide	Dandruff/seborrheic dermatitis	Shampoo is massaged into wet hair, left on for 2–3 min, and rinsed well. Apply twice a week until the dandruff is under control, usually within 2 wk, then once a week to maintain control	Avoid getting in eyes
	Cradle cap	Apply shampoo (1%) to the infant's scalp, massage in, and rinse well. Apply twice weekly. Resolution of cradle cap usually occurs after 2 wk of treatment	The shampoo should not be allowed to get in the infant's eyes, and it should be rinsed out well
Sulfacetamide sodium	Dandruff/seborrheic dermatitis	Apply lotion to affected areas at bedtime. Apply by parting the hair and squeezing a small amount of medication on the scalp. Once scalp is completely moistened, massage in medication for 2–3 min. Allow medication to remain on overnight, and rinse well or shampoo with a gentle cleanser Apply medication at bedtime for 8–10 nights. Once seborrhea is under control, lotion can be applied once or twice weekly to maintain control	If scalp is oily or greasy, shampoo hair before application of sulfacetamide sodium lotion. In severe cases (thick crusts or scaling), twice-daily application may be needed initially
Tar-derivative shampoos	Dandruff, seborrheic dermatitis, cradle cap, and other oily, itchy skin conditions	Refer to specific product labeling. Apply to wet hair, lather, rinse, and repeat, leaving on for 5 min the second time. Rinse well	Refer to product label for frequency of use. For severe cases, use daily until control is reached, then once or twice/wk

Table 23–13 ◆ **Available Dosage Forms: Antiseborrheic Medications**

Drug	Dosage Form	How Supplied	Cost
Ketoconazole shampoo			
• Nizoral (Rx)	2% shampoo	In 4 oz	$32.58
• Nizoral A-D (OTC)	1% shampoo	In 4, 7 oz	$15.49 (7 fl oz)
• Generic	2% shampoo		$27.53
Pyrithione zinc			
• Head & Shoulders	1% shampoo	In 120, 165, 210, 330, 450 mL	$7.99 (700 mL)
• Zincon	1% shampoo	In 118, 240 mL	$9.49 (236 mL)
• Danex	1% shampoo	In 120 mL	
• DHS Zinc	2% shampoo	In 180, 360 mL	
• Sebulon	2% shampoo	In 120, 240 mL	
• Tegrin	2% shampoo		$9.89
• Selsun Salon	1% shampoo	384 mL	$6.59
• ZNP Bar	2% shampoo	In 119-g bars	
Selenium sulfide shampoo			
• Selsun Blue (OTC)	1% shampoo	In 120, 240, 330 mL	$8.99 (325 mL)
• Selsun (Rx)	2.5% shampoo	In 120 mL	$17.29
• Head & Shoulders Intensive	1% shampoo	In 120, 240, 330 mL	
• Treatment (OTC)	2.5% shampoo	In 120 mL	
• Excel (Rx)	1% shampoo (Rx)	In 120 mL	
• Generic	2.5% shampoo (OTC)	In 120 mL	$15.29
Sulfacetamide sodium			
Sebizon (Rx)	10% lotion	In 85 g	$29.49
Tar-derivative shampoos (OTC)			
• Zetar	1% coal tar	In 6 oz	
• Theraplex T	1% coal tar	In 240 mL	
• Ional T Plus	2% coal tar	In 120, 240 mL	$29.99
• Neutrogena T/Gel Shampoo	2% coal tar	In 132, 255, 480 mL	$15.99 (473 mL)
• Neutrogena T/Gel Conditioner			$6.29
• Tegrin Medicated Shampoo	5% coal tar	Gel: In 71 g Lotion: In 110, 198 mL	$9.49
• Tegrin Medicated Extra Conditioning	7% coal tar	In 110, 198 mL	
• Denorex	9% coal tar	In 120, 240, 360 mL	$9.59 (237 mL)
• Extra Strength Denorex	12.5% coal tar	In 120, 240, 360 mL	$9.59 (237 mL)

should not be allowed to get in the infant's eyes, and it should be rinsed out well. Apply twice weekly, with resolution of cradle cap usually occurring after 2 weeks of treatment.

Rational Drug Selection

There are few clinical data to suggest that one antiseborrheic product is better than another. **Selenium sulfide** 2.5 percent shampoo is commonly prescribed or 1 percent shampoo purchased OTC. **Ketoconazole** shampoo is available OTC (**Nizoral A-D**) and has comparable results to **selenium sulfide** in the treatment of dandruff. Prescription **selenium sulfide** 2.5 percent (**Selsun** or generic) is approximately the same cost ($17 for a 120-mL bottle) as **ketoconazole (Nizoral)** ($16 for a 7-oz bottle) (http://www.drugstore.com). **Ciclopirox shampoo (Loprox)** is $220 for a 120-mL bottle (http://www.drugstore.com).

Monitoring

There is no laboratory monitoring necessary for any of the topical antiseborrheic agents.

Patient Education

Administration

The patient should be instructed to use the medication exactly as directed. Overuse increases adverse effects, without clinical improvement in seborrhea. Seborrheic dermatitis cannot be cured, only controlled; therefore, continued use of the medication will be necessary to maintain control. All of the medications should be rinsed well after use.

Adverse Reactions

Patients should be advised to notify their provider if they have an adverse reaction to the medication prescribed.

TOPICAL ANTIHISTAMINES AND ANTIPRURITICS

The topical antihistamine commonly used is **diphenhydramine (Benadryl)**. It may be combined with a variety of other ingredients such as **calamine** and **zinc oxide**

(Caladryl, Ziradryl) in OTC products used to treat itching associated with minor skin disorders. **Doxepin (Zonalon)** cream can be used for moderate to severe pruritus associated with atopic dermatitis.

Pharmacodynamics

Topical **diphenhydramine** provides local relief from pruritus and edema because its local effect on the H_1-receptors suppresses the formation of edema, flare, and pruritus. It may also provide local anesthetic activity by decreasing the permeability of the nerve cell membrane to sodium ions, thus blocking the transmission of nerve impulses.

Doxepin's topical mechanism of action is unclear but probably related to its H_1- and H_2-receptor blocking action. Histamine-blocking drugs appear to compete at histamine receptor sites and inhibit the activation of histamine receptors.

Pharmacokinetics

Absorption and Distribution

Diphenhydramine is not absorbed in sufficient quantities to produce measurable serum concentrations except in young children and infants when applied to large surface areas or denuded area.

Significant amounts of **doxepin** for topical use can be absorbed systemically if it is used over 10 percent of the body surface area or for long periods. Absorption is increased by occlusion. Serum levels may reach one-third the level of **doxepin** taken orally. It is unknown whether **doxepin** crosses the placenta. **Doxepin** is excreted in breast milk.

Metabolism and Excretion

Metabolism and excretion of topical **diphenhydramine** are unknown. Negligible amounts are absorbed.

Absorbed **doxepin** is metabolized in the liver, into an active metabolite, *N*-desmethyldoxepin. Parent drug and metabolite are excreted in gastric juice. *N*-desmethyldoxepin is reabsorbed and further metabolized. Primary excretion is renal. **Doxepin** and its metabolites are known to be excreted in breast milk.

Pharmacotherapeutics

Precautions and Contraindications

Topical **diphenhydramine** is contraindicated if the patient is sensitive to the medication in any form. It is for external use only, and contact with the eyes should be avoided. Prolonged use of topical **diphenhydramine** (more than 7 days) should be avoided. Topical **diphenhydramine** should not be used to treat chicken pox, poison ivy, or sunburn, or used on blistered or oozing skin in children. Applying **diphenhydramine** to denuded skin or to large surface areas increases the potential for toxic psychosis, especially in children (Taketomo et al, 2009). It is recommended that topical **diphenhydramine** be used in children 2 years and older. **Diphenhydramine** is Pregnancy Category B.

Drowsiness occurs in more than 20 percent of patients using **doxepin** cream, especially on more than 10 percent of body surface area. Patients with untreated narrow-angle glaucoma and urinary retention should not use **doxepin** orally or in topical form because of its anticholinergic effect, even in the topical form. **Doxepin** cream is contraindicated for use in children and is classified Pregnancy Category B. **Doxepin** should be used with caution in breastfeeding women; one case of apnea and drowsiness has occurred in an infant whose mother was taking oral **doxepin**.

Adverse Drug Reactions

Topical **diphenhydramine** may cause skin irritation if used for prolonged periods.

Topical **doxepin** cream may cause excessive drowsiness if used over more than 10 percent of the body surface area. It may also cause dry mouth and lips, thirst, headache, fatigue, or dizziness (occurring in 1% to 10% of patients). Up to 21 percent of patients report burning and stinging upon application of topical **doxepin**; 25 percent of those patients classify the burning as "severe." Pruritus, dry skin, and eczema exacerbation are reported in fewer than 10 percent of patients.

Drug Interactions

There are no known drug interactions with topical **diphenhydramine** (Table 23–14). Topical **diphenhydramine** should not be used concurrently with oral or systemic **diphenhydramine**, as doing so increases the likelihood of toxicity.

Doxepin cream interacts adversely with alcohol, cimetidine, and monoamine oxidase inhibitors (MAOIs), and these drugs should be avoided during therapy. **Doxepin** may also interact with any drug that is metabolized by the CYP450 2D6 enzymes.

Clinical Use and Dosing

Local Reactions to Insect Bites, Stings, and Minor Skin Disorders (Poison Ivy, Sumac, and Oak)

Topical **diphenhydramine** is applied to the affected area three to four times a day for up to 7 days (Table 23–15).

Severe Pruritus

Doxepin cream (**Prudoxin**) is applied in a thin layer four times a day in 3- to 4-hour intervals for up to 8 days of treatment. Treatment for longer than 8 days may result in higher systemic levels of **doxepin**. Other available topical antipruritics that are safer to use than **doxepin** are the emollients **Aveeno cream** (colloidal oatmeal based) and **Moisturel** emollient cream or lotion (petrolatum, glycerin based).

Table 23–14 ■ **Drug Interactions: Topical Antihistamine and Antipruritic Medications**

Drug	Interacting Drug	Possible Effect	Implications
Diphenhydramine	No known drug interactions		
Doxepin	Alcohol	Increased sedative effects of doxepin	Use together with caution. Advise patients to limit alcohol use when using topical doxepin
	Cimetidine	May affect serum doxepin levels	Avoid concurrent use
	MAOIs	Serious side effects and death reported with the use of MAOIs and drugs related to doxepin	Separate use of 2 medications by at least 2 wk
	Medications metabolized by CP450 2D6 enzymes	Decreased metabolism of doxepin, leading to increased plasma levels	Monitor closely. May need to adjust dosage of doxepin or other drug. Use together with caution

MAOIs = monoamine oxidase inhibitors.

Table 23–15 ● **Dosage Schedule: Topical Antihistamine and Antipruritic Medications**

Drug	Indication	Dosage	Comments
Diphenhydramine	Local reactions to insect bites, stings, and minor skin disorders (poison ivy, oak, sumac)	Apply to affected area 3 to 4 times/d for up to 7 d	
Doxepin	Short-term management of moderate to severe pruritus	Apply a thin film qid in at least 3- to 4-h intervals. May use for ≤8 d	If excessive drowsiness occurs, do one of the following: 1. Decrease body surface area treated 2. Reduce the number of applications/d

Rational Drug Selection

Selection of a topical **antihistamine** is based on the severity of the pruritus, with **doxepin** reserved for severe cases.

Monitoring

There is no laboratory monitoring necessary with the use of topical **diphenhydramine.**

There is no laboratory monitoring necessary with short-term use of topical **doxepin**, although serum **doxepin** levels may be necessary for use over prolonged periods.

Patient Education

Administration

The patient should be instructed to use the medication exactly as prescribed (Table 23–16). Overuse or incorrect use may increase the adverse effects of these topical medications.

Adverse Reactions

Parents should be cautioned against extensive use of topical **diphenhydramine** in infants and young children, as well as avoiding concurrent use of topical and oral products. Patients who are prescribed **doxepin** should be told about the potential for drowsiness and be warned against driving or operating hazardous machinery until they are reasonably certain that **doxepin** does not affect their ability to operate safely.

Table 23–16 ◆ **Available Dosage Forms: Topical Antihistamine and Antipruritic Medications**

Drug	Dosage Form	How Supplied	Cost
Diphenhydramine (OTC)			
• Benadryl	1% cream	In 15 g	$5.79
	1% spray	In 60 mL	$6.49
• Maximum Strength			
• Benadryl 2%	2% cream	In 15 g	
	2% spray	In 60 mL	$6.99
• Generic	1% cream	In 15, 45 g	$3.99
Doxepin			
Zonalon	5% cream	In 30 g	$144.29
		In 45 g	$200.13

Lifestyle Management

Patients should be encouraged to use nonpharmacological measures to control their pruritus, including avoidance of sensitizing agents and the use of OTC emollient products such as **Aveeno** to treat their pruritus.

MOISTURIZERS, EMOLLIENTS, AND LUBRICANTS

Moisturizers, **lubricants**, and **emollients** help to retain water in the skin. They are composed of petrolatum, lanolin, or other agents such as colloidal oatmeal in an emulsion.

Pharmacodynamics

Emollients, **moisturizers**, and **lubricants** are applied after the patient bathes. This procedure acts to trap the moisture in the skin. Ointments provide the most occlusive barrier; creams are the next best. Lotions offer the convenience of easy application over large areas of skin but are not as occlusive as ointments and creams.

Pharmacokinetics

Topical **emollients** interact only with the outermost layers of the skin and are not absorbed systemically.

Pharmacotherapeutics

Precautions and Contraindications

There are no true contraindications to **emollients**, other than to avoid getting them in the eyes. Patients who are allergic to wool should avoid **Eucerin** and other **lanolin**-containing products.

Adverse Drug Reactions

There are minimal to no adverse drug reactions reported with the use of **emollients**.

Drug Interactions

There are no known drug interactions with **emollients**.

Clinical Use and Dosing

Dry Skin

To treat dry skin, the **emollient** is applied one to four times per day, after patients bathe. Patients pat their skin dry and then liberally apply the lotion or cream to all affected areas. This procedure acts to trap the moisture in the skin. Ointments provide the most occlusive barrier; creams are the next best. Lotions offer the convenience of easy application over large areas of skin but are not as occlusive as ointments and creams. Before using a lotion, make sure it does not contain **alcohol**, which is drying and irritating.

There are many **emollient** products available, but many are eliminated from patient use by their additives of perfumes or other chemicals, to which many eczema patients are sensitive. Commonly used **emollients** are **Aveeno** cream or lotion, **Eucerin** cream or lotion, **Lubriderm** lotion, **Aquaphor** ointment, and **Moisturel** lotion. **White petrolatum (Vaseline)** or vegetable shortening **(Crisco)** can be used in severe cases, although the dermatological community varies in its members' opinions on the use of **petrolatum** and vegetable shortening.

Rational Drug Selection

Cost

Expense can play a role in choosing an **emollient**, as large amounts, over a long period, are needed to be effective. **White petrolatum** is inexpensive and a treatment option for eczema patients who have limited resources. Discussing the cost of **emollients** prior to recommending them to the patient will determine if the provider needs to assist the patient in finding resources to pay for **emollients**, which are usually not covered by health insurance plans. The use of generic equivalents will decrease the cost of **emollients**.

Monitoring

No laboratory monitoring is necessary with the use of **emollients**. Ongoing monitoring of clinical status is necessary to determine if the **emollient** is effective.

Patient Education

Administration

The patient should be instructed to apply liberal amounts of the **emollient** to the areas of dry skin. The **emollient** is most effective if applied just after bathing. Daily use offers the best results.

Lifestyle Management

Nonpharmacological measures used to treat dry skin include hydrating baths and avoidance of offending agents that cause exacerbations. Patients should be told to use rubber or plastic gloves when their hands may be exposed to harsh chemicals or detergents, which may increase dryness. They should avoid wearing irritating fabrics such as wool. Soft cotton clothing allows the skin to breathe.

Baths hydrate the skin. The patient should take a warm—not hot—bath for 20 minutes. The skin is patted dry, and **emollients** are applied immediately (within 3 min) to maintain the skin's hydration. The patient should use mild soap to cleanse the groin and axilla and avoid harsh deodorant soaps. After the bath is also a good time to apply **corticosteroid** creams or ointments, if needed.

AGENTS USED IN THE TREATMENT OF BURNS

In primary care, the most commonly prescribed preparation for partial-thickness burn is **silver sulfadiazine (Silvadene)**. Alternative treatment for a partial-thickness burn includes the topical **antibiotic bacitracin**. Other products used to treat second- and third-degree burns include **nitrofurazone (Furacin)** and **mafenide (Sulfamylon)**, although they are not commonly used in primary care and are not discussed in depth here.

Pharmacodynamics

Silver sulfadiazine is a topical anti-infective active against both bacteria and yeast. It is bactericidal, as it acts on the cell membrane and cell wall to produce a toxic effect on bacteria. It is active against both gram-positive and gram-negative organisms. The organisms that are generally susceptible to **silver sulfadiazine** include *S. aureus, S. epidermidis,* β-hemolytic streptococci, *C. albicans, Klebsiella* species, *Escherichia coli, Enterobacter* species, *Proteus, Pseudomonas, Clostridium perfringens, Morganella morganii, Serratia* species, and *Providencia* species.

Mafenide is bacteriostatic against many gram-positive and gram-negative bacteria, including *Pseudomonas.* It is active in the presence of pus and serum.

Nitrofurazone is a synthetic **nitrofuran,** with a broad spectrum of antibacterial activity, including the following organisms: *S. aureus, Streptococcus* species, *E. coli, C. perfringens,* and *Proteus.*

Reduction of bacterial growth after a deep partial-thickness burn promotes spontaneous healing by preventing conversion of partial-thickness burns to full thickness by sepsis.

Pharmacokinetics

Absorption and Distribution

Silver sulfadiazine is not absorbed through intact skin. On burns, up to 10 percent of the sulfadiazine may be absorbed from **silver sulfadiazine,** with only 1 percent of the silver absorbed. Serum concentrations of 10 to 20 mcg/mL of **sulfadiazine** have been reported when large surface areas have been treated. Once absorbed, **sulfadiazine** is distributed into most body tissues. It is not known whether it crosses the placenta or is excreted in breast milk.

Metabolism and Excretion

The portion of **sulfadiazine** that is absorbed is metabolized in the liver and excreted renally.

Pharmacotherapeutics

Precautions and Contraindications

Silver sulfadiazine is contraindicated in patients sensitive to any of the contents of the preparation, including **sulfa**-sensitive patients.

Silver sulfadiazine is Pregnancy Category B but is considered Pregnancy Category D in the near-term pregnancy. Pregnant women at or near term should not use **silver sulfadiazine.** It is also contraindicated in premature infants and infants 2 months or younger because the sulfonamide displaces bilirubin and causes kernicterus. Use with caution in breastfeeding women.

Silver sulfadiazine should be used cautiously in patients with G6PD deficiency because sulfonamides may cause hemolytic anemia in these patients.

Silver sulfadiazine should be used with caution in patients with hepatic or renal disease, as well as patients with thrombocytopenia, leukopenia, or other hematological disorders. **Sulfonamides** may worsen these disorders.

Sulfonamides should be used with caution in patients with porphyria, as they may precipitate porphyria.

Adverse Drug Reactions

Leukopenia (white blood cell [WBC] count less than 5,000) can occur in up to 20 percent of patients who use **silver sulfadiazine,** especially if large surface areas are treated. This occurs within 2 to 4 days of beginning therapy and resolves spontaneously upon discontinuation of the medication.

Patients may also experience burning or pruritus at the site of application. Skin discoloration may occur.

Systemic **sulfonamide** reactions have also been reported.

Clinical Use and Dosing

Silver sulfadiazine is applied to burns once or twice daily, in a sterile fashion. It is applied to a thickness of 1/16 inch. The wound should be clean and debrided. **Silver sulfadiazine** should cover the burn at all times; reapply if the medication is removed. Dressings are not necessary but are helpful to prevent the medication from getting on the patient's clothing. **Silver sulfadiazine** should be used until the burn is completely healed.

Monitoring

If the area that the **silver sulfadiazine** is applied to is large or if treatment is prolonged, the patient's CBC, platelet count, liver function, and renal function need to be monitored. The burn should also be monitored for signs of superinfection or delayed separation.

Patient Education

Administration

Patients can treat small partial-thickness burns themselves and apply the **silver sulfadiazine** at home, although the first one or two applications are best done by a trained health-care provider to teach the patient the proper technique for applying the medication in a sterile fashion.

Adverse Reactions

Patients should be informed of the possible adverse drug reactions that may occur with the use of **silver sulfadiazine** and report any adverse symptoms to their provider.

SCABICIDES AND PEDICULICIDES

Skin and hair infestation is a frequently seen problem in primary care, with arthropods, scabies, and lice the most common. The pharmacological management of scabies and lice consists of **ectoparasiticides.** The specific medication used varies according to the type of infestation and the age of the patient. There is a choice of OTC products (**permethrin, pyrethrins**) for the treatment of head lice. Prescription-strength **permethrin (Elimite)** and lindane are the commonly prescribed **ectoparasiticides**. The first new head lice product in many years, **benzoyl alcohol (Ulesfia)** was approved for use in 2009 and is the first non-neurotoxin FDA approved for head lice. **Malathion (Ovide)** is a pediculicide that is available OTC in the United Kingdom and has been reapproved as a treatment for infestations in the United States, and will be discussed here. **Ivermectin,** which has been used worldwide for scabies treatment, has been recently approved for treatment of immunocompromised patients with severe or crusted scabies. **Ivermectin** will not be discussed in this chapter, as it would not be prescribed in primary care. Nonpharmacological, environmental measures are a key part of the treatment of any infestation, as patients can reinfect themselves or other family members and restart the infestation cycle.

Pharmacodynamics

Pyrethrins are derived from chrysanthemums and are found in combination with piperonyl butoxide in OTC pediculicide products (**RID, Pronto, A-200**). **Pyrethrins** are 100 percent insecticidal and 70 to 80 percent ovicidal. **Pyrethrins** kill lice in 10.5 to 18.6 minutes. There is no residual activity.

Permethrin is a synthetic compound that is related to **pyrethrins.** It acts on the nerve cell membrane to disrupt the sodium channel current. This disrupts the sodium channel polarization, leading to paralysis. **Permethrin** is 97 percent insecticidal and 70 to 80 percent ovicidal. **Permethrin** cream rinse has residual activity against lice for up to 10 days.

Lindane is absorbed through the exoskeleton of parasites, causing CNS excitation, which leads to convulsions and death. It is 67 percent insecticidal and 45 to 70 percent ovicidal. **Lindane** has no residual activity against head lice.

Malathion is an organophosphate agent that acts as a pediculicide by inhibiting cholinesterase activity in vivo. It is very effective against head lice, with 96 percent mortality in 30 minutes (Downs, Narayan, Stafford, & Coles, 2005). Some residual remains and can kill newly hatched lice for up to 7 days.

The active ingredient in **benzoyl alcohol** appears to stun the breathing spiracles of the lice open, enabling the vehicle to penetrate the respiratory mechanism (spiracles), leading to asphyxiation.

Pharmacokinetics

The pharmacokinetics of **pyrethrins** is unknown.

Permethrin is absorbed in unknown amounts, although it is thought to be less than 2 percent of the dose. It is then rapidly metabolized by ester hydrolysis into inactive metabolites, which are excreted in the urine. It is unknown whether **permethrin** crosses the placenta or is excreted in breast milk.

Lindane is slowly and incompletely absorbed through intact skin. Absorption is increased though damaged or occluded skin. There are measurable amounts of lindane absorbed. **Lindane** is stored in the body fat. It is metabolized by the liver and excreted in the urine and feces. It is unknown whether **lindane** crosses the placenta. **Lindane** is excreted in breast milk.

Malathion (Ovide) is absorbed through the scalp when applied as a shampoo and left on for 12 hours. The amount absorbed is small (8%) when applied to the skin, the exact amount when applied to the scalp is not found in the literature. It is not know whether **malathion (Ovide)** crosses the placenta or whether it is excreted in breast milk.

Benzoyl alcohol is minimally absorbed after an exaggerated exposure of 3 times the recommended treatment length in studies of children age 6 months to 11 years.

Pharmacotherapeutics

Precautions and Contraindications

Hypersensitivity to any component of the products is a contraindication to their use. Sensitivity to chrysanthemums is a contraindication to the use of **permethrin.**

Although all of the head lice and scabies treatments are relatively safe, they are classified as neurotoxic agents, and they should be used exactly as directed. To limit exposure, the medication should be washed off at a sink, rather than in a shower. Cool or lukewarm water should be used to minimize absorption caused by vasodilatation (Chesney & Burgess, 1998).

Permethrin should not be used near the eyes. If it gets in the eyes, they should be flushed with water immediately.

Lindane should be avoided in patients with a known seizure disorder. **Lindane** should not be used on abraded or inflamed skin, which increases the absorption of the medication. **Lindane** is neurotoxic and should not be used in pregnant women more than twice during the pregnancy or in children younger than 2 years. **Permethrin** should not be used on infants younger than 2 months.

Malathion (Ovide) is contraindicated in neonates and infants due to the scalp being more permeable, and therefore this age group may have increased absorption of the lotion (see package label). Safety has not been established in children younger than 6 years. **Ovide** is flammable due to its high **alcohol** content and care should be taken not to expose the lotion or wet hair to open flames (including cigarettes) or electric heat sources such as hair dryers or curling irons.

The safety and efficacy of **benzoyl alcohol (Ulesfia Lotion)** was studied in a large multicenter trail in children age 6 months to 12 years. Safety in pediatric patients below the age of 6 months has not been established. **Ulesfia Lotion** is Pregnancy Category B.

Adverse Drug Reactions

All of the topical **ectoparasiticides** can cause skin irritation, some burning, or pruritus. Contact dermatitis can occur, usually the result of incorrect use.

CNS toxicity can occur with **lindane**, but this is almost always associated with ingestion or misuse of the product.

Organophosphate poisoning and severe respiratory distress may occur with ingestion of **malathion**. The product should be used by adults only and care taken to avoid prolonged exposure or over large surface areas.

The common adverse effects of **benzoyl alcohol (Ulesfia)** during clinical trials were pruritus (12%), erythema (10%), and pyoderma (7%).

Clinical Use and Dosing

Head Lice

Treat only those family members who are actively infected (lice or nits seen on head). Do not treat head lice prophylactically. The Centers for Disease Control and Prevention (CDC), Division of Parasitic Diseases recommends that a cream rinse, combination shampoo/conditioner, or conditioner should not be used before using lice medicine. Hair should not be washed for 1 to 2 days after lice treatment (CDC, 2008a). Dosing of **ectoparasiticides** is found in Table 23–17.

Table 23–17 ● **Dosage Schedule: Ectoparasiticides**

Drug	Indication	Dosage	Comments
Permethrin	Head lice	Apply permethrin 1% cream rinse after shampooing. Leave in hair for 10 min, then rinse off. Repeat treatment in 1 wk	It is important that the shampoo formula contain no conditioners, which make the permethrin less effective. Treatment should be repeated in 1 wk, regardless of whether signs of infestation are present
	Body lice	Permethrin 5% is massaged into skin from head to soles of feet and left on for 8 h (overnight), then showered off	Dispense 30 g for an average adult. Should not be used in children <2 mo
	Scabies	Apply 5% cream to entire body and leave on for 8–14 h, then shower off	All family members must be treated. Dispense 30 g per adult
Pyrethrins	Head lice	Pyrethrin shampoo is applied to ***dry hair*** and left on for 10–20 min, with the time varying by brand. Re-treat in 1 wk	It is important for the product to be applied to dry hair to enable the pediculicide to better enter the insect's body. The patient should be retreated in 1 wk regardless of whether there is evidence of infestation
Lindane	Head lice	Lindane is applied to dry hair, working small quantities of water in to create a good lather. Leave shampoo in hair for 4 min	The amount of shampoo prescribed for short hair is 1 oz; for long hair, prescribe 2 oz. The shampoo should be rinsed well
	Body lice	Apply cream or lotion to the total body and leave on for 8–12 h (overnight). Shower off	Dispense 2 oz for an adult
	Pubic lice	Use lindane cream, lotion, or shampoo. Apply a thin layer of cream or lotion to the hair and skin surrounding the pubic area, and leave on for 12 h. The shampoo is massaged into dry pubic hair and left on for 5–10 min. If axillary or thigh hair is also infested, use cream or lotion. Treat again in 7 d if there is evidence of live lice	Sexual partners should be treated concurrently. Bedding and clothing should be washed
	Scabies	Apply cream or lotion from the neck down, and leave on for 8–2 h Shower off	All family members should be treated. Dispense 2 oz per adult
Malathion	Head lice	Apply to dry hair, wet hair and scalp. Let dry naturally. Shampoo after 8–12 h	Flammable; do not use hair dryer

Benzoyl alcohol Head lice
Ulesfia Lotion Usage guideline: Apply to dry hair and scalp. Rinse well after 10 min. Repeat in 7 d.

- *Hair length 0–2 in.: 4–6 oz*
- *Hair length 2–4 in.: 6–8 oz*
- *Hair length 4–8 in.: 8–12 oz*
- *Hair length 8–16 in.: 12–24 oz*
- *Hair length 16–22 in.: 24–32 oz*
- *Hair length >22 in.: 32–48 oz*

Treat only family members who are actively infested (lice or nits seen on head). Do not treat head lice prophylactically.

Pyrethrin shampoo is applied to *dry* hair and left on for 10 to 20 minutes, with the time varying by brand. It is important for the product to be applied to dry hair to enable the **pediculicide** to enter the insect's body more efficiently. The patient should be retreated in 1 week, regardless of whether there is evidence of infestation.

Permethrin is a cream rinse that is applied after shampooing (Table 23–18). It is important that the shampoo not have any conditioners in its formula, which makes the **permethrin** less effective. The cream rinse is left in the hair for 10 minutes and then rinsed out. Treatment should be repeated in 1 week, regardless of whether signs of infestation are present.

Lindane is applied to dry hair, working small quantities of water in to create a good lather. The shampoo is left on for 4 minutes. The amount of shampoo prescribed for short hair is 1 oz; for long hair, 2 oz. The shampoo should be rinsed well.

Malathion (Ovide) is applied to dry hair in an amount sufficient to wet the hair and scalp. Hair should be allowed to dry naturally. Hands should be washed with soap after applying **Ovide. Ovide** is left on for 8 to 12 hours and then shampooed. After rinsing, use a nit (or fine-tooth) comb to remove dead lice and eggs. If lice are present in 7 days, **Ovide** may be repeated.

Benzoyl alcohol (Ulesfia Lotion) is applied to dry hair, completely saturating the hair and scalp and left on for 10 minutes. The lotion is rinsed off well with water. Treatment with another application of **Ulesfia** should be repeated in 7 days.

Nonpharmacological treatments for head lice are popular. With the growing problem of resistance and concern over exposing children to repeated doses of pediculicides, parents are looking for various nonmedicated therapies. Popular and safe remedies are mayonnaise (full-fat variety), olive oil, and petroleum jelly. These remedies likely asphyxiate the lice by blocking their breathing apparatus or immobilize them and affect their ability to feed. A small study of six home remedies found petroleum jelly had the highest egg mortality; only 6 percent of the eggs hatched (Takano-Lee, Edman, Mullens, & Clark, 2004). The authors suggested that none of the remedies they studied were as effective as are pediculicides, which are insecticidal and ovicidal. If a family would like to try these treatments, they should apply a thick layer of the product and cover with a shower cap. The product is left on from 1 hour to overnight, then shampooed out. Removal of nits and lice is critical to the success of treatment.

Body Lice

Because body lice live on clothing and underwear and come to the skin only to feed, instruct patients to wash all clothing and bedding in hot water to kill lice and nits that are on it, as well as treat their bodies with a **pediculicide** (CDC, 2008b). A low potency **corticosteroid** can be prescribed for the pruritus associated with body lice.

Permethrin 5 percent **(Elimite)** is massaged into skin from head to soles of feet, left on for 8 hours (overnight), and then showered off. Dispense 30 g for an average adult.

Lindane has more ADRs than **permethrin**, so it is second-line therapy. It is applied to the total body as a cream or lotion and left on 8 to 12 hours (overnight). The amount needed for an adult is 2 oz.

Pubic Lice

Pubic lice are treated with the same medications used to treat pediculosis capitis (head lice) which are **permethrin** 1 percent or **pyrethrin.** Thoroughly saturate

Table 23–18 ◆ **Available Dosage Forms: Ectoparasiticides for the Treatment of Scabies and Lice**

Drug	Dosage Form	How Supplied	Cost
Permethrin			
• Elimite (Rx)	5% cream	In 60 g	$83.61
• Nix (OTC)	1% cream rinse	In 60 mL with comb	$21.99
Pyrethrins (OTC)			
Generic shampoo		8 oz	$13.49
• RID	0.3% shampoo	In 60 mL	
		In 120 mL	
		In 240 mL	$21.99
• Pronto	0.33% shampoo	In 60 mL	
		In 120 mL	$13.76
• A-200	0.33% shampoo	In 60 mL	
		In 120 mL	
Lindane			
Generic	1% cream	In 60 g	
	1% lotion	In 30 mL, 60 mL, pint, gal	$142.33 (60 mL)
	1% shampoo	In 30 mL, 60 mL, pint, gal	$126 (60 mL)
Malathion (Ovide)	0.5% lotion	In 59-mL bottles	$109.55
Benzoyl alcohol (Ulesfia)	5% lotion	In 227 g bottles	$62.99

hair with lice medication and leave medication on for 10 minutes. **Lindane** is a second-line treatment that is not recommended for first-line therapy because of neurotoxicity (CDC, 2008c). If using **Lindane**, leave on for only 4 minutes. Thoroughly rinse off medication with water. Dry off with a clean towel (CDC, 2008c). Reapply in 7 days if there is evidence of live lice. Sexual partners should be treated concurrently, and bedding and clothing should also be washed. Infestation of eyelashes by pubic lice is treated with **petrolatum (Vaseline)** ointment applied three to four times daily for 8 to 10 days. Nits should be removed by hand from the pubic area, axilla, and eyelashes.

Scabies

All family members should receive treatment for scabies, even those who are asymptomatic. Family members may be in the incubation period, and so all members of the household need treatment to prevent recurrence. The CDC recommends that sexual and any close personal contacts who have had direct prolonged skin-to-skin contact with an infested person also be examined and treated (CDC, 2008d).

Permethrin 5 percent cream **(Elimite, Acticin)** is the drug of choice for the treatment of scabies in young children and pregnant women. It is 90 percent effective against the scabies mite and can be used in infants as young as 2 months and in pregnant women. The cream is massaged into the skin from the neck to the soles of feet. It should be left on for 8 to 14 hours and then washed off in the shower. Infants require special application of **permethrin** to the scalp, temple, forehead, hands, and feet. One ounce of **permethrin** per family member is prescribed.

Lindane 1 percent lotion or cream is used for scabies in children older than 6 months and in nonpregnant adult patients. It is applied in a thin layer from the neck down to the soles of the feet, left on for 8 to 12 hours (overnight), and then washed off thoroughly. If there are crusted lesions present, a tepid bath should be taken prior to application to soften the lesions. Patients should dry the skin thoroughly before applying **lindane**. Two ounces of **lindane** per family member are prescribed.

Topical **corticosteroids** are used *after scabies treatment* to treat the pruritus and inflammation associated with the scabies mite. **Hydrocortisone** 1 percent or 2.5 percent or a stronger **corticosteroid**, if indicated, is applied to affected areas twice a day until the lesions are healed.

Rational Drug Selection

Cost

The relative costs of the different OTC **ectoparasiticides** for head lice are similar, so cost is not usually a consideration in the treatment. **Benzoyl alcohol (Ulesfia)** is $63 per bottle, with up to four bottles needed for treatment if the patient has long hair. **Lindane shampoo** is $126 for 60 mL, the amount needed for one treatment.

Adverse Effects

The provider may choose the drug based on the patient's age and the toxicity of the agent. **Lindane** and **malathion** should be avoided in pregnant patients. **Lindane** is contraindicated in children younger than 2 years, and **malathion** in children younger than 6 years.

Monitoring

No specific laboratory monitoring is necessary with the use of **ectoparasiticides**.

Patient Education

Administration

Patients should be instructed to use the prescribed medication exactly as directed. Treatment failure due to incorrect use of the medication is common. Give *written* instructions about how to apply the medication and the length of time that the medication should be left on the skin or hair.

With the use of **malathion (Ovide)** careful instruction should be given regarding the flammability of the product. Lotion and wet hair should not be exposed to open flames or electric heat sources, including hair dryers and electric curlers. Do not smoke while applying lotion or while hair is wet. Allow hair to dry naturally and to remain uncovered after application of **Ovide Lotion**.

Adverse Reactions

When used as directed, there are minimal adverse effects from the use of **ectoparasiticides**. Skin irritation or toxicity may occur, but the incidence increases if patients use the medication incorrectly.

Lifestyle Management

Environmental measures should be discussed, and written instructions given to patients or family members to take home to refer to as they delouse the home.

CAUTERIZING AND DESTRUCTIVE AGENTS

The cauterizing agents used in primary care are **silver nitrate** and **chloroacetic acid**. There are three **chloroacetic acid** preparations: **monochloroacetic acid**, **dichloroacetic acid**, and **trichloroacetic acid**. **Podophyllum resin** (**Podophyllin**) and **podofilox** (**Condylox**) are used for genital warts.

Pharmacodynamics

Silver nitrate is a strong caustic agent and escharotic. The silver acts as antiseptic, astringent, and germicide. The silver attaches to the protein ion and decreases the protein's solubility. The local effects of silver are self-limiting, and the spread of damage occurs only when the dose of silver overwhelms the capacity of the tissues to fix the ion at the site of application.

Chloroacetic acid rapidly penetrates and cauterizes the skin, keratin, and other tissues.

Podophyllum resin contains podophyllotoxin, which binds to the microtubules in the cell, causing mitotic arrest in metaphase. **Podophyllum** is considered cytotoxic to the wart cells.

Pharmacotherapeutics

Precautions and Contraindications

Cauterizing agents should be used with great care because they damage any skin they touch.

Silver nitrate used for prolonged periods discolors the skin. It also stains any clothing or linens it contacts.

If wet dressings containing **silver nitrate** are used over large surface areas, electrolyte imbalances may occur, specifically hyponatremia and hypochloremia.

Chloroacetic acids are contraindicated in the treatment of malignant or premalignant lesions.

Only a health-care provider should apply **podophyllum resin**, a powerful caustic and severe irritant that must be handled carefully.

Podophyllum resin should not be used in pregnancy because it has led to birth defects, fetal death, and stillbirth. It is also contraindicated in breastfeeding women.

Podophyllum resin is contraindicated in diabetic patients and other patients with poor circulation. **Podophyllum resin** is also contraindicated in the treatment of malignant or premalignant lesions, bleeding warts, and warts with hair growing from them. The use of **podophyllum** should be avoided if the wart or surrounding tissue is inflamed or irritated.

Adverse Drug Reactions

Cauterizing agents are powerful keratolytics and cauterants. Use with caution to avoid contact with healthy skin. To prevent **chloroacetic acid** from spreading to healthy skin, apply petrolatum around the area to be treated as a barrier to the acid.

Irritation and ulcerative local reactions are the major side effects of **podophyllum. Podophyllum** may cause paresthesias. Serious neuropathy and death have occurred from the use of **podophyllum** in large amounts on multiple lesions.

Clinical Use and Dosing

Umbilical Granuloma

Use a **silver nitrate** stick and touch to granulomatous area. One treatment is usually curative.

Aphthous Ulcer, Vesicular, or Bullous Lesion

Touch lesion with a **silver nitrate** stick. One treatment is usually all that is necessary to provide styptic action.

Poorly Healing Wounds or Ulcers

Apply cotton pad dipped in **silver nitrate** solution to the affected area. A **silver nitrate** stick may also be used.

Verruca (Warts)

Remove the callus. Apply a layer of petrolatum to the normal skin around the wart. Apply either **bichloroacetic** or **trichloroacetic acid** to the wart, and cover with a bandage for 5 days. The wart should be removed with the bandage when it is removed.

If using **dichloroacetic acid**, apply it with a pointed wooden applicator or a cotton-tipped applicator. There should never be a large excess drop of acid on the applicator stick. Prevent this by drawing the stick over the lip of the acid container. Touch the applicator stick to the wart. Cauterization progress is determined by a change of the color of the wart to gray white. Three or four treatments may be necessary for heavy growths.

Podophyllum resin is applied by a health-care provider to genital warts. It is not to be dispensed to the patient. After the area is cleansed, **podophyllum** resin is applied sparingly to the lesion. Avoid contact with healthy skin. The first treatment should be left in place for 30 to 40 minutes and then washed off thoroughly with soap and water. Later treatments may require 1 to 4 hours of contact to produce the desired result. Do not treat numerous lesions or large areas in one treatment, which increases the incidence of neuropathy occurring from **podophyllum** use. Multiple treatments may be necessary.

Podofilox (Condylox) is used for the treatment of genital warts. The patient applies the medication twice daily to the wart for 3 days, then discontinues treatment for 4 days. Treatment may be repeated up to four times. It should not be used for warts on the mucous membranes.

KERATOLYTICS

Keratolytic agents are used to treat a variety of hyperkeratotic and scaling cutaneous lesions, such as corns, calluses, and warts. **Salicylic acid** is the only OTC product considered safe and effective by the FDA. **Lactic acid** is used to treat xerosis and ichthyosis vulgaris.

Pharmacodynamics

Salicylic acid produces desquamation of the horny layer of the skin without affecting the viable epidermis. It acts by dissolving the intercellular cement substance in the stratum corneum.

Lactic acid is thought to diminish corneocyte cohesion by interfering with the formation of ionic bonds.

Pharmacotherapeutics

Precautions and Contraindications

Salicylic acid products are contraindicated if the patient is sensitive to **salicylic acid**. Prolonged use in infants and patients with decreased renal or hepatic function is contraindicated, as it may lead to salicylism. Topical **salicylic acid** use is contraindicated patients with diabetes or impaired circulation.

Lactic acid should be used carefully on the face or in patients with fair skin, as irritation may occur. Minimize the exposure to UV light or sun when using lactic acid topically. Lac-Hydrin (12% lactic acid) lotion is Pregnancy Category C and is not recommended for use in nursing mothers. Lac-Hydrin (12% lactic acid) cream is Pregnancy Category B.

Adverse Drug Reactions

Local irritation can occur from salicylic acid contact with normal skin surrounding the wart or callus.

Transient stinging or burning has been reported with the use of topical Lac-Hydrin (12% lactic acid). Erythema, peeling, dryness, or hyperpigmentation may also occur. Lac-Hydrin (12% lactic acid) may cause an eczema flare.

Clinical Use and Dosing

Warts, Corns, and Calluses

There are many salicylic acid products available. Products that are 5 to 17 percent in collodion are used for safe, effective removal of common and plantar warts. Transdermal patches are available in 40 percent and 15 percent strengths for use on warts, corns, and calluses. Patients should refer to the individual product's label for instructions for use. To ensure successful treatment, patients should soak the affected area in warm water for at least 5 minutes before applying salicylic acid. Loose tissue or dried wart tissue is removed with a washcloth or emery board. In the treatment of warts, improvement should occur in 1 to 2 weeks, with complete resolution taking 4 to 6 weeks.

Xerosis, Dry Skin, and Ichthyosis

Lac-Hydrin (12% lactic acid) is applied to the affected area twice a day. The lotion or cream should be rubbed in when applied. Lac-Hydrin cream is not recommended in children younger than 2 years.

Patient Education

Administration

When instructing patients to use OTC salicylic acid, the provider should tell them to soak the affected area in warm water for at least 5 minutes or to bathe just before applying the medication. This will soften the area and allow better penetration of the medication. Improvement will take at least 1 to 2 weeks, and patients should be advised that total healing may take several weeks.

TOPICAL ANESTHETICS

This section discusses the use of EMLA (lidocaine-prilocaine), Synera (lidocaine-tetracaine), and LMX-4 (4% lidocaine cream) for local anesthesia. These products are unique in that they bridge the gap between topical and infiltration anesthesia. It is useful in preparing for painful procedures such as bone marrow biopsies, IV starts, and blood draws. A lidocaine 5 percent patch (Lidoderm) is available for the treatment of postherpetic neuralgia.

Pharmacodynamics

EMLA is a unique mixture of lidocaine 2.5 percent and prilocaine 2.5 percent. The combination has a lower melting point than does either agent alone. EMLA cream produces anesthesia to a depth of 5 mm. Local anesthetics inhibit conduction of nerve impulses from sensory nerves because of an alteration in the cell membrane permeability to ions. When applied to intact skin and covered with an occlusive dressing, local anesthesia is achieved in 1 hour.

Synera is a transdermal patch containing lidocaine 70 mg and tetracaine 70 mg used for local dermal analgesia for superficial venous access or superficial dermatological procedures. The patch is applied to skin 30 minutes before the procedure.

LMX-4 (previously ELA-Max) is a 4 percent lidocaine cream in a liposomal delivery system and is available OTC. Little information is available regarding this product although it is marketed for the treatment of minor cuts and abrasions. It has been used for cosmetic procedures such as dermal anesthesia for chemical peels.

Lidocaine patch 5 percent (Lidoderm) is composed of an adhesive material containing 5 percent lidocaine, which is applied to a nonwoven polyester felt backing and covered with a polyethylene terephthalate (PET) film release liner. Each adhesive patch contains 700 mg of lidocaine (50 mg per g adhesive) in an aqueous base. The penetration of lidocaine into intact skin after application of Lidoderm is sufficient to produce an analgesic effect, but less than the amount necessary to produce a complete sensory block (package labeling information). It is approved for pain associated with postherpetic neuralgia.

Pharmacokinetics

Absorption and Distribution

Lidocaine is absorbed systemically, with greater amounts absorbed based on the amount of medication applied to skin. Absorption is increased across abraded skin or mucous membranes. Once absorbed, lidocaine and prilocaine are widely distributed. They most likely cross the placenta and are excreted in breast milk.

Metabolism and Excretion

The metabolism and excretion of lidocaine and prilocaine are unknown.

Pharmacotherapeutics

Precautions and Contraindications

In the patient with methemoglobinemia, EMLA is contraindicated. EMLA increases the risk of methemoglobinemia if used in patients with G6PD deficiency or in young infants. It is contraindicated in patients with known hypersensitivity to **lidocaine** or other local anesthetics.

If instilled into the middle ear, **EMLA** can be ototoxic. Therefore, use in the ear near the tympanic membrane is contraindicated.

In patients with severe hepatic disease, older adults, or debilitated and acutely ill patients, topical **lidocaine** should be used with caution. The minimal effective dose should be used to prevent adverse effects. Topical **lidocaine** is Pregnancy Category B. It should be used with caution in nursing mothers.

Adverse Drug Reactions

Adverse reactions are generally dose related and usually result from high plasma levels of anesthetic due to excessive dosage or rapid absorption.

The patient may experience local adverse effects, such as paleness of the area, erythema, and changes in temperature sensation.

Drug Interactions

Do not prescribe topical **lidocaine** products to be used in children younger than 12 months who are concurrently taking methemoglobinemia-inducing drugs (**acetaminophen, sulfonamides, nitrates, phenytoin, phenobarbital**).

Class I antiarrhythmic agents (**tocainide** and **mexiletine**) may potentiate the toxicity of topical **lidocaine** products.

Clinical Use and Dosing

Topical Anesthetic

To provide local anesthesia for minor procedures such as IV cannulation, venipuncture, or circumcision, the dose of **EMLA** varies by the age of the patient. For adults and children older than 1 year, an **EMLA** disk can be applied for 1 hour or cream applied and occluded for 1 hour. If the patient is to self-administer the medication before a procedure, for ease of administration **EMLA** disks can be prescribed or a 5-mg tube dispensed and the patient instructed to apply half of the tube to the site or sites. For IV cannulation or venipuncture anesthesia, two sites may be treated. Dosing of cream for younger infants is determined by age, and the provider must refer to the dosing schedule for accurate dosing to prevent adverse effects. Higher dosing is used to harvest skin grafts, which is rarely done in primary care.

A **Synera** patch is applied to intact skin 20 to 30 minutes before venipuncture or 30 minutes before a dermatological procedure. **Synera** is approved for children age 3 years or older and adults. Patches are not to be cut. **Synera** patches contain iron powder and should be removed before a patient undergoes an MRI.

Lidoderm patch is applied to intact skin in the most painful postherpetic neuralgia sites. Up to three patches may be applied at once for up to 12 hours of a 24-hour period. To adjust dose cut patches before release liner is removed. Do not apply to broken or inflamed skin. Avoid eyes and mucous membranes.

Monitoring

The patient being treated with topical **lidocaine** products should be monitored for adverse effects, such as methemoglobinemia.

Patient Education

Administration

Patients who are to self-administer topical **lidocaine** products should have clear instructions as to the correct use. The patient should clearly understand how to apply the **EMLA** cream and occlude the area with the occlusive dressing or how to apply the **Synera patch**. If possible, the first dose can be applied by a health-care provider to demonstrate proper use.

MINOXIDIL

Topical **minoxidil** (**Rogaine**) is the first FDA-approved medication for stimulating hair growth. Alopecia androgenetica, also known as male pattern baldness, affects men and some women. It involves hair loss from the frontal, vertex, and occipital regions of the scalp in men and thinning of the hair in the frontoparietal area or diffuse hair loss in women.

Pharmacodynamics

The exact mechanism of action is unknown, but it does produce growth of epithelial cells near the base of the hair follicle. It may also induce vasodilatation of the scalp blood vessels, which also promotes hair growth. It does not appear to have an antiandrogen effect.

Pharmacokinetics

Absorption and Distribution

Topical **minoxidil** is poorly absorbed (2% of the dose) from an intact scalp. It is widely distributed in body tissues. It is not known whether **minoxidil** crosses the placenta or is distributed in breast milk.

Metabolism and Excretion

The small portion of topical **minoxidil** that is absorbed is extensively metabolized in the liver. Both the unchanged drug and the metabolites are excreted in the urine.

Pharmacotherapeutics

Precautions and Contraindications

Minoxidil topical solution used as directed has minimal cardiac effects, but if large amounts are applied, there is a potential for cardiac side effects, including hypotension.

Absorption of **minoxidil** is increased through abraded or irritated skin, leading to a slightly higher risk for cardiac side effects.

Minoxidil should not be used by pregnant patients (Pregnancy Category C) or by children younger than 18 years.

Adverse Drug Reactions

Minoxidil is generally well tolerated. The topical solution contains **alcohol** and therefore may be irritating upon application. Patients may be sensitive to **minoxidil** and develop contact dermatitis.

Drug Interactions

Topical steroids, retinoids, and other drugs that increase blood flow to the area may increase the absorption of **minoxidil**, leading to increased hypotension. Avoid using these topical medications concurrently on the scalp. **Guanethidine** use concurrently with **minoxidil** use may cause orthostatic hypotension. There is a possible additive effect if **minoxidil** is used concurrently with **antihypertensives**.

Clinical Use and Dosing

Alopecia Androgenetica

Minoxidil is available OTC for the treatment of alopecia androgenetica (male pattern baldness). It is important to note that **minoxidil** does not treat balding of the frontoparietal areas in men; it only treats this in women. **Minoxidil** is effective in treating balding on the *vertex* of the scalp in men.

Minoxidil 2 percent topical solution is applied to the scalp twice daily for the entire length of treatment. Men may use the 5 percent solution if needed. The patient applies 1 mL directly to the affected area of the scalp (vertex area in men and frontoparietal area in women). The medication should be applied to a dry scalp. Patients should be instructed to wash their hands after using their fingers to rub medication into the scalp. Twice-daily application for at least 4 months may be needed to obtain observable hair growth. If the medication is discontinued, the hair in the treated area will shed in 3 to 4 months.

Monitoring

There is no specific laboratory monitoring needed when topical **minoxidil** is used.

Patient Education

Realistic expectations of therapy should be addressed. **Minoxidil** does not treat patients with predominantly frontal hair loss. It may take 3 to 4 months for the effects of treatment to be noticed. Treatment needs to be continued for there to be a continued effect, and the new hair will shed if the medication is discontinued. Effectiveness is variable among patients. New hair may initially be fine and almost colorless. With continued treatment, the hair should be the same color and thickness as the hair on the rest of the scalp.

Administration

Caution the patient to use the medication exactly as prescribed or, for OTC **minoxidil**, as the instructions indicate.

Adverse Reactions

Adverse effects of the medication should be discussed, and the patient instructed to use the medication exactly as recommended to decrease adverse effects.

MISCELLANEOUS TOPICAL MEDICATIONS

Bath Dermatologicals

Bath dermatologicals contain colloidal solids and oils that act as **emollients** (Table 23–19). They are used to treat dry skin and the pruritus associated with dry skin and common dermatological conditions. Emollient baths that contain colloidal oatmeal solids (**Aveeno**) or oils (**Alpha Keri Bath Oil, Lubriderm Bath Oil**) can be used to provide relief from pruritus associated with contact dermatitis. These products are available OTC, and the patient

Table 23–19 ■ **Drug Interactions: Miscellaneous Topical Medications**

Drug	Interacting Drug	Possible Effect	Implications
EMLA	Methemoglobinemia-inducing drugs: • Acetaminophen • Sulfonamides • Nitrates • Phenytoin • Phenobarbital	Methemoglobinemia	Methemoglobinemia can occur in very young (<12 mo) or patients with G6PD deficit, so do not use concurrently. Monitor other patients closely if using concurrently
	Class I antiarrhythmic drugs: • Tocainide • Mexiletine	Additive toxic effects	Use concurrently with caution

Continued

Table 23–19 ■ **Drug Interactions: Miscellaneous Topical Medications—cont'd**

Drug	Interacting Drug	Possible Effect	Implications
Minoxidil	Topical steroids Topical retinoids Guanethidine Antihypertensives	Increased absorption of minoxidil Increased absorption of minoxidil Increased orthostatic hypertension Possible additive effect	Avoid concurrent use Avoid concurrent use Avoid concurrent use Monitor closely if using concurrently
Wet dressings and soaks	Collagenase	May be inhibited by aluminum acetate solution	Cleanse site with repeated washing of normal saline before applying the enzyme ointment
Aluminum chloride (Drysol)	No known drug interactions		
Bentoquatam	No known drug interactions		

should be instructed to use them according to the label instructions. Baths may be used as needed for comfort. Caution the patient to be careful when using bath oils to prevent slipping in the tub.

Wet Dressings and Soaks

Wet dressings and soaks are used to provide comfort from inflammatory conditions of the skin, such as contact dermatitis, insect bites, and athlete's foot. Burow's solution or Domeboro (aluminum acetate solution) is an astringent wet dressing for relief of the inflammation associated with contact dermatitis. It can be applied as a wet dressing for 30 minutes four times a day (Table 23–20).

Astringents

Aluminum chloride hexahydrate (Drysol) is an astringent used for the management of hyperhidrosis (Table 23–21). The solution is applied once daily to the

Table 23–20 ● **Dosage Schedule: Miscellaneous Topical Medications**

Drug	Indication	Dosage	Comments
Lidocaine-prilocaine (EMLA)	Topical anesthesia	***Adults:*** Minor dermal procedures: Apply 1 disk or 2.5 g cream in a thick layer with occlusion over 20–25 cm^2 for 1 h Major dermal procedures: Apply 2 g/10 cm^2 in a thick layer with occlusion for 2 h For male genital skin as adjunct before local anesthetic infiltration: Apply 1 g in thick layer with occlusion for 15 min	Apply to clean skin. Avoid eyes, mucous membranes, tympanic membrane, and application to large areas
Lidocaine and tetracaine (Synera)	Topical analgesia	Children ≥3 yr and adults: apply patch 20 to 30 min before venipuncture or 30 min before dermatological procedures.	Apply to intact skin. Remove before undergoing MRI (it contains iron powder)
		Children birth–3 mo (<5 kg): Maximum of 1 g applied/10 cm^2 for up to 1 h *Children 3–12 mo (>5 kg):* Maximum of 2 g applied/20 cm^2 for up to 4 h *Children 1–6 yr (>10 kg):* Maximum of 10 g applied/100 cm^2 for up to 4 h *Children 7–12 yr (>20 kg):* Maximum of 20 g applied/200 cm^2 for up to 4 h	Not recommended for children <37 weeks' gestation
Minoxidil	Male pattern baldness	Men: Use minoxidil 5%. Apply 1 mL with dropper or sprayer (6 sprays) bid directly to affected scalp areas	Do not exceed recommended dose. Continue use, or hair loss will begin again

Table 23–20 ● **Dosage Schedule: Miscellaneous Topical Medications—cont'd**

Drug	Indication	Dosage	Comments
	Diffuse hair loss or frontoparietal thinning in women	Women: Use minoxidil 2%. Apply 1 mL with dropper bid directly to affected scalp areas	
Wet dressings and soaks (Burow's solution, Domeboro)	Relief of inflammatory conditions of the skin (athlete's foot, poison ivy, allergy, insect bites)	Burow's solution: Apply wet dressing of 4 treatments/d, each lasting 30 min Domeboro: Dissolve 1–2 packets in 16 oz water. Apply wet dressing 4 times/d for 30 min each	
Aluminum chloride (Drysol)	Hyperhidrosis	Solution is applied once daily to the affected area at bedtime, then washed off in the morning. Excessive sweating may stop after 2 or more treatments	Once control of hyperhidrosis is achieved, the medication is applied once or twice weekly
Bentoquatam	Skin protection against rash caused by poison oak, ivy, and sumac	Apply as a wet film to exposed skin at least 15 min prior to possible exposure. Reapply every 4 h to maintain protective barrier. Remove with soap and water	Must be applied before contact with plant oils. Bentoquatam is not to be used in children <6 yr

Table 23–21 ◆ **Available Dosage Forms: Miscellaneous Topical Medications**

Drug	Dosage Form	How Supplied	Cost
Lidocaine 2.5%–prilocaine 2.5%	Cream	In 5 g with dressings	
		In 30 g	$47.79
EMLA	1-g disk	In 2s and 10s	$11.79
5% Lidocaine cream LMX-4	5% cream	In 15 g, 30 g	$30.99, $55.99
Minoxidil			
• Rogaine Extra Strength for Men	5% solution	In 60 mL	$49.99
• Rogaine for Women	2% solution	In 60 mL	$49.99
• Generic	5% solution	3-mo supply	$40.39
		3-mo supply	$48.99
		3-mo supply	$27.99
Wet dressings and soaks			
• Aluminum acetate solution (Burow's solution)	Solution	In 480 mL	
• Aluminum sulfate and calcium acetate (Domeboro)	Powder packets	In 12s, 100s	
Aluminum chloride			
Drysol	20% solution	In 35 mL	$16.99
Bentoquatam			
IvyBlock	5% lotion	In 120 mL	$10.99

affected area at bedtime and then washed off in the morning. Excessive sweating may stop after two or more treatments. Once control of hyperhidrosis is achieved, the medication is applied once or twice weekly. **Aluminum chloride hexahydrate** solution should be applied to clean, completely dry skin to prevent irritation. Avoid use on broken, irritated, or recently shaved skin.

Hair Growth Retardants

Eflornithine HCl (**Vaniqa**) is thought to inhibit hair growth by irreversibly inhibiting ornithine decarboxylase enzymes, which are necessary for the synthesis of polyamine. Polyamine inhibits cell division affecting the rate of hair growth. In clinical trials, 32 percent of women reported marked improvement in hair growth reduction (product label). Adverse effects of **eflornithine** include acne, pseudofolliculitis barbae, stinging, burning, and rash. **Vaniqa** is Pregnancy Category C and is not recommended for use in children. It has been labeled for use in women. **Vaniqa** cream is applied twice a day (at least 8 hours apart) to affected areas of face and adjacent areas under the chin. The medication is rubbed in thoroughly and the area should not be washed for at least 4 hours. **Vaniqa**

works for most women within 8 weeks when used consistently twice a day. Women need to understand that this product only slows hair growth and they will need to continue to use other hair-removal methods (tweezing, shaving, etc.).

Sunscreens

Sunscreens provide either a chemical or physical barrier to sunlight. Chemical **sunscreens** are transparent and absorb portions of ultraviolet light. Some chemical sunscreens block UVA (**avobenzone**) and others UVB (**PABA** and others). **Oxybenzone** and **dioxybenzone** block both UVA and UVB light. Multiple-chemical **sunscreens** are usually combined in commercial products to provide broad-spectrum coverage. Physical barrier **sunscreens** contain large particulate ingredients (**titanium dioxide, red petrolatum,** or **zinc oxide**) that reflect and scatter UVA, UVB, and visible light.

Efficacy of **sunscreens** is determined by their sunscreen protective factor (SPF). Theoretically, a sunscreen with an SPF of 15 should allow the person to remain out in the sun 15 times longer before burning than if the skin is unprotected. SPF is affected by sweating, reflection, and wind. Waterproof formulas maintain sunburn protection for 80 minutes in the water, whereas water-resistant formulas protect for only 40 minutes.

Sunscreens must be applied liberally 30 minutes before sun exposure to allow penetration and binding to skin and must be reapplied after swimming.

Do not use **sunscreens** on children younger than 6 months. Do not use sunscreen with an SPF as low as 2 or 3 on children 2 years or younger. Sensitivity to **sunscreen** can occur. Contact dermatitis may occur with the use of **PABA** or its esters. **PABA** may permanently stain clothing yellow.

Skin Protectant

Bentoquatam (IvyBlock) is an OTC product that provides a protective barrier against contact dermatitis caused by exposure to poison ivy, oak, or sumac when it is applied before contact. The lotion is applied as a wet film to exposed skin at least 15 minutes prior to possible exposure. Reapply every 4 hours to maintain the protective barrier. Remove with soap and water. **Bentoquatam** is not to be used in children younger than 6 years.

REFERENCES

American Academy of Dermatology. (2009). Acne. Retrieved from http://www.skincarephysicians.com/acnenet/index.html

American Academy of Pediatrics Committee on Infectious Diseases. (2009). *Pediculosis capitis. Red book* (26th ed.). Elk Grove Village, IL: Author. Available at *Red Book Online,* which features the full book content, http://aapredbook.aappublications.org/

Avner, S., Nir, N., & Henri, T. (2005). Combination of oral terbinafine and topical ciclopirox compared to oral terbinafine for the treatment of onychomycosis. *Journal of Dermatological Treatment, 16*(5–6), 327–330.

Baran, R., & Kaoukhov, A. (2005). Topical antifungal drugs for the treatment of onychomycosis: An overview of current strategies for monotherapy and combination therapy. *Journal of the European Academy of Dermatology and Venereology, 19*(1), 21–29.

Barber Starr, N. (2004). Dermatological diseases. In C. E. Burns, M. A. Brady, C. Blosser, C. N. Barber Starr, & A. M. Dunn (Eds.), *Pediatric primary care: A handbook for nurse practitioners* (pp. 1059–1133). Philadelphia: Saunders.

Bell, E. A. (2004). Update on pharmacotherapy of head lice. *Infectious Diseases in Children, September 2004.* Retrieved April 28, 2006, from http://www.idinchildren.com/logon/frameset.asp?article=logon.asp

Boguniewicz, M., Eichenfield, L. F., & Hultsch, T. (2003). Current management of atopic dermatitis and interruption of the atopic march. *Journal of Allergy and Immunology, 112*(6), S140–S150.

Brady, M. A. (2004). Atopic disorders and rheumatic diseases. In C. E. Burns, N. Barber, M. A. Brady, & A. M. Dunn (Eds.), *Pediatric primary care: A handbook for nurse practitioners.* Philadelphia: Saunders.

Centers for Disease Control and Prevention, Division of Parasitic Diseases. (2008a). Treating head lice infestation. Retrieved from http://www.cdc.gov/lice/head/treatment.html

Centers for Disease Control and Prevention, Division of Parasitic Diseases. (2008b). Body lice infestation. Retrieved from http://www.cdc.gov/lice/body/index.html

Centers for Disease Control and Prevention, Division of Parasitic Diseases. (2008c). Pubic lice infestation. Retrieved from http://www.cdc.gov/lice/pubic/index.html

Centers for Disease Control and Prevention, Division of Parasitic Diseases. (2008d). Scabies. Retrieved from http://www.cdc.gov/scabies/treatment.html

Charakida, A., Dadzie, O., Teixeira, F., Charakida, M., Evangelou, G., & Chu, A. C. (2006). Calcipotriol/betamethasone dipropionate for the treatment of psoriasis. *Expert Opinion on Pharmacotherapy, 7*(5), 597–606.

Chesney, P. J., & Burgess, I. F. (1998). Louse infestations, resistance and considerations for treatment. *Contemporary Pediatrics, 15,* 181–192.

Cooper, K. D., Menter, M. A., Ritchlin, C. T., Taylor, J. R., & Zanolli, M. D. (1999). Psoriasis: New clues to causation, new ways to treat. *Patient Care for the Nurse Practitioner, 2*(5), 42–50.

Del Roso Do, J. Q. (2006). Combination topical therapy for the treatment of psoriasis. *Journal of Drugs in Dermatology, 5*(3), 232–234.

Downs, A. M. R., Narayan, S., Stafford, K. A., & Coles, G. C. (2005). Effectiveness of Ovide against malathion-resistant head lice. *Archives of Dermatology, 141,* 1318.

Drug facts and comparisons. (2009). St. Louis, MO: Wolters Kluwer Health.

Feldman, S. R., Fleischer, A. B., Jr., & McConnell, R. C. (1998). Most common dermatologic problems identified by internists, 1990–1994. *Archives of Internal Medicine, 158*(7), 726–730.

Flinders, D. C., & De Schweinitz, P. (2004). Pediculosis and scabies. *American Family Physician, 69*(2), 341–348.

German, D., & Lee, A. (Eds.). (2006). *Nurse practitioner prescribing reference.* New York: Prescribing Reference.

Gupta A. K., Onychomycosis Combination Therapy Study Group. (2005). Ciclopirox topical solution, 8% combined with oral terbinafine to treat onychomycosis: A randomized, evaluator-blinded study. *Drugs Dermatology, 4*(4), 481–485.

Hansen, R. C., Krafchik, B. R., Lane, A. T., Odio, M. R., & Schachner, L. A. (1998). Dealing with diaper dermatitis. *Contemporary Pediatrics, 15*(May Suppl.), 5–10.

Kundu, S., & Archar, S. (2002). Principles of office anesthesia: Part II. Topical anesthesia. *American Family Physician, 66*(1), 99–102.

Lorch Dauk, K. C., Conroy, E., Blumer, J. L., O'Riordan, M. A., & Furman, L. M. (2010). Tinea capitis: Predictive value of symptoms and time to cure with griseofulvin treatment. *Clinical Pediatrics, 49*(3), 280–286.

Luba, K. M., & Stulberg, D. L. (2006). Chronic plaque psoriasis. *American Family Physician, 73*(4), 636–644.

Luhman, J., Hurt, S., Shootman, M., & Kennedy, R. (2004). A comparison of buffered lidocaine versus ELA-Max before peripheral intravenous catheter insertions in children. *Pediatrics, 113*(3), e217–e220.

Mallon, E., Newton, J. N., Klassen, A., Stewart-Brown, S. L., Ryan, T. J., & Finlay, A. Y. (1999). The quality of life in acne: A comparison with general medical conditions using generic questionnaires. *British Journal of Dermatology, 140*(4), 672–676.

Menter, A., Korman, N. J., Elmets, C. A., Feldman, S. R., Gelfand, J. M., Gordon, K. B., et al. (2009). Section 3. Guidelines of care for the management and treatment of psoriasis with topical therapies. *Journal of the America Academy of Dermatology, 60*(4), 643–659.

Naldi, L., & Rebora, A. (2009). Seborrheic dermatitis. *New England Journal of Medicine, 360*(4), 387–396.

Skevington, S. M., Bradshaw, J., Hopplewhite, A., Dawkes, K., & Lovell, C. R. (2006). How does psoriasis affect quality of life? Assessing an Ingram-regimen outpatient programme and validating the WHOQOL-100. *British Journal of Dermatology, 154*(4), 680–691.

Strauss, J. S., et al. (2007). Guidelines for acne vulgaris management. *Journal of the American Academy of Dermatology, 56*, (4) 651–63.

Suarez, S., & Friedlander, S. (1998). Antifungal therapy in children: An update. *Pediatric Annals, 27*, 177–185.

Takano-Lee, M., Edman, J. D., Mullens, B. A., & Clark, J. M. (2004). Home remedies to control head lice: Assessment of home remedies to control the human head louse, *Pediculus humanus capitis. Journal of Pediatric Nursing, 19*(6), 393–398.

Taketomo, C. K, Hodding, J. H., & Kraus, D. M. (2009). *Pediatric Dosage Handbook* (16th ed.). Lexi-Comp: Hudson, OH.

Walker, G. J. A., & Johnstone, P.W. (2006). Interventions for treating scabies. *The Cochrane Database of Systematic Reviews, 2,* 1–37.

U.S. Food and Drug Administration (2006). FDA Approves Updated Labeling with Boxed Warning and Medication Guide for Two Eczema Drugs, Elidel and Protopic. Retrieved from http://www.fda.gov/NewsEvents/Newsroom/PressAnnouncements/2006/ucm108580.htm

CHAPTER 24

DRUGS USED IN TREATING INFECTIOUS DISEASES

Teri Moser Woo

Chapter Outline

In 1928, Alexander Fleming discovered the first **antibiotic, penicillin.** In the ensuing years, a wide variety of **antibiotic, antifungal,** and **antiviral** classes and drugs have been developed. These **anti-infective agents** have made a significant difference in morbidity and mortality throughout the world. Many disease processes once incurable are now treatable with **antibacterial, antifungal,** or **antiviral drugs.**

ANTIMICROBIAL RESISTANCE

Within ten years of Fleming's discovery, group A *streptococci* and *pneumococci* had developed modes of resistance (Schumann & Nollette, 2000). This **antibiotic** resistance has continued with widespread acquisition of **penicillin** resistance in the 1950s and 60s, and outbreaks of resistant gram-negative organisms and beta-lactamase-producing bacteria in the 1970s. In the 1980s, new pathogens began to emerge, and organisms previously susceptible to therapy developed multidrug resistance (Thomas, 2005). The first known **penicillin**-nonsusceptible pneumococcus was identified in the 1960s; by the 1980s, there was a high prevalence of **antibiotic**-resistant pneumococci worldwide (Linares, Ardanuy, Pallares, & Fenoll, 2010). In the 1990s, **vancomycin**-resistance enterococci came on the scene. Factors that contribute to this phenomenon include increasing populations of immunocompromised patients, increases in the number and complexity of invasive medical procedures, and increased survival of patients with chronic diseases. Spread of resistant organisms in the community has been associated with day care for young children, overcrowding, and travel (Thomas, 2005). Thomas states the leading causes of drug resistance are recent use of **antibiotics,** age younger than 2 years or older than 65 years, day-care center attendance, exposure to young children, multiple medical comorbidities, and immunosuppression.

Excessive and inappropriate use of **anti-infective** agents is a major factor in drug resistance (Bishai, Morris, & Scanland, 2004; Centers for Disease Control and Prevention [CDC], 2009c; Linares et al, 2010). Such use includes increased empirical use of broad-spectrum **antibiotics** by providers who fear treatment failure or legal liabilities due to resistant organisms (CDC, 2009c; Schumann & Nollette, 2000). Thomas (2005) stresses the need to use pharmacokinetic and pharmacodynamic principles to make rational drug selections, and the CDC (http://www.cdc.gov/drugresistance) encourages using the knowledge of drug resistance patterns in the community to make these decisions, utilizing the local antibiogram. Bishai and colleagues (2004) remind the provider to "prescribe the most potent and narrowly targeted drugs from the outset in order to minimize the selection for resistance."

In the 21st century, *every* **antibiotic** class has resistant organisms. Unless novel drug mechanisms are developed, a prospect many experts find less than likely, providers will be dependent on the current classes of drugs to treat infectious disease.

There is one bright light in the drug resistance data. The resistance to *Streptococcus pneumoniae* peaked in 2000 and has been declining since. The reason for this decline appears to be the introduction of the **seven-valent pneumococcal conjugate vaccine (PCV-7),** which was licensed in 2000 and recommended for universal infant vaccination in the United States. This vaccine covered seven serotypes of the *S. pneumoniae* organism that accounted for the majority of isolates recovered from children in the prevaccine era. These seven serotypes were more likely to be resistant to **antibiotics** than the nonvaccine serotypes, so declines in the occurrence of these serotypes may explain the concurrent decrease in resistance (Thomas, 2005).

With successful vaccination come new patterns of resistance. In a longitudinal study of *S. pneumoniae* isolates in children younger than age 18 years from 2001 to 2007, 85 percent of the isolates were non-PCV-7 isolates, with **ceftriaxone**-resistant isolates accounting for approximately 20 percent of isolates particularly serotype 19A (Hsu, Shea, Stevenson, & Pelton, 2010). With the growing resistance in non-PCV-7 isolates, a **13-valent conjugate vaccine (Prevnar13)** was approved in 2010 that contains six additional strains of pneumococci (types 1, 3, 5, 6A, 7F, and 19A), responsible for 64 percent of invasive pneumococcal disease in children vaccinated with PCV-7 (CDC, 2010c). In 2008, 28 percent of the 41,500 cases of invasive pneumococcal disease were resistant to one drug, down from a high of 40 percent resistance in 2000 (CDC, 2010b). Yet the problem of resistant pneumococci continues to evolve, noting that a study finding 20 percent of invasive pneumococcal isolates in 2007 resistant to **ceftriaxone** (Hsu et al, 2010) and in 2008 28 percent of pneumococcal isolates were resistant to one drug (CDC, 2010b). Potential emergence of nonvaccine serotypes as drug-resistant strains requires that providers continue to be vigilant and evidence based in their prescribing practices. SP is the most common bacterial pathogen in upper respiratory infections such as otitis media and sinusitis.

This chapter focuses on systemic applications of drugs that are active against bacterial, fungal, viral, or parasitic organisms. Topical applications associated with dermatological conditions are presented in Chapter 23. Although many of these drugs are available in IV formulations, oral (PO) and intramuscular (IM) formulations are more commonly used in primary care and are the focus of this chapter.

ANTIBIOTICS: BETA-LACTAMS

The discovery of **penicillins** initiated the **antibiotic** era. **Penicillins** are classified as **beta-lactam** drugs because their chemistry includes a unique four-member lactam ring. They share features of chemistry, mechanism of action, and clinical effects with the other **beta-lactam antibiotics: cephalosporins, monobactams, carbapenems,** and **beta-lactamase inhibitors. Cephalosporins** are discussed in the next section, and **beta-lactamase inhibitors** are described with the **penicillins** because they are usually used together in combination products. **Monobactams** and **carbapenems** are used to treat serious infections in the hospital and are not included here.

PENICILLINS

Penicillins are characterized chemically by the 6-aminopenicillanic acid joined to the beta-lactam ring. Attachment of different substitutes to 6-aminopenicillanic acid in the chemical compound results in different pharmacological and antibacterial characteristics, which are the basis for four **penicillin** subclasses: (1) **penicillinase-sensitive** or **natural penicillins,** (2) **penicillinase-resistant** or **antistaphylococcal penicillins,** (3) **aminopenicillins,** and (4) **antipseudomonal** or **extended-spectrum penicillins.**

Pharmacodynamics

Penicillins hinder bacterial growth by inhibiting the biosynthesis of bacterial cell wall mucopeptide (also called murein or peptidoglycan). This action is dependent on the drug's reaching the **penicillin**-binding proteins (PBPs), which include transpeptidase, carboxypeptidase, and endopeptidase enzymes involved in the terminal stages of forming the cell wall. When **penicillins** bind to the PBPs, the wall is weakened, and lysis of the bacterial cell wall occurs. Because human cells lack a cell wall, there is virtually no action against host cells. **Penicillins** are bactericidal against sensitive organisms when adequate concentrations are achieved and are most effective during active cellular multiplication. Less than adequate concentrations may result in only bacteriostatic effects.

Sensitivity

The **natural penicillinase-sensitive** group is active against aerobic, gram-positive organisms, including *Streptococcus* species such as *pneumoniae* and group A beta-hemolytic (GABHS), some *Enterococcus* strains, and some nonpenicillinase-producing *Staphylococcus.* Only about 5 to 15 percent of community-acquired *Staphylococcus aureus* remains susceptible to natural penicillins, principally because the majority of strains produce penicillinase.

The concern about resistance of *S. pneumoniae* (SP) to **penicillins** has been somewhat decreased with less indiscriminate use of **antibiotics** and vaccination against pneumococcus. Resistant strains dropped from a high of 40 percent in 2000 to 20 percent in 2003 with the use of universal use of PCV-7 (Thomas, 2005). **Penicillin**-resistant strains are also commonly resistant to **cephalosporins, macrolides,** and **sulfonamides** and to a lesser extent to **clindamycin;** they are commonly called drug-resistant *S. pneumoniae* (DRSP) (Thomas, 2005).

The *Sanford Guide to Antimicrobial Therapy* (2010) recommends **natural penicillins** for *Streptococcus* group A, *S. pneumoniae, Enterococcus, Legionella, Neisseria meningitidis, Actinomyces, Clostridium, Peptostreptococcus,* and *Treponema pallidum.* **Penicillin** G is no longer listed as active against *Neisseria gonorrhoeae* (CDC, 2009a; see Chapter 44) or against and *Staphylococcus* species. Penicillinase-producing organisms have reduced the breadth of organisms that this group is used to treat.

The **penicillinase-resistant group,** also called **antistaphylococcal penicillins,** has a different spectrum of activity than the **natural penicillins.** They are active against *Salmonella, Shigella, Serratia marcescens, Proteus mirabilis, Proteus vulgaris, Morganella species* (**methicillin** only), *Brucella species* (**methicillin** only), and penicillinase-producing *S. aureus* and *Staphylococcus epidermidis* organisms. However, resistance mediated by a mechanism other than penicillinase production is manifested by **methicillin**-resistant *S. aureus* (MRSA) and *S. epidermidis* (MRSE). **Methicillin**-resistant strains are resistant to all drugs in the **penicillinase-resistant** group, as well as all **penicillins** and **cephalosporins. Vancomycin,** which is not a **penicillin,** is currently the only single **antibiotic** consistently effective against serious MRSA and MRSE infections. A new cephalosporin **ceftaroline** is active against MRSA, with similar results to **vancomycin** and was approved by the U.S. Food and Drug Administration (FDA) in 2010.

Aminopenicillins are broad-spectrum drugs that are active against many of the same organisms as both the **natural penicillins** and the **penicillinase-sensitive group**, but they have greater activity against gram-negative bacteria because of their enhanced ability to penetrate the outer membrane of these organisms. They are especially useful for gram-negative urinary and gastrointestinal (GI) pathogens such as *Escherichia coli, Proteus mirabilis, Salmonella,* some *Shigella* species, and *Enterococcus faecalis*. **Aminopenicillins** are also active against the common gram-negative respiratory pathogens *Moraxella catarrhalis* (formerly *Branhamella catarrhalis*) and *Haemophilus influenzae* type b. Many strains of *H. influenzae, Enterobacteriaceae, Salmonella,* and *Shigella* are beta-lactamase producers and therefore resistant to **aminopenicillins**, and resistance due to beta-lactamase production of *E. coli* is increasing. **Amoxicillin** is effective against the broadest number and type of organisms. It is one of the few **penicillins** with sufficient MIC-90 concentrations to be affective in otitis media, sinusitis, and community-acquired pneumonia.

The **antipseudomonal group** has enhanced activity against gram-negative bacilli, especially *Pseudomonas aeruginosa, Enterobacter, Morganella,* and *Providencia* species, and other gram-negative rods, while retaining activity against the organisms sensitive to the **aminopenicillins**, although they are less active against *Streptococcus* and *Enterococcus*. The **antipseudomonal mezlocillin** has the greatest activity against *Klebsiella* species and *Bacteroides fragilis*.

The combination of **beta-lactamase inhibitors** (e.g., **clavulanate, sulbactam,** and **tazobactam)** with certain **aminopenicillins** and **antipseudomonal penicillins** has broadened their spectrum to include beta lactamase–producing strains. The oral combination of **amoxicillin** and **clavulanate** is effective against beta lactamase–producing *S. aureus, N. gonorrhoeae, H. influenzae,* and *M. catarrhalis*.

Many texts and references, including the *Sanford Guide to Antimicrobial Therapy* (2010), have tables that list the organisms generally susceptible to various **penicillins**.

Resistance

Resistance to **penicillins** is due to (1) inactivation by beta-lactamases, (2) alteration in target PBPs on the bacterial cell wall, or (3) a permeability barrier preventing penetration of the **antibiotic** to the target cell. Beta-lactamase production is the most common mechanism. Beta-lactamases include a large group of enzymes called penicillinases and cephalosporinases. Beta-lactamases produced by *S. aureus, Haemophilus species,* and *E. coli* have narrow specificity for **penicillins**; those produced by *P. aeruginosa* and *Enterobacter species* have broader specificity and will hydrolyze both **penicillins** and **cephalosporins**. **Beta-lactamase inhibitors (clavulanate, sulbactam,** and **tazobactam)** have weak antibacterial activity but irreversibly inactivate beta-lactamase enzymes produced by bacteria by binding to their active site and protecting the **antibiotic** from inactivation.

Alteration in PBPs is responsible for **methicillin** resistance in staphylococci and **penicillin** resistance in pneumococci. Drug penetration problems are associated with the cellular outer membrane, which is present in gram-negative but not gram-positive organisms. This barrier becomes important only when beta-lactamase is also acting to hydrolyze the **antibiotic** as it slowly enters the membrane.

Pharmacokinetics

Absorption and Distribution

Oral **penicillin** formulations are generally well absorbed from the GI tract, but several are unstable in acid, resulting in the majority of the dose being destroyed in the stomach. To produce acceptable drug levels, the doses of these acid-labile drugs must be three to four times that of the parenteral formulation and be taken on an empty stomach. Thus, **oral penicillins** are not reliable enough to use for serious systemic infections.

Penicillin V has less individual variation in absorption than **Penicillin G** and is virtually the only oral **natural penicillin** in use. **Nafcillin's** oral absorption is so poor that the oral route is rarely used, whereas **dicloxacillin** is the best absorbed of the **penicillinase-resistant** group, producing blood levels twice that of **oxacillin** or **cloxacillin. Amoxicillin** is more completely absorbed than **ampicillin** and may be given without regard to food. **Carbenicillin**, the only oral **antipseudomonal penicillin**, is not adequately absorbed orally to attain blood levels effective for systemic infections, so it is indicated only for urinary tract and prostatic infections. It is not first-line for this indication.

All subclasses of **penicillin** have agents that can be given IM, but different **penicillin salts** have different absorption rates. The IM route is unreliable and erratic, as well as irritating to the tissue, and repeated dosing by this route should be avoided. Because the **penicillin G procaine** and **penicillin G benzathine** formulations are slowly absorbed, they are used as depot agents for deep IM use only. They are not to be injected near an artery or vein; to avoid intravascular administration, aspirate injection site. IV injection of these depot formulations of penicillin may cause cardiac arrest and death.

Penicillins are bound to plasma proteins to varying degrees and are well distributed to most tissues and body fluids. Inflammation enhances penetration of the meninges, joints, and eye fluids, which are otherwise poorly penetrated. **Penicillins** cross the placenta and enter breast milk.

Metabolism and Excretion

Excluding **nafcillin** and **oxacillin**, **penicillins** undergo negligible metabolism and are excreted primarily as unchanged drug in the urine, achieving high concentrations of active drug in the urine. Ninety percent of the renal excretion of **penicillin** is by active tubular secretion, and most other **penicillins** undergo extensive tubular secretion. **Probenecid,** which competes with **penicillins** for the tubular secretion carrier, will prolong the half-life and raise the peak plasma concentration of **penicillins**. Thus, concurrent administration of oral **probenecid** is used to treat some serious infections. Renal insufficiency prolongs the half-life and increases the risk for toxicity of **penicillins.** Table 24–1 shows the pharmacokinetic properties of each of the **penicillin** subclasses. Throughout this chapter, any change in dosing that is required based on renal impairment will be shown in the dosage schedule tables.

Pharmacotherapeutics

Precautions and Contraindications

Although less than 10 percent of patients taking these drugs have an allergic reaction, **penicillins** are the most likely class of drugs to cause an allergic reaction. History of a serious hypersensitivity reaction (e.g., anaphylaxis, serum sickness, exfoliative dermatitis, hemolysis, or other blood dyscrasia) to a **penicillin** contraindicates the use of any **penicillin** on account of the total cross-reactivity among the **penicillins.** A study of more than 3 million patients who had received at least one prescription of **penicillin** (Apter et al, 2004) found that the risk of an allergic-like event after **penicillin** is increased about 10-fold in those who have had a prior event. They also found that 48.5 percent of the patients in this study had been given a second prescription for **penicillin**! Luckily, the type of reaction in both the first and second prescription was urticaria in 75 percent of the patients, whereas anaphylaxis and other serious events accounted for 0.5 percent of the events. Allergic reactions to **cephalosporins, imipenem,** or **beta-lactamase inhibitors** may contraindicate use of **penicillins.** Cross-sensitivity between these drugs occurs in 5 to 16 percent of patients. Patients with a history of allergy to other substances (e.g., atopic skin conditions) should also use these drugs with caution.

Mezlocillin, carbenicillin (parenteral), and **piperacillin** may induce hemorrhagic manifestations, and they should be used with extreme caution by patients who have anemia, thrombocytopenia, granulocytopenia, or bone marrow depression or who are receiving **anticoagulants.**

Penicillins are Pregnancy Category B, but there are not adequate and controlled studies in women. They should be used only when clearly indicated. They are excreted in low concentrations in breast milk and may cause diarrhea, candidiasis, or allergic response in the nursing infant. **Ampicillin** is the most likely to cause this reaction and to sensitize the infant for future use of **penicillins.**

The safety and efficacy of **carbenicillin** and the **piperacillin-tazobactam** combination have not been established for children younger than 12 years. Dosage adjustment of **penicillins** may be required for infants because of their undeveloped renal function (see the Clinical Use and Dosing section for further discussion).

Adverse Drug Reactions

Serious and occasionally fatal immediate hypersensitivity reactions (type I hypersensitivity) have occurred, with an incidence of anaphylactic shock of 0.015 to 0.04 percent. These reactions usually occur within 2 to 30 minutes after administration and are characterized by nausea, vomiting, urticaria, pruritus, tachycardia, severe dyspnea, diaphoresis, stridor, vertigo, and eventually loss of consciousness and circulatory collapse. Treatment is the same as for any anaphylactic reaction. Skin testing may be used to identify those at risk for **penicillin** allergy. Radioallergosorbent test (RAST), or a combination of RAST and minor determinant skin testing may also be used. Patients should be referred to an allergist for skin testing. Patients with a known allergy or a positive skin test can be given desensitization therapy (Schafer, Mateo, Parlier, & Rotschafer, 2007). Other hypersensitivity reactions include skin rashes, a serum sickness–like reaction (skin rash, joint pain, fever), exfoliative dermatitis (red, scaly skin), and blood dyscrasias (hemolytic anemia, neutropenia, leukopenia).

A pruritic, maculopapular rash that does not represent a true allergy occasionally occurs with **ampicillin** (9%). It is more common with patients who have mononucleosis (43% to 100%), chronic lymphocytic leukemia (90%), or concurrent **allopurinol** therapy (15% to 20%). This measles-like, pruritic, generalized rash typically appears 7 to 10 days after initiation of therapy and remains for a few days to a week after the drug in discontinued. This rash does not contraindicate subsequent use of **aminopenicillins.**

As with many **antibiotics,** common adverse reactions include GI symptoms such as nausea, vomiting, diarrhea, and epigastric distress. **Amoxicillin** produces these symptoms less often than **ampicillin** and can be taken with food, which will further decrease incidence of these adverse effects. Addition of **clavulanate** to form **amoxicillin/clavulanate** doubles the incidence of diarrhea to 10 percent, but new formulations with lower concentrations of **clavulanate** have reduced this uncomfortable side effect. The **penicillinase-resistant penicillins** are the most likely group to cause hepatotoxicity, especially when administered with other hepatotoxic drugs.

Use of broader-spectrum **penicillins,** or prolonged or repeat therapy with any broad-spectrum **antibacterial,** may result in bacterial or fungal overgrowth (i.e., superinfection) of nonsusceptible organisms. The patient should be monitored for this possibility and treated with appropriate measures. *Clostridium difficile* colitis is a superinfection that manifests as severe abdominal cramps and pain, watery severe diarrhea that may be bloody, and fever, occurring up to several weeks after discontinuation of the drug. This pseudomembranous colitis or **antibiotic**-associated colitis is a serious sequela

Table 24–1 ▶ **Pharmacokinetics: Penicillins**

Drug	Onset	Peak	Duration	Protein Binding	Bioavailability	Half-Life	Penicillinase Resistance	Acid Stability	Elimination
Penicillinase Sensitive									
Penicillin G sodium (IM)	Rapid	0.5–3 h	4–6 h	60%	0	0.7 h	No	NA	70% unchanged by kidney
Penicillin G benzathine (IM)	Delayed	12–24 h	3 wk	UA	0	0.5–1 h	No	NA	70% unchanged by kidney
Penicillin G procaine (IM)	Delayed	1–4 h	12 h	UA	0	0.5–1 h	No	NA	70% unchanged by kidney
Penicillin G potassium (PO)	1 h	1 h	4–6 h	UA	UA	0.5–1 h	No	No	70% unchanged by kidney
(IM)	Rapid	15–30 min	4–6 h	UA	0	0.5–1 h	No	NA	70% unchanged by kidney
Penicillin V (PO)	Rapid	0.5–1 h	4–6 h	80%	60%	0.5 h	No	No	70% unchanged by kidney
Penicillinase Resistant									
Cloxacillin (PO)	30 min	0.5–1.5 h	6 h	93%–95%	49%	0.5 h	Yes	Yes	9%–22% by liver; 30%–45% by kidney
Dicloxacillin (PO)	30 min	1–2 h	6 h	96%–98%	UA	0.8 h	Yes	Yes	6%–10% by liver; 50% unchanged in urine
Methicillin (IM)	Rapid	0.5–1 h	4–6 h	40%	Minimal	0.4 h	Yes	NA	Unchanged by kidney
Nafcillin (PO) (IM)	Rapid Rapid	30 min 30 min	1–2 h 1–2 h	80%–90% 80%–90%	Low 0	0.5–1.5 h 0.5–1.5 h	Yes Yes	Yes NA	60% by liver; rest unchanged in urine
Oxacillin (PO) (IM)	Rapid	0.5–1 h Rapid	4–6 h 0.5 h	90%–94% 4–6 h	33% 90%–94%	0.5–1 h 0	Yes	Yes Yes	49% by liver; rest unchanged in urine NA
Aminopenicillins									
Amoxicillin (PO)	30 min	1–2 h	8 h	20%	80%	1–1.3 h	No	Yes	30% by liver; 70% unchanged in urine
Ampicillin (PO)	Rapid	1.5–2 h	4–6 h	20%	50%	1–1.5 h	No	Yes	60% in urine
(IM)	Rapid	1 h	4–6 h	20%	0	1–1.5 h	No	NA	50%–85% in urine
Antipseudomonals									
Carbenicillin (PO)	30 min	0.5–2 h	6 h	50%	UA	0.8–1 h	No	Yes	36% unchanged in urine
Mezlocillin (IM)	Rapid	1–1.5 h	4–6 h	16%–42%	0	0.7–1.3 h	No	NA	55%–60% unchanged in urine; 15%–30% in bile
Piperacillin (IM)	Rapid	0.5–1 h	4–6 h	16%	0	0.5–1.2 h	No	NA	90% unchanged in urine; 10% in bile
Combinations									
Amoxicillin/clavulanate (PO)	30 min	1–2 h	8 h	18%–25%	80%	1–1.3 h	Yes	Yes	30% by liver; 70% unchanged in urine
Ampicillin/sulbactam (IM)	Rapid	1 h	6–8 h	20%–38%	0	1–1.3 h	Yes	NA	Variable by liver and kidney
Piperacillin/tazobactam (IM)	Rapid	0.5–1 h	4–6 h	16%–30%	0	0.7–1.2 h	Yes	NA	Variable; tazobac tam 80% by kidney

NA = not applicable; UA = information unavailable.

that may abate with supportive therapy and discontinuance of the **antibiotic**, but severe cases require treatment with oral **metronidazole**, oral **vancomycin**, or **cholestyramine**.

Patients who are HIV-positive are more susceptible to hepatotoxicity resulting from **cloxacillin**, **dicloxacillin**, and **oxacillin** than are HIV-negative patients. Although interstitial nephritis was commonly seen with **methicillin**, which is no longer used, it still occurs occasionally with **oxacillin**, **nafcillin**, or any other **penicillin**. High doses of **procaine penicillin G** can cause transient mental disturbances, including combativeness, irritability, and hallucinations. Platelet dysfunction is primarily associated with parenteral **carbenicillin**, **piperacillin**, and **ticarcillin**. Irritability and seizures have occurred with high doses of **penicillin G**, especially in patients with renal insufficiency.

Drug Interactions

The main drug interactions with **penicillins** are shown in Table 24–2. Of interest is the potential for reduced efficacy of **oral contraceptives**, particularly with **aminopenicillins**. It is difficult to tie **contraceptive** failure to concurrent use of any **antibiotic**, in that no oral contraceptive is 100 percent efficacious. There are few case reports of such failures. When the slight risk of pregnancy is unacceptable to the patient, an additional form of **contraception** should be considered. For drug interactions specific to a particular **penicillin**, selecting a different **penicillin** may be acceptable, but often a different **antibiotic** class

Table 24–2 ■ **Drug Interactions: Penicillins**

Drug	Interacting Drug	Possible Effect	Implications
Penicillins	Diuretics	Potassium-wasting diuretics may have increased risk for hypokalemia; the reverse is true for potassium-sparing diuretics.	If they must be given together, monitor serum potassium levels and for indications of these electrolyte imbalances.
	Oral contraceptives	Evidence is contradictory. The efficacy of oral contraceptives may be reduced, and increased breakthrough bleeding may occur. Although infrequently reported, contraceptive failure is possible.	It is difficult to tie contraceptive failure directly to penicillin use because no oral contraceptive is 100% efficacious. The use of an additional form of contraception during penicillin therapy should be considered.
	Probenecid	Delays renal elimination and increases blood levels	Monitor for penicillin toxicity. Rarely used therapeutically.
	Tetracyclines	Bacteriostatic action of tetracyclines may impair bactericidal effects of penicillins	Avoid coadministration.
Ampicillin	Beta blockers	May reduce bioavailability of atenolol. Beta blockers may potentiate anaphylactic reactions of penicillin	Select a different penicillin if patient is taking atenolol.
	Allopurinol	Higher incidence of ampicillin-induced rash.	Avoid coadministration.
Mezlocillin, piperacillin	Lithium	May alter excretion of lithium.	Avoid concurrent administration.
Nafcillin	Cyclosporine	Concurrent administration produces subtherapeutic cyclosporine levels.	If they must be used concurrently, monitor cyclosporine levels more closely.
Nafcillin, oxacillin, cloxacillin, dicloxacillin	Food and acidic juices	Decreased absorption of these penicillins.	Avoid concurrent administration.
Penicillin G	Aspirin, phenylbutazone, sulfonamides, thiazide diuretics, indomethacin, furosemide	These drugs compete with penicillin G for renal tubular secretion and thus prolong the serum half-life of penicillin.	Consider altered pharmacokinetics when prescribing or select a different penicillin.
	Colestipol, cholestyramine	May decrease absorption of oral penicillin G.	Separate doses. Give penicillin G 1 h before or 4 h after colestipol or cholestyramine.

that will treat the infection is preferable. Food and acid juices decrease absorption of **penicillin V** and the **penicillinase-resistant group**.

Clinical Use and Dosing

Antibiotics are among the most frequently prescribed drugs in primary care practice, amounting to 12 to 14 percent of all outpatient prescriptions. An **antibiotic** from the **penicillin** family is usually the drug of choice for a susceptible organism because the toxicity of this class is minimal in the nonallergic individual. The most common infections treated with **penicillins** in ambulatory care have been upper respiratory infections (URIs) (pharyngitis, otitis media, sinusitis, bronchitis), pneumonia, sexually transmitted infections, urinary tract infections, and wound infections. Other important indications for **penicillins** are endocarditis prophylaxis, eradication of *Helicobacter pylori* in gastritis and peptic ulcer disease, and Lyme disease. Serious infections that require hospitalization for monitoring and IV therapy are not included in this discussion, although **penicillins** are an important component of treatment for the 30 to 50 percent of hospitalized patients who receive **antibiotics**.

Cold, Acute Bronchitis, and Upper Respiratory Infection

Over the past 15 years concern has been growing that overuse and misuse of **antibiotics** for URIs contribute to **antibiotic** resistance (Bucher et al, 2003; Schumann & Nollette, 2000; Thomas, 2005). The CDC (2005c) reported that up to 50 percent of patients treated for colds, bronchitis, and URIs received **antibiotics** inappropriately and launched a nationwide campaign to educate providers and patients regarding the inappropriate use of antibiotics titled "Get Smart: Know When Antibiotics Work" (http://www.cdc.gov/getsmart). In spite of almost 10 years of focusing on appropriate use of **antibiotics**, approximately 75 percent of **antibiotic** prescriptions written in pediatric practice are for otitis media, sinusitis, cough illness/bronchitis, pharyngitis, and the common cold (American Academy of Pediatrics, 2009). Because the common cold, URI, and acute bronchitis are seasonal, self-limiting illnesses usually caused by viruses, **antibiotics** have no role in management of uncomplicated cases (CDC, 2009c). Symptomatic treatment, rest, and proper nutrition should be instituted to support the patient while these self-limiting disorders progress through their natural course and is discussed in Chapter 46.

Cough illness of fewer than 3-weeks' duration seldom requires treatment in adults or generally well-appearing children (CDC, 2009c; Thomas, 2005). The American College of Chest Physicians produced an extensive guideline regarding the management of acute and chronic cough, with clear guidelines not to use **antibiotics** for acute bronchitis and to educate patients regarding the overuse of **antibiotics** for acute cough (Irwin et al, 2006). Bronchitis requires **antimicrobial** therapy only if there is prolonged cough with a diagnosed etiology of a specific infection, such as *Bordetella pertussis* or *Mycoplasma pneumoniae* (Irwin et al, 2006). **Penicillins** are generally not appropriate for the infecting organisms in these complicated cases of bronchitis. During the common cold, mucopurulent rhinitis (thick, opaque, or discolored nasal discharge) is not an indication for **antimicrobials** unless it persists without improvement for more than 10 to 14 days, at which point the symptoms meet the criteria for acute sinusitis, discussed in depth in Chapter 46 (American Academy of Allergy, Asthma, and Immunology [AAAAI], 2005; Rosenfeld et al, 2007).

Chronic Bronchitis

It is important to distinguish acute bronchitis from an acute exacerbation of chronic bronchitis. Chronic bronchitis, a condition largely confined to smokers, is defined as a recurrent daily cough with sputum production that persists for at least 3 months at a time in at least 2 consecutive years (Irwin et al, 2006). Patients with underlying chronic bronchitis may periodically become infected with a wide variety of organisms. The common organisms found in the sputum of patients with chronic bronchitis are most commonly viruses, as well as *H. influenzae, S. pneumoniae, M. pneumoniae,* and *M. catarrhalis* (Rabe et al, 2007). Gram's stain and culture are unreliable in patients with acute exacerbation of chronic bronchitis because the respiratory tract is normally colonized below the vocal cords. The decision to use **antimicrobial** drugs may be based on presence of at least two of the three cardinal symptoms: increased sputum volume, increased sputum purulence, and increased dyspnea. The patient reports feeling sicker than usual and may have a fever. A radiograph of the chest may be required to rule out bronchopneumonia. Recovery usually begins 3 to 4 days after antibiotics are initiated. **Amoxicillin/clavulanic acid, macrolides**, and double-strength **sulfamethoxazole/trimethoprim** are all appropriate first-line choices (Rabe et al, 2007). Resistant organisms require a change in **antibiotic** therapy after drug susceptibility studies are completed. Patients who don't respond to first-line therapy should be treated with a respiratory **fluoroquinolone (levofloxacin, moxifloxacin, gemifloxacin)**. Length of treatment is 7 to 14 days.

Otitis Media

Acute otitis media (AOM) is the most common indication for **antibiotic** prescribing in the United States and accounts for nearly half of all pediatric diagnoses and office visits. In assessing middle-ear symptoms, it is important to distinguish between AOM and otitis media with effusion (OME). AOM is defined as the presence of fluid in the middle ear in association with signs or symptoms of acute local illness (otalgia, otorrhea, immobile bulging tympanic membrane that may be red) and/or systemic illness (e.g., fever) (American Academy of

Pediatrics Subcommittee on Management of Otitis Media [AAP/OM], 2004; Thomas, 2005). OME is the presence of fluid in the middle ear in the absence of signs or symptoms of acute illness. OME often follows resolution of AOM and may not abate for several months after the infection. The American Academy of Pediatrics (AAP) and American Academy of Family Physicians (AAFP) developed a consensus guideline for the treatment of acute otitis media used in this text (AAP/AAFP, 2004). Chapter 46 discusses AOM.

Observation without use of **antibiotics** in a child with uncompleted AOM is an option (see Chapter 46). Even if the decision is made to treat with **antibiotics**, the treatment effect is small, with 80 to 90 percent of untreated cases resolving clinically by 7 to 14 days. Viral etiology is assumed for 35 percent of AOM, and the three most common bacterial etiologies are *S. pneumoniae* (30% to 35%), *H. influenzae* (20% to 25%), and *M. catarrhalis* (10% to 15%). Because culture of AOM requires tympanocentesis, AOM is usually treated empirically. **Amoxicillin** is the first-line drug of choice for AOM in the nonallergic patient in initial doses of 875 mg twice daily or 500 mg three times daily for adults. The pediatric dose is 80 to 90 mg/kg/day in two or three divided doses (AAP/AAFP, 2004). Patients with severe illness (fever of 39°C or higher, moderate to severe otalgia) and those who warrant coverage for beta lactamase–positive *H. influenzae* and *M. catarrhalis*, then **amoxicillin/clavulanate** (90 mg/kg/d of **amoxicillin** and 6.4 mg/kg/d of **clavulanate** in two divided doses) is the drug of choice (AAP/AAFP, 2004).

If the patient fails to respond within 48 to 72 hours, reassessment of the diagnosis is indicated to exclude other causes of the illness and decide if the **antibiotic** choice should be changed. In general, if high-dose **amoxicillin** was the initial choice, then **amoxicillin/clavulanate** should be tried before moving to a different drug class. Almost 100 percent of *M. catarrhalis* strains and 50 percent of *H. influenzae* strains produce beta-lactamase (AAP/AAFP, 2004), and 15 to 53 percent of *S. pneumoniae* are drug resistant (DRSP). However, **amoxicillin** is still highly effective, safe, and inexpensive for AOM, compared with other **antibiotics**. The AAP/AAFP guidelines (2004) recommend the length of treatment in children under age 6 years to be 10 days and in children age 6 years and older with moderate disease a 5- to 7-day course of **antibiotics**. These guidelines have not been updated, and remain the standard of care (Klein & Pelton, 2009). Perforated tympanic membrane requires at least 10 days of **antimicrobial** treatment with a combination of topical **antibiotic** and oral therapy.

Persistent OME after therapy for AOM is expected and does not require treatment. OME should be treated with **antimicrobials** only if bilateral effusions, accompanied by documented hearing loss, persist for 3 or more months, although insertion of tympanostomy tubes is probably more effective therapy.

Sinusitis

Sinus inflammation can be a response to viruses, allergy, pollution, or other irritation. Viral rhinosinusitis is 20 to 200 times more common than bacterial sinusitis, which complicates 0.5 to 2 percent of cases of viral URI (Thomas, 2005). Clinical diagnosis of acute bacterial sinusitis requires prolonged nonspecific upper respiratory signs such as rhinosinusitis and cough without improvement for more than 10 days, or more severe upper respiratory signs and symptoms such as substantial fever, facial swelling, or maxillary tooth or facial pain (usually unilateral) (AAAAI, 2005; Rosenfeld et al, 2007; Thomas, 2005). In children, the signs and symptoms are more subtle and difficult to diagnose. The CDC recommends not treating mucopurulent nasal discharge in children as a sinus infection until it has been present for at least 10 to 14 days, or if there are severe symptoms such as fever great than 39°C, or facial swelling or pain (CDC, 2009b). Acute bacterial sinusitis is caused by the same pathogens as otitis media (*S. pneumoniae, H. influenzae, M. catarrhalis*). **Antibacterial** resistance is an issue in sinusitis treatment, similar to otitis media treatment. The mechanism for **penicillin** resistance is alteration of **penicillin**-binding proteins and this phenomenon varies considerably according to geographic region (AAP [sinusitis], 2001). Health-care providers should consult their local antibiogram for data on resistance patterns in their area. **High-dose amoxicillin**, in doses listed for otitis media, is often successful for initial treatment since only the most resistant strains do not respond to it. If the patient is worsening or not improving in 7 days, bacterial resistance needs to be considered. It is important to discern between slow improvement and failure to improve as sinusitis may slowly resolve (Rosenfeld et al, 2007). Treatment should be continued 7 days beyond substantial improvement or resolution of signs and symptoms, usually 10 to 14 days (AAAAI, 2005). **Antimicrobial** drugs have little efficacy in treatment of chronic sinusitis. Sinusitis treatment is discussed in depth in Chapter 46.

Pharyngitis

The pathogen in pharyngitis is usually a virus, and concurrent rhinorrhea, cough, hoarseness, conjunctivitis, and diarrhea strongly suggest a viral etiology. Most bacterial pharyngitis is self-limiting and will subside without sequelae (AAP, 2009a). The exception is group A beta-hemolytic streptococci (GABHS; *Streptococcus pyogenes*), which is associated with rheumatic fever if not treated. It is important to note that only 5 to 15 percent of pharyngitis cases are produced by these organisms (Schumann & Nollette, 2000; Thomas, 2005) and the risk of rheumatic fever is now so rare in the United States that 3,000 to 4,000 patients with GABHS would need to be treated to prevent a single case (Thomas, 2005). An antigen detection ("rapid strep") test should be used to confirm the diagnosis, with negative results backed up with a throat culture. **Antibiotics** have no effect on the clinical course of patients with negative cultures. **Antibiotic** therapy started within 9 days of pharyngitis onset will avoid rheumatic fever.

The goal of therapy in GABHS pharyngitis is to use as narrow a spectrum agent as possible. Because this organism is still universally susceptible to **penicillin**, it remains the first choice in both adults and children (AAP, 2009a; CDC, 2009b). The drug of choice is **penicillin V** 250 mg two to three times a day for children weighing less than 27 kg (60 lb) and 500 mg two to three times a day for patients weighing more than 27 kg, including adolescents and adults (AAP, 2009a). To prevent acute rheumatic fever, **penicillin** should be given for a full 10 days, even if the patient is afebrile and feeling asymptomatic (AAP, 2009). Treatment failure is more likely to occur with oral **penicillin** than with **penicillin G benzathine** given IM due to poor adherence to oral therapy (AAP, 2009a). Because the taste of the suspension or solution of **penicillin V** may not be acceptable to some children, **amoxicillin** 50 mg/kg per day in one dose (maximum 1,000 mg/d) for 10 days may be used. Because the broader-spectrum drug may promote resistance, **penicillin V** is preferred over **amoxicillin.** If nonadherence is anticipated, **penicillin G benzathine** as a single IM dose of 1.2 million U for adults, or a pediatric dose of 25,000 U/kg, may be substituted. For patients who are allergic to **penicillin**, a narrow-spectrum, first generation **cephalosporin (cephalexin)** or a **macrolide (erythromycin, azithromycin)** may be substituted.

Urinary Tract Infections

Urinary tract infections (UTIs) are responsible for 8.27 million (1.41 million men; 6.86 million women) office visits per year (Litwin & Saigal, 2007). *Escherichia coli* is responsible for 85 percent of community-acquired UTIs and 50 percent of hospital-acquired UTIs. Empirical treatment with **trimethoprim/sulfamethoxazole (TMP/SMX, Septra, Bactrim)** is the first-line choice when no complicating factors are present. **Amoxicillin** can be prescribed as second-line therapy to patients who are allergic to **sulfa** drugs or the **fluoroquinolones** or as first-line treatment for women who are pregnant. Up to 25 to 70 percent of *E. coli* is resistant to **amoxicillin**; therefore, it should not be used as first-line therapy unless patient factors warrant its use. Because of its safety profile, **amoxicillin/clavulanate** 500 mg twice daily for 3 to 5 days is an acceptable therapy for treating asymptomatic bacteriuria or UTI during pregnancy (Hooton & Stamm, 2010). It is also useful in the elderly who have reduced renal function. Because **amoxicillin** concentrates in the urine and has a wide safety profile, and the usual first-line drugs to treat UTIs often create problems in the elderly, **amoxicillin** is a good choice to treat UTIs in this population

Sexually Transmitted Infections

Because of beta-lactamase production by many strains of *N. gonorrhoeae*, **penicillins** no longer have a role in treatment of gonococcal infections. However, *T. pallidum* retains susceptibility to **natural penicillins**, so recommended treatment for adults with early primary, secondary, or latent syphilis of less than 1 year's duration is one 2.4-million-U dose of **penicillin G benzathine IM** (CDC, 2010e). If latent syphilis is over 1 year's duration or of indeterminate duration, three doses at weekly intervals are required (CDC, 2010e). Because **penicillin G benzathine** does not attain adequate concentrations in the brain, neurosyphilis and congenital syphilis are treated with **IV penicillin G** or **IM penicillin G procaine** (2.4 million U daily for 10 d) plus **oral probenecid** (1 g daily for 10 d). An accepted use of **amoxicillin** is the treatment of chlamydial infections in pregnant women unable to tolerate **erythromycin** (CDC, 2010e).

Skin and Tissue Infections

Amoxicillin/clavulanate is indicated as first-line therapy for prophylaxis of infection following bites of a variety of mammals, including humans, and for infected postoperative or posttraumatic wounds. **Oral penicillinase-resistant penicillins, oxacillin,** and **dicloxacillin** are indicated for bullous impetigo caused by *S. aureus* and erysipelas of the extremities. **Penicillin V** and **penicillin G benzathine** are used in the treatment of impetigo caused by group A streptococci. Wounds accompanied by sepsis and severe tissue involvement require hospitalization and IV treatment.

Pneumonia

Although the pattern of causal organisms in pneumonia varies by age, whether community or hospital acquired, and other risk factors (e.g., smoking, HIV, **alcohol** abuse, IV drug abuse, airway obstruction, use of **corticosteroids**), the most common pathogens in community-acquired pneumonia (CAP) are *S. pneumoniae, M. pneumoniae, Chlamydia pneumoniae, H. influenzae,* and *M. catarrhalis. M. pneumoniae* lack a cell wall and are naturally resistant to **penicillins.** Acquired resistance is common in strains of the other organisms that cause pneumonia, so oral or IM **penicillins** have a minimal role in the empirical treatment of pneumonia. **High-dose amoxicillin** (80 to 90 mg/kg/d) is used for children under age 5 years, as *S. pneumonia* is the most likely pathogen causing their pneumonia. **Amoxicillin** can be combined with a **macrolide** as an alternative to respiratory **fluoroquinolones** for CAP. Management of pneumonia is fully described in Chapter 42.

Helicobacter Pylori Eradication

Antral gastritis and peptic ulcer of the stomach or duodenum are associated with colonization of *H. pylori:* 95 to 100 percent of duodenal ulcers are colonized by this organism. Once colonized, it remains in the body for life unless eradicated by **antibiotics.** Eradication of the organism decreases recurrence of ulcer and promotes resolution of gastritis. Although there are many treatment regimens for *H. pylori* eradication, treatment with **amoxicillin** 1 g given twice daily for 10 to 14 days in combination with two other drugs is standard therapy (Lew, 2009). Because there is greater than 90 percent eradication with 7-day therapy with these combinations, selection pressure for resistance and adverse effects are reduced by limiting therapy to 1 week. Other **antimicrobials** used in *H. pylori* eradication include **clarithromycin, metronidazole, tetracycline,** and **bismuth subsalicylate.** Some experts recommend *H. pylori* eradication prior to initiation of **NSAIDs** to prevent **NSAID**-induced peptic ulcers, but further research is needed to confirm the efficacy of this prophylaxis. Further discussion of *H. pylori* eradication is found in Chapter 34 and four treatment protocols are found in Table 34–6.

Lyme Disease

Lyme disease is caused by *Borrelia burgdorferi* and other *Borrelia* species, transmitted by tick bite. Diagnosis is primarily clinical, although serological testing of positive findings on both the enzyme-linked immunosorbent assay (ELISA) and Western blot tests provide confirmatory evidence. According to the Infectious Disease Society of America guidelines, **amoxicillin** 500 mg three times daily for 14 to 21 days may be used in early stages of the disease, characterized by erythema chronicum migrans, isolated facial nerve paralysis, or arthritis (Wormser et al, 2006). Children are treated with **amoxicillin** 50 mg/kg/day (maximum 500 mg/dose) for 14 to 21 days (Wormser et al, 2006). Alternative treatments for the early stage include **doxycycline, clarithromycin,** or **cefuroxime axetil.**

Bacterial Endocarditis Prophylaxis

Antibiotic administration has traditionally been recommended for susceptible patients prior to certain oral, GI, and pulmonary invasive procedures when bacteria may be released into the circulation. A joint task force from the American College of Cardiology and the American Heart Association recently published a joint document that updated prophylactic **antibiotic** therapy and currently recommends therapy only for those with prosthetic heart valves, previous infective endocarditis, certain patients with congenital heart disease, and cardiac transplant patients with valve regurgitation who are undergoing dental procedures that involve manipulation of either gingival tissue or the periapical region of the teeth (Nishimura et al, 2008). Patients with congenital heart disease (CHD) who require prophylaxis include those with unrepaired cyanotic CHD, completely repaired CHD repaired with prosthetic material or device during the first 6 months after repair, and repaired CHD with residual effects at the site of the prosthetic patch or device (Nishimura et al, 2008). **Penicillins** that are first-line therapy for prophylaxis include **amoxicillin** (adults 2 g and children 50 mg/kg orally 1 h before procedure) and **ampicillin** (adults 2 g and children 50 mg/kg IM or IV within 30 min before procedure). **Penicillin**-allergic patients should use **cephalosporins (cefazolin, ceftriaxone, cephalexin), clindamycin,** or the newer **macrolides (azithromycin, clarithromycin)** for prophylaxis (Nishimura et al, 2008).

Group B Streptococcal Disease Prevention

Group B streptococci (GBS) sepsis is the leading cause of neonatal morbidity and mortality within the United States (CDC, 2010d) . Updated guidelines in 2010 recommend all pregnant women be screened for GBS vaginal and rectal colonization with GBS at 35 to 37 weeks' gestation (CDC, 2010d). Women who have had previous GBS isolation either via urine screen or who had a previous infant with invasive GBS do not need screening; they receive intrapartum **antibiotic** prophylaxis. At time of labor or rupture of membranes, intrapartum **antibiotic** prophylaxis is given to all women who test positive for GBS (CDC, 2010d). The universal screening strategy includes **antimicrobial** therapy for all women with positive lower genital tract cultures obtained between 35 and 37 weeks' gestation, as well as for women with unknown culture results at the time of labor who have one or more risk factors (less than 37 wk gestation, rupture of membranes greater than 18 h, intrapartum temperature, intrapartum testing positive for GBS). Women in preterm labor are started on prophylactic **antibiotics** while awaiting culture results. For positive culture or risk factors in the woman with intact membranes, prophylaxis during labor is IV **aqueous crystalline penicillin G** 5 million-U loading dose and 2.5 to 3 million U every 4 hours until delivery or IV **ampicillin** 2-g loading dose and then 1 g every 4 hours until delivery (CDC, 2010d). Table 24–3 presents the dosage schedule of **penicillins** for their common indications.

Rational Drug Selection

Indication

The first consideration in drug selection is whether **antimicrobial** therapy is indicated. **Antibiotic** therapy is indicated only when the benefits of therapy (prevention of sequelae or death, more rapid recovery, patient comfort, limitation of transmission) outweigh the costs and risks of the treatment (e.g., **antibiotic** resistance, allergic response, adverse effects, economic burden). For self-limiting infections, the balance always favors symptomatic and supportive treatment, rather than **antibiotic** therapy. If the benefit-to-risk balance favors **antibiotic** therapy, there are two major approaches to drug selection. The definitive or directed method is based on defining tests to identify the organism and drug, and the empirical method is based on previous experience with similar cases (Table 24–4).

Four steps characterize both the empirical and definitive approaches, beginning with making the clinical diagnosis that identifies the infection, such as pharyngitis, urinary cystitis, or cervicitis. Collection of specimens for culture or laboratory test follows the clinical diagnosis. For some infections, such as otitis media or pelvic inflammatory disease, specimens are not available without invasive procedures, so they are usually not obtained. Additionally, specimens for culture are not helpful if the site is commonly

Table 24–3 ◉ **Dosage Schedule: Penicillins**

Drug	Indications	Initial Dose	Maximal Dose and Comments
Amoxicillin (Amoxil, Trimox, Polymox, Wymox, generic)	Antibacterial	*Adults:*	Maximal daily dose 4.5 g
		PO: 250–500 mg q8h, 875 mg q12h	Duration of therapy depends on site of infection
		Children >3 mo: 25–50 mg/kg/d in divided doses	Continue treatment 5–14 d, depending on site of infection
		PO:	Suspensions retain potency after reconstitution for up to 14 d at room temperature or refrigerated, depending on manufacturer
		High dose: 80 to 90 mg/kg/day in two divided doses	
	Exacerbation of chronic bronchitis	*Adults:* 500 mg tid	Usual duration of therapy 3–10 d
	Acute otitis media	*Adults:* 500 mg tid or 875 mg bid	Usual duration of therapy 5–7 d
		Children: 80–90 mg/kg/day in 2 to 3 divided doses	Usual duration of therapy 10 d
	Chlamydia and nongonococcal urethritis or cervicitis	*Adults:* 500 mg tid	Usual duration of therapy 7 d
	Helicobacter pylori eradication in peptic ulcer disease	*Adults:* 1 g bid *Children:* 90 mg/kg/d in 2 divided doses	Given as part of 3-drug regimen for 10–14 d
	Sinusitis	*Adults:* 500 mg tid or 875 mg bid	
		Children: 80–90 mg/kg/d in 2–3 divided doses	4 g/d in divided doses for patients at risk for DRSP 90 mg/kg/d doses for patients at risk for DRSP
	Suspected resistant *Streptococcus pneumoniae* (DRSP)	*Children:* PO: 80–90 mg/kg/d divided into 2–3 doses	
	Endocarditis prophylaxis, preprocedural	*Adults:* 2 g 1 h before procedure *Children:* 50 mg/kg 1 h before procedure	
	Lyme disease	*Adults:* 500 mg tid for 14–21 d *Children:* 50 mg/kg/day for 14–21 d	
	Urinary tract infections uncomplicated	*Pregnant women:* 500 mg tid for 7 d	
Amoxicillin and potassium clavulanate (Augmentin)	Antibacterial	*Children >40 kg and adults:* PO: 250 mg amoxicillin and 62.5 mg clavulanate q8h for 7–10 d	Suspensions maintain potency after reconstitution for 10 d if refrigerated
		Children <40 kg: PO: 20–40 mg/kg/d amoxicillin component q8h for 7–10 d *or* 25 to 45 mg/kg/d amoxicillin component q 12h. Use 200 mg/ 5mL or 400 mg/ 5 ml amoxicillin formulation or 200 mg or 400 mg chewable	Less diarrhea if daily dose in bid therapy because of lower amount of clavulanate Pediatric dose equivalent to 70–90 mg/kg amoxicillin/d in 2–3 divided doses. Using 600 mg amoxicillin and 42.9 mg clavulanate/5 mL formulation bid decreases clavulanate-related diarrhea
	Antibacterial, pneumonia, serious or resistant infections	*Children >40 kg and adults:* PO: 500 mg amoxicillin and 125 mg clavulanate q8h *or* 875 mg amoxicillin and 125 mg clavulanate q12h *Children ≥16 yrs and adults:* Extended release tablet = 2000 mg q12h	

Table 24–3 ◉ Dosage Schedule: Penicillins—cont'd

Drug	Indications	Initial Dose	Maximal Dose and Comments
		Children <40 kg: PO: 80–90 mg/kg/d of amoxicillin component, 7:1 bid formulation or ES-600 suspension	NOTE: children <40 kg should not receive the 250 mg film-coated tablets which contain a higher dose of clavulanic acid than the 250 mg chewable tablets
	Acute exacerbation of chronic bronchitis	*Adults:* 875/125 mg bid	Usual duration of therapy 10 d
	Acute otitis media and sinusitis	*Adults:* 875/125 mg bid *Children:* 80–90 mg/kg/d of amoxicillin component with 6.4 mg of clavulanate	Usual duration of therapy 5–7 d Do not exceed 6.4 mg clavulanate
	Animal bites (excluding spider)	*Adults:* 875/125 mg bid or 500/125 mg tid	Usual duration of therapy 5 d. For penicillin allergy, clindamycin may be substituted
Ampicillin (Polycillin, Principen, Totacillin, generic)	Antibacterial	*Children ≥20 kg and adults:* PO: 250–500 mg q6h	Maximum dose: parenteral 14 g/d; oral 4 g/d Take on empty stomach
		Children <20 kg: PO: 12.5–25 mg/kg q6h *or* 16.7–33.3 mg/kg q8h	Suspensions retain their potency after reconstitution for 7 d at room temperature or 14 d in refrigerator, depending on manufacturer
Ampicillin and sulbactam (Unasyn)	Antibacterial	*Adults:* IM: 1.5–3 g q6h	After reconstitution, the IM solution loses potency in 1 h Equivalent to 1–2 g amoxicillin and 0.5–1 g sulbactam
		Children <12 yr: IM: 300–600 mg/kg/d divided into 3–4 doses	Off-labeled dosage for children. Equivalent to 200–400 mg/kg/d amoxicillin and 100–200 mg/kg/d sulbactam
Carbenicillin indanyl sodium (Geocillin)	UTI and prostatitis	*Adults:* PO: 500–1,000 mg q6h	Not effective in severe renal impairment (creatinine clearance [CCr] <10 mL/min)
Cloxacillin sodium (Cloxapen, generic)	Antibacterial	*Children ≥20 kg and adults:* PO: 250–500 mg (base) q6h *Children <20 kg:* PO: 6.25–12.5 mg/kg (base) q6h	Maximum 6 g (base)/d Suspension stable 14 d in refrigerator. Shake suspension well before measuring Take on empty stomach, preferably 1 h before meals
Dicloxacillin sodium (Dynapen, Dycill, Pathocil, generic)	Antibacterial	*Children ≥40 kg and adults:* PO: 125–500 mg q6h *Children <40 kg:* PO: 3.125–6.25 mg/kg (base) q6h	Maximum adult dose 6 g (base)/d Shake suspension well before measuring Take on empty stomach, preferably 1 h before meals
	Infections in cystic fibrosis patients	*Children <40 kg:* PO: 12.5–25 mg/kg (base) q6h	
Oxacillin (Bactocill, Prostaphlin)	Antibacterial	*Children ≥40 kg and adults:* PO: 500 mg–1 g (base) q4–6h IM: 250 mg–1 g (base) q4–6h *Children <40 kg:* PO: 12.5–25 mg/kg (base) q6h IM: 12.5–25 mg/kg (base) q6h *or* 16.7 mg/kg q4h	Maximum adult daily dose 6 g Take oral forms on empty stomach, preferably 1 h before meals After reconstitution, IM solution retains potency for 4 d at room temperature or 7 d if refrigerated After reconstitution, oral solution retains potency for 7 d at room temperature or 14 d if refrigerated

Continued

Table 24–3 ◉ **Dosage Schedule: Penicillins—cont'd**

Drug	Indications	Initial Dose	Maximal Dose and Comments
Penicillin G, benzathine (Bicillin L-A)	Prophylaxis for streptococcal infections in patient with rheumatic fever history	*Adults:* IM: 1,200,000 U q3–4wk *Children: >27 kg:* IM: 1,200,000 U q2–3wk *Children <27 kg:* 600,000 U q2–3wk	For deep IM use only into large muscle mass. IV injection causes embolic or toxic reaction. Intra-arterial injection causes necrosis of extremity or organ, especially in children Maximum daily adult dose 2,400,000 U Inject at slow, steady rate to avoid blockage of the needle
	Pharyngitis, group A streptococci	*Adolescents and adults:* IM: 1,200,000 U as single dose *Children >27 kg:* IM: 1.2 million U as single dose *Children <27 kg:* IM: 600,000 U as single dose	
	Syphilis (primary, secondary, early latent)	*Adolescents and adults:* IM: 2,400,000 U as single dose *Children:* IM: 50,000 U/kg up to 2,400,000 units as single dose	
	Syphilis (late latent or latent of unknown duration)	*Adolescents and adults:* IM: 2,400,000 U weekly for 3 wk *Children:* IM: 50,000 U/kg weekly up to 2,400,000 U as single dose for 3 wk	
Penicillin G, procaine	Antibacterial	*Adults:* IM: 600,000–1,200,000 U/d	For deep IM use only into large muscle mass. After large doses, some patients may experience a CNS syndrome of transient anxiety, confusion, agitation, combativeness, depression, seizures, hallucinations, expressed fear of impending death
	Neurosyphilis	*Adults:* IM: 2,400,000 U and 500 mg probenecid qid for 10–14 d	
	Congenital syphilis	*Children:* 50,000 U/kg/d for 10–14 d	
	Diphtheria	*Adults:* IM: 300,000–600,000 U/d as adjunct to diphtheria antitoxin	
	Rat bite fever	*Adults:* IM: 600,000 U every 12 h	
Penicillin G benzathine and procaine combined (Bicillin-CR)	Antibacterial	*Children >27 kg and adults:* IM: 2,400,000 U as single dose *Children* 14–27 kg: IM: 900,000–1,200,000 U as single dose *Children <14 kg:* IM: 600,000 U as single dose	See comments for penicillin G benzathine and penicillin G procaine May be dosed with half of dose on day 1 and half on day 3 For deep IM use only into large muscle mass Continue until afebrile for 48 h
	Pneumococcal infections (excluding meningitis)	*Adults:* IM: 1,200,000 U every 2–3 d *Children:* IM: 600,000 U every 2–3 d	

Table 24–3 ◉ **Dosage Schedule: Penicillins—cont'd**

Drug	Indications	Initial Dose	Maximal Dose and Comments
Penicillin V (Beepen-VK, Betapen-VK, Ledercillin-VK, Pen Vee K, Veetids, V-Cillin K, generic)	Antibacterial	*Adults and children >12 yr:* 125–500 mg q6–8h *Children <12 yr:* 2.5–8.3 mg/kg q6h *or* 5–16.7 mg/kg q8h	Maximum adult dose 7.5 g/d. Solution retains potency for 14 d if refrigerated Shake solution well before measuring
	Continuous prophylaxis of streptococcal infection in patients with history of rheumatic heart disease	*Children >12 yr and adults:* 125–250 mg q12h	
	Erysipelas	*Children >12 yr and adults:* PO: 500 mg q6h *Children <12 yr:* See antibacterial	
	Gingivitis, acute necrotizing	*Adults:* PO: 500 mg q6h	
	Rat bite fever	*Children* >12 yr and adults: 500 mg q6h for 14 d *Children <12 yr:* See antibacterial	
	Lyme disease	*Children >12 yr and adults:* 250–500 mg 3–4 times daily for 3–4 wk *Children <12 yr:* 5–12.5 mg/kg qid for 3–4 wk	Duration dependent on response. Treatment failures have occurred and retreatment may be necessary
Penicillin V	Pharyngitis (GABHS)	<27 kg (60 lb): 250 mg PO 2 to 3 times/d >27 kg: 500 mg PO 2 to 3 times/d	Usual duration of therapy for both adult and child 10 d
Piperacillin (Pipracil)	Antibacterial	*Children >12 yr and adults:* IM: 3–4 g q4–6h	Maximum adult daily dose 24 g. CCr <40 mL/min requires reduced dosage and/or frequency IM injection should not exceed 2 g per site
	Urinary tract infection, uncomplicated	*Adults:* IM: 1.5–2 g q6h or 3–4 g q12h	

DRSP = drug-resistant *Streptococcus pneumoniae*; GABHS = Group A beta hemolytic streptococcus

Table 24–4 **Steps in Antimicrobial Drug Selection**

Step 1	Make clinical diagnosis
Step 2	Obtain cultures and/or specimens
Step 3	Make microbial diagnosis Results of culture and/or lab test *or* most likely pathogen, references
Step 4	Select drug Results of sensitivity *or* usual susceptibility

colonized, such as acute exacerbation of chronic bronchitis. Microbiological testing is an important tool in the rational prescribing of **antibiotics,** although delay in obtaining results, misinterpretation of colonization as infection, quality control (mislabeling of specimen or using wrong procedure), and cost are disadvantages of routine culture and sensitivity (Kolmos & Little, 1999). Near-patient testing procedures such as the group A streptococci antigen test, urine dipsticks, and microscopy are widely used and have the advantages of moderate cost and immediate results. When the result is negative and immediate, it is much easier for the prescriber to refuse to give in to patients' demands for an **antibiotic.** Urine dipsticks and microscopy are not considered definitive of the causal organism, and the definitive method is often an unrealized ideal in ambulatory practice. However, even with the empirical method, culture results can confirm the empirical diagnosis or allow appropriate adjustment of therapy.

The final two steps, making the microbial diagnosis and drug selection, differ for definitive and empirical therapy. In definitive therapy, the microbial diagnosis is based on valid and reliable tests such as culture or antigen assays, and drug selection is based on results of sensitivity testing or laboratory tests such as beta-lactamase assay. The goal of susceptibility testing is to identify a nontoxic **antibiotic** that will resolve the infection.

Although this goal is not always achieved, susceptibility testing can often identify a narrower spectrum or less toxic agent than would be identified by the empirical method of drug selection.

Susceptibility tests measure the concentration of the drug required in vitro to inhibit the growth of the organism (called minimum inhibitory concentration, or MIC) or the concentration required to kill the organism (minimum bactericidal concentration, or MBC). Usually only the MIC is determined, although when bactericidal action is required, such as for immunocompromised patients, endocarditis treatment, and meningitis treatment, the MBC is determined. The MIC or MBC can be correlated with concentrations of the drug attainable by various doses and routes in various compartments of the body where the organism may exist (e.g., middle-ear fluid, serum, synovial fluid, cerebrospinal fluid [CSF]).

There are two approaches to susceptibility testing: the disk or agar diffusion (Kirby-Bauer method) and the broth dilution method. In the agar diffusion approach, a disk containing a standard amount of the antimicrobial agent is placed on agar lightly seeded with the **antibiotic.** After incubation, susceptibility is determined by the diameter of the visible area of growth inhibition around the disk. The broth dilution method consists of inoculating the organism into a series of liquid media containing increasing concentrations of the **antibiotic.** The MIC is the lowest concentration that inhibits growth. The broth dilution method is preferred if there is no sharp distinction between sensitivity and resistance on the disk method. Sensitivity and resistance represent a continuum rather than a dichotomy. For example, *S. pneumoniae* strains are defined as **penicillin**-susceptible if the MIC is less than 0.1 mcg/mL, intermediate if the MIC is 0.1 mcg/mL to 1 mcg/mL, and resistant if the MIC is greater than 2 mcg/mL.

In empirical testing, the microbial diagnosis and drug regimen are determined based on epidemiological studies. References that compile and update these data annually or biannually include the *Sanford Guide to Antimicrobial Therapy*, the *Handbook of Antimicrobial Therapy*, periodic updates given in the biweekly *Medical Letter on Drugs and Therapeutics*, and material available on the CDC Web site at http://www.cdc.gov. These references identify the drug with the narrowest spectrum that covers the most likely microbiological pathogens for a specific clinical diagnosis. Clinicians should also consult local sources for the antibiogram of pathogens and susceptibility.

Allergy History

Susceptibility, whether empirically or definitively derived, is not the sole determinant of drug selection. Allergy history is important because cross-reactivity to **penicillins** is total; that is, the patient allergic to any **penicillin** will be allergic to all other **penicillins.** In addition, the risk for cross-allergy to related drugs, such as **cephalosporins** and **beta-lactamase inhibitors,** is a consideration. References for empirical therapy provide an alternative non**penicillin** agent whenever the drug of choice is a **penicillin.** For example, **erythromycin** is an alternative to **penicillin** V for treatment of pharyngitis caused by GABHS.

Age, Pregnancy, and Genetic Factors

Age is important in drug selection and dosing, primarily because renal elimination of **penicillins** changes with age. Neonates and elderly patients often have poor renal function and are more prone to drug toxicity. Highly plasma protein–bound drugs such as **sulfonamides** and the **penicillinase-resistant penicillins** should be avoided in late pregnancy and neonates because these agents may displace bilirubin from plasma proteins of the newborn, causing kernicterus, a central nervous system (CNS) disorder.

Pregnancy contraindicates several classes of **antibiotics,** such as **tetracyclines** and **fluoroquinolones,** so **aminopenicillins** may be used for gravid women, even though another agent is the drug of choice in the nonpregnant state.

For some drugs, genetic factors predispose patients to adverse effects. Pharmacogenomics are discussed in Chapter 8.

Site of Infection

The anatomical site of the infection affects drug selection, as well as dose, route, and duration of therapy. For example, **penicillins** enter CSF poorly, so a CNS infection may require a different agent, higher doses, IV and/or intraventricular administration, or prolonged therapy. When the meninges are inflamed, as in meningitis, **penicillin** attains higher concentrations in the CSF. By contrast, **penicillins** enter the respiratory tree in high concentrations, permitting single-dose or short-course therapy for susceptible organisms.

Immunocompromised Status

One of the most important factors in drug selection is the immunocompetence of the patient. Patients with immunodeficiency syndromes or neutropenia require bactericidal drugs and extended therapy.

Affordability

Affordability is another consideration in drug selection, although existing data contradict the common assumption that newer, more expensive agents are more effective than established, inexpensive agents. One reason **amoxicillin** is the preferred drug of choice for several common infections is its low cost, combined with its high efficacy and long history of safe use. Cost data are provided in the available dosage forms tables throughout the chapter.

Taste and Convenience

Taste is a significant factor in patient acceptance of a liquid product, affecting adherence to the prescribed regimen (Steele, Thomas, & Begue, 2001). The use of **amoxicillin** suspension rather than **penicillin V** suspension for group A streptococcal infections is an example of drug selection based on taste and convenience. Steele and colleagues (2001) provide comparative ratings on **antibiotic** suspensions based on overall taste and adjusts them for cost. In all categories in this study, no **antibiotic** scored significantly higher than **amoxicillin**.

Convenience is largely a matter of the number of times per day that a drug must be taken. **Amoxicillin** requires two or three doses daily, whereas **penicillin V** requires two to four doses per day. Frequent dosing decreases compliance and may be particularly problematic when the patient is away from home, such as at work or in day care, especially when the drug requires refrigeration or cannot be taken with food.

Monitoring

Both microbiological and clinical responses are used to evaluate the therapeutic outcome of **antimicrobial** therapy. Serial cultures of specimens from infected sites become sterile with successful treatment. Follow-up cultures may detect superinfection or development of resistance. All patients with early or congenital syphilis should have a quantitative Venereal Disease Research Laboratory (VDRL) test at 6 and 12 months after therapy.

For most infections treated in outpatient settings, it is sufficient to monitor clinical response alone. Local signs of heat, redness, swelling, tenderness, or discharge usually abate after 48 to 72 hours. Specific indicators of improvement such as the resolution of pulmonary infiltrates and normalization of pulse oximetry in pneumonia are important outcomes to monitor. Systemic signs such as fever, malaise, and leukocytosis also improve. The patient should be advised to call the prescriber if there is no improvement in 48 to 72 hours, when consideration should be given to adjusting the treatment; alternatively, the provider can initiate telephone contact to evaluate progress and improvement. Compliance is monitored throughout the course of therapy, particularly if there is therapeutic failure, as well as after symptoms resolve and the patient is less motivated to complete the therapy.

Signs of allergic reactions may occur from minutes to weeks after the **antibiotic** is initiated, and even after the course of therapy is completed. Although immediate hypersensitivity reactions are more likely to be life threatening, delayed reactions can also be serious. Superinfection often presents with subtle and nonspecific symptoms such as mouth or throat pain (oral candidiasis) or perineal itching or discharge (vaginal candidiasis), so it is important to attend to these minor complaints. Distinguishing between **antibiotic** diarrhea and pseudomembranous colitis is at times difficult, but more than four to six watery stools per day or blood in the stool warrants stool cytotoxin assay to detect *C. difficile*.

Other adverse effects are almost exclusively associated with high-dose parenteral therapy, protracted oral therapy, or impaired renal function. During parenteral therapy, periodic urinalysis, blood urea nitrogen (BUN), and creatinine determinations should be performed, especially with agents from the **penicillinase-resistant group** or the **antipseudomonal group**. However, most of the **penicillins**, especially **amoxicillin**, have a wide range of tolerance for renal impairment. This is an especially safe drug for the elderly, who commonly have decreased renal function. When combined with a **beta-lactamase inhibitor** closer monitoring is appropriate. Monitor serum potassium in patients receiving **piperacillin**, **potassium penicillin G**, or other parenteral agents. Patients with low potassium reserves, especially if they are taking **cytotoxic drugs** or **diuretics**, can develop hypokalemia. Hyperkalemia has occurred with high doses of **potassium penicillin G** in patients with impaired renal function. The partial thromboplastin time (PTT) and prothrombin time (PT) should be assessed at baseline and during therapy with parenteral **carbenicillin**, **piperacillin**, or **ticarcillin**, particularly for patients with renal impairment.

Patient Education

Administration

The most critical information to provide to patients who will self-administer **antibiotics** is the importance of completing the full course of therapy. They should understand that failure to complete therapy may result in resistant infections that can be passed on to family and friends or cause the patient to be more seriously ill. Doses of the medication should be spaced as evenly as possible without sleep disruption throughout the 24 hours of a day. Missed doses should be taken as soon as they are remembered, but the dose should not be doubled.

Oral penicillins that should be taken on an empty stomach, 1 hour before a meal or 2 hours after meals, include **ampicillin**, **carbenicillin**, and the **penicillinase-resistant agents cloxacillin**, **oxacillin**, **nafcillin**, and **dicloxacillin**. Chewable tablets must be crushed or chewed, or the drug may not absorb adequately. Oral tablets and chewable tablets of **amoxicillin/clavulanate** have different **clavulanate** content and should not be considered interchangeable. The available dosage forms are shown in Table 24–5.

Table 24–5 ◈ Available Dosage Forms: Penicillins

Drug	Dosage Form	How Supplied	Cost
Amoxicillin	Tablets: 500 mg		$47/1,000
	875 mg		$66/100
	Tablets (chewable): 125 mg	In bottles of 40, 60, 100, 500 tablets	$21/100
	(chewable): 250 mg	In bottles of 30, 40, 60, 100, 500 tablet	$31/100
	Capsules: 250 mg	In bottles of 21, 30, 100, 250, 500, 1,000 capsules	$8/100
	500 mg	In bottles of 21, 30, 50, 100, 250, 500 capsules	$4/30 $10/90
	Powder for oral suspension: 125 mg/5 mL (reconstituted), 250 mg/5 mL (reconstituted), 400 mg/5 mL	In 80-, 100-, 150-, 200-mL bottles	$4/80 mL $4/100 mL $4/150 mL (on Walmart list)
(Amoxil)	Tablets (chewable): 125 mg	In bottles of 60 (cherry-banana-peppermint flavor)	
	(chewable): 200 mg	In bottles of 30, 100 (cherry-banana-peppermint flavor)	$11/100
	Capsules: 250, 500 mg	In bottles of 100, 500 capsules	
	Powder for oral suspension: 50 mg/mL (drops) (reconstituted)	In 15-, 30-mL bottles (Drops)	$5/100
	200 mg/5 mL (reconstituted), 400 mg/5 mL (reconstituted)	In 80-, 100-, 150-mL bottles	$11/100 $11/100
	Tablets: 875 mg		$84/100
(Trimox)	Capsules: 250, 500 mg	In bottles of 30, 100, 500 capsules	$12/100
	Powder for oral suspension:	In 15-mL bottles	$14/100
	125 mg/5 mL (reconstituted); 250 mg/5 mL (reconstituted)	In 80-, 100-, 150-mL bottles	
	Drops: 50 mg/mL (reconstituted)	In 15-mL bottle	$3/15 mL $6/15 mL
Amoxicillin and potassium clavulanate (Augmentin)	Tablets: 250 mg amoxicillin/125 mg clavulanate	In 30, 100 tablets	$85/30
	500 mg amoxicillin/125 mg clavulanate	In 20, 100 tablets	$83/20
	875 mg amoxicillin/125 mg clavulanate	In 20, 100 tablets	$111/20
	Tablets (chewable): 125 mg amoxicillin/31.25 mg clavulanate	In 30 tablets (lemon-lime flavor)	$42/30
	(chewable): 200 mg amoxicillin/28.5 mg clavulanate	In 20 tablets (cherry-banana flavor)	$41/20
	(chewable): 250 mg amoxicillin/62.5 mg clavulanate	In 30 tablets (lemon-lime flavor)	$67/30
	(chewable): 400 mg amoxicillin/57 mg clavulanate	In 20 tablets (cherry-banana flavor)	$76/20
	Powder for oral suspension: 125 mg amoxicillin/31.25 mg clavulanate per 5 mL	In 75-, 100-, and 150-mL bottles (banana flavor)	$33/100 mL
	200 mg amoxicillin/28.5 mg clavulanate per 5 mL	In 50-, 75-, 100-mL bottles (orange-raspberry flavor)	$47/100 mL
	250 mg amoxicillin/62.5 mg clavulanate per 5 mL	In 75-, 100-, 150-mL bottles (orange flavor)	$61/100 mL
	400 mg amoxicillin/57 mg clavulanate per 5 mL	In 50-, 75-, 100-mL bottles (orange-raspberry flavor)	$76/100 mL
	Powder for oral suspension: 600 mg amoxicillin and 42.9 mg clavulanate (Augmentin ES)	In 75-, 125-, 200-mL bottles	$40/75-mL bottle

Table 24–5 ◆ **Available Dosage Forms: Penicillins—cont'd**

Drug	Dosage Form	How Supplied	Cost
Ampicillin sodium	Capsules: 250 mg	In bottles of 20, 30, 40, 100, 500, 1,000 capsules	$16/100
	500 mg	In bottles of 16, 20, 28, 40, 100, 500, 1,000 capsules	$26/100
	Powder for oral suspension: 125 mg/5 mL (reconstituted), 250 mg/5 mL (reconstituted)	In 80-, 100-, 150-, 200-mL bottles	$5/100
	Powder for injection: 125 mg, 250 mg, 500 mg, 1 g, 2 g	In multidose vials	$8/100
(Principen)	Capsules: 250, 500 mg	In bottles of 100, 500 capsules	
	Powder for suspension: 250 mg/5 mL (reconstituted), 250 mg/5 mL (reconstituted)	In 100-, 150-, 200-mL bottles	
Ampicillin sodium and sulbactam sodium (Unasyn)	Powder for injection: 1.5 g (1 g ampicillin/ 0.5 g sulbactam)	In multidose vials	$159/10 vials
	3 g (2 g ampicillin/1 g sulbactam)		
Carbenicillin (Geocillin)	Tablets: 382 mg	In bottles of 100 tablets	$226/100
Cloxacillin sodium	Capsules: 250 mg, 500 mg	In bottles of 100 capsules	$13/100
	Powder for oral solution: 125 mg/5 mL	In 100-, 200-mL bottles	
(Cloxapen)	Capsules: 250 mg	In bottles of 100 capsules	
	500 mg	In bottles of 30, 100 capsules	
Dicloxacillin sodium	Capsules: 250 mg	In bottles of 40, 100, 500 capsules	$45/100
	500 mg	In bottles of 30, 40, 50, 100, 500 capsules	$93/100
(Dynapen)	Capsules: 125 mg, 250 mg	In bottles of 24, 100 capsules	$14/100
	500 mg	In bottles of 50 capsules	
	Powder for oral suspension: 62.5 mg/5 mL (reconstituted)	In 100-, 200-mL bottles	
Oxacillin sodium	Capsules: 250, 500 mg	In bottles of 100 capsules	
	Powder for oral solution: 250 mg/5 mL (reconstituted)	In 100-mL bottles	
	Powder for injection: 250 mg, 500 mg, 1 g, 2 g, 4 g	In multidose vials	
Penicillin G, procaine (Wycillin)	Injection	600,000 U per dose in 1-mL Tubex	
		1,200,000 U per dose in 2-mL Tubex	
		2,400,000 U per dose in 4-mL disposable syringe	
Penicillin G, benzathine (Bicillin L-A)	Injection	300,000 U per mL in 10-mL vials	
		600,000 U per dose in 1-mL Tubex	
		1,200,000 U per dose in 2-mL Tubex	
		2,400,000 U per dose in 4-mL syringe	
(Permapen)	Injection	1,200,000 U per dose in 2-mL Isoject	

Continued

Table 24–5 ◆ **Available Dosage Forms: Penicillins—cont'd**

Drug	Dosage Form	How Supplied	Cost
Penicillin G, benzathine-procaine combined (Bicillin C-R)	Injection	300,000 U (150,000 U of each) per dose in 10-mL vials 600,000 U (300,000 U of each) per dose in 1-mL Tubex 1,200,000 U (600,000 U of each) in 2-mL Tubex 2,400,000 U (1,200,000 U of each) in 4-mL syringe 1,200,000 U (900,000 U of benzathine and 300,000 U of procaine) per dose in 2-mL Tubex	
Penicillin V (Penicillin VK)	Tablets: 250 mg 500 mg Powder for oral solution: 125 mg/5 mL (reconstituted) 250 mg/5 mL (reconstituted)	In bottles of 20, 30, 40, 80, 100, 500, 1,000 tablets In bottles of 20, 30, 40, 100, 500, 1,000 tablets In 80-, 100-, 150-, 200-mL bottles	$4/28 tabs $10/84 tabs $4/200 mL $10/600 mL $4/100 mL $10/300 mL
Penicillin V (Pen Vee K)	Tablets: 250, 500 mg Powder for oral solution: 125 mg/5 mL (reconstituted) 250 mg/5 mL (reconstituted)	In bottles of 100-mg and 500-mg scored tablets In 100- and 200-mL bottles In 100-, 150-, and 200-mL bottles	$20/100 $43/100
Piperacillin (Pipracil)	Powder for injection: 2, 3, 4 g	In multidose vials	

Many **penicillins** are available as solutions or suspensions. Suspensions must be shaken to disperse the particles of drug immediately before measurement. Refrigerated liquid formulations maintain full activity for 14 days after reconstitution, except **amoxicillin/clavulanate** suspension, which lasts for 10 days in the refrigerator. **Amoxicillin** suspension maintains full activity for 14 days whether refrigerated or not, although some manufacturers specify refrigerated storage. Instruct patients not to use **antibiotics** beyond the expiration date. Liquid formulations should always be dispensed with a calibrated measuring device.

Because household teaspoons vary from 2 mL to 10 mL in volume, they are unreliable for medication measurement. Clinicians should tell the patient whether there will be liquid remaining at the end of the course of therapy and urge disposal of unused medication.

Very concentrated oral forms of **amoxicillin** (50 mg/mL) or **ampicillin** (100 mg/mL) in suspension are called **antibiotic drops.** It is important to explain that the drops are for oral use, describe how to measure and administer the medication appropriate to the patient's developmental and physical capabilities, and specify that an appropriate measuring device be used.

Medications mixed for injection also lose potency with time, although refrigeration after reconstitution will extend the period of full potency. Consult the package insert for proper mixing and storage of reconstituted parenteral **penicillins.** Some of these agents (e.g., **piperacillin**) can be prepared with **lidocaine** to decrease pain on IM injection. Adhere to the manufacturer's limits on volume of injection at one site. IM injection should be slow and steady, extended over 12 to 15 seconds to minimize pain and avoid blockage of the needle, especially with **procaine** and **benzathine** preparations that are very thick. Because IV extravasation of **nafcillin** causes tissue necrosis, IM injection should be avoided, and Z-track injection technique used if this route is unavoidable.

Adverse Reactions

Patients should be taught to distinguish allergic reactions from other adverse effects, so that they can provide an accurate drug allergy history. Many patients claim **penicillin** allergy because they experienced diarrhea during therapy. Patients with immediate or type I allergies of the anaphylactic type should wear an identification bracelet.

If severe diarrhea occurs, the patient should contact the prescriber before initiating any treatment. For mild diarrhea, they can use **adsorbent antidiarrheal agents** containing **attapulgite** (e.g., **Donnagel**) but should avoid **antiperistaltic** agents that promote the retention of toxins.

Aminopenicillins and **clavulanate** cause false positives on glucose urine testing by the copper sulfate technique (Clinitest). Diabetics on these **penicillins** should use blood glucose monitoring or urine testing based on glucose enzymatic tests (Clinstix, TesTape).

Lifestyle Management

Most infections are self-limiting and resolve with symptomatic treatment, rest, fluids, and nutritious diet. Instead of seeking antibiotics for every minor illness, people must learn to trust the natural healing capacity of the human body. Prevention of infection by good hand washing, shunning crowded environments, avoiding cigarette smoke including passive smoke, practicing safe sex, and maintaining a generally healthy lifestyle will limit the need for antibiotics. Other risk-reduction counseling specific to otitis media includes breastfeeding of infants, avoidance of passive smoke, elimination of the pacifier in children older than 1 year, enrollment in day care with small class size if day care is unavoidable, and **pneumococcal and influenza vaccine** (Schumann & Nollette, 2000; Thomas, 2005). Because pain has been shown to inhibit the immune system, comfort measures and pain management of patients with infections will promote the **antibiotic** action.

CEPHALOSPORINS

Cephalosporins are **beta-lactam antibiotics**, structurally and chemically related to the **penicillins. Cefoxitin** and **cefotetan** are actually **cephamycins**, and **loracarbef** is a **carbacephem**, but they are usually included with the **cephalosporins** because of their clinical and chemical similarity.

This class of drugs is divided into four generations, based on the order of development and spectrum of **antibacterial** activity. In general, as the designation increases from first to fourth generation, there is increased activity against gram-negative organisms and anaerobes, less activity against gram-positive organisms, and increased ability to withstand destruction by beta-lactamases.

> **On The Horizon** — **FAROPENEM**
>
> **Faropenem (Orapem)** is an oral carbapenem for use with acute bacterial sinusitis, community-acquired pneumonia, acute exacerbation of chronic bronchitis and infections of the skin and skin structures. A New Drug Application was filed December 2005 and the FDA granted a non-approval letter in 2006. The manufacturer is working with the FDA to resubmit.

Pharmacodynamics

Cephalosporins inhibit mucopeptide synthesis in the bacterial cell wall, making the bacterium osmotically unstable. As with **penicillins**, this action involves **cephalosporins** binding with PBP involved in the terminal stages of cross-linking peptidoglycans at the cell wall. **Cephalosporins** are usually bactericidal, depending on organism susceptibility, dose, tissue concentration, and the rate of organism multiplication. They are most effective against rapidly growing organisms forming cell walls.

Sensitivity

First generation cephalosporins are active against gram-positive cocci, including *S. aureus* and *S. epidermidis*, excluding **methicillin-resistant strains.** Agents in this group are also active against group A beta-hemolytic *S. pyogenes* and *S. pneumoniae*, except DRSP. **First generation cephalosporins** have limited activity against aerobic gram-negative organisms, such as *E. coli, P. mirabilis*, and *Klebsiella pneumoniae,* and do not enter the CSF.

Second generation cephalosporins are active against the same organisms as the first generation, with increased activity against *Klebsiella, Proteus,* and *E. coli.* This group is active against beta lactamase–producing strains of *H. influenzae* and *M. catarrhalis,* as well as intermediate-resistant *S. pneumoniae.* Each of the drugs in this generation has a slightly different spectrum of activity, so susceptibility tests for each must be performed, rather than assuming consistency within the group. This group is not active against *Pseudomonas* and does not reach effective concentrations in the CSF.

Third generation cephalosporins are active against the same organisms as the first two generations, with added spectrum of activity against gram-negative organisms. They are also active against unusual strains of enteric organisms such as *Providencia,* and *Serratia,* with increased activity against *Enterobacter.* **Cefixime,** however, is not active against *Serratia* species and none in this group are effective against *Serratia marcescens.* Parenteral **cefoperazone, cefotaxime, ceftazidime, ceftizoxime,** and **ceftriaxone** are active against *P. aeruginosa.* Drug-resistant strains tend to develop, however, if these drugs are used as monotherapy to treat *Pseudomonas.* Several drugs in this group are active against beta-lactamase–producing strains of *N. gonorrhoeae.* **Ceftriaxone,** a parenteral formulation, is active against *chancroid, H. influenzae, N. gonorrhoeae, N. meningitidis,* and *Salmonella.*

Some agents in this group reach clinically effective concentrations in the CSF.

The **fourth generation cephalosporin cefepime** (Maxipime) has a broader spectrum of activity and is more resistant to beta-lactamases that inactivate many **third generation agents. Maxipime** is active against both gram-positive and gram-negative organisms and against resistant strains of *Enterobacter* and *Pseudomonas*.

Many texts and references (e.g., *Sanford Guide to Antimicrobial Therapy, Drug Facts and Comparisons*) have tables that list the organisms generally susceptible to various **cephalosporins** for each of the **cephalosporin** generations.

Resistance

First generation cephalosporins are generally inactivated by beta lactamase–producing organisms. **Cefonicid, cefdinir, loracarbef,** and **cefixime** have a high degree of stability to some beta-lactamases. **Cefoxitin, cefuroxime, ceftriaxone, cefotaxime, ceftizoxime, cefmetazole,** and **cefotetan** are highly stable even in the presence of both penicillinases and cephalosporinases produced by both gram-negative and gram-positive organisms. **Cefoperazone, cefpodoxime,** and **ceftazidime** are highly stable in the presence of beta-lactamases produced by gram-negative pathogens. **Cefaclor** is stable in the presence of some beta-lactamases. Changes of PBPs that prevent **cephalosporins** from binding to receptors are accountable for resistance of MRSA, DRSP, *E. faecalis,* and *Enterococcus faecium* to **cephalosporins. Cefepime** is active against most gram positive and gram-negative pathogens, including resistant strains.

Pharmacokinetics

Absorption and Distribution

Cephalosporins that have oral formulations are well absorbed from the GI tract. Except for **cefadroxil** and **cefprozil,** absorption is delayed by food, but the amount absorbed is not affected. The absorption of oral ester prodrugs **cefpodoxime proxetil** and **cefuroxime axetil** is increased when given with food. All IM formulations are well absorbed from muscle tissue. Differences in bioavailability exist for the suspension and tablet formulations of both **cefpodoxime proxetil** and **cefixime,** so the formulations should not be substituted.

All **cephalosporins** are widely distributed to most tissues and fluids. Protein binding varies, but **ceftriaxone** is so highly bound to albumin that it should be avoided in neonates at risk for hyperbilirubinemia, especially preterm infants. The penetration of CSF varies by generation. Except for **cefuroxime, first** and **second generation drugs** do not readily enter the CSF, even when the meninges are inflamed. **Third** and **fourth generation drugs** and **cefuroxime** readily enter the CSF in the presence of meningeal inflammation. The CSF levels of **cefoperazone,** however, are relatively low. Therapeutic levels are reached in bone at usual doses for most **cephalosporins,** and they are used prophylactically and therapeutically in orthopedic disorders. **Cefazolin** penetrates inflamed bone at higher concentrations than it penetrates normal bone, and it is the drug of choice in preventing and treating bone infection associated with orthopedic surgery.

High concentrations of **ceftriaxone** and **cefoperazone** are found in bile. Bile levels of **cefazolin** can exceed serum levels by up to five times in patients with obstructive biliary disease.

Metabolism and Excretion

Cephapirin is metabolized to less active compounds; however, one of its metabolites contributes to the drug's antibacterial activity. A metabolite of **cefotaxime** increases its spectrum of activity and extends the dosing intervals because of its prolonged metabolic half-life. **Cefuroxime** and **cefpodoxime** are pro-drugs metabolized to active metabolites.

Most **cephalosporins** are excreted via the kidney in varying degrees as unchanged drug. Increased **cephalosporin** plasma concentrations may occur when **probenecid** blocks renal tubular secretion of **cephalosporins.** The combination of oral **probenecid** and **cephalosporins** is used in serious infections and single-dose therapy of sexually transmitted infections. Renal impairment significantly extends the half-life of these drugs. **Cefoperazone** is excreted mainly in bile, and its half-life is unchanged, even in severe renal insufficiency. **Ceftriaxone** also includes an extra-renal route of excretion so that its half-life is affected to a limited degree by severe renal insufficiency. In hepatic dysfunction, the half-life and urinary excretion of both of these drugs are increased. The extra-renal excretion of some **cephalosporins** makes these drugs relatively safe in significant renal insufficiency.

Changes Related to Pregnancy and in Children

The pharmacokinetic properties of **cephalosporins** change during pregnancy, tending toward shorter half-lives, lower serum levels, larger volumes of distribution, and increased clearance.

In neonates, accumulation of these drugs because of undeveloped renal function results in prolonged half-lives. **Ceftriaxone** is contraindicated in neonates younger than 28 days of age with hyperbilirubinemia because of the displacement of bilirubin from plasma albumen, leading to more free bilirubin and possible bilirubin encephalopathy. In children older than 3 months, higher doses of **cefoxitin** have been associated with increased incidence of eosinophilia and elevated AST. In children older than 6 months, **ceftizoxime** has been associated with transient elevated levels of AST, ALT, and CPK.

Table 24–6 presents the pharmacokinetics of selected **cephalosporins.** Half-life alterations associated with end-stage renal disease are included.

Table 24–6 ▶ **Pharmacokinetics: Cephalosporins**

Drug	Onset	Peak	Duration	Protein Binding	Bioavailability	Half-Life NRF/ESRD*	Elimination (% unchanged in urine)
FIRST GENERATION							
Cefadroxil (PO)	Rapid	1.5–2 h	12–24 h	20%	90%	78–96 min/20–25 h	>80%
Cefazolin (IM)	Rapid	1–2 h	6–12 h	80%–86%	0	90–120 min/3–7 h	60%–80%
Cephalexin (PO)	15–30 min	1 h	6–12 h	10%	UA	50–80 min/19–22 h	>95%
Cephradine (PO)	Rapid	1–2 h	6–12 h	8%–17%	>90%	48–80 min/8–15 h	100%
(IM)	Rapid				>90%	48–80 min/8–15 h	100%
SECOND GENERATION							
Cefaclor (PO)	15 min	0.5–1 h	6–12 h	25%	>90%	35–54 min/2–3 h	60%–85%
Cefamandole (IM)	Rapid	0.5–2 h	4–8 h	65%–75%	0	30–60 min/2.1 h	UA
Cefotetan (IM)	Rapid	1–3 h	12 h	88%–90%	0	180–276 min/13–35 h	51%–81%
Cefoxitin (IM)	Rapid	0.5 h	4–8 h	73%	0	40–60 min/20 h	85%
Cefprozil (PO)	UA	1–2 h	12–24 h	36%	95%	78 min/5.2–5.9 h	60%
Cefuroxime (PO)	UA	2 h	8–12 h	50%	UA	80 min/16–22 h	66%–100%
(IM)	Rapid	15–60 min	6–12 h	50%		80 min/16–22 h	66%–100%
Loracarbef (PO)	Rapid	0.5–1.2 h	12 h	25%	79%	60 min/32 h	>90%
THIRD GENERATION							
Cefdinir (PO)	Slow	2–4 h	UA	60%–70%	20–25%	100 min/16 h	12%–18%
Cefixime (PO)	15–30 min	2–6 h	25 h	65%	30–50%	180–240 min/11.5 h	85%
Cefoperazone (IM)	Rapid	1–2 h	12 h	82%–93%	0	120 min/1.3–2.9 h	20%–30%
Cefotaxime (IM)	Rapid	0.5 h	4–12 h	30%–40%	0	60 min/3–11 h	60%
Cefpodoxime (PO)	UA	2–3 h	12 h	21%–29%	UA	120–180 min/9.8 h	29%–33%
Ceftazidime (IM)	Rapid	1 h	6–12 h	<10%	0	114–120 min/14–30 h	80%–90%
Ceftibuten (PO)	Rapid	2–3 h	24 h	65%	UA	144 min/13.4–22.3 h	70%
Ceftizoxime (IM)	Rapid	0.5–1.5 h	6–12 h	30%	0	102 min/25–30 h	80%
Ceftriaxone (IM)	Rapid	1–2 h	12–24 h	85%–95%	0	348–522 min/15.7 h	33%–67%
FOURTH GENERATION							
Cefepime (IM)	30 min	1–2 h	12 h	20%	0	102–138 min/17–21 h	85%

ESRD = end-stage renal disease; NRF = normal renal function; UA = information unavailable.

Pharmacotherapeutics

Precautions and Contraindications

Like the **penicillins**, **cephalosporins** may produce hypersensitivity reactions in a small percentage of patients. Cross-sensitivity with **penicillins** increases the risk and occurs in 5 to 16 percent of patients. **Cephalosporins** cannot be assumed to be an absolutely safe alternative to **penicillin** in the **penicillin**-allergic patient and are generally not recommended for those who have had a type I (immediate, anaphylactic) reaction to any **penicillin**. Skin testing is not helpful for identifying individuals likely to experience anaphylactic reactions to **cephalosporins**.

Cephalosporins and other broad-spectrum **antibiotics** should be prescribed with care for patients with a known history of GI disease, especially colitis, because of the risk for developing pseudomembranous colitis. Renal function impairment significantly affects the half-life of most of these drugs, and they may also be nephrotoxic. Use in the presence of markedly impaired renal function (creatinine clearance [CCr] 10 to 50 mL/min) is undertaken with extreme caution. Older adults and patients with known or suspected renal impairment are monitored carefully prior to and during therapy. Dosage adjustments of 50 percent are recommended for oral agents only after the glomerular filtration rate (gfr) reaches less than 10 mL/minute, a condition not usually seen in primary care patients in some sources, but *Drugs Facts and Comparisons* (2010) recommends titrated dosage adjustments for some **cephalosporins** for CCr less than 30 mL/minute. Dosage adjustments are usually not required based on renal function at higher levels.

Hepatic function impairment is a concern for **cefoperazone** and **ceftriaxone.** If doses above 4 g are used per day, serum concentrations must be monitored.

Cephalosporins are Pregnancy Category B; however, their use during pregnancy should always be based on a risk/benefit determination because relatively few controlled studies exist. All of these drugs cross the placenta with maternal to fetal serum ratios of 0.16 to 1. **Cefotetan,** however, reaches therapeutic levels in cord blood (see discussion about pharmacokinetic changes in pregnancy).

Most **cephalosporins** are excreted in breast milk in small quantities. The average breast milk plasma ratio is 0.01 to 0.5 after 500-mg to 2-g doses. **Cefdinir** has not been detected in breast milk and **ceftibuten** has not been studied.

The safety and efficacy in children vary by drug. Safety and efficacy have not been established for children younger than 1 month for **cefazolin, cefotaxime,** and **cefaclor;** younger than 2 months for **cefpodoxime;** younger than 3 months for **cefuroxime, cephapirin,** and **cefoxitin;** younger than 6 months for **cefdinir, loracarbef, cefixime, ceftizoxime,** and **cefprozil;** younger than 9 months for **oral cephradine;** and younger than 1 year for **cefepime** and **parenteral cephradine. Cefditoren** is not approved for use in children younger than 12 years.

Adverse Drug Reactions

In addition to type I immediate anaphylactic-type hypersensitivity, (see the Precautions and Contraindications section), serum sickness–like reactions, consisting of erythema multiforme, other skin rashes, arthralgia, and fever, have been reported. This type III delayed reaction usually occurs following a second course of therapy and may be delayed up to 10 or more days after initiation of the drug. Between 0.1 and 1 percent of patients who receive **cefaclor** have the reaction. **Antihistamines** and **corticosteroids** may help to manage symptoms.

Several parenteral **cephalosporins** have been associated with induction of seizure activity, especially in the presence of renal impairment when the dose was not adjusted downward. Discontinuance of the drug resolved the problem in most cases.

Coagulation abnormalities have occurred in conjunction with administration of **parenteral cephalosporins** containing a particular chemical group, **cefamandole, cefmetazole, cefoperazone,** and **cefotetan.** Patients at risk appear to be those with renal impairment, cancer, impaired vitamin K synthesis, malnutrition, or low vitamin K stores. These **cephalosporins** are also associated with the **disulfiram**-like reaction in patients who consume or, less frequently, inhale **alcohol** (such as aftershave or alcohol swabs).

Immune hemolytic anemia has also been observed with **cephalosporins** in rare instances. Patients who develop anemia within 2 to 3 weeks of the initiation of **cephalosporin** therapy should be evaluated for the role the **cephalosporin** may play in this disorder, and the drug should be stopped until the etiology is determined.

Pseudomembranous colitis is a potentially serious adverse reaction to **cephalosporins** and other broad-spectrum **antibiotics.** Detection and management are described in the discussion of the adverse effects of **penicillins.** Use of **cephalosporins,** especially prolonged or repeat therapy, may result in bacterial or fungal overgrowth of nonsusceptible organisms. The patient should be monitored for this superinfection and treated with appropriate measures.

Incidence of non–*C. difficile* diarrhea is high with some **oral cephalosporins,** including **cefdinir** (16%), **cefixime** (16%), and **cefpodoxime** (7%). There have been reports with **cefpodoxime** of acute liver injury, bloody diarrhea, and pulmonary infiltrates with eosinophilia. **Ceftriaxone** has caused accumulation of biliary sludge or pseudolithiasis, which clears on discontinuation of the drug.

Drug Interactions

Drug interactions vary by drug. Table 24–7 shows specific drugs and their interactions. Drugs that interact with all **cephalosporins** include **probenecid,** which increases plasma levels of **cephalosporins,** and **loop diuretics,** which increase the risk for nephrotoxicity.

Clinical Use and Dosing

Exacerbation of Chronic Bronchitis

The common organisms found in the sputum of patients with COPD with acute exacerbation of chronic bronchitis are viruses, *H. influenzae, S. pneumoniae, M. pneumoniae,* and *M. catarrhalis.* The most common organism is *S. pneumoniae* (Rabe et al, 2007). Although **penicillins** are among the first-line agents to treat this disorder, **oral cephalosporins** are also useful in mild to moderate disease based on their action with *S. pneumoniae, H. influenzae,* and *M. catarrhalis.* For severe disease, **macrolides** or respiratory **fluoroquinolones** have a broader spectrum that includes the likely organisms and is more effective against DRSP. When **cephalosporins** are used, treatment is continued for 5 to 10 days at dosages shown in Table 24–8.

Acute Otitis Media

Although **amoxicillin** is the recognized first-line drug of choice for otitis media (see discussion in the Clinical Use and Indications section for **penicillins**), **cephalosporins** play an important role in the management of this common infection. For therapeutic failures of **amoxicillin,** the AAP/AAFP guidelines recommend **amoxicillin/clavulanate,**

Table 24–7 ■ Drug Interactions: Cephalosporins

Drug	Interacting Drug	Possible Effect	Implications
All cephalosporins	Probenecid	Probenecid may increase and prolong cephalosporin plasma levels by competitively inhibiting renal tubular secretion.	Avoid concurrent administration unless planned for therapeutic reasons.
	Loop diuretics	Increased risk of nephrotoxicity.	Use with caution and monitor renal function.
Cefazolin, cefoperazone, cefotetan	Ethanol	Alcoholic beverages consumed concurrently or within 72 h after these cephalosporins may produce an acute disulfiram-like reaction within 30 min of alcohol ingestion. This reaction may occur ≤3 d after last antibiotic dose.	Warn patients to avoid concurrent ingestion of alcohol.
	Anticoagulants	Hypoprothrombinemic effects of anticoagulants may be increased. Bleeding complications may occur. This interaction is also reported with some other cephalosporins.	Select a different antibiotic class for patients taking anticoagulants. If they must be given together, monitor PT more closely.
Cefaclor, cefdinir, cefpodoxime	Antacids	Extended-release tablets may have reduced plasma concentration when given with antacids.	If both must be given, separate administration by at least 2 h. Cefprozil and ceftibuten do not appear to be affected by antacids and may be substituted if appropriate.
Cefpodoxime, cefuroxime	Histamine$_2$ blockers	Plasma concentrations of the cephalosporin may be reduced by coadministration.	Cefaclor does not appear to be affected and may be substituted if appropriate.
Cefdinir	Iron supplements	Iron supplements and foods fortified with iron reduce absorption of cefdinir by 80% and 30%, respectively.	If iron must be taken, separate administration by 2 h. Iron-fortified infant formula has no effect.

Table 24–8 ● Dosage Schedules: Cephalosporins

Drug	Indications	Initial Dose	Maximal Dose and Comments
		FIRST GENERATION	
Cefadroxil (Duricef)*	Endocarditis prophylaxis	*Adults:* PO: 2 g 1 h prior to surgery *Children:* PO: 50 mg/kg 1 h prior to surgery	Maximum adult daily dose 4 g. Decrease dose frequency if CCr <50 mL/min
	Pharyngitis/ tonsillitis, impetigo (children)	*Adults:* PO: 500 mg q12h *or* 1 g once daily for 10 d *Children:* PO: 15 mg/kg q12h *or* 30 mg/kg once/d for 10 d	
	Skin and soft tissue infection	*Adults:* PO: 500 mg q12h *or* 1 g once daily *Children:* PO: 15 mg/kg q12h	
	Urinary tract infection, uncomplicated	*Adults:* PO: 500 mg-1 g q12h *or* 1–2 g once daily *Children:* PO: 15 mg/kg q12h	

Continued

Table 24–8 ◉ **Dosage Schedules: Cephalosporins—cont'd**

Drug	Indications	Initial Dose	Maximal Dose and Comments
		FIRST GENERATION	
Cefazolin (Kefzol, Ancef)*	Endocarditis prophylaxis	*Adults:* IM: 1 g 30 min prior to surgery *Children:* IM: 25 mg/kg 30 min prior to surgery	Maximum adult daily dose 6 g, although up to 12 g/d have been used in rare instances Reconstituted IM solution stable for 24 h at room temperature and 10 d if refrigerated
	Urinary tract infection, uncomplicated	Adults: IM: 1 g q12h	
	Antibacterial, mild to moderate infections	*Adults:* IM: 250 mg–1 g q6–8h *Children:* IM: 6.25–25 mg/kg q6h *or* 8.3–33.3 mg/kg q8h	
Cephalexin (Keftab, Keflex)	Antibacterial, mild to moderate infection	*Children: >40 kg and adults:* PO: 250 mg q6h *Children* PO: 25–50 mg/kg/d divided q6–8h	Adult maximum daily dose 4 g. If adult dose >4 g/d is needed, substitute parenteral therapy. Shake suspension well before measuring Potency of suspension maintained after reconstitution for 14 d if refrigerated
	Antibacterial, severe infection	*Children >40 kg and adults:* PO: 1 g q6h *Children:* 50–100 mg/kg/d divided q6–8 h	
	Endocarditis prophylaxis (off-labeled use)	*Children >40 kg and adults:* PO: 2 g as single dose 1 h prior to surgery *Children ≥1 yr:* PO: 50 mg/kg as single dose 1 h prior to surgery	
	Pharyngitis, skin and soft tissue infections, tonsillitis	*Children > 40 kg and adults:* PO: 500 mg q12h *Children ≥1 yr:* PO: 25–50 mg/kg/d divided q12 h	
	Cystitis, uncomplicated	*Adolescents >15 yr and adults:* 50 mg q12h for 7–14 d	
Cephradine (Velosef)*	Antibacterial, serious or chronic infections	*Adults:* PO: 250–500 mg q6h *or* 500 mg-1 g q12h *Children ≥9 mo:* PO: 6.25–12.5 mg/kg q6h *or* 12.5–25 mg/kg q12h *Infants <9 mo:* PO: 6.25–12.5 mg/kg q6h	Maximum adult daily dose 4 g. Adults with impaired renal function (CCr <200 mL/min) require decreased dosage Shake suspension well before measuring After reconstitution, retains potency 7 d at room temperature or 14 d if refrigerated
	Urinary tract infections, uncomplicated	*Adults:* PO: 500 mg q12h	
	Skin and soft tissue infections and upper respiratory tract infections	*Adults:* PO: 250 mg q6h *or* 500 mg q12h *Children:* See mild to moderate bacterial infections	
	Prostatitis	*Adults:* PO: 500 mg q6h *or* 1 g q12h	

Table 24–8 ● **Dosage Schedules: Cephalosporins—cont'd**

Drug	Indications	Initial Dose	Maximal Dose and Comments
		SECOND GENERATION	
Cefaclor (Ceclor)	Bacterial infections, pharyngitis, pneumonia, skin infections due to *Staphylococcus. aureus* or *S. pyogenes* tonsillitis, or urinary tract infection Acute exacerbation of chronic bronchitis	*Adults:* PO: 250–500 mg q8h *or* 375–500 mg extended-release tablet q12h *Infants >1 mo:* PO: 6.7–13.4 mg/kg q8h *or* 10–20 mg/kg q12h 500 mg q8h or 500 mg q12h for CD form	Adult maximum dose 2 g/d, although 4 g/d have been used in rare cases. Extended-release formulation should be taken with food and not crushed or chewed Cefaclor extended-release 500 mg bid is equivalent to capsules 250 mg tid, but not to other formulations at doses of 500 mg tid Shake suspension well before measuring After reconstitution, the suspension maintains potency for 14 d if refrigerated
Cefamandole (Mandol)*	Skin and soft tissue infections	*Adults:* IM: 500 mg q6h	Maximum adult daily dose 12 g Adults with impaired renal function (CCr <80 mL/min) require decreased dosage and/or frequency of administration After reconstitution, the solution maintains potency for 24 h at room temperature and 96 h if refrigerated Carbon dioxide is formed after reconstitution and may cause leakage if syringes are not used immediately
	Urinary tract infections	IM: 500 mg–1 g q8h	
	Severe bacterial infections	*Adults:* IM: 1 g q4–6h *Infants >1 mo and children:* IM: 25–50 mg/kg q4–8h	
Cefprozil (Cefzil)	Pharyngitis, tonsillitis	*Children >12 yr and adults:* PO: 500 mg q24h for 10 d *Children 2–12 yr:* PO: 15 mg/kg/d divided q12h	
	Sinusitis, acute pneumonia	*Children >12 yr and adults:* PO: 250–500 mg q12h for 10 d *Children 6 mo–12 yr:* PO: 7.5–15 mg/kg q12h for 10 d	
	Skin and soft tissue infections	*Children >12 yr and adults:* PO: 500 mg q24h for 10 d *Children 2–12 yr:* PO: 20 mg/kg q24h for 10 d	
	Otitis media	*Children 6 mo–12 yr:* PO: 30 mg/kg q12h for 10 d	
	Urinary tract infection	*Children >12 yr and adults:* PO: 500 mg q24h for 10 d	
Cefotetan (Cefotan)*	Skin and soft tissue infections, mild to moderate	*Adults:* IM: 1–2 g q12h for 5–10 d	Lidocaine (0.5%–1%) without epinephrine can be used as diluent for preparing IM injection. Solutions maintain potency 24 h at room temperature, 96 h if refrigerated, and 1 wk if frozen. Dosage should be decreased if CCr <30 mL/min

Continued

Table 24–8 ● **Dosage Schedules: Cephalosporins—cont'd**

Drug	Indications	Initial Dose	Maximal Dose and Comments
		SECOND GENERATION	
	Urinary tract infections	*Adults:* IM: 500 mg q12h *or* 1–2 g q12–24h for 5–10 d	
	All other bacterial infections, mild to moderate	*Adults:* IM: 1–2 g q12h for 5–10 d	
Cefuroxime axetil (Ceftin)*	Pharyngitis, sinusitis, tonsillitis	*Children >12 yr and adults:* PO: 250 mg bid for 10 d *Children 3 mo–12 yr:* PO: 10 mg/kg q12h for 10 d	Studies indicate 4- to 6-day treatment effective for group A streptococcal pharyngitis
	Otitis media or impetigo	*Children 3 mo–12 yr:* PO: 30 mg/kg/d divided q12h up to 1,000 mg/d for 10 d	Suspension is not as well absorbed as tablets
	Bronchitis, skin and soft tissue infections	*Children >12 yr and adults:* PO: 250–500 mg bid for 10 d	Oral forms should be taken with food to increase absorption
	ABECB	250 to 500 mg q12h	Suspension does not require refrigeration and maintains potency for 10 d after reconstitution
	Lyme disease, early	*Children >12 yr and adults:* PO: 500 mg bid for 20 d	Single-dose packets for suspension can be mixed with 10 mL or more cold water; apple, grape, or orange juice; or lemonade. Mix and consume entire volume immediately. Low rating for palatability of suspension
	Pneumonia	500 mg bid	
	Urinary tract infection, uncomplicated	*Adults:* 125–250 mg for 7–10 d	
Loracarbef (Lorabid)	Bronchitis, exacerbation	*Adults:* PO: 400 mg q12h for 7 d	Shake suspension well before measuring
	Pharyngitis, streptococcal	*Adults:* PO: 200–400 mg q12h for 10 d *Children 6 mo–12 yrs:* 15 mg/kg/d in divided doses q12h for 10 d	Refrigeration of the suspension is not necessary Palatability of suspension is rated very high
	Pneumonia *(S. pneumoniae or Haemophilus influenzae)*	*Adults:* PO: 400 mg q12h for 14 d	Dosage reduction required if CCr <50 mL/min
	Sinusitis	*Adults:* PO: 400 mg q12h for 10 d	
	Urinary tract infection, uncomplicated cystitis	*Adults:* PO: 200 mg q24h for 7 d	
	Uncomplicated pyelonephritis	*Adults:* PO: 400 mg q12h for 14 d	
Cefdinir (Omnicef)	Sinusitis, otitis media	*Adults:* PO: 300 mg q12h *or* 600 mg q24h for 10 d *Children:* PO: 7 mg/kg q12h *or* 14 mg/kg q24h for 5–10 d	
	Community-acquired pneumonia, skin and soft tissue infections	*Adults:* PO: 300 mg q12h *or* 600 mg q24h for 10 d *Children:* PO: 7 mg/kg q12h for 10 d	
	Pharyngitis, tonsillitis	*Adults:* PO: 300 mg q12h for 5–10 d *or* 600 mg q24h for 10 d *Children:* PO: 7 mg/kg q12h for 5–10 d *or* 14 mg/kg q24h for 10 d	

Table 24–8 ● Dosage Schedules: Cephalosporins—cont'd

Drug	Indications	Initial Dose	Maximal Dose and Comments
		THIRD GENERATION	
Cefixime (Suprax)*	Bronchitis, exacerbation; pharyngitis; tonsillitis; or urinary tract infection	*Children >50 kg and adults:* PO: 400 mg q24h *Children 6 mo–12 yr, <50 kg:* PO: 4 mg/kg q12h *or* 8 mg/kg q24h	Palatability of suspension rated high Oral suspension results in higher blood level than tablets, so do not substitute tablets for suspension in otitis media Shake suspension well before measuring Refrigeration not required. After reconstitution, it maintains potency for 14 d at room temperature Dosage reduction required if CCr <60 mL/min
	Gonorrhea, cervical, urethral, rectum	*Adults:* PO: 400 mg as a single dose	
Cefoperazone (Cefobid)	Mild to moderate infection	*Adults:* IM: 1–2 g q12h	Adults with impaired liver function should not receive more than 4 g/d. Adults with combined hepatic and renal impairment should receive no more than 1–2 g/d Lidocaine without epinephrine may be added when preparing injection
Cefotaxime (Claforan)*	Antibacterial, uncomplicated infection	*Children >50 kg and adults:* IM: 1 g q12h *Children >1 mo <50 kg:* IM: 8.3–30 mg/kg q4h *or* 12.5–45 mg/kg q6h	After preparation, the solution retains potency for 12 h at room temperature and 5 d if refrigerated in syringe and 7 d if refrigerated in original container For pneumonia, only if MIC = 2 mcg/mL
Cefpodoxime proxetil (Vantin)	ABECB	200 mg q12h	Palatability of suspension rated low
	Sinusitis	*Adolescents and adults:* 200 mg q12h *Infants > 6 mo and children:* 10 mg/kg/d divided q12h max 200 mg/dose	Shake suspension well before measuring Take suspension with food or alone. Tablets should be taken with food After reconstitution, maintains potency for 14 d if refrigerated
	Urinary tract infection	*Adults:* PO: 100 mg q12h for 7 d	
	Pharyngitis, tonsillitis	*Children >12 yr and adults:* PO: 100 mg q12h for 5–10 d *Children 2 mo–12 yr:* PO: 5 mg/kg, up to 400 mg, q12h for 10 d	
	Otitis media	*Children 2 mo–12 yr:* PO: 10 mg/kg, up to 400 mg, q24h for 10 d *or* 5 mg/kg, up to 200 mg, q12h for 10 d	
	Pneumonia, community acquired	*Children >12 yr and adults:* PO: 200 mg q12h for 14 d	
	Skin and soft tissue infection	PO: 400 mg q12h for 7–14 d	

Continued

Table 24–8 ● Dosage Schedules: Cephalosporins—cont'd

Drug	Indications	Initial Dose	Maximal Dose and Comments
		THIRD GENERATION	
Ceftibuten (Cedax)*	Pharyngitis, tonsillitis	*Children >12 yr and adults:* PO: 400 mg q24h for 10 d *Children* 6 mo–12 yr: PO: 9 mg/kg q24h for 10 d	Maximal daily adult dose 400 mg Renal impairment (CCr <50 mL/min) requires dosage decrease Shake suspension well before measuring Maintains potency for up to 14 d if refrigerated
Ceftizoxime (Cefizox)	Gonorrhea, uncomplicated	*Children >12 yr and adults:* IM: 1 g as a single dose	After reconstitution, IM solution retains potency at room temperature for 24 h and for 48–96 h if refrigerated Yellow to amber discoloration does not affect potency. Renal impairment (CCr <80 mL/min) requires dosage decrease
	Urinary tract infection	*Children >12 yr and adults:* IM: 500 mg q12h	
	Antibacterial, mild to moderate infection	*Children >12 yr and adults:* IM: 1 g q8–12h *Children 6 mo–6 yr:* IM: 50 mg q6–8h	
Ceftriaxone (Rocephin)	Gonorrhea, uncomplicated; chancroid	*Adolescents and Adults:* IM: 250 mg as a single dose	Maximal daily dose is 4 g for adults and 2 g for children (except meningitis is 4 g) Dose should not exceed 2 g/d in patients with both hepatic and renal impairment After reconstitution, IM solution retains potency for 24 h at room temperature and 48–96 h if refrigerated Yellow to amber discoloration does not affect potency
	Syphilis, Early	1 gm daily IM or IV for 10 d to 14 d	
	Pelvic inflammatory disease	250 mg IM as a single dose	Must give with doxycycline 100 mg/d for 14 d
	Epididymo-orchitis	250 mg IM as a single dose	Must give with doxycycline 100 mg/d for 10 d
	Gonococcal conjunctivitis	1 g IM as a single dose	Adults only. Also saline lavage of eye
	Otitis media	*Children:* IM: 50 mg/kg, up to 1 g, daily × 3 d	
	Skin and soft tissue infections	*Children:* IM: 50–75 mg/kg q24h or 25–37.5 mg/kg q12h, up to 2 g/d	
	All other serious infections	*Adults:* IM: 1–2 g q24h or 500 mg–1 g q12h *Children:* 80–100 mg/kg/d in 1–2 divided doses (max 4 g/d)	
	Febrile neutropenia	*Children:* IM: 25–37.5 mg/kg q12h up to 2 g/d	

Table 24–8 ◉ **Dosage Schedules: Cephalosporins—cont'd**

Drug	Indications	Initial Dose	Maximal Dose and Comments
		FOURTH GENERATION	
Cefepime (Maxipime)	Complicated intra-abdominal infections	*Adults:* 2 g IV q8h	Combine with metronidazole
	Pneumonia	*Children:* 50 mg/kg/dose q8h *Adults:* 2 g IV q8–12h for 4 to 7 d	
	Skin and skin structure infections, uncomplicated	*Adults:* 1–2 g q8– 12h *Children:* 50 mg/kg/dose q 12 h for 10 d	
	Urinary tract infections	*Children:* 50 mg/kg/dose q 12 h for 10 d *Adults:* Mild to moderate 0.5 to 1 g q12h for 7 to 10 d Severe 2 g q12h for 10 d	

* Required dosage adjustments for renal impairment. Frequently it means extending the time between doses. If a drug must be used in the presence of renal impairment because there is no alternative, consult the package insert for specific dosage data.

and then high-dose **cefpodoxime** (10 mg/kg/d as single dose), **cefprozil** (30 mg/kg/d in two divided doses), **cefdinir** (7 mg/kg/dose twice daily) or **cefuroxime axetil** (30 mg/kg/d in two divided doses). Duration of therapy is 10 days for children younger than 2 years; 5 to 7 days for children older than 2 years. **Ceftriaxone** 50 mg/kg as a daily IM dose can be given for 3 days. **Ceftriaxone** is approved as a single injection for first-line therapy, but three daily doses are recommended for children who have recently failed therapy with another **antimicrobials**.

Sinusitis

The primary organisms involved in acute sinusitis are *S. pneumoniae* (31%), *H. influenzae* (21%), *M. catarrhalis* (2%), group A streptococci (2%), anaerobes (6%), viruses (15%), and *S. aureus* (4%). **Second and third generation cephalosporins** with beta-lactamase stability and activity against *S. pneumoniae* are effective against many of these organisms and are indicated for the treatment of bacterial sinusitis (see the discussion of guidelines for initiating treatment in the Clinical Use and Indications section for **penicillins**). If the patient has not had any **antibiotics** within the past 3 months and/or the risk for DRSP is less than 30 percent, **amoxicillin** or **amoxicillin/clavulanate** is the first-choice drug. Thereafter, **cefdinir** 300 mg twice daily, **cefpodoxime proxetil** 200 mg twice daily, or **cefprozil** 250 to 500 mg twice daily, all given for 10 days, are useful. If the patient is allergic to **penicillin**, respiratory **fluoroquinolone** (adults only) is recommended. **Fluoroquinolones** (**gatifloxacin**, **gemifloxacin**, **moxifloxacin**, or **levofloxacin**) are used for treatment failures after 3 days.

Pharyngitis

Penicillin V is the drug of choice for treatment of pharyngitis caused by group A streptococci (AAP, 2009a). A narrow-spectrum **first generation cephalosporin** (**cephalexin**) is indicated as an alternative for this infection as a 10-day course of treatment. Recommended pediatric dosages for this indication include 25 to 50 mg/kg/day divided every 12 hours. Adult dosage for **cephalexin** for streptococcal pharyngitis is 500 mg every 12 hours. Patients with a type I **penicillin** allergy should not be treated with a **cephalosporin** because of the risk of cross-sensitivity (AAP, 2009b). **Penicillin**-allergic patients should be treated with a **macrolide** (**erythromycin**, **azithromycin**).

Urinary Tract Infection

The **cephalosporins** (**cephalexin**, **cefpodoxime**, **cefixime**) can be prescribed as second-line therapy to patients who are allergic to **sulfa** drugs or the **fluoroquinolones** or as first-line treatment for women who are pregnant. Duration of therapy for cystitis-urethritis in adults is 3 days; uncomplicated pyelonephritis requires 14 days of treatment. Children require 10 days of therapy for UTI because it is difficult to distinguish cystitis and pyelonephritis in young children. **Cefpodoxime proxetil** is used in adult dosages of 100 mg twice daily for urethritis-cystitis, 200 mg twice daily for pyelonephritis, and pediatric dosages of 10 mg/kg/day divided into two doses. **Cefixime** is used in adult dosages of 400 mg once daily for urethritis-cystitis and pyelonephritis; pediatric dosages of 8 mg/kg/day divided into two doses. Dosage of other agents for adults and children are listed in Table 24–8.

UTI is a common cause of unexplained fever in infants and young children aged 2 months to 2 years. In this population, diagnosis requires culture obtained by catheterization. Febrile UTI is treated aggressively in infants and children, as fever is often an indication of pyelonephritis (Gaylord & Starr, 2009). Infants and children with febrile UTI should receive parenteral antibiotics for the first 24 hours or until afebrile. **Ceftriaxone** 50 to 75 mg/kg divided every 12 to 24 hours IV/IM is often used because of the convenience of 24-hour dosing. Another appropriate parenteral **antibiotic** choice is **cefotaxime** (50 to 200 mg/kg/d in divided doses every 6 to 8 h). The treatment of UTIs is discussed in depth in Chapter 47.

Sexually Transmitted Infections

Ceftriaxone and **cefixime** are the recommended antibiotics for the treatment of cervicitis, urethritis, pharyngitis, and proctitis due to *N. gonorrhoeae* (CDC, 2007). Recommended adult dosages are **ceftriaxone** 250 mg IM or **cefixime** 400 mg orally, both as single doses (CDC, 2010e). Acceptable alternative parenteral treatments include **ceftizoxime** 500 mg IM; or **cefoxitin** 2 g IM, administered with **probenecid** 1 g orally; or **cefotaxime** 500 mg IM (CDC, 2010e). An acceptable alternative single-dose oral therapy is **cefpodoxime** 400 mg or **cefuroxime axetil** 1 g (CDC, 2010e). **Ceftriaxone** 1 g IM or IV every 24 hours is used for disseminated gonococcal infections with **cefotaxime** (1 g IV every 8 h) or **ceftizoxime** (1 g IV every 8 h) alternative regimen (CDC, 2010e). Because *Chlamydia* is commonly associated with genital gonorrhea, **azithromycin** 1 g as a single dose or **doxycycline** 100 mg twice daily for 10 days should be prescribed concurrently (CDC, 2006a). **Ceftriaxone** is also used in the treatment of chancroid (250 mg as a single IM dose); early primary, secondary, or latent syphilis (1 g daily IM for 8 to 10 d); pelvic inflammatory disease (250 mg IM as a single dose plus **doxycycline** 100 mg daily for 14 d); epididymo-orchitis (250 mg IM as a single dose plus **doxycycline** 100 mg daily for 10 d); and gonococcal conjunctivitis in the adult (1 g IM as single dose plus saline lavage of eye) (CDC, 2006a; CDC, 2007). Treatment of STIs is discussed in depth in Chapter 44.

Skin and Tissue Infections

First generation cephalosporins are first-line agents in the treatment of primary and secondary skin infections, including cellulitis, erysipelas, impetigo, traumatic wound infection, and surgical incision infection. The most commonly used drug is **cephalexin.** Other first-line drugs include **amoxicillin/clavulanate** and **azithromycin** to cover other common skin organisms not covered by **cephalexin.** Dosages are listed in Table 24–8.

Coverage for methicillin-resistant *S. aureus* (MRSA) is indicated in areas of high prevalence and a clinical suspicion of MRSA. Antibiotic appropriate for MRSA include **TMP-SMZ, doxycycline,** or **clindamycin,** depending on local resistance patterns. Cat bites, 80 percent of which become infected with *Pasteurella multocida* and/or *S. aureus*, can be treated with **amoxicillin/clavulanate** or **cefuroxime axetil** 500 mg twice daily. **Cephalexin** and other **first generation cephalosporins** should not be used for cat bite infections.

Community-Acquired Pneumonia

Macrolides are the first line treatment for community-acquired pneumonia (CAP) in adults (Mandell et al, 2007) and high-dose **amoxicillin** is the first-line treatment for CAP in children under age 5 years (Cincinnati Children's Hospital Medical Center, 2005). **Cephalosporins (cefpodoxime, cefuroxime,** or parenteral **ceftriaxone** followed by oral **cefpodoxime)** combined with a **macrolide** are used as alternative therapy to respiratory **fluoroquinolones** in adults with CAP (Mandell et al, 2007). **Ceftriaxone** (50 mg/kg in one daily dose) is appropriate therapy for 1 to 2 days in toxic-appearing children who may not be able to take oral antibiotics. Treatment of pneumonia is discussed in Chapter 42.

Other Uses

Although an off-labeled use, oral and parenteral first generation **cephalosporins** are effective in dosages listed on Table 24–8 for endocarditis prophylaxis prior to surgery for patients with a history of rheumatic heart disease. **Cefuroxime axetil** in adult doses of 500 mg twice a day for 21 days is used in early Lyme disease characterized by erythema migrans. **Ceftriaxone** in adult doses of 2 g daily for 14 to 28 days has been used for facial nerve involvement and arthritis of Lyme disease.

Rational Drug Selection

The general principles of rational antimicrobial selection, using the definitive and empirical approaches, are

> **On The Horizon — CEFTOBIPROLE**
>
> **Ceftobiprole** is a new fifth generation cephalosporin active against MRSA and penicillin-resistant *Streptococcus* pneumoniae. It is intended for use with skin and skin structure infection and for nosocomial pneumonia. It was originally submitted to the FDA in May 2007 for the treatment of complicated skin and skin structure infections. In 2010 the FDA requested further information and studies before approving **ceftobiprole**.

presented in the section on **penicillins.** Because there is so much variability within each generation of the **cephalosporins,** sensitivity testing is valuable in drug selection. Selection of **cephalosporins,** like selection of any **antimicrobial,** is based on the organism that is present (in the definitive approach) or most likely present (in the empirical approach), site of infection, resistance patterns, adverse effects, pharmacokinetics, cost, and convenience.

The oral **first generation cephalosporins** are interchangeable in terms of efficacy and safety, although the wholesale price for **cephradine** is less than it is for **cephalexin** or **cefadroxil.** Parenteral **cefazolin** has good tissue penetration and is the drug of choice for surgical prophylaxis. Oral **first generation** agents are good alternatives to **penicillinase-resistant penicillins** in the **penicillin**-allergic patient, unless the allergy is a type I hypersensitivity reaction. An off-labeled use is endocarditis prophylaxis prior to surgical procedures; **first generation cephalosporins** have the advantage of a fairly narrow spectrum and may be used by most **penicillin**-allergic individuals.

Second generation oral cephalosporins are slightly less active against gram-positive cocci than **first generation oral cephalosporins,** so the latter are the preferred empirical treatment for skin and tissue infections. **Cefaclor** is more susceptible to beta-lactamases than other oral **second generation cephalosporins. Cefaclor** and **loracarbef** have less activity against *H. influenzae* than **amoxicillin** and are not recommended for the treatment of otitis media in current guidelines. **Cefuroxime axetil** has the most consistent activity of the **second generation cephalosporins** against **penicillin** intermediate-resistant pneumococci. Consequently, although all **second generation oral cephalosporins** are approved for URIs, the resistance pattern favors **cefuroxime axetil** for oral therapy for otitis media unresponsive to **amoxicillin,** for sinusitis, and for pneumonia if *S. pneumoniae* is suspected. For other indications including UTIs, all **second generation agents** apparently have comparable efficacy. Generic **cefuroxime axetil** is among the less expensive oral **cephalosporins,** but the suspension formulation has been rated one of the least palatable liquid preparations. In one study of **antibiotic** suspensions, **loracarbef** was the least expensive of the **cephalosporins** and had the highest palatability rating of all **cephalosporin** suspensions (Steele, Thomas, & Begue, 2001). **Cefixime** suspension was also low in cost and rated as moderate to high on palatability. With the exception of **cefaclor,** which requires three doses daily, the oral **second generation** agents are dosed twice daily. Extended-release **cefaclor** (Ceclor-CD) has the advantages of twice-daily dosing and daily cost comparable to other **second generation cephalosporins.** Cost information is provided in Table 24–9.

Table 24–9 ◆ **Available Dosage Forms: Cephalosporins**

Drug	Dosage Form	How Supplied	Cost*
		FIRST GENERATION	
Cefadroxil	Capsules: 500 mg Tablets: 1 g	In bottles of 100 capsules In bottles of 24, 50, 100, 500 tablets	$96 $277/50
(Duricef)	Capsules: 500 mg Tablets: 1 g Powder for oral suspension: 125 mg/5 mL 250 mg/5 mL 500 mg/5 mL	In bottles of 20, 50, 100 capsules In bottles of 50, 100 tablets In bottles of 50, 100 mL (orange-pineapple flavor) In bottles of 50, 75, 100 mL (orange-pineapple flavor)	$110/100 $86/100 mL
Cefazolin	Powder for injection: 250 mg, 500 mg, 1 g, 5 g	In multidose vials	
(Ancef, Kefzol)	Powder for injection: 500 mg, 1 g, 5 g	In multidose vials	
Cephalexin	Capsules: 250 mg 500 mg Tablets: 250 mg, 500 mg 1 g Powder for oral suspension: 125 mg/5 mL, 250 mg/5 mL	In bottles of 100, 500, 1,000 capsules In bottles of 100, 250, 500, 1,000 capsules In bottles of 20, 100, 500 tablets In bottles of 24 tablets In 100-, 200-mL bottles	$4/28 (Walmart list) $4/30 $57, $80 $11, $12
(Keflex)	Capsules: 250 mg 500 mg Powder for oral suspension: 125 mg/5 mL, 250 mg/5 mL	In bottles of 20, 100 capsules In bottles of 20 capsules In 100-, 200-mL bottles	$34/28 $48/21

Continued

Table 24–9 ◈ **Available Dosage Forms: Cephalosporins—cont'd**

Drug	Dosage Form	How Supplied	Cost*
FIRST GENERATION			
Cephradine	Capsules: 250 mg, 500 mg Powder for oral suspension: 125 mg/5 mL, 250 mg/5 mL	In bottles of 24, 40, 100, 500 capsules In 100-, 200-mL bottles	$21/24, $63/24
(Velosef)	Capsules: 250 mg, 500 mg Powder for oral suspension: 125 mg/5 mL, 250 mg/5 mL Powder for injection: 250 mg, 500 mg, 1 g	In bottles of 12 to 100 capsules In 100-mL bottles (fruit flavor) In multidose vials	$86, $167
SECOND GENERATION			
Cefaclor	Capsules: 250 mg 500 mg	In bottles of 30, 100, 500, 1,000 capsules In bottles of 15, 100, 500 capsules	$28 $57
Cefaclor ER	500 mg Powder for oral suspension: 125 mg/5 mL 187 mg/5 mL 250 mg/5 mL 375 mg/5 mL	 In 75-, 150-mL bottles In 50-, 150-mL bottles In 75-, 150-mL bottles In 50-, 100-mL bottles	$302 $9.50/75 mL $17/150 mL $11/75 mL $19/100 mL
(Ceclor)	Pulvules: 250 mg 500 mg CD extended-release: 375 mg, 500 mg Powder for oral suspension: 125 mg/5 mL 250 mg/5 mL 375 mg/5 mL	In bottles of 15, 100 capsules In bottles of 15, 30, 100 capsules In bottles of 60 tablets In 50- and 100-mL bottles (strawberry flavor) In 75- and 150-mL bottles (strawberry flavor) In 50-, 100-mL bottles (strawberry flavor)	$200 $61/15
(Raniclor)	125 mg, 187 mg, 250 mg, 375 mg		
Cefamandole (Mandol)	Powder for injection: 1 g 2 g	In 10-mL vials In 20-mL vials	
Cefotetan (Cefotan)	Powder for injection: 1 g, 2 g	In ADD-Vantage vials	
Cefprozil (Cefzil)	Tablets: 250 mg 500 mg Powder for oral suspension: 125 mg/ 5 mL, 250 mg/5 mL	In bottles of 100 film-coated tablets In bottles of 50, 100 film-coated tablets In 50-, 75-, 100-mL bottles (bubblegum flavor)	$416 $844
Cefuroxime	Powder for injection: 750 mg 1.5 g Tablets: 250 mg 500 mg	In 10-mL multidose vials In 20-mL multidose vials	 $17 $26
(Ceftin)	Tablets: 125 mg, 500 mg 250 mg Suspension: 125 mg/5 mL 250 mg/5 mL	In bottles of 20, 60 film-coated tablets In bottles of 10, 20, 60 film-coated tablets In 50-, 100-mL bottles (tutti-frutti flavor)	 $108/20
(Kefurox)	Powder for injection: 750 mg 1.5 g	In 10-, 100-mL multidose vials In 20-, 100-mL multidose vials	
(Zinacef)	Powder for injection: 750 mg, 1.5 g	In multidose vials	
Loracarbef	Pulvules: 200 mg, 400 mg	In bottles of 30 to 100 capsules	$387, $152/30
(Lorabid)	Powder for oral suspension: 100 mg/ 5 mL, 200 mg/5 mL	In 50-, 75-, 100-mL bottles, strawberry-bubblegum flavor	

Table 24–9 ◆ **Available Dosage Forms: Cephalosporins—cont'd**

Drug	Dosage Form	How Supplied	Cost*
THIRD GENERATION			
Cefdinir	Capsules: 300 mg	In bottles of 60 capsules	$254
(Omnicef)	Oral suspension: 125 mg/5 mL	In 60-, 100-mL bottles (strawberry flavor)	$44/60 mL
Cefixime	Tablets: 200 mg	In bottles of 100 scored tablets	
(Suprax)	400 mg Powder for oral suspension: 100 g/5 mL	In bottles of 50, 100 scored tablets In 50-, 75-, 100-mL bottles (strawberry flavor)	
Cefoperazone (Cefobid)	Powder for injection: 1 g, 2 g	In multidose vials	
Cefotaxime (Claforan)	Powder for injection: 500 mg, 1 g, 2 g	In multidose vials	
Cefpodoxime	Tablets: 100 mg, 200 mg	In bottles of 20, 100 tablets	100 mg = $85/20, 200 mg = $112/20
(Vantin)	Granules for suspension: 50 mg/5 mL, 100 mg/5 mL	In 50-, 75-, 100-mL bottles (lemon cream flavor)	
Ceftazidime	Powder for injection: 500 mg	In multidose vials	
(Fortaz)	1 g, 2 g	In multidose and ADD-Vantage vials	
(Tazidime)	Powder for injection: 500 mg 1 g 2 g	In 10-mL multidose vials In 20-, 100-mL ADD-Vantage vials In 50-, 100-mL ADD-Vantage vials	
(Ceptaz)	Powder for injection: 1 g, 2 g	In multidose vials	
(Tazicef)	Powder for injection: 1 g, 2 g	In multidose and ADD-Vantage vials	
Ceftibuten (Cedax)	Capsules: 400 mg Powder for oral suspension: 90 mg/5 mL 180 mg/5 mL	In bottles of 20, 100 capsules In 30-, 60-, 90-, 120-mL bottles (cherry flavor) In 30-, 60-, 120-mL bottles (cherry flavor)	$149/20 $76/120
Ceftizoxime (Cefizox)	Powder for injection: 500 mg 1 g, 2 g	In 10-mL single-dose fliptop vials In 20-mL single-dose fliptop vials	
Ceftriaxone (Rocephin)	Powder for injection: 250 mg, 500 mg, 1 g, 2 g	In multidose vials	
FOURTH GENERATION			
Cefepime (Maxipime)	500-mg/15-mL vial, 1-g/15-mL vial, 2-g/15-mL vial		

*Cost is per 100 units unless otherwise stated.

Because of the enhanced beta-lactamase resistance and extended gram-negative spectrum of **third generation cephalosporins**, agents in this class are indicated for infections where resistance mediated by beta-lactamase is a major consideration, such as gonorrhea infections and resistant otitis media. Although the incidence of GI intolerance would be expected to be lower with the parenteral route of single-dose IM **ceftriaxone**, diarrhea has been observed in up to 25 percent of patients who receive **ceftriaxone** for otitis media. Additionally, IM injections may be poorly accepted by children and their parents, so the convenience and improved compliance expected with **ceftriaxone** may be offset by these liabilities. **Cefdinir** and **cefpodoxime proxetil** are oral agents that share similar **antibacterial** activity. **Cefixime** and **ceftibuten** are much less active than **cefpodoxime proxetil** against pneumococci, are completely inactive against penicillin-resistant pneumococcal strains, and have poor activity against *S. aureus*. **Cefixime** and **cefpodoxime proxetil** are the most active oral agents against *N. gonorrhoeae*. Parenteral **ceftriaxone** and **cefotaxime** are effective against resistant strains of pneumococcus and are used empirically in serious infections presumed to be caused by these strains. Because they cross the blood–brain barrier, **third generation parenteral cephalosporins** are used to treat meningitis. Unfortunately, this class of drugs is commonly misused for infections that could be treated by a narrower-spectrum agent. Because of long half-lives, **ceftriaxone**, **ceftibuten**, and **cefixime** can be dosed once daily for most infections; **cefpodoxime proxetil** and **cefdinir** require two doses daily. **Third generation cephalosporins** are expensive relative to other **antimicrobials**. The palatability of **cefixime** suspension was rated moderate to high, whereas **cefpodoxime proxetil** suspension had one of the lowest ratings of all suspensions tested (Steele, Thomas, & Begue, 2001).

Monitoring

Monitoring for therapeutic and adverse responses to **antimicrobials** requires clinical, microbiological, and laboratory data (see the Monitoring section for the **penicillins**).

Because the **cephalosporins** have a broad spectrum, signs and symptoms of pseudomembranous colitis associated with *C. difficile*, as well as other superinfections, should be noted. Diarrhea is common with some **cephalosporins** and must be distinguished from pseudomembranous colitis. Obtain a *C. difficile* cytotoxin assay of the stool if there are more than six watery stools per day or if there is blood in the stool. Although hemolytic anemia is rare with the **cephalosporins**, signs of tiredness or weakness, yellow skin, or yellow eyes require a red blood cell (RBC) count with indices. During prolonged therapy, periodic urinalysis, BUN, and creatinine determinations should be performed to evaluate renal function. If the CCr indicates renal impairment, dosage should be decreased according to the schedule in the package insert or drug reference. The majority of older patients require dosage adjustment because of age-related decrements in renal function. Patients who are receiving protracted courses of **cefamandole**, **cefmetazole**, **cefoperazone**, or **cefotetan**, which are parenteral **cephalosporins** that affect clotting, require baseline and periodic assessment of PT. Administer exogenous vitamin K (phytonadione; AquaMephyton) 10 mg IM if PT time is prolonged. Patients taking these agents should also be observed for **disulfiram** reaction (abdominal cramping, facial flushing, headache, hypotension, palpitations, shortness of breath, sweating, tachycardia, vomiting) if exposed to **alcohol**.

Patient Education

Administration

Emphasize to the patient or caregiver the importance of completing the entire course of **antibiotic** therapy. Available dosage forms are shown in Table 24–9. IM **cephalosporins** may be irritating and painful. Inject the medication deep into a large muscle mass, and avoid repeated injection by initiating IV access for therapy requiring more than a few injections. Medications mixed for injection will lose potency with time, although refrigeration after reconstitution will usually extend the period of full potency. Consult the package insert for proper mixing and storage of reconstituted parenteral **cephalosporins**. Adhere to the manufacturer's limits on volume of injection at one site (see also Table 24–8).

Usually, **oral cephalosporins** should be taken with food or milk if they cause stomach irritation. **Ceftibuten** is the exception because it is poorly absorbed unless taken on an empty stomach; it should be taken 1 hour before or 2 hours after meals. **Cefuroxime axetil**, particularly the suspension formulation, and **cefpodoxime proxetil** should be taken with food to enhance absorption. Tablets and suspension forms of cefuroxime axetil and **cefixime** should not be used interchangeably because they have different bioavailability. **Cefuroxime** tablets are more completely absorbed than the suspension; however, the suspension of **cefixime** is better absorbed than the tablets. **Cefdinir** must be taken 2 hours before or 1 hour after **antacids** that contain **magnesium** or **aluminum**, which impairs its absorption. Patients with phenylketonuria should avoid **cefprozil**, which contains phenylalanine.

Suspensions and **antibiotic** solutions must be shaken to disperse or dissolve particles of drug immediately before measurement. Adhere to the manufacturer's specifications for storage after reconstitution, and advise the patient not to use the drug after the expiration date. Describe to the patient whether there will be liquid remaining at the end of the course of therapy and urge disposal of unused medication. Ask the pharmacist to dispense a measuring device with every liquid preparation.

Adverse Reactions

If severe diarrhea occurs, the patient should contact the prescriber before initiating any treatment. For mild diarrhea, **adsorbent antidiarrheal agents** containing **attapulgite** can be used, but **antiperistaltic agents** that would promote the retention of *C. difficile* toxins must be avoided.

Other signs and symptoms of adverse effects that patients should be advised to report include vaginal itching or discharge, sore mouth or throat, white patches on mucous membranes of mouth, easy bruising or bleeding, altered urine output, yellow skin or eyes, or unusual lethargy commencing after the drug is started. Development of skin rash, aching joints, hives, or respiratory problems may signal allergic response and should also be reported. **Cephalosporins** cause false positives on urine testing for glucose when the copper sulfate technique (Clinitest) is used. Diabetics taking **cephalosporins** should use blood glucose monitoring or urine testing based on the glucose enzymatic tests (e.g., Clinstix, TesTape). Anorexia, epigastric pain, nausea, and vomiting in a patient taking a course of **ceftriaxone** may indicate development of biliary sludge or pseudolithiasis, which abates when the drug is discontinued.

Lifestyle Management

Practicing infection control and good health hygiene, such as safe sex practices and a healthy lifestyle, helps to prevent infections. Supportive nutrition, adequate rest, appropriate fluids, and comfort measures promote recovery from an infection. Maintaining a clean, dry wound site free of excess necrotic tissue and foreign bodies is essential to resolution of a wound infection and wound healing.

FLUOROQUINOLONES

The **fluoroquinolones** are synthetic, broad-spectrum **antibiotics** chemically related to the **quinolone nalidixic acid** (NegGram), a narrow-spectrum **antibiotic** used to treat UTIs. **Fluoroquinolones** are a newer class of **antibiotics** introduced in the 1980s. The **fluoroquinolones** are divided into the older group (**ciprofloxacin** [Cipro], **norfloxacin** [Noroxin], **ofloxacin** [Floxin]) and the newer group (**gemfloxacin** [Factive], **levofloxacin** [Levaquin], **moxifloxacin** [Avelox]). The newer **fluoroquinolones** are often referred to as the respiratory **fluoroquinolones**. Two newer **fluoroquinolones** have been withdrawn from the market because of adverse effects: **trovafloxacin** (Trovan) because of liver toxicity and **gatifloxacin** (Tequin) because of hypoglycemia and hyperglycemia. **Sparfloxacin** is no longer available in the United States. An ophthalmic solution of **gatifloxacin** (Zymar) is still available.

Pharmacodynamics

Fluoroquinolones are bactericidal through interference with enzymes required for the synthesis and repair of bacterial DNA. Addition of two chemical moieties, including a fluorine-containing group and a piperazine group, to the structure of the **quinolone nalidixic acid** resulted in the greatly enhanced **antimicrobial** efficacy of the **fluoroquinolones**. The fluorine molecule added to create the **fluoroquinolones** provides increased potency against gram-negative organisms and broadens the spectrum to include gram-positive organisms as well. The added piperazine moiety is responsible for the antipseudomonal activity of **fluoroquinolones**. **Levofloxacin**, the pure L-isomer of racemic **ofloxacin**, has a broader gram-positive spectrum than the racemate.

Fluoroquinolones inhibit bacterial topoisomerase II (DNA gyrase) and topoisomerase IV. Inhibition of DNA gyrase prevents the relaxation of positively supercoiled DNA that is required for normal transcription and replication. Inhibition of topoisomerase IV probably interferes with separation of replicated DNA into the daughter cells during replication.

Sensitivity

Fluoroquinolones are notable for their extensive gram-negative activity against *Brucella* species, *C. pneumonia, S. aureus, S. epidermidis, E. coli, Klebsiella* species, *Enterobacter, Campylobacter, Salmonella, Shigella, Proteus vulgaris, S. marcescens, Haemophilus* species, *N. gonorrhoeae, N. meningitidis, M. catarrhalis, Legionella, Pseudomonas,* and many others. Newer **fluoroquinolones** are effective against **penicillin**-resistant *S. pneumoniae,* whereas resistance has developed to the older **fluoroquinolones**. Older **fluoroquinolones** have little activity against anaerobic organisms but are active against atypical organisms such as *Chlamydia, Mycobacterium,* and *Mycoplasma* species. Only **ciprofloxacin** and **levofloxacin** have full activity against *P. aeruginosa*.

Resistance

Resistance is mediated by mutations in the **quinolone**-binding region of the target enzyme or by a change in the permeability of the organism (Piddock, 1999). Many scientists and clinicians are concerned that overuse of these agents has already eroded the utility of this group of drugs. *Staphylococcus, Streptococcus,* and *Enterococcus* species once susceptible have now developed resistance. The CDC no longer recommends **ciprofloxacin** in the treatment of gonorrhea because of resistance (CDC, 2007). **Fluoroquinolone**-resistant tuberculosis is associated with previous exposure to **fluoroquinolones** (Devasia et al, 2009). To prevent increased development of resistance to this group of drugs, **fluoroquinolones** should not be used for upper and lower respiratory infections or for skin and soft tissue infections for which other inexpensive, safe, and narrower-spectrum drugs are still effective. Rather, **fluoroquinolones** should be reserved for uses for which the alternative is costlier and more hazardous.

Pharmacokinetics

Absorption and Distribution

All drugs in this class are well absorbed after oral administration. Food only marginally affects absorption of other drugs in this class, but not all agents have been studied for food effects on absorption. Therefore, the manufacturers recommend taking some of these drugs on an empty stomach.

All drugs in this class are widely distributed, with high tissue and urinary levels. For most **fluoroquinolones**, tissue concentrations are usually higher than plasma concentrations. Plasma protein binding is variable. **Fluoroquinolones** are also found in saliva, nasal and bronchial secretions, sputum, bile, lymph, and peritoneal fluid. They cross the blood–brain barrier poorly into

On The Horizon GARENOXACIN

Garenoxacin is a new addition to the quinolone group already approved for use in Japan. It is broad spectrum and effective against both gram + and gram – infections, including those caused by anaerobic bacteria. It carries the added advantage of once daily dosing. Its approval application was withdrawn from the FDA process in 2006 due to licensing issues and is expected to be resubmitted at some point.

uninflamed meninges, but **ciprofloxacin** and **ofloxacin** penetrate to a moderate extent in the presence of inflammation. All appear to cross the placenta. Although **ciprofloxacin** and **ofloxacin** are known to enter breast milk, this property has not been adequately studied for other **fluoroquinolones**.

Metabolism and Excretion

The predominant route of elimination varies widely between **fluoroquinolones**. **Ofloxacin**, **levofloxacin**, and **lomefloxacin** have predominant renal excretion with minimal (less than 10%) metabolism. In contrast, **nalidixic acid** and **moxifloxacin** undergo extensive metabolism (greater than 35%). The other drugs undergo modest metabolism but have significant renal excretion as well. A few of them are also excreted in feces. Renal impairment results in increased half-lives of those with substantial excretion of unchanged drug. For patients with CCr of 50 mL/minute or less, dosage adjustments may be needed. This is especially of concern with older adults, who are likely to have some degree of reduced renal function. **Moxifloxacin** pharmacokinetics are not significantly altered even in the presence of severe renal impairment. No dosage adjustment is needed. All other **fluoroquinolones** have some degree of dosage adjustment required for significant renal impairment. If they must be used based on no reasonable alternative, seek data on dosage adjustments for any patient, especially older adults, who may have renal impairment. Table 24–10 lists the pharmacokinetics of selected oral **fluoroquinolones**.

Pharmacotherapeutics

Precautions and Contraindications

All of the **fluoroquinolones** have a black box warning regarding the risk of tendon rupture and tendonitis. The risk is increased in older patients; in patients taking **corticosteroids**; and patients with heart, kidney, or lung transplant.

All **fluoroquinolones** produce slight prolongation of the QTc interval, the increase is not considered to be clinically significant and is rarely reported in **ciprofloxacin** and **levofloxacin**. Preexisting QTc prolongation or concurrent use of other drugs producing this cardiac conduction change produces additive effects with the **fluoroquinolones**.

Cautious use is required for patients with renal impairment. Dosage adjustments of all **fluoroquinolones** except **moxifloxacin** are needed for patients with impaired renal function. **Lomefloxacin** shows increased area under the curve (AUC) by 33 percent in older adults, in part due to reduced renal function.

Seizures, increased intracranial pressure, and toxic psychoses have occurred with this class. CNS stimulation, including tremors, restlessness, sleeplessness, tiredness, dizziness, lightheadedness, bad dreams, confusion, and hallucinations, may also occur. These symptoms are dose dependent and tend to resolve with continued use. Some studies indicate **fluoroquinolones** inhibit bonding of gamma-aminobutyric acid (GABA) to its receptor, which may be the mechanism of CNS stimulation. Slight decreases in magnesium concentration amplify the effect (*Sanford Guide*, 2010). Patients with known or suspected CNS disorders and other factors that predispose to seizures should use these agents with caution and careful monitoring.

Older adults and dialysis patients have increased risk of tendon rupture and adverse CNS reactions. Use **fluoroquinolones** cautiously with these populations.

Fluoroquinolones are Pregnancy Category C. Use is not recommended in pregnant women because there are no adequate, well-controlled studies in this population,

Table 24–10 ▶ **Pharmacokinetics: Fluoroquinolones**

Drug	Onset	Peak	Duration	Protein Binding	Bioavailability	Half-Life*	Elimination
Ciprofloxacin	1 h	1–2 h	12–24 h	20%–40%	70%	3–4.8 h	40%–50% unchanged in urine; remainder in feces
Gatifloxacin	Rapid	1–3 h	24 h	20%	96%	7–8.4 h	70% unchanged in urine
Levofloxacin	Rapid	1–2 h	24 h	24%–38%	99%	6–8 h	87% unchanged in urine; eliminated by tubular secretion
Lomefloxacin	Rapid	1.5 h	12–24 h	10%	95%–98%	6–8 h	60%–80% unchanged in urine; 5% metabolized; 28%–30% biliary excretion
Moxifloxacin	Rapid	1–3 h	24 h	30%–45%	86%	11–16 h	20% unchanged; 10% metabolized
Norfloxacin	Rapid	2–3 h	12 h	10%–15%	30%–40%	6.5 h	30% unchanged in urine; 30% in feces; 10% metabolized by liver
Ofloxacin	Rapid	1–2 h	12 h	20%–25%	89%	5–7 h	70%–80% unchanged in urine

*Half-life is increased in renal impairment, and dosage adjustments may be needed.

and teratogenesis has been demonstrated in animals. Use during pregnancy only if there is clear benefit that justifies the risk to the fetus.

Norfloxacin is not detected in breast milk following a 20-mg dose to nursing mothers; however, this dose is low. **Ciprofloxacin** is excreted in breast milk, but the dose ingested by the infant is small. Concentration of **ofloxacin** in breast milk is similar to maternal plasma, and it is presumed that its L-isomer, **levofloxacin**, also enters breast milk. **Moxifloxacin** is excreted in the breast milk of rats, but the drug has not been studied in humans. Because **fluoroquinolones** have caused cartilage lesions on weight-bearing joints in young animals, lactating women should use **fluoroquinolones** only if there is no safer alternative.

The safety and efficacy of this drug class have not been established in children. **Fluoroquinolones** are not recommended for children younger than 18 years. Arthropathy and osteochondrosis have been demonstrated in all species of immature animals tested. **Nalidixic acid, norfloxacin,** and **ciprofloxacin** have been used in children without evidence of arthropathy or osteochondrosis, but these three agents have poorer tissue penetration than other **fluoroquinolones.**

The only indications for which a **fluoroquinolone** is licensed by the FDA for use in patients younger than 18 years are complicated urinary tract infections, pyelonephritis, and post-exposure treatment for inhalation anthrax. The American Academy of Pediatrics (2006) recommends that the systemic use of **fluoroquinolones** in children should be restricted to situations in which there is no safe and effective alternative to treat an infection caused by multidrug-resistant bacteria or to provide oral therapy when parenteral therapy is not feasible and no other effective oral agent is available.

Adverse Drug Reactions

Pseudomembranous colitis has been reported with nearly all **antibacterial** agents, including **fluoroquinolones**, and may be mild to life threatening. It is important to consider this diagnosis in patients who present with diarrhea subsequent to administration of **fluoroquinolones**, especially if this diarrhea contains blood, pus, or mucus. Other common GI adverse reactions include abdominal pain, nausea, and altered taste, which are the most frequent adverse drug reactions.

Serious and occasionally fatal hypersensitivity reactions, including Stevens-Johnson syndrome, have occurred with **fluoroquinolones**. Some of the reactions occur following the first dose, presumably due to cross-allergy with other chemicals in the environment. Reactions that are anaphylactic in nature have also occurred.

Use of **fluoroquinolones**, especially in prolonged or repeat therapy, may result in bacterial or fungal overgrowth of nonsusceptible organisms. The patient should be monitored for this superinfection and treated with appropriate measures.

Unique, rare adverse effects have been associated with individual **fluoroquinolones**.

Ciprofloxacin has been associated with acidosis, renal failure, polyuria, urinary retention, and renal calculi. Cardiovascular adverse reactions including angina, atrial flutter, cardiopulmonary arrest, cerebral thrombosis, myocardial infarction, and ventricular ectopy have also been seen. None of these adverse reactions occurs commonly. **Norfloxacin** has rarely been associated with erythema multiforme, hepatitis, pancreatitis, and arthralgia.

Ofloxacin has been associated with vaginal discharge and genital pruritus. CNS symptoms such as sleep disorders, nervousness, and vertigo have also been seen uncommonly. Crystalluria has been reported with **ciprofloxacin** and other **fluoroquinolones**, especially in patients with alkaline urine (pH greater than 7). **Levofloxacin** and other **fluoroquinolones** have increased or decreased blood sugar in treated diabetics.

Phototoxicity has been observed with all **fluoroquinolones.** Clinical manifestations range from mild erythema to severe bullous eruptions in the sun-exposed areas. **Fluoroquinolones** with high phototoxic potential include **lomefloxacin** and **sparfloxacin.**

Fluoroquinolone tendinitis begins with inflammatory edema that manifests as painful and swollen tendons that are bilateral in 50 percent of cases. Failure to take appropriate measures to rest the tendon can result in rupture. Time from initiation of the drug to onset of tendinitis has varied up to 120 days, or even months after treatment (Stahlmann & Lode, 2010). The elderly are at high risk of developing tendon rupture (Stahlmann & Lode, 2010). This condition has led to the black box warning regarding the risk of tendonitis and tendon rupture with the use of **fluoroquinolones.**

Ophthalmological abnormalities, including cataracts and multiple punctate lenticular opacities, have occurred during therapy with some **fluoroquinolones**. A causal relationship has not been clearly established.

Additional adverse reactions are listed in the Precautions and Contraindications section.

Drug Interactions

Drug interactions vary somewhat by drug. Table 24–11 shows the various drug interactions. Several drugs interact with all to decrease their absorption. **Cimetidine** interferes with the elimination of **fluoroquinolones.** Some **fluoroquinolones** inhibit drug metabolism by cytochrome P450 (CYP) 3A4, one of the most important enzymes in hepatic drug metabolism. **Cyclosporine's** nephrotoxic effects are increased by concurrent administration with most **fluoroquinolones,** but especially with **ciprofloxacin** and **norfloxacin. Caffeine** interacts with several drugs in this class and, as with many other drugs that inhibit hepatic enzymes, **warfarin** has increased effects when administered to a patient receiving **fluoroquinolones.**

Table 24–11 ■ **Drug Interactions: Fluoroquinolones**

Drug	Interacting Drug	Possible Effect	Implications
All fluoroquinolones	Antacids, bismuth subsalicylate, iron salts, sucralfate, zinc salts	Interfere with GI absorption of the fluoroquinolone, resulting in decreased serum levels	Avoid simultaneous use; administer antacids 2–4 h before or after the fluoroquinolone
	Anticoagulants	Effects of anticoagulant may be increased	Monitor PT/INR
	Antineoplastic agents	Serum levels of fluoroquinolone may be decreased	Select different antibiotic or monitor serum levels
	Cimetidine	Cimetidine may interfere with elimination of fluoroquinolones	Select different histamine$_2$ blocker
	Cyclosporine	Nephrotoxic effects increased	Closely monitor renal function
	Glucocorticoids	Concurrent use may increase risk for tendon rupture	Select different antibiotic
	Theophylline	Decreased clearance, increased plasma levels, and toxicity of theophylline have occurred with concurrent use of ciprofloxacin and enoxacin. Data on norfloxacin and ofloxacin contradictory	Monitor theophylline levels
Ciprofloxacin	Caffeine	Total body clearance on caffeine reduced, with possible increased pharmacological effects	Avoid concurrent use
	Hydantoins	Phenytoin levels may be reduced, producing decreased therapeutic effects	Avoid concurrent use
	Probenecid	Renal clearance of ciprofloxacin reduced 50%; serum concentrations increased 50%	Avoid concurrent use
Norfloxacin	Caffeine	Total body clearance of caffeine reduced, with possible increased pharmacological effects	Ofloxacin does not appear to affect caffeine
	Nitrofurantoin	Antibacterial effect of norfloxacin in urinary tract may be antagonized	Avoid concurrent use
Levofloxacin	NSAIDs	Concurrent use increases CNS stimulation and seizures	Avoid concurrent use
	Antidiabetic drugs	Increase or decrease blood sugar	Carefully monitor blood sugar
Moxifloxacin	Amiodarone, disopyramide, quinidine, bepridil, sotalol	Increased risk of serious adverse cardiovascular effects	Avoid concurrent use

INR = international normalized ratio; PT = prothrombin time.

Food may decrease the absorption of **norfloxacin.** Food delays the absorption of **ciprofloxacin**, although total absorption is not changed. Dairy products reduce the absorption of **ciprofloxacin** and should not be used concurrently. **Antacids, bismuth subsalicylate, iron salts, sucralfate**, and **zinc salts** form an insoluble chelate with **fluoroquinolones**, preventing the absorption of the antimicrobial drug.

Clinical Use and Dosing

Exacerbations of Chronic Bronchitis

Because culture and sensitivity are unreliable due to bronchial colonization in acute exacerbation of chronic bronchitis, empirical therapy is selected to cover the most likely pathogens. The primary organisms are viruses (20% to 50%), *C. pneumoniae* (5%), and *M. pneumoniae* (less than 1%). The treatment of ABECB is described in the Clinical Use and Indications section for **penicillins**. Patients with moderate exacerbation who may require hospitalization or who do not respond to first-line therapy should be treated with a respiratory **fluoroquinolone (levofloxacin, moxifloxacin, gemifloxacin)**, using dosages summarized in Table 24–12. Treatment of acute exacerbations of chronic bronchitis is discussed in Chapter 30.

Community-Acquired Pneumonia

In dosages listed in Table 24–12, **fluoroquinolones** with enhanced gram-positive activity, such as **levofloxacin**, **moxifloxacin**, and **gemifloxacin**, are active against strains of *S. pneumoniae*. In addition, **fluoroquinolones** cover *Legionella*, as well as *M. pneumoniae* and *C. pneumoniae*, which are the most common pathogens in CAP patients without comorbidity. These organisms are resistant to **beta-lactam antibiotics** used for CAP, such as **ampicillin-clavulanate** and **second generation oral cephalosporins**, but susceptible to **macrolides**. A

Table 24–12 ◉ **Dosage Schedule: Fluoroquinolones**

Drug	Indications	Initial Adult Dose	Comments
Ciprofloxacin (Cipro)	Bone and joint infections, mild to moderate	PO: 500 mg q12h for at least 4–6 wk	Maximal adult daily dose 1.5 g Renal impairment (CCr <50 mL/min) requires dosage reduction Not recommended for children, but doses of 10–20 mg/kg q12h have been used where no alternative existed Oral suspension stable for 14 d at room temperature or in refrigerator Shake well before measuring Take with full glass of water Oral and parenteral routes are bioequivalent
	Bone and joint infections, severe or complicated	PO: 750 mg q12h for at least 4–6 wk	
	Bacterial diarrhea	PO: 500 mg	
	Inhalation anthrax	*Adults:* PO 500 mg q12h × 60 days post exposure *Children:* PO 15 mg/kg/dose q12h × 60 d post exposure	
	Intra-abdominal infections	PO: 500 mg q12h for 7–14 d in combination with oral metronidazole	
	Meningococcal carrier (off-labeled use)	500 mg as a single dose	
	Prostatitis	500 mg q12h for 28 d	
	Sinusitis	PO: 500 mg q12h 10 d	
	Typhoid fever	PO: 500 mg q12h for 10 d	
	Skin and soft tissue infections, mild to moderate	500 mg q12h for 7–14 d	
	severe or complicated	750 mg q12h for 7–14 d	
	Urinary tract infection, acute, uncomplicated	250 mg q12h for 3 d	
	mild to moderate	250 mg q12h for 7–14 d	
	Severe or complicated	*Adults:* 500 mg q12h for 7–14 d *Children:* 20–40 mg/kg/d divided q12h (max 2 g/d)	
(Ciloxan)	Bacterial conjunctivitis	Ophthalmic solution: >1 yr: 1–2 drops every 2 h while awake for 2 d, then 1–2 drops qid while awake for 5 d	
Gatifloxacin (Zymar)	Bacterial conjunctivitis	Ophthalmic solution: >1 yr: 1 drop every 2 h while awake for 2 d, then 1 drop qid while awake for 5 d	
Levofloxacin (Levaquin)	Bronchitis, acute exacerbation of chronic	500 mg q24h for 7 d	Not recommended for use by children Renal impairment (CCr <50 mL/min) requires dosage reduction Take with full glass of water Oral and parenteral routes are bioequivalent and interchangeable
	Community-acquired pneumonia; DRSP	500 mg q24h for 7–14 d	
	Nongonococcal urethritis and gonorrhea	500 mg daily for 7 d	Alternative regimen (CDC 2002)
	Multi–drug-resistant *Streptococcus pneumoniae* in community-acquired pneumonia	750 mg daily for 7–14 d	Can use oral or injectable form
	Pyelonephritis treatment	250 mg q12h for 10 d	
	Sinusitis	500 mg q24h for 10–14 d	
	Skin and soft tissue infection	500 mg q24h for 7–10 d	
	Urinary tract infection, complicated		

Continued

Table 24–12 ◉ **Dosage Schedule: Fluoroquinolones—cont'd**

Drug	Indications	Initial Adult Dose	Comments
(Quixin)	Bacterial conjunctivitis	Ophthalmic solution: >1 yr: 1 drop every 2 h while awake for 2 d, then 1 drop qid while awake for 5 d	
Lomefloxacin (Maxaquin)	Bronchitis, bacterial exacerbation	400 mg daily for 10 d	Not recommended for use by children Renal impairment (CCr <40 mL/min) requires dosage reduction Take with full glass of water with or without food
	Urinary tract infection, prophylaxis	400 mg as a single dose 1–8 h before surgery	
	Urinary tract infection, complicated uncomplicated due to *Escherichia coli* uncomplicated, due to *P. mirabilis, Klebsiella pneumoniae, S. saprophyticus*	400 mg daily for 14 d 400 mg daily for 3 d 400 mg daily for 10 d	
Moxifloxacin (Avelox)	Acute sinusitis Acute exacerbation of chronic bronchitis Community-acquired pneumonia	400 mg daily for 10 d 400 mg daily for 5 d 400 mg daily for 10 d	Not for use by children
(Vigamox)	Bacterial conjunctivitis	Ophthalmic solution: ≥ 1 yr: 1 drop tid for 7 d	
Norfloxacin (Noroxin)	Gonorrhea	800 mg as a single dose	Maximal adult daily dose 800 mg (1.2 g infectious diarrhea) Take on empty stomach with full glass of water (1 h before or 2 h after food or milk) Not recommended for use by children
	Gastroenteritis (off-labeled) Prostatitis, acute or chronic Urinary tract infection, uncomplicated, due to *E. coli, K. pneumoniae, P. mirabilis* uncomplicated, due to other organisms	400 mg q8–12h for 5 d 400 mg q12h for 28 d 400 mg q12h for 3 d 400 mg q12h for 7–10 d	
Ofloxacin (Floxin)	Bronchitis, bacterial exacerbations or community-acquired pneumonia	400 mg q12h for 10 d	Maximal adult daily dose 400 mg. Not recommended for use by children Renal impairment (CCr <50 mL/min) requires dosage reduction Take with a full glass of water
	Skin and soft tissue infections *Chlamydia*, endocervical or urethral Gonorrhea, uncomplicated; nongonococcal urethritis Pelvic inflammatory disease, acute Prostatitis Urinary tract infection, complicated Cystitis due to E. *coli, K. pneumoniae* Cystitis due to other organisms	400 mg q12h for 10 d 300 mg q12h for 7 d 33 mg bid × 7 d 400 mg q12h for 10–14 d 300 mg q12h for 6 wk 200 mg q12h for 10 d 200 mg q12h for 3 d 200 mg q12h for 7 d	
(Ocuflox)	Bacterial conjunctivitis	Ophthalmic solution: >1 yr: 1–2 drops every 2–4 h while awake for 2 d, then 1 drop qid while awake for 5 d	

respiratory fluoroquinolone such as moxifloxacin, gemifloxacin, or levofloxacin is used as first-line therapy when there are comorbidities, such as chronic heart, lung, liver, or renal disease; diabetes mellitus; alcoholism; malignancies; asplenia; immunosuppressing conditions or use of immunosuppressing drugs; or other risk for DRSP infection such as use of antimicrobials within the previous 3 months (Mandell et al, 2007). For older patients or those with underlying disease, levofloxacin may be the best choice of the first-line agents. Usual duration of therapy for CAP is 7 to 14 days. Higher dosages of some fluoroquinolones are required for more serious infections. Pneumonia treatment is discussed in depth in Chapter 42.

Urinary Tract Infection

Although empirical treatment with trimethoprim/sulfamethoxazole (TMP/SMX, Septra, Bactrim) is the first-line treatment for a UTI, an alternative first-line treatment is the fluoroquinolone ciprofloxacin (Griebling, 2007; Grover et al, 2007). Other fluoroquinolones that may be used as second-line therapy include gatifloxacin and evofloxacin. Moxifloxacin and gemifloxacin are not approved for use with UTIs because they have poor concentration in the urine. Cross-resistance occurs with the fluoroquinolones. Fluoroquinolone resistance has been steadily increasing with 24.2 percent of *E. coli* resistant to ciprofloxacin and 24 percent resistant to levofloxacin (Kashanian et al, 2008). Fluoroquinolones are not prescribed to children or pregnant women because of concern for adverse effects on joints and cartilage, which have been found in animal studies. The exception is ciprofloxacin, which has FDA approval as second-line therapy in complicated UTI or pyelonephritis in children.

Uncomplicated cystitis and urethritis are treated with oral fluoroquinolones for 3 days. Complicated UTI and pyelonephritis require 7 to 14 days of therapy. Dosages of some fluoroquinolones for acute cystitis are lower than dosages for more serious urinary tract and kidney infections. Treatment of UTIs is discussed in Chapter 47.

Sexually Transmitted Infections and Genital Infections

Previously the fluoroquinolones were recommended for treatment of uncomplicated gonorrhea manifested as cervicitis, urethritis, pharyngitis, or proctitis. Unfortunately, strains of gonococci resistant to fluoroquinolones have been identified worldwide and the CDC treatment guidelines no longer recommend the use of ciprofloxacin or other fluoroquinolones (CDC, 2007).

Oflaxacin or levofloxacin are recommended by the CDC as second-line therapy for chlamydia (CDC, 2010e). First-line therapy is azithromycin or doxycycline. If treating with a fluoroquinolone, oflaxacin 300 mg twice a day or levofloxacin 500 mg daily for 7 days is prescribed (CDC, 2010e).

The fluoroquinolones ofloxacin and levofloxacin are recommended for the treatment of acute epididymitis most likely caused by enteric organisms or with negative gonococcal culture or nucleic acid amplification test (CDC, 2006a). Dosing for the treatment of epididymitis with ofloxacin is 300 mg orally twice a day for 10 days and with levofloxacin is 500 mg orally once daily for 10 days.

Detailed discussion of treatment of sexually transmitted infections is found in Chapter 44.

Skin and Tissue Infections

Although approved for skin and tissue infections, use of fluoroquinolones in these infections should be avoided to decrease selection pressure for bacterial resistance. Most skin and tissue infections treated in outpatient settings respond to beta-lactam antibiotics, except wounds that have been exposed to fresh water, such as ponds, lakes, and swimming pools, which may be infected with *Pseudomonas* and *Aeromonas* species.

Infectious Diarrhea

Fluoroquinolones are first-line therapy in treatment of traveler's diarrhea and severe diarrhea not associated with antibiotic therapy. Recommended self-treatment for traveler's diarrhea is 3 days of twice-daily therapy with oral ciprofloxacin (500 mg), norfloxacin (400 mg), or ofloxacin (300 mg), combined with loperamide 4 mg initially and 2 mg after each stool.

For mild bacterial diarrhea not associated with antibiotics, characterized by three or fewer stools per day and minimal associated symptomatology, supportive therapy is usually adequate. For moderate infectious diarrhea, evidenced by four or more stools per day or fewer stools with systemic symptoms, an antiperistaltic drug (e.g., loperamide) may be added to supportive therapy. Severe infectious diarrhea not associated with antibiotics is manifested by six or more unformed stools per day and/or a temperature 38.8°C or more, tenesmus, blood, or fecal leukocytes. Presence of blood may be indicative of *E. coli* O157:H7 infection, which has serious sequelae and requires hospitalization. Most common pathogens in severe infectious diarrhea not associated with antibiotics are *Shigella, Salmonella, Campylobacter jejuni,* and *E. coli* (O157:H7 strains). Drugs of choice for severe bacterial diarrhea (not associated with antibiotics) are ciprofloxacin 500 mg every 12 hours or norfloxacin 400 mg every 12 hours. Therapy is continued for 3 to 5 days.

Other Uses

Ciprofloxacin is approved for bone and joint infections, but with the exception of bone infections in cystic fibrosis, many typical pathogens are no longer susceptible to this drug. Use should be reserved for proven susceptibility on culture and sensitivity. Although several fluoroquinolones are approved for use in sinusitis, these agents are probably best reserved for other indications because of the nature of this infection (see the Clinical Use and Dosing section for **penicillins**). **Ciprofloxacin** may be indicated for sinusitis resulting from nasogastric or nasotracheal intubation, in which gram-negative bacilli are the likely pathogens. **Levofloxacin** and **moxifloxacin** are indicated for treatment of sinusitis due to highly **penicillin**-resistant pneumococcal infections. Although an off-labeled use, **ciprofloxacin** as a single 750-mg dose is accepted for eradicating the meningococcal carrier state. **Ciprofloxacin** is also a first-line treatment of typhoid fever in doses of 500 mg twice daily for 10 days. If the patient is in shock or has impaired mental status, mortality will be decreased by initiating **dexamethasone** (3 mg/kg initially, followed by 1 mg/kg every 6 h for 8 doses) a few minutes prior to anti-infective therapy for typhoid.

Rational Drug Selection

Both definitive drug selection and empirical drug selection follow the same principles described in the Rational Drug Selection section for the **penicillins**, regardless of the infection or drug class involved. Specific implications to consider in selecting **fluoroquinolones** are cost, resistance, and adverse effect profile. Brand-name **fluoroquinolones** are relatively high-cost agents. **Ciprofloxacin** is on multiple $4 lists, making it a cost-effective choice if appropriate. The cost of **fluoroquinolones** is comparable to other newer broad-spectrum agents such as **amoxicillin/clavulanate**, **clarithromycin**, and **cefuroxime axetil** (see the available dosage forms table for these drug classes). Cost data are provided in Table 24–13.

Another reason to use **fluoroquinolones** judiciously is to prevent resistance. **Ciprofloxacin** is unique as an oral agent effective for *P. aeruginosa*, and the agents with enhanced gram-positive spectrum (**levofloxacin**, **gemifloxacin**, **moxifloxacin**) have activity against highly **penicillin**-resistant strains of *S. pneumoniae* that are also resistant to **cephalosporins**, **tetracyclines**, **macrolides**, and **sulfonamides**. It behooves us to guard these susceptibilities as long as possible by using definitive drug selection based on culture and sensitivity and by selecting agents with the narrowest spectrum. Within the **fluoroquinolones**, agents with an enhanced gram-positive spectrum are the most costly, and agents indicated primarily for genitourinary infections (e.g., **ciprofloxacin**) are least expensive.

Table 24–13 ◆ Available Dosage Forms: Fluoroquinolones

Drug	Dosage Form	How Supplied	Cost
Ciprofloxacin (Cipro)	Tablets: 250 mg (G);	In 20	$4
	500 mg (G);	In bottles of 100	$38.99
		In 20	$4
		In bottles of 30	$135.99
	750 mg (G)	In bottles of 30, 50, 100 and Cystitis Pak 6	$338
	100 mg (B);	In bottles of 50, 100 and UD 100	$450
	250 mg (B),	In bottles of 30, 50, 100 and UD 100	$177/30
	500 mg (B),	In 20	$187.53
	500 mg extended release (B)	In bottles of 50,100	$537
	750 mg (B)	In bottles of 50, 100 and UD 30	$385
	Tablet-XR: 500 mg (B); 1 g (B)	In bottles of 50, 100 and UD 30	$438/50
	Powder for oral suspension: 250 mg/5 mL (G); 500 mg/ 5 mL (G)	In 100-mL bottles	
	250 mg/5 mL (B);	In 100-mL bottles	$105
	500 mg/5 mL (B)	In 100-mL bottles	$122
Gemifloxacin (Factive)	Tablets: 320 mg	In UD 5 and 7	
Levofloxacin (Levaquin)	Tablets: 250 mg (B);	In bottles of 10, 50 and UD 100	$119.91/10
	500 mg (B)	In bottles of 10, 50 and UD 100	$158.98/10
	750 mg (B)	In bottles of 30, 50, UD 5 and UD 100	$779/30
Lomefloxacin (Maxaquin)	Tablets: 400 mg (B)	In bottles of 20	
Moxifloxacin (Avelox)	Tablets: 400 mg (B)	In bottles of 30, UD 50, ABC Packs of 5	$286/30
Norfloxacin (Noroxin)	Tablets: 400 mg (B)	In bottles of 100, UD 20 and UD 100	$341
Ofloxacin (Floxin)	Tablets: 200 mg (B)	In bottles of 50, UD 6 and UD 100	$241/50
	300 mg (B)	In bottles of 50 and UD 100	$287/50
	400 mg (B)	In bottles of 100 and UD 100q	$602

B = brand name; G = generic; XR = extended release.

Selection between agents with similar spectrums of bacterial activity may depend on the comparative adverse effects and drug interactions profile. **Norfloxacin** has much less effect on **caffeine** metabolism; **lomefloxacin** and **ofloxacin** appear devoid of effects on **caffeine** metabolism. Treated diabetics should avoid **fluoroquinolones** if other equally effective **antimicrobial** drugs are available. The patient with prolonged QTc interval or taking drugs that increase the QTc interval should be prescribed **fluoroquinolones** with caution. Unless there are compelling reasons, **fluoroquinolones** should not be used by children and pregnant women. Renal impairment requires decreased dosage of all agents except **moxifloxacin.** Other **antibacterial** drugs are also preferable for patients with severe cerebral arteriosclerosis or who are otherwise seizure prone (e.g., epilepsy, **alcohol** abuse, theophylline or **antipsychotic** drug use).

Monitoring

Monitoring for therapeutic response to **antimicrobial** drugs is described in the Monitoring section for **penicillins.** Patients on prolonged therapy with **fluoroquinolones** should have periodic assessment of organ function, including renal, hepatic, and hematopoietic function. Renal function should be measured or estimated with standard formulas prior to initiation of a **fluoroquinolone.** It is prudent to obtain a baseline electrocardiogram (ECG) prior to prescription of **moxifloxacin.** The drugs should be withheld and the ECG repeated if syncope occurs, which may indicate development of torsades de pointes, a potentially lethal arrhythmia. Patients taking **theophylline** and **cyclosporine** should have determinations of the plasma concentrations ("blood levels") of these agents, which are metabolized by CYP3A4, a hepatic drug-metabolizing enzyme inhibited by **fluoroquinolones.** Patients on **warfarin** who are started on **fluoroquinolones** should have their INR monitored closely. When either **ofloxacin** or **levofloxacin** is administered for gonorrhea, it may mask, but not cure, coexisting syphilis. Obtain serological testing for syphilis whenever a diagnosis of gonorrhea is made, with repeat testing at 3 months after treatment. Patients with epilepsy, **alcohol** abuse, or concurrent **theophylline** use should be monitored for CNS irritability (agitation, irritability) and seizure activity.

Patient Education

Administration

Available dosage forms are shown in Table 24–13. As with all **antimicrobial** drugs, the patient must understand the significance of taking all doses and completing the full course of therapy. Although the effect of food on absorption is unknown, the manufacturer suggests that the optimal time for administration of **ciprofloxacin** is 2 hours after meals. All **fluoroquinolones** should be taken with a full glass of water to help avoid dehydration, which can lead to crystalluria. **Fluoroquinolones** should not be taken within 2 to 6 hours of drugs that may chelate them (including **antacids, sucralfate, iron preparations,** and **zinc salts**) and prevent absorption. Dairy products hamper absorption of **norfloxacin.**

Adverse Reactions

Although **lomefloxacin** is most likely to cause photosensitivity or phototoxicity, all patients on **fluoroquinolones** should be taught to avoid direct sunlight, sun lamps, and tanning beds from the first dose until several days after therapy is completed. They should withhold the drug and report any blister, rash, or itching that occurs. With **lomefloxacin,** severe phototoxic reactions have occurred through glass and in spite of sunscreen use. Recovery is prolonged and the reaction tends to recur if the patient is exposed to sunlight again before recovery. Sunscreens, hats, and long-sleeved clothing should be suggested for even short-term exposure.

Fluoroquinolones often cause dizziness or lightheadedness, so driving and hazardous activities should be avoided until a patient's reaction is known. Adequate fluid intake to maintain urine output of 1,500 mL per day will avoid crystalluria. Minimize use of urinary alkalinizers such as citrus drinks and avoid baking soda and **antacids.** If tenderness or inflammation occurs in any tendon, the patient should immediately discontinue the **fluoroquinolone,** notify the prescriber, rest, and refrain from exercise of the affected joint. Diabetics should immediately report any signs or symptoms of hypoglycemia and should perform home blood glucose testing regularly. The drug should be discontinued at any sign of an allergic reaction (hives, itching, yawning, dyspnea) because serious anaphylactic reactions have occurred during first exposure to a **fluoroquinolone.**

Lifestyle Management

See the Lifestyle Modification section for the **penicillins.**

LINCOSAMIDES

The original drug in this class was **lincomycin.** Although structurally different from **erythromycin, lincomycin** resembled it in activity. Unfortunately, it was too toxic and is rarely used. It will not be discussed in this chapter. **Clindamycin (Cleocin)** is a chlorine-substituted derivative of **lincomycin** and the only other drug in the class. Although less toxic, its indications are still limited because of its potential to cause severe antibiotic-associated colitis.

Pharmacodynamics

Clindamycin binds to the 50S subunit of the bacterial ribosomes and suppresses protein synthesis. This is the same as the receptor for **macrolides,** so combined use with **erythromycin** and related drugs may decrease the effectiveness of both drugs. The action of **clindamycin** is usually bacteriostatic, but it may produce bactericidal effects if the target tissue is especially sensitive.

Sensitivity

Susceptible organisms are primarily gram-positive, including *S. pneumoniae, S. pyogenes,* and *Streptococcus viridans; S. aureus, S. epidermidis,* and *Staphylococcus albus;* and *Corynebacterium diphtheriae* and *Corynebacterium acnes.* It is also effective against selected anaerobic pathogens: *Bacteroides, Fusobacterium, Actinomyces, Peptococcus, Clostridium perfringens,* and *Clostridium tetani*. It is also effective against *Campylobacter jejuni* and *Gardnerella vaginalis,* so that it can be used to treat bacterial vaginosis. A primary indication of **clindamycin** is hospital treatment of serious intra-abdominal infections caused by anaerobic bacteria. In primary care, **clindamycin** is used for infections by gram-positive cocci in **penicillin**-allergic patients and infections by DRSP such as pneumonia, sinusitis, and otitis media. In some areas of the country MRSA is sensitive to **clindamycin.** Its spectrum of activity also makes it useful in infections of the mouth, including dental abscesses.

Resistance

Enterococci and gram-negative aerobic organisms are resistant to **clindamycin.** *C. difficile,* an important cause of **antibiotic**-associated pseudomembranous colitis (AAPMC), is resistant, which explains the prevalence of this disorder as an adverse effect of the drug. Mechanisms of resistance include mutation or modification of the ribosomal receptor site and enzymatic inactivation of **clindamycin.** Resistance to **clindamycin** commonly confers cross-resistance to **macrolides.**

Pharmacokinetics

Absorption and Distribution

Oral administration of **clindamycin** results in complete absorption, and it is not affected by gastric acid. It distributes to pleural and peritoneal fluids, with high concentrations in bile, bone, and urine, but poor penetration of CSF. It can achieve a CSF concentration of about 40 percent of serum levels when the meninges are inflamed.

This concentration, however, is not sufficient to treat meningitis effectively. Plasma protein binding is high. It readily crosses the placenta and is found in breast milk at 0.7 to 3.8 mcg/mL following doses of 150 to 600 mg.

Metabolism and Excretion

Clindamycin is metabolized by the liver to active and inactive metabolites. Both the parent drug and its metabolites are excreted in the bile and in urine. Dosage modification is not usually required for renal impairment unless it is very severe, but hepatic impairment may require a decreased dose. Table 24–14 shows the pharmacokinetics of this drug.

Pharmacotherapeutics

Precautions and Contraindications

Use with caution in patients with a history of asthma or significant allergies. Hypersensitivity may occur.

Cautious use is also recommended for the patient with severe renal or hepatic impairment accompanied by severe metabolic aberrations. The routes of excretion include both hepatic and renal.

Clindamycin is Pregnancy Category B. However, it crosses the placenta in amounts approximating 50 percent of maternal serum levels. It also appears in breast milk. According to LactMed, the National Institutes of Health Drug and Lactation Database, if **clindamycin** is required by a nursing mother, breastfeeding may continue, but an alternative drug may be a better choice in breastfeeding women.

Dosages are given for infants and children. Yet **clindamycin** should be used only for serious infections and when other, less toxic alternatives are not appropriate.

Adverse Drug Reactions

The main adverse reactions with this drug are GI, including nausea, vomiting, and a bitter or metallic taste. The most serious is the risk for AAPMC. The provider should consider antibiotic-associated pseudomembranous colitis in patients who present with diarrhea subsequent to administration of **clindamycin,** especially if the diarrhea involves six or more stools per day and contains blood, pus, or mucus. Older adults are less likely to tolerate any diarrhea and the drug should be used cautiously with that population.

Other adverse effects include dizziness, vertigo, headache, hypotension, and rare cardiac arrhythmias. Jaundice and other indications of hepatic dysfunction and oliguria and other indications of renal dysfunction occasionally occur.

Drug Interactions

There are few drug interactions with **clindamycin.** Table 24–15 lists them.

Clinical Use and Dosing

Because of its anaerobic activity, **clindamycin** is first-line therapy for several serious infections treated parenterally in the hospital. **Clindamycin** is appropriate first-line

Table 24–14 ▶ **Pharmacokinetics: Lincosamides**

Drug	Onset	Peak	Duration	Protein Binding	Bioavailability	Half-Life	Elimination
Clindamycin	Rapid	45 min	6–8 h	93%	>90%	2–3 h	>90% hepatic; 10% unchanged in urine; 3.6% in feces

Table 24–15 ■ **Drug Interactions: Lincosamides**

Drug	Interacting Drug	Possible Effect	Implications
Clindamycin	Erythromycin	Antagonistic effects have occurred for both oral and topical formulations	Avoid concurrent use
	Kaolin-pectin	GI absorption is delayed when coadministered	Give 2 h before or 3–4 h after clindamycin, or avoid concurrent use
	Neuromuscular blockers	Enhanced neuromuscular blockade that may cause severe respiratory depression	Avoid concurrent use

therapy for MRSA in areas of the country where there is low resistance; providers will need to know their local antibiogram to make an informed prescribing decision. Other uses of **clindamycin** in primary care are limited to second-line treatment of gram-positive cocci. Despite the controversy about whether **clindamycin** causes a higher incidence of AAPMC than other **antimicrobials**, research shows that limiting its use decreases prevalence of AAPMC and decreases **clindamycin** resistance.

Infections in Penicillin-Allergic Patients

Clindamycin is used for bacterial endocarditis prophylaxis as an alternative to **penicillins** in individuals allergic to **penicillin**. It also can be substituted for **penicillin** in treatment of pneumococcal pneumonia and skin and tissue infections, although there are other effective agents that patients with **penicillin** allergies can use.

Drug-Resistant Pneumococcal Infections

Although many strains of *S. pneumoniae* are resistant (DRSP) to **penicillins, cephalosporins, macrolides, tetracyclines**, and **sulfonamides, clindamycin** retains good activity against resistant strains of this organism. **Clindamycin** is recommended for second- or third-line therapy for upper and lower respiratory infections (pneumonia, sinusitis, otitis media) due to DRSP. Because it does not cover other common pathogens (*H. influenzae* and *M. catarrhalis*), **clindamycin** should be reserved for definitive therapy for DRSP or used in otitis media for nonresponse after at least 72 hours of therapy with a drug that covers *H. influenzae.*

Infections in Special Populations

Clindamycin is indicated for pregnant women and children to treat infections when the first-line agent may be harmful or is not tolerated. For example, **clindamycin** has been used for bacterial vaginosis in pregnancy in doses of 300 mg twice daily for 7 days. Because the first-line agent **metronidazole** is now recognized as safe for use in pregnancy, use of **clindamycin** will probably decline. **Clindamycin** is also used in treatment of malaria and other protozoal infections in pregnant women, children, and in patients unable to tolerate first-line therapy.

Odontogenic (Dental) Infections

Because of the organisms found in the mouth, **clindamycin** 300 to 450 mg given every 6 hours for 3 to 5 days has an indication and is first-line therapy to treat odontogenic infections. Pediatric dosing of **clindamycin** for dental infections is 10 to 20 mg/kg/day in 3 to 4 divided doses. It is especially helpful in dental abscesses. Table 24–16 presents the dosage schedules of lincosamides.

Table 24–16 ● **Dosage Schedule: Lincosamides**

Drug	Indication	Initial Dose	Comments
Clindamycin (Cleocin)	Serious bacterial infections	*Adults:* PO: 150–300 mg q6h *Children:* PO: 8–16 mg/kg/d in 3–4 equal doses	Maximal daily adult dose is 2.7 g. Take with food and a full glass of water to decrease esophageal irritation. Sit or stand for 30 min after dose. Dosing for clindamycin palmitate HCl (Cleocin Pediatric) oral solution varies slightly from tablets for children:

Continued

Table 24–16 ● **Dosage Schedule: Lincosamides—cont'd**

Drug	Indication	Initial Dose	Comments
			Severe infection: 8–12 mg/kg/d in 3–4 equal doses. *Serious infection:* 13–25 mg/kg/d in 3–4 equal doses. Shake solution well before measuring.
	Severe bacterial infection	*Adults:* PO: 300–450 mg q6h *Children:* PO: 16–20 mg/kg/d in 3–4 equal doses	Dispense with calibrated measuring device. Do not refrigerate solution because it will become thick and hard to pour.
	Endocarditis prophylaxis (off-labeled)	*Adults:* PO: 2 g 1 h before procedure *Children:* PO: 20 mg/kg 1 h before procedure	
	Malaria treatment	*Adults:* PO: 900 mg tid for 3 d *Children:* PO: 6.7–7.3 mg/kg tid for 3 d	
	Bacterial vaginosis in pregnancy (off-labeled)	*Adults:* PO: 300 mg bid for 7 d	
	Pneumocystis carinii pneumonia (off-labeled)	*Adults:* PO: 1,200–1,800 mg/d in divided doses with 15–30 mg primaquine daily	
	Toxoplasmosis of CNS treatment (off-labeled)	*Adults:* PO: 1,200–2,400 mg/d in divided doses with 50–100 mg pyrimethamine daily	
	Odontogenic (dental) infections	*Adults:* 300–450 mg q6h for 3–5 d *Children:* 10–20 mg/kg/d divided in 3 to 4 doses	Especially useful for dental abscesses.

Rational Drug Selection

Both definitive drug selection and empirical drug selection follow the same principles described in the Rational Drug Selection section for the **penicillins**, regardless of the infection or drug class involved. Specific implications for selection of **clindamycin** are spectrum of activity and adverse effects. Because **clindamycin** has a narrow spectrum of aerobic activity and lacks activity against *H. influenzae,* it cannot be substituted for other agents typically used to treat URIs, but must be used when there is reasonable certainty that the organisms are susceptible to **clindamycin.** Because of the high incidence of AAPMC associated with **clindamycin,** patients with a history of colitis and older patients who tolerate colitis poorly should probably not receive this agent. Severe hepatic impairment requires careful monitoring of drug response.

Monitoring

Monitoring for therapeutic response to antibiotics is described in the Monitoring section for **penicillins.** If significant diarrhea occurs (six or more stools daily and/or blood, mucus, or watery diarrhea), the drug should be discontinued. Cytotoxin assay may be used to detect the presence of *C. difficile* and its toxin. If the original infection for which **clindamycin** was prescribed is severe, therapy can continue with observation in the hospital and proctosigmoidoscopy. Mild colitis usually responds to stopping the drug, although fluid, electrolyte, and protein supplements may be required. Systemic **corticosteroids** or **corticosteroid** enemas have sped resolution of mild colitis. Severe AAPMC requires treatment with **metronidazole** or **oral vancomycin,** possibly combined with **cholestyramine** to adsorb the toxins.

Prolonged therapy with **clindamycin** requires assessment of liver function, renal function, and blood counts. Because **clindamycin** contains tartrazine, patients with asthma or **aspirin** allergy are at risk to develop an allergic response and should be assessed for allergic reaction.

Patient Education

Administration

Available dosage forms are given in Table 24–17. The patient should be advised of the necessity of completing the full course of therapy. Because **clindamycin** requires

Table 24–17 ◆ **Available Dosage Forms: Lincosamides**

Drug	Dosage Form	How Supplied	Cost
Clindamycin	Capsules: 75 mg, 150 mg	In bottles of 100 capsules 30, 100 capsules	$24.99/30
	300 mg	In 30, 100 capsules	$79.99/30
	Topical		
	1% lotion	60-mL bottle	$39.99
	1% gel	30-g, 60-g tube	$17.99/30 g
	1% solution	60-mL bottle	$16.99/60 mL
	1% swab	60 swab box	$39.99
Cleocin	Capsules: 75 mg	In bottles of 16, 100 capsules	
	150 mg		$127.04/30
	300 mg		
	Granules for oral suspension: 75 mg/5 mL	In 100-mL bottles	$75.70/100 mL
	Vaginal:		
	100 mg suppository	3 suppositories	$80.03/3
	2% cream	40 g	$81.56
Cleocin-T	Topical:		
	1% lotion	60-mL bottle	$86.09
	1% gel	30-g, 60-g tube	$62.98/30 g
	1% solution	60-mL bottle	$69.30
	1% swab	60-swab box	$76.00

multiple daily doses, the patient should be guided in planning mnemonic or other strategies to promote adherence. The drug can be taken without regard to meals, but taking the drug with food and a full glass of water will avoid esophageal irritation. Sitting or standing for a full 30 minutes after the dose will also decrease risk of esophageal irritation.

Adverse Reactions

If severe diarrhea develops, the patient should check with the prescriber before initiating any **antidiarrheal** treatment. **Antiperistaltic** agents, which may worsen the symptoms, should not be used. For mild diarrhea, the patient may use an **attapulgite**-containing **antidiarrheal** (e.g., **Kaopectate, Donnagel**) at least 2 hours before or 3 to 4 hours after the **clindamycin**. If surgery or general anesthesia is planned during or within a day or so after therapy, the anesthetist or anesthesiologist must be advised, in that **clindamycin** can intensify neuromuscular blockade.

Lifestyle Management

See the Lifestyle Management section for the **penicillins**.

MACROLIDES, AZALIDES, AND KETOLIDES

The **macrolides** are another early **antibiotic** group. The prototype drug in this group, **erythromycin**, was discovered in 1952. The drugs in the class (**erythromycin, clarithromycin** [**Biaxin**], **dirithromycin** [**Dynabac**], and **troleandomycin** [**Tao**]) are compounds characterized by a macrocyclic lactone ring with deoxy sugars attached. A closely related drug, **azithromycin (Zithromax)**, is chemically an **azalide** derived from **erythromycin** by the addition of a methylated nitrogen to the lactone ring. The latest addition to this group is **telithromycin (Ketek)**, which is chemically a **ketolide** derived from **erythromycin** by the lack of alpha-L-cladinose at position 3 on the erythronolide A ring. They are generally included with the **macrolide** group and are discussed in the same section here. **Troleandomycin** has little **antibacterial** activity and is not considered in this chapter.

Pharmacodynamics

This group of drugs reversibly binds to the P site of the 50S ribosome subunit of susceptible organisms and may inhibit RNA-dependent protein synthesis by stimulating the dissociation of peptidyl-tRNA from ribosomes. These drugs may be bacteriostatic or bactericidal, depending on drug concentration.

Macrolides are weak bases, and their activity increases in alkaline media.

Erythromycin is inactivated by acid, and **erythromycin base** is marketed in acid-resistant, enteric-coated form to retard gastric inactivation. **Erythromycin** is also formulated as acid-stable salts and esters to improve bioavailability. These salts include **erythromycin ethylsuccinate, erythromycin estolate,** and **erythromycin stearate. Dirithromycin** is a pro-drug that is converted nonenzymatically during intestinal absorption into a form of **erythromycin. Azithromycin, telithromycin,** and **clarithromycin** are semisynthetic derivatives of **erythromycin.**

Sensitivity

Macrolides are active against gram-positive organisms such as pneumococci and other *Streptococcus* species, methicillin-sensitive staphylococci, and *Corynebacterium.* Atypical and intracellular organisms commonly resistant to **beta-lactam antibiotics** are also susceptible, such as *Mycoplasma, Legionella, Chlamydia, Helicobacter, Listeria,* and certain strains of *Mycobacterium.* The gram-negative spectrum of the oral **macrolides** includes *Neisseria* species, *B. pertussis, Bartonella quintana,* some *Rickettsia* species, *T. pallidum,* and *Campylobacter* species. *H. influenzae* is somewhat less susceptible.

Among the **macrolides**, there is some variability of spectrum. **Azithromycin** has the greatest activity of the **macrolides** against gram-negative organisms such as *H. influenzae* and *M. catarrhalis.* It is more active than **erythromycin** against anaerobes and has activity similar to erythromycin against gram-positive organisms. **Clarithromycin** has broad anaerobic activity and greater activity than **erythromycin** or **azithromycin** against gram-positive organisms such as *Streptococcus* species and methicillin-sensitive *Staphylococcus.* Its activity against *H. influenzae* is greater than that of **erythromycin** but less than that of **azithromycin. Telithromycin** is also effective against multiple drug-resistant *S. pneumoniae* (MDRSP), including those resistant to **penicillin, cephalosporins, tetracycline, trimethoprim/sulfamethoxazole,** and other **macrolides.** Dirithromycin has the narrowest spectrum of the **macrolides.** The single best use for all these drugs is with infections in which organisms include those with high intracellular growth patterns.

Resistance

Resistance to **erythromycin** is usually plasmid encoded by (1) reduced permeability of the cell membrane or active efflux, (2) production of esterase by *Enterobacteriaceae* that hydrolyze **macrolides**, or (3) modification of the ribosomal binding site by chromosomal mutation or by a **macrolide**-inducible methylase. Cross-resistance is nearly complete between **erythromycin** and the other **macrolides.** It is less prominent with the **azalide. Macrolide**-resistant pneumococci range from 24.6 percent (Jacobs, Felmingham, Appelbaum, Gruneberg, for the Alexander Project Group, 2003) to 29.2 percent (Kays & Brown, 2004) in two large studies. **Telithromycin** is newer, but resistance has developed to *S. pyogenes* (Richter et al, 2008). Cross-resistance may also develop with other **antibiotics** that share the same ribosomal binding site, such as **clindamycin.**

Pharmacokinetics

Absorption and Distribution

The **macrolides, azalides,** and **ketolides** are all well absorbed from the duodenum following oral administration. Food decreases the amount of absorption of **azithromycin** tablets by 23 percent and the rate of suspension absorption by 56 percent, so these formulations should be taken on an empty stomach. Food does not affect the absorption of **telithromycin.** Absorption of enteric-coated products of **erythromycin** is delayed by food. Food also delays the absorption of **clarithromycin,** although bioavailability is not affected, so this drug may be taken without regard to meals. **Dirithromycin** is best absorbed when taken with food or within an hour of having eaten. **Erythromycin base** or **stearate** must be taken on an empty stomach, but the absorption of the **estolate** and **ethylsuccinate** forms are not affected by food intake. Minimal absorption occurs after topical or ophthalmic use.

Macrolides distribute readily to body tissues and enter pleural fluid, ascitic fluid, middle-ear exudates, and sputum. When meninges are inflamed, **macrolides** enter the CSF. Because of high intracellular concentrations, particularly in phagocytic cells, tissue levels are higher than serum levels and concentrations in white blood cells may remain high for many hours after the last dose of the drug.

Metabolism and Excretion

Macrolides, azalides, and **ketolides** are partially metabolized by the liver, and **clarithromycin, dirithromycin,** and **telithromycin** are converted to active metabolites. This class of drugs is excreted mainly unchanged in bile; the drug is also excreted unchanged in urine in varying degrees. **Clarithromycin** and its active metabolite are substantially eliminated by the kidneys. Because older adults often have renal impairment, dosage adjustment should also be considered for this population.

Erythromycin is heavily metabolized by CYP450 3A4, which explains many of its drug interactions and its cautious use in the presence of hepatic impairment. **Telithromycin** is 50 percent metabolized by CYP450 3A4, but the remaining 50 percent is CYP450 independent, so dosage adjustments are not required based on hepatic function. Table 24–18 presents the pharmacokinetics.

Pharmacotherapeutics

Precautions and Contraindications

Hypersensitivity to any of the **macrolides** and patients' use of **pimozide** contraindicate use of **macrolides.** The removal of **terfenadine** and **cisapride** from the market was related to serious dysrhythmic reactions that frequently were triggered by inhibition of cytochrome P450 3A4 drug metabolism by **erythromycin** and other drugs.

Known, suspected, or potential bacteremia contraindicates use of **dirithromycin** because serum levels are inadequate to provide **antibacterial** coverage of the plasma.

Table 24–18 ▶ **Pharmacokinetics: Macrolides, Azalides, and Ketolides**

Drug	Onset	Peak	Duration	Protein Binding	Bioavailability	Half-Life	Elimination
Azithromycin	Rapid	2.5–3.2 h	24 h	7%–50%	40%	11–14 h after single dose; 68 h after multiple doses	6% unchanged in urine; remainder unchanged in bile
Clarithromycin	UA	2 h	12 h	40%–70%	55%	3–4 h for 250-mg dose; 5–7 h or 500-mg dose	20%–30% unchanged in urine
Dirithromycin	UA	2–4 h	6–8 h	15%–30%	10%	2–36 h	81%–97% fecal/ hepatic
Erythromycin	1 h	1–4 h	UA	7%–90%	35–60%	1.4–2 h	5% unchanged in urine; remainder largely in bile
Telithromycin	Rapid	0.5–4 h	24 h	60%–70%	57%	7.16 h after single dose; 9.81 h after multiple doses	7% unchanged in feces; 13% unchanged in urine; 37% metabolized by liver

UA = information unavailable.

Patients with Renal and Hepatic Impairment

Azithromycin is principally excreted via the liver. Patients with impaired hepatic function require cautious use of this drug. There are no data about use with renal impairment, so cautious use is also recommended in decreased renal function.

Clarithromycin is excreted via the liver and the kidney. Dosage adjustments are not required for hepatic impairment in the presence of normal renal function. Renal impairment with CCr less than 30 mL/minute with or without hepatic impairment requires dosages be halved or the dosing interval doubled.

Erythromycin is contraindicated for patients with preexisting liver disease. **Erythromycin estolate** has been associated with the infrequent (1 case per 1,000 patients) occurrence of cholestatis hepatitis. This has also occurred with other **erythromycin salts** but is rarer in children. Laboratory findings include abnormal liver function tests, peripheral eosinophilia, and leukocytosis. Symptoms include malaise, nausea, vomiting, abdominal cramps, and fever. Jaundice may or may not be present. These symptoms tend to occur after 1 to 2 weeks of continuous therapy, disappear if the drug is discontinued, and reappear within 48 hours if the drug is readministered.

Telithromycin has not shown altered AUC for patients with hepatic impairment. In severe renal impairment (CCr less than 30 mL/min), AUC was increased. To date, no dosage adjustments are recommended.

Erythromycin may aggravate the weakness of patients with myasthenia gravis. This drug should be avoided in those patients.

Older Adults

Although maximum plasma concentrations and AUC of **clarithromycin** and **dirithromycin** increase in older adults, no specific dosage adjustments or precautions are recommended for older adults with normal renal and hepatic function. Adjustments are based on renal function and older adults with impaired renal function should be treated as any patient with that impairment. Younger and older adults appear to have the same pharmacokinetics for **azithromycin** and **telithromycin**.

Pregnant Women

Azithromycin and **erythromycin** are Pregnancy Category B and safe to use during pregnancy. **Clarithromycin**, **dirithromycin**, and **telithromycin** are Pregnancy Category C. Animal studies with **clarithromycin** have shown adverse effects on pregnancy outcome and on fetal development. Animal studies with **dirithromycin** have shown significantly decreased fetal weight and incomplete ossification of fetal bone. These latter two drugs should not be used during pregnancy except in clinical circumstances in which no alternative therapy is appropriate. **Telithromycin** was not teratogenic in animals, but there are no adequate, well-controlled studies in pregnant women.

The American Academy of Pediatrics considers **erythromycin** compatible with breastfeeding. **Telithromycin** is excreted in the breast milk of rats, and probably in human breast milk. Data are not available for the other drugs in this class, and they should be used with extreme caution in nursing mothers.

Pediatric Patients

Erythromycin has been used extensively in infants and children and is considered safe for children of all ages. **Azithromycin** was studied and relabeled in 2008 for safety and efficacy for children as young as age 6 months for otitis media, sinusitis, and CAP. Efficacy been established for children older than 2 years for pharyngitis-tonsillitis. Safety and efficacy of **azithromycin** in children younger than age 6 months have not been established. **Clarithromycin** has established safety and efficacy for children older than 6 months. The safety and efficacy of **dirithromycin** have not been established for children younger than 12 years. The safety and efficacy of **telithromycin** in children has not been established.

Adverse Drug Reactions

The most common adverse reactions to **macrolides** are dose-related GI symptoms, including nausea, vomiting, abdominal pain, cramping, and diarrhea, as well as headache. In general, these reactions are transient, mild to moderate, and reversible when the drug is discontinued. **Erythromycin** is most likely to produce them, whether given orally or parenterally, because it stimulates the motilin receptor in the GI tract. In fact, an off-labeled use of **erythromycin** for the treatment of gastroparesis derives from this receptor activity.

Diarrhea may also be secondary to pseudomembranous colitis, a serious superinfection that requires discontinuation of the drug that has been described for **penicillins, cephalosporins**, and **lincosamides**.

Hyperkinesia, dizziness, and agitation have occurred in fewer than 1 percent of children taking **azithromycin**. Stomatitis, dry mouth, and dysphagia have occurred in a small number of adults for all **macrolides**.

Erythromycin has been associated with urticaria, bullous eruptions, eczema, and Stevens-Johnson syndrome. Isolated cases of reversible hearing loss have also been reported with this drug, particularly with parenteral administration.

Laboratory abnormalities include elevated liver function studies (**azithromycin**), increased platelet counts (**dirithromycin** and **erythromycin**) and elevated potassium levels (**dirithromycin**). In each case, less than 6 percent of patients were affected. No laboratory abnormalities have been reported with **telithromycin**.

Drug Interactions

Clarithromycin, erythromycin, and **telithromycin** have more drug interactions than the other two drugs in this class because they are strong inhibitors of the CYP450 enzymes, particularly CYP450 3A4. Object drugs in these interactions include such common drugs as **warfarin, theophylline, carbamazepine, selected benzodiazepines**, and **digoxin**. Combination of either of these macrolides with **pimozide (Orap)** a drug used to treat Tourette syndrome can result in serious dysrhythmia; the inhibited metabolism causes prolonged QTc interval of the cardiac cycle, predisposing to potentially fatal cardiac dysrhythmias. Table 24–19 lists the various drug interactions by specific drug. Although **azithromycin** has fewer drug interactions than **macrolides**, confirmed interactions with drugs with narrow therapeutic margins include **digoxin, cyclosporine**, and **pimozide**, which have enhanced effects when given concurrently. In addition, **antacids** containing **aluminum** or **magnesium** slow absorption of **macrolides** and **azalides**, so they should be taken 1 hour before or 2 hours after the **antimicrobial drug**, particularly with **azithromycin**.

Antacids do not affect the pharmacokinetics of **telithromycin**, and neither does grapefruit juice. Also in terms of lack of adverse drug interactions with **telithromycin** are the following notations:

- Although **digoxin** levels increased, no increased toxicity was seen.
- No changes in pharmacokinetic or pharmacodynamic changes were seen with coadministration with **warfarin**.
- No interference occurs with the anti-ovulatory effects of **oral contraceptives**.

Clinical Use and Dosing

Macrolides are drugs of choice only for primarily empirical treatment of CAP due to increased prevalence of intracellular organisms and resistant strains from extracellular organisms in this disorder and for infections by *Chlamydia*, which is an intracellular organism. They are first- or second-line agents for numerous infections. Relative safety in children and convenient dosing schedules have made the newer **macrolides, azithromycin** and **clarithromycin**, popular in primary care practice. In particular, **azithromycin** has both a 3-day dosing schedule and a 5-day dosing schedule with a loading dose on the first day and single daily doses for the subsequent 4 days. **Clarithromycin** usually requires twice-daily dosing but is available in a delayed-release formulation that can be administered once daily. Although bioavailability varies by **erythromycin salt**, the dosage of **base, stearate**, and **estolate salts** are the same for any indication. The dosage of **erythromycin ethylsuccinate** is higher because of the mass of the **ethylsuccinate** component. The equivalent of 250-mg base is 400-mg **ethylsuccinate**. Specific dosages are included in Table 24–20.

Community-Acquired Pneumonia

Pathogens in CAP that are naturally resistant to **beta-lactam antibiotics** are the atypical organisms *C. pneumoniae, M. pneumoniae*, and *Legionella pneumophila*. Other

(Text continues on page 797)

Table 24–19 ■ **Drug Interactions: Macrolides and Azalides**

Drug	Interacting Drug	Possible Effect	Implications
All macrolides	Pimozide	Two sudden deaths occurred when clarithromycin was added to ongoing pimozide therapy	Coadministration is contraindicated
Azithromycin, dirithromycin, erythromycin	Antacids	Aluminum and magnesium based antacids reduce peak serum levels but not extent of absorption of azithromycin; when given immediately following antacids, dirithromycin absorption is slightly enhanced; when given immediately prior to antacids, elimination rate of erythromycin may be slightly decreased	Consider outcomes in patient education
Azithromycin, clarithromycin, erythromycin	HMG-CoA reductase inhibitors	Increased risk of severe myopathy or rhabdomyolysis	Avoid concurrent use
	Cyclosporine	Elevated cyclosporine concentration with increased risk for toxicity	Dirithromycin is not expected to react
	Digoxin	Digoxin levels may be elevated based on effect of macrolide on gut flora that metabolizes digoxin in 10% of patients	Carefully monitor digoxin levels in any patient taking a macrolide
Clarithromycin, erythromycin	Rifabutin, rifampin	Antibiotic effects of macrolide reduced; adverse GI effects increased	Select different macrolide
	Alprazolam, diazepam, midazolam, triazolam	Plasma levels of benzodiazepine elevated, increasing and prolonging CNS depression effects	Azithromycin and dirithromycin not expected to react
	Buspirone	Plasma levels of buspirone elevated, increasing pharmacological and adverse effects	Azithromycin and dirithromycin not expected to react
	Carbamazepine	Increased concentration of carbamazepine	Azithromycin and dirithromycin not expected to react
	Disopyramide	Plasma levels of disopyramide increased. Arrhythmias and prolonged QTc have occurred	Avoid concurrent administration
	Ergot alkaloids	Acute ergot toxicity, characterized by severe peripheral vasospasm and dysesthesia, has occurred	Carefully monitor any patient receiving both drugs
	Oral anticoagulants	Potentiates anticoagulant effects	Carefully monitor anticoagulant effects for patients receiving any macrolide
	Theophylline	Concurrent use associated with increased serum theophylline levels	Avoid concurrent use Azithromycin and dirithromycin not expected to interact
Clarithromycin	Fluconazole	Increased mean steady-state trough levels (33%) and AUC (18%) of clarithromycin	Avoid concurrent use
	Omeprazole	Increased plasma levels of both drugs and 14-OH clarithromycin	Select different drug combination
Dirithromycin	Histamine$_2$ blockers	Dirithromycin absorption slightly enhanced when given immediately after H_2 blocker	Separate doses by at least 1 h or select different macrolide
Erythromycin	Alfentanil	Alfentanil clearance decreased and elimination half-life increased	Select different macrolide

Continued

Table 24–19 ■ **Drug Interactions: Macrolides and Azalides—cont'd**

Drug	Interacting Drug	Possible Effect	Implications
	Bromocriptine	Bromocriptine levels increased; increased pharmacological and adverse effects	Select different macrolide
	Felodipine	Felodipine levels increased; increased pharmacological and adverse effects	Select different macrolid
	Clindamycin, penicillins	Antagonistic effects. Synergism also reported for penicillins	Select different macrolide
	Methylprednisolone	Clearance of methylprednisolone greatly reduced	May be used therapeutically to reduce methylprednisolone dose
Telithromycin	Itraconazole, ketoconazole	Significant increase in telithromycin AUC	Select different antifungal
	Simvastatin; possibly atorvastatin and lovastatin	Significant increase in simvastatin AUC; possible increased risk for rhabdomyopathy	Avoid concurrent use
	Midazolam; BDZs metabolized by CYP3A4	Increased risk for sedation and adverse effects of midazolam and BDZs	Adjust dose of interacting drug if concurrent use cannot be avoided
	Digoxin	Peak and trough levels of digoxin increased by 73% and 21%, respectively. No increased risk for digoxin toxicity seen in research	Monitor digoxin level closely
	Rifampin, phenytoin, carbamazepine, phenobarbital	Decreased levels of telithromycin and loss of effect	Avoid concurrent use

Table 24–20 ● **Dosage Schedule: Macrolides, Azalides, and Ketolides**

Drug	Indication	Dose	Comments
Azithromycin (Zithromax)	Community-acquired pneumonia, otitis media, uncomplicated skin and soft tissue infections, acute bacterial exacerbation of chronic bronchitis	*Adults:* 500 mg as single dose on day 1, followed by 250 mg daily on days 2–5; or 500 mg daily for 3 d *Children:* 10 mg/kg as a single dose on day 1 (not to exceed 500 mg/d), followed by 5 mg/kg as a single dose on days 2–5	Take capsules and pediatric suspension on empty stomach. Tablets and adult single-dose packets may be taken without regard to meals. Store pediatric oral suspension at room temperature after reconstitution. Stable for 10 d. Discard excess after dosing is complete. Shake suspension before measurement, using calibrated dosing device. Pediatric dosing limits: 500 mg daily for pharyngitis, tonsillitis, and first day of dosing for otitis media and pneumonia; 250 mg daily for days 2–5 for otitis media and pneumonia. Do not use adult single-dose packet formulation for doses >1,000 mg.
	Pharyngitis/tonsillitis	*Adults:* Same as community-acquired pneumonia *Children:* 12 mg/kg daily for 5 d (not to exceed 500 mg daily)	As above

Table 24–20 ◉ **Dosage Schedule: Macrolides, Azalides, and Ketolides—cont'd**

Drug	Indication	Dose	Comments
	Chancroid, genital ulcer disease, nongonococcal urethritis caused by *Chlamydia trachomatis*	*Adults:* Single 1-g dose	As above
	Gonococcal urethritis or cervicitis	*Adults:* Single 1-g dose	As above. Also safe for use in pregnancy.
	Mycobacterium avium complex (MAC)	*Adults:* 1.2 g/wk	As above
Clarithromycin (Biaxin)	Pharyngitis, tonsillitis, otitis media, or skin and soft tissue infections	*Adults:* 250 mg bid for 10 d *Children:* 15 mg/kg/d in 2 divided doses	May be given without regard to food. If CCr <30 mL/min, dose should be halved or dosing interval doubled. Store suspension at room temperature after reconstitution. Stable for 14 d. Do not refrigerate. Shake suspension well before measurement with calibrated measuring device.
	Acute maxillary sinusitis	*Adults:* 500 mg bid for 14 d *Children:* Same as above for 10–14 d	As above
	Acute exacerbation of chronic bronchitis caused by *Streptococcus pneumoniae or Moraxella catarrhalis*	*Adults:* 500 mg q12h for 7 d or ER formulation 1 g daily for 7 d	As above
	Acute exacerbation of chronic bronchitis caused by *Haemophilus influenzae*	*Adults:* 500 mg bid for 7–14 d	As above
	M. avium complex (MAC) treatment	*Adults:* 500 mg twice daily *Children:* 7.5 mg/kg up to 500 mg bid; give in conjunction with other antimycobacterial drugs	As above
	MAC prophylaxis	*Adults:* 500 mg bid	As above
	Community-acquired pneumonia	*Adults:* 250 mg q12h for 7–14 d	As above
	Active duodenal ulcer associated with *Helicobacter pylori* infection in combination with bismuth citrate	*Adults:* 500 mg tid with ranitidine bismuth citrate 400 mg bid for days 1–14; followed by bismuth citrate 400 mg/d days 15–28	As above
	Active duodenal ulcer associated with *H. pylori* infection in combination with omeprazole	*Adults:* 500 mg tid with omeprazole 40 mg bid for 4 d	As above
	Active duodenal ulcer associated with *H. pylori* infection, in combination with amoxicillin and lansoprazole	*Adults:* 500 mg clarithromycin, 1,000 mg amoxicillin, and 30 mg lansoprazole q12h for 7 d	As above

Continued

Table 24–20 ◉ Dosage Schedule: Macrolides, Azalides, and Ketolides—cont'd

Drug	Indication	Dose	Comments
Erythromycin dose in mg erythromycin base	Antibacterial, mild infection, usual dose		
Estolate (Ilosone)		*Adults:* 250 mg base (400 mg ethylsuccinate) q6h; or 500 mg (800 mg ethylsuccinate) q12h; or 333 mg q8h	Take with 180–240 mL of water Maximum adult daily dose is 4 g.
Ethylsuccinate (EryPed, E.E.S.)			
Base (E-Mycin, E-Base, Ery-Tab, Eryc) Stearate (Erythrocin Stearate)		*Children:* 30–50 mg/kg/d of base in divided doses (or 50–80 mg/kg/d ethylsuccinate)	Taking with food may decrease effectiveness of erythromycin stearate and certain formulations of erythromycin base. Check package insert for erythromycin base. Take erythromycin stearate and most erythromycin base at least 2 h before or after a meal. Erythromycin estolate, erythromycin ethylsuccinate, and some enteric-coated formulations of base can be taken without regard to meals. Should be taken with meals if GI upset occurs. Do not chew or crush erythromycin base. Suspensions should be shaken before measurement, using a calibrated dispensing spoon.
	Erysipelas or nonbullous impetigo due to *Streptococcus pyogenes*	*Adults:* 250–500 mg qid for 10 d *Children:* 20–50 mg/kg/d in divided doses for 10 d	As above
	Bullous impetigo or cellulitis due to *Staphylococcus aureus*	*Adults:* 250 mg q6h or 500 mg q12h to maximum of 4 g/d *Children:* 20–50 mg/kg/d in divided doses	As above
	Community-acquired pneumonia, mild to moderate	*Adults:* 250–500 mg q6h for 10–14 d; treat severe mycoplasma pneumonia with higher dose up to 21 d *Children:* 20–50 mg/kg/d in divided doses for 10–14 d	As above
	Upper respiratory tract infection, mild to moderate due to *S. pyogenes or S. pneumoniae*	*Adults:* 250–500 mg qid for 10 d *Children:* 20–50 mg/kg/d in divided doses for 10 d	As above
	Pertussis (whooping cough) due to *Bordetella pertussis*	*Adults:* 500 mg qid for 10 d *Children:* 40–50 mg/kg/d in divided doses for 10 d	As above

Table 24–20 ● **Dosage Schedule: Macrolides, Azalides, and Ketolides—cont'd**

Drug	Indication	Dose	Comments
	Newborn conjunctivitis, pneumonia of infancy due to *C. trachomatis*	*Children:* 50 mg/kg/d in 4 divided doses for 14 d (conjunctivitis) or 21 d (pneumonia)	As above
	Urethral, endocervical, or rectal infections due to *C. trachomatis*	*Adults:* 500 mg qid for 7 d or 250 mg qid for 14 d (in pregnancy)	As above
	Nongonococcal urethritis; urethral, endocervical, or rectal infections due to *Neisseria gonorrhoeae*	*Adults:* 500 mg qid for at least 7 d	As above
	Primary syphilis	*Adults:* 20 g in divided doses over 10 d or 500 mg qid for 14 d	As above
	Endocarditis prophylaxis	*Adults:* 1 g 2 h before procedure, 500 mg 6 h after procedure *Children:* 20 mg/kg 2 h before procedure, 10 mg/kg 6 h after procedure	As above
Dirithromycin (Dynabac)	Acute bacterial exacerbations of chronic bronchitis; uncomplicated skin and soft tissue infections due to methicillin-sensitive *S. aureus*	*Adults:* 500 mg/d for 7 d	Take with food or within 1 h of eating. Do not crush or chew tablets.
	Community-acquired pneumonia caused by *M. catarrhalis or S. pneumoniae* (not for empirical therapy)	*Adults:* 500 mg/d for 14 d	As above
	Pharyngitis/tonsillitis caused by *S. pyogenes*	*Adults:* 500 mg/d for 10 d	
Erythromycin ethylsuccinate and sulfisoxazole (Pediazole, Eryzole)	Acute otitis media	*Children:* 50 mg/kg/d erythromycin and 150 mg/kg/d (to a maximum of 6 g/d) sulfisoxazole in 4 evenly divided doses for 10 d	May be taken without regard to meals. Not for use in infants <2 mo.
Telithromycin	Acute exacerbation of chronic bronchitis	800 mg daily for 5 d	Tablets should be swallowed whole and may be taken with or without food.
	Acute bacterial sinusitis	800 mg daily for 5 d	
	Community-acquired pneumonia	800 mg daily for 7–10 d	

common pathogens in CAP are *S. pneumoniae, H. influenzae,* and *M. catarrhalis,* some of which are increasingly resistant to many **antibiotics.** *S. aureus* is occasionally the pathogen in postbronchitic pneumonia. Initial empirical therapy to treat CAP in the previously healthy older child (older than age 5 years), adolescent, or adult outpatient with no cardiopulmonary disease, no antibiotics in the past 3 months (no risk for DRSP), and no modifying factors is to treat with an **advanced-generation macrolide** (level I evidence), such as **azithromycin** or **clarithromycin** (Mandell et al, 2007). Usual dosages are **azithromycin** 500 mg once on day 1, followed by 250 mg daily on days 2 to 5, or 500 mg daily for 3 days (children 10 mg/kg day 1, then 5 mg/kg on days 2 to 5); or **clarithromycin** 500 mg twice daily for 7 to 14 days (children **clarithromycin** 7.5 mg/kg twice daily). Outpatient treatment of infants and children for CAP may also be **erythromycin** 10 mg/kg orally four times daily. It is desirable to obtain sputum for culture and Gram's stain so that the treatment may be more directed, but it is impossible to identify a pathogen in up to 50 percent of patients with CAP. Consequently, treatment often proceeds empirically. **Macrolides** have high cross-resistance (50%) for highly penicillin-resistant *S. pneumoniae* strains. If the patient's condition deteriorates or is not improving by 48 to 72 hours, a switch to a **respiratory fluoroquinolone** with extended gram-positive spectrum (e.g., **levofloxacin**) is indicated if the patient is an adult. Detailed discussion of pneumonia and its management is found in Chapter 42.

Sexually Transmitted Infections

Nongonococcal and postgonococcal urethritis or cervicitis is most commonly caused by *C. trachomatis* (50%) or *Mycoplasma hominis*. Other etiologies such as *Ureaplasma, Trichomonas, Mycoplasma genitalium*, and viruses account for 10 to 15 percent of cases. **Azithromycin** 1 g as a single oral dose is a drug of choice for nongonococcal urethritis and cervicitis (CDC, 2010e). If the urethritis is recurrent or persistent, therapy includes **metronidazole** 2 g as a single oral dose to cover *Trichomonas*, plus **azithromycin** 1 g as a single dose if not used for the initial episode. If cervicitis is recurrent or persistent the women should be reevaluated for possible reexposure to an STI (CDC, 2010e). **Azithromycin** is also first-line treatment of chancroid as a single oral dose of 1 g. An alternative is **erythromycin base** 500 mg orally four times daily for 7 days (CDC, 2010e). **Azithromycin** is commonly prescribed as part of the treatment of gonococcal urethritis and cervicitis as a 1-g oral dose to cover the chlamydial infections that often coexist with gonorrhea. **Azithromycin** is no longer indicated in the treatment of pelvic inflammatory disease due to *C. trachomatis, M. hominis*, or *N. gonorrhoeae* because of resistance (CDC, 2010e). **Azithromycin** 2 g as a single dose may be used as a second-line therapy for penicillin-allergic patients with early syphilis, although this has not been well studied and treatment failure has been noted (CDC, 2010e). Sexually transmitted infections are discussed in more detail in Chapter 44.

Mycobacterium avium Complex

Infections with the nontuberculous mycobacterial organism *Mycobacterium avium* complex (MAC) occur in up to 40 percent of patients with AIDS. Advanced immunosuppression is the major risk factor for MAC. Patients with AIDS are thought to acquire this organism, usually resident in water and soil, by respiratory or GI routes. The syndrome presents with high fever, diarrhea, night sweats, weight loss, anemia, and neutropenia. Diagnosis is usually based on blood culture, although it is sometimes identified on biopsy of the liver, bone marrow, or lymph nodes. MAC prophylaxis is now strongly recommended for HIV-infected adults with a mean CD4 lymphocyte count of fewer than 50 mcg/mL. The first-line drug is **clarithromycin** at dosages listed in Table 24–20. An alternative treatment is **azithromycin** if **clarithromycin** is not tolerated (Benson, Kaplan, Masur, Pau, & Holms, 2004). Before prophylaxis is initiated, patients should be evaluated to assure they do not have active MAC or *Mycobacterium tuberculosis*. National guidelines indicated that treatment of MAC should include at least two **antimicrobials** to prevent or delay resistance, one of which should be either **clarithromycin** or **azithromycin** (Benson et al, 2004). Of these, **clarithromycin**, 500 mg twice daily, has the greatest evidence for efficacy. **Ethambutol** is commonly the second drug, and many expert clinicians add **rifabutin** as a third agent (Benson et al, 2004). HIV infection and its management are discussed in Chapter 37.

Peptic Ulcer Disease

Most patients with peptic ulcer who are not taking NSAIDs, as well as many who are taking **NSAIDs**, have evidence of *H. pylori*. Eradication of *H. pylori* is recommended for all peptic ulcer disease patients with an active ulcer, a history of ulcer complications, or a need for maintenance therapy. Duodenal and gastric ulcers recur in up to 80 percent of patients treated with drugs to reduce gastric acid but not treated for eradication of *H. pylori* infection. Multiple treatment regimens for *H. pylori* eradication are available, including combining a **proton pump inhibitor (PPI)** and two antibiotics for 14 days (Lew, 2009). **Antimicrobial** agents used include **clarithromycin, tetracycline, amoxicillin, levofloxacin**, and **metronidazole**. They are given in three or four drug regimens with **PPIs** and **bismuth subsalicylate**. Approved combinations are included in Table 34–8 (Chapter 34). Two regimens include the **macrolide antibiotic clarithromycin** (500 mg twice daily).

Endocarditis Prophylaxis

The American Heart Association and the American College of Cardiology published joint updated guidelines for endocarditis prophylaxis in 2008, narrowing the recommendation for therapy to only those with prosthetic heart valves, previous infective endocarditis, certain patients with congenital heart disease, and cardiac transplant patients with valve regurgitation who are undergoing dental procedures that involve manipulation of either gingival tissue or the periapical region of the teeth (Nishimura et al, 2008). For patients who can take oral medications but are allergic to **penicillins**, a single dose of 500 mg of **azithromycin** or **clarithromycin** for adults or 15 mg/kg for children is indicated for endocarditis prophylaxis 1 hour before the procedure.

Exacerbations of Chronic Bronchitis

If a patient with chronic obstructive pulmonary disease (COPD) is producing purulent sputum, treatment with antibiotics is warranted. Any of the **macrolides** are active against the most common pathogens (see discussion in penicillin section for pathogen list) and are appropriate first-line choices (Rabe et al, 2007). Length of treatment is 7 to 14 days. Asthma and bronchitis and their management are discussed in Chapter 30.

Upper Respiratory Infections

The common bacterial infections in the upper respiratory tract include acute otitis media (AOM), sinusitis, and pharyngitis. *S. pneumoniae, H. influenzae,* and *M. catarrhalis* are the most common pathogens found in AOM and sinusitis in both children and adults. **Amoxicillin** is the recommended first-line treatment for both AOM and sinusitis. *S. pneumoniae* is resistant to the common **macrolides erythromycin** (35.3% resistance), **azithromycin** (35.3% resistance), and **clarithromycin** (35.2% resistance) (Jenkins & Farrell, 2009). Thus the **macrolides** are no longer considered first-line agents for AOM or sinusitis. In **penicillin**-allergic patients **azithromycin** may be used; in children a combination of **erythromycin** and **sulfisoxazole (Pediazole)** may be used. The **macrolides** are also used for treatment of GABHS pharyngitis in **penicillin**-allergic patients. Dosages are shown in Table 24–20.

Skin or Soft Tissue Infections

Macrolides are primarily indicated for skin and soft tissue infections in **penicillin**-allergic patients, although they are not first-line treatment because of resistance. Oral and topical **erythromycin** has been used in the treatment of acne (see Chapter 32).

Other Uses

An accepted off-labeled use for **erythromycin** is Lyme disease in individuals who are allergic to **penicillin** and in children younger than age 9 years. However, **erythromycin** may be less effective than **amoxicillin** or **doxycycline**, possibly because of erratic absorption. Other accepted off-labeled uses for **erythromycin** include treatment of actinomycoses, anthrax, lymphogranuloma venereum, and relapsing fever caused by *Borrelia* species. **Erythromycin** and **azithromycin** are considered drugs of first choice for *C. jejuni.* **Erythromycin** is indicated in the treatment of listeriosis caused by *L. monocytogenes* and in diphtheria prophylaxis and treatment. It has been used in conjunction with oral-local **neomycin** for preoperative preparation of the bowel. **Erythromycin** is also approved for treatment of erythrasma caused by *Corynebacterium minutissimum.* **Erythromycin** is an agonist at the motilin receptor and has been effective in the treatment of gastroparesis.

Erythromycin ophthalmic ointment 0.5 percent is administered to all newborns to prevent ophthalmic neonatorum. During a shortage of **erythromycin** ointment in 2009, the CDC recommended **azithromycin** ophthalmic drops as an alternative, off-labeled treatment, but when the shortage ended the CDC issued a statement that alternatives to **erythromycin** ointment no longer be used (CDC, 2010a). **Erythromycin** is indicated in chlamydial conjunctivitis in newborns and chlamydial pneumonia in infants caused by *C. trachomatis.*

Rational Drug Selection

Both definitive drug selection and empirical drug selection follow the same principles described in the Rational Drug Selection section for the **penicillins**, regardless of the infection or drug class involved. **Macrolides, azalides,** or **ketolides** are often selected for susceptible organisms as alternatives in **penicillin**-allergic patients. **Azithromycin** and **clarithromycin** have a slightly broader spectrum than **erythromycin** and additional indications, such as MAC. Because of its long history, **erythromycin** has accumulated indications for which the newer agents have not been tested. Increasing resistance of *H. influenzae, Staphylococcus,* and *S. pneumoniae* may increasingly limit the utility of **macrolides** for common bacterial infections. In addition to spectrum of action, the indications for selection of a specific **macrolide, azithromycin,** or **telithromycin** are cost, convenience, and adverse effect profile. **Erythromycin salts** are substantially less expensive than the newer drugs but have more GI adverse effects. The good bioavailability and milder GI effects of the **erythromycin estolate salt** are offset by the risk of cholestatic jaundice in adults. This agent should not be prescribed for individuals with liver impairment. Patients with history of cardiac arrhythmia or QT prolongation should avoid **erythromycin** or be carefully monitored. **Azithromycin** may be selected over **erythromycin, clarithromycin,** or **telithromycin** if the patient is taking interacting drugs whose hepatic metabolism is subject to inhibition. **Erythromycin** is generally preferred over the newer agents during pregnancy and for very young infants because of greater accumulated clinical experience. A major reason for selection of **azithromycin** over other drugs is the enhanced compliance caused by its convenient dosing schedule. However, with its once-per-day dosing and short duration of 3 to 5 days, a single missed dose could jeopardize the successful outcome. There are no indications for **dirithromycin** over other drugs.

Monitoring

Monitoring for therapeutic response to antibiotics is described in the Monitoring section for **penicillins.** Because **erythromycin, clarithromycin,** and **telithromycin** inhibit the metabolism of many drugs, observation for altered response to concurrent medications metabolized by CYP450 3A4 or 2C9 is essential, beginning with the first dose and continuing for several half-lives of the drugs after it is discontinued. Patients taking drugs with narrow therapeutic margins require extra scrutiny if they are taking any **macrolides, clarithromycin,** or **telithromycin.** Individuals with a history of hearing loss may be at increased risk for further hearing loss, especially if they have hepatic or renal impairment and are taking high doses (more than 4 g/d) of **erythromycin.** These risk factors may indicate audiometric testing at baseline and whenever there is clinical evidence of hearing loss (e.g., dizziness, fullness in the ears). The hearing loss is usually reversible; it occurs from 36 hours to 8 days after treatment is initiated and begins to recover 1 to 14 days after the drug is discontinued. ECG monitoring of QT interval is particularly recommended for high-dose parenteral therapy. If the patient develops malaise, nausea, vomiting, skin rash, abdominal pain, or jaundice within 1 to 2 weeks after therapy is initiated, the drug should be discontinued and liver function tests initiated to assess for cholestatic jaundice.

Patient Education

Administration

Doses of **macrolides** should be evenly spaced for the best effect. **Azithromycin** and **telithromycin** are given once daily. The available dosage forms are shown in Table 24–21. Suspensions must be shaken thoroughly before administration, and excess medication should be discarded after the prescribed therapy is administered and never used by another individual or by the same patient for a different episode. Because it is irritating to the GI mucosa, **erythromycin** should be taken with a full 8-oz glass of water by adults and with at least 4 to 6 oz by children.

Food interactions are complex for these drugs. **Azithromycin tablets**, the adult **single-dose azithromycin** packet, **clarithromycin**, **erythromycin estolate**, and **telithromycin** can be taken without regard to meals. **Erythromycin stearate**, most brands of **erythromycin base**, **erythromycin ethylsuccinate**, **azithromycin capsules**,

Table 24–21 ◆ **Available Dosage Forms: Macrolides and Azalides**

Drug	Dosage Form	How Supplied	Cost
Azithromycin (Zithromax)	Tablets: 250 mg	In bottles of 30 tablets and Z-pak with tablets	$222/30, $134/18 Z-pak $71 generic $26/6
	500 mg	In bottles of 30, UD 50, and TRI-PAK 3	$134/9
	600 mg	In bottles of 30 tablets	TRI-PAK $74
	Powder for oral suspension: 100 mg/5 mL	In 300-mg bottles (cherry, creme de vanilla, and banana flavors)	$531/30
	200 mg/5 mL	In 600-, 900-, 1,200-mg bottles (same flavors)	$39/30 mL generic $33/15 mL
	1 g-packet	In single-dose packets of 3, 10	$124/3
Clarithromycin (Biaxin)	Tablets: 250 mg, 500 mg Granules for oral suspension: reconstituted	In bottles of 60 film-coated tablets: UD 100	250 mg $361/60
	125 mg/5 mL, 250 mg/5 mL	In 50- and 100-mL bottles (fruit punch flavor)	
Dirithromycin (Dynabac)	Tablets: 250 mg	In bottles of 60 and D5-pak 10	$224/160, $113/30
Erythromycin base	Tablets: 250 mg	In bottles of 40, 100, 500 and UD 100	250 mg = $36/30
	500 mg	In bottles of 100 film-coated tablets	500 mg = $46/30
	Capsules: 250 mg	In bottles of 60, 100, 500 delayed-release capsules	250 mg cap = $46/30
(E-Base)	Tablets: 333 mg	In bottles of 100, 500, 1,000 delayed-release, enteric-coated tablets	
	500 mg	In bottles of 100, 500 enteric-coated tablets	
(Eryc)	Capsules: 250 mg	In bottles of 100 delayed-release capsules	
(E-Mycin)	Tablets: 250 mg	In bottles of 40, 100, 500 enteric-coated tablets	
	333 mg	In bottles of 100, 500 enteric-coated tablets: UD 100	
(Ery-Tab)	Tablets: 250, 333 mg	In bottles of 100, 500 delayed-release, enteric-coated tablets: UD 100	
(PCE Dispertab)	Tablets: 333 mg	In bottles of 60 tablets with polymer-coated particles	
	500 mg	In bottles of 100 tablets with polymer-coated particles	

Table 24–21 ◆ **Available Dosage Forms: Macrolides and Azalides—cont'd**

Drug	Dosage Form	How Supplied	Cost
Erythromycin estolate	Capsules: 250 mg Suspension: 125 mg/5 mL, 250 mg/5 mL	In bottles of 100 capsules In 480-mL bottles	
(Ilosone)	Tablets: 500 mg Capsules: 250 mg Suspension: 125 mg/5 mL 250 mg/5 mL	In bottles of 50 tablets In bottles of 100 capsules In 480-mL bottles (orange flavor) In 100- and 480-mL bottles (cherry flavor)	
Erythromycin stearate	Tablets: 250 mg 500 mg	In bottles of 100, 500, 1,000 film-coated tablets In bottles of 100, 500 film-coated tablets	250 mg = $30/30 $4/28 (Walmart list) $10/84 (Walmart)
Erythromycin ethylsuccinate	Tablets: 400 mg Suspension: 200 mg/5 mL, 400 mg/5 mL	In bottles of 100, 500 tablets In 480-mL bottles	$31/100
(EryPed)	Tablets: 200 mg Suspension: 200 mg 400 mg Drops/suspension: 100 mg/2.5 mL	In bottles of 40 chewable tablets (fruit flavor) In 100, 200-mL bottles (fruit flavor) In 60-, 100-, 200-mL bottles (banana flavor) In 50-mL bottle (fruit flavor)	
(E.E.S.)	Tablets: 400 mg Suspension: 200 mg/5 mL, 400 mg/5 mL Granules/powder for oral suspension: 200 mg/5 mL (reconstituted)	In 100, 500, 1,000 film-coated tablets In 100-, 480-mL bottles (orange flavor) In 100-, 200-mL bottles (cherry flavor)	$21/100
Erythromycin ethylsuccinate and sulfisoxazole	Granules for oral suspension: 200 mg erythromycin base activity and 600 mg sulfisoxazole/5 mL	In 100, 150, 200 mL	
(Eryzole)	Granules for oral suspension: 200 mg erythromycin base activity and 600 mg sulfisoxazole/5 mL	In 100, 150, 200 mL (strawberry flavor)	
(Pediazole)	Granules for oral suspension: 200 mg erythromycin base activity and 600 mg sulfisoxazole/5 mL	In 100, 150, 200 mL (strawberry-banana flavor)	$21/100 mL $46/150 mL $53/200 mL
Telithromycin (Ketek)	Tablets: 400 mg	In bottles of 60 Ketek Pak (blister with 2 tablets in each cavity) 10 cards UD 100 blister pak	$ 296.21/60

and **azithromycin suspension** must be taken on an empty stomach, 1 hour before or 2 hours after eating. **Dirithromycin** should be taken with food or within an hour of a meal. **Erythromycin ethylsuccinate** has improved bioavailability if taken with food. Because the requirements for administration with respect to food may vary by brand, the package insert is the best guide for **erythromycin base.** Tablets of **erythromycin base, erythromycin stearate,** and **dirithromycin** should not be chewed or crushed. If chewable tablets of **erythromycin ethylsuccinate** are prescribed, the necessity for chewing the dosage form should be stressed. If pediatric drops of **erythromycin estolate** (100 mg/mL) or **erythromycin ethylsuccinate** are prescribed, the prescription should specify dispensing a calibrated dropper, and the parent should be instructed on proper measurement and oral administration technique; parents have occasionally assumed drops were meant to be administered in the ear. The adult **single-dose azithromycin** packet should be thoroughly mixed with 2 oz (60 mL) of water and consumed immediately. An additional 2 oz of water should be added to the container, mixed, and ingested to ensure consumption of the entire dose. This form should not be used for doses greater than 1,000 mg.

Adverse Reactions

Taking **erythromycin** with a full glass of water decreases the GI symptoms that are the most common adverse effects. Because patients often discontinue the medication if adverse effects are intolerable, they should be urged to call the prescriber if GI distress becomes severe so that an alternative drug can be prescribed. Patients who experience signs of liver impairment (malaise, nausea, vomiting, abdominal cramps, skin rash, fever, with or without jaundice) should discontinue the **macrolide** and call the prescriber immediately. Syncope may indicate torsades de pointes related to cardiac QT interval prolongation and should also be reported. Other patient education includes information about symptoms of superinfection that is part of the education for all **antibacterial** drugs.

Lifestyle Management

See the Lifestyle Management section for the **penicillins**.

OXAZOLIDINONES

Linezolid (Zyvox), approved in the United States in 2000, is the first drug in a new class of **antibiotics**, the **oxazolidinones**. Each **antibiotic** developed within the past 60 years has seen the emergence of resistant organisms. Recently, there has been a specific need to develop drugs effective against **methicillin**-resistant, **penicillin**-resistant, and **vancomycin**-resistant strains of bacteria that have produced serious illness. Unfortunately, although new variants of drugs within a class have created subclasses (e.g., **azalides** and **ketolides**), no entirely new class of **antibiotics** has been developed since the 1980s (Mollering, 2003). The **oxazolidinones** represent a unique class of totally synthetic antibiotics, which make the development of naturally occurring resistance mechanism less likely.

Pharmacodynamics

The **oxazolidinones** are inhibitors of bacterial ribosomal protein synthesis, but unlike other **antibiotics** they stop the first step in which bacteria assemble ribosomes from their dissociated subunits. **Linezolid** does this by binding to the 50S ribosomal subunit near its surface with the 30S subunit, thus preventing the formation of a 70S initiation complex required for protein synthesis. No other known antibiotic uses this process, so there is no cross-resistance.

Sensitivity

Linezolid is bacteriostatic against some organisms and bacteriocidal against others. It is most effective against aerobic gram-positive bacteria. The in vitro spectrum of activity also includes certain gram-negative and anaerobic bacteria. The main susceptible organisms include group A and B *Streptococcus, S. pneumoniae, E. faecalis, E. faecium, S. aureus* (both MSSA and MRSA), *S. epidermidis, Clostridium jeikeium*, and *L. monocytogenes*. It also exhibits good in vitro activity against *M. tuberculosis* and *M. avium* complex.

It is weakly effective against *H. influenzae* and *M. catarrhalis* and not effective against *M. pneumoniae*.

Resistance

Although resistance is not widespread, reports of **linezolid** resistance emerged as early as 2002 (Auckland et al, 2002; Bersos, Maniati, Kontos, Petinaki, & Maniatis, 2004). Resistance has been reported to enterococci (*E. faecalis* and *E. facecium*) (Kainer et al, 2007) and rarely to MRSA (Garcia et al, 2010). **Linezolid** resistance is associated with previous use of **antibiotics** for MRSA and hospitalization leading to nosocomial transmission (Bersos et al, 2004).

Pharmacokinetics

Absorption and Distribution

Linezolid is rapidly and completed absorbed after oral administration. Food slightly delays its uptake, but does not affect total amount of drug absorbed. **Linezolid** may be taken without regard to meals. It is only 31 percent protein bound and the binding is concentration dependent. Distributed to well-perfused tissues, including breast milk, it has a volume of distribution of 40 to 50 L.

Metabolism and Excretion

There are two inactive metabolites of **linezolid** created by oxidation of the morpholine ring. Because this is a nonenzymatic oxidation, this drug does not induce the CYP450 system. Nonrenal excretion accounts for 65 percent of the total clearance; of the remainder, 30 percent is excreted unchanged in urine. A small degree of nonlinearity in clearance is observed with increasing doses; however, the difference is small and not clinically significant. No dosage adjustments are required for impaired hepatic or renal function.

Clearance is altered by age; it is most rapid in the youngest age group (age 1 week to 11 years). As the age of the child increases, the clearance decreases and reaches that of the adult population during adolescence. Once again, no dosage adjustments are required, except for preterm neonates younger than 7 days because they have lower clearance values. Table 24–22 presents the pharmacokinetics of this drug.

Table 24–22 ▶ **Pharmacokinetics: Oxazolidinones**

Drug	Onset (h)	Peak (h)	Duration (h)	Protein Binding	Bioavailability	Half-life (h)	Elimination
Linezolid	Rapid	1–2	12	31%	100%	4.4–5.5	30%–35% in urine; 65% nonrenal elimination

Pharmacotherapeutics

Precautions and Contraindications

Myelosuppression (anemia, leucopenia, pancytopenia, and thrombocytopenia) have been reported in patients receiving **linezolid.** Blood counts return to normal after **linezolid** is discontinued. Complete blood counts should be monitored weekly if a patient is on **linezolid** for longer than 2 weeks.

Lactic acidosis has been reported with the use of **linezolid.** Patients with recurrent nausea or vomiting, unexplained acidosis, or low bicarbonate level should be evaluated.

Linezolid is Pregnancy Category C. In animal studies, fetal toxicities were seen only at ranges that produced maternal toxicity. There are no adequate, well-controlled studies in pregnant women, so use during pregnancy only if the potential benefit clearly outweighs the potential risk to the fetus.

Because this drug is excreted in breast milk in concentrations similar to those in maternal plasma, consider the benefit to the mother in choosing to continue the drug and/or to discontinue breastfeeding.

Linezolid is approved for use in children from birth. Preterm infants and neonates require reduced dosing per 24 hours because of reduced clearance.

Adverse Drug Reactions

The most common adverse reactions reported were diarrhea (2.8% to 11%), headache (0.5% to 11.3%), and nausea (3.4% to 9.6%). Although uncomfortable, none created serious medical consequences. Pseudomembranous colitis has been reported with nearly all **antibiotics.** If this is the suspected cause of the diarrhea, discontinuance of the drug is effective in mild to moderate cases, and severe cases may require treatment of *C. difficile* infection.

Myelosuppression has been reported, but it resolves with discontinuance of the drug. This adverse event seems to be related to duration of therapy (longer than 2 wk). Consider discontinuing the drug if the patient develops or has worsening myelosuppression.

Drug Interactions

Linezolid was originally developed as a **monoamine oxidase inhibitor** (MOI) and has properties of that inhibition. **Indirect-acting sympathomimetics, vasopressors,** or **dopaminergic** drugs may have increased effects when given concurrently, requiring decreased doses of these drugs. Because **linezolid** is a reversible, nonselective inhibitor of monoamine oxidase, it also has potential interactions with **serotonergics.** Signs and symptoms of **serotonin** syndrome (e.g., hyperpyrexia and cognitive dysfunction) should be watched for if concomitant therapy is required. There is also potential interaction with tyramine-rich foods and drinks. They do not need to be eliminated entirely, but should not be eaten in large quantities (Table 24–23).

Clinical Use and Dosing

Pneumonia and Complicated Skin and Skin Structure Infections

The adult dose is 600 mg every twelve hours for 10 to 14 days. In pediatric patients (birth to 11 yr) the dose is

Table 24–23 ■ **Drug Interactions: Oxazolidinones**

Drug	Interacting Drug	Possible Effect	Implications
Linezolid	Adrenergic (sympathomimetic) drugs (e.g., dopamine and epinephrine)	Increased action of the interacting drug	Reduce and titrate initial doses of interacting drug
	Serotonergics (e.g., SRIs)	Development of serotonin syndrome	Watch for serotonin syndrome indications. Avoid concurrent use unless no appropriate alternative
	Food interactions Tyramine-rich foods and drinks	Significantly increased blood pressure	No need to delete entirely from diet, but quantities of tyramine eaten should not exceed 100 mg/meal

10 mg/kg every 8 hours for 10 to 14 days. In each case it is useful only for susceptible bacteria and only after older, less expensive agents have been tried and are found to be ineffective. The goal is to keep any new **antibiotic** free from resistant strains of bacteria as long as possible. It should be remembered that **linezolid** has poor activity against *H. influenzae* and none against *M. pneumoniae*, two common pneumonia organisms. The FDA approval for CAP is for **penicillin**-susceptible strains of *S. pneumoniae* or *S. aureus* only.

Uncomplicated Skin and Skin-Structure Infections

The dosage is less for these uncomplicated infections and it varies with age. For adults it is 400 mg every 12 hours; for adolescents it is 600 mg every 12 hours; for children aged 5 to 11 years it is 10 mg/kg every 12 hours. For young children (younger than 5 yr), the dose is 10 mg/kg every 8 hours due to the renal clearance issues discussed above. Once again, it is not first-line therapy and is intended for resistant organisms.

Vancomycin-Resistant Enterococcus faecium Infections

Probably the most useful indication for this drug is dealing with **vancomycin** resistance. The dose for this indication is 600 mg every 12 hours for 14 to 28 days in adults and 10 mg/kg every 12 hours for children birth to 11 years. It should be noted that the 28 days' length of therapy is the outer limit that has been evaluated in clinical trials and is the duration of therapy associated with more adverse effects. Dosage schedules are found in Table 24–24.

Rational Drug Selection

This drug, which is the only one in the class, is not first-line therapy or even second-line therapy for any of its indications. The drug's cost is prohibitive as first-line therapy ($1,152 for 20 of the 600-mg tablets) unless absolutely needed and using **linezolid** selectively will decrease the development of widespread resistance.

Monitoring

Because of the risk for myelosuppression, a complete blood count should be done prior to therapy as baseline and as symptoms suggest.

Patient Education

Administration

Patient counseling for all **antibiotics** includes advice to complete the entire course of therapy, take the drug as prescribed on an evenly spaced schedule, and do not double missed doses. **Linezolid** may be taken with or without food, but should be taken with a full glass of water. Because significantly elevated blood pressure may occur if taken with tyramine-rich foods, the amount of tyramine consumed at any one meal should be limited (less than 100 mg/meal). Oral suspensions should be gently inverted 3 to 5 times to mix; do not shake. The drug should be stored at room temperature. Available dosage forms are shown in Table 24–25.

Adverse Reactions

The main adverse reactions are diarrhea, headache, and nausea. Diarrhea should be reported to the health-care

Table 24–24 ◉ **Dosage Schedules: Oxazolidinones**

Drug	Indication	Dose	Comments
Linezolid	Community-acquired pneumonia and complicated skin and skin-structure infections	*Adults:* 600 mg q12h for 10–14 d *Children birth–11 yr:* 10 mg/kg q8h for 10–14 d	May be administered without regard to food, but amount of tyramine-rich food in any meal should be kept low (<100 mg/meal)
	Uncomplicated skin and skin-structure infections	*Adults:* 400 mg q12h for 10–14 d *Adolescents:* 600 mg q12h for 10–14 d *Children 5–11 yr:* 10 mg/kg q12h	Oral suspensions should be gently inverted 3–5 times to mix; do not shake
		Children <5 yr: 10 mg/kg q8h	Store at room temperature
	Vancomycin-resistant *Enterococcus faecium* infections	*Adults:* 600 mg q12h for 14–28 d *Children birth–11 yr:* 10 mg/kg q8h for 14–28 d	Longer duration of therapy associated with more adverse effects

Note: Most preterm neonates <7 d of age (gestational age <34 wk) have lower systemic linezolid clearance values and larger AUC values than many full-term neonates and older infants. These neonates should be initiated with a dosing regimen of 10 mg/kg q12h. Consideration may be given to the use of 10 mg/kg q8h regimen in neonates with a suboptimal clinical response. All neonatal patients should receive 10 mg/kg q8h by 7 days of life (Zyvox label).

Table 24–25 ◆ **Available Dosage Forms: Oxazolidinones**

Drug	Dosage Form	How Supplied	Cost
Linezolid (Zyvox)	Tablets: 400, 600 mg Powder for oral suspension: 100 mg/5 mL	In bottles of 20, 100 and UD 30	600 mg = $1,152/20

provider. Blood, pus, or mucus in the stool may indicate a serious problem that requires treatment. Otherwise, an **antidiarrheal** medication may be suggested by the provider.

Lifestyle Management

Lifestyle management is the same as discussed in **penicillins**.

SULFONAMIDES, TRIMETHOPRIM, AND NITROFURANTOIN

The **sulfonamides** were once major **antibacterials**, but the development of resistant strains of bacteria and the incidence of allergic reactions to **sulfa** drugs resulted in their largely being relegated to treatment of UTIs, otitis media, and some sexually transmitted infections. **Sulfasalazine (Azulfidine)** is used in the treatment of ulcerative colitis and rheumatoid arthritis for its **anti-inflammatory** properties rather than for treatment of infection. **Mafenide (Sulfamylon)** and **silver sulfadiazine (Silvadene)** are used to prevent infection in patients with burns. Topical applications such as those for burns are not discussed in this chapter. Included in this section are drugs commonly used in combination with **sulfonamides**, such as **trimethoprim (Proloprim, Trimpex)**, and agents used to treat UTIs, such as **nitrofurantoin (Furadantin, Macrodantin)**. The combination formulation **trimethoprim-sulfamethoxazole (Bactrim, Septra, TMP-SMZ)** is also considered in this section.

Pharmacodynamics

Sulfonamides and **trimethoprim** both have distinctive pharmacodynamic properties, which are enhanced when combined.

Sulfonamides

Sulfonamides exert their bacteriostatic action by competitive antagonism of para-aminobenzoic acid (PABA), required by susceptible organisms for an essential step in the production of purines and the synthesis of nucleic acids, thereby blocking folic acid synthesis. Microorganisms that use exogenous folic acid and do not synthesize folic acid are not susceptible to **sulfonamides**.

Sensitivity

Sulfonamides inhibit both gram-positive and gram-negative bacteria. Susceptible organisms include *E. coli, S. pyogenes, S. pneumoniae, H. influenzae, Actinomyces, Nocardia, C. trachomatis, N. gonorrhoeae,* and some protozoa (*Pneumocystis carinii* and toxoplasmosis).

Resistance

The increasing frequency of resistant organisms limits the use of these drugs in chronic and recurrent UTI. Mutations that result in excessive production of PABA cause organisms to develop resistance. Dihydropteroate synthetase with a low **sulfonamide** affinity may be encoded on a plasmid that is transmissible and can be disseminated rapidly and widely. Cross-resistance between **sulfonamides** is common. Initiating therapy promptly with adequate doses for sufficient time can minimize resistance.

Trimethoprim

Trimethoprim inhibits bacterial dihydrofolic acid reductase. Dihydrofolic acid reductases convert dihydrofolic acid to tetrahydrofolic acid, a stage leading to the synthesis of purine and ultimately to DNA. Given with **sulfonamide**, it produces a sequential blocking in the metabolic sequence, resulting in synergistic activity of both drugs. This combination is often bactericidal. The widely used formulation **trimethoprim- sulfamethoxazole** (TMP-SMZ) illustrates the synergy of the combination.

Sensitivity

Trimethoprim is active against both gram-positive and gram-negative organisms. Gram-positive organisms include *S. pneumoniae,* some staphylococci, and *Enterococcus.* Its spectrum of gram-negative organisms includes *Acinetobacter, Citrobacter, Enterobacter, E. coli, K. pneumoniae, P. mirabilis, Salmonella,* and *Shigella.* Some *Serratia* and the protozoon *P. carinii* are also susceptible.

Resistance

Resistance results from reduced cell permeability, overproduction of dihydrofolate reductase, or production of an altered reductase with less drug-binding ability. Mutation is possible, but the most common cause is plasmid-encoded resistant reductases. As with the **sulfonamides**, dissemination of resistance is rapid and widespread.

Nitrofurantoin

Nitrofurantoin is a **synthetic nitrofuran** that is bacteriostatic in low concentrations and bactericidal in high concentrations. The mechanism of action for this drug is not clearly known, but it may inhibit acetyl coenzyme A, interfering with bacterial carbohydrate metabolism. It may also disrupt bacterial cell wall formation.

Sensitivity

Nitrofurantoin is active against most gram-positive cocci and gram-negative bacilli that cause UTIs. These include *E. coli, Klebsiella* and *Enterobacter* species, *E. faecalis,* and *S. aureus.* Some strains of *Enterobacter* and *Klebsiella* are resistant. It has no activity against *Pseudomonas* species or *Staphylococcus saprophyticus.*

Although in vitro susceptibility of *Salmonella, Shigella, Neisseria, S. pneumoniae,* and many anaerobes has been demonstrated, **nitrofurantoin** does not appear to have clinically significant activity against these organisms.

Resistance

Among susceptible organisms, resistant mutants are rare. Some plasmid-mediated resistance transferable to susceptible organisms has been demonstrated. There is no cross-resistance between this drug and other **antibacterial** agents.

Pharmacokinetics

Absorption and Distribution

Oral **sulfonamides** are absorbed readily from the GI tract. They are distributed widely throughout the body and found in all body tissues, and they readily enter the CSF, pleura, synovial fluids, and the eye. They cross the placenta and enter breast milk. They are bound to plasma proteins in varying degrees. "Free" serum levels of 5 to 15 mg/dL are therapeutically effective for most infections.

Trimethoprim is also well absorbed following oral administration. It is widely distributed in body tissues and crosses the placenta. Distribution into breast milk occurs with high concentrations.

Nitrofurantoin is readily absorbed via oral administration. The macrocrystalline form is absorbed more slowly because of slower dissolution and causes less GI distress, and the monohydrate crystals are so slowly absorbed that twice-daily dosing is effective. Bioavailability is enhanced by taking **nitrofurantoin** with food. Because it undergoes rapid tubular secretion, therapeutic serum and tissue concentrations are achieved only in the urinary tract at usual oral doses. It is not effective in patients with severe renal impairment.

Metabolism and Excretion

Metabolism of **sulfonamides** occurs in the liver by conjugation and acetylation to inactive metabolites. Patients who are slow acetylators have increased risk for toxicity.

Renal excretion is mainly by glomerular filtration, with some acetylated metabolites being less soluble. Acetylated metabolites may produce crystalluria unless the urine is sufficiently alkaline and adequate fluid intake (more than 2,500 mL/d) is maintained. **Sulfadiazine** is especially prone to this problem. Small amounts are excreted in feces, bile, breast milk, and other secretions.

Liver metabolism of **trimethoprim** is less than 20 percent. Eighty percent of this drug is excreted unchanged in the urine. Because it is so dependent on the kidney for excretion, elimination is delayed and its half-life is increased in patients with renal impairment.

Approximately 50 to 70 percent of **nitrofurantoin** is rapidly metabolized by body tissues. Distribution is to most body tissues, and it crosses the placenta and enters breast milk. Renal excretion is via glomerular filtration and tubular secretion. Acid urine enhances **antibacterial** activity in urine and enhances tubular reabsorption, which increases its activity in renal tissues. Serum half-life is increased in patients with severe renal impairment. Usual doses produce therapeutic urinary levels in patients with normal renal function. If CCr is less than 40 mL/minute, urinary concentrations are not therapeutic, and the increased serum levels may produce toxicity.

Table 24–26 presents the pharmacokinetics of **sulfonamides, trimethoprim,** and **nitrofurantoin.**

Pharmacotherapeutics

Precautions and Contraindications

There are a number of patients in which the **sulfonamides, trimethoprim,** and **nitrofurantoin** should be used cautiously. Such patients include those with glucose-6-phosphate dehydrogenase deficiency, renal impairment, and folate deficiency.

Blood Dyscrasias and Glucose-6-Phosphate Dehydrogenase Deficiency

Sulfonamides are contraindicated for patients who have blood dyscrasias and G6PD deficiency. Serious adverse reactions secondary to direct toxic effects on the bone marrow have sometimes resulted in death. They include agranulocytosis, aplastic anemia, and other blood dyscrasias. Acute hemolytic anemia resulting in increased destruction of RBCs has resulted in patients whose RBCs have been sensitized because of G6PD deficiency. Sore throat, fever, pallor, purpura, or jaundice may be early indications of these serious blood disorders. These problems occur only rarely with **trimethoprim** and with **nitrofurantoin** only in conjunction with G6PD deficiency.

Renal Impairment

Sulfonamides are used cautiously for patients with mild renal impairment and are contraindicated if CCr is less than 50 mL/minute. The more soluble drugs in this class (**sulfisoxazole** and **sulfamethoxazole**) are less likely to result in renal complications. Adequate hydration (more than 2,500 mL/d) helps to prevent crystalluria and stone formation. Cautious use of **trimethoprim** is recommended for patients with renal

Table 24–26 ▶ **Pharmacokinetics: Sulfonamides, Trimethoprim, and Nitrofurantoin**

Drug	Onset	Peak	Duration	Protein Binding	Bioavailability	Half-Life	Elimination
Nitrofurantoin	UA	0.5 h	6–12 h	60%	UA	20 min*	30%–50% unchanged in urine
Sulfadiazine	Varies	3–6 h	6–12 h	32%–56%	70%–100%	13 h	Mainly in urine, small amount in feces
Sulfamethoxazole	1 h	2–4 h	12 h	65%	70%–100%	7–12 h	Mostly by liver; 20% unchanged in urine
Sulfamethoxazole/ trimethoprim	Rapid	2–4 h	6–12 h	65%/50%	UA	8–13 h	20% by liver; remainder unchanged in urine
Sulfisoxazole	1 h	2–4 h	4–6 h	90%	70%–100%	5–8 h	Mostly by liver
Trimethoprim	Rapid	1–4 h	12–24 h	50%	UA	8–11 h	80% unchanged in urine; 20% by liver

UA = information not available.
*Increased in renal impairment.

impairment. Renal impairment increases the risk of toxicity of **nitrofurantoin**, which is not effective in severe renal impairment.

Folate Deficiency

Because of its effect on folic acid synthesis, **trimethoprim** should be used with caution for patients with folate deficiency. Folate supplementation may be administered concomitantly without interfering with antibacterial action.

Pregnancy

Sulfonamides are Pregnancy Category C. These drugs cross the placenta, and fetal levels average 70 to 90 percent of maternal serum levels. Significant levels may persist if they are given near term. **Sulfonamides** are highly bound to plasma albumin and compete for binding sites with bilirubin, resulting in increased free bilirubin concentrations. In utero, the fetus clears free bilirubin through the placental circulation. After birth, this route is no longer available, and unbound bilirubin may cross the blood–brain barrier. Do not use near term. Jaundice, hemolytic anemia, and kernicterus have occurred. Teratogenicity has occurred in animal studies.

Trimethoprim is also Pregnancy Category C. It crosses the placenta, producing similar levels in fetal and maternal plasma. Teratogenicity has occurred in animal studies. Because it may interfere with folic acid metabolism, it should be used only when its benefits clearly outweigh fetal risks.

Nitrofurantoin is Pregnancy Category B. Use for women of childbearing potential only when it is clearly needed. The incidence of fetal changes in animal studies was low and the alterations minor. It should not be given, however, to pregnant patients with G6PD deficiency because of the risk of hemolysis for both mother and fetus. It should not be used at term because it may induce hemolytic anemia in the newborn because of immature enzyme systems. For this reason, **nitrofurantoin** is contraindicated in infants less than 1 month.

Lactation

Because **sulfonamides** are excreted in breast milk in low concentrations and milk:plasma ratios are as low as 0.5 to 0.6, the American Academy of Pediatrics considers breastfeeding safe during administration of **sulfonamides**. However, premature infants or those with hyperbilirubinemia or G6PD deficiency should not be breastfed while the mother is taking the drugs. **Trimethoprim** milk:plasma ratios are 1.25, indicating the drug concentrates in breast milk. Because it may interfere with folic acid metabolism, it should be used cautiously for nursing women. **Nitrofurantoin** is excreted in breast milk in very low concentrations. Infants with G6PD deficiency, however, should not nurse while the mother is receiving this drug.

Children

Sulfonamides are contraindicated in infants less than 2 months of age (except as adjunctive therapy with pyrimethamine for congenital toxoplasmosis). Insufficient clinical data are available on prolonged or recurrent therapy with **sulfamethoxazole** in children under 6 years with chronic renal disease. It is best to avoid its use in these patients.

Safety for use in infants less than 2 months has not been established for **trimethoprim**, and efficacy has not been established for children younger than 12 years. **Nitrofurantoin** is contraindicated in infants less than 1 month.

Adverse Drug Reactions

As with most **antibiotics**, the most common adverse reactions for all these drugs are in the GI tract. Anorexia, nausea, vomiting, diarrhea, stomatitis, and abdominal pain are the main adverse reactions.

Rashes and generalized skin eruptions are also common adverse reactions for **sulfonamides** and trimethoprim. The incidence is dose related and may include exfoliative dermatitis and Stevens-Johnson syndrome.

Hypersensitivity reactions may occur with **sulfonamides.** Cholestatic jaundice is the indication of the adverse reaction. For the **sulfonamides**, cross-hypersensitivity may occur with chemically related drugs such as **sulfonylureas**, **thiazide** and **loop diuretics**, **carbonic anhydrase inhibitors**, and **sunscreens with PABA**.

Photosensitivity reactions can occur with **sulfonamides**. Measures such as sunscreens and protective clothing may reduce these problems.

Peripheral neuropathy may develop and become severe and irreversible with **nitrofurantoin**. Predisposing conditions include renal impairment, anemia, diabetes, electrolyte imbalances, vitamin B deficiency, and debilitating disease. Less severe peripheral neuropathy has also occurred with **sulfonamides**. CNS adverse effects, including headache, dizziness, and drowsiness, have occurred with both of these drug classes.

Other serious adverse reactions are discussed in the Precautions and Contraindications section.

Drug Interactions

Trimethoprim and **nitrofurantoin** have very few drug interactions. **Sulfonamides** interact with several commonly used drugs, including **salicylates**, **warfarin**, and **hydantoins**. Specific drug interactions are listed in Table 24–27.

Clinical Use and Dosing

Urinary Tract Infections

Lower tract UTIs are most commonly caused by gram-negative bacteria (95%), with *E. coli* the most prevalent organism (equal to or greater than 80%) (Wagenlehner, Weidner, & Naber, 2005). Among community-acquired infections, *S. saprophyticus*, *Klebsiella*, and gram-negative enteric bacilli cause almost all UTIs not caused by *E. coli*. In children, additional organisms include *Klebsiella* in

Table 24–27 ■ **Drug Interactions: Sulfonamides, Trimethoprim, and Nitrofurantoin**

Drug	Interacting Drug	Possible Effect	Implications
Nitrofurantoin	Anticholinergics	Increase nitrofurantoin bioavailability by delaying gastric emptying and increasing absorption.	Monitor for adverse reactions and toxicity.
	Magnesium salts	May delay or decrease nitrofurantoin absorption.	Avoid concurrent administration.
	Probenecid	High doses decrease renal clearance and increase serum levels of nitrofurantoin.	Monitor for increased risk for toxicity.
All sulfonamides	Oral anticoagulants	Enhance action of warfarin. Hemorrhage could occur.	Monitor PT/INR closely.
	Cyclosporine	Increased cyclosporine concentration and risk of nephrotoxicity.	Select different antibacterial.
	Hydantoins	Increased serum hydantoin levels.	Monitor serum levels closely
	Sulfonylureas	Increased sulfonylureas half-life and risk of hypoglycemia.	Avoid concurrent use or monitor blood glucose closely.
	Probenecid and other uricosurics, salicylates, indomethacin	Sulfonamides may be displaced from plasma albumin resting in increased free drug. Sulfonamides may potentiate action of uricosurics.	Unless planned for therapeutic reasons, avoid concurrent administration.
	Thiazide diuretics	May cause increased incidence of thrombocytopenia with purpura.	Avoid coadministration.
Trimethoprim	Phenytoin	Inhibition of hepatic metabolism may result in increased effects of phenytoin.	Avoid concurrent administration or monitor phenytoin levels closely.

INR = international normalized ratio; PT = prothrombin time.

neonates and *Proteus* in boys. All of the **antibiotics** mentioned have a spectrum of activity that covers these organisms.

Trimethoprim-sulfamethoxazole is the most effective drug when no complicating factors are present; the recommended dose for adults is one double-strength tablet twice daily for 3 days if local *E. coli* resistance is less than 20 percent (Griebling, 2007; Grover et al, 2007). If 3-day empirical therapy fails, urine should be sent for culture and subsequent therapy continued for 14 days. The American Academy of Pediatrics (AAP) (1999) recommends 6 to 12 mg **trimethoprim** and 30 to 60 mg **sulfamethoxazole** per kg/day in two divided doses (1 mL suspension per kg/d). Children should be treated with a 10-day regimen. Resistance to **TMP-SMZ** is seen in patients who have had antibiotic therapy for any reason in the past three months or if they have been hospitalized recently.

Nitrofurantoin is an effective treatment for UTIs, with a low *E. coli* resistance rate of 2.1 percent in a recent study comparing it to **TMP-SMZ**, **ciprofloxacin**, and **levofloxacin** (Kashanian et al, 2008). The dose of **nitrofurantoin** is 50 to 100 mg twice a day. This drug can also be used prophylactically in adults and children who have recurrent UTIs more often than three times per year. **Nitrofurantoin** is useful in pregnant women because it is Pregnancy Category B. During pregnancy, the dose must be given for 7 days. **Nitrofurantoin** should be avoided in pregnancy near term, in labor, and during lactation when the infant is less than 1 month of age because of the risk for the infant's developing hemolytic anemia. The pediatric dose is 5 to 7 mg/kg/day divided every 6 hours for 7 to 10 days. Shortened therapy should not be used.

Recurrent infections (more than three infections in 1 yr) may be treated with prophylactic antibiotics. Low-dose **nitrofurantoin** at bedtime (50 to 100 mg) or **TMP-SMZ** (40 mg **TMP** and 200 mg **SMZ** or 1 single-strength tablet) at bedtime and postcoitally to prevent recurrent UTIs in women.

Pregnant women with asymptomatic bacteriuria detected during routine screening during the first trimester can be treated with **TMP-SMZ**, **nitrofurantoin**, or **trimethoprim**, as well as **amoxicillin** or oral **cephalosporins**. Other genitourinary indications for **TMP-SMZ** are treatment of acute prostatitis in men older than 35 years, chronic prostatitis, recurrent UTI (more than three in a year), and prophylaxis before and after invasive urological procedures. Although infrequently used, the **sulfonamides sulfadiazine**, **sulfamethizole**, **sulfamethoxazole**, and **sulfisoxazole** are approved for treatment of cystitis and uncomplicated pyelonephritis. A more detailed discussion of UTI and its management is found in Chapter 47. For dosage schedules see Table 24–28.

Table 24–28 ● Dosage Schedule: Sulfonamides, Trimethoprim, and Nitrofurantoin

Drug	Indication	Dose	Comments
Nitrofurantoin (Furadantin) Nitrofurantoin macrocrystals (Macrodantin)	Urinary tract infection	*Adults:* 50–100 mg qid with meals and at bedtime for 3–7 d or more	Maximum daily dose 600 mg for adult or 10 mg/kg for children. Take all nitrofurantoins with food or milk to decrease GI distress.
		Children: 5–7 mg/kg/d in 4 divided doses for at least 7 d	All nitrofurantoins are contraindicated in infants under age 1 mo. Suspension should be shaken well before measurement, using a calibrated measuring device. Store at room temperature. The oral suspension can be mixed with water, milk, fruit juice, or infant formula, although it may discolor.
	Long-term suppression of urinary tract infection	*Adults:* 50–100 mg at bedtime *Children:* 1 mg/kg/24 h in 1 or 2 divided doses	As above
	Urinary tract infection: If *Escherichia coli* resistance ≥20% or sulfa allergy	*Adults:* 50–100 mg qid with meals and at bedtime for 7 d	

Continued

Table 24–28 ● Dosage Schedule: Sulfonamides, Trimethoprim, and Nitrofurantoin—cont'd

Drug	Indication	Dose	Comments
Monohydrate macrocrystals (Macrobid)	Urinary tract infections	*Adults:* 100 mg q12h for 3–7 d	As above
	Urinary tract infection: If *E. coli* resistance ≥20% or sulfa allergy	*Adults:* 50–100 mg bid for 7 d	
Sulfadiazine	Antibacterial or antiprotozoal	*Adults:* 2–4 g as initial dose, then 1 g q4–6h *Children:* 75 mg/kg as initial dose, then 37.5 mg/kg q6h or 25 mg/kg q4h	Take with a full glass of water.
Sulfamethoxazole (Gantanol)	Antibacterial or antiprotozoal, mild to moderate infections	*Adults:* Initial dose of 2 g, followed by 1 g q8–10h *Children >2 mo:* 50–60 mg/kg to maximum of 2 g initially, followed by 25–30 mg/kg q12h	Maximum dose for children is 75 mg/kg. Fluid intake should be sufficient to maintain urine output of at least 1,200 mL/d. Most crystalluria-prone sulfonamide. Take with full glass of water.
Sulfisoxazole (Gantrisin)	Recurrent acute otitis media	*Children:* 50 mg/kg/d in 2 divided doses q12h	Maximum adult daily dose 8 g; maximum daily pediatric dose 6 g. Take with full glass of water. Fluid intake should be sufficient to maintain urine output of at least 1,200 mL/d. Shake suspension well before measurement, using calibrated dosing device. Store at room temperature.
	Rheumatic fever prophylaxis (secondary)	*Adults:* With carditis, 1 g/d for 10 y or until age 25 Without carditis, 1 g/d for 5 y or until aged 18	As above
	Antibacterial or antiprotozoal	*Adults:* 2–4 g initially, then 750 mg–1.5 g q4h; 1–2 g q6h *Children >2 mo:* 75 mg/kg or 2 g/m² initially, followed by 25 mg/kg q4h or 37.5 mg/kg q6h	As above
Trimethoprim (Polytrim, Trimpex)	Urinary tract infection, treatment	*Adults:* 100 mg q12h for 10 d or 200 mg daily *Children >2 mo:* 3 mg/kg bid for 10 d	May be taken on an empty stomach or with food to decrease GI distress. Doses >600 mg daily have been used to treat *Pneumocystis carinii.*
	Urinary tract infection, prophylaxis	*Adults:* 100 mg/d	As above
Trimethoprim (TMP)/ Sulfamethoxazole (SMZ) (Bactrim, Septra)	Urinary tract infection: If *E. coli* resistance < 20%	*Adults:* 160 mg TMP/800 mg SMZ bid for 3 days *Children >2 mo:* 6–12 mg TMP/30–60 mg SMZ per kg/d in two divided doses × 10 d	If empirical 3-d treatment fails, culture urine for treatment decision. For pyelonephritis duration of therapy is 7–14 d; in pregnancy duration of therapy is 7 d.
	MRSA	*Adults:* 160 mg TMP/800 mg SMZ for 7 to 10 d *Children >2 mo:* 4–6 mg TMP mg 1 kg/dose TMP/ 20–30 mg/kg/dose SMZ for 7–10 d	

Table 24–28 ◉ **Dosage Schedule: Sulfonamides, Trimethoprim, and Nitrofurantoin—cont'd**

Drug	Indication	Dose	Comments
	Chronic suppression of urinary tract infection in women	*Adults:* 40 mg TMP/200 mg SMZ at bedtime a minimum of 3 times wk and postcoitally	Dose is ½ of a single-strength tablet.
	Otitis media: For children with penicillin allergies	*Children:* 8 mg TMP/40 mg SMZ per kg/d in two divided doses q12h	Not first-line therapy. Only for penicillin allergy.
	Acute exacerbation of chronic bronchitis	*Adults:* 160 mg TMP and 800 mg SMZ q12h for 14 d	As above
	P. carinii pneumonia prophylaxis	*Adults:* 160 TMP and 800 SMZ orally q24h *Children:* 150 mg/m^2 TMP and 750 mg/m^2 SMZ/d in 2 divided doses on 3 consecutive d	As above

Upper Respiratory Infection

TMP-SMZ is considered an alternative first-line therapy in patients with sinusitis who are allergic to penicillin (Rosenfeld et al, 2007). TMP-SMZ is no longer recommended in the treatment of AOM. Although TMP-SMZ is effective in vitro against group A beta-hemolytic *S. pyogenes,* it does not eradicate the organism or protect against rheumatic fever. Thus, it should not be used to treat streptococcal pharyngitis.

Exacerbations of Chronic Bronchitis

Although treatment of ABECB is controversial, TMP-SMZ may be a good choice for patients who have not taken **antibiotics** recently and therefore are less likely to be infected with a resistant strain and for those with a persistent cough (Rabe et al, 2007). Treatment is one DS tablet twice daily for 14 days. Another advantage of this formulation is low cost. However, with repeated use of TMP-SMZ, resistant organisms are likely to prevail and it is not first-line therapy.

MRSA

Methicillin-resistant *Staphylococcus aureus* (MRSA) has emerged as a common pathogen in both hospital-acquired and community-acquired infections. Depending on local resistance patterns, TMP-SMZ is an inexpensive treatment for community-acquired MRSA (CA-MRSA) (CDC, 2006b; Oregon Health Sciences University, n.d.).

Other

TMP-SMZ is approved for treatment of shigellosis enteritis in adults and children. It also is used for the prevention and treatment of pneumonia caused by the protozoon *Pneumocystis jiroveci* (PCP) in immunocompromised patients, particularly HIV patients (Benson et al, 2004; Mofeson et al, 2009). Malaria is another protozoal infection that **sulfonamides** are used to treat as part of multidrug therapy. **Sulfonamides** are inexpensive agents used primarily outside North America to treat trachoma, inclusion conjunctivitis, toxoplasmosis, chancroid, and meningitis.

Rational Drug Selection

Both definitive drug selection and empirical drug selection follow the same principles described in the Rational Drug Selection section for the **penicillins**, regardless of the infection or drug class involved. Although no longer primary agents for any infectious disease, the **sulfonamides**, **trimethoprim**, and **nitrofurantoin** are useful, low-cost alternatives for pregnancy, children, and individuals with **penicillin** allergy. Because **trimethoprim** and **nitrofurantoin** are indicated as monotherapy only for UTI, use of these agents does not contribute as much to selection pressure that promotes resistance to drugs used for other infections. **Sulfonamides** are the most allergenic drug group and should be avoided in those with hypersensitivity to other **sulfonamides** (e.g., **loop diuretics**, **thiazide diuretics**, **sulfonylurea antidiabetic drugs**) and used with caution in patients with severe allergy or bronchial asthma.

Nitrofurantoin is available as microcrystals, macrocrystals, and monohydrate macrocrystals. **Microcrystals** (**Furadantin**) cause excessive GI irritation and should not be used. **Monohydrate macrocrystals** (**Macrobid**) form a gel that gradually releases the drug, requiring only twice-daily dosing, whereas **macrocrystals** (**Macrodantin**) require administration every 6 hours. **Nitrofurantoin** should be used with caution in those predisposed to its adverse effects: older patients and patients with anemia, renal impairment, electrolyte imbalance, diabetes, vitamin B deficiency, and debilitating diseases.

Monitoring

Monitoring for therapeutic response to **antibiotics** is described in the Monitoring section for **penicillins**. Culture of the urine to follow up a UTI will verify eradication of the infection. If a patient is on long-term therapy of **nitrofurantoin**, **trimethoprim**, or a **sulfonamide**, periodic assessment of the complete blood cell (CBC) count, hepatic function, and renal function should be conducted. For **nitrofurantoin**, there should also be periodic evaluation of pulmonary function for signs of fibrosis, physical examination for indications of peripheral neuropathy, and urine culture; superinfections with *Pseudomonas* or *Candida* sometimes occur with chronic therapy. Elderly patients on **nitrofurantoin** should be monitored closely because serious adverse effects such as acute pneumonitis and peripheral neuropathy occur more commonly in this population. Any patient on **nitrofurantoin** who develops cough, dyspnea, chest pain, or fever should receive a chest x-ray, sedimentation rate, and CBC to detect the signs of hypersensitivity and pulmonary fibrosis. Patients on long-term sulfonamide therapy should also have periodic urinalysis to check for crystalluria or urinary calculi formation. Patients with AIDS are prone to adverse effects of **sulfonamides**.

Patient Education

Administration

Patient counseling for all **antimicrobials** includes advice to complete the entire course of therapy, take the medications as prescribed on a regular schedule, and abstain from sharing medications with others. Available dosage forms are shown in Table 24–29. **Sulfonamides** and solid or liquid forms of **trimethoprim-sulfamethoxazole** should be taken with a full glass of water and sufficient daily fluid intake to maintain 1,200 mL urine output in the adult. **Nitrofurantoin** causes less GI distress and is better absorbed if taken with food or milk. Suspensions should be shaken before measurement and taken with a specially marked measuring spoon or comparable device.

Adverse Reactions

Patients taking **sulfonamides** and **trimethoprim** or combinations containing these agents should be counseled to avoid photosensitivity or photoallergy by wearing protective clothing and sunscreens. They should not expose their skin to ultraviolet light from sun or tanning lamps more than a few minutes until tolerance is determined. The patient who develops a rash while taking these

Table 24–29 ◆ **Available Dosage Forms: Sulfonamides, Trimethoprim, and Nitrofurantoin**

Drug	Dosage Form	How Supplied	Cost*
Nitrofurantoin (Furadantin)	Oral suspension: 25 mg/5 mL	In 60- and 470-mL bottles	
Nitrofurantoin macrocrystals	Capsules: 50 mg, 100 mg	In bottles of 100, 500, 1,000 capsules	$128, $104
(Macrodantin)	Capsules: 25 mg 50 mg, 100 mg	In bottles of 100 capsules In bottles of 100, 500, 1,000 capsules	$87 $114, $192
(Macrobid) Sulfadiazine	Capsules: 100 mg Tablets: 500 mg	In bottles of 100 capsules In bottles of 100, 1,000 tablets	$209
Sulfamethoxazole (Gantanol)	Tablets: 500 mg	In bottles of 100 tablets	
Trimethoprim and sulfamethoxazole	Tablets: 400 mg/80 mg 800 mg/160 mg Oral suspension: 200 mg/ 40 mg/5 mL	In bottles of 100, 500 tablets In bottles of 100, 500 double-strength tablets In 150-, 240-, 480-mL bottles	$4/20 $15.99/30 $4/20 $15.99/30 $4/120 mL $18.99/200 mL $10/360 mL
(Bactrim)	Tablets: 400 mg/80 mg 800 mg/160 mg Oral suspension: 200 mg/ 40 mg/5 mL	In bottles of 100 tablets In bottles of 150, 250, 500 tablets In 480-mL bottles (cherry flavor)	$51.07/30 $92.87/30
(Cotrim)	Tablets: 400 mg/80 mg 800 mg/160 mg Oral suspension: 200 mg/ 40 mg/5 mL	In bottles of 100, 500 tablets In bottles of 100, 500 double-strength tablets In 473-mL bottles	

Table 24–29 ◆ **Available Dosage Forms: Sulfonamides, Trimethoprim, and Nitrofurantoin—cont'd**

Drug	Dosage Form	How Supplied	Cost*
(Septra)	Tablets: 400 mg/80 mg 800 mg/160 mg Oral suspension: 200 mg/ 40 mg/5 mL	In bottles of 100 tablets In bottles of 100, 250 double-strength tablets In 20-, 100-, 150-, 200-, 473-mL bottles (cherry flavor); in 473-mL bottles (grape flavor)	$105 $178 $206
(Sulfatrim)	Oral suspension: 200 mg/ 40 mg/5 mL	In 473-mL bottles	$78
Sulfisoxazole (Gantrisin)	Tablets: 500 mg	In bottles of 100, 500 tablets	
Trimethoprim	Tablets: 100 mg 200 mg	In bottles of 14, 30, 100 tablets In bottles of 100 tablets	$44
(Proloprim)	Tablets: 100 mg, 200 mg	In bottles of 100 tablets	
(Trimpex)	Tablets: 100 mg	In bottles of 100 tablets	

*Cost per 100 units unless otherwise stated.

agents should discontinue the drug and contact the health-care provider; rash may develop into Stevens-Johnson syndrome. Patients on **sulfonamides** should also report signs of crystalluria (blood in urine) and blood dyscrasias (sore throat, fever, chills, pale skin, unusual bleeding or bruising). **Sulfonamides** may cause dizziness that can make operation of machinery and automobiles dangerous.

Counseling for patients on **nitrofurantoin** includes similar cautions for signs of blood dyscrasias (sore throat, fever, chills, pale skin, unusual bleeding or bruising). Patients should know that the drug may cause brownish discoloration of the urine and elicit a false positive on copper sulfate urine tests for glucose. Patients should call the health-care provider if there are signs of acute pulmonary fibrosis (sudden onset of chest pain, dyspnea, cough, fever) or subacute pulmonary fibrosis (dyspnea, nonproductive cough, malaise after 1 to 6 mo of therapy). Because rechallenge with **nitrofurantoin** could cause rapid return of the pulmonary condition, the patient should be provided with written information to warn future health-care providers of the reaction. Other symptoms to report are signs of peripheral neuropathy (numbness, tingling, pain in extremities) and intolerable GI upset.

Lifestyle Management

See the Lifestyle Management section for the **penicillins**.

TETRACYCLINES

Tetracyclines are broad-spectrum **antibiotics** that are used extensively throughout the world. Originally introduced in 1948, they are used in the United States mainly for uncommon infections because newer **antibiotics** can treat common susceptible infections with fewer adverse reactions and drug–drug and drug–food interactions. The second generation drug **doxycycline (Doxy, Doxychel, Vibramycin)** has fewer problems with drug–food interactions and is frequently used to treat sexually transmitted infections and as one of four drugs in the treatment of *H. pylori* infection. **Tetracycline** is used both topically and orally to treat acne. Topical application is discussed in Chapters 23 and 32.

Pharmacodynamics

Tetracyclines include a group of drugs with a common basic structure and activity. Hydrochloride forms of these drugs are more soluble, and **doxycycline** and **minocycline (Dynacin, Minocin)** are highly lipid soluble. The hydrochloride forms are acidic and fairly stable. **Tetracyclines** chelate divalent and trivalent ions, which can interfere with their absorption and activity.

These drugs enter microorganisms by passive diffusion and energy-dependent active transport. Susceptible cells concentrate the drug intracellularly. Once inside the cell, they bind reversibly to the 30S subunit of the bacterial ribosome, eventually preventing the addition of amino acids to growing peptides. They are bacteriostatic for many gram-positive and gram-negative organisms, including anaerobes, *Rickettsia,* Chlamydia, mycoplasmas, and some protozoa, including amoebae.

Sensitivity

Tetracyclines are active against *Rickettsia* (Rocky Mountain spotted fever, typhus, Q fever, rickettsial pox, and tick fever); *M. pneumoniae, Borrelia recurrentis* (relapsing fever); and the agents responsible for psittacosis, lymphogranuloma venereum, and granuloma inguinale.

Gram-negative organisms that **tetracyclines** are effective against include *Haemophilus ducreyi* (chancroid), *Yersinia pestis, Francisella tularensis, Bartonella bacilliformis, Bacteroides* species, *Acinetobacter, Vibrio cholerae,* and *Brucella*. Although not first-line therapy, they also are active against *E. coli*, *Shigella*, *H. influenzae*, and *Klebsiella* respiratory and urinary infection.

When **penicillin** is contraindicated, **tetracycline** may be used as an alternative for treatment of infections due to *N. gonorrhoeae*, *T. pallidum*, *Treponema pertenue* (yaws), *Clostridium*, and *Bacillus anthracis*.

Because extensive use of **tetracyclines** in the past has resulted in bacterial resistance that may be as high as 74 percent in some organisms, these drugs should not used for common infections unless the organism has been shown by culture and sensitivity testing.

Doxycycline is considered first-line therapy for *C. trachomatis*, and *Ureaplasma urealyticum*. **Minocycline** is used for treatment of asymptomatic nasopharyngeal carriers of *N. meningitidis*. **Tetracycline** and **minocycline** appear to inhibit the growth of *Propionibacterium acnes* on the skin surface and reduce the concentration of free fatty acids in sebum.

Resistance

The mechanisms of resistance to **tetracyclines** are (1) decreased intracellular accumulation due to impaired influx or increased efflux of an active transport protein pump, (2) ribosome protection by proteins that interfere with drug binding, and (3) enzymatic inactivation. The most important is the pump activity. The pump protein is encoded on a plasmid and may be transmitted to other organisms. Cross-resistance may occur with **aminoglycosides**, **sulfonamides**, and **chloramphenicol**.

Pharmacokinetics

Absorption and Distribution

Tetracyclines are adequately but incompletely absorbed in the fasting state. The percentage of oral dose absorbed is highest for **doxycycline** and **minocycline** (95% to 100%) and intermediate for **oxytetracycline** (**Terramycin**) and **tetracycline** (60% to 70%). Achlorhydria has no effect on absorption of **tetracyclines**. Food and polyvalent cations (Ca++, Mg++, Fe+++, and Al++) decrease absorption of **tetracycline** and **oxytetracycline** but have little effect on **doxycycline** or **minocycline**.

Doxycycline and **minocycline** are highly lipid soluble; readily penetrate the CSF, brain, eye, and prostate; and cross placental membranes. Fetal plasma concentrations reach 60 percent of maternal serum levels. **Minocycline** displays good penetration of saliva. **Tetracycline** has intermediate lipid solubility, and **oxytetracycline** has the least.

Oxytetracycline readily diffuses across the placenta into fetal circulation and into pleural fluid.

Metabolism and Excretion

This class of drugs undergoes enterohepatic recirculation, is concentrated by the liver in the bile, and is excreted in both urine and feces, largely unchanged. Because renal clearance is by glomerular filtration, excretion is significantly affected by renal function. Dosage adjustments of **tetracycline** and **oxytetracycline** are required for renal impairment. **Doxycycline** is secreted in inactive form into the intestinal lumen and eliminated in feces.

Some is excreted unchanged in the urine. Its half-life does not significantly increase in renal impairment, so no dosage adjustments are required. **Minocycline** is metabolized by the liver and its half-life is prolonged in oliguria. Because it also uses nonrenal routes of excretion, however, dosage adjustments are not required in renal impairment. Table 24–30 describes the pharmacokinetics of selected **tetracyclines**.

Table 24–30 ▶ **Pharmacokinetics: Tetracyclines**

Drug	Onset	Peak	Duration	Protein Binding	Bioavailability	Half-Life	Elimination
Doxycycline	1–2 h	1.5–4 h	12 h	80%–95%	93%	18–22 h	30%–42% unchanged in urine; some inactivation in intestine; remainder excreted in bile and feces
Minocycline	Rapid	2–3 h	6–12 h	70%–80%	90%	11–22 h	5%–10% unchanged in urine; some metabolism by liver; remainder excreted in bile and feces
Oxytetracycline	1–2 h	2–4 h	6–12 h	20%–40%	UA	6–12 h	10%–35% unchanged in urine
Tetracycline	1–2 h	2–4 h	6–12 h	65%	60%–80%	6–12 h	20%–55% unchanged in urine

UA = Information unavailable.

Pharmacotherapeutics

Precautions and Contraindications

There are a number of patients for whom the **tetracyclines** should be prescribed cautiously; such patients include those with renal impairment, those with hepatic impairment, pregnant women, lactating women, and children.

Renal Impairment

Extreme caution should be used in the presence of renal impairment. Even usual doses of **tetracyclines** (except **doxycycline** and **minocycline**) may lead to excessive accumulation of the drugs and possible hepatotoxicity, so lower-than-normal doses are required in renal impairment. If therapy is prolonged, assay of drug serum concentration may be advisable. The antianabolic actions of **tetracyclines** (except **doxycycline**) may cause an increase in BUN and lead to azotemia, hyperphosphatemia, and acidosis in the presence of severe renal impairment.

Hepatic Impairment

There are serious concerns related to hepatotoxicity for IV forms of **tetracycline**. This is not a major concern with oral administration, but liver function studies are advisable during long-term management with **doxycycline** or **minocycline**.

Hepatotoxicity has been reported with **minocycline**, and it should be used with caution in patients with hepatic dysfunction.

Pregnancy

Doxycycline is Pregnancy Category D. Others are Pregnancy Category X and should not be used during pregnancy. They readily cross the placenta in concentrations up to 60 percent of maternal plasma. **Tetracyclines** are found in fetal tissue and can produce retardation of skeletal development in the fetus and staining of deciduous teeth.

Lactation

Tetracyclines are excreted in breast milk. A dosage of 2 g/day for 3 days has achieved a milk:plasma ratio of 0.6 to 0.8. Because of the potential for serious adverse reactions, these drugs are not recommended during lactation.

Children

Children younger than 8 years generally should not use any **tetracycline**. These drugs form a stable calcium complex in any bone-forming tissue, decreasing bone growth. They also may cause permanent yellow/gray/brown discoloration of deciduous and permanent teeth. Enamel hypoplasia has also been reported. **Doxycycline** is less likely to produce these problems, but the risk outweighs any potential benefit for most indications.

Adverse Drug Reactions

As with other **antibiotics**, the most common adverse reactions are associated with the GI tract. Anorexia, nausea, vomiting, and diarrhea are caused by direct irritation of the intestinal mucosa. Taking the drug with food (note food interactions above), reducing the dose, or discontinuing the drug usually controls them. Esophageal ulcers have occasionally occurred but can be avoided by taking the drug with a full glass of water and remaining upright for at least 1 to 2 minutes after taking the drug. As broad-spectrum **antibiotics**, **tetracyclines** can cause AAPMC, previously discussed in the sections on **penicillins**, **cephalosporins**, and **clindamycin**.

Lightheadedness, dizziness, and vertigo have been reported in 35 to 70 percent of patients taking **minocycline** and in some patients taking **doxycycline**. Pseudotremor cerebri (benign intracranial hypertension) has also been associated with **tetracycline** and **minocycline** use. Symptoms are headache and blurred vision and bulging fontanels in infants. Discontinuing the drug usually resolves these problems, but the possibility for permanent sequelae exists.

Dermatological adverse reactions include photosensitivity manifested by an exaggerated sunburn reaction, as well as maculopapular and erythematous rashes. Blue gray pigmentation of skin and mucosa has been reported with **minocycline**.

Under no circumstances should outdated **tetracyclines** be administered. The degradation products of these drugs are highly nephrotoxic, and reversible nephrotoxicity including a Fanconi-like syndrome has been reported.

Drug Interactions

The main drug–drug and drug–food interactions associated with **tetracyclines** are with **antacids**, **iron salts**, and **dairy products**, based on the formation of poorly soluble chelated compounds. The result is a decrease in **antibiotic** activity. Separation of these products from the administration of **tetracyclines** by at least 2 hours, taking the **tetracycline** first, is recommended. **Doxycycline** and **minocycline** have less affinity for these products and are not significantly affected. Whether **tetracyclines** cause a decrease in efficacy of **oral contraceptives** is controversial, but the alleged mechanism is related to the enterohepatic recirculation of **tetracycline** and **oral contraceptives**. It does seem prudent to suggest the use of a barrier contraceptive method while the patient is taking the **tetracycline** and until the next menses. These and other interactions of the **tetracyclines** are shown in Table 24–31.

Clinical Use and Dosing

The **tetracyclines** are prescribed for sexually transmitted infections, acne, *H. pylori*, and other less common infections.

Genitourinary Infections

One of the most important indications for **doxycycline** is treatment of genital *C. trachomatis* infections and

Table 24–31 ■ **Drug Interactions: Tetracyclines**

Drug	Interacting Drug	Possible Effects	Implications
Tetracyclines	Antacids, dairy foods, iron salts, and sodium bicarbonate	Impair absorption because of formation of a poorly soluble chelate	Take on empty stomach or separate doses by 2 h and take tetracycline first. Doxycycline and minocycline have low affinity for these and are not significantly affected by food or dairy products.
	Oral anticoagulants	Tetracyclines may increase hypoprothrombinemic effects	Avoid concurrent administration or monitor PT/INR closely.
	Barbiturates, carbamazepine, hydantoins	Increase metabolism and decrease half-life and serum levels of doxycycline	Antibacterial activity decreased. Avoid concurrent administration.
	Cimetidine	Decreased GI absorption of tetracyclines because of pH-dependent inhibition of dissolution	Antibacterial activity decreased. May be true for other histamine$_2$ blockers. Avoid concurrent administration.
	Digoxin	Serum levels of digoxin increased in 10% of patients with risk for toxicity	Effects last for months after tetracycline discontinued. Select different antibiotic class.
	Insulin	May reduce insulin requirements	Further study needed. Monitor blood glucose closely.
	Lithium	May increase or decrease lithium levels	Monitor serum levels closely.
	Oral contraceptives	May decrease effectiveness; breakthrough bleeding may occur	Controversial. Suggest barrier method for women taking tetracyclines.
	Penicillin	May interfere with bactericidal action of penicillins	Avoid concomitant administration.

INR = international normalized ratio; PT = prothrombin time.

nongonococcal urethritis and cervicitis. **Doxycycline** in doses of 100 mg twice daily for 7 days is a first-line agent because of its low cost, but it may have lower compliance than the more expensive **azithromycin**, which requires a single dose in these infections (CDC, 2010e). Sexual partners should be evaluated and treated. **Doxycycline** is contraindicated in pregnancy; the drug of choice for pregnant women is **amoxicillin** or **azithromycin** (CDC, 2010e). In **penicillin**-allergic patients, **doxycycline** (100 mg orally twice daily) or **tetracycline** (500 mg orally four times daily), for 14 days is the only recommended alternative treatment of early primary, secondary, or latent syphilis of less than 1 year's duration (CDC, 2010e). For latent syphilis of more than 1 year's duration without neurosyphilis, a longer course of treatment (28 d) is required.

Doxycycline (100 mg twice daily for 10 d) combined with **ceftriaxone** (250 mg IM) is indicated for empirical treatment of epididymo-orchitis in heterosexual men less than 35 years of age where the likely pathogens are *C. trachomatis* or *N. gonorrhoeae* (CDC, 2010e).

Men with acute proctitis who practice receptive anal sex should be treated with a combination of antibiotics that cover for *N. gonorrhoeae* and *C. trachomatis*. The CDC guidelines (2006a) recommend **ceftriaxone** 250 mg IM combined with **doxycycline** 100 mg twice daily for 7 days. Chronic prostatitis, the most common form, is a chronic pain syndrome of unknown etiology. Studies suggest it may have a microbial etiology, and **doxycycline** (100 mg twice daily for 14 d) is used empirically for treatment.

Acne

Patients with moderate, inflammatory acne who show no improvement with 6 to 8 weeks of topical therapy may be treated with oral **antibiotics** to treat the *P. acnes* that cause inflammatory papules and pustules. Treatment is **tetracycline (Achromycin)** 500 mg twice daily for 1 to 2 months; then, when acne control is achieved, the dose is lowered to 500 mg per day for 1 to 2 months, after which a maintenance dose of 125 to 500 mg daily is taken. **Minocycline** is an alternative, although more expensive treatment. Dosing of **minocycline** is 100 mg twice daily; then the patient is weaned to 50 mg daily. In comparing the cost for 100 capsules, **tetracycline** 500-mg capsules are $19.99, and **minocycline** is $75 for 100-mg capsules. **Doxycycline** is an oral alternative to topical **metronidazole** in the treatment of acne rosacea.

Peptic Ulcer Disease

Tetracycline is one component of the quadruple drug regimen used for the eradication of *H. pylori* associated with peptic ulcer disease (PUD). **Tetracycline** 500 mg four times a day is combined with **metronidazole** 250 mg four times a day, **bismuth subsalicylate** 525 mg four times a day and a **proton pump inhibitor** to treat PUD. The quadruple drug therapy is more complex than the triple drug therapy. Full prescribing information for PUD is found in Chapter 34.

Lyme Disease

The International Lyme and Associated Diseases Society (ILADS) has released evidence-based guidelines recommending early and aggressive **antibiotic** treatment to prevent Lyme disease from becoming persistent or recurrent (Cameron et al, 2006). **Doxycycline,** 100 mg twice daily, is the first-line drug of choice for early treatment of Lyme disease, a tickborne infection caused by *B. burgdorferi.* Duration of oral treatment varies by the presenting signs: early erythema migrans (14 to 21 d), mild cardiac involvement (21 d), arthritis (28 d), and isolated facial paralysis (21 to 28 d). **Amoxicillin** is the alternative for pregnant women and children younger than 8 years, for whom **doxycycline** is contraindicated (*Sanford Guide,* 2010). The ILADS recommends early empirical treatment for patients with a likely diagnosis of Lyme disease, while waiting for laboratory confirmation (Cameron et al, 2006).

Other

Doxycycline is an alternative for **penicillin**-allergic patients for prophylaxis of rat, bat, raccoon, and skunk bites (*Sanford Guide,* 2010). The primary drug of choice for ehrlichiosis and rickettsial infections (e.g., Rocky Mountain spotted fever, typhus, Q fever, trench fever caused by *B. quintana*) is **doxycycline. Minocycline,** 100 mg twice daily for 6 to 8 weeks, is the drug of first choice for infections by *Mycobacterium marinum,* an infection associated with contamination by water from aquariums. **Minocycline** is also recommended for treating the meningitis carrier state, as an alternative to **sulfonamides** in nocardiosis, and in the treatment of rheumatoid arthritis (100 mg twice daily). **Tetracyclines** are first-line therapy for a number of diseases rarely seen in North America, including trachoma, cholera, and granuloma inguinale. **Doxycycline** 100 mg twice daily for 6 days is an alternative therapy for post-exposure prophylaxis to anthrax (*Sanford Guide,* 2010). **Doxycycline** is also used in prophylaxis and treatment of falciparum malaria and as an adjunct in treatment of intestinal amebiasis. Table 24–32 presents the dosage schedule of **tetracyclines**.

Rational Drug Selection

Both definitive drug selection and empirical drug selection follow the same principles described in the Rational Drug Selection section for the **penicillins**, regardless of the infection or drug class involved. When a patient with renal impairment requires a **tetracycline, doxycycline** is

Table 24–32 ◉ **Dosage Schedule: Tetracyclines**

Drug	Indication	Dose	Comments
Doxycycline (Vibramycin)	Antibacterial	*Adults:* 50–100 mg q12h *Children >8 yr:* 2.2–4.4 mg/kg/d divided into 2 doses q12h	Maximal daily adult dose 500 mg for 5 d for acute gonococcal infection; 300 mg for all other infections. Shake suspension well before measurement with calibrated device. Store at room temperature for up to 14 d. Do not take this drug within 1 h of other medicines; separation of 3 h preferable. May be administered without regard to meals.
Anthrax (post-exposure prophylaxis)		*Children <8 yr:* 2.2 mg/kg q12h (max 100 mg/dose) *Children ≥ 8 yr and adults:* 2.2 mg/kg q12h (max 100 mg/dose)	
	Endocervical, rectal, or urethral infection caused by *Chlamydia trachomatis*	*Adults:* 100 mg q12h for 7 d	As above
	Epididymo-orchitis caused by *C. trachomatis* or *Neisseria gonorrhoeae;* nongonococcal urethritis	*Adults:* 100 mg q12h for 10 d	As above

Continued

Table 24–32 ◉ Dosage Schedule: Tetracyclines—cont'd

Drug	Indication	Dose	Comments
	Gonococcal infections, uncomplicated	*Adults:* 100 mg q12h for 7 d	Ceftriaxone is 1st line treatment.
	Lyme disease	*Adults:* 100 mg q12h *Children >8 yr:* 1–2 mg/kg q12h	As above
	Malaria prophylaxis	*Adults:* 100 mg daily beginning 1–2 wk before travel, continued through visit and for 4 wk after traveler leaves the malarious area *Children >8 yr:* 2 mg/kg daily, up to 100 mg daily on same schedule as adult	As above
	Early syphilis in penicillin-allergic patient	*Adults:* 100 mg q12h for 14 d (extend to 4 wk if >1 y duration)	As above
	Acne vulgaris	*Adolescents and adults:* 100 mg bid for inflammatory form	May wean
	Acne rosacea	*Adults:* 100 mg q12h	As above
	Acute exacerbation of chronic bronchitis	*Adults:* 100 mg q12h for 5–10 d	As above
	Bite of rat, bat, raccoon (prophylaxis)	*Adolescents and adults:* 100 mg q12h	As above
Minocycline (Dynacin, Minocin)	Antibacterial, other infections	*Adults:* 200 mg base initially, then 100 mg q12h; *or* 100–200 mg initially, then 50 mg q6h *Children >8 yr:* 4 mg base/kg initially, then 2 mg/kg q12h	As above
	Acne	*Adolescents ≥12 yr:* 100 mg bid for 1 to 2 months then wean to 50 mg/d	Treat for at least 12 wks.
Oxytetracycline (Terramycin)	Brucellosis	*Adults:* 500 mg q6h for 6 wk, given concurrently with 1 g streptomycin IM q12h the first wk and once/d the second wk	Maximum daily adult dose 4 g; maximum daily pediatric dose 250 mg. Take with full glass of water. Keep container tightly closed in a dry place. Store at room temperature. Parenteral dose must be given by deep IM injection; do not administer IV. Change to oral form as soon as possible.
Tetracycline (Achromycin V)	Acne	*Adults:* 500 mg–2 g/d in divided doses for severe cases; gradually reduce to maintenance dose of 125 mg–1 g/d in divided doses. Alternate-day dosing or intermittent therapy possible if in remission.	Shake suspension well before measurement with calibrated device. Not for children <8 yr. Keep container tightly closed in a dry place. Store at room temperature. Heed expiration date. Dispose of excess or leftover drug.

Table 24–32 ● **Dosage Schedule: Tetracyclines—cont'd**

Drug	Indication	Dose	Comments
			Do not take within 1–3 h of other drugs. Take with full 8-oz glass of water, and stand for at least 90 sec after swallowing. Take drug at least 1 h before bedtime.
	Brucellosis	*Adults:* 500 mg qid for 3 wk in combination with streptomycin 1 g bid for the first wk and 1 g/d for second wk	As above
	Lyme disease (off-labeled use)	*Adults:* 250–500 mg qid *Children >8 yr:* 6.25–12.5 mg/kg qid	As above
	Syphilis	*Adults:* 30–40 g over 10–15 d	As above
	Uncomplicated rectal, urethral, or endocervical infections by *C. trachomatis*	*Adults:* 500 mg qid for at least 7 d	As above
	Other bacterial infections	*Adults:* 250–500 q6h *or* 500 mg–1 g q12h *Children >8 yr:* 6.25–12.5 mg/kg q6h *or* 12.5–25 mg q12h	As above

preferred; it does not require dosage adjustment and lacks the antianabolic effects that increase azotemia when other **tetracyclines** are used. Another advantage of **doxycycline** and **minocycline** is decreased chelation with polyvalent cations, which allows them to be taken with meals if necessary. Additionally, these two agents also require fewer daily doses than other **tetracyclines.** Unfortunately, **tetracyclines** are contraindicated in children younger than 8 years and during pregnancy because of bone and teeth abnormalities in the fetus and young child, as well as increased risk of hepatotoxicity during pregnancy. Besides age and pregnancy, reasons to choose alternative agents over **tetracyclines** are concurrent administration of other hepatotoxic drugs and risk of noncompliance with the complex scheduling required to avoid drug–food interactions.

Monitoring

Monitoring for therapeutic response to antimicrobial drugs is described in the Monitoring section for **penicillins.** Long-term therapy with **tetracyclines** exceeding several weeks requires periodic hematopoietic, hepatic, and renal function tests. Because **doxycycline** is metabolized by CYP450-dependent enzymes, other drugs can induce or inhibit its metabolism. Patients should be assessed for potential interactions of other drugs with **doxycycline,** particularly inducers such as **rifampin, phenytoin, carbamazepine,** and **barbiturates** that accelerate **doxycycline** metabolism and may result in therapeutic failure. Additionally, **digoxin** assays should be obtained when a patient takes broad-spectrum **antibiotics** concurrent with **digoxin.**

Patient Education

Administration

Available dosage forms are given in Table 24–33. Oral solid dosing forms of **tetracyclines** should be stored in a tightly closed container in a dry environment to avoid accelerated decomposition that might result in toxic constituents. The patient should note the expiration date and dispose of outdated **tetracycline** that can cause serious toxicity. The entire prescription should be taken, with doses evenly spaced.

Suspension products should be shaken before measurement of the dose with a calibrated dosing device. Although some **tetracyclines** come in liquid formulations for use by adult patients who cannot swallow solids, it should not be assumed they are indicated for children younger than 8 years. Administer **tetracyclines** 1 hour before or 2 hours after meals and give **tetracyclines** 2 hours before **antacids.** However, **doxycycline** and **minocycline** can be taken with meals if they cause GI upset when taken on an empty stomach. To avoid esophageal irritation, take **tetracyclines** at least 1 hour before meals with a full 8 ounce glass of water and remain standing for at least 90 seconds after swallowing the drug.

Table 24–33 ◈ **Available Dosage Forms: Tetracyclines**

Drug	Dosage Form	How Supplied	Cost*
Doxycycline	Capsules: 50 mg	In bottles of 50, 60, 100, 500 capsules	$4/30
	100 mg	In bottles of 10, 11, 14, 20, 50, 100, 200, 500 capsules	$4/20
	Tablets: 100 mg	In bottles of 20, 28, 30, 32, 50, 200, 500 tablets	$4/20
(Doxy Caps)	Capsules: 25 mg, 100 mg	In bottles of 50 capsules	
(Vibramycin)	Capsules: 50 mg	In bottles of 50 capsules	
	100 mg	In bottles of 50, 100, 500 capsules	$466
	Tablets: 100 mg	In bottles of 50, 100, 500 film-coated tablets	$466
	Powder for oral suspension: 25 mg/5 mL (reconstituted)	In 60-mL bottles (raspberry flavor)	
	Syrup: 50 mg/5 mL	In 60-mL bottles	
Minocycline	Capsules: 50 mg	In bottles of 100 capsules	$50
	100 mg	In bottles of 50, 100 capsules	$94
(Dynacin)	Capsules: 50 mg	In bottles of 100 capsules	$334
	100 mg	In bottles of 50, 100 capsules	$582
(Minocin)	Capsules: 50 mg	In bottles of 100 pellet-filled capsules	$221
	100 mg	In bottles of 50 pellet-filled capsules	$364
	Oral suspension: 50 mg/5 mL	In 60-mL bottles (custard flavor)	
Oxytetracycline	Capsules: 250 mg	In bottles of 100, 1,000 capsules	
(Terramycin)	Capsules: 250 mg	In bottles of 100, 500 capsules	
Tetracycline	Oral suspension: 125 mg/5 mL	In 60-, 480-mL bottles	
	Capsules: 100 mg	In bottles of 1,000 capsules	
	250 mg	In bottles of 20, 28, 30, 40, 60, 100, 500, 1,000 capsules	$4/60 $10/180
	500 mg	In bottles of 20, 28, 40, 50, 100, 500, 1,000 capsules	$4/60 $10/180
	Tablets: 250 mg, 500 mg	In bottles of 30, 60 tablets	
(Sumycin)	Oral suspension: 125 mg/5 mL	In 473-mL bottles (fruit flavor)	
	Capsules: 250 mg	In bottles of 100, 1,000 capsules	
	500 mg	In bottles of 100, 500 capsules	
	Tablets: 250 mg	In bottles of 100, 1,000 tablets	
	500 mg	In bottles of 100, 500 tablets	

*Cost in 100 units unless otherwise stated.

Tetracyclines can be particularly dangerous during pregnancy and should be avoided in children younger than 8 years.

Adverse Reactions

Tetracyclines can cause phototoxicity, so sunlight and tanning lights should be avoided. Wear sunscreen, hats, and protective clothing if it is necessary to be in the sun for more than a few minutes. Avoid hazardous activities and driving if dizziness, lightheadedness, or unsteadiness develops, which is most common with **minocycline.** Contact the prescriber if these symptoms interfere with activities of daily living. The patient should stop taking the **tetracycline** and contact a health-care provider if headache and blurred vision develop; these are the symptoms of pseudotumor cerebri. Signs of superinfection that should be reported to the prescriber include pruritus, hoarseness, glossitis, sore throat, dysphagia, or vaginal itching and discharge. The patient should also report symptoms of hepatotoxicity that include upper abdominal pain, nausea, vomiting, dark urine, clay-colored stools, or yellowing of skin or eyes. Diarrhea involving six or more stools per day and blood or mucus in the stool could indicate AAPMC and require discontinuation of the **tetracycline** and consultation with the prescriber. Women of childbearing age would be prudent to use a backup barrier method of contraception during **tetracycline** therapy and until the next menses. Women on **hormone replacement**

should know that broad-spectrum **antibiotics** can cause exacerbation of hot flashes and menopausal symptoms during therapy. **Tetracyclines** can cause reversible pigmentation of skin and mucous membranes, which is more common with **minocycline.**

Lifestyle Management

See the Lifestyle Management section for the **penicillins.**

LIPOGLYCOPEPTIDES

The **lipoglycopeptides** are a group of **antibiotics** consisting of **vancomycin, telavancin (Vibativ)**, and a drug in phase III trials, **dalbavancin (Zeven)**. This group of **antibiotics** is used for severe gram-positive infections such as MRSA resistant to first-line **antibiotics.**

Vancomycin is a narrow-spectrum **antibiotic** that is the first drug in this class. Use of **vancomycin** has increased because of the development of organisms resistant to other drugs. Unfortunately, its widespread use led to the development of strains of **vancomycin**-resistant *Enterococcus* (VRE) and **vancomycin**-intermediate *S. aureus* (VISA), greatly reducing treatment options for some infections, especially nosocomial infections in hospitals.

Telavancin was approved in 2009 for use in complicated skin and skin structure infections (cSSSI) caused by susceptible gram-positive bacteria. It is used IV for skin infections resistant to less powerful antibiotics.

Pharmacodynamics

Vancomycin is a **tricyclic glycopeptide antibiotic** that inhibits cell wall synthesis by binding firmly to the D-A1a-D-A1a terminus of nascent peptidoglycan pentapeptide. The end result is a weakened cell wall susceptible to lysis. The cell membrane is also damaged, contributing to the antibacterial effects.

Telavancin is a lipoglycopeptide antibacterial that is a synthetic derivative of **vancomycin. Telavancin** inhibits cell wall synthesis by binding the bacterial membrane and disrupting membrane barrier function.

Sensitivity

Vancomycin is bactericidal for gram-positive organisms (streptococci, pneumococci, *Corynebacterium, Listeria, Lactobacilli, Actinomyces,* and *Clostridium*) and most pathogenic staphylococci, including those producing beta-lactamase and those resistant to **nafcillin** and **methicillin** (MSSA and MRSA), are killed by a concentration of 4 mcg/mL or less. It kills staphylococci relatively slowly and only if cells are actively dividing.

Telavancin is active against gram-positive organisms including *S. aureus* (including **methicillin**-resistant isolates), *S. pyogenes, E. faecalis* (**vancomycin**-susceptible isolates only), *Streptococcus agalactiae,* and *Streptococcus anginosus* group (includes *S. anginosus, S. intermedius,* and *S. constellatus*). Additionally, *E. faecium* (**vancomycin**-susceptible isolates only), *Staphylococcus haemolyticus,* and *Staphylococcus epidermidis* are more than 90 percent susceptible to **telavancin.**

Resistance

Resistance is due to a modification of the binding site of the peptidoglycan building block. This results in loss of a critical hydrogen bond that facilitates high-affinity binding of **vancomycin** to the target organism. To reduce the development of resistant strains, the CDC has recommended limiting this drug to the following uses only:

1. Avoid or minimize use in the empirical treatment of febrile patients with neutropenia unless the prevalence of MRSA or MRSE is high.
2. **Metronidazole** is the preferred initial treatment for *C. difficile* colitis.
3. Avoid or minimize use of **vancomycin** as surgical prophylaxis and for low-birth-weight infants, intravascular catheter colonization or infection, and peritoneal dialysis.

Although most of these recommendations are related to hospitalized patients, primary care providers should also limit the use of this drug.

There is some cross-resistance between VRE strains with high vancomycin MIC with **telavancin.**

Pharmacokinetics

Absorption and Distribution

Absorption of **vancomycin** from the GI tract is poor, although clinically significant serum concentrations have occurred. Onset of action is rapid, with peak concentrations in 1 hour and a duration of 12 hours. It is 52 to 56 percent protein bound and has less than 1 percent bioavailability by the oral route. Its half-life is 4 to 6 hours in adults and 2 to 3 hours in children. Distribution is wide, with 20 to 30 percent penetration of the CSF. The drug crosses the placenta.

Telavancin is administered IV and is 90 percent protein bound. Its single-dose half-life is 8 hours. Concentrations of **telavancin** in skin blister fluid were 40 percent of those in plasma.

On The Horizon **DALBAVANCIN**

A new glycopeptide antibiotic, **dalbavancin (Zeven)** is in phase III trials. The only other drug structurally related to **dalbavancin** is **vancomycin.** This once-weekly antibiotic is effective against MRSA and MRSE. In 2008 Pfizer withdrew its global applications to conduct further studies on **dalbavancin**. In 2010 Pfizer out-licensed **dalbavancin** to Durata Therapeutics, which will continue phase III trials.

Metabolism and Excretion

Oral doses of **vancomycin** are excreted primarily in feces, but some is excreted in the urine and serum half-life is increased in renal impairment. IV forms are eliminated more than 90 percent by glomerular filtration.

Telavancin is primarily excreted in the urine (76%). Clearance is increased in patients with renal impairment.

Pharmacotherapeutics

Precautions and Contraindications

Because of poor absorption, oral forms of **vancomycin** are unlikely to cause systemic adverse effects. However, clinically significant serum concentration may occur in some patients who have inflammatory conditions of the intestinal mucosa. Extreme care should be taken if this drug must be administered to these patients. **Vancomycin** is ototoxic, with increased risk for these problems in older adults, who may have an underlying hearing loss. It should be used with extreme caution in this population.

Oral vancomycin is listed as Pregnancy Category B, and IV forms are Pregnancy Category C. **Telavancin** is Pregnancy Category C; there are no data on the use of **telavancin** in pregnant women. The VIBATIV pregnancy registry should be contacted to monitor outcomes of **telavancin** exposure during pregnancy at 1-888-658-4228.

Vancomycin is excreted in breast milk, although concentrations in breast milk during oral administration are low. It is unknown whether **telavancin** is excreted in human milk. Exercise caution when giving either drug to a nursing mother. **Vancomycin** has been used in serious infections in neonates and children and there are published doses for neonates, infants, and children. **Vancomycin** use in children is best confined to serious infections during which the child is hospitalized. **Telavancin** has not been studied and is not approved for children younger than age 18 years.

Adverse Drug Reactions

Vancomycin therapy can lead to serious ototoxicity that may be transient or permanent. It has occurred most often in patients with high IV doses, who have underlying hearing loss, or who are receiving concomitant therapy with another ototoxic drug. Serial tests of auditory function may be helpful to minimize this adverse reaction. Reversible neutropenia has occurred. Skin rash is the most common adverse effect with oral therapy.

The significant adverse reaction to **telavancin** is nephrotoxicity, especially in patients who are at risk for decreased renal function (preexisting renal disease, diabetes mellitus, congestive heart failure) and *C. difficile* diarrhea.

If **telavancin** or **vancomycin** is infused too fast the patient may develop Red Man syndrome, a flushing of the upper body, urticaria, pruritus, or rash. Stopping or slowing the infusion usually leads to resolution of the rash. Slow infusion over 60 minutes may decrease the likelihood of developing the syndrome.

Drug Interactions

The only significant interaction between **vancomycin** and drugs used in primary care occur with drugs that also have ototoxic or neurotoxic effects **(aminoglycosides)**. The concomitant administration increases the risk and is to be avoided.

The adverse effects of **telavancin** may be increased by drugs that may affect renal function, such as ACE inhibitors, loop diuretics, and NSAIDS. Renal function should be monitored and the patient observed for adverse effects.

Clinical Use and Dosing

Vancomycin (Vancocin) is used to treat AAPMC caused by *C. difficile;* however, it is recommended that **metronidazole** be tried first. It is also used to treat staphylococcal enterocolitis. It is not effective in any other intestinal infections or in systemic infections unless used in combination with an **aminoglycoside**. Adult dosages are 125 to 500 mg every 6 hours for 7 to 10 days. The maximum daily adult dosage is 2 g. Studies have indicated that higher dosages result in fecal concentrations far in excess of MIC and that the 125-mg dose is as effective as higher doses. Dosage for children is 10 mg/kg, up to 125 mg, every 6 hours. Recurrences, which develop in approximately 25 percent of treated patients, may be treated with a second course of **oral vancomycin, oral metronidazole,** or **oral bacitracin.**

Because of the cost and potential for resistance with vancomycin, the CDC recommends **metronidazole** as the first choice for treating AAPMC. **Cholestyramine resin** has been shown to bind *C. difficile* toxins in vitro and may be used as monotherapy or in conjunction with **antibiotics.**

Vancomycin is available for oral administration in pulvules at 125-mg and 250-mg formulations. It is also available as a powder for reconstitution as a solution of 250 mg/5 mL or 500 mg/6 mL. The more concentrated solution contains ethanol. The solution must be refrigerated after reconstitution and will maintain potency for 14 days. It should be dispensed with a calibrated measuring device.

IV **vancomycin** dose is 2 to 3 g per day (30 to 60 mg/kg/d) in divided doses every 8 to 12 hours, with a dosage adjustment for decreased renal function. The usual dose for infants older than 1 month and children is 10 to 15 mg/kg every 6 hours.

Telavancin dose for complicated skin and skin structure infections is 10 mg/kg IV every 24 hours for 7 to 14 days. Infuse over 60 minutes. In patients with renal function impairment, dosing is adjusted accordingly: CrCl 30 to 50 mL/minute, give 7.5 mg/kg every 24 hours; CrCl 30 to 10 mL/minute, give 10 mg/kg every 48 hours.

Monitoring

For oral **vancomycin**, positive response to therapy will be manifested in cessation of diarrhea and associated symptoms. Proctosigmoidoscopy and/or colonoscopy may be useful to document the presence of pseudomembranous colitis or relapse in patients with persistent symptoms. Enzyme immunoassay of stool samples for the presence of *C. difficile* toxins may remain positive after treatment, so follow-up cultures and toxin assays are not recommended if clinical improvement is complete. Renal function determinations may be warranted periodically during either oral or IV **vancomycin** therapy in patients with renal function impairment or inflammatory disorders of the intestinal mucosa. White blood cell (WBC) count or audiometry may also be monitored during extended or repeat therapy.

Renal function should be measured prior to starting **telavancin** and during treatment at 48 to 72 hour intervals. Pregnancy testing should be done on all women of childbearing age before start of therapy.

Patient Education

Administration

If **cholestyramine** is used in conjunction with **vancomycin**, the medications should be administered several hours apart because **cholestyramine** also binds **oral vancomycin** and prevents its effectiveness. The oral solution can cause a bitter or unpleasant taste and mouth irritation and should be followed by a full glass of water. **Oral vancomycin** can be taken without regard to meals. If the patient is too ill for oral therapy, **vancomycin** solution may be administered by enema, long intestinal tube, or directly into a colonoscopy or ileostomy. **Vancomycin** can also be administered IV for colitis because 6 to 15 percent of parenteral **vancomycin** is excreted in the feces. However, IV **vancomycin** is considerably more dangerous than oral-local use.

Adverse Reactions

Skin rashes may occur and, if serious, should be reported to the health-care provider. Patients with renal impairment or inflammatory colitis should report evidence of ototoxicity (loss of hearing; ringing, buzzing, or fullness in ears; dizziness), neutropenia (chills, coughing, difficult breathing, sore throat, fever), or nephrotoxicity (altered frequency or amount of urine, nausea or vomiting, increased thirst, difficulty breathing, weakness).

Lifestyle Management

Mild cases of *C. difficile* colitis may respond to discontinuation of medication alone. Moderate to severe cases require fluid, electrolyte, and protein replacement. If diarrhea is present, administration of an **antiperistaltic antidiarrheal** (e.g., **atropine** and **diphenoxylate, loperamide, opioids**) is contraindicated because it may delay the elimination of toxins from the colon, thereby prolonging or worsening the condition. Good perianal hygiene will improve patient comfort during this illness.

Patients should be educated about how to prevent spread of skin infections, including hand washing and covering open skin lesions.

ANTIMYCOBACTERIALS

Mycobacterial infections are among the most difficult to cure because mycobacteria (1) grow slowly and are relatively resistant to drugs that are largely dependent on how rapidly cells are dividing, (2) have a lipid-rich cell wall relatively impermeable to many drugs, (3) are usually intracellular and inaccessible to drugs that do not have good intracellular penetration, (4) have the ability to go into a dormant state, and (5) easily develop resistance to any single drug. Tuberculosis, an example of mycobacterial infection, is a worldwide public health issue. In addition to drug–organism issues, adherence is often poor to treatment regimens that include multiple drugs and last for months.

Despite these problems, drug combinations have proved effective in the treatment of mycobacterial disease. Drugs used to treat tuberculosis include first-line drugs (**isoniazid** [INH], **rifampin** [RIF, **Rifadin, Rimactane**], **ethambutol** [EMB, **Myambutol**], **pyrazinamide** [PZA], and **streptomycin**) and second-line drugs used for retreatment or recurrent disease (**para-aminosalicylic acid** [PASA], **ethionamide** [**Trecator-SC**], **capreomycin** [**Capastat**], **cycloserine** [**Seromycin**], **kanamycin** [**Kantrex**], **ciprofloxacin** [**Cipro**], **ofloxacin** [**Floxin**], **levofloxacin** [**Levaquin**], and **sparfloxacin** [**Zagam**]). **Rifabutin** (**Mycobutin**) is used mainly to treat or prevent MAC. Each of these drugs not already discussed in previous sections of this chapter is discussed in this section. The focus is on those whose main indication is mycobacteria. Management of tuberculosis is further discussed in Chapter 45, and HIV infection is discussed in Chapter 37.

Pharmacodynamics

Sensitivity

Isoniazid is the most active drug for the treatment of tuberculosis. It interferes with lipid and nucleic acid biosynthesis in growing organisms. It is also thought that **isoniazid** and **ethambutol** inhibit synthesis of mycolic acids. These acids are important constituents for mycobacteria cell walls but are not found in mammalian cells, which explains this high selectivity. This drug is bactericidal against susceptible mycobacteria.

Rifampin binds to the beta subunit of mycobacteria DNA-dependent RNA polymerase and inhibits RNA synthesis. **Antimycobacterial** action results in destruction of both multiplying and inactive bacilli. It readily penetrates most tissues and can kill bacteria that are poorly accessible to many other drugs. This drug is bactericidal against susceptible mycobacteria. **Rifampin** also has activity against *N. gonorrhoeae, Staphylococcus, Mycobacterium leprae* (the cause of leprosy), MAC, and *H. influenzae* type b.

Ethambutol inhibits synthesis of arabinogalactan, an essential component of mycobacteria cell walls. It also arrests cell multiplication, causing cell death. **Ethambutol** enhances the activity of lipophilic drugs such as **rifampin** and **ofloxacin** that cross the mycobacteria cell wall primarily in lipid portions of this wall. It is bacteriostatic against susceptible mycobacteria.

Pyrazinamide, an analogue of **nicotinamide**, is among the least expensive of the drugs in this class. The mechanism of action is unknown, but, although inactive in a neutral pH, at a pH of 5.5 it is bactericidal against tubercle bacilli and some other mycobacteria at concentrations of approximately 20 mcg/mL.

Streptomycin is an **aminoglycoside** used now almost exclusively to treat *M. tuberculosis* infections. It is added as a fourth drug to the treatment regimen because up to 80 percent of patients treated with this drug harbor resistant bacilli after 4 months of treatment. Other mycobacteria except MAC and *Mycobacterium kansasii* are resistant to **streptomycin**. This drug is an irreversible inhibitor of protein synthesis. It penetrates cells poorly but is bactericidal in an alkaline extracellular environment.

Para-aminosalicylic acid, structurally similar to **para-aminobenzoic acid** (PABA) and the **sulfonamides**, is a **folate synthesis antagonist** that is active almost exclusively against *M. tuberculosis.* It is bacteriostatic. It is not used frequently because primary resistance is common and newer drugs are better tolerated. It will not be discussed further.

Ethionamide is chemically related to **isoniazid** and also blocks the synthesis of mycolic acids. It is bacteriostatic against *M. tuberculosis,* and this drug also inhibits some other *Mycobacterium* species.

Capreomycin, a peptide antibiotic, inhibits RNA synthesis, thereby decreasing the replication of tubercle bacilli. Because resistance easily develops when it is given alone, it is given as part of a multidrug regimen. It is bactericidal to susceptible mycobacteria.

Rifabutin is a **semisynthetic ansamycin antibiotic** derived from **rifamycin.** It inhibits DNA-dependent RNA polymerase in susceptible mycobacteria and some other organisms. Prevention of disseminated MAC in HIV-infected patients is its main use. Up to 25 percent of **rifampin**-resistant strains of *M. tuberculosis* will be susceptible to **rifabutin**, and it may also be used in this instance.

Resistance

Resistance to **isoniazid** has been associated with excessive production of the product of the *inhA* gene and with mutation or deletion of *katG,* which encodes mycobacterium catalase. *InhA* mutants have low-level resistance and cross-resistance to **ethionamide.** The *katG* mutants have high-level resistance but no cross-resistance. Resistant mutants occur with a frequency of about 1 per 10^6 bacilli. Resistant mutants are selected out if this drug is given alone. Single-drug therapy with **isoniazid** has resulted in 10 to 20 percent prevalence of resistant strains in clinical isolates from the Caribbean and Southeast Asia. Only about 8 to 10 percent of organisms in the United States are resistant to this drug.

Resistance to **rifampin** and **rifabutin** results from point mutations that prevent binding to RNA polymerase. Cross-resistance often exists between these **rifamycins.**

The mechanism of resistance is unknown for **ethambutol**, but it develops rapidly when used as monotherapy. Resistance to **ethionamide** also develops rapidly when it is used as monotherapy.

Resistance also develops rapidly to **pyrazinamide**, but there is no cross-resistance to other **antimycobacterial drugs** so that it can be given to patients exposed to a case of multidrug-resistant tuberculosis. **Capreomycin** is also useful for treatment of drug-resistant tuberculosis because of its lack of cross-resistance to first-line drugs.

Point mutation that alters the ribosomal binding site is the mechanism of resistance for **streptomycin.**

Pharmacokinetics

Absorption and Distribution

All oral **antimycobacterials** are rapidly and well absorbed in the GI tract after oral administration. **Rifampin** and **rifabutin** need to be taken on an empty stomach. High-fat meals slow the rate of absorption but not the extent of absorption. The injectable drugs are rapidly absorbed in muscle tissue but not from the GI tract.

Isoniazid readily diffuses into all body fluid including CSF (90% of serum levels), pleural, and ascitic fluid; tissues; organs; and saliva, sputum, and feces. It also crosses the placenta and enters breast milk.

Rifampin and **ethambutol** also penetrate and concentrate in most body fluids. Adequate penetration of CSF occurs only in the presence of inflamed meninges. They both cross the placenta and enter breast milk.

Pyrazinamide is widely distributed in body tissues and fluids including the liver and lung, and it reaches high concentrations in CSF. It enters breast milk.

Streptomycin and **capreomycin** are widely dis ributed through extracellular fluid, cross the placenta, and enter breast milk in small amounts. They have poor CSF penetration except in the presence of inflamed meninges.

Ethionamide is widely distributed to body tissues and fluids. CSF concentrations are equal to those in the serum.

Rifabutin is highly lipophilic and distributes in most body fluids and intracellular tissues.

Metabolism and Excretion

The metabolism of **isoniazid** is highly variable and dependent on acetylator status. The liver, in a process that is genetically controlled, primarily acetylates it. Fast acetylators metabolize this drug five to six times faster than slow acetylators do. Approximately 50 percent of both blacks and whites are slow acetylators, and the rest are rapid acetylators. The majority of Alaskan natives and Asians are rapid acetylators. The rate of acetylation does not alter effectiveness but may increase the risk for toxic reactions in slow acetylators. Rapid clearance is of no consequence when the drug is given daily but may result in subtherapeutic doses when given once weekly. **Isoniazid** metabolites and unchanged drug are excreted in the urine. Elimination is largely independent of renal function.

Rifampin is also metabolized in the liver by deacetylation, and the metabolite is also active against *M. tuberculosis*. With repeated administration, the half-life decreases. It is excreted mainly through the liver into bile; then, through enterohepatic recirculation, the remainder is excreted in feces, with a small amount excreted in urine.

About 20 percent of **ethambutol** is metabolized by the liver, and it is mainly excreted as unchanged drug in the urine. Marked accumulation may occur in renal failure.

Pyrazinamide is hydrolyzed by the liver to a metabolite that also has **antimycobacterial** activity. Its half-life may be significantly prolonged in the presence of impaired renal or hepatic function. Approximately 70 percent of the oral dose is excreted in urine by glomerular filtration. **Streptomycin** and **capreomycin** are excreted almost exclusively by the kidney.

Approximately 35 percent of **ethionamide** is metabolized by the liver, and the majority of the drug is excreted in urine as inactive metabolites. Less than 1 percent is excreted as unchanged drug.

Hepatic insufficiency or the age of the patient alters the pharmacokinetics of **rifabutin** only slightly. Somewhat reduced drug distribution and faster drug elimination are seen in renal insufficiency and may result in decreased drug concentrations. Table 24–34 presents the pharmacokinetics of selected **antimycobacterials.**

Pharmacotherapeutics

Precautions and Contraindications

Cautious use in renal impairment is recommended for **isoniazid**, **ethambutol**, **streptomycin**, and **capreomycin.** Dosage adjustments may be required and are discussed in the Clinical Use and Dosing section.

Cautious use in the presence of hepatic impairment is recommended for **isoniazid**, **rifampin** (hepatotoxic),

Table 24–34 ▶ **Pharmacokinetics: Selected Antimycobacterials**

Drug	Onset	Peak	Duration	Protein Binding	Bioavailability	Half-Life	Elimination
Capreomycin (IM)	Rapid	1–2 h	UA	UA	UA	4–6 h	52% unchanged in urine within 12 h
Ethambutol	Rapid	2–4 h	24 h	UA	69%–85%	3–4 h*	50% metabolized by liver; 50% unchanged in urine
Ethionamide	Rapid	3 h	UA	10%	100%	2–3 h	Metabolized by liver; <1% unchanged in urine
Isoniazid (PO/IM)	Rapid	1–2 h	24 h	80%	UA	1–4 h	50% metabolized by liver; 50% unchanged in urine
Pyrazinamide	Rapid	2 h	UA	UA	UA	9–10 h*	70% metabolites in urine within 24 h
Rifampin	Rapid	2–4 h	24 h	88%–90%	90%–95%	1–5 h†	40%–60% in bile and by enterohepatic circulation
Rifabutin	Rapid	2–4 h	24 h	85%	20%	45 h	30% in feces; 53% as metabolites in urine
Streptomycin (IM)	Rapid	0.5–1.5 h	UA	34%–62%	UA	2–3 h*	>90% in urine

UA = information unavailable.
*Increased in renal or hepatic impairment.
†Varies by dose and averages 2–3 h after repeated doses.

pyrazinamide, and **ethionamide** (hepatotoxic). Black and Hispanic women, women postpartum, and patients older than 50 years are at special risk for development of hepatitis while taking **isoniazid**.

Ethionamide should be given cautiously to patients with diabetes mellitus. Management may be more difficult and hepatitis is more likely in these patients.

Hematologic alterations including various anemias and thrombocytopenia have been seen with the use of **isoniazid** and **rifampin. Ethambutol** and **pyrazinamide** each may precipitate gouty arthritis attacks and should be used cautiously in the presence of this disorder.

Pregnancy categories vary by drug. **Ethambutol** is Pregnancy Category B and has been used in pregnant women without adverse effects on the fetus. The others are Pregnancy Category C. Often the effect of the drug on the fetus is unknown, or the adverse effect has occurred in animal studies only. Using any of the Pregnancy Category C drugs requires consideration of the benefit to the woman patient versus the potential risk to the fetus. **Streptomycin** may cause congenital deafness if given to pregnant women and is Pregnancy Category D.

The infant should be observed for any evidence of adverse effects from drugs that appear in breast milk. Discontinuing the drug must take into account the importance of the drug for the mother. The drugs that enter breast milk in smaller amounts include **rifampin** and **pyrazinamide. Capreomycin** is excreted in such small amounts as to be undetectable in some women.

Use in children varies by drug. Pediatric doses are listed for all of these drugs, but the age under which they should not be used varies. No age restrictions are provided for **isoniazid, rifampin,** and **pyrazinamide. Ethambutol** is not FDA approved for use by children younger than 13 years. Safety and optimal dosage have not been determined for children for **ethionamide** and **capreomycin.** Ototoxicity risk precludes use of **streptomycin** in neonates and in older adults or patients with diminished hearing.

Adverse Drug Reactions

All of the **antimycobacterial** drugs have risks for hypersensitivity reactions, some of which may be severe. The usual management associated with these reactions applies here as well.

Peripheral neuropathy is the most common adverse reaction with **isoniazid.** It occurs in about 2 percent of patients taking 5 mg/kg/day. Prevalence is higher for patients taking higher doses, up to about 44 percent for patients taking 24 mg/kg/day. The symptoms include symmetrical numbness and tingling in the extremities. Patients predisposed to this adverse reaction include the malnourished, slow acetylators, pregnant women, older adults, diabetics, and patients with chronic liver disease, including alcoholics. **Pyridoxine** (B_6) prevents the development of peripheral neuropathy and is recommended for patients in these at-risk categories. Some providers use **pyridoxine** for all patients on **isoniazid.** Recommended prophylactic doses range from 10 to 50 mg daily. Treatment of established neuropathy requires 50 to 200 mg daily.

Hepatotoxicity occurs in 10 to 20 percent of patients taking **isoniazid.** Patients at risk were discussed previously. The symptoms are those usually associated with the development of hepatitis, including abnormal liver function studies, jaundice, and fatigue. The frequency of progressive liver damage increases with age. Concurrent **alcohol** use increases the risk. When **rifampin** is given concurrently, the risk is increased 4-fold.

Other adverse reactions associated with **isoniazid** include blood dyscrasias, metabolic acidosis, gynecomastia, and hypocalcemia related to altered vitamin D metabolism.

The most common adverse reactions associated with **rifampin** are GI in nature: anorexia, nausea, vomiting, diarrhea, flatulence, and abdominal pain. Although hepatotoxicity is less common than it is with **isoniazid**, hepatotoxicity leading to hepatitis occurs with **rifampin.** A harmless orange red discoloration of body fluids including tears, saliva, urine, sweat, CSF, and feces also occurs. Hematuria should not be confused with this discoloration because hematuria may be an indication of a hypersensitivity reaction.

Other adverse reactions associated with **rifampin** include blood dyscrasias, headache, drowsiness and inability to concentrate, a pruritic rash (1% to 5% of patients), visual disturbances, and exudative conjunctivitis.

Ethambutol also has the usual GI disturbances, but the most serious adverse reaction is optic neuritis, which appears to be dose-related. Signs and symptoms include decreased visual acuity, red green color blindness, diminished visual fields, and sometimes loss of vision. These adverse reactions are generally reversible when the drug is discontinued promptly. In rare cases, recovery may take up to 1 year. Vision testing should be done before and throughout therapy.

Other adverse reactions include precipitation of gouty arthritis related to elevated uric acid levels, transient impairment of liver function, and infrequent peripheral neuropathy.

The principal adverse reaction with **pyrazinamide** is dose-related hepatotoxicity that may appear anytime during therapy. Patients at risk for this adverse reaction are the same ones mentioned in the Precautions and Contraindications section. Discontinuing the drug may be required. Because this drug inhibits the renal excretion of urates, hyperuricemia also often occurs. It is often asymptomatic but may precipitate acute gouty arthritis. Baseline serum uric acid levels should be drawn.

The most serious adverse effect associated with **streptomycin** and **capreomycin** is ototoxicity. Damage to the eighth cranial nerve results in vertigo, nausea, vomiting, and loss of hearing. The risk is increased with higher doses and longer duration of therapy. Nephrotoxicity is also a serious risk for patients on any **aminoglycoside.** Risk for this adverse reaction increases for patients with renal insufficiency and for older adults with age-related decreased renal function. Dosage adjustments are made based on renal function studies to reduce the risk for this adverse reaction. Doses taken two or three times weekly rather than daily also reduce the risk for toxicity.

Ethionamide has few adverse reactions, but it is often poorly tolerated because of its most common adverse reaction, GI distress. Some patients develop a metallic taste in their mouth. Other common adverse reactions include hepatitis (rare), optic neuritis, and peripheral neuritis (common). Neurological symptoms can be alleviated by pyridoxine.

Rifabutin has been associated with neutropenia and thrombocytopenia. Other adverse reactions include rash (4%) and GI intolerance (3%).

Drug Interactions

Drug interactions and drug–food interactions vary by drug. Many are associated with increasing the common adverse reactions for the particular **antimycobacterial**. Some are associated with reduced effectiveness of the interacting drug. **Rifampin** is an inducer of CYP450 enzyme system and speeds the metabolism of many drugs, resulting in therapeutic failure. Table 24–35 provides a list of the drug interactions.

Clinical Use and Dosing

Resistance to **antimycobacterial** drugs has a frequency of about 1 bacillus in 10^6.

However, with 10^8 bacilli lesions in an infected person, resistant mutants are selected out when only one drug is given. Because of the relatively high proportion of adult patients with tuberculosis caused by organisms that are resistant to **isoniazid**, four drugs are necessary in the initial phase of therapy for the 6-month regimen to be maximally effective (CDC, 2003). Multiple drugs with independent actions lower the prevalence of resistance.

Table 24–35 ■ Drug Interactions: Selected Antimycobacterials

Drug	Interacting Drug	Possible Effect	Implications
Capreomycin	Aminoglycosides and other ototoxic and nephrotoxic drugs	Additive ototoxicity and nephrotoxicity	Avoid concurrent use If symptoms occur, discontinue one of the drugs
	Isoniazid, ethionamide	Additive CNS effects; increased risk for peripheral neuropathy	
	Phenytoin	Inhibition of phenytoin metabolism; increased toxicity risk	Monitor serum levels of phenytoin
Ethambutol	Other neurotoxic drugs	Additive neurotoxicity	Avoid concurrent use
	Aluminum salts	Reduced absorption of ethambutol	Administer ethambutol 1–2 h before aluminum salt
Isoniazid	Alcohol	Daily ingestion increases risk for hepatitis	Avoid concurrent use
	Aluminum salts	Reduced oral absorption of isoniazid	Administer isoniazid 1–2 h before aluminum salts
	Oral anticoagulants	Enhanced anticoagulant activity	Avoid concurrent use or monitor PT/INR
	Benzodiazepines (BDZs)	Isoniazid may inhibit metabolic clearance of BDZs that undergo oxidative metabolism (e.g., diazepam, triazolam)	Avoid concurrent use
	Carbamazepine	Toxicity or hepatotoxicity may occur	Monitor carbamazepine drug levels and liver function
	Disulfiram	Acute behavioral and coordination changes	Avoid coadministration
	Hydantoins	Increased serum hydantoin levels because of inhibition of CYP-450 enzymes. Most significant in slow acetylators	Monitor hydantoin levels and adjust doses as needed
	Ketoconazole	Decreased serum ketoconazole levels; decreased antifungal activity	Select different antifungal
	Meperidine	Hypotension or CNS depression	Select different pain management
	Rifampin	Increased risk for hepatotoxicity	If alterations in liver function tests, discontinue one of these drugs

Continued

Table 24–35 ■ **Drug Interactions: Selected Antimycobacterials—cont'd**

Drug	Interacting Drug	Possible Effect	Implications
	Tyramine-containing foods	Isoniazid has slight monoamine oxidase inhibition activity	Teach patient foods to avoid
	Histamine-containing foods	Diamine oxidase may be inhibited	Teach patient foods to avoid (e.g., tuna, sauerkraut, yeast extract)
Pyrazinamide	Laboratory interactions	Has been reported to interfere with Acetest and Ketostix urine tests to produce a pink brown color	Select different method of determining ketoacidosis
Rifampin, rifabutin	Acetaminophen, oral anticoagulants, barbiturates, BDZs, beta blockers, chloramphenicol, clofibrate, oral contraceptives, corticosteroids, cyclosporine, digitoxin, disopyramide, estrogens, hydantoins, methadone, mexiletine, quinidine, sulfonylureas, theophylline, tocainide, verapamil	Rifampin induces CYP-450 enzyme systems that metabolize these drugs. Therapeutic effects of these drugs decreased	If patient must take one of the interacting drugs, select different antimycobacterial
	Digoxin	Decreased serum levels of digoxin	Monitor serum levels or select different antimycobacterial
	Enalapril	Significant increase in blood pressure	Occurred in 1 patient. Monitor
	Isoniazid	Increased risk for hepatotoxicity	See isoniazid above
	Ketoconazole	Decreased ketoconazole levels; decreased antifungal activity	Select different antifungal
	Laboratory interactions	Therapeutic levels of rifampin interfere with standard assays of serum folate and B_{12}	Consider alternative methods for determining concentrations
Streptomycin	Cephalosporins, vancomycin	Increased risk of nephrotoxicity	Monitor renal function
	Loop diuretics	Increased risk for ototoxicity. Hearing loss may be irreversible	Avoid concurrent use
	Polypeptide antibiotics	Increased risk of respiratory paralysis and renal dysfunction	Avoid concurrent use. Select different antimycobacterial

CNS = central nervous system; INR = international normalized ratio; PT = prothrombin time.

Patients with HIV infection are especially at risk for tuberculosis and their disease is more likely to be a resistant form. Treatment regimens include initial phase and continuation phases. Initial phases have four drugs (**isoniazid** [INH], **rifampin** [RIF], **pyrazinamid** [PZA], and **ethambutol** [EMB]) given for 2 months followed by continuation phases, usually with two drugs (INH and another drug, most often RIF) given for 4 to 7 months.

The first-line **antimycobacterial** drugs should be administered together; split dosing should be avoided. Fixed-dose combination preparations may be more easily administered than single-drug tablets and may decrease the risk for acquired drug resistance and drug errors. Two combination formulations have been approved for use in the United States: INH/RIF (**Rifamate**) and INH/RIF/PZA (**Rifater**). It should be noted that for patients weighing more than 90 kg, the dose of PZA in the three-drug combination is insufficient and additional PZA tablets are necessary.

Some continuation phase protocols are designed for mainly HIV-infected individuals. These combinations are discussed in Chapter 37. Initial phase and continuation phase drug combinations and dosing for tuberculosis are discussed in Chapter 45. Table 24–36 presents the dosage schedule for selected **antimycobacterials**.

Rational Drug Selection

Rifampin is also used to treat several nonmycobacterial infections. It is used as prophylaxis for close contacts of people with meningococcal infections caused by *N. meningitidis*, including household members, children and personnel in nurseries and day-care centers, and closed populations such as in college dormitories and military barracks. Health-care personnel with intimate

Table 24–36 ◉ **Dosage Schedule: Selected Antimycobacterials**

Drug	Indication	Initial Dose	Comments
Capreomycin (Capastat)	Tuberculosis, as part of combined drug therapy	1 g IM daily for 60–120 d, then 1 g 2–3 times/wk	Maximum adult daily dose 20 mg/kg. Monitor renal function tests, audiograms, vestibular function, and sites of injection at baseline and at least weekly. Serum potassium should be measured at baseline and monthly during daily therapy. Administer deep IM into large muscle mass because superficial injections are associated with pain and sterile abscess. Administer within 24 h of reconstitution. Store in refrigerator after reconstitution. Darkening of reconstituted drug from initial nearly colorless or straw color does not affect potency. Renal impairment requires decreased dose (see package insert). Educate patients to report altered hearing, dizziness, imbalance; altered urination, nausea, vomiting, or thirst. Patients should advise prescribers they are taking capreomycin because of its potential for drug interactions.
Ethambutol (Myambutol)	Tuberculosis, as part of combined drug therapy	*Adults:* Orally 15–25 mg/kg/d; *or* 50 mg/kg up to 2.5 g twice/wk; *or* 25–30 mg/kg 3 times/wk *Children <13 yr:* No dosage established, but should be considered for children with organisms resistant to other drugs and susceptible to ethambutol; not recommended for children <6 yr in whom visual acuity cannot be monitored	Maximum adult daily dose 2.5 g. Impairment of renal function may require a decreased dosage. Monitor visual fields and red and green discrimination prior to and monthly during treatment, especially for prolonged therapy or >15 mg/kg daily. Periodic uric acid and renal function tests. Educate about importance of vision monitoring. Blurred vision, eye pain, vision loss, or problems with red and green discrimination should be reported. Other reportable symptoms include evidence of peripheral neuropathy (numbness, tingling, burning pain, weakness in hands or feet), gout (chills, pain and swelling of joints, hot skin over affected joints), and hypersensitivity (rash, fever, joint aches). Take drug with food if GI irritation occurs.
	Atypical mycobacterial infections (off-labeled)	Orally 15–25 mg/kg/d	As above
Ethionamide (Trecator-SC)	Tuberculosis, as part of combined drug therapy	*Adults:* 250 mg q8–12h for 1–2 yr or more *Children:* 4–5 mg/kg q8h	Maximal daily adult dose 1 g. Children have required 20 mg/kg/d, but maximal daily dose for children is 750 mg. For the approximately 30% of patients unable to tolerate therapeutic dose, dosage is reduced by 2 to 1. Monitor liver function tests periodically. Ophthalmic examinations if symptoms of visual impairment. Orthostatic blood pressure checks. Thyroid function tests if signs of hypothyroidism; serum glucose if signs of hypoglycemia. Neurological exam for peripheral neuritis.

Continued

Table 24–36 ◉ **Dosage Schedule: Selected Antimycobacterials—cont'd**

Drug	Indication	Initial Dose	Comments
			Pyridoxine decreases risk of peripheral neuropathy. Report signs of hepatitis (yellow eyes or skin, upper abdominal pain, malaise), peripheral neuritis (numbness, tingling, burning pain, weakness in hands or feet), optic neuritis (blurred vision, eye pain), hypoglycemia (poor concentration, tachycardia, hunger, shakiness), or hypothyroidism (weight gain; dry, puffy skin; coldness; irregular menses). Administer with or after meals if GI irritation occurs. Usually administered after evening meal or at bedtime as a single dose. Serum concentrations may be higher with divided doses, but GI irritation may worsen. Rectal suppositories cause fewer adverse effects, but may cause local irritation.
	Atypical mycobacterial infections (off-labeled) or leprosy (off-labeled)	*Adults:* 250 mg q8–12h	As above
Isoniazid (Laniazid)	Tuberculosis prophylaxis	*Adults:* PO or IM 300 mg/d *Children:* 10 mg/kg, up to 300 mg, once daily	Maximal adult daily dose 300 mg. Renal impairment does not usually require dosage adjustment if serum creatinine is <6 mcg/dL and patient is fast acetylator. For slow acetylators, adjust dose to maintain plasma concentration <1 mcg/mL at 24 h after last dose. Monitor liver function tests monthly, or more often if liver impairment or clinical signs of hepatitis or prodromal symptoms. CBC and platelet count periodically or at signs of blood dyscrasia (fever, sore throat, bleeding or bruising, tiredness). Ophthalmic exam if signs of optic neuritis. Educate to report signs of clinical hepatitis (dark urine, yellow eyes or skin), hepatitis prodromal symptoms (anorexia, nausea and vomiting, unusual tiredness), optic neuritis (blurred vision or loss of vision, with or without eye pain), or peripheral neuropathy (numbness, clumsiness, burning pain of hands or feet). High risk for peripheral neuropathy (pregnant, high alcohol use, taking anticonvulsants, poor diet, malnourished, history of neuritis, chronic renal failure, diabetes, and over 65) indicates 25 mg pyridoxine/d. May be taken with meals or antacids if GI irritation occurs, but do not take within 1 h of aluminum-ontaining cantacid. Measure syrup with calibrated measuring device. Crystals may form at low temperatures, but they redissolve upon warming to room temperature.

Table 24–36 ◉ **Dosage Schedule: Selected Antimycobacterials—cont'd**

Drug	Indication	Initial Dose	Comments
	Tuberculosis, as part of combined drug therapy	*Adults:* PO or IM 300 mg once daily *or* 15 mg/kg, up to 900 mg, given 2–3 times/wk *Children:* 10 mg/kg, up to 300 mg, once daily, *or* 20–40 mg/kg, up to 900 mg, given 2–3 times/wk	As above.
Pyrazinamide	Tuberculosis, as part of combined drug therapy	*Adults and children:* 15–30 mg/kg once daily or 50–70 mg/kg 2–3 times/wk; patients with HIV take 20–30 mg/kg/d for first 2 mo	Maximal adult and pediatric daily dosage is 2 g when taken daily, 3 g when taken 3 times/wk, 4 g when taken twice/wk. Monitor liver function tests prior to and every 2–4 wk during treatment. Uric acid determinations may be needed. Educate that arthralgia is usually mild and self-limiting and to report signs of hepatotoxicity (dark urine, anorexia, nausea, vomiting, yellow skin or eyes) and gout (pain, swelling, heat over joints). May be taken without regard to meals.
Rifampin	Tuberculosis, as part of combined drug therapy	*Adults:* 600 mg PO once daily *or* 10 mg/kg up to 600 mg 2–3 times/wk *Infants <1 mo:* 10–20 mg/kg PO once daily *or* 10–20 mg/kg 2–3 times/wk	Maximum adult or pediatric daily oral dose should not exceed 600 mg. Severe hepatic impairment requires 50% reduction in dosages. Monitor hepatic function prior to and at least monthly during treatment; CBC if signs of blood dyscrasia (sore throat, bleeding, bruising). Advise patients to report signs of hepatotoxicity (dark urine, anorexia, nausea, vomiting, yellow skin or eyes), flu-like syndrome, or blood dyscrasias. Reddish orange or reddish brown discoloration may stain clothes or soft contact lenses but is harmless. Avoid alcohol, which can increase hepatotoxicity. Advise health-care providers of rifampin use because of high risk of drug interactions. May be taken without regard to meals. Shake suspension before measurement, using calibrated dosing device. Store suspension at controlled room temperature and discard remaining liquid 30 d after reconstitution.
	Meningococcal meningitis prophylaxis	*Adults:* 600 mg PO once/d for 4 d *Children:* 5 mg/kg q12h for 2 d	As above.
	Haemophilus influenzae meningitis prophylaxis (off-labeled)	*Adults:* 600 mg PO once/d for 4 d *Children:* 20 mg/kg once daily for 4 d (10 mg/kg if infant <1 mo)	As above.
Rifabutin (Mycobutin)	MAC disease prophylaxis	*Adults:* 300 mg once daily	May need to monitor platelet count and WBC. Before rifabutin increases rate of metabolism of many drugs, including anti-HIV agents, monitor drug response and/or blood levels, if available. Also, dose of rifabutin may need to be adjusted up or down because of drug interactions.

Continued

Table 24–36 ◉ **Dosage Schedule: Selected Antimycobacterials—cont'd**

Drug	Indication	Initial Dose	Comments
			Counsel patient to report allergic reaction, GI intolerance, or asthenia. May turn secretions reddish brown that can stain clothing and soft contact lenses. May be administered without regard to food. If unable to tolerate single dose, split into 2 equal doses with food. May need to adjust dose up or down for patient taking antiretrovirals.
Streptomycin	Tuberculosis, as part of combined drug therapy	*Adults:* 1 g once daily IM. Reduce to 1 g 2–3 times/wk as soon as clinically feasible *Children:* 20 mg/kg once daily IM, not to exceed 1 g/d *Elderly:* 500–750 mg once daily IM Duration of therapy may be 1–2 y	Maximum adult daily dose 4 g daily. Maximum pediatric daily dose 1 g. Renal impairment requires reduced dosage. Monitor serum concentrations: peak concentrations >50 mcg/mL are associated with nephrotoxicity and should not be >20–25 mcg/mL in patients with preexisting renal damage. Caloric stimulation tests may be required before, during, and after prolonged therapy to detect vestibular toxicity. Do audiograms and renal function tests periodically and frequent urinalysis to detect albumin, casts, cells, and decreased specific gravity. Educate patient to report signs of hypersensitivity (skin itching, rash, swelling), vestibular ototoxicity (clumsiness, dizziness, nausea, vomiting), auditory ototoxicity (hearing loss; fullness, ringing, buzzing in ears), peripheral neuritis (burning of face or mouth, numbness, tingling), and nephrotoxicity (altered frequency or amount of urination, thirst, anorexia, nausea and vomiting). Administer deep IM, alternating injection sites. Concentration of solution should not exceed 500 mg/mL. After reconstitution, solution retains potency for 2–28 days at room temperature and 14 days in refrigerator, depending on manufacturer. See package insert. Darkening of solution does not affect potency.

exposure to index cases (such as mouth-to-mouth resuscitation) should receive prophylactic therapy. Prophylaxis for adults is oral **rifampin** 600 mg every 12 hours for four doses. The dose for children is 10 mg/kg every 12 hours for four doses.

Rifampin is also indicated for prophylaxis for close contacts of people with actual or suspected infections with *H. influenzae* type b. If one of the contacts in a household is an unvaccinated child 4 years or younger, it is recommended that all contacts in the household except pregnant women receive prophylaxis. In a day-care center attended by unvaccinated children younger than 2 years, prophylaxis with **rifampin** 20 mg/kg up to 600 mg for four doses for all contacts and vaccination of all unvaccinated children should be considered. If all contacts are older than 2 years, prophylaxis is not indicated. If there have been two or more cases in the center within 60 days and unvaccinated children attend, prophylaxis is recommended for children and personnel.

Finally, **rifampin** has an off-labeled use in the treatment of leprosy and concurrently with other **antistaphylococcal agents** in the treatment of serious infections in hospitalized patients caused by *Staphylococcus,* including methicillin-resistant and multidrug-resistant strains.

Patient Education

Administration

Because of the long duration of therapy and complexity of the protocols in tuberculosis infections, instruction and support are essential. Multidrug therapy, essential to prevent development of resistance, presents serious challenges for adherence. Some protocols are given daily for 8 weeks (56 doses) or 5 days/week for 8 weeks (40 doses) in the initial phase and then given twice weekly for 18 weeks (36 doses) during the continuation phase. To maintain this complex two- to four-drug regimen requires commitment on the part of the patient and usually outside help. This is especially true for lower-socioeconomic populations and other high-risk groups that normally have limited contact with the health-care system. Directly observed therapy (DOT), in which each dose is observed by a health-care provider or other designated person, has proved very effective in promoting compliance and improving response to therapy. Lifestyle implications of tuberculosis include general health promotion strategies such as good nutrition, rest, and appropriate exercise.

Adverse Reactions

Adverse effects, especially GI upset, are relatively common in the first few weeks of initial phase therapy. However, first-line drugs, particularly **rifampin,** must not be discontinued because of minor adverse effects. Although taking the drug with food may delay or moderately decrease the absorption, the effects of food have little clinical significance. Patients who have epigastric distress or nausea with this drug should be told that they can take their whole drug protocol with meals or that the hour of dosing can be changed. Administration with food is preferable to splitting a dose or changing to a second-line drug.

Lifestyle Management

Lifestyle management is discussed in the Chapter 37 related to HIV infection and Chapter 45 related to tuberculosis. Dosages, monitoring, and patient education are summarized in Table 24–36; available dosage forms are given in Table 24–37.

ANTIVIRALS

Viral infections range from the annoying but short-lived and self-limiting "common cold" to the progressive and, to date, incurable HIV. Discussion in this section focuses on nucleoside analogues used to treat herpes virus infections and agents used to prevent and treat influenza. Chapter 37 discusses drugs to treat HIV. Drugs used to treat cytomegalovirus (CMV) retinitis and other CMV disease in HIV patients (e.g., **foscarnet, ganciclovir, valganciclovir)** are also discussed Chapter 37.

Viruses are obligate intracellular parasites that depend on use of the host cell's genetic material for replication. As a result, antiviral drugs must either block entry into the cells or be active inside host cells to be effective. The activity of these drugs is usually nonselective to viral components, and so damage to host cells as well as virus results. To further complicate treatment, replication of the virus peaks at or before clinical symptoms appear in many viral

Table 24–37 ◆ **Available Dosage Forms: Selected Antimycobacterials**

Drug	Dosage Form	How Supplied	Cost*
Capreomycin (Capstat)	Powder for injection: 1 g	In 10-mL multidose vials	
Ethambutol (Myambutol)	Tablets: 100 mg 400 mg	In bottles of 100 coated tablets In bottles of 100, 1,000 and UD 100 scored, film-coated tablets	$157
Ethionamide (Trecator-SC)	Tablets: 250 mg	In bottles of 100 sugar-coated tablets	
Isoniazid	Tablets: 100 mg 300 mg Syrup: 50 mg/5 mL Injection: 100 mg/mL	In bottles of 100, 1,000 tablets In bottles of 30, 100, 1,000 tablets In pint (orange flavor) In 10-mL multidose vials	$8.50 $11 $25
(Nydrazid)	Injection: 100 mg/mL	In 10-mL multidose vials	
Isoniazid combinations (Rifater)	Tablets: 120 mg rifampin, 50 mg isoniazid, 300 mg pyrazinamide	In bottles of 60, 100 tablets	$200
(Rifamate)	Capsules: 150 mg isoniazid, 300 mg rifampin	In bottles of 50, 100 tablets	$268
Rifabutin (Mycobutin)	Capsules: 150 mg	In bottles of 100 capsules	$638
Rifampin (Rifadin)	Capsules: 150 mg 300 mg	In bottles of 30 capsules In bottles of 30, 60, 100 capsules	$96/30 $157
(Rimactane)	Capsules: 300 mg	In bottles of 30, 60, 100 capsules	
Pyrazinamide	Tablets: 500 mg	In bottles of 100, 500 scored tablets	
Streptomycin sulfate	Injection: 400 mg/mL	In 2.5-mL ampules	

*Cost per 100 units unless otherwise stated.

infections, so that optimal clinical efficacy depends on early recognition and treatment or prevention. Finally, many viruses depend on enzymes to reproduce and can quickly mutate in the presence of drug therapy.

Viral replication consists of several steps: (1) adsorption to and penetration into susceptible cells; (2) uncoating of viral nucleic acid; (3) synthesis of early, regulatory proteins; (4) synthesis of RNA or DNA; (5) synthesis of late, structural proteins; (6) assembly of viral particles; and (7) release from the cell. **Antiviral** drugs are targeted at these steps. Many of the currently available **antiviral** agents act on synthesis of purine and pyrimidine (step 4).

NUCLEOSIDE ANALOGUES

Pharmacodynamics

The **nucleoside analogues** are used mainly to treat herpes infections. **Acyclovir (Zovirax)** is an **acyclic guanosine derivative** that requires three phosphorylation steps for activation. It is first converted to the monophosphate derivative by the virus-specific thymidine kinase and then to the di- and triphosphate compounds by the host's cellular enzymes. Because it requires the viral kinase for the first step, it is selectively activated only in infected cells. The final step, acyclovir triphosphate, inhibits viral DNA synthesis.

Valacyclovir (Valtrex) is the **L-valyl ester of acyclovir.** It is rapidly converted after oral administration to **acyclovir.** Its mechanism of action is then that of **acyclovir.** Serum levels, however, are three to five times higher than those achieved with **acyclovir** and approximate those achieved by IV administration of **acyclovir.**

Famciclovir (Famvir) is the **diacetyl ester pro-drug** of 6-deoxy penciclovir, an **acyclic guanosine analogue.** It is rapidly converted to **penciclovir** by first-pass metabolism. **Penciclovir** has similar pharmacodynamics to **acyclovir.** Activation is catalyzed by virus-specified thymidine kinase in infected cells, resulting in competitive inhibition of the viral DNA polymerase and inhibition of DNA synthesis. It has lower affinity for the viral DNA polymerase than acyclovir, but it achieves higher intracellular concentrations and has a more prolonged intracellular effect.

Ganciclovir (Cytovene) is phosphorylated to a substrate that competitively inhibits the binding of deoxyguanosine triphosphate to DNA polymerase, causing inhibition of DNA synthesis.

Another **nucleoside analogue, ribavirin (Virazole),** is active against a wide range of DNA and RNA viruses, including influenza A and B, parainfluenza, respiratory syncytial virus (RSV), paramyxoviruses, herpes C virus (HCV), and HIV-1. Oral doses of **ribavirin,** however, have not proved beneficial for RSV, HCV, or HIV-1 infections. It is given via a SPAG-2 aerosol treatment, usually in the hospital. It is not discussed further in this chapter.

Sensitivity

Acyclovir is active against herpes simplex virus (HSV) 1 and 2; varicella-zoster virus (VZV); and, to a lesser extent, Epstein-Barr virus (EBV), CMV, and herpes virus 6, which is implicated as the cause of roseola and other febrile diseases in childhood. **Famciclovir** is active against HSV-1 and HSV-2, VZV, EBV, and hepatitis B virus. **Valacyclovir** is converted to **acyclovir** after oral administration and is active against the same viruses. **Ganciclovir** is active against CMV.

Resistance

Resistance to **acyclovir** can develop in HSV and VZV, through alteration is either the viral thymidine kinase or viral DNA polymerase. Because most resistance is based on deficient thymidine kinase activity, cross-resistance occurs with **valacyclovir** and **famciclovir.** CMV resistance to **ganciclovir** has been observed in individuals with AIDS and CMV retinitis who have never received **ganciclovir** therapy.

Pharmacokinetics

Absorption and Distribution

Absorption following oral administration varies by drug. **Acyclovir** is poorly absorbed orally (15% to 20%), although therapeutic levels are achieved. Topical formulations produce local concentrations that may exceed 10 mcg/kg in herpetic lesions, but systemic concentrations are undetectable. **Famciclovir** is absorbed in the intestine for conversion to its active form, **penciclovir. Penciclovir** is marketed as a topical preparation only. **Valacyclovir** is a pro-drug converted to **acyclovir** and is 54 percent bioavailable as **acyclovir** after oral administration. Oral **ganciclovir** has increased bioavailability when given with a fatty meal (5% when taken fasting versus 28% to 31% with a fatty meal).

Acyclovir, famciclovir, and **valacyclovir** are widely distributed. CSF concentrations are 50 percent of plasma for **acyclovir** and **valacyclovir.** All cross the placenta and are known to enter breast milk.

Metabolism and Excretion

Acyclovir is 90 percent eliminated in the urine as unchanged drug, primarily by glomerular filtration and tubular secretion. The liver metabolizes the rest. The kidneys also excrete the active metabolite of **famciclovir (penciclovir). Valacyclovir** is rapidly converted to **acyclovir** and has the same excretion pattern. Dosage adjustments are required for each of these drugs in the presence of renal impairment because of prolonged half-lives. **Ganciclovir** is excreted by the kidneys as 80 to 99 percent unchanged drug.

Table 24–38 presents the pharmacokinetics of **nucleoside analogues** for herpes virus infections.

Table 24–38 ▶ **Pharmacokinetics: Nucleoside Analogues for Herpesvirus Infections**

Drug	Onset	Peak	Duration	Protein Binding	Bioavailability	Half-Life	Elimination
Acyclovir	UA	1.5–2.5 h	4 h	9%–33%	15%–20%	3–4 h; 20 h in anuria	>90% in urine; rest metabolized by liver.
Famciclovir	Rapid	1 h	8–12 h	20%	77%	2–3 h; prolonged in renal impairment	Mostly in urine.
Ganciclovir	UA	UA	UA	1%–2%	5%	3.5–4.8 h	Unchanged in urine.
Valacyclovir	UA	1.5–2.5 h	8–24 h	13%–18%	54%	2.5–3h; 14 h in anuria	>90% in urine; rest metabolized by liver.

UA = information unavailable.

Pharmacotherapeutics

Precautions and Contraindications

For all drugs in this group, cautious use for patients with renal impairment is recommended, with dosage adjustments based on CCr. This caution is also important in older adults, who commonly have diminished renal function. They should also be used with caution by patients with serious hepatic or electrolyte abnormalities. Although dosage adjustments are not required, alterations in pharmacokinetics have been observed in the presence of hepatic impairment.

Acyclovir is listed as Pregnancy Category C; however, there are no adequate well-controlled studies in pregnant women. **Famciclovir** and **valacyclovir** are listed as Pregnancy Category B; however, **valacyclovir** converts to **acyclovir** and should be used with the same precautions as **acyclovir**. To monitor maternal-fetal outcomes of pregnant women exposed to **valacyclovir**, Glaxo Wellcome maintains a pregnancy registry. Providers can register their patients by calling 800-722-9292, extension 58465. **Ganciclovir** is listed as Pregnancy Category C, but it should be avoided in pregnancy. **Ganciclovir** has a black box warning, stating it was teratogenic in animal studies and may cause spermatogenesis. Contraceptive precautions are recommended while the patient is on **ganciclovir** and for 90 days after therapy.

Acyclovir (from the parent drug and from the metabolite of **valacyclovir**) concentrations in breast milk following oral administration have varied from 0.6 to 4.1 times maternal plasma levels. These concentrations could potentially expose the infant to doses of up to 0.3 mg/kg a day. It is appropriate to exercise caution in prescribing these drugs to nursing mothers. **Famciclovir** has been associated with tumorigenicity. The decision to discontinue nursing or avoid the drug is based on the importance of the drug to the mother.

Among these drugs, **acyclovir** is the safest for children and can be used in children older than 2 years. **Famciclovir** does not have established safety and efficacy for children younger than 18 years. The safety and efficacy of **valacyclovir** have not been established for children.

Adverse Drug Reactions

Adverse drug reactions vary by drug. **Acyclovir** has few reactions when given orally. Those associated with short-term administration include headache (0.6%), skin rash (0.3%), nausea and vomiting (2.7%), and diarrhea (0.3%). The prevalence of each of these reactions increases with long-term use. The most frequent adverse reactions associated with **famciclovir** are headache (9%), dizziness (1%), somnolence, and paresthesias (both 1%). Because it is converted to **acyclovir**, the adverse reactions for **valacyclovir** are the same as for **acyclovir. Valacyclovir** does have a higher incidence of adverse reaction, including serious ones (thrombocytopenia purpura, hemolytic uremic syndrome) in immunocompromised patients. **Ganciclovir's** most significant adverse reaction is that it may be carcinogenic. Patients taking **ganciclovir** may experience granulocytopenia (neutropenia), anemia, and thrombocytopenia. In animal studies, **ganciclovir** caused inhibition of spermatogenesis and infertility, irreversible at higher doses. As noted above, **ganciclovir** is a teratogen.

Drug Interactions

Drug interactions are minimal for **acyclovir, famciclovir,** and **valacyclovir.** Table 24–39 presents the few drug interactions that exist for **nucleoside analogues.**

Clinical Use and Dosing

The most important variable in selecting the dosage of **nucleoside analogues** is renal function. The dosing interval, dosage, or both are adjusted for patients with impaired renal function, depending on the dosage and degree of impairment. For example, the usual dose of **valacyclovir** for herpes zoster treatment in a patient with CCr greater

Table 24–39 ■ **Drug Interactions: Nucleoside Analogues**

Drug	Interacting Drug	Possible Effect	Implications
Acyclovir, famciclovir	Probenecid	Increased bioavailability and terminal half-life of acyclovir; decreased renal clearance.	Avoid concurrent use
	Nephrotoxic drugs	Increased risk for renal toxicity	Avoid concurrent use or monitor renal function closely.
Famciclovir	Cimetidine	Penciclovir AUC and urinary recovery increased 18% and 12%, respectively	No clinical significance
	Theophylline	Penciclovir AUC increased 22%. Renal clearance decreased 12%	No clinical significance
	Digoxin	C_{max} of digoxin increased 19% in healthy male volunteers	Probably of no clinical significance, but to be prudent, monitor digoxin levels closely.

than 50 mL/minute is 1 g every 8 hours, whereas the dosage for a CCr less than 10 mL/minute is 500 mg every 24 hours; for **acyclovir** the usual dose is 800 mg every 4 hours (5 times/d). If CCr is less than 10 mL/min, the dose is 200 mg every 12 hours. The prescriber should consult the package insert or a comprehensive reference for specific dosing guidelines.

The **nucleoside analogues** are recommended for the treatment of infections by the herpes simplex virus commonly seen in primary care, specifically genital herpes, herpes zoster (shingles), varicella (chickenpox), and gingivostomatitis in children. The **nucleoside analogues** do not cure herpes infections but may shorten duration, decrease severity, and reduce the incidence of sequelae of the infection. Oral forms of **acyclovir, valacyclovir,** and **famciclovir** are all indicated for primary genital herpes; they increase the rate of healing but do not prevent recurrences. Although **topical acyclovir** is also approved for treatment of initial herpes genitalis infections, it is less effective than the **oral nucleoside analogues** and is not recommended. The **oral nucleoside analogues** should be initiated as soon as possible after the onset of a recurrent episode. Patients are usually provided with a prescription that can be filled at the first sign of recurrence. **Topical acyclovir** has no benefit in recurrent disease in immunocompetent patients, although it has some value in suppression of mucocutaneous herpes in immunocompromised individuals. Patients with frequent recurrences can be placed on suppression therapy, which decreases subclinical shedding between active episodes and the number of symptomatic recurrences. Suppressive therapy is costly, averaging an annual cost between $300 for **acyclovir** 400 mg twice a day, $3,600 for 1 g/day and $2,100 for 500 mg/day for **valacyclovir**, and $3,700 for **famciclovir** 500-mg tablets. In untreated patients, the number of recurrences tends to decrease over time during the first 5 years of the disease. By 3 to 5 years after the initial episode, the number of recurrences may have declined to the point that episodic treatment of recurrences may be preferable. Therefore, the need for suppressive therapy should be reconsidered annually.

Oral acyclovir is indicated for the treatment of varicella in immunocompetent patients when started within 24 hours of the chickenpox rash. For immunocompromised patients, **parenteral acyclovir** should be used. The American Academy of Pediatrics does not recommend **acyclovir** for the treatment of uncomplicated chickenpox in healthy children. **Acyclovir** is recommended for healthy, nonpregnant patients 13 years and older; children older than 12 months with a chronic cutaneous or pulmonary disorder; and children receiving short, intermittent, or aerosolized courses of **corticosteroids**. If possible, the **steroids** should be discontinued after known exposure to varicella. The CDC recommends aggressive treatment of varicella in adults 20 years and older, in that the majority of deaths from chickenpox occur in this age group. **Varicella-zoster immune globulin** should be given within 96 hours of known exposure of a susceptible adult. If prophylaxis fails, early initiation of **acyclovir** within 24 hours of onset of varicella rash is urged. Susceptible adults at high risk (e.g., immunosuppressed, HIV, corticosteroid users) should be vaccinated. Varicella is the leading cause of vaccine-preventable deaths in the United States, so vaccination of children is recommended (see Chapter 19 for the latest immunization schedule or go to http://www.cdc.gov).

Therapy with **nucleoside analogues** should be initiated within 3 days of the outbreak of the rash in herpes zoster. Therapy is most effective if initiated within 48 hours of the outbreak of the rash. Drug therapy speeds healing and reduces the duration of postherpetic neuralgia.

Other recommended uses of **oral acyclovir** include prophylaxis of herpes simplex and herpes zoster in immunocompromised patients, Bell's palsy, and primary gingivostomatitis in children. **Parenteral acyclovir** is used to treat herpes encephalitis, perinatal herpes simplex of mother and neonate, herpes pneumonia, and herpes simiae from a monkey bite.

Ganciclovir injection is used to treat CMV retinitis in immunocompromised patients, including patients with AIDS. **Ganciclovir** for injection is also indicated for the prevention of CMV disease in transplant recipients at risk for CMV disease. Table 24–40 presents the dosage schedule for **nucleoside analogues** for herpes virus infections.

Rational Drug Selection

Three of the **nucleoside analogues** used to treat herpes simplex infections have shown equal efficacy in the treatment of genital herpes; hence, the selection of the specific agent is based on cost and convenience. **Acyclovir** is available as a generic preparation and is generally less expensive than the other **nucleoside analogues**. However, it must be dosed three to five times daily, which may be disruptive and promote noncompliance. **Famciclovir** is dosed two to four times daily, and **valacyclovir** requires one to two doses daily, depending on the indication. However, both of the latter drugs are much more expensive.

Table 24–40 ◉ **Dosage Schedule: Nucleoside Analogues for Herpesvirus Infections**

Drug	Indication	Initial Dose	Comments
Acyclovir (Zovirax)	Genital herpes, initial episode (mild to moderate)	*Adults:* 200 mg q4h while awake, 5 times/d for 10 d; accepted off-labeled dose: 400 mg PO 3 times/d for 10 d	Severe cases and infections in immunocompromised patients require hospitalization and IV therapy. Acute or chronic renal impairment may require dosage adjustment, depending on CCr and dose. Suspension should be well shaken before measurement, using a calibrated device. Take with water. Suspension retains its potency for 24 mo from date of manufacture. Does not require reconstitution or refrigeration. May be taken without regard to meals. Cross-allergy to valacyclovir.
	Genital herpes, intermittent therapy for recurrent infections (<6 episodes/yr)	*Adults:* 200 mg q4h while awake, 5 times/d for 5 d; accepted off-labeled dose: 400 mg PO 3 times daily for 5 d or 500 mg bid for 5 d	As above.
	Genital herpes, chronic suppressive therapy (≥6–10 episodes/yr)	*Adults:* 400 mg PO twice/d or 200 mg 3–5 times/d for up to 12 mo	As above.
	Herpes zoster (shingles)	*Adults:* 800 mg PO q4h while awake, 5 times/d, for 7–10 d	As above.
	Gingivostomatitis, primary, in children	*Children 2–12 yr and <40 kg:* 15 mg/kg 5 times/d for 7 d or 20 mg/kg qid for 5 d	
	Oral labial (fever blister) in normal host (off-labeled)	400 mg 5 times/d for 5 d	Duration of symptoms decreased by ½ d.
	Herpes simplex (Whitlow)	400 mg tid for 10 d	Risks and benefits to fetus and mother still unknown. Experts recommend treatment, especially during third trimester.
	Varicella during pregnancy	800 mg 5 times/d for 5 d	May add VZIG.
	Varicella (chickenpox) Initiate at earliest sign of the infection (treatment of chickenpox in children 2–12 yr not recommended by American Academy of Pediatrics)	*Adolescents and adults:* 800 mg PO q4h for 5 d	As above.

Continued

Table 24–40 ◉ Dosage Schedule: Nucleoside Analogues for Herpesvirus Infections—cont'd

Drug	Indication	Initial Dose	Comments
	Herpes simplex, mucocutaneous prophylaxis (off-labeled)	*Adults:* 400 mg PO q12h	As above
	Bell's palsy due to herpes simplex virus 1 or 2	*Adults:* 400 mg PO 5 times/d for 10 d	As above
Famciclovir (Famvir)	Genital herpes, initial episode (mild to moderate)	*Adults:* (off-labeled) 250 mg PO 3 times/d for 7–10 d	Renal impairment may require decreased dosage. May be taken without regard to meals. Initiate as soon as possible after onset of signs or symptoms.
	Genital herpes, intermittent therapy for recurrent infections (<6 episodes/yr)	*Adults:* 125 mg twice/d for 5 d	
	Genital herpes, chronic suppressive therapy (≥6–10 episodes/yr)	*Adults:* 250 mg PO twice/d or 500 mg once/d for up to 1 yr	
	Oral labial (fever blisters) in normal host	500 mg bid for 7 d	Duration of symptoms decreased by 2 d.
	Varicella (chickenpox) (off-labeled)	*Adolescents and young adults:* 500 mg tid for 5 d	
	Herpes zoster (shingles)	750 mg daily for 7 d or 500 mg bid for 7 d or 250 mg tid for 7 d	Adjust dose for renal failure. CCr 10–50 mL/min change tid dose to bid and bid dose to q24h. No 750-mg dose. For CCr <10 mL/min dose is 250 mg daily.
Ganciclovir (Cytovene)	CMV retinitis in immunocompromised patients	*Adults:* Induction therapy: 5 mg/kg/dose every 12 h for 14 to 21 d, followed by maintenance therapy Maintenance therapy: 5 mg/kg/day as a single dose once a day for 7 days/week Oral: 1,000 mg tid with food or 500 mg 6 times a day with food Prevention of CMV in patients with advanced HIV: Oral 1,000 mg tid with food Prevention of CMV infection in transplant patients: 5 mg/kg/dose for 7 to 14 days then maintenance	Patients with normal renal function.
Valacyclovir (Valtrex)	Genital herpes, initial episode (mild to moderate)	*Adults:* 1 g PO twice/d for 10 d	Renal impairment may require dosage adjustment. Hepatic impairment may slow rate, but not extent, of conversion to acyclovir, but dosage adjustment is not required for hepatic impairment. Not indicated for immunocompromised patients (bone marrow transplant, human immunodeficiency syndrome, renal transplantation) because of risk of thrombotic thrombocytopenic purpura/hemolytic uremic syndrome. May be taken without regard to meals. Cross-allergy to acyclovir.

Table 24–40 ◉ **Dosage Schedule: Nucleoside Analogues for Herpesvirus Infections—cont'd**

Drug	Indication	Initial Dose	Comments
	Genital herpes, intermittent therapy for recurrent infections (<6–10 episodes/yr)	*Adults:* 500 mg PO twice/d for 3 d	
	Genital herpes, chronic suppressive therapy (>6 episodes/yr)	*Adults:* 1 g PO once/d for up to 1 y 500 mg PO daily with 1 g given instead if breakthrough lesions	
	Herpes zoster (shingles)	1 g PO 3 times/d for 7 d	
	Oral labial (fever blisters) in normal host	2 g q12h for 1 d	Duration of symptoms decreased by 1 d.
	Varicella (chickenpox) (off-labeled)	*Adolescents and young adults:* 1 g tid for 5 d	

Topical applications are discussed in Chapters 23 and 32.
CCr = creatinine clearance; VZIG = varicella-zoster immune globulin; CMV = cytomegalovirus

Because of long experience and more extensive research, only **acyclovir** is approved for some indications, such as use by children, varicella treatment, and prevention of oral labial mucocutaneous lesions in immunocompromised patients. Many experts consider **valacyclovir** to be the drug of choice for treatment of herpes zoster because clinical trials have indicated that it decreased the duration of postherpetic neuralgia in patients older than 50 years more than **acyclovir** did.

Ganciclovir is used for CMV retinitis in immunocompromised patients.

Monitoring

The characteristic herpetic lesions of genital herpes, herpes zoster, and chickenpox should be evaluated for resolution or signs of secondary bacterial infection. Temperature and general condition also reflect resolution. BUN and serum creatinine may be assessed prior to therapy in those with risk factors for renal impairment and periodically during prolonged therapy to detect changes in renal function.

Patient Education

Administration

The **nucleoside analogues** can all be taken without regard to meals, in that food does not alter absorption. The available dosage forms are shown in Table 24–41. All forms should be taken with a full glass of water. It is important that the drug be initiated at the earliest sign of recurrence of genital herpes simplex, so the patient must be taught

Table 24–41 ◈ **Available Dosage Forms: Nucleoside Analogues for Herpesvirus Infections**

Drug	Dosage Form	How Supplied	Cost*
Acyclovir (Zovirax)	Tablets: 400, 800 mg (G)	In bottles of 100, 500, 1,000	400 mg = $17; 800 mg = $30
	400, 800 mg (B)	In bottles of 100	400 mg = $307; 800 mg = $595
	Capsules: 200 mg (G)	In bottles of 100	$17
	200 mg (B)	In bottles of 100 and UD 100	$159
	Suspension: 200 mg/5 mL (G)	In 473-mL bottles	$120/473 mL
	200 mg/5 mL (B)	In 473-mL bottle (banana flavor)	
Famciclovir (Famvir)	Tablets: 125, 250 mg (B)	In bottles of 30	125 mg = $111/30; 250 mg = $120/30
	500 mg (B)	In bottles of 30 and UD 50	$240/30
Valacyclovir (Valtrex)	Tablets: 500 mg (B),	In bottles of 30 and UD 100	$133/30
	1 g (B)	In bottles of 21	$169/21
Ganciclovir (Cytovene)	Tablets: 500 mg	In 60, 100	$549/60 tablets

B = brand name; G = generic.
*Cost per 100 units unless otherwise stated.

the symptoms of recurrence and how to self-initiate the medication. Early initiation of drug therapy also increases its efficacy for treatment of varicella and herpes zoster, so public education needs to emphasize the treatability of these infections. It is particularly important for adolescents or adults with chickenpox to seek treatment at the first sign of rash or in the prodromal period if they know they are susceptible and have been exposed.

Adverse Reactions

Although acute renal failure from precipitation of **acyclovir** in the tubules is most common with parenteral **acyclovir**, patients on oral agents have developed acute renal failure and should drink sufficient fluids to remain well hydrated during therapy. Signs of declining renal function that should be reported include abdominal pain, decreased frequency or amount of urination, thirst, anorexia, and nausea or vomiting. Other reportable signs and symptoms include encephalopathic changes (coma, confusion, hallucinations, seizures, tremor), blood dyscrasias (unusual tiredness, chills, fever, sore throat, black stools, unusual bleeding, pinpoint red spots on skin, bruising), and skin reactions like Stevens-Johnson syndrome (peeling, blistering, or loosening of skin; muscle cramps, pain, or weakness; red eyes; rash, itching, or hives).

Lifestyle Management

Keeping herpetic lesions clean and dry promotes healing. Wearing loose clothing that does not rub on the lesions decreases pain and enhances healing. Herpes genitalis may be sexually transmitted even if the partner is asymptomatic. Sexual activity should be avoided whenever either partner has symptoms of herpes genitalis. Oral or topical drug therapy does not prevent transmission of the virus. A male or female condom may decrease the risk of transmission, but spermicides and diaphragms have no effect on transmission. Women with a history of genital herpes are more likely to develop cervical cancer; annual or more frequent Pap tests are required. Those who develop postherpetic neuralgia following herpes zoster should be provided with appropriate pain management for this neuropathic pain syndrome.

OTHER ANTIVIRALS FOR INFLUENZA

Amantadine (Symmetrel) and **rimantadine** (Flumadine) are used for prevention and treatment of respiratory infections due to influenza A virus. **Zanamivir** (Relenza) and **oseltamivir phosphate** (Tamiflu) are approved for treatment of acute illness in adults. **Zanamivir** has been approved for children older than 7 years, and **oseltamivir** has been approved for children older than 1 year who have been symptomatic less than 48 hours. **Oseltamivir** has been approved for the prevention of influenza in patients age 1 year or older. Each of these drugs is reserved for patients at high risk for complications from influenza infections, when vaccination is contraindicated, or to protect the patient until active immunity can develop following vaccination. These drugs should not be considered a substitute for vaccination.

Pharmacodynamics

The pharmacodynamics varies among the **antivirals**. Sensitivity and resistance to the influenza **antivirals** vary year to year, depending on the circulating influenza virus.

Sensitivity

The exact mechanism of **antiviral** action by **amantadine** and **rimantadine** is not fully understood. It appears to be the prevention of uncoating and release of infectious viral nucleic acid into the host cells. The reaction is virus-specific to influenza A subtypes H1N1, H2N2, and H3N2. It does not appear to interfere with the immunogenicity of inactivated influenza A vaccine and has little or no activity against influenza B virus isolates.

The proposed mechanism of action for **zanamivir** is selective inhibition of influenza A and B virus neuraminidase. This enzyme is essential for viral replication, allows viral release from infected cells, prevents viral aggregation, and possibly decreases the ability of the respiratory mucus to inactivate the influenza virus. Vaccination does not appear to alter the activity of **zanamivir** or **oseltamivir**.

Resistance

Emergence of resistance to **amantadine** and **rimantadine** is common in treated patients, with a prevalence of 50 percent within 4 to 6 days. The mechanism of resistance appears to be mutations in the RNA sequence coding for the structural M2 protein.

Transmission of resistance to household contacts has been demonstrated.

Resistance to **zanamivir** and **oseltamivir** is associated with mutations that result in amino acid changes in the viral neuraminidase or viral hemagglutinin or both. In the 2008–2009 influenza season, the circulating influenza A virus was highly resistant to **oseltamivir**. This mutation reduced the neuraminidase response to **zanamivir** by 1,000-fold. There is cross-resistance with **oseltamivir**.

On The Horizon PERAMIVIR

During the 2009 H1N1 influenza pandemic, the FDA issued an emergency authorization for the use of **peramivir**, an antiviral drug in phase III trials for the treatment of influenza. When the pandemic was declared to be over, the drug reverted back to its NDR (new drug request) status.

CLINICAL PEARL

Cdc Influenza Antiviral Recommendations

The Centers for Disease Control and Prevention (CDC) tracks influenza worldwide to determine circulating and emerging strains of influenza. Weekly updates on flu activity and surveillance provides information on what strains are circulating in each state. The CDC also provides recommendations for the use of **antivirals** during influenza season, including updates as resistance patterns emerge. Providers can refer to "Information for Health Professionals," accessible at http://www.cdc.gov/flu, for the latest information.

Pharmacokinetics

Absorption and Distribution

Amantadine, rimantadine, and **oseltamivir** are well absorbed after oral administration. **Oseltamivir** is a pro-drug of the active compound GS4071. Approximately 4 to 17 percent of the inhaled dose of **zanamivir** is systemically absorbed. **Amantadine** is widely distributed to various body tissues including saliva and nasal secretions, and it concentrates in lung tissue. CSF concentrations are half of those in the serum. It crosses the placenta and enters breast milk. Distribution of the other drugs is not known. Protein binding is highest for **amantadine** (67%), midrange for **rimantadine** (40%) and **oseltamivir** (42%), and low for **zanamivir** (10%).

Metabolism and Excretion

Amantadine, oseltamivir, and **GS4071**, the active form of **oseltamivir**, are renally excreted as unchanged drug, and no metabolites have been detected. Children 12 years and younger cleared both the pro-drug and the active metabolite of **oseltamivir** faster than adult patients. **Rimantadine** is metabolized by the liver, and less than 25 percent is excreted as unchanged drug in the urine. **Zanamivir** is excreted as unchanged drug in the urine. Unabsorbed drug is excreted in the feces. Table 24–42 presents the pharmacokinetics of **antivirals** for influenza.

Pharmacotherapeutics

Precautions and Contraindications

Most of the adverse reactions to **amantadine** and **rimantadine** are CNS or psychic disturbances. This drug should be used cautiously for patients with seizure disorders or psychoses. Heart failure (HF) and peripheral edema have developed in patients taking **amantadine.** Careful observation and dosage titration are required for patients with cardiac disease. Because **amantadine** is extensively excreted by the kidney, renal impairment can result in significant accumulations in plasma and body tissues. Dosage adjustments are required based on CCr and it should be used with caution by patients with renal dysfunction.

These cautions are especially true for older adults, who may have age-related diminished renal function.

The liver metabolizes **rimantadine,** and apparent clearance of the drug in patients with severe liver dysfunction was 50 percent lower than that reported for healthy subjects. Because of the potential for accumulation of this drug and its metabolites, it should be used cautiously in the presence of severe hepatic impairment. Although it is less dependent on renal excretion, dosage adjustments are still required and cautious use is recommended for patients with renal impairment, including older adults.

Amantadine and **rimantadine** are Pregnancy Category C. Embryotoxicity and teratogenesis have been observed in animal studies, and there are no adequate well-controlled studies in pregnant women. Use only when clearly needed and when the potential benefits outweigh the fetal risks. **Zanamivir** is listed as Pregnancy Category B. Although **zanamivir** crosses the placenta, fetal blood

Table 24–42 ▶ **Pharmacokinetics: Antivirals for Influenza**

Drug	Onset	Peak	Duration	Protein Binding	Bioavailability	Half-Life	Elimination
Amantadine	48 h	1–4 h	UA	67%*	67%	9–37 h	Excreted unchanged in urine
Oseltamivir	Rapid	2.5–6 h	UA	UA	80%	6–10 h	Pro-drug; active metabolite GS4071 excreted unchanged in urine
Rimantadine	Rapid	6–7 h	UA	40%	UA	20–65 h	<25% unchanged in urine
Zanamivir	Rapid	1–2 h	UA	<10%	UA	2.5–5.1 h	Excreted unchanged in urine

UA = information unavailable.
*In hemodialysis patients, 59%.

concentrations in animal studies were significantly lower than those of maternal plasma. **Oseltamivir** is Pregnancy Category C. With no adequate well-controlled studies in pregnant women, cautious use of both agents is recommended.

Amantadine is excreted in breast milk. Use caution when administering to a nursing mother. It is not known whether **zanamivir** or **oseltamivir** is excreted in human milk, although they were excreted in breast milk in animal studies. Caution is also recommended with these agents. **Rimantadine** has been associated with adverse effects in the offspring of animals treated with this drug during the nursing period. The drug concentrates in breast milk at approximately twice the levels that it does in maternal serum. It should not be given to nursing mothers.

The safety and efficacy of **amantadine** and **rimantadine** for children younger than 1 year have not been established. For **zanamivir** and **oseltamivir**, safety and efficacy have been established for children older than 7 years for **zanamivir**, and for children older than 1 year for **oseltamivir**.

Adverse Drug Reactions

The most frequent adverse reactions for all of these drugs are GI (nausea, vomiting, constipation) and CNS-related (dizziness, depression, insomnia). **Amantadine** has a higher incidence than do the others. **Amantadine** is also approved for treatment of Parkinson's disease because it increases the availability of dopamine in certain areas of the brain. This is thought to be the mechanism for the high incidence of CNS symptoms and nausea with **amantadine**.

Amantadine is also associated with a less frequent (1% to 5%) incidence of an unusual skin disorder (livedo reticularis) in which there is a semipermanent bluish mottled appearance of the skin of the legs and hands that may result from abnormal capillary permeability associated with vasoconstriction. Occasionally, orthostatic hypotension, peripheral edema, and leukopenia have been reported.

Bronchitis, cough, and shortness of breath are associated with **rimantadine** and **zanamivir**. For **zanamivir**, these problems are related to irritation from inhalation of the drug. **Zanamivir** also is associated with ear, nose, and throat infections. For **oseltamivir** the most common adverse effects were nausea, vomiting, and diarrhea. For all of these drugs, adverse reactions are most common and more severe in older adults.

Drug Interactions

Drug interactions are minimal. **Zanamivir** is not a substrate, nor does it affect any of the CYP450 isoenzyme systems. No drug interactions are reported for **oseltamivir** and **zanamivir**. Table 24–43 lists the few existing drug interactions.

Clinical Use and Dosing

Rimantadine, **amantadine**, and **oseltamivir** are approved for the prophylaxis and treatment of influenza type A, whereas **zanamivir** is approved for the treatment of both influenza types A and B. Indications for prophylactic therapy include short-term prophylaxis in institutions such as nursing homes, as an adjunct to immunization after the influenza season has commenced, as a supplement to vaccination for those with impaired immunity, to reduce the spread of influenza by unvaccinated health-care workers, to prevent the disease in workers in critical service positions such as firefighters and police, and as chemoprophylaxis in those who cannot take the vaccine because of allergy to one of the vaccine constituents.

In times of pandemic, the **neuraminidase inhibitors** may be recommended for prophylaxis, particularly when an unvaccinated high-risk patient is exposed to influenza. The individual is vaccinated immediately and started on **neuraminidase inhibitors** to allow the antibody response to the vaccine to achieve protective concentrations.

Indications for treatment include unvaccinated individuals who contract influenza. However, vaccinated individuals can also get influenza and should be offered treatment, particularly if they are at high risk for pneumonia and other sequelae of influenza.

Lower dosages of **amantadine** and **rimantadine** are required for patients with renal impairment and for older patients who are likely to have an age-related decrement in renal function, such as those who reside in nursing homes. The recommended dosage for adults older than

Table 24–43 ■ Drug Interactions: Antivirals for Influenza

Drug	Interacting Drug	Possible Effect	Implications
Amantadine	Anticholinergic drugs (antihistamines, phenothiazines, quinidine, disopyramide, and tricyclic antidepressants)	Increased anticholinergic effects (dry mouth, blurred vision, constipation)	Reduce dose of amantadine or the interacting drug
	Hydrochlorothiazide with triamterene	Decreased urinary excretion of amantadine with increased plasma concentrations	Avoid concurrent use
Rimantadine	Acetaminophen, aspirin, cimetidine	Peak concentrations and AUC of rimantadine decreased by 10% to 16%	Probably not clinically significant

65 years is half the dosage for younger adults. The active components of both **zanamivir** and **oseltamivir** are excreted primarily unchanged in the urine. Recommendations for dosage reduction in renal impairment are not available for either agent. However, because **zanamivir** is an inhaled drug that is only 20 percent absorbed systemically, the risk of accumulation is slight. The active metabolite of **oseltamivir** is excreted in the urine, so renal impairment will impede its excretion and predispose a patient to toxicity. However, this drug is new, and the clinical significance of accumulation in older and debilitated patients is unknown.

The CDC maintains an updated Web site with information regarding recommendations for antivirals based on the circulating influenza strain (http://www.cdc.gov/flu). These recommendations are updated based on emerging resistance patterns; therefore, the provider is wise to refer to the recommendations multiple times during the influenza season. Table 24–44 presents the dosage schedule for **antivirals** used for influenza.

Table 24–44 ◉ Dosage Schedule: Antivirals for Influenza

Drug	Indications	Initial Dose	Comments
Amantadine (Symmetrel)	Influenza A prophylaxis or treatment	No renal impairment: *Children 1–9 yr:* 4.4–4.8 mg/kg/d once daily or divided twice daily. Not to exceed 150 mg/d. *Children 9–12 yr:* 100 mg bid *Children and adults 13–64 yr:* 200 mg once daily or divided twice daily *Adults >65 yr:* 100 mg once daily Renal function impairment: CCr (mL/min) 30–50: 200 mg first d; 100 mg daily thereafter 15–29: 200 mg first d; 100 mg on alternate d <15: 200 mg every 7 d	Maximum daily dose for children 1–9 yr, 150 mg; for children 9–12 yr, 100 mg; for adults >65 yr, daily doses > 100 mg should be used with caution, and reduced further if there is renal impairment, seizure disorder, altered mental/behavioral function. Renal impairment at any age may require dosage reduction. Syrup should be stored at room temperature and dispensed with a calibrated liquid measuring device. May be taken without regard to meals.
Oseltamivir (Tamiflu)	Influenza A and B treatment and prophylaxis	*Adults:* 75 mg PO twice daily for 5 d; start within 48 h of onset of symptoms *Children:* (oral suspension dosing by body weight) ≤15 kg: 30 mg bid (2.5 mL) <15–23 kg: 45 mg bid (3.8 mL) >23–40 kg: 60 mg bid (5 mL) >40 kg: 75 mg bid (6.2 mL)*	For prophylaxis after exposure, immunize with flu vaccine and administer 75 mg PO once daily for 4 wk. Less nausea if taken with food.
Rimantadine (Flumadine)	Influenza A prophylaxis	*Children >10 yr and adults:* 100 mg PO twice daily *or* 200 mg PO once daily *Children <10 yr:* 5 mg/kg PO once daily, not to exceed 150 mg per dose	In adults with impaired renal function (CCr ≤10 mL/min), severe hepatic dysfunction, *or* elderly nursing home patients, a dose of 100 mg once daily is recommended. After exposure, give flu vaccine followed by 4 wk at prophylactic doses. Although the manufacturer recommends twice-daily dosing, the half-life is sufficiently long that once-daily dosing has proved effective.

Continued

Table 24–44 ◉ **Dosage Schedule: Antivirals for Influenza—cont'd**

Drug	Indications	Initial Dose	Comments
			May be taken without regard to meals. The syrup should be measured with a calibrated liquid dosing device.
	Influenza A treatment	*Adults:* 100 mg PO twice/d *or* 200 mg PO once/d for 5–7 d after initial onset of symptoms	
Zanamivir (Relenza)	Influenza A or B treatment	*Children ≥7 yrs and adults:* 2 (5-mg) inhalations twice daily for 5 d; take 2 doses on day 1 if at least 2 h apart, and start within 48 h of initial onset of symptoms	Not FDA-approved for influenza prophylaxis, although studies have indicated efficacy. For prophylaxis after exposure, immunize with flu vaccine and administer 2 inhalations once/d for 4 wk.

CCr = Creatinine clearance
*Oral dosing dispenser with 30-, 45-, and 60-mg graduations is provided with the oral suspension.

Rational Drug Selection

The benefit of influenza drugs is tempered by the need to initiate treatment within 48 hours of the onset of the illness. Although the presence of fever, cough, myalgia, and known influenza activity in the community provide the basis for clinical diagnosis, these symptoms are not definitive. Rapid testing for influenza should be conducted if available. These tests take no more than 20 minutes, cost between $15 and $20, and have acceptable sensitivity and specificity.

The selection of an anti-influenza agent depends on the spectrum, adverse effect profile, cost, and convenience. The cost of **rimantadine** and **amantadine** is considerably lower than the cost of the **neuraminidase inhibitors**, but they cover only influenza A. Another problem with these agents has been the rapid emergence of resistance. Although **rimantadine** has considerably fewer central nervous system effects than **amantadine**, both appear to have more adverse drug reactions that the **neuraminidase inhibitors**. Because **zanamivir** and **oseltamivir** are both relatively new drugs, the full extent of adverse effects and drug interactions may be unknown. The inhaled route of administration of **zanamivir** has the advantage of decreased systemic effects compared with **oseltamivir**, but the inhalation procedure may contribute to noncompliance.

Monitoring

Baseline evaluation of renal function should be considered for older and debilitated patients who are taking anti-influenza prophylactic therapy, which averages several weeks rather than the 5 to 7 days required for treatment. All patients taking **amantadine** or **rimantadine** should be assessed for irritability and seizure activity, and older patients should also be evaluated for confusion, hallucinations, and cognitive impairment. For older and debilitated patients, monitoring should include breath sounds (for evidence of heart failure or development of pneumonia), heart sounds, and weight. Vital signs will also evidence resolution of the influenza and development of adverse effects or sequelae.

Patient Education

Administration

As with all **antivirals**, the importance of taking the full course of therapy and following the labeled directions should be stressed. The available dosage forms are shown in Table 24–45. Patients on **zanamivir** require instruction on the proper use of the diskhaler. The oral anti-influenza drugs can be taken without regard to food.

Adverse Reactions

If asthmatics on **zanamivir** experience severe bronchospasm after using the diskhaler, an alternative treatment may be needed. Because the **neuraminidase inhibitors** represent a relatively new drug group, patients should be encouraged to report their experiences with these agents. As with all drugs, serious occurrences should be reported to MedWatch (http://www.fda.gov/safety/medwatch), the FDA's voluntary reporting system for adverse events and product problems.

Amantadine and, to a lesser extent, **rimantadine** have potentially serious adverse effects. Patients should be advised that the drugs can cause dizziness and blurred vision and that patients should defer hazardous activities until they know how they react to the medication. **Alcohol** should be avoided during therapy, as it would compound hypotension and dizziness. Patients and family members

Table 24–45 ◆ **Available Dosage Forms: Antivirals for Influenza**

Drug	Dosage Form	How Supplied	Cost*
Amantadine (Symmetrel)	Tablets: 100 mg (B) Capsules: 100 mg (G) Syrup: 50 mg/5 mL (G) 50 mg/5 mL (B)	In bottles of 100, 500 In bottles of 100, 500 and UD 100 In 480 mL In 480 mL	$126 $35
Oseltamivir (Tamiflu)	Capsules: 75 mg (B) Powder for oral suspension: 12 mg/mL (reconstituted) (B)	In blister packs of 10 In 25 mL (tutti-frutti flavor) with bottle adapter and oral dispenser	$67/10 $35/25 mL
Rimantadine (Flumadine)	Tablets: 100 mg (B) Syrup: 50 mg/5 mL (B)	In bottles of 100 In 240 mL (raspberry flavor)	$217
Zanamivir (Relenza)	Blisters of powder for inhalation: 5 mg	In 4 blisters with 5 Rotadisks and 1 diskhaler	$52/20 disks/box

B = brand name; G = generic.
*Cost per 100 units unless otherwise stated.

should be advised to report signs of CHF (swelling of feet or legs, shortness of breath), neurological and mental status changes (depression, suicidal ideation, hallucinations, confusion, seizures, clumsiness), and anticholinergic effects (dry mouth, blurred vision, constipation, difficult urination). Dry mouth can be relieved by sucking on ice or sugarless candy, practicing good oral hygiene, and using an over-the-counter (OTC) saliva substitute.

By the time a patient gets influenza, it is too late to educate him or her about the importance of taking the medication within the first 36 hours after onset of symptoms.

Therefore, this has to be part of the anticipatory guidance given at the time of the annual influenza shot. Duration of influenza therapy is 5 days for the **neuraminidase inhibitors** and about 5 to 8 days for **amantadine** and **rimantadine**.

Lifestyle Management

The single most important factor in influenza prevention is the annual vaccination of individuals at risk and those in service positions. Public health officials are increasingly promoting influenza vaccine for broader segments of the population. Most candidates for prophylactic therapy should probably have received vaccination. The wholesale cost of a course of therapy with a **neuraminidase inhibitor** is approximately $45 to $67, exclusive of diagnostic testing, whereas the cost of annual vaccination is $7. Other components of prevention include good hand washing, disposing of contaminated tissues properly, and encouraging infected individuals to convalesce at home rather than in crowded schools and workplaces.

SYSTEMIC AZOLES AND OTHER ANTIFUNGALS

Fungi are free-living, highly organized cells with a nucleus bound by a nuclear membrane and a rigid cell wall. Their life cycle includes a dormant spore stage. They occur naturally in soil, water, and air, and on plants. Few of them are capable of causing disease in humans, but the incidence of human fungal infections has increased dramatically in recent years, largely because of increased use of immunosuppressive drugs and antibiotics.

Candida albicans, a member of the yeast family of fungi, is now the fourth most common organism found in blood cultures in the United States.

Most fungi are completely resistant to conventional **antibiotics**, and new classes of drugs have been created to treat them. There are four main classes of **antifungal drugs**. The first class, **polyene macrolides**, includes **amphotericin B** and **nystatin (Mycostatin, Nilstat)**. The second main class, the **azole** group, includes two subgroups. The **imidazoles** include **butoconazole** (Femstat, Gynazole, Mycelex-3), **clotrimazole** (Gyne-Lotrimin, Lotrimin, Mycelex), **econazole** (Spectazole), **ketoconazole** (Nizoral), **miconazole** (Micatin, Monistat), **terconazole** (Terazol), and **tioconazole** (Vagistat). The **triazoles** include **fluconazole** (Diflucan) and **itraconazole** (Sporanox). The third main class, **allylamines**, includes **naftifine** (Naftin) and **terbinafine** (Lamisil). The fourth main class, **nuclear acid synthesis inhibitors**, consists of only one drug, **flucytosine** (Ancobon). **Posaconazole** (Noxafil) was approved in September 2006 for the management of invasive aspergillosis, fusariosis, and zygomycosis in patients with refractory disease. Its use in planned for patients who have undergone bone marrow transplants or chemotherapy for cancer. It is unlikely that it will be used is primary care practice and so it is not discussed further in this chapter. **Voriconazole** (Vfend) was approved by the FDA in May 2002. It is indicated for invasive aspergillosis and other serious fungal infections not responsive or intolerant to other treatments. Because the oral form is used only after a loading dose is given IV and it is not likely to be used in generalist primary care practice, it is not included in this chapter.

On The Horizon ISAVACONAZOLE

Isavaconazole is a novel, broad-spectrum azole intended to treat most yeasts and molds, including **fluconazole**-resistant *Candida* strains, *Aspergillus*, and *Zygomyces*. It is currently in phase III trials.

Griseofulvin is a **miscellaneous antifungal.** Other **antifungals** used topically include **ciclopirox (Loprox), haloprogin (Halotex), oxiconazole (Oxistat),** and **tolnaftate (Tinactin, Absorbine, Aftate).** The topical use of **antifungals** to treat dermatological infections is discussed in Chapters 23 and 32, and their use in treating vaginal infections is discussed in Chapter 44. This section discusses the systemic use of **antifungals** and the oral route of administration. The classes used in primary care by this route are three **azoles** and **terbinafine**, the oral **allylamines.**

Pharmacodynamics

Both subgroups of **azoles** (**imidazoles** and **triazoles**) reduce fungal ergosterol synthesis in cell membranes by inhibition of fungal CYP450 enzymes. The specificity of these drugs results from greater affinity for fungal CYP450 rather than human CYP450. **Imidazoles** are less specific than **triazoles**, resulting in a higher incidence of drug interactions and adverse reactions.

Among the **imidazoles**, **ketoconazole** is the least specific to fungal CYP450, resulting in more drug interactions and adverse reactions than the other **azoles**, and **fluconazole** is the most specific. In general, the **azoles** are fungistatic in low to moderate doses and fungicidal in higher doses.

Human cells and fungal cells share many anatomical and functional characteristics, so it is difficult to identify drugs that will harm the fungal pathogen without harming the human host. However, because fungi contain ergosterol as the essential lipid in the cell membrane and because in human cells this vital function is fulfilled by cholesterol, many antifungal agents are directed at ergosterol. The **allylamines**, represented by **terbinafine** as an agent in the class with an oral formulation, interfere with the synthesis of ergosterol in the cell membranes of fungi at an earlier step than the **azoles** do by inhibiting the enzyme squalene epoxide. This results in an intracellular accumulation of squalene, disruption of cell membrane function and cell wall synthesis, and fungal cell death.

Sensitivity

The **azoles** have a broad spectrum of activity that includes *Candida* species, *Cryptococcus neoformans*, the endemic mycoses (blastomycosis, coccidioidomycosis, histoplasmosis), and the dermatophytes. **Itraconazole** is also active against *Aspergillus.*

Terbinafine (Lamisil) has in vitro activity against yeasts and a wide range of dermatophyte, filamentous, and dimorphic fungi. It is fungicidal against dermatophytes, such as *Trichophyton* species, *Microsporum* species, and *Epidermophyton floccosum.* It is fungistatic only against *C. albicans*, although it is 65 percent effective in mycological cure of skin infections by this organism. **Terbinafine** is approved only for treatment of onychomycosis (fungal infection of the nails) but is used off-labeled for tinea capitis (ringworm of the scalp), tinea corporis (ringworm of the body), tinea pedis (ringworm of the feet; athlete's foot), and tinea cruris (ringworm of the groin; jock itch). **Terbinafine** is not effective in the treatment of pityriasis versicolor; the concentrations attained by oral **terbinafine** in the stratum corneum are not adequate to treat this infection.

Resistance

Resistance to **azoles** occurs through a variety of mechanisms. Although still rare, the incidence of resistance is increasing as these drugs are used for prophylaxis as well as therapy. Resistant strains of *C. albicans* have been recovered from patients with AIDS.

Pharmacokinetics

The pharmacokinetics of the different **azoles** and of **terbinafine** vary significantly. Table 24–46 presents these pharmacokinetic differences.

Absorption and Distribution

Fluconazole is well absorbed after oral administration, with excellent bioavailability (greater than 90%). It is widely distributed with good penetration into CSF, the eye, and the peritoneum.

The absorption of **itraconazole** is enhanced when it is taken with food, resulting in a bioavailability of 55 percent. The absorption of the oral solution is not affected by food, and it is given without regard to food. The bioavailability of the oral solution is different from that of the capsule, and they should not be used interchangeably. Tissue concentrations are higher than plasma concentrations. **Itraconazole** does not enter the CSF but does enter breast milk.

Absorption of **ketoconazole** from the GI tract is pH dependent, with increasing pH resulting in decreasing absorption. Administration with food may decrease absorption. It is widely distributed, but CSF penetration is unpredictable and minimal. Detectable concentrations are found in urine, saliva, sebum, and cerumen. **Ketoconazole** crosses the placenta and enters breast milk.

Terbinafine is well absorbed after oral administration, with bioavailability of 70 to 85 percent, and is not affected by the presence of food. It is lipophilic and extensively distributed. It concentrates in the stratum corneum, attaining concentrations 25 times that in plasma. It is also distributed via the sebum to hair follicles, skin, and nails. It is not

Table 24–46 ▶ **Pharmacokinetics: Systemic Antifungal Agents**

Drug	Onset	Peak	Duration	Protein Binding	Bioavailability	Half-Life	Elimination
Fluconazole	Slow	1–2 h	24 h	11%–12%	>90%	30 h*	>80% unchanged in urine; 11% as metabolites in urine
Itraconazole†	Rapid	1.5–5 h	12–24 h	99%	55%	21 h–64 h	40% in urine as inactive metabolites; 3%–18% in feces
Ketoconazole	Rapid	1–4 h	24 h	99%	75%	8 h	85%–90% in bile and feces; 10%–15% in urine
Terbinafine	Slow	2 h	UA	>99%	70%–80%	11–17 h	80% in urine as metabolites; 20% in feces

*Increased in renal impairment.
†First number represents capsule, and second number represents oral solution.

known whether **terbinafine** crosses the placenta, but it does enter breast milk.

Metabolism and Excretion

Fluconazole is cleared primarily by renal excretion, with 80 percent appearing as unchanged drug in the urine and 11 percent as metabolites. **Fluconazole** is an inhibitor of CYP450 3A4 and 2C9. Half-life is markedly affected by renal impairment, with an inverse relationship between the elimination half-life and CCr. Dosage adjustments are required for patients with impaired renal function.

Itraconazole is extensively metabolized by the liver into several active metabolites, and fecal excretion varies from 3 to 18 percent of the dose. **Itraconazole** and its metabolites are inhibitors of CYP450 3A4. About 40 percent of the dose is excreted in urine as metabolites.

Ketoconazole is also extensively metabolized by the liver, but to inactive metabolites. It is a potent inhibitor of CYP450 3A4. Excretion is mainly in feces via bile. Renal failure does not alter dosing requirements.

Terbinafine undergoes extensive first-pass metabolism. Metabolism involves only a small fraction (less than 5%) of the hepatic CYP450 capacity, so the drug interactions that are common with the **azoles** do not affect **terbinafine.** Fifteen metabolites have been identified, but none is active. About 80 percent of a dose is excreted in the urine as metabolites, and 20 percent is eliminated in the feces. Both liver impairment and renal impairment require dosage reduction. Table 24–46 depicts the pharmacokinetics of these selected systemic **antifungals.**

Pharmacotherapeutics

Precautions and Contraindications

All of the **azoles** and **terbinafine** have been associated with hepatotoxicity and with rare cases of hepatitis that are usually reversible with discontinuance of the drug. The **azoles** and **terbinafine** are used cautiously for patients with hepatic impairment. For the ones excreted primarily by the kidney, cautious use is required for patients with renal impairment. With both hepatic and renal impairment, dosage adjustments may be required. Both **fluconazole** and **itraconazole** doses are cut in half if the CCr is less than 30 mL/minute. Because of the burden on the liver, **terbinafine** should be used with caution by patients with alcoholism, either active or in remission.

Ketoconazole should not be given to patients with prostatic cancer. High doses of **ketoconazole** are known to suppress adrenal cortical function, and patients with prostatic cancer have died when given this drug. This drug is used with caution for patients with a history of achlorhydria or hypochlorhydria because of the effect of pH on its absorption.

All of the **azoles** are Pregnancy Category C. Both **ketoconazole** and **itraconazole** have teratogenic effects in animals. There are no adequate well-controlled studies in pregnant women. These drugs should be used during pregnancy only when the potential benefits to the mother clearly outweigh the risks to the fetus and there is no reasonable alternative drug. **Terbinafine** is Pregnancy Category B; animal studies show no effects on fertility or fetal toxicity, but adequate studies in humans have not been conducted.

All of the **azoles** and **terbinafine** are excreted in breast milk. After a single 500-mg dose of **terbinafine,** 0.2 to 0.7 mg of **terbinafine** was detected in breast milk. In spite of these low concentrations, it is prudent to avoid administration of **antifungal** drugs to nursing mothers.

The safety and efficacy of these drugs in children vary. **Ketoconazole** is contraindicated for children younger than 2 years and is not recommended as first choice among **azoles** for any pediatric patient. The safety and efficacy of **itraconazole** have not been established for children. Children aged 3 to 16 years, however, have been treated with 100 mg/day for systemic fungal infections without report of serious adverse reactions. One study with the oral solution was conducted on 26 pediatric patients receiving doses of 5 mg/kg a day for 2 weeks. **Fluconazole** has safe and effective doses for infants and children. Experience with neonates is limited, but there is a dosage schedule. Although the safety and efficacy of **terbinafine** have not been established in children, it has been used in a small number of children aged 3 to 16 years and was well tolerated.

Adverse Drug Reactions

Azoles are relatively nontoxic, and the most common adverse reactions are relatively minor GI symptoms. Patients taking **fluconazole** and **itraconazole** have rarely developed exfoliative skin disorders. Patients who develop rashes should be carefully monitored, and the drug discontinued if the lesion progresses. The inhibition of human CYP450 enzymes by **ketoconazole** interferes with the biosynthesis of adrenal and gonadal steroid hormones, producing gynecomastia, infertility, and menstrual irregularities.

The most common adverse reactions with **terbinafine** are also GI and include nausea, vomiting, and diarrhea. Reversible loss or change of taste has occurred after 5 to 8 weeks of therapy, requiring 2 to 6 months to recover after the drug was discontinued. Other adverse effects reported include hypersensitivity, hepatitis, blood dyscrasias, and Stevens-Johnson syndrome (Amichai & Grunwald, 1998).

Drug Interactions

Drug interactions are more common for the drugs with greater human CYP450 activity. All of these drugs are inhibitors of CYP450 3A4 and some of other isoenzyme systems as well (see above). **Ketoconazole** interacts with drugs that increase gastric pH to produce decreased absorption of **ketoconazole.** Additive hepatotoxicity is also possible with other hepatotoxic drugs.

Itraconazole has many drug interactions including **rifampin, histamine$_2$ blockers,** and **warfarin. Fluconazole** has slightly fewer drug interactions but also interacts with **rifampin** and **warfarin.**

Additive hepatotoxicity may occur with concurrent administration of **terbinafine, alcohol,** or other hepatotoxins. Because **terbinafine** is hepatically metabolized by CYP450, drugs that induce or inhibit these enzymes may alter the clearance of **terbinafine.** Those interactions that have been documented for the **azoles** and **terbinafine** are listed in Table 24–47.

Table 24–47 ◆ Drug Interactions: Selected Systemic Antifungal Agents

Drug	Interacting Drug	Possible Effect	Implications
Fluconazole	Cimetidine	Reduced fluconazole AUC	Separate doses
	Hydrochlorothiazide	Significant increase in fluconazole AUC, possibly because of reduced renal clearance	Avoid concurrent use
	Phenytoin	Increased phenytoin AUC	Monitor serum phenytoin levels.
	Rifampin	A single dose of fluconazole after chronic rifampin resulted in a decrease in AUC and a shorter half-life for fluconazole	If both must be taken, monitor effectiveness of fluconazole and adjust dose if needed.
	Sulfonylureas	Significant increase in AUC of tolbutamide, glyburide, and glipizide. Several patients experienced hypoglycemic episodes, some requiring oral glucose treatment	If both must be used, monitor blood glucose levels closely while azole is taken.
	Theophylline	Theophylline AUC and half-life increased and clearance decreased. Increased toxicity risk	Monitor serum theophylline levels. Dosage adjustment may be needed.
	Warfarin	A single warfarin dose after 14 d of fluconazole resulted in an increase in PT/INR	Monitor PT/INR closely while taking azole.
Itraconazole	Benzodiazepines	Elevated plasma concentrations of oral midazolam and triazolam. Prolonged sedative/hypnotic effects	Select different benzodiazepine.
	Buspirone	May elevate buspirone levels, increasing the pharmacological and adverse effects	Closely monitor clinical response to buspirone. Prudent to start with conservative dose and adjust dose of buspirone as needed.

Table 24–47 ◈ **Drug Interactions: Selected Systemic Antifungal Agents—cont'd**

Drug	Interacting Drug	Possible Effect	Implications
	Calcium channel blockers	Edema with concurrent use of dihydropyridines	Monitor cardiac status
	Phenytoin, phenobarbital, isoniazid, carbamazepine	Increased metabolism of itraconazole. Decreased metabolism of phenytoin	Increased dosage of azole may be needed. Monitor phenytoin levels; dosage adjustments may be needed.
	Cyclosporine, tacrolimus, oral hypoglycemic agents, and warfarin	Itraconazole decreases metabolism of these drugs. Increased risk for toxicity, hypoglycemia, and anticoagulant effect	Monitor cyclosporine levels. Monitor for indications of hypoglycemia. Monitor PT/INR.
	Digoxin	Increased digoxin levels	Monitor digoxin levels closely.
	Antacids, histamine$_2$ blockers, and other drugs that increase gastric pH	Reduced plasma itraconazole levels	Much less of a problem with oral solution than with capsules.
Ketoconazole	Antacids, histamine$_2$ blockers, proton-pump inhibitors, and other drugs that increase gastric pH	Inhibit ketoconazole absorption	Avoid concurrent use. Fluconazole absorption is not affected.
	Rifampin, isoniazid	Bioavailability and serum levels of either drug may be affected.	Avoid concurrent use.
	Hepatotoxic drug	Additive hepatotoxicity	Avoid concurrent use.
	Cyclosporine, corticosteroids, warfarin	Ketoconazole decreases metabolism of these drugs. Increased risk for toxicity, anticoagulant effect	Monitor serum levels. Monitor PT/INR more closely. Because the effect on cyclosporine levels is consistent and predictable, this combination has been used therapeutically to reduce cyclosporine dosage.
	Theophylline	Decreased serum theophylline levels	Monitor theophylline levels. Dosage adjustment may be needed.
Terbinafine	Alcohol, hepatotoxins	Additive liver damage	Avoid concurrent use or monitor hepatic function closely.
	Cimetidine	Decreased metabolism of terbinafine	Avoid concurrent use.
	Phenytoin, rifampin	Increased metabolism of terbinafine	Avoid concurrent use or monitor response to terbinafine.
	Caffeine	Decreased metabolism of caffeine	Prudent use of caffeinated beverages.
	Cyclosporine	Increased clearance of cyclosporine, possibly leading to organ rejection	Avoid concurrent use or monitor cyclosporine levels.

INR = international normalized ratio; PT = prothrombin time.

Clinical Use and Dosing

Because of its long half-life, **fluconazole** does not achieve steady state for 5 to 10 days with the usual oral doses, but steady state can be achieved in 2 days with a loading dose of twice the usual dose on the first day. Hence, most dosage regimens for **fluconazole** include a loading dose. Because it may undergo saturation metabolism at higher plasma concentrations, the initial dose of **itraconazole** is often doubled, resulting in a 3-fold increase in the plasma concentration. However, patients with hepatic or renal insufficiency may need reduced maintenance doses of **fluconazole** and **terbinafine**.

Oral antifungal drugs are used to treat superficial infections by yeasts (*Candida,* pityriasis versicolor) and dermatophytes (tinea infections) and to treat invasive systemic mycoses (e.g., paracoccidioidomycosis, blastomycosis, histoplasmosis, aspergillosis, candidiasis). Indications and dosages of the **oral antifungal** drugs are summarized in Table 24–48.

Table 24–48 ◉ **Dosage Schedule: Selected Systemic Antifungal Agents**

Drug	Indication	Initial and Maintenance Dose	Comments
Fluconazole (Diflucan)	Vaginal candidiasis	*Adults:* 150 mg as single PO dose	Maximal daily pediatric dose 600 mg. Shake suspension well before measurement, using calibrated liquid dosing device. Store suspension in refrigerator or at room temperature. Dispose of unused suspension 2 wk after reconstitution.
	Oropharyngeal candidiasis	*Adults:* 200 mg PO on first day, followed by 100 mg once daily for 2 wk *Children:* 6 mg/kg PO on first day, followed by 3 mg/kg once daily for at least 2 wk	May be taken without regard to meals.
	Esophageal candidiasis	*Adults:* 200 mg PO on first day, followed by 100 mg once daily for 2 wk; doses up to 400 mg may be used based on patient response *Children:* 6 mg/kg PO on first day, followed by 3 mg/kg once daily for at least 3 wk and 2 wk beyond resolution of symptoms; doses up to 12 mg/kg/d have been used	Doses are reduced by 50% for CCr <30 mL/min. Older adults may have impaired renal function and require lower dose.
	Other *Candida* infections	*Adults:* 50–400 mg/d PO *Children:* 6–12 mg/kg/d PO have been used	
Ketoconazole (Nizoral)	Candidiasis, vulvovaginal	*Adults:* 200–400 mg PO once daily for 5 d *Children >2 yr:* 3.3–6.6 mg/kg/d as a single dose *Children <2 yr:* Dosage not established	Maximal adult daily dosage is 1 g. Therapy should be continued 1–2 wk in candidiasis (3–5 d in vaginal candidiasis); for 1–8 wk in dermatophytic infections and mycoses of hair and scalp; for 3 mo–1 yr for paracoccidioidomycosis; and for 6 mo in other systemic mycoses. Chronic mucocutaneous candidiasis following a remission usually requires indefinite maintenance treatment to prevent relapse. Take with food to promote absorption and decrease GI irritation. In patients with hypochlorhydria or achlorhydria take with acid drink. May be dissolved in cola or seltzer water or taken with these fluids. Shake suspension well before measurement using a calibrated liquid measuring device. Store at room temperature.

Table 24–48 ◉ **Dosage Schedule: Selected Systemic Antifungal Agents—cont'd**

Drug	Indication	Initial and Maintenance Dose	Comments
	Paronychia	*Adults:* 400 mg PO once daily *Children >2 yr:* 5–10 mg/kg PO once daily *Children <2 yr:* Dosage not established	
	Pityriasis versicolor	*Adults:* 200 mg PO once daily for 5–10 d	
	Fungal pneumonia or septicemia	*Adults:* 400 mg-1 g PO once daily *Children >2 yr:* 5–10 mg/kg PO once daily *Children <2 yr:* Dosage not established	
	All other antifungal indications	*Adults:* 200–400 mg PO once daily *Children >2 yr:* 3.3–6.6 mg/kg PO once daily *Children <2 yr:* Dosage not established	
Itraconazole (Sporanox)	Onychomycosis	*Adults:* 200 mg PO once daily with meal for 12 consecutive wk	Safety and efficacy not established for children. A small number of children aged 3–16 yr with systemic infections have taken itraconazole capsules, 100 mg daily, without serious adverse effects. In life-threatening conditions a loading dose of 200 mg 3 times/d (600 mg/d) is given for first 3 d. Continue treatment for minimum of 3 mo until clinical parameters indicate fungal infection has subsided. Take capsules with food or cola beverage for better absorption. Oral solution should be vigorously swished in mouth, 10 mL at a time, for several sec and swallowed. Solution should be taken on an empty stomach. Dispense solution with calibrated liquid measuring device.
	Onychomycosis, fingernail	*Adults:* 200 mg bid for 1 wk; repeat after 3-wk period without itraconazole	Doses are reduced by 50% for CCr <30 mL/min. Older adults may have impaired renal function and require lower dose.
	Onychomycosis, toenail	200 mg once daily for 12 consecutive wk	Do not use injectable form in patients with CCr <30 mL/min.
	Aspergillosis	*Adults:* 200–400 mg PO once daily with meal	
	Blastomycosis or histoplasmosis	*Adults:* 200 mg PO once daily with meal; if no improvement or progression, increase in 100-mg increments to 400-mg maximum daily dose. Give doses >200 mg daily in 2 divided doses	

Continued

Table 24–48 ◉ **Dosage Schedule: Selected Systemic Antifungal Agents—cont'd**

Drug	Indication	Initial and Maintenance Dose	Comments
	Candidiasis, esophageal	*Adults:* For solution: 100 mg PO (swish and swallow) once daily for minimum of 3 wk (2 wk after resolution of symptoms); off-labeled: 100–200 mg capsules PO once daily after a meal for 14 d; dose for AIDS and neutropenic patients is 200 mg for 4 wk	
	Candidiasis, oropharyngeal	*Adults:* For solution: 200 mg PO (swish and swallow) once daily for 7–14 d; if refractory to fluconazole, use 100 mg twice/d for 2–4 wk; off-labeled: 100–200 mg capsules PO once daily after a meal for 14 d; dose for AIDS and neutropenic patients is 200 mg for 4 wk	
	Candidiasis, vulvovaginal (off-labeled)	*Adults:* 200 mg PO once daily with meal for 3 d	
	Coccidioidomycosis (off-labeled)	*Adults:* 200 mg PO twice daily with meals for 6 wk	
	Histoplasmosis suppression (off-labeled)	*Adults:* 200 mg PO twice daily with meals	
	Paracoccidioidomycosis (off-labeled)	*Adults:* 100 mg PO once daily with meal for 6 wk	
	Tinea corporis or cruris (off-labeled)	*Adults:* 100 mg PO once daily with meal for 15 d	
	Tinea manus or pedis (off-labeled)	*Adults:* 100 mg PO once daily with meal for 30 d	
Terbinafine (Lamisil)	Onychomycosis, fingernail	*Adults:* 250 mg PO once daily for 6 wk	May be taken without regard to meals Patients with preexisting stable liver disease, impaired renal function (CCr <50 mL/min), or serum creatinine <3.4 mg/dL should receive 50% reduction in dosage Safety and efficacy for children and children's dosage not established. Following dosages have been use in treatment of children age 3–16 yr: Children 12.5–18.5 kg: oral 62.5 mg once daily Children 18.5–25 kg: 125 mg once daily Children >25 kg: 250 mg once daily
	Onychomycosis, toenail	*Adults:* 250 mg PO once daily for 12 wk; extensive toenail infections may take longer	
	Tinea capitis (off-labeled)	*Adults:* 250 mg PO once daily for 4–6 wk	
	Tinea corporis or cruris (off-labeled)	*Adults:* 250 mg PO once daily for 2–4 wk	
	Tinea pedis (plantar or interdigital) (off-labeled)	*Adults:* 250 mg PO once daily for 2–6 wk	

CCr = creatinine clearance.

Rational Drug Selection

Antifungal drug selection is based on susceptibility, pharmacokinetics, and adverse effects. The spectrum of **terbinafine** includes dermatophytes, and it is recommended for treatment of onychomycosis and tinea infections. The spectrum of the **azoles** includes dermatophytic and superficial fungi, as well as invasive systemic fungi. **Fluconazole** has more reliable bioavailability than the other **azoles** and is generally recommended for the treatment of mild to moderate systemic fungal infections. **Fluconazole** also has fewer drug interactions than other **azoles**, has a single-dose regimen for some indications, and is preferred by many clinicians for these reasons. It is also the drug of choice for treating vaginal yeast infections in patients with diabetes.

Monitoring

Prompt recognition of liver injury is essential with **oral antifungal** drugs, particularly **ketoconazole.** AST, ALT, alkaline phosphatase, and bilirubin should be monitored prior to initiation of therapy, monthly for 3 to 4 months, and frequently thereafter during treatment. Even modest elevations in liver enzymes require discontinuation of **ketoconazole.** Because of the numerous drug interactions with **azoles**, it is important to monitor the drug response of concurrent medications. Therapeutic response should be evaluated at 6 to 8 weeks after initiation of drug therapy for tinea infections, 4 to 6 months for fingernail onychomycosis, and 8 to 9 months for toenail mycoses.

Patient Education

Administration

The available dosage forms are shown in Table 24–49. **Itraconazole** capsules and **ketoconazole** should be taken with food to alleviate GI symptoms and promote absorption. **Antacids** should not be used in conjunction with these agents. **Itraconazole** solution should be taken on an empty stomach; **fluconazole** and **terbinafine** can be taken without regard to meals. Because these drugs have many drug interactions, any time that a new drug is added to the patient's treatment regimen, it should be reviewed for possible interactions.

Adverse Reactions

Ketoconazole can cause drowsiness, so patients should not perform hazardous tasks until their response to the medication is established. Because hepatotoxicity is common to all the **oral antifungals**, concurrent use of **alcohol** is discouraged. **Ketoconazole** may cause phototoxicity, so sunscreen and protective clothing are advisable outdoors. Patients should report signs of liver toxicity (unusual tiredness, anorexia, nausea and vomiting, jaundice, pale stools, dark urine), Stevens-Johnson syndrome (rash, blisters, loosening of skin, red joints), and leukopenia (sore throat or fever). Patients on **terbinafine** should know that loss of taste is a reversible adverse effect.

Lifestyle Management

Factors that have contributed to the rise of fungal infections are overuse of **antibiotics**, increased numbers of

Table 24–49 ◆ **Available Dosage Forms: Selected Systemic Antifungals**

Drug	Dosage Form	How Supplied	Cost
Fluconazole (Diflucan)	Tablet: 50 mg (B)	In bottles of 30 tablets	$169/30
	100 mg (B)	In bottles of 30 and UD 100 tablets	$264/30
	150 mg (B)	In UD 1 tablets	$169/12
	200 mg (B)	In bottles of 30 and UD 100 tablets	$431/30
	Powder for oral suspension: 10 mg/mL (B);	In 35 mL	$43/35 mL
	40 mg/mL (B)	In 35 mL	$144/35 mL
Itraconazole (Sporanox)	Capsule: 100 mg (G)	In bottles of 28, 30, 100, 500 and UD 28 and 30 capsules	
	100 mg (B)	In bottles of 30, UD 30 and PulsePak 28 capsules	$264/30; $248 for BlisterPak 28
	Oral solution: 10 mg/mL (B)	In 150 mL	$127/150 mL
Ketoconazole (Nizoral)	Tablets: 200 mg (G)	In bottles of 30, 50, 100, 250, 500, 1,000 and blister packs of 10; UD 30, 50, 100 tablets	$35/100
	200 mg (B)	In bottles of 100 tablets	$405/100
Terbinafine (Lamisil)	Tablet: 250 mg	In bottles of 30, 100 tablets	$995/100

B = brand name; G = generic.

immunocompromised patients, and increased environmental exposure. Patients and providers should try to limit **antibiotic** use, which will decrease emergence of bacterial resistance, and fungal superinfection.

ANTHELMINTICS

Infestation with parasitic worms is a major health problem throughout the world infecting billions and killing millions annually (World Health Organization, 2010). In the United States, approximately 60 million people are estimated to harbor a helminthic parasite (VandeWaa, Henderson, White, & Nowatzke, 1998). The worms are divided into four groups: intestinal nematodes (roundworms), tissue nematodes (roundworms), cestodes (flatworms and tapeworms), and trematodes (flukes). The only common helminthic infections in the United States are intestinal nematodes: *Enterobius vermicularis* (pinworm), *Trichuris trichiura* (whipworm), *Ascaris lumbricoides* (roundworm), *Strongyloides stercoralis* (threadworm), and the hookworms *Ancylostoma duodenale* and *Necator americanus.* Only those drugs used to treat these infections are discussed in this chapter.

Pharmacodynamics

The **benzimidazoles (mebendazole [Vermox], thiabendazole [Mintezol], albendazole [Albenza])** act in different ways directly on the parasite. **Mebendazole** inhibits the formation of the worm's microtubules and irreversibly blocks glucose uptake, depleting endogenous glycogen storage. The worm "starves to death." **Thiabendazole** suppresses production of eggs or larvae and their subsequent development. **Albendazole** inhibits tubulin polymerization, resulting in loss of cytoplasmic microtubules.

Pyrantel (Pin-Rid, Reese's Pinworm, Antiminth) is a depolarizing neuromuscular blocking agent that creates spastic paralysis in the worm. It also inhibits cholinesterases. **Ivermectin (Stromectol)** increases the permeability of the cell membrane, resulting in loss of extracellular calcium and increase in intracellular calcium and also producing massive contractions and paralysis of the worm's neuromusculature.

Drugs of choice for treating intestinal nematodes include **mebendazole, pyrantel,** and **thiabendazole.** Tissue nematodes are best treated with **mebendazole, thiabendazole, albendazole,** or **ivermectin.**

Pharmacokinetics

Absorption and Distribution

Thiabendazole is well absorbed from the GI tract after oral administration. The other drugs are poorly absorbed following oral administration. The oral bioavailability of **albendazole** and **mebendazole** appears to be enhanced (up to 5-fold) when taken with a fatty meal.

Albendazole is widely distributed and has been detected in urine, bile, liver, cyst wall, cyst fluid, and CSF. **Ivermectin** has a wide tissue distribution. It apparently enters the eye slowly and to a limited extent. The distribution of **mebendazole, pyrantel,** and **thiabendazole** is not known.

Metabolism and Excretion

Albendazole is rapidly converted by the liver to the primary metabolite, **albendazole sulfoxide,** which is further converted to other metabolites. These metabolites are excreted primarily in the urine.

Ivermectin is metabolized by the liver. The parent drug and its metabolites are excreted almost exclusively in feces over an estimated 12 days.

Absorbed **mebendazole** is mostly metabolized by the liver. More than 95 percent is excreted in feces, and the remainder by the kidney. **Thiabendazole** is also extensively metabolized by the liver, and the inactive metabolites are excreted in the urine.

Pyrantel pamoate undergoes limited metabolism, and more than 50 percent is excreted as unchanged drug in the feces. Less than 7 percent is found in urine as parent drug and metabolites. Table 24–50 presents the pharmacokinetics of selected **anthelmintics.**

Pharmacotherapeutics

Precautions and Contraindications

Because the activity of these drugs is specific to the parasites, precautions and contraindications are minimal. Drugs extensively metabolized by the liver require cautious administration to patients with hepatic impairment. Drugs excreted extensively by the kidney may require careful monitoring of renal function.

Pregnancy Category C is given to all of these. There are no adequate well-controlled studies in pregnant women, however, for any of these drugs. **Albendazole** and **ivermectin** have demonstrated teratogenic and embryotoxic effects in some animal studies and should not be given to pregnant women.

It is not known whether **albendazole, mebendazole, pyrantel pamoate,** or **thiabendazole** is excreted in breast milk. Caution should be exercised when giving them to a nursing mother. Deciding to discontinue the drug or the nursing should take into account the importance of the drug to the mother. **Ivermectin** is known to be excreted in breast milk. Nursing can begin 1 week after the last dose of **ivermectin.**

The safety and efficacy of these drugs in children vary by drug. **Mebendazole** and **pyrantel pamoate** are not recommended for children younger than age 2 years, and **albendazole** is not recommended for children younger than 6 years (although no adverse reactions have been found in studies of children as young as 1 year). Weight is the determination for some drugs, with **thiabendazole** not recommended for children less than 13.5 kg and **ivermectin** contraindicated for children less than 15 kg.

Table 24–50 ▶ **Pharmacokinetics: Selected Anthelmintics**

Drug	Onset	Peak	Protein Binding	Bioavailability	Half-Life	Elimination
Albendazole	UA	2–5 h	70%	UA	8–12 h	Mainly in urine; small amount in feces
Ivermectin	UA	4 h	UA	UA	16 h	Fecal elimination; <1% in urine
Mebendazole	UA	2–4 h	95%	2%–3%	2.5–5.5 h	>90% fecal elimination; 2% in urine
Pyrantel pamoate	UA	1–3 h	UA	UA	UA	50% unchanged drug in feces; <7% in urine
Thiabendazole	Rapid	1–2 h	UA	UA	1.2 h	5% in feces; 90% in urine

Duration of action of all of these drugs is unknown.
UA = information unavailable.

Adverse Drug Reactions

Adverse reactions vary by drug, with the most common being nausea, vomiting, diarrhea, transient abdominal pain, fever, pruritus, and skin rash. Reversible neutropenia has occurred with **mebendazole**, and CNS symptoms has occurred with **thiabendazole**.

Some patients taking **ivermectin** experience the Mazzotti reaction (fever, headache, dizziness, somnolence, weakness, rash, pruritus, diarrhea, joint pain and muscle spasms, hypotension, tachycardia, lymphadenitis, and peripheral edema), which starts the first day and peaks the second day of therapy. It is due to the killing of the microfilariae and not to toxicity. This reaction diminishes with repeated dosing. **Corticosteroids** may be needed for several days to suppress the inflammatory response.

Drug Interactions

There are few drug–drug interactions with any of these drugs. Table 24–51 lists these interactions.

Clinical Use and Dosing

The five common intestinal helminthic infections in the United States are described here, with indication of the usual **antimicrobial** agents. Dosages of the **anthelmintic** drugs are summarized in Table 24–52.

Enterobius Vermicularis (Pinworm)

The pinworm is named for the morphology of the posterior of the female. As many as 50 million people in the United States, primarily children, are infected with pinworm. The primary symptoms of pinworm, perianal itching and sleep disruption, are related to the fact that

Table 24–51 ■ **Drug Interactions: Selected Anthelmintics**

Drug	Interacting Drug	Possible Effect	Implications
Albendazole	Dexamethasone	Steady state trough of main metabolite 50% higher	Avoid coadministration
	Cimetidine	Metabolite concentrations in bile and cystic fluid higher	May be used therapeutically
Mebendazole	Carbamazepine, phenytoin	May reduce plasma levels of mebendazole; possible decrease in therapeutic effects	Avoid concomitant use
	Cimetidine	Increased plasma concentrations of mebendazole	May be used therapeutically
Pyrantel pamoate	Theophylline	May increase serum levels of theophylline	Further study needed. Only one case noted
Thiabendazole	Xanthines	Thiabendazole may compete with these drugs for metabolism sites; may elevate serum levels of xanthine with increased toxicity risk	Monitor serum levels of xanthine closely

Table 24–52 ◉ **Dosage Schedule: Selected Anthelmintics**

Drug	Indication	Initial Dose	Comments
Albendazole (Albenza)	Ascariasis	*Children >2 yr and adults:*	Maximal daily dose for adults and adolescents <60 kg is 800 mg.
	Enterobiasis Hookworm infections	400 mg PO once daily for 3 d; may repeat in 3 wk	Take with food containing fat. Swallow tablets whole with small amount of liquid.
	Trichuriasis	*Children <2 yr:* 200 mg PO as single dose; may repeat in 3 wk	Shake suspension well before measurement with calibrated liquid measuring device. Store at room temperature.
	Strongyloidiasis	*Children >2 yr and adults:* 400 mg PO once daily for 3 d; may repeat in 3 wk *Children <2 yr:* 200 mg PO once daily for 3 d; may repeat in 3 wk	
	Giardiasis	*Adults:* 400 mg PO daily for 5 d	
Ivermectin (Stromectol)	Strongyloidiasis	*Children >15 kg and adults:* 200 mcg/kg as single dose	Take with full glass of water 1 h before breakfast. Repeat in 1 to 2 wk.
	Scabies in immunocompromised patients	*Adults:* 200 mcg/kg as a single dose	
Mebendazole (Vermox)	Ascariasis Trichuriasis Hookworm Roundworms Enterobiasis	*Children >2 yr and adults:* 100 mg PO twice daily, morning and evening, for 3 d; may repeat in 2–3 wk if required *Adults:* 100 mg PO as single dose; may repeat in 2–3 wk if required	Take with high-fat meals. Tablets may be chewed, crushed, or swallowed whole.
Mebendazole	Pinworms	*Children and Adults:* One single 100 mg chewable tablet; repeat in 2 wk	
Pyrantel pamoate (Pin-Rid)	Enterobiasis	*Children and adults:*	Maximum daily dose 1 g.
	Ascariasis Trichuriasis Hookworm	11 mg/kg as single dose	May be taken with milk, food, or juice at any time of day Shake suspension well, and measure with calibrated liquid measuring device. Store at room temperature.
Thiabendazole (Mintezol)	Strongyloidiasis, uncomplicated	*Children >13.6 kg and adults:* 25 mg/kg twice daily for 2 d	Maximum adult daily dose 3 g. Chew or crush tablets before swallowing. Take after meals. Shake suspension well before measurement with calibrated liquid dosing device. Take after meals.
	Strongyloidiasis, hyperinfection	*Children >13.6 kg and adults:* 25 mg/kg twice daily for 5–7 d; may be repeated if required	

the female lays eggs nocturnally in the perianal area. Drugs used to treat pinworms include **pyrantel pamoate, albendazole,** and **mebendazole.**

Trichuris Trichiura (Whipworm)

Some 80 million people worldwide and 2.2 million in the United States are infected with whipworm. People acquire whipworm by ingesting uncooked vegetables grown in soil contaminated by human feces. The infection is usually asymptomatic, although heavy infestations may produce anemia, bloody diarrhea, and growth retardation. Drugs used for whipworm infections include **pyrantel pamoate, albendazole,** and **mebendazole.**

Ascaris Lumbricoides (Roundworm)

The roundworm is the most common helminthic parasite worldwide and affects 4 million people in the United States, primarily in the Southeast. Infection generally is derived from eating feces-contaminated raw vegetables. The parasite has a larval stage that migrates through the lungs, causing seasonal pneumonitis, but GI symptoms are more common. Massive infections can cause intestinal obstruction. The drug used for roundworm infections is **mebendazole**.

Ancylostoma Duodenale or *Necator Americanus* (Hookworm)

Hookworms comprise pathogens from two genera, *A. duodenale* and *N. americanus.* The larvae live in the soil and must penetrate the skin to enter the circulation, where they are carried to the lungs. Here they penetrate the alveoli, crawl up the pharynx, and are swallowed. They attach to the intestinal wall and can cause anemia. A recent phenomenon is the use of hookworms to treat allergies and asthma. Although there is little evidence regarding the effectiveness of this treatment, patients can purchase hookworms via the Internet and self-medicate. Drugs used for hookworm infections include **pyrantel pamoate**, **albendazole**, and **mebendazole**.

Strongyloides Stercoralis (Threadworm)

The larvae of the threadworm are found in warm, moist soil in the tropics and the southern United States. The larvae may penetrate the skin or be ingested. Pulmonary and GI symptoms are common. The drugs used for threadworm infections are **ivermectin** and **thiabendazole**. **Ivermectin** is the drug of choice because it has fewer adverse effects, but **thiabendazole** has the added benefit of promoting immune function in patients with AIDS.

Scabies

Ivermectin may be prescribed off-labeled to selected patients with scabies (Currie & McCarthy, 2010). It is particularly effective in treating scabies in patients who are immunocompromised. The dose is 200 mcg/kg given as a single dose (Currie & McCarthy, 2010). Because **ivermectin** is not ovicidal, it should be repeated in 1 to 2 weeks.

Rational Drug Selection

Drugs are selected for helminthic infections based on research and previous clinical experience, published by the CDC. Drug selection is modified by specific patient characteristics. For example, **albendazole** is contraindicated in pregnancy. Because it is available as a liquid formulation, **pyrantel pamoate** may be preferred for children when the organism is susceptible. It is also available OTC, which may reduce inconvenience and promote adherence.

Monitoring

Evaluation of the efficacy of the **anthelmintic** drugs includes assessing the eradication of the helminth. For *E. vermicularis,* cellophane tape swabs of the perianal area should be obtained before starting and 1 week after drug therapy, especially in patients with persistent symptoms. The swab should be obtained every morning prior to defecation and bathing for at least 3 days to determine proof of cure.

For roundworms, hookworms, ascariasis, trichuriasis, and whipworms, stool samples are obtained before and 1 to 3 weeks after treatment to determine proof of cure. For strongyloidiasis, routine stool examinations and special examinations such as the Baermann technique may be required prior to treatment and repeated at intervals of 3 months, beginning at 6 weeks after treatment, to establish proof of cure.

Patients taking prolonged therapy with these agents should have periodic evaluation of hepatic function and CBCs. These tests should also be repeated whenever there is clinical evidence of hepatotoxicity or blood dyscrasias.

Patient Education

Administration

The available dosage forms are shown in Table 24–53. **Albendazole** should be swallowed whole with a small amount of water and a high-fat meal to decrease GI effects and increase absorption. **Mebendazole** is also taken with a high-fat meal, but it can be chewed or crushed before it is swallowed. **Ivermectin** must be taken with a full glass of water on an empty stomach 1 hour before breakfast. **Pyrantel pamoate** can be taken without regard to meals, at any time of the day. **Thiabendazole** must be chewed or crushed before swallowing and taken after a meal.

Adverse Reactions

Women of childbearing capacity should take **albendazole** after a negative pregnancy test in the first 7 days following the onset of menses and should use a backup barrier method of contraception for 1 month after completing the therapy. **Albendazole** should not be used in conjunction with OTC or prescription **cimetidine**, which decreases clearance of **albendazole**. Patients who have recently taken **albendazole** should also report signs of neutropenia (sore throat, fever, unusual tiredness). **Mebendazole** should also be avoided during pregnancy.

Ivermectin and **thiabendazole** can cause lightheadedness, so hazardous activities should be avoided during therapy. Patients should be warned of the asparagus-like odor of urine during **thiabendazole** therapy, which may be unpleasant but is harmless. Both of these agents may be associated with a skin rash or itching during treatment of strongyloidiasis because of the death of microfilariae in the skin. If serious, this syndrome may require short-term therapy with **corticosteroids** to suppress the inflammatory response. Patients on **thiabendazole** should report any evidence of neurotoxicity (numbness or tingling of the hands, delirium, disorientation, hallucinations), crystalluria (back pain, burning on urination), or Stevens-Johnson

Table 24–53 ◆ **Available Dosage Forms: Selected Anthelmintics**

Drug	Dosage Form	How Supplied	Cost
Albendazole (Albenza)	Tablets: 200 mg	In bottles of 112 tablets	$40/12
Ivermectin (Stromectol)	Tablets: 6 mg	In 10-unit doses	
Mebendazole (Vermox)	Chewable Tablets: 100 mg	In 12 tablets	$16/1 tablet
Pyrantel pamoate (Pin-Rid)	Capsules: 180 mg (62.5 mg of pyrantel base) Liquid: 50 mg/mL	In bottles of 24 soft-gel capsules In 60-mL bottles (cherry flavor)	
(Pin-X)	Liquid: 50 mg/mL	In 30-mL bottles (caramel flavor)	
(Reese's Pinworm)	Capsules: 180 mg (62.5 mg of pyrantel base) Liquid: 50 mg/mL	In bottles of 24 soft-gel capsules In 30-mL bottles	
(Antiminth)	Oral suspension: 50 mg/mL	In 30-mL bottles	
Thiabendazole (Mintezol)	Tablets: 500 mg Oral suspension: 50 mg/mL	In bottles of 36 scored, chewable tablets (orange flavor) In 120-mL bottles	

syndrome (rash, blistering, loose skin, peeling, aching joints and muscles, chills, fever).

Lifestyle Management

Patients with hookworm and whipworm infections may require **iron** replacement therapy. Eradication of pinworm infections usually requires simultaneous treatment of all household contacts; a vigorous hygiene program of cleaning bed linens, nightwear, and underwear; and good hand-washing habits. Contrary to popular belief, treatment of helminthic infections does not require special diets or purging with **laxatives** before or after the **antimicrobial** drug.

METRONIDAZOLE AND NITAZOXANIDE

Metronidazole (Flagyl, Metric 21, Protostat) is a drug that crosses classes—that is, it is effective in both parasitical and bacterial infections—so its systemic use is discussed in this separate section. Topical applications are discussed in Chapters 23 and 32 for skin conditions and in Chapter 44 for vaginal disorders. **Nitazoxanide (Alinia)** is used in treating *Giardia lamblia* and for its role in treating *Cryptosporidium parvum* infections. **Tinidazole (Tindamax)** is approved for treatment of amebiasis, giardiasis, and trichomoniasis.

Pharmacodynamics

Metronidazole is a **nitroimidazole** that disrupts DNA and protein synthesis of susceptible organisms. With anaerobic bacteria and sensitive protozoal cells, the nitro group of this drug is chemically reduced to ferredoxin, which is bactericidal by reacting with intracellular macromolecules.

Metronidazole possesses direct trichomonacidal and amebicidal activity against *Trichomonas vaginalis* and *Entamoeba histolytica.* It is also active against *H. pylori* and against anaerobic bacteria including *Bacteroides* and *Clostridium.* Although an off-labeled use, it is active against *G. lamblia* and *Gardnerella vaginalis.* It is now the recommended drug for treatment of pseudomembranous colitis associated with *C. difficile* overgrowth secondary to use of **antibiotics.**

Nitazoxanide interferes with the pyruvate-ferredoxin oxidoreductase (PFOR) enzyme-dependent electron transfer reaction, which is essential to anaerobic energy metabolism in the protozoa. It is also active in vitro in inhibiting the growth of sporozoites and oocytes of *C. parvum* and *G. lamblia.*

Tinidazole is an **antiprotozoal** agent similar to **metronidazole.** The nitro group of **tinidazole** is reduced but cell extracts of *Trichomonas.* The mechanisms by which it exhibits activity against *Giardia* and *Entamoeba* is not known. It has shown activity against *T. vaginalis, G. lamblia,* and *E. histolytica*.

Pharmacokinetics

Absorption and Distribution

Oral metronidazole is readily absorbed and widely distributed into most tissue and fluids, including CSF, breast milk, alveolar bone, liver abscesses, vaginal secretions, and seminal fluid. It also crosses the placenta. Intracellular concentrations approach extracellular levels. **Nitazoxanide** is well absorbed orally. When **nitazoxanide** tablets are administered with food, the AUC for the two metabolites increases 2-fold and the C_{max} is increased by approximately 50 percent. Administration of the oral solution results in a 45 to 50 percent increase in AUC and the C_{max} increases only 10 percent or less. Both formulations should be taken with food. Ninety-nine percent of the first metabolite is bound to plasma proteins for distribution. **Tinidazole** is rapidly and completely absorbed after oral administration. Administration with food delays T_{max} by approximately 2 hours and C_{max} declines by approximately 70 percent; however, it does not affect overall bioavailability of the drug. It is widely distributed to virtually all tissues, crosses the blood–brain barrier and the placental barrier, and is secreted in breast milk.

Metabolism and Excretion

Metronidazole is partially metabolized by the liver (30% to 60%); the drug and its metabolites are excreted in feces (6% to 15%), with the rest excreted in urine. **Nitazoxanide** is rapidly metabolized after oral administration to an active metabolite, **tizoxanide**, which then undergoes conjugation, primarily by glucuronidation to a second active metabolite, **tizoxanide glucuronide**. The parent compound is not detected in the plasma. Despite its extensive metabolism by the liver, the CYP450 system does not appear to be affected by **nitazoxanide**. **Tinidazole** is metabolized similarly to **metronidazole**. It is metabolized mainly by the CYP3A4 isoenzyme system. **Tinidazole** is excreted by both the liver and kidneys. Table 24–54 presents the pharmacokinetics of these three drugs.

Pharmacotherapeutics

Precautions and Contraindications

Cautious use is recommended with **metronidazole** for patients with a history of blood dyscrasias. Seizures have occurred as an adverse reaction, and patients with a history of seizure disorder or neurological problems should use this drug with caution. Severe hepatic dysfunction may decrease plasma clearance, and metronidazole should be used cautiously with these patients. **Tinidazole** is also a **nitroimidazole** and has the same precautions and contraindications.

The pharmacokinetics of **nitazoxanide** in patients with compromised renal or hepatic function have not been studied. It must be administered with caution to patients with hepatic and biliary disease and to patients with renal disease or a combination of the two. Older adults often have renal impairment and it should be used cautiously in that population for that reason.

Metronidazole is listed as Pregnancy Category B, but many experts believe it should not be used in the first trimester of pregnancy. It has been used to treat trichomoniasis in the second and third trimesters of pregnancy, but not as a single-dose regimen. Although this drug has been used for more than 20 years with no increase in congenital abnormalities, stillbirths, or low birth weight reported, as with any drug given during pregnancy, prudence suggests that it be used only when clearly indicated. **Nitazoxanide** is also listed as Pregnancy Category B. Animal studies have been done and show no evidence of impaired fertility or harm to the fetus. However, there are no adequate, well-controlled studies in humans and this drug is relatively new on the market. It should be used only when clearly indicated and when there is no other reasonable drug. **Tinidazole** is Pregnancy Category C. It has not been studied in pregnant patients, but is known to cross the placental barrier. It should not be given to pregnant patients in the first trimester. Given the long history of use of **metronidazole**, it is a better drug choice for treatment of *G. lamblia* in pregnancy.

A nursing mother who needs **metronidazole** or **tinidazole** should interrupt nursing for 24 hours and use a single-dose regimen. Safety and efficacy in young children have not been established. It is not known if **nitazoxanide** is excreted in breast milk and the choice to use it for a lactating mother should be made with extreme caution.

Safety and efficacy of **metronidazole** in children have been established only for treatment of amebiasis, although there are also drug dosages published for trichomoniasis and giardiasis. Elimination relates inversely to age. A single tablet of **nitazoxanide** contains more drug than is

Table 24–54 ▶ Pharmacokinetics: Metronidazole, Nitazoxanide, and Tinidazole

Drug	Onset (h)	Peak (h)	Duration (h)	Protein Binding	Bioavailability	Half-Life	Elimination
Metronidazole	Rapid	1–3	8	<20%		7.5 h	20% unchanged in urine; 6%–15% in feces
Nitazoxanide	UK*	1–4 ; 2–8**	12	99%	Tablet: 100%; oral suspension: 70%	UK	As metabolites
Tinidazole	UK	1.6 h	72 h	12%		12–14 h	12% excreted in feces; 20%–25% unchanged in urine

UK = unknown.
*Onset of antidiarrheal activity is 24–48 hours.
**The first number is for the tizoxanide metabolite; the second number is for the tizoxanide glucuronide metabolite.

allowed for pediatric patients 11 years or younger; only oral suspension should be used for children aged 1 to 11 years. It should not be used for children younger than 1 year. **Nitazoxanide** is approved for treatment of *G. lamblia* and *C. parvum* in children. No adult doses are provided. **Tinidazole** is approved for treatment of intestinal amebiasis and giardia in both adults and children 3 years of age or older.

Adverse Drug Reactions

Anorexia, nausea, abdominal pain, dizziness, and headache commonly occur with **metronidazole**. Dry mouth and a metallic taste may also develop. Although irritating, these adverse reactions are mild and transient. Infrequent adverse reactions include diarrhea, glossitis, rashes, leukopenia, and peripheral neuropathy. Taking the drug with meals lessens the GI irritation. One rare but serious adverse reaction is seizures.

GI irritation with abdominal pain, nausea, and diarrhea are the main adverse reactions for **nitazoxanide** as well. In clinical trails, they occurred in less than 8 percent of the patients.

Adverse effects associated with **tinidazole** are similar to those for **metronidazole**.

Drug Interactions

Drug interactions with all three drugs are few. **Cimetidine** may decrease the plasma clearance of **metronidazole**, increasing serum levels; **phenobarbital** and **phenytoin** may accelerate excretion, decreasing serum levels. **Metronidazole** potentiates the **anticoagulant** effects of **warfarin** so that close monitoring of prothrombin time/international normalized ratio (PT/INR) is required. A **disulfiram**-like reaction may occur with **alcohol** ingestion, and patients are warned not to consume alcohol while taking this drug and for 48 hours after completing it. Leukopenia risk is increased if it is given concurrently with **fluorouracil** or **azathioprine**. Concurrent use should be avoided. Drug interactions are similar for **tinidazole. Nitazoxanide** is heavily bound to plasma proteins, and may interact with other drugs that are also heavily protein bound (competition for binding sites), especially those with narrow therapeutic ranges (e.g., **warfarin**).

Clinical Use and Dosing

Metronidazole and **tinidazole** have antiparasitic and antibacterial properties. They are used against the common protozoal infections by *T. vaginalis, G. lamblia,* and *E. histolytica*. **Metronidazole** is also used to treat less common parasites, such as the protozoon *Balantidium coli* (with an oral dose of 750 mg three times daily for 5 d), as an alternative to **tetracycline**, and to treat the helminth *Dracunculus medinensis*, or guinea worm (with an oral dose of 250 mg three times daily for 10 d). **Antibacterial** uses of **metronidazole** include treatment of anaerobic bacterial infections, bacterial vaginosis, AAPMC, and eradication of *H. pylori* in gastritis and peptic ulcer disease. Most of the anaerobic bacterial infections treated with **metronidazole** are serious, even life threatening, and are treated in the hospital. Dosages of **metronidazole** for these diverse conditions are summarized in Table 24–55. In severe hepatic disease, the dosage of **metronidazole**

Table 24–55 ● **Dosage Schedule: Metronidazole, Nitazoxanide, and Tinidazole**

Drug	Indication	Initial Dose	Comments
Metronidazole (Flagyl, Metric 21, Protostat)	Anaerobic bacterial infection	*Adults* 7.5 mg/kg PO q6h for 7 d or longer *Children:*	Maximum adult daily dosage is 4 g. Reduction in dosage may be required for patients with severe hepatic impairment.
		7.5 mg/kg PO q6h *or* 10 mg/kg q8h	May be taken with meals or a snack to decrease GI irritation. Avoid alcoholic beverages during therapy and for 48 h after completing it. Sexual partners of patients with *Trichomonas vaginalis* should be treated even if asymptomatic. Abstain from sexual contact or use condom for 7 d after therapy begins. Antimicrobial drugs used with metronidazole to eradicate *Helicobacter pylori* include bismuth subsalicylate, amoxicillin, tetracycline, plus acid-reducing drug if disease is active.

Table 24–55 ◉ **Dosage Schedule: Metronidazole, Nitazoxanide, and Tinidazole—cont'd**

Drug	Indication	Initial Dose	Comments
			Oral forms: Generic: 250 mg in bottles of 100, 250, 500, and 1,000 tablets; 500 mg in bottles of 100, 200, 250, and 500 tablets. Flagyl: 250 mg in bottles of 50, 100, 250, 1,000, and 2500 tablets; 500 mg in bottles of 50, 100, and 500 tablets; 375 mg in bottles of 50 and 100 capsules. Metric 21: 250 mg in bottles of 100 tablets. Protostat: 250 mg in bottles of 100 scored tablets; 500 mg in bottles of 50 scored tablets.
	Antibiotic-associated pseudomembranous colitis *(Clostridium difficile)* (off-labeled)	*Adults*: 500 mg PO 3 times daily *or* 250 mg PO 4 times daily for 10–14 d	
	Bacterial vaginosis associated with *T. vaginalis* (off-labeled)	*Adults* 500 mg PO twice daily for 7 d	
	Giardiasis *(Giardia lamblia)* (off-labeled)	*Adults* 250 mg PO 3 times daily for 5–7 d *Children:* 5 mg/kg/dose PO 3 times daily for 5–7 d	
	Amebiasis *(Entamoeba histolytica)* dysentery	*Adults* 750 mg PO 3 times daily for 5–10 d *Children:* 35–50 mg/kg/24 h PO in 3 divided doses for 10 d *or* 11.6–16.7 mg/kg/dose PO 3 times daily for 10 d	
	Amebiasis *(E. histolytica)* liver abscess	*Adults*: 500–750 mg PO 3 times daily for 5–10 d *Children:* 35–50 mg/kg/24 h PO in 3 divided doses for 10 d *or* 11.6–16.7 mg/kg/dose PO 3 times daily for 10 d	
	Balantidiasis (off-labeled) *(Balantidium coli)*	Adults: 500–750 mg PO 3 times/d for 5–10 d *Children:* 11.6–16.7 mg/kg/dose 3 times daily for 10 d	
	Gastritis or peptic ulcer, *H. pylori*–associated	*Adults*: In combination with antibiotic therapy (see Comments): 500 mg PO 3 times daily for 7–14 d	
	Trichomoniasis *(T. vaginalis)*	*Adults*: 2 g PO as a single dose or 2 divided doses in 1 d; alternative: 250 mg PO 3 times/d for 7 d *Children:* 5 mg/kg/dose PO 3 times daily for 7 d	

Continued

Table 24–55 ◉ **Dosage Schedule: Metronidazole, Nitazoxanide, and Tinidazole—cont'd**

Drug	Indication	Initial Dose	Comments
	Anthelmintic	*Adults:* 250 mg PO 3 times daily for 10 d *Children:* 8.3 mg/kg/dose PO, up to a maximum of 250 mg, 3 times/d for 10 d	
Nitazoxanide	*G. lamblia*	*Children 1–3 yr:* 5-mL oral suspension* *q12h 4–11 yr:* 10-mL oral suspension q12h *≥ 12 yr:* 1 tablet (500 mg) q12h or 25-mL oral suspension q12h	Take with food. Duration of therapy is 3 d.
	Cryptosporidium parvum	*Children 1–3 yr:* 5-mL oral suspension q12h *4–11 yr:* 10-mL oral suspension q12h	
Tinidazole	Intestinal amebiasis	*Adults* 2 g/d *Children ≥3 yr:* 50 mg/kg/d	Duration of therapy is 3 d.
	Giardiasis	*Adults*: 2 g *Children ≥3 yr:* 50 mg/kg	Single dose.
	Trichomoniasis	*Adults*: 2 g	Single dose. Partner should also be treated.

*Oral suspension is 100 mg/5 mL.

may need to be decreased; increased dosages might be required for successful therapy of patients taking inducers of hepatic CYP450, such as **phenobarbital** and **phenytoin**.

Nitazoxanide has only two indications and **tinidazole** has three. They are discussed below.

Trichomonas Vaginitis

Trichomonas vaginal infection often occurs during or shortly after menses and is characterized by copious foamy discharge with a pH greater than 5, positive "whiff test," punctate hemorrhages of vaginal mucosa, and vaginal irritation. Although it is generally sexually transmitted, the organism can live for weeks on wet towels and toilet seats, so fomite transfer is theoretically possible. In the male, the infection may cause urethral discharge, but it is usually mild, if present at all. Both partners should be treated and a condom used during intercourse for a week to prevent reinfection. Short treatment with **metronidazole** requires 2 g as a single dose or in 2 divided doses of 1 g each given in the same day; long treatment is 250 mg three times a day for 7 days. If the infection occurs in the first trimester of pregnancy, deferral of treatment is recommended. Experts disagree over whether the long or short treatment is preferable during pregnant and nonpregnant states. Single-dose therapy promotes compliance, especially if administered under supervision. However, the 7-day therapy may be more effective and may minimize reinfection of the woman long enough to treat sexual contacts. For children, the dose is 5 mg/kg every 8 hours for 7 to 10 days.

Tinidazole is also used for this indication. The dose is 2 g as a single dose. Both partners should be treated. This drug is Pregnancy Category C, so **metronidazole** is the preferred drug in those circumstances.

Giardiasis

The life cycle of the protozoon *G. lamblia* involves two stages: a cyst and a trophozoite. The cyst form can live in cold water for months and is ingested by the human hosts. It can also be transmitted during sexual activity. The trophozoite—or actively metabolizing, motile form—lives in the upper two-thirds of the small intestine, and can be so numerous that it can mechanically interfere with digestion. *Giardia* infections may be asymptomatic or cause disease ranging from self-limiting diarrhea to a severe chronic syndrome with malnutrition.

In the United States, **metronidazole**, 250 mg three times a day for 5 to 7 days in adults and 11.6/16.7 mg/kg every 8 hours for 5 to 10 days in children, is used to treat giardiasis, although it is not approved for this indication. Asymptomatic cyst passers should also be treated. **Nitazoxanide** is FDA approved for treatment of *G. lamblia* in children older than 1 year. It is available in an oral suspension to make administration easier and more accurate in very young children. **Tinidazole** is used to treat giardiasis in adults and children older than 3 years. Doses are provided in Table 24–56.

Amebiasis

Several species of *Entamoeba* infect humans, but *E. histolytica* is the only species known to cause disease. Like many protozoa, *Entamoeba* has two life stages: the cyst and the trophozoite. Infection of the human usually involves ingestion of cysts from fecally contaminated food, water, or hands. Transmission of cysts and trophozoites can also occur with fecal exposure during sexual contact. In the intestine, cysts undergo excystation into the trophozoite form and multiply. In many cases, the cysts remain in the intestinal lumen (noninvasive infection), resulting in asymptomatic carriers and cyst passers. In some patients, the cysts invade the intestinal lumen (invasive intestinal disease), resulting in diarrhea or dysentery. Trophozoites also can travel through the bloodstream to form abscesses in the liver, brain, or lung (extraintestinal disease) that are manifested by local signs such as hepatomegaly or cholestasis. Drugs administered for presumptive treatment (broad-spectrum **antibiotics, kaolin, bismuth**, soapsuds enema, barium) can suppress shedding of amebas into the stool and delay diagnosis. For invasive intestinal amebiasis, **metronidazole**, 750 mg orally three times daily for 5 to 10 days, is the drug of choice.

Metronidazole can be used to treat the extraintestinal form of the disease IV or orally.

Metronidazole is so well absorbed that it is not effective against the noninvasive infection, and it may be necessary to add a luminal agent like **paromomycin** (**Humatin**), 500 mg orally three times daily for 7 days. **Paromomycin** is an **unabsorbable aminoglycoside** similar to **neomycin.** If the intestinal mucosa is not intact, as in concomitant inflammatory bowel disease, **paromomycin** can be absorbed and cause ototoxicity and nephrotoxicity.

Tinidazole 2 g orally each day for 3 days is also approved for treatment of amebiasis in adults. In children older than 3 years, the dose is 50 mg/kg/day for 3 days. The advantage of this drug is the once-daily dosing.

Bacterial Vaginosis

Bacterial vaginosis develops when the bacterial flora are altered, with loss of the normally predominant lactobacilli and overgrowth of strict and facultative aerobic species such as *Bacteroides, Peptococcus, Mobiluncus, Gardnerella, Streptococcus,* and *Mycoplasma.* The infection manifests with foul-odored, clear, copious vaginal discharge with a pH greater than 4.5, positive "whiff test," and few WBCs. Untreated bacterial vaginosis has been associated with pelvic inflammatory disease, cervicitis, abnormal Pap smear cytology, preterm labor, and low birth weight. During pregnancy, symptomatic women are screened and treated

Table 24–56 ◆ **Available Dosage Forms: Oral Metronidazole, Nitazoxanide, and Tinidazole**

Drug	Dosage Form	How Supplied	Cost*
Metronidazole (Flagyl, Protostat)	Tablets: 250 mg (G)	In bottles of 25, 100, 500, 1,000, UD 32, 100 tablets	$4/28 $10/84
	250 mg (F)	In bottles of 50, 100, 250, 1,000, 2500, UD 100 tablets	$228
	250 mg (P)	In bottles of 100 tablets	
	500 mg (G)	In bottles of 25, 50, 100, 250, 500, UD 32, 100 tablets	$4/14 $10/28
	500 mg (F)	In bottles of 50, 100, 500 and UD 100 tablets	$406
	500 mg (P)	In bottles of 50 tablets	
	Tablet, extended release: 750 mg (G) 750 (F)	In bottles of 30 tablets	$197
		In bottles of 30 tablets	$254
	Capsules: 375 mg (F)	In bottles of 50, 100 and UD 100 capsules	$175
Nitazoxanide (Alinia)	Tablets: 500 mg (B) Powder for oral suspension: 100 mg/5 mL	In bottles of 60 and UD 6 tablets In 60 mL	$1349/60 tablets
Tinidazole	Tablets: 250 mg, 500 mg	In bottles of 40 and 100 (scored tablets) In bottles of 20 and 60 (scored tablets)	No data available No data available

G = generic; F = Flagyl; P = Protostat.
*Cost per 10 units unless otherwise stated.

if they are at high risk for preterm delivery. Treatment of low-risk and symptomatic women during pregnancy is controversial. **Metronidazole,** 500 mg orally twice daily for 7 days, or **metronidazole intravaginal gel,** 1 full applicator twice daily for 5 days, is the drug of first choice for bacterial vaginosis. The 2-g single dose is not as effective for bacterial vaginosis as these two regimens. **Metronidazole** is avoided in the first trimester of pregnancy, although the alternative for bacterial vaginosis, **clindamycin,** has not been shown to prevent preterm birth and is no longer recommended by the CDC. It is not necessary to treat sexual partners of women with bacterial vaginosis unless balanitis is present. Doses are provided in Table 24–55.

Cryptosporidium Parvum

Nitazoxanide is the only drug in this group approved for treatment of the diarrhea caused by *C. parvum* in children 11 years old or less. Its safety and efficacy have not been established for older children or adults, but doses are provided in the literature for these age groups. Its action appears to be caused by interference with the PFOR enzyme-dependent electron transfer reaction essential for anaerobic energy metabolism in the organism. This protein sequence is similar to the one used by *G. lamblia.* Dosing for each age group is found in Table 24–55.

Rational Drug Selection

For most of the infections for which **metronidazole** is used, it is the drug of choice because it is clearly more efficacious than the alternatives. **Metronidazole** is on many retail $4 lists, so cost is not an issue. Issues in drug selection for these conditions are the lack of effective alternatives for use in the first trimester of pregnancy, comparative efficacy of the long- and short-term oral dosing regimen, and the choice between topical and oral forms for vaginal infections. These issues have been covered in previous sections.

For *G. lamblia,* **nitazoxanide** and **tinidazole** have FDA approval for this indication in children; **metronidazole** use is off-labeled. Only **nitazoxanide** has approval for treatment of *C. parvum* infections.

Monitoring

For most of the conditions treated with **metronidazole,** resolution of symptoms indicates effective treatment, and further evaluation is not required. For giardiasis treated with any of these drugs, symptoms may persist for weeks or months after the organism is eradicated because of the lactose intolerance brought on by the infection. If symptoms persist, three stool samples should be collected several days apart about 3 to 4 weeks after completion of treatment. If signs of leukopenia develop (sore throat and fever), a WBC count should be collected.

Patient Education

Administration

Although oral **metronidazole** can be taken without regard to meals, it should be taken with food or snacks to decrease GI irritation. **Nitazoxanide** should be taken with food and the oral suspension should be shaken well before administration. **Tinidazole** should also be taken with food. If vaginal or topical preparations of **metronidazole** are used, the patient should be provided with instruction and the opportunity to manipulate a model applicator in the office. Use of the extended-release form of **metronidazole** that can be administered once daily should be considered if nonadherence is an issue, although the vaginal gel and delayed-release oral form are considerably more expensive than other oral forms.

Adverse Reactions

Chewing sugarless gum or sucking on ice or candy can help to overcome the dry mouth and metallic taste that **metronidazole** can cause. Alcoholic beverages should be avoided during therapy with **metronidazole** or **tinidazole** and for 48 hours after the last dose because of the **disulfiram**-like reaction that about 40 percent of patients on the drug experience if exposed to **alcohol.** Because the drug can cause dizziness or lightheadedness, hazardous activities should be avoided until the patient's response to the medication is established. Headache is a common adverse effect that can be treated with **acetaminophen** or an NSAID.

Metronidazole causes a harmless darkening of urine. Female patients should be counseled about the symptoms of vaginal candidiasis superinfection, which can complicate therapy and could be mistaken for recurrence of the original infection. The patient and family members should know to report CNS symptoms (ataxia, mood and mental changes, clumsiness, ataxia, seizures), peripheral neuropathy (numbness, tingling, pain, or weakness in hands or feet), and leukopenia (sore throat or fever).

Lifestyle Management

Many of the infections treated with **metronidazole** and **tinidazole** are sexually transmitted. Male or female condom usage may decrease transmittal of some, but not all, infections. For amebiasis and giardiasis, which are not usually considered sexually transmitted, identification of a sexual mode of transmission is helpful in preventing recurrent infections caused by the "ping-pong" of the infection between partners. Patients should be advised of the route of transmission and practices that promote transmittal of the infection. Concurrent treatment and refraining from sexual activity until the treatment is complete may be necessary to resolve the infections. Foreign travel and wilderness travel are other sources of exposure to *Giardia* and amebas that should be considered in the history for diagnosing these conditions.

REFERENCES

American Academy of Allergy, Asthma, and Immunology (AAAAI); Slavin, R. G., Spector, S. L., & Bernstein, I. L. (Eds.). (2005). The diagnosis and management of sinusitis: A practice parameter update. *Journal of Allergy and Clinical Immunology, 116*(6), S13–S47.

American Academy of Pediatrics. (1999). Practice parameter: The diagnosis, treatment, and evaluation of initial urinary tract infections in febrile infants and young children. Committee on Quality Improvement: Subcommittee on Urinary Tract Infections. *Pediatrics, 103*(4), 843–852.

American Academy of Pediatrics. (2001). Clinical practice guideline: Management of sinusitis. *Pediatrics, 108*(3), 798–808.

American Academy of Pediatrics. (2006). The use of systemic fluoroquinolones. *Pediatrics, 118*(3), 1287–1292. Retrieved from http://www.pediatrics.org/cgi/content/full

American Academy of Pediatrics. (2009a). Group A streptococcal infections. In L. K. Pickering (Ed.), *Red book: 2009 report of the Committee on Infectious Disease* (28th ed., pp. 616–628). Elk Grove Village, IL: American Academy of Pediatrics. Retrieved September 2, 2010, from http://aapredbook.aappublications.org/cgi/content/full/2009/1/3.125

American Academy of Pediatrics. (2009b). Principles of appropriate use for upper respiratory tract infections. In L. K. Pickering (Ed.), *Red book: 2009 report of the Committee on Infectious Disease* (28th ed., pp. 740–742). Elk Grove Village, IL: American Academy of Pediatrics. Retrieved August 23, 2010, from http://aapredbook.aappublications.org/cgi/content/ full/2009/1/4.2.1

American Academy of Pediatrics (AAP) and American Academy of Family Physicians (AAFP). (2004). Clinical Practice Guidelines: Diagnosis and management of acute otitis media. *Pediatrics, 113*(5), 1451–1465.

American Academy of Pediatrics Subcommittee on Management of Acute Otitis Media (AAP/OM]. (2004). Diagnosis and management of acute otitis media. *Pediatrics, 113*(5), 1451–1465.

Amichai, B., & Grunwald, M. H. (1998). Adverse drug reactions and the new oral antifungal agents: Terbinafine, fluconazole, and itraconazole. *International Journal of Dermatology, 37,* 410–415.

Apter, A., Kinman, J., Bilker, W., Herlim, M., Margolis, D. J., Lautenbach, E., et al. (2004). Represcription after allergic-like events. *Journal of Allergy and Clinical Immunology, 113,* 764–770.

Auckland, C., Teare, L., Cooke, F., Kaufmann, M. E., Warner, M., Johnson, A. P., et al. (2002). Linezolid-resistant enterococci: Report of the first isolates in the United Kingdom. *Journal of Antimicrobial Chemotherapy, 50,* 743–746.

Benson, C. A., Kaplan, J. E., Masur, H., Pau, A., & Holms, K. K. (2004). Treatment of opportunistic infections among HIV-infected adults and adolescents. *Morbidity and Mortality Weekly Report, 53*(RR15), 1–112.

Bersos, Z., Maniati, M., Kontos, F., Petinaki, E., & Maniatis, A. N. (2004). First report of a linezolid-resistant vancomycin-resistant Enterococcus faecium strain in Greece. *Journal of Antimicrobial Chemotherapy, 53,* 685–686.

Bishai, W., Morris, C., & Scanland, S. (2004). *Treatment of community acquired pneumonia.* New York: Jobson Publishing.

Bucher, H., Tschudi, R., Young, J., Periat, P., Welge-Lussen, A., Zust, H., et al. (2003). Effect of amoxicillin-clavulanate in clinically diagnosed acute rhinosinusitis: A placebo controlled, double-blind, randomized trial in general practice. *Archives of Internal Medicine, 163,* 1793–1798.

Cameron, D., Gaito, A., Harris, N., Bach, G., Bellovin, S., Bock, K., et al. (2004). The International Lyme and Associated Diseases Society: Evidence-based guidelines for the management of Lyme disease. Retrieved from http://www.ilads.org/files/ILADS_Guidelines.pdf

Campos-Outcalt, D. (2003). Sexually transmitted disease: Easier screening tests, single dose therapies. *Journal of Family Practice, 52*(12), 965–969.

Centers for Disease Control and Prevention (CDC). (2003). Treatment of tuberculosis, American Thoracic Society, CDC, and Infectious Diseases Society of America. *Morbidity and Mortality Weekly Report, 52*(RR-11), 1–77.

Centers for Disease Control and Prevention (CDC). (2005a) Multi-level antimicrobial susceptibility test resources (MASTER). Retrieved July 29, 2005, from http://www.cdc.gov/drugresistance

Centers for Disease Control and Prevention (CDC). (2005b). *Pseudomonas aeruginosa, Staphylococcus aureus* and fluoroquinolone use. *Emerging Infectious Disease, 11*(8). Retrieved July 29, 2005, from http://www.cdc.gov/drugresistance

Centers for Disease Control and Prevention (CDC). (2006a). Sexually transmitted diseases: Treatment guidelines 2006. Retrieved from www.cdc.gov/std

Centers for Disease Control and Prevention (CDC). (2006b). Strategies for clinical management of MRSA in the community: Summary of an experts' meeting convened by the Centers for Disease Control and Prevention. Retrieved from http://www.cdc.gov/ncidod/dhqp/pdf/ar/CAMRSA_ExpMtgStrategies.pdf

Centers for Disease Control and Prevention (CDC). (2007). Updated recommended treatment regimens for gonococcal infections and associated conditions—United States, April 2007. Retrieved from http://www.cdc.gov/std/treatment/2006/updated-regimens.htm

Centers for Disease Control and Prevention (CDC). (2009a). Basic information about antibiotic-resistant gonorrhea (ARG). Retrieved from http://www.cdc.gov/std/Gonorrhea/arg/basic.htm

Centers for Disease Control and Prevention (CDC). (2009b). Careful antibiotic use: Pediatric appropriate treatment summary. Retrieved from http://www.cdc.gov/getsmart

Centers for Disease Control and Prevention (CDC). (2009c). Get smart: Know when antibiotics work. Treatment guidelines for upper respiratory tract infections. Retrieved from http://www.cdc.gov/getsmart/campaign-materials/treatment-guidelines.html

Centers for Disease Control and Prevention (CDC). (2009d). Guidelines for the prevention and treatment of opportunistic infections among HIV-exposed and HIV-infected children: Recommendations from CDC, the National Institutes of Health, the HIV Medicine Association of the Infectious Diseases Society of America, the Pediatric Infectious Diseases Society, and the American Academy of Pediatrics. *Morbidity and Mortality Weekly Report, 58*(RR11), 1–166.

Centers for Disease Control and Prevention (CDC). (2010a). CDC guidance on shortage of erythromycin (0.5%) ophthalmic ointment. Retrieved from http://www.cdc.gov/std/treatment/2006/erythromycinOintment Shortage.htm

Centers for Disease Control and Prevention (CDC). (2010b). Drug-resistant *Streptococcus pneumoniae* disease. Retrieved from http://www.cdc.gov//ncidod/dbmd/diseaseinfo/drugresisstreppneum_t.htm

Centers for Disease Control and Prevention (CDC). (2010c). Invasive pneumococcal disease in young children before licensure of 13-valent pneumococcal conjugate vaccine—United States, 2007. *Morbidity and Mortality Weekly Report, 59*(09), 253–257.

Centers for Disease Control and Prevention (CDC). (2010d). Recommendations for the prevention of perinatal group B streptococcal disease. *MMWR Recommendations and Reports, 59*(RR10), 1–32. Retrieved from http://www.cdc.gov/mmwr/preview/mmwrhtml/rr5910a1.htm

Centers for Disease Control and Prevention (CDC, 2010e). Sexually transmitted treatment guidelines, 2010. *Morbidity and Mortality Weekly Report, 59*(RR-12), 1–116. Retrieved from www.cdc.gov/std

Cheung, O., Chopra, K., Yu, T., & Nalesnik, M. (2004). Gatifloxacin-induced hepatotoxicity and acute pancreatitis. *Annals of Internal Medicine, 140*(1), 73–74.

Cincinnati Children's Hospital Medical Center. (2005). Evidence-based clinical practice guideline of community-acquired pneumonia in children 60 days to 17 years of age. Cincinnati, OH: Cincinnati Children's Hospital Medical Center. Retrieved from http://www.cincinnatichildrens.org/assets/0/78/1067/2709/2777/2793/9199/1633ae60-cbd1-4fbd-bba4-cb687fbb1d42.pdf

Currie, B. J., & McCarthy, J. S. (2010). Permethrin and ivermectin for scabies. *New England Journal of Medicine, 362,* 717–725.

Devasia, R. A., Blackman, A., Gebretasadik, T., Griffin, M., Shintani, A., May, C., et al. (2009). Fluoroquinolone resistance in mycobacterium tuberculosis: The effect of duration and timing of fluoroquinolone exposure. *American Journal of Respiratory and Critical Care Medicine, 180*(4), 365–370.

Drug facts and comparisons 2010. St. Louis, MO: Wolters Kluwer Health.

Garcia, M. S., De la Torre, M. A., Morales, G., Pelaez, B., Tolon, M. J., Domingo, S., et al. (2010). Clinical outbreak of linezolid-resistant *Staphylococcus aureus* in an intensive care unit. *Journal of the American Medical Association, 303*(22), 260–2264.

Gaylord, N. M., & Starr, N. B. (2009). Genitourinary disorders. In C. E. Burns, A. M. Dunn, M. A. Brady, N. B. Starr, & C. G. Blosser (Eds.), *Pediatric primary care* (pp. 866–905). St. Louis, MO: Saunders.

Gold, B., Colletti, R., Abbot, M., Czinn, S., Elitsur, Y., Hassall, E., et al. (2000). *Helicobacter pylori* infection in children: Recommendations for diagnosis and treatment. *Journal of Pediatric Gastroenterology, 31*(5), 490–497.

Gotfried, M. (2004). Appropriate outpatient macrolide use in community acquired pneumonia. *Journal of the American Academy of Nurse Practitioners, 16*(4), 146–157.

Griebling, T. L. (2007). Urinary tract infection in women. In M. S. Litwin & C. S. Saigal (Eds.), *Urologic diseases in America* (NIH Publication No. 07–5512, pp. 588–617). U.S. Department of Health and Human Services, Public Health Service, National Institutes of Health, National Institute of Diabetes and Digestive and Kidney Diseases. Washington, DC: U.S. Government Printing Office.

Grover, M. L., Bracamonte, J. D., Kanodia, A. K., Bryan, M. J., Donahue, S. P., Warner, A. M., et al. (2007). Assessing adherence to evidence-base guidelines for the diagnosis and management of uncomplicated urinary tract infection. *Mayo Clinic Proceedings, 82*(2), 181–185.

Hooton, T. M., & Stamm, W. E. (2010). Urinary tract infections and asymptomatic bacteriuria in pregnancy. *UpToDate*. Retrieved from http://www.uptodate.com/online/content/topic.do?topicKey=uti_infe/7516&source=see_link

Hsu, K. K., Shea, K. M., Stevenson, A. E., & Pelton, S. I. (2010). Changing serotypes causing childhood invasive pneumococcal disease: Massachusetts, 2001–2007. *Pediatric Infectious Disease Journal, 29*(4), 289–293.

Institute for Clinical Systems Improvement (ICSI). (2003). *Community-acquired pneumonia in adults.* Bloomington, MN: Institute for Clinical Systems Improvement, Dec. 2003. Retrieved August 1, 2005, from http://www.guideline.gov/summary/summary.aspx

Institute for Clinical Systems Improvement (ICSI). (2004a). *Dyspepsia and GERD.* Bloomington, MN: Institute for Clinical Systems Improvement, July 2004. Retrieved June 15, 2005, from http://www.guideline.gov/summary/summary.aspx

Institute for Clinical Systems Improvement (ICSI). (2004b). *Uncomplicated urinary tract infection in women.* Bloomington, MN: Institute for Clinical Systems Improvement, July 2004. Retrieved June 15, 2005, from http://www.guideline.gov/summary/summary.aspx

Irwin, R. S., Bauman, M. H., Bolser, D. S., Boulet, L. P., Braman, S. S., Brightling, C. E., et al. (2006). Diagnosis and management of cough: Executive summary. ACCP evidence-based clinical practice guidelines. *Chest, 129*(1 suppl), 1S–23S.

Jacobs, M. R., Felmingham, D., Appelbaum, P. C., Gruneberg, R. N., for the Alexander Project Group. (2003). The Alexander Project 1998–2000: Susceptibility of pathogens isolated from community-acquired respiratory tract infection to commonly used antimicrobial agents. *Journal of Antimicrobial Chemotherapy, 52,* 229–246.

Jenkins, S. G., & Farrell, D. J. (2009). Increase in pneumococcus macrolide resistance, United States. *Emerging Infectious Diseases, 15*(8), 1260–1264. Retrieved from http://www.cdc.gov/EID/content/15/8/1260.htm

Kainer, M. A., Devasia, R. A., Jones, T. F., Simmons, B. P., Melton, K., Chow, S., et al. (2007). Response to emerging infection leading to outbreak of linezolid-resistant enterococci. *Emerging Infectious Diseases, 13*(7), 1024–1030.

Kashanian, J., Hakimian, P., Blute, M., Wong, J., Khanna, H., Wise, G., & Shabsigh, R. (2008). Nitrofurantoin: The return of an old friend in the wake of growing resistance. *British Journal of Urology International, 102,* 1634–1637.

Kays, M. B., & Brown, S. (2004). Prevalence of antimicrobial resistance among *Streptococcus pneumoniae* isolates in the USA: PROTEKT US Years 1–3 [Abstract 354]. Abstracts of the Infectious Diseases Society of America annual meeting, Boston, MA.

Keren, R., & Chan, E. (2002). A meta-analysis of randomized, controlled trials comparing short- and long-course antibiotic therapy for urinary tract infections in children. *Pediatrics, 109*(5), e70.

Klein, J. O., & Pelton, S. (2009). Acute otitis media in children: Treatment. *UpToDate Online*. Retrieved from http://www.uptodate.com

Kolmos, H. J., & Little, P. (1999). Should general practitioners perform diagnostic tests on patients before prescribing antibiotics? *BMJ, 318,* 799.

Lew, E. (2009). Peptic ulcer disease. In N. J. Greenberger (Ed.), *Current diagnosis & treatment gastroenterology, hepatology, & endoscopy* (3rd ed.). McGraw Hill: New York.

Linares, J., Ardanuy, C., Pallares, R. & Fenoll, A. (2010). Changes in antimicrobial resistance, serotypes and genotypes in *Streptococcus pneumoniae* over a 30-year period. *Clinical Microbiology and Infection, 16*(5), 402–410.

Litwin, M. S., & Saigal, C. S. (2007). Introduction. In M. S. Litwin & C. S. Saigal (Eds.), *Urologic diseases in America* (NIH Publication No. 07–5512:3–7). Washington, DC: U.S. Government Printing Office.

Locksmith, G. J., Clark, P., & Duff, P. (1999). Maternal and neonatal infection rates with three different protocols for prevention of group B streptococcal disease. *American Journal of Obstetrics and Gynecology, 180,* 416–422.

Mandell, L. A., Wunderink, R. G., Anzueto, A., Bartlett, J. G., Campbell, G. D., Dowell, S. F., et al. (2007). Infectious Diseases Society of America/American Thoracic Society consensus guidelines on the management of community-acquired pneumonia in adults. *Clinical Infectious Disease, 44*(Suppl. 2), S27–S72.

Mangione-Smith, R., McGlynn, E. A., Elliott, M. N., Krogstad, P., & Brook, R. H. (1999). The relationship between perceived parental expectations and pediatrician antimicrobial prescribing behavior. *Pediatrics, 103,* 711–718.

Mofeson, L. M., Brady, M. T., Danner, S. P., et al. (2009). Guidelines for the prevention and treatment of opportunistic infections among HIV-exposed and HIV-infected children: Recommendations from CDC, the National Institutes of Health, the HIV Medicine Association of the Infectious Diseases Society of America, the Pediatric Infectious Diseases Society, and the American Academy of Pediatrics. *MMWR Recommendations & Reports, 58* (RR-11), 1–166.

Mollering, R. (2003). Linezolid: The first oxazolidinone antimicrobial. *Annals of Internal Medicine, 138*(2), 135–142.

Neff, M. (2003). ATS, CDC and IDSA update recommendations of the treatment of tuberculosis. *American Family Physician, 68*(9), 1854–1862.

Nicolle, L., Bradley, S., Colgan, R., Rice, J., Schaffer, A., & Hootne, T. (2005). Infectious Diseases Society of America guideline for the diagnosis and treatment of asymptomatic bacteriuria in adults. *Clinical Infectious Disease, 40*(5), 643–654.

Nishimura, R. A., Carabello, B. A., Faxon, D. P., Freed, M. D., Lytle, B. W., O'Gara, P. T., et al. (2008). ACC/AHA 2008 guideline update on valvular heart disease: Focused update on infective endocarditis. *Journal of the American College of Cardiology, 52,* 676–685.

North of England Dyspepsia Guideline Development Group. (2004). *Dyspepsia: Managing dyspepsia in adults in primary care.* Center for Health Services Research. Newcastle Upon Tyne (UK): University of Newcastle. Retrieved June 15, 2005, from http://www.guideline.gov/summary/summary.aspx

O'Dell, J. R. (1999). Is there a role for antibiotics in the treatment of patients with rheumatoid arthritis? *Drugs, 57,* 279–282.

Oregon Health Sciences University. (n.d.). Oral trimethoprim-sulfamethoxazole for MRSA infections. Retrieved from http://www.ohsu.edu/academic/medicine/residency//handouts/pharmpearls/Infectious%20Disease/OralTMP-SMXForMRSA.pdf

Patterson, D., Ko, W., Gottberg, A., Mohapatra, S., Casellas, J., Goossens, H., et al. (2004). International prospective study of *Klebsiella pneumoniae* bacteria: Implications of extended-spectrum β-lactamase production in nosocomial infections. *Annals of Internal Medicine, 140*(1), 26–32.

Piddock, L. J. V. (1999). Mechanisms of fluoroquinolone resistance: An update 1994–1998. *Drugs, 58*(Suppl. 2), 11–18.

Prais, D., Straussberg, R., Avitzur, Y., Nussinovitch, M., Harel, L., & Amir, J. (2003). Bacterial susceptibility to oral antibiotics in community acquired urinary tract infection. *Archives of Disease in Childhood, 88,* 215–218.

Rabe, K. F., Hurd, S., Anzueto, A., Barnes, P. J., Buist, S. A., Calverley, P., et al. (2007). Global strategy for the diagnosis, management, and prevention of chronic obstructive pulmonary disease. *American Journal of Respiratory Critical Care Medicine, 176,* 532–555.

Richter, S. S., Heilmann, K. P., Dohrn, C. L., Beekman, S. E., Riahi, F., Garcia-de-Lomas, J., et al. (2008). Increasing telithromycin resistance among

Streptococcus pyogenes in Europe. *Journal of Antimicrobial Chemotherapy, 61*(3), 603–611.

Rosenfeld, R. M., Andes, D., Bhattacharyya, N., Cheung, D., Eisenburg, S., Ganiats, T. G., et al. (2007). Clinical practice guideline: Adult sinusitis. *Otolaryngology—Head and Neck Surgery, 137,* S1–S31.

Sanford Guide to Antimicrobial Therapy (40th ed.). (2010). Gainesville, FL: U.S. Biomedical Information Systems.

Schafer, J. A., Mateo, N., Parlier, G. L., & Rotschafer, J. C. (2007). Penicillin allergy skin testing: What do we do now? *Pharmacotherapy, 27*(4), 542–545.

Schrag, S. J., Zywicki, S., Farley, M. M., Reingold, A. L., Harrison, L. H., Lefkowitz, L. B., et al. (2000). Group B streptococcal disease in the era of intrapartum antibiotic prophylaxis. *New England Journal of Medicine, 342,* 15–20.

Schumann, L., & Nollette, K. (2000). Antimicrobial resistance. *Journal of the American Academy of Nurse Practitioners, 12*(7), 286–296.

Schussheim, A. E., & Fuster, V. (1999). Antibiotics for myocardial infarction: A possible role of infection in artherogenesis and acute coronary syndromes. *Drugs, 57,* 283–291.

Schwartz, B., Mainous, A. G., & Marcy, S. M. (1998). Why do physicians prescribe antibiotics for children with upper respiratory tract infections? *Journal of the American Medical Association, 279,* 881–882.

Singapore Ministry of Health. (2004). *Management of* Helicobacter pylori *infection.* Singapore. Author. Retrieved June 15, 2005, from http://www.guideline.gov/summary/summary.aspx

Snow, V., Mottur-Pilson, C., & Gonzales, R. (2001). Principles of appropriate antibiotic use for treatment of acute bronchitis in adults. *Annals of Internal Medicine, 134*(6), 518–520.

Stahlmann, R., & Lode, H. (2010). Safety considerations of fluoroquinolones in the elderly: An update. *Drugs & Aging, 27*(3), 193–209.

Steele, R. W., Thomas, M. P., Begue, R. E., & Despinasse, B. P. (1999). Selection of pediatric antibiotic suspensions: Taste and cost. *Infection Medicine, 16,* 197–200.

Steele, R. W., Thomas, M. P., & Begue, R. (2001). Compliance issues related to the selection of antibiotic suspensions for children. *Pediatric Infectious Disease Journal, 20*(1), 1–5.

Thomas, A. (2005). *Judicious use of antibiotics* (2nd ed.). Oregon Alliance. Working for Antibiotic Resistance Education (AWARE) and Oregon Department of Human Services. Salem, Oregon. Retrieved from http://www.healthoregon.org/antibiotics.ctm

Towers, P. (2000). Urinary tract infections. *Journal of the American Academy of Nurse Practitioners, 12*(4), 149–154.

VandeWaa, E. A., Henderson, J. D., White, G. L., & Nowatzke, T. J. (1998). Common helminthic infections: Treating wormlike parasites in primary care. *Clinician Reviews, 8*(5), 75–92.

Wagenlehner, F., Weidner, W., & Naber, K. (2005). Emerging drugs for bacterial urinary tract infections. *Expert Opinion on Emerging Drugs, 10*(2), 275–298.

World Health Organization. (2010). Parasitic diseases. Retrieved from http://www.who.int/vaccine_research/diseases/soa_parasitic/en/index.html

Wormser, G. P., Dattwyler, R. J., Shapiro, E. D., Halperin, J. J., Steere, A. C., Klempner, M. S., et al. (2006). The clinical assessment, treatment, and prevention of Lyme disease, human granulocytic anaplasmosis and babesiosis: Clinical practice guidelines by the Infectious Diseases Society of America. *Clinical Infectious Diseases, 43,* 1089–1134.

CHAPTER 25

DRUGS USED IN TREATING INFLAMMATORY PROCESSES

Teri Moser Woo

Chapter Outline

Inflammation is a common symptom of many diseases, including arthritis, with an estimated 46 million adults reporting they have some form of arthritis, rheumatoid arthritis, gout, lupus, or fibromyalgia according to the 2003–2005 National Health Interview Survey (Centers for Disease Control and Prevention [CDC], 2006). This chapter discusses the medication used to treat inflammation—specifically inflammation associated with gout—and the nonspecific anti-inflammatory drugs. The anti-inflammatory actions of the corticosteroids are reviewed as well as the nonsteroidal anti-inflammatory drugs (NSAIDs) and the salicylates.

ANTIGOUT AND URICOSURIC AGENTS

Gout was the first form of arthritis to be recognized as crystal induced. An estimated 1.5 million adults had gout in 2005, and 6.1 million adults over age 20 years have had at least one episode of gout (Lawrence et al, 2008). The peak incidence occurs in patients 70 to 79 years old, and it is much more common in men than in women (Lawrence et al, 2008). Gout in women occurs exclusively postmenopause and is associated with hypertension, renal insufficiency, and exposure to **diuretics**. The gout syndrome is caused by an alteration in purine metabolism, the end product of which is uric acid. This alteration results in hyperuricemia and in the deposition of urate crystals in various tissues. The four phases of gout are asymptomatic hyperuricemia, acute gouty arthritis, intercritical gout, and chronic tophaceous gout. Patients with asymptomatic hyperuricemia do not require treatment, but efforts are made to lower their urate levels by encouraging them to make changes in diet and lifestyle. Acute gout is characterized by the sudden onset of pain, erythema, limited range of motion, and swelling in the involved joint, with approximately 50 percent of cases involving the first metatarsal join of the great toe, but other joints can be involved (CDC, 2010). The key elements in treatment of the latter three phases of this disorder are management of the acute pain and use of **antigout** and **uricosuric agents**. The drugs used to manage the pain are most often **NSAIDs** and **corticosteroids**, which are discussed later in the chapter. The three **antigout drugs**, **allopurinol** (**Zyloprim**), **colchicine**, and **febuxostat** (**Uloric**), and the two **uricosuric agents**, **probenecid** (**Benemid**) and **sulfinpyrazone** (**Anturane**), are the focus of this section.

Pharmacodynamics

Antigout Drugs

Antigout drugs act to reduce the inflammatory process or to prevent the synthesis of uric acid. **Allopurinol** and **febuxostat** inhibit xanthine oxidase, the enzyme responsible for the conversion of hypoxanthine and xanthine to uric acid. **Allopurinol** has a metabolite (**alloxanthine**), which is also an inhibitor of xanthine oxidase. **Allopurinol** acts directly on purine metabolism, reducing the production of uric acid, without disrupting the biosynthesis of vital purines. **Allopurinol** and **febuxostat** are the only drugs that act directly on the pathophysiological cause of gout.

Administration of **allopurinol** generally leads to a fall in both serum and urinary uric acid in 2 to 3 days. The magnitude of this decrease is dose dependent. A week or more of treatment may be necessary before the full effects of the drug can be seen.

Febuxostat is used to treat hyperuricemia in patients with gout. The goal is to have a serum uric acid level of less than 6 mg per dL. It may take 2 weeks or more to see the effect of **febuxostat**.

Unlike **allopurinol**, **colchicine** does not affect purine metabolism. It binds to microtubular proteins to interfere with the function of the mitotic spindles and inhibit the migration of granulocytes to the inflamed area. It reduces lactic acid production by granulocytes, which decreases deposition of uric acid, and it interferes with kinin formation and reduces phagocytosis. Taken together, these actions decrease the inflammatory response to the deposited urate crystals.

Although it relieves pain in acute attacks, **colchicine** is not an analgesic. It is also not uricosuric and does not prevent gout from progressing to chronic gouty arthritis. Its prophylactic, suppressive effect helps reduce the incidence of acute attacks and relieves the patient's occasional residual pain and mild discomfort.

Uricosuric Drugs

Uricosuric drugs, unlike **antigout drugs**, increase the rate of uric acid secretion. Both **probenecid** and **sulfinpyrazone** inhibit renal tubular reabsorption of urate and thus increase the renal excretion of uric acid and decrease serum uric acid levels. Effective uricosuria reduces the miscible urate pool, retards urate deposition, and promotes reabsorption of urate deposits. **Sulfinpyrazone** also competitively inhibits platelet prostaglandin synthesis, which prevents platelet aggregation and gives the drug an antithrombotic effect. Both drugs lack **anti-inflammatory** activity. They are most useful for patients with reduced urinary excretion of uric acid. They are not intended for treatment of acute attacks.

Pharmacokinetics

Absorption and Distribution

All gout drugs are well absorbed after oral administration (Table 25–1). **Febuxostat** absorption is decreased with a high fat meal, but there is not a clinically significant change in serum uric acid concentration, so it may be taken without regard to food. **Allopurinol** is widely distributed to tissues. **Colchicine** concentrates mainly in white blood cells. **Probenecid** crosses the placenta without producing adverse effects in the fetus or infant. **Sulfinpyrazone** also crosses the placenta but may be hazardous to the fetus. Both **probenecid** and **sulfinpyrazone** are highly protein bound and tend to displace other drugs that have a high affinity for the same binding sites.

Table 25–1 ▶ **Pharmacokinetics: Antigout and Uricosuric Agents**

Drug	Onset	Peak (in plasma)	Duration	Protein Binding	Half-Life	Elimination
Allopurinol	2–3 d*	1.5 h allopurinol 4.5 h oxipurinol	1–2 wk*	NA	1–2 h allopurinol 15 h oxypurinol	20% in feces; remainder in urine
Colchicine	12 h†	0.5–2 h	UK	50%	60 min in plasma <60 h in leukocytes	10%–20% in urine; remainder in bile and feces
Febuxostat	NA	1–1.5 h	UK	99.2%	5–8 h	Urine; 49% as metabolites, feces; 45% as metabolites
Probenecid	30 min*	2–4 h	8 h	85%–95%	5–8 h dose- dependent	In urine; primarily as metabolite
Sulfinpyrazone	NA	4 h	UK	98%–99%	4 h	50% in urine: 90% of this as unchanged drug; 10% as metabolite

UK = unknown.
*Hypouricemic action.
†Anti-inflammatory action.

Metabolism and Excretion

The liver metabolizes all five drugs used in gout treatment. All have active metabolites. Both biliary and renal routes excrete **allopurinol, colchicines,** and **febuxostat.** However, **colchicine** is not effective in the presence of renal failure. The other two drugs are excreted primarily in urine, and the dose of **probenecid** may need to be reduced in the presence of renal impairment.

Pharmacotherapeutics

Precautions and Contraindications

Allopurinol (Zyloprim), colchicines, probenecid (Benemid), and **sulfinpyrazone** (Anturane) are associated with poor urate clearance in the presence of renal impairment. They should be used cautiously, and renal function tests should be performed regularly to determine appropriate dosage of the drug. Data are insufficient regarding the use of **febuxostat** in patients with renal impairment.

Allopurinol and **colchicine** are associated with hepatotoxicity. They are not recommended for patients with severe hepatic dysfunction. If patients taking these drugs develop anorexia, weight loss, or pruritus, evaluation of liver function should be part of the diagnostic workup. For milder hepatic disorders, close monitoring of liver function is required.

Colchicine, probenecid, and **sulfinpyrazone** are all used cautiously in the presence of peptic ulcer disease or spastic colon. Gastrointestinal (GI) adverse reactions from these drugs are likely to make these disorders worse. Because **probenecid** and **sulfinpyrazone** are **sulfa-based drugs,** patients with known or suspected **sulfa** allergies should not use them.

Febuxostat, a xanthine oxidase inhibitor, is contraindicated in patients being treated with drugs requiring xanthine oxidase for metabolism (**azathioprine, mercaptopurine,** or **theophylline**) because of increased risk for toxicity.

There is a risk of gout flare up when **febuxostat** is started. Patients should be concurrently treated with an NSAID or **colchicine** for up to 6 months.

Pregnancy categories vary by drug. **Allopurinol** is Pregnancy Category C, but there are no adequate, well-controlled studies in pregnant women. Use only when benefits clearly outweigh potential risks to the fetus. **Colchicine** is Pregnancy Category C when given orally, D when given parenterally. This drug can cause fetal harm when administered to pregnant women and should be used only when benefits clearly outweigh risks to the fetus and other drugs are not effective. **Probenecid** is Pregnancy Category B. It crosses the placenta, but it has been used during pregnancy without producing harmful effects in the fetus. **Sulfinpyrazone** is Pregnancy Category D, but there are no adequate, well-controlled studies in pregnant women. Its use should be avoided in pregnancy unless no other drug is effective and reduction in urate levels is essential. **Febuxostat** is Pregnancy Category C. There are no adequate and well-controlled studies in pregnant women. **Febuxostat** should only be used if the benefits outweigh the risks.

Allopurinol has been found in breast milk. It is not known whether the other three drugs are excreted in breast milk. Exercise caution when prescribing these drugs for nursing women. **Febuxostat** is excreted in the milk of rats; it is unknown whether it is excreted in human milk.

These drugs are generally not indicated for use in children, except in hyperuricemia associated with the treatment of malignancy, and this disorder would likely be followed by a specialist. Dosage schedules are published for children only for the indication discussed and the use of **probenecid** for retarding **penicillin** or **cephalosporin** excretion in selected infections.

Adverse Drug Reactions

Urates tend to crystallize out in acid urine. Fluid intake of more than 3,000 mL/day, along with sufficient **sodium bicarbonate** (3–7.5 g/d) or **potassium citrate** (7.5 g/d), maintains alkaline urine. Continue alkalization until the serum uric acid level returns to normal limits and the tophaceous deposits disappear.

Colchicine, probenecid, and **sulfinpyrazone** are associated with adverse reactions affecting the GI tract. Symptoms include nausea, vomiting, diarrhea, and abdominal pain. These symptoms are particularly troublesome for patients with a history or peptic ulcer disease or active peptic ulcer disease.

Probenecid and **sulfinpyrazone** are **sulfa-based drugs.** They have been associated with hypersensitivity reactions related to this base. Severe, anaphylactic reactions are rare and usually occur within several hours after administration of the first dose of a restart regimen, following prior use of the drug. The appearance of a hypersensitivity reaction requires immediate discontinuance of the drug.

Allopurinol is associated with a maculopapular skin rash that sometimes is scaly or exfoliative. The incidence of this adverse reaction is increased in the presence of renal disorders. Because skin reactions may be severe and sometimes fatal, the drug should be discontinued at the first sign of rash. The most severe reactions include fever, chills, arthralgia, cholestatic jaundice, eosinophilia, mild leukocytosis, or leukopenia.

Patients on standard therapy with **colchicine** who have elevated plasma levels because of renal function have developed myopathy and neuropathy that result in weakness. This problem is often unrecognized and misdiagnosed as polymyositis or uremic neuropathy. Proximal weakness and elevated serum creatinine kinase are generally present. The condition resolves 3 to 4 weeks after drug withdrawal.

Colchicine also induces reversible malabsorption of vitamin B_{12}, perhaps because it alters the function of the ileal mucosa.

There is a risk of liver function abnormalities in patients taking **febuxostat** (6.6% in patients taking 40 mg/d and 4.6% taking 80 mg/d). A small number of patients (1.1%) experience nausea and arthralgia when taking 40 mg/day of **febuxostat**.

Drug Interactions

Colchicine has very few drug interactions. **Probenecid**, **allopurinol**, and **sulfinpyrazone** have many drug interactions. **Probenecid** inhibits the tubular secretion of most **penicillins** and **cephalosporins** and increases plasma levels by any route these **antibiotics** are given. **Sulfinpyrazone** reduces renal tubular secretion of organic anions (e.g., **antimicrobials** and **sulfonamides**) and displaces other anions bound extensively to plasma proteins (e.g., **tolbutamide, warfarin**).

Salicylates have a mutually antagonistic effect with both of these drugs. Because these drugs, with the exception of **colchicine**, have many drug interactions, checking drug interactions before prescribing them is important. **Febuxostat** should not be administered with drugs that are metabolized by xanthine oxidase, including **theophylline, mercaptopurine**, and **azathioprine**, as toxicity may occur. Table 25–2 lists the drug interactions.

Table 25–2 ■ **Drug Interactions: Antigout and Uricosuric Agents**

Drug	Interacting Drug	Possible Effect	Implications
Allopurinol	Angiotensin-converting enzyme inhibitors	Higher risk of hypersensitivity reaction	Avoid concurrent use
	Aluminum salts	Decreased effects of allopurinol	Separate administration
	Ampicillin	Rate of ampicillin-induced rash much higher	Warn patients
	Anticoagulants	Anticoagulant effect of some drugs enhanced; not warfarin	Use warfarin for anticoagulation; conflicting data
	Cyclophosphamide	Myelosuppressive effects enhanced; increased risk for bleeding	If must be used together, monitor for bleeding risk
	Theophylline	Theophylline clearance decreased with large doses of allopurinol; increased toxicity risk	Select different respiratory drug
	Thiazide diuretics	Increased incidence of hypersensitivity reactions	Avoid concurrent use or monitor for hypersensitivity
	Thiopurines	Clinically significant increases in pharmacological and toxic effect of thiopurines	Avoid concurrent use
	Uricosuric agents	Uricosuric agents that increase excretion of urate also likely to increase excretion of oxypurinol and lower degree of inhibition of xanthine oxidase; avoid concurrent use	Dosage adjustments may be needed if uricosuric added to treatment regimen
Colchicine	NSAIDs	Additive adverse GI effects	Avoid concurrent use; monitor for GI bleeding
Febuxostat	Drugs that are metabolized by xanthine oxidase: theophylline, mercaptopurine, azathioprine	Febuxostat may cause increased plasma levels	Concurrent use is contraindicated
Probenecid	Acyclovir	Decreased acyclovir renal clearance and increased bioavailability	Associated with IV use of drug; avoid this route
	Allopurinol	Increased blood levels for allopurinol	Beneficial effect; may be used therapeutically
	Barbiturates	Increased blood levels	Monitor central nervous system (CNS) effects
	Benzodiazepines (BDZs)	More rapid and prolonged BDZ effect	Monitor BDZ effects
	Clofibrate	Accumulation of clofibric acid; higher steady-state serum concentrations	Select different antilipidemic
	Dapsone	Possible accumulation of dapsone and its metabolites	Monitor for adverse effects or avoid concurrent use
	Dyphylline	Increased half-life, decreased clearance	May be used therapeutically to extend dyphylline dosing interval
	Methotrexate	Increased plasma level; therapeutic effects and toxicity increased	Avoid concurrent use
	NSAIDs	Increased plasma levels and toxicity	Avoid concurrent use

Table 25–2 ■ **Drug Interactions: Antigout and Uricosuric Agents—cont'd**

Drug	Interacting Drug	Possible Effect	Implications
	Pantothenic acid	Renal transport inhibited; plasma levels increased	No specific action required
	Penicillamine	Effects of penicillamine attenuated	Avoid concurrent use
	Penicillins, cephalosporins	Inhibits tubular secretion of most penicillins and cephalosporins; usually increases plasma levels by any route these antibiotics are given	Monitor for adverse effects
	Salicylates	Mutually antagonistic	Avoid concurrent use
	Sulfonamides	Renal transport inhibited; plasma levels increase	Select different antimicrobial
	Sulfonylureas	Half-life of sulfonylurea increased	Monitor blood glucose closely
	Zidovudine	Increased zidovudine bioavailability; cutaneous eruptions accompanied by malaise, myalgia, or fever have occurred	Avoid concurrent use
Sulfinpyrazone	Acetaminophen	Risk of hepatotoxicity may be increased	Conflicting data
	Anticoagulants, oral	Anticoagulant activity of warfarin enhanced: increased bleeding risk	Use probenecid if warfarin must be used
	Niacin	Reduce uricosuric activity of sulfinpyrazone	Avoid concurrent use
	Salicylates	Mutually antagonistic	Avoid concurrent use
	Theophylline	Increased theophylline clearance and decreased plasma levels	Avoid concurrent use or adjust dosage based on serum levels
	Tolbutamide	Decreased clearance and increased half-life of tolbutamide; hypoglycemia may result	Glyburide not affected; change hypoglycemic drug
	Verapamil	Increased clearance; decreased bioavailability	Select different calcium channel blocker

Clinical Use and Dosing

Gout

Colchicine given orally is the time-honored drug for treatment of acute gouty attacks, but its efficacy is limited by the adverse reactions that commonly occur with doses adequate to manage the symptoms. In addition, dosages must be adjusted for patients with impaired renal or hepatic function, and it must be administered with caution to older adults. When **colchicine** is given, the usual regimen is an initial dose of 1.2 mg at the first sign of flare, followed by 0.6 1 hour later (maximum 1.8 mg over 1 h). Historically, a non-FDA approved schedule of dosing is to administer 0.6 to 1.2 mg every 1 to 2 hours, until relief is obtained or until adverse reactions (usually diarrhea, nausea, and vomiting) develop, with 4 to 8 mg total administered. A randomized, double-blind, placebo-controlled, parallel-group, dose-comparison trial of low dose (1.8 mg total over 1 h) and high dose (4.8 mg total over 6 h) of **colchicine** found that low-dose **colchicine** had a better treatment response at 24 hours than did high dose (37.8% vs. 32.7%), with fewer adverse effects such as diarrhea (Terkeltaub et al, 2010). The low-dose **colchicines** group had adverse effects similar to placebo. Therefore, the historic treatment regimen of high-dose **colchicine** is not recommended by this author. Articular pain and swelling usually abate within 12 hours and are usually gone in 24 to 48 hours.

Preventive therapy for patients who have fewer than one acute attack per year is 0.6 mg/day of **colchicine** for 3 or 4 days a week. For patients who have more than one acute attack per year, the dose is 0.6 mg every day. Serious cases may require 1.2 to 1.8 mg/day.

Allopurinol, the drug of choice for patients with a history of urinary calculi, renal insufficiency, chronic tophaceous gout, or high levels of serum urate, is given in doses of 200 to 300 mg/day for mild gout and 400 to 600 mg/day for moderately severe tophaceous gout. The minimum effective dose is 100 to 200 mg/day, and the maximum dose is 800 mg/day. Doses greater than 300 mg/day must be divided. Dosage adjustments for patients with renal insufficiency are based on creatinine clearance (Ccr) values. These adjustments are listed in Table 25–3.

Febuxostat is indicated for the chronic management of hyperuricemia in patients with gout. The starting dose of **febuxostat** is 40 mg per day, once daily. If serum uric acid is not lowered to below 6 mg/dL after 2 weeks, then the dose is increased to 80 mg/day, once daily. **Febuxostat** is taken without regard to food or meals and no dosage adjustment is needed for renal or hepatic impairment.

Table 25–3 ◉ **Dosage Schedule: Antigout and Uricosuric Agents**

Drug	Indication	Initial Dose	Maintenance Dose
Allopurinol	Management of gout	*Adults:*	Minimum effective dose is 100–200 mg/d; maximum dose is 800 mg/d
		Mild disease: 200–300 mg/d	Doses >300 mg/d must be divided
		Moderately severe, tophaceous: 400–600 mg/d	Dosage adjustments for renal insufficiency in adults: CCr 60 mL/min: 200 mg/d CCr 40 mL/min: 150 mg/d CCr 20 mL/min: 100 mg/d CCr 10 mL/min: 100 mg every other day CCr <10 mL/min: 100 mg 3 times/wk
	Hyperuricemia associated with treatment of malignancy	*Adults:* 600–800 mg/d for 2–3 d with a high fluid intake	After 48 h titrate dose in all age groups according to serum uric acid levels
		Children 6–10 yr: 300 mg/d (100 mg tid) *Children <6 yr:* 150 mg/d (50 mg tid)	Another recommended regimen for children: 1 mg/kg/d in 4 divided doses given q6h; maximum dose 600 mg/d
	Recurrent calcium oxalate stones	*Adults:* 200–300 mg/d in single or divided doses	Dosage adjusted up or down based on control of hyperuricemia according to 24-h urinary urate determinations
Colchicine	Acute gouty attacks	*Adults:* 1.2 mg followed by 0.6–1.2 mg every 1–2 h up to 16 doses	Total needed during acute attack is usually 4–8 mg Wait 3 days before starting another course
	Management of gout		Adults with <1 acute attack/y: 0.6 mg/d for 3–4 d/wk Adults with >1 acute attack/y: 0.6 mg/d Serious cases: 1.2–1.8 mg/d
Febuxostat	Management of hyperuricemia in patients with gout	*Adults:* Start at 40 mg once daily. If uric acid levels not <6 mg/dL after 2 wk, increase dose to 80 mg once a day.	40 or 80 mg/d. NSAIDs or colchicine is needed in the first 6 mo of therapy to prevent acute gout attack.
Probenecid	Management of gout*	*Adults:* 0.25 g bid for 1 wk	0.5 g bid; if no acute attack in >6 mo, reduce dose by 0.5 g/d every 6 mo
Sulfinpyrazone	Management of gout	*Adults:* 200–400 mg/d in 2 divided doses	400 mg/d in 2 divided doses; doses as low as 200 mg/d and as high as 800 mg/d have been used

CCr = creatinine clearance.
*Probenecid is not effective for management of gout in the presence of chronic renal failure with CCr <30 mL/min.

Periodic uric acid levels are drawn, the first at 2 weeks of therapy. Liver function should be tested at 2 months and 4 months after starting therapy. It is recommended that **NSAIDS** or **colchicine** be administered prophylactically for the first 6 months of **febuxostat** therapy to prevent acute gout flare.

Inhibitors of uric acid synthesis are more toxic, especially in older adults, and should be reserved for patients who "overproduce" urate (e.g., those who excrete more than 800 mg in 24 h). **Probenecid** is the **uricosuric** agent of choice because of its well-established safety and its relatively long duration of action. Therapy should not be initiated until the acute attack has completely resolved, because rapid decrease in serum urate levels has been shown to exacerbate a gouty attack.

Doses of **probenecid** are 250 mg (1/2 tablet) twice daily for 1 week and then 500 mg twice daily. Doses may be increased by 500 mg/month to a maximum of 2 to 3 g/day. Gastric intolerance may indicate overdose, and decreasing the dosage may ease it. The dosage that maintains normal serum uric acid levels is continued for maintenance. When the patient has had no acute attacks for 6 months, the dose is decreased by 500 mg every 6 months. Do not reduce the maintenance dose to the point at which serum uric acid levels begin to rise.

In the presence of renal impairment, a once-daily dose of 1 g **probenecid** may be used. The daily dose may be increased in 500 mg increments every 4 weeks (usually to less than 2 mg/d) if symptoms are not controlled or the 24-hour urate excretion is less than 700 mg. **Probenecid** is not effective in chronic renal failure if the glomerular filtration rate is 30 mL/minute or less. Patients must maintain hydration and adequate sodium bicarbonate (2 to 7.5 g daily) or potassium citrate (7.5 mg daily) to maintain an alkaline urine while on **probenecid** to prevent formation of uric acid crystals. Alkalization of the urine is recommended until uric acid level is in the normal range.

Sulfinpyrazone is a potent **uricosuric agent**, but it must be given several times daily, is more likely than the other drugs to cause gastric adverse reactions, and can cause platelet dysfunction. For these reasons, it is prescribed only when **probenecid** and **allopurinol** are not tolerated. Initial dosage is 200 to 400 mg daily in two divided doses. Taking the drug with meals or milk reduces its adverse GI reactions. The dose is gradually increased to a maintenance dose of 400 mg daily in two divided doses. Doses can be as low as 200 mg/day or as high as 800 mg/day to control blood urate levels. Therapy is continued, even in the presence of acute exacerbations. This drug can be used concomitantly with **colchicine**. Patients previously controlled on **probenecid** may be transferred to **sulfinpyrazone** at the full maintenance dose.

For all of these drugs, the goal of treatment is a urate level less than 6 mg/dL. Doses are titrated upward until that goal is reached.

Hyperuricemia Associated With Malignancies

Allopurinol is approved for use in hyperuricemia associated with malignancies. Doses of 600 to 800 mg daily for 2 or 3 days, with a high fluid intake, have proved effective. Dosage is similar to the dose given for gout.

Children age 6 to 10 with hyperuricemia secondary to malignancy are given 10 mg/kg/day in two to three divided doses. Younger children are generally given 150 mg/day in three divided doses. Another suggested dosing regimen is 300 mg/day in two to three divided doses in children aged 6 to 10 years.

Recurrent Calcium Oxalate Calculi

Allopurinol 200 to 300 mg/day in single or divided doses is given to prevent recurrent calcium oxalate renal stones. Patients also benefit from dietary modifications such as increases in oral fluids and dietary fiber and reductions in animal protein, sodium, refined sugars, oxalate-rich food, and excessive calcium intake.

Off-Labeled Uses

Colchicine also has several off-labeled uses. These purposes and the recommended doses are the following:

1. Hepatic cirrhosis: 1 mg/day for 5 days each week.
2. Primary biliary cirrhosis: 0.6 mg twice daily.
3. Refractory idiopathic thrombocytopenic purpura: 1.2 to 1.8 mg/day for 2 weeks or more.
4. Skin manifestations of scleroderma: 1 mg/day.
5. Familial Mediterranean fever: 1.2 to 2.4 mg/day in one to two divided doses. Increase or decrease dose in 0.3 mg increments, to a maximum of 2.4 mg/daily.

Rational Drug Selection

Specific disease processes, for which each of these drugs is most appropriate, have already been mentioned. In general, **allopurinol** or **febuxostat** is best for patients who overproduce uric acid; **probenecid** is best for patients who undersecrete uric acid and have adequate renal function; **sulfinpyrazone** is best for patients who undersecrete uric acid when on a regular diet and those who need antiplatelet activity. Additional considerations in choosing the appropriate drug are shown in Table 25–3. Table 25–4 discusses available dosage forms of gout medications.

Renal Insufficiency

Because **allopurinol** blocks urate production, it is especially useful for patients with a history of urinary calculi, with renal insufficiency, or with excessive basal urinary

Table 25–4 ◆ **Available Dosage Forms: Antigout and Uricosuric Agents**

Drug	Dosage Form	How Supplied
Allopurinol (Zyloprim)	Tablets: 100 mg Tablets: 300 mg	In bottles of 100 tablets In bottles of 100, 500 tablets
(Generic)	Tablets: 100 mg, 300 mg	In bottles of 100, 500, 1,000 tablets
Colchicine	Tablets: 0.5 mg, 0.6 mg	In bottles of 100 tablets
Febuxostat (Uloric)	Tablets: 40 mg, 80 mg	30, 90, 100 tablets
Probenecid (Benemid)	Tablets: 0.5 mg	In bottles of 100 tablets
(Generic)	Tablets: 0.5 mg	In bottles of 100, 1,000 tablets
Sulfinpyrazone (Anturane)	Tablets: 100 mg Capsules: 200 mg	In bottles of 100 tablets In bottles of 100 capsules
(Generic)	Tablets: 100 mg Capsules: 200 mg	In bottles of 100, 500 tablets In bottles of 100, 500, 1,000 capsules

uric acid excretion (750 to 800 mg/24 h). Serious adverse reactions occur in fewer than 2 percent of patients, typically within the first 2 months of therapy. Patients should be kept under close surveillance during this period. Toxicity seems more likely when **allopurinol** is given concomitantly with **thiazide diuretics**.

Peptic Ulcer Disease

IV **colchicine** rapidly provides a therapeutic plasma level and does not cause GI adverse reactions. It is useful for patients who cannot take the drug orally, have peptic ulcer disease, or have contraindications to **NSAIDs**. Diluted in 20 mL of normal saline and given over 10 minutes, 2 mg usually provides relief within 6 to 8 hours. Care must be used to prevent extravasation because **colchicine** may cause tissue necrosis.

High Levels of Serum Urate Associated With Secondary Gout

Allopurinol is the drug of choice because it is the only drug in this group that blocks urate production.

Monitoring

All patients receiving these drugs require serum uric acid level monitoring. A baseline assessment is done at initiation of therapy. Uric acid levels should be normal after 1 to 3 weeks of therapy, and serum levels should be drawn again then and periodically throughout therapy or in the presence of exacerbations. The upper limit of normal for men and postmenopausal women is 7 mg/dL; for premenopausal women, it is 6 mg/dL.

For **allopurinol**, liver and renal function must be assessed prior to initiation of therapy and periodically during the first few months of therapy, particularly for patients with preexisting liver disease. Perform blood urea nitrogen (BUN), serum creatinine, and Ccr tests, and reassess dosages based on the results.

Probenecid and **sulfinpyrazone** both have blood dyscrasias (anemia, hemolytic anemia) as adverse reactions. Patients taking these drugs should have periodic complete blood counts (CBCs).

Patients whose urine is being alkalinized to prevent crystallization of urates in the urine should have their acid–base balance monitored.

Patient Education

Administration

Each drug should be taken exactly as prescribed. A dose that is missed should be taken as soon as the patient remembers but without doubling doses. For **allopurinol**, if the dosing schedule is once daily, do not take it until the next day. If the dosing schedule is more than once a day, take up to 300 mg for the next dose. None of these drugs should be discontinued without first consulting the health-care provider. Uric acid levels rise when the drug is stopped.

In the event of an acute attack during maintenance therapy, **allopurinol**, **febuxostat**, **probenecid**, and **sulfinpyrazone** should be continued while **colchicine** is added to the regimen to treat the acute attack. Dosage adjustments of the maintenance drugs may be necessary.

Allopurinol can be crushed and given with fluid or mixed with food for patients who have difficulty in swallowing.

Patients should avoid taking **aspirin** or **salicylates** while taking **probenecid** or **sulfinpyrazone**. These drugs are mutually antagonistic.

Adverse Reactions

The main adverse reaction for all these drugs is GI distress. Taking these drugs with food or milk may minimize gastric irritation.

Probenecid and **sulfinpyrazone** are **sulfa-based drugs** that have been associated with hypersensitivity reactions related to this base. Patients should be asked about **sulfa** allergies and taught the indications of a hypersensitivity reaction and the importance of reporting it. A hypersensitivity reaction requires immediate discontinuance of the drug. Other symptoms to report with these drugs include sore throat, fatigue, yellowing of the skin or eyes, and unusual bleeding or bruising. These drugs have been associated with blood dyscrasias and hepatotoxicity.

Allopurinol has been associated with a maculopapular rash that sometimes is scaly or exfoliative. Because this skin reaction can be severe or even fatal, patients should report to their health-care provider the first indication of a rash. They should be seen to evaluate this rash, and discontinuance of the drug should be considered.

Drowsiness and dizziness have occasionally affected patients who are taking **allopurinol**. Caution patients to avoid driving or other activities requiring alertness until their response to the drug is known.

Patients taking standard doses of **colchicine** have developed proximal muscle weakness related to myopathy and neuropathy. Patients should be warned to report these symptoms to their health-care provider. Stopping the drug usually reverses the symptoms within 3 to 4 weeks.

Lifestyle Management

To reduce available urates, an alkaline diet may be prescribed that includes reductions in sodium, refined sugars, oxalate-rich foods (e.g., liver, kidney, anchovies, sardines, herring, mussels, bacon, codfish, scallops, trout, haddock, veal, venison, turkey), and excessive calcium intake, as well as increases in oral fluids and dietary fiber. Fluid intake in excess of 3,000 mL/day also reduces the risk for renal calculi. Because large amounts of **alcohol** increase uric acid concentrations and may decrease the effectiveness of medications, **alcohol** should be avoided or consumed in very small amounts.

CORTICOSTEROIDS

Cortisol, the endogenous glucocorticoid in the body, is produced and secreted on the basis of feedback mechanisms of the hypothalamus-pituitary-adrenal (HPA) axis. The adrenal cortex synthesizes and secretes the steroid hormones that include mineralocorticoids and glucocorticoids and, to a lesser extent, androgens. Figure 25–1 depicts this feedback system. Exogenously administered adrenal cortex hormones (**corticosteroids**) affect this feedback mechanism.

Corticosteroids have a major role in the management of a variety of disease processes. In primary or secondary adrenal cortex insufficiency, they are used for replacement therapy. In rheumatic disorders, they may be short-term adjunctive therapy for acute episodes or exacerbation. These drugs are also used to treat collagen disease, dermatological conditions, asthma, allergic rhinitis, neoplastic disorders, inflammatory bowel disease, and idiopathic thrombocytopenia purpura. The role of **inhaled corticosteroids** in management of respiratory disorders is covered in Chapter 17. **Topical corticosteroids** used to manage dermatological conditions are covered in Chapter 23. This chapter focuses on the use of **systemic corticosteroids** to manage inflammatory conditions in primary care situations.

Pharmacodynamics

Glucocorticoids have metabolic, anti-inflammatory, and growth-suppressing effects. **Cortisol** is the "wake-up" hormone, and altered levels result in changes in levels of awareness and sleep patterns. Central nervous system (CNS) effects also result in labile emotional states, and high levels of **cortisol** are associated with decreased recent memory recall. They increase blood glucose concentration by stimulating gluconeogenesis in the liver and by decreasing uptake of glucose into muscle, lymphatic, and adipose cells. In extrahepatic tissues, they stimulate protein catabolism and inhibit amino acid uptake and protein synthesis. Decreased proliferation of fibroblasts in connective tissue in concert with the poor protein synthesis leads to poor wound healing (McCance & Huether, 2010). **Glucocorticoids** inhibit the immune and inflammatory systems by their actions at

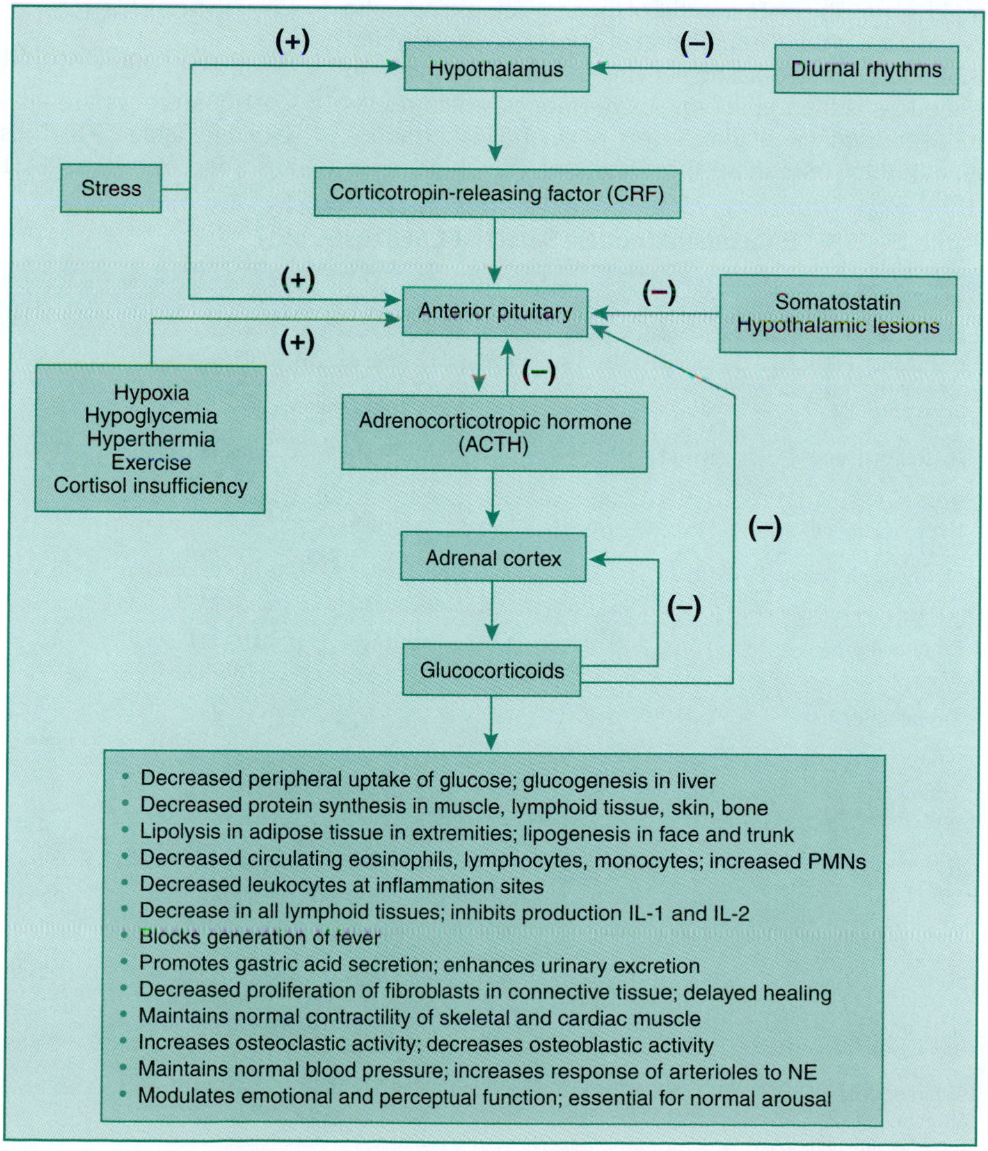

Figure 25–1. Hypothalamus-pituitary-adrenal axis and feedback control of cortisol.

several sites: depressing proliferation of T lymphocytes, including those that produce the antiviral protein interferon; decreasing natural killer cell activity; reversing macrophage activity; and suppressing the synthesis, secretion, and actions of chemical mediators involved in inflammatory and immune responses. These chemical mediators include interleukins, prostaglandins, leukotrienes, bradykinin, serotonin, and histamine.

Glucocorticoids also increase circulating erythrocytes; increase appetite; promote fat deposits in the face and cervical areas, while promoting lipolysis in the extremities; increase uric acid excretion; and decrease serum calcium levels, possibly by inhibiting GI absorption of calcium and phosphate (American College of Rheumatology, 2001 update). They also promote gastric acid secretion. In the urinary tract, they enhance urinary excretion. Their feedback activity on the HPA axis suppresses secretion and synthesis of adrenocorticotropic hormone (ACTH) and suppresses prostaglandin E production of insulin-like growth hormone secretion so that somatic growth is inhibited. Skeletal wasting also occurs and is most rapid during the first 6 months of therapy. This osteoporotic process is a result of stimulation of osteoclastic activity and inhibition of osteoblastic activity. An additional factor in bone loss is their effect on sex hormones, which results in decreased circulating levels of anabolic hormones. Finally, they potentiate the effects of catecholamines, thyroid hormone, and growth hormone on adipose tissue. Figure 25–1 depicts the control of cortisol secretion.

Mineralocorticoids (predominantly **aldosterone**) are also secreted by the adrenal cortex under the control of the renin-angiotensin-aldosterone system. The main role of **aldosterone** is to retain sodium and water and excrete potassium. Naturally occurring adrenocorticosteroids have both **cortisol** and **aldosterone** properties in varying amounts. This difference in percentage of hormone may be a factor in the choice of **corticosteroid. Hydrocortisone** and **cortisone** are naturally occurring **glucocorticoids** with predominant **cortisol** activity and are used as replacement therapy in adrenocortical deficiency states and may be used as **anti-inflammatory** drugs. **Prednisone, prednisolone,** and **fludrocortisone** are synthetic steroids with mixed **cortisol** and **aldosterone** activity but are used mainly for their **cortisol** effects. **Triamcinolone, dexamethasone, methylprednisolone,** and **betamethasone** are also synthetic compounds that have almost no **aldosterone** activity and are used for their potent **anti-inflammatory** activity.

Pharmacokinetics

Absorption and Distribution

Corticosteroids are all well absorbed from the upper jejunum (Table 25–5). Those with IM formulations are well absorbed from IM sites. Injections of suspensions and

Table 25–5 ▶ **Pharmacokinetics: Selected Corticosteroids**

Drug	Onset (hours)	Peak (hours)	Duration (days)	Protein Binding	Half-Life	RAP	RMP	Elimination
Cortisone* PO	Rapid	2	1.25–1.5	Very high	30 min P 8–12 h B	0.8	2	1% unchanged in urine
Cortisone* IM	Slow	20–48	1.25–1.5	Very high	—	0.8	2	1% unchanged in urine
Hydrocortisone* PO	Rapid	1	1.25–1.5	High	80–118 min P 8–12 h B	1	2	1% unchanged in urine
Hydrocortisone† IM	Slow	4–8	Varies	High	—	1	2	1% unchanged in urine
Methylprednisolone†	UK	1–2	1.25–1.5	High	78–188 min P 18–36 h B	5	0	1% unchanged in urine
Prednisolone†	1	1–2	1.25–1.5	High	115–211 min P 18–36 h B	4	1	1% unchanged in urine
Prednisone†	1	1–2	1.25–1.5	Very high	60 min P 18–36 h B	4	1	1% unchanged in urine
Triamcinolone†	UK	1–2	2.25	High	200 + min P 18–36 h B	5	0	1% unchanged in urine
Dexamethasone‡ PO	UK	1–2	2.75	High	110–210 min P 36–54 h B	20–30	0	1% unchanged in urine
Dexamethasone‡ IM	Rapid	8	6	High	—	20–30	0	1% unchanged in urine
Betamethasone‡ PO	UK	1–2	3.25	High	300 + min P 36–54 h B	20–30	0	1% unchanged in urine
Betamethasone‡ IM	1–3	UK	7	High	—	20–30	0	1% unchanged in urine

B = biological half-life; P = plasma half-life; RAP = relative anti-inflammatory potency; RMP = relative mineralocorticoid potency; UK = unknown.
*Short acting.
†Intermediate acting.
‡Long acting.

esters produce greatly altered onset and duration times. Absorption is rapid for esters (**sodium phosphates** and **sodium succinate**) and relatively slow for other derivatives (**acetates, acetonides,** and **tebutates**). Absorption from local sites (e.g., intra-articular or intrasynovial) is slower than from IM sites. Because onset, peak, and duration of action vary, these drugs are classified into short-, intermediate-, and long-acting forms.

Corticosteroids are reversibly bound to corticosteroid-binding proteins.

Corticosteroids have significantly altered pharmacological effects on patients with altered protein-binding capacities. Pregnancy, for example, is a hyperproteinemic state in which the total plasma level of steroid would be elevated. All these drugs are widely distributed, cross the placenta, and probably enter breast milk.

Metabolism and Excretion

The liver metabolizes **hydrocortisone (Cortef)**, and this is the rate-limiting step in its clearance. The metabolism and excretion of other **corticosteroids** generally parallel those of **hydrocortisone.** Induction of hepatic enzymes increases the metabolic clearance of all **corticosteroids.** The liver converts **cortisone (Cortone)** to **hydrocortisone**, and **prednisone (Deltasone)** is converted to **prednisolone (Delta-Cortef, Prelone).** These metabolites are then clinically active and metabolized by the liver for clearance. Approximately 1 percent of the daily dose of the drug is excreted unchanged in urine. Renal clearance is increased when plasma levels are increased.

Table 25–5 depicts that pharmacokinetics of selected **corticosteroids**, including their relative **anti-inflammatory** and **mineralocorticoid** activity.

Pharmacotherapeutics

Precautions and Contraindications

The wide range of contraindications and warnings about cautious use associated with **corticosteroids** is a factor of their numerous actions. They are contraindicated in the presence of active untreated infections because they may mask the indications of infection, and new infections may appear during their use. A patient may also have decreased resistance, and the host defense mechanisms may be unable to prevent dissemination of the infection. **Corticosteroids** may exacerbate systemic fungal infections and activate latent amebiasis or tuberculosis. Although they have been advocated for the treatment of chronic active hepatitis, they may be harmful in hepatitis positive for hepatitis B surface antigen.

For many disorders, these drugs should be used cautiously. Average and large doses of drugs with high relative mineralocorticoid potency (e.g., **cortisone** and **hydrocortisone**) can cause elevated blood pressure, salt and water retention, and increased excretion of potassium. These effects can be especially problematic for patients with hypertension and cardiovascular disorders (e.g., congestive heart failure [CHF]). Sodium restriction and potassium supplementation may be necessary. Edema can occur in the presence of renal disease with a fixed or decreased glomerular filtration rate (GFR). These drugs should be used with caution in renal insufficiency, acute glomerulonephritis, or chronic nephritis.

All **corticosteroids** increase calcium excretion, which creates problems for postmenopausal women and others at risk for osteoporosis.

Patients with diabetes mellitus may have difficulty maintaining glycemic control because **corticosteroids** alter the liver's glucose regulation. The relationship between peptic ulceration and **corticosteroid** therapy is unclear. Patients with ulcerative colitis or peptic ulcer disease or with concomitant use of gastric irritants (e.g., **NSAIDs**) and stress have an increased probability of GI bleeding and perforation.

Some of these products contain **tartrazine** or **sodium bisulfite**, both of which can cause severe allergic reactions. Patients with these allergies should notify their health-care provider, and the label of the drug should be read carefully for these inclusions.

Corticosteroids cross the placenta (**prednisone** has the least transport), and most are Pregnancy Category C. In animal studies, large doses resulted in cleft palate, stillborn fetuses, and decreased fetal size. Chronic ingestion during the first trimester in humans has shown a 1 percent incidence of cleft palate. In considering use of these drugs during pregnancy or in women with childbearing potential, the benefits must be carefully weighed against the potential risks to the fetus. Infants of mothers who have taken these drugs are observed closely for signs of hypoaldosteronism.

Corticosteroids appear in breast milk and could retard the nursing infant's growth, interfere with endogenous corticosteroid production, or cause other unwanted effects. Several studies suggest that the amount excreted in breast milk is negligible with **prednisone** or **prednisolone** doses 20 mg or less per day and **methylprednisolone (Medrol)** doses 8 mg or less per day. For mothers who want to nurse, waiting 3 to 4 hours after taking the drug and using one of these drugs within these doses may be tried (LactMed, 2011).

When given **corticosteroids**, children may experience altered growth and development, and they require careful monitoring if they must be on prolonged therapy. Some of these products contain benzyl alcohol, which has been associated with a fatal "gasping syndrome" in infants.

Older adults often have chronic disorders that are worsened by **corticosteroids.** Consider the risk/benefit factors of **steroid** use. Lower doses and careful monitoring of blood pressure, blood glucose, and electrolytes at least every 6 months are appropriate.

Adverse Drug Reactions

Adverse reactions can be discussed by the body system that is affected.

Muscle and Skin

Common skin changes reported with **systemic corticosteroids** include atrophy and thinning of the skin, alopecia, acneiform eruptions, poor healing, purpura, striae, hirsutism, and desquamation. Myopathy is also seen, with marked muscle wasting. No relationship between dose or duration of therapy and these adverse reactions is apparent. Alteration in body fat is also noted, particularly in patients who take **corticosteroids** for more than 60 days, with the most common changes being truncal obesity, buffalo hump, and moon facies.

Skeletal Tissues

Osteoporosis develops in 11 to 20 percent of patients treated for more than 1 year. Skeletal fractures, mainly of the spine, ribs, and pelvis, may occur secondary to the reduced bone density. **Glucocorticoid therapy** at doses of 7.5 mg/day or greater of **prednisone** for 6 or more months results in a rapid loss of trabecular bone in the spine, hip, and forearm. Bone mineral density should be measured in all individuals who are likely to be on this therapy long term (American College of Rheumatology, 2001 update).

Ocular Tissues

Prolonged use may produce subcapsular cataracts, glaucoma with possible damage to the optic nerve, and increased risk for secondary ocular infections due to fungi or viruses.

Gastrointestinal System

Corticosteroids have been implicated in the induction of peptic ulcer disease. Patients who appear to be at risk are those being treated for nephrotic syndrome or hepatic disease; are taking a total dose of **prednisone** exceeding 1 g; or have a history of ulcer disease, concomitant use of a known gastric irritant, or stress. Combining **corticosteroids** and **NSAIDs** or **aspirin** increases the risk of peptic ulcer disease. Prophylaxis with **proton pump inhibitors (PPIs)** or **H_2 blockers** is suggested for patients with two or more of these risk factors (Feldman & Das, 2010; Saag & Furst, 2010). Patients also taking **NSAIDs** may require **misoprostol (Cytotec)**; **misoprostol's** use is described in Chapter 34.

Cardiovascular System

Hypertension is the most common adverse reaction. This and other cardiovascular problems (e.g., fluid and electrolyte disturbances) are discussed in the Precautions and Contraindications section.

Central Nervous System

Delirium, agitation, insomnia, mood swings, and severe depression characterize steroid psychosis. The onset of symptoms is usually within 15 to 30 days. Predisposing factors include doses above 40 mg of **prednisone** or its equivalent dose in another drug, female gender, and a family history of psychiatric disorder. The incidence is correlated with dose. If the **steroid** cannot be stopped, **psychotropic drugs** are effective in relieving the symptoms.

Endocrine System

Prolonged therapy with **corticosteroids** may lead to adrenal suppression. The degree of suppression depends on dosage, relative **glucocorticoid** (anti-inflammatory) potency, biological half-life, and duration of therapy. As a general rule, suppression occurs with doses above the physiological range that are given for more than 1 month. It can be minimized by using intermediate-acting agents on an alternate-day dosing schedule. Abrupt withdrawal after adrenal suppression has occurred may result in a withdrawal syndrome, with symptoms similar to those seen in adrenal insufficiency. To minimize this adverse reaction, the dose of **corticosteroids** used for prolonged therapy should be tapered. Recovery from HPA suppression can take up to 12 months.

The effect on glucose metabolism and regulation is discussed in the Precautions and Contraindications section. Amenorrhea, postmenopausal bleeding, and other menstrual irregularities have also been seen.

Drug Interactions

Additive hypokalemia may occur with drugs that also produce this adverse reaction. This hypokalemia increases the risk for toxicity in **digoxin.** Several drugs stimulate the metabolism of **corticosteroids,** and **oral contraceptives** decrease their metabolism. **NSAIDs** increase the risk for GI adverse reactions. Other drug interactions are in Table 25–6.

Clinical Use and Dosing

Adrenocortical Insufficiency

In primary adrenocortical insufficiency, **glucocorticoid** and **mineralocorticoid** properties are lost; however, in secondary adrenocortical insufficiency, **mineralocorticoid** function is preserved. In the United States, primary adrenocortical insufficiency is an uncommon disorder. Widespread **corticosteroid** use has made secondary adrenocortical insufficiency due to **steroid** withdrawal much more common. Approximately 6 million persons are considered to have undiagnosed adrenocortical insufficiency only during times of physiological stress. The key to treatment of primary or secondary disease is replacement of the missing hormones. The drugs of choice are **hydrocortisone, cortisone,** and **prednisone** because each has both **glucocorticoid** and **mineralocorticoid** effects and requires no additional **mineralocorticoid.**

Initial doses for **hydrocortisone** are 50 mg every 8 hours for 48 hours for adults; then the dose is tapered to 30 to 50 mg/day in divided doses. In children the dose is 2.5 to 10 mg/kg/day for children under age 12, in three to four divided doses, and then the dose is tapered to the maintenance dose over 14 days. Children over 12 years are dosed as adults. For **cortisone,** the initial adult dose is 25 to 300 mg/day in two divided doses, and the pediatric

Table 25–6 ■ **Drug Interactions: Selected Corticosteroids**

Drug	Interacting Drug	Possible Effect	Implications
Betamethasone, cortisone	Insulin, oral hypoglycemics	Decreased effectiveness, resulting in altered glycemic control	Monitor blood glucose levels more closely if drugs must be given concurrently
Hydrocortisone	Cholestyramine	Hydrocortisone area under the curve (AUC) decreased	Separate dose by 4 h and give hydrocortisone first
	Insulin, oral hypoglycemics	Decreased effectiveness, resulting in altered glycemic control	Monitor blood glucose levels more closely if drugs must be given concurrently
Dexamethasone	Ephedrine	Decreased half-life and increased clearance of dexamethasone	Avoid concurrent administration
	Insulin, oral hypoglycemics	Decreased effectiveness, resulting in altered glycemic control	Monitor blood glucose levels more closely if drugs must be given concurrently
Prednisone	NSAIDs, other GI irritants	Increased risk for GI bleed	Avoid concurrent use
	Insulin, oral hypoglycemics	Decreased effectiveness, resulting in altered glycemic control	Monitor blood glucose levels more closely if drugs must be given concurrently
Methylprednisolone	Macrolide antimicrobials (e.g., erythromycin, clarithromycin)	Significant decrease in methylprednisolone clearance	Has been used therapeutically to decrease methylprednisolone dose
	Insulin, oral hypoglycemics	Decreased effectiveness, resulting in altered glycemic control	Monitor blood glucose levels more closely if drugs must be given concurrently
All corticosteroids	Barbiturates	Decrease the pharmacological effects of the corticosteroid	Avoid concurrent use
	Oral contraceptives	Corticosteroid half-life and concentration increased; clearance decreased	May require dosage adjustment
	Estrogens	Corticosteroid clearance decreased	May require dosage adjustment
	Hydantoins, rifampin	Corticosteroid clearance increased; reduced therapeutic effects	May require dosage adjustment
	Ketoconazole	Corticosteroid clearance decreased; AUC increased	Select different imidazole
	Digoxin	May increase risk of digitalis toxicity	Avoid coadministration
	Isoniazid	Isoniazid serum concentrations decreased	If must be used together, dosage adjustments may be needed; monitor therapy closely
	Potassium-depleting agents (e.g., thiazide and loop diuretics, mezlocillin, piperacillin, ticarcillin)	Additive hypokalemia	Avoid concurrent use; monitor serum potassium levels
	Salicylates	Reduced serum salicylate levels; decreased therapeutic effectiveness	Avoid concurrent use
	Somatrem	Inhibits growth-promoting effect of somatrem	Consult with endocrinologist for best action

dose is 0.25 to 0.35 mg/kg/day IM in two divided doses. Once again, the drug is tapered over 14 days to the maintenance dose. **Prednisone** is started at 5 to 60 mg/day in two divided doses for adults and 1 to 2 mg/kg/day in a once- or twice-daily dose for children. This drug is tapered in the same way (Klauer, 2009).

For maintenance replacement of **cortisol**, under normal circumstances patients are given 15 to 20 mg of **cortisol** or its equivalent daily. Dosage schedules vary, but the simplest and least expensive in adults is **cortisone** 25 mg daily. **Hydrocortisone** 20 mg or **prednisone** 5 to 20 mg may also be used on the same schedule. To approach diurnal rhythms, the dose is given in the morning before 9 a.m. Equivalent doses of another **corticosteroid** may be used but have no specific advantage. In addition, other **corticosteroids** have less relative **mineralocorticoid** potency, and an additional drug to provide **mineralocorticoid** activity might be required if they are used.

The response to any of these drugs is highly variable. Doses are highly individualized, and much higher doses given in divided doses may be needed. Specific doses and ranges for each of the **corticosteroids** for this indication, for both adults and children, are provided in Table 25–7.

Inflammation

Any of the **corticosteroids** may be used to reduce or prevent inflammation. Because the need for **mineralocorticoid** activity is low to absent in this indication, drugs with more **anti-inflammatory** activity—**methylprednisolone**, **prednisone**, and **triamcinolone (Aristocort)**—are appropriate. **Betamethasone** also has only **anti-inflammatory** activity, but it is four to five times more potent than the other drugs, which increases the risk for adverse reactions. **Dexamethasone** is used most often in acute care to relieve the inflammation that causes intracranial pressure after closed head injury or cranial surgery. Doses are shown in Table 25–7.

Table 25–7 ◉ **Dosage Schedule: Selected Corticosteroids**

Drug	Indication	Dose	Notes
Betamethasone	Inflammation, immunosuppression	*Adults:* 0.6–7.2 mg/d PO as single or divided doses *Children:* 62.5–250 mcg/kg/d PO in 3 divided doses	Long-acting. Suppresses HPA at doses >0.6 mg/d
Cortisone	Adrenocortical insufficiency	*Adults:* Initial dose 25–300 mg. Maintenance dose is 10–37 mg/d in single or divided dose *Children:* Initial dose 25–300 mg orally or 0.25–0.35 mg/kg/d IM in 2 divided doses. Maintenance dose is 0.56 mg/kg/d	Has mineralocorticoid activity but may need additional drug; short-acting; suppresses HPA at doses >20 mg/d. Taper initial dose to maintenance dose over 14 d
	Inflammation, immunosuppression	*Adults:* 25–300 mg/d PO in single or divided doses *Children:* 2.5–10 mg/kg/d PO as single or divided doses	Has mineralocorticoid activity but may need additional drug; short-acting; suppresses HPA at doses >20 mg/d
Dexamethasone	Adrenocortical insufficiency	*Children:* 23.3 mcg/kg/d PO in 3 divided doses	Not commonly used for this indication in adults; required addition of mineralocorticoid.
	Inflammation, immunosuppression	*Adults:* 0.5–9 mg/d PO in single or divided doses *Children:* 83.3–333.3 mcg/kg/d PO in 3–4 divided doses	Long-acting. Suppresses HPA at doses >0.75 mg/d
Hydrocortisone	Adrenocortical insufficiency	*Adults:* Initial dose 50 mg q8h for 48 h Maintenance dose 20–240 mg/d in single or divided doses	Has mineralocorticoid activity; short-acting; suppresses HPA at doses >20 mg/d. Taper initial dose to maintenance dose over 14 d
	Inflammation, immunosuppression	*Adults:* 20–240 mg/d PO in 1–4 divided doses *Children:* 2–8 mg/kg/d in single or divided doses	Has mineralocorticoid activity; short-acting; suppresses HPA at doses >20 mg/d
	Inflammatory bowel disease	*Adults:* 100 mg nightly in retention enema for 21 d or until remission	Has mineralocorticoid activity; short-acting; suppresses HPA at doses >20 mg/d
Methylprednisolone	Inflammation, immunosuppression	*Adults:* 4–48 mg/d PO in single or divided doses initially; up to 240 mg/d for maintenance *Children:* 0.117–1.67 mg/kg/d PO in 3–4 divided doses	Intermediate-acting; suppresses HPA at doses of 4 mg/d
	Multiple sclerosis	*Adults:* 160 mg/d for 7 d; then 64 every other day for 1 mo	Intermediate-acting; suppresses HPA at doses of 4 mg/d
Prednisolone	Adrenocortical insufficiency	*Adults:* Initial dose and maintenance dose 5–60 mg *Children:* 1–2 mg/kg/d initial and maintenance doses	Intermediate-acting; suppresses HPA at doses >5 mg/d. Taper over 14 d

Table 25–7 ● **Dosage Schedule: Selected Corticosteroids—cont'd**

Drug	Indication	Dose	Notes
	Inflammation, immunosuppression	*Adults:* 5–60 mg/d PO in single or divided doses *Children:* 0.5–2 mg/kg/d PO in 3–4 divided doses	Intermediate-acting; suppresses HPA at doses >5 mg/d
	Multiple sclerosis	*Adults:* 200 mg/d for 7 d; then 80 mg every other day for 1 mo	Intermediate-acting; suppresses HPA at doses >5 mg/d
Prednisone	Adrenocortical insufficiency	*Adults:* 5–60 mg/d PO in single or divided doses	Minimal mineralocorticoid activity; intermediate-acting; suppresses HPA at doses >5 mg. Taper over 14 d
	Inflammation, immunosuppression	*Adults:* 5–60 mg/d PO in single or divided doses *Children:* 0.14–2 mg/kg/d PO in 4 divided doses	Minimal mineralocorticoid activity; intermediate-acting; suppresses HPA at doses >5 mg
	Nephrotic syndrome	*Children:* Initial dosing 2 mg/kg/day in 1 to 3 divided doses (maximum 80 mg/day) until urine is protein free. Maintenance dose 2 mg/kg/dose administered every other day. Taper and discontinue after 4 to 6 weeks.	Minimal mineralocorticoid activity; intermediate-acting; suppresses HPA at doses >5 mg
Triamcinolone	Adrenocortical insufficiency	*Adults:* 4–12 mg/d PO in single or divided doses *Children:* 117 mcg/kg/d in single or divided doses	No mineralocorticoid activity; requires addition of mineralocorticoid drug. Intermediate-acting; suppresses HPA at doses >4 mg/d.
	Rheumatic disorders	*Adults:* 8–12 mg/d PO	No mineralocorticoid activity; requires addition of mineralocorticoid drug. Intermediate-acting; suppresses HPA at doses >4 mg/d.
	Systemic lupus erythematosus	*Adults:* 20–32 mg/d PO	No mineralocorticoid activity; requires addition of mineralocorticoid drug. Intermediate-acting; suppresses HPA at doses >4 mg/d.
	Other inflammatory diseases or for immunosuppression	*Adults:* 4–48 mg/d PO in single or divided doses *Children:* 0.416–1.7 mg/kg/d PO in single or divided doses	No mineralocorticoid activity; requires addition of mineralocorticoid drug. Intermediate-acting; suppresses HPA at doses >4 mg/d.

HPA = hypothalamus-pituitary-adrenal axis.
For parenteral doses, see other sources.

Immunosuppression

Although all **corticosteroids** have immunosuppressive capability, the most commonly used is **prednisone.** It has a short half-life, low cost, and negligible **mineralocorticoid** activity, and it is available in 5- and 20-mg tablets that make dosage changes simple for the patient to manage. Tapering doses can be complex, with different doses every day or every other day. When patients are being tapered from high doses (e.g., after organ rejection episodes), the tapering schedule may last for weeks. Patients can be instructed to take a specific number of tablets on day 1 and then reduce the dose by one tablet each day as a simple taper, without their having to keep track of the number of milligrams they are to take on any given day. **Prednisolone,** the active hepatic metabolite of **prednisone,** is useful in the presence of hepatic dysfunction. Other drugs in this class may also be used for this indication, and their dosing schedule is presented in Table 25–7.

Rheumatoid Arthritis

Rheumatoid arthritis (RA) is a system inflammatory disorder and treatment to reduce inflammation is appropriate. First-line therapy is with **NSAIDs;** however, low-dose oral **glucocorticoids** (e.g., less than 7.5 mg/d of **prednisone** or its equivalent as single dose) may be considered for short-term use. It has been shown to decrease progression or erosions for the first 2 years (Simon et al, 2002). When an oral **glucocorticoid** is used, prophylaxis with a **bisphosphonate,** along with **calcium supplementation** and daily **supplemental vitamin D,** has been shown to the lower the risk of **glucocorticoid**-induced osteoporosis (American College of Rheumatology, 2001 update; Simon et al, 2002). New treatment guidelines are under development by the American College of Rheumatology (http://www.rheumatology.org).

Regardless of the disease process for which the drug is given, several overall dosing guidelines apply (Table 25–8). The following guidelines are adapted from *Drug Facts and Comparisons* (2010) and McCance and Huether (2010).

1. The maximum activity of the adrenal cortex in producing cortisol is between 2 and 8 a.m. To best match this natural body rhythm, daily doses are best taken in the morning before 9 a.m.
2. The initial dose depends on the specific disease being treated. Maintain or adjust the dose until an acceptable response is achieved. Establish a time frame within which to expect this response. If such a response does not occur within that time frame, discontinue the **corticosteroid** and consult or refer the patient for other therapy.
3. After an acceptable response is achieved, determine the maintenance dose by decreasing the dosage in small amounts at intervals until the lowest dosage

Table 25–8 ◈ **Available Dosage Forms: Selected Corticosteroids**

Drug	Dosage Form	How Supplied	Cost
Betamethasone (Celestone)	Tablets: 0.6 mg	In bottles of 100 and UD 21 tablets	
	Syrup: 0.6 mg/5 mL	In 118 mL	
Cortisone (Generic only)	Tablet: 25 mg	In bottles of 8, 100, 500, 1,000, and UD 100 tablets	$33/100
Dexamethasone (Decadron) (Generic)	Tablets: 0.25 mg, 0.5 mg	In bottles of 100 and 1,000 tablets (Decadron brand scored)	0.75 mg = $10.66/12
	0.75 mg	In bottles of 100, 500, 1,000, and UD 100 tablets (Decadron brand in 12 and 100 scored)	0.5 mg = $57/100
	Tablets: 1 mg	In bottles of 100 and UD 100 scored tablets	0.25 mg = No data
	1 mg	In bottles of 50, 100, 500, 1,000, and UD 100 tablets	$20/30
	1.5 mg	In bottles of 100 and UD 100 scored tablets	$13/30
	2 mg	In bottles of 50, 100, 500, 1,000, and UD 100 tablets	$22/30
	4 mg		$23/90
	6 mg	In bottles of 50, 100 and UD 100 tablets	$23/30
	Elixir: 0.5 mg/5 mL	In 100- and 237-mL bottles	$50/120 mL
	Oral solution: 0.5 mg/5 mL	In 500 mL and UD 5 mL, 20 mL, 237 mL	
	Oral solution concentrate: 1 mg/mL	In 30 mL w/dropper	
Hydrocortisone (Cortef)	Tablet: 5 mg, 10 mg, 20 mg		5 mg = $13/50 10 mg = $38/100 20 mg = $71/100
	Oral suspension: 10 mg/5 mL	In 120 mL	Susp. = No data
(Generic)	Tablets: 10 mg, 20 mg	In bottles of 100 tablets	
Methylprednisolone (Medrol)	Tablets: 2 mg	In bottles of 100 scored tablets	2 mg = $57/100
	4 mg	In bottles of 30, 100, 500 scored tablets	4 mg = $24/21
	8 mg	In bottles of 25 scored tablets	8 mg = $39/25
	16 mg	In bottles of 50 scored tablets	16 mg = $116/50
	24 mg, 32 mg	In bottles of 25 scored tablets	24 mg = No data 32 mg = $87/25
(Generic)	Tablets: 4 mg	In bottles of 21, 100 tablets	
	16 mg	In bottles of 50 tablets	
Prednisolone (Delta-Cortef, Generic)	Tablets: 5 mg	In bottles of 100, 500, 1,000 tablets (Delta-Cortef tablets are scored)	$14/100
(Prelone)	Syrup: 15 mg/5 mL	In 240 mL, 480 mL	$16.40/240 mL
	Syrup: 5 mg/5 mL, 15 mg/5 mL	In 120 mL, 240 mL (cherry flavor)	5 mg/5 mL = $16.40/120 mL
Prednisone (Deltasone)	Tablets: 2.5 mg		
	5 mg	In bottles of 100, 500 and UD 100 and Dosepak 21 scored tablets	
	10 mg	In bottles of 100, 500 and UD 100 scored tablets	
	20 mg	In bottles of 100, 500 and UD 100 scored tablets	
	50 mg	In bottles of 100 scored tablets	

Table 25–8 ◆ **Available Dosage Forms: Selected Corticosteroids—cont'd**

Drug	Dosage Form	How Supplied	Cost
(Liquid Pred)	Syrup: 5 mg/5 mL	In 120, 240 mL	
(Generic)	5 mg	In bottles of 100, 500, 1,000, 5,000 tablets	\$6/100 = 2.5 mg
	10 mg	In bottles of 100, 1,000 tablets	\$6/100 = 5 mg
	20 mg	In bottles of 100, 500, 1,000 tablets	\$9/100 = 10 mg
	50 mg	In bottles of 100 tablets	\$11/100 = 20 mg
	Oral solution: 5 mg/5 mL	In 500 mL	
	Prednisone concentrate: 5mg/mL	In 30 mL	
Triamcinolone (Aristocort)	Tablets: 4 mg (generic)	In bottles of 100, 500 tablets	
	4 mg (Aristocort)	In bottles of 30, 1,000 and Aristo-Pak 16 tablets	
	4 mg (Kenacort)	In bottles of 100 tablets	
	8 mg (Aristocort)	In bottles of 50, scored tablets	
	8 mg (Kenacort)	In bottles of 50 tables	
	Syrup: 4 mg/5 mL (Kenacort)	In 120 mL	
(Kenacort)	Tablets: 8 mg	In bottles of 50 tablets	
	Syrup: 4 mg/5 mL	In 120 mL	
(Generic)	Tablets: 4 mg	In bottles of 100, 500 tablets	

UD = unit dose.
*Injectable forms are not shown on this table. Only oral forms are listed.

that maintains an adequate clinical response is reached. The lowest possible dose is always best, especially with long-term therapy, to avoid or reduce adverse reactions. In the presence of increased stress (e.g., trauma, surgery, or infection), a temporarily increased dosage may be needed.

4. If, after long-term therapy or because of spontaneous remission, the drug is to be stopped, withdraw it gradually to prevent an adrenal insufficiency crisis. Tapering is generally not necessary after short-term therapy (e.g., 1 to 2 wk) because adrenal suppression has not occurred.
5. Most conditions that require chronic **corticosteroid** therapy can be well controlled on alternate-day therapy, although the therapy must usually be started with daily dosing. For alternate-day dosing, twice the daily dose is given every other morning before 9 a.m. It works best if the patient is taking an intermediate-acting drug but may be used with short-acting drugs as well. The purpose of this schedule is to provide the patient on long-term therapy the benefits of the drug while minimizing the HPA-axis suppression, withdrawal symptoms, and for children, growth retardation. Long-acting agents may still produce HPA suppression, even with alternate-day dosing. The regimen is only for patients on long-term therapy who can be trusted to follow this schedule without needing the prompting of daily therapy. In the advent of a flare-up in the disease process, a return to daily dosing may be necessary, at least until the flare-up clears.
6. Unlike a tapering schedule, alternate-day scheduling retains the same total steroid dose. Switching is carried out by gradually increasing the dose on the first day and then decreasing it on the second day until a double dose is taken every other day with no drug on the in-between days. A rough guideline for switching is to make changes in increments of 10 mg of **prednisone** (or its equivalent) when the daily dose is more than 40 mg, and in 5-mg increments when the daily dosage is 20 to 40 mg. Below 20 mg, the change is made in increments of 2.5 mg. The interval between changes varies from 1 day to several weeks and is empirically based on the clinical response.
7. The schedule for tapering and withdrawing is different. The goal is to reduce the drug to physiological levels or to eliminate the drug altogether. For doses above 40 mg, the dose is reduced by 10 mg of **prednisone** (or its equivalent) every 1 to 3 weeks. Doses below 40 mg require reductions of 5 mg every 1 to 3 weeks. Once the physiological dose is reached (5 to 7.5 mg/d), the patient can be switched to 1-mg tablets so that dosage reductions can be continued. Weekly or biweekly reductions can then be done 1 mg at a time.

Rational Drug Selection

Length of Therapeutic Activity

Corticosteroids are classified according to their therapeutic effects into short-, intermediate-, and long-acting forms. Short-acting agents are less likely to produce HPA suppression, especially when taken only in the morning and in low doses on an alternate-day schedule. Long-acting agents are preferred if the effects of high doses must be sustained (e.g., increased intracranial pressure or organ transplant rejection).

Relative Potency

Mineralocorticoid activity is desirable in adrenocortical insufficiency but not if the primary goal of therapy is **anti-inflammatory** or **immunosuppressive**. Drugs with higher relative **mineralocorticoid** potency (RMP) are selected for adrenal insufficiency. Drugs high in relative **anti-inflammatory** potency (RAP) are selected when the goal is to reduce inflammation or suppress the immune system.

Monitoring

Monitoring is based on the common adverse reactions associated with the use of **corticosteroids**: weight gain, edema, hypertension, and indications of excessive potassium loss and negative nitrogen balance associated with protein catabolism. Bone mineral density testing is also appropriate for patients on long-term therapy in which osteoporosis is a significant risk. Carefully monitor the growth and development of children on prolonged therapy.

Laboratory monitoring begins with an initial assessment of serum electrolytes, glucose, and CBC. For patients on long-term therapy or high doses, annual monitoring of these parameters, as well as guaiac testing of stools and serum lipid analysis, is appropriate. For patients at risk for or with indications of GI adverse reactions, upper GI x-rays are desirable.

Systemic corticosteroids may produce subcapsular cataracts in as many as 30 percent of patients, and patients who have or are at risk for increased intraocular pressure (IOP) may experience increases in IOP while on these drugs. A slit-lamp examination is recommended every 6 to 12 months for patients on long-term **corticosteroid** therapy.

Patient Education

Administration

Instruct the patient to take the drug exactly as prescribed. Missed doses should be taken as soon as the patient remembers, unless it is almost time for the next dose. Doses should not be doubled. If the patient is being switched from daily to alternate-day therapy or is on a tapering or withdrawal protocol, make the changes as simple as possible and provide written instructions.

Corticosteroids should not be discontinued or the dosage changed without first consulting the health-care provider. Adrenal insufficiency (anorexia, nausea, weakness, fatigue, dyspnea, hypotension, and hypoglycemia) may result when the drug is stopped suddenly. If these signs appear, then the health-care provider should be notified immediately. Adrenal insufficiency can be life threatening.

In the event of an acute attack during maintenance therapy, the drug should be continued and the health-care provider notified. Dosage or schedule adjustments of the maintenance drugs or the addition of another drug may be necessary. Determining the cause of the exacerbation is important because removal of that cause may be the main treatment.

Adverse Reactions

Corticosteroids cause immunosuppression and may mask symptoms of infection. Instruct the patient to avoid people with known contagious illnesses and to report possible infections immediately. Patients should avoid vaccinations without first consulting their health-care provider.

Review the probable adverse reactions with the patient. Patients should immediately report severe abdominal pain or tarry stools to their health-care provider. They should also report unusual swelling, weight gain, tiredness, bone pain, nonhealing sores, visual disturbances, and behavioral or mood changes.

Discuss possible changes in body image, and explore coping mechanisms for them.

Advise patients to wear medical identification that describes their disease process and drug regimen in the event of a medical emergency that prevents patients from relating their medical history. They should also inform any health-care professional who provides care that they are taking **corticosteroids**.

Lifestyle Management

A diet high in protein, potassium, and calcium and low in sodium and carbohydrates can counteract some of the adverse reactions associated with **corticosteroids. Multivitamins with minerals** are appropriate. Caloric management to prevent obesity should also be implemented. Alcohol should be avoided during therapy. Osteoporosis risk can be reduced not only with calcium intake but also with regular exercise. Because stress can be a source of HPA stimulation, stress management techniques are used.

NONSTEROIDAL ANTI-INFLAMMATORY DRUGS (NSAIDS)

Inflammation, pain, and fever are common manifestations of many diseases. **NSAIDs** offer the advantage of having activity in all three areas, which allows a less complex and less costly regimen. They also reduce the need for **opioid analgesics**, which are associated with chemical dependency and addiction. These advantages have resulted in **NSAIDs** becoming the most widely used prescription and over-the-counter (OTC) drugs in use today.

Aspirin and other **salicylates** that are members of this class are discussed in the next section. **Acetaminophen (Tylenol)**, although not an **anti-inflammatory** drug by chemistry, is often used to treat pain and fever and so is included in this section.

Pharmacodynamics

The inflammatory response is the same, regardless of the injury. Destruction of cell membranes results in release of chemical mediators, including histamine, prostaglandins, leukotrienes, cytokines, oxygen radicals, and enzymes. The cascade of events is depicted in Figure 25–2. Two major enzymes, lipo-oxygenase and cyclo-oxygenase, are required to produce these mediators. Although the exact mode of action of **NSAIDs** is not known, the major mechanism is thought to be inhibition of cyclo-oxygenase activity and prostaglandin synthesis. Inhibition of lipo-oxygenase, leukotriene synthesis, lysosomal enzyme release, neutrophil aggregation, and various cell membrane functions may also occur. These agents may also suppress rheumatoid factor.

Two cyclo-oxygenase isoenzymes have been identified: COX-1 and COX-2. COX-1 is expressed systemically and synthesized continuously so that it is present all the times in all tissues and cells, especially platelets; endothelial cells; the GI tract; and renal microvasculature, glomeruli, and collecting ducts. It has roles in homeostatic maintenance, such as platelet aggregation, the regulation of blood flow to the kidney and stomach, and the regulation of gastric acid secretion and production of protective mucus, especially in the stomach. Inhibition of these activities by **NSAIDs** accounts for their adverse reactions, especially on the renal and GI tracts.

COX-2 is an "inducible" enzyme that is synthesized mainly in response to pain and inflammation. However, there is some synthesis in the kidney, brain, bone, female reproductive system, and GI tract. Nonspecific **NSAIDs** inhibit both COX-1 and COX-2. Most **NSAIDs** (e.g., **aspirin**, **ketoprofen** [Actron, Orudis], **flurbiprofen** (Ansaid), **indomethacin** [Indocin], **piroxicam** [Feldene], **sulindac** [Clinoril]) are mainly COX-1 selective. Some (e.g., **ibuprofen** [Advil, Motrin], **naproxen** [Aleve, Naprosyn], **diclofenac** [Cataflam, Voltaren]) are slightly selective for COX-1, and others (e.g., **etodolac** [Lodine], **nabumetone** [Relafen], **meloxicam** [Mobic]) are slightly selective for COX-2.

Three COX-2 selective drugs (e.g., **celecoxib** [Celebrex], **rofecoxib** [Vioxx], **valdecoxib** [Bextra]) have been developed that appear not to inhibit COX-1. These drugs were used for patients who had higher risks for GI bleeding. However, in 2004, research indicated that the overall risk for GI bleeding was not sufficient to compensate for the increased risk for cardiovascular events that occurred with these drugs. In September 2004, **rofecoxib** was voluntarily removed from the market. In April 2005, the U.S. Food and Drug Administration (FDA) requested that **valdecoxib** be removed from the market. At that time, a black box warning was placed on all **NSAIDs** and on **celecoxib** related to this risk. All OTC **NSAIDs** also had their labeling revised to include more specific information about potential GI and cardiovascular risks. In 2005, the FDA requested that sponsors of all **NSAIDs** and **celecoxib**, both prescription and OTC, add to the labeling a boxed warning about cardiovascular risk events and the well-described, serious, potentially life-threatening GI bleeding associated with their use. In addition, a Medication Guide must now be provided with each prescription.

The **NSAIDs** are primarily used for their **anti-inflammatory** activity, but they are effective **analgesics** useful for the relief of mild to moderate pain. They also have **antipyretic** properties. Because the mechanism of antiplatelet activity is reversible binding to thromboxane, antiplatelet activity exists only while the NSAID is in the blood. For this reason, NSAIDs are not used for **antiplatelet** therapy.

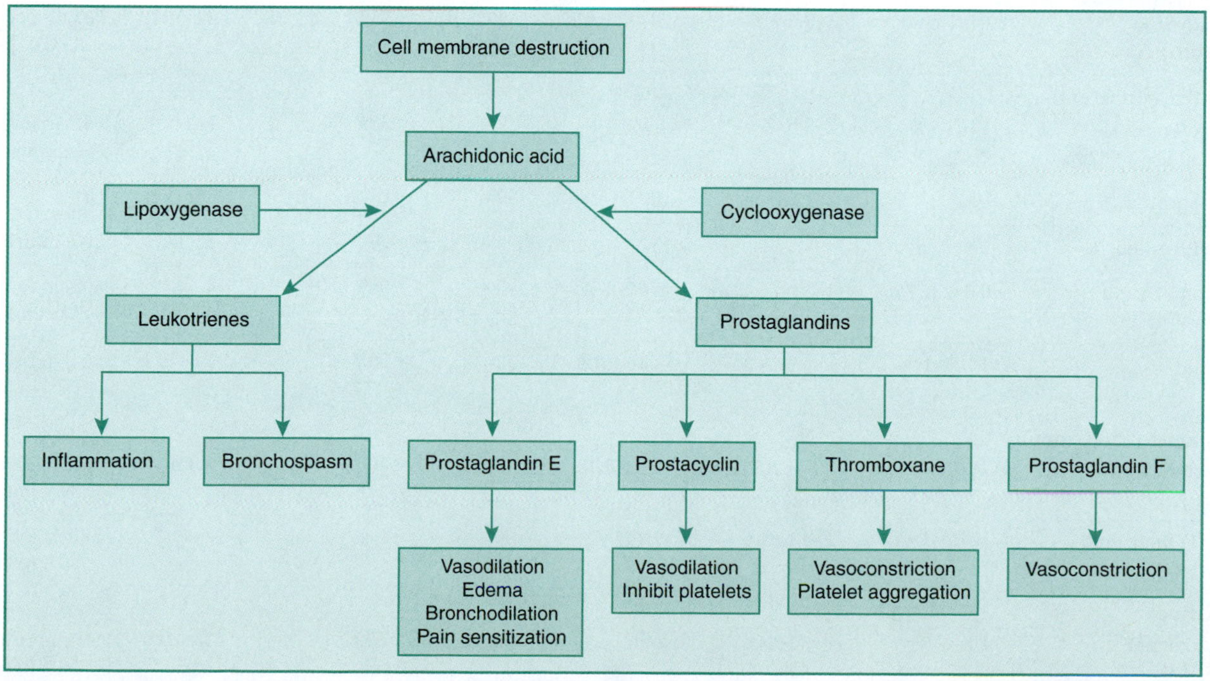

Figure 25–2. Sequence of events in inflammatory response. The sequence of events is the same, regardless of the source of injury.

Acetaminophen is an analgesic and antipyretic with limited anti-inflammatory activity. Although its mechanism of action is not known, it is thought to act by inhibiting central and peripheral prostaglandin synthesis. The central inhibition is almost as potent as that of aspirin, but its peripheral action is minimal. It reduces fever by direct actions on the hypothalamic heat-regulating centers, which increase dissipation of body heat via vasodilation and sweating. It has the advantages of minimal GI irritation and of not affecting bleeding times, uric acid levels, or respiration.

Pharmacokinetics

Absorption and Distribution

After oral administration, NSAIDs are rapidly and almost completely absorbed (Table 25–9). Naproxen sodium (Naprosyn) is more rapidly absorbed than naproxen and is used when rapid analgesia is desired. Diclofenac potassium (Cataflam) is formulated to release the drug in the stomach, whereas the sodium formulation (Voltaren) is released in the higher pH environment of the duodenum. In general, food delays absorption of all NSAIDs but does not affect the total amount absorbed. Administration with food reduces GI adverse reactions. Ketorolac (Toradol) is the only drug in the class with an IM route of absorption.

All NSAIDs are more than 90 percent protein bound. They are widely distributed in tissues, cross the placenta, and enter breast milk in low concentrations.

Acetaminophen is also rapidly and almost completely absorbed after oral administration. Rectal absorption is variable. Serum protein binding is low at therapeutic concentrations but varies from 20 to 50 percent with toxic concentrations. It is relatively uniformly distributed in body tissues, crosses the placenta, and enters breast milk.

Metabolism and Excretion

The NSAIDs are all metabolized by the liver and excreted by the kidney, primarily as metabolites. Sulindac and nabumetone are inactive pro-drugs converted by the liver to active metabolites.

Table 25–9 ▶ **Pharmacokinetics: Selected NSAIDs and Acetaminophen**

Drug	Onset Anal/ AntiR	Peak Anal/ AntiR	Duration Anal/AntiR	Protein Binding	Bioavailability	Half-Life	Elimination
Propionic Acid Group							
Ibuprofen	0.5 h/7 d	1–2 h/1–2 wk	4–6 h/UK	90%–99%	>80%	1.8–2.5 h	45%–79% in urine
Ketoprofen	0.5 h/NA	0.5–2 h/NA	4–8 h/NA	99%	90%	2.1 h	80% in urine
Ketoprofen ER		ER: 6–7 h	ER: 24 h			ER: 5 h	
Naproxen	1 h/14 d	2–4 h/2–4 wk	7–12 h/UK	99%	95%	12–15 h	95% in urine
Naproxen sodium	1 h/14 d	1–2 h/2–4 wk	7–12 h/UK	99%	95%	10–20 h	95% in urine
Oxaprozin	1 h/7 d	3–5 h/UK	24–48 h/UK	>99%	95%	42–50 h	65% in urine; 35% in feces
Acetic Acid Group							
Diclofenac	1 h/1 wk	2–3 h/2 wk	4–8 h/UK	99%	50%–60%	1–2 h	65% in urine (metabolites)
Fenoprofen	UK	2 h	UK	99%	UK	3 h	Urine
Flurbiprofen	UK	1.9 h	UK	99%	UK	7.5 h	70% in urine
Indomethacin	0.5–2 h/7 d	1–2 h /1–2 wk SR: 2–4 h/NA	4–6 h/UK	99% SR: 4.5–6 h	98%	4.5 h	60% in urine; 33% in feces
Sulindac	1 h/7 d	2–4 h/2–3 wk	7–16 h/UK	93–98%	90%	7.8–16 h	50% in urine; 25% in feces
Fenamic Acid Group							
Meclofenamate	1 h/few days	0.5–1 h/2–3 wk	4–6 h/UK	>99%	100%	1.3 h	70% in urine; 30% in feces
Mefenamic acid	Varies/NA	2–4 h/NA	6 h/NA	90%	UK	2–4 h*	52% in urine; 20% in feces
Oxicams							
Meloxicam	UK	4–5 h/NA	24 h	99.4%	89%	15–20 h	50% in urine; 50% in feces

Table 25–9 ▶ **Pharmacokinetics: Selected NSAIDs and Acetaminophen—cont'd**

Drug	Onset Anal/ AntiR	Peak Anal/ AntiR	Duration Anal/AntiR	Protein Binding	Bioavailability	Half-Life	Elimination
Piroxicam	15–30 min/ 7–12 d	3–5 h/2–3 wk	48–72 h/UK	99%	UK	50 h	Minimal amounts unchanged in urine
Naphthylalkanone group							
Nabumetone	1–2 h/1–2 d	5 h/2 wk	24–48 h/UK	99%	>80	22.5–30 h*	80% in urine; 9% in feces
Pyrrolizine carboxylic acid group							
	UK/NA	2–3 h	4–6 h	99%	100%	5–6 h	91% in urine; 6% in feces
Ketorolac	IM: 10 min	IM: 1–2 h	IM: ≥6 h				
Pyranocarboxylic acid group							
Etodolac	0.5h/d	1–2 h/UK	4–12 h/ 6–12 h	>99%	>80	7.3 h	72% in urine; 16% in feces
COX-2 Inhibitor							
Celecoxib	UK	3 h	12–24 h	97.5%	UK	11 h	27% in urine; 57% in feces
Acetaminophen	PO: 0.5–1 h	1–3 h	3–8 h	20%–50%		1–4 h	90–100% in urine (metabolites)
	Rect: 0.5–1 h	1–3 h	3–4 h				

Anal. = analgesic action; AntiR = antirheumatic action; NA = no action; not used for this indication; UK = unknown.
*Prolonged in older adults and impaired renal function.

Acetaminophen is extensively metabolized by the liver and excreted by the kidney primarily as inactive metabolites. When it is taken regularly or in large doses, the stores of one hepatic conjugate (glutathione) become depleted, and hepatic necrosis may occur. Half-life is prolonged in neonates, and severe hepatic dysfunction is related to its dependence on a liver function for metabolism.

Table 25–9 provides pharmacokinetic information on **NSAIDs**, including the one remaining **COX-2 inhibitor**, **celecoxib**, and **acetaminophen**.

Pharmacotherapeutics

Precautions and Contraindications

The only relative contraindications are for **ketorolac**, **mefenamic acid (Ponstel)**, **flurbiprofen**, and **nabumetone** in the presence of preexisting renal impairment. Because **NSAID** metabolites are excreted primarily by the kidneys, all others should be used with caution in the presence of renal function impairment. Renal function should be assessed prior to initiation of therapy and during therapy.

The liver extensively metabolizes **NSAIDs**. **Naproxen** may exhibit an increase in unbound fraction and reduced clearance of free drug in cirrhotic patients. A reduced dose may be necessary. The area under the curve (AUC) of **sulindac** may be increased in patients with cirrhosis because of alterations in sulfide formation and metabolism. In patients treated with a single 15-mg dose of **meloxicam**, there was no marked difference in plasma concentrations in patients with mild to moderate hepatic impairment compared with healthy subjects. Protein binding was also not affected in these patients. Because the effects of hepatic disease on other **NSAIDs** are not known, they should be used cautiously in patients with hepatic impairment.

The liver also extensively metabolizes **acetaminophen**. High doses or long-term use and chronic alcoholism have been associated with hepatotoxicity. Avoid high doses or long-term use. For patients with chronic alcoholism, no safe dose has been determined. It should not be used for these patients.

GI adverse reactions are the most common reasons for cautious use. Serious GI bleeding, ulceration, and perforation can occur at any time without warning symptoms. Studies have not identified any subset of patients not at risk for these problems. A history of serious GI events, alcoholism, and smoking are the only specific factors associated with increased risk. Based on these data, active or chronic inflammation or ulceration of the GI tract relatively contraindicates use of all **NSAIDs**, especially **indomethacin** and **sulindac**. Other **NSAIDs** are sometimes used concurrently with a **cytoprotective agent** such as **sucralfate** (Carafate) or **misoprostol** (Cytotec).

Diclofenac is produced in a combination with **misoprostol** under the brand name **Arthrotec. Cytoprotective agents** are discussed in Chapter 20. Wherever possible, however, these patients should be treated with **nonulcerogenic drugs.**

Indomethacin may aggravate depression or other psychiatric disturbances. A different **NSAID** should be chosen in this situation.

Age appears to increase the risk for adverse reactions to **NSAIDs.** The risk for serious ulcer disease is greater in adults over age 65. This risk appears to be dose-dependent, and reduced dosages may be necessary. **Ketorolac** is cleared more slowly in older adults. **Nabumetone** shows no difference in overall efficacy and safety between older adults and younger patients.

The **NSAIDs** are Pregnancy Category B (**ketoprofen, naproxen, diclofenac, ibuprofen, indomethacin, meclofenamate [Meclomen], piroxicam [Feldene], sulindac**) or Pregnancy Category C (**etodolac [Lodine], flurbiprofen, ketorolac, mefenamic acid, nabumetone, oxaprozin [Daypro]**). There are no adequate and well-controlled studies in pregnant women, so use during pregnancy must be carefully weighed in terms of risks and benefits. Agents that inhibit prostaglandin synthesis may cause closure of the ductus arteriosus and other untoward effects in the fetus. Use in the first trimester is less troublesome; **NSAIDs** should be avoided during the last trimester.

Acetaminophen is Pregnancy Category B. Although it crosses the placenta, it has been routinely used during all stages of pregnancy. At therapeutic doses, it appears safe for short-term use.

Most **NSAIDs** are excreted in breast milk. In studies, **ibuprofen** was not detected in breast milk, **naproxen** was detected at 1 percent of maternal concentration, and **ketorolac** was detected at a maximum milk:plasma ratio of 0.037. In general, nursing mothers should not use **NSAIDs** because of their potential effect on the infant's cardiovascular system. If they are used, **ibuprofen, naproxen,** or **ketorolac** should be selected.

Acetaminophen is excreted in breast milk in low concentrations with reported milk:plasma ratios of 0.91 to 1.42 at 1 and 12 hours, respectively. No adverse effects on nursing infants have been reported.

Mefenamic acid and **meclofenamate** are not recommended for children under age 14 years. Children under age 14 years should not take **indomethacin** except in circumstances that clearly warrant the risk. Closely monitor the liver function of children between ages 2 and 14 years who take it. Cases of hepatotoxicity, including fatalities, have been reported in children with juvenile rheumatoid arthritis. **Flurbiprofen** is not approved for use in children. Other **NSAIDs** may be used to treat children, and pediatric doses are published for these drugs. **Acetaminophen** is also safe for infants and children.

Adverse Drug Reactions

The most common adverse reactions with **NSAIDs** are GI disturbances, in particular nausea, vomiting, constipation, and diarrhea. Taking the drug with food can reduce these reactions. GI bleeding and ulceration were discussed in the Precautions and Contraindications section and in the Pharmacodynamics section.

Acute renal insufficiency has occurred in patients with preexisting renal disease or compromised renal perfusion. Patients at greatest risk are older adults, premature infants, those taking diuretics, and those with heart failure, systemic lupus erythematosus, or chronic glomerulonephritis. Stopping the drug usually brings recovery. Interstitial nephritis has occurred with increasing frequency in patients who take **NSAIDs,** and it may be due to altered prostaglandin metabolism.

Hematological effects are less common but can be related to the actions of the drugs. **NSAIDs** inhibit platelet aggregation and may increase bleeding time. Decreased hemoglobin and hematocrit levels have occurred rarely. Patients with initial values below 10 g/dL who are to receive long-term therapy should have these values regularly monitored.

Fluid retention and peripheral edema are not severe but can be problematic for patients with compromised cardiovascular function. Patients with severe heart failure may have significant deterioration in hemodynamic function, presumably related to inhibition of prostaglandin-dependent compensatory mechanisms.

Cholestatic hepatitis, jaundice, and abnormal liver function tests have occurred rarely. Pancreatitis has developed in patients who take **sulindac.**

Adverse reactions associated with **acetaminophen** are few; however, those that do exist are significant. Acute hepatic necrosis occurs with doses of 10 to 15 g. Doses above 25 g are usually fatal. Children appear less susceptible to toxicity than adults because they have less capacity for glucuronidation, the metabolic pathway for **acetaminophen.** Acute poisoning is manifested by nausea, vomiting, drowsiness, confusion, liver tenderness, and renal failure, which occur within the first 24 hours and may persist for more than 1 week. Acute renal failure may also occur.

Acetaminophen Poisoning

Acetaminophen is a common cause of poisoning, either intentional or accidental due to the lay public underestimating the toxicity of the drug. A single dose of 150 mg/kg in children or 7.5 gm to 10 gm of **acetaminophen** may be toxic. Drugs that induce CYP2E1 enzymes (**carbamazepine, phenobarbitol, phenytoin, isoniazid,** and **rifampin**) may cause hepatotoxicity when combined with **acetaminophen.** The course of **acetaminophen** poisoning is divided into four stages:

1. 0.5 to 24 hours: Nausea, vomiting, diaphoresis, pallor, and anorexia. Some patients may be asymptomatic initially.
2. 24 to 72 hours: Clinically improved; aspartate transaminase (AST), alanine transaminase (ALT), bilirubin, and prothrombin levels begin to rise.
3. 72 to 96 hours: Peak hepatotoxicity; jaundice, confusion, AST of 10,000 not unusual.

4. 4 to 14 days: Death or recovery. Patients who survive enter a recovery phase.

Acute acetaminophen poisoning should be referred to a poison control center hospital. If this is not possible, the following treatment regimen may be followed. If the acute ingestion is more than 150 mg/kg or the dose cannot be determined, obtain a serum **acetaminophen** assay 4 hours after ingestion. If the level is more than 300 mg/mL, hepatic damage has occurred in 90 percent of patients. Minimum hepatic damage results from a level below 120 mg/mL. Treatment is by gastric lavage in all cases, preferably within 4 hours of ingestion. Oral ***N*-acetylcysteine** is a specific antidote for **acetaminophen** toxicity. Contact a poison control center for correct dosing of the antidote.

Anemia, neutropenia, pancytopenia, and thrombocytopenia also occur but are not severe. The skin eruptions and urticarial skin reactions that may develop are also transient and not severe.

Drug Interactions

Both **NSAIDs** and **acetaminophen** have many drug interactions. **NSAIDs** decrease the effectiveness of **antihypertensive drugs** because of their tendency to cause fluid retention and increased extracellular fluid volume. Coadministration with **anticoagulants** may prolong prothrombin time because both drugs affect platelet aggregation. Drugs that have adverse reactions associated with increased risk for GI bleeding or ulceration have an even higher risk if taken with **NSAIDs**. Drugs that require glucuronidation for metabolism may affect the metabolism of **acetaminophen** by competing for metabolic sites. These and other interactions are listed in Table 25–10.

Table 25–10 ■ **Drug Interactions: Selected NSAIDs and Acetaminophen**

Drug	Interacting Drug	Possible Effect	Implications
Acetaminophen	Alcohol	Increased risk for hepatotoxicity	Avoid alcohol intake
	Anticholinergics	Delayed onset of action of acetaminophen; ultimate pharmacological effects not altered	No action required
	Beta-adrenergic blockers	Propranolol inhibits the enzyme systems responsible for glucuronidation and oxidation of acetaminophen, resulting in increased pharmacological effects	Select different beta adrenergic blocker
	Contraceptives, oral	Increased glucuronidation, resulting in increased plasma clearance and decreased half-life of acetaminophen	Select NSAID for treatment if long-term therapy; not a problem with single dose
	Probenecid	Increases the therapeutic effectiveness of acetaminophen	Used therapeutically
	Loop diuretics	Decreased effectiveness of diuretic because acetaminophen may decrease renal prostaglandin excretion and decrease plasma renin activity	Avoid concurrent use
	Zidovudine	Decreased pharmacological effects of zidovudine related to enhanced nonhepatic or renal clearance of zidovudine	Avoid concurrent use; select NSAID for long-term use
All NSAIDs	Anticoagulants	May prolong prothrombin time (PT)	Avoid coadministration; monitor PT and patients closely; instruct patients to watch for indications of bleeding
	Beta adrenergic blockers	Antihypertensive effect impaired; sulindac and naproxen do not affect atenolol	Select appropriate drug match
	Hydantoins	Serum levels of phenytoin increased, resulting in increased pharmacological and toxic effects of phenytoin	If they must be used together, monitor serum levels and adjust dose accordingly
	Lithium	Serum lithium levels increased; sulindac has no effect or decreases levels	Avoid concurrent use or select sulindac; monitor serum levels
	Loop diuretics	Decreased effects of loop diuretics	Avoid concurrent use for long-term therapy or select different diuretic
	Probenecid	Probenecid may increase concentrations and toxicity risk of NSAIDs	Avoid concurrent use
	Salicylates	Decreased plasma concentrations of NSAIDs	Avoid concurrent use; offers no therapeutic advantage and significantly increases incidence of GI adverse reactions

Continued

Table 25–10 ■ **Drug Interactions: Selected NSAIDs and Acetaminophen—cont'd**

Drug	Interacting Drug	Possible Effect	Implications
Indomethacin	Digoxin	May decrease digoxin serum levels; ibuprofen has similar effect	Select different NSAID
	Phenylpropanolamine	Increased blood pressure	Avoid coadministration
	Dipyridamole	Additive fluid retention	Select different NSAID
Indomethacin, naproxen	Thiazide diuretics	Decreased antihypertensive and diuretic action; sulindac may enhance effects	Avoid concurrent use; select sulindac if enhanced effect is desired

Clinical Use and Dosing

Rheumatoid Arthritis

The ultimate goals in managing RA are to prevent and control joint damage, prevent loss of function, and decrease pain. **NSAIDs**, **glucocorticoid** joint injection, and/or low-dose **prednisone** may be used for control of symptoms (American College of Rheumatology, 2002 update.) The initial drug treatment involves the use of **salicylates**, **NSAIDs**, or **celecoxib** to reduce joint pain and swelling and to improve joint function. They have analgesic and anti-inflammatory properties but do not alter the course of the disease or prevent joint destruction, so they should not used as the sole treatment for RA. Although most **NSAIDs** have been used for this indication, no one NSAID has demonstrated a clear advantage for the treatment of RA (*Drug Facts and Comparisons,* 2010). Only **ketorolac** and **mefenamic acid** do not have a labeled indication for treatment of RA. Doses of the drugs with this indication are presented in Table 25–11. These drugs do not significantly differ in their efficacy. Choice is determined by adverse reactions, cost, duration of action, and patient preference. For women of childbearing age, Pregnancy Category may affect choice. **Nabumetone**, **piroxicam**, and **oxaprozin** have longer durations of action than the other drugs commonly used. **Ibuprofen** is

Table 25–11 ● **Dosage Schedule: Selected NSAIDs and Acetaminophen**

Drug	Indication	Dosage Schedule	Comments
Acetaminophen	Mild to moderate pain and/or fever	***Oral Doses***	Not to exceed 4 g/d
		Adults and children >14 yr: 325–650 mg every 4–6 h *or* 1 g tid or qid	For all ages of children, doses not to exceed 5 doses in 24 h
		Children 10 to 15 mg/kg/dose every 4 h	Max dose 650 mg/dose
		Suppositories	Not to exceed 4 g/d
		Adults and children >12 yr: 650 mg every 4–6 h	Not to exceed 720 mg/d
		Children 3–11 mo: 80 mg up to every 6 h	Not to exceed 2.6 g/d
		Children 1–3 yr: 80 mg up to every 4 h	Not to exceed 4 g/d
		Children 3–6 yr: 120–125 every 4–6 h	
		Children 6–12 yr: 325 mg every 4–6 h	
	Osteoarthritis	*Adults:* Up to 1 g qid	
Etodolac	Osteoarthritis, rheumatoid arthritis	*Adults:* 800–1,200 mg/d in divided doses, followed by dosage adjustments within the range of 600–1,200 mg/d in divided doses	Not to exceed 1,200 mg/d; for patients ≤60 kg, do not exceed 20 mg/kg
	Analgesia	*Adults:* 200–400 mg every 6–8 h as needed	Not to exceed 1,200 mg/d; for patients ≤60 kg, do not exceed 20 mg/kg
Diclofenac	Rheumatoid arthritis	*Adults:* 100–200 mg/d in divided doses (50 mg tid–qid or 75 mg bid)	Doses above 225 mg/d not recommended
		Chronic therapy with extended-release tablets: 100 mg/d	
	Osteoarthritis	*Adults:* 100–200 mg/d in divided doses (50 mg bid–tid or 75 mg bid)	Doses above 200 mg/d are not recommended
		Chronic therapy with extended-release tablets: 100 mg/d	

Table 25–11 ● **Dosage Schedule: Selected NSAIDs and Acetaminophen—cont'd**

Drug	Indication	Dosage Schedule	Comments
	Ankylosing spondylitis	*Adults:* 100–125 mg/d delayed-release tablets (25 mg qid with an extra dose at bedtime if needed)	Doses above 125 mg not recommended
	Analgesia, primary dysmenorrhea	*Adults:* 50 mg tid; some patients may need 100 mg tid initially, followed by 50 mg tid	After first day, maximum dose 200 mg; doses generally should not exceed 150 mg
Fenoprofen	Rheumatoid arthritis, osteoarthritis	*Adults:* 300–600 mg 3 to 4 times a day	Not approved for use in children <18 years.
	Mild-to-moderate pain	*Adults:* 200 mg q4 to 6 hr	Not recommended in patients with advanced renal disease
Flurbiprofen	Rheumatoid arthritis, osteoarthritis	*Adults:* 200–300 mg/ day in 2, 3 or 4 divided doses. Maximum of 100 mg in a single dose	Not approved for use in children <18 years.
Ibuprofen	Rheumatoid arthritis, osteoarthritis	*Adults*: 1.2–3.2 g/d (300 mg qid or 400, 600, or 800 mg tid–qid)	Not to exceed 3.2 g/d; higher doses usually needed for rheumatoid arthritis
	Juvenile arthritis	*Children:* 30–70 mg/kg/d in 3–4 divided doses; 20 mg/kg/d may be adequate in milder disease	
	Acute gouty arthritis	*Adults:* 800 mg qid; taper to eliminate as soon as pain is relieved	Not to exceed 3.2 g/d
	Mild to moderate pain	*Adults:* 400 mg every 4–6 h as needed	Not to exceed 1,200 mg/d
	Muscle sprain, strain (anti-inflammatory, analgesic)	*Adults:* 600 mg qid or 800 mg tid for 5 d	Not to exceed 3,600 mg/d
		Children: 20–40 mg/kg/d in divided doses	Not to exceed 50 mg/kg/d
	Primary dysmenorrhea	*Children* >12 yr and adults: 400 mg every 4 h as needed	Not to exceed 1,200 mg/d
	Fever reduction	*Adults:* 200–400 mg every 4–6 h	Not to exceed 1,200 mg/d
		Children 6 mo–12 yr: 5 mg/kg for temperature <39.1°C (102.5°F) or 10 mg/kg for higher temperatures; may be repeated every 4–6 h	Not to exceed 40 mg/kg/d
	OTC use for pain and/or fever	*Adults:* 200 mg every 4–6 h while symptoms persist; if response is not adequate, may use 400 mg	Not to exceed 1,200 mg/d; do not take for >10 d for pain or >3 d for fever
		Children ≥ 6 mo: 5 mg to 10 mg every 6 to 8 hr	Do not administer to children <6 mo
Indomethacin	Moderate to severe rheumatoid arthritis, ankylosing spondylitis, and osteoarthritis	*Children >14 yr and adults:* 25 mg bid–tid initially; increase dose by 25–50 mg at weekly intervals until satisfactory response Sustained release: 75 mg can be taken daily as alternative to 25 mg tid or bid as alternative to 50 mg tid	Not to exceed 200 mg/d; for patients with persistent night pain or morning stiffness, give larger portion of dose at bedtime (up to 100 mg)
	Acute gouty arthritis	*Adults:* 25 to 50 mg qid; taper to eliminate as soon as pain is relieved	Not to exceed 200 mg/d
	Acute painful shoulder (bursitis or tendinitis)	*Children >14 yr and adults:* 75–100 mg/d in 3–4 divided doses for 7–14 d	
	Acute gouty arthritis	*Adults:* 50 mg tid; taper to eliminate drug as soon as pain is relieved	Do not use sustained-release form

Continued

Table 25–11 ◉ **Dosage Schedule: Selected NSAIDs and Acetaminophen—cont'd**

Drug	Indication	Dosage Schedule	Comments
Ketoprofen	Rheumatoid arthritis, osteoarthritis	*Adults:* 75 mg tid *or* 50 mg qid initially Maintenance dose is 150–300 mg/d in 3–4 divided doses Extended release: 200 mg once daily	Reduce dose by 1/2–1/3 for older adults and those with renal impairment; not to exceed 300 mg/d
	Acute gouty arthritis	*Adults:* 75 mg qid; taper to eliminate as soon as pain is relieved	Not to exceed 300 mg/d
	Mild to moderate pain, primary dysmenorrhea	*Adults:* 25–50 mg every 6–8 h as needed	Doses >50 mg have not increased efficacy; not to exceed 300 mg/d
	OTC use for pain	*Children >16 yr and adults:* 12.5 mg with full glass of liquid every 4–6 h; if pain or fever persists after 1 h, follow with 12.5 mg	Not to exceed 25 mg in a 4–6 h period or 75 mg/24 h
Ketorolac	Acute, moderately severe pain	*Adults <65 yr:* 60 mg IM single dose or 30 mg every 6 h (not to exceed 120 mg/d); then 20 mg PO initially, followed by 10 mg every 4–6 h as needed (not to exceed 40 mg/d) *Adults >65 yr or <50 kg or with renal impairment:* 30 mg IM single dose or 15 mg every 6 h (not to exceed 60 mg/d); then 10 mg PO every 4–6 h as needed (not to exceed 40 mg/d)	Not intended for >5 d combined IM and PO, or for minor or chronic pain; oral therapy is intended only as continuation from IM therapy
Meclofenamate	Rheumatoid arthritis, osteoarthritis	*Adults:* 200–400 mg/d in 3–4 equally divided doses	Not to exceed 400 mg/d
	Mild to moderate pain	*Children >14 yr and adults:* 50–100 mg every 4–6 h	Not to exceed 400 mg/d
	Excessive menstrual bleeding, dysmenorrhea	*Children >14 yr and adults:* 100 mg tid for up to 6 d, starting with first day of menstrual flow	Not to exceed 400 mg/d
Mefenamic acid	Acute pain	*Children >14 yr and adults:* 500 mg, then 250 mg every 6 h as needed	Not to exceed 1 wk
	Primary dysmenorrhea	*Children >14 yr and adults:* 500 mg, then 250 mg every 6 h as needed starting at onset of bleeding or symptoms	Should not be necessary for more than 2–3 d
Nabumetone	Rheumatoid arthritis, osteoarthritis	*Adults:* 1,000 mg daily; may increase to 1,500–2,000 mg/d	Not to exceed 2,000 mg/d
Naproxen	Rheumatoid arthritis, osteoarthritis, ankylosing spondylitis	*Adults:* 250–500 mg bid; may increase to 1.5 g/d for limited periods Delayed release: 375–500 mg bid Controlled release: 750–1,000 mg once daily Naproxen sodium: 275–550 mg bid; may increase to 1.65 mg for limited periods	Morning and evening doses do not need to be equal; more than twice-daily dosing does not improve efficacy
	Juvenile arthritis	*Children:* 10 mg/kg/d in 2 divided doses Suspension: 13-kg child = 2.5 mL bid; 25-kg child = 5 mL; 38-kg child = 7.5 mL	
	Acute gouty arthritis	*Adults:* 500 mg bid; taper to eliminate as soon as pain is relieved Controlled release: Same Naproxen sodium: Same	Not to exceed 1 g/d
	Acute gout	*Adults:* 750 mg, then 250 mg every 8 h until attack subsides Controlled release: 1,000–1,500 mg once daily on first day, then 1,000 mg once daily until the attack subsides Naproxen sodium: 825 mg, then 275 mg every 8 h until attack subsides	
	Mild to moderate pain, dysmenorrhea, acute tendinitis or bursitis	*Adults:* 500 mg, then 250 mg every 6–8 h as needed Controlled release: 1,000 mg once daily; 1,500 mg/d may be used for limited period	Not to exceed 1.25 g/d

Table 25–11 ● **Dosage Schedule: Selected NSAIDs and Acetaminophen—cont'd**

Drug	Indication	Dosage Schedule	Comments
		Naproxen sodium: 550 mg, then 275 mg every 6–8 h as needed *Children:* Naproxen suspension, 5 mg/kg/d in 2 divided doses	Not to exceed 1.375 g/d
	OTC use for pain	*Adults:* 200 mg with full glass of liquid every 8–12 h while symptoms persist; dose of 400 mg initially, then 200-mg doses, may be necessary *Adults >65 yr:* Do not take >200 mg every 12 h *Children:* Do not give to children <12 yr, except under advice/supervision of HCP	Not to exceed 600 mg/d
Oxaprozin	Rheumatoid arthritis, osteoarthritis	*Adults:* 1,200 mg once daily; patients with low body weight or milder disease may use 600 mg once daily	Not to exceed 1,800 mg/d or 26 mg/kg, whichever is lower; doses >1,200 mg/d should be divided
Piroxicam	Rheumatoid arthritis, osteoarthritis	*Adults:* 20 mg once daily; may divide dose *Adults >65 yr:* 10 mg once daily initially	
	Dysmenorrhea	*Adults:* 40 mg first day, then 20 mg/d	
Sulindac	Rheumatoid arthritis, osteoarthritis, ankylosing spondylitis	*Adults:* 150 mg bid	
	Acute gout, painful shoulder (tendinitis, bursitis)	*Adults:* 200 mg bid	Therapy usually not longer than 7 d

HCP = health-care provider; OTC = over the counter.

the least expensive and is available OTC. **Diclofenac** comes in a combination with a **cytoprotective agent (misoprostol)** to reduce the risk for GI bleeding and ulceration, but this combination is quite expensive.

Patients with RA are nearly twice as likely as patients with osteoarthritis (OA) to have a serious complication with **NSAID** treatment. Risk factors for the development of **NSAID**-associated gastroduodenal ulcers include advanced age (older than 75 years), history of ulcer, concomitant use of **glucocorticoids** or **anticoagulants**, higher doses of **NSAIDs**, use of multiple **NSAIDs**, or a serious underlying disease (American College of Rheumatology, 2002 update). Age appears to be less of a risk for adverse reactions with **nabumetone**, which shows no difference in overall efficacy and safety between older adults and younger patients. The American College of Rheumatology suggests the following approaches for patients with RA who would benefit from an **NSAID** but are at increased risk of serious adverse GI effects:

- Use low-dose **prednisone** instead of an **NSAID**.
- Use a **nonacetylated salicylate** (see later).
- Use **celecoxib**.
- Use a combination of an **NSAID** and a **cytoprotective agent**. **Gastroprotective agents**, which are effective, include high-dose **H_2 blockers**, **proton pump inhibitors**, and **oral prostaglandin analogues (misoprostol)**.
- If antiplatelet therapy is indicated (e.g., as risk reduction for cardiovascular disease), low-dose **aspirin** (75 to 160 mg/d) should be used.

If a good clinical response occurs without signs of inflammation, the treatment regimen is continued. More advanced disease or patients with partial or poor response to **NSAIDs** require a change of drug therapy.

Osteoarthritis

OA is the most common form of arthritis in the United States. Patients have joint pain that typically worsens with weight-bearing and activity and improves with rest as well as stiffness and swelling of the involved joint after periods of inactivity. Although there is no known cure for OA, treatment can help to maintain or improve joint mobility and limit functional impairment. With OA, nonpharmacological modalities are as important as drug therapy. They include weight loss; aerobic, range-of-motion, and muscle-strengthening exercises; appropriate footwear; and assistive devices for ambulation and activities of daily living when necessary. Drug therapy includes **acetaminophen**, **NSAIDs**, and **COX 2 inhibitors**. Topical agents such as **capsaicin** and **methyl salicylate** may also be used (American Academy of Orthopedic Surgeons, 2008; American College of Rheumatology, 2000).

The patient's pain, disability, and comorbidities provide the guidelines for management of OA. Initially, **acetaminophen** in doses up to 1 g four times a day are given to manage joint pain. Daily doses should not exceed 4 g. Although it is analgesic, there is little evidence that **acetaminophen** provides any benefit when peripheral inflammation is a causative factor for the pain (Simon et al, 2002). If this drug fails to control pain, **NSAIDs** are prescribed (American Academy of Orthopedic Surgeons, 2008; American College of Rheumatology, 2000; Simon et al, 2002). For many patients with OA, the relief of mild to moderate joint pain is comparable with both **acetaminophen** and **NSAIDs**; however, with severe pain, studies have shown **NSAIDs** to be more effective (American College of Rheumatology, 2000). Although **NSAIDs** have both **analgesic** and **anti-inflammatory** actions, they do not alter the course of the disease or prevent joint destruction. All **NSAIDs** except **ketorolac** and **mefenamic acid** have an indication for treatment of OA. Doses are presented in Table 25–11. As in RA, the choice of **NSAID** to be used is determined by adverse reactions, cost, duration of action, and patient preference. There is no significant difference in efficacy, and patient response is variable. For patients who experience adverse effects on the GI tract, adjunctive administration of H_2 **blockers** or **cytoprotective agents** may be needed. Both of these drug classes are discussed in Chapter 20.

The use of both **glucosamine** (1,500 mg daily) and **chondroitin** (1,200 mg daily) for joint pain due to knee OA is a common practice among patients who are self-prescribing for OA. The evidence on the use of **glucosamine** and **chondroitin** does not consistently show improvement in pain; therefore, the Agency for Healthcare Research and Quality (AHRQ) clinical guidelines do not recommend either for knee arthritis (2009). Because these two agents are available OTC and encouraged in many health food establishments, providers should ask the patient about their use and effectiveness for that patient.

Gout

NSAIDs have largely replaced **colchicines** for management of acute episodes of gouty arthritis. **Indomethacin**, **naproxen**, and **sulindac** have acute gout listed as an indication. **Ibuprofen** and **ketoprofen** have also been used. Table 25–11 provides dosage schedules for these five drugs.

Mild to Moderate Pain

Almost every individual at some time experiences an episode of mild to moderate pain. Regardless of the source of the pain, **nonopioid analgesia** is the primary choice for management, especially if inflammation accompanies or is the cause of the pain. Although any NSAID may be used for this indication, several have been routinely used and proved effective. **Ibuprofen** is the most commonly used because it is inexpensive, available OTC, and short acting so that acute pain can be managed without long-term effects and adverse reactions. For women of childbearing age, it is Pregnancy Category B, and for nursing women it is not detected in breast milk. **Naproxen sodium** is used as an **analgesic** because it reaches its peak more rapidly. Other drugs used for this indication include **ketoprofen**, **ketorolac**, **meclofenamate**, and **mefenamic acid**. When an injectable NSAID is needed, only **ketorolac** has such a formulation.

As with other indications, there is no clear difference in efficacy. Taking the drug around the clock, rather than as necessary, is most effective. Choice is based on adverse reactions, cost, duration of action, and patient preference. Health-care providers often choose one short-acting drug (**ibuprofen**, **diclofenac**, **ketoprofen**, **ketorolac**, **meclofenamate**), an intermediate-acting one (**naproxen**), and a long-acting drug (**ketoprofen ER**) and use the same drugs repeatedly. Experience with a limited number of drugs provides more clinical knowledge, and there is no clear benefit to using more than a few. Because different patients seem to respond better to different **NSAIDs**, if one drug does not produce the desired effect, another one can be tried.

Acetaminophen is useful in treating mild to moderate pain that is not accompanied by or caused by inflammation. It is not intended for pain management for more than 5 days in children or 10 days in adults because of the increased risk for hepatic adverse reactions. For adults, a dose of 325 to 650 mg every 4 to 6 hours usually suffices. Children's doses are based on weight; 10 to 15 mg/kg per dose every 4 to 6 hours. After age 14 years, the adult dose is used. These doses are shown in Table 25–11.

Primary Dysmenorrhea

Ibuprofen, **diclofenac potassium**, **ketoprofen**, **meclofenamate**, **mefenamic acid**, and **naproxen** are the drugs used for this indication. Doses are shown in Table 25–11.

Tendinitis and Bursitis

Indomethacin SR, **naproxen**, and **sulindac** are used for this indication. **Naproxen** and **sulindac** both are intermediate acting and provide longer duration of action than **indomethacin**, even in its sustained-release form. They also have fewer drug interactions. **Naproxen** is less likely to produce GI adverse reactions. These same three drugs are used to manage the pain in gout because it is associated with inflammation. Treatment choices are determined on the same basis.

Fever

Ibuprofen is the NSAID of choice for fever for children over age 6 months and adults. Doses are published for both adults and children. **Acetaminophen** may also be used for this purpose, but not for longer than 3 days. It is best used in those patients with **aspirin** allergy; blood coagulation disorders; upper GI disease; and the fever that accompanies the common cold, flu, and other viral illnesses in children. Patients should be well hydrated if using **ibuprofen** for fever to decrease renal toxicity.

Rational Drug Selection

There is no clear difference in efficacy between NSAIDs. The rationale for choices is provided in the Clinical Use and Dosing section. Acetaminophen is used only for fever and for mild to moderate pain not associated with inflammation.

Monitoring

Monitoring is required only for long-term therapy. Because these drugs may produce acute renal insufficiency, assess renal function (serum creatinine) before initiation of therapy and annually throughout long-term therapy. A CBC prior to initiation of therapy and annually thereafter is appropriate because of the risk for GI bleeding. Any other monitoring is related to the disease being treated.

Patient Education

Administration

Take the drug exactly as prescribed (Table 25–12). A missed dose should be taken as soon as the patient remembers unless it is almost time for the next dose. For drugs taken more than once daily, ideally take the missed dose within 1 to 2 hours of the time it was scheduled. Do not double doses. Taking higher doses than those prescribed does not increase efficacy and may increase adverse reactions.

Table 25–12 ◆ Available Dosage Forms: Selected NSAIDs and Acetaminophen

Drug	Dosage Form	How Supplied	Cost
Acetaminophen (Tylenol)	Tablets: 325 mg, 500 mg 500 mg extra strength	In bottles of 10, 24, 50, 100, 200 tablets In bottles of 100 tablets	325 mg = $8.99/100 500 mg = $9.99/100
	Chewable tablets: 80 mg	In bottles of 30, 48, 96 bubble gum and cherry-flavored chewable tablets	80 mg chew = $4.99/30
	160 mg	In bottles of 24 grape- and fruit-flavored chewable tablets	160 mg chew = $6.29/24
	Caplets: 325 mg	In bottles of 24, 50, 100 caplets	
	650 mg extended relief	In bottles of 100 caplets	
	Gelcaps: 500 mg extra strength	In bottles of 24, 50, 100 gelcaps	$13.99/100
	Elixir: 160 mg/5 mL	In 60 and 120 mL (grape and cherry flavors)	
	Liquid: 500 mg/15 mL	In 240 mL; with dosing cup	$160 mg/5 mL liquid = 6.99/100 mL
	Infant drops: 100 mg/mL	In 7.5, 30 mL; with 0.8-mL dropper	
Generic	Tablets: 325 mg	In bottles of 50, 100, 1,000 tablets	325 mg = $4.99/100
	500 mg	In bottles of 100, 1,000 tablets	500 mg = $7.29/100
	650 mg	In bottles of 1,000 tablets	
	Chewable tablets: 80 mg	In bottles of 30, 100 chewable tablets	80 mg chew = $1.75/30
	500 mg	In bottles of 50, 100, 1,000 capsules	160 mg chew = $3.99/24
	Elixir: 160 mg/5 mL	In 118 and 120 mL, pint and gallon	
	Liquid: 160 mg/5 mL	In 120 and 500 mL	$3.49/120 mL
	500 mg/15 mL	In 237 mL	
	Solution: 100 mg/mL	In 15 mL	$5.99/30 mL
	Suppository: 120 mg, 300 mg, 325 mg, 650 mg	In 12 individually foil-wrapped suppositories	120 mg supp = $6.49/6 325 mg supp = $$8.29/6
Celecoxib (Celebrex)	Capsules: 100 mg, 200 mg, 400 mg	In bottles of 100, 500 and UD 100 capsules	100 mg = $277/100 200 mg = $449/100 400 mg = $668/100
Diclofenac (Voltaren)	Tablets: 25 mg, 50 mg, 75 mg	In bottles of 60, 100 tablets In bottles of 60, 100, 1,000 tablets	75 mg = $211/60
	Extended release: 100 mg	In bottles of 100 tablets	$635/90
(Cataflam)	Tablets: 50 mg	In bottles of 100 and UD 100 tablets	$396/100
(Generic)	Delayed release: 25 mg, 50 mg, 75 mg	In bottles of 60, 100, 1,000 tablets	50 mg = $66/100
Fenoprofen (Nalfon)	Capsules: 200 mg	100	$87/100
(Generic)	Tablets: 600 mg	30, 90, 100	$89/100
Flurbiprofen (Ansaid)			
(Generic)	Tablets: 50 mg, 100 mg	100	50 mg = $29/100 100 mg = $37/100

Continued

Table 25–12 ◆ **Available Dosage Forms: Selected NSAIDs and Acetaminophen—cont'd**

Drug	Dosage Form	How Supplied	Cost
Etodolac (Lodine)	Tablets: 400 mg, 500 mg	In 100 and UD 100 tablets	
	Tablets, extended release: 400 mg, 500 mg, 600 mg	In bottles of 100 and UD 100 tablets	400 mg = $147/100 500 mg = $153/100
	Capsules: 200 mg, 300 mg	In bottles of 100 and UD 100 tablets	200 mg = $134/100 300 mg = $151/100
(Generic)	Tablets: 400 mg and 500 mg	In bottles of 100, 500, 1,000 tablets	400 mg = $65/100 500 mg = $126/100
	Tablets, extended release: 400 mg 500 mg and 600 mg	In bottles of 100, 500 tablets In bottles of 100 tablets	400 mg = $94/90 500 mg = $98/90 600 mg = $180/90
	Capsules: 200 mg and 300 mg	In bottles of 100, 500, 1,000 capsules	200 mg = $37/100 300 mg = $53/100
Ibuprofen (Advil)	Tablets: 200 mg	In bottles of 4, 8, 24, 50, 100, 165, 250 tablets	200 mg tables = $9.99/100
	Caplets: 200 mg	In bottles of 24, 50, 100, 154, 250 caplets	200 mg caplets = $9.99/100
	Suspension: 100 mg/5mL	In 119 and 473 mL (fruit flavor)	100 mg/5 mL = $7.99/120 mL
	Pediatric drops: 100 mg/5mL	In 7.5 mL	50 mg/1.25 mL = $6.49/ 15 mL
	Children's tablets, chewable: 50 mg	In bottles of 24 and 50 tablets (fruit and grape flavor)	
	Junior strength tablets, chewable: 100 mg	In bottles of 24 tablets (fruit and grape flavor)	
	Liqui-gel capsules: 200 mg	In packets of 4, and bottles of 20, 40, 80 capsules	200 mg Liqui-gel = $15.79/120
(Motrin)	Tablets: 100 mg	In 100 scored, film-coated tablets	100 mg = $12.49/100
	200 mg	In bottles of 24, 50, 100, 130, 165	200 mg = $9.99/100
	300 mg, 500 mg, 600 mg, 800 mg	In bottles of 500 tablets	
	Junior strength tablets: 100 mg	In bottles of 24 tablets	
	Chewable tablets: 50 mg, 100 mg	In bottles of 100 citrus-flavored chewable tablets	
	Gelcaps: 200 mg	In bottles of 24, 50 gelcaps	
	Suspension: 100 mg/5 mL	In 60, 120, 480 mL (berry flavor)	
	Oral drops: 40 mg/mL	In 15 mL (berry flavor)	
(Generic)	Tablets: 200 mg	In bottles of 50, 100, 500 tablets	
	400 mg, 600 mg	In bottles of 50, 100, 250 tablets	
	800 mg	In bottles of 12, 15, 21, 30, 40, 50, 60, 100, 360, 500 tablets	
	Suspension: 100 mg/5 mL	In 118 mL	
Indomethacin (Indocin)	Capsules: 25 mg	In bottles of 100, 1,000 capsules	25 mg = $29/100
	50 mg	In bottles of 100 capsules	50 mg = $32/100
	Sustained release: 75 mg	In 60s	75 mg = $208/90
	Suspension: 25 mg/5 mL	In 237 mL (pineapple-coconut-mint flavor)	
	Suppository: 50 mg	In 30 individually foil-wrapped suppositories	
(Generic)	Capsules: 25 mg	In bottles of 60, 100, 500, 1,000 capsules	
	50 mg	In bottles of 23, 72, 100, 250, 500 capsules	
	Sustained release: 75 mg	In bottles of 60, 100 capsules	
	Suspension: 25 mg/5 mL	In 500 mL (fruit-flavor)	
Ketoprofen (Orudis)	Tablets: 12.5 mg	In bottles of 24, 50 tablets	
	Capsules: 25 mg, 50 mg	In bottles of 100 tablets	
	75 mg	In bottles of 100, 500 tablets	
(Oruvail)	Extended release: 100 mg, 150 mg, 200 mg	In bottles of 100 capsules	$290/100
(Generic)	Capsules: 50 mg	In bottles of 100 capsules	$23/100
	75 mg	In bottles of 100, 500 capsules	$25/100
	Extended release: 100 mg, 200 mg		200 mg = $216/90
Ketorolac (Toradol)	Tablets: 10 mg 10 mg	In bottles of 100 film-coated tablets	

Table 25–12 ◈ Available Dosage Forms: Selected NSAIDs and Acetaminophen—cont'd

Drug	Dosage Form	How Supplied	Cost
	Injection: 15 mg/mL 30 mg/mL	In bottles of 100, 500 tablets In 1-mL Tubex syringes In 1- and 2-mL Tubex syringes	$114/100
(Generic)	Tablets: 10 mg	30, 90, 100	$71/100
Meclofenamate (Meclomen)	Capsules: 50 mg, 100 mg	In bottles of 100, 500, 1,000	
(Generic)	Capsules: 50 mg, 100 mg	In bottles of 100, 250, 500 capsules	50 mg = 73/100 100 mg = $195/100
Mefenamic acid (Ponstel)	Capsules: 250 mg	In bottles of 100 capsules	$126/100
Meloxicam (Mobic)	Tablet: 7.5 mg, 15 mg	In bottles of 30, 100 and UD 100	7.5 mg = $452/100 15 mg = $667/100
(Generic)	Tablet: 7.5 mg, 15 mg	30, 100	7.5 mg = $47/100 15 mg = $19/100
	Suspension: 7.5 mg/15 mL	100 mL	$87/100 mL
Nabumetone (Relafen)	Tablets: 500 mg, 750 mg	In bottles of 100, 500 film-coated tablets	$160/100, $190/100
(Generic)	Tablets: 500 mg, 750 mg	In bottles of 100	500 mg = $67/100 750 mg = $110/100
Naproxen (Aleve) (Naprelan)	Tablets: 200 mg	In bottles of 24, 50, 100 tablets	
	Controlled release: 375 mg 500 mg	In bottles of 100 tablets In bottles of 75 tablets	
(Naprosyn)	Tablets: 250 mg, 375 mg, 500 mg Enteric coated: 375 mg, 500 mg Tablets, delayed release: 375 mg and 500 mg Suspension: 125 mg/5 mL	In bottles of 100, 500 tablets In bottles of 100 enteric-coated tablets In bottles of 100, 500 enteric-coated tablets In 474 mL (pineapple-orange flavor)	 $28/100, $29/100
(Naproxen)	Tablets: 250 mg, 375 mg, 500 mg Suspension: 125 mg/5 mL	In bottles of 100, 500, 1,000 tablets In 5 and 500 mL (pineapple-orange flavor)	$11/100, $12/100, $15/100 No data
(Naproxen sodium)	Tablets: 275 mg, 550 mg	In bottles of 100, 200, 500, 1,000 tablets	$12.99/200
Oxaprozin (Daypro)	Caplets: 600 mg	In bottles of 100, 500 film-coated caplets	$291/100
(Generic)	Tablet: 600 mg	100	$29/100
Piroxicam (Feldene)	Capsules: 10 mg	In bottles of 100 tablets	
	20 mg	In bottles of 100, 500 tablets	$469/100
(Generic)	Capsules: 10 mg, 20 mg	In bottles of 100, 500, 1,000 capsules	20 mg = $229
Sulindac (Clinoril)	Tablets: 150 mg, 200 mg	In bottles of 100 tablets	100 mg = $106/100 200 mg = $151/100
(Generic)	Tablets: 150 mg, 200 mg	In bottles of 60, 100, 500 tablets	100 mg = $29/100 200 mg = $33/100

There are many brand names for several of these drugs. Only the most commonly used are presented here.

For some **NSAIDs**, there is a prescribed length of time beyond which the drug may not be taken. Patients should be informed of this time limitation. Taking the drug with food or a full glass of fluid and remaining in an upright position for 15 to 30 minutes may reduce GI discomfort and adverse reactions. Remind patients to avoid **aspirin**, **alcohol**, or other GI irritants while taking these drugs.

Adverse Reactions

Advise patients about probable adverse reactions, and what they should do if reactions occur. The most common adverse reaction is GI bleeding. They should contact their health-care provider if they experience coffee-ground emesis or black, tarry stools. The provider should also be notified of skin rash, itching, visual disturbances, weight gain, edema, or persistent headache. With **meclofenamate** and **mefenamic acid**, if rash, diarrhea, or other digestive problems occur, patients should discontinue the drug and contact their health-care provider.

These drugs may cause drowsiness. Patients should avoid activities requiring mental alertness until their response to the drug is known.

Lifestyle Management

Lifestyle modifications are only those related to the disease being treated.

ASPIRIN AND NONACETYLATED SALICYLATES

Aspirin is the prototype drug for this class, which makes it one of the most used drug classes for the treatment and prevention of a wide variety of disorders. Although **salicylates** are prescribed for conditions similar to those that the **NSAIDs** are used for, in addition to the **analgesic**, **anti-inflammatory**, and **antipyretic** properties common to the **NSAIDs**, the **salicylates** also possess antiplatelet properties to varying degrees. This latter property accounts for some of their adverse reactions but also for the increased breadth of their use beyond those for which **NSAIDs** are prescribed. The ability of **aspirin** to reduce platelet aggregation has given it a role in managing rheumatic fever, transient ischemic attacks (TIAs), coronary artery disease, and deep vein thrombosis. The **antiplatelet** role of **aspirin** is discussed in Chapter 18. Its nonspecific anti-inflammatory effect is invaluable in reducing cardiac workload for patients with severe carditis and heart failure. **Aspirin** has been shown to reduce the incidence of myocardial infarction (MI) and the incidence of death in all patients with unstable angina. These roles are discussed in Chapters 28, 33, 36, and 40. **Salicylates** are also used topically as keratolytic agents and counterirritants. This role is discussed in Chapters 23 and 32.

Pharmacodynamics

All **salicylates** have analgesic, anti-inflammatory, antipyretic, and antiplatelet actions. The pharmacological effects are qualitatively similar. **Salicylates** lower body temperature through its effect on the hypothalamic thermostat and vasodilation of peripheral vessels, thus enhancing dissipation of heat. The **anti-inflammatory** and **analgesic** activities are mediated through inhibition of prostaglandin synthesis in the same manner as **NSAIDs**. However, **aspirin** more potently inhibits prostaglandin synthesis and has greater **anti-inflammatory** activity than the **NSAIDs**. The acetyl group of the **aspirin** molecule is thought to be responsible for these differences. **Aspirin** acetylates the cyclo-oxygenase enzyme in the prostaglandin biosynthesis pathway; therefore, it may be theoretically classified as a COX inhibitor.

Aspirin also irreversibly inhibits platelet aggregation. Single analgesic-level doses prolong bleeding time. Acetylation of platelet cyclo-oxygenase prevents synthesis of thromboxane A, which is a potent vasoconstrictor and inducer of platelet aggregation for the life of the platelet (7 to 10 d). This drug has shown success as an **antiplatelet** agent for patients with thromboembolic disease. For this indication, low doses appear to be more effective than higher ones. Further discussion is found in Chapter 18.

The **nonacetylated salicylates (salsalate [Disalcid], choline magnesium trisalicylate [Trilisate]**, and **choline salicylate [Arthropan])** and **diflunisal (Dolobid)** are salicylic acid derivatives not metabolized to salicylic acid, are not as potent as **aspirin**, and do not possess the same degree of **antiplatelet** activity.

Pharmacokinetics

Absorption and Distribution

Salicylates are rapidly and completely absorbed after oral administration (Table 25–13). Bioavailability depends on the dosage form, gastric emptying time, gastric pH, presence of antacids or buffering agents, and particle size. The bioavailability of enteric-coated products may be erratic. The presence of food in the gut slows absorption, and absorption from rectal suppositories is also slower, resulting in lower salicylate levels.

Aspirin is partially hydrolyzed to salicylic acid during absorption and is distributed to all body tissues and fluids, including fetal tissue, breast milk, and the CNS. The highest concentrations are in plasma, the liver, the renal cortex, the heart, and lung tissues.

Protein binding of **salicylates** is concentration dependent. At low concentrations (100 mcg/mL), 90 percent is bound; at higher concentrations (400 mg/mL), only 76 percent is bound.

Diflunisal is also rapidly and completely absorbed after oral administration. It crosses the placenta and enters breast milk. The first dose tends to have slower onset of pain relief than other drugs but achieves comparable peak effects. More than 99 percent is bound to plasma proteins.

Metabolism and Excretion

Salicylic acid is eliminated by renal excretion of **salicylic acid** and by oxidation and conjugation of metabolites by

Table 25–13 ▶ **Pharmacokinetics: Salicylates**

Drug	Onset	Peak	Duration	Protein Binding	Half-Life	Elimination
Acetylsalicylic acid	15–20 min	1–3 h	3–6 h	90%–91%; 25%–76%*	15–20 min; 2–3 h; 15–30 h*	In urine and by liver*
Choline salicylate	5–30 min	1–3 h	3–6 h	90%–91%; 25%–76%*	15–20 min; 2–3 h; 15–30 h*	In urine and by liver*
Choline magnesium salicylate	5–30 min	1–3 h	3–6 h	90%–91%; 25%–76%*	15–20 min; 2–3 h; 15–30 h*	In urine and by liver*
Salsalate	5–30 min	1–3 h	3–6 h	90%–91%; 25%–76%*	15–20 min; 2–3 h; 15–30 h*	In urine and by liver*
Diflunisal	1 h	2–3 h	8–12 h	>99%	8–12 h	90% in urine; <5% in feces

*See discussion in text.

the liver. The amount excreted depends on urine pH. As urine pH increases from 5 to 8, renal clearance of free ionized **salicylate** increases from 2 to 3 percent to more than 80 percent. Alteration of urine pH is used in the treatment of **salicylate** poisoning to increase excretion.

Aspirin has a half-life of 15 to 20 minutes. **Salicylic acid's** half-life is 2 to 3 hours at low doses; at higher doses, it ranges from 6 to 12 hours. Plasma levels increase disproportionately as **salicylate** doses increase.

Diflunisal has a long half-life and nonlinear pharmacokinetics so that time to steady state is 3 to 4 days with 125 mg twice daily and 7 to 9 days with 500 mg twice daily. A loading dose shortens the time to steady state. Because 90 percent of each dose is eliminated by the kidneys, the half-life increases with renal impairment.

Pharmacotherapeutics

Precautions and Contraindications

Taking **salicylates**, especially **aspirin**, by children or adolescents with influenza or chickenpox has been associated with the development of Reye syndrome, a rare but life-threatening condition characterized by vomiting, lethargy, and eventually delirium and coma. The mortality rate is 20 to 30 percent, and permanent brain damage has been reported in survivors. Children or adolescents with influenza or chickenpox should not take **salicylates. Salicylates** probably should not be taken by anyone with any viral upper respiratory infection (URI).

Aspirin should be avoided for 1 week before any surgery because of the increased risk for postoperative bleeding because of its **antiplatelet** effects. For similar reasons, **salicylates** in general are contraindicated for patients with active peptic ulcer disease or other GI bleeding–related disorders or a history of such disorders. **Salsalate** and **choline salicylate** may cause less GI irritation and bleeding than **aspirin.** The **antiplatelet** effects contraindicate **salicylate** use for patients who are taking **anticoagulants** or who have anemia or a history of blood coagulation defects.

Salicylates should be used cautiously for patients with hepatic impairment. Reversible hepatic encephalopathy has occurred after even therapeutic doses for RA. Cautious use is also required for patients with renal insufficiency because **salicylates** may cause a transient decrease in renal function and aggravate chronic kidney diseases. **Magnesium salicylates** are contraindicated in the presence of renal insufficiency because the kidney cannot eliminate the magnesium, and hypermagnesemia results.

Salicylates affect uric acid accumulation. In low doses (less than 2 g/d), they decrease urate excretion and raise serum uric acid levels. At high doses (3 to 5 g/d), they have a uricosuric effect; however, they are rarely tolerated at this high a dose. They should be used with caution in the presence of gout.

Aspirin is Pregnancy Category D; **salsalate** and **magnesium salicylate** are Pregnancy Category C. Ingestion during pregnancy may produce anemia in the mother and increase the risk for postpartum hemorrhage. Inhibition of prostaglandin synthesis may cause constriction of the ductus arteriosus and other possible untoward effects in the fetus. Avoid use in pregnancy, especially during the third trimester. **Diflunisal** is Pregnancy Category C. Although its safety during pregnancy has not been established, it should not be used, especially during the last trimester.

Salicylates are excreted in breast milk in low concentrations. Adverse effects on nursing infants have not been reported. **Diflunisal** is excreted in breast milk in concentrations of 2 to 7 percent of the maternal plasma. Because of potential adverse effects, discontinuing either this drug or nursing is recommended.

The safety and efficacy of **magnesium salicylate** and **salsalate** have not been established in children. **Aspirin** should not be used in children with acute febrile illness. Children with dehydration appear more at risk for **salicylate** toxicity.

Adverse Drug Reactions

The most common adverse reaction to **salicylates** is GI irritation and bleeding. Although fecal blood loss is lower with enteric-coated products, these drugs have erratic absorption and still must be used cautiously by patients with GI disorders. The amount of blood lost from GI bleeding secondary to **salicylate** use is usually clinically insignificant, but with prolonged use it can result in **iron** deficiency anemia. Patients who have developed peptic ulcers while taking **salicylates** have healed these ulcers with the use of **proton pump inhibitors**, **H_2 blockers**, and **antacids**, despite continued **salicylate** use. Only 20 to 25 percent of patients on chronic **aspirin** therapy for RA develop mucosal injury.

Hypersensitivity reactions have occurred with **salicylates.** Hypersensitivity to **salicylates** or **NSAIDs** contraindicates **aspirin** use and requires extremely cautious use of the other **salicylates.** Cross-sensitivity exists between **aspirin** and NSAIDs and between **aspirin** and **tartrazine dye.** This cross-sensitivity does not appear to occur with **choline salicylate. Aspirin** sensitivity is more prevalent in patients with asthma, nasal polyps, or chronic urticaria.

Salicylates are ototoxic at increased blood levels. They should be discontinued if dizziness, tinnitus, or impaired hearing develops. Temporary hearing loss disappears gradually when the drug is stopped.

Toxicity

The acute lethal dose of **salicylates** in adults is 10 to 30 g, and in children it is 4 g. Chronic **salicylate** toxicity can occur when more than 100 mg/kg is ingested daily for 2 or more days. Signs of **salicylate** poisoning appear at serum levels of 200 mcg/mL. Severe toxicity may occur at levels of 400 mcg/mL. Respiratory alkalosis is seen initially. Hyperpnea and tachypnea occur as a result of increased CO_2 production and a direct stimulatory effect of the **salicylate** on the respiratory center in the brain. Other symptoms include nausea, vomiting, hypokalemia, tinnitus, disorientation, irritability, seizures, dehydration, hyperthermia, thrombocytopenia, and other hematological disorders.

Treatment for **salicylate** toxicity includes induction of emesis or gastric lavage to remove any unabsorbed drug from the stomach. Activated charcoal diminishes **salicylate** absorption if it is given within 2 hours of ingestion. **Salicylate** levels and acid–base, fluid, and electrolyte balances are carefully monitored. The rest of therapy is supportive. Forced alkaline diuresis increases **salicylate** excretion. Hemodialysis is reserved for those patients with severe poisoning.

Drug Interactions

Aspirin may potentiate the **anticoagulant** action of **heparin, warfarin,** or **thrombolytic agents** (Table 25–14). It may increase the risk for bleeding with **cefamandole, cefoperazone, cefotetan, valproic acid,** or **plicamycin.**

All **salicylates** may enhance the activity of **penicillins, phenytoin, methotrexate, valproic acid, sulfonylureas,** and **sulfonamides.** They may antagonize the beneficial effects of **probenecid** or **sulfinpyrazone** and blunt the

Table 25–14 ■ **Drug Interactions: Salicylates**

Drug	Interacting Drug	Possible Effect	Implications
Acetylsalicylic acid	Angiotensin-converting enzyme inhibitors, beta adrenergic blockers	Decreased antihypertensive effect because of prostaglandin inhibition	Consider discontinuing salicylate or selecting different antihypertensive
	Heparin, warfarin	Prolonged bleeding time, impaired platelet function	Avoid concurrent use
	Nitroglycerin	Unexpected hypotensive effects	Reduce nitroglycerin dose
	NSAIDs	Aspirin may decrease serum concentrations	Avoid concomitant use; no therapeutic advantage and may increase risk for GI bleed
All salicylates	Alcohol, cefamandole, cefoperazone, cefotetan, valproic acid, plicamycin	Increased risk for GI bleeding	Avoid alcohol while taking salicylates; select different antimicrobial or avoid use of salicylate
	Loop diuretics, aminoglycosides, bumetanide, ethacrynic acid	May increase risk for ototoxicity	Avoid concurrent use or monitor for tinnitus, hearing loss
	Probenecid, sulfinpyrazone	Salicylates antagonize uricosuric effects	Avoid concurrent use
	Spironolactone	Salicylates inhibit diuretic effects	Avoid concurrent use
	Sulfonylureas	Salicylates in doses >2 g/d have hypoglycemic effect; potentiate glucose-lowering effect	Select different drug combination
	Penicillins, phenytoin, methotrexate, valproic acid, sulfonamide	May enhance effects of these drugs	Monitor for potential dosage adjustments
	Foods that acidify urine*	Decreases renal excretion and increases serum levels of salicylates	May increase risk for toxicity
	Foods that alkalinize urine*	Increases renal excretion and decreases serum levels of salicylates	May be used therapeutically to treat overdose

Table 25–14 ■ **Drug Interactions: Salicylates—cont'd**

Drug	Interacting Drug	Possible Effect	Implications
Diflunisal	Acetaminophen	Concurrent administration may result in 50% increase in acetaminophen levels	Increased risk for hepatotoxicity; avoid concurrent use
	Heparin, warfarin	Competitively displaces warfarin from protein binding sites; increased risk for bleeding	Avoid concurrent use; monitor PT/INR closely
	Hydrochlorothiazide (HCTZ)	Significantly decreased HCTZ plasma levels	Avoid concurrent use
	Aspirin, NSAIDs, colchicine, glucocorticoids, alcohol	Additive risk for GI bleeding	Avoid concurrent use
	Lithium	May increase serum lithium levels	Select different salicylate
	Probenecid	Increased risk of diflunisal toxicity	Avoid concurrent use or monitor closely for indications of toxicity
	Antacids	Concurrent administration decreases absorption of diflunisal	Separate administration by at least 1 h
	Indomethacin	Decreased renal clearance and significantly increased indomethacin serum levels	Avoid concurrent use
	Sulindac	Increased renal clearance and significantly decreased sulindac serum levels	Avoid concurrent use

INR = international normalized ratio; PT = prothrombin time.
*Foods that alkalinize urine: all fruits except cranberries, prunes, plums; all vegetables; milk. Foods that acidify urine: cheeses, cranberries, eggs, fish, grains, meats, plums, poultry, and prunes.

therapeutic response to **diuretics, antihypertensives,** and some **NSAIDs. Glucocorticoids** decrease serum **salicylate** levels.

There is an increased risk for GI bleeding when **aspirin** is taken with any other drug with any other GI irritant, such as **ethanol**. The risk for ototoxicity is increased when it is taken with any other drug that causes ototoxicity (e.g., **aminoglycosides, loop diuretics**).

Some foods contain **salicylate**. Foods and spices high in **salicylate** include curry, paprika, licorice, Benedictine liqueur, prunes, raisins, tea, and gherkins. Foods that acidify the urine may increase serum **salicylate** levels, and those that alkalinize the urine may have the opposite effect.

Clinical Use and Dosing

Fever

Aspirin is the **salicylate** of choice for reduction of fever in adults. It is contraindicated for use with pregnant patients, however. To be used with children, the cause of the fever must first be determined. It is contraindicated in children and adolescents if the cause of the fever is influenza or chickenpox. Although not clearly stated in the literature, this warning may extend to other viral URIs. Many providers do not use it as an antipyretic for any children because there are other drugs that do not carry the concern about Reye syndrome. **Acetaminophen** or **ibuprofen** is probably better for fever management in children. Adults' and children's doses of **aspirin** are shown in Table 25–15.

Diflunisal is not recommended as an antipyretic. In single doses, it reduces fever in some patients but not in a clinically significant amount.

Mild to Moderate Pain

Pain associated with inflammation is especially well managed with **salicylates** or **NSAIDs. Aspirin, choline salicylate, choline magnesium salicylate,** and **diflunisal** are all approved for this indication. **Aspirin** is the gold standard against which others are judged. It is

Table 25–15 ● **Dosage Schedule: Salicylates**

Drug	Indication	Dose	Comments
Acetylsalicylic acid	Fever, pain, headache, dysmenorrhea	*Adults:* 325–650 mg every 4 h; with extra strength may use 500 mg every 3 h *or* 1 g every 6 h; not to exceed 4 g/d	
		Children 2–11 yr: 65 mg/kg/d in 4–6 divided doses*	*Use cautiously in children
	Rheumatoid arthritis, osteoarthritis	*Adults:* 3.2–6 g/d in divided doses	Toxicity risk increased at this dose

Continued

Table 25–15 ◉ Dosage Schedule: Salicylates—cont'd

Drug	Indication	Dose	Comments
	Juvenile rheumatoid arthritis	*Children <25 kg:* 60–110 mg/kg/d in divided doses (every 6–8 h); start with 60 mg/kg/d and increase by 20 mg/kg/d after 5–7 d, then increase by 10 mg/kg/d after another 5–7 d *Children >25 kg:* 50–60 mg/kg/d with a similar dosing increase schedule	Maintain a serum salicylate level of 15–30 mg/mL for anti-inflammatory effects
	Acute rheumatic fever	*Adults:* 5–8 g/d initially in 3–4 divided doses; increase dose to reach serum salicylate level of 15–30 mg/mL; not to exceed 8 g/d *Children:* 100 mg/kg/d for 2 wk, then decrease to 75 mg/kg/d for 4–6 wk; not to exceed 130 mg/kg/d	
	Transient ischemic attack	*Adults:* 50–325 mg/d	Aspirin combined with extended release dipyridamole is recommended over aspirin alone
	Myocardial infarction prophylaxis	*Adults:* 81–160 mg/d	
Choline salicylate	Fever, pain	*Adults and children >12 yr:* 870 mg every 3–4 h; maximum 6 times/d	Has fewer adverse reactions than aspirin
	Rheumatoid arthritis	*Adults:* 870–1,740 mg up to qid	
Choline magnesium salicylate	Fever, pain, rheumatoid arthritis	*Adults:* 2–3 g/d in divided doses or 150 mg bid *Children >37 kg:* 2.2 g/d in 2 divided doses* *Children <37 kg:* 50 mg/d in 2 divided doses*	
Salsalate	Rheumatic conditions	*Adults:* 1,500 mg bid *or* 750 mg qid; not to exceed 4 g/d	
Diflunisal	Mild to moderate pain	*Adults:* 1 g initially, followed by 500 mg every 8–12 h	Half this dose initially and following may be effective
	Osteoarthritis	*Adults:* 500 mg–1 g/d in 2 divided doses; not to exceed 1.5 g/d	

* Dosing schedules are published for analgesia and fever reduction. Use cautiously. Not recommended for children with influenza or chickenpox because of risk for Reye syndrome.

inexpensive, available OTC, the most potent analgesic in the class, and short acting, so that acute pain can be managed without long-term effects and adverse reactions. It is has limitations, however. It is Pregnancy Category D, especially in the third trimester, and contraindicated in children with influenza or chickenpox.

Diflunisal offers the advantage of analgesia comparable with that of **aspirin**, with longer-lasting responses. Like the other drugs in this group, it can be used for this indication, but all four are more often used to treat arthritic conditions.

Rheumatoid Arthritis

Salicylates or **NSAIDs** can be used to treat RA. Once again, **aspirin** is the gold standard. Serum levels can easily be measured to determine adherence and therapeutic efficacy, and it is the least expensive **salicylate. Nonacetylated salicylates** are less potent anti-inflammatory agents, but they have fewer adverse reactions than **aspirin**. The main disadvantages of **aspirin** are the high incidence of GI intolerance (take with food or use enteric-coated tablets), the inconvenience of taking four or five doses daily, and the relatively long interval (4 to 7 d) before a full anti-inflammatory effect is reached. A trial of therapy of 3 to 4 g/day for 4 to 6 days is recommended, because 70 to 80 percent of patients who will respond will do so within this time frame. Older adults are predictably less tolerant to the adverse GI reactions, and their trial dose should be 2 to 3 g/day. If the response is inadequate and adherence has been good, a **salicylate** level should be drawn before changing drugs. If the drug level is within therapeutic parameters (20 to 25 mg/dL in adults; 15 to 20 mg/dL in older adults) without adequate response, or if the drug is not tolerated, another drug should be tried. If the **salicylate** level is too low, but the patient has been adherent and tolerates the **aspirin**, the dose should be increased by 325 to 650 mg/day until the desired **anti-inflammatory** level of the drug is reached.

The margin is narrow between a good therapeutic level and toxicity in treating patients with RA because the dose is higher than that used for fever or **analgesia**. The earliest manifestation of toxicity is tinnitus or mild deafness. **Aspirin** should be stopped immediately if these symptoms occur. Once they abate, it may be restarted at a lower dose, or an **NSAID** may be chosen. Toxicity is discussed in the Adverse Reactions section.

For patients whose main reason for discontinuing **aspirin** is GI intolerance, **salsalate** is a good alternative. It can be given in twice-daily dosing and has a much lower incidence of GI bleeding. **Choline salicylate** and **choline magnesium salicylate** can also be used and may be given in two times to four times daily dosing.

Osteoarthritis

Patients with OA may present occasionally with acute or subacute painful episodes in which the underlying problem is inflammation. No drugs have proven efficacy in altering the course of OA, but both **salicylates** and **NSAIDs** are used successfully to treat the pain associated with these exacerbations. **Aspirin** is an effective **analgesic** and **anti-inflammatory** that is usually well tolerated in divided doses of 1.2 to 2.4 g/day. **NSAIDs** tend to have more adverse reactions with no better pain relief when given at **anti-inflammatory** doses over the course of more than a few days. **Acetaminophen** is helpful for **analgesia** but has no **anti-inflammatory** effects.

The **nonacetylated salicylates** are also effective and have fewer GI adverse reactions than **aspirin**. **Diflunisal** has the advantage of twice-daily dosing but may take up to 2 weeks to achieve full anti-inflammatory effects. Although it is more expensive than **aspirin**, the cost may approach that of many of the **NSAIDs**. Discussion of **NSAIDs** is in the section preceding this one.

Juvenile Rheumatoid Arthritis

Juvenile RA is an autoimmune disease that occurs in four different forms, all of which are characterized by joint inflammation. Pediatric specialists generally follow children with the disorder and determine their treatment protocol. **Salicylates** and **NSAIDs** are commonly part of this protocol.

Aspirin is prescribed in daily doses of 60 to 110 mg/kg for children. **NSAIDs** are prescribed if the child does not respond to or cannot tolerate **aspirin** therapy.

Nonacetylated salicylates are not indicated for treatment of juvenile forms of RA.

Acute Rheumatic Fever

Acute rheumatic fever is usually a sequela of group A beta-hemolytic streptococcal infection. Rheumatic fever incidence is 0.1 to 0.2 cases per 100,000 persons in Canada, the United States, and western Europe (Madden & Kelly, 2009). There is a higher incidence (10 to 20 cases/100,000) of rheumatic fever in emerging economies, indigenous peoples, and tropical regions (Madden & Kelly, 2009). Acute rheumatic fever is treated with **antimicrobials**, but the inflammatory manifestations are treated with **aspirin**. Although this disorder is more common in children, it can also occur in adults. Dosage schedules for both are presented in Table 25–15.

Myocardial Infarction Prophylaxis

Daily treatment of 81 to 325 mg **aspirin** in patients with MI has been associated with a 20 percent reduction in risk of subsequent and nonfatal reinfarction. In the International Study of Infarct Survival (Baigent et al, 1998), patients who received a combination of **aspirin** 160 mg/day and **streptokinase** after the onset of a suspected MI had significantly fewer reinfarctions, strokes, and deaths than those who received placebo. The combination was also better than either drug alone. This result has led to the recommendation that, at the first sign of an MI (chest pain and other symptoms), patients should take one 325-mg **aspirin** tablet (Anderson et al, 2007; Bolooki & Askari, 2009).

The American Heart Association (AHA) recommends low-dose **aspirin** in patients with higher risk for coronary heart disease. The AHA recommends 75 to 160 mg/day of **aspirin** for prophylaxis (Pearson et al, 2002). Low-dose **aspirin** (75 to 160 mg/d) is as effective as higher doses for cardiovascular risk reduction (Pearson et al, 2002). **Nonacetylated salicylates** do not have adequate **antiplatelet** activity for this indication and have not been subjected to research to support their use. Extensive discussion of the use of **aspirin** for this indication is found in Chapters 28, 33, 36, and 40.

Transient Ischemic Attacks

The American Heart Association/American Stroke Association recommends the use of **aspirin** for the prevention of stroke in patients with stroke and transient ischemic attack (Adams et al, 2008). **Aspirin** (50 to 325 mg/d) monotherapy or a combination of **aspirin** and extended-release **dipyridamole** are accepted therapy options for stroke prevention (Adams et al, 2008). The combination of **dipyridamole** and **aspirin** is preferred over **aspirin** alone (Adams et al, 2008). Patients who are allergic to **aspirin** may be treated with **clopidogrel**. **Clopidogrel** and its dosing for this indication are discussed in Chapter 18.

Dosing schedules for **aspirin** for each indication are presented in Table 25–15.

Rational Drug Selection

Rational drug selection is based largely on indication, cost, and convenience of therapy (Table 25–16). All of these are discussed in the Clinical Use and Dosing section.

Monitoring

A random **salicylate** level should be drawn 7 to 10 days after initiation of chronic therapy. Periodic **salicylate**

Table 25–16 ◆ **Available Dosage Forms: Salicylates**

Drug	Dosage Form	How Supplied
Acetylsalicylic acid (Bayer aspirin*)	Tablets: 325 mg	In bottles of 12, 24, 50, 100, 200, 300 tablets
	Chewable tablets: 81 mg	In bottles of 36
	Enteric-coated tablets: 325 mg	In bottles of 50, 100 tablets
	Timed-release tablets: 650 mg	In bottles of 30, 72, 125 tablets
	Caplets: 325 mg	In bottles of 40 100, 200 caplets
	500 mg	In bottles of 30, 60 caplets
(Generic)	Tablets: 325 mg	In bottles of 100, 200, 250, 500, 1,000 tablets
	500 mg	In bottles of 100 tablets
	Enteric-coated tablets: 325 mg	In bottles of 30, 60, 90, 100, 1,000 tablets
	650 mg	In bottles of 100, 1,000 tablets
	975 mg	In bottles of 100 tablets; prescription only
	Suppository: 120 mg, 200 mg, 300 mg, 600 mg	In 12 individually foil-wrapped suppositories
Choline salicylate (Arthropan)	Liquid: 870 mg/5 mL	In 240 and 480 mL (mint flavor)
Choline magnesium salicylate (Trilisate)	Tablets: 500 mg, 750 mg	In bottles of 100 scored tablets
	1 g	In bottles of 60 scored tablets
	Liquid: 500 mg/5 mL	In 237 mL (cherry flavor)
Salsalate (Disalcid)	Capsules: 500 mg	In bottles of 100 capsules
	Tablets: 500 mg, 750 mg	In bottles of 100, 500 tablets
(Generic)	500 mg, 750 mg	In bottles of 100, 500 tablets
Diflunisal (Dolobid)	Tablets: 250 mg, 500 mg	In bottles of 60 tablets

*There are many different brands of aspirin. Bayer was selected because it has several different forms.

levels should be drawn during long-term management to check maintenance of therapeutic levels and monitor for toxic manifestations.

Because all of these drugs are eliminated by the kidney and dosage adjustments may be required based on renal function, serum creatinine levels should be assessed before therapy is begun and annually throughout long-term therapy. Urinary pH should also be monitored regularly. Sudden acidification of urine can more than double the plasma **salicylate** level, resulting in toxicity.

Salicylates interfere with homeostasis. A CBC should be drawn prior to initiating therapy and at least annually throughout long-term therapy. A CBC should also be drawn and fecal occult blood studies should be done as well if there is any indication of GI bleeding.

Hepatic function should be monitored prior to antirheumatic therapy and if hepatotoxicity symptoms occur. These problems are more likely in patients with rheumatic fever, juvenile RA, or preexisting hepatic diseases, especially children.

Ophthalmic effects have been reported in patients taking **diflunisal**. Ophthalmic studies are appropriate for patients who develop eye complaints during therapy.

Patient Education

Administration

Instruct the patient to take **salicylates** exactly as prescribed. Taking with food or a full glass of water and remaining in an upright position for 15 to 30 minutes after administration can reduce GI irritation. Food slows absorption but does not alter the total amount absorbed.

Remind patients not to crush or chew enteric-coated tablets or take **antacids** within 1 hour of enteric-coated tablets. Chewable tablets may be chewed, dissolved in liquid, or swallowed whole. Tablets with a vinegar-like odor (acetic acid) should be discarded.

Instruct patients not to increase the dose beyond that prescribed. Increased doses increase the risk for **salicylate** poisoning. For patients taking **aspirin** for MI or TIA prophylaxis, increasing the dose has not proved to provide additional benefits but does increase the risk for adverse reactions.

Adverse Reactions

The most common adverse reactions are ototoxicity and GI irritation and bleeding. Advise patients to report tinnitus; unusual bleeding from the gums; bruising; black, tarry stools; or fever lasting longer than 3 days. Patients who are taking **salicylates** should not use **alcohol** or other substances that increase GI irritation.

Reye syndrome practically disappeared after the Centers for Disease Control and Prevention (CDC) started warning against giving **aspirin** to children or adolescents with influenza, influenza-like syndromes, or chickenpox (varicella) because of a possible association with Reye syndrome, a "public health triumph" (Monto, 1999).

Parents should be informed of the risk of Reye syndrome and educated regarding not giving **aspirin** to a child with a viral illness.

Lifestyle Management

Rest, heat, exercise, and other lifestyle modifications are part of the management of arthritic conditions. The modifications are as important as the pharmacological management and should be stressed.

REFERENCES

Adams, R. J., Albers, G., Alberts, M. J., Benavente, O., Furie, K., Goldstein, L. B., et al. (2008). Update to the AHA/ASA recommendations for the prevention of stroke in patients with stroke and transient ischemic attack. *Stroke, 39,* 1647–1652.

Agency for Healthcare Research and Quality. (2009). *Three treatments for osteoarthritis of the knee: Evidence shows lack of benefit* [AHRQ Publication No. 09-EHC001-3]. Rockville, MD: AHRQ Publications Clearinghouse. Retrieved from http://www.effectivehealthcare.ahrq.gov/ehc/index.cfm/search-for-guides-reviews-and-reports/?pageAction=displayProduct&productID=134#512

American Academy of Orthopedic Surgeons. (2008). Guideline on the treatment of osteoarthritis (OA) of the knee. American Association of Orthopedic Surgeons. Retrieved from http://www.aaos.org/research/guidelines/guidelineoaknee.asp

American College of Rheumatology. (2000). Recommendations for the medical management of osteoarthritis. *Arthritis and Rheumatism, 43*(9), 1905–1915.

American College of Rheumatology. (2001 update). Recommendations for the prevention and treatment of glucocorticoid-induced osteoporosis. Retrieved July 8, 2005, from http://www.rheumatology.org/publications/guidelines

American College of Rheumatology. (2002 update). Guidelines for the management of rheumatoid arthritis. *Arthritis and Rheumatism, 46*(2), 328–346.

Anderson, J., Adams, C., Antman, E., Bridges, C., Califf, R., Casey, D., et al. (2007). ACC/AHA 2007 guidelines for the management of patients with unstable angina/non-ST-elevation myocardial infarction: A report of the American College of Cardiology/American Heart Association Task Force on Practice Guidelines (Writing Committee to Revise the 2002 Guidelines for the Management of Patients With Unstable Angina/Non-ST-Elevation Myocardial Infarction) developed in collaboration with the American College of Emergency Physicians, the Society for Cardiovascular Angiography and Interventions, and the Society of Thoracic Surgeons endorsed by the American Association of Cardiovascular and Pulmonary Rehabilitation and the Society for Academic Emergency Medicine. *Journal of the American College of Cardiology, 50*(7), e1–e157. Retrieved from MEDLINE database.

Baigent, C., Collins, R., Appleby, P., Parish, S., Sleight, P., & Peto, R. (1998). ISIS-2: 10-year survival among patients with suspected acute myocardial infarction in randomized comparison of intravenous streptokinase, oral aspirin, both, or neither. *British Medical Journal, 316*(7141), 1337–1343.

Bolooki, H. M., & Askari, A. (2009). Acute myocardial infarction. *Cleveland Clinic Center for Continuing Education.* Retrieved from http://www.clevelandclinicmeded.com/medicalpubs/diseasemanagement/cardiology/acute-myocardial-infarction/#s0080

Centers for Disease Control and Prevention (CDC). (2006). Prevalence of doctor-diagnosed arthritis and arthritis-attributable activity limitation—United States, 2003–2005. *Morbidity and Mortality Weekly Report, 55*(40), 1089–1092.

Centers for Disease Control and Prevention (CDC). (2010). Arthritis: Gout. Retrieved from http://www.cdc.gov/arthritis/basics/gout.htm

Drug Facts and Comparisons (2010). Wolters Kluwer Health. Retrieved from http://www.factsandcomparisons.com/

Feldman, M., & Das, S. (2010). NSAIDs (including aspirin): Primary prevention of gastroduodenal toxicity. *UpToDate Online.* Retrieved from http://www.uptodate.com/online/content/topic.do?topicKey=acidpep/9491&selectedTitle=10~150&source=search_result#H12

Harris, M., Siegel, L., & Alloway, J. (1999). Gout and hyperuricemia. *American Family Physician, 59*(4). Retrieved July 8, 2005, from http://www.aafp.org/afp/990215ap

Klauer, K. M. (2009). Adrenal insufficiency and adrenal crisis: Treatment & medication. *eMedicine.* Retrieved from http://emedicine.medscape.com/article/765753-treatment

LactMed. (2011). Prednisone. *Drug and Lactation Database: LactMed.* National Library of Medicine: Bethesda, MD. Retrieved from http://toxnet.nlm.nih.gov/cgi-bin/sis/search/f?./temp/~c4DOOJ:1

Lawrence, R. C., Felson, D.T., Helmick, C. G., Arnold, L. M., Choi, H., Deyo, R. A., et al, for the National Arthritis Data Workgroup. (2008). Estimates of the prevalence of arthritis and other rheumatic conditions in the United States. *Arthritis & Rheumatism, 58*(1), 26–35.

Madden, S., & Kelly, L. (2009). Update on acute rheumatic fever: It still exists in remote communities. *Canadian Family Physician, 55,* 475–478.

McCance, K., & Huether, S. (2010). *Pathophysiology: The biological basis for disease in adults and children* (6th ed.). St. Louis, MO: Elsevier Mosby.

Monto, A. S. (1999). The disappearance of Reye's syndrome—a public health triumph. *New England Journal of Medicine, 340,* 1423–1424.

Pearson, T. A., Blair, S. N., Daniels, S. R., Eckel, R. H., Fair, J. M., Frotman, S. P., et al. (2002). AHA guidelines for primary prevention of cardiovascular disease and stroke: 2002 update. Consensus panel guide to comprehensive risk reduction for adult patients without coronary or other atherosclerotic vascular diseases. *Circulation, 106,* 388–394.

Saag, K. G., & Furst, D. E. (2010). Major side effects of systemic glucocorticoids. *UpToDate.* Retrieved from http://www.uptodate.com/online/content/topic.do?topicKey=treatme/6535&selectedTitle=1~150&source=search_result#H11

Simon, L., Lipman, A., Jacox, A., Caudill-Slosberg, M., Gill, L., et al. (2002). *Pain in osteoarthritis, rheumatoid arthritis and juvenile chronic arthritis.* Glenview, IL: American Pain Society.

Terkeltaub, R. A., Furst, D. E., Bennett, K. A., Crockett, R. S., & Davis, M. W. (2010). High versus low dosing of oral colchicines for early acute gout flare: Twenty-four-hour outcomes of the first multicenter, randomized, double-blind, placebo-controlled, parallel-group, dose-comparison colchicines study. *Arthritis and Rheumatism, 62*(4), 1060–1068.

CHAPTER 26

DRUGS USED IN TREATING EYE AND EAR DISORDERS

Teri Moser Woo

Chapter Outline

This chapter discusses the medications used to treat eye and ear disorders, including the common **anti-infective agents** for conjunctivitis, the medications used for allergic conjunctivitis, and common **anti-inflammatory agents** used for ocular inflammation. Although primary care providers may not prescribe some of the glaucoma medications, many drugs interact with these ophthalmic medications, and therefore, a basic understanding of these agents is necessary and included. **Eye lubricants** and **vasoconstrictors** are discussed here. The use of **fluorescein**, a diagnostic agent commonly used in primary care, is addressed in this chapter. The ear medications discussed in this chapter include the **anti-infectives**, **analgesics**, and **ceruminolytics**.

DRUGS USED IN TREATING EYE DISORDERS

Ophthalmic Anti-Infectives

Common eye infections that are treated by primary care providers include bacterial conjunctivitis, viral conjunctivitis, blepharitis, and hordeolum. Acute conjunctivitis is the most common disorder of the eye seen by the primary care provider (Wald, 1997). An estimated 4 million cases of bacterial conjunctivitis occur in the United States annually (Smith & Waycaster, 2009). The commonly used **antibacterial agents** for conjunctivitis are **sulfacetamide sodium** (Bleph-10), **erythromycin** (Ilotycin), **tobramycin** (Tobrex), **gentamicin** (Garamycin), **azithromycin** (AzaSite), and the **fluoroquinolones norfloxacin** (Noroxin), **ciprofloxacin** (Ciloxan), and **ofloxacin** (Ocuflox). The combination drugs **Polytrim** and **Polysporin Ophthalmic** may also be used and are discussed here. **Chloramphenicol** (Chloroptic) is rarely used in primary care because of its adverse effects. More serious infectious eye disorders such as herpes simplex virus (HSV) infection, keratitis, and corneal ulcers are treated by ophthalmologists and, therefore, are not covered at great length in this chapter, although the **antiviral agents** that may be used to treat viral eye infections are briefly discussed.

Pharmacodynamics

Ophthalmic antibiotics may be bacteriostatic or bactericidal. **Bacitracin** is **bacteriostatic** and inhibits the incorporation of amino acids and nucleotides into the cell. It is active against many gram-positive (staphylococci, streptococci, clostridia, corynebacteria, and anaerobic cocci) and gram-negative (gonococci, meningococci, and fusobacteria) organisms.

Erythromycin is a **bacteriostatic macrolide antibiotic** that is active against a wide range of organisms. It binds to the 50S ribosomal subunit, inhibiting bacterial protein synthesis. The gram-positive organisms that are susceptible to **erythromycin** include *Staphylococcus aureus, Streptococcus pyogenes, Streptococcus pneumoniae,* the *Streptococcus viridans* group, and *Corynebacterium diphtheriae.* **Erythromycin** has limited gram-negative coverage. It is also active against *Chlamydia trachomatis.*

Sulfacetamide is a **synthetic sulfonamide** that inhibits bacterial dihydrofolate synthetase. It is active against the following susceptible organisms: streptococci, staphylococci, *Escherichia coli, Klebsiella pneumoniae, Pseudomonas pyocyanea, Neisseria gonorrhoeae,* and *C. trachomatis.*

Tobramycin is a **broad-spectrum aminoglycoside.** The exact mechanism by which it is bactericidal is unknown. It is active against staphylococci, streptococci, *Corynebacterium* species, *K. pneumoniae, Moraxella* species, *Proteus* species, beta-hemolytic streptococci, and *Haemophilus influenzae.* **Tobramycin ophthalmic** is not active against *N. gonorrhoeae* or *C. trachomatis.*

Gentamicin is a **broad-spectrum antibiotic** that is active against a wide range of gram-positive and gram negative organisms. It is unclear how **gentamicin** causes cell death. It is active against staphylococci, *S. pneumoniae,* beta-hemolytic streptococci, *E. coli, H. influenzae, N. gonorrhoeae,* and *Enterobacter* species.

Azithromycin (AzaSite) is a macrolide antibiotic active against both gram-positive and gram-negative organisms. The manufacturer's premarketing studies indicated that **azithromycin** drops eradicated 88 percent of gram-positive bacteria and 92 percent of gram-negative bacterial in randomized controlled trials (RCT), including 93 percent of *H. influenzae,* a common pathogen in pediatric conjunctivitis (Inspire Pharmaceuticals, 2008).

The **fluoroquinolones ciprofloxacin, garifloxacin, levofloxacin, moxifloxacin, norfloxacin,** and **ofloxacin** are bactericidal via inhibition of DNA gyrase. It is unclear how inhibition of DNA gyrase leads to cell death. The **fluoroquinolones** are active against staphylococci, *S. pneumoniae, H. influenzae, K. pneumoniae, Proteus* species, *Enterobacter* species, and *Pseudomonas aeruginosa.*

Polytrim is an **ophthalmic antibacterial preparation** that combines **polymyxin B** and **trimethoprim. Polymyxin B** binds to cell membranes with high affinity, specifically the phospholipids in the cell wall. This causes increased cellular permeability. **Polymyxin B** is generally active against gram-negative bacteria *(E. coli, P. aeruginosa, H. influenzae).* **Trimethoprim** inhibits bacterial dihydrofolate reductase. **Trimethoprim** has both gram-positive and gram-negative activity. **Trimethoprim** is active against *S. aureus, S. pneumoniae,* and *S. pyogenes.*

Polysporin Ophthalmic contains **polymyxin B** and **bacitracin.** This combination provides activity against gram-positive and gram-negative bacterial organisms, as discussed previously.

Two **antiviral ophthalmic agents** that may be prescribed by an ophthalmologist are **vidarabine (Vira-A)** and **trifluridine (Viroptic). Vidarabine** inhibits viral DNA replication, although the exact mechanism of action is not known. **Vidarabine** has antiviral activity against HSV types 1 and 2, varicella-zoster virus, cytomegalovirus, vaccinia, and hepatitis B. The exact mechanism of action of **trifluridine** is not known, although it is thought to interfere with DNA synthesis. **Trifluridine** is active against HSV-1 and HSV-2, adenovirus, and vaccinia virus.

Pharmacokinetics

Ophthalmic antibiotic and **antiviral preparations** generally penetrate only the ocular fluid and tissues. Systemic absorption is minimal, although there may be enough absorption for sensitization to occur, specifically with **sulfacetamide.** There is no information regarding the metabolism and excretion of **ophthalmic anti-infectives.**

Pharmacotherapeutics

Precautions and Contraindications

Hypersensitivity to any component of the preparation is a contraindication to its use. There may be cross-sensitivity between the individual **aminoglycosides (tobramycin** and **gentamicin).** The same is found with the **fluoroquinolones.**

The vehicles used in **ophthalmic ointments** may retard corneal healing after ocular trauma or ocular surgery. Improvements in **ophthalmic ointment vehicles** have improved this situation, but manufacturers still warn that many preparations may retard corneal healing.

Purulent exudates that contain **para-aminobenzoic acid** may inactivate **sulfacetamide** antibacterial activity.

Antibacterial agents are not effective against fungal infection, viral infection, or all types of bacterial infection. If the patient is not responding to therapy, reevaluation, including appropriate cultures, is indicated.

Erythromycin, azithromycin, and **tobramycin** ophthalmic preparations are Pregnancy Category B. **Gentamicin, ciprofloxacin, gatifloxacin, levofloxacin, moxifloxin, norfloxacin, ofloxacin, polymyxin B,** and **sulfacetamide** are Pregnancy Category C. The **antiviral ophthalmic agents vidarabine** and **trifluridine** are both Pregnancy Category C. Safety for use during pregnancy has not been determined.

The use of the **sulfacetamides** and the **fluoroquinolones** should be avoided during lactation because they are harmful to the infant and breast milk excretion is unknown.

Erythromycin and **tobramycin** are safe and effective in children. The safety of the **fluoroquinolones (ciprofloxacin, gatifloxacin, moxifloxacin, levofloxacin, norfloxacin, ofloxacin,** and **besifloxacin)** and **azithromycin** in children under age 1 has not been established. **Sulfacetamide** and **polymyxin B/bacitracin** should not be prescribed to infants younger than 2 months.

Adverse Drug Reactions

All of the **ophthalmic anti-infective preparations** may cause local irritation, which is usually transient. Irritation may include burning, itching, and inflammation. Superinfection may occur with prolonged or repeated use of **ophthalmic anti-infectives.**

Bacitracin may cause blurred vision, which usually lasts only a few minutes.

Sulfacetamide ophthalmic preparations may cause a hypersensitivity reaction in patients who have previously exhibited sensitivity to **sulfonamides.** Stevens-Johnson syndrome is a rare adverse reaction that has been reported with **sulfacetamide ophthalmic ointment** use. Fever, bone marrow depression, and lupus erythematosus may rarely occur with **sulfonamides,** including topical preparations. There may be intense burning and stinging, especially with the 30 percent **sulfacetamide sodium solution (Sulamyd 30%).**

Aminoglycosides may cause localized ocular toxicity and hypersensitivity.

The **fluoroquinolones** may cause a white crystalline precipitate to form in the superficial portion of the cornea. This was observed in about 17 percent of the patients on **ciprofloxacin.** Lid margin crusting, crystals, scales, and the sensation of a foreign body in the eye are also reported with **ophthalmic fluoroquinolones.** Patients also report a bitter or bad taste in the mouth, specifically with **ciprofloxacin solution. Fluoroquinolones** may also cause photophobia, tearing, nausea, decreased vision, conjunctival hyperemia, and corneal staining.

The **ophthalmic antiviral preparations** may cause burning and irritation on instillation into the eye. **Vidarabine** may also cause photophobia, pruritus, erythema, ocular pain, and, less commonly, increased lacrimation. Patients who are using **ophthalmic vidarabine** may develop superficial punctate keratitis after exposure to ultraviolet (UV) light, and they should wear sunglasses to protect their eyes when exposed to bright light. **Trifluridine** has adverse reactions similar to those of **vidarabine,** with the addition of reported increases in intraocular pressure (IOP).

Drug Interactions

There are no drug interactions reported for **ophthalmic preparations** of **bacitracin, gentamicin, tobramycin, polymyxin B, azithromycin,** and **erythromycin.**

Sulfacetamide is incompatible with **silver-containing preparations** and should not be used in conjunction with **ophthalmic products containing silver salts, including silver nitrate.** Concomitant use of **ophthalmic sulfacetamide** with **zinc sulfate** causes a precipitate to form. **Ester-type local anesthetics** including **benzocaine, chloroprocaine, cocaine, procaine, propoxycaine,** and **tetracaine** should not be used concurrently with **sulfacetamide** because they can antagonize the therapeutic actions of the **sulfonamide.**

The **fluoroquinolones (ciprofloxacin, gatifloxacin, moxifloxacin, levofloxacin, norfloxacin,** and **ofloxacin)** may increase **theophylline** levels and potentiate **oral anticoagulants.** These interactions are theoretical with ophthalmic use of **fluoroquinolones,** in that little is known regarding the amount of medication that is systemically absorbed, and whether enough is absorbed to cause a drug interaction. Table 26–1 presents drug interactions with **ophthalmic anti-infectives.**

Table 26–1 ■ **Drug Interactions: Ophthalmic Anti-Infectives**

Drug	Interacting Drug	Possible Effect	Implications
Sulfacetamide sodium	Silver preparations	Incompatibility	Do not use concurrently
Erythromycin	None reported		
Tobramycin	None reported		
Gentamicin	None reported		
Gatifloxacin	Theophylline, caffeine, oval anticoagulants	May raise serum levels	Monitor PT/INR levels
Levofloxacin	Theophylline, caffeine, oval anticoagulants	May raise level of these drugs	Monitor INR/PT levels
Moxifloxacin	None reported		
Norfloxacin	Warfarin, theophylline, cyclosporine	May raise levels of these systemic drugs	Monitor theophylline level and PT/PTT times
Ciprofloxacin	Warfarin, theophylline, cyclosporine	May raise levels of these systemic drugs; may increase renal toxicity from cyclosporine	Monitor theophylline level

Continued

Table 26–1 ■ **Drug Interactions: Ophthalmic Anti-Infectives—cont'd**

Drug	Interacting Drug	Possible Effect	Implications
Ofloxacin	Warfarin, theophylline, caffeine, cyclosporine	May raise levels of these systemic drugs; may increase renal toxicity from cyclosporine	Monitor PT/INR levels closely
Polymyxin B–trimethoprim	None reported		
Polymyxin B-bacitracin ophthalmic	None reported		

PT = prothrombin time; PTT = partial thromboplastin time; INR = international normalized ratio.

Clinical Use and Dosing

Conjunctivitis

The common organisms that are associated with bacterial conjunctivitis vary with the age of the patient. Newborns should be evaluated for ophthalmia neonatorum. Preschool children most commonly have bacterial conjunctivitis, with viral etiology (adenovirus) more likely in schoolchildren. *N. gonorrhoeae* conjunctivitis should be excluded in sexually active adolescents and adults. Adults may have viral or bacterial conjunctivitis. *Chlamydia* is seen in the neonate and sexually active teen and adult. Table 26–2 presents the clinical and laboratory features of conjunctivitis.

Ophthalmia Neonatorum

Any infant younger than 1 month who presents with conjunctivitis should have Gram's stain, antigen detection tests, and cultures of the eye discharge to rule out gonococcal, chlamydial, or HSV origin. Chlamydia is the most common cause of neonatal conjunctivitis. Gonococcal conjunctivitis is the most serious cause of ophthalmia neonatorum owing to concerns of the bacteria causing blindness (American Academy of Pediatrics, 2009b). In the newborn, gonococcal conjunctivitis requires intramuscular (IM) **ceftriaxone** (50 mg/kg, maximum 125 mg). If there are extraocular manifestations, a 7-day course of IM or IV **ceftriaxone** is warranted. **Ceftriaxone** is not given to neonates with hyperbilirubinemia; **cefotaxime** (50 to 100 mg/kg/d divided bid for 7 d) is an alternative. To prevent ophthalmia neonatorum, the Centers for Disease Control and Prevention (CDC) recommends prophylactic administration of antibiotic eye medication within 1 hour of delivery. The recommended antibiotic is **erythromycin** ointment 0.5 percent (0.25 to 0.5 in. to each eye). If **erythromycin** is

Table 26–2 **Clinical and Laboratory Features of Conjunctivitis**

Type	Common Patient Group	Common Pathogens	Clinical Features
Ophthalmia neonatorum	Infants <1 mo	*Neisseria gonorrhoeae, Chlamydia*	Erythema, purulent exudate, chemosis
Bacterial conjunctivitis	Most common in children between 3 mo and 8 yr; can happen at any age	*Haemophilus influenzae* *Staphylococcus aureus* *Streptococcus pneumoniae*	Erythema, purulent discharge, itching, burning, matted eyelashes
Conjunctivitis-otitis syndrome	Predominantly in children <6 yr	*H. influenzae* (~73% of patients)	Bacterial conjunctivitis accompanied by otitis media
Gonococcal conjunctivitis	Newborns, sexually promiscuous teens, and adults	*N. gonorrhoeae*	Eye is markedly inflamed, with copious discharge and swollen lids
Blepharitis	Any age group	May be infected with *S. aureus*	Chronic or acute inflammation of the eyelash follicles
Hordeolum	Any age group	*S. aureus*	Tender, swollen red furuncle along eyelid margin
Viral conjunctivitis	Any age group, most common in children	Adenovirus Herpes simplex virus	Redness, chemosis, photophobia

not available, as happened in a recent shortage situation, the CDC states **azithromycin (AzaSite)** may be used, although there are no clinical efficacy data (CDC, 2009). The recommended dose of **azithromycin** is 1 to 2 drops placed in the conjunctival sac of each eye. Because this is a solution rather than an ointment, it is important to assure that drops are placed properly. **Gentamicin** ophthalmic ointment 0.3 percent may be used but cases of eyelid swelling and dermatitis have been reported (CDC, 2009). If **erythrymycin** ointment is not available, other options include **tobramycin** ophthalmic ointment or one of the fluoroquinolones. Because clinical efficacy for any of the acceptable alternatives has not been established, the CDC recommends a posthospital visit 48 to 72 hours postdischarge (2009).

Chlamydial conjunctivitis in the newborn requires treatment with **systemic erythromycin** (30–50 mg/kg/d) for 2 to 3 weeks; topical treatment is ineffective (American Academy of Pediatrics, 2009a). A short course of **azithromycin** 20 mg/kg per day for 3 days may also be effective (Hammerschlag et al, 1998). Chlamydial conjunctivitis is not prevented by prophylactic use of **erythromycin** at birth; therefore, any mucopurulent eye discharge in the first few weeks of life should be evaluated for chlamydia.

Bacterial Conjunctivitis

Children between ages 3 months and 8 years are most likely to have staphylococcal, streptococcal, or *Haemophilus* conjunctivitis. Nontypable *H. influenzae* is seen more in warmer climates between May and October. *S. pneumoniae* is seen in colder climates and during the winter. *S. aureus* shows no geographic or seasonal pattern. In studies of children with acute bacterial conjunctivitis, *H. influenzae* is the most common organism isolated in children less than 7 years (Hautala, Hautala, & Koskela, 2008; Smith & Waycaster, 2009). *Staphylococcus aureus* and *Pseudomonas aeruginosa* are the most common pathogens in the elderly (older than age 70) (Hautala, Hautala, & Koskela, 2008).

Although bacterial conjunctivitis is considered a self-limited disease (unless caused by gonorrhea), patients who receive **topical antibiotic therapy** have faster clinical improvement. When conjunctivitis prevents the patient from going to school or work, **antibiotics** can speed the recovery. Most schools require treatment for the child to return to school.

Uncomplicated conjunctivitis may be treated with **sulfacetamide** 10 percent **ophthalmic solution** or **ointment, erythromycin ointment, trimethoprim/polymyxin B (Polytrim),** or **bacitracin/polymyxin B (Polysporin). Sulfacetamide** has no coverage against *H. influenzae*, a fact that should be considered in choosing an antibiotic. Gram's stain or culture can further guide the choice of **antibiotic.** Other choices for uncomplicated bacterial conjunctivitis include **tobramycin, gentamicin, azithomycin,** or any of the **fluoroquinolones.** See Table 26–3 for dosing information.

Table 26–3 ● **Dosage Schedule: Ophthalmic Anti-Infectives**

Drug	Indication	Dose	Comments
Sulfacetamide sodium	Conjunctivitis Trachoma	Solution: 1–2 drops q2–3h during the day, less often at night Trachoma: 2 drops q2h with systemic therapy Ointment: Small amount tid-qid and qhs	Not recommended for infants <2 mo
Erythromycin	Conjunctivitis and flare-ups of chronic blepharitis Prophylaxis of ophthalmia neonatorum	Ointment: 0.25- to 0.5-in. ribbon 2–3 times/d Ointment: 0.5-in. ribbon of ointment in each conjunctival sac no later than 1 h after birth	Safe in infants Use a new tube in each infant
Azithromycin	Bacterial conjunctivitis	Age ≥1 yr: 1 drop in affected eye(s) bid (8–12 h apart) for 2 d and then once daily for the next 5 d	Not recommended for children < age 1 year
Gentamicin	Conjunctivitis	Severe infections: 2 drops q1h or 0.5-in. ointment q3–4h; may prolong interval as infection improves Mild/moderate infections: 0.5 drop q4h *or* 0.5 in. of ointment bid–tid	May be used in children
Tobramycin	Susceptible infections of conjunctiva and cornea	Severe infections: 2 drops q1h or 0.5-in. ointment q3–4h; may prolong interval as infection improves Mild to moderate infections: 1–2 drops q4h *or* 0.5 in. of ointment bid–tid	Safe and effective in children >1 mo

Continued

Table 26–3 ◉ **Dosage Schedule: Ophthalmic Anti-Infectives—cont'd**

Drug	Indication	Dose	Comments
Ciprofloxacin	Susceptible infections of conjunctiva and corneal ulcer	Solution: Corneal ulcer: day 1, 2 drops q15min, then 2 drops q30min; day 2, 2 drops q1h; days 3 to 14, 2 drops q4h; treat for 14 d or until corneal epithelialization occurs Conjunctivitis: 1–2 drops q2h while awake × 2 d; then 1–2 drops q4h while awake for next 5 d Ointment: For conjunctivitis: 0.5 in. tid × 2 d, then bid × 5 d	Solution not recommended for children <1 yr Ointment not recommended for children <2 yr
Gatifloxacin	Bacterial conjunctivitis	*Adults and Children ≥1 yr:* 1 drop q2h while awake (max 8 times/day) on days 1 and 2; then 1 drop q4h while awake for next 5 d	Not recommended for children <1 yr
Levofloxacin	Bacterial conjunctivitis	*Adults and Children ≥1 yr:* 1–2 drops in affected eye q2h while awake on days 1 and 2; then 1–2 drops q4h while awake, up to 4 doses/d on d 3–7	Not recommended for children <1 yr
Moxifloxacin	Bacterial conjunctivitis	*Adults and Children ≥1 yr:* 1 drop in affected eye tid for 7 d	Not recommended for children <1 yr
Norfloxacin	Susceptible infections of conjunctiva and cornea	1–2 drops qid for up to 7 d; may administer q2h while awake on day 1	Not recommended for children <1 yr
Ofloxacin	Susceptible infections of conjunctiva and corneal ulcer	Corneal ulcer: days 1 and 2, 1–2 drops q20min while awake and 4 and 6 h after retiring; days 3 to 9, 1–2 drops q1h while awake; thereafter, 1–2 drops qid Conjunctivitis: 1–2 drops q2–4h while awake × 2 d, then 1–2 drops qid while awake for next 5 d	Not recommended for children <1 yr
Polymyxin-trimethoprim	Susceptible infections of conjunctiva and cornea	1 drop q3h for 7–10 d, up to 6 doses/d	Not recommended for infants <2 mo Contraindicated in ophthalmia neonatorum
Polymyxin B–bacitracinophthalmic	Susceptible infections of conjunctiva and cornea	Ointment: Apply 0.5-in. ribbon q3–4 h	May be used safely in children
Trifluridine	Herpes simplex Type 1 and 2 keratoconjunctivitis	1 drop every 2 hours while awake (max 9 drops a day). After reepithelialization, 1 drop q4h for 7 d.	Do not exceed recommended dose. Not recommended for children <6 yrs

Bacterial conjunctivitis caused by dacryostenosis may be treated with **erythromycin ointment** (Blosser, 2009).

Conjunctivitis-Otitis Syndrome

The syndrome of conjunctivitis accompanied by otitis media predominantly occurs in children younger than age 6 years. *H. influenzae* is the causative organism in the majority (73%) of patients with conjunctivitis-otitis syndrome (Wald, 1997). Treatment is **systemic antibiotics** that are effective against *H. influenzae.* **Amoxicillin** dosed at 80 to 90 mg/kg a day is the first-line drug of choice. If **systemic antibiotics** are prescribed, **topical ophthalmic treatment** is usually not needed. See Chapter 45 for management of otitis media.

Gonococcal Conjunctivitis

Purulent bacterial conjunctivitis usually responds to **topical antibiotic therapy.** An exception is hyperpurulent gonococcal conjunctivitis, which is usually found in the newborn and in sexually promiscuous teenagers and adults. The eye discharge should be gram stained and cultured to confirm the diagnosis. Treatment consists of **parenteral antibiotics** and **sterile saline irrigations** to clear the exudate. Use of a **beta-lactamase–resistant cephalosporin** such as **ceftriaxone** is warranted. Because untreated gonococcal infection can penetrate the intact eye, treatment should begin as soon as the diagnosis is suspected.

Blepharitis

Blepharitis is an acute or chronic inflammation of the eyelash follicles and meibomian glands of the eyelids. Treatment consists of scrubbing the eyelashes with gentle, no-tears shampoo and applying **erythromycin ophthalmic ointment** (0.25-in. ribbon to each eye twice a day) until the symptoms clear and then for an additional 7 days. Ointment is preferred in the treatment of blepharitis due to the increased contact with the ocular tissue. The patient should not wear contact lenses during treatment, and the contacts should be sterilized before reinserting. Eye makeup should be discarded to prevent reinfection (Blosser, 2009).

Hordeolum

Hordeolum, commonly called a *sty,* is an infection of the sebaceous gland of the eyelash or eyelid. The causative organism is *S. aureus.* Treatment consists of warm, moist compresses four times a day for 15 minutes each time. **Antibiotic eyedrops (sulfacetamide 10%)** or **ointment (erythromycin 0.5%)** should be applied four times a day until the symptoms subside and then for an additional 2 to 3 days. The hordeolum usually spontaneously ruptures; if it does not, the patient should be referred to an ophthalmologist. Multiple or recurrent hordeolum may require systemic antibiotic treatment with **erythromycin** or **dicloxacillin.**

Viral Conjunctivitis

Viral conjunctivitis is usually caused by an adenovirus, HSV, or herpes zoster. Simple viral conjunctivitis caused by adenovirus is treated with **sulfacetamide 10 percent solution** or **ointment** four times a day or a **broad-spectrum antibiotic,** such as **tobramycin,** to prevent secondary bacterial infection. The course of the conjunctivitis runs 12 to 15 days. Herpes keratitis is a potentially serious consequence of infection with HSV. If herpes keratitis is suspected, a referral to an ophthalmologist for diagnosis and treatment is indicated. Two commonly used **antiviral agents** are **trifluridine** and **vidarabine.** Table 26–3 presents the dosage schedule of **ophthalmic anti-infectives.**

Rational Drug Selection

Efficacy

A determination of the suspected organism guides the choice of an **ophthalmic antibiotic.** If *H. influenzae* is high on the list of suspected organisms, then **sulfacetamide** should not be the first choice for treatment because it has poor coverage for *H. influenzae.* A combination product such as **Polysporin** or **Polytrim** provides good coverage for the common organisms that cause bacterial conjunctivitis. In infants, **erythromycin** is usually the drug of choice because of its good coverage, and ointment is more easily administered than drops (Table 26–4).

Table 26–4 ◆ **Available Dosage Forms: Ophthalmic Anti-Infectives**

Drug	Dosage Form	How Supplied	Cost
Sulfacetamide Sodium			
Bleph-10	10% solution	In 2.5, 5, 10 mL	$22.70/5 mL
	10% ointment	In 3.5 g	
Sodium Sulamyd	10% solution	In 5 and 15 mL	$29.29/15 mL
	30% solution	In 15 mL	
	10% ointment	In 3.5 g	
Generic	10% solution	In 5 and 15 mL	$12.99/15 mL
	30% solution	In 15 mL	
	10% ointment	In 3.5 g	
Erythromycin			
Ilotycin, Generic	Ointment: 5 mg/g	In 3.5 g	$12.99/3.5 gm
Azithromycin			
Azasite	Solution: 1%	2.5 mL	$90.28/2.5 mL
Tobramycin			
Tobrex	Solution: 0.3%	In 5-mL dropper bottle	$63.40/5 mL
	Ointment: 3 mg/g	In 3.5 g	$80.02/3.5 g
Generic	Solution: 0.3%	In 5-mL dropper bottle	$15.99/5 mL
Gentamicin			
Garamycin, Genoptic	Solution: 3 mg/mL	In 5-mL dropper bottle	$8.99/1 mL
	Ointment: 3 mg/g	In 3.5 g	$24.99
Generic	Solution: 3 mg/mL	In 5-mL dropper bottle	11.99/5 mL
	Ointment: 3 mg/g	In 3.5 g	

Continued

Table 26–4 ◈ **Available Dosage Forms: Ophthalmic Anti-Infectives—cont'd**

Drug	Dosage Form	How Supplied	Cost
Gatifloxacin			
Zymar	0.3% solution	In 2.5 mL In 5 mL	$87.53/5 mL
Levofloxacin			
Quixin	0.5% solution	In 5 mL	$56.99/5 mL
Moxifloxacin			
Vigamox	0.5% solution	In 3 mL	$90.72/3 mL
Norfloxacin			
Chibroxin	Solution: 3 mg/mL	In 5-mL Ocumeters	$46.99
Ciprofloxacin			
Ciloxan	Solution: 3 mg/mL	In 2.5- and 5-mL dropper bottles	$68.33/5 mL
Ofloxacin			
Ocuflox	Solution: 3 mg/mL	In 5- and 10-mL dropper bottles	$57.32/5 mg $91.61/10 mg
Polymyxin B-Trimethoprim			
Polytrim Ophthalmic	Solution: polymyxin B 10,000 U/g, trimethoprim 1 g/mL	In 10 mL	$43.25/10 mL
Polymyxin B-Bacitracin Ophthalmic			
Polysporin Ophthalmic, Generic	Ointment: polymyxin B 10,000 U/g, bacitracin 500 U/g	In 3.5 g	$34.99/3.5 gm
Trifluridine			
Viroptic	Solution: 1%	7.5 mL	$139.01/7.5 mL

Cost

The least expensive **ophthalmic** is generally generic **erythromycin, bacitracin,** or **sulfacetamide 10 percent. Azithromycin** and the **fluoroquinolones** are more expensive, up to ten times the cost of erythromycin.

Monitoring

There is no laboratory monitoring necessary with **ophthalmic anti-infectives.**

Patient Education

Administration

Administration of ophthalmic medications can be challenging for patients. The patient should be instructed in the importance of keeping the tip of the dropper or tube from touching the eye, fingertips, or any other surface to prevent contamination. Hands should be washed before and after instillation of eye medications. Eye medications should not be shared.

Ophthalmic ointment should be transferred from the tube onto a moistened cotton swab, then rolled into each conjunctival sac. Use one swab for each eye to prevent contamination.

Eyedrops are self-administered by holding the bottle of solution in the dominant hand and using the pointer finger of the other hand to gently pull down the lower eyelid to form a "pocket" for the solution to be dropped into. The patient can use this method for both eyes.

For children who may resist the "bull's-eye" method of instilling eyedrops, one of three methods may be used. School-age children can assist with the instillation by pulling down their own lower eyelid, while the parent or care provider instills the eyedrop into the pocket formed. If this method doesn't work, a child may lie down on his or her back and close the eyes, keeping the head still. A drop of the antibiotic or antiviral is placed on the inner canthus. After the eyedrops are placed on the internal canthus, the child should slowly open his or her eyes without moving the head. The eyedrops instill into the eyes. Younger children require immobilization to instill eyedrops or ophthalmic ointment. This can be accomplished by two people, one to hold the child and the other to administer the medication.

Adverse Reactions

The patient should be instructed that there might be transient burning or stinging with most of the **ophthalmic anti-infective agents.** If burning is severe or prolonged, the patient should contact the provider. Other adverse effects should be discussed with the patient, with instructions to report any unusual symptoms.

CLINICAL PEARL

Proper Instillation of Eye Medications

Proper Instillation of Eyedrops

- Wash hands before administering eyedrops.
- Tilt head back or lie on back.
- Gently pull down lower eyelid to form a "pocket" to place the drop of medication into.
- Squeeze the medication onto the eye without touching eye with the dropper.
- Close eye. Do not rub. Try not to blink.
- To prevent cross-contamination, do not use medication labeled for another patient.
- Wait at least 5 minutes between administration if administering more than one eye medication.

Proper Instillation of Eye Ointment

- Wash hands prior to administering eye medications.
- Warm the ointment by holding it in the hand for 1 to 2 minutes.
- With first use of a new tube, squeeze out and discard the first 0.25 inch of medication.
- Angle head back or lie on back.
- Gently pull down lower eyelid to form a "pocket" to place the drop of medication into.
- Squeeze 0.25 to 0.5 inch of medication onto the eye without touching eye with tip of tube.
- Close eye for 1 to 2 minutes. Do not rub.
- Wipe excess medication from around the eye with a tissue.
- To prevent cross-contamination, do not use medication labeled for another patient.
- Wait at least 10 minutes between administrations if administering more than one eye medication.
- Temporary blurred vision is typical after administration of ophthalmic ointment.

Lifestyle Management

The most important nonpharmacological measure is for the patient and family members to wash their hands thoroughly whenever the infected eyes are touched and before instilling medication. Hand washing will decrease spread of the infection to other contacts.

The patient with an eye infection should not share hand towels with the rest of the family. The patient with an eye infection should use a separate towel or paper towels to prevent the spread of infection to family members.

Eye makeup needs to be thrown away after an eye infection because mascara and other makeup can harbor bacteria or viruses, and the patient can become reinfected.

Crusty, purulent discharge can be irritating and may be distressing to children whose eyes become "glued shut" with the dried discharge. Purulent discharge can be removed with cotton balls moistened with warm water. The cotton ball is wiped gently from the interior canthus to the external canthus to remove discharge. A clean cotton ball should be used for each wipe and for each eye. If a washcloth is used, patients or parents should be instructed to use a clean area of the cloth for each swipe of the eye and to use a clean washcloth every time.

Antiglaucoma Agents

Glaucoma is a group of disorders in which IOP damages the optic nerve. In the United States, glaucoma affects 4 million people and is the leading cause of blindness in African Americans (Glaucoma Research Foundation, 2009). Glaucoma can affect a patient of any age; one in 10,000 newborns is diagnosed with congenital glaucoma and 8 percent of adults over age 70 years are diagnosed with glaucoma (Glaucoma Research Foundation, 2009). The patient may have open-angle glaucoma, in which a block at the level of the trabecular meshwork impairs aqueous humor reabsorption, or the patient may have angle-closure glaucoma, which develops when the normal path of the aqueous flow is interrupted in an eye with a shallow anterior chamber. Current medical therapies are aimed at decreasing the production of aqueous humor at the ciliary body and at increasing the outflow of this fluid from the angle structures. Glaucoma or the suspicion of glaucoma requires evaluation and treatment by an ophthalmologist. Primary care providers need to be aware of the medications that are prescribed, the drug interactions that may occur, and the adverse effects of the prescribed medications.

Pharmacodynamics

The **antiglaucoma agents** can be roughly divided into the following categories: **beta blockers**, **adrenergic agonists**, **miotics**, **carbonic anhydrase (CA) inhibitors**, **sympathomimetics**, and the **prostaglandin agonist latanoprost** (Xalatan).

CLINICAL PEARL

Tips for Administering Eye Medications to a Child

If only one adult is available to administer eyedrops, then the adult can sit on the floor with the child between his or her legs, with the child's legs in the same direction as the adult's. The child's head can be immobilized between the adult's thighs and the arms held firmly down under the adult's thighs. This leaves the adult's hands free to instill the medication. The child may kick, but this will not affect the administration of the medication. Although this method may sound drastic, trying to administer eye medication to a squirming toddler or preschooler can be almost impossible, and with this method the eyedrops can be effectively administered in less than 1 minute.

Beta Blockers

Beta-adrenergic antagonists, also known as **beta blockers**, reduce IOP by interference with the cyclic adenosine monophosphate (cAMP) induced production of aqueous humor by the ciliary processes in the eye, although the exact mechanism of action is not known. IOP is reduced in patients with either elevated or normal IOP. Visual acuity, pupil size, and accommodation do not appear to be affected by **ophthalmic beta blockers**.

Miotics, Cholinesterase Inhibitors

Cholinesterase inhibitors are indirect-acting agents that inhibit the cholinesterase enzyme. Topical application to the eye causes intense miosis and muscle contraction. The IOP is reduced by a decreased resistance to aqueous outflow. The **cholinesterase inhibitors** are divided into reversible and irreversible agents. The **reversible agents physostigmine** and **demecarium** combine with cholinesterase, and as the resulting union is hydrolyzed, the cholinesterase regenerates over a number of hours. **Echothiophate iodide (Phospholine)** is considered an **irreversible agent** that binds to cholinesterase in a covalent bond that does not hydrolyze. Cholinesterase must be synthesized or drawn from other parts of the body in order for ophthalmic action to return to normal.

Miotics, Direct-Acting

The **direct-acting miotics** are **parasympathomimetic (cholinergic) drugs** with muscarinic effects. When applied topically, these drugs produce pupillary constriction, stimulate the ciliary muscles, and increase aqueous humor outflow. They also reduce outflow resistance by contraction of the iris sphincter. IOP is decreased with the increase in outflow.

Carbonic Anhydrase Inhibitors

CA inhibitors decrease aqueous humor secretion by slowing the formation of bicarbonate ions. This leads to reduction in sodium and fluid transport, leading to decreased aqueous humor production and subsequent decreased IOP.

Sympathomimetics

Sympathomimetics applied topically cause vasoconstriction, papillary dilation, and reduction of IOP. It is believed that sympathomimetics reduce IOP by reducing the production of aqueous humor and by increasing aqueous humor outflow.

Alpha-Adrenergic Agonists

Alpha-adrenergic agonists reduce IOP by reducing the production of aqueous humor and by increasing uveoscleral outflow.

Prostaglandin Agonists

Latanoprost is a selective agonist of a prostaglandin receptor known as the FP receptor. **Latanoprost** increases the outflow of aqueous humor by acting on the FP receptor. This leads to decreased IOP. **Bimatoprost (Lumigan)** is a **prostamide**, a synthetic prostaglandin. **Bimatoprost** lowers IOP by increasing aqueous humor outflow. **Unoprostone (Rescula)** and **Travoprost (Travatan)** are **synthetic prostaglandin $F_{2\alpha}$ analogues** whose exact mechanism of action is unknown, although they are thought to reduce IOP by decreasing uveoscleral outflow. **Bimatoprost** is also marketed as **Latisse** for treatment of eyelash hypotrichosis. Patients should experience thicker and darker eyelashes after 2 months of treatment.

Pharmacokinetics

Little is known about the specific pharmacokinetic parameters of the **beta blockers**. Duration of action is noted in Table 26–5. What is known is determined by clinical observation of pharmacodynamic responses. An unknown amount of absorption occurs, but systemic absorption is known to occur because both cardiac and pulmonary signs of **beta blocker** activity can occur. **Beta blockers** are metabolized in the liver and excreted in the urine and feces.

The pharmacokinetics of **cholinesterase inhibitors** and the **direct-acting miotics** are not known. Duration of action is noted in Table 26–5.

Following topical administration into the eye, **brinzolamide (Azopt)** is absorbed systemically, although plasma concentrations remain low and generally below the level of detection. It is widely distributed, including into the breast milk in animal studies. It may cross the placenta. **Brinzolamide** is metabolized to *N*-desthyl brinzolamide and excreted primarily in the urine.

Dorzolamide (Trusopt), when applied topically to the eye, has some systemic absorption, although no free drug is measured in the plasma. **Dorzolamide** is excreted primarily unchanged in the urine.

Methazolamide (Neptazane) is an oral **CA inhibitor.** It is well absorbed from the gastrointestinal (GI) tract. **Methazolamide** is distributed throughout the body, including the plasma, cerebrospinal fluid, aqueous humor of the eye, red blood cells, bile, and extracellular fluid. Its exact metabolism is not described. Excretion is primarily renal, with 25 percent of the drug excreted unchanged in the urine.

The pharmacokinetics of the **sympathomimetics** is not known.

Following ophthalmic administration of **brimonidine (Alphagan)**, peak serum levels occur in 1 to 4 hours. **Brimonidine** is extensively metabolized in the liver and eliminated in the urine.

Latanoprost is absorbed through the cornea, where it is hydrolyzed to become biologically active. Plasma levels of **latanoprost** can be measured. Distribution is unknown. It is not known whether **latanoprost** crosses the placenta, although in animal studies adverse fetal effects were found. It is not known whether **latanoprost** is excreted in breast milk. **Latanoprost** is metabolized via fatty-acid beta oxidation in the liver. The metabolites are

Table 26–5 ▶ **Pharmacokinetics: Antiglaucoma Agents**

Drug	Duration
Beta Blockers	
Betaxolol, carteolol	12 h
Levobunolol, metipranolol, timolol	12–24 h
Miotics	
Carbachol	6–8 h
Pilocarpine	4–8 h
Echothiophate	Days/weeks
Carbonic Anhydrase Inhibitors	
Acetazolamide	8–12 h
Brinzolamide	NA
Dorzolamide	About 8 h
Methazolamide	10–18 h
Sympathomimetics	
Epinephrine, dipivefrin	12 h
Alpha-Adrenergic Agonists	
Apraclonidine	7–12 h
Brimonidine	12 h
Prostaglandin Analogues	
Latanoprost	24 h
Bimatoprost	1.5 h
Unoprostone	<1 h
Travoprost	<1 h

NA = information not available.

excreted primarily in the urine (88%). **Bimatoprost** is absorbed and reaches a steady state in the plasma, with 12 percent remaining unbound in human plasma. It is metabolized by oxidation and is excreted in the urine (67%) and feces (25%). **Travoprost** is rapidly absorbed from the cornea and peaks in the plasma within 30 minutes. **Travoprost** is hydrolyzed by esterases in the cornea into free acid. Elimination of **travoprost** is rapid with unmeasurable levels within an hour of administration. **Unoprostone** is rapidly absorbed from the cornea and hydrolyzed into unoprostone-free acid, which is eliminated rapidly in the urine. Table 26–5 presents the pharmacokinetics of **antiglaucoma agents**.

Pharmacotherapeutics

Precautions and Contraindications

Although primary-care providers do not prescribe **ophthalmic antiglaucoma agents**, the medications are absorbed and systemic levels reached in great enough amounts to cause complications of chronic conditions. Coordination of care with the ophthalmologist will ensure the optimal care for the patient's glaucoma and other medical problems.

The **beta blocker ophthalmic medications** are contraindicated in patients with asthma, a history of asthma, chronic obstructive pulmonary disease (COPD), or other pulmonary disease. There may be bronchospasm associated with the use of **topical beta blockers**, which may prove fatal to patients with respiratory disease.

Beta Blockers

Beta blockers suppress conduction through the atrioventricular (AV) node; therefore, **topical beta blockers** are contraindicated in patients with bradycardia or advanced AV block. **Beta blockers** should not be used in patients with compromised ventricular dysfunction, patients in cardiogenic shock, or patients with systolic congestive heart failure. Discontinue **topical beta blockers** at the first sign of cardiac failure. **Beta blockers** are contraindicated for patients with hypotension (standing blood pressure [SBP] less than 100 mm Hg).

Beta blockers should be used with caution in patients with poorly controlled diabetes mellitus because **beta blockers** can prolong or enhance hypoglycemia by interfering with glycogenolysis. **Beta blockers** may also mask the signs and symptoms of acute hypoglycemia. Because they may mask the clinical signs of hypothyroidism, **beta blockers** should be used with caution in patients with hyperthyroidism.

Patients using **beta blockers** during surgery should be monitored closely for signs of cardiac failure. Severe, protracted hypotension and difficulty in restarting the heart have been reported. **Beta blockers** may need to be withdrawn before surgery, with the last dose 2 days prior to surgery.

Beta blockers are contraindicated in patients with Raynaud's disease or peripheral vascular or cerebrovascular disease because decreased cardiac output can exacerbate symptoms.

Ophthalmic beta blockers are Pregnancy Category C. Fetal anomalies and fetotoxicity have been observed in animal studies. Most of the **ophthalmic beta blockers** are excreted in breast milk and are contraindicated in breastfeeding. **Ophthalmic beta blocker agents** are used in children, but they must be monitored closely.

Miotics

The **miotics** are contraindicated when active inflammation of the eye is present. They are also contraindicated when constriction is not wanted, for example, in iritis, uveitis, and some forms of secondary glaucoma.

The **miotics** are Pregnancy Category C, with **demecarium (Humorsol)** given the classification of Pregnancy Category X. Use with caution in lactating women. Use with extreme caution in children.

Carbonic Anhydrase Inhibitors

Dorzolamide and **brinzolamide** contain **sulfonamide** and are absorbed in amounts great enough to cause hypersensitivity reactions in patients with sulfonamide sensitivity. **Dorzolamide** and **brinzolamide** are Pregnancy Category C. They are contraindicated in lactation, and their safety for use in children is not known.

Methazolamide is contraindicated in patients with hyponatremia, hypokalemia, renal disease, liver disease, suprarenal gland failure, hyperchloremic acidosis, adrenocortical insufficiency, and severe pulmonary obstruction. It is Pregnancy Category C and not recommended for use in children.

Sympathomimetics

Apraclonidine (Iopidine) is contraindicated in patients with clonidine hypersensitivity. **Dipivefrin (AKPro, Propine)** is contraindicated in patients with narrow-angle glaucoma and aphakic patients. **Apraclonidine** is Pregnancy Category C, and **dipivefrin** is Pregnancy Category B. They are not recommended for use by nursing mothers or by children.

Alpha-Adrenergic Agonists

Brimonidine is contraindicated in patients taking **monoamine oxidase inhibitors (MAOIs). Brimonidine** should be used with caution in patients with cardiac, renal, or liver disease. **Brimonidine** should not be instilled with contact lenses in place. The patient should wait 15 minutes after instilling **brimonidine** before replacing contacts. **Brimonidine** is Pregnancy Category B. **Brimonidine** should be avoided in children and lactating women.

Prostaglandin Agonists

Latanoprost should not be administered while the patient is wearing contact lenses. **Latanoprost** should be used with caution in patients with intraocular inflammation (iritis) and aphakic patients. It is Pregnancy Category C. It is not recommended for use during lactation or by children. **Brimatoprost** is Pregnancy Category C. If **brimatoprost (Latisse)** is being prescribed for hypotrichosis, it may lower IOP in patients with normal IOP, but the magnitude of change is not clinically significant.

Adverse Drug Reactions

All of the **antiglaucoma medications** may cause transient discomfort or tearing. Blurred vision, photophobia, and hyperemia may also occur. Allergic conjunctivitis may occur with any of the **topical ophthalmic medications.**

Headaches and dizziness may occur with the use of **beta blockers.** Patients may exhibit **systemic beta blocker** effects with the use of **ophthalmic preparations.** Symptoms include bradycardia, hypotension, bronchospasm, and, rarely, AV block.

Miotics may cause corneal clouding, ciliary spasm, headache, induced myopia, and retinal detachment. Patients may have systemic anticholinergic effects if excessive absorption occurs. These symptoms include headache, hypertension, salivation, sweating, nausea, and vomiting. Iris cysts may be seen with cholinesterase inhibitors.

Many patients (about 25%) report dysgeusia, or bitter taste in the mouth, after ocular administration of **CA inhibitors.** Superficial punctate keratitis is reported in 10 to 15 percent of patients using **ophthalmic preparations.**

Systemic CA inhibitors (methazolamide) may cause melena and GI upset, such as anorexia, nausea, and vomiting. Glycosuria and urinary frequency have been reported. Weakness, malaise, fatigue, bone marrow depression, thrombocytopenia, leukopenia, and hemolytic anemia have been reported with use of **methazolamide.** Renal calculi and nephrotoxicity have also been reported. Fever is a rare adverse effect of **methazolamide.**

The local effects of the **sympathomimetics** include conjunctival or corneal pigmentation. Systemic effects of **topical sympathomimetic** use include headache, hypertension, tachycardia, and cardiac arrhythmias (with excessive absorption).

The local effects of **alpha agonists** that occur in 10 to 30 percent of patients include the sensation of a foreign body in the eye and ocular pain. Systemic adverse effects include dry mouth, drowsiness, and headache. Corneal staining may occur.

The local adverse effects reported in 5 to 15 percent of patients using **prostaglandin agonists** include foreign body sensations, keratopathy, and iridal discoloration. The iridal discoloration may be gradual (many months) and is caused by an increase in the amount of brown pigmentation in the iris because of an increased number of melanosomes in melanocytes. The color change may be permanent. **Bimatoprost (Latisse)** may cause permanent brown iris pigmentation and hair growth outside the treatment area and must be applied only to the upper eyelid, using the sterile applicator supplied, and not allowed to drip down onto the cheek or other skin area.

Drug Interactions

Beta Blockers

The use of **ophthalmic beta blockers** with **systemic beta blockers** may cause additive beta blockade effects. Coadministration of **ophthalmic timolol** has caused bradycardia and asystole.

Miotics

Carbachol and **pilocarpine solution** have no reported drug interactions. **Pilocarpine ocular sustained-release inserts (Ocusert Pilo)** potentiate the absorption of epinephrine. **Echothiophate** may potentiate the effects of succinylcholine, leading to respiratory and possibly cardiovascular collapse. **Echothiophate** may have additive effects when used with **systemic anticholinesterases** used in the treatment of myasthenia gravis. There is additive toxicity (increased parasympathomimetic effects) if organic pesticides or carbamate is absorbed by someone using **ophthalmic echothiophate.**

Carbonic Anhydrase Inhibitors

Concurrent use of **CA inhibitors (topical brinzolamide, dorzolamide, and systemic methazolamide)** and high-dose **salicylates** may lead to metabolic acidosis and salicylate toxicity, which allow greater penetration of salicylate into the central nervous system (CNS). This interaction is theoretical with the **topical CA inhibitors. CA inhibitors** may inhibit excretion of basic drugs and promote excretion of acidic drugs. The concurrent use of **oral** and **topical CA inhibitors** is not recommended.

Sympathomimetics

There are no known drug interactions with **ophthalmic dipivefrin. Apraclonidine** may interact with **cardiovascular drugs. Apraclonidine** should not be used by patients who are using **MAOIs** because concurrent use may cause a hypertensive crisis.

Alpha-Adrenergic Agonists

The **alpha-adrenergic agonists** are contraindicated with the use of **MAOIs**. There may be additive CNS depression if **topical alpha-adrenergic agonists** are used concurrently with **CNS depressants. Tricyclic antidepressants** can affect the metabolism and uptake of circulating amines. Medications that may cause bradycardia (**beta blockers, antihypertensives,** and **cardiac glycosides**) may have additive depression of pulse and blood pressure if used concurrently with **alpha-adrenergic agonists.**

Prostaglandin Agonists

The only reported drug interaction noted with **latanoprost** is **thimerosal,** which can cause precipitation if administered concurrently. Advise the patient to wait at least 5 minutes between administration of two ophthalmic medications if one contains thimerosol.

Table 26–6 presents drug interactions with **antiglaucoma agents.**

Table 26–6 ■ **Drug Interactions: Antiglaucoma Agents**

Drug	Interacting Drug	Possible Effect	Implications
Beta Blockers			
Betaxolol, carteolol, metipranolol	Oral beta blockers	Additive effects, excessive hypotension, increased reduction of IOP	Use with caution
	Antihypertensive agents	Additive antihypertensive effects	Monitor BP
	Antiarrhythmics (diltiazem, verapamil, amiodarone, digoxin)	Additive effects; may cause significant effects on AV node conduction; may cause complete heart block	Use with caution, monitor closely
	Beta agonist bronchodilators (albuterol, metaproterenol [Alupent], salmeterol)	Beta blocker may antagonize the effects of beta agonists	Use with caution; avoid concurrent use if possible
Levobunolol	Oral beta blockers	Additive effects, excessive hypotension, increased reduction of IOP	Use with caution
	Cimetidine	Interferes with hepatic metabolism of levobunolol, potentially increasing its effects	Avoid concurrent use
	Sympathomimetics, including inhaled beta agonists	Antagonism of desired therapeutic effects	Avoid concurrent use
Timolol	Oral beta blockers	Additive effects, excessive hypotension, increased reduction of IOP	Use with caution
	Antihypertensive agents	Additive antihypertensive effects	Monitor BP
	Antiarrhythmics (diltiazem, verapamil, amiodarone, digoxin)	Additive effects; may cause significant effects on AV node conduction; may cause complete heart block	Use with caution; monitor closely
	Verapamil	Coadministration of ophthalmic timolol has caused bradycardia and asystole	Do not use concurrently
	Beta agonist bronchodilators (albuterol, metaproterenol [Alupent], salmeterol)	Timolol may antagonize the effects of beta agonists	Use with caution; avoid concurrent use if possible
	Quinidine	Quinidine can potentiate timolol-induced bradycardia	Use with caution; monitor closely

Continued

Table 26–6 ■ **Drug Interactions: Antiglaucoma Agents—cont'd**

Drug	Interacting Drug	Possible Effect	Implications
Miotics			
Carbachol, pilocarpine	No significant interactions		
Echothiophate	Succinylcholine (anesthetic)	May potentiate succinylcholine, leading to possible respiratory and cardiovascular collapse	Do not use concurrently; consider stopping echothiophate before surgery
	Systemic anticholinesterases	Additive effects	Coadminister cautiously
	Carbamate or organophosphate insecticides and pesticides	Increased parasympathomimetic effects	Warn patients who are gardeners or workers who may be exposed to these chemicals to protect themselves with masks, frequent washing of skin, and clothing changes
Carbonic Anhydrase Inhibitors			
Acetazolamide	Barbiturates, aspirin, lithium	Excretion decreased	May lead to decreased effectiveness of interacting drugs
	Amphetamines, quinidine, procainamide, tricyclic antidepressants	Excretion decreased	May result in toxicity to interacting drugs
Brinzolamide	No known drug interactions		
Dorzolamide	Oral CA inhibitors	Potential additive effects	Concurrent use not recommended
Methazolamide	Diflunisal	Significant decrease in IOP	Avoid concurrent use
	Salicylates	Accumulation of methazolamide, resulting in CNS depression and metabolic acidosis	Avoid concurrent use
	Topiramate	Increased risk of renal stone formation	Avoid concurrent use
	Basic pH drugs	Inhibited renal excretion of basic drugs	
	Acidic pH drugsc	Promotes excretion of acidic drugs	Monitor potassium
	Corticosteroids, potassium-depleting diuretics	Hypokalemia	Monitor potassium
Sympathomimetics			
Epinephrine	Anesthetics (cyclopropane, halogenated hydrocarbons)	May cause cardiac arrhythmias	Discontinue epinephrine prior to surgery
Dipivefrin	No significant interactions		
Alpha-Adrenergic Agonists			
Apraclonidine	Cardiovascular agents: antihypertensives, cardiac glycosides, beta blockers	Apraclonidine may reduce pulse and BP	If using concurrently, monitor pulse and BP frequently
	MAOIs		Concurrent use contraindicated
Brimonidine	CNS depressants: alcohol, barbiturates, opiates, sedatives, or anesthetics	Additive CNS depression	Use with caution
	Beta blockers, antihypertensives	Brimonidine may reduce pulse pressure and BP	Use with caution; monitor cardiac status

Table 26–6 ■ Drug Interactions: Antiglaucoma Agents—cont'd

Drug	Interacting Drug	Possible Effect	Implications
	Tricyclic antidepressants	Tricyclic antidepressants can lower circulating amines	Monitor IOP closely if necessary to administer concurrently
	MAOIs		Use contraindicated
Prostaglandin Analogues			
Latanoprost	Thimerosal	Precipitation of latanoprost occurs when used concurrently	Administer at least 5 to 10 min apart
Bimatoprost	No significant interactions		Allow 5 min between application of other topical ophthalmic agents
Unoprostone	No significant interactions		Allow 5 min between application of other topical ophthalmic agents
Travoprost	No significant interactions		Allow 5 min between application of other topical ophthalmic agents

IOP = intraocular pressure; BP = blood pressure; AV = atrioventricular; CA = carbonic anhydrase; CNS = central nervous system; MAOIs = monoamixe oxidase inhibitors.

Clinical Use and Dosing

Glaucoma

Antiglaucoma medications are prescribed by ophthalmologists. Dosage is determined by the clinical condition of the patient.

Rational Drug Selection

The ophthalmologist determines what medication should be used, based on the patient's glaucoma type and underlying medical conditions.

Monitoring

The patient who is prescribed antiglaucoma medications may require monitoring of blood pressure and cardiovascular status. IOP is measured and monitored by the ophthalmologist. No laboratory monitoring is necessary.

Patient Education

Administration

The patient should be instructed to administer the medication exactly as the ophthalmologist has prescribed (Table 26–7). Abruptly stopping the medication can increase adverse effects.

Adverse Reactions

The patient should have been instructed by the ophthalmologist regarding the adverse effects of the medication. Reinforcement may be necessary. If the patient is experiencing adverse effects from the medication, the primary care provider can facilitate a referral back to the ophthalmologist.

Ocular Antiallergic and Anti-Inflammatory Agents

There are several ocular antiallergic and anti-inflammatory drugs. The antiallergic medications include the mast cell stabilizers lodoxamide (Alomide) and cromolyn sodium (Crolom). Levocabastine (Livostin), antazoline (Vasocon-A, Antazoline-V), ketotifen (Zaditor), pheniramine (Naphcon-A), and emedastine (Emadine) are antihistamines. The NSAIDs are flurbiprofen (Ocufen), suprofen (Profenal), diclofenac (Voltaren ophthalmic solution), nepafenac (Nevanac), and ketorolac (Acular). Corticosteroid ophthalmic agents are used as anti-inflammatories, although they are rarely used in primary care because of the serious adverse effects. Anti-inflammatory agents are found in single formula or in combination with antibiotics.

Pharmacodynamics

Ophthalmic Antiallergic Agents

The mast cell stabilizers limit hypersensitivity reactions by inhibiting the degranulation of sensitized mast cells that occur after exposure to specific antigens. They also inhibit the release of histamine and SRS-A (slow-reacting substance of anaphylaxis). They have no intrinsic antihistamine activity.

Table 26–7 ◆ **Available Dosage Forms: Antiglaucoma Agents**

Drug	Dosage Form	How Supplied
Beta Blockers		
BETAXOLOL		
Betoptic*	Solution: 5.6 mg/mL	In 2.5, 5, 10, 15 mL
Betoptic S*	Suspension: 2.8 mg/mL	In 2.5, 5, 10, 15 mL
CARTEOLOL		
Ocupress	1% solution	In 5-, 10-mL dropper bottles
Generic	1% solution	In 5-, 10-, 15-mL bottles
LEVOBUNOLOL		
Betagan	0.25% solution	In 5-, 10-mL bottles
	0.5% solution	In 2-, 5-, 10-, 15-mL bottles
AKBeta, Generic	0.25% solution	In 5-, 10-mL bottles
	0.5% solution	In 5-, 10-, 15-mL bottles
METIPRANOLOL		
OptiPranolol	0.3% solution	In 5-, 10-mL dropper bottle
TIMOLOL		
Timoptic	0.25%, 0.5% solution	In 2.5-, 5-, 10-, 15-mL bottles
		In 2.5, 5 mL
Timoptic-XE	0.25%, 0.5% gel	In 5-, 10-, 15-mL bottles
Betimol	0.25%, 0.5% solution	In 5-, 10-, 15-mL bottles
Generic	0.25%, 0.5% solution	In 5-, 10-, 15-mL bottles
COMBINATION PRODUCTS		
β blocker timolol & Carbonic anhydrase inhibitor dorzolamide Cosopt	Solution: Timolol 0.5% & dorzolamide 2%	10 mL
Miotics		
CARBACHOL		
Isopto Carbachol	0.75% solution, 1.5% solution	In 15-, 30-mL dropper bottles
	2.25% solution	In 15-mL bottles
	3% solution	In 15-, 30-mL dropper bottles
Carboptic	3% solution	In 15-mL bottle
PILOCARPINE		
Isopto Carpine	Solution: 0.25%, 0.5%, 1%, 2%, 3%, 4%, 5%, 6%, 10%	In 15-, 30-mL dropper bottles
		In 15-, 30-mL dropper bottles
Pilocar	Solution: 0.5%, 1%, 2%, 3%, 4%, 6%	In 3.5 g
Pilopine HS	Gel: 4%	In 15-, 30-mL dropper bottles
Generic	Solution: 0.5%, 1%, 2%, 4%, 6%, 8%	
ECHOTHIOPHATE		
Phospholine iodide	Powder for solution: 0.03%, 0.06%, 0.125%, 0.25%	In 5 mL diluent
Carbonic Anhydrase Inhibitors		
ACETAZOLAMIDE		
Diamox	Tablets: 125 mg, 250 mg	In 100 s
BRINZOLAMIDE		
Azopt*	1% suspension	In 10, 15 mL
DORZOLAMIDE		
Trusopt*	2% solution	In 5, 10 mL
METHAZOLAMIDE		
Neptazane	Tablets: 25 mg, 50 mg	In 100s
Generic	Tablets: 25 mg, 50 mg	In 100s

Table 26–7 ◆ **Available Dosage Forms: Antiglaucoma Agents—cont'd**

Drug	Dosage Form	How Supplied
Sympathathomimetics		
EPINEPHRINE		
Epifrin*†	0.5% solution	In 15-mL dropper bottle
	1% solution	In 10-mL dropper bottle
	2% solution	In 15-mL dropper bottle
Glaucon*†	1% solution, 2% solution	In 10-mL dropper bottle
DIPIVEFRIN		
Propine, generic	0.1% solution	In 5-, 10-, 15-mL bottle
Alpha-Adrenergic Agonists		
APRACLONIDINE		
Iopidine	1% solution	In 0.25-mL dispenser
	0.5% solution	In 5-mL droptainer
BRIMONIDINE		
Prostaglandin Analogues		
LATANOPROST		
Xalatan	0.005% solution	In 2.5 mL
Latisse	0.03% solution	In 3 mL
UNOPROSTONE		
Rescula	0.15% solution	In 5 mL
TRAVOPROST		
Travatan	0.004%	In 2.5 mL, 5 mL
Travatan Z	0.004%	In 2.5 mL

*Contains benzalkonium chloride, which cannot be administered with soft contact lenses in place.
†Contains sulfites.

Ocular antihistamines are selective for the H_1 histamine receptor. They block the H_1 histamine receptors and inhibit histamine-stimulated vascular permeability in the conjunctiva. This relieves ocular pruritus associated with allergic conjunctivitis.

Ocular Anti-Inflammatory Agents

The **ocular NSAIDs** have analgesic, antipyretic, and anti-inflammatory activity. The **ophthalmic NSAIDs** reduce prostaglandin E_2 in aqueous humor by inhibition of prostaglandin biosynthesis. It is thought to be through the inhibition of cyclo-oxygenase enzyme, which is essential to the synthesis of prostaglandins.

Topical steroids exert an anti-inflammatory action. The exact mechanism of action for **ocular corticosteroids** is not known. They are thought to act by the induction of phospholipase A_2 inhibitory proteins. These proteins control the mediators of inflammation, such as prostaglandins and leukotrienes. Corticosteroids can increase IOP; the mechanism is not clear.

Pharmacokinetics

Limited systemic absorption occurs with the use of **ophthalmic anti-inflammatory** and **antiallergic agents.**

The metabolism and excretion of **ophthalmic antiallergic** and **anti-inflammatory agents** are unknown.

Pharmacotherapeutics

Precautions and Contraindications

Hypersensitivity to any component of the product is a contraindication of any of the **ophthalmic medications.** Use caution with patients with known sensitivity to **acetylsalicylic acid** when prescribing NSAIDs because cross-sensitivity may occur.

Ophthalmic Antiallergic Agents

Patients should not wear soft contact lenses while inserting any ophthalmic product that contains **benzalkonium chloride (cromolyn sodium, lodoxamide, ketotifen, emedastine, levocabastine).** Wear can be resumed within a few hours of discontinuing **cromolyn, levocabastine, lodoxamide,** and **nepanfenac.** Patients who are using **ketotifen** and **emedastine** may wear their soft contacts if they wait at least 10 minutes after instilling the eyedrops to insert their contacts.

Emedastine, cromolyn sodium, and **lodoxamide** are Pregnancy Category B. **Antazoline, ketotifen, levocabastine,** and **nepafenac** are Pregnancy Category C, although no studies have been done on pregnant women. Safe use in lactation has not been established, although such minimal amounts are absorbed that use during lactation is probably safe.

Lodoxamide is safe in children as young as age 2. **Cromolyn sodium ophthalmic** can be prescribed to children older than age 4. The safety of **emedastine** and **ketotifen** in children younger than age 3 has not been established. **Nepanfenac** is not recommended for children younger than 10 years of age.

Ocular Anti-Inflammatory Agents

Referral to an ophthalmologist is warranted for patients who appear to need **corticosteroid therapy**. They require slit-lamp examination to rule out herpes keratitis prior to initiating therapy.

Corticosteroid eye medications should not be administered to patients with acute, untreated purulent bacterial, viral, or fungal ocular infection. Prescribing **ophthalmic corticosteroids** to a patient with herpes keratitis can lead to serious complications, including blindness. This may also occur with **ocular NSAIDs**; therefore, a referral is indicated before treatment.

The **ocular NSAIDs** are Pregnancy Category C, and the **ocular corticosteroids** are also Pregnancy Category C. Safety in children has not been established.

Adverse Drug Reactions

All **ophthalmic antiallergic** and **anti-inflammatory medications** may cause transient discomfort or tearing. Blurred vision, photophobia, and hyperemia may also develop. Allergic conjunctivitis may occur with any of the **topical ophthalmic medications.**

Other adverse reactions reported (1% to 5%) with the use of the **mast cell stabilizer lodoxamide** include dry eye, foreign body sensation, ocular itching and pruritus, and crystalline deposits. **Cromolyn sodium** may also cause itchy eyes, eye dryness and puffiness, and styes.

The most frequent adverse reaction reported with the use of **ocular H_1 histamine blockers** is headache. Conjunctival injection and rhinitis are reported in 10 to 25 percent of patients treated. The adverse reactions that occur in fewer than 5 percent of patients include asthenia, blurred vision, corneal staining, dysgeusia, hyperemia, keratitis, pruritus, rhinitis, and sinusitis.

Naphazoline may precipitate narrow-angle glaucoma. It may also cause mydriasis, increased IOP, and allergic dermatitis. Systemic adrenergic or antihistamine effects may occur with excessive use.

The **ocular NSAIDs** may cause minor ocular irritation on instillation (less than 40% incidence). The other reported adverse reactions noted in 1 to 10 percent of patients using **ocular NSAIDs** include superficial ocular infection, superficial keratitis, ocular inflammation, corneal edema, and iritis. Reactions reported less frequently include corneal infiltrates, corneal ulcer, keratitis, and mydriasis.

The severe adverse reactions that can occur with the use of **ocular corticosteroids** include glaucoma (elevated IOP) with optic nerve damage, loss of visual acuity and field defects, cataract formation, secondary infection of the eye, exacerbation of existing infections, and perforation of the globe. Systemic side effects may develop with extensive use.

Drug Interactions

There are no drug interactions noted with any of the **ocular antiallergic medications.**

Ocular NSAIDs may potentiate oral anticoagulants; the patient should be monitored for prolonged bleeding times if the drugs are used concurrently.

Ophthalmic steroids have no known drug interactions.

Clinical Use and Dosing

Allergic or Vernal Conjunctivitis

Allergic conjunctivitis can occur in response to a variety of allergens; vernal conjunctivitis refers to conjunctivitis that occurs primarily in the spring, usually because of an allergen. The **mast cell stabilizers (lodoxamide, cromolyn sodium)** may be used to treat vernal conjunctivitis. They may be used safely for up to 3 months.

The **ophthalmic H_1 blocker ketotifen** can be prescribed for allergic conjunctivitis and ocular pruritus. The dose used in adults and children over age 3 is 1 drop in the affected eye every 8 to 12 hours. The dosage for **levocabastine**, another prescription **ophthalmic H_1 blocker**, is 1 drop in the affected eye four times a day.

The over-the-counter (OTC) products available to treat allergic conjunctivitis combine a **decongestant** with an **antihistamine.** Products that combine **antazoline** and **naphazoline** (Vasocon-A) or **naphazoline** and **pheniramine** (Opcon-A, Naphcon-A) are used for temporary relief of the minor eye symptoms of itching and redness caused by pollen and other allergens such as animal hair. Patients may self-prescribe these products; therefore, the primary care provider needs to monitor the patient for proper use and the adverse effects associated with the use of these medications.

Ocular Inflammation

Consultation with an ophthalmologist is indicated in the treatment of ocular inflammation. The patient requires a slit-lamp examination to rule out herpes keratitis or other infectious disease before beginning therapy with **ocular anti-inflammatory agents.** The dosing of these agents may be found in Table 26–8.

Rational Drug Selection

Safety

The **ophthalmic mast cell stabilizers** are quite safe to use, even in children and in pregnant patients. The **ocular antihistamines** are safe and can be used in children as young as 2 (lodoxamide). The **ophthalmic H_1 blockers** are safe for use in adults, with **ketotifen** safe for use in children as young as 3 years.

The **ocular NSAIDs** are safe for treating a clear case of vernal conjunctivitis. If the diagnosis is unclear, an

Table 26–8 ◉ **Dosage Schedule: Selected Ocular Antiallergic and Anti-Inflammatory Agents**

Drug	Indication	Dose	Notes
Mast Cell Stabilizers			
Cromolyn sodium	Allergic or vernal conjunctivitis	*Adults and children ≥4 yr:* 1–2 drops each eye 4–6 times daily	Safety in children <4 yr is not known Advise the patient not to wear soft contact lenses while using ophthalmic cromolyn sodium
Lodoxamide	Vernal conjunctivitis, keratoconjunctivitis, vernal keratitis	*Adults and Children >2 yr:* 1–2 drops qid for up to 3 mo	Not recommended in children <2 yr
Pemirolast	Allergic conjunctivitis	*Children ≥ 3 yr:* 1–2 drops each eye qid	Not recommended in children <3 yr
Nedo cromil	Allergic conjunctivitis	*Children ≥ 3 yr:* Instill 1–2 drops in each eye bid at regular intervals	Continue treatment throughout period of exposure (e.g., until pollen season is over) Not recommended in children <3 yr
Antihistamines			
Antazoline/ naphazoline	Allergic conjunctivitis	*Adults:* 1–3 drops into eyes q3–4h	OTC; use for temporary relief of allergic conjunctivitis symptoms
Azelastine	Allergic conjunctivitis	*Adults and children ≥ 3 yr:* Instill 1 drop each eye bid	Not recommended in children <3 yr
Epinastine	Allergic conjunctivitis	*Adults and children ≥ 3 yr:* Instill 1 drop each eye bid	Not recommended in children <3 yr
Emedastine	Allergic conjunctivitis	*Adults and children ≥ 3 yr:* 1 drop qid	Not recommended in children <3 yr Soft contact wearers may reinsert lens 10 min after administration of emedastine
Ketotifen	Temporary prevention of ocular itching due to allergic conjunctivitis	*Adults and children ≥ 3 yr:* 1–2 drops q8–12h	Not recommended in children <3 yr Soft contact wearers may reinsert lens 10 min after administration of ketotifen
Levocabastine	Seasonal allergic conjunctivitis	*Adults and children ≥ 12 yr:* 1 drop into affected eye qid for up to 2 wk	Not recommended for use in children
Pheniramine/ naphazoline	Allergic conjunctivitis	*Adults:* Instill 1–2 drops q3–4h	OTC; use for temporary relief of allergic conjunctivitis symptoms
Olopatadine	Temporary prevention of ocular itching due to allergic conjunctivitis	*Adults and children ≥3 yr:* 1–2 drops bid, at least 6–8 h interval	Not recommended in children <3 yr Soft contact wearers may reinsert lens 10 min after administration of olopatadine
NSAIDs			
Diclofenac	Post-op inflammation after cataract surgery	After surgery, instill 1 drop into affected eye qid for 2 wk, beginning 24 h after surgery	Prescribed by ophthalmologists
Flurbiprofen	Post-op inflammation after cataract surgery	On day of surgery, instill 1 drop into eye every 30 min, beginning 2 h prior to surgery	Prescribed by ophthalmologists

Continued

Table 26–8 ● Dosage Schedule: Selected Ocular Antiallergic and Anti-Inflammatory Agents—cont'd

Drug	Indication	Dose	Notes
Ketorolac	Seasonal allergic conjunctivitis	*Adults and children ≥12 yr:* 1 drop in affected eye(s) qid	Patients wearing hydrogel soft contact lenses may experience ocular irritation when using concurrently Advise patients not to wear contacts while using this drug
Nepafenac	Post-op pain and inflammation following cataract surgery	Adults ≥10 yrs: 1 drops in affected eye TID beginning the day before surgery	Prescribed by ophthalmologists
Suprofen	Post-op inflammation after cataract surgery	On day of surgery, instill 2 drops into eye at 3, 2, and 1 h prior to surgery; after surgery, instill 2 drops into affected eye q4h for 1 d	Prescribed by ophthalmologists

ophthalmological consult is indicated before prescribing to clarify the diagnosis and rule out herpes keratitis.

The **ophthalmic corticosteroid preparations** have serious adverse effects. They should be prescribed only by an ophthalmologist.

Monitoring

The primary care provider needs to monitor the patient for effectiveness of therapy. There is no specific laboratory monitoring necessary with these medications. IOP should be periodically monitored by a trained eye professional if using medications that may increase IOP, **ocular corticosteroids**, and **naphazoline.**

Patient Education

Administration

The patient should be instructed to use the medication exactly as prescribed (Table 26–9). Overuse or underuse can adversely affect the outcome of the clinical condition. Advise the patient to avoid touching the dropper to the eye or other surface, which may contaminate the medication. To prevent cross-contamination, neither prescription nor OTC products should be shared with another person.

Adverse Reactions

Alert the patient to the adverse reaction of transient stinging and burning that may occur with the use of **ocular medications.** If the burning or stinging is intense or prolonged or if there is any other adverse reaction, the patient should contact the primary care provider.

Ocular Lubricants

Ocular lubricants offer tearlike lubrication for the relief of dry eyes and eye irritation. **Ocular lubricants** are also referred to as *artificial tears.* An artificial tear insert consisting of **hydroxypropyl cellulose (Lacrisert)**, which may be prescribed by an ophthalmologist or optometrist, is not discussed in this chapter. The immunomodulator/anti-inflammatory **cyclosporine (Restasis)** is used to treat dry eye and is prescribed by an ophthalmologist.

Pharmacodynamics

Ocular lubricants contain a balanced solution of salts to maintain ocular tonicity, buffers to adjust pH, viscosity to prolong eye contact time, and preservatives.

Pharmacokinetics

Ocular lubricants are not absorbed in measurable amounts.

Pharmacotherapeutics

Precautions and Contraindications

There are no true contraindications to the use of **ocular lubricants.**

Products that contain **benzalkonium chloride (Teargen, Akwa Tears, Puralube Tears, Comfort Tears, Dry Eyes, HypoTears, Ultra Tears, Isopto Plain, Isopto Tears, Just Tears, LubriTears, Moisture Drops, Murine, Nature's Tears, Nu-Tears, Nu-Tears II, Tearisol, OcuCoat, Tears Naturale, Tears Renewed)** should not be used with soft contacts.

Adverse Drug Reactions

The **ocular lubricants** may cause mild stinging and temporary blurred vision.

Drug Interactions

There are no significant drug interactions with the **ocular lubricants.**

Table 26–9 ◆ **Available Dosage Forms: Ocular Antiallergic and Anti-Inflammatory Agents**

Drug	Dosage Form	How Supplied	Cost
Mast Cell Stabilizers			
Cromolyn sodium			
Crolom*	4% solution	In 10 mL	$45.99
Opticrom*	4% solution	In 10 mL	$31.99
Lodoxamide			
Alomide	0.1% solution	In 10 mL	$102.67
Pemirolast (Alamast)	0.1% solution	In 10 mL	$113.61
Nedocromil (Alocril)	2% solution	In 5 mL	$93.01
Antihistamines			
Antazoline-naphazoline			
Vasocon-A*	Solution: antazoline 0.5%, naphazoline 0.027%	In 5, 15 mL	
Generic	Solution: antazoline 0.5%, naphazoline 0.027%	In 15 mL	
Epinastine (Elestat)	0.05% solution	In 5 mL	$116.58/5 mL
Azelastine (Optivar)	0.05% solution	In 6 mL	$109.60/6 mL
Emedastine			
Emadine*	0.05% solution	In 5 mL	$78.75/5 mL
Ketotifen			
Zaditor* (OTC)	0.025% solution	In 5 mL	$14/5 mL
Levocabastine			
Livostin	0.05% suspension	In 2.5 mL, 5 mL, 10 mL	$55.39/5 mL
Pheniramine-naphazoline			
Naphcon-A* (OTC)	Solution: 0.3% pheniramine, 0.025% naphazoline	In 15 mL	$10.99/15 mL
Naphazoline Plus,*			
Generic			$5
Olopatadine			
Patanol*	0.1% solution	In 5 mL	$106.80/5 mL
NSAIDs			
Diclofenac			$51/2.5 mL
Voltaren	0.1% solution	In 2.5 mL, 5 mL	$76.99/5 mL $20
Generic	0.1% solution	2.5 mL 5 mL	$26
Flurbiprofen			
Ocufen	0.03%	In 2.5 mL	$22.70/2.5 mL
Generic		In 2.5 mL	$18.99/50 mg tablets x 60
Ketorolac			
Acular*	0.5% solution	In 3 mL, 5 mL, 10 mL	$59.34/3 mL $122.36/5 mL $229.15/10 mL
Acular PF	0.5% solution, preservative free	Single-use vials: 12 × 0.4 mL	$60.17/12 vials
Suprofen			
Profenal†	1% solution	In 2.5 mL	

*Contains benzalkonium chloride, which cannot be administered with soft contact lenses in place.
†Contains thimerosal.

Clinical Use and Dosing

Dry Eye Syndrome

Ocular lubricants or artificial tears are used as needed to provide relief of dry eyes and ocular irritation. They can also be used as lubricants for artificial eyes. The patient should be instructed to instill 1 or 2 drops into the eye(s) three to four times a day or as needed. Table 26–10 presents the dosing schedule.

Monitoring

There is no laboratory monitoring needed with the use of artificial tears.

Patient Education

Administration

Advise the patient to avoid touching the dropper to the eye or another surface, which may contaminate the medication.

Adverse Reactions

Advise the patient that transient mild stinging and blurred vision may occur. The patient should contact the primary care provider if headache, eye pain, vision changes, prolonged redness, or discharge occurs.

Ophthalmic Vasoconstrictors

Ophthalmic vasoconstrictors are used in primary care to provide temporary relief of redness of the eye due to minor eye irritants. There are ophthalmic vasoconstrictors that are used by eye-care specialists to dilate the pupil (hydroxyamphetamine Hbr, 2.5% and 10% phenylephrine) and are not covered in this chapter.

Pharmacodynamics

The ophthalmic vasoconstrictors are sympathomimetic agents that act by constricting the conjunctival blood vessels. The products used for eye redness are generally weak sympathomimetic solutions.

Pharmacokinetics

Information regarding the pharmacokinetics of the ophthalmic vasoconstrictors is not available, other than duration of action. The duration of action of naphazoline is 3 to 4 hours. Oxymetazoline's duration of action is 4 to 6 hours, and tetrahydrozoline's duration of action is 1 to 4 hours.

Pharmacotherapeutics

Precautions and Contraindications

The ophthalmic vasoconstrictors are contraindicated if the patient is sensitive to any of the components of the

Table 26–10 ● **Dosage Schedule: Miscellaneous Ophthalmic Products**

Drug	Indication	Dose	Comments
Ocular Lubricants			
Artificial tears	Ocular irritation, xerophthalmia	*Adults and children:* Instill 1–2 drops into affected eye(s) 3–4 times/d as needed	
Ophthalmic Vasoconstrictors			
Naphazoline	Relief of eye redness	Instill 1–2 drops qid as needed	Treatment should not continue for longer than 3 to 4 d without the supervision of an ophthalmologist
Oxymetazoline	Relief of eye redness	*Adults and children:* 1–2 drops in affected eye(s) bid-qid but no more frequently than every 6 h	OTC
Tetrahydrozoline	Relief of eye redness	*Adults:* Instill 1–2 drops into the affected eye(s) up to 4 times/d	OTC
Ophthalmic Diagnostic Products			
Fluorescein	Detection of corneal abrasion or defect	2% solution: Instill 1–2 drops into the eye; use Wood's lamp to detect staining of defect Strips: Moisten strip with sterile water and place at fornix in the lower cul-de-sac; the patient should close lid tightly and blink several times; use Wood's lamp to detect defect	After examination, excess stain can be removed with sterile saline solution Soft contact lenses can be reinserted 1 h after the eyes are flushed with saline to remove fluorescein

product. They are also contraindicated in any patient who has narrow-angle glaucoma.

The **ophthalmic vasoconstrictors** are Pregnancy Category C; the safety of their use in pregnancy has not been established.

Adverse Drug Reactions

The patient may experience transient stinging or burning on instillation. Blurring of vision may occur and is temporary, passing within minutes. Patients may experience mydriasis. Increased lacrimation, irritation, and discomfort may occur.

The most serious adverse reaction that may occur is increased IOP.

Rebound congestion or redness can develop with frequent or extended use of **ophthalmic vasoconstrictors**.

Drug Interactions

There are no significant drug interactions with the use of **oxymetazoline** or **tetrahydrozoline**.

Tricyclic antidepressants and **maprotiline (Ludiomil)** may potentiate the pressor effects of **naphazoline**. If **MAOIs** are used with **ophthalmic sympathomimetics**, exaggerated adrenergic effects may result. Do not use **MAOIs** within 21 days of the **ophthalmic sympathomimetics**.

Systemic adverse effects may more easily occur if **ophthalmic sympathomimetics** are used with **beta blockers**.

Clinical Use and Dosing

Relief of Eye Redness

Ophthalmic vasoconstrictors that are used for temporary relief of eye redness due to irritation or allergic conjunctivitis include **tetrahydrozoline**, **oxymetazoline**, **naphazoline**, and **phenylephrine**. The usual adult dose is 1 or 2 drops instilled in the eyes four times a day. Use in children is not recommended.

Rational Drug Selection

Tetrahydrozoline, **oxymetazoline**, **naphazoline** (0.012%, 0.02%, 0.03%), and **phenylephrine** 0.12 percent are available OTC (Table 26–11). **Naphazoline 0.1 percent** is available only by prescription. **Phenylephrine 2.5 and 10 percent** are used only for pupil dilation and are instilled by eye-care specialists.

Monitoring

There is no laboratory monitoring necessary with the use of **ophthalmic vasoconstrictors**.

Patient Education

Administration

Advise the patient to avoid touching the dropper to the eye or another surface, which may contaminate the medication. The patient should avoid prolonged or excessive

Table 26–11 ◆ **Available Dosage Forms: Miscellaneous Ophthalmic Products**

Drug	Dosage Form	How Supplied	Cost
Ocular Lubricants			
ARTIFICIAL TEARS (MANY AVAILABLE)			
Bion Tears	Preservative-free solution: dextran, hydroxypropyl methylcellulose	Single-use containers—28	$16.99
Duratears Naturale	Ointment: lanolin, mineral oil	In 3.5 g	
Hypotears	Solution: polyvinyl alcohol	In 15, 30 mL	$14.99
	Preservative-free ointment: light mineral oil, white petrolatum	In 3.5 g	
Lacri-Lube	Ointment: petrolatum, mineral oil	In 3.5, 7 g	$18.99/7 g
Muro 128	Solution: sodium chloride	In 2, 15, 30 mL	$16.99/15 mL $28.99/30 mL
Ophthalmic Vasoconstrictors			
NAPHAZOLINE			
Bausch & Lomb Allergy Drops	0.012% solution	In 15 mL	
Bausch & Lomb Maximum Strength Allergy Drops	0.03% solution	In 15 mL	$7.19
Clear Eyes	0.012% solution	In 15 mL	$6.02/30 mL
Comfort Eye Drops	0.03% solution	In 15 mL	
Naphcon	0.012% solution	In 15 mL	$10.99
Naphcon Forte	0.1% solution	In 15 mL	
Vasocon Regular	0.1% solution	In 15 mL	
Vasoclear	0.02% solution	In 15 mL	

Continued

Table 26–11 ◆ **Available Dosage Forms: Miscellaneous Ophthalmic Products—cont'd**

Drug	Dosage Form	How Supplied	Cost
OXYMETAZOLINE			
OcuClear	0.025% solution		$5.39/30 mL
Visine LR	0.025% solution	In 30 mL	$1.99/8 mL
		In 15, 30 mL	
TETRAHYDROZOLINE			
Visine	0.05% solution		$5.39/30 mL
		In 15, 22.5, 30 mL	$1.99/8 mL
Murine Plus, Generic	0.05% solution		$5.99/15 mL
		In 15, 30 mL	
Ophthalmic Diagnostic Products			
FLUORESCEIN	2% solution		
	Strips: 0.6, 1, 9 mg	In 1, 2, 15 mL	

use of **ocular vasoconstrictors** because rebound congestion or redness may occur.

Adverse Reactions

Advise the patient that transient mild stinging and blurred vision may occur.

Ophthalmic Diagnostic Products

The **ophthalmic diagnostic** that is used in primary care is **topical fluorescein sodium.** It is used to detect corneal epithelial defects or abrasions. The **injectable form of fluorescein** is used by ophthalmologists as a diagnostic aid in ophthalmic angiography. Only the topical form is discussed in this chapter.

Pharmacodynamics

Fluorescein is a yellow, water-soluble dibasic acid xanthine dye. It produces an intense fluorescent green color in alkaline (pH 0.5) solution. **Fluorescein** detects defects in the corneal epithelium. A corneal abrasion or corneal epithelial defect will uptake the dye and appear bright green under ultraviolet light (Wood's lamp). **Fluorescein** does not stain the intact cornea.

Pharmacokinetics

When used for the detection of corneal abrasion, topical **fluorescein** is not absorbed.

Pharmacotherapeutics

Precautions and Contraindications

Hypersensitivity to **fluorescein** is a contraindication to its use.

Do not use **fluorescein** with soft contact lenses, which become stained. Lenses can be reinserted after the eyes are flushed with sterile saline and the patient waits an hour.

Fluorescein is Pregnancy Category C, although there are no reports of fetal complications or anomalies.

Adverse Drug Reactions

There are no adverse drug reactions reported with **topical fluorescein** use, other than staining of soft contact lenses.

Drug Interactions

There are no drug interactions with the use of **topical fluorescein.**

Clinical Use and Dosing

Detection of Corneal Epithelial Defects

If a corneal abrasion or foreign body is suspected, the provider instills 1 or 2 drops of **fluorescein 2 percent solution** into the eye. After a few seconds, epithelial defects will stain. The use of a Wood's lamp enhances detection of defects. **Fluorescein** strips may be used. The strip is moistened with sterile water and placed at the fornix in the lower cul-de-sac close to the punctum. The patient should close the lid tightly over the strip until the desired amount of staining occurs. Have the patient blink several times to distribute the stain. After examination, excess stain can be removed with sterile saline solution. An anesthetic eyedrop can be administered before instilling the **fluorescein** if the patient is experiencing discomfort from the initial injury.

Monitoring

There is no specific laboratory monitoring necessary with the use of **topical fluorescein.**

Patient Education

Administration

Advise the patient that the staining of the cornea is temporary and will resolve within a few hours. The patient should not be wearing soft contact lenses during the examination. Advise the patient to wait at least 1 hour before reinserting the contact lenses.

DRUGS USED IN TREATING EAR DISORDERS

Otic Anti-Infectives

Otitis externa (OE) is an acute, painful inflammatory condition of the external auditory canal. Commonly known as *swimmer's ear,* OE affects people of all ages, and it is the most common cause of visits for ear pain. It can easily be treated by a primary care provider, yet it can have serious, even life-threatening complications, especially in diabetic or immunocompromised patients.

OE occurs when there is a breakdown in several protective mechanisms. The normally acidic environment creates a hostile climate for bacterial growth. Cerumen is bacteriostatic and provides a protective layer that protects the epithelium against hyperhydration. Factors that alter these defenses and contribute to OE include an abrasion in the ear canal, water in the ear canal, and maceration of the skin from heat and moisture. With OE, the acidic environment in the ear canal is changed to neutral or basic, usually by retained moisture. Itching and a sense of fullness develop from damage to the epithelium caused by hyperhydration. Organisms invade wet intact skin as well as damaged epithelium.

Pharmacodynamics

The medications used in the treatment of OE include **combination products** (Cortisporin, Pediotic, Ciprodex) that contain a **corticosteroid** (hydrocortisone) and **antibiotic(s)** (neomycin, polymyxin B, ciprofloxacin); a combination of **corticosteroid** (hydrocortisone), an **antibiotic/antifungal** (chloroxylenol) and a **topical anesthetic** (pramoxine) (Cortane-B Aqueous); **antibiotic alone** (gentamycin, ofloxacin), and **acid** or **alcohol drops** (Otic Domeboro, Burow's Otic, VoSol, VoSol HC) (Tables 26–12 and 26–13)

Table 26–12 **Dosage Schedule: Drugs Used in Treating Ear Disorders**

Drug	Indication	Dose	Comments
Otic Anti-Infectives			
Gentamicin	Otitis externa	Use ophthalmic drops: 4 drops in affected ear qid for 7–10 d	Broad-spectrum coverage
Ofloxacin	Otitis externa Chronic suppurative otitis media with perforated tympanic membrane Otitis media in children with tympanostomy tubes	*Children 6 mo–12 yr:* 5 drops in affected ear once daily for 10 d *Children ≥12 yr:* 10 drops in affected ear once daily for 10 d	To prevent dizziness, warm bottle in hand for 1–2 min prior to administering Not recommended for use in children <6 mo
Otic Anti-Infective-Steroid Combination			
Ciprofloxacin-hydrocortisone	Acute otitis externa	*Children ≥1 yr:* 3 drops in affected ear bid for 7 d	To minimize dizziness warm suspension by holding bottle in hand for 1–2 min before use Not recommended in children <1 yr Contraindicated if tympanic membrane ruptured
Ciprofloxacin-dexamethasone	Acute otiti media in pediatric patients with tympanostomy tubes Acute otiti externa	*Children ≥6 mo:* 4 drops in affected ear bid for 7 d	Not recommended in children <6 mo
Hydrocortisone-neomycin-polymyxin B	Otitis externa Chronic suppurative otitis media with perforated tympanic membrane	*Children: 3* drops of suspension in affected ear 3–4 times/d *Adults*: 4 drops of suspension in affected ear 3–4 times/d	Suspension is less ototoxic than solution; solution is contraindicated if TM is perforated
Hydrocortisone-ciprofloxacin	Acute otitis externa	*Children ≥1 yr:* 3 drops in affected ear bid for 7 d	To prevent dizziness, warm bottle in hand for 1–2 min prior to administering Not recommended for use in children <1 yr
Hydrocortisone-neomycin-colistin	Otitis externa	4 drops of suspension in affected ear 3–4 times/d	Contraindicated if TM perforated

Continued

Table 26–12 ◉ **Dosage Schedule: Drugs Used in Treating Ear Disorders—cont'd**

Drug	Indication	Dose	Comments
Acid–Alcohol Solutions			
Acetic acid-aluminum acetate	Otitis externa	Clean ear canal; instill 4 drops 3–4 times/d for 7–10 d If canal swollen: Insert wick saturated with solution; instill 4–6 drops q2–3h; keep moist for 24 h	Contraindicated if TM perforated
Acetic acid-propylene glycol	Otitis externa	Clean ear canal; instill 5 drops 3–4 times/d for 7–10 d If canal swollen: Insert wick saturated with solution; instill 4–6 drops q2–3h; after 24 h, remove wick and instill 5 drops qid	Contraindicated if TM perforated Not recommended in children ≤3 yr
Acetic acid-propylene glycol-hydrocortisone	Otitis externa	Clean ear canal, and instill 5 drops 3–4 times daily for 7–10 d May use cotton wick for first 24 h	Contraindicated if TM perforated Not recommended in children ≤3 yr
Isopropyl alcohol-glycerine	Drying solution for ear canal	Instill 4–6 drops in each ear after swimming or bathing	
Isopropyl alcohol-propyleneglycol	Drying solution for ear canal	Instill 6–8 drops in each ear after swimming or bathing bid	
Otic Analgesics			
Benzocaine-antipyrine-glycerin	Analgesia in acute otitis media Adjunct in cerumen removal	Otitis media: Fill affected canal and insert cotton plug; may repeat every 1–2 h if needed Cerumen removal: Fill ear canal tid for 2–3 d	Contraindicated if TM perforated
Benzocaine-antipyrine-propylene glycol	Analgesia in acute otitis media	Fill ear canal and insert cotton plug; repeat q2–4h as needed	Contraindicated if TM perforated
Ceruminolytics			
Carbamide peroxide	Cerumen removal	Instill 5–10 drops in ear canal, keep drops in for several minutes, and repeat bid for up to 4 d	Contraindicated if TM perforated Not recommended in young children
Triethanolamine	Cerumen removal	Fill ear canal, insert cotton plug, allow to remain for 15–30 min, and flush ear	Contraindicated if TM perforated

TM = tympanic membrane

Table 26–13 ◈ **Available Dosage Forms: Drugs Used in Treating Ear Disorders**

Drug	Dosage Form	How Supplied	Cost
Otic Anti-Infectives			
Gentamicin ophthalmic			
Garamycin, Genoptic	Solution: 3 mg/mL	In 5-mL dropper bottle	$11.99/5 mL
Generic	Solution: 3 mg/mL	In 5- and 15-mL dropper bottles	
Ofloxacin			
Floxin Otic	0.3% solution	In 5 mL, 10 mL	$79.79/5 mL $142.91/10 mL
Generic		In 5 mL, 10 mL	$59.99/5 mL $92.99

Table 26–13 ◆ **Available Dosage Forms: Drugs Used in Treating Ear Disorders—cont'd**

Drug	Dosage Form	How Supplied	Cost
Otic Anti-Infective Steroid Combination			
Ciprofloxacin-hydrocortisone (Cipro HC Otic)	Suspension: Ciprofloxacin 2 mg/mL hydrocortisone 10 mg/mL	In 10 mL	$117.17/10 mL
Ciprofloxacin-dexamethasone (Ciprodex)	Suspension: ciprofloxacin 0.3% dexamethasone 0.1%	In 5 mL In 7.5 mL	$126.43/7.5 mL
Hydrocortisone-neomycin-polymyxin B	Suspension: hydrocortisone 1%, neomycin 5 mg/mL, polymyxin B 10,000 U/mL	In 10 mL	$21.99/10 mL
Cortisporin Otic, Generic	Solution: hydrocortisone 1%, neomycin 5 mg/mL, polymyxin B 10,000 U/mL	In 10 mL	$79.55/10 mL
Pediotic	Suspension: hydrocortisone 1%, neomycin 5 mg/mL, polymyxin B 10,000 U/mL	In 7.5 mL	$57.33/7.5 mL
Hydrocortisone-neomycin-colistin Coly-Mycin S Otic	Suspension: hydrocortisone 1%, neomycin 5 mg/mL, colistin 3 mg/mL	In 5 mL	$44.73/5 mL
Acid–Alcohol Solutions			
Acetic acid-aluminum acetate Otic Domeboro, Burow's Otic	Solution	In 60 mL	
Acetic acid-propylene glycol VoSol Otic	Solution	In 15 mL and 30 mL	$8.80/30 mL
Acetic acid-propylene glycol-hydrocortisone VoSol HC Otic	Solution	In 15 and 30 mL	
Isopropyl alcohol-glycerin Swim-Ear	Liquid: 95% isopropyl alcohol, 5% anhydrous glycerin	In 30 mL	$4.99/30 mL
Isopropyl alcohol-propylene glycol EarSol	Drops: 44% isopropyl alcohol, propylene glycol	In 50 mL	$14.50
Otic Analgesics			
Benzocaine-antipyrine-glycerin Auralgan	Solution	In 10 mL with dropper	$16.20/15 mL
Generic	Solution	In 15 mL with dropper	
Benzocaine-antipyrine-propylene glycol Tympagesic	Solution	In 13 mL with dropper	
Ceruminolytics			
Carbamide peroxide			$7.49/15 mL
Debrox	6.5% drops	In 15 mL with dropper	$5.99/15 mL
Murine Ear	6.5% drops	In 15 mL with dropper In 15 mL with dropper and ear syringe	$8.29
Auro Ear Drops	6.5% drops	In 15 mL	
Triethanolamine Cerumenex Drops	10% solution	In 6 and 12 mL with dropper	$15.99

Prices retrieved from www.drugstore.com or www.costco.com.

Hydrocortisone reduces the inflammation caused by OE. The exact mechanism of action for **topical corticosteroids** is not known. They are thought to act by the induction of phospholipase A_2 inhibitory proteins. These proteins control the mediators of inflammation, such as prostaglandins and leukotrienes.

Neomycin is active against *S. aureus* and *Proteus* and *Enterobacter* species. **Polymyxin B** is generally active against gram-negative bacteria *(P. aeruginosa, E. coli, H. influenzae).* **Gentamicin** is a **broad-spectrum aminoglycoside** that is active against *P. aeruginosa*, staphylococci, *S. pneumoniae*, beta-hemolytic streptococci, and *Enterobacter* species. The **fluoroquinolones (ciprofloxacin, ofloxacin)** are active against staphylococci, *S. pneumoniae, Proteus* and *Enterobacter* species, and *P. aeruginosa.*

Acid and **alcohol solutions** such as **Otic Domeboro** and **Burow's Otic** contain 2 percent acetic acid in aluminum acetate solution. Another **acid solution, VoSol Otic**, contains 2 percent acetic acid solution and 3 percent propylene glycol. These solutions reduce inflammation and are antibacterial and antifungal.

Pharmacokinetics

Information regarding the pharmacokinetics of **otic preparations** is not available.

Pharmacotherapeutics

Precautions and Contraindications

Hypersensitivity to any component of the product is a contraindication to its use.

Ciprofloxacin is contraindicated if the tympanic membrane (TM) is perforated. **Cortisporin otic solution** is contraindicated if the TM is perforated. **Cortisporin otic** suspension may be used. **Cortane-B Aqueous (chloroxylenol, pramoxine, hydrocortisone)** is contraindicated if the TM is perforated or if the patient has tympanostomy tubes.

Prolonged use of **topical antibiotics** may lead to superinfection and overgrowth of nonsusceptible organisms and fungi.

Adverse Drug Reactions

Local reactions, such as contact dermatitis, may occur with any of the **otic preparations.** Superinfection may develop with prolonged use. **Ofloxacin otic** may cause taste alteration. Dizziness, vertigo, and paresthesias have also been reported with **otic ofloxacin** use. Ototoxicity may occur with prolonged use of **Pediotic** and **Cortisporin otic solution.**

Drug Interactions

There are no known drug interactions for the **topical otic preparations.**

Clinical Use and Dosing

Acute Otitis Externa (Swimmer's Ear)

On presentation of OE, the canal is swollen and full of discharge. The organisms found in OE (swimmer's ear) are usually gram-negative rods, *P. aeruginosa, Enterobacter* species, and *Proteus mirabilis. Pseudomonas* is the most common organism found in OE. Mycotic OE is less common, usually caused by *Aspergillus, Trichophyton,* or *Candida.* Occasionally, a furunculosis (small abscess) of the external canal may be caused by *S. aureus* or *S. pyogenes*, carried there by dirty fingers.

Once it has been determined that the TM is intact, the canal can be gently cleaned with warm saline or 3 percent hydrogen peroxide. If the TM cannot be visualized, irrigation should not be performed.

Topical medication is the treatment of choice.

A **steroid/antibiotic drop** that combines **hydrocortisone** with **neomycin** and **polymyxin B (Cortisporin Otic, Pediotic), colistin** (**Coly-Mycin S Otic**), a **hydrocortisone/ciprofloxacin** (**Ciloxan HC**) **suspension**, or the combination of an antibiotic/topical anesthetic/hydrocortisone (**Cortane-B**) is instilled in the affected ear four times a day. The usual dose is 4 drops, and treatment should continue for 7 to 10 days. **Gentamicin** and **ofloxacin** provide good coverage for the common organisms, but the combination products decrease inflammation faster. **Ciprofloxacin** and **Cortane-B** cannot be used if the TM is perforated.

A **topical acid** or **alcohol solution** (**Otic Domeboro, Burow's Otic, VoSol**) can be instilled into the ear four times a day if the TM is intact. A 1:1 mixture of vinegar and rubbing alcohol is just as effective, but it can be painful to administer. If excessive inflammation is present, a combination of **acid** with **hydrocortisone** (**VoSol HC**) may be effective.

If the canal is too swollen to allow the drops to be instilled, a wick of 0.25-inch gauze or cotton may be inserted into the swollen external canal for 24 to 36 hours. The medication can be dropped onto the wick. To evaluate progress, the patient will need to be reexamined 48 hours after the wick has been placed.

Chronic Otitis Externa

Chronic OE can be inflammatory or infectious. Psoriasis, eczema, or seborrhea can cause inflammatory chronic OE. Chronic infectious OE may be caused by infected sinus tracts, cysts, or fungi.

The treatment for inflammatory chronic OE is determined by the severity of presentation. If the patient is complaining of chronic itching, accompanied by dry skin elsewhere on the body, the treatment consists of placing 2 or 3 drops of baby oil or mineral oil in the canal daily. If the patient has psoriasis in the external canal, it can be treated with **steroid** cream or lotion (see Chap. 32). Seborrhea can cause a scaly inflammation in the external auditory canal and behind the ears, usually accompanied by seborrhea of the forehead, eyelids, and face. Treatment is the use of **selenium sulfide shampoo** and **topical corticosteroids** (see Chap. 23, Drugs Affecting the Integumentary System).

If the ear canal is greatly inflamed, treatment includes cleansing the external canal of debris and using a **steroid** otic solution (Decadron) two or three times a day until the swelling decreases. If needed to relieve the inflammation, a wick can be placed and **Otic Domeboro or Burow's Otic** dropped onto the wick for 24 to 48 hours.

Malignant Otitis Externa

Malignant OE is a rare but potentially lethal infection caused by *P. aeruginosa.* Malignant OE occurs mainly in older patients with diabetes (90%). It develops when OE extends and invades the surrounding tissues, causing osteomyelitis of the base of the skull and purulent meningitis, accompanied by multiple cranial nerve palsies. Standard treatment includes **parenteral antibiotics** with an **aminoglycoside** and **carbenicillin** for 4 to 6 weeks, plus surgical debridement.

Prevention of Swimmer's Ear

Most cases of acute OE (swimmer's ear) can be prevented by instilling **isopropyl ear drops (Swim-Ear, EarSol)** or 1 or 2 drops of rubbing alcohol into the ear canal to dry the ear after swimming. A combination of 1:1 isopropyl alcohol and white vinegar may also be used. The commercial preparations have the advantage of less stinging with application if the skin is slightly macerated.

Table 26–12 presents the dosage schedule of drugs used in treating ear disorders.

Monitoring

There is no laboratory monitoring necessary with these medications. The patient with a severely inflamed external canal requiring a wick should be reassessed 48 hours after treatment is begun and at the end of treatment to determine clinical cure. Patients with chronic EO need cleansing of the canal and reassessment every 2 to 3 weeks and may require alterations in topical medications, depending on clinical status.

Patient Education

Administration

Advise the patient to hold the bottle of medication in the hand for a few minutes to warm the medication before instilling. The patient should lie on her or his side with the affected ear up, instill the drops, and keep the ear up for 2 minutes or insert a soft cotton plug to prevent the medication from draining out.

Adverse Reactions

Advise patients to notify their primary care provider if adverse effects occur.

Otic Analgesics

Topical anesthetics are used in the ear to treat pain associated with otitis media. The **local anesthetic antipyrine** and **benzocaine (Auralgan)** is used to provide pain relief until **systemic antibiotics** can take effect. **Analgesic eardrops** are instilled into the affected ear three to four times daily or up to once every 1 to 2 hours as needed for pain. The tympanic membrane should be examined to ensure it is intact before prescribing **topical anesthetic** agents.

Ceruminolytics

Some patients have an excessive accumulation of cerumen, which can lead to conductive hearing loss, impaction, and an environment for OE to develop. Patients who use cotton-tipped applicators (Q-Tips) to try to remove the cerumen actually push the cerumen farther into the canal. The cerumen often forms a hard plug that is painful to remove. Treatment includes instillation of mineral oil, which softens the wax, or the use of **carbamide peroxide (Debrox, Dent's Ear Wax, Murine Ear Wax Removal)**, which softens and emulsifies the wax. Dosage of **carbamide peroxide** is to instill 1 to 5 drops (depending on the size of the ear canal) twice daily for up to 4 days. Once the cerumen is softened, the ear canal can be irrigated with *warm* water or saline. If the canal is excoriated, application of **antibiotic** or **steroid eardrops** for 7 to 10 days will prevent the development of OE.

REFERENCES

American Academy of Pediatrics. (2009a). *Chlamydia trachomatis.* In L. K. Pickering (Ed.), *Red book: 2009 report of the committee on infectious diseases* (28th ed., pp. 255–259). Elk Grove Village, IL: American Academy of Pediatrics. Retrieved February 15, 2010, from http://aapredbook.aappublications.org/cgi/content/full/2009/1/3.27.3

American Academy of Pediatrics. (2009b). Gonococcal infections. In L. K. Pickering (Ed.), *Red book: 2009 report of the committee on infectious diseases* (28th ed., pp. 305–313). Elk Grove Village, IL: American Academy of Pediatrics. Retrieved February 15, 2010, from http://aapredbook.aappublications.org/cgi/content/full/2009/1/3.45

American Academy of Pediatrics. (2009c). Haemophilus influenzae infections. In L. K. Pickering (Ed.), *Red book: 2009 report of the committee on infectious diseases* (28th ed., pp. 314–321). Elk Grove Village, IL: American Academy of Pediatrics. Retrieved February 15, 2010, from http://aapredbook.aappublications.org/cgi/content/full/2009/1/3.47

Blosser, C.G. (2009). Eye problems. In C. E. Burns, A. M. Dunn, AM Brady, N. Barber, & C.G. Blosser (Eds.), *Pediatric primary care: A handbook for nurse practitioners* 4th Ed. (pp. 673–704). Philadelphia: Saunders.

Centers for Disease Control and Prevention (CDC). (2006). STD treatment guidelines. *MMWR Morbidity and Mortality Weekly Report, 55*(RR11), 1–94.

Centers for Disease Control and Prevention (CDC). (2009). CDC guidance on shortage of erythromycin (0.5%) ophthalmic ointment—September 2009. Retrieved from http://www.cdc.gov/std/treatment/2006/erythromycinOintmentShortage.htm

Gitinger, J. W. (1996). Eye diseases. In J. C. Bennett & F. Plum (Eds.), *Cecil textbook of medicine* (20th ed., pp. 2174–2183). Philadelphia: Saunders.

Glaucoma Research Foundation. (2009). Glaucoma facts and stats. Retrieved from Retrieved February 15, 2010, from http://www.glaucoma.org/learn/glaucoma_facts.php

Hammerschlag, G. M., Gelling, M., Roblin, P.M., Kutlin, A., & Jule, J. E.. (1998). Treatment of neonatal chlamydial conjunctivitis with azithromycin. *Pediatric Infectious Disease Journal, 17*(11), 1049–1050.

Hautala, N., Hautala, T., & Koskela, M. (2008). Major age group-specific differences in conjunctival bacteria and evolution of antimicrobial resistance revealed by laboratory data surveillance. *Current Eye Research, 33,* 907–911.

Inspire Pharmaceuticals. (2008). AzaSite: Proven action against common ocular pathogens. Retrieved July 18, 2010 from http://www.azasite.com/ AzaSiteWebPages/AntimicrobialActivity.aspx

LaRosa, S. (1998). Primary care management of otitis externa. *Nurse Practitioner, 23*(6), 125–128, 131–133.

Moroi, S. E., & Lichter, P.R. (1996). Ocular pharmacology. In J. G. Hardman & L. E. Limbard (Eds.), *Goodman & Gilman's the pharmacological basis of therapeutics* (9th ed., pp. 1619–1645). New York: McGraw-Hill.

Murphy, J. L. (Ed.). (1999). *Nurse practitioner prescribing reference*. New York: Prescribing Reference.

Nard, J. A. (2000). Otitis externa. In M. R. Dambro & J. A. Griffith (Eds.), *Griffith's 5 minute clinical consultant* (8th ed.). Baltimore: Williams & Wilkins.

Petersen-Smith, A. M. (1996). Ear disorders. In C. E. Burns, N. Barber, A. M. Brady, & A. M. Dunn (Eds.), *Pediatric primary care: A handbook for nurse practitioners* (pp. 593–607). Philadelphia: Saunders.

Rosenfield, J. A., & Clarity, G. (1998). The ear, nose and throat. In R. B. Taylor, A. K. David, T. A. Johnson, D. M. Phillips, & J. E. Scherger (Eds.), *Family medicine principles and practice* (5th ed.). New York: Springer.

Smith, A. F., & Waycaster, C. (2009). Estimate of the direct and indirect annual cost of bacterial conjunctivitis in the United States. *BMC Ophthalmology, 9,* 13.

Wald, E. R. (1997). Conjunctivitis in infants and young children. *Pediatric Infectious Disease Journal, 16*(2), S17–S20.

Weiss, A. H. (2003). Conjunctivitis in the neonatal period (ophthalmia neonatorum). In S. S. Long (Ed.), *Principles and practice of pediatric infectious diseases* (2nd ed.). St. Louis, MO: Elsevier.

Yetman, R. J., & Coody, D. K. (1997). Conjunctivitis: A practice guideline. *Journal of Pediatric Health Care, 11*(5), 238–241.

UNIT III

Pharmacotherapeutics With Multiple Drugs

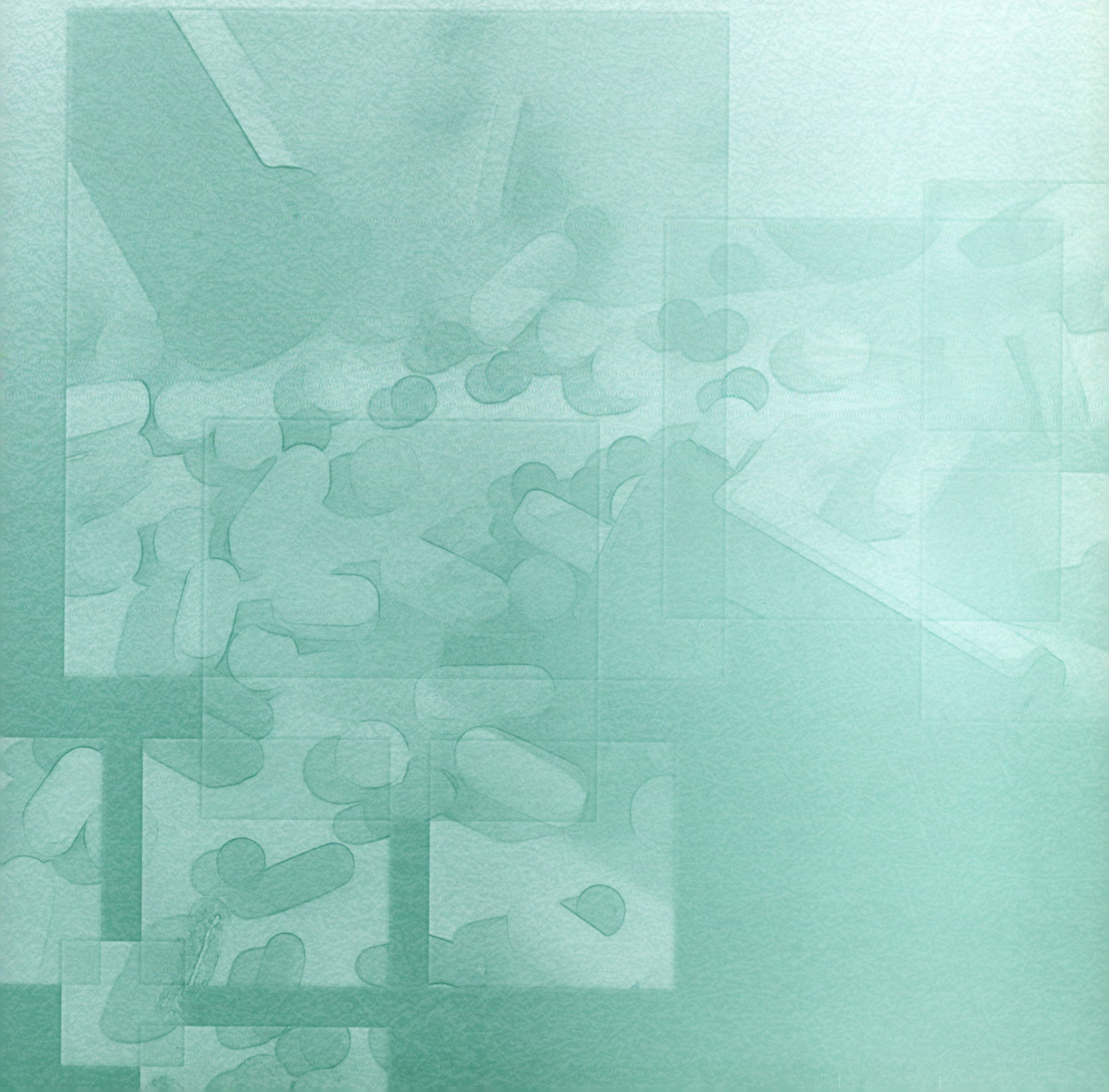

CHAPTER 27

ANEMIA

Teri Moser Woo

Chapter Outline

Anemias are extremely common in primary care practice; there are 5.5 million ambulatory care visits annually that list anemia as the primary diagnosis (Schappert & Rechtsteiner, 2008). The World Health Organization (WHO) estimates that 1.62 billion people worldwide have anemia (2008). Anemia is a sign of disease rather than a disease itself. Iron deficiency anemia (IDA) is the most common type of anemia, with a prevalence of 12 percent in women age 12 to 49 years (Centers for Disease Control and Prevention [CDC], 2002). Anemia of chronic disease (ACD) develops secondary to a chronic disease, cancer, or long-term infection and is the second most common form of anemia, The third major form of anemia is sickle cell disease (SCD), which affects 70,000 to 100,000 Americans, mainly of African ancestry, with SCD occurring in approximately 1 in every 500 African American births (Centers for Disease Control, 2010). Other forms of anemia discussed in this chapter are folic acid deficiency and pernicious anemia.

Diagnosis and treatment of the various forms of anemia entail interpretation of blood studies and peripheral smears to correctly diagnose the type of anemia. Normal blood count values are found in Table 27–1. Treatment consists of lifestyle modifications in the form of diet and energy conservation, and prescription of drugs specific to each disorder. This chapter reviews the relevant pathophysiology of the common anemias seen in primary care, as well as management or comanagement of the disorder.

PATHOPHYSIOLOGY COMMON TO ALL ANEMIAS

The underlying pathophysiology in all types of anemia is a decrease in the oxygen-carrying capacity of the blood. Figure 27–1 depicts the progression and manifestations of anemia. The reasons for this decrease vary by type of anemia. Anemias are classified by erythrocyte size and hemoglobin (Hgb) content. Size is referred to by the terms microcytic (small), macrocytic (large), and normocytic. Hgb content is referred to by the terms hypochromic (low Hgb) or normochromic.

Regardless of the disease process, the decreased oxygen transport to tissues carries the same results. Decreased mitochondrial oxygenation at the cellular level leads to decreased ATP production and reliance on the glycolytic process, resulting in poor energy generation and the formation of lactic acid, which affects the body's acid–base balance. It also affects the functioning of the body's largest energy consumer, the sodium-potassium-ATPase pump. As this pump works less efficiently, fluid and electrolyte shifts occur. Activation of the renin-angiotensin-aldosterone system augments the fluid shifts, with resultant sodium and water retention.

A reduction in the number of circulating red blood cells (RBCs) affects the consistency and volume of blood. Less viscous blood flows faster and more turbulently and may cause ventricular dysfunction, cardiac dilation, and heart valve insufficiency. Increased venous

Table 27–1 **Normal Blood Values by Age and Gender**

Age/Gender	Hemoglobin (g/100 mL)	Hematocrit	RBC Count (million/mm^3)	Mean Corpuscle Volume (mcg^3) Concentration (pg/cell)	Mean Corpuscle Hemoglobin Concentration (pg/cell)	RBC Distribution Width
Infants 3 mo	9.5–14.5 Mean 12	32%–41%	2.7–4.9	78	30–33	
Infants 6 mo to children 6 yr	10.5–14	32–41%	3.7–5.3	77–81	31–34	
Children 9–12 yr	12–15	34%–43%	4.0–5.2	83–86	31–34	
Adolescents 12–14 yr Male Female	 12–16 11.5–15	 35%–45% 34%–44%	 4.5–5.3 4.1–5.1	 78–88 78–90	 31–34	
Adolescents 15–17 yr Male Female	 12.3–16.6 11.7–15.3	 37%–48% 34%–44%	 4.5–5.3 4.1–5.1	 Adult levels Adult levels	 31–34	
Adults 18 + yr Male	 13.2–17.3	 40%–54%	Both genders: 4.2–5.4	Both genders: Microcytic = <87	Hypochromic = <32	Both genders: 11.5%– 14.5% CU
Female	11.7–15.5	35%–47%	3.6–5.0	Normocytic = 87–103 Macrocytic = >103	Normochromic = 32–36 Hyperchromic = >36	

CU = conventional units.

return to the heart stimulates the heart to pump harder and faster, resulting in tachycardia and the risk of heart failure. To better oxygenate the reduced number of RBCs, the respiratory rate and depth increase. If the anemia is severe enough to overcome the usual compensatory mechanisms, the patient experiences shortness of breath, a rapid pounding pulse, dizziness, and fatigue, even at rest. Laboratory values with anemias are found in Table 27–2.

Iron Deficiency Anemia

The World Health Organization (WHO) considers iron deficiency the most common and widespread nutritional disorder in the world (2010). IDA decreases oxygen-carrying capacity because of a low hemoglobin concentration that is due to reduced RBC production (lack of adequate **iron** intake, poor absorption of **iron** by the body, or lead poisoning) or acute or chronic blood loss. This produces a microcytic-hypochromic anemia that develops slowly after the normal stores of iron have been depleted in the body and particularly the bone marrow.

IDA affects 2 to 5 percent of women of childbearing age and 4 to 10 percent of minority women, related largely to **iron** loss secondary to blood loss from menstruation. About 50 percent of pregnant women also have IDA based in part on the use of **iron** by the fetus. This type of IDA can be easily managed by the use of **vitamins** that contain additional **iron** (Dunphy & Winland-Brown, 2001; Office of Dietary Supplements [ODS], 2010a). IDA also affects about 4 percent of males.

Pathological iron loss occurs most often from gastrointestinal (GI) bleeding. Gastric and duodenal ulcers, diverticula, hemorrhoids, and ulcerative colitis are common sources of this bleeding. Less common causes include malabsorption syndromes, achlorhydria, steatorrhea, and unrelenting diarrhea (Montoya, Wink, & Sole, 2002). Individuals with renal failure, especially those being treated with dialysis, are at high risk for developing IDA because their kidneys do not secrete sufficient erythropoietin. Erythropoietin and **iron** can both be lost in dialysis. The National Kidney Foundation (2006) has a clinical practice guideline specifically addressing this issue. Lead exposure can also lead to IDA because high blood lead levels impair **iron** uptake and prevent Hgb formation.

Finally, some drugs that reduce acid secretion by the parietal cells (e.g., **histamine-2 blockers** and **proton pump inhibitors**) may produce IDA because acid is necessary for the uptake of iron in the GI tract. **Sulfonamides** can also decrease plasma iron levels by binding to plasma stores of iron. **Vitamin A** mobilizes iron from its storage sites, so a deficiency in vitamin A limits the body's ability to use stored iron and may also lead to IDA.

IDA develops slowly over three overlapping stages. In stage 1, the body's **iron** stores are depleted. Erythropoiesis proceeds normally with the Hgb content of RBCs

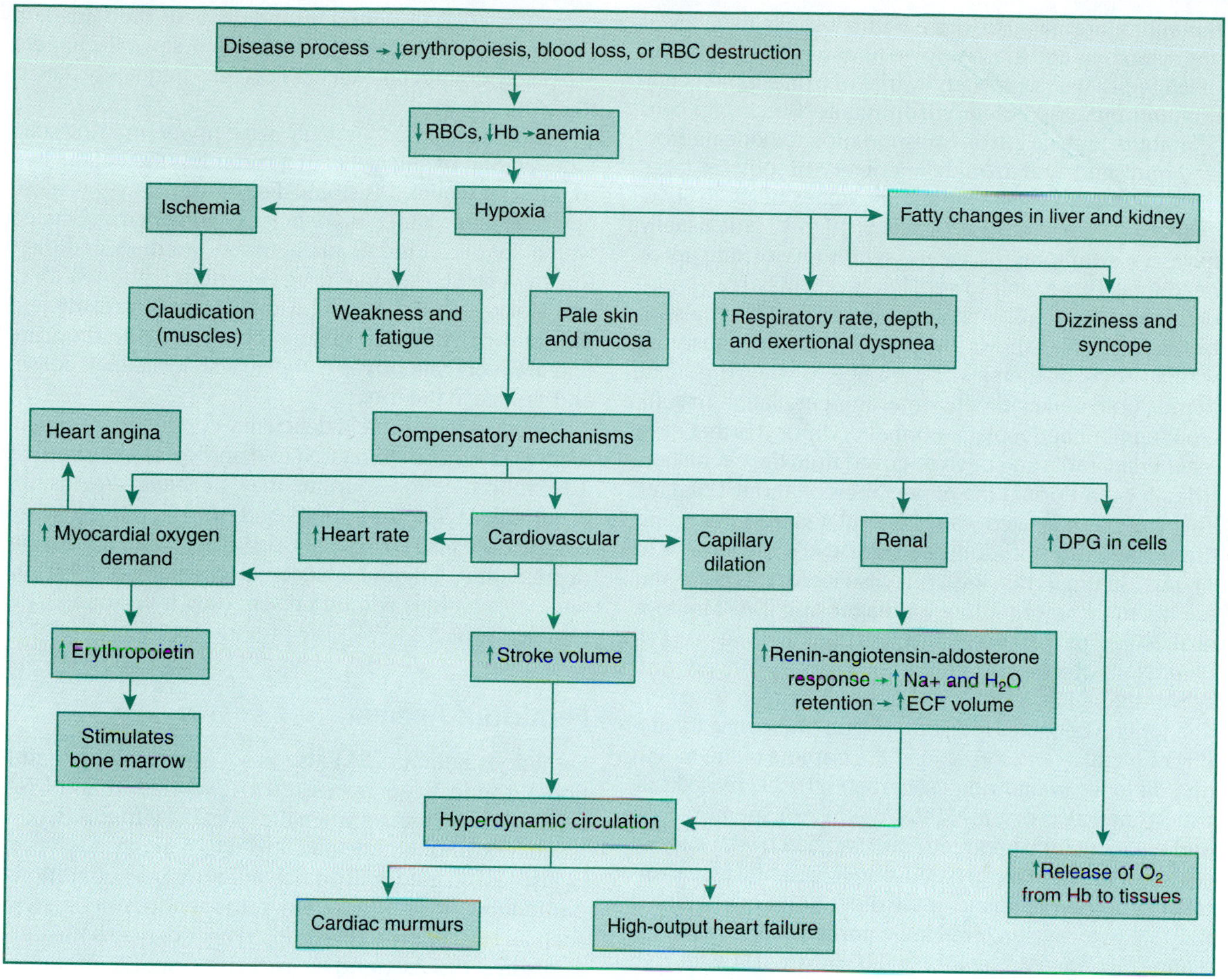

Figure 27–1. Progression and manifestations of anemia.

Table 27–2 **Laboratory Findings in Selected Anemias**

Test	Iron Deficiency Anemia	Folic Acid Deficiency Anemia	Pernicious Anemia	Anemia of Chronic Disease	Sickle Cell Anemia
Hemoglobin	Low	Low	Low	Low	Low (5–11 g/dL)
Hematocrit	Low	Low	Low	Low	Low (about 20%)
Reticulocyte count	Normal	Low	Low	Normal	Low (5%–20%)
Plasma iron	Low	High	High	Normal or low	Normal
Total iron-binding capacity	High	Normal	Normal	Normal or low	Normal
Ferritin	Low	High	High	Normal	Normal
Transferrin	Low	Slightly high	Slightly high	Slightly low	Normal
Mean corpuscular volume (MCV)	Low	High	High	Normal or low	Normal to low*
Serum B_{12}	Normal	Normal	Low	Normal	Normal
Folate	Normal	Low	Normal	Normal	Normal

*MCV will be low if a combination of sickle cell disease (SCD) and beta thalassemia are present, and normal if only SCD is present.

remaining normal also. The patients usually have few, if any, symptoms and those who do have a vague expression of fatigue. Diagnosis is often by trial of **iron** supplementation and increased dietary **iron** intake, which improves symptoms. In stage 2, **iron** transportation to bone marrow is diminished and **iron**-deficient erythropoiesis takes place. During this stage laboratory values begin to show changes. Patients with Hgb levels of 10 to 12 g/dL usually have no symptoms or vague symptoms of fatigue or headache. Those with lower Hgb levels may have more definitive symptoms, such as weakness and shortness of breath. Table 27–2 shows the laboratory values consistent with a variety of anemias. Stage 3 begins when the small, hemoglobin-deficient cells enter the circulation in sufficient number and replace normal erythrocytes that have reached maturity and been removed from the circulation. RBCs have a normal life expectancy of about 120 days. This stage is associated with IDA, depleted **iron** stores, and diminished Hgb production. Hgb levels are now 7 to 11 g/dL. Serum ferritin levels are also low at this point and are the most powerful tool for diagnosing IDA (Montoya et al, 2002). The earlobes, palms, and conjunctivae become pale. Nails become brittle, thin, coarsely ridged, and spoon-shaped as a result of impaired oxygen transport. The tongue becomes red, sore, and painful owing to atrophy of papillae. Dry, sore skin at the corners of the mouth and difficulty swallowing exacerbated by decreased salivation may also occur. Mental confusion, memory loss, and disorientation frequently are associated with anemia secondary to poor oxygen transport to cerebral tissue. This is especially problematic in the older adult population if they are wrongly perceived to be normal events related to aging (McCance & Huether, 2006). Severe IDA with Hgb levels below 7 g/dL may result in postural hypotension, dizziness, weakness, gastritis, irritability, numbness, and lethargy.

Folic Acid Deficiency Anemia

Folic acid deficiency anemia (FOA) decreases oxygen-carrying capacity because of a low Hgb concentration. **Folic acid** is necessary for the normal maturation and functioning of RBCs. Folic acid deficiency produces a macrocytic-normochromic anemia within 3 months of the start of an inadequate diet, because **folate** stores are rapidly depleted.

The primary biochemical function of folate coenzymes is the synthesis of purines and pyrimidines, the bases for DNA and RNA. These coenzymes also are involved in the synthesis of thymidylate, which is also a precursor of DNA. Symptoms of folic acid deficiency become apparent when the synthesis of thymidylate is critically impaired. Apoptosis of RBCs in the late stages of differentiation is thought to occur with this disorder. Because of its role in DNA and RNA synthesis, **folate** is a critical component of the diet of pregnant women and **folate** supplementation is recommended (Institute for Clinical Systems Improvement [ICSI], 2004). Along with anemia, **folate** deficiency is associated with neural tube defects of the fetus and heart disease. It is also implicated in several cancers, especially colorectal cancers. FDA also frequently affects the older adult.

Folate is absorbed primarily in the upper small intestine independent of any facilitating factor. It is then circulated to the liver where it is stored. **Folate** deficiency is more common than vitamin B_{12} deficiency and often associated with alcoholics, chronic malnutrition, fad diets, and diets low in vegetables. Some drugs interfere with the cobalamin-folate–dependent pathway (e.g., **methotrexate** and **fluorouracil**). **Dilantin, sulfamethoxazole/trimethoprim,** and **oral contraceptives** compete with folate metabolism and storage in the liver.

Patients with folic acid deficiency commonly complain of glossitis, stomatitis, nausea and anorexia, and diarrhea. A systolic ejection murmur may be heard. A positive Romberg's sign and increased or decreased deep tendon reflexes (DTRs) may also occur. Mild confusion, depression, apathy, and intellectual loss may occur. Peripheral neuropathies will be present only if **vitamin B_{12}** is also deficient.

Pernicious Anemia

Pernicious anemia (PA) also has a low Hgb concentration. **Vitamin B_{12}** is necessary for maturation and DNA synthesis in RBCs, and when the cause of **vitamin B_{12}** deficiency is autoimmune and linked to heredity, it is PA. PA is also associated with other autoimmune conditions, particularly those that affect the endocrine system such as Hashimoto's thyroiditis, type 1 diabetes mellitus, Addison's disease, and Graves' disease. PA produces a macrocytic-normochromic anemia that develops slowly, often over years, and it is frequently severe before it is diagnosed. In the absence of genetic mutations, **vitamin B_{12}** deficiency is practically nonexistent because there are rich dietary sources in animal proteins. However, other patients who are prone to consume too little **vitamin B_{12}** are vegetarians, particularly vegans, and those with Crohn's disease, in which a section of the small intestine may be destroyed.

Gastric parietal cells secrete intrinsic factor, which binds to dietary **vitamin B_{12}** during digestion and absorption of nutrients. Adequate intrinsic factor, along with hydrochloric acid, is needed to permit this vitamin to be absorbed. Patients with PA have a genetic absence of intrinsic factor. Other causes include gastrectomy and gastric atrophy of parietal cells associated with type A chronic gastritis.

Vague early symptoms of PA (e.g., infections; mood swings; and GI, cardiac, or kidney problems) are often ignored. The classic symptoms of anemia are not seen until Hgb approaches 7 to 8 g/dL. Neurological symptoms are the result of nerve demyelination, and the patient may experience loss of position and vibratory sense, ataxia, and spasticity. Concomitant symptoms include a beefy red tongue secondary to glossitis, and peripheral neuropathy; the latter is often used to clinically differentiate between FDA and PA. The liver may be enlarged, especially in older adults, indicating right-sided heart failure.

Anemia of Chronic Disease

ACD is also associated with low Hgb, but it is caused by destruction of RBCs by a hyperactive reticuloendothelial system, decreased production of RBCs by hypoactive bone marrow, or altered **iron** metabolism, with defective transfer of **iron** from stores to the plasma. Overall, ACD appears to be produced by the activation of the cellular immune system. Specific cytokines that have been implicated in ACD include tumor necrosis factor alpha, interferon delta, interleukin-1 beta, and interleukin-6. Microvascular eruptions occur in the GI tract in response to the inflammatory mediators. This results in occult blood escaping into the intestines. Chronic use of **NSAIDs**, such as **aspirin** or **ibuprofen**, must also be considered as the source of occult bleeding. ACD produces a normocytic-normochromic anemia in 75 percent of cases, but is microcytic in 25 percent of cases. It develops slowly and is often mild or asymptomatic.

Sickle Cell Anemia

The National Heart, Lung, and Blood Institute (NHLBI, 2004) recommends universal screening for SCD. More than 98 percent of children born in the United States are screened for sickle cell anemia (SCA) as part of the routine newborn screening for preventable diseases (CDC, Division of Laboratory Services, 2009).

Patients with SCA have a normal amount of Hgb (normocytic-normochromic), but their RBCs contain an abnormal type of Hgb, hemoglobin S (HbS). SCD is actually a group of autosomal recessive genetic disorders characterized by the predominance of this Hgb. These disorders include SCA, a homozygous form that is the most severe; sickle cell thalassemia syndromes and sickle cell HbC disease are heterozygous forms in which the child also inherits another type of abnormal Hgb from one parent. Sickle cell trait, in which the child inherits HbS from one parent and normal hemoglobin (HbA) from the other parent, is a heterozygous carrier state. It does not cause abnormalities in the blood count, and it does not produce vaso-occlusive symptoms under physiological conditions.

These disorders are found in people of African, Mediterranean, Indian, and Middle Eastern heritage. In the United States, SCD occurs more commonly in African Americans, with a reported incidence ranging from 1 in 400 to 1 in 500 live births. Sickle cell HbC disease is less common (1 in 800 births), and sickle cell thalassemia is the least common (1 in 1,700 births). Sickle cell trait occurs in 7 to 13 percent of African Americans, but the incidence among East Africans may be as high as 45 percent. This trait may provide some protection against lethal forms of malaria that are endemic in the areas that provide the gene pool of African Americans, but it provides no genetic advantage to persons living in the United States.

Sickle cell Hgb is produced by a recessive allele of the gene encoding the beta chain of the protein hemoglobin. A single amino acid, glutamic acid, is replaced by valine at the sixth position of the chain producing HbS. There are two cardinal pathophysiological features of SCD: chronic hemolytic anemia and vaso-occlusion, which results in ischemic tissue injury. Low oxygen tensions in the blood from ischemia or decreased partial pressures of oxygen in the air cause HgbS to crystallize, which distorts the RBCs into a sickle shape and makes them fragile and easily destroyed. The degree of deoxygenation required to produce sickling varies with the percentage of HbS in the cells. Sickle trait cells will sickle at oxygen tensions of about 15 mm Hg, whereas those with SCD will sickle at about 40 mm Hg.

Sickling is rarely permanent, and most sickled RBCs regain a normal shape when reoxygenated and rehydrated. Some irreversible sickling occurs based on damage to the plasma membrane of the RBC. Hemolytic anemia may be related to repeated cycles of sickling and unsickling. Tissue injury is usually produced by hypoxia secondary to the obstruction of blood vessels by sickled erythrocytes. The sickled cells are unable to squeeze through the smaller blood vessels, and tissues supplied by these blood vessels undergo ischemia. The organs at greatest risk for damage are those with venous sinuses in which blood flow is low and oxygen tension and pH are low (spleen and bone marrow) and those with a limited terminal arterial blood supply (eye and head of the femur and humerus). The kidney is also at risk, especially as the patient ages. Specific discussion of the complications associated with SCD and SCA are presented in the *Management of Sickle Cell Disease* (NHLBI, 2004). Additional information may also be found on several organizations' Web sites, including the American Sickle Cell Anemia Association (http://www.ascaa.org/); National Heart Lung and Blood Institute Sickle Cell Anemia (http://www.nhlbi.nih.gov/health/dci/Diseases/Sca/SCA_WhatIs.html); and the Sickle Cell Anemia Center (http://www.scinfo.org), a program sponsored by a partnership between Emery University School of Medicine, Grady Health System, Morehouse School of Medicine, and others, that offers extensive information on SCA for patients, families, and health-care providers. An expert panel is updating the NHLBI SCA guidelines, to be published in Fall 2011.

GOALS OF TREATMENT

The ultimate goal of treatment for all types of anemia is to provide adequate oxygen transport to body tissues. For patients with IDA, FDA, and PA, this may be seen in a return to normal in the number and character of RBCs and to normal Hgb values. ACD is normocytic and normochromic, so the goal is a return to the normal number of RBCs and to normal Hgb values. Table 27–1 shows the normal blood indices for each age and sex grouping. The goal of treatment for SCA is prevention of the morbidity and mortality associated with this disease and reduction in the percentage of HgbS in the blood.

RATIONAL DRUG SELECTION

Iron Deficiency Anemia

Risk Stratification and Screening

Growth, development, and gender factors play important roles in risk stratification. The fetus stores **iron** during the last trimester, providing the infant with stores that usually last about 6 months. Maternal conditions during pregnancy, including anemia, hypertension or diabetes can lead to low fetal iron stores (Baker, Greer, and the Committee on Nutrition, 2010). Preterm infants may have only 3 months of **iron** stores, and they grow at a more rapid rate, compounding the problem of poor **iron** stores.

The diet is the major source of **iron.** Human milk contains 0.35 mg/L of **iron** (Baker et al, 2010). The **iron** in breast milk is well absorbed (50% absorbed), as opposed to the **iron** in cow's milk which is 10% absorbed. Breastfeeding reduces the risk for IDA in infants by providing a minimum of 0.27 mg/day of **iron** term infants younger than age 6 months need (Baker et al, 2010). Due to waning iron stores between age 4 and 6 months of age, the American Academy of Pediatrics recommends exclusively breastfed infants be supplemented with 1 mg/kg per day of oral **iron** until **iron**-fortified foods (**iron**-fortified cereal) are introduced into the diet (Baker et al, 2010). Preterm infants who are breast fed should have 2 mg/kg per day of supplemental elemental **iron** daily until age 12 months (Baker et al, 2010). Infants, including preterm infants who are formula fed should receive **iron**-fortified formula for the first 12 months of life. Partially breast fed infants (more than half their nutrition from breast milk), should receive 1 mg/kg per day of **iron.** The early addition of solid foods to the infant's diet may impair the ability to absorb **iron**, and solid foods should be introduced slowly, with conscious inclusion of foods high in **iron.** Cow's milk should not be introduced into the diet before age 12 months (Baker et al, 2010). Conducting a good history of **iron** intake is a guide for whether screening for IDA should occur at the routine 9- or 12-month well visit. The American Academy of Pediatrics recommends all children have hemoglobin measured to screen for IDA at approximately age 12 months (Baker et al, 2010). Prematurity, low birth weight, lead exposure or low **iron** diet may indicate a need for earlier screening.

The Institute for Clinical Systems Improvement (ICSI) (2004) and the American Academy of Pediatrics (Baker et al, 2010) recommend an **iron**-rich diet for all children from birth to 6 years of age. Children between ages 1 and 2 are particularly prone to IDA (CDC, 2002). Toddlers require 7 mg per day of **iron** (Baker et al, 2010). Typically, toddlers may have somewhat picky eating habits and may consume large quantities of milk. Children age 1 to 3 years who do not have adequate dietary intake of **iron**, should receive daily supplementation with **iron** in liquid, chewable, or if in Canada, sprinkle form (Baker et al, 2010). If toddlers or preschoolers exhibit signs and symptoms consistent with anemia (tiredness, irritability, loss of appetite) or have a history of inadequate **iron** intake or drinking more than 32 oz of milk a day, they should be screened with Hgb and Hct tests (Baker et al, 2010). Lead poisoning can also contribute to IDA in young children; therefore, high-risk children should be screened for lead.

Iron needs increase during periods of rapid growth. Teenage girls are in a high-risk group because of their growth spurt, the onset of menstruation, and poor dietary intake of **iron**-containing foods (less than 15 mg of **iron** per day). Although IDA is more common in females, adolescent boys may be at risk during their growth spurt if they don't have adequate intake of **iron** (11 mg/d). Adolescents should be screened with Hgb and Hct tests at ages 12 to 14 years, based on a history of their risk factors including dietary intake, vegan or vegetarian diet, skipping meals or disordered eating, history of heavy menstrual periods, participation in endurance sports, or intensive physical training (National Anemia Action Council, 2009).

Although anemia is common in older adults, in this population it is usually due to GI blood loss associated with ulcers, the use of **aspirin** or **NSAIDs**, or chronic disease rather than to **iron** deficiency. A study of carefully selected older adults (screened for health status, socioeconomic status, race, nutritional status, and altitude of residence) revealed that no older women had Hgb values of less than 12 g/dL, and only 2.3 percent of older men had values below 14 g/dL. Another study of healthy, very old people revealed little fluctuation in Hgb values, even into the ninth decade. With the exception of older adults with lower socioeconomic status, African Americans, and patients with concomitant diseases that place them at risk, screening for IDA is not appropriate in the elderly.

Women generally have smaller stores of **iron** than do men and have increased loss through menstruation, and their balance between intake and loss of **iron** is precarious. IDA occurs more frequently in nonpregnant women who experience menorrhagia. Pregnancy places a woman at risk of IDA because their **iron** stores have to serve the increased blood volume of the mother and also be a source of Hgb for the growing fetus. Women at risk should be screened for IDA at annual physical examinations, and pregnant women should have screening included as part of their regular prenatal care.

Algorithm

Treatment of IDA begins with prevention, but **iron** deficiency cannot be overcome with increased dietary intake alone. **Iron supplements** are always required.

Lifestyle Modification

The primary goal of management for IDA is prevention. The key to prevention of IDA not due to a disease process is adequate nutrition. Prevention, for infants, starts with breastfeeding. The American Academy of Pediatrics (AAP) recommends exclusive breastfeeding for the first 4 to 6 months of life (Baker et al, 2010). The AAP recommends **iron** fortification of 1 mg/kg per day of **iron** be started at age 4 months and **iron**-rich foods be introduced at age 6 months (Baker et al, 2010). Preterm infants require **iron** supplementation of 2 mg/kg per day starting at age 1 month and continuing until age 12 months (Baker et al, 2010). Low-birth-weight infants, or infants with hematological disorders require **iron** supplementation before age 6 months. The American Academy of Pediatrics recommends liquid or chewable forms of **iron** (Baker et al, 2010). **Iron** sprinkles are available in Canada. Formula-fed infants should use an **iron**-fortified formula. Children and adults need to eat sufficient amounts of **iron**-rich foods. Foods rich in **iron** that the body can readily absorb include raisins, lean meats, fish, poultry, eggs, legumes, soybeans, dark green leafy vegetables, blackstrap molasses, fortified cereals, and whole grain rice. The **iron** in many vegetables is poorly absorbed, so vegetarians must pay special attention to their intake of legumes and rice. Table 27–3 presents **iron** intake recommendations for the prevention and treatment of IDA.

Learning energy conservation techniques, such as planning rest periods, pacing activities, keeping objects within reach when performing tasks, and sitting down when doing chores, are other important lifestyle modifications for the patient with IDA.

Drug Therapy

Once the decision is made to begin drug therapy, the choice of drug is based on age and gender variables. Figure 27–2 delineates the drug treatment algorithm for IDA. See Table 27–3 for the dosages of **iron** recommended for infants, children, adolescents, adults, and during pregnancy and lactation. Doses ranging from 60 to 185 mg of **elemental iron** have been used. Oral formulations of 325 mg (60 mg of **elemental iron**) are usually taken by mouth with each meal tid. Chapter 18 has a more detailed discussion of **iron formulations**, including their cost. Although Chapter 18 includes **ferrous sulfate, gluconate,**

Table 27–3 **Iron Intake Recommendations for the Prevention and Treatment of Iron Deficiency Anemia**

Risk Group	Prevention	Treatment
Infants	• Breastfeeding for first yr or iron-fortified formula • Preterm infants: 2 mg/kg of iron from 1 mo in 12 months Breast fed infants 1 mg/kg per day of iron until adequate dietary intake of iron from foods • Begin iron-rich cereals or supplement at 6 mo • Screen for IDA at approximately 12 months	Mild to moderate deficiency: 3 mg/kg/d in 1–2 divided doses Severe anemia: 6 mg/kg/d of elemental iron in 3 divided doses
Children 1–3 yr: 3 to 12 yr: Male 12–18 yr: Female 12-18 yr: All adolescents:	 7 mg/d of iron in diet 10 mg/d of iron in diet 11 mg/d of iron in diet 15 mg/d of iron in diet Diet should include iron-rich foods	1–3 yr: 6 mg/kg/d of elemental iron in 3–4 divided doses 3–12 yr: 3 mg/kg/d of elemental iron in 3–4 divided doses 12–21 yr: 150–250 mg of elemental iron/d Ferrous sulfate is best choice for oral iron Absorption enhanced by taking it on an empty stomach or with vitamins C and E; milk, antacids, tea, and food interfere with absorption
Adults 19–50 yr Male: Female:	 8 mg/d of iron 18 mg/d of iron Diet should be high in iron-rich foods	150–250 mg of elemental iron/d (e.g., ferrous sulfate 300–325 mg tid or qid)
Adults 51+ yr:	8 mg/d	
Pregnant and lactating women	30 mg of elemental iron daily during last two trimesters and while lactating	Ferrous sulfate 300–325 mg/d

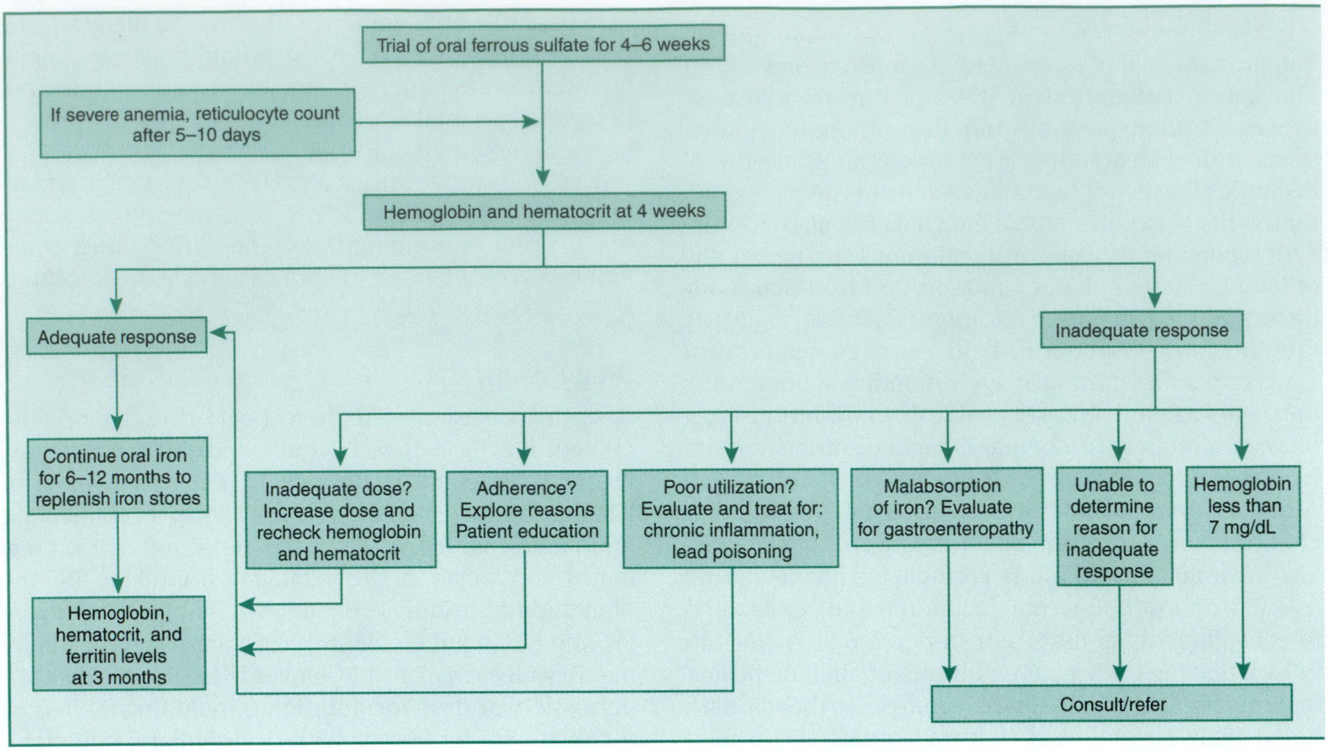

Figure 27–2. Drug treatment algorithm for iron deficiency anemia.

and **fumarate formulations, ferrous sulfate** is the least expensive and the most easily absorbed. Slow-release and enteric-coated compounds have been advertised to reduce GI distress, and they require only once-daily dosing. However, they dissolve slowly and can bypass the proximal small bowel, where most absorption of **iron** takes place. Slow-release formulas are also significantly more expensive ($24.99 for 90 tablets of Slow Fe Slow Release Iron with 50 mg of elemental iron versus $4.49 for 100 tablets of generic ferrous sulfate with 65 mg of iron at http://drugstore.com). There is no evidence to suggest that these formulations are worth the extra cost. If patients experience GI upset, it can be reduced by adjusting the dosage and by taking the drug with food.

Monitoring

The response to **iron** therapy is apparent within 10 days of initiating therapy. The first change noted in blood values is an increase in the reticulocyte count as soon as 4 days after treatment is started, followed by a rise in Hgb concentration of 1 to 2 g/dL per day. If the anemia is severe (Hgb less than 8 g/dL), a reticulocyte count can be obtained 5 to 10 days after initiating therapy. If the anemia is not severe, Hgb, Hct, and ferritin levels are checked at 4 weeks. If the IDA is mild (Hgb 10 to 12 g/dL and Hct 30% to 60%), follow-up every 4 to 6 months is appropriate. Referral is almost never required unless there is an inadequate response to therapy in which the Hgb remains very low (Hgb less than or equal to 7 g/dL); there is a question of possible malabsorption that requires special GI testing; or the reason for the inadequate response is unclear.

Outcome Evaluation

Several weeks of therapy are required to bring Hgb levels back into the normal range, and replenishing iron stores may take months. Speed is not the issue, however, unless there is rapid blood loss. In that case, consultation or referral to a physician is appropriate. Hgb, Hct, and RBC indices should be evaluated at 4 weeks, 3 months, and annually. If the Hgb level does not return to normal limits within 6 weeks, the inadequate response should be evaluated. If the dose is inadequate, it may be increased. Starting with a lower dose and gradually increasing it reduces the likelihood of adverse reactions that may hamper adherence to the treatment regimen. Persistent, unrecognized blood loss should be sought with stool specimens for occult blood and ova and parasites. Referral to a gastroenterologist for x-rays and endoscopy may be necessary. The source of the blood loss should then be treated. If there is a history of poor weight gain, diarrhea and other GI symptoms, or surgery on the GI tract, malabsorption syndromes should be ruled out.

Poor **iron** utilization can result from chronic inflammation, lead poisoning, or sideroblastic anemia. Chronic inflammation can be demonstrated with elevated sedimentation rates, elevated iron and total iron-binding capacity levels, low percentage of iron saturation, and high ferritin levels. Lead poisoning is demonstrated with increased serum lead levels and basophilic stippling on

RBC morphology. Sideroblastic anemia is usually found in infancy. Laboratory values reveal high ferritin levels, normal or high iron and total iron-binding capacity levels, and elevated bone marrow stores of iron. Each of these disorders must be treated before **iron** therapy can be successful. When the history, physical examination, and standard laboratory analyses do not lead to a determination of the cause of the inadequate response, or the initial Hgb level is less than 7 g/dL, consultation with or referral to a hematology specialist is appropriate.

Patient Education

Patient education related to IDA should focus on:

1. Understanding the pathophysiology of IDA and its potential long-term effects.
2. Recognizing the importance of prevention and the role of diet and energy conservation.
3. Understanding the necessity of adherence to the treatment regimen.
4. Understanding the need for follow-up visits with the primary care provider because IDA can recur.

Stress to the patient that a diet with sufficient amounts of **iron**-rich foods may avoid the need for supplemental **iron** therapy, but only after the IDA has been resolved.

When diet alone is inadequate or when **iron** needs are very high, as in pregnancy, drug therapy is initiated. Patient education specific to drug therapy includes the following:

1. The reason for taking **iron**.
2. Doses and schedules for the drug.
3. Potential drug interactions and the need to inform other providers that they are taking **iron**.
4. Possible adverse reactions and ways to reduce them. The most common adverse reactions that lead to nonadherence are GI problems such as nausea and constipation. Taking **iron** with food reduces the total amount absorbed but can also reduce the nausea. Adequate fluids and fiber can prevent constipation. Stool softeners may be needed to treat constipation associated with **iron** therapy.

Additional patient education related to **iron** therapy is presented in Chapter 18.

Folic Acid Deficiency Anemia

Risk Groups

Several patient populations, including age-based, gender-based, and concomitant disease–based groups, are at risk for **folic acid** deficiency. Certain drugs are also associated with effects on dihydrofolate reductase, an enzyme critical to **folate** synthesis.

Infants who are fed powdered milk products or goat's milk develop this deficiency because these products are deficient in both **folic acid** and **vitamin B_{12}**. Older children who are exclusively vegetarian or who have severe nutritional deficiencies, absorption problems, or tapeworm infestations are also at risk. Prolonged cooking of vegetables destroys **folates** and can result in deficiency if such foods are the only source of this vitamin. Older adults whose diets lack vegetables, eggs, and meat often develop **folic acid** deficiency.

Women are not especially at risk unless they become pregnant. Pregnant women have increased **folate** requirements (800 μg daily versus 50 to 100 μg per day) and may become deficient, especially if their diets are lacking in **folic acid**–containing foods such as dark green vegetables. Evidence suggests that maternal **folic acid** deficiency is associated with increased risk for neural tube defects in the fetus.

Disease states associated with **folic acid** deficiency caused by impaired absorption include sprue, Crohn's disease, giardial infections, and short bowel syndrome. Disease states that result in deficiency because of increased demand include hyperthyroidism, hemolytic anemia, malignancy, and other chronic debilitating disorders. Alcoholics and patients with liver disease develop deficiency because of poor diet and reduced hepatic storage of **folates**. There is also evidence that **alcohol** interferes with the absorption and metabolism of **folates**. Patients undergoing renal dialysis lose **folates** from the plasma during dialysis, and that results in deficiency.

Drugs that interfere with folate absorption or metabolism include **phenytoin (Dilantin)** and some other **anticonvulsants, methotrexate (Folex), oral contraceptives, isoniazid (INH), triamterene (Dyrenium), trimethoprim (Trimpex)**, and **pyrimethamine (Daraprim)**. Patients who take these drugs, especially on a long-term basis, should be monitored for folate deficiency.

Lifestyle Modifications

Patients should be instructed to eat foods high in **folic acid**. Such foods include dark green leafy vegetables, bran, yeast, dried beans, fortified cereals, and nuts. They should also be educated about the increased needs for **folic acid** prior to and during pregnancy. The U.S. Preventive Services Taskforce recommends **folic acid supplements** of 400 to 800 μg daily for all female planning or capable of becoming pregnant (2009).

Drug Therapy

Oral folic acid is well absorbed, and doses of 1 to 2 mg/day result in correction of the deficiency in 4 to 5 weeks. Hgb levels begin to rise within the first week, and the anemia is completely corrected in 1 to 2 months. Because of the potential teratogenic effects of **folate** deficiency in pregnant women, women of childbearing age should take prophylactic doses of 0.4 to 0.8 mg/day and continue this dose throughout any pregnancy. **Folic acid supplementation** to prevent deficiency should also be considered in the other high-risk patients mentioned previously. Detailed discussion of clinical use and dosing of **folic acid** is provided in Chapters 9 and 18.

Monitoring

Response to treatment is assessed after 2 weeks and then monthly until the condition stabilizes. A rapid rise in reticulocytes follows the initial treatment, with a peak in 5 to 8 days, an improving Hgb and Hct within 1 week, and a normal Hct within 2 months. The only monitoring required is to follow Hgb and Hct levels at regular intervals. The timing of such assessment is based on the acute versus chronic nature of the cause of the deficiency.

Patient Education

Patient education focuses on prevention as well as treatment. Diet and appropriate cooking methods are central to prevention, especially for strict vegetarians. Women of childbearing age should have the need for **folic acid supplementation** discussed. Alcoholics require special attention and help in correcting this addiction. When diet alone is inadequate or **folate** needs are very high, as in pregnancy, drug therapy is initiated. Patient education specific to drug therapy includes the following:

1. The reason for taking **folic acid.**
2. The doses and schedule for the drug.
3. The fact that some drugs may potentially interfere with **folate** metabolism.
4. The need to inform their providers that they are taking supplemental **folic acid.**

More specific discussion of patient education is found in Chapter 18.

Pernicious Anemia

Risk Groups

The underlying disorder in PA is usually defective secretion of gastric intrinsic factor, which is necessary for **vitamin B_{12}** absorption. It is most common in northern Europeans, but can occur in any age or ethnic group. **Vitamin B_{12}** malabsorption occurs in 10 to 30 percent of adults over the age of 50 because they have reduced pepsin activity and gastric acid secretion. This reduced activity interferes with the cleavage of **vitamin B_{12}** from dietary protein before it is absorbed. Partial or total gastrectomy and small bowel resection are the two most common iatrogenic causes of this problem. The former surgery removes the parietal cell–containing portion of the stomach that secretes intrinsic factor, and the latter surgery removes a portion of the bowel that absorbs the vitamin B_{12}–intrinsic factor complex. Diseases of the terminal ileum, fish tapeworm, thyroid diseases, and bacterial overgrowth in the small bowel from stasis can also cause PA. Nutritional deficiency is rare but may be seen in strict vegetarians after several years without meat, eggs, or dairy products.

Screen for PA any of these risk groups and other patients who present with the neurological symptoms of peripheral neuropathy, symmetrical paresthesias in the hands and feet progressing to ataxia from loss of vibratory and position sense, memory loss, depression, agitation, personality change, or central visual scotomata. This is especially true for older adults, in which some of these changes may be confused with senile dementia.

Lifestyle Modifications

The underlying problem in PA is **vitamin B_{12}** deficiency. Patients should be taught to eat foods high in this vitamin, such as mollusks (e.g., clams), fortified breakfast cereals, liver, trout, salmon, milk, and eggs. These foods are listed in the order of highest to lowest amount of **vitamin B_{12}** (ODS, 2010b).

Drug Therapy

Because the underlying problem in almost all cases of PA is malabsorption, therapy with **vitamin B_{12}** is required. Oral, IM, and intranasal replacements are available. **Oral vitamin B_{12}** is useful only for the rare case of nutritional deficit and for patients who cannot take the parenteral form. If the **vitamin B_{12}** deficiency is a nutritional deficit and not PA, 1,000 mcg of **oral cobalamin** is given until normal B_{12} levels are achieved, usually in 6 to 12 weeks. **Intranasal cyanocobalamin (Nascobal)**, a synthetic **vitamin B_{12}**, may be used for maintenance therapy of patients with hematological remission after initial treatment. Once-weekly dosing of intranasal **cyanocobalamin** (one spray in one nostril) gives a 500-mcg dose. For PA, the parenteral route is often used, although oral therapy may also be effective (Oh & Brown, 2003). **Vitamin B_{12} therapy** is initiated with 1,000 mcg IM daily for 1 week followed by 100 to 1,000 mcg IM weekly for a month. Doses of 1,000 mcg may be used, as excess **vitamin B_{12}** is excreted in the urine. Because PA is not correctable, the patient must take **vitamin B_{12}** for life.

Parental, nasal, or oral therapy may be used once a patient's B_{12} levels return to normal. Parenteral therapy consists of 1,000 mcg of **vitamin B_{12}** monthly. Nasal therapy consists of 500 mcg of **cyanocobalamin** weekly. Oral therapy consists of 1,000 mcg daily for life. Oral therapy should be tried because of administration ease and cost.

The hematological response to **parenteral vitamin B_{12}** is rapid. The bone marrow usually returns to normal within 48 hours. Reticulocytosis begins on the second or third day and is usually maximum by the fifth to the tenth day. Patients usually show some other hematological improvements in 5 to 7 days, with deficiency resolving in 3 to 4 weeks. Hgb and Hct levels should return to normal within 1 to 2 months. It may take up to 6 months to resolve neurological symptoms. Correctable conditions require treatment of the underlying problem, and parenteral therapy continues temporarily. Sudden drops in serum potassium levels have been reported with **vitamin B_{12}** therapy. Serum potassium levels should be monitored and **supplemental oral potassium** given if needed.

Chapter 18 has a detailed discussion of rational drug selection and dosing for **vitamin B_{12}**. Although it is not urgent to treat most cases of PA, the reversibility of neurological deficits is, to some extent, dependent on their duration. Patients with neurological symptoms should have this disorder promptly diagnosed and treated. When neurological symptoms are present, twice-monthly dosing is recommended for 6 months prior to beginning the usual monthly dose.

Monitoring

Reticulocyte counts, Hgb and Hct, iron, folic acid, and vitamin B_{12} serum levels are obtained prior to treatment, between the fifth and the seventh day of therapy, and then frequently until the Hgb and Hct are normal. Relapse of symptoms is not uncommon in the presence of continuing therapy. Blood counts should continue at regular intervals throughout the patient's lifetime, based on individual response to therapy.

Because of the potential for sudden drops in serum potassium levels, these should also be monitored at the same time as Hgb and Hct levels are drawn. Liver function tests (LFTs) should also be done. If LFTs (aspartate transaminase [AST] and alanine transaminase [ALT]) are elevated before the start of **cobalamin** therapy, they should be evaluated every 2 to 4 weeks to monitor for liver dysfunction. If LFTs elevate after the start of therapy, more frequent testing might be required to assess for hepatotoxicity. The Schilling test is used for diagnosis but not as a monitoring tool. Referral to or consultation with a hematologist and gastroenterologist should occur with the diagnosis of PA.

Patient Education

Patient education related to PA should focus on:

1. Understanding the pathophysiology of PA and its potential long-term effects.
2. The importance of adherence to the treatment regimen.
3. The need for follow-up visits with the primary care provider in that PA and its symptoms can recur, even with continuing therapy.

Patient education specific to the drug therapy includes the following:

1. The reason for taking **vitamin B_{12}**.
2. The fact that the oral **vitamin B_{12}** found in multivitamin tablets is not sufficient to treat the problem.
3. The doses and schedule for the drug.
4. The fact that patients need to take the drug for the rest of their lives.

Anemia of Chronic Disease

Risk Stratification and Screening

ACD is the most common form of anemia in older adults and is associated with several specific chronic diseases, including osteomyelitis, tuberculosis, rheumatoid diseases, hepatitis, carcinoma, myeloma, lymphoma, and leukemia. Anemias associated with renal failure occur secondary to erythropoietin deficiency, and the National Kidney Foundation (2006) has produced a separate guideline for diagnosis and management of this subset of ACD. Anemias associated with endocrine deficiency (e.g., thyroid, adrenal, or pituitary deficiency) reduce bone marrow responsiveness by not stimulating erythropoietin secretion. These disorders also have their own management.

Older adults with any chronic illness and patients of any age with these illnesses should be evaluated for the presence of anemia. ACD may also coexist with IDA. In these patients, ACD is usually mild and asymptomatic, but some patients may present with fatigue, shortness of breath, loss of appetite, weight loss, or light-headedness after mild activity. Because these symptoms may be the same as those seen with the underlying chronic illness, it is important to include evaluation for anemia in the workup for these disorders.

Hct in patients with ACD is rarely less than 25 percent, and other laboratory findings are shown in Table 27–2. The criterion for the coexistence of ACD and IDA is a serum ferritin level of 20 to 50 nanogram (ng)/mL. Serum ferritin, however, may elevate in the presence of an acute inflammatory reaction and may not accurately reflect total body iron stores.

Algorithm

There is no effective therapy directed specifically at ACD. Treatment of the underlying chronic disease is necessary to resolve the anemia. Sometimes, patients have a concomitant IDA that is amenable to treatment with **iron**, but otherwise, **oral iron** is not necessary. The main focus of therapy for ACD, besides treatment of the underlying disease, is energy conservation.

When ACD is caused by chronic renal failure, the cause is probably associated in part with decreased production of erythropoietin by the kidney. The target for successful treatment of this form of anemia is an Hgb level of 11 to 12 g/dL and an Hct level of 33 to 36 percent. To achieve this level, sufficient **iron** should be administered to maintain greater than 20 percent transferrin saturation and a serum ferritin level of 100 ng/mL or higher. In this case, administration of **epoetin alfa (Epogen, Procrit)** may lead to an increase of 6 to 10 percent in the Hct within 6 weeks. During the initiation of **epoetin alfa therapy** and while increasing the dose in order to achieve an increase in Hgb and Hct, the percentage of transferrin saturation and the serum ferritin level should be checked every month in patients not receiving **iron** and every 3 months in patients receiving **iron** until target Hgb and Hct are reached (National Kidney Foundation, 2006).

For patients with anemia associated with chronic renal failure or zidovudine-treated HIV **epoetin alpha** is started at 50 to 100 units/kg in adults and 50 units/kg in children, and dosed three times a week. **Epoetin alpha** dose is titrated to keep Hgb level between 10 and 12 g/dL. Dosage is increased by 25 percent if Hgb is less than 10 g/dL and has not increased by 1 g/dL after 4 weeks of therapy or if

Hgb decreases below 10 g/dL. **Epoetin alpha** dose is decreased by 25 percent if hemoglobin approaches 12 g/dL or Hgb increases more than 1 g/dL in any 2-week period. The maintenance dose for patients on dialysis is individualized for each patient. The malignant diseases causing ACD may also require the use of this drug, which is discussed in Chapter 18.

Sickle Cell Anemia

This chapter does not discuss the total management of SCD. The reader is referred to NHLBI Publication No. 04-2117 (2004) for a complete discussion and guidelines for management of common problems, such as pain and infection (updated guidelines will be published Fall 2011). However, it is important to remember that treatment of pain with **NSAIDs** carries with it the risk for GI bleeding, which may be a source of anemia beyond that associated with sickling. Hematuria can also occur secondary to renal abnormalities in SCD, and may also contribute to anemia. This chapter focuses on management of the anemia and precipitants of sickling and the resultant ischemia.

Prevention

Prevention of the morbidity and mortality associated with the hemolytic anemia of SCD is focused on avoidance of the precipitants of a sickling crisis. Serious bacterial infections, especially those due to *Streptococcus pneumoniae, Haemophilus influenzae,* and *Mycoplasma pneumoniae,* are a major cause of sickling. Patients and their parents need to be taught early recognition of signs and symptoms of these infections, and early aggressive treatment is critical. Children with SCD should also receive pneumococcal and influenza vaccines and all other childhood immunizations. Dehydration is another precipitant. Adequate hydration (2 qt/d or more in children and adults) should be stressed, especially during periods of elevated environmental temperature and physical activity. Exposure to cold, with its resultant vasoconstriction, can precipitate a sickling event and should be avoided. Although strenuous exercise may precipitate a sickling event, there is no evidence that most exercise is harmful, and the beneficial effects of exercise are well known. Patients with SCD are encouraged to participate in physical activities and set their own limits. Exercise capacity is reduced by as much as 50 percent in adults with SCD. Participation in noncompetitive recreational activities that do not involve strenuous exercise should be encouraged. Any activity, whether recreation or employment, resulting in exhaustion should be discouraged. Exercise under adverse conditions, such as cold weather, high altitude, or cold water exposure, should also be avoided.

Dietary Counseling

Dietary counseling is an important part of patient care. Mothers should be encouraged to breastfeed their infants, although **iron**-fortified formulas are an acceptable alternative. Foods high in **iron** and **folic acid** should be encouraged in children and adults. Chapter 9 has more information on foods high in these nutrients.

Drug Therapy

Sickle cell patients have a greater need for **folic acid** owing to increased erythropoiesis. A daily dose of 1 mg of **folic acid** is recommended to avoid decreased serum folate levels and megaloblastic anemia (NHLBI, 2004). A daily multivitamin supplement is also recommended (Tanyi, 2003). Dunphy and Winland-Brown (2001) also recommend a diet rich in complex B **vitamins** and **vitamin** C and stress the importance of eight glasses of water daily to maintain hydration.

Patients with SCA do not usually have concurrent IDA. **Supplemental iron** should not be prescribed unless the patient is documented to have reduced iron stores by specific assessments of the serum ferritin level or measurement of serum iron and iron-binding capacity. Children with SCA are often microcytic in the absence of iron deficiency. The incidence of alpha thalassemia trait is also quite high in African Americans and may produce microcytosis in the absence of iron deficiency. Routine administration of **supplemental folic acid** is also not necessary unless the diet history reveals inadequate folate intake, for example, low intake of green leafy vegetables. Most patients eat poorly during painful crises, and daily supplements of 1 mg of **folic acid** should be prescribed during those times if not already being taken. The danger of masking a vitamin B_{12} deficiency is small, but African American patients are at risk. There is no evidence that any other form of vitamin supplementation is of value in SCD.

Infections also enhance susceptibility to vaso-occlusive events and their subsequent ischemia. Prophylactic **penicillin** is so effective in reducing the number of life-threatening episodes of pneumococcal sepsis in children under age 5 that most states screen newborns for SCD so they can be placed on the drug by age 2 to 3 months. Oral **penicillin VK** 125 mg bid is given until age 3 years, then 250 mg bid is given until age 5 (NHLBI, 2004). Prophylaxis in older children has not been shown to be beneficial and may be unnecessary after *S. pneumoniae* and *H. influenzae* immunizations are complete and antibody titers are protective (NHLBI, 2002). *Streptococcus pneumoniae* vaccination is also recommended for adults with SCD. **Penicillin** is discussed in more detail in Chapter 24.

A consensus statement from the NIH published in 2008 states that evidence is strong for the use of **hydroxyurea** in the treatment of SCD in adults (Brawley et al, 2008) Although there is no drug to cure SCD, **hydroxyurea (Droxia, Hydrea)** has been shown to reduce the frequency of sickle cell crisis in adults by as much as 50 percent (Bonds, 1995, as cited in NHLBI, 2004). SCD patients requiring **hydroxyurea** are usually managed by a specialist in hematology. The dosing schedule varies, but patients are usually started on

10 mg/kg initially, with the dose increased by 5 mg/kg every 12 weeks until the maximum dose of 25 to 35 mg/kg per day is reached, unless toxicity was observed. Toxicity is defined as absolute neutrophil counts lower than 2,000/mm^3, absolute reticulocyte counts lower than 80,000/mm^3, platelet counts lower than 80,000/mm^3, or a fall in Hgb from greater than or equal to 7 g/dL to 4.5 to 5 g/dL if reticulocytes are lower than 320,000 or Hgb is lower than 4.5 g/dL. The NIH consensus statement found variable evidence regarding the use of **hydroxyurea** in children with SCD and recommends further study (Brawley et al, 2008).

Hydroxyurea may not be appropriate for all patients and should not be used for patients likely to become pregnant or those unwilling or unable to follow instructions regarding treatment. This drug is a cytotoxic agent and has the potential to cause life-threatening cytopenia. The onset of leukopenia and thrombocytopenia may occur within 10 days of beginning therapy. White blood cell and platelet counts should be monitored prior to and periodically during therapy. Because it attacks rapidly growing cells, stomatitis, anorexia, nausea, vomiting, and diarrhea may occur. Good oral hygiene and monitoring of nutritional status are important. If the decision is made to try this drug, referral to or consultation with a hematologist is suggested. Patients and caregivers should be instructed not to handle the tablets with bare hands; gloves should be worn when handling tablets.

Experimental drug therapy is being tried with **erythropoietin** to determine its capability in augmenting the production of fetal Hgb (HgbF). HgbF interferes with the polymerization of HgbS in solution and with the sickling of HgbS RBCs. Butyrate, a simple fatty acid widely used as a food additive, is also being investigated as an agent that may increase HgbF production. Their role in therapy, alone or in combination with **hydroxyurea**, is still unclear. **Erythropoietin** is discussed in Chapter 18.

Transfusions

With the mild to moderate anemia common to SCD, body systems except the eye and the spleen adapt fairly well to the reduced oxygen-carrying capacity of the blood. Most patients with SCD are relatively asymptomatic from their anemia and do not require transfusions to improve oxygen-carrying capacity. Transfusions may be used for specific indications when the anemia is severe or to prevent chronic complications. According to the NHLBI (2004), indications for RBC transfusions include the following:

1. In severely anemic patients, simple transfusions without exchange when:
   a. Patients are so anemic that they have physiological derangement that is manifested by impending or overt high-output cardiac failure, dyspnea, postural hypotension, angina, or cerebral dysfunction.
   b. Patients have had a sudden diminution in Hgb concentration, particularly patients who are having an acute splenic or hepatic sequestration crisis, manifested by rapid spleen or liver enlargement and rapidly falling Hct.
   c. Patients exhibit fatigue and dyspnea, usually at Hgb levels lower than 5 g/dL and a Hct less than 15 percent.
2. When there is a need to improve microvascular perfusion by decreasing the proportion of erythrocytes containing HgbS, an exchange transfusion is indicated unless the patient is severely anemic and has good cardiac function. Conditions for exchange transfusion include the following:
   a. Acute or suspected stroke or transient ischemic attack (TIA). The STOP Trial (Adams, 2000) found that first-time stroke can be prevented in children found to be at risk by periodic blood transfusion to suppress HgbS concentration to less than 30 percent.
   b. Multiorgan failure syndrome, including fat embolization.
   c. Acute chest syndrome or other acute lung disease, when arterial oxygen cannot be maintained at near-normal levels or when the process progresses despite antibiotic and other indicated therapy.
   d. Acute priapism unresponsive to therapy.
   e. Surgery on the posterior segment of the eye, even if done under local anesthesia or preparation for general anesthesia.
3. Chronic transfusion programs, usually initiated by exchange transfusion, when:
   a. Children have had stroke, to prevent further complications.
   b. Chronic congestive heart failure exists in conjunction with other treatment.

In any case, the goal is a percentage of HgbS between 20 and percent (NHLBI, 2004). This usually requires repeated transfusion every 3 to 4 weeks. Maintaining this percentage has reduced the rate of cerebral infarction in children by 90 percent. These serious conditions often require hospitalization.

Conditions that are not indications or are contraindications for transfusion therapy include chronic steady-state anemia, uncomplicated acute painful crises, infections, minor surgery not requiring prolonged general anesthesia (e.g., myringotomy), aseptic necrosis of the hip or shoulder not requiring surgery, and uncomplicated pregnancy.

Transfusions are not without complications. Volume overload may require administration of **furosemide (Lasix)**, especially if the patient has cardiac dysfunction or minimum cardiac reserve. Iron overload can occur with chronic transfusions, usually after 1 to 3 years of therapy. Serum ferritin levels should be measured periodically. If the level is above 2,000 ng/mL and transfusions are still required, chronic chelation therapy using nightly subcutaneous injections of **deferoxamine (Desferal)**

5 nights each week over several months is recommended by the NHLBI. Complications of this therapy include ototoxicity, ophthalmic toxicity, allergic reactions, growth failure, unusual infections, and pulmonary hypersensitivity. Annual visits to ophthalmological and audiological specialists for early detection of possible adverse reactions should be arranged. Ongoing education and support are usually necessary to maintain adherence to therapy. **Deferoxamine** should be discontinued during acute bacterial infections.

Monitoring

Hgb, Hct, reticulocyte counts, platelet counts, and white blood cell counts should be done frequently during the first year of life to establish the patient's baseline. After the first year, Hgb and Hct are relatively stable and need to be checked only once or twice a year in stable patients. Stable patients also require annual urinalysis, blood urea nitrogen (BUN), creatinine, and liver enzyme studies to monitor for evidence of organ damage. Before administration of transfusions, RBC antigens are needed. Patients with SCD are often difficult to crossmatch.

Most adults with SCD should have regular medical evaluations every 3 to 6 months. Blood counts, urinalysis, and routine chemistry tests should be done annually. With advancing age, complications such as chronic organ failure often require more frequent visits and more extensive laboratory evaluations. Attention focuses primarily on abnormalities in renal function and complications such as gallstones, aseptic necrosis, leg ulcers, and priapism.

Outcome Evaluation

The overall goal of therapy is the reduction in the number of sickling crises and prevention of organ damage. Hgb level goals are 9 g/dL or greater, but levels of at least 7 g/dL may be acceptable in asymptomatic patients. The goal for percentage of HgbS is 30 percent or less. Outcomes for chronic transfusion therapy were presented previously.

Patient Education

Patient and parental information related to SCA should focus on the following:

1. Understanding the pathophysiology of SCD and the organs commonly damaged.
2. Recognizing the importance of prevention, especially the central role of prevention of infection and avoidance of precipitants of sickling.
3. Learning how to administer prophylactic **antibiotics** and other drugs.
4. Understanding the necessity of adherence to the treatment regimen.
5. Recognizing need for regular follow-up visits with a primary care provider to manage this chronic disease.
6. Understanding the role of genetic counseling.

Prevention of sickling requires the parents and the patient to learn specific assessment skills. Any sign of illness in a child with SCD can be serious.

Patient education related to the administration of **penicillin** is discussed in Chapter 24.

Measures to minimize the risk of vaso-occlusive events beyond prevention of infection were discussed previously. The hazards of cigarette smoking and excessive **alcohol** intake and the benefits of a well-planned exercise program should be included.

Although IDA is not common for patients with SCD, prevention of IDA with a diet that includes sufficient amounts of **iron**-rich foods should be discussed. When **iron** is required, follow the patient education instructions for IDA.

Patient education specific to the use of **hydroxyurea** includes the following:

1. Take the drug exactly as prescribed, even if nausea, vomiting, or diarrhea occurs.
2. If a dose is missed, do not take it at all; do not double dose.
3. Notify the health-care provider of fever; chills; sore throat; loss of appetite; nausea; vomiting; diarrhea; bleeding gums; bruising; petechiae; or blood in the urine, stool, or emesis.
4. Avoid alcoholic beverages, **aspirin**, and **NSAIDs**, which may increase risk of bleeding.
5. Inspect oral mucosa for erythema and ulceration. If it occurs, use a sponge brush and rinse mouth with water after eating and drinking. If mouth pain interferes with eating, contact the health-care provider for lidocaine-based mouthwash.
6. Encourage fluid intake of 2,000 to 3,000 mL of noncaffeinated fluid daily.
7. Review need for contraception during therapy because of the teratogenic potential of this drug.

Patient education related to the other drugs used in treatment of SCD and its complications is presented in the Unit II chapters that include these drugs. Patient education related to the other complications of SCD is detailed in the NIH publications in the References section.

REFERENCES

Adams, R. J. (2000). Lessons from the Stroke Prevention Trial in Sickle Cell Anemia (STOP) study. *Journal of Child Neurology, 15*(5), 344–349.

American Academy of Family Physicians. (2004). *Summary of policy recommendations for periodic health examinations.* Lenwood, KS: American Academy of Family Physicians.

Baker, R. D., Greer, F. R., and The Committee on Nutrition (2010). Clinical report—Diagnosis and prevention of iron deficiency and iron-deficiency anemia in infants and young children (1–3 years of age). *Pediatrics, 126*(5), 1040–1050.

Brawley, O. W., Cornelius, L. J., Edwards, L. R., Gamble, V. N., Green, B. L., Inturrisi, C., James, A. H., Laraque, D., Mendez, M., Montoya, C. J., Pollock, B. H., Robinson, L., Scholnik, A. P., & Schori, M. (2008). National Institutes of Health Consensus Development Conference Statement: Hydroxyurea treatment for sickle cell disease. *Annals of Internal Medicine, 148*(12), 932–938.

Burns, C., Dunn, A., Brady, M., Barber-Starr, N., & Blooser, K. (2009). *Pediatric primary care* (4th ed.). Philadelphia: Saunders.

Centers for Disease Control and Prevention (CDC). (1998). CDC recommendations to prevent and control iron deficiency in the United States. *Morbidity and Mortality Weekly Report, Recommendations Report, 47*, 1–29.

Centers for Disease Control and Prevention (CDC). (2002). Iron deficiency—United States 1999–2000. *Morbidity and Mortality Weekly Report, 51*(40), 897–899.

Centers for Disease Control and Prevention (CDC), Division of Laboratory Services. (2009). Quality assurance and proficiency testing for newborn screening. Retrieved from http://www.cdc.gov/nceh/dls/newborn.htm

Centers for Disease Control and Prevention (CDC). (2010). Sickle cell disease. Retrieved from http://www.cdc.gov/ncbddd/sicklecell/data.html

Dunphy, L., & Winland-Brown, J. (2001). *Primary care: The art and science of advanced practice nursing.* Philadelphia: F.A. Davis.

Institute for Clinical Systems Improvement (ICSI). (2004). *Preventive counseling and education—by topic.* Bloomington, MN: Institute for Clinical Systems Improvement.

McCance, K., & Huether, S. (2006). *Pathophysiology: Biological basis for disease in adults and children* (5th ed.). St. Louis, MO: Mosby.

Montoya, V., Wink, D., & Sole, M. (2002). Adult anemia: Determine clinical significance. *Nurse Practitioner, 27*(3), 38–53.

National Anemia Action Council. (2009). Anemia in adolescents—the teen scene. National Anemia Action Council. Retrieved from http://www.anemia.org/patients/feature-articles/content.php?contentid=000348

National Heart, Lung, and Blood Institute (NHLBI). (2004). *Management of sickle cell disease* (NIH Publication No. 04-2117). Rockville, MD: National Institutes of Health.

National Kidney Foundation. (2006). *NKF-K/DOQI clinical practice guidelines and clinical practice recommendations for anemia of chronic kidney disease.* Retrieved November 9, 2010 from http://www.kidney.org/professionals/kdoqi/guidelines_anemia/index.htm

Office of Dietary Supplements. (2010a). Dietary supplement fact sheet: Iron. National Institutes of Health. Retrieved from http://ods.od.nih.gov/factsheets/Iron-HealthProfessional/

Office of Dietary Supplements. (2010b). Dietary supplement fact sheet: Vitamin B_{12}. National Institutes of Health. Retrieved from http://ods.od.nih.gov/factsheets/VitaminB12-HealthProfessional/

Oh, R. C., & Brown, D. L. (2003). Vitamin B_{12} deficiency. *American Family Physician, 67*(5), 979–986.

Pass, K., Lane, P., Fernhoff, P., Hinton, C. F., Panny, S. R., Parks, J. S., et al. (2000). Newborn screening system guidelines II: Follow-up of children, diagnosis, management, and evaluation. Statement of the Council of Regional Networks for Genetic Services. *Journal of Pediatrics, 137*(Suppl.), S1–S46.

Richer, S. (1997). A practical guide for differentiating between iron deficiency anemia and anemia of chronic disease in children and adults. *Nurse Practitioner, 22*(4), 82–103.

Schappert, S. M., & Rechtsteiner, E. A. (2008). *Ambulatory medical care utilization estimates for 2006* (National Health Statistics Reports No. 8). Hyattsville, MD: National Center for Health Statistics.

Stoltzfus, R. (2001). Defining iron-deficiency anemia in public health terms: Reexamining the nature and magnitude of the public health problem. *Journal of Nutrition, 131,* 565S–570S.

Tanyi, R. (2003). Sickle cell disease: Health promotion and maintenance and the role of primary care nurse practitioners. *Journal of the American Academy of Nurse Practitioners, 15*(9), 389–397.

U.S. Department of Health and Human Services. (2005). *Dietary guidelines for Americans, 2005.* Washington, DC: U.S. Department of Health and Human Services, U.S. Department of Agriculture.

U.S. Preventive Services Task Force. (2006). *Screening for iron deficiency anemia—including iron supplementation for children and pregnant women: Recommendation statement* (Publication No. AHRQ 06-0589). Rockville, MD: Agency for Healthcare Research and Quality.

U.S. Preventive Services Task Force. (2009). Folic acid for the prevention of neural tube defects: U.S. Preventive Services Task Force recommendation statement. *Annals of Internal Medicine, 150*(9), 626–631.

World Health Organization. 2008. Worldwide Prevalence of Anaemia 1993–2005. WHO Global Database on Anaemia. Retrieved from http://www.who.int/nutrition/publications/micronutrients/anaemia_iron_deficiency/9789241596657/en/index.html

World Health Organization. 2010. Micronutrient deficiencies: Iron deficiency anemia. Retrieved from http://www.who.int/nutrition/topics/ida/en/index.html

CHAPTER 28

CHRONIC STABLE ANGINA AND LOW-RISK UNSTABLE ANGINA

Anita Lee Wynne and Sharon Maxey

Chapter Outline

Angina is a clinical syndrome typically characterized by deep, poorly localized chest or arm discomfort that is reproducibly associated with physical exertion or emotional stress and promptly relieved by rest or **nitroglycerin.** The pathophysiology behind it is an imbalance between myocardial oxygen supply and demand (ischemia) associated with coronary artery disease (CAD). Several million Americans suffer from ischemic heart disease, and more than 600,000 die each year from this disorder or its complications. Chronic stable angina is the form most commonly seen in primary care, but even these patients have a mortality risk of 2 to 12 percent annually. The lifetime risk of death from CAD is 49 percent for males and 32 percent for females.

Treatment includes lifestyle modifications and pharmacological and surgical interventions. Pharmacological management includes the use of **aspirin, nitrates, beta-adrenergic blockers, long-acting calcium channel blockers (CCBs), angiotensin-converting enzyme (ACE) inhibitors, ranolazine, and low-density lipoprotein (LDL)** cholesterol lowering with a **3-hydroxy-3-methylglutaryl coenzyme A (HMG CoA) reductase inhibitor (statin).** These drugs are discussed in detail in Chapters 14, 16, and 18. Concomitant disorders often include diabetes mellitus, hyperlipidemia, and hypertension, so that the treatment regimen can be quite complex. Chapters 33, 39, and 40, respectively, discuss management of these specific disorders. The focus of this chapter is the long-term management of chronic stable angina and low-risk unstable angina that is usually done by primary care providers.

Several guidelines have been written about this management. The central guideline to which others refer or with which others are consistent is the American College of Cardiology/American Heart Association (ACC/AHA) guideline, originally published in 1999 and updated in 2002. Institute for Clinical Symptoms Improvement (ICSI) guidelines published in 2007 and 2008 and American College of Physicians guidelines published in 2004 all refer to the 2002 ACC/AHA guideline as a scientifically valid, high-quality review of evidence and agree with the findings of that guideline. The recommendations in this chapter are consistent with that guideline. Where other guidelines add to or differ from this guideline, this is discussed.

PATHOPHYSIOLOGY

CAD, myocardial ischemia, and myocardial infarction (MI) form a pathophysiological continuum that impairs the pumping ability of the heart by depriving it of sufficient oxygen and nutrients. Figure 28–1 depicts the physiological

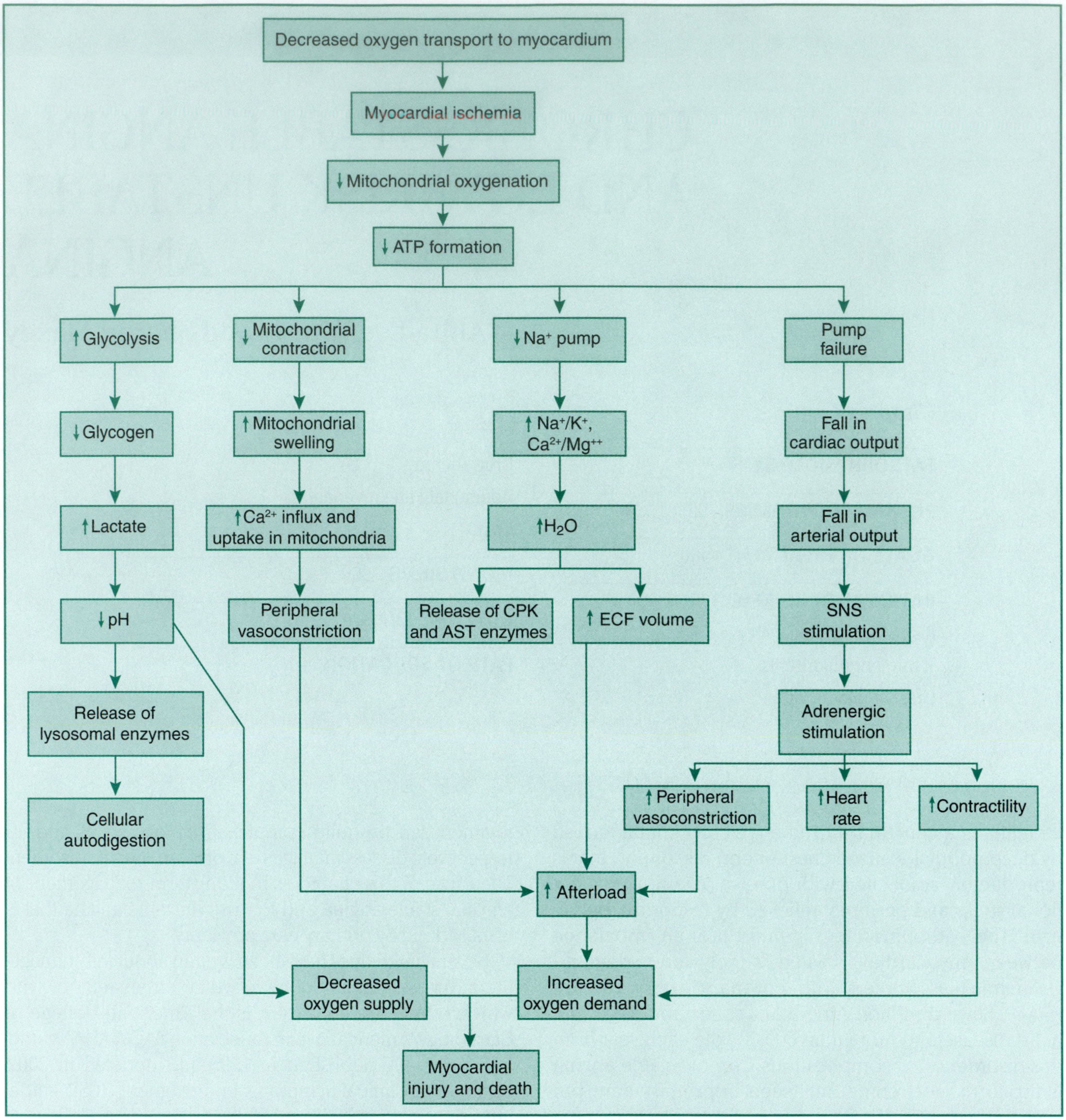

Figure 28–1. Pathophysiology of myocardial ischemia.

changes that occur when the myocardium is deprived of oxygen. The coronary arteries supply oxygen to the myocardium. Oxygen extraction from these vessels is at maximum efficiency at all times, and there is no oxygen reserve during periods of increased oxygen demand. Ischemia occurs when demand exceeds supply. One mechanism available to increase oxygen supply is to dilate the coronary arteries and bring more blood flow to the myocardium. Nitrates can do this in patients with normal hearts. Unfortunately, in CAD, usually associated with atherosclerosis and plaque formation, the coronary arteries are often maximally dilated already. Most of the drugs available to treat angina decrease myocardial oxygen demand by decreasing the workload of the heart. The drugs accomplish this by decreasing afterload, preload, or both. The one exception to these mechanisms is **ranozaline**, whose mechanism is not completely elucidated at this point but does seem to involve effects on preload and afterload.

In patients with ischemia, **nitrates** do not increase total coronary blood flow but redistribute the blood to the ischemic areas. Although they have some ability to dilate the coronary arteries, **nitrates** are also able to facilitate movement of oxygen across the arterial–myocardial membrane and their use in CAD relates as much to this action as it does to vasodilation.

The most common cause of CAD and resultant myocardial ischemia is atherosclerosis. The growing mass of plaque, platelets, fibrin, and cellular debris eventually narrows the lumen enough to impede blood flow. The growth of this mass is related in part to the action of angiotensin II, which acts as a growth factor for vascular cells. **ACE inhibitors** prevent the formation of angiotensin II and thus reduce this growth. The link between CAD and elevated plasma lipoprotein concentrations is well documented (see Chaps. 29, 39, and 40). The fatty streaks that will eventually form the plaque have a lipoprotein/cholesterol base, the main component of which is LDL cholesterol. **Statins** have a major role in reducing LDL cholesterol concentrations and preventing plaque formation. Platelet aggregations release the prostaglandin thromboxane A_2, a potent vasoconstrictor capable of causing spasms of the coronary arteries. The use of **aspirin** in patients with CAD is associated with its role in irreversibly blocking thromboxane A_2.

Imbalances between myocardial supply and demand can result from a variety of conditions. Supply is reduced by the following:

- Hemodynamic factors such as increased resistance in coronary vessels, hypotension, and decreased blood volume. **ACE inhibitors, beta blockers,** and the **dihydropyridine CCBs** decrease peripheral resistance through their vasodilatory actions.
- Cardiac factors such as decreases in diastolic filling time, increases in heart rate, and valvular incompetence. **Beta blockers** and **non-dihydropyridine CCBs** decrease heart rate. The **beta blockers** have the further advantage of preventing the recurrence of MIs.
- Hematological factors such as the oxygen content of the blood, the acid–base status of the blood, and anemia.
- Systemic disorders, such as shock, which reduce blood flow or the availability of oxygen.

Demand is increased by the following:

- High systolic blood pressure, which increases the work the heart has to do to move blood from the left ventricle to the systemic circulation. One focus of anginal management is control of blood pressure. **ACE inhibitors, beta blockers,** and both types of **CCBs** decrease blood pressure.
- Increased ventricular volume, which increases the work the heart has to do because the left ventricle must move more blood. **ACE inhibitors** reduce sodium and water retention.
- Increased thickness of the myocardium (ventricular hypertrophy). The same mechanism that facilitated growth of the vessel walls in atherosclerosis also increases the thickness of the myocardium. **ACE inhibitors** play a major role here to decrease the remodeling.
- Increased heart rate resulting from exercise, stress, hyperthyroidism, fever, anemia, or hyperviscosity of the blood.
- Conditions that heighten the myocardium's contractile response. **Beta blockers** and **CCBs** both have negative inotropic effects.

Ischemia caused by the imbalance between myocardial oxygen supply (MOS) and myocardial oxygen demand (MOD) produces pain referred to as angina. There are three types of angina: chronic stable angina, unstable angina, and Prinzmetal's angina. Chronic stable angina (exertional angina) is caused by narrowing of the arterial lumen and hardening of the arterial walls, so that the affected vessels cannot dilate in response to the increased MOD associated with physical exertion or emotional stress. Research indicates that up to 90 percent of ischemia is asymptomatic (silent ischemia). Diabetes mellitus and hypertension are associated with an increased prevalence of silent ischemia. Ischemia with or without pain has the same prognosis. In both cases, the myocardium is at risk.

On the cellular level, the myocardium becomes cyanotic within the first 10 seconds of impaired oxygen supply, and electrocardiographic (ECG) changes occur. Deprived of oxygen, the myocardial cells convert to anaerobic metabolism, and lactic acid accumulates. Myocardial nerve fibers are irritated by this lactic acid and transmit a pain message to the cardiac nerves and upper thoracic posterior nerve roots. Under ischemic conditions, cardiac cells are viable for about 20 minutes. The supply–demand imbalance must be resolved during this time to prevent permanent damage.

PHARMACODYNAMICS

Nitrates affect the supply–demand equation on both sides. Low doses of nitroglycerin preferentially dilate the veins more than the arterioles. The resulting decrease in venous return to the heart decreases left ventricular end-diastolic pressure (preload), resulting in decreased wall tension and an increased transmyocardial gradient. This increased gradient improves perfusion between the coronary arteries on the outside of the heart and the subendocardium on the inside of the heart and increases oxygen supply to the myocardium. Higher doses of **nitrates** dilate arterial vessels, which results in decreased systemic vascular resistance (afterload). Additionally, the higher doses cause further dilation of venous vessels, which results in venous pooling, and decreased venous return to the heart. MOD is reduced by the reduced cardiac workload. **Nitrates** also dilate coronary arteries to some extent, but doing so is difficult in severe atherosclerotic arteries, and this effect is now thought to be only a small part of their action in relieving ischemia.

Beta blockers affect the supply–demand equation on the demand side. Both **beta$_1$-selective agents** and **nonselective beta blockers** decrease the force of myocardial contractility and decrease heart rate and conduction velocity. **Beta blockers** also decrease systemic vascular resistance and blood pressure (afterload). All of these effects reduce myocardial oxygen demand and thus relieve anginal pain.

CCBs primarily affect the supply–demand equation on the demand side of the equation. By blocking calcium influx into cells, the **dihydropyridines** cause arterial smooth muscle relaxation, which results in peripheral vasodilation and decreased afterload and ultimately decreased MOD. They also accomplish this at doses that do not affect cardiac smooth muscle. The **dihydropyridines** have the potential to cause coronary vasodilation, but again, because the coronary arteries are usually already maximally dilated in patients with angina, this will result in only a small, if any, increase in MOS. The **nondihydropyridine calcium channel blockers (Verapamil** and **diltiazem)** depress the rate of sinoarterial (SA) node depolarization and slow atrioventricular (AV) conduction, resulting in a decreased heart rate as well as decreased contractility in cardiac smooth muscle.

These two actions result in negative chronotropic and inotropic effects and ultimately decrease MOD. They accomplish this at doses that have only a small impact on vascular smooth muscle and consequently little effect on vasodilation.

ACE inhibitors also affect both the MOS and the MOD sides of the equation. Through their action on the renin-angiotensin-aldosterone system, **ACE inhibitors** prevent the formation of angiotensin II, a potent vasoconstrictor. This action decreases peripheral vascular resistance and thereby MOD, as the heart has decreased afterload against which it must pump. Reduced formation of angiotensin II also decreases the thickening of coronary artery walls, resulting in increased MOS (McCance & Huether, 2006), and decreases the thickening of ventricular walls, resulting in decreased MOD. They also reduce the secretion of aldosterone, which reduces the retention of sodium and water, thereby reducing extracellular fluid volume and preload.

Ranolazine has antianginal and anti-ischemic effects that do not depend on reduction in heart rate or blood pressure. Although the exact mechanism of action has not been determined, at therapeutic levels it can inhibit the cardiac late sodium current. The relationship of this inhibition to angina symptoms is uncertain.

Aspirin inhibits the synthesis of thromboxane A_2 in the production of platelets. This action reduces platelet aggregation to stop the cycle of vasoconstriction and platelet buildup. Research has clearly demonstrated a role for this drug in primary prevention of MI as an adjunct to risk factor management.

Finally, **statins** are a recent addition to the treatment regimen for angina. Their role is on the MOS side of the equation as reduction in LDL cholesterol levels plays a significant role in decreasing the formation of atherosclerotic plaque. This plaque is central to the narrowing of the arterial lumen.

GOALS OF TREATMENT

The immediate goals are to treat to complete, or near complete, elimination of anginal chest pain and return to normal activities; maintain the patient at a symptom level of Canadian Cardiovascular Society (CCS) classification of angina class I with minimum adverse effects; and keep blood pressure less than 130/85 mm Hg and pulse less than 70 beats per minute (Veterans Health Administration, Department of Defense [VA/DoD], 2003). The ultimate goals of therapy are to reduce the risks of MI and death. Although the clinical course of some patients may extend for 15 or 20 years, most patients with chronic stable angina are still at increased risk for cardiovascular morbidity and mortality. Their prognosis is strongly affected by the number and locations of coronary artery stenoses, the severity of the ischemia, and the presence of other CAD risk factors, such as smoking, hypertension, hypercholesterolemia, low high-density lipoprotein (HDL) cholesterol, diabetes mellitus, and age and gender considerations. Achievement of these goals is accomplished through improving oxygen supply and decreasing oxygen demand.

RATIONAL DRUG SELECTION

Angina is associated with MI and sudden cardiac death in the mind of provider and public alike. This presents a two-edged sword in therapeutic management: recognition of the potential complications, leading to consistent adherence to the treatment regimen, versus denial of the seriousness of the disorder, leading to lack of adherence to the treatment regimen. The health-care provider can improve adherence by placing angina in a realistic perspective and tailoring treatment options to each patient's needs. For effective management, the choice of treatment should be low cost, limited in complexity, and with the fewest possible adverse reactions. To achieve this treatment protocol, lifestyle modifications and pharmacological therapy are chosen based on risk stratification, grade of angina, and specific patient variables. For each of these variables, the therapy discussed includes lifestyle modifications, initial monotherapy, and two- and three-drug therapy.

Risk Stratification

Major Risk Factors

The major risk factors for CAD are age, family history, smoking, hypertension, hypercholesterolemia, low HDL cholesterol, and diabetes mellitus (discussed in Chap. 39 and shown in Table 39–3). These risk factors are used in the Framingham equations for calculating 10-year risk for the development of coronary heart disease (Anderson et al, the American College of Cardiology/American Heart Association Task Force on Practice Guidelines, 2007). In addition, conditions that decrease oxygen supply and increase oxygen demand are also major risk factors for ischemic heart disease. These include heart failure (see Chap. 36), anemia (see Chap. 27), hypertension (see Chap. 40), hyperthyroidism (see Chap. 41), valvular heart disease, and morbid obesity.

Noncardiac Factors

There are also noncardiac disorders that mimic angina because their primary symptom is chest pain. These include pulmonary embolism, pneumonia, pneumothorax, gastroesophageal spasm or reflux, cholecystitis, peptic ulcer, pancreatitis, rib fractures, herpes zoster, and panic disorder. Some of these disorders also decrease oxygen supply and can cause angina. These disorders should be ruled out before deciding a patient has angina.

Women often have symptoms of angina that are atypical and may include fatigue, shortness of breath without chest pain, nausea and vomiting, back pain, jaw pain, dizziness and weakness (ICSI, 2007). A study of cardiovascular outcomes in women with nonobstructive CAD (Gulati et al, 2009) found that women with symptoms and signs suggestive of ischemia, even if they were atypical symptoms, but without obstructive CAD were still at elevated risk for cardiovascular events compared with asymptomatic women. This elevated risk for females should not be overlooked.

Classification System for Grading Angina

The New York Heart Association (NYHA) and the CCS have devised a classification system for grading the severity of angina (Table 28–1). The lower the class, the more likely the patient's angina can be controlled by lifestyle modification and intermittent **nitroglycerin** (Table 28–2). The higher the class, the more likely the patient will require multiple drug therapy. The ACC/AHA guidelines have a classification system that incorporates the NYHA/CCS system and additional data. Table 28–3 depicts this classification system.

Treatment Algorithms

It is not within the scope of this book to discuss the testing involved in the diagnosis and grading of angina; however, a thorough history including questions about symptoms and when they occur related to exercise, about smoking, a physical examination, laboratory testing for possible causes of the symptoms (e.g., anemia or thyroid disorders), and a resting 12-lead ECG should be obtained. For those with abnormal ECG findings, referral to or consultation with a cardiologist is recommended. The treatment protocol discussed in this chapter assumes accurate diagnosis of angina with the appropriate diagnostic tools. Once the diagnosis is made, protocols are based on the grade or class of angina and the risk profile.

All patients with angina should be on **aspirin** 81 to 325 mg/day (ACC/AHA, 2002; ICSI, 2007; Scottish Intercollegiate Guidelines Network [SIGN], 2001; Snow et al, 2004; VA/DoD, 2003). **Aspirin** is known to be effective for reducing mortality in patients with CAD and has been associated with a decrease in nonfatal MI, nonfatal stroke, and vascular death (ICSI, 2007; Italiano per lo Studio della Sopravvivenza nell'Infarto Miocardio, 1990). In these studies, **aspirin** was associated with preventing reinfarction and significantly reduced recurrent ischemic events. In another trial, the use of **aspirin** was associated with a significant reduction in admissions to the hospital for unstable angina.

Table 28–1 **Grading of Angina by the New York Heart Association and the Canadian Cardiovascular Society**

Class	New York Heart Association	Canadian Cardiovascular Society
Class I	Proven coronary artery disease without symptoms	Ordinary physical activity, such as walking or climbing stairs, does not cause angina. Angina occurs with strenuous, rapid, or prolonged exertion at work or recreation.
Class II	Angina only with unusually strenuous physical exertion	Slight limitation of ordinary activity. Angina occurs on walking or climbing stairs rapidly; walking uphill; walking or stair climbing after meals; in cold wind; under emotional stress; or only during the few hours after awakening. Walking more than two blocks on the level and climbing more than one flight of ordinary stairs at a normal pace and in normal conditions does not cause angina.
Class III	Angina during routine physical activity	Marked limitations of ordinary activity. Angina occurs on walking one to two blocks on the level and climbing one flight of stairs in normal conditions and at a normal pace.
Class IV	Angina during minimal activity or rest	Inability to carry on any physical activity without discomfort. Angina may occur at rest.

Table 28–2 Risk Profiles Associated With Angina

Risk	Lifestyle Risk	Physiological Risk
Low	• Nonsmoker • Normotensive • Low cholesterol • Negative family history	• Mild stable angina (class I–II) • Good exercise tolerance tests • Normal ventricular function on echocardiography
High	• Smoker • Hypertensive • Hypercholesterolemia • Positive family history	• Severe angina (class III–IV) • Unstable angina • Poor exercise test performance • Impaired ventricular function
Uncertain	• Obesity • Sedentary lifestyle • Type A personality • Emotional stress	• Silent ischemia

Table 28–3 American College of Cardiology/American Heart Association Risk Stratification in Patients With Chronic Stable Angina

Class	Description
Class I	• Disabling (CCS III and IV) chronic stable angina despite medical therapy • High-risk criteria on noninvasive testing regardless of anginal severity • Angina and have survived sudden cardiac death or serious ventricular dysrhythmias • Angina and symptoms of CHF • Clinical characteristics that indicate a high likelihood of severe CAD
Class IIa	• Significant LV dysfunction (ejection fraction <45%). CCS Class I or II angina and demonstrable ischemia but less than high-risk criteria on noninvasive testing • Inadequate prognostic information after noninvasive testing
Class IIb	• CCS Class I or II angina, preserved LV dysfunction (ejection fraction >45%) and less than high-risk criteria on noninvasive testing • CCS Class III or IV angina, which improves to Class I or II with medical therapy • CCS Class I or II angina, but intolerance to adequate medical therapy
Class III	• CCS Class I or II angina who respond to medical therapy and have no evidence of ischemia on noninvasive testing • Patients who prefer to avoid revascularization

CHF = congestive heart failure; LV = left ventricular.

If the **aspirin** is contraindicated, **clopidogrel (Plavix)** 75 mg daily may be substituted, but it is much more expensive (Kaiser Permanente Care Management Institute, 2006). One large (19,000 patients) randomized controlled study of patients with a history of ischemic heart disease, MI, or atherosclerotic peripheral arterial disease found **clopidogrel** demonstrated a relative-risk reduction of 8.7 percent when compared with **aspirin** 325 mg daily (VA/DoD, 2003).

Patients with angina only on exertion, a normal resting ECG, and symptoms that can be controlled by rest and intermittent **nitroglycerin** (ACC/AHA class III) should be started on lifestyle modifications and have any concurrent aggravating factors or disease processes treated. For example, hypertension itself can cause angina, and elevated cholesterol contributes to the continued development of atherosclerosis. Their treatment is critical. Patients with known CAD, age 60 and older, with ECG changes on exertion, and with diabetes are considered high risk for unstable angina and should be started on both lifestyle modifications and drug therapy.

Lifestyle Modification

Fundamental to the management of all types and grades of angina is the reduction of risk factors through lifestyle modification. Lifestyle modifications may prevent the development of complications commonly associated with myocardial ischemia and have little cost. Even when they cannot control angina alone, they may reduce the number and dosage of drugs required for angina management and prevent the need for surgical intervention. All patients should be advised to stop smoking, maintain appropriate levels of blood pressure and cholesterol; follow the

Dietary Approaches to Stop Hypertension (DASH) diet for control of hypertension, including the recommendation for cholesterol management (see Chaps. 39 and 40); and achieve, to the extent possible, their ideal body weight. Table 28–4 discusses the main lifestyle modifications appropriate for patients with angina. They are similar to those appropriate for patients with hypertension and hypercholesterolemia.

Concurrent with lifestyle modifications, patients with angina should have any concomitant diseases—such as hypertension, hypercholesterolemia, severe anemia, hyperthyroidism, hypoxic lung disorders, diabetes mellitus, and critical valvular stenosis—treated and brought under control. When these initial therapies have not resulted in improved exercise tolerance or decreased episodes of angina, or when the patient is ACC/AHA class I or IIa on the grading scale, initial drug therapy is begun. Figure 28–1 delineates the drug treatment protocol for chronic stable angina and low-risk unstable angina.

Drug Therapy

Initial Therapy for Symptomatic Patients

Nitrates, ACE inhibitors, beta-adrenergic blockers, and **CCBs** are the mainstays of initial drug therapy for patients with angina (Kaiser Permanente Care Management Institute, 2006; Snow et al, 2004). Each has a group of patients for whom they are best suited and a group for whom they are contraindicated. Detailed discussions of each of these classes of drugs are given in Chapters 14 and 16. The focus here is on their role in angina management.

ACE inhibitors are recommended by the American College of Physicians (Snow et al, 2004) and in other guidelines (ICSI, 2007; Kaiser Permanente Care Management Institute, 2006) for all symptomatic patients with chronic stable angina to prevent MI or death and to reduce symptoms. ACC/AHA (2002) and the Veterans Health Administration (2003) also recommend this drug class, but limit it to CAD patients who also have diabetes or left ventricular dysfunction. They recommend that **ACE inhibitors** be considered in CAD patients even without left ventricular dysfunction. They have been shown to improve outcomes for CAD patients through their ability to both increase MOS and decrease MOD. **ACE inhibitors** are discussed in more detail in Chapter 17. Table 28–5 shows concomitant diseases for which they are more useful and for which they are contraindicated.

Angiotensin II receptor blocker (ARB) therapy is recommended for patients with CAD and diabetes with hypertension, and those with left ventricular systolic dysfunction

Table 28–4 **Lifestyle Modifications**

Attain Ideal Body Weight. Excess weight increases cardiac workload and increases oxygen demand. It is also associated with hypertension, and loss of as little as 10 lb can significantly reduce blood pressure.
Increase Aerobic Physical Activity Within the Limitations of Angina. The overall goal of anginal therapy is to restore optimal exercise capacity. The presence of angina, however, indicates an imbalance in oxygen supply and demand and denotes possible damage to the myocardium. Start with a level of activity that does not produce pain, and gradually increase the activity level by 1 min each day as long as there is no angina. Even limited activity is preferred to no activity. Daily activity is preferred to intermittent activity.
Reduce Sodium Intake to No More Than 2,400 mg of Sodium or 6 g of Sodium Chloride. Sodium helps the body retain water, which increases the amount of blood volume. This increases cardiac workload and increases oxygen demand. It is also associated with hypertension. Reduced intake of this level can often be achieved by not adding salt during cooking or on the table and by watching hidden sources of salt, such as canned foods.
Maintain Adequate Intake of Dietary Potassium (Approximately 60 mEq/d). The heart is heavily dependent on potassium for contractility.
Reduce Intake of Dietary Saturated Fats and Cholesterol. Cholesterol and saturated fats are implicated in the development of atherosclerosis, which narrows coronary arteries and makes angina worse. The level of reduction depends on serum cholesterol levels. Hypercholesterolemia requires lower levels than those required for patients with normal cholesterol levels. Start with the American Heart Association Step 1 diet.
Stop Smoking. Nicotine is implicated in several ways in making angina worse. Absorbed nicotine increases blood pressure and heart rate, thus increasing myocardial oxygen demand. Nicotine also causes vasospasm, and the rise in carboxyhemoglobin from smoke inhalation reduces oxygen supply. Even passive smoke inhalation can reduce exercise tolerance in patients with angina. The low doses of nicotine found in nicotine replacement therapy (NRT) do not significantly elevate blood pressure or heart rate, and NRT may be used to aid in smoking cessation.
Limit Alcohol Intake. For men and heavier patients, alcohol intake should be no more than 1 oz (30 mL) of ethanol (e.g., 24 oz beer, 10 oz wine, 2 oz 100-proof whiskey)/d. For women and lighter-weight patients, the intake should be no more than 0.5 oz/d.

Table 28–5 **Drug Choice Based on Concomitant Disease States**

	EFFECT ON CONCOMITANT DISEASE STATES	
Drug Choice	**Favorable Effects**	**Unfavorable Effects**
Nitrates	Heart failure Hypertension	Migraine headaches MI
Beta-Adrenergic Blockers	Heart failure Arrhythmias, atrial tachycardia Hypertension "Stage fright" Migraine headaches Hyperthyroidism	Advanced AV block Reactive airway disease Claudication/Raynaud's disease (can use $beta_1$-selective drug) Diabetes mellitus (may try $beta_1$-selective drug)
	Post-MI	Depression
ACE Inhibitors	Diabetes mellitus Heart failure Hyperlipidemia Hypertension	Contraindicated in: Pregnancy Bilateral renal artery stenosis Angioedema history
HMG-Co-A Reductase Inhibitors (Statins)	Hyperlipidemia Hypertension	Contraindicated in pregnancy Myopathy history
Calcium Channel Blockers Dihydropyridines	Hypertension, isolated systolic hypertension Systolic heart failure Raynaud's disease, peripheral vascular disease	Peripheral edema
Verapamil	Atrial tachycardias Hypertension Migraine headache MI	Advanced AV block Constipation Heart failure Concurrent use with beta blockers may cause additive bradycardia
Diltiazem	Atrial tachycardia Diabetes mellitus MI	Advanced AV block Heart failure
Amlodipine	Atherosclerosis Heart failure	

ACE = angiotensin-converting enzymes; AV = atrioventricular; HMG-Co-A = 3-hydroxy-3-methyl glutaryl coenzyme A; MI = myocardial infarction.

when these patients are intolerant to **ACE inhibitors**. For other patients who are tolerant to **ACE inhibitors**, there is insufficient evidence to recommend for or against **ARB** therapy (Kaiser Permanente Care Management Institute, 2006). **ARBs** can be added to **ACE inhibitor** therapy for clinical reasons, such as uncontrolled hypertension or insufficient vasodilation, but it is not recommended as a routine addition.

Beta blockers with no intrinsic sympathomimetic activity (ISA) properties are recommended as initial therapy by all the guidelines for all patients, with or without previous MI, unless specifically contraindicated. They especially decrease MOD and are the drugs of choice for exertional angina (ACC/AHA all classes). Because they do not improve myocardial oxygen supply, their main role is in preventing recurrence of MIs in patients with CAD. They are especially useful for patients with exertional angina whose lifestyle involves frequent vigorous activity, patients with resting tachycardia (e.g., hyperthyroidism), and for patients who have concomitant diseases that might benefit from beta blockade. The Kaiser guidelines (2006) make a strong recommendation for giving a **beta blocker** to CAD patients with left ventricular systolic dysfunction (NYHA classes I through IV). Table 28–5 shows these concomitant diseases. **Beta blockers** are contraindicated for patients with severe, uncontrolled reactive airway diseases, and vasospastic angina. For patients with mild to moderate reversible airway disease or chronic obstructive pulmonary disease, cardioselective **beta blockers** maybe used as long as the airway disease is stable and well controlled (Kaiser Permanente Care Management Institute, 2006). The most cost-effective and convenient

beta blocker is **atenolol (Tenormin)**, with its once-daily dosing, low adverse reactions profile, and $beta_1$ selectivity. **Beta blockers** are discussed in more detail in Chapter 14.

Most guidelines recommend lipid-lowering therapy with **statins** for all CAD patients who have LDL cholesterol levels greater than 100 mg/dL except the Veterans Health Administration (2003), which does not mention LDL levels, and Kaiser guidelines, which call for LDL less than 70 mg/dL. ICSI (2007; updated in 2009) guidelines recommend **statin** therapy for all CAD patients regardless of their lipid level unless contraindicated. Treatment of elevated LDL cholesterol is discussed extensively in Chapter 39, and the drugs themselves are discussed in Chapter 16.

Nitrates and **CCBs** are appropriate for symptoms management and specific indications. **Nitrates** are the oldest and best studied of the **antianginals**, are cost effective, and have a variety of routes of administration that allow flexibility for the patient. They are more effective than **beta blockers** in relieving and preventing anginal episodes in patients with vasospastic angina. **Nitroglycerin** 0.3 to 0.4 mg sublingual tablets or translingual spray is used for immediate symptom relief. All patients with angina should carry some form of rapid-acting **nitrate** with them at all times. They should be instructed to use this medication at the first sign of angina, even if they are uncertain if the symptoms are angina. If symptoms persist after three doses of this drug have been taken at 5-minute intervals, the patient should go to the hospital for medical attention. One recent study showed that only 35 percent of patients with CAD are **nitrate** responsive for the diagnosis of active CAD (Henrikson et al, 2003). Gibbons (2003), however, questions the validity of the one study and suggests we continue to use the protocol above because **nitrates** decrease MOD by decreasing preload and afterload during acute coronary syndromes, and they may dilate large coronary arteries and collateral vessels that would improve oxygen supply. Chapter 16 has specific information on the treatment protocol and storage of **nitroglycerin** in its various forms.

For patients who respond well to sublingual or translingual **nitroglycerin** and who experience angina episodes more than "rarely," and who are intolerant of **beta blockers**, long-acting oral or transdermal **nitrates** are generally indicated. Among the available drugs, the most cost-effective is **isosorbide dinitrate (Isordil)** given bid or tid, with a 10- to 12-hour **nitrate**-free interval to prevent **nitrate** tolerance. The timing of the **nitrate**-free interval should coincide with the time of fewest episodes of angina, which is typically at night. The administration schedule that seems most effective is 7 a.m. and 2 p.m. daily. Headache is the most common adverse reaction, but tachyphylaxis to this problem also develops, and the headaches resolve. Starting with low doses and slowly increasing the dose reduces the incidence of headache.

CCBs, like the **nitrates**, decrease MOD. They are the initial drugs of choice when coronary artery vasospasm is suspected to be a contributing mechanism to the angina. They are also effective for patients with exertional angina who have fixed atherosclerotic CAD; when optimal doses of **beta blockers** or **nitrates** are ineffective, contraindicated, or poorly tolerated; and when a concomitant disease might benefit from the use of a **CCB**. Table 28–5 shows these concomitant diseases. Studies have also shown one **CCB**, **amlodipine (Norvasc)**, to be effective in inhibiting vascular smooth muscle cell proliferation in atherosclerosis, and it may have a protective mechanism in preventing or retarding the progression of atherosclerosis (Stepien et al, 1998). It also has the advantage of a long half-life that allows once-daily dosing without resorting to a sustained-release form.

There have been concerns raised about the potential for **CCBs** to negatively affect long-term survival in patients post-MI. Studies have shown that this problem is specific to the dramatic lowering of blood pressure associated with the use of short-acting **nifedipine (Adalat)**. Other studies did not support an association between long-acting forms of **nifedipine** or other **CCBs** and decreased long-term survival in this population. In contrast, one study (Reicher-Reiss et al, 1998) did find that low-dose, short-acting **nifedipine** therapy used in a randomized clinical trial for 1 year was not associated with increased mortality during a 5-year follow-up.

When initial therapy with low to moderate doses of these drugs is not adequate to control angina or to reduce the grade from a lower class (ACC/AHA class I or IIa) to a higher one (ACC/AHA class IIb or III), two choices are possible. One is to increase the dose of at least one of the drugs. This is always done with consideration for the potential adverse reactions associated with that drug. In some cases, the addition of another drug to minimize the adverse reactions and provide an additive effect to maximize benefits may be more appropriate than significant increases in the initial drug. The second option is to substitute a drug from a different class. **Nitrates** and **CCBs** are both effective, for example, in vasospastic angina, but not all patients respond well to **nitrates**. **Ranolazine** has been evaluated in patients with chronic symptomatic angina despite treatment with the maximum dose of other antianginal agents. Statistically significant decreases in angina attacks were observed. This drug may be used concurrently with any of the antianginal classes discussed above and with antiplatelet and lipid-lowering drugs.

Multidrug Therapy

Combinations of **beta blockers** and **calcium channel blockers** have been shown to be more effective than the individual drugs used alone. Both **amlodipine** and **felodipine (dihydropyridine CCBs)** work especially well in this group of patients. Their effects on reducing MOD are complementary, making it possible to use lower doses of both drugs, and many of their adverse reactions cancel out. Lower doses also reduce the risk of hypotension. Patients not adequately controlled by either drug alone tend to benefit from the addition of the second drug. They are a questionable combination for patients with left ventricular dysfunction because they may induce heart failure or bradycardia in these patients. **Verapamil** and **diltiazem** should be avoided in this combination.

Combinations of a long-acting **nitrate** and a **beta blocker** are also safe, effective, and low in cost. Their effects are additive, permitting lower doses of both drugs, and their adverse reactions often cancel out. The **beta blocker** slows any reflex tachycardia caused by the **nitrate**, which helps to reduce MOD.

Combinations of long-acting **nitrates** and **CCBs** are rarely used because of the high risk for hypotension and because their adverse reaction profiles are additive. This combination is usually reserved for refractory cases of vasospastic angina.

When the drug combination greatly improves angina, it is worthwhile to attempt gradual reduction of prior drug doses over time. For example, if the addition of a **beta blocker** to high-dose **nitrate** therapy greatly improves angina, gradual reduction in the **nitrate** doses can be tried.

Patients with severe (classes III–IV) angina frequently require at least three drugs from different classes. When this level of regimen is required, referral to a cardiologist is appropriate.

Drug Therapy for Asymptomatic Patients

The focus of drug therapy for asymptomatic patients is prevention of MI and death. For these patients, **aspirin** is prescribed as for all patients with CAD. Lipid lowering with **statins** is also appropriate to achieve LDL cholesterol of less than 70 mg/dL. Factors that favor a decision to reduce LDL-C levels to less than 70 mg/dL are those that place patients in the category of *very high risk*. Among these factors are the presence of established cardiovascular disease (CVD) plus (1) multiple major risk factors (especially diabetes); (2) severe and poorly controlled risk factors (especially continued cigarette smoking); (3) multiple risk factors of the metabolic syndrome (especially high triglycerides greater than or equal to 200 mg/dL plus non-HDL-C greater than or equal to 130 mg/dL with low HDL-C [40 mg/dL]); and (4) on the basis of PROVE IT (a research trial), patients with acute coronary syndromes. To avoid any misunderstanding about cholesterol management in general, it must be emphasized that the optional goal of achieving an LDL cholesterol level of less than 70 mg/dL does not apply to individuals who are not high risk (National High Blood Pressure Education Program [NHBPEP], 2003). **Beta blockers** are recommended for ACC/AHA classes I and IIa. **ACE inhibitors** are recommended for ACC/AHA classes I and IIa who also have diabetes or systolic dysfunction.

Table 28–6 presents the drugs commonly used to treat angina, whether alone or in combination with other drugs.

In general, all patients with CAD should consume a diet rich in fruits, vegetables, legumes, nuts, whole grains, and omega-3 polyunsaturated fat. An increase in intake of **omega-3 polyunsaturated fatty acids** to a level of about 1 g/day, and the elimination of intake of *trans*-fatty acids are recommended by several studies (Kaiser Permanente Care Management Institute, 2006; Mente, deKoning, Shannon, & Anand, 2009).

Table 28–6 Drugs Commonly Used: Angina

Drug	Brand Name
ACE Inhibitors	
Captopril	Capoten
Enalapril	Vasotec
Lisinopril	Prinivil, Zestril
Ramipril	Altace
Trandolapril	Mavik
Beta-Adrenergic Blockers	
Atenolol	Tenormin
Propranolol	Inderal
Calcium Channel Blockers	
Amlodipine	Norvasc
Diltiazem	Cardizem
Felodipine	Plendil
Nifedipine sustained release	Procardia XL
Nitrates	
Isosorbide dinitrate	Isordil
Isosorbide mononitrate	Imdur
Nitroglycerin (sublingual)	Nitrostat

ACE = angiotensin-converting enzyme; XL = extended release.

Drug Therapies That Are Not Helpful and/or Are to Be Avoided

According to ACC/AHA (2002) and Kaiser (2006), the following therapies are not helpful in treating angina based on evidence: vitamins C and E supplementation, chelation therapy, garlic, acupuncture, and **coenzyme Q_{10}**. Kasier guidelines (2006) also mention **folic acid, coenzyme Q_{10}, vitamin B_6**, and **vitamin B_{12}** as being ineffective. Studies reviewed by Mente, deKoning, Shannon, and Anand (2009) showed varying degrees of evidence of causal links between dietary factors and coronary heart disease. No other guidelines specifically mention therapies that are ineffective.

Additional Patient Variables

Older Adults

The treatment protocol for angina is the same for older adults as it is for other adults, with consideration for the usual changes in pharmacokinetics in this age group. Lifestyle modifications are always first-line therapy because of their safety and cost. When drugs are chosen, consideration should be given to the risks for CAD and MI, which are higher in older adults. Older adults, however, may have chronic airway diseases, and nonselective **beta blockers** are contraindicated with this concomitant disease. Congestive heart failure is also common and particularly lethal in older patients. **ACE inhibitors** and **beta blockers** have important roles in this disease process, whereas the negative inotropic effects of some non-dihydropyridine **CCBs** may make this disorder worse. The dihydropyridine CCBs **amlodipine** and **felodipine** do not have the negative inotropic effect and therefore do not seem to worsen heart failure in older adults. Hypertension and hypercholesterolemia are also more common in older adults. Table 28–5 shows the appropriate drug class selection for each of these disease processes.

Women

Initiation of **hormone replacement therapy** in postmenopausal women for the purpose of reducing cardiovascular risk is no longer appropriate. Data from the Women's Health Initiative indicated that this therapy may increase risk for some and was not helpful in others. The Heart and Estrogen/Progestin Replacement Study (HERS) (Miller & Oparil, 2003; Vittinghoff et al, 2003) concluded that women with coronary disease are at high risk for MI even in the absence of other risk factors. Their risk increases up to 6-fold when many risk factors are present. Established drugs for secondary preventions, including **aspirin, beta blockers,** and **lipid-lowering agents (statins)**, are underutilized in these women, especially those at highest risk. The authors recommend the use of these established drugs rather than **hormone replacement** as a means to reduce cardiovascular risk.

Women of all ages are at higher risk for silent myocardial ischemia. Studies that have included significant percentages of female patients have found that taking **aspirin** produced the same lowering of all-cause mortality and lower incidence of nonfatal MI and stroke as found in men (Harpaz, Benerely, Goldbourt, Kishon, & Behar, 1996). There is no gender-based difference in the treatment protocol for angina. There may be differences based on concomitant disease states such as hypertension and hypercholesterolemia (discussed in Chaps. 39 and 40). Premenopausal women are at higher risk for anemia that may affect MOS. Treatment for anemia is discussed in Chapter 27.

Concomitant Diseases

Drugs used to treat angina may improve the management of some diseases and worsen others. Selection of an angina drug that treats a concomitant disease can simplify the overall therapeutic regimen, reduce cost, and increase the likelihood of adherence. It is not within the scope of this book to discuss all possible concomitant disease states, but those most common in patients with angina who might benefit from appropriate drug selection to treat the angina are discussed here.

Myocardial Infarction

Angina is usually associated with CAD, the major underlying mechanism behind MI. Both **aspirin** and **beta blockers** have been associated with MI prophylaxis and have the strongest evidence for their use. **Diltiazem (Cardizem)** in its long-acting form has been shown to decrease mortality for patients with non–Q wave MIs. Non-dihydropyridine **CCBs** should be avoided after MI for patients with poor ejection fractions (less than 40%) because of their negative inotropic effects. **Nitrates** tend to cause reflex tachycardia. The increased MOD associated with this tachycardia cannot be adjusted for with coronary arteries that are blocked and unable to effectively dilated. They should be used with caution. **ACE inhibitors** are useful after MI to prevent heart failure and mortality. They are drugs of choice to treat angina in patients with diabetes or left ventricular dysfunction. Their action on angiotensin II produces antiatherogenic effects, and they diminish MOD and increase nitric oxide through their action on the bradykinin system. Post-MI patients who are given **ACE inhibitors** may also benefit from reduced angina. Both **ACE inhibitors** and **beta blockers** have been shown to decrease the cardiac remodeling that occurs with MI.

Heart Failure

Heart failure is commonly associated with higher grades of angina. Several drugs used to treat angina also reduce blood pressure and improve myocardial function to reduce the risk for development of heart failure. **ACE inhibitors** are associated with decreased morbidity and mortality from heart failure and are first-line therapy for that disorder. Clinical benefits in heart failure include less dyspnea, improved exercise tolerance, reduced need for emergency care, and improved survival. A meta-analysis of 32 randomized controlled trials of **ACE inhibitors** for symptomatic heart failure found an overall decrease in mortality of 28 percent. The greater benefit was found in NYHA class IV failure, left ventricular ejection fractions less than 25 percent, and congestive heart failure due to ischemic heart disease (VA/DoD, 2003). Their "cousins," the **angiotensin II receptor blockers (ARBs)**, are being tested for use with heart failure as well. The negative inotropic effects of **beta-adrenergic blockers** were thought to make heart failure worse and were avoided in the past. More recent data about their role in reducing sympathetic nervous system discharge have moved some of them into first-line therapy in heart failure. The **beta blockers** that are indicated or approved for use in patients with reduced (less than 45%) left ventricular function are **carvedilol, metoprolol succinate,** and **bisoprolol.** The **dihydropyridines amlodipine** and **felodipine (Plendil)** are the only **CCBs** demonstrated to be safe in treating angina with concomitant heart failure caused by advanced left ventricular dysfunction. Non-dihydropyridine **CCBs** should be avoided in heart failure based on their negative inotropism. Lifestyle modifications are also central to heart failure prevention and management. Drugs and lifestyle modifications are discussed in Chapter 36.

Hypertension

All patients with angina should have their blood pressure assessed and managed consistent with the JNC 7 guidelines (NHBPEP, 2003) to a goal of less than 140/90 mm Hg, or 130/80 mm Hg if diabetic. Lifestyle modifications are the first approach to treatment of both hypertension and angina. Emphasis is placed on control of weight; reduced intake of sodium, saturated fat, cholesterol, and **alcohol**; and increased physical activity for both disease processes. All drug classes used to treat angina are helpful in the treatment of hypertension. **ACE inhibitors** are useful in blood pressure control based on their vasodilating effects and their ability to reduce extracellular fluid volume. Both of these actions also assist in the treatment and prevention of angina. **Beta blockers** are first-line therapy in hypertension because of cost and MI prophylaxis. **CCBs** are also acceptable for patients with hypertension. Chapter 40 discusses the concomitant use of these drugs in more detail.

Hypercholesterolemia

Because hyperlipidemia contributes to atherosclerosis and the narrowing of blood vessels that result in angina, all patients with angina should have their cholesterol checked by a lipid panel with a goal of less than 100 mg/dl for most patients and less than 70 mg/dL for those in the very-high-risk category. As with hypertension, lifestyle modifications are the first-line approach to treatment. Treatment with a **statin** is now recommended for all CAD patients and is discussed above. The only class of antianginal drugs that negatively affects hypercholesterolemia is the **beta blockers.** They increase triglycerides and cholesterol transiently and reduce the level of HDL. Because this alteration in lipid levels is transient, these drugs should not be avoided when there are other compelling reasons for the use of a **beta blocker**, such as MI prophylaxis.

Peripheral-Vascular Diseases

The vasoconstrictive effects of nonselective **beta blockers** have an adverse effect on peripheral blood flow that contraindicates their use for patients with concomitant peripheral-vascular disease (PVD). The peripheral vasodilating effects of the **dihydropyridine group** of **CCBs** have resulted in their having an off-labeled use in the treatment of Raynaud's disease. They are the drugs of choice for patients with concomitant PVD.

Diabetes Mellitus

Diabetic patients with angina should make every effort to optimize glycemic control with a goal of fasting blood glucose levels less than 126 mg/dL. **ACE inhibitors** are the drugs of choice for patients with diabetes. Not only are they recommended by all the treatment guidelines used in this chapter, but they are also recommended by JNC 7 and the American Diabetes Association (ADA) guidelines. **CCBs** are also useful because of their lower effects on glucose metabolism. They have also been shown to have some degree of renal protection. **Beta-adrenergic blockers** decrease insulin secretion and may mask the signs of hypoglycemia. The one sign of hypoglycemia that is not masked is diaphoresis, and patients with diabetes who are taking these drugs should be taught to test their blood glucose levels in the event of a diaphoretic episode. If a **beta blocker** must be used to treat angina for compelling reasons, blockade of these warning signs are associated with $beta_2$ blockade, and use of a **$beta_1$-selective drug** reduces but does not eliminate this issue. Management of diabetes is discussed in detail in Chapter 33. The use of **beta blockers** is important enough in the treatment of CAD in diabetic patients that its use in this group should not be avoided.

Elevated levels of plasma homocysteine were demonstrated to be a strong and independent risk factor for congestive heart disease events in a study of a large cohort of patients with type 2 diabetes (Soinio, Marniemi, Laasko, Lehto, & Ronnemaa, 2004). To date, there are no specific drugs to treat this risk factor, but lifestyle modifications, especially dietary, may be helpful. To date there has been no compelling evidence to indicate that **folate** therapy is helpful, although it was once thought to be so.

Asthma and Chronic Airway Diseases

Beta blockers in both oral and topical ophthalmic forms may exacerbate asthma and other chronic airway diseases. They should be avoided unless the reasons for their use are compelling. If they are to be used, the choice of a **$beta_1$-selective** oral agent and the occlusion of the nasal-lactrimal duct while administering the ophthalmic form minimize this issue. Management of asthma and chronic obstructive pulmonary disorder is discussed in Chapter 30. Appropriate **calcium channel blockers** are a good alternative.

Other disease processes that are affected positively or negatively by the drugs commonly used to treat angina are shown in Table 28–5.

Cost

The cost of **antianginal drug therapy** should be considered in drug selection, especially because patients are often on multiple drugs and a significant proportion of patients who are older may be on fixed incomes. In general, generic formulations are acceptable and cheaper than brand-name drugs.

Nitrates are the cheapest of the **antianginals.** Among the **nitrates, nitroglycerin sublingual** is significantly cheaper than the translingual spray. For patients with dry mouth, however, the sublingual tablet may not dissolve completely. As a result the spray, which does not have this problem, may be more appropriate regardless of cost. The spray has a much longer shelf life and may actually be closer in price if the patient uses the drug rarely. **Isosorbide dinitrate** comes in a generic form that is almost ten times less expensive than **isosorbide mononitrate.** Despite bioavailability differences between the two drugs, there appears to be no clear advantage to the more expensive **mononitrate.** If a once-daily dosing schedule is needed, the simplified regimen may make cost less of an issue.

The **beta blockers** are in the middle in cost. An older drug, **propranolol (Inderal),** is relatively inexpensive, but its lipid solubility increases the adverse reactions profile, and it must be taken two to four times each day. It is a nonselective **beta blocker,** along with **labetalol, nadolol,** and **timolol.** Lack of selectivity results in more adverse reactions. In patients without reduced left ventricular systolic function, the drug of choice is **atenolol.** It is among the least expensive; is **beta$_1$ selective;** has a long half-life, enabling daily dosing; and has low lipid solubility, which results in a low adverse reaction profile.

CCBs and ACE **inhibitors** are the most expensive **antianginals.** Both classes have generic forms of some of the drugs that are less expensive. Short-acting forms are also less expensive but must be taken several times each day. Generically available, **captopril** is the only short-acting **ACE inhibitor.** Research suggests an increased mortality risk for short-acting **nifedipine** (a dihydropyridine CCB). It should be prescribed only in its long-acting form. **Diltiazem** in its short-acting form is among the least expensive CCB; its sustained-release form is significantly more expensive. **Verapamil** is the least expensive, but it has limited use, and almost 100 percent of patients who take it develop constipation. This constipation usually requires an additional medication **(stool softener)** to treat the problem, and by the time the cost of the second drug is added in, all cost savings are lost. **Amlodipine** is a newer formulation that is also available in generic formulation. The expense needs to be weighed against its range of uses, once-daily dosing, reduced peripheral edema, decreased incidence of reflex tachycardia, and antiatherogenic properties. These drugs are discussed in Chapters 14 and 16, and cost indices are listed in the available drugs tables.

Aspirin brands do not appear to have significant advantages over generics. Enteric coating makes this drug more expensive, and there have been recent questions about inconsistent bioavailability with enteric coating. Therefore, use of the generic nonenteric-coated **aspirin** will be the most efficacious and cost-effective preparation.

MONITORING

The most important monitoring parameters are the presence, characteristics, and timing of angina episodes. Precipitating factors such as exercise, effort that involves use of the arms above the head, cold environment, walking after a meal, emotional stress, anger or anxiety, or coitus need to be reviewed. Patients should be evaluated every 4 to 6 months during the first year of therapy. After the first year, annual evaluations are recommended if the patient is stable and reliable enough to call or make an appointment when anginal symptoms become worse or other symptoms occur. The American College of Physicians (Snow et al, 2004) recommends that patients who are comanaged by the primary care provider and a cardiologist may alternate visits but stresses the need for good communication between the two so that all appropriate issues are addressed at each visit.

The ACC/AHA (2002) and the American College of Physicians (Snow et al, 2004) recommend five questions that should be answered during the follow-up of any patient receiving treatment for chronic stable angina:

- Has the patient's level of physical activity decreased since the last visit?
- Have the patient's anginal symptoms increased in frequency or become more severe since the last visit? If they have, has the patient decreased physical activity to avoid precipitating angina?
- How well is the patient tolerating therapy?
- How successful has the patient been in modifying risk factors and improving knowledge about ischemic heart disease?
- Has the patient developed any new comorbid illnesses or has the severity or treatment of known comorbid illnesses worsened the patient's angina?

Answers to these questions are as important as any diagnostic testing in determining whether the management plan needs alteration. Check with the patient first.

Initial laboratory studies should include an ECG and fasting lipid profile. Further tests are based on history and physical findings and may include chest x-ray (Woodard et al, the Expert Panel on Cardiac Imaging, 2008); complete blood count (CBC); and tests for diabetes, thyroid function, and renal function (ICSI, 2007). Any further laboratory tests are largely based on the need to monitor concomitant disease states.

For ACC/AHA class III, low-risk angina patients, initial diagnostic tests may involve exercise treadmill testing and exercise echocardiography. After laboratory data and other monitoring parameters specific to the drugs they are taking have been taken and assessed, an annual 12-lead ECG, CBC, and blood chemistry tests are probably enough. For ACC/AHA class I or II or high-risk angina patients, monitoring parameters should be determined in collaboration with a cardiology specialist. There is no clear evidence that routine, periodic testing of any sort is useful without a change in history or physical examination (Snow et al, 2004). The ACC/AHA (2002) consensus is that nine specific diagnostic tests be done when specific changes occur in anginal symptoms, cardiac rhythms, congestive heart failure, or valvular heart disease. All of these tests require referral to a cardiologist, so it seems prudent that any significant changes in the areas mentioned trigger a consultation with a cardiologist to see if this testing is needed.

OUTCOME EVALUATION

Figure 28–2 shows the drug treatment protocol for angina management. Evaluation for angina control occurs throughout the protocol. The main indication for substitution of a drug from a different class or the addition of more drugs is inadequate control of angina or failure to reduce the grade or class to a lower grade or class of angina.

There are situations in which to worry about treating an angina patient and times when referral to a specialist is appropriate:

1. When chronic stable angina becomes unstable—Unstable angina means that it is new or accelerating or has become unpredictable in its characteristics or precipitating factors. It is important to rule out the possibility that it is still stable angina but that

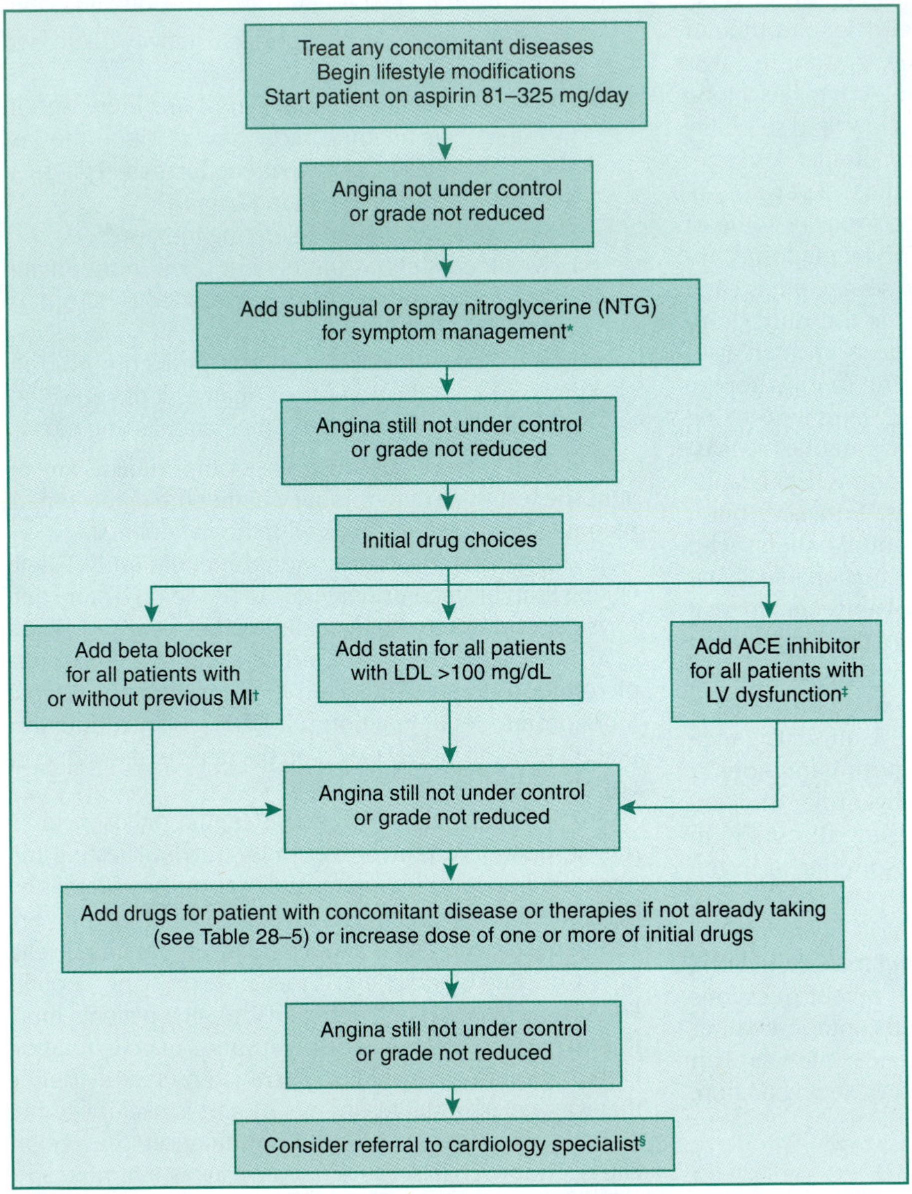

* If patient nitrate intolerant, may use calcium channel blocker for symptom relief.

† If beta blocker contraindicated or has unacceptable side effects, may use calcium channel blocker or long-acting nitrate.

‡ ACC/AHA recommends ACE inhibitors for diabetics and patients with LV dysfunction; American College of Physicians recommends for all with no restrictions.

§ ACC/AHA class I patients may require initial referral to cardiology specialist; consultation should occur whenever needed in planning care for all classes.

Figure 28–2. Drug treatment protocol for chronic stable angina and low-risk unstable angina.

changes in lifestyle or the onset of a concomitant illness is causing changes in the anginal symptoms. However, the time taken to rule this out should be very short, especially if ECG changes are noted. In general, patients with new-onset unstable angina should be referred to a specialist for urgent work-up.

2. When the patient has "ominous" findings on an exercise tolerance test—These tests are usually administered by a specialist, who would probably be the first to notice the findings.
3. When a post-MI patient develops new-onset angina, especially with ECG changes—The more recent the MI, the higher the risk is. Urgent referral is required.
4. When an MI is suspected, based on anginal and other symptoms—Obtain an ECG, draw appropriate laboratory studies, and obtain a consultation with a physician.
5. When standard therapy is not successful in improving exercise tolerance and reducing the incidence of angina symptoms, when a secondary cause of the angina that may require surgical intervention is suspected, or when the patient has complex concomitant disease processes—Consultation is appropriate. This may result in a referral, but it is generally not urgent.

PATIENT EDUCATION

Patient education should include a discussion of information related to the overall treatment plan as well as that specific to the drug therapy, reasons for taking the drug, drugs as part of the total treatment regimen, and adherence issues.

PATIENT EDUCATION

PATIENT EDUCATION

Angina Related to the Overall Treatment Plan/Disease Process

- ☐ Pathophysiology of angina and its prognosis
- ☐ Role of lifestyle modifications in improving prognosis and keeping down the number and cost of required drugs
- ☐ Importance of adherence to the treatment regimen
- ☐ Indications of complications that need to be reported and the need for regular follow-up visits with the primary care provider

Specific to the Drug Therapy

- ☐ Reason for taking the drug(s) and the anticipated action of the drug(s) on the disease process
- ☐ Doses and schedules for taking the drugs
- ☐ Possible adverse reactions and what to do when they occur
- ☐ Interactions between lifestyle modification and these drugs

Reasons for Taking the Drug(s)

Patient education about specific drugs used to treat angina is provided in Chapters 14 and 16. Specific information related to angina includes reasons for the drugs being given. Antianginal drugs are given to reduce cardiovascular morbidity (especially MI) and mortality. Some drugs do both of these things; most do either one or the other. The expectation should be clear about what these drugs can and cannot do. Stable angina is a chronic condition that requires lifelong treatment, and so the regimen should be incorporated into the daily life of the patient. Even well-managed angina can become unstable and may require urgent management. Knowledge of when and how to use sublingual or translingual **nitroglycerin** is important.

Drugs as Part of the Total Treatment Regimen

Angina therapy is based on lifestyle modification. These modifications are not always easy to maintain, but they are equally as important as drugs in successful control of symptoms and prevention of complications. Among the lifestyle modifications is sodium restriction to reduce extracellular fluid volume, decrease afterload, and reduce MOD. Care should be taken not to reduce salt and fluid too quickly, which may result in fluid volume deficit, leading to hypotension and a reduction in MOS. Patients should be taught signs and symptoms of fluid volume deficit to report. None of the **antianginal drugs** directly reduces fluid volume, but all except **aspirin** have vasodilating actions that may make fluid volume deficit worse. Sodium reduction may also lead some patients to seek salt substitutes that have potassium as part of their contents. Changes in potassium levels can significantly affect myocardial functioning, so these substitutes should be used sparingly. Use of nonsalt herbal seasoning is encouraged.

Another central lifestyle modification is regular aerobic exercise, such as walking or cycling. The amount and type of exercise must be carefully monitored and targeted to anginal symptoms. Patients can be referred to a cardiac rehabilitation program at the start of their exercise program so that their response can be monitored. Later, they can monitor their own response and determine the pace and amount of exercise that works for them. The key is gradually increasing, regular aerobic exercise. Several of the **antianginal drugs,** especially the **nitrates,** have the potential to cause orthostatic hypotension. Exercise should be timed to avoid this adverse reaction, and adequate fluids should be taken while exercising.

REFERENCES

American College of Cardiology/American Heart Association (ACC/AHA). (2002). *ACC/AHA guideline update for the management of patients with chronic stable angina: A report to the American College of Cardiology/American Heart Association Task Force on Practice Guidelines.* Bethesda, MD: American College of Cardiology Foundation.

Anderson, J., Adams, C. Antman, E., Bridges, C., Califf, R., Casey, D., Jr., et al, the American College of Cardiology/American Heart Association Task Force on Practice Guidelines (ACC/AHA). (2007). ACC/AHA 2007 guidelines for the management of patient with unstable angina/ non-ST-elevation myocardial infarction. *Journal of the American College of Cardiology, 50*(7), e1–e157.

Gibbons, R. (2003). Nitroglycerine: Should we still ask? *Annals of Internal Medicine, 139*(12), 1036–1037.

Gulati, M., Cooper-DeHoff, R., McClure, C., Johnson, D., Shaw, L., Handberg, E., et al. (2009). Adverse cardiovascular outcomes in women with nonobstructive coronary artery disease: A report from the Women's Ischemia Syndrome Evaluation Study and the St. James Women Take Heart Project. *Archives of Internal Medicine, 169*(9), 843–850.

Harpaz, D., Benderly, M., Goldbourt, U., Kishon, Y., & Behar, S. (1996). Effect of aspirin on mortality in women with symptomatic or silent myocardial ischemia. *American Journal of Cardiology, 78*(11), 1215–1219.

Henrikson, C., Howell, E., Bush, D., Miles, J., Meininger, G., Friedlander, T., et al. (2003). Chest pain relief by nitroglycerine does not predict active coronary artery disease. *Annals of Internal Medicine, 139*, 979–986.

Institute for Clinical Symptoms Improvement (ICSI). (2007, April). Stable coronary artery disease with 2009 update as addendum. Bloomington, MN: Institute for Clinical Symptoms Improvement (ICSI). 45 pp. Retrieved June 16, 2009, from http://www.guideline.gov/ summary/summary.aspx

Institute for Clinical Symptoms Improvement (ICSI). (2008, October). Diagnosis and treatment of chest pain and acute coronary syndrome (ACS). Bloomington, MN: Institute for clinical Symptoms Improvement (ICSI). 69 pp. Retrieved June 6, 2009, from http://www.guideline.gov/ summary/summary.aspx

Italiano per lo Studio della Sopravvivenza nell'Infarto Miocardio. (1990). GISSI-2: A factorial randomized trial of alteplase versus streptokinase and heparin versus no heparin among 12,490 patients with acute myocardial infarction. *Lancet, 336*, 65–71.

Kaiser Permanente Care Management Institute. (2006). Secondary prevention of coronary artery disease clinical practice guidelines. Oakland, CA: Kaiser Permanente Care Management Institute. 117 pp. Retrieved June 16, 2009, from http://www.guideline.gov/summary/ summary.aspx

Krumholz, H., Radford, M., Ellerbeck, E., Hennen, J., Meehan, T., Petrillo, M., et al. (1996). Aspirin for secondary prevention after acute myocardial infarction in the elderly: Prescribed use and outcomes. *Archives of Internal Medicine, 124*(3), 292–298.

McCance, K., & Huether, S. (2006) *Pathophysiology: The biological basis for disease in adults and children.* St. Louis, MO: Mosby.

Mente, A., deKoning, L., Shannon, H., & Anand, S. (2009). A systematic review of the evidence supporting a causal link between dietary factors and coronary heart disease. *Archives of Internal Medicine, 169*(7), 659–669.

Miller, A., & Oparil, S. (2003). Secondary prevention of coronary heart disease in women: A call to action. *Annals of Internal Medicine, 138*(2), 150–151.

National High Blood Pressure Education Program (NHBPEP). (2003). *The seventh report of the Joint National Committee on Prevention, Detection, Evaluation, and Treatment of High Blood Pressure (JNC 7).* Rockville, MD: National Institutes of Health, National Heart, Lung, and Blood Institute.

Reicher-Reiss, H., Behar, S., Boyko, V., Mandelzweig, L., Kaplinsky, E., & Goldbourt, U. (1998). Long-term mortality follow-up of hospital survivors of a myocardial infarction randomized to nifedipine in the SPRINT study. *Cardiovascular Drugs and Therapy, 12*, 171–176.

Scottish Intercollegiate Guidelines Network (SIGN). (2001). *Management of stable angina: A national guideline.* Scottish Intercollegiate Guidelines Network (SIGN) Pub. No. 51.

Snow, V., Barry, P., Fihn, S., Gibbons, R., Owens, D., Williams, S., et al. (2004). Primary care management of chronic stable angina and asymptomatic suspected or known coronary artery disease: A clinical practice guideline from the American College of Physicians. *Annals of Internal Medicine, 141*(7), 562–567.

Soinio, M., Marniemi, J., Laasko, M., Lehto, S., & Ronnemaa, T. (2004). Elevated plasma homocysteine level is an independent predictor of coronary heart disease events in patients with type 2 diabetes mellitus. *Annals of Internal Medicine, 140*(2), 94–100.

Stepien, O., Gogusev, J., Zhu, D., Iouzalen, L., Herembert, T., Drueke, T., et al. (1998). Amlodipine inhibition of serum-, thrombin-, or fibroblast growth factor-induced vascular smooth-muscle cell proliferation. *Journal of Cardiovascular Pharmacology, 31*, 786–793.

Veterans Health Administration, Department of Defense (VA/DoD). (2003). *VA/DoD clinical practice guidelines for the management of ischemic heart disease.* Washington, DC: Veterans Health Administration, Department of Defense.

Vittinghoff, E., Shiplak, M., Varosy, P., Furberg, C., Ireland, C., Khan, S., et al. (2003). Risk factors and secondary prevention in women with heart disease: The Heart and Estrogen/Progestin Replacement Study. *Annals of Internal Medicine, 138*(2), 81–89.

Williams, S., Fihn, S., & Gibbons, R. (2001). Guidelines for the management of patients with chronic stable angina: Diagnosis and risk stratification. *Annals of Internal Medicine, 135*, 530–547.

Woodard, P., Yucel, E., Khan, A., Atalay, M., Haramate, L., Ho., V., et al., the Expert Panel on Cardiac Imaging. (2008). ACR Appropriateness Criteria chronic chest pain—low to intermediate probability of coronary artery disease. Reston, VA: American College of Radiology (ACR). 5 pp. Retrieved June 29, 2009, from http://www.guideline.gov/summary/summary/aspx

CHAPTER 29

ANXIETY AND DEPRESSION

Margaret Scharf

Chapter Outline

Primary care providers are often the first health-care professionals whom patients consult when they are struggling with symptoms of anxiety and depression. They may not clearly state the problem as such but rather present a combination of physical, emotional, and social symptoms intertwined with nonspecific health problems. The advanced practice nurse must rule out physiological causes for these symptoms in making a diagnosis of anxiety or depression.

Mind and body work together and can affect physical, cognitive, emotional, behavioral, and social functioning. Psychosocial stressors can stimulate cortisol secretion that depletes serotonin (5-HT) and norepinephrine (NE) neurotransmitter (NT) resources. With fewer of these NTs available in the brain, depending on the location of the NT reduction in the brain, physiological symptoms of emotional disorders occur. For example, with decreased 5-HT in the frontal cortex and in the hypothalamus, the most common symptoms are poor concentration and decision making, decreased appetite, decreased libido, and difficulty in sleeping. Consequently, the patient might not be able to perform as well at work, might have difficulty maintaining sexual intimacy, and feel fatigue and decreased self-esteem. Medications can treat only physiologically based symptoms, and the primary care provider needs to know how to rationally prescribe for mental health problems.

Using a single mode of treatment for major depressive or anxiety disorders (i.e., only medications or only psychotherapy) is much less effective than using a multimodal approach (Black, 2006; Eddy, Dutra, Bradley, & Westen, 2004; Mitte, 2005; Thase et al, 2007), and adherence to medication is highly associated with concurrent psychotherapy (Pampallona, Ballini, Tibaldi, Kupalnick,

& Munizza, 2004). The primary care provider can best serve the patient by explaining how medications can help with the physiological aspects of the symptoms and how therapy or counseling can assist in learning new skills in handling stress. This chapter describes the pathophysiology of anxiety and depression; the physiological, psychological, and behavioral manifestations; and pharmacotherapy and nonpharmacotherapy treatment approaches. It is not within the scope of this book to discuss the diagnosis of these disorders in any depth. For further discussion of the diagnostic process, see management texts and the *Diagnostic and Statistical Manual of Mental Disorders,* fourth edition, text revision *(DSM-IV-TR)* (American Psychiatric Association, 2000) for diagnostic criteria. The treatment protocols presented here assume appropriate diagnosis of anxiety or depression.

PATHOPHYSIOLOGY

Anxiety and depressive symptoms result from an interaction of the central nervous, peripheral nervous, and endocrine systems, as well as the generalized stress response. Usually, the generalized stress response is mediated by the immune system in producing cortisol to activate the fight, flight, or freeze response, which is a function of the peripheral nervous system. For review of the various functions of the brain and their anatomical locations, see a basic physiology text. They are summarized briefly in this section.

Nervous System

The main structures of the brain involved in the anxiety and mood symptoms include the frontal cortex, the diencephalons, the brainstem and cerebellum, and the limbic system. The frontal lobe is responsible for higher integrative functions such as executive control, personality traits, expression of emotionality, problem solving, decision making, and conceptualization. The diencephalon acts as a relay center for sensory input and motor output between the cerebral cortex and the deeper areas of the brain. The hypothalamus maintains the internal milieu, such as appetite, sleep and wakefulness, sex drive, body temperature, and endocrine functions through the hypothalamic-pituitary-endocrine axes. The vegetative symptoms of depression, such as poor appetite, difficulty in sleeping (including insomnia and hypersomnia), and low sex drive, arise from inadequate functioning of the hypothalamus.

The brainstem contains the three nuclei where essential NTs are produced: the locus ceruleus for 5-HT, the raphe nucleus for NE, and the substantia nigra for dopamine (DA). Also within the brainstem lies the reticular activating system, which maintains attentiveness. Interconnecting all these structures is the limbic system, a network of neuronal fibers connecting the basal ganglia, thalamus, hypothalamus, cingulate gyrus, hippocampus, amygdala, and eventually, the frontal cortex. The hippocampus and amygdala store memories, especially those with intense emotional overtones, and are responsible for learning and formation of emotions. The limbic system, therefore, serves to connect most of the major structures involved in emotion, perception, learning, cognition, and behavior. Clearly, it is of vital importance in understanding and intervening in mental health problems. The endocrine system becomes involved in mental health symptoms by virtue of activation of the hypothalamic-pituitary-endocrine axes. These axes are discussed in more detail in Chapter 15. The significance in mental health of the hypothalamic-pituitary-endocrine axes is the need for the clinician to distinguish between the hormonal influences on behavior and which is primary. That is, is the mood and energy disturbance due to hypothyroidism or depression, or both? Sometimes, depression contributes to decreased hypothalamic function, resulting in lowered thyroid levels.

Neurotransmitters

NTs are biochemicals that permit neurons to communicate with each other for a whole-body response. The primary NTs involved in most behavioral symptoms, including anxiety and depression, are serotonin (5-HT), norepinephrine (NE), dopamine (DA), gamma-aminobutyric acid (GABA), and acetylcholine (ACh). There are other NTs involved in psychiatric symptoms, but their mechanisms are still exploratory and are not discussed in this chapter. Each NT has a specific neuroreceptor to which it can bind. The receptors may have several subtypes. For example, 5-HT has at least 15 receptor subtypes to which binding of 5-HT_2 may contribute to improved appetite but diminished sexual response. Blocking 5-HT_2 postsynaptic receptors and blocking 5-HT reuptake presynaptically (with consequential increase of NTs available to bind with receptors) will result in improved depressive symptoms without interfering with sexual response because the NTrs cannot enter 5-HT_2. Table 29–1 depicts the various receptors and the effects of receptor activity.

5-HT and NE follow very similar pathways; however, NE acts more as an arousing or activating agent, and 5-HT acts on mood or the general tenor of emotion. Epinephrine and NE activity are discussed in more detail in Chapter 15.

GABA is a different kind of NT in that it acts on the chloride channel of the neural membrane to produce an extended hyperpolarization of the neuron, thereby inhibiting additional impulses briefly. The highest concentration of GABA receptors is found in the amygdala. GABA has two types of receptors: GABA-A affects mostly anxiety symptoms and GABA-B affects anxiety and seizure activity. The GABA receptor is very complex, with several subunits permitting many different binding sites. **Benzodiazepines (BZDs)**, for example, bind to and enhance the action of the GABA-A receptors and indirectly modulate the chloride ion channel of the GABA receptor. As neuroscience continues to evolve, much more knowledge is forthcoming

Table 29–1 **Effects of Neurotransmitter Receptor Activation**

Receptor Activity	Effects of Receptor Activity
Acetylcholine blockade	• Second most potent action of cyclic antidepressants • Potentiation of effects of drugs with anticholinergic properties, including OTC cold medications • Adverse reactions: dry mouth, blurred vision, constipation, urinary retention, sinus tachycardia, lengthening of QT interval, memory disturbances
$Alpha_1$-adrenergic blockade	• Potentiation of antihypertensives acting by way of $alpha_1$ blockade • Adverse reactions: postural hypotension, dizziness, reflex tachycardia, sedation
$Alpha_2$-adrenergic blockade	• Antagonism of antihypertensives acting as $alpha_2$ stimulants (e.g., clonidine, methyldopa) • Adverse reactions: sexual dysfunction
Dopamine reuptake blockade	• Antidepressant, antiparkinsonian effect • Adverse reactions: psychomotor activation, aggravation of psychosis
$Dopamine_1$ blockade	• May mediate antipsychotic effect
$Dopamine_2$ blockade	• In mesolimbic area, antipsychotic effect correlates with clinical efficacy in controlling positive symptoms of schizophrenia; an inverse relationship exists between $dopamine_2$ blockade and therapeutic antipsychotic dosage • In nigrostriatal tract, contributes to extrapyramidal adverse reactions (rigidity, tremor) • In hypothalamus-pituitary area, contributes to endocrine adverse reactions (galactorrhea, gynecomastia) and sexual dysfunction in men
$Dopamine_3$ blockade	• May mediate antipsychotic effect on negative symptoms of schizophrenia
$Dopamine_4$ blockade	• May mediate antipsychotic effect on positive symptoms of schizophrenia
$Histamine_1$ blockade	• Most potent action of cyclic antidepressants and mirtazapine • Potentiation of effects of other CNS drugs • Adverse reactions: sedation, drowsiness, postural hypotension, weight gain
Norepinephrine reuptake blockade	• Antidepressant effect • Potentiation of pressor effects of norepinephrine • Interaction with guanethidine (interferes with antihypertensive effect) • Adverse reactions: tremors, tachycardia, sweating, insomnia, erectile and ejaculation problems
Serotonin reuptake blockade	• Antidepressant, antiobsessive effect • Can increase or decrease anxiety, depending on dose • Potentiation of drugs with serotonergic properties (e.g., L-tryptophan, phentermine); watch for serotonin syndrome
$Serotonin_1$ blockade	• Antidepressant, anxiolytic, and antiaggressive action
$Serotonin_2$ blockade	• Anxiolytic, antidepressant, antipsychotic, antimigraine effect • May correlate with clinical efficacy in decreasing negative symptoms of schizophrenia; may compensate for (decrease) extrapyramidal effects caused by $dopamine_2$ blockade • Adverse reactions: hypotension, ejaculatory problems, sedation

OTC = over the-counter; CNS = central nervous system.

about the complexity of the GABA receptor, and new drugs will likely have remarkably different pharmacodynamics.

Neuroconduction-neurotransmission cascade

Communication between neurons is accomplished through a cascade of electrical and neurochemical events, depicted in Figure 29-1. Initially, the electrical current of the cell at rest is –70 mV (1). When there is an electrical wave depolarizing the neural membrane, the action potential (2) progresses down the axon into the nerve terminal. This depolarization is caused by the opening of Na+ channels in the neural membrane. Na+ ions enter, causing the interior of the axon to depolarize (become less negative or even positive +35 mV). When the action potential reaches the axon terminal, it opens voltage gated Ca++ channels (3) in the axon terminal membrane, allowing Ca++ influx. The calcium influx causes the vesicles containing the NT to move over to the terminal neuronal membrane and release their contents by exocytosis (fusing the membrane with the axon terminal) into the synaptic cleft (4). The neuron repolarizes by moving the Na+ ions back out of the axon, which requires ATP.

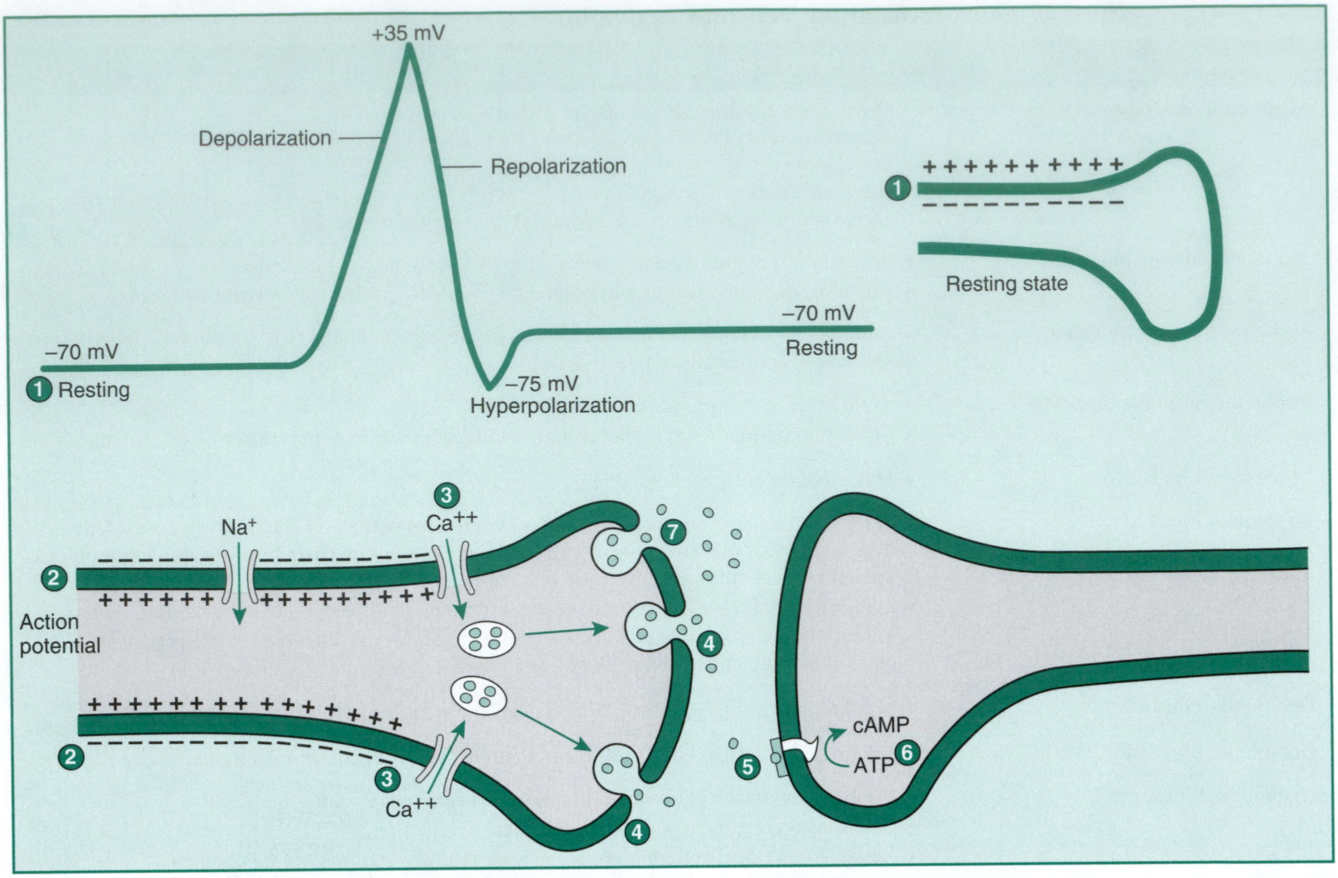

Figure 29–1. Neuroconduction-neurotransmission cascade.

At this point, the voltage of the cell drops back to resting stage and may even drop to less than –75 mV, which is referred to as hyperpolarization. While the cell is in this hyperpolarized state, it is resistive to another impulse; therefore, the cell cannot fire again for a few milliseconds. At the terminal membrane, the NT can then bind with a postsynaptic receptor (5) causing a change in ionic conductance of the cell and activating intracellular processes in the receptive cell. Once the NT is bound to its receptor, it generates either an excitatory postsynaptic potential (EPSP) or an inhibitory postsynaptic potential (IPSP). The net effect of the ESPSs and ISPSs from the synapses determine whether or not the postsynaptic neuron will generate an action potential. Some NT receptors also release second messengers which change cellular chemistry in the postsynaptic neuron (6). If the NT does not bind to a postsynaptic receptor, the action of the NT may be terminated through a reuptake transporter system (7) that carries it back into the presynaptic cell, by diffusion out of the synapse or by destruction by enzymes in the synapse.

PHARMACODYNAMICS

All the current **psychoactive drugs** act on this neuroconduction-neurotransmission cascade in some way. Drugs may inhbit the uptake or transport into the presynaptic cell, thereby making more of the NT available for eventual binding to a receptor. This, in turn, places a demand on the postsynaptic cells to produce or reduce receptors on the cell membrane and improve receptor binding. Another mechanism interferes with the ionic action of conduction through blocking the calcium or sodium channels, thereby slowing down or speeding up conduction and movement of the vesicle to the cell membrane. Neuroscientists are already beginning to develop drugs that act on the second messenger system, thereby influencing actual message replication.

Nine classes of drugs are used for anxiety and depression: **nonselective norepinephrine-serotonin reuptake inhibitors (tricyclics and heterocyclics), serotonin-selective reuptake inhibitors (SSRIs), serotonin-norepinephrine reuptake inhibitors (SNRIs), norepinephrine- dopamine reuptake inhibitors (NDRIs), serotonin-agonist reuptake inhibitors (SARIs), norepinephrine- serotonin specific agonists (NaSSAs), norepinephrine-selective reuptake inhibitors (NRIs), MAO inhibitors (MAOIs), and BZDs.** Each class acts on NTs in a different way. Currently all **antidepressants** have an FDA black box warning regarding an increased risk of suicidal thinking and behavior in children, adolescents, and young adults to age 24. Because depression itself is associated with an increase in suicidal ideation, the chances of such ideation must be considered when making a choice about appropriate treatment. All patients—who are prescribed an **antidepressant**, including the parents of children, adolescents, or young adults—should be educated to monitor for an increase in suicidal ideation or behavior.

Nonselective Norepinephrine-Serotonin Reuptake Inhibitors

Nonselective norepinephrine-serotonin reuptake inhibitors were previously referred to as *tricyclic antidepressants (TCAs)* and include such drugs as the following:

- **imipramine** (Tofranil)
- **desipramine** (Norpramin)
- **amitriptyline** (Elavil)
- **doxepin** (Sinequan)

They affect the NE, 5-HT, ACh, and histamine receptors to increase availability of NE and 5-HT to bind to postsynaptic receptors. They do this by inhibiting their transport back into the presynaptic neuron when the postsynaptic receptors have failed to pick up the NT in the synaptic cleft. These drugs are all equally efficacious in treating depression as the other classes, less expensive, but with a greater side effect profile.

Serotonin-Selective Reuptake Inhibitors

SSRIs act by blocking the transport mechanism that returns unbound 5-HT left in the synaptic cleft into the presynaptic neuron, thereby terminating the transmission of the message carried by that receptor. When the transport mechanism is blocked, more 5-HT is available to bind to the postsynaptic 5-HT receptor. Common **SSRIs** include the following:

- **fluoxetine** (Prozac, Sarafem, Prozac Weekly)
- **paroxetine** (Paxil, Paxil CR)
- **sertraline** (Zoloft)
- **fluvoxamine** (Luvox)
- **citalopram** (Celexa)
- **escitalopram** (Lexapro)

The **SSRIs** demonstrate equal efficacy to the **nonspecific SNRIs** with a safer and more tolerable side effect profile.

Serotonin-Norepinephrine Reuptake Inhibitors

SNRIs block the reuptake mechanism of NE and 5-HT, thus permitting greater availability of these NTs to bind with the respective neuroreceptors. Three **SNRIs** are available in the United States: **venlafaxine** (Effexor and Effexor XR), **duloxetine** (Cymbalta), and **desvenlafaxine** (Pristiq). Use of single drug compounds that target two or more NTs shows promise for treating complex depressions including the "double depression" of both chronic and acute depression and melancholic depression.

Norepinephrine-Dopamine Reuptake Inhibitors

Only one NDRI is available in the United States: **bupropion** (Wellbutrin, Wellbutrin SR, Wellbutrin XL). **Bupropion** affects the frontal cortex, the limbic system, the caudate, and the brainstem by increasing NE and DA. Also important is what it does *not* affect. It does not block 5-HT reuptake or inhibit MAO. It does provide a mild degree of DA reuptake blockade; more important, however, the active metabolites of bupropion block the reuptake of NE. It is likely that the NE reuptake blockade, especially in the frontal cortex, serves to activate and calm at the same time. **Bupropion** possibly acts on the serotonergic neurons indirectly through the DA blockade and, therefore, creates a compensatory increase in 5-HT release in the synaptic space. Another action that introduces alternative clinical use includes occupying the DA receptors in the nucleus acumbens (also referred to as the reward center). When these receptors are occupied, there is a sense of well-being and satisfaction. Other ligands that bind in this site include cocaine, nicotine, caffeine, and xanthine derivatives such as chocolate. Therefore, **bupropion** can be useful in treating smoking cessation and as an adjunct to substance abuse recovery.

Serotonin Agonist Reuptake Inhibitor

There are two SARIs: **nefazadone** and **trazadone** (Desyrel). They not only inhibit the reuptake of 5-HT but also block the 5-HT_2 and 5-HT_3 receptor subtypes. Because these receptors are implicated in sexual and weight gain side effects, blocking 5-HT binding there and diverting the 5-HT to the 5-HT_{1A} receptor increases the antidepressant and anxiolytic properties with fewer side effects. Because 5-HT_{1A} receptors densely populate the limbic system, increasing 5-HT binding here probably accounts for modulating emotions such as sadness, aggression, and anxiety. **Nefazadone** has an FDA black box warning related to hepatotoxicity; the drug is available only in generic form at this time.

Norepinephrine- and Serotonin-Specific Agonist

Mirtazepine (Remeron) is a unique addition to **psychotropics** used to treat anxiety and depression. It is a 5-HT agonist and reuptake inhibitor that blocks the reuptake of NE and the somatodendritic reuptake of 5-HT, resulting in an increase in 5-HT available for release from the presynaptic neuron and more NE available in the synaptic cleft. Unfortunately, it also blocks histamine, contributing to drowsiness and weight gain at some doses.

On The Horizon **ON THE HORIZON**

What to look for during the next 5 years in psychopharmacology:

- New mechanisms of action, especially receptor-specific modulation and antagonism of the somatordendritc autoreceptors for 5-HT and NE
- Development of single drug compounds affecting two or more NTs in a deliberate way (similar to **venlafaxine, duloxetine**, and **fluoxetine/olanzapine)**
- Development of drugs targeting the second messenger system for faster response rates and possibly neuroprotective qualities in preventing further depression
- Targeting antagonism of the glutamate receptor to treat depression
- Corticotropin-releasing factor antagonists to mediate effects of stress on the pathophysiology of depression

Norepinephrine-Specific Reuptake Inhibitors

Atomoxetine (Strattera) is the only **NE-specific reuptake inhibitor** available in the United States, although **reboxetine** is available in Canada, England, and most other European countries. **Atomoxetine** is predominantly marketed for the treatment of attention deficit disorder because it is a nonstimulant approach to treating this disorder. By increasing the availability of NE in the frontal cortex, executive functions improve, including organization, attentiveness, decision making, and problem solving. Furthermore, NE is a major NT involved in depression, making this an effective mechanism for depression characterized by hypersomnia, amotivation, poor decision making, and melancholia.

Monoamine Oxidase Inhibitors

MAOIs such as **phenelzine (Nardil)** and **tranylcypromine (Parnate)** inhibit MAO, the enzyme that contributes to degradation of the monoamines (DA, 5-HT, and NE). In doing so, more of these NTs are available for postsynaptic binding. Because there are dietary restrictions with these drugs that, if neglected, can contribute to lethal side effects, these drugs are used less often than are other **antidepressants** and should be prescribed by a psychiatric specialist. An MAOI inhibitor, the **selegeline transdermal patch (Ensam)**, is now available with fewer food restrictions if the transdermal dose remains below the 9 mg/24 hours patch.

Benzodiazepines/GABA-ergics

The last class of **psychotropics**, **BZDs**, is used to treat anxiety. They are divided into short-acting agents: **clorazepate (Tranxene)**, **halazepam (Paxipam)**, and **Prazepam (Centrex)**; intermediate-acting agents: **alprazolam (Xanax)**, **lorazepam (Ativan)**, **oxazepam (Serax)**, and **chlordiazepoxide (Librium)**; and long-acting agents: **diazepam (Valium)** and **clonazepam (Klonopin)**. **BZDs** act on the chloride ion channel of GABA-A receptors when they are bound to their adjacent **BZD** receptor. In doing so, they enhance GABA neurotransmission, which then lengthens hyperpolarization of the impulse, thus slowing down responses to successive impulses. The net effect is to decrease reactivity of the brain. **BZDs** have four main effects: anxiolytic, anticonvulsant, muscle relaxation, and sedation. The advantages of **BZDs** are rapid onset of action, tolerability, few drug–drug interactions, inexpensive in generic form, and little effect on the cardiovascular system. The disadvantages are dependence and withdrawal, sedation, interaction with alcohol, impaired motor coordination, and impaired cognition.

Buspirone (Buspar) is a **nonbenzodiazepine** GABA agonist that is used to treat anxiety. It is does not act directly on the GABA receptor but acts as an agonist to the 5-HT_{1A} and DA_2 receptors. The effect on DA is not yet understood, but the action on 5-HT occurs primarily in the hippocampus and, to a lesser extent, the frontal cortex. This unusual combination of actions places it in a class of its own. By its main action on the limbic system, it reduces anxiety, and its lesser effect on the frontal cortex prevents cognitive impairment. It has minimal side effects but the 2- to 3-week therapeutic lag time, multiple daily dosing, and subtle effects make it less popular among patients than are other **anxiolytic agents**.

GOALS OF TREATMENT

Anxiety

The goals for treatment of anxiety disorders are resolution of symptoms and prevention of relapse. Major errors in psychopharmacological treatment of these disorders are the following:

- not achieving full remission of symptoms but instead accepting partial response
- not providing an adequate trial of medications (8 to 12 wk) before switching, discontinuing, or augmenting
- not optimizing the dosage range and providing regular follow-up with patients to ensure medication adherence

To meet the goals of treatment requires lifestyle modifications through counseling as well as drug therapy. The goals of treatment are very similar as those for depression: relief of symptoms, stabilization of mood, and prevention of relapse. Specific expected outcomes related to work with the therapist are individualized to the patient but may include the following:

- practicing relaxation exercises for 20 to 30 minutes a day every day for 6 weeks

- participating with friends in both entertainment and support
- exercising for at least 15 minutes daily
- using affirmations to replace negative thinking
- identifying contributing events in the past and present and working with the therapist to reach some peaceful balance and resolution
- learning effective expressions of feelings with significant others

Depression

The specific goals for treating depression are the following:

- reducing the symptoms
- improving quality of life and daily functioning
- eliminating suicidal ideation
- minimizing adverse treatment effects
- preventing relapse of depression

Maximizing pharmacological treatment is necessary to achieve full recovery from depression. At the same time, attention to suicidal ideation, which may be present with the depression or occur as a result of antidepressant treatment, is essential. The goals of depression treatment may be reached through medication, psychotherapy, or a combination of both. The psychosocial interventions listed earlier for anxiety apply equally to depression treatment.

RATIONAL DRUG SELECTION

Anxiety

Anxiety is a normal emotion in response to threat or anticipation of harm. The total body responds to threat through the autonomic system by preparing the body to flee the situation, remain and fight, or remain and freeze. The central nervous system (CNS) activates the frontal lobe, to enable problem solving and thinking about the situation, as well as the memory centers, to consider previous situations and responses. Finally, the rest of the cortex reacts interactively to enable the person to ask for help from others and use environmental resources to deal with the situation. Clearly, anxiety serves an adaptive purpose, and to automatically medicate anxiety may be countertherapeutic. When a patient maladaptively responds to stress, the provider should consider medication. In deciding to prescribe medication, first identify the target symptoms and then determine if they meet the criteria for a diagnosis. Many managed health-care insurers do not cover medications without a diagnosis establishing medical necessity. *DSM-IV-TR* describes specific categories of anxiety disorders, with criteria for each diagnosis. If the client's symptoms do not fully meet the criteria or present a mixed picture, it is advisable to refer the client to an advanced practice psychiatric–mental health nurse or mental health professional. Figure 29–2 presents the algorithm for treatment of anxiety.

The primary neural pathways involved in anxiety include 5-HT, NE, and GABA. Therefore, pharmacological intervention can use **nonselective norepinephrine-serotonin reuptake inhibitors, SSRIs,** and/or **SNRIs,** or **serotonin agonists. BZDs** and **beta-adrenergic blockers** have minor roles. **Beta-adrenergic blockers** are discussed in Chapter 14.

Nonselective norepinephrine-serotonin reuptake inhibitors can be used for these anxiety symptoms as well as for panic attacks and chronic pain. They usually take 2 to 4 weeks to produce the full therapeutic effect, with gradual improvement beginning with the vegetative symptoms, then arousal symptoms, before relief of mood symptoms. Unfortunately, these drugs have adverse reactions because of their action on the cholinergic and histamine receptors, and a patient can easily overdose on these drugs and die from cardiac consequences They are not first-line therapy; there are better and safer drugs.

SSRIs can be used for depression, anxiety, obsessive-compulsive disorders, and panic attacks. They also usually take 2 to 4 weeks to provide the full therapeutic effect, with similar progression as the **nonselective norepinephrine-serotonin reuptake inhibitors.** Anxiety symptoms resolve much earlier than depressive symptoms; however, they usually require a higher dosage than do depressive symptoms. They have fewer adverse reactions than the nonselective drugs and are often first-line therapy.

SNRIs affect both of these NTs. The complementary blocking of 5-HT and NE permits targeting symptoms of both mood and arousal; therefore, they are useful for treating depression, sleep and pain disorders, and anxiety disorders such as generalized anxiety and social phobia, as well as attention deficit and eating disorders. **Venlafaxine** demonstrates some unique effects on the G-coupling mechanism after postsynaptic receptor binding, which may explain the decrease in the time needed to reach full therapeutic effect.

In the past, **GABA agonists** and **BDZs** have been used to treat anxiety; however, they have potential for cognitive impairment, tolerance, and dependence. Because the **SSRIs** and **SNRIs** have not been found to be addicting, they can be given with less serious consequences.

Psychiatrists and advanced practice psychiatric–mental health nurses prescribe **BZDs** least often, and many of the clinical specialties and primary care providers prescribe them the most often. This is probably because the BZDs provide relatively immediate relief from anxiety symptoms. Over time, however, patients may need a higher dosage to bring about the same effect, and when they abruptly stop taking them, they experience symptoms of anxiety and even panic. Long-acting BZDs are much less likely to produce tolerance and are prescribed initially while introducing an **SSRI** for long-term management.

Other drugs that can be advantageous in anxiety are those that affect the ion channels of neurons, such as **beta-adrenergic blockers** such as **propranolol (Inderal)** and **atenolol (Tenormin)**, the **serotonin partial agonist,**

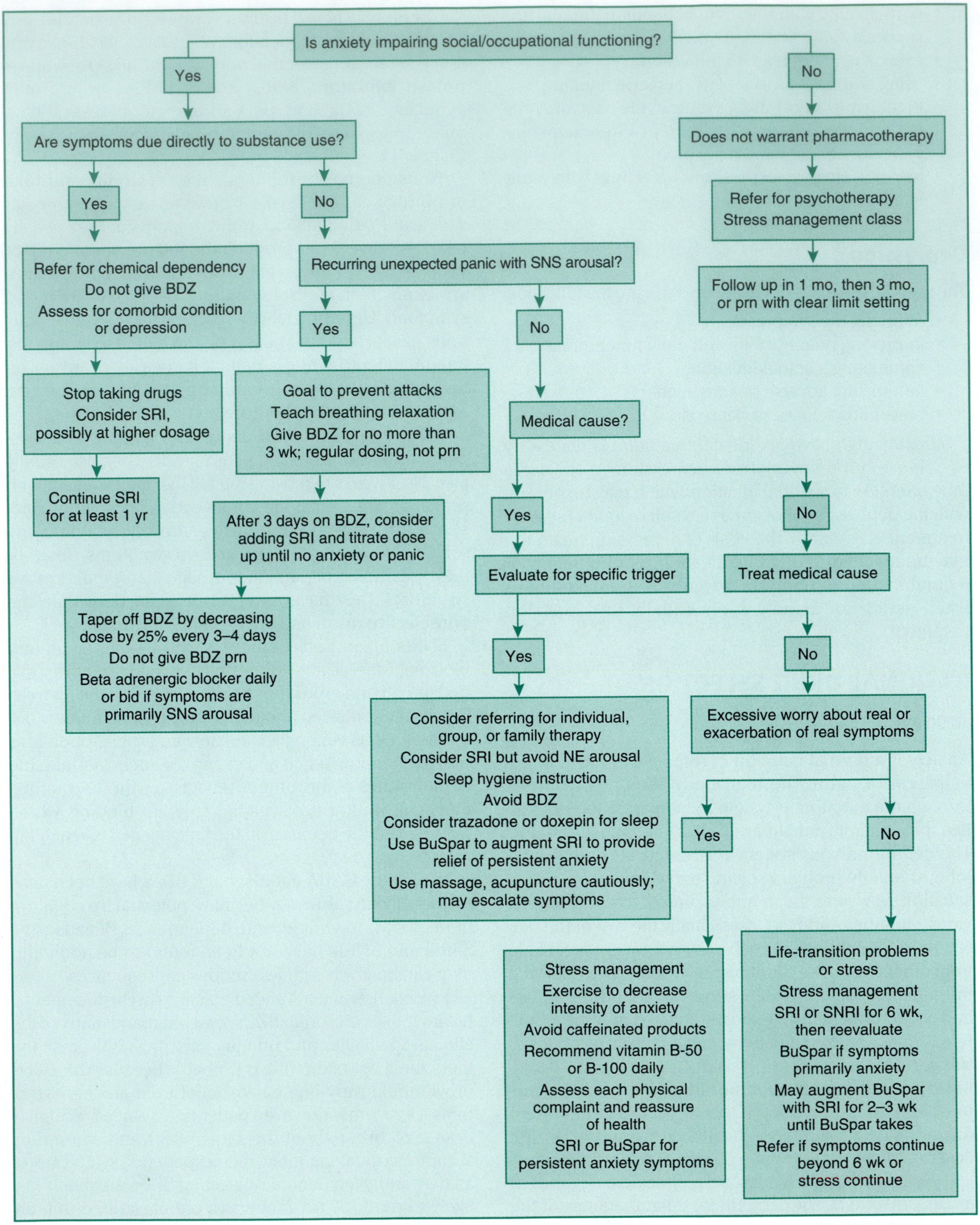

Figure 29–2. Treatment algorithm for anxiety.

buspirone (Buspar), and the **non-BZD GABA-ergics valproate (Depakote)** and **lamotrigine (Lamictal)**. **Beta-adrenergic blockers** are particularly effective with panic disorders when the predominant symptoms are sympathetic nervous system arousal (shortness of breath, rapid heart rate, clammy skin, blurred vision).

Buspirone does not produce tolerance or dependency. It requires about 2 weeks to reach full therapeutic level, which may be intolerable to those with severe anxiety. Behavioral strategies can complement the medication effect, especially while waiting for the full therapeutic medication effect. It cannot be taken as needed and must be taken on a regular basis, usually more than once a day. **Buspirone** seems to be especially effective with patients who have generalized anxiety disorder but is not at all effective with panic or anxiety attacks. **Buspirone** is also helpful in augmenting the **SSRIs** and **SNRIs** and in treating patients with agitated or anxious depression. Because there seems to be no cross-tolerance, **buspirone** is a helpful drug to use with clients in alcohol or drug recovery. The drug must be taken every day to be effective and cannot be used to relieve immediate anxiety.

Panic and Adjustment Disorders

Long-acting **BZDs** (e.g., **clonazepam** or **diazepam**) are the first-line drugs of choice for panic disorder because the anxiety is so acute that the patient seeks relief in whatever way possible. Taking the medication only when the panic is occurring inadvertently conveys to the client that the panic is inevitable and can be relieved only with the medication. Instead, it is best to identify any particular patterns to the panic (e.g., nighttime panic or situationally determined anxiety) and prescribe anticipatory to the event and to take the medication on a regular basis (once or twice a day). In this way, the medication prevents severe anxiety rather than treats it after the fact by an as-needed dose. The drug is prescribed at bedtime if the panic is nighttime or at lunchtime if the panic is midday. After a week on the BZD, if the symptoms are adequately relieved, the prescriber can introduce an SSRI, such as **citalopram**, along with the BZD at an ordinary initial dosage and titrate the SSRI upward as the BZD is titrated downward. In this case, tapering off the BZD is more for symptom coverage while the prescriber introduces the SSRI than for prevention of withdrawal symptoms. For many patients, this is an effective way of treating panic or adjustment disorder with anxiety or mixed anxiety and depression. The BZD may need to be reinstated if breakthrough panic symptoms occur. The drug should be short-term with patients with adjustment disorder, but patients with panic disorder may need to stay on some medication plan for up to a year. The patient with adjustment disorder is likely to spontaneously get better within 6 weeks or when the situation is resolved and not need a referral for psychotherapy. The patient with panic disorder may benefit from a referral for psychotherapy to learn stress management strategies.

Depression

Depression is an interesting phenomenon among Americans in that there is an implicit stigmatizing notion that people who are depressed have weak characters and, therefore, depression needs to be denied. Yet the English language has many terms and idioms to describe the gamut of severity of depression such as *the blues, having a funky day, down in the dumps, doldrums, low, sad, gloomy, despairing, disheartened,* and *despondent.* In fact, the rate for diagnosed depression has steadily increased since World War II with an impressive peak between 1960 and 1975. Major depression is the fourth leading cause of disease burden in 1990, and by 2020 is likely to be the leading cause of disease burden (Greenberg et al, 2003; Kessler et al, 2005; Kilbourne, Daugherty, & Pincus, 2007). Until recently, depression was seen as a disorder of adults, but recent studies indicate that it is important to recognize and treat childhood and teenage depression as a protection against future, more severe and more frequent bouts. A genetic predisposition is implied because the risk for depression among first-degree relatives is two to ten times higher than it is among unrelated or distantly related people (Sadock, Sadock, & Ruiz, 2009).

There are different kinds and degrees of depression. *DSM-IV-TR* identifies major depressive disorder as the acute form (onset of symptoms for at least 2 wk) and dysthymia (symptom duration greater than 2 yr) as the chronic form. The spectrum of depression may also be considered from the degree of severity of symptoms spanning from mild, moderate, severe, and with psychotic features although the predominant symptoms include depressed mood, diminished interest and motivation, fatigue and loss of energy, diminished concentration, and feelings of worthlessness and hopelessness. Another presentation includes irritability, sensitivity to rejection, agitation, hostility, and anxiety (American Psychiatric Association, 2000).

Instead of, or in addition to, exhibiting emotional and behavioral symptoms of depression, patients may present with a myriad of somatic symptoms. Prepubertal children complain of gastrointestinal symptoms or may say they are sick to avoid going to school. Adults, especially those older than 65 years, commonly express depression through cardiovascular, gastrointestinal, and genitourinary systems and low back pain or other muscular pain. Especially in older adults, cognitive deficits may predominate to falsely lead the clinician to diagnosis dementia.

A frustrating problem for primary care providers is the relative frequency with which depression accompanies other mental disorders. Patients with panic attacks are often also depressed. Studies show they have a higher lifetime risk for suicide than those without any mental disorder. These patients often experience marriage and family conflicts, occupational difficulties and unemployment, financial strain, and drug and alcohol abuse (Sadock, Sadock, & Ruiz, 2009). With friends becoming burned out and greater constriction in social support due to fear and embarrassment about having repeat panic attacks, the person begins to experience symptoms of major depressive disorder.

People with personality disorders, especially borderline, avoidant, and dependent disorders, have associated intermittent depression. Those with borderline personality disorder may fear rejection and abandonment by friends and family; when they do experience inevitable disappointment, they feel it much more strongly than others would. In trying to cope with the perceived loss, they feel an abandonment type of depression. Similarly, those with dependent personality disorder may have exhausted their social resources and respond with depression and immobility. These patients often unconsciously turn to their primary care providers for nurturing. They may use outpatient, primary care, and even emergency care excessively with what seem to be minor problems. The primary care provider should recognize the behavior as a clumsy or misguided attempt to have someone care for them instead of interpreting the behaviors as manipulative or malingering. In this case, the primary care provider would have better results by treating the problems as a masked depression.

Medical disorders may underlie depressive symptoms and confuse both the advanced practice psychiatric–mental health nurse and the primary care nurse practitioner. Because the symptoms of depression overlap extensively with hypothyroidism, ruling out thyroid dysfunction with appropriate laboratory studies is essential. In addition, unrecognized malignancies (including brain tumors) may be disguised as depression. Other conditions include chronic renal failure, autoimmune disorders, and biochemical lesions in the midbrain and brainstem such as Parkinson's disease and Huntington's disease. Similarly, some medical treatments may induce depression, most notably antihypertensive medications that antagonize the biogenic NTs. Figure 29–3 presents the algorithm for depression.

Keeping in mind the basic neurophysiological mechanisms that contribute to the target symptoms of depression and anxiety, providers can more accurately and deliberately assess and treat the condition. Conceptually, both anxiety and depression can be medicated with the same groups of drugs. Drugs that are commonly used to treat depression compounded by anxiety include **NDRIs**, **SARIs**, and **MAOIs**.

Bupropion is currently the only **norepinephrine-dopamine agonist.** Because it affects the frontal cortex, limbic system, caudate, and brainstem, it has many uses in treating target symptoms of depression, attention deficit disorder, and social phobia, as well as disturbances in satiety such as eating disturbances, substance abuse, and nicotine dependency. In fact, **bupropion** is being increasingly used to help with smoking cessation, weight loss, depression, and postopioid addiction because of its activity in the hypothalamus at the reward and satiety center.

Because of the slow onset of therapeutic effects, it sometimes helps to start a client on low doses of an **SSRI**, add the **bupropion** 3 or 4 days later, gradually increase the **bupropion** dose until therapeutic effects become evident, and then taper off the dose of the **SSRI**. In additon, **bupropion** is an early choice of medications to augment the effects of **SSRIs** in patients with refractory depression.

Mirtazapine, the only **norepinephrine-selective serotonin agonist**, is very effective in reducing anxiety and depressive symptoms without contributing to 5-HT_2- and 5-HT_3-receptor activity resulting in anxiety, insomnia, sexual dysfunction, or gastrointestinal effects. Two major problems with **mirtazapine** include weight gain and drowsiness due to significant histamine blockade. Oddly enough, more adverse reactions occur at the lower or higher doses. The best outcomes result when patients take a middle-range dose of 30 to 45 mg, and drowsiness occurs most often in the 7.5- to 15-mg range.

The **MAOIs** have been available since the early 1960s and have only recently fallen out of use because of the newer and safer drugs that are now available. **MAOIs** block monoamineoxidase by binding to the enzyme and permanently inactivating it. Synthesis of replacement MAO requires about 2 weeks. This allows for levels of the catecholamines (DA and NE) and 5-HT to rise, but it also decreases MAO availability for two other amines found in human diets, tyramine and phenylethylamine. MAO is a natural rate-limiting substance needed to detoxify tyramine in the human body before it causes such severe events as a sudden rise in pulse and blood pressure. Therefore, use of the **MAOIs** requires dietary restrictions of tyramine-containing foods such as any aged meats and cheeses and fermented products (e.g., wine, beer, sauerkraut, soy sauce).

Although studies show the **MAOIs** to be particularly effective with atypical depression, mixed anxiety and depression, panic disorder, eating disorders, and depression accompanying borderline personality disorder, they can also be very difficult to manage with a potentially suicidal person. It is safest and most prudent for the advanced practice nurse to avoid using **MAOIs** and to consider **SSRIs** and **SNRIs** as the first-line drugs to treat depression and anxiety.

Lifestyle Modifications

If the patient is highly self-critical, has low self-esteem, and lacks assertiveness, medication will not directly improve these symptoms. Improved thinking and reduced sensitivity through medications and therapy will improve the psychological symptoms. When patients experience some relief of anxiety, sadness, insomnia, and anorexia, they become more motivated to address deeper emotional and

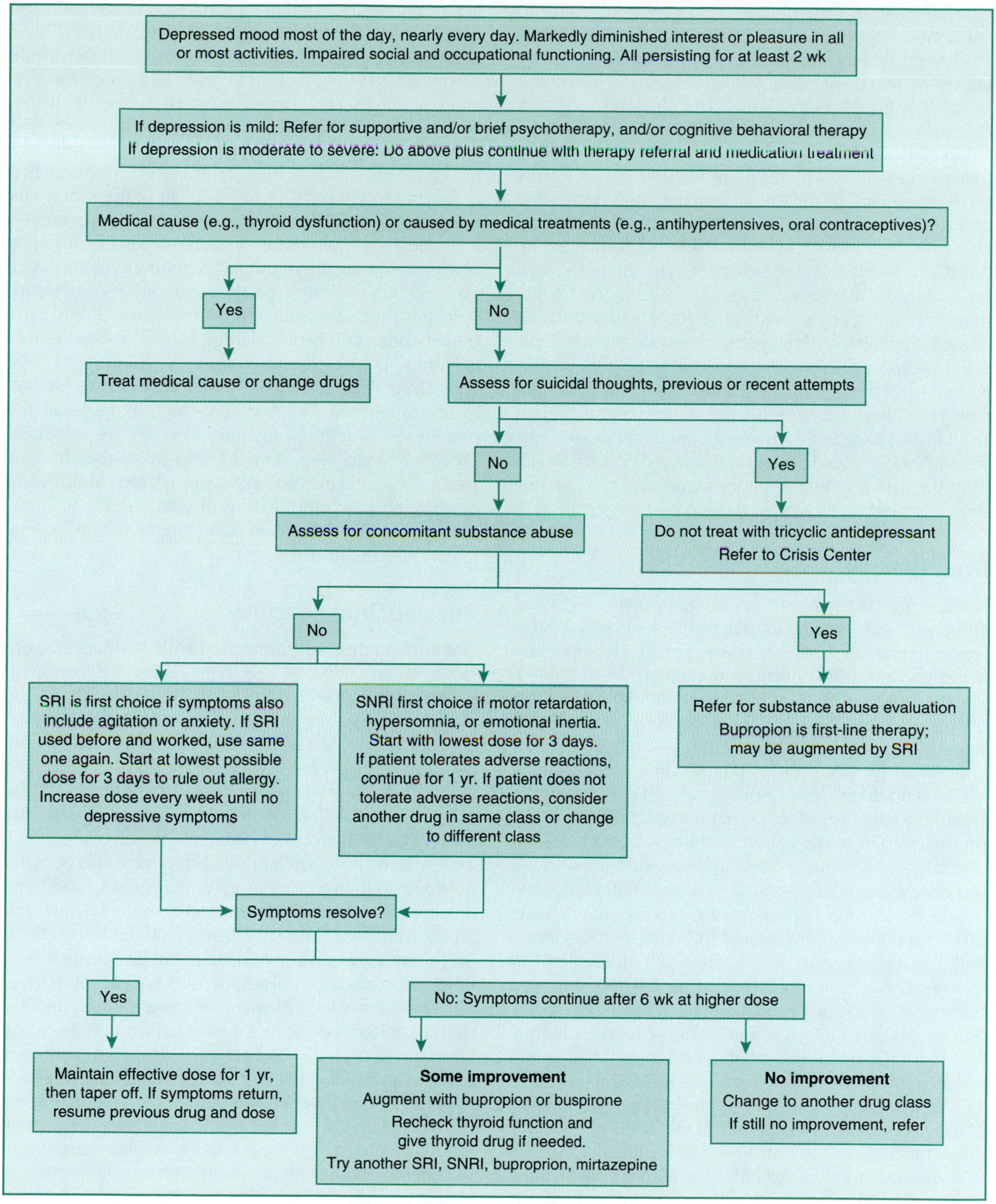

Figure 29–3. Treatment algorithm for depression.

interpersonal issues. If they are in therapy, they are able to learn more and grapple with their conflicts meaningfully. The therapist can augment the medication effects by teaching stress management skills such as deep breathing, progressive muscle relaxation, and meditation. In addition, cognitive skills such as challenging thought distortions, developing assertiveness, and problem solving enhance the patient's self-efficacy. At this point, the medication repairs the biochemical disturbance of anxiety and depression and the psychotherapeutic skills provides long-term recovery. Because the brain heals slowly, medication to correct the neurochemical changes needs to remain in place for a considerably longer time after remission of symptoms. Remaining on the medication for at least a year after complete remission of symptoms ensures enduring recovery. However, with every recurrence of symptoms, there is a higher risk of additional episodes, especially of depression. Possibly, with later return of symptoms, the patient would need to return to the medication that worked previously. The advanced practice nurse needs to review with the patient what target symptoms signal a return of depression and ways to respond to those symptoms early.

Drug Therapy

Lifestyle modifications brought about through counseling alone are rarely enough to treat moderate to severe anxiety or depression. A recent meta-analysis by Fournier and investigators (2010) questions the effectiveness of medication treatment in mild and moderate depression, but depressed patients should not be deprived of the opportunity to try medication treatment, especially when other contextual factors, such as patient preference, therapy availability, and insurance reimbursement may prohibit or lessen the effectiveness of psychotherapy. Selection of appropriate drugs is also central to therapy and is based on several variables. Symptoms improve gradually, with full responsiveness taking about 2 to 4 weeks at steady-state dosage if the primary symptoms are depression. Anticipate relief of anxiety within the first 2 to 3 days; then expect appetite and concentration to improve within the first 1 to 2 weeks. The last symptoms to improve are sleep and then dysphoric mood and consequential behaviors. It is important to monitor the symptoms of depression frequently and to increase the dosage of the drug until the patient reaches full therapeutic effect. This is likely to take 8 to 12 weeks. If the patient still does not show full remission of symptoms at the maximum dosage of the medication, the clinician needs to consider augmenting the medication with another drug, switching to another class of drugs, or referring to a psychiatric specialist for further psychopharmacology.

Treatment algorithms that include lifestyle modifications and drug therapy are presented in Figures 29–2 for anxiety and 29–3 for depression. Understanding the biochemistry of the brain and how drugs act on it permits clinicians to prescribe in a deliberate and thoughtful manner instead of simply following a protocol. Because the terms **antidepressant** and **anxiolytic** do not distinctively describe the NT action of these drugs, it helps to consider what NTs are involved in order to predict response and adverse drug reactions. The focus of prescribing then becomes clear identification of the target symptoms that are distressing, determining if those symptoms are amenable to biological therapy, and selecting a drug that is specific to the putative mechanism of the symptoms. Knowing the regions of the brain and tissue interaction that mediate symptoms also aids in selecting appropriate pharmacotherapy. If symptoms are predominantly cognitive (e.g., indecisiveness, poor motivation) and vegetative (e.g., poor appetite, difficulty sleeping, low libido), the frontal cortex and hypothalamus are involved, and probably there is some dysfunction in the NE and 5-HT systems. Drugs that increase the levels of these two NTs are most appropriate. The treatment algorithms assist the provider in beginning to think through the treatment process. Patients often do not follow these algorithms as well as we would like. Recently, **aripiprizole (Abilify)** and **quetiapine (Seroquel XR)**, antipsychotic medications have gotten FDA indication as an augmentation strategy for use with an **antidepressant.**

Adverse Drug Reactions

The adverse drug reactions seen with **antidepressants** can often be explained by understanding their action on the receptors in the CNS. The **SSRIs** are not specific for the receptor subtype to which 5-HT binds. Instead, all the available **SSRIs** can bind with any 5-HT receptor subtype. The binding of 5-HT to the 5-HT_2 receptor may be implicated in the adverse sexual reactions of the SSRIs. With 5-HT_2 antagonists (e.g. **nefazodone** and **trazodone**) and the 5-HT_{14} agonist **buspirone (BuSpar)**, however, the sexual dysfunction effects are minimal. **Buspirone** also does not produce cognitive or memory impairment or disinhibition euphoria like the **BZDs** do and does not interact with alcohol. Because the **SSRIs** have minimum to no effects on NE, DA, histamine, or ACh, there are few adverse reactions associated with blockade of these receptors (e.g., anxiety, restlessness, drowsiness, constipation, and orthostasis). Reduced sexual desire, delayed or absent orgasm, premature ejaculation, and erectile disturbance occur in about 35 percent of patients. Clinical experience suggests that men have fewer sexual dysfunction adverse reactions with **paroxetine** and women have fewer problems with **sertraline.** These adverse reactions usually do not become evident for about a month, which may be due simply to relief of depression and, therefore, recognition of sexual dysfunction. It is important to advise patients of these adverse reactions and ask them to report these problems, which can be corrected. The most direct correction is lowering the dose or changing to another **SSRI** or **SNRI.** If the patient does not want to try a different medication and the lowered dose does not help, other strategies might include adding **bupropion** or considering a **5-HT antagonist** (e.g., **amantadine** or **cyproheptadine**) prior to anticipated symptoms. Another option might be skipping a dose (except **fluoxetine**) if the patient is not bothered by withdrawal effects. **Citalopram** may have fewer sexual dysfunction adverse reactions and would be the first choice of change, or consider **nefazadone, venlafaxine,** or **duloxetine.** Changing to a different SSRI can occur by substituting the equivalent dosage at the next dose time.

Table 29–2 lists the dose equivalents for all **antidepressants**, including **SSRIs**. In changing from an SSRI to **bupropion**, it is advisable to first add the **bupropion** and then titrate off the SSRI after 3 weeks. Changing from an SSRI to an SNRI can be the same direct change to the equivalent dose, but there may be NE-mediated adverse reactions, especially restlessness and anxiety. Chapter 15 presents dosage schedules for each of these drugs.

Bupropion has a dose-dependent increased risk for seizures in patients with bulimia; therefore, it should not be given in single doses over 150 mg. The lowered seizure threshold and relatively short half-life require **bupropion** to be administered in two or three daily doses. The **slow-release preparation** (Wellbutrin SR) helps with a more even distribution, but because of the seizure potential, it still requires multiple daily dosing. The **extended-release preparation** (Wellbutrin XL), however, provides even distribution with single dosing possible. It has a benign adverse reaction profile because it does not affect the cholinergic pathways and has even been used to reverse the sexual dysfunction adverse reactions of **SSRIs** because it blocks 5-HT_2 receptors.

SNRIs have adverse reactions similar to those of **SSRIs**, including insomnia, somnolence, and nausea. Like the SSRIs, drugs in this class could contribute to sexual dysfunction.

Table 29–2 **Dose Equivalents for Antidepressants**

Generic Drug Name	Equivalent Dose in mg
Amitriptyline	100
Bupropion	150
Citalopram	20
Desipramine	150
Doxepin	150
Fluoxetine	20
Imipramine	150
Maprotiline	75
Mirtazapine	30
Nefazodone	150
Nortriptyline	50
Paroxetine	20
Protriptyline	20
Sertraline	50
Trazodone	150
Trimipramine	100
Venlafaxine	100

Drug Interactions

To a significant degree, the **SSRIs** interact with many other drugs. They are highly protein bound and inhibit the cytochrome P450 (CYP450) isoenzyme system to varying extents, leading to many drug interactions. Patients who are taking several other drugs may benefit from a drug choice that has fewer drug interactions. **SNRIs** show less protein binding than the **SSRIs**, are weak inhibitors of the CYP450 2D6 isoenzyme system, and have fewer drug–drug interactions. **MAOIs** can have dangerous interactions with many medications, including over-the-counter medications and herbal remedies.

The CYP450 enzymes are responsible for the metabolism of many **psychotropic drugs** and have drug interactions based on this metabolism. Table 29–3 summarizes the major drug interactions based on CYP450.

Additional Patient Variables

Patients who abuse other substances (drugs or **alcohol**) are more likely to develop tolerance to and dependency on **psychotropics**, especially **BZDs**. When the clinician identifies that the patient has developed a tolerance to the BZD, it is time to consider a withdrawal plan. Of special notice should be the patient who is taking very large doses of medication, such as 60 to 120 mg of **diazepam** a day. If the patient is taking a short-acting or intermediate-acting BZD, a long-acting drug such as **clonazepam** can be substituted at a comparable dosage before beginning the taper. Usually, tapering by 25 percent a week adequately prevents withdrawal symptoms and rebound anxiety. A patient who has difficulty with tapering should be referred to a drug treatment program, a psychiatrist, or an advanced practice psychiatric–mental health nurse for discontinuance.

MONITORING

Patients need to know that the provider is concerned and does not think they are weak or bad for having symptoms of depression or anxiety. It is important to follow up on the recommendations within the first week after the initiation of therapy, which can usually be handled by a telephone consultation or 15-minute face-to-face appointment. It is especially important to assess for suicidality through the first 3 weeks of initiating

Table 29–3 ■ **Four Cytochrome P-450 Isoenzymes and Potential Drug Interactions**

Isoenzyme	Substrates	Inhibitors	Comments
1A2	Acetaminophen, caffeine, theophylline, trimipramine, doxepin, clomipramine, amitriptyline, tacrine, propranolol, clozapine, phenacetin, trazodone, mirtazapine, alprazolam	Citalopram, fluoxetine, fluvoxamine, nefazodone, moclobemide, fluoroquinolones, grapefruit juice	
2D6	Fluoxetine, sertraline, amitriptyline, clomipramine, desipramine, imipramine, nortriptyline, trimipramine, maprotiline, venlafaxine, nefazodone, trazodone, paroxetine, bupropion, flurazepam, type I antiarrhythmics, dextromethorphan, oxycodone, codeine, haloperidol, perphenazine, risperidone, thioridazine, propranolol, alprenolol, timolol, metoprolol, indoramin	Citalopram, fluoxetine, fluvoxamine, paroxetine, sertraline, nefazodone, trazodone, venlafaxine, amitriptyline, clomipramine, quinidine, fluphenazine, haloperidol, perphenazine, thioridazine, methadone	Not the most abundant isoenzyme but important for metabolism of many psychotropic medications 7%–10% of whites have limited or absent capacity ("poor metabolizers") to metabolize
2C19	Citalopram, moclobemide, clomipramine, nortriptyline, desipramine, trimipramine, diazepam, hexobarbital, omeprazole, phenytoin, fluoxetine, venlafaxine, phenelzine	Citalopram, fluvoxamine, fluoxetine, paroxetine, sertraline, venlafaxine, mirtazapine, imipramine, moclobemide, tranylcypromine, diazepam, cimetidine, felbamate, omeprazole	All 2C subfamily comprises 20% of P-450 system Significant polymorphism in 18% Japanese, 19% African Americans, 8% Africans, and 3%–5% whites
3A4	Astemizole, loratadine, alprazolam, clonazepam, diazepam, midazolam, triazolam, estazolam, flurazepam, carbamazepine, ethosuximide, amitriptyline, imipramine, clomipramine, bupropion, nefazodone, sertraline, trazodone, venlafaxine, citalopram, calcium channel blockers, amiodarone, disopyramide, lidocaine, propafenone, quinidine, erythromycin, acetaminophen, alfentanil, codeine, androgens, dexamethasone, estrogens	Fluvoxamine, fluoxetine, paroxetine, sertraline, nefazodone, venlafaxine, mirtazapine, diltiazem, verapamil, clarithromycin, itraconazole, ketoconazole, cimetidine, dexamethasone, grapefruit juice	Potentially dangerous arrhythmias for those taking antihistamines, tricyclic antidepressants Accounts for 30% of all P-450 isoenzymes

treatment and consider hospitalization if the patient persists in suicidal thinking. Once the patient shows relief from the original symptoms and response and adverse reactions are tolerable, progress should be monitored in 6 months and again in 1 year. After 1 year, it is reasonable to consider tapering the drug for possible discontinuance. If symptoms return within 3 weeks, drug therapy needs to be reinstituted at the effective dose for another 6 months. When planning with the patient to discontinue **antidepressant medication**, it is important to select a target time when ordinary stresses are low; holidays, major family events, or return to school are *not* good times to discontinue medication.

OUTCOME EVALUATION

Outcome evaluation and appropriate referral points are presented in the algorithms. Advance practice primary care nurses are likely to see patients with depressive and anxiety symptoms in their practice, whether or not the patients directly identify their concerns as depression or anxiety. Therefore, it is important to assess possible explanations for multiple somatic symptoms, especially those that involve the autonomic system, poor concentration, insomnia or hypersomnia, loss of appetite and libido, fatigue, restlessness, irritability, and increased or absent emotionality. Because many medical problems may mimic depression and anxiety, as well as the reverse, a thorough examination including laboratory studies can help the practitioner narrow the clinical options and therefore treat appropriately.

Medications target physiological symptoms only and all the **psychotropic medications** act specifically on neural pathways in different parts of the brain. The psychological and social symptoms, such as low self-esteem, social withdrawal, and poor communication, can be better treated with psychotherapy. Because the physiological, psychological, and social symptoms occur together in depression and anxiety, the advanced practice primary care nurse would serve the patient best by not only prescribing medications but also discussing psychotherapy and referring the patient to a therapist to learn some new ways of coping with stress. When making a referral, it is equally important to inquire about the effectiveness of the referral at later appointments. If the patient has not followed up on the referral, the clinician should ask about this and offer additional referrals if necessary.

Comorbidity of Medical and Psychiatric Disorders

Reversing the picture of anxiety and depression presenting in primary care patients to that of primary care patients with chronic diseases, there is a clear pattern of anxiety and depression complicating medical diagnoses and management of chronic diseases and contributing to poor outcomes. Various studies indicate that migraines; pulmonary diseases such as asthma, pulmonary hypertension, chronic obstructive pulmonary disease (COPD), and chronic bronchitis; rheumatoid arthritis; fibromyalgia; seizure disorders; cardiovascular diseases such as myocardial infarction, ceratoid atherosclerosis, and cardiomyopathy; and irritable bowel disease all have remarkable association with depression and anxiety (Cooper et al, 2007; Frasure-Smith & Lesperance, 2005; Goodwin, Kroenke, Hoven, & Spitzer, 2003; Howard, El-Mallakh, Rayens, & Clark, 2007; Jones, Bromberger, Sutton-Tyrrel, & Matthews, 2003; Lake, Rains, Penzien, & Lipchik, 2005; Mussell et al, 2008; Thieme, Turk, & Flor, 2004). Furthermore, frequent users of primary care and emergency services are twice as likely to have anxiety, depressive, and somatoform disorders than are mid- and low-range users (Ford, Trestman, Steinberg, Tennen, & Allen, 2004; Roy-Byrne & Wagner, 2004). Work disability has a greater association with severity of depressive symptoms than with physical health state or function (Lowe et al, 2004). Such research clearly demonstrates that depression and anxiety symptoms are an essential element of patients' general health state, their ability to cope with physical illnesses, and their quality of life with chronic illness. Primary care providers are the gatekeepers for these patients and recognition of the comorbidity can influence the outcomes for these patients if they recognize and treat the mental health features along with the physical health features.

The choice of medication in treating depression and anxiety depends on the prominent symptoms the patient presents, comorbid conditions, other medications the patient is taking, and tolerance to adverse reactions. In addition, because mental disorders are often familial, it helps to know if anyone else in the family has similar symptoms and what medications worked for them. When several choices are reasonable, select the medication that other blood relatives have had success with because they are likely to affect the patient in the same manner.

Clinical guidelines recommend that symptoms of depression and anxiety are best treated with a combination of medications and psychotherapy (Black, 2006; Eddy et al, 2004; Mitte, 2005; Rush et al, 2006; Thase et al, 2007). The primary care advanced practice nurse is in a pivotal position in initiating pharmacological treatment and in assisting the patient to find a mental health therapist for behavioral treatments. It is important, therefore, to have readily available a list of therapists of both genders who are culturally diverse. When recommending therapy, the primary care nurse should provide two or three names of therapists. Discussing with the patient the therapists' features that would make the patient feel the most comfortable (e.g., gender, discipline, geographical area, ethnicity) invites the patient to follow up on the referral. It is also helpful to tell the patient a little about each referral specific to therapeutic style (e.g., interactive, a good listener), theoretical orientation (e.g., cognitive-behavioral, interpersonal), and special interests (e.g., family conflicts, developmental transitions, sexual orientation). Of course, this requires that the nurse know something about the therapists, and that information is acquired through networking and collaboration.

Frequently, the primary care provider takes on the prescribing and medication management role while the patient is in therapy and after therapy is concluded. Maintaining an open line of communication between the therapist and the PCP, with a patient's signed authorization for the release of information, reduces confusion in treatment direction.

Working with the patient who is depressed and/or anxious is challenging and hard work. Respectful and collaborative consulting with mental health professionals yields rewarding outcomes for both patient and provider. Probably the greatest reward is seeing and hearing about the improvement the patient is making. It is tempting for both patient and primary care provider to attribute success to the medications, but to do so invalidates the power and capacity of patients. Medications can only help the brain return to its normal functioning. It is the whole person who makes the changes necessary for recovery to mental health.

PATIENT EDUCATION

Patient education is critical in attaining the patient's cooperation and participation in taking the medications.

Compliance is least likely to be an issue with well-informed patients who understand the biology of their symptoms as well as the biology of how the medications work. The various pharmaceutical companies that produce **psychotropic medications** have informative patient education that can supplement the clinician's teaching. The Internet also has several helpful and reliable Web sites as patient resources, including:

- WebMD.com.
- Mentalhealth.com.
- Healthyplace.com.
- National Institute of Mental Health (www.nimh.nih.gov) (publications in English and Spanish for patients to download)

One of the most frequent errors in treating depression is ending medication treatment prematurely. When patients begin to feel better, they believe they no longer need the medication. However, the medications focus on correcting the brain's functioning, and the brain's resumption of proper function may take up to a year or longer, depending on how long the patient has been depressed. Undertreatment of depression leaves the patient vulnerable to future depressive episodes that are more severe than were any previous episodes. Patients need to know that they will be taking the medication for at least a year and then will need to taper off the medication to see if the symptoms resume. Another error in prescribing **psychotropic medication** is maintaining a dose insufficient to treat the symptoms adequately. The goal is reasonable and attainable if the dosage is raised to treat the symptoms completely. Because all the medications that are now available for depression and anxiety have a 2- to 4-week lag time for therapeutic effects, the trial of any medication requires 4 to 6 weeks before deciding it is ineffective unless the patient cannot tolerate the adverse effects of the drug. It helps to tell the patient that some symptoms remit earlier than others; usually, anxiety with or without depression is the first to remit, whereas improvements of mood and sleep disturbance are likely to happen later.

Last, remember that prescribing for patients who have anxiety and depressive symptoms hinges on how the provider relates to the patient. A caring relationship in which the patient feels he or she is being heard, believed, and taken seriously allows complete assessment, accurate medication decisions, and effective medication monitoring in collaboration with the patient. The placebo effect of **psychotropic medication** is about 35 percent, which means that the patient's belief that the medication will help is a powerful tool in having the medication work. Therefore, the provider should tell the patient that this medication will help, explain what to look for as the improvement occurs, and ask that the patient to keep the prescriber informed of how the medication affects the patient, both positively and negatively.

CLINICAL PEARL

Tapering Patients Off Antidepressants

1. Reduce dose by 50 percent for 3 to 4 days.
2. Then reduce another 50 percent for 3 to 4 days and discontinue.
3. If withdrawal symptoms occur (dizziness, nausea, diarrhea, sweating, irritability, anxiety), raise dose to stop symptoms. Then, slowly taper the rate—for example, give 40 mg to 30 mg for 5 days, then give 20 mg for 5 days, and so forth.
4. If dosing cannot be reduced in this fashion because the medication is available in capsule form only or because of low dosing, try to dose every other day for 10 days and then discontinue.
5. **Fluoxetine** may not need to be tapered because of its long half-life.

After tapering dosing to determine possible termination of long-term **antidepressant** treatment, a return of depressive symptoms requires a return to treatment regimen.

Do not start **monoamine oxidase inhibitors (MAOIs)** within 14 days of stopping other **antidepressants;** do not start another **antidepressant** until 14 days after stopping an **MAOI**.

CONCLUSIONS

Primary care providers carry a major responsibility in providing overall health care for the majority of patients within the health-care system. This is a heavy burden that is complicated by the need to control costs, time efficiency, and range of services. Because many patients first seek help for any health problem from their primary care provider, the primary care provider also has an essential role in identifying mental health issues that influence health care and quality of life. By collaborating with mental health–care providers, including advanced practice psychiatric–mental health nurses, the primary care providers can lessen their own burden of care for these patients. Some primary care settings include mental health–care providers as consultants and providers within the same clinic. This enhances collaboration and coordination of care and provides more satisfaction for providers and patients.

REFERENCES

American Psychiatric Association. (2000). *Diagnostic and Statistical Manual of Mental Disorders* (4th ed., text revision). Washington, DC: Author.

Barsky, A. J., Orav, E. J., & Bates, D. W. (2005). Somatization increases medical utilization and costs independent of psychiatric and medical comorbidity. *Archives of General Psychiatry, 62*(8), 903–910.

Black, D. (2006). Efficacy of combined pharmacotherapy and psychotherapy versus monotherapy in the treatment of anxiety disorders [Review]. *CNS Spectrums, 11*(Suppl. 12), 29–33.

Cooper, C., Parry, G., Morice, S., Hutchcrof, B., Moore, J., & Esmonde, L. (2007). Anxiety and panic fear for adults with asthma: Prevalence in primary care. *BMC Family Practice, 8,* 162.

Eddy, K. T., Dutra, L., Bradley, R., & Westen, D. (2004). A multidimensional meta analysis of psychotherapy and pharmacotherapy for obsessive-compulsive disorder. *Clinical Psychology Review, 24*(8), 1011–1030.

Ford, J. D., Trestman, R. L., Steinberg, K., Tennen, H., & Allen, S. (2004). Prospective association of anxiety, depressive, and addictive disorders with high utilization of primary, specialty and emergency medical care. *Social Science & Medicine, 58*(11), 2145–2148.

Frasure-Smith, N., & Lesperance, F. (2005). Reflections on depression as a cardiac risk factor. *Psychosomatic Medicine, 67*(Suppl. 1), 19–25.

Fredman, S. J., & Korn, M. L. (2001). On the horizon: New antidepressants. *154th Annual Meeting of the American Psychiatric Association.* Retrieved January 3, 2006, from http://www.Medscape.com

Fournier, J., DeRubeis, R., Hollon, S., Dimidjian, S., Amsterdam, J., Shelton, R., et al. (2010). Antidepressant drug effects and depression severity: A patient-level meta-analysis. *Journal of the American Medical Association, 303*(1), 47–53.

Goodwin, R. D., Kroenke, K., Hoven, C. W., & Spitzer, R. L. (2003). Major depression, physical illness, and suicidal ideation in primary care. *Psychosomatic Medicine, 65*(4), 501–505.

Greenberg, P. E., Kessler, R. C., Birnbaum, H. C., Leong, S. A., Lowe, S. W., Berglund, P. A., et al. (2003). The economic burden of depression in the U.S.: How did it change between 1990 and 2000? *Journal of Clinical Psychiatry, 64*(12), 1465–1475.

Howard, P., El-Mallakh, P., Rayens, M., & Clark, J. (2007). Comorbid medical illnesses and perceived general health among recipients of Medicaid mental health services. *Issues in Mental Health, 28,* 255–274.

Jones, D. J., Bromberger, J. T., Sutton-Tyrrel, K., & Matthews, K. A. (2003). Lifetime history of depression and carotid atherosclerosis in middle-aged women. *Archives of General Psychiatry, 60*(2), 153–160.

Kessler, R., Demler, O., Frank, R., Olfson, M., Pincus, H. A., Walters, E. E., Zaslavsky, A. M., et al. (2005). Prevalence and treatment of mental disorders, 1990–2003. *New England Journal of Medicine, 352*(24), 2515–2523.

Kilbourne, A., Daugherty, B., & Pincus, H. (2007). What do general medical guidelines say about depression care? Depression treatment recommendations in general medical practice guidelines. *Current Opinion in Psychiatry, 20,* 626–631.

Lake, A. E., III, Rains, J. C., Penzien, D. B., & Lipchik, G. L. (2005). Headache and psychiatric comorbidity: Historical context, clinical implications, and research relevance. *Headache, 45*(5), 493–506.

Lowe, B., Willand, L., Eich, W., Zipfel, S., Ho, A. D., Herzog, W., et al. (2004). Psychiatric comorbidity and work disability in patients with inflammatory rheumatic diseases. *Psychosomatic Medicine, 66*(3), 395–402.

Mitte, K. (2005). A meta-analysis of the efficacy of psycho- and pharmacotherapy in panic disorder with and without agoraphobia. *Journal of Affective Disorders, 88,* 27–45.

Mussell, M., Kroenke, K., Spitzer, R., Williams, J., Herzog, W., & Lowe, B. (2008). Gastrointestinal symptoms in primary care: Prevalence and association with depression and anxiety. *Journal of Psychosomatic Research, 64*(6), 605–612.

Pampallona, S., Ballini, P., Tibaldi, G., Kupalnick, B., & Munizza, C. (2004). Combined pharmacotherapy and psychological treatment for depression: A systematic review. *Archives of General Psychiatry, 61*(7), 714–719.

Roy-Byrne, P. P., & Wagner, A. (2004). Primary care perspectives on generalized anxiety disorder. *Journal of Clinical Psychiatry, 65*(Suppl. 12), 20–26.

Rush, A., Trivedi, M., Wisniewski, S., Nierenberg, A. A., Stewart, J. W., Warden, D., et al. (2006). Acute and longer-term outcomes in depressed outpatients requiring one or several treatment steps: A STAR*D report. *American Journal of Psychiatry, 163,* 1905–1917.

Sadock, B., Sadock, V., & Ruiz, P. (2009). *Comprehensive Textbook of Psychiatry* (9th ed.). Philadelphia: Lippincott, Williams and Wilkins.

Thase, M., Friedman, E., Biggs, M., Wisniewski, S. F., Trivedi, M. H., Luther, J. F., Rush, A. J., et al. (2007). Cognitive therapy versus medication in augmentation and switch strategies as second-step treatments: A STAR*D report. *American Journal of Psychiatry, 164*(5), 739–752.

Thieme, K., Turk, D. C., & Flor, H. (2004). Comorbid depression and anxiety in fibromyalgia syndrome: Relationship to somatic and psychosocial variables. *Psychosomatic Medicine, 66*(6), 837–844.

CHAPTER 30

ASTHMA AND CHRONIC OBSTRUCTIVE PULMONARY DISEASE

Teri Moser Woo

Chapter Outline

Asthma and chronic obstructive pulmonary disease (COPD) are two of the most common chronic respiratory illnesses worldwide. According to the National Heart, Lung, and Blood Institute (NHLBI) and the World Health Organization (WHO), asthma affects more than 300 million people worldwide (Global Initiative for Asthma, 2009). COPD affects 5 percent of the adult U.S. population, is the fourth-leading cause of death, and is the 12th-leading cause of morbidity (Qaseem et al, 2007). It is predicted that COPD will become the third-leading cause of death worldwide by 2020 (Global Initiative for Chronic Obstructive Lung Disease [GOLD], 2009). This chapter discusses the pharmacological management of these two diseases.

ASTHMA

More than 22 million Americans, including 6 million children have asthma (National Asthma Education and Prevention Program [NAEPP], 2007). Canada has similar statistics with 2.3 million Canadians diagnosed with asthma in 2009 (Statistics Canada, 2010). This chapter focuses on the pharmacological management of asthma according to the current guidelines established by the NAEPP *Expert Panel Report 3: Guidelines* (2007). The chapter briefly discusses the pathophysiology of asthma to help explain the rationale for selecting appropriate medications. Monitoring and outcome evaluations are essential in asthma therapy, as adjustments can have a significant impact on a patient's activity level, and patient education is the key to having patients with asthma feel that they have control over a chronic illness. The overall goal of the asthma portion of the chapter is to enable the health-care provider to render optimal care for patients with asthma.

Pathophysiology

In the past, asthma was seen as episodic bronchospasm occurring in response to specific and nonspecific stimuli. It is now known that asthma is a chronic inflammatory disorder of the airways. The airway inflammation is present even between flare-ups and can significantly alter lung function. Based on this information, the NAEPP offers the following definition: "Asthma is a chronic inflammatory disorder of the airways in which many cells and cellular elements play a role: in particular, mast cells, eosinophils, neutrophils (especially in sudden onset, fatal exacerbations, occupational asthma, and patients who smoke), T lymphocytes, macrophages, and epithelial cells. In susceptible individuals, this inflammation causes recurrent episodes of coughing (particularly at night or early in the morning), wheezing, breathlessness, and chest tightness. These episodes are usually associated with widespread but variable airflow obstruction that is often reversible either spontaneously or with treatment" (NAEPP, 2007, p. 9). When asthma therapy is adequate, inflammation can be decreased over the long term, thereby preventing most asthma-related problems.

Chronic Inflammation

The lungs of patients who have died from asthma are visually noted to be overinflated. Both large and small airways are plugged with mucus and a mixture of cell debris, inflammatory cells, and serum proteins. Microscopic examination reveals extensive infiltration of the airway lumen and wall with eosinophils, mononuclear cells accompanied by vasodilation, evidence of microvascular leakage, and epithelial disruption (NAEPP, 2007). The airway smooth muscle is often hypertrophied, with new vessel formation, increased numbers of epithelial goblet cells, mucous gland hyperplasia and deposition of interstitial collagen beneath the epithelium. These changes further support the theory of chronic inflammation in asthma.

A series of interrelated cellular mechanisms, mast cells, eosinophils, epithelial cells, macrophages, and activated T cells have been shown to cause inflammation and affect lung function (Fig. 30–1). These cells can influence airway function by a number of routes. The release of histamine and leukotrienes can lead directly to bronchoconstriction. The release of proinflammatory cytokines from the mast cells, macrophages, and T cells activates the neutrophils, eosinophils, and macrophages, and this activation leads to the chronic inflammation associated with asthma. Cytokines can also cause the changes found on autopsy in patients with asthma: smooth muscle hypertrophy, increased vascular permeability, and mucus secretion.

Airway Hyperresponsiveness

Airway hyperresponsiveness is a hallmark of asthma, leading to the clinical symptoms of wheezing, chest tightness, and dyspnea after exposure to stimuli such as allergens, environmental irritants, viral infections, exercise, and cold

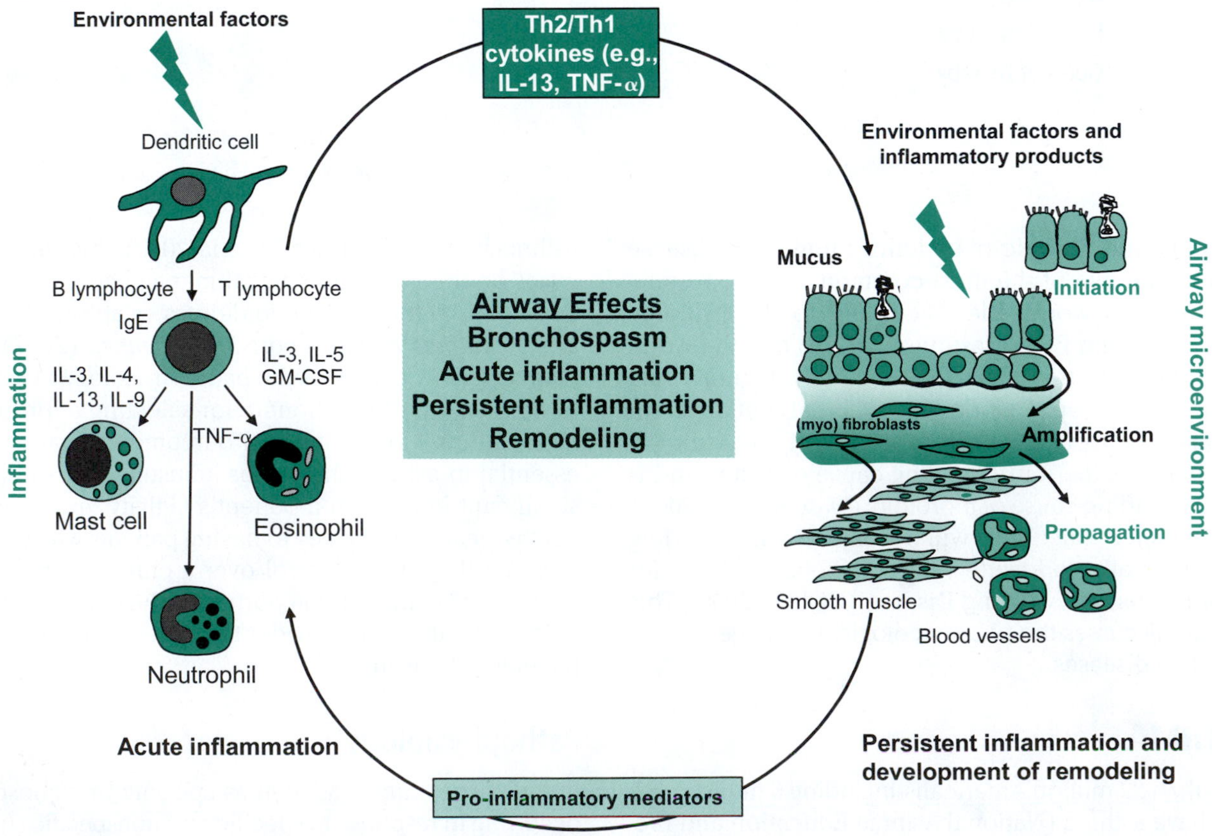

Figure 30–1. Factors limiting airflow in acute and persistent asthma. Key: GM-CSF, granulocyte-macrophage colony-stimulating factor; IgE, immunoglobulin E; IL-3, interleukin 3 (and similar); TNF-α, tumor necrosis factor-alpha. *(Source: Holgate, S. T., & Polosa, R. [2006]. The mechanisms, diagnosis, and management of severe asthma in adults.* Lancet, 368, *780–793.)*

air. The inclination of airways to narrow too easily and too much is a major aspect of asthma, along with the chronic inflammation noted previously. In the past, treatment of asthma focused on treating acute attacks with **bronchodilator** therapy. It is now known that the underlying inflammation influences the airway in such a way as to cause airway hyperresponsiveness. An allergen may trigger the release of a multitude of cellular mediators, cytokines, and chemokines, which result in increased smooth muscle responsiveness. Therefore, treating only the bronchoconstriction without treating the underlying inflammation leads to treatment failure if inflammation is present. Treatment of asthma and decreasing airway inflammation not only reduces symptoms but also decreases airway hyperresponsiveness.

Airflow Obstruction

Airflow obstruction is caused by a variety of changes in the airway. Acute bronchoconstriction and airway edema are two causes already discussed. Chronic mucous plug formation caused by increased mucus secretion can also influence airflow. It is now known that in some patients, airway changes are only partially reversible. Chronic inflammation leads to airway remodeling. Histological evidence indicates that there is an alteration in the amount and composition of the extracellular matrix in the airway wall. This change is not fully understood but suggests a rationale for early, aggressive treatment with **anti-inflammatory** therapy.

Understanding the role of inflammation and the cellular mechanisms involved has led to new treatment strategies. Understanding the multiple mechanisms involved in airway inflammation has led to treatment aimed at either multiple components (**inhaled corticosteroids**) or specific mediators of inflammation. For example, **leukotriene modifiers** are a treatment aimed at specific mediators. Leukotrienes are responsible, in part, for increased mucus production, bronchoconstriction, and eosinophil infiltration. **Leukotriene modifiers**, as described in Chapter 17, are either **Leukotriene receptor agonists** (**LTRAs**) (**zafirlukast** and **montelukast**) or **5-lipoxygenase pathway** (**zileuton**). Research continues to develop a better understanding of the pathology of asthma and treatment targeted at controlling the cellular changes that occur in acute and chronic asthma.

Classification of Asthma

According to the *Expert Panel Report 3: Guidelines*, asthma severity in children 12 years or older and adults is determined by clinical features before treatment. There are four classifications of severity, based on need for medication to relieve symptoms, nighttime symptoms, and lung function:

1. Mild intermittent asthma: Symptoms occur less often than twice a week and the patient is asymptomatic between exacerbations; nighttime symptoms occur less than twice a month; and peak expiratory flow (PEF) is greater than 80 percent predicted. The use of **short-acting beta$_2$ agonists** (SABA) should be less than twice a week, unless using it for exercise-induced bronchospasm (EIB).
2. Mild persistent asthma: Symptoms occur more often than twice a week but less often than once a day and exacerbations may affect activity; nighttime symptoms occur three to four times a month; and PEF is greater than 80 percent predicted. Patients with mild persistent asthma may use their **short-acting beta$_2$ agonists** more than twice a week but not daily, and not more than once daily.
3. Moderate persistent asthma: The patient is having daily symptoms; requires daily use of a **beta$_2$ agonist**; exacerbations affect normal activity; nighttime symptoms occur more often than once a week; and PEF is greater than 60 percent to less than 80 percent.
4. Severe persistent asthma: The patient has some degree of symptoms all the time; extremely limited physical activity and frequent exacerbations; frequent nighttime symptoms, often 7 days a week; and decreased lung function (PEF less than 60% predicted). Table 30–1 outlines the classifications of asthma severity in patients aged 12 years or older.

In children, classification of asthma is based on severity and frequency of symptoms (NAEPP, 2007). Table 30–2 discusses classification of asthma severity and initiating therapy in children.

1. Mild intermittent asthma: Symptoms occur less often than twice a week and the patient is asymptomatic between exacerbations. Children aged 0 to 4 years have no nighttime symptoms, and children aged 5 to 11 years have nighttime symptoms less than twice a month and PEF is greater than 80 percent predicted. The use of short-acting beta$_2$ agonists should be less than twice a week, unless using for EIB. Exacerbations requiring oral systemic corticosteroids occur no more than once a year.
2. Mild persistent asthma: Symptoms occur more often than twice a week but less often than once a day and exacerbations may affect activity. In children aged 0 to 4 years, nighttime symptoms occur one to two times a month, and in children aged 5 t[...] 11 years, nighttime symptoms three to fou[...] month; PEF is greater than 80 pe[...] Patients with mild persist[...] **short-acting bet[...]** week but not da[...] Children younger t[...] ent asthma have [...] in 6 months requiri[...] episodes of wheezing [...] day and risk factors fo[...] aged 5 to 11 with mild p[...] erbations two or more ti[...]

Table 30–1 Classification of Asthma Severity ≥12 Years of Age

Assessing severity and initiating treatment for patients who are not currently taking long-term control medications

Components of Severity		Classification of Asthma Severity ≥12 years of age			
			Persistent		
		Intermittent	Mild	Moderate	Severe
Impairment	Symptoms	≤2 days/week	> 2 days/week but not daily	Daily	Throughout the day
	Nighttime awakenings	≤2x/month	3–4x/month	>1x/week but not nightly	Often 7x/week
	Short-acting $beta_2$-agonist use for symptom control (not prevention of EIB)	≤2 days/week	>2 days/week but not daily, and not more than 1x on any day	Daily	Several times per day
Normal FEV_1/FVC:	Interference with normal activity	None	Minor limitation	Some limitation	Extremely limited
8–19 yr 85% **20–39 yr 80%** **40–59 yr 75%** **60–80 yr 70%**	Lung function	• Normal FEV_1 between exacerbations • FEV_1 >80% predicted • FEV_1/FVC normal	• FEV_1 >80% predicted • FEV_1/FVC normal	• FEV_1 >60% but <80% predicted • FEV_1/FVC reduced 5%	• FEV_1 <60% predicted • FEV_1/FVC reduced >5%
Risk	**Exacerbations requiring oral systemic corticosteroids**	**0–1/year (see note)**	**≥2/year (see note) →**		
		← Consider severity and interval since last exacerbation. → Frequency and severity may fluctuate over time for patients in any severity category. Relative annual risk of exacerbations may be related to FEV_1.			
Recommended Step for Initiating Treatment (See "Stepwise Approach for Managing Asthma" for treatment steps.)		Step 1	Step 2	Step 3 and consider short course of oral systemic corticosteroids	Step 4 or 5
		In 2–6 weeks, evaluate level of asthma control that is achieved and adjust therapy accordingly.			

Key: EIB, exercise-induced bron-chospasm, FEV1, forced expiratory volume in 1 second; FVC, forced vital capacity; ICU, intensive care unit

Notes:

- The stepwise approach is meant to assist, not replace, the clinical decisionmaking required to meet individual patient needs.
- Level of severity is determined by assessment of both impairment and risk. Assess impairment domain by patient's/caregiver's recall of previous 2–4 weeks and spirometry. Assign severity to the most severe category in which any feature occurs.
- At present, there are inadequate data to correspond frequencies of exacerbations with different levels of asthma severity. In general, more frequent and intense exacerbations (e.g., requiring urgent, unscheduled care, hospitalization, or ICU admission) indicate greater underlying disease severity. For treatment purposes, patients who had ≥2 exacerbations requiring oral systemic corticosteroids in the past year may be considered the same as patients who have persistent asthma, even in the absence of impairment levels consistent with persistent asthma.

Source: From National Asthma Education and Prevention Program (NAEPP). (2007). *The Expert Panel Report 3: Guidelines for the diagnosis and management of asthma.* Bethesda, MD: National Heart, Lung, and Blood Institute, National Institutes of Health.

3. Moderate persistent asthma: The child is having daily symptoms; requires daily use of a **beta$_2$ agonist**; exacerbations affect normal activity. In children aged 4 years or younger, nighttime symptoms occur [illegible]ree or four times a month, and in children aged 5 [illegible]1 years nighttime symptoms occur more than [illegible] a week but not nightly; PEF is greater than [illegible]ent to less than 80 percent. Children with moderate persistent asthma have exacerbations two or more times a year.
4. Severe persistent asthma: The patient has some degree of symptoms all the time; extremely limited physical activity; frequent nighttime symptoms (more than once a week in children younger than age 4 years and in older children they often occur 7 days a week; and decreased lung function (PEF

Classifying Asthma Severity and Initiating Therapy in Children

	Components of Severity	Intermittent		Persistent: Mild		Persistent: Moderate		Persistent: Severe	
		Ages 0–4	Ages 5–11	*Ages 0–4*	Ages 5–11	*Ages 0–4*	Ages 5–11	*Ages 0–4*	Ages 5–11
Impairment	Symptoms	≤2 days/week		>2 days/week but not daily		Daily		Throughout the day	
	Nighttime awakenings	0	<2x/month	1–2x/month	3–4x/month	3–4x/month	>1x/week but not nightly	>1x/week	Often 2x/week
	Short-acting beta$_2$-agonist use for symptom control	≤2 days/week		>2 days/week but not daily		Daily		Several times per day	
	Interference with normal activity	None		Minor limitation		Some limitation		Extremely limited	
	Lung function • FEV_1 (predicted) or peak flow (personal best) • FEV_1/FVC	N/A	Normal FEV_1 between exacerbations >80% >85%	N/A	>80% >80%	N/A	60–80% 75–80%	N/A	<60% <75%
Risk	Exacerbations requiring oral systemic corticosteroids (consider severity and interval since last exacerbation)	0–1/year (see notes)		≥2 exacerbations in 6 months requiring oral systemic corticosteroids, or ≥4 wheezing episodes/1 year lasting > 1 day AND risk factors for persistent asthma	≥2x/year (see notes) Relative annual risk may be related to FEV_1				
Recommended Step for Initiating Therapy (See "Stepwise Approach for Managing Asthma" for treatment steps.) **The stepwise approach is meant to assist, not replace, the clinical decision making required to meet individual patient needs.**		Step 1 (for both age groups)		Step 2 (for both age groups)		Step 3 and consider short course of oral systemic corticosteroids	Step 3: medium-dose ICS option and consider short course of oral systemic corticosteroids	Step 3 and consider short course of oral systemic corticosteroids	Step 3: medium-dose ICS option OR step 4 and consider short course of oral systemic corticosteroids
		In 2–6 weeks, depending on severity, evaluate level of asthma control that is achieved. • Children 0–4 years old: If no clear benefit is observed in 4–6 weeks, stop treatment and consider alternative diagnoses or adjusting therapy. • Children 5–11 year old: Adjust therapy accordingly.							

Key: FEV_1, forced expiratory volume in 1 second; FVC, forced vital capacity; ICS, inhaled corticosteroids; ICU, intensive care unit; N/A, not applicable

Notes:

- Level of severity is determined by both impairment and risk. Assess impairment domain by caregiver's recall of previous 2–4 weeks. Assign severity to the most severe category in which any feature occurs.
- Frequency and severity of exacerbations may fluctuate over time for patients in any severity category. At present, there are inadequate data to correspond frequencies of exacerbations with different levels of asthma severity. In general, more frequent and severe exacerbations (e.g., requiring urgent, unscheduled care, hospitalization, or ICU admission) indicate greater underlying disease severity. For treatment purposes, patients with ≥2 exacerbations described above may be considered the same as patients who have persistent asthma, even in the absence of impairment levels consistent with persistent asthma.

Source: From National Asthma Education and Prevention Program (NAEPP). (2007). *The Expert Panel Report 3: Guidelines for the diagnosis and management of asthma.* Bethesda, MD: National Heart, Lung, and Blood Institute, National Institutes of Health.

less than 60% predicted). Children aged 5 to 11 with severe persistent asthma have exacerbations two or more times a year.

Goals of Therapy

The Expert Panel Report 3Guidelines (NAEPP,2007) clearly define the goals of asthma therapy:

Reduce Impairment

1. Prevent chronic and troublesome symptoms (e.g., coughing or breathlessness in the night, in the early morning, or after exertion).
2. Require infrequent use (less than twice a week) of inhaled **short-acting beta$_2$ agonists** for relief of symptoms (not including use for EIB).
3. Maintain (near) "normal" pulmonary function.
4. Maintain (near) normal activity levels.
5. Meet patients' and families' expectations of and satisfaction with asthma care.

Reduce Risk

1. Prevent recurrent exacerbations of asthma and minimize the need for emergency department visits or hospitalizations.
2. Prevent loss of lung function; for children, prevent reduced lung growth.
3. Provide optimal pharmacotherapy with minimal or no adverse effects.

Rational Drug Selection

Asthma Step Therapy

The Expert Panel Report 3: Guidelines (NAEPP, 2007) recommend a stepwise approach to the pharmacological management of asthma. Management can begin at a higher level and gradually step down or start low and move up, depending on the patient's status when beginning treatment. The panel recommends that medications be categorized into two general classes: long-term-control medications to achieve and maintain control of persistent asthma and quick-relief medications to treat acute symptoms and exacerbations. Asthma severity determines the amount and frequency of medication, with suppression of airway inflammation the goal. One essential component of asthma treatment is the patient's cooperation in keeping a log of asthma symptoms. This patient self-assessment enables the provider to track the effectiveness of therapy and make treatment decisions based on medication use, nighttime symptoms, and PEF. Although step therapy is a helpful framework, the clinician must individualize therapy based on a patient's individual circumstances and response to therapy.

Initiating Control of Asthma

The *Expert Panel Report 3: Guidelines* prefer an aggressive approach of gaining quick control with a higher level of therapy and then stepping down the care (NAEPP, 2007). A stepwise approach for managing asthma incorporates assessment of severity to initiate therapy or assessment of control to monitor or adjust therapy. New to the 2007 *Expert Panel Report 3: Guidelines* is the recommendation to assess asthma control and adjust therapy accordingly at regular intervals (NAEPP, 2007). Asthma control is "the degree to which the manifestations of asthma are minimized by therapeutic intervention and the goals of therapy are met" (NAEPP, 2007). Once patients have received initial treatment for their asthma, they need ongoing monitoring to assess the degree of control. Control is based on level of impairment (symptoms, nighttime awakenings, interference with normal activity, SABA use and spirometry or peak flows. Validated questionnaires can be used to measure level of impairment found in the *Expert Panel 3 Report: Guidelines* (Asthma Therapy Assessment Questionnaire, Asthma Control Questionnaire and Asthma Control Test). Patients should be assessed regarding risk in relation to exacerbations. Table 30–3 outlines assessment of control in youths 12 years of age or older and adults, Table 30–4 is the assessment of control for children. The stepwise approach to treating asthma in adults is found in Table 30–5 and in children is found in Table 30–6. Drugs commonly used to treat asthma are shown in Table 30–7. Additional components of care include patient education and environmental control measures. See also Tables 30–7 and 30–8.

Mild Intermittent Asthma

Treatment for mild intermittent asthma symptoms consists of using **short-acting inhaled beta$_2$ agonists** as needed for symptoms. Patients with mild intermittent asthma have asthma symptoms only when exposed to their asthma triggers (e.g., allergens, viral respiratory illness, chemical inhalants), people who have only exercise-induced asthma, and infants and children who wheeze with viral upper respiratory infections (NAEPP, 2007). Using **short-acting beta$_2$ agonists** more than twice a week may indicate a need to step up to step 2 therapy or to initiate long-term-control therapy. Education at this step is introducing the patient and family to the use of medication and teaching them about asthma, proper inhaler technique if appropriate, care during exacerbation of symptoms, and environmental controls to known allergens.

Drazen and colleagues (1996) conducted a comparison study of 255 patients with mild asthma in which patients followed for 16 weeks were to administer their **inhaled albuterol** either on a regular schedule (126 patients) or as needed (129 patients). The study concluded that there were no significant differences between the study groups' peak flow variability, forced expiratory volume (FEV), the number of puffs of supplemental **albuterol** needed, asthma symptoms, asthma quality-of-life score, or airway responsiveness to **methacholine.** This study underscores the *Expert Panel Report 3 Guidelines* recommendation that patients with

(Text continues on page 999)

Table 30–3 Assessing Asthma Control and Adjusting Therapy in Youths >12 Years and Adults

Components of Control		Classification of Asthma Control (≥12 years of age)		
		Well Controlled	*Not Well Controlled*	*Very Poorly Controlled*
Impairment	Symptoms	≤2 days/week	>2 days/week	Throughout the day
	Nighttime awakenings	≤2x/month	1-3x/week	>4x/week
	Interference with normal activity	None	Some limitation	Extremely limited
	Short-acting $beta_2$-agonist use for symptom control (not prevention of EIB)	≤2 days/week	>2 days/week	Several times per day
	FEV_1 or peak flow	>80% predicted/ personal best	60-80% predicted/ personal best	<60% predicted/ personal best
	Validated questionnaires ATAQ ACQ ACT	 0 ≤0.75* ≥20	 1-2 ≥1.5 16-19	 3-4 N/A ≤15
Risk	Exacerbations requiring oral systemic corticosteroids	0–1 year	≥2/year (see note)	
		Consider severity and interval since last exacerbation		
	Progressive loss of lung function	Evaluation requires long-term followup care.		
	Treatment-related adverse effects	Medication side effects can vary in intensity from none to very troublesome and worrisome. The level of intensity does not correlate to specific levels of control but should be considered in the overall assessment of risk.		
Recommended Action for Treatment **(See "Stepwise Approach for Managing Asthma" for treatment steps.)**		• Maintain current step. • Regular followup at every 1–6 months to maintain control. • Consider step down if well controlled for at least 3 months.	• Step up 1 step. • Reevaluate in 2–6 weeks. • For side effects consider alternative treatment options.	• Consider short course of oral systemic corticosteroids. • Step up 1–2 steps. • Reevaluate in 2 weeks. • For side effects, consider alternative treatment options.

*ACQ values of 0.76–1.4 are indeterminate regarding well-controlled asthma.

Key: EIB, exercise-induced bronchospasm; ICU, intensive care unit

Notes:

- The stepwise approach is meant to assist, not replace, the clinical decision making required to meet individual patient needs.
- The level of control is based on the most severe impairment or risk category. Assess impairment domain by patient's recall of previous 2–4 weeks and by spirometry/or peak flow measures. Symptom assessment for longer periods should reflect a global assessment, such as inquiring whether the patient's asthma is better or worse since the last visit.
- At present, there are inadequate data to correspond frequencies of exacerbations with different levels of asthma control. In general, more frequent and intense exacerbations (e.g., requiring urgent, unscheduled care, hospitalization, or ICU admission) indicate poorer disease control. For treatment purposes, patients who had ≥2 exacerbations requiring oral systemic corticosteroids in the past year may be considered the same as patients who have not-well-controlled asthma, even in the absence of impairment levels consistent with not-well-controlled asthma.

ATAQ = Asthma Therapy Assessment Questionnaire©

ACQ = Asthma Control Questionnaire©

ACT = Asthma Control Test ™

Minimal Important

Difference: 1.0 for the ATAQ; 0.5 for the ACQ; not determined for the ACT.

Before step up in therapy:

— Review adherence to medication, inhaler technique, environmental control, and comorbid conditions.

— If an alternative treatment option was used in a step, discontinue and use the preferred treatment for that step.

Source: From National Asthma Education and Prevention Program (NAEPP). (2007). *The Expert Panel Report 3: Guidelines for the diagnosis and management of asthma.* Bethesda, MD: National Heart, Lung, and Blood Institute, National Institutes of Health.

Table 30–4 Assessing Asthma Control and Adjusting Therapy in Children

	Components of Control	Well Controlled: Ages 0–4	Well Controlled: Ages 5–11	Not Well Controlled: Ages 0–4	Not Well Controlled: Ages 5–11	Very Poorly Controlled: Ages 0–4	Very Poorly Controlled: Ages 5–11
Impairment	Symptoms	≤2 days/week but not more than once on each day		>2 days/week or multiple times on ≤2 days/week		Throughout the day	
	Nighttime awakenings	≤1x/month		>1x/month	≥2x/month	>1x/week	≥2x/week
	Interference with normal activity	None		Some limitation		Extremely limited	
	Short-acting beta$_2$-agonist use for symptom control (not prevention of EIB)	≤2 days/week		>2 days/week		Several times per day	
	Lung function • FEV_1 (predicted) or peak flow personal best • FEV_1/FVC	N/A	>80% >80%	N/A	60–80% 75–80%	N/A	<60% <75%
Risk	Exacerbations requiring oral systemic corticosteroids	0–1x/year		2–3x/year	≥2x/year	>3x/year	≥2x/year
	Reduction in lung growth	N/A	Requires long-term followup	N/A		N/A	
	Treatment-related adverse effects	Medication side effects can vary in intensity from none to very troublesome and worrisome. The level of intensity does not correlate to specific levels of control but should be considered in the overall assessment of risk.					
Recommended Action for Treatment (See "Stepwise Approach for Managing Asthma" for treatment steps.) The stepwise approach is meant to assist, not replace, the clinical decision making required to meet individual patient needs.		• Maintain current step. • Regular followup every 1–6 months. • Consider step down if well controlled for at least 3 months.		Step up 1 step	Step up at least 1 step	• Consider short course of oral systemic corticosteroids. • Step up 1–2 steps	
				• Before step up: Review adherence to medication, inhaler technique, and environmental control. If alternative treatment was used, discontinue it and use preferred treatment for that step. • Reevaluate the level of asthma control in 2–6 weeks to achieve control; every 1–6 months to maintain control. Children 0–4 years old: If no clear benefit is observed in 4–6 weeks, consider alternative diagnoses or adjusting therapy. Children 5–11 years old: Adjust therapy accordingly. • For side effects, consider alternative treatment options.			

Key: EIB, exercise-induced bron-chospasm, FEV_1, forced expiratory volume in 1 second; FVC, forced vital capacity; ICU, intensive care unit; N/A, not applicable

Notes:

- The level of control is based on the most severe impairment or risk category. Assess impairment domain by patient's or caregiver's recall of previous 2–4 weeks. Symptom assessment for longer periods should reflect a global assessment, such as whether the patient's asthma is better or worse since the last visit.
- At present, there are inadequate data to correspond frequencies of exacerbations with different levels of asthma control. In general, more frequent and intense exacerbations (e.g., requiring urgent, unscheduled care, hospitalization, or ICU admission) indicate poorer disease control.

Source: From National Asthma Education and Prevention Program (NAEPP). (2007). *The Expert Panel Report 3: Guidelines for the diagnosis and management of asthma.* Bethesda, MD: National Heart, Lung, and Blood Institute, National Institutes of Health.

Table 30–5 **Stepwise Approach for Managing Asthma in Youths > 12 Years and Adults**

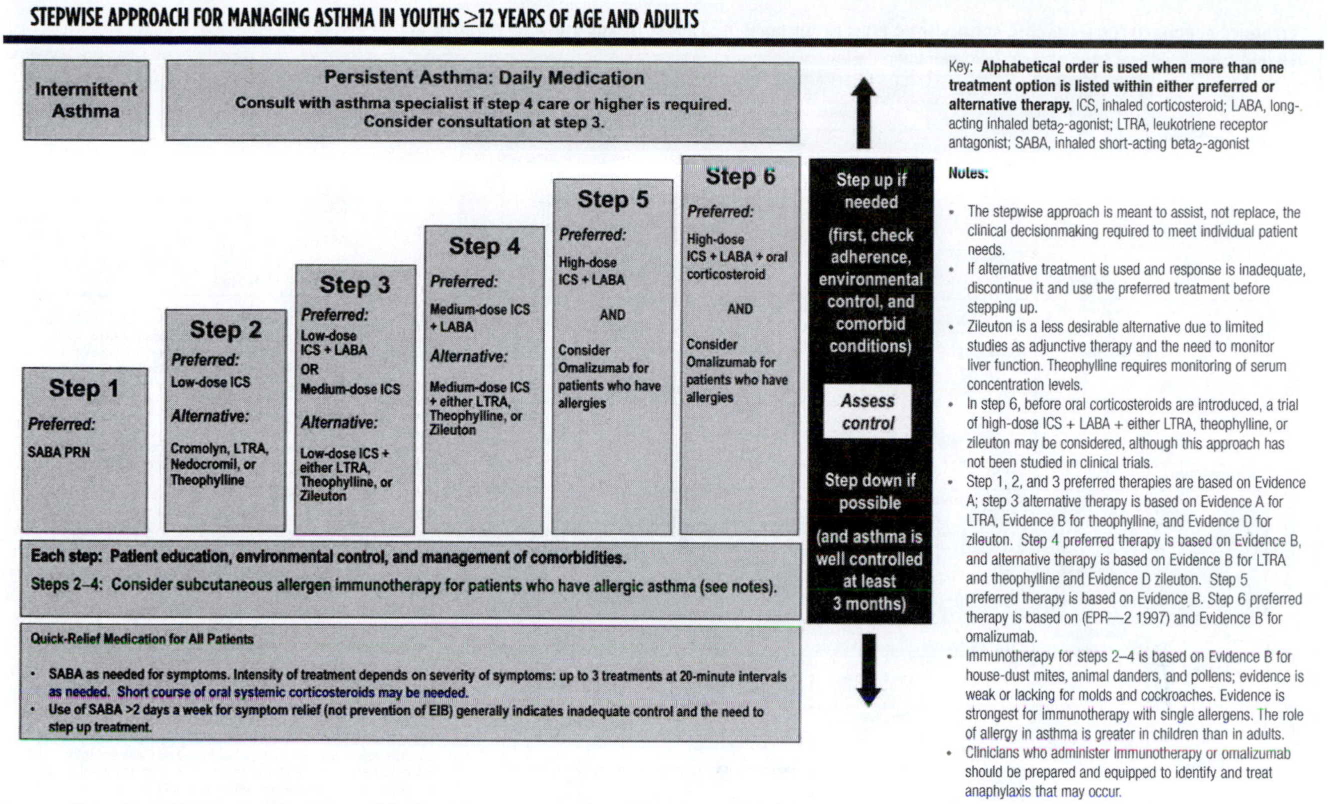

Source: From National Asthma Education and Prevention Program (NAEPP). (2007). *The Expert Panel Report 3: Guidelines for the diagnosis and management of asthma.* Bethesda, MD: National Heart, Lung, and Blood Institute, National Institutes of Health.

mild asthma use their **albuterol** inhaler on an as-needed basis, which enables patients to feel that they have some control over their asthma. Mild intermittent asthma is not inconsequential, as attacks can be severe, and it varies from patient to patient.

Mild Persistent Asthma

The recommended treatment for patients with mild persistent asthma is one long-term-control medication daily. The primary treatment is inhaled **anti-inflammatory** medication. Treatment is started with **inhaled low-dose corticosteroids** for all age groups. **Cromolyn (Intal)**, a **leukotriene modifier**, and **nedocromil (Tilade)** are alternative treatments. The suggested beginning dose of **inhaled steroids** is 80 to 240 mcg/day of **beclomethasone HFA (QVAR)** or **budesonide (Pulmicort Turbuhaler)** 180 to 600 mcg/day or the equivalent. Sustained-release **theophylline** to serum concentrations of 5 to 15 mcg/mL is an alternative therapy, but it should be used with caution and with close monitoring of serum **theophylline** levels. **Inhaled short-acting beta$_2$ agonists** are used as needed to relieve symptoms. If symptoms persist, **inhaled corticosteroids** should be increased to 240 to 480 mcg/day of **beclomethasone HFA (QVAR)**, which is three to six puffs per day of 80 mcg/puff or the equivalent. If a patient is requiring daily use of **inhaled beta$_2$ agonists** and is using the medications correctly, then step 3 therapy is indicated. Patient education at this step is teaching self-monitoring and developing and reviewing the self-management plan.

Moderate Persistent Asthma

Patients with moderate persistent asthma require long-term preventive medication to maintain control of their asthma. The dose of **inhaled corticosteroids** should be 240 to 480 mcg of **beclomethasone HFA** (three to six puffs per day of 80 mcg/puff) or low-dose **inhaled corticosteroids** combined with a **long-acting beta-agonist bronchodilator (Advair)**. The **long-acting beta-agonist salmeterol (Serevent)** should not be prescribed without the concurrent use of **inhaled corticosteroids** because of increased risks of catastrophic events (asthma related intubations and death), as discussed in Chapter 17. Quick relief of symptoms is obtained with **short-acting inhaled beta$_2$ agonists.** A more severe exacerbation may require **oral corticosteroids.** If control of symptoms is not achieved and the patient is adhering to the asthma plan, including correct inhaler technique, then increasing the treatment to step 4 is indicated. Having patients record their medication use and symptoms is essential at all steps but critical at step 3 because documentation is helpful in determining whether referral to an asthma specialist is indicated if the patient needs step 4 therapy.

(Text continues on page 1005)

Table 30–6 Stepwise Approach for Managing Asthma Long Term in Children

STEPWISE APPROACH FOR MANAGING ASTHMA LONG TERM IN CHILDREN, 0–4 YEARS OF AGE AND 5–11 YEARS OF AGE

Step up if needed (first check inhaler technique, adherence, environmental control, and comorbid conditions)

Assess control

Step down if possible (and asthma is well controlled at least 3 months)

Children 0–4 Years of Age

	Step 1	Step 2	Step 3	Step 4	Step 5	Step 6
	Intermittent Asthma	Persistent Asthma: Daily Medication Consult with asthma specialist if step 3 care or higher is required. Consider consultation at step 2.				
Preferred	SABA PRN	Low-dose ICS	Medium-dose ICS	Medium-dose ICS + LABA *or* Montelukast	High-dose ICS + LABA *or* Montelukast	High-dose ICS + LABA or Montelukast + Oral corticosteriods ICS
Alternative		Cromolyn *or* Montelukast				
	Each Step: Patient Education and Environmental Control					
Quick-Relief Medication	• SABA as needed for symptoms. Intensity of treatment depends on severity of symptoms. • With viral respiratory symptoms: SABA q 4–6 hours up to 24 hours (longer with physician consult). Consider short course of oral systemic corticosteroids if exacerbation is severe or patient has history of previous severe exacerbations. Caution: Frequent use of SABA may indicate the need to step up treatment. See text for recommendations on initiating daily long-term-control therapy.					

Notes

- The stepwise approach is meant to assist, not replace, the clinical decisionmaking required to meet individual patient needs.
- If an alternative treatment is used and response is inadequate, discontinue it and use the preferred treatment before stepping up.
- If clear benefit is not observed within 4–6 weeks, and patient's/family's medication technique and adherence are satisfactory, consider adjusting therapy or an alternative diagnosis.
- Studies on children 0–4 years of age are limited. Step 2 preferred therapy is based on Evidence A. All other recommendations are based on expert opinion and extrapolation from studies in older children.
- Clinicians who administer immunotherapy should be prepared and equipped to identify and treat anaphylaxis that may occur.

Key: Alphabetical listing is used when more than one treatment option is listed within either preferred or alternative therapy. ICS, inhaled corticosteroid; LABA, inhaled long-acting beta$_2$-agonist; LTRA, leukotriene receptor antagonist; oral corticosteroids, oral systemic corticosteroids; SABA, inhaled short-acting beta$_2$-agonist

Children 5–11 Years of Age

	Step 1	Step 2	Step 3	Step 4	Step 5	Step 6
	Intermittent Asthma	Persistent Asthma: Daily Medication Consult with asthma specialist if step 4 care or higher is required. Consider consultation at step 3.				
Preferred	SABA PRN	Low-dose ICS	Low-dose ICS + LABA, LTRA, *or* Theophylline *OR* Medium-dose ICS	Medium-dose ICS + LABA	High-dose ICS + LABA	High-dose ICS + LABA + Oral corticosteroids
Alternative		Cromolyn, LTRA, Nedocromil, *or* Theophylline		Medium-dose ICS + LTRA *or* Theophylline	High-dose ICS + LTRA *or* Theophylline	High-dose ICS + LTRA *or* Theophylline + oral corticosteroids
	Each Step: Patient Education, Environmental Control, and Management of Comorbidities Steps 2–4: Consider subcutaneous allergen immunotherapy for patients who have persistent, allergic asthma.					
Quick-Relief Medication	• SABA as needed for symptoms. Intensity of treatment depends on severity of symptoms: up to 3 treatments at 20-minute intervals as needed. Short course of oral systemic corticosteroids may be needed. Caution: Increasing use of SABA or use >2 days a week for symptom relief (not prevention of EIB) generally indicates inadequate control and the need to step up treatment.					

- The stepwise approach is meant to assist, not replace, the clinical decisionmaking required to meet individual patient needs.
- If an alternative treatment is used and response is inadequate, discontinue it and use the preferred treatment before stepping up.
- Theophylline is a less desirable alternative due to the need to monitor serum concentration levels.
- Steps 1 and 2 medications are based on Evidence A. Step 3 ICS and ICS plus adjunctive therapy are based on Evidence B for efficacy of each treatment and extrapolation from comparator trials in older children and adults—comparator trials are not available for this age group; steps 4–6 are based on expert opinion and extrapolation from studies in older children and adults.
- Immunotherapy for steps 2–4 is based on Evidence B for house-dust mites, animal danders, and pollens; evidence is weak or lacking for molds and cockroaches. Evidence is strongest for immunotherapy with single allergens. The role of allergy in asthma is greater in children than adults.
- Clinicians who administer immunotherapy should be prepared and equipped to identify and treat anaphylaxis that may occur.

Key: Alphabetical listing is used when more than one treatment option is listed within either preferred or alternative therapy. ICS, inhaled corticosteroid; LABA, inhaled long-acting beta$_2$-agonist; LTRA, leukotriene receptor antagonist; SABA, inhaled short-acting beta$_2$-agonist

Source: From National Asthma Education and Prevention Program (NAEPP). (2007). *The Expert Panel Report 3: Guidelines for the diagnosis and management of asthma.* Bethesda, MD: National Heart, Lung, and Blood Institute, National Institutes of Health.

Table 30–7 Drugs Commonly Used: Asthma and COPD

Drug	Dosage	How Supplied	Comments
Short-Acting Bronchodilators			
Albuterol HFA (Ventolin HFA, Proventil HFA, ProAir HFA)	***Inhaler*** 2 puffs q4–6h 2 puffs 15 min prior to exercise	***Metered-Dose Inhaler*** 90 mcg/puff	• May repeat dose in 5–10 min during exacerbations
Albuterol	***Nebulizer*** (run over 10–15 min) *Adults:* Dilute 0.5 mL of 0.5% solution in 3-mL normal saline *or* give 1 unit dose Tablets: 2 mg, 4 mg *Children:* 0.01–0.03 mL/kg of 0.5% solution diluted in 2-mL normal saline ***Oral*** *Adults:* 2–4 mg tid or qid up to a max of 32 mg/d	***Solution for Nebulizer*** 0.5% (5 mg/mL) 0.083 in unit-dose vial ***Oral*** Extended-release tabs: 4 mg, 8 mg Syrup: 2 mg/5 mL	• Check proper inhaler technique with every clinic visit

Table 30–7 **Drugs Commonly Used: Asthma and COPD—cont'd**

Drug	Dosage	How Supplied	Comments
	Children 6–12 yr: 2 mg tid or qid *Children <6 yr:* 0.1 mg/kg divided tid		
Levalbuterol (R-albuterol, Xopenex)	***Nebulizer*** 0.31 mg/3 mL 0.63 mg/3 mL 1.25 mg/3 mL *Adults:* 0.63 mg–2.5 mg q 4–8 h *Children:* 0.025 mg/kg (min 0.63 mg, max 1.25 mg) q4–8h ***Inhaler*** *Children ≥5 yr and adults:* 2 puffs every 4 to 6 h *Children <5 yr:* not FDA approved	***Nebulizer Solution*** 0.63 mg of levalbuterol is equivalent in efficacy and side effects to 1.25 mg of racemic albuterol. The product is a sterile-filled preservative-free unit dose vial ***Inhaler*** 45 mcg/puff	Levalbuterol has not been evaluated for continuous nebulization therapy
Terbutaline (Brethine)	***Oral*** *Children >15 yr and adults:* 5 mg tid; maximum 15 mg/24 h *Children 12–15 yr:* 2.5 mg tid; maximum 7.5 mg/24 h ***Parenteral*** *Adults:* 0.5 mg SC in the lateral deltoid; may repeat in 15–30 min; maximum dose 0.5 mg in 4 h	***Oral*** Tablets: 2.5 mg, 5 mg ***Parenteral*** 1 mg/mL	• Not recommended for children younger than 12 yr • Terbutaline is used to control premature contractions in pregnant women; use with care in the patient in the third trimester nearing her expected date of confinement (EDC), as it may affect labor
Bitolterol (Tornalate)	***Inhaler*** *Children >12 yr and adults:* For bronchospasm: 2 puffs 1–3 min apart, followed by a third puff if needed For prevention of bronchospasm: 2 puffs every 8 h	***Inhaler*** 0.37 mg/puff	Not recommended for children younger than 12 yr
Pirbuterol (Maxair inhaler)	***Inhaler*** *Children >12 yr and adults:* 1–2 puffs q 4–6 h; maximum 12 puffs/day	***Inhaler*** 0.2 mg/puff	Not recommended for children younger than 12 yr
Long-Acting Bronchodilator Salmeterol (Serevent Diskus)	***Diskus Inhaler*** *Children >4 yr and adults:* For asthma and control of bronchospasm: 1 inhalation bid For exercise-induced asthma: 1 inhalation 30–60 min prior to exercise	***Discus Inhaler*** 50 mcg/inhalation	**Not to be prescribed as monotherapy for persistent asthma.** Not to be used for short-term relief. Patients need to have a short-acting bronchodilator also prescribed for short-term relief and told not to

Continued

Table 30–7 **Drugs Commonly Used: Asthma and COPD—cont'd**

Drug	Dosage	How Supplied	Comments
			use drug for acute exacerbations. If using salmeterol twice a day, do not use another dose for exercise-induced asthma; a short-acting bronchodilator or cromolyn should be used.
Formoterol (Foradil)	DPI 12-mcg/single-use capsule *Children ≥5 years and adults:* Inhale 1 capsule q12h Note: capsule is not to be swallowed	12-mcg capsule	Each capsule is for single use only; additional doses should not be administered for at least 12 h Capsules should be used only with the Aerolizer inhaler and should not be taken orally. Efficacy and safety have not been studied in children <5 yr
Anticholinergic Agents			
Ipratropium bromide (Atrovent, Atrovent HFA)	***Inhaler*** *Children >12 yr and adults:* 2–3 puffs qid; maximum 12 puffs/24 h 500 mcg per unit-dose vial *or* 0.25 mg/mL *Children:* 1–2 puffs q6h ***Nebulizer*** 1 unit dose *Adults:* 0.5 mg q30 minutes for 3 doses then 0.25 mg q6h *Children:* 0.25 mg q 20 min for 3 doses, then 0.25 mg q6h 0.5 mg/3 mL ipratropium bromide and 2.5 mg/3 mL albuterol *Adults:* 2–3 puffs q6h *Adults:* 3 mL q4–6h *Children:* 1.5–3 mL q8h	***Inhaler*** 17 mcg/puff ***Solution for Nebulizer*** • Contraindicated in patients with soybean or peanut allergy.	• Can be mixed with albuterol 0.5% solution for nebulizer use if used within 1 h.
Tiotropium (Spiriva)	***HandiHaler*** *Adults with COPD:* 2 inhalations of the powder contents of a single capsule once daily	DPI capsule: 18 mcg/capsule	Not approved for use in children. Approved for use in COPD.
Combination Inhaled Medications			
Albuterol/ipratropium bromide (Combivent)	***Inhaler*** *Children:* 1–2 puffs q8h *Adults:* 2 puffs qid	***Inhaler*** Ipratropium 18 mcg/puff combined with albuterol 90 mcg/puff	• Primarily used for COPD patients
	Nebulizer *Adults:* 3 mL every 30 min for 3 doses, then q 2–4 hours prn *Children:* 1.5 mL q 20 min for 3 doses then every 2–4 h	***Solution for Nebulizer*** Each 3 mL vial contains 0.5 mg ipratropium bromide and 2.5 mg albuterol	• Simplifies medication regimen by combining two commonly prescribed medications • Not recommended for children

Table 30–7 **Drugs Commonly Used: Asthma and COPD—cont'd**

Drug	Dosage	How Supplied	Comments
Fluticasone/Salmeterol (Advair Diskus)	DPI 100 mcg, 250 mcg, or 500 mcg/50 mcg *Adults:* 1 inhalation bid: dose depends on severity of asthma *Children:* 1 inhalation bid; dose depends on severity of asthma	Not FDA approved in children <12 yr. 100/50 for patient not controlled on low-to-medium dose inhaled corticosteroids. 250/50 for patients not controlled on medium-to-high dose inhaled corticosteroids	
Budesonide and formoterol (Symbicort)	***Inhaler*** *Children 5 to 11 yr:* Symbicort 80/4.5, 2 inhalation bid *Children ≥12 yr and adults:* Symbicort 80/4.5, 2 inhalations bid *or* Symbicort 160/4.5, 2 inhalations bid (medium dose steroid)	***Inhaler*** Symbicort 80/4.5 containing 80 and 4.5 mcg of formoterol fumarate dihydrate per inhalation Symbicort 160/4.5 containing 160 mcg of budesonide and 4.5 mcg of formoterol fumarate dihydrate per inhalation.	
Systemic Corticosteroids			
Prednisone	*Adults:* "Burst" therapy 40–60 mg/d in 1 or 2 doses *Children:* "Burst" 1–2 mg/kg/d in 1–2 doses; maximum of 60 mg/d	***Tablets*** 5 mg, 10 mg, 20 mg	If given in short "bursts" of 3–10 d, dose does not have to be tapered
Prednisolone (Prelone, Pediapred syrup)	*Children:* "Burst" 1–2 mg/kg/d in 1–2 doses; maximum of 40–50 mg/d	***Syrup*** Pediapred 5 mg/5 mL Prelone 15 mg/5 mL	Same as for prednisone
Inhaled Anti-Inflammatory Agents			
Cromolyn (Intal)	***Nebulizer*** *Children >2 yr and adults:* 1-unit dose qid, weaning down to bid	***Solution for Nebulizer*** 20 mg/2-mL ampule	• Must be used continuously for 3–4 wk before maximum effect is achieved • Very safe to use in children, with fewer adverse reactions than inhaled steroids
Nedocromil (Tilade)	***Nebulizer*** *Adults and children >2 yr:* 1 ampule via nebulizer qid	***Solution for Nebulizer*** 11 mg/2.2-mL ampule	
Inhaled Corticosteroids			
Beclomethasone dipropionate Beclomethasone HFA (QVAR)	*Adults:* *Low dose:* 80–240 mcg *Medium dose:* 240–480 mcg *High dose:* >480 mcg *Children:* *Low dose:* 80–160 mcg *Medium dose:* 160–320 mcg *High dose:* >320 mcg	QVAR MDI 40 mcg/puff 80 mcg/puff	
Budesonide (Pulmicort Flexihaler)	*Adults:* *Low dose:* 180–600 mcg daily (1 or 2 inhalations daily) *Medium dose:* 600–1200 mcg daily (2–3 inhalations daily)	***Turbohaler DPI*** 90 mcg/puff 180 mcg/puff 200 mcg/puff	

Continued

Table 30–7 **Drugs Commonly Used: Asthma and COPD—cont'd**

Drug	Dosage	How Supplied	Comments
	High dose: >1,200 mcg daily (>3 inhalations daily) *Children:* *Low dose:* 200 mcg daily (1 inhalation daily) *Medium dose:* 200–400 mcg daily (2–3 inhalations daily) *High dose:* >400 mcg/d (>2 inhalations daily)		
Budesonide Inhalation suspension (Pulmicort Respules) for nebulization (child dose)	*Children 4 yr:* *Low dose:* 0.25 to 0.5 mg/d *Medium dose:* 0.5 mg to 1.0 mg/d *High dose:* 2.0 mg *Children 5 to 11 yr:* *Low dose:* 0.5 mg/d *Medium dose:* 1.0 mg/d *High dose:* 2.0 mg/d	***Suspension for Nebulizer*** 0.25 mg/mL 0.5 mg/mL	
Flunisolide (Aerobid)	*Children ≥12 years and adults:* *Low dose:* 500–1,000 mcg daily (2–4 puffs daily divided in bid dose) *Medium dose:* 1,000–2,000 mcg daily (4–8 puffs divided bid) *High dose:* >2,000 mcg daily (>8 puffs divided bid) *Children 5 to 11 yr:* *Low dose:* 500–750 mcg (2–3 puffs daily) *Medium dose:* 1,000–1,250 mcg daily (4–5 puffs daily divided bid) *High dose:* >1,250 mcg daily (>5 puffs divided bid)	***Inhaler*** 250 mcg/puff	Rinse mouth after use.
Fluticasone (Flovent)	*Adults:* *Low dose:* 88–264 mcg daily (2–6 puffs of 44 mcg divided bid) *Medium dose:* 264–660 mcg daily (2–6 puffs of 110 mcg daily divided bid) *High dose:* >660 mcg (>6 puffs 110 mcg *or* >3 puffs 220 mcg) *Children 5 to 11 yr:* *Low dose:* 88–176 mcg daily (2–4 puffs of 44 mcg divided bid) *Medium dose:* 176–440 mcg daily (2–4 puffs 110 mcg divided bid) *High dose:* >440 mcg (>4 puffs 110 mcg *or* >2 puffs 220 mcg)	***Inhaler*** 44 mcg/puff 110 mcg/puff 220 mcg/puff	

Table 30–7 **Drugs Commonly Used: Asthma and COPD—cont'd**

Drug	Dosage	How Supplied	Comments
Fluticasone dry powder inhaler (Advair Diskus)	*Adults:* *Low dose:* 100–300 mcg *Medium dose:* 300–600 mcg *High dose:* >600 mcg *Children:* *Low dose:* 100–200 mcg *Medium dose:* 200–400 mcg *High dose:* >400 mcg	DPI: 50, 100, or 250 mcg/inhalation 50 mcg/puff 100 mcg/puff 250 mcg/puff	
Leukotriene Modifiers			
Montelukast (Singulair)	*Adults:* 10 mg once daily in the p.m. *Children 6–14 yr:* 5 mg once daily in the P.M. *Children 6 mo–5 yr:* 4 mg qhs	***Oral*** 10-mg tablets 5-mg chewable tablets 4-mg chewable tablets Granules: 4 mg/packet	Not recommended for children younger than 6 mo Exhibits a flat dose response curve. Doses >10 mg do not produce a greater response in adults. Chewable tablets contain phenylalanine
Zafirlukast (Accolate)	*Children ≥12 years and adults:* 20 mg bid *Children 5–11 yr:* 10 mg bid	***Oral*** 20-mg tablets 10-mg tablets For zafirlukast, administration with meals decreases bioavailability; take at least 1 h before or 2 h after meals	• Not recommended for children <5 yr • Must be taken on an empty stomach
Zileutin (Zyflo)	*Adults:* 600 mg qid	***Oral*** 600-mg tablets 300-mg tablets	• Not recommended for children • Evaluate liver function prior to initiating therapy and routinely during therapy; contraindicated in acute liver disease

*Children ≤12 yr

Severe Persistent Asthma

Treatment for patients with severe persistent asthma symptoms requires step 4, 5, or 6 therapy. Step 4 therapy is daily medium-dose **inhaled corticosteroids** (240 to 480 mcg/d of **beclomethasone HFA** or the equivalent) and a **long-acting beta-agonist (Serevent)**. An alternative approach is a medium dose **inhaled corticosteroid** and a **leukotriene modifier** or **theophylline**. Step 5 therapy is daily **inhaled high-dose corticosteroids** combined with daily **long-acting bronchodilators**. The **inhaled corticosteroid** dose should be in the high range, which is greater than 480 mcg of **beclomethasone HFA** (more than 6 puffs/d at 80 mcg/puff) or the equivalent. Step 6 therapy for severe persistent asthma consists of **high-dose corticosteroids** combined with daily **long-acting bronchodilators** and oral **corticosteroids**. If long-term **oral corticosteroids** are required, the lowest dose possible to achieve results should be used and on an alternate-day schedule if possible. **Oral steroids** are dosed at 2 mg/kg per day, not to exceed 60 mg/day. **Inhaled corticosteroids** are preferable to **systemic corticosteroids**, and the maximum dose should be used before long-term systemic therapy is initiated. Exacerbations require short bursts of high-dose **systemic corticosteroids**. Severe persistent asthma requiring step 5 or step 6 therapy and associated with allergies may benefit from **omalizumab (Xolair)** therapy, which is a recombinant humanized mouse monoclonal antibody that binds to free immunoglobulin E (IgE) in the circulation and prevents them from responding to relevant allergens (dust mite, cockroach, cat, or dog) (NAEPP, 2007). It is administered every 2 to 4 weeks via subcutaneous route and has been demonstrated to reduce exacerbations and total emergency visits

Table 30–8 **Comparative Daily Dosages for Inhaled Corticosteroids**

	Low Daily Dose			Medium Daily Dose			High Daily Dose		
Drug	*Child 0–4 Years of Age*	*Child 5–11 Years of Age*	*≥12 Years of Age and Adults*	*Child 0–4 Years of Age*	*Child 5–11 Years of Age*	*≥12 Years of Age and Adults*	*Child 0–4 Years of Age*	*Child 5–11 Years of Age*	*≥12 Years of Age and Adults*
Beclomethasone HFA 40 or 80 mcg/puff	NA	80–160 mcg	80–240 mcg	NA	>160–320 mcg	>240–480 mcg	NA	>320 mcg	>480 mcg
Budesonide DPI 90, 180, or 200 mcg/inhalation	NA	180–400 mcg	180–600 mcg	NA	>400–800 mcg	>600–1,200 mcg	NA	>800 mcg	>1,200 mcg
Budesonide Inhaled Inhalation suspension for nebulization	0.25–0.5 mg	0.5 mg	NA	>0.5–1.0 mg	1.0 mg	NA	>1.0 mg	2.0 mg	NA
Flunisolide 250 mcg/puff	NA	500–750 mcg	500–1,000 mcg	NA	1,000–1,250 mcg	>1,000–2,000 mcg	NA	>1,250 mcg	>2,000 mcg
Flunisolide HFA 80 mcg/puff	NA	160 mcg	320 mcg	NA	320 mcg	>320–640 mcg	NA	≥640 mcg	>640 mcg
Fluticasone **HFA/MDI:** 44, 110, or 220 mcg/puff	176 mcg	88–176 mcg	88–264 mcg	>176–352 mcg	>176–352 mcg	>264–440 mcg	>352 mcg	>352 mcg	>440 mcg
DPI: 50, 100, or 250 mcg/inhalation	NA	100–200 mcg	100–300 mcg	NA	>200–400 mcg	>300–500 mcg	NA	>400 mcg	>500 mcg
Mometasone DPI 200 mcg/inhalation	NA	NA	200 mcg	NA	NA	400 mcg	NA	NA	>400 mcg
Triamcinolone acetonide 75 mcg/puff	NA	300–600 mcg	300–750 mcg	NA	>600–900 mcg	>750–1,500 mcg	NA	>900 mcg	>1,500 mcg

Key: DPI, dry power inhaler; HFA, hydrofluoroalkane; MDI, metered-dose inhaler; NA, not available (either not approved, no data available, or safety and efficacy not established for this age group)

Source: From National Asthma Education and Prevention Program (NAEPP). (2007). *The Expert Panel Report 3: Guidelines for the diagnosis and management of asthma.* Bethesda, MD: National Heart, Lung, and Blood Institute, National Institutes of Health.

(Abramowicz, 2005; Bousquet et al, 2005; Chiang, Clark, & Casale, 2005). All patients who require step 4 treatment need referral to an asthma specialist.

Monitoring Control

Once control is achieved, patients need to be monitored every 1 to 6 months to determine if a step up or step down in therapy is indicated. Step therapy is meant to be a dynamic program of therapy in which changes in a patient's symptoms require movement up or down. For appropriate treatment decisions to be made, it is essential that patients be monitored frequently and that they maintain a self-assessment record. The *Expert Panel Report 3: Guidelines* say that the dose of **inhaled corticosteroids** may be reduced about 25 to 50 percent every 2 to 3 months to the lowest dose possible to maintain asthma control (NAEPP, 2007). Most patients with persistent asthma require daily medication to suppress underlying airway inflammation, and they may relapse if **inhaled corticosteroids** are withdrawn completely.

If at any time control of asthma symptoms is not achieved and sustained, the health-care provider has a number of actions to take. First and most important, the provider must review and observe the patient's medication administration. Improper inhaler technique can create havoc in the management of asthma, as the patient is not getting relief at increasing "doses" of medication. This problem can lead to unnecessary changes in therapy. The patient's inhaler technique should be reviewed at every visit because research has shown that technique deteriorates between visits. The provider needs to be aware that the prescribed regimen may not be followed at home, and intensive education may be needed to ensure compliance.

Managing Exacerbations

A temporary increase in **anti-inflammatory** therapy may be needed to reestablish control or treat exacerbations. The need for **oral steroids** is characterized by increased need for **short-acting bronchodilators** or decreased PEF (20% or greater), reduced tolerance to activity, and increased nocturnal symptoms. A short "burst" of **oral prednisone** is often effective. The appropriate dose is 40 to 60 mg/day as a single or divided (twice a day) dose (1 to 2 mg/kg in children to a maximum of 60 g/d) for 5 to 10 days in adults and 3 to 10 days in children. If the steroid burst is successful (the PEF returns to normal and symptoms improve), then no other treatment is necessary. If the **prednisone** burst does not control symptoms, then a step up to a higher level is indicated. If frequent bursts of **steroids** are required, then higher-level care is needed. Doubling the dose of **inhaled corticosteroids** is not effective in treating asthma exacerbations (NAEPP, 2007).

Maintaining Control of Asthma

Factors that influence maintaining control of asthma include exposure to allergens, barriers to care (e.g., financial), and self-management issues. Allergy testing and referral to an allergy specialist may be necessary to maintain effective control of asthma symptoms. Families in crisis have difficulty in maintaining a complex medication regimen, and every effort should be made to simplify the treatment for all patients regardless of their resources.

Home Management of Exacerbations of Asthma

Home management of asthma exacerbations is an integral part of asthma management. Patients need to be educated to recognize early symptoms of decreasing lung function and to adjust their medications accordingly. The *Expert Panel Report 3: Guidelines* (NAEPP, 2007) recommend the following home pharmacological therapy, which is described in detail in Figure 30–2:

First, assess severity. Patients at high risk for a fatal asthma attack require immediate attention after initial treatment. Patients at risk include those having previous severe exacerbations requiring intubation or intensive care unit (ICU) admission for asthma, two or more hospitalizations or more than three emergency department visits in the past year, use of more than two **short-acting beta-agonist** canisters per month, difficulty perceiving airway obstruction or worsening asthma, or low socioeconomic status or inner-city residence.

Initial home treatment consists of increased frequency of **inhaled beta$_2$ agonists**, up to two treatments (two to six puffs of MDI) 20 minutes apart or nebulizer treatment. If the response is good, the patient should continue the **inhaled short-acting beta agonists**, and contact the provider to discuss whether a short course of **oral corticosteroids** is required. If the response is incomplete to initial therapy and persistent wheezing or tachypnea is present, the patient should be started on **systemic oral corticosteroids**, continue the **short-acting beta agonists**, and contact the provider urgently (the same day). If the response is poor to initial therapy, determined by marked wheezing and dyspnea, the patient should repeat the **short-acting beta agonist** immediately and start **oral corticosteroids**. If the distress is severe, the patient should be transported to the emergency department (consider calling 911).

Patients with good response to therapy need to continue more intensive therapy (step up in care) for several days until the PEF returns to normal. Patients should contact their health-care provider any time they begin **oral steroids** if the attack is severe, or if emergent treatment is necessary.

Patient Variables

Pregnancy

Asthma affects between 3.5 and 8.4 percent of pregnant women in the United States (Kwon, Belanger, & Bracken, 2003). Pregnant women with asthma need to be monitored closely for changes in lung function as the effects of pregnancy on the course of asthma is unpredictable and the asthma may worsen, improve, or remain unchanged

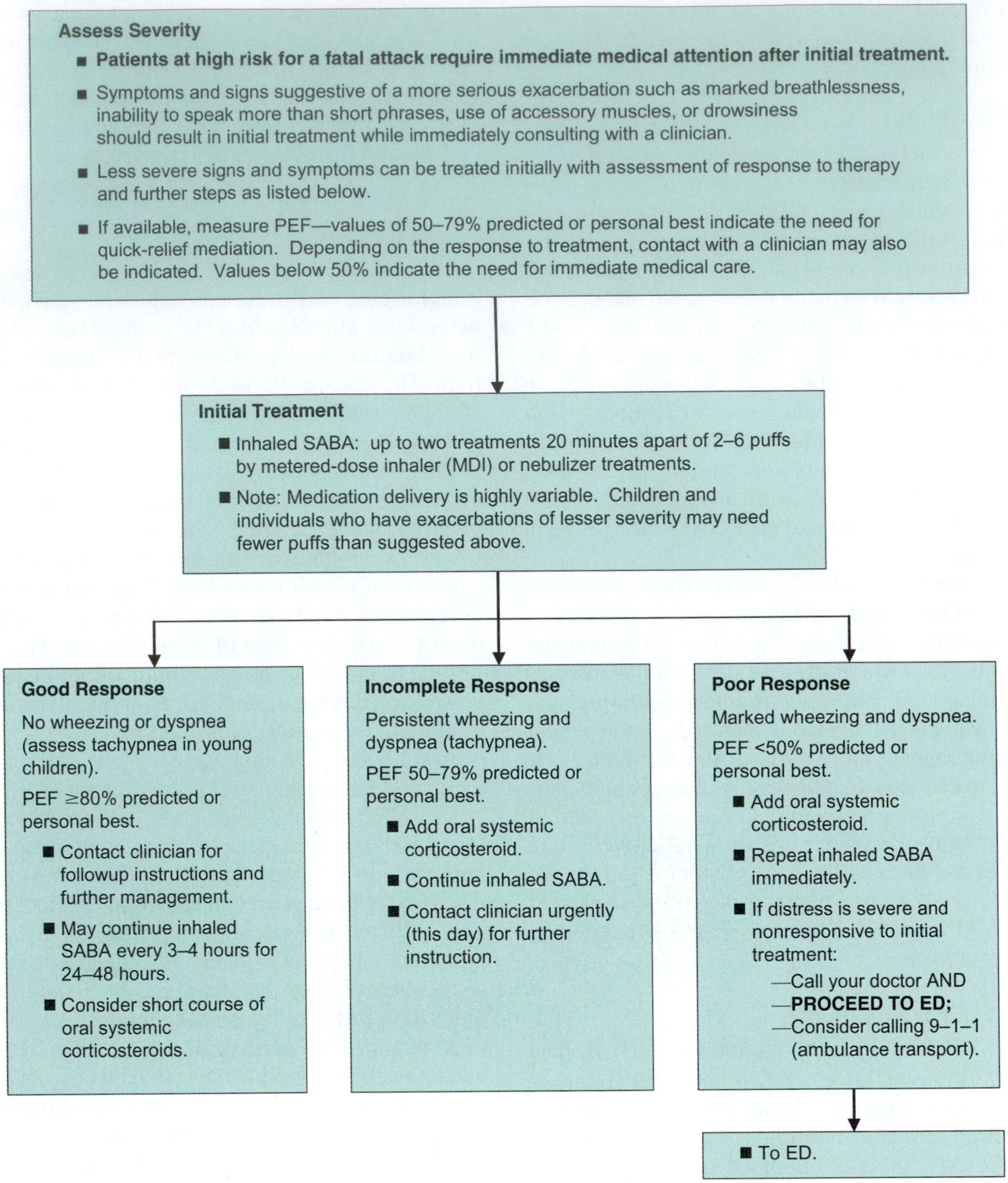
Assess Severity
Patients at high risk for a fatal attack require immediate medical attention after initial treatment.
Symptoms and signs suggestive of a more serious exacerbation such as marked breathlessness, inability to speak more than short phrases, use of accessory muscles, or drowsiness should result in initial treatment while immediately consulting with a clinician.
Less severe signs and symptoms can be treated initially with assessment of response to therapy and further steps as listed below.
If available, measure PEF—values of 50–79% predicted or personal best indicate the need for quick-relief mediation. Depending on the response to treatment, contact with a clinician may also be indicated. Values below 50% indicate the need for immediate medical care.
Initial Treatment
Inhaled SABA: up to two treatments 20 minutes apart of 2–6 puffs by metered-dose inhaler (MDI) or nebulizer treatments.
Note: Medication delivery is highly variable. Children and individuals who have exacerbations of lesser severity may need fewer puffs than suggested above.
Good Response
No wheezing or dyspnea (assess tachypnea in young children).
PEF ≥80% predicted or personal best.
Contact clinician for followup instructions and further management.
May continue inhaled SABA every 3–4 hours for 24–48 hours.
Consider short course of oral systemic corticosteroids.
Incomplete Response
Persistent wheezing and dyspnea (tachypnea).
PEF 50–79% predicted or personal best.
Add oral systemic corticosteroid.
Continue inhaled SABA.
Contact clinician urgently (this day) for further instruction.
Poor Response
Marked wheezing and dyspnea.
PEF <50% predicted or personal best.
Add oral systemic corticosteroid.
Repeat inhaled SABA immediately.
If distress is severe and nonresponsive to initial treatment:
—Call your doctor AND
—PROCEED TO ED;
—Consider calling 9–1–1 (ambulance transport).
To ED.

Figure 30–2. Management of asthma exacerbations: Home treatment. Key: ED, emergency department; MDI, metered-dose inhaler; PEF, peak expiratory flow; SABA, short-acting beta$_2$ agonist (quick-relief inhaler). *(Source: From National Asthma Education and Prevention Program [NAEPP]. [2007].* The Expert Panel Report 3: Guidelines for the diagnosis and management of asthma. *Bethesda, MD: National Heart, Lung, and Blood Institute, National Institutes of Health.)*

(Hanania & Belfort, 2005). Adequate oxygenation is essential for the fetus to develop normally. Poorly controlled asthma can lead to low birth weight, increased perinatal morbidity, and prematurity. In general, asthma therapy is the same for pregnant women as for other patients with asthma. They need to be educated and monitor their PEF throughout the pregnancy, with the *Expert Panel Report 3: Guidelines* recommending monitoring of asthma status at prenatal visits. Any changes in PEF require prompt treatment and modification in pharmacological therapy. Most medications used to treat asthma are Pregnancy Class C, as noted in Chapter 17. Oral forms of **beta$_2$ agonists** should be used selectively in patients who are in labor, as **terbutaline** is a tocolytic (off-labeled use). Inhaled forms of **beta$_2$ agonists** are less likely to affect uterine contractions, and **albuterol** is the **beta agonist** of choice because of its safety profile (NAEPP, 2007). **Inhaled corticosteroids (ICS)** are the long-term control medications of choice, with **budesonide** the ICS with the most data available in pregnant women (NAEPP, 2007). Minimal data are available regarding the safety of **leukotrienes** in pregnant women, but animal data do not indicate a concern for use during pregnancy (NAEPP, 2007).

Pediatric Patients

Approximately 6.3 million children in the United States have asthma (Covar & Spahn, 2003). The Global Initiative for Asthma (2009) describes three categories of wheezing in children younger than age 5 years: transient early wheezing, persistent early onset wheezing, and late-onset wheezing/asthma. Transient early wheezing is associated with prematurity and parental smoking and is often outgrown by age 3 years. Persistent early onset wheezing occurs before age 3 years and is characterized by recurrent episodes of wheezing associated with viral upper respiratory infections. The symptoms usually persist through school age and early adolescence. Children with early onset wheezing have no evidence of atopy. Late-onset wheezing/asthma is often associated with atopy, often eczema.

Pediatric patients under age 5 years require special management strategies. *Expert Panel Report 3: Guidelines* break out the treatment of children younger than age 5 years to address the needs of the population. First, diagnosing asthma in infants and young children is difficult. Asthma is often underdiagnosed and undertreated in this age group because objective measures of lung function are difficult to obtain and treatment decisions are made on clinical assessment. Some health-care providers are reluctant to label children as having asthma, and often the child is given a label of chronic bronchitis, wheezy bronchitis, "happy wheezer," or the like and, therefore, does not receive adequate treatment. Note that not all wheezing and coughing are asthma, and the patient may have less common conditions such as cystic fibrosis, vascular ring, tracheomalacia, congenital heart disease, foreign body aspiration, and primary immunodeficiency.

As noted, among children younger than 5 years, the most common cause of asthma symptoms is viral respiratory infection. As most infants and toddlers contract repeated viral respiratory infections, susceptible children may have repeated episodes of asthma symptoms. Parents are often frightened and frustrated with these repeated exacerbations. Parental stress associated with frequent health-care visits, uncertain diagnosis, missed work because of the child's illness, or parental guilt about needing to work instead of being at home with the child can make working with these families a challenge for the provider. Ladebauche (1997) suggests that "development of a partnership with parents of an infant with asthma should begin as soon as the diagnosis is established. Open communication between health care provider and parents should be used to clearly define roles and expectations of care." The *Expert Panel Report 3: Guidelines* stress collaborating with parents and meeting their expectations regarding the care of their child with asthma.

Lieu and colleagues (1997) found that having a written asthma management plan and starting medications at the onset of cold or flu lowered the odds of an emergency department visit in a case-control study of children up to age 14 with asthma in a large regional health management organization. Parents can be taught how to identify and anticipate asthma symptoms, such as the beginning of a child's upper respiratory infection symptoms. Parents can learn to identify objective parameters of concern, such as respiratory rate or use of accessory muscles for breathing. Asthma education must be written and frequently repeated to stressed and often fatigued parents. It is best to provide in-depth teaching when the child is well so the parents can be at their optimal and not distracted by the child's condition.

The *Expert Panel Report 3: Guidelines* recommend that all children with asthma symptoms be given a therapeutic trial of **bronchodilators**, specifically inhaled short-acting **beta$_2$ agonists.** The *Expert Panel Report 3: Guidelines* include a stepwise approach for managing infants and young children 0 to 4 years with asthma symptoms. Use of **bronchodilators** more than twice a week is an indication of the need for step 2 therapy: daily **anti-inflammatory** medication. Daily long-term therapy should begin with **low-dose inhaled corticosteroids** delivered via nebulizer or metered-dose inhaler (MDI) with holding chamber with or without mask. Alternative medications include **cromolyn** (nebulizer is preferred) or **montelukast.** Step 3 therapy is indicated for moderate persistent asthma (symptoms daily or more than 3 to 4 nights/mo) requires therapy with **medium-dose inhaled corticosteroids.** Poor response to step 3 regimen indicates a need to step up to step 4 therapy a combination of **low-dose inhaled corticosteroids** and a **montelukast.** If step 3 therapy is required, the *Expert Panel Report 3: Guidelines* say that control should be established quickly with higher doses of **inhaled corticosteroids** and that therapy should be stepped down after 2 to 3 months to the lowest dose required to maintain control. Referral to an asthma specialist is essential for all children who require step 3 or higher care. Poor control at step 2 may also be a reason to consider referral. Exacerbations caused by viral upper respiratory infections can be quite severe, and **systemic corticosteroids** may be needed often in this age group because of the number of viral upper respiratory infections that children get in infancy. A short burst of **oral corticosteroids** may be needed to establish control of asthma in children with moderate or severe asthma (NAEPP, 2007). A "burst" dose is 1 to 2 mg/kg/day (maximum 30 mg/d) of **prednisone** in two divided doses for 3 to 10 days. Table 30–6 discusses the stepwise approach to managing children with asthma.

Delivery of medication to infants and young children can be a challenge. There are several delivery devices available, but the dose of medication received can vary considerably among devices and age groups. Nebulizer therapy is preferred for children younger than 2 years. Nebulizers may be used in older children who are unable to use MDIs well enough to get therapeutic effects.

MDIs with either a spacer or a face mask can be used. An MDI and spacer with face mask is an alternative strategy in infants if there is a need for portable treatment, such as for traveling or day care. It is also a good choice if the family is financially stressed and the cost of a nebulizer and medication is prohibitive. Prior to changing or stepping up therapy, patients and parents must be assessed for proper use of delivery devices. It should be noted that **Pulmicort Respules (budesonide inhalation suspension)** should be administered with a compressed-air-driven jet nebulizer, NOT an ultrasonic nebulizer.

The *Expert Panel Report 3: Guidelines* added a separate diagnosis and management category for children aged 5 to 11 years (NAEPP, 2007). The management of school-age children is similar to that of younger children, with the addition of **theophylline** as alternative long-term control medication in step 2 therapy and the use of **long-acting beta-agonists** combined with **inhaled corticosteroids** in step 3 or higher therapy (see Table 30–6). The U.S. Food and Drug Administration (FDA, 2010) recommends **long-acting beta agonists** not be prescribed without **inhaled corticosteroids** to children, and preferably a combination product **(Advair)** is prescribed.

Older children and adolescents often have to manage symptoms at school or otherwise away from parents, and the *Expert Panel Report 3: Guidelines* recommend a written asthma action plan be shared with the school or day care (NAEPP, 2007). School-age children are developmentally interested in learning and mastering new skills. Including school-age children in decisions regarding their care and allowing them to accept responsibility for their asthma management can increase their sense of accomplishment and self-confidence (Ladebauche, 1997). School-age and adolescent children need to be able to effectively administer inhaled medications. Therefore, as children with asthma get older and gain independence, the provider needs to observe the child's inhaler technique and make adjustments as necessary. Many schools do not allow students to carry and self-administer medications. The NAEPP (2007) has endorsed a resolution allowing students to carry and self-administer medications if the provider and parent consider it appropriate. The plan has to be worked out among the parent, the school, and the health-care provider.

Sports and physical activities are essential to a healthy lifestyle for children. Every attempt should be made to control asthma symptoms so that children can participate in physical activities. Treatment just prior to activity may prevent the cough and wheeze some children experience with exercise. Poor exercise tolerance is an indication of poorly controlled asthma and the need to modify the asthma management plan. Adding a long-term-control medication usually improves exercise tolerance. Guidance from the health-care provider can assist parents and children in choosing appropriate sports. Often, children allergic to pollens cannot play outdoor sports such as baseball or soccer yet can participate in swimming, basketball, and gymnastics without problems. Restricting physical activity should be a last resort.

Older Adults

Older adults with asthma symptoms often present with a variety of other disease processes. The provider must first determine how much of the airflow obstruction is reversible and how much is due to other obstructive lung disease (chronic bronchitis, emphysema). Often a trial of 2 to 3 weeks of **systemic corticosteroids** is necessary to determine the extent of reversibility of airway disease. Inhaled long-term-control medications can then be introduced if indicated.

The medications used to treat asthma have increased adverse effects in the older patient. Those with preexisting ischemic heart disease may also be more sensitive to **beta$_2$ agonist** adverse effects, including tremor and tachycardia. Concomitant use of **anticholinergics** and **beta$_2$ agonists** may be beneficial in the older patient. **Theophylline** clearance is reduced, causing increased serum **theophylline** levels. Frequent monitoring of blood levels is necessary if **theophylline** is used for the older patient. **Systemic corticosteroids** can cause confusion, agitation, and changes in glucose metabolism. There is also a dose-dependent reduction in bone mineral content that may be associated with **inhaled corticosteroid** use. Low to medium doses appear to have no major effect on bone density. Older patients may be at more risk because of preexisting osteoporosis, lower estrogen levels (in women), and a sedentary lifestyle. Consider treatment with **calcium** and **vitamin D** supplements and, as appropriate, **estrogen replacement** for older patients on **high-dose inhaled corticosteroid** therapy.

Another concern in older patients is that the medications used to treat other chronic diseases may cause asthma exacerbations or require medication adjustments. Patients who are taking **theophylline** need to be assessed for medications that affect **theophylline** clearance. The **nonselective beta blockers**, including some **beta blockers** in eyedrops used to treat glaucoma, can result in mutual inhibition of therapeutic effects if used with **beta$_2$ agonists**. **NSAIDs** used to treat arthritis may cause asthma exacerbation. At each visit for asthma-related symptoms, it is essential to assess the patient's complete history, including all medications the patient takes.

Special Situations

Seasonal Asthma

Seasonal asthma is identified when patients appear to have asthma symptoms only in relationship to certain pollens and molds. Seasonal asthma is managed in the same stepwise approach to long-term management of asthma that was previously discussed. If the patient has predictable seasonal asthma—each spring, for example—**long-term anti-inflammatory** treatment should be initiated approximately 1 month before the anticipated onset of symptoms and continued through the season.

Cough Variant Asthma

Cough variant asthma is seen especially in young children. Cough variant asthma is diagnosed when cough, usually at night, is the principal symptom. Daytime examination may be normal, thereby often delaying or confusing the diagnosis. A therapeutic trial of **bronchodilator** medication is often diagnostic of cough variant asthma. Monitoring PEF changes between morning and evening readings may also assist in the diagnosis. Management is according to the stepwise approach to long-term management of asthma.

The **montelukast** demonstrated in a small double-blind randomized controlled study to reduce cough 75.7 percent from baseline by week 4 in the treatment group, whereas the placebo group had a 20.7 percent reduction in cough (Spector & Tan, 2004). Larger trials are indicated, but this shows promise for the treatment of cough variant asthma.

Exercise-Induced Bronchospasm

EIB should be anticipated in all patients with asthma, with 50 to 90 percent of asthmatics having airways that are hyperreactive to exercise (Parsons & Mastronarde, 2005). Some patients (less than 10%) exhibit asthma symptoms only when exercising. Bronchospasm is due to hyperventilation of air that is cooler and dryer than that of the respiratory system, which causes loss of heat and water from the lungs. The diagnosis of EIB is made first by history of cough, shortness of breath, chest pain or tightness, or wheezing during or right after exercise. Formal diagnosis can be made in a laboratory or by having patients exercise strenuously enough to increase their heart rate to 80 percent of maximum for 4 to 6 minutes. Otherwise healthy patients can run in the hallway or stairway of the clinic if appropriate. The PEF measurements are taken before and at 5-minute intervals for 20 to 30 minutes. A 15 percent decrease in PEF is compatible with EIB.

The goal of EIB therapy is for patients to be able to participate in any activity they choose without asthma symptoms. Teachers and coaches need to be notified that a child or an athlete has EIB. The *Expert Panel Report 3: Guidelines* (NAEPP, 2007) recommend the following treatment strategies:

1. **Short-acting beta$_2$ agonists** used just prior to exercise prevent EIB in 80 percent of patients for 2 to 3 hours. **Salmeterol** has been shown to prevent EIB for 10 to 12 hours. **Long-acting beta agonists** used daily will have decreased effectiveness; therefore, if daily pretreatment for exercise is needed, an alternative should be used.
2. **Cromolyn** and **nedocromil** inhaled shortly before exercise are also effective in preventing EIB, but are not as effective as **short-acting beta$_2$ agonists**.
3. A lengthy warm-up before exercise may decrease the need for repeated medications if the patient can tolerate continuous exercise without symptoms.
4. Long-term-control therapy with **inhaled anti-inflammatory** medication may be indicated and helpful in reducing airway responsiveness and therefore decreasing EIB. **Inhaled corticosteroids** are recommended as first-line therapy for athletes who have persistent asthma to prevent worsening of symptoms during exercise.
5. A mask or scarf over the mouth may attenuate cold-induced EIB.
6. **Leukotriene modifiers** may attenuate EIB in up to 50 percent of patients (NAEPP, 2007).

Surgery

Surgery places patients with asthma at risk for complications both during and after a procedure. These complications include acute bronchoconstriction triggered by intubation, hypoxemia, and possible hypercapnia; impaired cough effectiveness; atelectasis; and respiratory infections. The more severe the patient's asthma before surgery, the higher the likelihood of complications will be. Prior to surgery, the asthmatic patient should have an evaluation that includes symptoms, review of medications, and pulmonary function testing. If possible, patients ought to be at their personal best PEF. A short burst of **systemic corticosteroids** may be necessary to reach ideal lung function. Patients who have received **systemic corticosteroids** in the past 6 months require **IV hydrocortisone** during the surgical period.

Monitoring

Monitoring patients with asthma is a continuous process, beginning with the initial diagnosis. The *Expert Panel Report 3: Guidelines* recommend ongoing monitoring of the following six areas: signs and symptoms, pulmonary function, quality of life and functional status, history of asthma exacerbations, pharmacotherapy, and patient–provider communication and patient satisfaction.

Monitoring Signs and Symptoms of Asthma

All patients should be taught to monitor and recognize their asthma symptoms. Recording symptoms and PEF on a self-assessment diary enables the patient and the provider to track asthma symptoms and determine if there is adequate control. Clinical signs of asthma should be assessed at each visit through physical examination and appropriate questioning of the patient. Questions should be asked about the recent past (e.g., In the past 2 weeks, how many times have you had nighttime symptoms?). Questions about longer periods give a more generalized response (e.g., Have your symptoms been better or worse since your last visit?). Assessment of symptoms should differentiate between daytime symptoms, nighttime symptoms, and symptoms that occur in the early morning and that do not improve after inhaling a **short-acting beta$_2$ agonist**.

Monitoring Pulmonary Function

Monitoring lung function is essential to diagnosis and management of asthma. Lung function can be monitored by spirometry and peak flow monitoring. The *Expert Panel Report 3: Guidelines* (NAEPP, 2007) recommend that spirometry tests be done at the time of initial assessment, after treatment is initiated and PEF has stabilized to determine "normal" airway function for the individual patient, and then every 1 to 2 years to assess the maintenance of airway function. Spirometry may also be needed to check the accuracy of PEF readings before making major treatment decisions if there is a question about the reliability of the PEF. Peak flow meters are used for ongoing monitoring, not diagnosis, of asthma. Patients who have frequent exacerbations or require long-term therapy need to have a peak flow meter at home and be comfortable with its use. Monitoring PEF is essential to management of moderate to severe asthma in order to determine the severity of exacerbations and to guide treatment decisions. Daily PEF readings help to detect early changes in asthma status, help to evaluate response to changes in medication therapy, and provide a quantitative measure of airflow obstruction. The *Expert Panel Report 3: Guidelines* do not recommend long-term daily peak flow monitoring of patients with mild intermittent or mild persistent asthma, although PEF may be helpful during exacerbations. Patients should be given in-depth teaching regarding peak flow meter use, which may require more than one visit or referral to a nurse clinician who can teach proper peak flow meter use. Patients need to establish their personal best PEF and use that reading as the basis of their action plan. The patient should use the same brand of peak flow meter or reestablish personal best PEF if changing brands because there is no universal normative value for peak flow meters and the PEF may vary between brands. Peak flow meters are usually covered by insurance if the provider writes a prescription for the item.

Monitoring Quality of Life and Functional Status

Monitoring quality of life and functional status is essential to determine if the goals of asthma therapy are being met. The *Expert Panel Report 3: Guidelines* (NAEPP, 2007) recommend that the following areas of quality of life be periodically assessed:

1. Missed work or school because of asthma.
2. Reduction in usual activities.
3. Any disturbances in sleep due to asthma.
4. Any change in caregiver activities due to child's asthma (for caregivers of children with asthma).

Monitoring History of Asthma Exacerbations

Monitoring the history of asthma exacerbation is essential at every visit. The provider must question the patient and evaluate self-monitoring records to determine exacerbation, both self-treated and those treated by other health-care providers (e.g., emergency department visit, hospitalization). Changes in drug treatment are based on the exacerbation history.

Monitoring Pharmacotherapy

Monitoring the effectiveness of pharmacological therapy is key to successful asthma treatment. The following should be monitored: patient adherence to the regimen, inhaler technique, level of usage of as-needed **inhaled short-acting beta$_2$ agonist**, frequency of **oral corticosteroid** "burst" therapy, and changes in dosages of **inhaled anti-inflammatory** or other long-term-control medication. The provider must also determine if the patient is at the appropriate level of step therapy and if changes need to be made. At each visit, an up-to-date asthma action plan has to be reviewed and revised as appropriate.

Monitoring Patient-Provider Communication and Patient Satisfaction

Patient satisfaction and patient–provider communication should be assessed routinely. Two aspects of patient satisfaction should be assessed and addressed as appropriate: satisfaction with asthma control and satisfaction with quality of care (NAEPP, 2007).

Outcome Evaluation

Evaluating the effectiveness of asthma therapy is an ongoing process, as described in the Monitoring section. The best outcome for asthma patients is being able to accomplish their activities of daily living, whatever their lifestyle, with minimum asthma symptoms.

The *Expert Panel Report 3: Guidelines* (NAEPP, 2007) recommend that referral to an asthma specialist be made if there are difficulties in achieving or maintaining control, if immunosuppressive therapy is being considered, or if a patient requires step 4 care (step 3 if patient is an infant or young child).

Patient Education

Patient education should include a written asthma action plan, which includes a discussion of information related to the overall treatment plan as well as that specific to the drug therapy, reasons for taking the drug, drugs as part of the total treatment regimen, and adherence issues. The *Expert Panel Report 3: Guidelines* provide a systematic review of the evidence related to written asthma action plans compared with medical management alone and clearly recommends the use of a written plan based on the evidence to date in decreasing emergency department visits and hospitalizations (NAEPP, 2007).

The key to asthma patient education is to establish and maintain a partnership among the patient, the family, and the health-care team. Patients and families are being asked to manage complex medical regimens, detect and self-treat most exacerbations (unless severe), and communicate appropriately with the team. Asthma education is cost effective and can reduce morbidity for both adults and children.

ASTHMA

PATIENT EDUCATION

Related to the Overall Treatment Plan and Disease Process

BASIC FACTS ABOUT ASTHMA

Use a variety of teaching methods such as illustrations, video, written pamphlets or books, and models. Repeat key facts at every visit until the patient and/or family demonstrates an understanding of asthma. An example would to be to show the patient a drawing of a normal airway and an airway affected by asthma. The provider can then demonstrate how different medications act on different components of asthma (**bronchodilator** relaxes smooth muscle, **anti-inflammatory** decreases inflammation, etc.). This information can be repeated when reviewing medications at each visit until a clear understanding is demonstrated.

MEDICATION SKILLS

This includes proper inhaler use, spacer use if appropriate, when to take quick-relief medications, and nebulizer use if appropriate.

SELF-MONITORING SKILLS

This includes self-assessment of symptoms, peak flow monitoring, and how to record symptoms and peak expiratory flow (PEF) on self-assessment diary. Recognizing early signs of declining lung function is essential knowledge for the patient and family.

Environmental control and avoidance strategies will enable the patient and family to avoid possible asthma triggers. Discussion of how environmental exposure to allergens and irritants can worsen asthma symptoms and how to avoid triggers at home, work, and school will assist patients in learning self-management.

Specific to the Drug Therapy

Reason for the drug being given and its anticipated action in the disease process.
Doses and schedules for taking the drug.
Coping mechanisms for complex and costly drug regimens.
Interactions between other treatment modalities and these drugs.

Reasons for the Drug(s) Being Taken

Patient education about specific drugs is provided in Chapter 17.

Drugs as Part of the Total Treatment Regimen

Information should be provided concerning drugs as part of the total treatment regimen and individualized to the patient's age and asthma severity.

Many educational resources are available, the best of which are from the National Institutes of Health (NIH) and the Global Initiative for Asthma. These documents include the following:

National Asthma Education Prevention Program. (2007). *The Expert Panel Report 3: Guidelines for Management of Asthma.* Includes copy-ready patient handouts on use of peak flow meter, inhalers, and asthma action plans.

Global Initiative for Asthma. (2009). Global strategy for asthma management and prevention. http://www.ginasthma.org. Includes a patient guide to asthma and interactive learning modules on asthma in adults and children.

Internet-Based Patient Education Resources on Asthma

The *Expert Panel Report 3: Guidelines* can be found at http://www.nhlbi.nih.gov/guidelines/asthma/index.htm and the NIH/WHO Global Initiative for Asthma documents can be found at http:/www.ginasthma.com
Other resources include the following:
Allergy and Asthma Network, Mothers of Asthmatics. http://www.aanma.org/
American Academy of Allergy, Asthma, and Immunology. http://www.aaaai.org
Asthma and Allergy Foundation of America. http://www.aafa.org
Canadian Network for Respiratory Care. http://www.cnrchome.net/
National Asthma Education and Prevention Program. NHLBI http://www.nhlbi.nih.gov/health/public/lung/index.htm#asthma
National Institutes of Health National Heart Lung and Blood Institute. Asthma. http://www.nhlbi.nih.gov/health/dci/Diseases/Asthma/Asthma_WhatIs.html

CHRONIC OBSTRUCTIVE PULMONARY DISEASE

Chronic obstructive pulmonary disease (COPD) is the term commonly used to refer to conditions of chronic airflow limitation that is not fully reversible. The airflow restriction is usually progressive and involves both the airways and lung parenchyma. Other terms used include chronic obstructive airway disease and chronic obstructive lung disease. The primary risk factor is cigarette smoking, although occupational exposure (grain, coal, asbestos) and air pollution are also known factors. Not all cigarette smokers develop COPD, so genetic factors may influence who will develop the disease. Four professional organizations have published guidelines regarding COPD, the American Thoracic Society (ATS), the European Respiratory Society (ERS), the Global Initiative for Chronic Obstructive Lung Disease (GOLD), and the American College of Physicians (ACP).

COPD is a heterogeneous disorder that includes primarily chronic bronchitis and emphysema but also comprises peripheral airway disease and asthmatic bronchitis. The diagnosis of obstructive lung disease is determined by spirometry tests of lung function. A positive diagnosis of COPD is made when the FEV in 1 second (FEV_1) and the ratio to the forced vital capacity (FVC) is less than 70 percent. COPD can be classified as mild, moderate, severe, or very severe by the ATS and the ACP (see Table 30–9).

The differences between the clinical presentations of emphysema and of chronic bronchitis are clear, although patients can have components of both diseases. Patients with emphysema are older at diagnosis and often thinner than patients with chronic bronchitis (Table 30–10). The pathological changes in emphysema consist of permanent enlargement of the airspaces distal to the terminal bronchioles and destruction of the bronchiole wall. The primary symptom seen in emphysema is dyspnea. Chronic

Table 30–9 **Stages of COPD**

Classification	Definition by Spirometry
At Risk Patients who: smoke or have exposure to pollutants have cough, sputum or dyspnea have family history of respiratory disease	$FEV_1/FVC > 0.70$ $FEV_1 >= 80\%$ predicted
Mild	$FEV_1/FVC < 0.70$ $FEV_1 >= 80\%$ predicted
Moderate	$FEV_1/FVC < 0.70$ $50\% <= FEV_1 < 80\%$ predicted
Severe	$FEV_1/FVC < 0.70$ $30\% <= FEV_1 < 50\%$ predicted
Very Severe	$FEV_1/FVC < 0.70$ $FEV_1 <30\%$ predicted, or $FEV_1 <50\%$ predicted plus chronic respiratory failure

Source: Derived from American Thoracic Society, 2004; Qaseem et al, 2007.

Table 30–10 **Clinical Features of Chronic Bronchitis and Emphysema**

Characteristic	Chronic Bronchitis	Emphysema
Age at onset of symptoms	40–50 yr	50–60 yr
Primary symptoms	Cough	Dyspnea
Sputum	Copious, usually purulent	Scant, usually mucoid
Chest x-ray	Peribronchial thickening, often evidence of old inflammatory disease diaphragm	Hyperlucent, overinflated lung, flattened
Weight	Frequently obese	Thin, often marked weight loss
Total lung capacity	Normal or slightly decreased	Increased
Chest examination	Noisy chest, slight hyperinflation	Clear, may have slight end-expiration wheeze, marked hyperinflation
Cor pulmonale with heart failure	Common	Infrequent until end stages of disease

bronchitis is defined by chronic cough with copious sputum production for 3 months in 2 successive years (American Thoracic Society [ATS]/European Respiratory Society Task Force, 2004). Physical presentation differs in that patients with emphysema are typically barrel chested and breathe through pursed lips ("pink-puffers"), whereas patients with chronic bronchitis are typically obese and suffer from significant hypoxemia, cyanosis, and carbon dioxide retention ("blue-bloaters").

Pathophysiology

The pathophysiology of COPD is characterized by both acute and chronic inflammation. There are also changes in cellular proliferation, leading to tissue destruction, loss of structural ciliated columnar cells, squamous and goblet cell metaplasia, glandular and smooth muscle hypertrophy, and scarring. Clinically, these changes lead to worsened obstruction, hyperinflation of the lungs, increased sputum production, recurrent respiratory infections, and altered gas exchange. As the disease progresses, the patient experiences respiratory muscle fatigue, ventilatory disorders, cardiovascular compromise, and poor quality of life.

Emphysema

Emphysema is closely linked to cigarette smoking and the damage to the respiratory tract from the chronic cellular changes smoking produces. The chronic, progressive destruction of the alveolar structures found in emphysema is thought to be caused by an imbalance between proteases and antiproteases in the lower respiratory tract. Proteases, specifically polymorphonuclear neutrophil (PMN) elastase and pulmonary alveolar macrophage (PAM) elastase, work unchecked to destroy alveolar structures and their elastin network. Cigarette smokers have increased numbers of PMNs and PAMs in their lungs, which results in the loss of elastic recoil and structural support found in the lungs of smokers with emphysema. These findings are also found in patients with genetic $alpha_1$ antitrypsin deficiency, which accounts for 2 percent of patients with emphysema. $Alpha_1$ antitrypsin functions as an antiprotease in the lung to inhibit neutrophil elastase. Therefore, the same structural changes occur in these patients as occur in smokers with emphysema.

Chronic Bronchitis

Cigarette smoking is also the major contributor to the development of chronic bronchitis. Other inhaled irritants are also known to cause chronic bronchitis, among them dust, grain dust, fumes, and asbestos. Three direct effects of inhaling bronchial irritants contribute to the development of chronic bronchitis: (1) stimulation of mucus secretion in the airways, (2) impaired mucus clearance due in part to interference with ciliary activity, and (3) decreased resistance to bronchopulmonary infection because of altered alveolar macrophage function. Clinically, the patient presents with a chronic cough that is due to accumulation of the secretions. Airflow obstruction is due to inflammation of the airways and the thick secretions. The increased mucus is an excellent medium for recurrent bronchial infections, which cause further damage to the airways.

Goals of Therapy

The major goals of treatment for patients with COPD are to slow the disease process and maintain quality of life. Although medications such as **antibiotics, bronchodilators**, and **corticosteroids** are part of the treatment, other nonpharmacological measures have just as much impact. Most important, the patient must quit smoking. Nutrition and infection protection are key in maintaining optimal health. Exercise and pulmonary rehabilitation improve function and quality of life for the patient with COPD. A well-managed regimen of medication and nonpharmacological therapies enhances the outcome for patients with COPD.

Rational Drug Selection

The medication regimen for the COPD patient often includes different medications, each treating a different aspect of the disease. The ACP conducted an evidence-based review of therapies and made recommendations for treatment: maintenance monotherapy (**long-acting beta agonists, long-acting inhaled anticholinergics**, or **inhaled corticosteroids**) for symptomatic patients with COPD and FEV_1 less than 60 percent predicted; consider combination inhaled therapies for symptomatic patients with COPD and FEV_1 less than 60 percent of predicted (Qaseem et al, 2007). Drugs commonly used to treat COPD are shown in Table 30–7.

Bronchodilators

Bronchodilators are the mainstay of pharmacological therapy for COPD patients. They treat the reversible component of COPD and maximize airflow by relaxing the airway smooth muscle and improving lung emptying during tidal breathing (ATS/European Respiratory Society Task Force, 2004). Three types of **bronchodilators** are used in COPD management: **$beta_2$ agonists, anticholinergic drugs**, and **methylxanthines (theophylline)**.

Inhaled $beta_2$ agonists have been the mainstay for COPD therapy. The ACP recommends **long-acting beta agonists** as monotherapy or in combination with an inhaled **anticholinergic** or inhaled **corticosteroid** (Qaseem et al, 2007). **The long-acting beta agonists** are effective in reducing COPD exacerbations and as of this writing may still be used for monotherapy in COPD patients, whereas they have received a black box warning not to be used as monotherapy in asthma (U.S. Food and Drug Administration, 2010). The **long-acting beta agonists, salmeterol**

(Serevent) or **formoterol** (Perforomist) can be prescribed singly or in combination with an inhaled **corticosteroid** (Advair or Symbicort). The combination of a **short-acting beta agonist** (albuterol) and **ipratropium** (an inhaled **anticholinergic**) reduces exacerbations of COPD compared to **albuterol** alone (Qaseem et al, 2007).

Theophylline is not included in the ACP 2007 recommendations, but are in the GOLD 2009 guidelines as a second-line drug, noting low-dose **theophylline** reduces exacerbations of COPD. The GOLD guidelines further note high doses of **theophylline** have bronchodilator effects, but because of toxicity potential inhaled **bronchodilators** should be used.

Anticholinergic agents such as **ipratropium bromide (Atrovent)** and **tiotropium (Spiriva)** reduce the volume of sputum without changing the viscosity, which in addition to their bronchodilation effects, may make them the drug of choice in COPD. **Tiotropium (Spiriva HandiHaler)**, a dry inhalation powder, has been found to reduce exacerbations and hospitalizations of COPD patients compared with placebo and ipratropium (ATS/European Respiratory Society Task Force, 2004; Qaseem et al, 2007). **Tiotropium** additionally has the convenience of once-a-day dosing. One caution is that the inhaled **anticholinergics** are not effective for immediate relief of bronchospasm because of their slow onset of action; therefore, regular dosing is necessary. Combining agents such as **albuterol** and **ipratropium** (Combivent) or **formoterol** and **tiotropium (Symbicort)** produces a greater change in spirometry over 3 months than either agent alone. The ACP recommendations note clinicians may consider combination inhaled medications for COPD if FEV_1 is less than 60 percent of predicted (Qaseem et al, 2007). Combination medications may be more convenient and economical for patients with COPD who require both medications. The combination of **albuterol** and **ipratropium** is also available in solution for nebulizer use (DuoNeb).

Corticosteroids

Corticosteroids have nonspecific anti-inflammatory activity at multiple points in the inflammatory process. Because of the cellular level airway changes that define COPD, **corticosteroids'** effects are less dramatic in COPD than seen in asthma. Yet **corticosteroids** are key components in the management of stable COPD and COPD exacerbations.

The use of daily **inhaled steroids** in the COPD patient has mixed results in clinical studies (ATS/European Respiratory Society Task Force, 2004; Global Initiative for Chronic Obstructive Lung Disease [GOLD], 2009; Man & Sin, 2005; Qaseem et al, 2007). The consensus of the expert panel groups based on the evidence to date is that **inhaled corticosteroids** do not modify the long-term decline in FEV_1 seen in COPD, but as both monotherapy and in combination with **inhaled bronchodilators** they decrease exacerbations and improve health status in patients with symptomatic COPD (GOLD, 2009; Qaseem et al, 2007). Therefore, the current ACP and GOLD guidelines recommend starting a patient on moderate- to high-dose **inhaled corticosteroids** (see Table 30–1). Combination therapy of **inhaled corticosteroids** and a **long-acting beta agonist**, such as **Advair (salmeterol/fluticasone)**, is more effective in decreasing exacerbations than either agent alone (level A evidence in GOLD report); therefore, combination therapy should be considered in any patient with moderate to severe COPD defined by FEV_1 less than 60 percent predicted (GOLD, 2009; Qaseem et al, 2007).

Education about the slow onset of **inhaled corticosteroids** is necessary so patients do not become frustrated as the **inhaled steroids** are introduced. Patients need to be cautioned to rinse their mouths after **inhaled steroid use** to prevent oral candidiasis. **Corticosteroids** are useful in the short-term treatment of acute COPD exacerbation (ATS/European Respiratory Society Task Force, 2004; GOLD, 2009). There is level A evidence for the use of oral **corticosteroids** because they shorten recovery time, improve lung function, and decrease hypoxemia during the exacerbation (GOLD, 2009). If, in spite of maximum therapy with **bronchodilators**, the patient continues to have significant airway obstruction, a course of **systemic corticosteroids** is indicated. **Prednisone** is given as a dose of 30 to 40 mg daily for 10 days (ATS/European Respiratory Society Task Force, 2004; GOLD, 2009). At that time, the patient should have a 20 to 30 percent increase in pulmonary function (FEV_1). Some patients respond to a 10-day burst of **corticosteroids**, and the medications can be discontinued. Other patients require a taper of medication to the lowest **prednisone** level required to prevent recurrent attacks and relieve bronchospasm. The **prednisone** dose is tapered over 1 to 2 weeks and then to 5 mg over 5 days. Tapering may lead to recurrence of symptoms, and patients should be educated regarding monitoring their symptoms and PEF during tapering. Long-term treatment with **oral corticosteroids** is not recommended in COPD (level A evidence) and patients should be transitioned to **inhaled corticosteroids** either as monotherapy or in combination with **inhaled long-acting beta agonists** (GOLD, 2009).

Oxygen

In some patients, home **oxygen** therapy is necessary. **Oxygen** therapy can be used short term during acute exacerbations or long term in chronically hypoxemic patients. The goals of supplemental **oxygen** therapy are to correct arterial hypoxemia and prevent secondary organ damage; ideally, oxygen saturation should be greater than 90 percent. In patients experiencing an acute exacerbation of COPD, a drop in partial pressure of oxygen in arterial blood (Pao_2) to below 55 mm Hg is an indication for short-term supplemental **oxygen**. These patients should be monitored to determine when **oxygen** therapy can be discontinued. For the chronically hypoxemic COPD patient, continuous home **oxygen** therapy for 15 hours or more per day is associated with increased survival rate in patients with severe airway obstruction (Qaseem et al, 2007). Patients should be started on continuous **oxygen** therapy if they demonstrate persistent hypoxemia at rest (Pao_2 less than 55 mmHg and less than 88% oxygen saturation). Patients with cor pulmonale or polycythemia with Pao_2 less than 59 mm Hg and less than 89 percent oxygen saturation require supplemental **oxygen.** Patients on continuous **oxygen** therapy require arterial blood gas studies after 1, 3, and 6 months of therapy. Supplemental **oxygen** improves exercise tolerance, neuropsychological function, and quality of life, all key factors in the patient's emotional health in learning to live with this chronic disease.

Antibiotics

Patients with COPD have an excess of thick pulmonary mucus and decreased ciliary clearance of secretions; therefore, they are susceptible to repeated bronchial infections. Infection is considered present when the patient is producing a purulent sputum. The common organisms found in the sputum of patients with COPD patients are *Haemophilus influenzae, Streptococcus pneumoniae, Mycoplasma pneumoniae,* and *Moraxella catarrhalis.* The most common organism is *S. pneumoniae* (Rabe et al, 2007). **Antibiotic** choices have to cover these organisms until sputum cultures are available to determine sensitivity. **Amoxicillin/clavulanic acid, macrolides,** and double-strength **sulfamethoxazole/trimethoprim** are all appropriate first-line choices (Rabe et al, 2007). Resistant organisms require a change in **antibiotic** therapy after drug susceptibility studies are completed. Patients with moderate exacerbation who may require hospitalization or who don't respond to first-line therapy should be treated with a respiratory **fluoroquinolone (levofloxacin, moxifloxacin, gemifloxacin).** Length of treatment is 7 to 14 days.

Leukotrienes

There are no data to support the use of **leukotriene receptor antagonists** in the treatment of COPD.

> **CLINICAL PEARL**
>
> **Oxygen Therapy**
>
> One note of caution in providing oxygen therapy to some patients with COPD who have poor ventilatory capacity: These patients, known as "carbon dioxide retainers," no longer rely on rises in $Paco_2$ as the primary drive to breathe. If these patients receive too much oxygen, raising their Pao_2 above their normal baseline, hypoventilation may occur. This results in CO_2 retention and the somnolence, lethargy, and coma that occur with carbon dioxide narcosis. Monitoring arterial blood gases is essential in all patients receiving oxygen therapy.

Alpha-Trypsin Augmentation Therapy

Patients who have emphysema related to genetic alpha$_1$ antitrypsin deficiency may benefit from augmentation therapy with an **alpha$_1$-proteinase inhibitor (Prolastin, Aralast, Zemaira).** These medications are administered weekly via IV. Patients with alpha$_1$ antitrypsin deficiency should be referred to a specialist for therapy.

Immunizations

Infection prevention is essential in management of patients with COPD, and vaccination against respiratory infections is an integral component in preventing illness in these patients. Protection against influenza virus is recommended annually. Optimally, the **influenza vaccine** should be administered between October and January, the earlier in the influenza season the better, to allow adequate antibody response. Patients with COPD also require a **pneumococcal vaccine** every 6 years regardless of age. Patients should be taught the importance of these vaccines, so they remember to get them.

Smoking Cessation

Smoking is a major contributor to COPD. Cigarette smoking results in severe destruction of lung tissue, and the damage is largely irreversible. To halt the progression of COPD, the patient must stop smoking. The benefits of smoking cessation include an eventual return to a nearly normal age-related rate of ventilatory function.

There are many new medications that can help the patient stop smoking. Smoking cessation is discussed in depth in Chapter 43.

Monitoring

Monitoring patients with COPD has four aspects related to pulmonary function and quality of life: signs and symptoms of COPD, pulmonary function, pharmacotherapy, and quality of life.

All patients should be taught how to monitor their symptoms for worsening pulmonary function. Patients with chronic bronchitis need to monitor their sputum for changes in color from their baseline to more purulent. Any symptoms of respiratory infection must be reported to their health-care provider so that appropriate antibiotic therapy can be started. During times of poor outdoor air quality, these patients need to remain indoors and report

> **CLINICAL PEARL**
>
> **Influenza Vaccine Reminders**
>
> The health-care provider should keep a tickler file of chronic respiratory patients (those with asthma and COPD), so the patients can be reminded each fall to get their influenza vaccine.

any signs of respiratory distress to their health-care provider. Patients with COPD may require increased use of bronchodilators or oxygen during these times.

Monitoring pulmonary function is done by spirometry, peak flow meter, oxygen saturation (pulse oximetry), and arterial blood gases. Patients can be taught to use a peak flow meter to monitor lung function at home and determine their need for changes in their medication regimen in times of illness or poor air quality. All patients with COPD need objective monitoring of lung function on a regular basis to identify worsening of function and, therefore, need for a change in their treatment regimen.

Patients should bring their medications to every visit to the health-care provider. MDI use should be reviewed and technique monitored with each visit. Patients who use more than the recommended amounts of **beta$_2$ agonists** need to be assessed closely to determine the reason for the increased use. Is the patient using the inhaler incorrectly, or is the disease progressing? Increased use of **inhaled bronchodilators** is an indication for reevaluation of the medication regimen and a possible need for **systemic steroids.** Patients on supplemental **oxygen** therapy require arterial blood gases, as previously mentioned, at 1, 3, and 6 months after beginning therapy. Any change in respiratory status is an indication for repeat arterial blood gas determination. All patients require a written medication management plan that is reviewed at every visit.

Monitoring quality of life at every visit can determine if the treatment regimen is successful. Is the patient able to tolerate activities of daily living without assistance? Exercise tolerance, activity level, and nutrition all need to be evaluated. The financial burden of a chronic illness such as COPD is significant, and referral to a social worker may be necessary to help the patient pay for prescribed treatment.

Outcome Evaluation

Successful management of patients with COPD includes their self-assessment of quality of life, as well as physical parameters of optimal treatment. As COPD is chronic and for the most part irreversible, outcome evaluation is based on the patient's having the best quality of life for the disease state. The successfully managed patient with COPD has optimal activity tolerance, which varies for each patient. Pharmacological management is aimed at decreasing bronchospasm and secondary infections. Therefore, the amount of bronchospasm and the number of infections determine if treatment is successful.

Patient Education

Patient education should include a discussion of information related to the overall treatment plan as well as that specific to the drug therapy, reasons for taking the drug, drugs as part of the total treatment regimen, and adherence issues.

Patient education for the COPD patient centers on maintaining optimal pulmonary function and quality of life. Teaching self-management is the basis of successful treatment.

CHRONIC OBSTRUCTIVE PULMONARY DISEASE

PATIENT EDUCATION

Related to the Overall Treatment Plan and Disease Process

The patient needs to be taught the following areas of self-management:

SMOKING CESSATION

This is a difficult area of education because of the physical and psychological addiction to cigarettes. Many patients have attempted to quit smoking previously and need to be encouraged to try again, using some of the pharmacological interventions available to aid in tobacco cessation.

PATHOPHYSIOLOGY OF CHRONIC OBSTRUCTIVE PULMONARY DISEASE

A basic understanding of the changes in the pulmonary system that occur with COPD will assist the patient in understanding the role that the different medications play in the treatment regimen.

MEDICATION SKILLS

Patients with COPD often have other chronic illnesses that require routine medications. Administering a complex regimen of multiple medications can be overwhelming, especially to older patients. Written schedules (in large print) and divided pill boxes are two strategies for medication management. Providing the patient with the generic and trade names of medications will decrease medication confusion. Having the patient bring all medications in for review will prevent medication errors. Often, the patient may be seeing other providers, including specialists who may also be prescribing medications. It is the role of the primary care provider to coordinate between specialty providers and monitor medications the patient is taking. Encourage patients to use a magnifying glass to read the generic names on the meter dose inhaler (MDI) canisters, as the canister color may change with different brands of the same medication.

CHRONIC OBSTRUCTIVE PULMONARY DISEASE—cont'd

PATIENT EDUCATION

Specific to the Drug Therapy

Reason for the drug being given and its anticipated action in the disease process.
Doses and schedules for taking the drug.
Coping mechanisms for complex and costly drug regimens.
Interactions between other treatment modalities and these drugs.

Reasons for the Drug(s) Being Taken

Patient education about specific drugs is provided in Chapter 17.

Drugs as Part of the Total Treatment Regimen

The total treatment regimen also includes teaching self-monitoring skills, including, if indicated, proper use of a peak flow meter.

Infection control measures are also taught. Patients with COPD are at high risk for respiratory infections. They need to be taught the importance of annual influenza vaccine and the need for a pneumococcal pneumonia vaccine every 6 years. They need to avoid crowds and people, especially children, with respiratory infections.

Adherence Issues

Health-care providers should be aware of the potential problem of nonadherence with the treatment regimen and should discuss the importance of adherence with the patient and family members.

REFERENCES

Abramoqicz, M. (Ed.). (2005). Drugs for asthma. *Treatment Guidelines From the Medical Letter, 3*(33), 33–38.

American Medical Association. (1997). *Managing asthma today: Integrating new concepts.* Chicago, IL: American Medical Association.

American Thoracic Society (ATS)/European Respiratory Society Task Force. (2004). *Standards for the diagnosis and management of patients with COPD* (Version 1.2). New York: American Thoracic Society. Retrieved from http://www.thoracic.org/clinical/copd-guidelines/resources/copddoc.pdf

Autio, L., & Rosenow, D. (1999). Effectively managing asthma in young and middle adulthood. *Nurse Practitioner, 24*(1), 100–111.

Boehringer Ingelheim Pharmaceuticals. (2009). SPIRIVA Handihaler prescribing information. Retrieved from http://bidocs.boehringer-ingelheim.com/BIWebAccess/ViewServlet.ser?docBase=renetnt&folderPath=/Prescribing+Information/PIs/Spiriva/Spiriva.pdf

Bousquet, J., Cabrera, P., Berkman, N., Buhl, R., Holgate, S., Wenzel, S., et al. (2005). The effect of treatment with omalizumab, an anti-IgE antibody, on asthma exacerbations and emergency medical visits in patients with severe persistent asthma. *Allergy, 60*(3), 302–308.

Chiang, D. T., Clark, J., & Casale, T. B. (2005). Omalizumab in asthma: Approval and postapproval experience. *Clinical Reviews in Allergy and Immunology, 29*(1), 3–16.

Colice, G. L. (1996). Nebulized bronchodilators for outpatient management of stable chronic obstructive pulmonary disease. *American Journal of Medicine, 100*(Suppl. 1A), 11S–18S.

Covar, R. A., & Spahn, J. D. (2003). Treating the wheezing infant. *Pediatric Clinics of North America, 50*(3), 631–654.

Drazen, J. M., Israel, E., Boushey, H. A., Chinchilli, V. M., Fahy, J. V., Fish, J. E., et al. (1996). Comparison of regularly scheduled with as-needed use of albuterol in mild asthma. *New England Journal of Medicine, 335*(12), 841–847.

Drombrowski, M., Thom, E., & McNellis, D. (1999). Maternal-fetal medicine units (MFMU) studies of inhaled corticosteroids during pregnancy. *Journal of Allergy and Clinical Immunology, 103*(2, Part 2), S356–S359.

Georgitis, J. W. (1999). The 1997 asthma management guidelines and therapeutic issues relating to the treatment of asthma. *Chest, 115*(1), 210–217.

Global Initiative for Asthma. (2009). Global strategy for asthma management and prevention. Retrieved from http://www.ginasthma.org

Global Initiative for Chronic Obstructive Lung Disease [GOLD]. (2009). Global Strategy for the Diagnosis, Management, and Prevention of Chronic Obstructive Pulmonary Disease: Updated 2009. Medical Communications Resources. Retrieved from www.goldcopd.org

Halbert, R. J., Isonaka, S., George, D., & Iqbal, A. (2003). Interpreting COPD estimates: What is the true burden of disease? *Chest, 123*(5), 1684–1692.

Hanania, N. A., & Belfort, M. A. (2005). Acute asthma in pregnancy. *Critical Care Medicine, 33*(Suppl. 10), S319–S324.

Johannsen, J. M. (1994). Chronic obstructive pulmonary disease: Current comprehensive care for emphysema and bronchitis. *Nurse Practitioner, 10*(1), 59–67.

Konig, P., & Shaffer, J. (1996). The effect of drug therapy on long-term outcome of childhood asthma: A possible preview of the international guidelines. *Journal of Allergy and Clinical Immunology, 98*(6), 1103–1111.

Kwon, H. L., Belanger, K., & Bracken, M. B. (2003). Asthma prevalence among pregnant and childbearing-aged women in the United States: Estimates from national health surveys. *Annals of Epidemiology, 13,* 317–324.

Ladebauche, P. (1997). Managing asthma: A growth and developmental approach. *Pediatric Nursing, 23*(1), 37–44.

Lieu, T. A., Quesenberry, C. P., Capra, A. M., Sorel, M. E., Martin, K. E., & Mendoza, G. R. (1997). Outpatient management practices associated with reduced risk of pediatric asthma hospitalization and emergency department visits. *Pediatrics, 100*(3), 334–341.

Luskin, A.T. (1999). An overview of the recommendation of the working group on asthma and pregnancy. *Journal of Allergy and Clinical Immunology, 103*(2), S350–S353.

Man, S. F. P., & Sin, D. D. (2005). Inhaled corticosteroids in chronic obstructive pulmonary disease: Is there a clinical benefit? *Drugs, 65*(5), 579–591.

National Asthma Education and Prevention Program (NAEPP). (2007). *The Expert Panel Report 3: Guidelines for the diagnosis and management of asthma.* Bethesda, MD: National Heart, Lung, and Blood Institute, National Institutes of Health. Retrieved from http://www.nhlbi.nih.gov/guidelines/asthma/

National Heart, Lung, and Blood Institute (NHLBI). (1995). *Global strategy for asthma management and prevention. NHLBI/WHO Report* [NIH Publication No. 95–3659]. Bethesda, MD: National Institutes of Health.

Parsons, J. P., & Mastronarde, J. G. (2005). Exercise-induced bronchoconstriction in athletes. *Chest. 128*(6), 3966–3974.

Qaseem, A., Snow, V., Shekelle, P., Sherif, K., Wilt, T. J., Weinberger, S., et al. (2007). Diagnosis and management of stable chronic obstructive pulmonary disease: A clinical practice guideline from the American College of Physicians. *Annals of Internal Medicine, 147,* 633–638.

Rabe, K. F., Hurd, S., Anzueto, A., Barnes, P. J., Buist, S. A., Calverley, P., et al. (2007). Global strategy for the diagnosis, management, and prevention of chronic obstructive pulmonary disease. *American Journal of Respiratory Critical Care Medicine, 176*(6), 532–555.

Simmons, M. S., Nides, M. A., Rand, C. S., Wise, R. A., & Tashkin, D. P. (1996). Trends in compliance with bronchodilator inhaler use between follow-up visits in a clinical trial. *Chest, 109*(4), 963–968.

Spector, S. L., & Tan, R. A. (2004). Effectiveness of montelukast in the treatment of cough variant asthma. *Annals of Allergy, Asthma, and Immunology, 9*(3), 232–236.

Statistics Canada (2010). Asthma, by sex, provinces and territories. Retrieved from http://www40.statcan.ca/l01/cst01/health50a-eng.htm

Tashkin, D. P., Bleecker, E., Braun, S., Campbell, S., DeGraff, A. C., Hudgel, D. W., et al. (1996). Results of a multicenter study of nebulized inhalant bronchodilator solutions. *American Journal of Medicine, 100*(Suppl. 1A), 62S–69S.

U.S. Food and Drug Administration. (2010). FDA drug safety communication: New safety requirements for long-acting inhaled asthma medications called long-acting beta-agonists (LABAs). Retrieved from http://www.fda.gov/Drugs/DrugSafety/PostmarketDrugSafetyInformationforPatientsandProviders/ucm200776.htm

VanAndel, A. E., Reisner, C., Menjoge, S. S., & Witek, T. J. (1999). Analysis of inhaled corticosteroid and oral theophylline use among patients with stable COPD from 1987 to 1995. *Chest, 115*(3), 703–707.

Wendel, P. J., Ramin, S. M., Barnett-Hamm, C., Rowe, T. F., & Cunningham, F. G. (1996). Asthma treatment in pregnancy: A randomized controlled study. *American Journal of Obstetrics and Gynecology, 175*(1), 150–154.

Williams, D. M. (1995). Chronic obstructive airways disease. In L. Y. Young & M. A. Koda-Kimble (Eds.), *Applied therapeutics.* Vancouver: Applied Therapeutics.

CHAPTER 31

CONTRACEPTION

Teral Gerlt

Chapter Outline

Choosing a method of **contraception (birth control)** is an intimate process and one in which patients, male and female, often seek advice from their health-care provider. Unintended pregnancy rates remain high in the United States. In 2001, 49 percent of all pregnancies in women age 15 to 44 were unplanned (Finer & Henshaw, 2006). Considerations that must be addressed include the safety of the method chosen, age of the patient, the health and medical conditions of the patient, ability to comply with method use, frequency of sexual relations, risk of sexually transmitted infections, and cost. The most important of these considerations after safety is compliance; any method that offers safety to the patient offers very little protection from pregnancy if use of the method does not fit their lifestyle.

Many contraceptive options are available with varying efficacy rates (Hatcher et al, 2007). These options and their efficacy rates for first year of use are presented in Table 31–1. This chapter focuses on the pharmacological methods of **contraception** that offer the highest rates of effectiveness. Over the past several years, novel modes of delivery for **contraceptive hormones** have been introduced. The new delivery modes offer potentially lower rates of failure due to user error because they involve less frequent administration intervals, therefore increasing the user's ability to comply with proper use. Pharmacological methods include **oral contraceptives** (OCs), topical patches, vaginal rings, subdermal implants, injections, and intrauterine devices (IUDs). These methods include **progestin**-only preparations, and preparations that include various combinations of **estrogen** and **progestin**.

PHYSIOLOGY OF THE NORMAL MENSTRUAL CYCLE

The menstrual cycle is regulated by positive and negative feedback in the hypothalamic-pituitary-ovarian axis. The pituitary gland releases stimulating and inhibiting hormones. Release of these hormones is regulated by pulses of gonadotropin-releasing hormone (GnRH) from the hypothalamus. GnRH pulses regulate follicle-stimulating hormone (FSH) and luteinizing hormone (LH) that in turn regulate the secretion of estrogen and progesterone from the ovary. The most obvious manifestation of this complex system is cyclic menstrual bleeding.

Table 31–1 **Contraceptive Options**

Method	Advantages	Disadvantages	Perfect Use Efficacy	Typical Use Efficacy
		Estrogen/Progestin Combination Contraception		
Pills	Menstrual cycle control	Daily administration may be difficult for some users	99%	92%
Patch	Menstrual cycle control Weekly administration	Patch may cause some local irritation Patch may fall off partially or completely		
Ring	Menstrual cycle control Once per cycle administration	User must be comfortable with vaginal administration		
		Progestin Only		
Oral contraception	No estrogen; may be useful for users in whom estrogen is contraindicated	Daily administration may be difficult for some users Unpredictable bleeding pattern	99%	92%
Progestin injectable contraception	Administration once every 12 wk Use of method discreet from others	Administration requires office visit Unpredictable bleeding pattern	99%	97%
Progestin implant	Offers contraception for 3 yr	Insertion and removal requires office procedure Unpredictable bleeding pattern	99%	99%
		Intrauterine Device (IUD)		
Copper	Hormone free Offers contraception for 10 yr	Insertion and removal requires office visit Dysmenorrhea and menstrual flow may be increased in first few months after insertion	99%	99%
Progestin-releasing	Decreased menstrual flow Offers contraception for 5 yr	Requires office visit for insertion and removal		
		Barrier Methods		
Male condom	Protection from most STIs Available without prescription	Use linked to coitus and partner dependant	98%	85%
Female condom	Protection from most STIs Available without prescription	Use linked to coitus	95%	79%
Spermicide	Available without prescription	Use linked to coitus	82%	71%
Diaphragm	May be inserted several hours before intercourse	Available only with provider fitting and prescription Must be used with spermicide User must be comfortable with vaginal insertion technique	94%	84%

Table 31–1 **Contraceptive Options—cont'd**

Method	Advantages	Disadvantages	Perfect Use Efficacy	Typical Use Efficacy
Cervical cap	May be inserted several hours before intercourse	Available only with provider fitting and prescription Must be used with spermicide User must be comfortable with vaginal insertion technique Lower efficacy for parous women	74%–91%	68%–84%
Vaginal sponge	Available without prescription Contains spermicide May be inserted several hours before intercourse	Lower efficacy for parous women	80%–91%	68%–84%

STIs = sexually transmitted infections.

The menstrual cycle is divided into four phases: follicular, ovulatory, luteal, and menstrual. During the follicular phase, FSH stimulates several follicles to develop, with one ultimately becoming dominant. The dominant follicle synthesizes enough estradiol to create negative feedback and decrease FSH levels. During the ovulatory phase, estradiol levels peak and exert positive feedback to induce an LH surge, which in turn facilitates release of the mature ovum. Estrogen also promotes proliferation of the endometrium, and development of progesterone receptors in the endometrium. During the luteal phase, progesterone dominates; it is produced predominantly by the corpus luteum and prevents new follicle development as well as differentiation of the endometrium. If pregnancy does not occur, the corpus luteum degenerates. Once the corpus luteum degenerates, estrogen and progesterone levels decline, resulting in endometrial shedding or menstrual bleeding. Other gynecological organs are also influenced by estrogen and progesterone. The fallopian tubes exhibit increased proliferation, differentiation, and tubular contractility under the influence of estrogen; these processes are inhibited under the influence of progesterone. Cervical mucus water content is increased and penetration of sperm is facilitated by estrogen, whereas it is decreased by progesterone.

Estrogen exerts effects on other body systems, including positive effects on bone mass, increasing serum triglycerides, improving high-density lipoprotein (HDL) to low-density lipoprotein (LDL) ratios, and stimulating coagulation and fibrinolytic pathways. Progesterone increases body temperature, increases insulin levels, and may slightly depress the central nervous system (Katzung, 2009).

PHARMACODYNAMICS

The major difference between endogenous **estrogen** and **progestins** and pharmacological preparations is their oral bioavailability. All orally available **estrogen** and **progestins** undergo first-pass metabolism in the liver. Currently two formulations of **estrogen** are available in contraceptive preparations, **ethinyl estradiol** (EE) and **mestranol. Mestranol** is the weaker of the two preparations, and must be metabolized into EE before it is able to bind with **estrogen** receptors. Fifty mcg of **mestranol** is equivalent to 35 mcg of EE. The **estrogen** used in the vast majority of hormonal contraceptive formulations in use today is **ethinyl estradiol,** with most preparations containing between 20 and 35 mcg of EE.

Most **progestins** used in **hormonal contraception** are derivatives of testosterone. The alteration of testosterone not only makes them bioavailable, but also changes their activity from androgenic to much more selective progestational activity. Currently several different androgen-derived **progestins** are available in **oral contraceptive** preparations. **Norethindrone, norethindrone acetate,** and **ethynodiol diacetate** are first generation **progestins.** Both **norethindrone acetate** and **ethynodiol diacetate** are converted to **norethindrone** in the body. As the amount of these **progestins** used in the formulations decreased, women experienced more spotting and breakthrough bleeding. In response, the second generation **progestins, norgestrel** and **levonorgestrel,** were developed. **Levonorgestrel** is the levorotatory form of **norgestrel** and its active metabolite. These **progestins** had increased androgenic activity, thereby decreasing breakthrough bleeding; however, increasing the androgenic activity led to problems with acne, hirsutism, and dyslipidemia (Hatcher et al, 2007).

Desogestrel and **norgestimate** are considered newer **progestins,** or third generation; the main difference is a decrease in androgenicity. **Desogestrel** undergoes conversion to its active metabolite **etonogestrel,** which is the progestin used in the vaginal ring and the subdermal implant. **Norelgestromin** is the primary metabolite of **norgestimate,** and available in the contraceptive patch. Decreased androgenicity theoretically reduced adverse effects on carbohydrate and lipid metabolism found in previous formulations, as well as lessening acne and hirsutism. **Medroxyprogesterone acetate** is available for injectable **contraception**.

The latest progestin developed is a derivative of **spironolactone, drospirenone**. As a derivative of **spironolactone** it has a mild diuretic effect as well as antimineralocorticoid effects. **Drospirenone** may cause hyperkalemia and should be used cautiously in women who are using drugs that cause a potassium-sparing effect such as angiotensin-converting enzyme (ACE) **inhibitors** (Speroff & Darney, 2005).

Mechanism of Pregnancy Prevention

Progestins are primarily responsible for the contraceptive effect in hormonal preparations. **Progestins** exhibit a negative effect in the hypothalamic-pituitary-ovarian axis, essentially suppressing the LH surge necessary for ovulation. They also cause thickening of cervical mucus, making penetration by sperm difficult. Tubal motility is slowed, delaying transport of the ovum and sperm. Finally, **progestins** cause atrophy of the endometrium, preventing implantation.

The **estrogen** component of hormonal contraception improves efficacy by suppressing FSH release, and therefore development of a dominant follicle. **Estrogen** also adds to cycle control, decreasing irregular bleeding patterns commonly found with progestin-only methods (Katzung, 2009).

GOALS OF TREATMENT

Treatment goals of pharmacological **contraception** are to use the safest, best-tolerated, and most effective method that the patient desires. In order to help the patient determine which **contraception** method may be best for her, the provider needs to be aware of any cultural or religious determents, as well as partner acceptance.

On The Horizon — NEW OCS

In May 2010, the FDA approved the first **OC** to contain **estradiol valerate,** a synthetic prodrug of 17ß-estradiol and a new **progestin, Dienogest,** which displays properties of 19-**nortestosterone** derivatives as well as properties associated with **progesterone** derivatives. **Natazia,** which should be available for prescription in August 2010, will also be the first four-phasic oral contraceptive to be marketed in the United States.

In December 2010, the FDA approved the first chewable **OC** which combines 0.8 mg **norethindrone** and 0.025 mg **ethinyl estradiol** in chewable form, with four 75-mg **ferrous fumarate** placebo tablets. The 24/4 regimen, marketed by Watson Pharmaceuticals, Inc, is intended to decrease breakthrough bleeding and provide short, light, predictable periods. The product is expected to be available in the second quarter of 2011.

Safety

The fear over increased risk of breast cancer with **oral contraceptive** use is largely media induced. A meta-analysis of breast cancer data (Kahlenborn, Modugno, Potter, & Severs, 2006) suggests a small overall increase in breast cancer risk (OR = 1.19) across different use patterns. In studies that controlled for parity, the data indicated that the risk of breast cancer in nulliparous women was OR equal to 1.24 and length of **hormonal contraceptive** use did not increase risk. The most interesting finding was the increased risk of breast cancer in parous women who used **OCs** for more than 4 years prior to their first full-term pregnancy (OR = 1.52). However, Speroff and Darney (2005) put this in perspective by pointing out that because most of the women using **OCs** are in an age bracket during which breast cancer is very rare, the overall increase in breast cancer cases is relatively small. Other data show breast cancer risk is not increased by current or past use of **OCs,** even in women who have previously used pills containing more than 50 mcg of **estrogen** (Marchbanks et al, 2002).

Current studies find no increase in the frequency of liver cancer in women who use **OCs.** Studies do show a negligible increase in the incidence of gallstones in current users, but the data point to this in women who have underlying asymptomatic disease and its acceleration, rather than an actual increase in the population.

Cardiovascular disease risk related to lipid metabolism is difficult to quantify because so many other risk factors are involved. Formulations with less than 50 mcg of **estrogen** seem to have no detrimental effects. In general, the cardiovascular risk factors other than OC use play the predominant role in the occurrence of ischemic stroke and myocardial infarction. Patients who smoke share an increased risk for heart attack, stroke, and thromboembolic phenomena (deep venous thrombosis [DVT] and pulmonary embolism) as they approach 35 years of age (Speroff & Darney, 2005). Findings from the Women's Health Initiative are discussed in Chapter 38 as they relate to hormone replacement therapy. These findings should be considered in prescribing **OCs,** but the risk for these low doses of **estrogen** and progesterone were not part of this study.

Tolerance

More than 40 years of experience in prescribing **OCs** have provided much data with which to knowledgeably help patients decide to choose an OC. Current **OCs** have less **estrogen**; therefore, they cause fewer of the pregnancy-like symptoms that had earlier been so distressing. The third and fourth generation **progestins** show fewer weight changes, improved complexion, and reduced mood swings. Improved packaging has also improved compliance by providing cues in the packaging as to the day of the week each pill should be taken.

Effectiveness

The theoretical effectiveness is 99 percent or greater with most hormonal therapies. Patients have lower discontinuation rates and therefore fewer unwanted pregnancies if they are well educated about **emergency hormonal contraception** and use a backup method such as **spermicide** and condoms. Vomiting and diarrhea as seen with gastrointestinal illnesses can decrease **oral contraceptive** effectiveness by decreasing absorption; women should be advised to use a backup method for at least 7 days after a gastrointestinal illness (Speroff & Darney, 2005).

RATIONAL DRUG SELECTION

Guidelines

A good place to start in helping a patient choose a new **hormonal contraceptive** is to exclude those methods that are absolutely or relatively contraindicated because of existing health concerns and patient age. Deciding whether the patient has any contraindications to the use of **estrogen** narrows the choices considerably. Then review which delivery mode appeals to the patient based on her perceived ability to comply with the dosing regimen. Fine-tuning choices can then be made based on acceptability of likely changes in bleeding pattern and side effect profile. The provider should also discuss the theoretical and typical use failure rates with the patient to ascertain if these are congruent with the patient's desire to avoid pregnancy. Other factors to consider are a patient's need for discreetness in the use of her method; a patient may wish to conceal her contraceptive method from partners or other family members and taking a daily pill or wearing a patch may preclude these as choices. Timing of a subsequent pregnancy should also be considered; for some methods a return to fertility is delayed after cessation of use. For patients who are satisfied with their current **hormonal contraceptive** choice, and for whom no new contraindications because of health issues are present, changing to a product or method to one that is newer to the market is unnecessary.

More than four dozen formulations of monophasic combined **oral contraceptives** (COCs), about two dozen multiphasic COCs, and several formulations of **progestin-only pills** (POPs), as well as several non-**oral contraceptive** hormone delivery methods are available. Table 31–2 summarizes the name brand and generic hormone formulas currently available (*Drug Facts and Comparisons*, 2009; Hatcher et al, 2007; Shrader & Dickerson, 2008).

Table 31–2 **Oral Contraceptives**

Brand Name	Estrogen Dose (mcg)	Progestin Dose (mg)
PROGESTIN-ONLY TABLETS		
Camilla, Errin, Jolivette, Micronor, Nor-QD		Norethindrone 0.35
MONOPHASIC COMBINATION TABLETS		
Karvia, Mircette	Ethinyl estradiol 20	Desogestrel 0.15
Yaz 24/4	Ethinyl estradiol 20	Drospirenone 3
Alesse, Aviane, Lessina, Levlite, Lutera	Ethinyl estradiol 20	Levonorgestrel 0.1
Junel 21 1/20, Loestrin 1/20, Loestrin 24 Fe, Microgestin 1/20	Ethinyl estradiol 20	Norethindrone acetate 1
Watson Pharmaceutical (chewable)	Ethinyl estradiol 25	Norethindrone 0.8
Apri, Desogen, Ortho-Cept, Reclipsen	Ethinyl estradiol 30	Desogestrel 0.15
Ocella ,Yasmin,	Ethinyl estradiol 30	Drospirenone 3
Jolessa, Levlen, Levora, Nordette, Portia, Quasense	Ethinyl estradiol 30	Levonorgestrel 0.15
Junel 21 1/30	Ethinyl estradiol 30	Norethindrone acetate 1
Loestrin 1.5/30, Microgestin 1.5/30	Ethinyl estradiol 30	Norethindrone acetate 1.5
Cryselle, Lo/Ovral, Low-Ogestrel	Ethinyl estradiol 30	Norgestrel 0.3
Demulen 1/35, Kelnor, Zovia 1/35	Ethinyl estradiol 35	Ethynodiol diacetate 1
Balziva, Femcon Fe, Ovcon 35, Zenchent	Ethinyl estradiol 35	Norethindrone 0.4

Continued

Table 31–2 **Oral Contraceptives—cont'd**

Brand Name	Estrogen Dose (mcg)	Progestin Dose (mg)
MONOPHASIC COMBINATION TABLETS		
Brevicon, Modicon, Necon 0.5/35, Nortrel 0.5/35	Ethinyl estradiol 35	Norethindrone 0.5
Necon 1/35, Norethin 1/35, Norinyl 1/35, Nortrel 1/35, Ortho-Novum 1/35	Ethinyl estradiol 35	Norethindrone 1
MonoNessa, Ortho-Cyclen, Sprintec	Ethinyl estradiol 35	Norgestimate 0.25
Necon 1/50, Norinyl 1/50, Ortho-Novum 1/50	Mestranol 50 (equivalent to 35 ethinyl estradiol)	Norethindrone 1
Demulen 1/50, Zovia 1/50	Ethinyl estradiol 50	Ethynodiol diacetate 1
Ovcon 50	Ethinyl estradiol 50	Norethindrone 1
Ogestrel 28, Ovral 21	Ethinyl estradiol 50	Norgestrel 0.5
EXTENDED CYCLE PACKS		
Seasonale	Ethinyl estradiol 30 (84 d)	Levonorgestrel 0.15 (84 d)
Seasonique	Ethinyl estradiol 30 (84 d)	Levonorgestrel 0.15 (84 d)
	Ethinyl estradiol 10 (7 d)	
LoSeasonique	Ethinyl estradiol 20 (84 d)	Levonorgestrel 0.1 (84 d)
	Ethinyl estradiol 10 (7 d)	
Lybrel (Continuous dosing)	Ethinyl estradiol 20	Levonorgestrel 0.09
BIPHASIC COMBINATION TABLETS		
Necon 10/11	Ethinyl estradiol 35	Norethindrone 0.5 (10 d)
	Ethinyl estradiol 35	Norethindrone 1 (11 d)
TRIPHASIC COMBINATION TABLETS		
Mircette, Kariva	Ethinyl estradiol 20	Desogestrel 0.15 (21 d)
	Placebo (2 d)	
	Ethinyl estradiol 10 mcg (5 d)	
Caziant , Cyclessa, Velivet	Ethinyl estradiol 25	Desogestrel 0.1 (7 d)
	Ethinyl estradiol 25	Desogestrel 0.125 (7 d)
	Ethinyl estradiol 25	Desogestrel 0.15 (7 d)
Ortho-Tri-Cyclen Lo, Tri-Lo-Sprintec	Ethinyl estradiol 25	Norgestimate 0.18 (7 d)
	Ethinyl estradiol 25	Norgestimate 0.215 (7 d)
	Ethinyl estradiol 25	Norgestimate 0.25 (7 d)
Tri-Sprintec, TriNessa	Ethinyl estradiol 35	Norgestimate 0.18 (7 d)
	Ethinyl estradiol 35	Norgestimate 0.215 (7 d)
	Ethinyl estradiol 35	Norgestimate 0.25 (7 d)
Estrostep	Ethinyl estradiol 20	Norethindrone acetate 1 (7 d)
	Ethinyl estradiol 30	Norethindrone acetate 1 (7 d)
	Ethinyl estradiol 35	Norethindrone acetate 1 (7 d)

Table 31–2 **Oral Contraceptives—cont'd**

Brand Name	Estrogen Dose (mcg)	Progestin Dose (mg)
TRIPHASIC COMBINATION TABLETS		
Enpresse, —, Trivora	Ethinyl estradiol 30	Levonorgestrel 0.05 (6 d)
	Ethinyl estradiol 40	Levonorgestrel 0.075 (5 d)
	Ethinyl estradiol 30	Levonorgestrel 0.125 (10 d)
Necon 7/7/7, Nortrel 7/7/7, Ortho-Novum 7/7/7	Ethinyl estradiol 35	Norethindrone 0.5 (7 d)
	Ethinyl estradiol 35	Norethindrone 0.75 (7 d)
	Ethinyl estradiol 35	Norethindrone 1 (7 d)
Aranelle, Tri-Norinyl	Ethinyl estradiol 35	Norethindrone 0.5 (7 d)
	Ethinyl estradiol 35	Norethindrone 1 (7 d)
	Ethinyl estradiol 35	Norethindrone 0.5 (7 d)
Tri-Previfem, Ortho Tri-Cyclen	Ethinyl estradiol 35	Norgestimate 0.18 (7 d)
	Ethinyl estradiol 35	Norgestimate 0.215 (7 d)
	Ethinyl estradiol 35	Norgestimate 0.25 (7 d)
Tilia Fe, TriLegest	Ethinyl estradiol 20	Norethindrone acetate 1 (5 d)
	Ethinyl estradiol 30	Norethindrone acetate 1 (7 d)
	Ethinyl estradiol 35	Norethindrone acetate 1 (9 d)

If all OCs are similar in effectiveness and well tolerated, then choosing among them may seem difficult. In general, using a **hormonal contraceptive** with the lowest dose while still offering cycle control is best. Many experienced practitioners have a few favorite formulations that they use in clinical practice; they only venture from these choices if a patient has a particular side effect that may be improved by switching to another formulation based on increasing or decreasing the dose of its component drugs. This is also a good place for new practitioners to start when becoming comfortable with contraceptive counseling and prescribing. A short list should include one preparation that does not contain **estrogen**, an ultra-low dose, or 20-mcg EE pill (e.g., to use for women older than 35 years of age or those who smoke more than 15 cigarettes per day), a monophasic COC, a multiphasic COC, and a nondaily administration method for women who have difficulty with daily regimens. One factor that may influence what is on the short list is the availability of samples or products for purchase at the clinical site. Another influence may be patient request for a particular brand-name product because of direct-consumer advertising practices of the drug companies. Additionally, the provider should be aware of what OCs are covered by the patient's insurance and what OCs are available on the $4 retail plans locally.

Cost

Cost can be a major barrier to contraceptive use for patients who do not have health insurance or prescription drug coverage. Most communities have county or private not-for-profit contraceptive centers with a sliding-scale fee schedule based on income to assist women without health insurance. The average cost for most forms of cyclical **hormonal contraception** is $30 to $70 per cycle. Generic substitutions at lower prices are now available for many formulations, including formulations on the $4 retail plans. The cost of **injectable contraception** could be higher because of the office visit required for administration.

The initial cost of an IUD insertion may prohibit this from being an easy choice, but the cost spread over the life of the device may be less than that of other forms. Not all drug prescription plans cover IUDs; some may require a co-payment that is more than that for a single prescription. Even for women who have prescription drug coverage, cost can be an issue. Many insurance companies have implemented two- or three-tier co-payment schedules, resulting in higher costs for the client if a drug is not on the first-line formulary. The insurance companies are to provide formulary information to patients and providers to assist in decision making.

Patient Variables

Differences in a woman's physiological and psychological responses to **estrogens** and **progestins** make choosing OCs more art than science. However, taking a thorough personal and family history, performing a complete physical examination, and performing screening laboratory tests appropriate for patient age will identify patients for whom OCs should not be prescribed. Patient variables that require withholding OCs or monitoring more closely are listed in Table 31–3.

The primary indication for using hormonal contraceptive preparations is to prevent pregnancy. These methods offer effectiveness and reversibility. In addition, users may experience the following noncontraceptive benefits (Hatcher et al, 2007).

- Decreased dysmenorrhea, menstrual irregularities, and menstrual blood loss
- Lessening of acne and hirsutism
- Fewer ovarian cysts
- Significantly reduced endometrial and ovarian cancer risk
- Lower incidence of benign breast conditions such as fibrocystic changes and fibroadenoma
- Reduced risk of hospitalization for gonorrheal pelvic inflammatory disease (PID)
- Suppression of endometriosis for women who do not currently desire pregnancy

Drug Variables

Drug Interactions

Hormonal contraception that is administered orally undergoes first-pass metabolism in the liver; therefore, drugs that induce liver enzymes will decrease their contraceptive efficacy. Agents that treat tuberculosis, **barbiturates**, **anticonvulsants**, and the herbal preparation St. John's wort have all been shown to increase liver

Table 31–3 **WHO Contraindications to Initiation of Combined Contraception with 35 mcg EE or Less**

Risk	Contraindication
WHO Category 2 Contraceptive benefits usually outweigh risks; may require more frequent monitoring	Age >40 yr
	Smoker <35 yr
	BMI >30 due to increased VTE risk
	Hx HTN during pregnancy, BP now normal
	Known hyperlipidemia
	First-degree relative with DVT/PE
	Major surgery without prolonged immobilization
	Superficial thrombophlebitis
	SLE on immunosuppressive therapy or with severe thrombocytopenia
	Sickle cell
	Valvular heart disease, uncomplicated
	Non-migraine headaches
	Migraine without neurological aura, age <35 yr
	Unexplained vaginal bleeding, suspicious for serious underlying condition
	Cervical intraepithelial neoplasia
	Cervical cancer, awaiting treatment
	Undiagnosed breast mass
	Diabetes, insulin dependent or non-insulin dependent, without vascular disease
	Asymptomatic gallbladder disease, or postcholecystectomy
	Benign focal nodular hyperplasia of the liver
	Hx of cholestasis in pregnancy
WHO Category 3 Risks usually outweigh contraceptive benefits	Postpartum <3 wk
	Age >35 yr and smoker <15 cigarettes/d
	Multiple risk factors for coronary artery disease (based on age, smoking, diabetes, hypertension)
	Hypertension, adequately controlled and monitored Systolic 140–159 or diastolic 90–99
	Migraine without neurological aura, age >35 yr
	Hx of breast cancer, no disease >5 yr
	Diabetic with nephropathy, neuropathy, retinopathy
	Diabetic with vascular disease

Table 31–3 **WHO Contraindications to Initiation of Combined Contraception with 35 mcg EE or Less—cont'd**

Risk	Contraindication
	Diabetic >20 yr Symptomatic gallbladder disease Past COC-related cholestasis
WHO Category 4 Unacceptable risk	Age >35 yr and smoker >15 cigarettes/d HTN, not controlled or with vascular disease Systolic ≥160 or diastolic ≥100 Current or hx of DVT/PE Major surgery with prolonged immobilization Known thrombogenic mutations Current or hx of ischemic heart disease Current or hx of stroke Valvular heart disease, complicated Migraine with neurological aura SLE with positive or unknown antiphospholipid antibodies Current breast cancer Active viral hepatitis Cirrhosis, severe/decompensated Benign hepatocellular adenoma or malignant liver tumor

BMI = body mass index; BP = blood pressure; COC= combined oral contraceptives; DVT/PE = deep venous thrombosis/pulmonary embolism; EE = ethinyl estradiol; Hx = history; HTN = hypertension; SLE = systemic lupus erythematosus; WHO = World Health Organization.

metabolism of OCs; irregular bleeding and a decrease in contraceptive effectiveness may occur (*Drug Facts and Comparisons*, 2009). Common broad-spectrum antibiotics have not been shown to decrease serum concentrations of OCs (Helms et al, 1997). **Penicillin** and **tetracycline** are known to alter steroid metabolism in the gut because of changes in intestinal flora; this may potentially reduce their absorption and effectiveness. Therefore, product labeling and *Drug Facts and Comparisons* (2009) still advise caution and the use of a backup method of contraception during and for 7 days after their use. However, both Hatcher and colleagues (2007) and Speroff and Darney (2005) agree that a backup method is not necessary.

Another area of concern has been the effect of OCs on laboratory values. Previous thyroid test methods were affected by protein binding, but the new TSH is not. Lipid levels (cholesterol, triglycerides, and high-density lipoprotein cholesterol) may be affected by OCs (Katzung, 2009). A baseline lipid profile should be performed in women who have a significant family history or other risk factors for cardiovascular disease.

Adverse Effects/Contraindications

Many studies have investigated the incidence of venous thromboembolism (VTE) in COC users. The incidence of VTE is low in young women, one to three cases per 10,000 per year. VTE risk is increased by two to five times in COC users without other significant risk factors. The increase in risk is attributable to the **estrogen** component of **COCs**, which influences clotting factors and is dose dependant. The incidence of VTE is extremely low; therefore, for any individual user this increase in risk still represents a very low chance of an adverse event. Risk factors such as inherited clotting disorders, strong family history of inherited clotting disorders, being older than 35 years, smoking more than 10 cigarettes per day, or obesity (body mass index [BMI] greater than 30) increase the risk three to ten times. Such factors illustrate the need for screening patients diligently by taking a detailed family history before prescribing hormonal contraception (Lidegaard, Edström, & Kreiner, 2002).

In a recent MEGA (multiple environmental and genetic assessment of risk factors for venous thrombosis) case-controlled study, van Hylckama Vlieg, Helmerhorst, Vandenbroucke, Dogen, and Rosendaal (2009) found that over all, the use of COCs increases the risk of DVTs 5-fold over that of nonusers. The data also showed a significant difference in odds ratios in formulations using different **progestins**, but all using low-dose **estrogens**. **Norethindrone** and **levonorgestrel** had the lowest odds ratios of 3.9 and 3.6, respectively, whereas the odds ratio for **norgestimate** was 5.9, **drospirenone** 6.3, and **desogestrel** 7.3. These are third and fourth generation **progestins** that allow greater estrogenic activity, thereby increasing the risk. The authors' conclusion is "the safest option with regard to the risk of venous thrombosis is an **oral contraceptive** containing **levonorgestrel** combined with a low dose of **estrogen**" (van Hylckama Vlieg et al, 2009, p. 7).

Other major, but rare, adverse effects can occur with **hormonal contraception**: cholestatic jaundice, benign hepatic neoplasms, myocardial infarction, stroke, and neurological migraines. Patients should be counseled about the symptoms associated with these events, and instructed to call their provider immediately if they experience them. Table 31–3 lists absolute and relative contraindications to **hormonal contraceptives** with 35 mcg of EE or less, as recommended by the World Health Organization (2009).

On The Horizon **DOSING OPTIONS**

Numerous studies are under way experimenting with various dosing schedules, not only for **COCs,** but also the patch and vaginal ring. The traditional monophasic 21/7 dosing schedule may soon be a thing of the past.

Dosing Regimens

Combined Contraceptives

Oral contraceptive pills are traditionally dispensed in packages containing 28 pills, with the first 21 pills containing active synthetic hormone; the last 7 pills contain inert ingredients (or **iron**), during which withdrawal bleeding occurs. Several brands are available containing only the 21 active pills; the user then takes no pill for 7 days, during which withdrawal bleeding occurs. **COCs** come in many different formulations. The primary difference between brand names is the type and dose of **progestin** used. Monophasic preparations use the same dose of **estrogen** and **progestin** for each of the active pills. Biphasic preparations vary the dose of **progestin**, with an increase in the amount of **progestin** in the latter half of the active pills; these are rarely used today. More popular today are triphasic preparations, which vary the dose of **estrogen**, **progestin**, or both.

Several products now offer extended menstrual cycling. **Seasonale**, which contains active pills for 84 days, with 7 days off, produces withdrawal bleeding once every 3 months. Two newer products, **Seasonique** and **LoSeasonique**, are classified as monophasic but contain 10 mcg of EE in the last week of one cycle of dosing. **Lybrel** uses a continuous cycle without any hormone-free weeks for 1 year. Although these are the only U.S. Food and Drug Administration (FDA) approved pills using an extended cycle dosing schedule, other monophasic pills may be used similarly to space or manipulate the timing of menstrual periods, using the active pills continuously with less frequent intervals of inert pills (*Drug Facts and Comparisons*, 2009). The newest dosing regimen is monophasic **COCs**, having 24 active and 4 nonactive pills per cycle. The Watson Pharmaceuticals chewable **OC** has 24 active, hormone-containing pills and 4 tablets of **ferrous fumarate** tablets. The goal is to have lighter and shorter withdrawal bleeds and to decrease breakthrough spotting (Shrader & Dickerson, 2008).

Starting Methods

COCs may be started in several different ways, each offering different advantages in the timing of starting the first and subsequent packs.

First Day Start. The first pill is taken on the first day of the menstrual cycle. No backup method is needed using this initiation method, as ovulation will be suppressed with the first cycle. Many pill packages include the ability to mark the start day to help the user keep track of pill taking, although for many pill packages Sunday is the default start day marked.

Sunday Start. The first pill is taken on the Sunday following the start of menses; a backup method is recommended for the first 7 days. Starting on Sunday may offer the user the convenience of having menses occur only during the week.

Quick Start. The first pill is taken on the day of the office visit; a backup method is recommended for the first 7 days. This method can be used if the clinician is reasonably sure that the user is not currently pregnant (Hatcher et al, 2007).

Side effect tolerance and compliance with daily pill taking are important factors in a woman's success with **oral contraception**. Missed pills occur much more frequently than either the user or prescriber realize. One study showed that 23 percent of women missed a pill the previous cycle; most were missed in the first week of the pack (Aubeny et al, 2002, 2004). Another study showed that 48 percent of women missed two or more pills in a 3-month period; the most common reasons were being away from home, forgetting, or not having a new pill available (Smith & Oakley, 2005). Helping the patient choose a time to take the pill when she is most likely going to be near the pill pack, and helping her to associate pill taking with another daily activity may help increase compliance. The patient should also be instructed on what to do if pills are missed. Table 31–4 gives instructions for what

CLINICAL PEARL

Multiphasic Pills

Triphasic pill packs with pills of various colors maybe confusing to some patients. If confusion is a concern, start with a monophasic **OC** for simple instructions.

CLINICAL PEARL

LMP Notation

Last menstrual period (LMP) should be considered a vital notation to be displayed at the top of each chart note in a patient's medical record.

Table 31–4 **Instructions for Missed Oral Contraceptives**

Missed 1 active pill	Take pill as soon as you remember, taking two pills in 1 d if missed pill was d prior	Use backup contraception for 7 d
Missed 2–4 active pills	Take two pills for 2–3 d	Use backup contraception for 7 d
Missed 5 or more active pills	Start new pack on next start day (e.g., Sunday for Sunday starters)	Use backup contraception until 7 d of active pills taken

to do about missed pills. Instructions are also found in the patient information included in each pill package (*Drug Facts and Comparisons,* 2009).

Side effects women experience may lead to discontinuation of OCs. Rosenberg and Waugh (1998) found that 50 percent of women who discontinue do so because of side effects, and many do so in the first 2 months. More recent studies found that discontinuation rates because of side effects are more in the range of 17 to 34 percent and access issues are the most common reasons for discontinuation (Frost, Singh, & Finer, 2007; Westhoff et al, 2007). The majority of the side effects resolve with continued use (Hatcher et al, 2007). Therefore, education about expected side effects, especially in new pill takers, may increase continuation rates.

Topical Patch

Ortho Evra is a topical patch that releases 20 mcg of EE and 150 mcg of **norelgestromin**, which is the primary active metabolite of **norgestimate**. **Norelgestromin** still undergoes liver metabolism; however, the resulting metabolite, **levonorgestrel**, is highly bound to sex hormone-binding globulin, limiting its biological impact (Speroff & Darney, 2005). The patch is applied once a week for 3 weeks, with one week being patch free, during which withdrawal bleeding occurs. Patch use should be initiated on the first day of menses; if it is started on any other day, a backup method should be used for 7 days. Patch location should be rotated with each patch change; it should be placed on skin that is clean and dry. It may be placed on the abdomen, upper torso, outer arm, or buttock. Side effect profiles for the patch are similar to **COCs**, with the exception of skin irritation, which may occur at the application site (*Drug Facts and Comparisons,* 2009). Efficacy studies indicate that women weighing more than 198 pounds may have an increased risk of failure; although the overall number of failures is low, a significant number occurred in this group (Zieman et al, 2002).

CLINICAL PEARL

New-User Spotting

Use conjugated **estrogen,** 1.25 mg or **estradiol,** 2 mg for 7 days in addition to **COCs** to stop spotting during active pills, and avoid changing to another OC brand.

Vaginal Rings

NuvaRing is a soft, flexible plastic ring that releases 15 mcg of EE and 120 mcg of **etonogestrel** daily. The ring is placed in the vagina, left in place for 3 weeks, and then removed for a week when withdrawal bleeding occurs. It does not require fitting by a provider and is easily placed by the user. In addition, it releases steady, low doses of hormones, which offer better cycle control in the form of decreased breakthrough bleeding when compared to OCs (Oddsson et al, 2005). The primary advantage is the convenience of once-monthly self-administration, which may be particularly useful for the patient who has difficulty remembering to take a pill daily.

Other features of this method are the lower systemic exposure to EE, which is approximately 50 percent of what is typically seen in COCs with 30 mcg of EE (Timmer & Mulders, 2000), and 30 percent of those levels measured with patch use (van den Heuvel, van Bragt, Alnabawy, & Kaptein, 2005). Despite lower systemic levels of EE, ovulation is completely suppressed (Mulders & Dieben, 2001). As with **COCs**, evidence indicates that serum concentrations of EE are not affected by concomitant use of **amoxicillin** or **doxycycline** (Dogterom, van den Heuvel, & Thomsen, 2005).

As with all **hormonal contraceptives**, neither **estrogens** nor **progestins** should be used by women who have medical conditions that preclude their use. Other possible contraindications to use of **NuvaRing** are in women who have significant pelvic prolapse (Hatcher et al, 2007).

Progesterone-Only Contraceptives

Progestin-Only Pills

Two brand-name **progestin**-only pills are currently available: **Micronor** and **Nor-QD**. Three generics also contain 0.35 mg **norethindrone**. These pills contain no **estrogen** and are primarily used with special populations in which **estrogen** is contraindicated because of medical conditions or breastfeeding. Because these pills contain very low levels of hormone, users need to be particularly diligent with accurate pill taking. The primary contraceptive effect is through thickening of cervical mucus and prevention of sperm penetration, which occurs 2 to 4 hours after administration, and diminishes after 22 hours of administration. If a pill is taken even a few hours late, a backup method is recommended for the following 48 hours. As with other progestin-only methods, common side effects are changes in bleeding patterns and breast tenderness (Speroff & Darney, 2005).

Injectable Progestins

Depot medroxyprogesterone acetate (DMPA), Depo-Provera, is a long-acting, injectable progestin-only contraceptive. One injection of 150 mg IM is effective at suppressing ovulation for 12 to 13 weeks. DMPA also thickens cervical mucus and atrophies the endometrium (Hatcher et al, 2007). In 2005, Pfizer released a 104-mg SQ dose of DMPA that offers a lower overall hormone dose with no change in efficacy, even in patients with a high BMI. SQ administration can be done by the user without an office visit (Jain et al, 2004).

Injection offers the advantage of dosing once every 12 weeks, with very reliable efficacy. User errors can occur if the patient does not return for doses within the prescribed time, although it is acceptable to give a repeat dose up to 1 week late without clinical assessment to exclude pregnancy. DMPA will change a woman's bleeding pattern, causing an increased number of days of spotting or amenorrhea. This side effect may be unacceptable for some users, and is the primary reason women discontinue use. Women in our society are socialized to believe that they need to have a monthly period. Patient education regarding expected bleeding pattern changes can increase acceptability of these changes and contribute to the patient's success with this method. Weight gain may also be of concern for some patients; average weight gain is several pounds per year of use. Users of DMPA may also have a delay of return to fertility, on average 9 to 10 months (Hatcher et al, 2007).

Before initiating Depo-Provera the provider should exclude the possibility that the patient is currently pregnant. If a client discovers that she is pregnant after the drug's administration, the intramuscular injection cannot be reversed. The drug can be started while the client is menstruating, or if the client has had two negative urine pregnancy tests spaced 2 weeks apart only if the client has not had unprotected intercourse during that time.

In 2004, the FDA issued a black box warning for Depo-Provera users in response to data showing a decrease in bone density with longer-term use. The warning states that it should not be used for more than 2 years consecutively if other alternatives are acceptable. Of particular concern is use in adolescents when bone accretion is still under way. Recommendations were made to assess bone density if women were to continue use for longer than 2 years (Omar, 2005). The black box warning applied to the lower SQ dose prior to published data. However, in a randomized 2-year study comparing IM DMPA with sub-Q DMPA the authors found similar to slightly less bone loss in the first two years of use (Kauntiz, Darney, Ross, Wolter, & Speroff, 2009). Increasingly, however, data suggest that most if not all of the bone mineral density changes are reversed after discontinuation of the drug (Kauntiz, Arias, & McClung, 2008) and that increasing calcium intake and stopping smoking can significantly modify bone loss (Rahman & Berenson, 2010).

Intrauterine Progestin

Mirena is an intrauterine device that releases 20 mcg of levonorgestrel daily and can be left in place for 5 years. The local release of progestin creates only small levels of systemic circulating hormone and incidence of systemic side effects is small. Mirena causes thickening of cervical mucus and endometrial atrophy, but has only a minimal effect on ovulation suppression. Changes in menstrual bleeding are common; many women experience a notable difference in menstrual flow or amenorrhea that may be more pronounced over time. Normal endometrial function typically returns within 1 to 3 months after discontinuation (Jensen, 2005).

Progestin Implants

Implanon provides contraception for up to 3 years and is the only implant currently available in the United States. It consists of one rod that contains 68 mg of etonogestrel, an active metabolite of desogestrel (Hatcher et al, 2007). Implanon has an overall serum progestin concentration that is lower than Norplant, which is no longer available in the United States, and has less variation (Speroff & Darney, 2005). Because it is only one rod, insertion and removal is simpler than Norplant.

Emergency Contraception

Emergency contraception (EC) is a term used to describe methods of pregnancy prevention after an episode of improperly protected intercourse. EC should be taken as soon as possible, within 72 hours, but may be initiated within 120 hours (5 days). Improperly protected intercourse may occur if no method of pregnancy prevention was used, if the method used failed (condom broke or slipped off; diaphragm/cap/sponge became dislodged), or if the method was used improperly (missed pills). Multiple COCs or a copper IUD may be used.

CLINICAL PEARL

Depo-Provera and Osteoporosis

Counsel patients using **Depo-Provera** to increase dietary calcium intake and weight-bearing exercise. These interventions along with stopping smoking will mitigate bone mineral density changes.

Other products are **Plan B** and **Next Choice** (two pills of 0.75-mg **levonorgestrel**), which are **progestin**-only products packaged specifically for use as EC. The use of high-dose **progestins** is more effective than using multiple **COCs** and is better tolerated. The traditional dosing is to take one tablet 12 hours apart, but taking both doses at the same time does not decrease efficacy and is easier to take (Speroff & Darney, 2005). Existing pregnancy is the only contraindication to EC use; therefore, a urine pregnancy test should be performed before EC use. Nausea and vomiting are the most common side effects; nonprescription **antiemetics** can be used for prevention or treatment of these effects (Trussell, Ellertson, Stewart, Raymond, & Shochet, 2004).

MONITORING

Traditionally, **hormonal contraception** is provided during an annual examination, consisting of detailed personal and family histories, blood pressure measurement, general physical examination, breast and pelvic examinations, Pap smear, and sexually transmitted infection (STI) screening. These are vital for evaluation of a woman's health; but blood pressure measurement and personal and family histories provide the clinically relevant information necessary to initiate **hormonal contraception** safely. Physical examination, breast examination, pelvic examination, and Pap smear may be deferred to facilitate access to **contraception** (Stewart et al, 2001).

Monitoring for the adverse effects of **OCs** should be done initially at 3 months, and then annually. Serious effects that could be caused by **OCs** include abnormal vaginal bleeding; hypertension; amenorrhea; unilateral numbness, weakness, or tingling, indicating possible cerebral spasm or occlusion; breast pain or mass; leg pain; chest pain; sudden loss of vision from possible thromboembolic phenomena; and jaundice (Hatcher et al, 2007).

In addition to screening for adverse drug effects, the provider should use these well-patient visits to screen for asymptomatic STIs and reinforce barrier protection for patients at risk for disease. Use of **tobacco** and **alcohol** are the two most common lifestyle habits that contribute to morbidity and mortality at all ages. Both have interaction effects on the organ systems of patients who use an OC. Patients with a chronic disease such as diabetes, seizure disorder, or migraine headache require more frequent monitoring visits based on their conditions.

> **CLINICAL PEARL**
>
> **Emergency Contraception**
>
> During each office visit, provide patients with an **emergency contraception** prescription and instructions for use in case their primary contraception method fails.

OUTCOME EVALUATION

Symptoms of serious adverse effects require immediate evaluation and discontinuation of **OCs** until the cause of the adverse symptom rules out OC etiology. Symptoms that can be handled less urgently are irregular vaginal bleeding, amenorrhea, and mild-to-moderate blood pressure elevation. Breakthrough bleeding frequently occurs in the initial cycles of use of any **OC** formulation, is most common in the first three cycles, and usually resolves with continued use. If the patient has not missed any doses, reassure her that breakthrough bleeding has not been associated with reduced efficacy. Some women may experience breakthrough bleeding after longer use; this is due to the decidualization and fragility of the endometrium, which is a progestational effect. Stopping the dosing regimen is unnecessary while resolving the problem. Use 1.25 mg conjugated **estrogens** or 2 mg **estradiol** for 7 days no matter where in the cycle spotting occurs. If this treatment is not effective, schedule an examination to rule out infection or other pathological causes. Amenorrhea is a common concern that may result after several months or years of OC use. **Progestins** atrophy the endometrium, and some women welcome scanty or no menses. Amenorrhea caused by **DMPA** may be a result of low **estrogen** levels (less than 30 pg) (Speroff & Darney, 2005). For many women, no monthly cycle produces anxiety, which is usually relieved by a negative pregnancy test.

> **CLINICAL PEARL**
>
> **Report of Bleeding**
>
> Patient reports of irregular or abnormal bleeding should be quantified with a menstrual calendar; have the patient differentiate between days on which spotting occurs and days on which bleeding is as heavy as her menses. Keeping a count of sanitary napkins or tampons used per day of bleeding may help further quantify bleeding. Bleeding may be excessive if a patient is using tampons and pads together and experiencing bleeding accidents. Serial hematocrit measurement several days or a week apart may assist in evaluating excessive bleeding. Excessive bleeding should be evaluated for underlying etiology such as uterine cancer or polyps, thyroid disorders, or bleeding dyscrasias (Hatcher et al, 2007).

PHARMACOLOGICAL CONTRACEPTION RELATED TO THE OVERALL TREATMENT PLAN/PHYSIOLOGICAL PROCESS

PATIENT EDUCATION

- Physiology of normal menstrual cycle.
- Need for follow-up visits: BP monitoring 3 months after initiation of methods containing **estrogen,** then annually. Annual breast and pelvic examinations, with annual Pap smears starting 3 years after sexual debut, or at age 21.
- Monthly breast self-examination beginning age 20.
- Safe-sex practices, including male or female condom use in conjunction with hormonal contraception for STI prevention.
- Emergency contraception access and use, which can be used with failures of all methods.

Specific to the Drug Therapy

- How contraceptives prevent pregnancy through suppression of ovulation in the hypothalamic-pituitary-ovarian axis or endometrial and cervical changes.
- Doses and schedules for taking the drug. Specifically start method, active vs. inactive pills, when to expect menses, what to do if pills are missed, suggestions for optimizing compliance with dosing schedule.
- Anticipated menstrual changes because of method use, such as lighter or shorter menses, amenorrhea, or irregular bleeding patterns.
- Common side effects with method use, such as breakthrough bleeding in first few cycles of **OC** use, breast tenderness, nausea, possible weight changes.
- Serious side effects, their symptoms, and how to access care in an emergency.
- Interactions between hormonal contraception and other treatment modalities or lifestyle habits. Emphasize the dangers of smoking with combined hormonal contraception at any age, and the increased risk in women over age 35. Also advise patients to stop combined hormonal contraception 4 weeks before and 2 weeks after major surgery to prevent thrombus formation.
- Review time frame for return to fertility after discontinuation for specific method.

Reasons for Taking the Drug(s)

Hormonal contraception offers very high efficacy; this may be particularly important for women between 15 and 35 years of age when fertility is highest. Use of methods can be used for long- or short-term deferment of childbearing, allowing control over timing and spacing of pregnancies.

Drugs as Part of the Total Treatment Regimen

- Women who use hormonal contraception may also enjoy noncontraceptive benefits such as less menstrual discomfort or lighter flow, and the ability to predict or manipulate timing of menses for vacation or other social events.
- Use of hormonal contraception also confers protection against uterine and ovarian cancer (Speroff & Darney, 2005).

Adherence Issues

- Noncompliance with pill taking occurs frequently for a variety of reasons (Aubeny et al, 2002, 2004).
- Access to clinic appointments and prescription refills is one of the reasons for gaps in **OC** use. If medically indicated, give the patient a full year of refills.
- Counseling, education, and use of written materials can increase a patient's success with any method. Thorough patient education is the cornerstone of contraceptive success.
- The following are most important for patients taking **OCs**—they should take a pill every day in the correct order, and they should never just stop. If there are questions or concerns, they should always call the clinic first.

REFERENCES

Aubeny, E., Buhler, M., Colau, J. C., Vicaut, E., Zadikian, M., & Childs, M. (2002). Oral contraception: Patterns of non-compliance. The Coraliance study. *European Journal of Contraception & Reproductive Health Care, 7*(3), 155–161.

Aubeny, E., Buhler, M., Colau, J. C., Vicaut, E., Zadikian, M., & Childs, M. (2004). The coraliance study: Non-compliant behavior. Results after a 6-month follow-up of patients on oral contraceptives. *European Journal of Contraception & Reproductive Health Care, 9,* 267–277. doi: 10.1080/13625180400017776

Dogterom, P., van den Heuvel, M. W., & Thomsen, T. (2005). Absence of pharmacokinetic interactions of the combined contraceptive vaginal ring NuvaRing with oral amoxicillin or doxycycline in two randomised trials. *Clinical Pharmacokinetics, 44*(4), 429–438.

Drug facts and comparisons. (2009). St. Louis, MO: Wolters Kluwer Health.

Finer, L. B., & Henshaw, S. K. (2006). Disparities in rates of unintended pregnancy in the United States, 1994 and 2001. *Perspectives on Sexual*

and Reproductive Health, 38(2), 90–96. Retrieved from http://www.guttmacher.org/pubs/psrh/full/3809006.pdf
Frost, J. J., Singh, S., & Finer, L. B. (2007). U.S. women's one-year contraceptive use patterns, 2004. *Perspectives on Sexual and Reproductive Health, 39*(1), 48–55. doi: 10.1363/3904807
Hatcher, R. A., Trussell, J., Nelson, A. L., Cates, W., Jr., Stewart, F. H., & Kowal, D. (2007). *Contraceptive technology* (19th ed.). New York: Ardent Media.
Helms, S. E., Bredle, D. L., Zajic, J., Jarjoura, D., Brodell, R. T., & Krishnarao, I. (1997). Oral contraceptive failure rates and oral antibiotics. *Journal of the American Academy of Dermatology, 36*(5 Pt. 1), 705–710.
Jain, J., Dutton, C., Nicosia, A., Wajszczuk, C., Bode, F. R., & Mishell, D. R. (2004). Pharmacokinetics, ovulation suppression and return to ovulation following a lower dose subcutaneous formulation of Depo-Provera. *Contraception, 70*(1), 11–18.
Jensen, J. T. (2005). Contraceptive and therapeutic effects of the levonorgestrel intrauterine system: An overview. *Obstetrical Gynecological Survey, 60*(9), 604–612.
Kahlenborn, C., Modugno, F., Potter, D. M., & Severs, W. P. (2006). Oral contraceptive use as a risk factor for premenopausal breast cancer: A meta-analysis. *Mayo Clinic Proceedings, 81*(10), 1290–1302.
Katzung, B. G. (2009). *Basic & clinical pharmacology* (11th ed.). New York: McGraw-Hill.
Kaunitz, A. M., Arias, R., & McClung, M. (2008). Bone density recovery after depot medroxyprogesterone acetate injectable contraception use. *Contraception, 77*, 67–76. doi: 10.1016/j.contraception.2007.10.005
Kaunitz, A. M., Darney, P. D., Ross, D., Wolter, K. D., & Speroff, L. (2009). Subcutaneous DMPA vs. intramuscular DMPA: A 2-year randomized study of contraceptive efficacy and bone mineral density. *Contraception, 80*, 7–17. doi: 10.1016/j.contraception.2009.02.005
Lidegaard, Ø., Edström, B., & Kreiner, S. (2002). Oral contraceptives and venous thromboembolism: A five-year national case-control study. *Contraception, 65*(3), 187–196.
Marchbanks, P. A., McDonald, J. A., Wilson, H. G., Folger, S. G., Mandel, M. G., Daling, J. D., et al. (2002). Oral contraceptives and the risk of breast cancer. *New England Journal of Medicine, 346*(26), 2025–2032.
Mulders, T. M., & Dieben, T. O. (2001). Use of the novel combined contraceptive vaginal ring NuvaRing for ovulation inhibition. *Fertility and Sterility, 75*(5), 865–870.
Oddsson, K., Leifels-Fischer, B., de Melo, N. R., Wiel-Masson, D., Benedetto, C., Verhoeven, C. H., et al. (2005). Efficacy and safety of a contraceptive vaginal ring (NuvaRing) compared with a combined oral contraceptive: A 1-year randomized trial. *Contraception, 71*(3), 176–182.
Omar, H. (2005). Depot medroxyprogesterone acetate (DMPA, Depo-Provera) in adolescents: What is next after the FDA black box warning. *Journal of Pediatric and Adolescent Gynecology, 18*(3), 183–188.
Rahman, M., & Berenson, A. B. (2010). Predictors of higher bone mineral density loss and use of depot medroxyprogesterone acetate. *Obstetrics & Gynecology, 115*(1), 35–40. doi: 10.1097/AOG.0b013e3181c4e864
Rosenberg, M. J., & Waugh, M. S. (1998). Oral contraceptive discontinuation: A prospective evaluation of frequency and reasons. *American Journal of Obstetrics and Gynecology, 179*(3 Pt. 1), 577–582.
Shrader, S. P., & Dickerson, L. M. (2008). Extended- and continuous-cycle oral contraceptives. *Pharmacotherapy, 28*(8), 1033–1040. doi: 10.1592/phco.28.8.1033
Smith, J. D., & Oakley, D. (2005). Why do women miss oral contraceptive pills? An analysis of women's self-described reasons for missed pills. *Journal of Midwifery & Women's Health, 50*(5), 380–385.
Speroff, L., & Darney, P. D. (2005). *A clinical guide for contraception* (4th ed.). Philadelphia: Lippincott Williams & Wilkins.
Stewart, F. H., Harper, C. C., Ellertson, C. E., Grimes, D. A., Sawaya, G. F., & Trussell, J. (2001). Clinical breast and pelvic examination requirements for hormonal contraception: Current practice vs evidence. *Journal of the American Medical Association, 285*(17), 2232–2239.
Timmer, C. J., & Mulders, T. M. (2000). Pharmacokinetics of etonogestrel and ethinylestradiol released from a combined contraceptive vaginal ring. *Clinical Pharmacokinetics, 39*(3), 233–242.
Trussell, J., Ellertson, C., Stewart, F., Raymond, E. G., & Shochet, T. (2004). The role of emergency contraception. *American Journal of Obstetrics and Gynecology, 190*(Suppl. 4), S30–S38.
van den Heuvel, M. W., van Bragt, A. J., Alnabawy, A. K., & Kaptein, M. C. (2005). Comparison of ethinylestradiol pharmacokinetics in three hormonal contraceptive formulations: The vaginal ring, the transdermal patch and an oral contraceptive. *Contraception, 72*(3), 168–174.
van Hylckama Vlieg, A., Helmerhorst, F. M., Vandenbroucke, J. P., Doggen, C. J. M., & Rosendaal, F. R. (2009). The venous thrombotic risk of oral contraceptives, effects of estrogen dose and progestogen type: Results of the MEGA case-control study. *British Medical Journal*, 339:b2921. doi: 10.1136/bmj.b2921
Westhoff, C. L., Heartwell, S., Edwards, S., Zieman, M., Stuart, G., Cwiak, C., et al. (2007). Oral contraceptive discontinuation: Do side effects matter? *American Journal of Obstetrics & Gynecology, 196*, 412.e1–412.e7. doi: 10.1016/j.ajog.2006.12.015
World Health Organization (WHO). (2009). *Medical eligibility criteria for contraceptive use* (4th ed.). Geneva, Switzerland: Author.
Zieman, M., Guillebaud, J., Weisberg, E., Shangold, G. A., Fisher, A. C., & Creasy, G. W. (2002). Contraceptive efficacy and cycle control with the Ortho Evra/Evra transdermal system: The analysis of pooled data. *Fertility and Sterility, 77*(2 Suppl. 2), S13.

CHAPTER 32

DERMATOLOGICAL CONDITIONS

Teri Moser Woo

Chapter Outline

The skin is the body's largest organ, and it is uniquely accessible for diagnosis and treatment. Primary care providers see patients with dermatological problems on a daily basis, with skin-related problems accounting for 9 percent of clinic visits.

The most common dermatological diagnosis reported in National Ambulatory Medical Care Survey, 1993–2005, is dermatitis (13 million office visits per year), with skin and soft tissues infections diagnosed at 6.3 million visits per year (Pallin, Espinola, Leung, Hooper, & Camargo, 2009). This chapter addresses the pharmacological management of common dermatological conditions seen in primary care. Accurate diagnosis of the condition is assumed.

DERMATITIS

Eczema (atopic dermatitis), contact dermatitis, diaper dermatitis, and seborrheic dermatitis are four common forms of dermatitis seen in primary care.

Eczema is a chronic skin disorder that affects all ages. It often begins in infancy and affects 10 to 15 percent of children. It may resolve during puberty, only to recur in adolescence or adulthood. The pattern of rash with eczema varies with age. Infants have the rash on the face, scalp, trunk, and the extensor surface of the extremities. In infants, the rash is usually acute or subacute, red, and vesicular. Eczema in adolescents and adults is usually chronic, with scaling, dryness, and lichenification on the flexure surfaces of the extremities, face, neck, hands, and upper chest. Eczema tends to worsen during the winter months.

Contact dermatitis is an acute inflammatory reaction of the skin to an irritant or allergen. It can be differentiated from eczema because it is generally not chronic or recurring and is usually distributed on exposed skin.

Diaper dermatitis (diaper rash) can occur in any patient who is incontinent and uses an occlusive barrier type of garment or diaper; however, it is most commonly seen in infants and toddlers.

Seborrheic dermatitis is a common inflammatory dermatitis characterized by erythematous, eczematous patches with yellow, greasy scale. It is usually localized to hairy areas and to areas with high concentrations of sebaceous glands. It can be found on the forehead, eyebrows, nasolabial folds, ear canals, neck, chest, intertriginous areas, the diaper or groin area, and intergluteal fold. In infants younger than 6 months, the scaling on the scalp without inflammation is commonly called cradle cap, and in adolescents and adults it is called dandruff.

Pathophysiology

Eczema

The exact etiology of eczema is unknown. Patients with eczema have high immunoglobulin E (IgE) antibody levels, but an exact immune cause has not been proved. A predisposition to pruritus and a reduced threshold of irritant responsiveness are believed to be key elements. Pruritus leads to increased scratching, which increases skin trauma, leading to increased itching (itch-scratch-itch cycle). Stroking the skin causes an abnormal reaction of dermatographism, a white line.

A high correlation exists between eczema and other atopic diseases, with 50 to 80 percent of children with eczema later developing asthma, allergic rhinitis, or hay fever. Often a positive family history for allergic disorders or asthma exists as well.

Contact Dermatitis

Contact dermatitis has two types: irritant and allergic. Both are usually confined to the point of contact with the irritant or allergen. This contact usually produces erythema, papules, and/or vesicles.

Irritant contact dermatitis is caused by contact of the skin with an irritating substance. The effect may be mild to severe. Irritating substances can be acid or alkali, solvents, or detergents. There is no immunological response as part of the inflammatory response in irritant contact dermatitis.

Allergic contact dermatitis is a delayed hypersensitivity response to an allergen. The allergen can be a variety of items in the environment, usually a small-molecular-weight substance that binds to the proteinaceous components of the skin to form a sensitizing antigen. Sensitization to the substance or allergen takes 10 to 14 days to develop after the first exposure. Dermatitis occurs within 1 to 7 days of subsequent exposure to the allergen. The most common allergens causing allergic contact dermatitis are certain plants (poison oak, ivy, and sumac), metals (especially in snaps, zippers, and jewelry), clothing (wool), cosmetics (fragrance or preservatives), topical medications (neomycin, anesthetics such as benzocaine, topical antihistamine), hair dyes, and soaps. Avoidance usually prevents the allergic response.

Diaper Dermatitis

Diaper dermatitis is an inflammatory disorder of the skin caused by a breakdown of the skin's natural barrier in the perineal or "diaper" area. The rash is often striking for its clear borders that coincide with the borders of the diaper or protective undergarment.

Forms of diaper dermatitis include irritant dermatitis, caused by chemical or mechanical irritation. Chemical irritation is caused by contact with urine and feces. Mechanical irritation is due to chafing of the diaper or undergarment on the skin folds. If the irritant dermatitis becomes chronic, the skin may appear dry. The rash may become more generalized and inflammatory, involving the creases and all the area that the diaper covers. The skin can become ulcerated or eroded with chronic irritation.

Infectious dermatitis may be caused by *Candida albicans* (candidiasis) and is usually a superinfection that can occur after a patient has had irritant dermatitis in the diaper area for 3 to 5 days. Candidiasis is suspected when there is a beefy red confluent rash with satellite lesions that are either red papules or pustules.

Other forms of diaper dermatitis include seborrheic dermatitis, psoriasiform napkin dermatitis, and atopic dermatitis. These disorders in the diaper area are treated the same as dermatitis on other parts of the body.

Seborrheic Dermatitis

The exact cause of seborrheic dermatitis is unknown. It is possibly related to increased production of sebum or an abnormal lipid composition of sebum. Seborrheic dermatitis is rare in children older than 6 to 12 months and in those who are prepubertal because the sebaceous glands are involuted and dormant during this time and become active again with puberty. Saprophytic *Malassezia* colonizes the skin of many patients with seborrhea, with the inflammation of seborrhea thought to be a host response to the fungal infection (Weston & Howe, 2010).

Goals of Treatment

With all forms of dermatitis, the primary goals are to decrease the inflammation and discomfort caused by the dermatitis.

Rational Drug Selection

With all forms of dermatitis, rational drug selection is based first on decreasing the symptoms of an acute exacerbation and then on preventing, decreasing, and/or controlling the frequency and severity of further exacerbations.

Eczema

Acute Exacerbations

Topical Corticosteroids

Topical corticosteroids are adrenocorticosteroid derivatives incorporated into a vehicle suitable for application to the skin. The anti-inflammatory effect of **topical steroids** is nonspecific and acts against most causes of inflammation. At the cellular level, they appear to inhibit the formation, release, and activity of the endogenous mediations of inflammation. When applied to inflamed skin, steroids inhibit the migration of macrophages and leukocytes into the area by reversing vascular dilation and permeability. This decreases edema, erythema, and pruritus.

Variable amounts of the drug are absorbed through the skin, depending on the drug used, the vehicle used, the amount of skin surface area the medication is applied to, and the condition of the skin. Absorption is enhanced by increased skin temperature, hydration, and application to denuded areas, intertriginous areas, or skin surfaces with thin stratum corneum layer (face or scrotum). Occlusive dressings enhance skin penetration and therefore increase drug absorption. Infants and children have a higher proportion of body surface area to body weight, and therefore they absorb proportionally more medication. Following topical administration, **corticosteroids** enter the bloodstream and are metabolized and excreted the same as **systemic steroids**. Therefore, in infants and young children, the lowest effective strength of topical steroid is used to prevent systemic corticosteroid effects. **Topical corticosteroids** are Pregnancy Category C. In pregnant patients, do not use **corticosteroids** extensively, for long periods, or in large amounts. Many topical **steroids** have been relabeled in the past few years due to newer studies indicating many formulations cause hypothalamic-pituitary-adrenal (HPA) axis suppression in children, providers need to stay current with labeling changes which may be found at the U.S. Food and Drug Administration (FDA) Web site, http://www.fda.gov.

The penetration of the **topical steroid** varies with the medication's vehicle. Ointments are more occlusive and usually more potent, and are good for scaly areas. Creams are less occlusive and usually less potent. Lotions are usually the least potent and contain the most water. Table 32–1 presents the common **topical steroids** used for eczema. The potency of any **steroid** can be increased approximately tenfold by occlusion with plastic wrap. Therefore, to increase the effects of a **steroid**, apply an occlusive dressing over the area. Do not use occlusive dressings more than 12 hours per day, or systemic steroid effects may occur. In young children, occlusive dressings are rarely used. A diaper is considered occlusive, and **steroid** use should be avoided in the diaper area unless a low-potency **steroid** is needed for short periods (e.g., 2 d).

There are many **topical steroid** preparations available, and it is impossible for any practitioner to be familiar with all of them. Familiarity with one or two agents in each category is reasonable. The most commonly used low-potency **topical steroid** is 1 percent **hydrocortisone**. Intermediate-potency topical steroids include **hydrocortisone butyrate** 0.1 percent (**Locoid**) and **triamcinolone acetonide** 0.1 percent (**Kenalog**). High-potency steroids include **betamethasone dipropionate**, augmented 0.05 percent (**Diprolene lotion, Diprolene AF**), and **triamcinolone acetonide** 0.5 percent (**Kenalog**). Super high potency topical steroids include **betamethasone dipropionate**, augmented 0.05 percent (**Diprolene** ointment or gel), and **halobetasol propionate** 0.05 percent (**Ultravate**). Providers need to know what medications are allowed from each category in the formulary or formularies they are using.

Oral Corticosteroids

Oral corticosteroids are occasionally used to treat severe eczema. Patients with eczema who receive **oral corticosteroids** for another disease, such as asthma, see a striking improvement in their skin. Improvement in acute exacerbations is often dramatic, a mixed blessing in the treatment of this chronic illness. Patients often feel so good that they may have the false impression that the steroids "cured" their eczema. Given the major adverse effects observed with prolonged or frequently repeated **corticosteroid** therapy, routine use of **oral steroids** for eczema is contraindicated. If oral **steroid** therapy for severe eczema is considered, consultation with a dermatology specialist is indicated. A patient who is using **oral steroids** must understand that the effects are short-term and that **oral steroid** preparations cannot be used frequently. When the oral preparation is started, patients must be started on a comprehensive prevention routine to prevent severe exacerbations. They need to be warned that their eczema will return after the steroid effect wears off.

Immunomodulators

The **immunomodulators** are a class of topical medications used in the short-term or intermittent long-term treatment of atopic dermatitis. **Pimecrolimus (Elidel)** and **tacrolimus (Protopic)** are a second line therapy after **topical corticosteroid** treatment failure for atopic dermatitis. They act by interrupting the inflammatory process. **Tacrolimus** has been found to inhibit T cells, Langerhans cells, mast cells, and keratinocytes in the epidermal cells. **Pimecrolimus** was specifically developed to treat inflammatory skin conditions; it inhibits the release of inflammatory cytokines and mediators from mast cells. The **immunomodulator** cream is chosen based on the severity of the eczema; **tacrolimus (Protopic)** is prescribed for moderate to severe eczema and **pimecrolimus (Elidel)** is prescribed for mild to moderate eczema. Neither product is to be used in children younger than 2 years, in immunocompromised patients, or in pregnant or lactating women (Pregnancy Category C). The **immunomodulators** have no steroid effects.

The **immunomodulator** creams are applied twice a day to the affected area(s). Patients are to be instructed not to occlude the area. It may take 2 to 3 weeks for patients to notice improvement. Providers need to reexamine patients every 6 weeks. If using **tacrolimus (Protopic)** in children aged 2 to 15 years the 0.03 percent strength should be prescribed. See Table 32–1 for full prescribing information.

Both **pimecrolimus** and **tacrolimus** have received a FDA black box warning regarding the long-term safely of topical immunosuppressant calcineurin inhibitors due to rare cases of malignancy (skin and lymphoma) have been reported in patients using the topical forms of these medications. The FDA advisory states the following: "Animal studies have shown that three different species of animals developed cancer following exposure to these drugs applied topically or given by mouth, including mice, rats, and a recent study of monkeys" (U.S. Food and Drug Administration, 2005).

Antipruritics

Antipruritics are used to control the itching associated with eczema and to break the itch-scratch-itch cycle. Commonly used oral agents are the antihistamines **diphenhydramine (Benadryl)** and **hydroxyzine (Atarax)**. These drugs have antipruritic and sedative actions. Pruritus can disrupt sleep; therefore, mild sedation can be helpful to prevent nocturnal itching, especially in children. **Cetirizine (Zyrtec)**, a metabolite of **hydroxyzine** without its sedative effects, can be used during the day to achieve an antipruritic effect without sedation. Another **antipruritic** is the tricyclic compound **doxepin (Sinequan)**, which has potent histamine$_1$- and histamine$_2$-blocking action.

Topical **antipruritics** can be used and should be considered if severe pruritus is present. **Doxepin cream (Zonalon)** can be used for moderate to severe pruritus associated with eczema. Care should be taken when prescribing **doxepin** for topical use because significant amounts can be absorbed systemically if it is used over 10 percent of the body surface area or if used for a long time. Drowsiness occurs in more than 20 percent of patients using **doxepin** cream, especially if it is used on more than 10 percent of body surface area.

Available topical **antipruritics** that are safer to use than **doxepin** are **Aveeno** cream (colloidal oatmeal-based) and **Moisturel** emollient cream or lotion **(petrolatum, glycerine based)**. These over-the-counter (OTC) agents can be used liberally on large surface areas with no harmful effects.

Emollients

Emollients play a key role in both acute exacerbations of eczema and in long-term therapy. Wet dressings and emollients can be used to soothe the skin, reduce redness, and treat pruritus caused by eczema (Weston & Howe, 2010). **Emollients** are applied to the skin and a wet cotton dressing applied; then the dressing is covered with dry cloths or clothing. This can be done nightly to decrease pruritus and redness.

The use of **emollients** is further discussed in the Long-Term Therapy section.

Antibiotics

Antibiotics may be necessary to treat secondary infections of *Staphylococcus aureus*, beta-hemolytic streptococci, a virus, or a fungus. If a bacterial infection is suspected, a culture should be obtained prior to beginning treatment. The likelihood of community-acquired methicillin-resistant *S. aureus* (MRSA) needs to be considered. For a patient with a localized infection, **mupirocin** ointment can be used. Most infected eczema will require treatment with an **oral antibiotic** that is effective against *S. aureus* and streptococci. **Cephalexin (Keflex), amoxicillin/ clavulanate (Augmentin)**, and **cefprozil (Cefzil)** are all effective; treatment should be for 7 to 10 days. If there is recurrent bacterial infection, a 3-week course of treatment is necessary.

Long-Term Therapy

Eczema is a chronic disorder, and the patient often cycles between mild to moderate dry skin and exacerbations that can be mild to severe. Once an exacerbation quiets, patients must continue to care for their skin to prevent further exacerbations. The keys to long-term therapy are adequate hydration of the skin and avoidance of agents that cause exacerbations.

Emollients

Moisturizers, lubricants, and **emollients** help retain water in the skin. They are composed of petrolatum, lanolin, or other agents such as colloidal oatmeal in an emulsion. The **emollient** is applied one to four times per day after patients bathe. They pat their skin dry and then apply the lotion or cream liberally to all affected areas within 3 minutes after bathing. This procedure traps the moisture in the skin. Ointments provide the most occlusive barrier; creams are the next best option. Lotions offer the convenience of easy application over large areas of skin but are not as occlusive as ointments and creams. Patients often decrease their use of **emollients** between exacerbations, and a review and reinforcement of their use during each clinic visit will increase compliance.

Of all the **emollient** products available, many are eliminated because they have additives such as perfumes or other chemicals, to which many patients with eczema are sensitive. Commonly used **emollients** are Aveeno cream or lotion, **Eucerin** cream or lotion, **Lubriderm** lotion, and **Moisturel** lotion. If the patient uses a lotion, make sure it does not contain alcohol, which is drying and irritating. Occasionally, patients are sensitive to the lanolin in **Eucerin**, which is a natural product derived from sheep's wool. Because large amounts are needed to be effective, expense can play a role in choosing an **emollient. White petrolatum** is inexpensive and a treatment option for patients with limited resources.

Nonpharmacological Measures

Nonpharmacological measures include hydrating baths and avoiding skin irritation and offending agents that cause exacerbations. Patients should be told to wear plastic or nitrile gloves when their hands may be exposed to harsh chemicals or detergents. They should avoid irritating fabrics such as wool. Soft cotton clothing allows the skin to breathe. Careful avoidance of perfumed lotions and soaps prevents flare-ups related to the additives in these products. Some patients have food sensitivities that exacerbate their eczema.

Baths are used to hydrate the skin. The patient should take a warm—not hot—bath for 20 minutes. The skin is patted dry, and emollients are applied immediately to maintain the skin's hydration. The patient should use a mild soap for cleansing the groin and axillae, not harsh deodorant soaps. After a bath is also a good time to apply corticosteroid creams or ointments, if needed.

Contact Dermatitis

The treatment for both types of contact dermatitis is the same. If a small area of skin is affected, a **topical corticosteroid** cream is usually effective. If more than 10 percent of the skin surface must be treated or if the allergic contact dermatitis is severe, oral corticosteroids are used. Wet dressings or baths are soothing to the inflamed skin. Oral **antihistamines** may help control pruritus.

Topical Corticosteroids

Topical **corticosteroid** creams or ointments are effective in treating mild to moderate contact dermatitis. A low-potency (**hydrocortisone** 1% or 2.5% cream) or intermediate-potency (**hydrocortisone valerate** 0.2% or **triamcinolone acetonide** 0.1%) cream can be used. Intermediate or high-potency **corticosteroids** should be used for plant dermatitis from poison ivy or oak (Prok & McGovern, 2010). See Table 32–1 for prescribing information. The patient should begin to experience relief in 2 to 3 days, with complete healing in 2 to 3 weeks.

Oral Corticosteroids

Oral **corticosteroids** (**prednisone** or **methylprednisolone**) are used if the contact dermatitis is severe or if a large skin surface area is involved. A 2- to 3-week course of therapy may be needed for severe cases, with 2 weeks usually the minimum length of therapy required for severe poison oak or ivy dermatitis. A too short course, such as the 6-day course in a **Medrol dose** pack, may lead to rebound dermatitis when treating poison oak or ivy dermatitis (Prok & McGovern, 2010). See Table 32–1 for prescribing information.

> **CLINICAL PEARL**
>
> **Dermatitis**
>
> - Occluding the surface with plastic wrap will increase penetration of the **topical corticosteroid.** Do not do this in children, as it will increase the systemic absorption of the **steroid.**
> - For contact dermatitis, caution the patient using bath oils against slipping in the tub. Children should be supervised at all times when using bath dermatologicals, which can all cause the tub to be slippery. Older adults should also be monitored.
> - For the patient with hand dermatitis, wearing cotton gloves overnight after applying a thick layer of **emollient** will increase absorption, and the patient will often see a significant improvement overnight.

Wet Dressings or Baths

Wet dressings or baths provide comfort. **Aluminum acetate solution (Burow's, Domeboro)** is an astringent wet dressing applied for 30 minutes four times a day for relief of inflammation associated with contact dermatitis. **Emollient** baths that contain colloidal oatmeal solids (**Aveeno**) or oils (**Alpha Keri Bath Oil, Lubriderm Bath Oil**) can be used to provide relief from pruritus associated with contact dermatitis. Baths may be used as needed for comfort.

Diaper Dermatitis

Drug therapy in the treatment of diaper dermatitis is aimed at protecting the skin, decreasing inflammation, and treating *Candida* infection. Nonpharmacological interventions are also used to prevent irritant diaper dermatitis.

Barrier Medications

Barrier medications are used to protect the skin from the irritant effects of contact with urine and feces. Plain **white petrolatum** is an effective and inexpensive barrier agent. Vitamins A and D are added to petrolatum to create a barrier OTC medication, **A&D Ointment. Zinc oxide** is a commonly used barrier that has a drying effect as well. It is combined with a variety of other agents such as petrolatum (**Diprotex, Diaparene, Bottom Better**), **cod liver oil** and **talc** (**Desitin**), and **balsam of Peru** (**Balmex**), which is thought to promote wound healing. Plain **zinc oxide** is an effective barrier that is less expensive than the many diaper rash products. Barrier medications should be used at the first sign of irritation.

Anti-Inflammatory Medications

Anti-inflammatory medications are used to decrease the inflammation associated with diaper dermatitis. Because of the occlusive nature of diapers and undergarments, a low-dose **hydrocortisone** (0.5% or 1%) should be used for a brief period. Low-dose **hydrocortisone** can be used for 2 to 3 days in the diaper area safely if it is applied sparingly (pea-sized amount) and used two to three times a day. Stronger **corticosteroid** preparations or combination medications containing midpotency **steroids** with an **antifungal** (**Lotrisone**) should not be used in the diaper area.

Antifungal Medications

Candidiasis is treated with a topical antifungal agent that is effective against *C. albicans*. Commonly used medications are **nystatin** (**Mycostatin**), **miconazole** (**Monistat-Derm**), and **clotrimazole** (**Lotrimin**). All of these medications are applied twice daily until the *Candida* infection is clear. **Miconazole** and **clotrimazole** are available OTC and are usually not covered by insurance plans. **Nystatin** is available by prescription only and is usually covered by insurance. If a patient does not respond to the OTC products, a trial of **nystatin** is warranted.

Wet Soaks

Wet soaks or sitz baths are used to decrease inflammation and provide comfort from diaper dermatitis. **Burow's solution** soaks or compresses can be used if the rash is weepy. Commercial diaper wipes often contain alcohol, which stings, and they should be avoided during diaper dermatitis. A spray bottle of clean water allows adequate cleansing without further irritating the area.

Nonpharmacological Management

Nonpharmacological management includes exposure to air, frequent diaper changes, and changing the brand of diaper or protective garment. Expose the affected area to air by leaving the diaper off, or blow-dry the area with a hair dryer on low/cool setting held several inches away from the skin two to three times a day.

Seborrheic Dermatitis

The mainstay of treatment for seborrheic dermatitis is topical antiseborrheic shampoos. Topical corticosteroids may also be used for nonhairy areas such as the face.

Antiseborrheic Shampoos

Antiseborrheic shampoos should be used as prescribed to control dandruff. A variety of preparations are available to treat scalp seborrhea or dandruff. **Selenium sulfide** 1 percent shampoos (**Selsun Blue, Head & Shoulders Intensive**) and **ketoconazole** (**Nizoral**) are the most commonly prescribed shampoos for seborrhea, and are available OTC. **Selenium sulfide** prescription formulas (**Exsel, Selun**) contain 2.5 percent **selenium sulfide**. **Coal tar** shampoos are available OTC and range in strength from 0.5 percent (**DHS Tar**) to 12 percent (**Extra Strength Denorex**) coal tar. **Pyrithione zinc**, the active ingredient in OTC shampoos such as **Head & Shoulders**, may also be used to treat seborrheic dermatitis. Bar soap containing **pyrithione zinc** is available for use on body areas with scalp seborrhea (**ZNP Bar**). Shampoos that combine **sulfur** and **salicylic acid** can also be used (**Sebulex, Fostex**). For treating cradle cap, low-strength **selenium sulfide** (1%) is generally recommended, and care should be taken to keep the shampoo out of the infant's eyes and to rinse the hair well. Table 32–1 presents prescribing information.

Table 32–1 Drugs Commonly Used: Dermatitis and Psoriasis

Drug	Indication	Strengths Available	Dose	Comments
		TOPICAL CORTICOSTEROIDS		
Low Potency				
Hydrocortisone (Hytone, Cortisporin, Cortaid)	Dermatitis	Cream, lotion, ointment: 1%, 2.5%, 0.5%	Apply a thin layer 2–4 times/d until healed	Available OTC
Triamcinolone acetonide (Aristocort, Aristocort A, Kenalog)	Dermatitis	Cream, lotion, ointment: 0.025%	Apply a thin layer 3–4 times/d until healed	Prescription required
Intermediate Potency				
Hydrocortisone valerate (Westcort)	Dermatitis	Cream, ointment: 0.2%	Apply a thin layer 2–3 times/d until healed	Should be used with caution on the face; choose lower potency on face
Hydrocortisone butyrate 0.1% (Locoid)	Dermatitis	Cream, ointment solution: 0.1%	Apply thin layer 2–3 times/d until clear	Should be used with caution on the face; choose lower potency on face

Table 32–1 **Drugs Commonly Used: Dermatitis and Psoriasis—cont'd**

Drug	Indication	Strengths Available	Dose	Comments
TOPICAL CORTICOSTEROIDS				
Mometasone furoate 0.1% (Elocon)	Dermatitis	Cream, ointment, lotion: 0.1%	Apply thin layer once daily. Maximum 3 wk therapy in children	Cream & ointment for children ≥2 yr. Lotion not to be used in children <12 yr
Triamcinolone acetonide (Aristocort, Kenalog)	Dermatitis	Cream, lotion, ointment: 0.1%	Apply a thin layer 3–4 times/d until healed	Should be used with caution on the face; choose lower potency on face
High Potency				
Betamethasone dipropionate, augmented (Diprolene)	Dermatitis	Emollient cream, lotion: 0.05%	Apply a thin film 1–2 times/d until healed; maximum of 45 g of cream or 50 mL of lotion/wk	Avoid abrupt cessation if used for chronic conditions; not recommended in children ≤12 yr due to documented HPA suppression
Triamcinolone acetonide (Aristocort A, Kenalog)	Dermatitis	Cream: 0.5%	Apply sparingly to affected area 2–3 times daily until healed	Avoid abrupt cessation if used for chronic conditions; use with caution and sparingly in children
Super-High Potency				
Betamethasone dipropionate augmented 0.05% (Diprolene AF)	Dermatitis	Ointment, cream: 0.05%	Apply thin film 1–2 times daily. Maximum: ointment 45g/wk gel 50 g/wk	Not recommended in children ≤12 yr. HPA axis suppression documented in children using this product (32%)
TOPICAL IMMUNOMODULATORS				
Pimecrolimus (Elidel)	Short-term or intermittent long-term treatment of mild to moderate atopic dermatitis	Cream: 1%	Apply to affected area twice daily	Not recommended in children <2 yr Pregnancy Category C Not recommended in nursing mothers Long-term safety has not been established Not a first-line therapy
Tacrolimus (Protopic)	Short-term or intermittent long-term treatment of moderate to severe atopic dermatitis	Ointment: 0.03%, 0.1%	Apply to affected area twice daily Apply to dry skin. Do not occlude *Children 2–15 yr:* use 0.03% strength	Not recommended in children <2 yr Pregnancy Category C Not recommended in nursing mothers Long-term safety has not been established Do not use as first-line therapy
ORAL CORTICOSTEROIDS				
Prednisone	Contact dermatitis (severe or if large skin surface area is involved)		*Adults:* 0.5–1 mg/kg/d (40–60 mg/d; maximum 60 mg/d)	Dose is usually tapered after the first 10–14 d, with tapering taking 1–2 wk

Continued

Table 32–1 **Drugs Commonly Used: Dermatitis and Psoriasis—cont'd**

Drug	Indication	Strengths Available	Dose	Comments
ORAL CORTICOSTEROIDS				
			Children: 1 mg/kg/d; maximum 40 mg/d	Severe cases may need a 2- to 3-wk course; 2 wk is the minimum length of treatment for severe poison oak or ivy dermatitis
Methylprednisolone (Medrol Dosepak)	Contact dermatitis (severe or if large skin surface area is involved)		Premeasured dose pack; dose is preset at 24 mg on day 1, tapering 4 mg/d to a dose of 4 mg on day 6	Allows for easy tapering over 6 d 6-d course may not be long enough for some patients
ANTIPRURITIC AGENTS				
Diphenhydramine (Benadryl)	Pruritus associated with dermatitis	Elixir: 12.5 mg/5 mL Chewable tablets: 12.5 mg Tablets: 25 mg	*Adults:* 25–50 mg every 4–6 h *Children 2–6 yr:* 6.25 mg; maximum 37.5 mg/24 h *Children 6–12 yr:* 12.5–25 mg q4–6h; maxi-mum 150 mg/24 h	May cause drowsiness
Hydroxyzine (Atarax)	Pruritus associated with dermatitis	Syrup: 10 mg/5 mL Tablets: 10, 25, 50, 100 mg	*Adults:* 25 mg 3–4 times/d *Children <6 yr:* 12.5 mg 3–4 times/d; maximum 50 mg/24 h *Children ≥6 yr:* 12.5–25 mg 3–4 times/d; maximum 50–100 mg/24 h	May cause drowsiness
Cetirizine (Zyrtec)	Pruritus associated with dermatitis	Syrup: 1 mg/mL Tablets: 5, 10 mg	*Adults:* 5–10 mg once daily *Children 6–24 mo:* 2.5 mg once daily *Children 2–5 yr:* 2.5 mg initially; can increase dose to 5 mg/d either as one 5-mg dose or 2.5 mg q12h *Children ≥6 yr:* 5–10 mg once daily	Less sedation than other antihistamines Should not be used concurrently with alcohol or other CNS depressants as it may potentiate the depressant effect

Table 32–1 **Drugs Commonly Used: Dermatitis and Psoriasis—cont'd**

Drug	Indication	Strengths Available	Dose	Comments
ANTIPRURITIC AGENTS				
Doxepin (systemic: Sinequan)	Pruritus associated with dermatitis	Capsules: 10, 25, 50, 75, 100, 150 mg	Dose range in 25–150 mg/d in single or divided doses; suggested starting dose is 75 mg/d, then titrate up or down as indicated Use dose that achieves effect with fewest adverse effects	Not recommended in children Do not use within 14 day of monoamine oxidase inhibitors (MAOIs). May potentiate drugs metabolized by CYP2D6 (cimetidine, tricyclic antidepressants, SSRIs, phenothiazines, carbamazepine, quinidine, etc.) avoid these drugs during therapy Contraindicated in patients with acute myocardial infarction (MI), urinary retention, or glaucoma. Pregnancy Category C; not recommend during pregnancy
Doxepin (topical: Zonalon)	Moderate to severe pruritus associated with atopic dermatitis (eczema)	Cream: 5%	Apply a thin film to affected areas 4 times/d in 3- to 4-h intervals	Interacts adversely with alcohol and MAOIs; Contraindicated in children Pregnancy Category B Patients with untreated narrow angle glaucoma and urinary retention should not use PO or topical form
SHAMPOOS FOR SEBORRHEIC DERMATITIS				
Ketoconazole shampoo (OTC: Nizoral)	Seborrheic dermatitis	2% shampoo	Apply to wet scalp, massage for 1 min, rinse, and repeat; leave on scalp for 3 min, then rinse well	See package Pregnancy Category C Not recommended in children
Selenium sulfide shampoo (Selsun Blue, Head & Shoulders Intensive Treatment, Excel)	Seborrheic dermatitis	OTC: 1% shampoo Rx: 2.5% shampoo	Apply to wet hair and massage in for 2–3 min before rinsing completely; apply twice a wk until control is achieved, then weekly thereafter For cradle cap: Apply 1% shampoo to scalp, avoiding eyes; rinse thoroughly	See package Advise patient that the shampoo will loosen crusted scales and that these scales may appear loose in the hair after the first few shampoos; brush to remove the scales from the hair; this will resolve after a few treatments

Continued

Table 32–1 **Drugs Commonly Used: Dermatitis and Psoriasis—cont'd**

Drug	Indication	Strengths Available	Dose	Comments
		SHAMPOOS FOR SEBORRHEIC DERMATITIS		
Coal tar shampoo (OTC: Zetar, Neutrogena T/Gel, Tegrin Medicated, Denorex, Theraplex T, lonal T Plus)	Seborrheic dermatitis	1% Zetar, Theraplex T 2% lonil T Plus, Ionil-T Therapeutic 1% coal tar shampoo, Neutrogena T/Gel 5%: Tegrin Medicated 7% Tegrin Medicated Extra conditioning 9% Denorex 12.5%: Extra Strength Denorex	Rub into wet hair and scalp and then rinse: repeat and leave shampoo in for 5 min, rinse well; may be used daily–weekly; follow package directions	See package Do not use if there are open infected lesions May cause sun sensitivity for 24 h after application
Pyrithione zinc (OTC: Head & Shoulders shampoo, Zincon, Danex, DHS, Sebulon, ZNP Bar)	Seborrheic dermatitis	1% shampoo: Head & Shoulders, Zincon, Danex 2% shampoo: DHS Zinc, Sebulon 2% soap: ZNP Bar	Shampoo: apply, lather, rinse, and repeat; use once or twice weekly Soap: wet skin, lather, rinse, and repeat; use once or twice a wk	See package
Sulfur and salicylic acid shampoo (Fostex, Sabex, Sebulex)	Seborrheic dermatitis	5% sulfur and 3% salicylic acid: Maximum Strength Meted 3% salicylic acid and 5% colloidal sulfur: MG400 2% sulfur and 2% salicylic acid: Fostex Medicated Cleansing, Sebex, Sebulex	Follow package directions	See package
Coal tar (OTC: Zetar, Medotar, Pentrax MG217 Medicated, MG217 Dual Treatment, Fototar, Tegrin for Psoriasis, Oxipor VHC)	Psoriasis	Emulsion: 30% (Zetar)	Follow package directions	May cause staining
		Ointment: 1% (Medotar, Taraphilic), 2% (MG217 Medicated) Cream: 2% (Fototar) Lotion: 5% (MG217 Dual Treatment, Tegrin for Psoriasis); 48.5% (Oxipor VHC) Various generics: 20%	Rinse well after use	Contraindicated if patient is taking tetracycline, psoralens, and topical retinoids May cause contact irritant dermatitis Pregnancy Category C

Table 32–1 **Drugs Commonly Used: Dermatitis and Psoriasis—cont'd**

Drug	Indication	Strengths Available	Dose	Comments
TOPICAL ANTIPSORIATICS				
Anthralin (Dithrocreme, Anthra-Derm, Dithro-Scalp)	Psoriasis	Cream: 0.1%, 0.25%, 0.5%, 1% Scalp cream: 0.25%, 0.5%	Begin with a low concentration (0.1%); apply a small amount to affected areas; rub in gently, avoiding healthy surrounding skin; leave on for 10 min, then wash off; after 1 wk, may increase to 15–20 min Increase strength in incremental steps until lesions are healed and skin looks and feels normal Scalp cream: begin with low concentration (0.25%); apply to scalp after combing hair to remove scales; leave on for 10–20 min; use daily for at least 1 wk; increase strength if needed	May stain skin and clothes Pregnancy Category C; safety in young children unknown May alternate with other therapies (retinoids, topical steroids, UV light)
Calcipotriene (Dovonex)	Psoriasis	Ointment, solution, cream: 0.0005%	Apply twice daily to affected area; rub in gently and completely Treat for 6–8 wk; improvement usually noted after 1–2 wk	Pregnancy Category C; should not be used during pregnancy or in children Older patients have a higher incidence of adverse skin reactions Rare reports of rapid onset of hypercalcemia
Calcitriol (Vectical Ointment)	Psoriasis	3 mcg/g ointment	Apply twice a day a.m. & p.m. to affected areas. Maximum dose is 200 g/wk	Pregnancy Category C; should not be used during pregnancy or in children. Hypercalcemia may occur.

OTC = over the counter; UV = ultraviolet; CNS = central nervous system; HPA = hypothalamic-pituitary-adrenal axis; SSRI = selective serotonic reuptake inhibitor

Topical Corticosteroids

Topical **corticosteroids** are used for inflammatory seborrhea that does not respond to medicated shampoo. Low-potency **steroid** lotion or gel is applied two to three times daily to affected areas. Ongoing use of topical **steroids** may be needed when seborrheic dermatitis recurs. Table 32–1 presents prescribing information.

Monitoring

Monitoring for all forms of dermatitis includes assessing the patient for effectiveness of therapy and determining if the patient has experienced any adverse effects or developed a secondary infection.

Outcome Evaluation

For all forms of dermatitis, effective management controls exacerbations and provides comfort measures to decrease pruritus or other symptoms. If the initial therapy has not controlled the exacerbation, increasing the potency of the initial medication or switching to another medication may be indicated. However, before switching to another medication, the provider should observe the patient's medication administration technique, which may be the problem. Secondary skin infections, if they occur, should be treated promptly. Referral to a dermatologist may be necessary if therapy is not managing the dermatitis, if **high-potency topical corticosteroids** are indicated, or if the patient has an unusual presentation.

Patient Education

Patient education should include a discussion of information related to the overall treatment plan as well as that specific to the drug therapy, reasons for taking the drug, drugs as part of the total treatment regimen, and adherence issues.

PSORIASIS

Psoriasis is a chronic skin condition that affects 2 percent of the population worldwide (Menter et al, 2009). It is characterized by sharply defined, symmetrical, erythematous patches with a distinctive silver scale. There are two peak age ranges of onset: from 16 to 22 years and from 57 to 60 years. However, it may occur at any age. Men and women are equally affected, but it is more common in whites than in darker-skinned people. There is a positive family history for the disease in 30 percent of patients. The disease may remain localized to a few areas, or it may become generalized. The condition is lifelong and may occur in an intermittent or a continuous pattern.

Pathophysiology

The exact pathogenesis of psoriasis is unclear although it is thought to be an immune-mediated disease (Feldman & Pearce, 2010a). There is a significant decrease in the amount of time that it takes for a psoriatic epidermal

DERMATITIS

PATIENT EDUCATION

Related to the Overall Treatment Plan/Disease Process

- ☐ Pathophysiology
- ☐ Role of preventive and nonpharmacological measures if appropriate
- ☐ Importance of adherence to the treatment regimen
- ☐ Self-monitoring of symptoms
- ☐ What to do when symptoms worsen
- ☐ Need for follow-up visits with the primary care provider

Specific to the Drug Therapy

- ☐ Reason for taking the drug and its anticipated action on the disease process
- ☐ Doses and schedules for taking the drug
- ☐ Possible adverse effects and what to do if they occur
- ☐ Interactions between other treatment modalities and these drugs

Reasons for Taking the Drug(s)

- ☐ Patient education about specific drugs is provided in the appropriate chapter

Specifically for Eczema

- ☐ Pathophysiology of eczema, that it is a chronic disorder requiring ongoing care, and that there is an itch-scratch-itch cycle that needs to be addressed, but that it is a recurring disease that can be controlled.
- ☐ Avoidance of offending agents that cause exacerbations.
- ☐ Appropriate use of **topical corticosteroids** should be demonstrated. With a sample, the provider can demonstrate how far a pea-sized amount of topical medication can be spread. The patient or caregiver applying the medication should be aware of the adverse effects of overuse of **topical corticosteroids.**

DERMATITIS—cont'd

PATIENT EDUCATION

- ☐ Avoidance of irritants or agents that cause exacerbation of the eczema should be taught, with a written list of common irritants provided to the patient
- ☐ Long-term therapy (skin hydration and **emollient** use) versus acute therapy

Specifically for Contact Dermatitis

- ☐ Pathophysiology
- ☐ Appropriate application of **topical corticosteroids** should be demonstrated
- ☐ Appropriate use of **antipruritic medication**

Specifically for Diaper Dermatitis

- ☐ The parent or patient should be educated about the underlying pathophysiology of diaper dermatitis, in that it is usually an irritant dermatitis caused by chemical irritation from urine or feces, complicated by mechanical irritation of the diaper or undergarment rubbing and chafing the skin.
- ☐ Describing the characteristics of a secondary infection with *Candida* will assist with early identification and treatment of this common complication in diaper dermatitis.
- ☐ Nonpharmacological management such as sitz baths, air drying, and frequent diaper changes should be discussed.
- ☐ If properly treated, the skin should return to normal in the area in 3 to 4 days. If the patient is not responding to treatment in 48 hours, then a reevaluation is necessary.

Specifically for Seborrheic Dermatitis

- ☐ The patient should know that seborrheic dermatitis cannot be cured and can only be controlled and that treatment will probably need to be continued long-term in adolescents and adults. In infants with cradle cap, it will usually resolve around age 6 months.
- ☐ The patient should contact the health-care provider if signs and symptoms of a secondary infection occur.

Drugs as Part of the Total Treatment Regimen

- ☐ The total treatment regimen includes pharmacological and nonpharmacological measures. Be sure the patient and/or family members are aware of the specific measures to be taken.

Adherence Issues

- ☐ Health-care providers should be aware of the potential problem of nonadherence and should discuss the importance of completing the entire treatment regimen with the patient and/or family members.

cell to travel to the skin surface and be cast off. A normal skin cell travels to the surface in 26 to 28 days; with psoriasis, the cells take only 3 to 4 days. This decreased time does not allow normal cell maturation to take place.

Lesions of active psoriasis can develop in areas of epidermal trauma. Surgical incisions, a sunburn, or scratch marks can all heal, leaving psoriatic lesions in their place (Koebner phenomenon). Exacerbations may be triggered by beta-hemolytic streptococcal infections, as well as by some medications (e.g., **lithium, beta-adrenergic antagonists, angiotensin-converting enzyme inhibitors, antimalarial drugs, and indomethacin**).

Extensor surfaces are affected more commonly, with other common sites being the intergluteal fold, the eyebrows, and around the ears. Nails may develop pits and ridges, may be thick and discolored, and have splinter hemorrhages.

Goals of Treatment

Although psoriasis is a chronic, lifelong, recurrent disease, the goal of therapy should be control of symptoms and clearing of psoriatic lesions. It should be emphasized to the patient that psoriasis is a treatable disease and that control is possible with continued, conscientious use of medication.

Rational Drug Selection

The management of psoriasis consists of topical medication and phototherapy for mild to moderate psoriasis (less

CLINICAL PEARL

Psoriasis

Psoriasis may affect a patient's self-esteem and may exacerbate depression. The patient's mood should be monitored. Referral to a support group or an organization such as the National Psoriasis Foundation (http://www.psoriasis.org) may be helpful.

than 5% of the body involved) and the addition of systemic medications for severe psoriasis (more than 5% to 10% of the body involved) (Feldman & Pearce, 2010b; Menter et al, 2009). Systemic treatments with **immunosuppressants (alefacept [Amevive], efalizumab [Raptiva], cyclosporine [Neoral], ustekinumab [Stelara]), retinoids (acitretin [Soriatane]), methotrexate** and **tumor necrosis factor blocker (etanercept [Enbrel], adalimumab [Humira], infliximab [Remicade])** are not covered in this chapter as they are prescribed only by dermatology specialists.

Topical Therapy

Topical therapy for psoriasis consists of **topical steroids, coal tar,** or **keratolytic shampoos** for scalp involvement, **keratolytic agents** for thick plaques, **anthralin,** and **calcipotriene. Topical immunomodulators** may also be used.

Topical Steroids

Topical steroids are used to treat psoriasis because of their anti-inflammatory effects on the plaques. Moderate- to high-potency **steroids** are used because the lesions are generally steroid-resistant (Menter et al, 2009). The **steroid** cream or ointment is applied two to three times per day (see Table 32–1). Chronic **topical corticosteroid** use can cause tachyphylaxis and may have adverse effects such as atrophy and telangiectasia. Intermittent or "pulse" therapy minimizes some of these effects. If **topical corticosteroids** are used in the intertriginous areas or on the face, a low-potency medication should be chosen. Regardless of the **topical steroid** used, 2 to 4 weeks of continuous use is the limit, with gradual reduction in frequency of application to prevent rebound (Feldman & Pearce, 2010b). Patients should be discouraged from using steroids for longer periods. **Topical corticosteroids** should be reserved for psoriasis flare, and another medication used for ongoing therapy.

Coal Tar

Coal tar (Zetar, Medotar, Tegrin for Psoriasis) affects psoriasis by enzyme inhibition and antimitotic action. Tar preparations include creams, shampoos, ointments, lotions, gels, and oils. They range in strength from 1 to 20 percent. Tar has few adverse effects and is safer to use than **topical steroids** and **anthralin,** although their use has decreased in the United States (Menter et al, 2009). The major problem is that they are messy and can stain the skin and clothes. The tar preparation is applied to the affected areas once or twice daily. If using **coal tar** shampoo or bath emulsion, the patient should be instructed to rinse well after use. Tar preparations make the patient photosensitive; therefore, the patient should be instructed to avoid sunlight and ultraviolet light (see Table 32–1).

Anthralin

Anthralin (Dithrocreme, Dithro-Scalp) is an antimitotic agent that is used for chronic psoriasis. It has an antiproliferative effect. Although it is effective, **anthralin** has the disadvantages of being irritating and of staining skin and clothing. **Anthralin's** use has decreased over the past few years with the availability of preparations that are more cosmetically acceptable (Menter et al, 2009). Careful instructions for use increase the likelihood of a successful outcome with this difficult-to-administer medication.

When prescribing **anthralin** to a patient who has never used the medication, choose a low-concentration product (0.1%). The medication is applied to the psoriatic lesions and rubbed gently until the medication is absorbed. Take care not to get the **anthralin** on the healthy surrounding skin. It is important not to apply excessive medication, which increases the staining of skin and clothes. After the medication is rubbed in, it is left on 10 to 20 minutes; then it is washed off in the shower. After 1 week, the length of time the medication is in contact with the skin can be increased to 15 to 20 minutes. The strength of **anthralin** can be increased in increments (0.25%, 0.5%, 1%) as tolerated. Some patients require the medication to be applied and left on for 60 minutes to have improvement in their psoriatic lesions. Treatment should be continued until the lesionsare completely healed (when nothing is felt with the fingers and the texture of the skin is completely normal). Table 32–1 presents prescribing information for **anthralin.**

Vitamin D_3 Derivatives

Calcipotriene (Dovonex) is a vitamin D_3 derivative that regulates cell differentiation and proliferation and suppresses lymphocyte activity. **Calcipotriene** is available in a cream, ointment, or solution preparation. It is effective and safe for short- or long-term treatment. **Calcipotriene** is applied in a thin film to the affected psoriasis plaques and rubbed into the skin gently and completely. In adults, the ointment is applied twice daily in the morning and evening. It is important that the patient does not exceed 100 g/week of **calcipotriene** applied to the skin. Safety and efficacy in children have not been established.

For the treatment of mild to moderate scalp psoriasis, the patient applies the topical solution twice daily. Improvement will be noted as soon as 1 to 2 weeks after treatment has begun. The patient should be reevaluated after 6 to 8 weeks. **Calcipotriene** may be used in combination with **topical steroids**, which is more effective than either treatment alone. Table 32–1 presents prescribing information for **calcipotriene**.

Topical **calcitriol (Vectical Ointment)** is a vitamin D_3 derivative similar to **calcipotriene**. **Calcitriol** inhibits keratinocyte proliferation and inhibits T cell proliferation and other inflammatory mediators (Feldman & Pearce, 2010b). **Calcitriol** is applied to affected psoriatic plaques twice a day. The maximum weekly dose should not exceed 200 grams. Hypercalcemia may occur and **calcitriol** should be discontinued until normocalcemia returns.

Phototherapy

Patients with psoriasis respond very well to phototherapy. Phototherapy with ultraviolet-B (UVB) light is effective in managing psoriasis by reducing DNA synthesis of epidermal cells. UVB light treatment is easy for the patient to use and can produce long-lasting remissions of 2 to 4 months. UVB therapy is usually prescribed by a dermatologist. The use of commercial tanning beds is not recommended.

Systemic Medications

Systemic medications used for psoriasis are **methotrexate**, **oral retinoids**, **immunosuppressants (alefacept [Amevive], efalizumab [Raptiva], cyclosporine [Neoral], ustekinumab [Stelara])**, **retinoids (acitretin [Soriatane])**, and **tumor necrosis factor blockers (etanercept [Enbrel], adalimumab [Humira], infliximab [Remicade])**. They have serious adverse effects and therefore should be prescribed only by a dermatologist and only if the patient meets criteria determined by the American Academy of Dermatology. To try to decrease the adverse effects, the medications may be prescribed intermittently or on a rotational basis. Patients should be advised to avoid pregnancy before, during, and for a period of time after taking these drugs. The primary care provider will need to consult with the dermatologist and observe the patient for adverse effects if any of these medications are prescribed.

Monitoring

The patient who is being treated for psoriasis should be monitored for effectiveness of therapy and for adverse effects of the medication.

Outcome Evaluation

Psoriasis lesions should eventually clear, with the skin returning to the patient's normal look and feel. If the patient is using the medication correctly and there is unsatisfactory clinical response, or if skin irritation occurs, then either the medication needs to be changed or the strength increased. Skin irritation is a common adverse effect of psoriasis medications, especially if the patient gets the medication on the surrounding skin. Review proper administration technique prior to changing the therapy.

Patient Education

Successful treatment of psoriasis requires educating the patient on the following key points:

1. The patient should understand the pathophysiology of psoriasis: that it is a chronic disease but that remission is possible if adequately treated.
2. Proper application of topical medications will not only optimize treatment but also decrease adverse effects of the medications.
3. Many of the medications stain the skin and clothing. The patient should be aware of this problem and instructed on how to minimize the staining.
4. Some medications cause photosensitivity; therefore, the patient needs to understand the hazards of sun exposure and use protective clothing and sunscreen.

ACNE AND ACNE ROSACEA

Acne affects an estimated 17 to 28 million Americans, accounting for 4.4 percent of internist visits. It is the number one condition seen by dermatologists, accounting for 18 percent of visits (Fleischer, Herbert, Feldman, & O'Brien, 2000). Approximately 85 to 100 percent of adolescents have acne to some degree, although acne can also occur in patients in their twenties to forties. Adolescent acne is more common in boys than in girls; however, adult acne is more common in women than in men. Males have a higher incidence of severe acne at all ages.

Although acne may be a minor problem from a medical standpoint, multiple studies have determined that acne has a significant impact on the patient's quality of life (Dalgard, Gieler, Holm, Bjertness, & Hauser, 2008; Lasek & Chren, 1998; Mallon et al, 1999). The adolescent is stereotyped as being the most concerned about acne, but studies have indicated that the older the patient is, the more the impact acne has on quality-of-life scores, regardless of severity (Lasek & Chren, 1998). Acne patients reported levels of social, psychological, and emotional problems that were as great as those reported by patients with chronic disabling asthma, epilepsy, diabetes, back pain, or arthritis (Mallon et al, 1999). The practitioner needs to address the patient's concerns about acne with this in mind.

Pathophysiology

The underlying cause of acne is multifactorial. A genetic susceptibility appears to predispose some people to acne. Acne begins below the skin surface in the pilosebaceous unit of the sebaceous glands. In acne, the sebaceous glands are enlarged and sebum production is increased, probably because of adrenogenic hormones. In patients with acne, there is an alteration in the keratinization process in the follicular infrainfundibulum. This causes the extra sebum to occlude the hair follicle and produce microcomedones. These may enlarge with time and form closed comedones (whiteheads) or open comedones (blackheads). *Propionibacterium acnes (P. acnes)* organisms colonize the follicles and convert the triglycerides in the sebum into free fatty acids. Free fatty acids are a factor in the synthesis of chemoattractants that draw inflammatory elements, leading to the inflammation associated with acne. The patient may have superficial papules and/or pustules or deeper nodules, depending on the intensity of the inflammatory process.

Goals of Treatment

At this time, acne has no cure. The goal is to control the acne and keep visible lesions and medication adverse effects to a minimum. Management goals that will control acne are (1) to control the inflammatory process associated with acne by altering the bacterial flora, and (2) to decrease the obstruction of the sebaceous ducts.

Rational Drug Selection

Acne treatment should be approached in a stepwise manner. If the acne is mild or moderate, a beginning therapy might include **topical retinoids** and/or **topical antibiotics.** If after 6 to 8 weeks this is not completely effective, an oral **antibiotic** might be added or a change in topical therapy initiated. For moderate to somewhat severe acne, the patient is usually started on an oral **antibiotic** and topical preparations combined. For severe, recalcitrant, nodular acne, the patient is prescribed **isotretinoin (Accutane).**

Figure 32–1 presents an algorithm of the pharmacological management of acne.

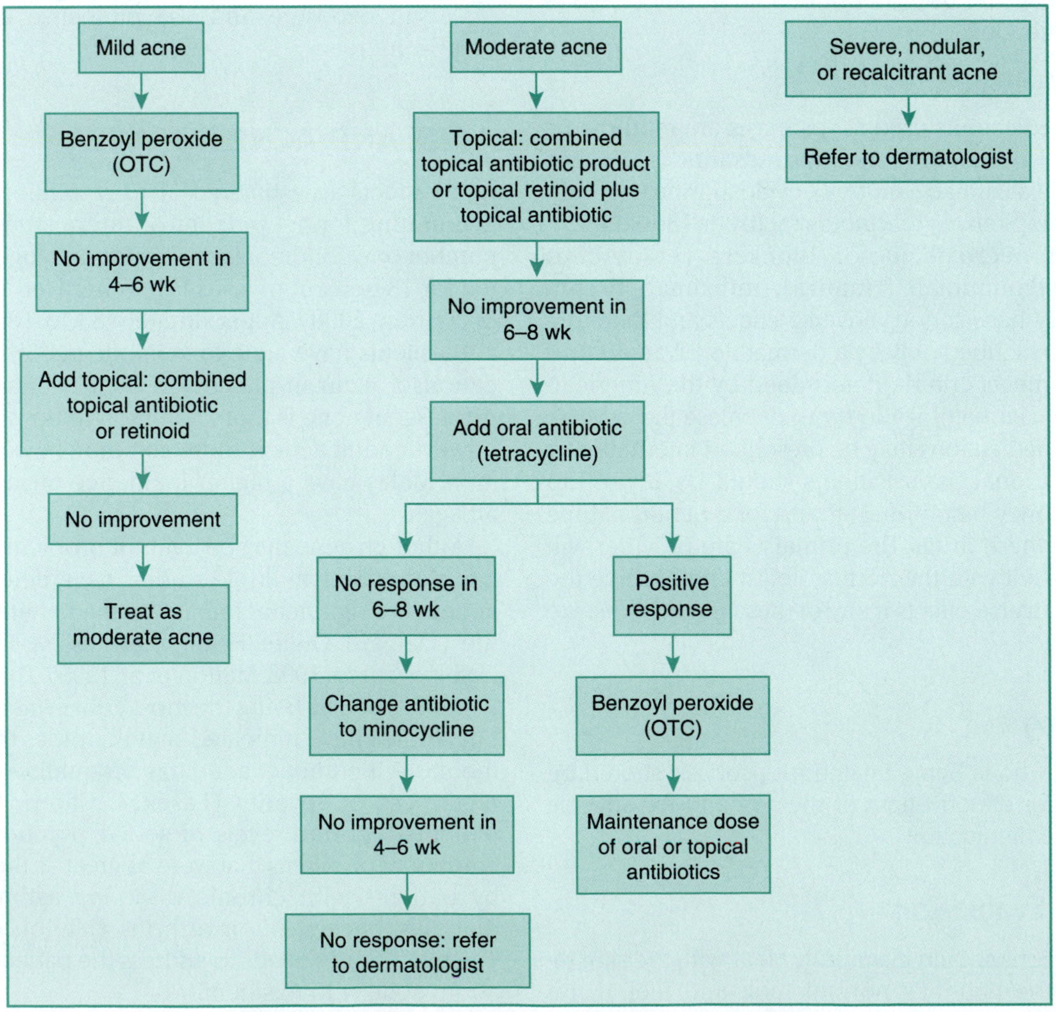

Figure 32–1. Algorithm: Pharmacological management of acne.

Topical Agents

The topical agents used for acne can be divided into two categories: **topical retinoids** and **topical antibiotics**.

Topical Retinoids

Topical retinoids (tretinoin [Retin-A]), **retinoid-like compounds** (adapalene [Differin]), or **retinoid prodrugs** (Tazarotene [Tazorac]) are used to treat inflammatory and noninflammatory acne. They act to alter the abnormal keratinization process of acne that leads to microcomedo formation. Additionally, they stimulate mitotic activity and increase the turnover of follicular epithelial cells, causing extrusion of the comedones. Clinically, this causes an initial worsening of acne, as comedones that were previously under the skin are extruded. This worsening is not a reason for discontinuation of treatment. Patients should be reassured that their faces will clear after approximately 6 to 8 weeks of treatment.

All **retinoid** preparations can cause some skin irritation, especially in fair-skinned patients or patients with sensitive skin. Atopic people can be quite sensitive to these products. The patient should not use any harsh **toners, astringents, scrubs,** or **cleansers** while on **topical retinoid** therapy because these increase irritation. The patient's skin is more photosensitive when **topical retinoids** are used, and the patient should be advised to use noncomedogenic **sunscreen** for any sun exposure.

The patient should avoid the eyes and mucous membranes when applying these products. There may be transient stinging, burning, or pruritus immediately after applying topical retinoids. Redness and peeling may occur with excessive application. If **topical retinoids** are used more than recommended, a dramatic increase in skin irritation occurs, but no improved response.

Table 32–2 presents the drugs commonly used to treat acne.

Topical Antibiotics

Topical **antibiotics** are thought to act to control acne by their bacteriostatic or bactericidal activity against *P. acnes*.

Table 32–2 **Drugs Commonly Used: Acne**

Drug	Indication	Strengths Available	Dose	Comments
Topical Retinoids				
Tretinoin (Retin-A)	Acne	Cream: 0.025%, 0.05%, 0.1% Gel: 0.025%, 0.01% Liquid: 0.05%	Apply to affected areas once daily after washing face with a mild cleanser; begin with 0.025% cream and increase strength or to bid if needed Sensitive-skin patients may need to dose every other night	Wash hands after application Normal use of cosmetics is permissible, but instruct patient to use noncomedogenic products Pregnancy Category C; pregnant women should be switched to another product
Adapalene (Differin)	Acne	Gel: 0.1% (alcohol free) Lotion: 0.1% (30% alcohol)	Apply to affected areas once daily (HS) after washing with a gentle cleanser; avoid eyes, lips, and mucous membranes	Avoid harsh soaps, cleansers, or alcohol-containing products, which increase skin irritation while using adapalene Pregnancy Category C May be used in children >12 yr
Adapalene and benzoyl peroxide (Epiduo)	Acne	Adapalene 0.1% and benzoyl peroxide 2.5% gel	*Adults and children >12 yr:* Apply thin film once daily after washing. Reduce frequency if irritation occurs	Avoid harsh soaps, cleansers, or alcohol-containing products, which increase skin irritation while using adapalene Pregnancy Category C May be used in children >12 yr
Topical Antibiotics				
Benzoyl peroxide (Rx: Benzac, Desquam-X Desquam-E) (OTC: Dryox, Fostex, Neutrogena Acne Mask, Clearasil)	Acne	Liquid wash: 2.5%, 5%, 10% Bar: 5%, 10%	For cleansers, wash once or twice daily; rinse well and pat dry	Has a drying action causes comedolysis, and has a mild desquamation effect (irritating to the skin)

Continued

Table 32–2 **Drugs Commonly Used: Acne—cont'd**

Drug	Indication	Strengths Available	Dose	Comments
		Mask: 5% Lotion: 5%, 5.5%, 10% Cream: 5%, 10%	For other forms; apply once daily; gradually increase to 2–3 times daily if needed; apply after cleansing skin	Pregnancy Category C; topical application during pregnancy is generally considered safe
		Gel: 2.5%, 4%, 5%, 10%, 20%		May be used in children >12 yr Bleaches fabrics Inactivates tretinoin and cannot be applied simultaneously
Benzoyl peroxide/ clindamycin (Benzaclin, Duac)	Acne	5% Benzoyl peroxide 1% Clindamycin gel	Benzaclin: Apply to affected areas bid Duac: Apply to affected areas once daily	Has a drying action, causes comedolysis, and has a mild desquamation effect (irritating to the skin) Pregnancy Category C; topical application during pregnancy is generally considered safe May be used in children >12 yr Bleaches fabrics Inactivates tretinoin and cannot be applied simultaneously Rare reaction: colitis
Erythromycin (Staticin, Akne-Mycin, A/T/S, Eryderm, Erymax, Ery-Sol, T-Stat, Erygel)	Acne	Solution: 1%, 2% Gel: 2% Ointment: 2%	Apply to affected areas bid after washing face with a mild cleanser	Pregnancy Category B Do not use concurrently with clindamycin
Benzoyl peroxide/ erythromycin (Benzamycin)	Acne	Gel	Apply to affected areas once or twice/d (gel dries to a crusty white appearance; therefore, patient may prefer evening application; patient may use plain benzoyl peroxide in the morning if this is concern)	Pregnancy Category C Bleaches fabrics Must be kept refrigerated; stable for only 3 mo after mixed Adverse effects include skin irritation and sun sensitivity
Clindamycin (Cleocin, Clinda-Derm, C/T/S)	Acne	Gel, lotion, topical solution	Apply thin layer to affected areas bid	Use with caution in patients with eczema Although rare, there are reports of colitis with topical administration If patient develops diarrhea, stop medication and investigate cause Pregnancy Category B Do not use in children <12 yr Adverse effects include skin dryness and irritation, burning, and peeling

Table 32–2 **Drugs Commonly Used: Acne—cont'd**

Drug	Indication	Strengths Available	Dose	Comments
Tetracycline (Topicycline)	Acne	Topical solution: 2.2 g/mL	Apply to affected areas bid; apply until skin is thoroughly wet (stinging and burning may occur but subside after a few minutes)	Pregnancy Category B May be staining to clothes; yellowing of skin may be removed by washing Assess patient for sulfite sensitivity Topicycline contains sodium bisulfite
Metronidazole (Metro-Gel, Noritate)	Acne rosacea	Gel: 0.75% Emollient cream: 1%	Apply a thin film bid to entire affected area after washing	Improvement should be noted within 3 wk, but there may be continued improvement through 9 wk of treatment Pregnancy Category B Some mild skin irritation may be noted
Oral Antibiotics				
Tetracycline (Achromycin)	Acne (long-term treatment)	Capsules: 250, 500 mg Tablets: 250, 500 mg	Initially, 500 mg bid for 1–2 mo After control is achieved, dose may be lowered to 500 mg daily for 1–2 mo; then determine maintenance dose of 125–500 mg daily	Must be taken on an empty stomach; poorly absorbed if taken with calcium containing foods, milk, or antacids Pregnancy Category D; do not prescribe to lactating women or children under age 8 (may cause staining of teeth)
Erythromycin base (E-Mycin, Ery-Tab), erythromycin estolate (llosone), erythromycin ethylsuccinate (EryPed, E.E.S.)	Acne (long-term treatment)	Erythromycin base: capsules: 250, 333, 500 mg Erythromycin estolate: tablets: 250, 500 mg suspension 125 mg/5 mL, 250 mg/5 mL Erythromycin ethyl succinate: chewable tablets: 200 mg; tablets: 400 mg; suspension: 200 mg/5 mL, 400 mg/5 mL	Initially; 1,000 mg/d in divided doses (usually qid) After control is achieved, dose can be decreased to 250–500 mg/	Some dermatologists prescribe a "burst" of 750 mg for 7–10 d if acne is cyclical such as menstrual associated acne Inexpensive Pregnancy Category B May cause gastrointestinal (GI) upset; take with food or milk
Minocycline (Minocin)	Acne (acne resistant to tetracycline and erythromycin)	Capsules: 50, 100 mg Tablets: 50, 100 mg	Initially, 100 mg bid, then wean to 50 mg daily after control is achieved	Expensive Must be taken on an empty stomach Pregnancy Category D; do not prescribe to lactating women or children <8 yr

They control the inflammatory process, probably by decreasing the free fatty acids that *P. acnes* produces. Applied topically, **antibiotics** have an uneven, erratic penetration into the follicles. Therefore, they are usually used in mild acne, for maintenance after a course of oral **antibiotics**, or in conjunction with topical retinoids. There is a concern that resistant *P. acnes* may develop if topical **antibiotics** are overused. The topical **antibiotics** that are approved for use include **benzoyl peroxide**, available by prescription (Benzac, Desquam-X, Desquam-E) or OTC (Dryox, Fostex, Neutrogena Acne Mask, Clearasil), **erythromycin** (Staticin, Akne-Mycin, A/T/S, Eryderm, Erymax, Ery-Sol, T-Stat, Erygel), **clindamycin** (Cleocin, Clinda-Derm, C/T/S), and **tetracycline** (Topicycline). A combination of **benzoyl peroxide** and **adapalene** (Epiduo Gel) is available. The combination of benzoyl peroxide and an antibiotic erythromycin (Benzamycin) or clindamycin (Benzaclin, Duac) is superior to either agent alone. Prescribing information is given in Table 32–2.

Oral Agents

Oral agents used for acne are divided into three categories: oral **antibiotics**, **hormonal** therapy, and **isotretinoin** (an oral **retinoid**). Oral **antibiotics** are prescribed for moderate to severe acne and are within the scope of practice of primary care providers. **Isotretinoin** is prescribed for severe nodulocystic acne but only by dermatologists because of its adverse effects.

Oral Antibiotics

Oral **antibiotics** are active against *P. acnes*, which helps transform comedones into inflammatory pustules and papules. Oral **antibiotics** do not affect existing lesions, but they prevent future lesions by decreasing sebaceous fatty acids by decreasing *P. acnes* colonization. They may also have an anti-inflammatory effect independent of their action against *P. acnes*. There is level I evidence for the use of **tetracycline, doxycycline, minocycline, erythromycin, trimethoprim-sulfamethoxazole, trimethoprim,** and **azithromycin** in the treatment of acne (Strauss et al, 2007). **Azithromycin** is effective against acne, but its routine use may lead to increased resistance (Ofori, 2010). Table 32–2 presents prescribing information for **tetracycline (Achromycin V), erythromycin (erythromycin base [E-Mycin, Ery-Tab], erythromycin estolate [Ilosone], erythromycin ethylsuccinate [EryPed, E.E.S.],** and **minocycline [Minocin]**).

Hormonal Therapy

Hormonal therapy can be prescribed to women who require birth control who also have mild to moderate acne. Multiple **oral contraceptives** currently have FDA approval for use in acne: **Ortho Tri-Cyclen, Ortho-Cyclen, Estrostep Fe,** and **Tri-Sprintec**. The **oral contraceptives** appear to control the inflammatory component of acne. The patient is prescribed a premeasured dose pack and takes one pill daily. Effects on acne are seen in 3 to 6 months of continued use. For full prescribing information, see Chapter 31.

Isotretinoin

Isotretinoin (Accutane) is the most potent agent for treating acne. It is reserved for severe recalcitrant cystic acne. Its exact mechanism of action is unknown but thought to be related to decreased sebum production (by 90%) and **isotretinoin's** ability to decrease abnormal keratinization. **Isotretinoin** is prescribed for a period of 15 to 20 weeks and may need to be repeated. The toxicity profile and its ability to cause fetal malformations require that the prescriber provide extensive education and close monitoring throughout therapy. The adverse effects of dry skin, cheilitis, and pruritus are seen in almost all patients taking the drug. Patients may experience elevated serum triglycerides and clinical hepatitis, including elevated liver enzymes. Therefore, liver enzyme and lipid levels should be obtained before beginning therapy and monitored throughout therapy. Patients may develop depression or suicide ideation; all patients taking **isotretinoin** should have their mood monitored. The major concern is the use of the drug in women who may become pregnant; therefore, there are very stringent requirements and consent that must be met before the drug is prescribed. For female patients, a pregnancy test needs to be performed before beginning therapy and then monthly throughout therapy. **Isotretinoin** is Pregnancy Category X. It should not be prescribed to teenagers who have not completed their linear growth. Because of the toxic effects of **isotretinoin**, it is rarely prescribed by a primary care provider and is usually prescribed only by a dermatologist. All providers and female patients need to be registered with iPledge, a pregnancy-prevention program committed to preventing pregnancy while patients are taking **isotretinoin**. To register, go to http://www.iPledgeprogram.com.

Acne Rosacea

Acne rosacea, commonly referred to as rosacea, is a skin condition that usually affects middle-aged patients. It is a chronic inflammatory disorder that affects the blood vessels and pilosebaceous glands of the face. The patient often has a characteristic red-colored nose. An important hallmark characteristic is easy facial flushing and blushing associated with the ingestion of alcohol, spicy foods, or caffeine-containing beverages.

Patients with acne rosacea have papules and pustules superimposed on diffuse erythema and telangiectasia over the central portion of the face. Hyperplasia of the sebaceous glands, connective tissue, and vascular bed can lead to a large bulbous red nose, called rhinophyma. The patient may also have ocular involvement that may require the care of an ophthalmologist.

Topical **metronidazole (Metro-Gel, Noritate)** is used to treat acne rosacea. The mechanism by which **metronidazole** works to improve the inflammation of rosacea is unknown but is probably related to its antibacterial effect. Rosacea usually responds well to **metronidazole**, but the antibiotic must be continued for life, as the rosacea will recur if the medication is discontinued. Table 32–2 presents prescribing information.

CLINICAL PEARL

ACNE

Tell patients using **benzoyl peroxide** products that **benzoyl peroxide** can bleach clothes and towels. Advise them to use an old or white pillowcase on their bed and an old or white towel to dry their hands after using these agents.

Monitoring

The patient needs to be monitored for effectiveness and adverse effects of the acne medication.

Laboratory testing before and during therapy may be indicated for some patients. The primary care provider may be involved in obtaining and monitoring these tests. For female patients, especially those taking **tetracycline**, **minocycline**, and **isotretinoin**, pregnancy testing is recommended prior to beginning treatment and as indicated throughout therapy.

Outcome Evaluation

The patient needs to use an acne medication for at least 6 to 8 weeks before effectiveness can be determined. If there is no response after that time, then a change in therapy can be considered—either adding another medication or changing the regimen completely. Before determining the medication is not effective, review administration of the medication with the patient. The adverse effects associated with topical acne treatments include skin irritation and some redness and peeling. Mild symptoms usually improve if the frequency of administration is decreased slightly. If possible, the strength of the topical medication can be decreased if there is mild to moderate irritation. Severe skin irritation warrants discontinuing the medication and switching to another.

Patient Education

Patient education should include a discussion of information related to the overall treatment plan as well as that specific to the drug therapy, reasons for taking the drug, drugs as part of the total treatment regimen, and adherence issues.

ACNE

PATIENT EDUCATION

Related to the Overall Treatment Plan/Disease Process

- ☐ Pathophysiology
- ☐ Role of preventive and nonpharmacological measures if appropriate
- ☐ Importance of adherence to the treatment regimen
- ☐ Self-monitoring of symptoms
- ☐ What to do when symptoms worsen
- ☐ Need for follow-up visits with the primary care provider

Specific to the Drug Therapy

- ☐ Reason for the drug's being given and its anticipated action on the disease process
- ☐ Doses and schedules for taking the drug
- ☐ Possible adverse effects and what to do if they occur
- ☐ Interactions between other treatment modalities and these drugs

Reasons for Taking the Drug(s)

- ☐ Patient education about specific drugs is provided in the appropriate chapter.

Specifically for Acne

- ☐ The patient should understand that it will take at least 6 weeks to determine if treatment is effective. Tying this into the explanation of normal skin growth will help the patient understand why it takes so long for the medication to work.
- ☐ Whatever level of treatment the patient is started on, the patient needs to understand what alternatives there are if the chosen treatment is not effective.

Drugs as Part of the Total Treatment Regimen

- ☐ The total treatment regimen includes pharmacological and nonpharmacological measures. Be sure the patient and/or family members are aware of the specific measures to be taken.

Adherence Issues

- ☐ Health-care providers should be aware of the potential problem of nonadherence and should discuss the importance of completing the entire treatment regimen with the patient and/or family members.

SKIN INFECTIONS

Skin infections commonly seen in primary care include bacterial, viral, and fungal skin infections.

Bacterial skin infections are common and seen in patients of any age. The skin infections seen in primary care include impetigo, a furuncle (boil or abscess), perianal streptococcal infection, and cellulitis. All require prompt treatment with the appropriate antibiotic.

Many viral skin infections can affect the skin, often causing rashes. Herpes simplex virus infection, herpes zoster (shingles), and varicella (chickenpox) are the common viral infections seen in primary care.

Fungal skin infections can be divided into two types: *Candida* infections and dermatophyte infections. Dermatophyte or tinea infections include tinea of the scalp (tinea capitis or ringworm of the scalp), tinea of the skin (tinea corporis or ringworm), tinea cruris ("jock itch"), tinea of the feet (tinea pedis or athlete's feet), and tinea versicolor. Onychomycosis, a fungal infection of the nails, is another type of fungal skin infection.

Pathophysiology

Bacterial Skin Infections

The most common bacterial organisms found in skin infections are *S. aureus* and *Streptococcus pyogenes*. The organism usually enters the skin through a break in the skin. The bacteria cause an inflammatory infectious process to begin.

Viral Skin Infections

Viral skin infections include herpes viral infections, varicella, and herpes zoster.

Herpes viral infections are spread by intimate contact between a person shedding the virus and a susceptible host. With inoculation into the skin or mucous membrane, herpes simplex virus (HSV) begins to replicate. The incubation period is 4 to 6 days. As replication continues, local inflammation and cell lysis lead to the distinctive vesicle with an erythematous region. The virus generally ascends the peripheral sensory nerves to the dorsal root ganglia. HSV replicates in the dorsal root ganglia and then enters an inactive or latent stage. The herpesvirus is unique in that it establishes latency for varying periods of time. HSV can be reactivated and enter a replication cycle at any time. There are two HSV infections, HSV-1 and HSV-2, with HSV-1 generally associated with nongenital infection and HSV-2 associated with genital infection.

Varicella (chickenpox) is a highly contagious disease caused by the varicella-zoster virus, a herpesvirus. It is spread by direct contact, in droplets, and by airborne transmission. The virus infects individuals by the conjunctivae or respiratory tract, replicating in the nasopharynx and upper respiratory tract. It spreads systemically to cause a viremia, resulting in a disseminated vesicular rash after an incubation period of 10 to 14 days. The patient is contagious for 1 to 2 days prior to the rash eruption and until all the lesions are dry. After the rash clears, the virus enters a latent phase and remains inactive in the dorsal root ganglia.

Herpes zoster (shingles) is caused by reactivation of latent varicella-zoster virus. The reason for the reactivation is unknown, although stress seems to have some impact. The incidence of the disease increases with age and immunosuppression. The patient usually experiences burning and pain along the dermatome prior to the vesicles erupting. The lesions are generally unilateral and appear along a dermatome, although there may occasionally be scattered lesions. The diagnosis is confirmed with Tzanck smear or viral culture.

Fungal Skin Infections

Candida infections are caused by *C. albicans,* which is commonly found on the skin and mucosal tissues in the oral, intestinal, and vaginal areas. Considered a normal flora in these areas, an overgrowth can lead to infection and erythema, ulceration, and characteristic white plaques. In the mouth, oral candidiasis is known as thrush. In women, a vaginal *Candida* infection is often referred to as a "yeast infection." *Candida* is diagnosed by examination of scrapings from the area, using potassium hydroxide (KOH) preparation.

Dermatophytes are a group of fungi that live on the keratin of the stratum corneum, nails, and hair. Symptoms of dermatophyte infection include pruritus, scaling, occasional vesicles, and, in tinea corporis, characteristic annular lesions with raised edges and clearing in the center. Tinea versicolor can have clinical findings of multiple scaling, discrete macules that can be hypopigmented or hyperpigmented.

Onychomycosis is a fungal infection of the fingernails or toenails.

Goals of Treatment

The goals of treatment for skin infections are to decrease the severity of the infection or eradicate it (as appropriate), alleviate symptoms, and heal the skin area and return it to normal (as appropriate).

Rational Drug Selection

Bacterial Skin Infections

Impetigo

Impetigo is a bacterial infection *(S. aureus* or *S. pyogenes)* of the superficial layers of the skin, which begins as vesicles that rupture, leaving a hallmark golden or honey-colored crust. Topical **mupirocin** ointment (**Bactroban**) or **retapamulin** (**Altabax**) is used if the impetigo is mild (up to five singular lesions). The OTC ointments **bacitracin** and combinations of **bacitracin, polymyxin B sulfate,** and **neomycin (Polysporin, Neosporin, Double Antibiotic Ointment,** and **Triple Antibiotic Ointment)** may be used if there are one or two lesions. Topical **antibiotic** ointments that do not contain **neomycin** are preferred, as **neomycin** sensitivity is a concern.

Oral **antibiotics**, such as **cephalexin (Keflex)** or **amoxicillin/clavulanate (Augmentin), dicloxacillin,** or **clindamycin,** are indicated if the patient has more than five lesions or if the lesions continue to worsen after 2 to 3 days of topical therapy.

Furuncle

Treatment of a small furuncle, which is usually caused by *S. aureus,* may respond to warm packs and not need systemic **antibiotics.** A larger boil or abscess may require incision and drainage, as well as systemic **antibiotics.** Gram's stain and culture of the drainage will determine if the organism will be sensitive to the antibiotic of choice. Prior to Gram's stain results, an appropriate first-line **antibiotic** would be **cephalexin, amoxicillin/clavulanate,** or **dicloxacillin.** Empiric therapy should include coverage for methicillin-resistant *S. aureus* (MRSA) in areas of high prevalence. Antibiotic appropriate for MRSA include **TMP/SMZ, doxycycline,** or **clindamycin,** depending on local resistance patterns. Length of treatment should be 7 to 10 days, unless longer treatment is indicated by clinical progress.

Perianal Streptococcal Infection

Perianal streptococcal infection, a localized infection of the perianal area, usually occurs in children. The rash is caused by group A beta-hemolytic streptococci. The diagnosis is confirmed by a perianal swab and culture. The treatment of choice is **penicillin,** with **erythromycin** prescribed to penicillin-allergic patients.

Cellulitis

Cellulitis is a painful, erythematous, spreading bacterial infection involving the soft tissue. The patient can become quite ill if untreated, including developing sepsis. The causative organisms are most commonly *Streptococcus pneumoniae, S. aureus,* or, in children, *Haemophilus influenzae.* Treatment is with systemic **antibiotics** that are effective against these organisms. If the clinical assessment warrants it, an initial dose of an intramuscular or intravenous **antibiotic (ceftriaxone, cefazolin, oxacillin)** can be given, followed by oral **antibiotic** treatment. Oral **antibiotic** treatment with a broad-spectrum **antibiotic** such as **amoxicillin/clavulanate** or a **cephalosporin** is indicated. Blood and tissue aspirate cultures will guide the practitioner in determining if the organism is sensitive to the **antibiotic** of choice. Close follow-up, usually within 24 hours, is indicated to determine if the clinical status is improving or worsening. The provider should consider MRSA if patients are not responding to initial therapy or have risk factors for MRSA. If MRSA is suspected oral **TMP/SMZ, clindamycin,** or **doxycycline** (child younger than age 8 years) are the drugs of choice. Parenteral **antibiotics** may be needed if cellulitis is severe or the patient does not respond to oral **antibiotics** within 24 to 48 hours.

Viral Skin Infections

HSV Infections, Varicella, and Herpes Zoster

The treatment of HSV infections, varicella, and herpes zoster includes the use of **acyclovir (Zovirax)**, which can be used topically or systemically. **Acyclovir** has inhibitory action against HSV-1, HSV-2, and varicella-zoster virus. It decreases the duration of acute infections in HSV-2 infections and, when used to treat herpes zoster, shortens the time to lesion scabbing and decreases the length of viral shedding. When prescribed for patients with varicella, **acyclovir** decreases the number of vesicular lesions, shortens the time to healing, and decreases fever by the second day.

Other antiviral agents that may be prescribed include **famciclovir (Famvir)** and **valacyclovir (Valtrex)**, which are the drugs of choice for recurrent outbreaks of HSV infection. **Famciclovir** can also be used for treatment of herpes zoster. It decreases the healing time by shortening the time to crusting and healing and decreases the length of viral shedding. **Valacyclovir** is a hydrochloride salt of L-valyl ester of **acyclovir;** is rapidly converted to **acyclovir;** and is active against HSV infections, varicella, and herpes zoster. See Table 32–3 for prescribing information.

Three topical antiviral medications are available: **acyclovir (Zovirax), penciclovir (Denavir),** and the OTC product **docosanol (Abreva). Acyclovir** is indicated in the management of initial episodes of herpes genitalis and in limited, non–life threatening, mucocutaneous HSV infections in immunocompromised patients. There is no clinical evidence for the benefit of using **acyclovir** in the immunocompetent patient, although decreased viral shedding may be noted. Topical **acyclovir** is applied to cover all lesions every 3 hours six times a day for 7 days. **Penciclovir** is indicated in the treatment of recurrent herpes labialis (cold sores) on the lips and face. Application to mucous membrane is not recommended. In adults, **penciclovir** 1 percent cream is applied every 2 hours while awake, with treatment started as early as possible (during the prodrome or when lesions appear). **Docosanol (Abreva)** is the only OTC product available for the treatment of herpes labialis. It is applied to the cold sore 5 times a day until healed. Treatment should begin at first sign of treatment. All of the topical products are most effective if started as early as possible, in the prodrome phase and need to be applied with a glove or finger cot to prevent spread to other areas.

Comfort measures with **antipruritics**, such as **antihistamines**, and wet soaks are also part of the treatment plan for viral skin infections. Table 32–3 presents prescribing information.

Fungal Skin Infections

Oral Candidiasis

Oral candidiasis (thrush) is commonly found in infants and immunocompromised patients. Prompt treatment is essential to maintain adequate nutrition and for patient comfort. The treatment of choice is a topical application of an antifungal agent, such as **nystatin (Mycostatin)**, **clotrimazole (Mycelex)**, or **gentian violet**, or oral administration of the systemic **antifungal fluconazole (Diflucan)**. Table 32–3 presents prescribing information.

Tinea Capitis

With tinea capitis (ringworm of the scalp), the patient presents with a characteristic bald patch, with crusting or scaling. *Microsporum* species usually present with broken hairs and a fine gray scale. *Trichophyton tonsurans* (black dot tinea) presents with tiny black dots that are the remains of broken hair shafts.

Treatment of tinea capitis consists of oral antifungal therapy with **griseofulvin (Grifulvin V, Grisactin)** and biweekly shampooing with a sporicidal shampoo (**selenium sulfide** or **ketoconazole**). Tinea capitis should always be treated with a systemic **antifungal**, never a topical agent. Treatment should continue for 6 to 8 weeks or until 2 weeks after KOH or culture is negative. Close contacts should be empirically treated with sporicidal shampoo twice a week. Resistant cases can be treated with **terbinafine**, **fluconazole**, or **itraconazole**, based on the sensitivity as determined by culture. Table 32–3 presents prescribing information.

Tinea Corporis and Tinea Cruris

Tinea corporis (ringworm) is commonly caused by *Microsporum canis, T. tonsurans,* or *Epidermophyton floccosum.* The classic presentation is an annular lesion with raised borders and a clear center. There may be scaling and usually some erythema. The infection spreads by direct contact with an infected person or animal, with household pets being a common source of infection.

Tinea cruris ("jock itch") affects the skin of the groin, upper thighs, and intertriginous folds. It is more common in males and rarely occurs before adolescence. It is caused by the dermatophytes *E. floccosum, Trichophyton rubrum, Trichophyton mentagrophytes,* and *C. albicans.* Tinea cruris is worse in hot, humid weather. The lesions are scaly with a raised border, erythematous, and slightly brown in color. Treatment for both tinea corporis and tinea cruris is topical antifungal cream, with **miconazole (Micatin, Monistat-Derm)**, **tolnaftate (Tinactin)**, and **clotrimazole (Lotrimin, Mycelex)** the least expensive and most commonly prescribed. Other topical **antifungals** that may be used include **terbinafine (Lamisil)**, **sulconazole (Exelderm)**, **ciclopirox (Loprox)**, **ketoconazole (Nizoral)**, **econazole (Spectazole)**, and **oxiconazole (Oxistat)**. Table 32–3 presents prescribing information.

> **CLINICAL PEARL**
>
> **Thrush**
>
> Infants (and some older or very ill patients) are unable to hold **nystatin** suspension in their mouth. To achieve better results with **nystatin** administration, instruct the parents or caregivers to dip a clean cotton-tipped applicator into the **nystatin** solution, then rub the medication into the areas of thrush on the inner cheeks. Use a clean swab for each side and do not redip the applicator into the **nystatin.** After swabbing on the **nystatin,** the parent or caregiver can then administer 1 to 2 mL to each cheek.

Tinea Pedis

Tinea pedis (athlete's foot) is caused by the dermatophytes *E. floccosum, T. rubrum, T. mentagrophytes,* and *C. albicans.* It is more common in males and rarely presents before puberty. It can present in three forms: interdigital maceration, scaling, and fissuring; a "moccasin" distribution of persistent dry scale with minimal inflammation; or scattered pustules and vesicles on the sole and lateral aspects of the feet. The nonpharmacological management includes measures to keep the feet dry and well aired such as wearing sandals whenever possible, wearing clean cotton socks, and drying the feet carefully after bathing. Pharmacological management is with topical **antifungals**, similar to those used for tinea corporis: **miconazole**, **clotrimazole**, **tolnaftate**, **terbinafine**, **sulconazole**, **ciclopirox**, **ketoconazole**, **econazole**, and **oxiconazole**. However, the length of treatment is usually longer than for tinea cruris. Table 32–3 presents prescribing information.

Tinea Versicolor

Tinea versicolor (pityriasis versicolor) is caused by *Pityrosporum orbiculare* (formerly called *Malassezia furfur*). Clinically, the infection appears as multiple scaling, discrete, oval-shaped macules that may be hypopigmented or hyperpigmented. The color of the macules ranges from salmon to brown, and they are usually seen on the trunk, neck, and shoulders. The infection is associated with warm, humid weather. Treatment consists of topical application of **selenium sulfide shampoo (Selsun)** or a topical **antifungal**, commonly one of the **imidazoles (miconazole, clotrimazole, econazole)**. The patient should be educated to observe for recurrence, which up to 50 percent of patients experience. The shampoo is applied to the affected area and left on for 10 to 15 minutes every day for 1 week. It may also be used prophylactically once a month. The topical **antifungal** is used for 2 to 4 weeks and is rubbed into the affected area twice a day.

Onychomycosis

Onychomycosis is a fungal infection of the nail, either fingernail or toenail. The common dermatophyte that is found in onychomycosis is tinea unguium, with *Candida* infections also a cause. Effective treatment usually involves months of a systemic antifungal medication, commonly **griseofulvin**, **ketoconazole**, **itraconazole**, or **terbinafine**. Topical treatment is usually not effective with the exception of **ciclopirox nail lacquer (Penlac)**. Recent studies have demonstrated added effectiveness when topical **ciclopirox** and systemic **antifungals** are combined. Clearing of onychomycosis takes months of treatment regardless of treatment modality. Table 32–3 presents prescribing information.

Table 32–3 **Drugs Commonly Used: Skin Infections**

Drug	Indication	Strengths Available	Dose	Comments
Topical Antibiotics				
Mupirocin (Bactroban)	Bacterial skin infections	2% ointment (15, 30 g) (available Rx only)	Apply to affected area tid until healed	Pregnancy Category B Safe in children
Polymyxin B/neomycin/ bacitracin (Neosporin, Triple Antibiotics Ointment)	Bacterial skin infections	Triple antibiotic combination (available OTC)	Apply a small amount to affected area 1–3 times/d until healed	Do not use if the patient has a neomycin sensitivity Topical use is safe in pregnancy and in young children
Polymyxin B/bacitracin (Polysporin, Double Antibiotic Ointment)	Bacterial skin infections	Double antibiotic combination (available OTC)	Apply a small amount to affected area 1–3 times/d until healed	Topical use is safe in pregnancy and in young children
Bacitracin (Baciguent)	Bacterial skin infections	Bacitracin only ointment (available OTC)	Apply to affected area 1–3 times/d until healed	May use in patients with neomycin sensitivity Safe during pregnancy and in young children
Retapamulin (Altabax)	Bacterial skin infections	1% ointment	*Children age ≥9 mo and adults*: Apply to skin lesion twice a day for 5 days. May cover with gauze or bandage.	Safe during pregnancy and in infants age 9 mo and older. Not for intranasal use. Reevaluate if no improvement in 3 to 4 weeks after starting therapy.
Systemic Oral Antibiotics				
Cephalexin (Keflex)	Bacterial skin infections	Capsules: 250, 500 mg Suspension: 125 mg/ 5 mL, 250 mg/5 mL	*Adults:* 500 mg every 12 h for 7–10 d *Children:* 25–50 mg/kg/d divided qid or tid; treat for 7–10 d	Inexpensive Pregnancy Category B Safe in children Well tolerated
Amoxicillin/ clavulanate (Augmentin)	Bacterial skin infections	Tablets: 250 mg amoxicillin with 125 mg clavulanate; 500 mg with 125 mg	*Adults:* 500 mg of amoxicillin every 12 h *or* 250 mg every 8 h for 7–10 d	Broad-spectrum coverage Moderately expensive Pregnancy Category B

Continued

Table 32–3 **Drugs Commonly Used: Skin Infections—cont'd**

Drug	Indication	Strengths Available	Dose	Comments
		Chewable tablets: 125 mg amoxicillin with 31.25 mg clavulanate; 200 mg with 28.5 mg; 250 mg with 62.5 mg; 400 mg with 57 mg; 125 mg with 31.25 mg/ 5 mL; 200 mg with 28.5/5mL 250 mg with 62.5 mg/ 5 mL; 400 mg with 57 mg/5 mL	*Children >3 mo:* 25–45 mg/kg/d of amoxicillin divided every 12 h (use 200 mg/5 mL or 400 mg/5 mL strength suspension) or 20–40 mg/kg/d of amoxicillin if using 125 mg/ 5 mL or 250 mg/ 5 mL strength suspension; treat for 7–10 d; use higher amounts with more severe infections	May cause gastrointestinal (GI) upset, especially at higher doses Children's dose in based on amoxicillin content Due to clavulanate content, two 250-mg tablets are not the same as one 500-mg tables; suspension doses are also not equivalent Children should not be given the 250-mg tablet until they weigh >40 kg
Cefadroxil (Duricef)	Bacterial skin infections	Tablets: 1 g Capsules: 500 mg Suspension: 125 mg/ 5 mL, 250 mg/5 mL, 500 mg/5 mL	*Adults:* 1 g once/d for 10 d *Children:* 30 mg/kg/d divided into 2 doses every 12 h	Pregnancy Category B First generation cephalosporin Convenient. dosing
Cefprozil (Cefzil)	Bacterial skin infections	Tablets: 250, 500 mg Suspension: 125 mg/ 5 mL, 250 mg/5 mL	*Children ≥12 yr and adults:* 250–500 mg every 12 h for 7–10 d	Broad-spectrum coverage Expensive Pregnancy Category B *Children 2–12 yr:* 20 mg/kg/d divided into 2 doses 12 h apart for 7–10 d
		Erythromycin estolate: 250-, 500-mg tablets; 125 mg/ 5 mL, 250 mg/5 mL suspension Erythromycin ethylsuccinate: 200-mg chewable tablets; 400- mg tablets; 200 mg/5 mL, 400 mg/5 mL suspension	*Children:* 20–50 mg/kg/d qid for 10 d	May cause GI upset: take with food or milk
Clindamycin (Cleocin)	Bacterial skin infections (MRSA)	Capsules: 75, 150, 300 mg	*Adults:* 150–300 mg qid	Pregnancy Category B
		Pediatric granules for oral solution: 75 mg/5 mL	*Children:* 8 mg/kg/d divided in 3–4 doses	May cause severe and possibly fatal colitis Discontinue drug if significant diarrhea occurs
Doxycycline (Doryx, Monodox) (Vibramycin)	Bacterial skin infections (MRSA)	Capsules: 50 mg, 75 mg, 100 mg	*Adults:* 100–200 mg/d in 1–2 divided doses	Contraindicated in children <8 yr
		Suspension: 25 mg/ 5 mL	*Children >8 yr:* 2–4 mg/kg/d in 1–2 divided doses maximum 200 mg/d	Pregnancy Category D Photosensitivity may occur

Table 32–3 **Drugs Commonly Used: Skin Infections—cont'd**

Drug	Indication	Strengths Available	Dose	Comments
Antivirals				
Acyclovir (Zovirax), topical	HSV infection, herpes zoster, varicella	3% ointment (3, 15 g)	Apply to lesion every 3 h 6 times/d for 7 d	Pregnancy Category C Use a finger cot or glove when applying ointment to prevent spread of virus
Acyclovir (Zovirax), oral	HSV infection, herpes zoster, varicella	Tablets: 400, 800 mg	*Adults:*	Pregnancy Category C
		Suspension: 200 mg/5 mL	Genital herpes: Initial: 200 mg every 4 h 5 times/d for 10 d Chronic: 400 mg bid or 200 mg 3–5 times/d for up to 12 mo Intermittent: 200 mg q4h 5 times/d for 5 d; begin at first sign of occurrence Herpes zoster: 800 mg q4h 5 times/d for 7–10 d Varicella: 20 mg/kg 4 times/d for 5 d maximum 800 mg/dose, begin within 24 h of first lesion Children ≥2 yr: Varicella: 20 mg/kg 4 times/day for 5 day; maximum 800 mg/dose; begin within 24 h of first lesion	Decrease dose in renal patients
Famciclovir (Famvir B)	HSV infection, herpes zoster	Tablet: 135, 250, 500 mg	Genital herpes: Initial episode: 125 mg q12h for 5 d; begin as soon as symptoms appear Recurrent episodes: 125 mg q12h for 5 d Suppression therapy: 250 mg q12h for up to 12 mo	Not recommended in patients <18 yr Decrease dose in renal patients Pregnancy Category B Register pregnant patients exposed by famciclovir by calling 800-366-8900 ext 5231

Continued

Table 32–3 **Drugs Commonly Used: Skin Infections—cont'd**

Drug	Indication	Strengths Available	Dose	Comments
			Herpes zoster; 500 mg q8h for 7 d; begin within 72 h of lesions appearing	
Valacyclovir (Valtrex)	HSV infection, herpes zoster	Caplet: 500 mg, 1 g	Genital herpes: Initial episode: 1 g daily for 10 d Recurrent episodes; 500 mg q12h for 5 d started within 24 h of first symptom of outbreak Herpes zoster: 1g q8h for 7 d; begin within 48–72 h of first lesions appearing	Not recommended in children Decrease dose in renal patients Pregnancy Category B Register pregnant patients exposed by valacyclovir by calling 800-722-9292, ext 39437
Antifungals				
Nystatin (Mycostatin, Nilstat)	Oral *Candida* infection	Suspension: 100,000 U/mL Pastilles: 200,000 U each	*Children and adults*: 2–3 mg in each inner cheek qid (total dose 4–6 mL); have patient hold medication in mouth as long as possible before swallowing; treat for 48 h after clinical cure to prevent relapse *Infants:* 1 mL each cheek qid (2 mL/dose total) until 48 h after clinical cure; may apply medication to inner cheeks and tongue with cotton swab prior to administering the 1-mL dose via dropper	Safe in pregnancy and in young children and even in debilitated infants Well tolerated, even with prolonged administration
Nystatin (Mycostatin, Nilstat, Nystex)	Cutaneous *Candida* infection	Cream, ointment, powder	Apply to affected areas 2–3 times/d until healed	Safe in pregnancy and in children

Table 32–3 **Drugs Commonly Used: Skin Infections—cont'd**

Drug	Indication	Strengths Available	Dose	Comments
Clotrimazole (Mycelex)	Oral *Candida* infection	Troches: 10 mg	*Adults and children >3 yr and adults:* 1 troche 5 times/d for 14 d; dissolve slowly in mouth	Not recommended in children Pregnancy Category C; not recommended for use in pregnancy May cause elevated liver function tests
Clotrimazole (Lotrimin, Mycelex)	Dermatophyte infections of the skin	1% cream (Rx and OTC); 1% solution (Rx and OTC); 1% lotion (Rx)	Apply to affected area bid for 2 wk Tinea pedis: treat for 4 wk	Pregnancy Category B Safe in children
Gentian violet	Oral *Candida* infection	Solution: 1%, 2% (available OTC)	Apply with cotton swab to entire inner surface of the mouth 2 times/d until healed	Stains every thing it touches purple; warn patient/parents about staining of mouth; stain resolves within a couple of days of discontinuing therapy
Fluconazole (Diflucan)	Oral *Candida* infection	Tablets: 50, 100, 150, 200 mg Suspension: 10 mg/mL 40 mg/mL	*Adults:* 200 mg first day, then 100 mg daily for 2 wk minimum *Infants and children:* 6 mg/kg on the first day, then 3 mg/kg daily for 2 wk minimum	Pregnancy Category C Interacts with cimetidine, hydrochlorothiazide, rifampin cyclosporine, phenytoin, and theophylline; monitor closely if patient is taking one of these medications with fluconazole
Miconazole (Micatin, Monistat-Derm, Micatin)	Dermatophyte infections of the skin	2% cream (Micatin, Monistat-Derm); 2% powder (Micatin); 2% spray (Micatin Liquid) (available OTC)	Apply to affected area 2–3 times/d for 2 wk Tinea pedis: treat for 4 wk	Topical use safe in pregnancy and in children
Tolnaftate (Tinactin, Ting, Aftate, Absorbine)	Dermatophyte infections of the skin, Tinea pedis	1% cream, solution, gel, powder, spray powder, spray liquid (available OTC)	Apply to affected area bid for 2–3 wk; if skin is thickened, treatment may take 4–6 wk	Safe for topical use in pregnancy Not recommended for use in children <2 yr
Terbinafine (Lamisil)	Dermatophyte infections of the skin	Cream	Apply to affected and immediate surrounding areas 1–2 times/d until symptoms are significantly improved (usually 1–4 wk) Tinea pedis: apply to affected and immediate surrounding areas until symptoms are significantly improved	Pregnancy Category B; safety in children <12 yr has not been established Clinical improvement may continue for 2–4 wk after therapy is stopped

Continued

Table 32–3 **Drugs Commonly Used: Skin Infections—cont'd**

Drug	Indication	Strengths Available	Dose	Comments
Sulconazole (Exelderm)	Dermatophyte infections of the skin	1% cream; 1% solution (Rx required)	Massage medication into affected area 2 times/d for 2 wk For tinea pedis, apply for 4 wk	Pregnancy Category C; use only if clearly needed
Ciclopirox (Loprox)	Dermatophyte infections of the skin	1% cream; 1% lotion (Rx required)	Massage medication into affected area 1–2 times/d for 3 wk For tinea pedis, apply bid for 4 wk	Pregnancy Category C; safety in children <10 yr has not been established
Ciclopirox (Penlac)	Onychomycosis of fingernails or toenails	8% topical solution (nail lacquer)	*Adults:* Apply thin layer to entire nail and surrounding 5 mm Leave on 8 h before washing once a week remove with alcohol. Trim and file nails while free of drug. Repeat for 48 wk	Not recommended in children Pregnancy Category B Product is flammable
Ketoconazole (Nizoral)	Dermatophyte infections of the skin	2% cream	Massage medication into affected area once/d for 2 wk For tinea pedis, apply for 6 wk	Pregnancy Category C May be used to treat cutaneous *Candida* infections
Econazole (Spectazole)	Dermatophyte infections of the skin	1% cream (Rx required)	Massage medication into affected area once/d for 2 wk minimum For tinea pedis, apply for 4-wk minimum	Pregnancy Category C; do not use in first trimester; use in second and third trimesters only if clearly needed
Oxiconazole (Oxistat)	Dermatophyte infections of the skin	1% cream; 1% lotion (Rx required)	Massage medication into affected area 1–2 times/d for 2 wk For tinea pedis, apply for 4 wk	Pregnancy Category B; use only if clearly needed
Griseofulvin Microsize (Fulvicin, U/F, Grifulvin V, Grisactin)	Tinea capitis, onychomycosis	Tablets: 250, 500 mg	Tinea capitis:	Pregnancy Category C; safe in children >2 yr
		Capsules: 125, 250 mg	*Adults:* 500 mg daily for 4–6 wk	

Table 32–3 **Drugs Commonly Used: Skin Infections—cont'd**

Drug	Indication	Strengths Available	Dose	Comments
		Suspension: 125 mg/ 5 mL	*Children:* 11 mg/kg/d for 4–6 wk Onychomycosis: *Adults:* 750–1,000 mg daily in divided doses; treat fingernail infection for 4 mo; toenail infection for 6 mo *Children:* 11 mg/kg/d; treat fingernail infection for 4 mo; toenail infection for 6 mo	Renal, liver, and hematopoietic function tests need to be drawn and monitored every 8 wk if on prolonged therapy Best absorbed if taken with a high-fat meal
Griseofulvin Ultramicro-size (Fulvicin P/G, Grisactin Ultra, Gris-PEG)	Tinea capitis, onychomycosis	Tablets: 125, 165, 250, 330 mg	Tinea capitis: *Adults:* 330–375 mg daily for 4–6 wk	Pregnancy Category C; safe in children >2 yr
			Children: 7.3 mg/kg/d for 4–6 wk Onychomycosis: *Adults:* 660–750 mg daily in divided doses; treat fingernail infection for 4 mo; toenail infection for 6 mo	Renal, liver, and hematopoietic function tests need to be drawn and monitored every 8 wk if on prolonged therapy
			Children: 7.3 mg/kg/d; treat fingernail infection for 4 mo; toenail infection for 6 mo	Best absorbed if taken with a high-fat meal
Ketoconazole (Nizoral)	Tinea capitis, onychomycosis	Tablets: 200 mg	*Adults:* 200 mg daily; may increase to 400 mg daily if inadequate clinical response; minimum length of treatment is 4 wk	Monitor hepatic function prior to initiating therapy and monthly during therapy
			Children ≥2 yr: 3.3–6.6 mg/kg/d	Pregnancy Category C; may be prescribed to children 2 yr and older Not first-line treatment for onychomycosis because of possible hepatotoxicity Use with caution if patient is taking medications that are primarily metabolized by the liver

Continued

Table 32–3 **Drugs Commonly Used: Skin Infections—cont'd**

Drug	Indication	Strengths Available	Dose	Comments
				Coadministration with astemizole is absolutely contraindicated because of secondary cardiotoxic effects
Itraconazole (Sporanox)	Onychomycosis	Capsules: 100 mg	*Adults:* Daily dosing schedule: toenails: 200 mg daily for 12 wk Pulse schedule: toenails: 400 mg daily for 1 wk/mo for 3–4 mo; for fingernails: 200 mg bid for 7 d, then 3 wk without medication, then 200 mg bid for 7 more days *Children:* Pulse schedule: 5 mg/kg/d for 1 wk/mo for 3–4 consecutive mo	If used for more than 8 consecutive weeks, liver enzymes and electrolytes should be drawn prior to and every 8 wk during treatment Pregnancy Category C; do not administer to pregnant women or women considering pregnancy In children use griseofulvin as first-line therapy Coadministration with astemizole is absolutely contraindicated because of secondary cardiotoxic effects Coadministration with cisapride, midazolam, triazolam, simvastatin, and lovastatin is also contraindicated
Terbinafine (Lamisil)	Onychomycosis	Tablets: 250 mg	Fingernail infection: 250 mg daily for 6 wk Toenail infection: 250 mg daily for 12 wk	Not recommended for use in children; safety not established Liver enzymes and complete blood count (CBC) should be monitored every 6 wk Pregnancy Category B; delay treatment until after pregnancy

HSV = herpes simplex virus; MRSA = methicillin-resistant *Staphylococcus aureus;* OTC = over the counter.

Monitoring

For all skin infections, the patient should be monitored to determine the effectiveness of the medication in treating the infection, compliance with the prescribed therapy, adverse effects, and the development of secondary infection.

Outcome Evaluation

For skin infections, improvement should be noted, usually within 24 to 48 hours. If not, a change in therapy may be indicated, with resistance suspected. Secondary skin infections, if they occur, should be treated promptly. Referral to a dermatologist may be necessary if therapy is not managing the infection.

Patient Education

Patient education should include a discussion of information related to the overall treatment plan as well as that specific to the drug therapy, reasons for taking the drug, drugs as part of the total treatment regimen, and adherence issues.

SKIN INFESTATIONS

Skin and hair infestation with arthropods, most commonly lice and scabies, is a frequently seen problem in primary care. Head lice infestation is at epidemic levels in school-age children, with 6 to 12 million people in the United States affected each year. Scabies is common at all ages and is more common when poor hygiene or crowded living conditions are present.

Pathophysiology

Lice

Pediculosis is infestation of the body with lice. The affected body area helps to determine what arthropod is

SKIN INFECTIONS

PATIENT EDUCATION

Related to the Overall Treatment Plan/Disease Process

- ☐ Pathophysiology
- ☐ Role of preventive and nonpharmacological measures if appropriate
- ☐ Importance of adherence to the treatment regimen
- ☐ Self-monitoring of symptoms
- ☐ What to do when symptoms worsen
- ☐ Need for follow-up visits with the primary care provider

Specific to the Drug Therapy

- ☐ Reason for taking the drug and its anticipated action on the disease process
- ☐ Doses and schedules for taking the drug
- ☐ Possible adverse effects and what to do if they occur
- ☐ Interactions between other treatment modalities and these drugs

Reasons for Taking the Drug(s)

- ☐ Patient education about specific drugs is provided in the appropriate chapter.

Specifically for Bacterial Skin Infections

- ☐ Explanation regarding the suspected cause of the infection and the rationale for the **antibiotic** treatment chosen
- ☐ Hand washing should be stressed to prevent spread of the skin infection to the patient or others
- ☐ Clear guidelines regarding notifying the practitioner if the infection is getting worse
- ☐ Improvement should be noted in 24 to 48 hours; if not, a change in therapy may be indicated

Specifically for Viral Infections

Expectations of the medication. The healthy patient will have resolution of the vesicular lesions even without pharmacological intervention. Effective antiviral therapy decreases the time to scabbing and healing of lesions and decreases viral shedding time. In immunocompromised patients, the medication will help decrease the severity of the outbreak.

- ☐ How the virus can become dormant and recur at a later time, even many years later.
- ☐ Patients using topical antivirals need to be instructed to use a glove or finger cot to apply the ointment to prevent getting the virus on their hands and spreading it; also, the patient may experience a transient burning when the medication is applied.
- ☐ It should be stressed to the patient and/or family members that the patient is contagious until the lesions are healed or scabbed over, even if antiviral agents are being taken; the patient should avoid contact with immunocompromised individuals and avoid sexual intercourse if the patient has genital herpes lesions.

Specifically for Fungal Infections

- ☐ The patient and/or family members should understand how the fungal infection is spread and how contagious the infection is.
- ☐ Family members and pets should be checked for signs of infection and treated if indicated.
- ☐ The provider should stress the possibility of relapse if the medication regimen is not followed correctly and for the full treatment time.

Drugs as Part of the Total Treatment Regimen

- ☐ The total treatment regimen includes pharmacological and nonpharmacological measures. Be sure the patient and/or family members are aware of the specific measures to be taken.

Adherence Issues

- ☐ Health-care providers should be aware of the potential problem of nonadherence and should discuss the importance of completing the entire treatment regimen with the patient and/or family members.

present. The skin signs seen with pediculosis are pruritus, excoriation from scratching, adenopathy (occasionally) in the affected region, and the presence of lice or nits.

The common name for infestation with *Pediculus humanus capitis* is head lice (pediculosis capitis). The mite of head lice is usually visible, and the nits or eggs are visualized attached to the hair shaft. The female louse lays approximately four eggs per day and has a lifespan of 2 to 4 weeks. Head lice are spread by direct contact with another infected person or by indirect contact with a hairbrush, hat, or article of clothing that the lice or nits have been transferred to. Outbreaks in schools are seen when children share hats or hairbrushes. When outer garments are hung in a close group, which is often the case in school, the lice can travel from coat to coat and spread to an unsuspecting new household. Diagnosis is made by observing mites or nits.

Body lice (pediculosis corporis), the common name for infestation with *P. humanus corporis,* are uncommon. They usually are not seen on the body but on the seams of clothing and undergarments. They come onto the body to feed and leave hemorrhagic pinpoint macules where they extract blood. There is often excoriation from scratching. The common sites for body lice are the belt line, collar, and underwear areas. Diagnosis is made by examining the clothing and underwear for the presence of mites and nits.

Infestation with *Phthirus pubis* is commonly called pubic lice (pediculosis pubis). Patients often refer to it as crabs. The mites are quite small and may need to be examined under a handheld magnifying glass, as they may be mistaken for a freckle. The mites and nits are found on the pubic hair and the hair of the perianal region. They may extend up to the hair on the abdomen and to the hair on the upper thighs. The eyelashes and axillary hair may also be involved. Pubic lice are never seen before pubertal hair development. They are often sexually transmitted. Diagnosis is made by observing the mite or nits in the pubic hair.

Scabies

Scabies is a highly contagious infestation with *Sarcoptes scabiei.* The female scabies mite burrows under the skin and lays eggs as she tunnels. The eggs hatch in about 2 weeks. The surface of the skin has characteristic curving burrows and excoriated papules. The burrows are in the horny layer of the skin and are seen most frequently on the sides of the fingers; the interdigital webs; flexor surfaces of the wrists, elbows, axillae, and genitalia. In infants, the scabies mite can often be found on the entire body, including the trunk and face. There may be a secondary infection present.

The incubation period is 1 to 2 months after contact with another infested person or with unwashed clothing recently worn by an infected person. Bed partners can be infected even if there is no body contact. Often the first sign of infestation with scabies is intense pruritus, which occurs 2 to 6 weeks after the first exposure to the mite. The itching is caused by sensitization to the mite feces. Definitive diagnosis is made by scraping a burrow that reveals mites or eggs.

Goals of Treatment

The goals of treatment are to completely eradicate the arthropods and to educate the patient and family about the disease and how to prevent further infestations.

Rational Drug Selection

Pharmacological management of lice and scabies consists of the use of **ectoparacides.** The specific medication used varies by the type of infestation and the age of the patient. For head lice, there is a choice of OTC products and, in the case of resistance to OTC products, prescription **lindane** or **malathion. Benzoyl alcohol (Ulesfia)** was approved for use in 2009 and is the first non-neurotoxin FDA approved for head lice. There is also variety of nonpharmacological remedies for head lice. For body lice, the treatment of choice is **lindane** or **permethrin** 5 percent **(Elimite)** and washing infested clothing and bedding. Pubic lice are treated with **lindane** shampoo. Scabies is treated with **permethrin** or **lindane.** Nonpharmacological, environmental measures are a key part of the treatment of any infestation because patients can reinfect themselves or other family members and restart the infestation cycle.

Head Lice

Head lice can cause great distress to the family. It is necessary to treat head lice aggressively and completely to prevent recurrence. Unfortunately, resistance to some **pediculicides** has made treating head lice at times a clinical challenge. The OTC products available for treating head lice include **pyrethrins** and **permethrin. Benzoyl alcohol (Ulesfia)** may be prescribed for head lice. **Lindane** and **malathion (Ovide)** are prescription drugs used as a second-line agents for resistant head lice (Centers for Disease Control and Prevention, Division of Parasitic Diseases [CDC], 2008d).

Although all of the head lice treatments are relatively safe, they are classified as neurotoxic agents (except **benzoyl alcohol**), and they should be used exactly as directed on the package or prescription. To limit exposure, the medication should be washed off at a sink, rather than in a shower. Cool or lukewarm water should be used to minimize absorption caused by vasodilation. After treatment, the hair should be combed to remove all the nits. There are special combs available for this, or slow, patient combing can be effective. Advise parents to comb hair a minimum of 20 minutes, dividing hair in sections. Treat only family members who are actively infested. Do not treat head lice prophylactically.

With the use of **malathion (Ovide)** careful instruction should be given regarding the flammability of the product.

Lotion and wet hair should not be exposed to open flames or electric heat sources, including hair dryers and electric curlers. Do not smoke while applying lotion or while hair is wet. Allow hair to dry naturally and to remain uncovered after application of **Ovide** lotion.

Pyrethrins

Pyrethrins are combined with **piperonyl butoxide (RID, Pronto, A-200)** and are available OTC. **Pyrethrins** are 100 percent insecticidal and 70 to 80 percent ovicidal. The shampoo is applied to dry hair and left on for 10 to 20 minutes, with the time varying by brand. It is important for the product to be applied to dry hair to enable the **pediculicide** to enter the insect's body better. The patient should be retreated in 1 week regardless of whether there is evidence of infestation. **Pyrethrins** have no residual activity and can be used in young children and pregnant women if used as directed.

Permethrin

Permethrin is a synthetic compound related to **pyrethrins**. It is available OTC in 1 percent cream (**Nix**) or prescription strength 5 percent cream (**Elimite**). Only **Nix** has FDA approval for use on head lice. **Nix** is 97 percent insecticidal and 70 to 80 percent ovicidal. **Permethrin** is a cream rinse that is applied after shampooing. It is important that the shampoo not have any conditioner in the formula, which makes the **permethrin** less effective. The cream rinse is left in the hair for 10 minutes before rinsing off. Treatment should be repeated in 1 week, regardless of whether signs of infestation are present. **Permethrin** cream rinse has residual activity against lice for up to 10 days.

Lindane

Lindane is a prescription product used as a second-line agent for head lice. The popular brand of **lindane, Kwell**, is no longer on the market, but multiple generic brands of the product are available. **Lindane** is 67 percent insecticidal and 45 to 70 percent ovicidal. **Lindane** is neurotoxic and should not be used in pregnant women or in infants. **Lindane** is applied to dry hair, working in small quantities of water to create a good lather. The shampoo is left on for 4 minutes. The amount of shampoo prescribed for short hair is 1 oz, and for long hair, 2 oz. The shampoo should be rinsed well. **Lindane** has no residual activity against head lice.

Malathion

Malathion (**Ovide**) is a pediculicide that is available OTC in the United Kingdom and has been recently reapproved as a treatment for head lice in the United States. **Malathion** is an organophosphate agent that acts as a pediculicide by inhibiting cholinesterase activity in vivo. It is very effective against head lice, with 96 percent mortality in 30 minutes (Downs, Narayan, Stafford, & Coles, 2005). Some residual remains and can kill newly hatched lice for up to 7 days.

Ovide is applied to dry hair in an amount sufficient to wet the hair and scalp. Hair should be allowed to dry naturally. Hands should be washed with soap after applying **Ovide**. **Ovide** is left on for 8 to 12 hours and then shampooed. After rinsing, use a nit (or fine-tooth) comb to remove dead lice and eggs. If lice are present in 7 days, **Ovide** may be repeated.

With the use of **Ovide**, careful instruction should be given regarding the flammability of the product. Lotion and wet hair should not be exposed to open flames or electric heat sources, including hair dryers and electric curlers. Do not smoke while applying lotion or while hair is wet. Allow hair to dry naturally and to remain uncovered after application of **Ovide** lotion.

Benzoyl Alcohol

Benzoyl alcohol (Ulesfia) is the first non-neurotoxin treatment for head lice. The active ingredient in **benzoyl alcohol** appears to stun the breathing spiracles of the lice open, enabling the vehicle to penetrate the respiratory mechanism (spiracles) leading to asphyxiation.

Benzoyl alcohol (Ulesfia lotion) is applied to dry hair, completely saturating the hair and scalp and left on for 10 minutes. The lotion is rinsed off well with water. Treatment with another application of **Ulesfia** should be repeated in 7 days.

Nonpharmacological Treatments

With the growing problem of resistance and concern over exposing children to repeated doses of pediculicides, there are anecdotal reports about the success of various nonmedicated therapies. Popular and safe remedies are mayonnaise (full-fat variety), olive oil, and petroleum jelly. It is thought that they asphyxiate the lice by blocking their breathing apparatus or immobilize them and affect their ability to feed. A patient who would like to try these treatments should apply a thick layer of the product and cover with a shower cap. The product is left on from 1 hour to overnight, then shampooed out.

The provider may be asked by a frustrated parent about other nonpharmacological remedies. It is important to give the parent clear guidelines regarding the use of unproven and possibly dangerous interventions, such as using lamp oil or other flammable liquid. Products developed for animals, such as dog lice shampoo, are also not advised.

Body Lice

The treatment for body lice is topical **pediculicides: lindane** and **permethrin** (CDC, 2008a). Body lice live on clothing and underwear and come to the skin only to feed, so it is important to instruct the patient to wash all clothing and bedding in hot water to kill lice and nits that are on the clothing.

Lindane

Lindane is applied to the total body as a cream or lotion and left on for 8 to 12 hours (overnight). The amount needed for an adult is 2 oz. **Lindane** should not be used in infants. It is Pregnancy Category B but should not be used as a first-line medication in pregnant patients because there have been no adequate studies in pregnant patients. If it is prescribed during pregnancy, then it should not be used more than twice during a pregnancy.

Permethrin

Permethrin 5 percent (**Elimite**) may be used for body lice. It is slightly safer in pregnant patients and can be used in children as young as 2 months. **Permethrin** is applied from head to toe and left on for 8 hours (overnight), then showered off.

Pubic Lice

Lindane

Pubic lice are treated with an application of **lindane** 1 percent cream, lotion, or shampoo. A thin layer of cream or lotion is applied to the hair and skin surrounding the pubic area and left on for 12 hours. If **lindane** shampoo is used, the shampoo is massaged into dry pubic hair and left on for 5 to 10 minutes. If axillary or thigh hair is also infested, then use the cream or lotion. Reapply in 7 days if there is evidence of live lice. Sexual partners should also be treated concurrently. Bedding and clothes should be washed.

Pyrethrins

Pubic lice may also treated with **pyrethrins** which are **permethrin** 1 percent, **pyrethrin** lotion, or shampoo. Advise the patient to thoroughly saturate hair with lice medication. Leave medication on for 10 minutes then thoroughly rinse off medication with water. Dry off with a clean towel (CDC, 2008b). Reapply in 7 days if there is evidence of live lice.

Sexual partners should be treated concurrently, and bedding and clothes should also be washed. Infestation of eyelashes by pubic lice is treated with petrolatum (**Vaseline**) ointment applied 3 to 4 times daily for 8 to 10 days. Nits should be removed by hand from the pubic area, axillae, and eyelashes.

Scabies

When treating scabies, the provider may choose between **permethrin** and **lindane.** The provider may choose the drug based on patient age and toxicity of the agent. All family members should receive treatment, even if asymptomatic. Family members may be in the incubation period (4 wk), and so all members of the household need treatment to prevent recurrence. Although one treatment is curative, the inflamed burrows and pruritus may last for up to 3 weeks after treatment with a scabicide. Families need to be educated regarding this prolonged healing phase. Patients should not be re-treated unless living mites are observed.

Permethrin

Permethrin 5 percent cream (**Elimite, Acticin**) is the drug of choice for the treatment of scabies in young children and pregnant women. It is 90 percent effective against the scabies mite and can be used in infants as young as 2 months old and in pregnant women. The cream is massaged into the skin from the neck to the soles of feet. It should be left on for 8 to 14 hours and then washed off in the shower. Infants require special application of **permethrin** to the scalp, temple, forehead, hands, and feet. One to two oz of **permethrin** per family member are prescribed.

Lindane

Lindane 1 percent lotion or cream is used for scabies in children older than 6 months and in nonpregnant adult patients. It is applied in a thin layer from the neck down to the soles of the feet and left on for 8 to 12 hours (overnight) and then washed off thoroughly. If there are crusted lesions present, a tepid bath should be taken prior to application to soften the lesions. The patient should dry the skin thoroughly before applying **lindane.** Two oz of **lindane** per family member are prescribed.

Topical Corticosteroids

Topical **corticosteroids** are used after scabies treatment to treat pruritus and inflammation associated with the scabies mite. **Hydrocortisone** 1 or 2.5 percent or a stronger **corticosteroid**, if indicated, is applied to affected areas twice a day until lesions are healed.

Monitoring

Patients and families need to be monitored for appropriate use of the medication and for effectiveness of treatment. The patient should be monitored for sensitivity to the medication prescribed. If medications are used appropriately, there is rarely an adverse reaction from them, although skin irritation or sensitivity may occur.

Outcome Evaluation

If effective treatment has been implemented, then the lice or scabies should be eradicated. Before resistance is assumed, the provider should review how the patient or family used the medication and if environmental measures were adequate.

Patient Education

Patient and family education is the key to effective eradication of lice and scabies. In prescribing treatment for lice or scabies, the following are key areas of education that need to be covered:

1. Explanation of how the patient was most likely infected with the lice or scabies and how they can be passed on to other family members or, in the case of pubic lice, sexual partners. The incubation period and early symptoms should be discussed to identify other contacts that may be infected, such as school contacts.

2. Proper use of the prescribed medication and environmental measures that may be taken. Written instructions should also be provided. Environmental measures that should be taken for lice and scabies include washing sheets, towels, clothing, and headgear worn recently in hot water and laundry soap. They need to be tumbled in a hot dryer for at least 20 minutes to kill any remaining nits or scabies that may be on the clothing. Clothing that cannot be put in a hot water wash must be dry-cleaned or pressed with a hot iron. Remind parents to wash coats and car seat covers if indicated. Items that cannot be washed or dry-cleaned, such as stuffed animals, should be placed in a plastic bag for 3 to 4 weeks; for scabies, only 4 days is needed. Brushes and combs should be washed in hot water and soaked for 1 hour in disinfectant such as Lysol or rubbing alcohol and then rinsed with hot water. Vacuuming play areas, floors, rugs, and furniture will pick up any nits or lice that may have been transferred to these areas. Parents should be told that insecticidal sprays or bombs are not necessary.

ALOPECIA ANDROGENETICA (MALE PATTERN BALDNESS)

Alopecia androgenetica (male pattern baldness) affects men and some women. It involves hair loss from the frontal, vertex, and occipital regions of the scalp in men and thinning of the hair in the frontoparietal area or diffuse hair loss in women.

Pathophysiology

Common male pattern baldness is genetically determined. The process can begin at any time after puberty. There is not actual hair loss, but a conversion of thick hair to fine, unpigmented vellus hairs, which are poorly seen.

The process is androgen dependent. A male who has a disorder that lowers testosterone production will never go bald, regardless of genetics; a woman who has a masculinizing disorder that raises androgen levels will develop classic male pattern baldness.

Goals of Treatment

A realistic goal is to achieve moderate to dense hair growth with continued use of topical **minoxidil** (**Rogaine**) for at least 4 months. If treating with **finasteride** (**Propecia**), a realistic goal would be increased hair growth after 3 months of continued treatment.

Rational Drug Selection

Alopecia androgenetica can be treated topically with **minoxidil** or systemically with **finasteride**. Choosing between the two medications can often be a simple task based on the patient profile. If the patient is also being treated for benign prostatic hypertrophy (BPH), then **finasteride** is the drug of choice. For a female patient, **minoxidil** is the only choice available.

Minoxidil

Minoxidil, the first drug approved by the FDA to treat male pattern baldness, is available OTC. The patient may be seeking a recommendation from the prescriber or self-prescribing and seeking information regarding its use. It is important to note that **minoxidil** does not treat balding of the frontoparietal areas in men, only in women. **Minoxidil** is effective in treating balding on the vertex of the scalp in men.

Minoxidil 2 percent topical solution is applied to the scalp twice daily for the entire length of treatment. The patient applies 1 mL directly to the affected area of the scalp (vertex area in men and frontoparietal area in women). The medication should be applied to a dry scalp. Patients should be instructed to wash their hands after using their fingers to rub the medication into the scalp. Twice-daily application for at least 4 months may be needed to obtain observable hair growth. If the medication is discontinued, the hair in the treated area will shed in 3 to 4 months.

Minoxidil should not be used by pregnant patients (Pregnancy Category C) or by children under age 18 years. **Minoxidil** is generally well tolerated. The topical solution contains alcohol and therefore may be irritating upon application. Patients may be sensitive to **minoxidil** and develop contact dermatitis. **Minoxidil** topical solution used as directed has minimal cardiac effects, but if large amounts are applied there is a potential for cardiac adverse effects.

Finasteride

Finasteride is a type II 5-alpha reductase–specific inhibitor that inhibits the conversion of testosterone into 5-alpha dihydrotestosterone (DHT). Development of alopecia androgenetica is dependent on DHT, as is the prostate gland. **Finasteride** is also used in treatment of BPH. **Finasteride** is effective in treating vertex and anterior midscalp baldness in men. Hair regrowth is noted after 3 months of daily treatment, with full treatment effect achieved after 6 to 12 months of use.

The dose of **finasteride** is 1 mg once daily with or without food. Continued use is necessary to have continued benefit. If treatment is stopped, hair will return to untreated levels within 12 months.

Finasteride should be prescribed with caution in patients with hepatic dysfunction because the drug is metabolized extensively in the liver. It causes a decrease in serum prostate specific antigen (PSA) levels, even in the presence of prostate cancer. It is Pregnancy Category X. **Finasteride** exposure during pregnancy, even in small quantities, may produce abnormalities of the external genitalia in male offspring. Pregnant women or a woman planning a pregnancy should not handle crushed tablets. **Finasteride** may be potentially absorbed from the semen. When a male patient's sexual partner is pregnant or may become pregnant, the patient should either avoid exposing his partner to his semen or discontinue **finasteride**. There is a small possibility (3% or less) of developing decreased libido, erectile dysfunction, or ejaculation disorder while taking **finasteride**.

Monitoring

The patient being treated for male pattern baldness needs to be monitored for effectiveness of treatment and adverse effects of the medication. The major adverse effect seen with **minoxidil** is dermatitis or sensitivity to the topical solution, which is treated by discontinuing the medication. Topical steroids should not be used concurrently with **minoxidil**. The patient should also be observed for possible cardiac adverse effects. **Finasteride** is generally well tolerated, and adverse effects are usually mild. If the patient experiences sexual dysfunction, then the drug should be discontinued. The patient should be monitored for prostate cancer with a digital rectal examination and PSA levels because **finasteride** causes a low PSA level, even in the presence of prostate cancer. If the patient's sexual partner is of childbearing age, he should be warned about the severe effects that **finasteride** can have on the developing fetus. Monitoring for use of birth control, with condoms used to prevent semen exposure, is necessary if there is a possibility of the patient's partner becoming pregnant.

Outcome Evaluation

It may take 3 to 4 months to determine if **minoxidil** or **finasteride** is effective. The provider should schedule a follow-up appointment with the patient for 3 to 4 months after beginning therapy to determine effectiveness.

Patient Education

In treating a patient with alopecia androgenetica, the following key points should be covered in patient education:

1. The pathophysiology and cause of male pattern baldness.
2. Realistic expectations of therapy, including what type of hair loss the drug treats; how long therapy takes until effects are noticed; that if treatment is stopped, hair shedding will occur; and that the new hair initially may be fine and almost colorless, but with continued treatment the hair should develop the same color and texture as the rest of the hair on the scalp.
3. Caution that the patient should take the medication exactly as prescribed or as indicated by the instructions if taking OTC **minoxidil**.
4. Adverse effects of the medications, especially the hazards to women from **finasteride** exposure.

REFERENCES

Avner, S., Nir, N., & Henri, T. (2005). Combination of oral terbinafine and topical ciclopirox compared to oral terbinafine for the treatment of onychomycosis. *Journal of Dermatological Treatment, 16*(5–6), 327–330.

Baran, R., & Kaoukhov, A. (2005). Topical antifungal drugs for the treatment of onychomycosis: An overview of current strategies for monotherapy and combination therapy. *Journal of the European Academy of Dermatology and Venereology 19*(1), 21–29.

Barber Starr, N. (2004). Dermatological diseases. In C. E. Burns, M. A. Brady, C. Blosser, N. Barber Starr, & A. M. Dunn (Eds.), *Pediatric primary care: A handbook for nurse practitioners* (pp. 1059–1133). Philadelphia: Saunders.

Bell, E. A. (2004, September). Update on pharmacotherapy of head lice. *Infectious Diseases in Children,* Retrieved April 28, 2006, from http://www.idinchildren.com/logon/frameset.asp?article=logon.asp

Boguniewicz, M., Eichenfield, L. F., & Hultsch, T. (2003). Current management of atopic dermatitis and interruption of the atopic march. *Journal of Allergy and Immunology, 112*(6), S140–S150.

Brady, M. A. (2004). Atopic disorders and rheumatic diseases. In C. E. Burns, M. A. Brady, C. Blosser, N. Barber Starr, & A. M. Dunn (Eds.), *Pediatric primary care: A handbook for nurse practitioners*. Philadelphia: Saunders.

Centers for Disease Control and Prevention, Division of Parasitic Diseases (CDC). (2008a). Body lice infestation. Retrieved from http://www.cdc.gov/lice/body/index.html

Centers for Disease Control and Prevention, Division of Parasitic Diseases (CDC). (2008b). Pubic lice infestation. Retrieved from http://www.cdc.gov/lice/pubic/index.html

Centers for Disease Control and Prevention, Division of Parasitic Diseases (CDC). (2008c). Scabies. Retrieved from http://www.cdc.gov/scabies/treatment.html

Centers for Disease Control and Prevention, Division of Parasitic Diseases (CDC). (2008d). Treating head lice infestation. Retrieved from http://www.cdc.gov/lice/head/treatment.html

Charakida, A., Dadzie, O., Teixeira, F., Charakida, M., Evangelou, G., & Chu, A. C. (2006). Calcipotriol/betamethasone dipropionate for the treatment of psoriasis. *Expert Opinion on Pharmacotherapy, 7*(5), 597–606.

Clore, E. R., & Longyear, L. A. (1993). A comparative study of seven pediculicides and their nit removal combs. *Journal of Pediatric Health Care, 7*(2), 55–60.

Dalgard, F., Gieler, U., Holm, J. O., Bjertness, E., & Hauser, S. (2008). Self-esteem and body satisfaction among late adolescents with acne: Results from a population survey. *Journal of the American Academy of Dermatology, 59*(5), 746–751.

Del Roso Do, J. Q. (2006). Combination topical therapy for the treatment of psoriasis. *Journal of Drugs in Dermatology, 5*(3), 232–234.

Downs, A. M. R., Narayan, S., Stafford, K. A., & Coles, G. C. (2005). Effectiveness of Ovide against malathion-resistant head lice. *Archives in Dermatology, 141,* 1318.

Feldman, S. R., & Pearce, D. J. (2010a). Epidemiology, pathophysiology, and diagnosis of psoriasis. *UpToDate Online 18.1* Retrieved from http://www.uptodate.com/online/content/topic.do?topicKey=papulos/4405&selectedTitle=1~150&source=search_result

Feldman, S. R., & Pearce, D. J. (2010b). Treatment of psoriasis. *UpToDate Online 18.1* Retrieved from http://www.uptodate.com/online/content/topic.do?topicKey=papulos/5539&selectedTitle=1~150&source=search_result

Fleischer, A. B., Jr., Herbert, C. R., Feldman, S. R., & O'Brien, F. (2000). Diagnosis of skin disease by nondermatologists. *American Journal of Managed Care, 6*(10), 1149–1156.

Flinders, D. C., & De Schweinitz, P. (2004). Pediculosis and scabies. *American Family Physician, 69*(2), 341–348.

German, D., & Lee, A. (Eds.). (2006). *Nurse practitioner prescribing reference.* New York: Prescribing Reference.

Gupta, A. K., Onychomycosis Combination Therapy Study Group. (2005). Ciclopirox topical solution, 8% combined with oral terbinafine to treat onychomycosis: A randomized, evaluator-blinded study. *Drugs in Dermatology, 4*(4), 481–485.

Hansen, R. C., Krafchik, B. R., Lane, A. T., Odio, M. R., & Schachner, L. A. (1998). Dealing with diaper dermatitis. *Contemporary Pediatrics, 5*(Suppl. May), 5–10.

Landow, K. (1997). Dispelling myths about acne. *Postgraduate Medicine, 102*(2), 94–112.

Lasek, R. J., & Chren, M. M. (1998). Acne vulgaris and the quality of life of adult dermatology patients. *Archives of Dermatology, 134*(4), 454–458.

Luba, K. M., & Stulberg, D. L. (2006). Chronic plaque psoriasis. *American Family Physician, 73*(4), 636–644.

Mallon, E., Newton, J. N., Klassen, A., Stewart-Brown, S. L., Ryan, T. J., & Finlay, A. Y. (1999). The quality of life in acne: A comparison with general medical conditions using generic questionnaires. *British Journal of Dermatology, 140*(4), 672–676.

Menter, A., Korman, N. J., Feldman, S. R., Gelfand, J. M., Gordon, K. B., Gottlieb, A., et al. (2009). Section 3. Guidelines of care for the management and treatment of psoriasis with topical therapies. *Journal of the American Academy of Dermatology, 60*(4), 643–659.

Ofori, A. O. (2010). Treatment of acne vulgaris. *UpToDate Online 18.1.* Retrieved from http://www.UpToDate.com

Pallin, D. J., Espinola, J. A., Leung, D. Y., Hooper, D. C., & Camargo, C. A. (2009). Epidemiology of dermatitis and skin infections in United States physicians' offices, 1993–2005. *Clinical Infectious Diseases, 49*(6), 901–907.

Prok, L., & McGovern, T. (2010). Poison ivy *(Toxicodendron)* dermatitis. *UpToDate 18.1.* Retrieved from http://www.UpToDate.com

Strauss, J. S., Krowchuk, D. P., Leyden, J. J., Lucky, A.W., Shalita, A. R., Siegfried, E.C., et al. (2007). Guidelines for acne vulgaris management. *Journal of the American Academy of Dermatology, 56*(4), 651–663.

Walker, G. J. A., & Johnstone, P. W. (2006). Interventions for treating scabies. *The Cochrane Database of Systematic Reviews, 2.*

Weston, W. L., & Howe, W. (2010). Overview of dermatitis. *UpToDate Online 18.1.* Retrieved from http://www.uptodate.com/online/content/topic.do?topicKey=dermat/2450&selectedTitle=1~150&source=search_result

U.S. Food and Drug Administration (2005). FDA Approves Updated Labeling with Boxed Warning and Medication Guide for Two Eczema Drugs, Elidel and Protopic. Retrieved January 25, 2011 from http://www.fda.gov/ NewsEvents/Newsroom/PressAnnouncements/2006/ucm108580.htm

CHAPTER 33

DIABETES MELLITUS

Anita Lee Wynne and Kathryn A. Hanavan

Chapter Outline

Diabetes and its complications remain a major cause of morbidity and mortality in the United States and around the world. In 2005 through 2006, the estimated crude prevalence of diabetes mellitus in the United States in people older than 20 years was 12.9 percent, 40 percent of which was undiagnosed (Cowie et al, 2009). The crude prevalence of pre-diabetes in the form of impaired fasting glucose was 25.7 percent and the rate of impaired glucose tolerance was 13.8 percent. Almost 33 percent of older adults had diabetes and 75 percent had either diabetes or pre-diabetes. Recently, a disturbing increase in the incidence of diabetes (both diabetes and pre-diabetes) has occurred, and it is more prevalent in several ethnic groups: African Americans, Hispanics, Native Americans, and Asian Americans have a 2- to 5-fold higher rate of diabetes than does the rest of the population.

The annual cost of diabetes care is estimated to be greater than $174 billion (Cowie et al, 2009). The disease is the leading cause of blindness and end-stage renal disease, and it accounts for approximately 67,000 lower extremity amputations annually.

Diabetes mellitus is actually a heterogeneous group of complex metabolic disorders that share common alterations in glucose metabolism. The disorders differ in age at onset, genetic predisposition, treatment options, and the complications developed. Table 33–1 provides a brief comparison of the differences between the two major forms of diabetes: type 1 and type 2. For a detailed discussion of all the permutations of diabetes, readers are referred to pathophysiology and management-related texts. Such a discussion is not within the scope of this book. This chapter focuses on the pharmacological management of type 1 and type 2 diabetes mellitus. Gestational diabetes, which requires consultation with the obstetrical provider, is briefly mentioned here.

Diabetes mellitus has been clearly interrelated with hyperlipidemia, hypertension, and coronary heart disease. The pathophysiology of these disorders is intertwined with diabetes mellitus and treatment protocols now include management of all these disorders as part of diabetes management. Chapter 28 discusses coronary heart disease, Chapter 39 discusses hyperlipidemia, and Chapter 40 discusses hypertension; each chapter discusses disease management. This chapter discusses where these disorders cross-link with diabetes mellitus.

Table 33–1 **Comparison of Type 1 and Type 2 Diabetes Mellitus**

Characteristic	Type 1	Type 2
Age at onset	Usually during childhood or adolescence, but can occur at any age, even in eighth and ninth decades	Usually after age 40 and risk for it increases with age, obesity, and lack of physical activity
Type of onset	Signs and symptoms abrupt, but disease process may be present for years	Insidious and gradual
Genetic susceptibility	HLA-DR3 and DR4 and others; 50% concordance in monozygotic twins	Frequent genetic background, but no relation to HLA; almost 100% concordance in monozygotic twins
Environmental factors	Viruses, toxins	Obesity, nutrition; more common in women with prior gestational diabetes and in patients with hypertension or hyperlipidemia
Etiology	Unknown; postulated causes include heredity, autoimmune disease, and viral infections	Unknown; heredity is highly associated
Islet cell antibody and pancreatic cell—mediated immunity	Present at onset	Absent
Endogenous insulin	Secretion is markedly diminished early in disease; may be totally absent later	Levels may be low (insulin deficiency), normal, or high (insulin resistance)
Nutritional status	Thin, catabolic state	Obesity is common
Symptoms	Polydipsia, polyphagia, polyuria, fatigue, and weight loss	May be asymptomatic; polydipsia or polyuria may be present
Ketosis	Prone at onset or during insulin deficiency	Resistant except during infection or stress
Control of diabetes	Often difficult with wide glucose fluctuations	Variable
Dietary management	Essential	Essential; sometimes controlled with diet and exercise
Insulin	Insulin therapy is mandatory	Required for 30%–40% of patients as disease progresses
Metformin, sulfonylureas, and other oral agents	Not efficacious	Efficacious
Complications	Occur in a majority of patients after >5 yr, but reduced incidence for those with tight control	Frequent, but reduced incidence for those with tight control

PATHOPHYSIOLOGY

Type 1 Diabetes Mellitus

Several pathogenic processes are involved in the development of diabetes mellitus. Type 1 diabetes, which accounts for 10 percent of total diabetes, results from an autoimmune destruction of the beta cells of the islet of Langerhans of the pancreas, which leads to insulin deficiency (American Diabetes Association, 2009a). Type 1 diabetes has two subtypes: immune mediated (autoimmune disease) and nonimmune (idiopathic). The latter occurs secondary to other diseases such as pancreatitis and is not discussed in this chapter. Autoantibodies to tyrosine phosphatases IA-2 and IA-2 beta, to islet cells, to **insulin,** and to glutamic acid decarboxylase (GAD65) are seen in 85 to 90 percent of patients with the immune-related subtype of type 1 diabetes (American Diabetes Association, 2009b). The other 10 to 15 percent of patients with type 1 diabetes have no known etiology (idiopathic). Most patients with idiopathic type 1 diabetes are African American or Asian American (American Diabetes Association, 2009b). This chapter focuses on the immune-related form.

Abnormalities at six genetic loci associated with type 1 diabetes have been identified to date. The most common is associated with mutation of the hepatic transcription factor (hepatocyte nuclear factor [HNF]-1 alpha) on chromosome 12. A second form involves the glucokinase gene on chromosome 7p. The latter form results in a defective glucokinase molecule. Because glucokinase converts glucose to glucose-6-phophate, which then stimulates insulin secretion, defects in this gene result in increased levels of glucose needed to elicit normal levels of insulin secretion (American Diabetes Association, 2009b). Less common forms result from mutations in other transcription factors: HNF-4alpha, insulin promoter factor (IPF)-1, and NeuroD-1.

Genetic mutations that result in the inability to convert pro-insulin to insulin and some that affect insulin action rather than production have also been identified.

Type 1 diabetes susceptibility has been linked to these genetic mutations. Current theories hold that islet-cell destruction occurs predominantly in persons who are genetically susceptible. Because twin studies have shown only 50 percent concordance, environmental factors, chemical agents, and dietary agents are likely contributing factors. Genetic counseling for parents is based on statistical risk. If one child has type 1 diabetes, siblings have a 5 to 10 percent chance of developing type 1 diabetes. The risk is 45 percent if the sibling is an identical twin. The offspring of a father with type 1 diabetes has a 4 to 6 percent risk, and the offspring of a mother with type 1 diabetes has a 2 to 3 percent risk. Theoretically, when a person with the appropriate genetic characteristics is exposed to an environmental agent such as a viral infection, the beta cells are destroyed directly, or an autoimmune process is triggered, which in turn destroys the beta cells. (For a more detailed discussion of these genetic defects, the reader is referred to a pathophysiology text.)

Previous thinking was that the onset and progression of hyperglycemic symptoms were rapid and acute in type 1 diabetes. Type 1 diabetes actually has a long preclinical period. Research has demonstrated the presence of islet-cell autoantibodies (ICA) for years before the occurrence of symptoms. ICAs precede beta cell deficiency and have been found in 85 to 90 percent of type 1 diabetes at the time of onset of clinical symptoms. Autoantibodies against insulin (IAA) have also been found. ICAs and IAA are probably the result of the beta cell destruction rather than its cause. They tend to disappear with time. Anti-GAD antibodies are more persistent and can be useful in determining the etiology of diabetes (e.g., type 1 vs. type 2) (McCance & Huether, 2006). This need to differentiate has been raised, in part, because type 1 diabetes sometimes has an onset in older adults because of a longer than usual preclinical period; and type 2 diabetes has been found in children as young as 4 years old (maturity onset diabetes of the young [MODY]). These children may have a monogenetic defect in beta-cell function that is inherited in an autosomal-dominant pattern, resulting in impaired insulin secretion but no defects in insulin action (American Diabetes Association, 2009b). Absence of these autoimmune markers may not indicate type 2 diabetes, according to Hathout, Thomas, El-Shahawy, Nahab, and Mace (2009), nor should their presence exclude its diagnosis. However, differentiating between the two types is usually more of a clinical diagnosis. Some patients, particularly children and adolescents, may present with ketoacidosis as the first manifestation of the disease. Adults with type 1 diabetes may retain residual beta cell function sufficient to prevent ketoacidosis for many years (American Diabetes Association, 2009b).

The presence of ICAs is strong evidence for an autoimmune pathogenesis of type 1 diabetes. Research suggests an organ-specific suppressor deficit may be the direct cause, but the exact sequence of events that triggers attachment of immune cells to islet cells is not yet known. Environmental factors are thought to play a role. Specific factors that have been linked to type 1 diabetes include certain drugs and chemicals (**alloxan, streptozocin, pentamidine**), nutritional intake (cow's milk, high levels of nitrosamines), and viruses (mumps, coxsackievirus, rubella [40% of persons with congenital rubella infection develop type 1 diabetes later], and cytomegalovirus) (McCance & Huether, 2006).

Before hyperglycemia occurs, 80 to 90 percent of the function of insulin-secreting beta cells must be lost. Beta cell abnormalities are present long before the acute clinical onset of type 1 diabetes and the event that precipitates the acute onset of symptoms may be far removed from the one that started the pathology.

Regardless of the cause, considerable evidence suggests that the pathology is probably disequilibrium between the relative excess production of glucagon by the pancreatic A cells and the lack of insulin produced by the B cells. This ratio of insulin to glucagon in the portal vein—not the concentration of each hormone—controls hepatic glucose and fat metabolism, two major problems in type 1 diabetes. The recognition that the totality of the metabolic pathology is a factor of both of these hormones is leading to a different approach to diabetes management. Figure 33–1 depicts the pathological cause of the various symptoms of type 1 diabetes.

Because insulin production by the beta cells of the islet of Langerhans is lacking, successful treatment requires **insulin** replacement. If the disease progresses without treatment, diabetic ketoacidosis (DKA), weight loss, and muscle wasting may develop. Once treatment is initiated, the patient may enter temporary partial remission, despite the continued destruction of beta cells ("honeymoon phase"). Different definitions of this partial remission have involved the amount of **insulin** required or the HbA_{1c} level of the patient. Mortensen and colleagues (2009) have suggested that the definition of the partial remission period in children and adolescents use a combination of the two in the following formula: HbA_{1c} (%) + [4 × **insulin** dose (units/kg/24 hr)], with a number less than 9 indicating partial remission. This is a practical measurement that may be useful as the management of type 1 diabetes begins to focus more on drugs and other interventions to preserve beta cell function early in the disease process. Under current treatment models, beta cell destruction eventually reaches a point at which hyperglycemia occurs again, and **insulin** therapy is required throughout the rest of the disease process.

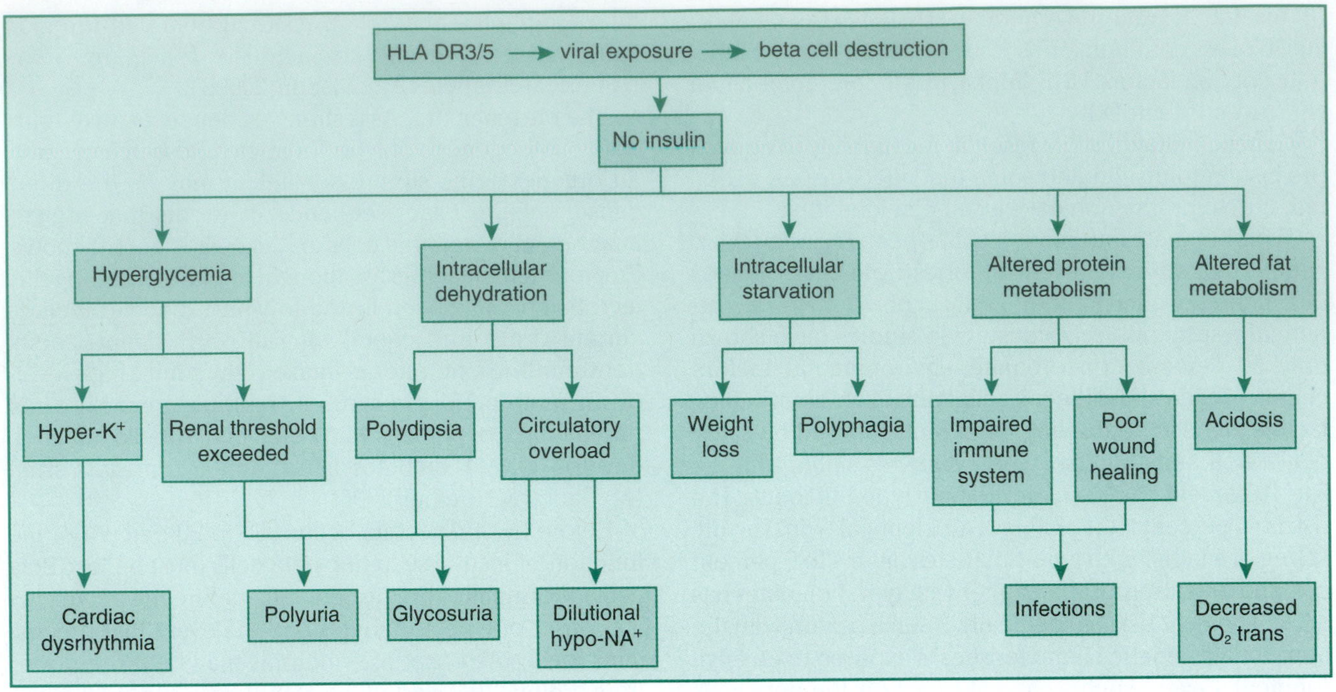

Figure 33–1. Pathophysiology of type 1 diabetes.

Type 2 Diabetes Mellitus

Type 2 diabetes is much more common than type 1; approximately 90 percent of diabetics are type 2 (American Diabetes Association, 2009b). As with type 1, prevalence varies by ethnic group; the condition is more common in Native Americans, Hispanics, and African Americans in the United States (Anand et al, 2000; Cowie et al, 2009).

The pathogenesis of type 2 diabetes is complex, and manifestations vary greatly across patients. Genetics have a strong influence, and a locus has been found on chromosome arm 7q that may be related to insulin resistance, one underlying alteration in type 2 diabetes (Bloomgarden, 2003). For type 2 diabetes, genetic counseling is based on known familial risk. Siblings of a person with type 2 diabetes have a 7 to 14 percent risk for developing type 2 diabetes. The offspring of parents who both have type 2 diabetes have a 15 to 45 percent chance of developing it. Children and young adults with type 2 diabetes have a 50 percent chance of transmitting the disease to their offspring.

Plasma insulin levels in type 2 diabetes may by low, normal, or high. Although the specific etiology of this form of diabetes is unknown, autoimmune destruction of beta cells does not occur (American Diabetes Association, 2009b). The main physiological alteration in type 2 diabetes is insulin resistance, a suboptimal response of insulin-sensitive tissues (especially in the liver, muscle, and adipose tissue) to insulin. The result is an increased rate of endogenous glucose production secondary to increased glucagon levels. The gastrointestinal system also plays a role in regulating the secretion of insulin. Incretin peptides secreted from endocrine cells in the intestinal tract are released in response to the ingestion of food. Glucagon-like peptide-1 (GLP-1) is one of two peptides produced, and it regulates glucose homeostasis in the postprandial period by stimulation of insulin synthesis, inhibition of glucagon secretion, delay of gastric emptying and promotion of satiety (Chahal & Chowdhury, 2007). In type 2 diabetes, the level of GLP-1 is decreased following a meal. If the pancreas is the major organ involved in type 1 diabetes, the liver and the incretin system are the major organs in type 2. Type 2 diabetics have few and nonspecific pancreatic changes. Many years of compensatory hyperinsulinemia may occur before the onset of clinical symptoms of diabetes. Eventually the beta cell responsiveness to glucose stimulus diminishes and hyperglycemia prevails. Adipose tissue also does not take up glucose in response to insulin, resulting in obesity. Increased visceral fat shows an inverse relationship with insulin sensitivity (American Diabetes Association, 2009b; Bloomgarden, 2003). Many type 2 diabetics are obese and obesity triples the risk for insulin resistance. Patients who are not obese by traditional weight standards may have an increased percentage of body fat distributed predominantly in the abdominal region (American Diabetes Association, 2009b). Finally, type 2 diabetes is associated with down-regulation of insulin receptors in skeletal muscle. The gradual onset and progression of type 2 diabetes allows patients to adapt to the symptoms without realizing that the disease process is producing them.

Insulin resistance has also been linked to three other important disorders: hyperlipidemia, hypertension, and coronary artery disease. The Framingham Offspring Study (Bloomgarden, 2003) was among the first to suggest a central metabolic syndrome with high triglyceride levels, low high-density lipoprotein (HDL) levels, obesity, and hyperglycemia, which was also associated with hypertension. Thus, dyslipidemia and hypertension are closely linked with type 2 diabetes. Because both dyslipidemia and hypertension are also linked with atherogenesis, diabetes has also become an independent risk factor for coronary heart disease. Individuals with any one of these disorders should be screened for the others. Screening is discussed below.

Insulin resistance and the metabolic syndrome are also associated with a prothrombotic state that contributes to the vascular complications seen in this disorder. Insulin has a direct antiplatelet effect and loss of insulin results in increased adhesiveness and exaggerated aggregation and thrombus generation (Randriamboavonjy & Fleming, 2009). Some of the newer oral drugs (e.g., **glitazones** and **gliptins**) have been reported to improve platelet function.

Because a sufficient endogenous insulin supply inhibits the development of DKA, insulin is not mandatory. Formerly insulin was used later in the disease process or during acute illness or stress. Newer guidelines suggest that **insulin** may have a role earlier in the disease process, especially in light of the prevention of the three complications: dyslipidemia, hypertension, and atherogenesis. Patients can, however, develop hyperglycemic, hyperosmolar nonketosis (HHNK). **Oral hypoglycemic agents** and other **oral antidiabetic agents** are effective in addressing one or more of the metabolic defects in type 2 diabetes.

Complications

Long-term complications of both types of diabetes are based on target organ damage. The organs most commonly involved are the eyes, heart, kidneys, and nervous system. Retinopathy with potential loss of vision; nephropathy leading to renal failure; peripheral neuropathy with risk of foot ulcers, amputation, and Charcot's joint; and autonomic neuropathy with gastrointestinal, genitourinary, and cardiovascular symptoms and sexual dysfunction may occur. Patients with diabetes have an increased incidence of atherosclerotic cardiovascular, peripheral vascular, and cerebrovascular diseases. They are at increased risk for hypertension, abnormalities of lipid metabolism, abnormalities of platelet function, and periodontal disease (American Diabetes Association, 2009a). The management of each of these complications is discussed in the following sections.

Diagnosis and Screening

Diagnostic Criteria for Diabetes and Pre-Diabetes

The diagnostic criteria for diabetes mellitus and pre-diabetes are shown in Table 33–2. Three ways to diagnose diabetes are possible, and each must be confirmed on a subsequent day by a different one of the three methods. For example, one instance of symptoms with a casual plasma glucose of 200 mg/dL or more, confirmed on a subsequent day by a fasting plasma glucose of 126 mg/dL or more, warrants the diagnosis of diabetes.

An intermediate group of patients whose glucose levels, although not meeting the criteria for diabetes, are nevertheless too high to be considered normal is also recognized. These patients are said to have impaired glucose tolerance (IGT) or impaired fasting glucose (IFG). Patients with these two disorders are at risk for diabetes and cardiovascular disease and probably have **insulin-resistance syndrome**. They are considered to have pre-diabetes (American Diabetes Association, 2009a, 2009b; Bloomgarden, 2008a; Gahagan & Silverstein, 2003). The United States Diabetes Prevention Program (Diabetes Prevention Program Research Group, 2002, 2003; Gahagan & Silverstein, 2003; Klein et al, 2004; Schmidt et al, 2003) has shown that lifestyle modification and, for adults, the administration of **metformin (Glucophage)** may prevent the development of type 2 diabetes in patients with pre-diabetes. This is a major impetus for screening at risk persons for diabetes.

The American Diabetes Association (2009a) has proposed a separate classification for pre-diabetes and given criteria for its diagnosis. These criteria, which include the former impaired fasting glucose and impaired glucose tolerance criteria, are the following:

- Fasting blood glucose of 100 to 125 mg/dL (impaired fasting glucose) or
- 2-hour blood glucose of 140 to 199 mg/dL (impaired glucose tolerance)

Table 33–2 **Diagnostic Criteria for Diabetes Mellitus and Pre-Diabetes**

Diagnostic Category	Diagnostic Criteria
Diabetes mellitus	Symptoms of diabetes plus casual plasma glucose concentration ≥200 mg/dL. *Casual* is defined as any time of day without regard to time since last meal. The classic symptoms of diabetes are polyuria, polydipsia, and unexplained weight loss. OR Fasting plasma glucose ≥126 mg/dL. *Fasting* is defined as no caloric intake for at least 8 h. OR 2-h postload plasma glucose in an oral glucose tolerance test ≥200 mg/dL. The test should be performed as described by the World Health Organization, using a glucose load containing the equivalent of 75 g anhydrous glucose dissolved in water.
Pre-diabetes	Fasting plasma glucose 100–125 mg/dL (IFG) Plasma glucose 140–199 mg/dL (IGT) 2-h postingestion of standard glucose load (75 g).

IFG = impaired fasting glucose; IGT = impaired glucose tolerance.

Both of these are considered risk factors for future diabetes and for cardiovascular disease. The American Diabetes Association recommends testing to detect pre-diabetes in asymptomatic people who are overweight or obese and who have one or more additional risk factors for diabetes. In those without these risk factors, testing should begin at age 45 years.

Balkau and colleagues (2008) did an epidemiological study on the insulin-resistant syndrome and the ability to predict the development of diabetes. The researchers found that the best clinical predictor of future diabetes was adiposity and the baseline glucose level was the best biological predictor. Genetic polymorphisms added little to predicting future diabetes.

The American College of Endocrinology held a consensus conference in July 2008, to discuss the criteria for the diagnosis of pre-diabetes and the goal and treatment modalities for it (Bloomgarden, 2008a, 2008b). Although the participants all seemed to agree that preventing individuals who have pre-diabetes from developing actual diabetes is a lofty goal, several problems arise in trying to do this:

- Pre-diabetes is an asymptomatic state, and using an illness model may not be appropriate.
- Movement to diabetes is a "relative risk" based on many factors than it is a guaranteed outcome if nothing is done.
- Proving that a specific intervention resulted in a delay in or prevention of diabetes development raises questions of suitable end points in research studies to show this.

Although discussion and research continue concerning the appropriate way to manage pre-diabetes, it is prudent to suggest lifestyle changes where needed and to prescribe therapies that have shown to effectively manage known risk factors for diabetes development (e.g., obesity) and the complications of diabetes (e.g., antihypertensives). The American Diabetes Association (2009a) also recommends that **metformin** be considered for those at high risk for developing diabetes and who are obese and under 60 years of age.

Screening Recommendations for Diabetes and Pre-Diabetes

Screening recommendations vary by the group presenting them and the reasons they have for doing so, but the most respected and used recommendations come from the American Diabetes Association, which is presented.

The American Diabetes Association (2009a) recommends testing to detect pre-diabetes and type 2 diabetes in asymptomatic adults of any age who are overweight or obese (body mass index [BMI] greater than 25 kg/m^2) and who have one or more additional risk factors for diabetes. The criteria for such testing are listed in Table 33–3.

People with type 1 diabetes present with acute symptoms of diabetes and markedly elevated blood glucose levels. Evidence from type 1 prevention studies suggests that measurement of islet autoantibodies identifies individuals who are at risk for developing type 1 diabetes. High-risk individuals, such as those with transient hyperglycemia or those who have relatives with type 1 diabetes, may be appropriate for this type of testing (American Diabetes Association, 2009a). Widespread screening of symptomatic low-risk individuals is not recommended.

The incidence of type 2 diabetes in adolescents has increased dramatically in the past 10 years, especially in minority populations. Asymptomatic children who meet the following criteria should be tested within the health-care setting:

- Overweight (BMI above the 85th percentile for age and sex, weight for height above the 85th percentile, or weight greater than 120% of ideal weight for height)

Plus any two of the following risk factors:

- Family history of type 2 diabetes in first or second-degree relative

Table 33–3 **Criteria for Testing Asymptomatic Adults for Diabetes**

Individuals ≥45 yr and who have a BMI ≥25 kg/m^2 should be tested. If normal, the test should be repeated at 3-yr intervals.
Individuals <45 yr and who have a BMI ≥25 kg/m^2 and have additional risk factors should have more frequent testing.
Additional risk factors are the following: • Habitually physically inactive • First-degree relative with diabetes • Members of high-risk ethnic group (African American, Hispanic, Native American, Asian American, Pacific Islander) • Delivered a baby weighing >9 lb or previously diagnosed with GDM • Hypertensive (B/P ≥140/90 mm Hg) • HDL cholesterol ≤35 mg/dL and/or triglyceride level ≥250 mg/dL • Have PCOS • IGT or IFG on previous testing • Have other clinical conditions associated with insulin resistance (PCOS or acanthosis nigricans) • History of vascular disease

BMI = body mass index; BP = blood pressure; GDM = gestational diabetes mellitus; HDL = high-density lipoprotein; IFG = impaired fasting glucose; IGT = impaired glucose tolerance; PCOS = polycystic-ovary syndrome.

Source: Adapted from American Diabetes Association. (2003). Standards of medical care for patients with diabetes mellitus. *Diabetes Care, 26*(1), S35.

- Race/ethnicity (Native American, African American, Latino, Asian American, Pacific Islander)
- Signs of insulin resistance or conditions associated with it.
- Maternal history of diabetes or gestational diabetes during the child's gestation.

Such testing should begin at age 10 years and occur every 3 years thereafter (American Diabetes Association, 2009a).

The test recommended for screening all age groups is the fasting plasma glucose (FPG). The oral glucose tolerance test (OGTT) is impractical and expensive for this purpose; however, it is used to diagnose gestational diabetes. Recent discussion within the American Diabetes Association suggests the possible future use of HbA_{1c} as an initial screening test; however, no guidelines have formally recommended such use. The cutoff values have yet to be determined.

The Atherosclerosis Risk in Communities Study group (Schmidt et al, 2003) also supports screening. The patients that the study group suggests screening are those at high risk for cardiovascular disease, because such patients are the most likely to benefit from early detection and treatment. The study group agrees with using the FPG as the main screening tool, but suggests the addition of clinical detection rules, and the OGTT when FPG results are positive. Their article in *Diabetes Care* provides a detailed table of diagnostic strategies to be used based on fasting glucose results and clinical factors with sensitivity and specificity data.

The Canadian Task Force on Preventive Health Care (Feig, Palda, & Lipscombe, 2005) suggests screening for those individuals with hypertension, hyperlipidemia, or previous impaired glucose tolerance (IGT). For patients who do not meet those criteria, but whose overall cardiovascular disease risk is more than 10 percent, screening may also be a benefit. The task force also supports the use of the FPG test as the primary test, but the OGTT is also acceptable. Tests should be done on two different occasions before a diagnosis can be made. The task force provides no data on screening frequency.

Diagnostic Criteria for Pregnant Women

Diagnosis of gestational diabetes (GDM) is presented in detail in several American Diabetes Association documents (American Diabetes Association, 2009a). Each document recommends either the one-step approach to performing a diagnostic OGTT between the 24th and 28th week of pregnancy or a two-step approach to performing an initial screening with a 50-g glucose challenge (GCT), and then a diagnostic OGTT if the GCT is outside normal parameters. The American Diabetes Association provides diagnostic criteria for each of the testing times in the OGTT, the association also suggests that no glucose testing is required for low-risk women, such as those younger than 25 years with normal weight before pregnancy, those who are not members of an ethnic group with high-risk status, and those who have no history of first-degree relatives with diabetes or abnormal glucose tolerance or poor obstetrical outcome. Women with GDM should be screened for diabetes 6 to 12 weeks postpartum and should be followed up with subsequent screening for the development of diabetes or pre-diabetes (American Diabetes Association, 2009a).

> **On The Horizon**
>
> **NOVEL NONINVASIVE BREATH TEST FOR DIABETIC SCREENING**
>
> Diagnosis of pre-diabetes and early-stage diabetes occurs primarily by means of invasive blood tests. A study by Dillon and colleagues (2009) collected blood and breath samples from study subjects after ingestion of a standard glucose dose. The researchers found correlations between the blood and breath tests. The results of that study suggest that the novel breath test used may assist in recognition of pre-diabetes or early-stage diabetes in at-risk individuals without the need for invasive blood sampling, thus making the test an attractive option for large-scale test of at-risk populations, such as children.

Screening Criteria for Children

The American Academy of Pediatrics (Gahagan & Silverstein, 2003) recommends screening of children with one or more risk factors. These risk factors include the following:

- Family history of type 2 diabetes in first- or second-degree relative
- Race or ethnicity of high-risk group (see Table 33–3)
- Presence of a condition associated with insulin resistance (acanthosis nigricans, hypertension, dyslipidemia, or polycystic-ovary syndrome [PCOS])
- BMI between the 85th and 95th percentiles for age and sex or weight greater than 20 percent of ideal weight for height

These children should be monitored closely, but no specific screening or monitoring interval is provided in the 2003 article.

Additional data on diagnosis of diabetes are provided in American Diabetes Association documents in the References section. The material in this chapter assumes an appropriate diagnosis of diabetes.

PHARMACODYNAMICS

Insulin

Insulin is used in the management of both types of diabetes. Naturally occurring **insulin** promotes the storage of fat as well as glucose and influences cell growth and metabolic functions in a wide variety of tissues. Its action on glucose transporters is discussed in detail in Chapter 21. In summary, these receptors "open the gate" to allow glucose to enter the cell. The total number of **insulin** receptors can be down-regulated by such factors as obesity and long-standing hyperglycemia, which may explain why weight loss can be a significant factor in diabetes management.

Insulin and its analogues lower blood glucose levels by stimulating peripheral glucose uptake, especially by skeletal muscle and fat, and by inhibiting hepatic glucose production. **Insulin** inhibits lipolysis in the adipocyte, inhibits proteolysis, and enhances protein synthesis.

Insulin acts on the liver to increase storage of glucose as glycogen and resets the liver after food intake by reversing the amount of catabolic activity. It also decreases urea production, protein catabolism, and cyclic adenosine monophosphate (cAMP) in the liver; promotes triglyceride synthesis; and increases potassium and phosphate uptake by the liver.

Insulin promotes protein synthesis by increasing amino acid transport and by stimulating ribosomal activity. It also promotes glycogen synthesis to replace glycogen stores used during muscle activity.

Finally, **insulin** reduces the circulation of free fatty acids and promotes the storage of triglycerides in adipose tissue. This process is accomplished, in part, by suppression of cAMP production and dephosphorylation of the lipases in fat cells.

Administration of the drug **insulin** produces the same effect as the naturally occurring hormone. Although **insulin** is given largely to control blood glucose in patients with diabetes, that is not its only effect on the body.

Insulin preparations are divided into categories based on onset, duration, and intensity of action following subcutaneous injection. Five relatively new **insulin** formulations deserve specific discussion.

- **Insulin lispro**, created by reversing two amino acids on the insulin B-chain. It is a very rapid-acting **insulin** with a short half-life and is compatible with **NPH.**
- **Insulin aspart**, homologous with **regular human insulin** except for one amino acid. It has a rapid onset of action similar to **insulin lispro.**
- **Insulin glulisine**, created by replacing lysine and glutamic acid on the **insulin** B chain. Its profile is similar to **lispro**, except that its duration is shorter.
- **Insulin glargine**, created by substituting glycine and arginine for other amino acids in **human insulin.** It has a unique area under the curve (AUC) profile that has no pronounced peak, as small amounts of **insulin** are released slowly, resulting in a constant concentration/time profile over 24 hours. This profile has resulted in improved glycemic control in large, diverse populations with longstanding type 2 diabetes. One large study (Davies, Storms, Shutler, Bianchi-Biscay, & Gomis, 2005) showed a low incidence of severe hypoglycemia even in a simple subject-administered titration algorithm.
- **Insulin detemir** is an **insulin** analogue that differs from **human insulin** by a single amino acid deletion and the acylation of myristic acid to the B terminus of the molecule. These changes prolong absorption from the subcutaneous depot, resulting in a more prolonged, less peaked absorption than that of **NPH insulin.** It has a pharmacokinetic profile similar to that of **insulin glargine** (Porcellati et al, 2007).

Although **insulin** is the drug of choice in managing pregnant diabetics, among these newer formulations only **insulin lispro** has been studied in pregnant women and is listed as Pregnancy Category B. The use of **insulin aspart**, **insulin glulisine**, **insulin glargine**, and **insulin detemir** during pregnancy is on a risk/benefit basis. These last four drugs are listed as Pregnancy Category C, and they are also not compatible with other **insulins** and must be given in a separate syringe. Work is under way on the development of combinations using these insulins. This research is discussed in Chapter 21. Average **insulin** doses are 0.3 to 0.7 U/kg for type 1 and 0.5 to 1.0 U/kg or larger doses for type 2 per day. Obese patients may require more than 100 units per day. Further discussion of each of these drugs is found in Chapter 21.

Oral Antihyperglycemic Agents

Sulfonylureas

Oral agents are efficacious for only type 2 diabetes, and most drugs act on different aspects of the metabolic defects. **Sulfonylureas** increase endogenous insulin secretion by the beta cells and may improve the binding between insulin and insulin receptors or increase the number of receptors. Hypoglycemic effects appear to be due to increased endogenous insulin production and to improved beta-cell sensitivity to blood glucose levels or suppression of glucose release by the liver. **Sulfonylureas** were the first class used to treat type 2 diabetes. Although they are still important for that indication, their risk for hypoglycemia and their limited action on **insulin** resistance has resulted in their now being a Step 2 therapy status (Nathan et al, 2009).

Biguanides

Biguanides are oral antihyperglycemic drugs. Their pharmacology and chemistry are different from the **sulfonylureas. Metformin (Glucophage, Fortamet, Glumetza)** was first released in its short-acting formulation in the United States in December 1994, and to date is the only drug in this class used clinically. **Metformin** increases peripheral glucose uptake and utilization, improves hepatic response to blood glucose levels so that the liver produces appropriate amounts of glucose, and decreases intestinal absorption of glucose. Together, these actions improve glucose tolerance and lower both basal and postprandial plasma glucose levels. Unlike the **sulfonylureas, metformin** does not stimulate **insulin** release from the pancreatic beta cells, so the risk for hypoglycemia is minimal. The drug also does not produce hyperinsulinemia.

In contrast to patients taking **sulfonylureas,** patients taking **metformin** do not gain weight. In fact, they often lose weight. Because obesity is a major factor in the pathogenesis of type 2 diabetes, weight loss is an important action of this drug.

Metformin also inhibits platelet aggregation and reduces blood viscosity. Increased platelet viscosity and aggregation form a major course of the macrovascular complications seen in both type 1 and type 2 diabetes. Because of its ability to affect several of the defects in type 2 diabetes, **metformin** has moved to tier 1 therapy in adults as well as children older than age 10 years. The Diabetes Prevention Program Research Group (2002) tested **metformin** and lifestyle modifications as methods for preventing the conversion of pre-diabetes to type 2 diabetes. Lifestyle interventions reduced the incidence of conversion by 58 percent, and **metformin** by 31 percent. To prevent one case of diabetes during a period of three years, 13.9 patients would have to receive **metformin.** The Diabetes Prevention Program Research Group also looked at the cost effectiveness of intervention (2003) and found that both **metformin** and lifestyle interventions were cost effective across subjects, regardless of age, ethnicity, or gender and affordable in routine clinical practice. The American Diabetes Association now recommends the use of **metformin** for the prevention of the development of diabetes in patients with diagnosed pre-diabetes.

Alpha-Glucosidase Inhibitors

Alpha-glucosidase inhibitors are also oral **antihyperglycemic** drugs, but their pharmacodynamics are different from the **sulfonylureas** and the **biguanides. Acarbose (Precose)** was first released in January 1996. **Miglitol (Glyset)** was approved by the U.S. Food and Drug Administration (FDA) in 1998 and released to the public in 1999. **Alpha-glucosidase inhibitors** do not act directly on any of the defects in metabolism seen in type 2 diabetes mellitus. They competitively inhibit and delay the absorption of complex carbohydrates (CHO) from the small bowel. **Alpha-glucosidase inhibitors** have no inhibitory activity against lactase and do not induce lactose intolerance. They lower blood glucose levels after meals. Unlike the **sulfonylureas,** they do not enhance pancreatic beta-cell secretion of **insulin.** Like **metformin,** they are not associated with weight gain and diminish the weight-increasing effects of **sulfonylureas** when given in combination with them. **Alpha-glucosidase inhibitor** activity is effective on any CHO food intake, including liquid diets taken via a nasogastric tube. They have a limited role as adjunct therapy and are listed in ADA/EASD guidelines under "other therapy" (Nathan et al, 2009).

Thiazolidinediones

Another class of drugs used to treat type 2 diabetes mellitus is the **thiazolidinediones (TDZ).** They are oral **antihyperglycemic** drugs. **Troglitazone (Rezulin)** was first released in March 1997. It was removed from the market in 1999 because of the adverse reactions associated with liver damage. **Pioglitazone (Actos)** and **rosiglitazone (Avandia)** were both FDA-approved in 1999. They have been associated with less risk of liver damage. **Thiazolidinediones** activate a nuclear receptor that regulates gene transcription, resulting in expression of proteins that improve **insulin** action in the cell. This action leads to increased utilization of available insulin by the liver and muscle cells and also in adipose tissue. In addition, these drugs reduce hepatic glucose production so that the liver produces appropriate amounts of glucagon. Taken together, these actions improve glucose tolerance and lower both basal and postprandial plasma glucose levels. Unlike the **sulfonylureas, thiazolidinediones** do not produce hypoglycemia in diabetic or nondiabetic patients, except in special situations, and do not cause hyperinsulinemia because they do not stimulate **insulin** release from the pancreatic beta cells. Like **metformin, thiazolidinediones** have a modest impact on lipids because of their actions in the liver.

TDZs are shown in the American Diabetes Association and the European Association for the Study of Diabetes guidelines as "less well validated" drugs (tier 2), but only **pioglitazone** is recommended. The potential for cardiovascular problems associated with the use of these drugs, especially with the use of **rosiglitazone,** is controversial. Chapter 21 discusses this controversy in some detail, including the removal of **rosiglitazone** from the American Diabetes Association and the European Association for the Study of Diabetes recommended list of drugs and the Canadian Diabetes Association's disagreement with this recommendation.

Meglitinides

The next class of drugs, the **meglitinides,** has a different mechanism of action from any of the other drugs used to treat type 2 diabetes. The **meglitinides** are short-acting **insulin secretagogues. Repaglinide (Prandin)** was first released in April 1998 and **nateglinide (Starlix)** was released in December 2000. Both drugs close adenosine triphosphate (ATP) dependent potassium channels in the beta-cell membrane by binding at specific receptor sites. This potassium channel blockade depolarizes the beta cell and leads to an opening of calcium channels. The resultant influx of calcium increases the secretion of **insulin.** Because their time in the plasma is less than 2 hours, the effect is very short. Plasma insulin levels fall to baseline by 4 hours after dosing. The end result of their stimulation of insulin secretion is a lowering in postprandial blood glucose levels. To achieve this effect, they are dosed three times daily no more than 20 minutes before meals. They do not directly affect fasting blood glucose levels or any of the other defects in metabolism seen in type 2 diabetes. They are most useful in patients whose primary glucose alteration is postprandial hyperglycemia. These drugs are not commonly used as adherence is difficult and they are expensive. The American Diabetes Association and the European Association for the Study of Diabetes guidelines place them in the "other therapy" category.

Dipeptidyl Peptidase-4 Inhibitors

The last class of drugs is the **dipeptidyl peptidase-4 inhibitors,** commonly called **gliptins.** They are the newest class of **antidiabetic agents; sitagliptin,** the first drug in the class, was approved in 2006. Their action is different from all other **antidiabetic agents** because they act on the incretin hormone system to have an indirect effect to increase insulin production. While the improvement in glycemic control is moderate and no more than with **metformin**, the **gliptins** are well tolerated, have a low risk for hypoglycemia, do not cause weight gain, and can be given orally once a day. Guidelines place them in the "other therapy" section, perhaps in part because they are so new and long-term safety has not been established. They are also expensive. Each of these drug classes is discussed in detail in Chapter 21.

GOALS OF TREATMENT

The overall goals for the treatment of diabetes are (1) near normalization of blood glucose (tight glycemic control), (2) prevention of acute complications such as hypoglycemia, (3) prevention of progression of the disease to target organ damage, and (4) appropriate patient-oriented self-management. Although these overall goals have not changed, the results of the Diabetes Control and Complications Trial (DCCT) (American Diabetes Association, 1993) have altered the glycemic targets. These new targets are outlined in Table 33–4 and now include blood pressure (BP) and lipid targets as well as glycemic control. Although the 2009 American Diabetes Association and the European Association for the Study of Diabetes guidelines have targeted a HbA_{1c} of less than 7, the most recent glycemic goal set by the International Diabetes Federation is a HbA_{1c} level of less than 6.5 (Nathan et al, 2009). The DCCT (1993), the Stockholm Diabetes Study of type 1 diabetes (Reichard, Nilsson, & Rosenqvist, 1993), the UK Prospective Diabetes Study (UKPDS) (1998), as well as the Kumamoto study (Ohkubo et al, 1995) conclusively demonstrated that in patients with type 1 diabetes, the risk for development or progression of retinopathy, nephropathy, and neuropathy is reduced by intensive treatment regimens when compared with conventional regimens. This implies that complete normalization of glycemic levels may prevent complications. Both types of diabetes are highly likely to benefit from tight glycemic control. The 2009 American Diabetes Association recommendations state that not only will lowering HbA_{1c} reduce microvascular and neuropathic complications, it may also lower the risk for myocardial infarction and cardiovascular death, and reduce morbidity in severe acute illness and perioperatively. Table 33–5 shows the relationship between HbA_{1c} levels and plasma glucose levels.

Table 33–4 American Diabetes Association Control Targets for Persons With Diabetes

Glycemic Control	
HbA_{1c}	<7%
Preprandial plasma glucose	90–130 mg/dL
Peak postprandial plasma glucose	<180 mg/dL
Blood Pressure	<130/80 mm Hg
Lipids	
LDL	<100 mg/dL
Triglycerides	<150 mg/dL
HDL	>50 mg/dL
Key Concepts in Setting Goals	
• Individualize goals	
• Special considerations for children, pregnant women, and older adults	
• Less intensive glycemic goals for patients with severe or frequent hypoglycemia	
• More intensive glycemic goals may further reduce microvascular complications at the risk of increasing hypoglycemia	
• Postprandial glucose may be targeted if HbA_{1c} goals are not met despite reaching preprandial glucose goals	

HDL = high-density lipoprotein; LDL = low-density lipoprotein.
Source: Adapted from American Diabetes Association. (2009). Standards of medical care in diabetes. *Diabetes Care, 32*(1), S13–S61.

Table 33–5 Correlation Between HbA_{1c} Level and Mean Plasma Glucose Level

Hemoglobin A_{1c} Levels	Mean Plasma Glucose (mg/dL)
6	135
7	170
8	205
9	240
10	275
11	310
12	345

RATIONAL DRUG SELECTION

Diabetes is a lifelong disease that may be asymptomatic until target organ damage occurs. For this reason, health-care providers often find themselves prescribing lifestyle modifications or drugs to treat a problem that patients have no clear evidence that they have and at a point when they do not feel acutely ill. For effective management, the choice of treatment should be low cost, limited in complexity, and have the fewest possible adverse reactions. This is especially important because diabetes is a largely self-managed disease. To achieve this treatment protocol, management is chosen based on the type of diabetes, the desired glycemic target, the severity of hyperglycemia, and specific patient variables. These management variables are discussed here in terms of stepped therapy, including lifestyle modification, initial monotherapy, and stepping up to multiple drugs.

Several professional groups have written guidelines for diabetes management. The most commonly used guidelines are the ones by the American Diabetes Association and the European Association for the Study of Diabetes (ADA/EASD), which were updated in January 2009. This chapter will use the ADA/EASD recommendations as the basis for its algorithms. Where other guidelines differ, those will be mentioned.

Algorithms

Type 1 Diabetes

Patients with type 1 diabetes have an absolute lack of insulin and must be given exogenous **insulin** to sustain life and prevent diabetic ketoacidosis DKA. Once a glycemic target is established, the algorithm for type 1 diabetes begins simultaneously with lifestyle modifications (medical nutrition therapy [MNT], exercise) and the administration of **insulin.** Patterns of administration and adjustments in dosage are based on blood glucose levels and assessment of glycosylated hemoglobin (HbA_{1c}) testing every 3 months. The recommended insulin therapy for type 1 diabetes consists of the following:

- Use multiple dose **insulin** injections (3 or 4/d) of basal and prandial **insulin.**
- Match prandial **insulin** to carbohydrate intake, premeal blood glucose levels and anticipated activity.
- Use **insulin analogues**, especially if hypoglycemia is a problem for the individual patient.

Make adjustments individually after reviewing patterns of control over at least 3 days and taking into consideration food and activity. Hypoglycemia is addressed first and then hyperglycemia. Make adjustments up or down in increments of only 1 U until sensitivity to insulin is well understood. Table 33–6 shows the commonly used **insulin** regimens.

Initial and annual assessments of BP and lipids are also done. If hypertension or hyperlipidemia are found, drugs to treat these conditions are also started early in diabetes management. These drugs are discussed in Chapters 40 and 39. Monitoring is discussed later. Figure 33–2 shows the algorithm for management of type 1 diabetes.

Table 33–6 **Lifestyle Modifications for Patients With Diabetes**

Nutrition	
Type 1	• Eat at consistent times synchronized with the action of the insulin preparation and the consumption of carbohydrate.
Type 1 and type 2	• Moderate caloric restriction if needed. • Space meals, spreading nutrient intake, especially carbohydrates, throughout the day. • In the presence of reduced kidney function, total protein intake 0.7–0.8 g/kg/d with 10%–20 % of caloric intake from protein. • 7% of calories from saturated fats and minimum *trans* fat intake • <200 mg of cholesterol • Total carbohydrate content is more important than type of carbohydrate. Fruits and milk have a lower glycemic response than most starches, and sucrose produces a glycemic response similar to bread, rice, and potatoes. Sucrose should be substituted 1:1 for other carbohydrates and not added to the meal plan. • Fiber recommendations are the same as for persons without diabetes. High fiber content in meals may slow the rate for glucose rise postprandially. • Sodium restriction, if any, is related to any concomitant hypertension. • Abstention from alcohol is advised. If consumed, it is best done with meals and no more than 2 drinks of alcohol/d for men and no more than 1/d for women (1 alcoholic beverage = 12 oz beer, 5 oz wine, or 1.5 oz distilled spirits).
Exercise	
Type 1 and type 2	• Exercise affects uptake of glucose by muscle and fat tissue; it can affect plasma glucose levels. Time the exercise to coincide with caloric intake. May need to decrease basal and bolus insulin for extended exercise (e.g., all-day hike, ski, etc.). Ideally, type 1 diabetics should exercise at the same time daily. Carbohydrate-based food should be readily available during and after exercise. • Increase aerobic activity to 50%–70% of maximum heart rate for 30 min 5 d/wk. Obese or low-activity patients may need to start with as little as 3 min of activity/d and increase the activity by 1 min/d until the desired 20–30 min is achieved. • Resistance training 3 X/wk can also be done and is especially good for older adults and type 2 diabetics. • Do not exercise if ketones are present. Monitor blood glucose before and after exercise. • Patients should learn their own glycemic response to different exercise conditions. They should keep records until they understand what their glycemic response is.
Weight Loss	
Type 1 and type 2	• Moderate caloric restriction (250–500 calories less than average daily intake as calculated from a food history). • Moderate weight loss (5–9 kg or 10–20 lb), regardless of starting weight, has been shown to affect insulin sensitivity.

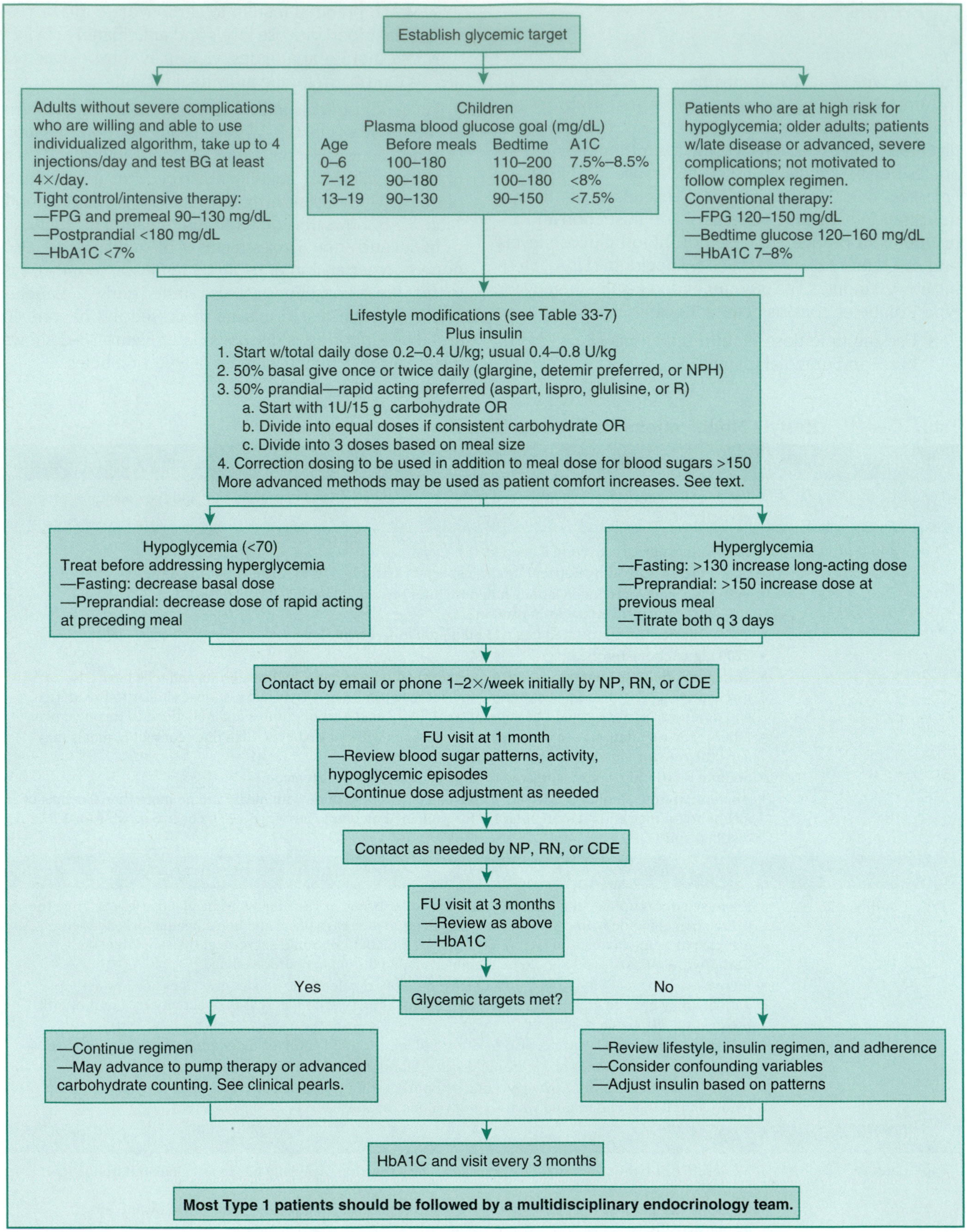

Figure 33–2. Treatment algorithm for type 1 diabetes.

CLINICAL PEARL

Pointers For Managing Type 1 Diabetes Mellitus

Most patients should see a diabetic specialist and treatment team as treatment is challenging and a team approach works best. At minimum, a Certified Diabetes Educator needs to be involved.

Make small changes gradually with close follow-up (every 1 to 2 wk) until good control is achieved. Some follow-up can be done by phone.

Reduce hypoglycemia before tackling hyperglycemia. Hypoglycemia can be life threatening.

It is normal to have wide variability in blood glucose levels even with adherence to the treatment plan. Variability does not necessarily mean nonadherence.

Consistency as to meal times, injection sites, and timing and frequency of exercise is vital, but difficult for most patients to achieve 24/7.

Individualize the treatment plan!!

CLINICAL PEARL

Rules For Fine-Tuning Insulin Doses

To tune insulin dose more finely, the provider can determine a correction factor (CF) and insulin: carbohydrate ratio (I:C) for patients with either type 1 or 2 taking insulin.

The rule of 1,500 enables the provider to find the CF or how much 1 U of insulin will drop blood sugar for high blood glucose levels (usually greater than 140 to 150). First, calculate the total daily dose (TDD) of insulin as basal + bolus—about 50 percent of each. Then divide 1,500 by the TDD. For example, 1,500 divided by 30 U per day of insulin equals 50. One unit RA insulin will drop glucose 50 pts.

The rule of 500 enables the provider to find the I:C ratio. Divide 500 by TDD. For example, 500 divided by 30 U per day of insulin equals 16.7. One unit will cover 16 to 17 g CHO (for ease of use, round down to 1 U:15 g\).

Type 2 Diabetes

Type 2 diabetes is a more complex disease than type 1 diabetes, and some endogenous insulin is present. Once a glycemic target is set, the algorithm for type 2 diabetes begins with lifestyle modifications (MNT, exercise, and so forth). Table 33–6 lists the appropriate lifestyle modifications for both type 1 and type 2 diabetes. Intensive glycemic targets are often difficult to reach with lifestyle modifications alone, and drug therapy (**insulin** or **metformin**) should be started in the initial step. To reduce the GI adverse reactions that are common with **metformin**, the dose is titrated up from 500 mg taken once or twice daily to the maximum effective dose, which is often 850 to 1,000 mg twice daily. A long-acting formulation is available in some countries and can be given once daily. The titration formula is found in Chapter 21, along with the discussion of **metformin**.

Oral hypoglycemic agents have limited ability to reduce hyperglycemia; therefore, for patients who initially present with blood glucose levels above 300, **insulin** may be needed to lower plasma glucose to less than 180 before oral agents are begun. When insulin is added, the dose of **insulin** is typically started with an intermediate-acting insulin at 10 U or 0.2 U/kg administered at bedtim. The dose is increased by 2 U every 3 days until daily FPG levels are consistently in glycemic goal range. If the FPG is

Table 33–7 **Commonly Used Insulin Regimens**

Regimen	Types of Insulin	Schedule	Advantages	Disadvantages
Multiple doses	Very rapid acting (analogue) and glargine	Glargine to = 50% of daily insulin dose at bedtime and then split VRA for before each meal *or* Use same dosing but give glargine at breakfast *or* Use same dosing but give glargine at dinner.	Consistent insulin dose throughout the day with glargine and added insulin only when food present.	Requires 4 injections and premeal + bedtime blood glucose checks. Glargine not compatible with other insulin, so requires separate syringe.
Split-mixed dose	Intermediate and short acting	Both at breakfast; short acting at dinner and intermediate acting at bedtime.	Three injections provide coverage for 24 h. Risk for 3 a.m. hypoglycemia reduced.	Requires three injections.
Multiple doses	Intermediate and short acting	Intermediate at bedtime and short acting before each meal.	More flexibility at mealtimes for amount of food intake.	Four injections required and premeal glucose checks. Requires highly individualized algorithm.

continued

Table 33–7 **Commonly Used Insulin Regimens—cont'd**

Regimen	Types of Insulin	Schedule	Advantages	Disadvantages
Multiple doses	Glargine and 70/30 mixed	Glargine to = 50% of daily insulin dose at bedtime; then split remainder of dose of 70/30 mixed insulin at bedtime and breakfast.	Consistent insulin dose throughout day with glargine. Two injections for 24-h coverage with other insulins.	Two injections required. Glargine not compatible with other insulin; needs separate syringe.
Type 2 only regimens				
Single dose	Intermediate acting	Start at 10 U or 0.2 U/kg at bedtime to initiate insulin therapy.	Start with low dose to reduce hypoglycemic risk.	Except for initiation of therapy, rarely used because not physiological.
Split-mixed dose (70/30 pre-mix)	Intermediate and short acting	Both given at breakfast and dinner.	Two injections provide 24-h coverage.	Two injections required. Patient must adhere to set meal pattern.
Multiple doses	Glargine and oral agent	Glargine at breakfast with the oral agent.	Once-daily dosing of both agents. Consistent insulin dose throughout day.	Requires injection as well as oral agent.

Short-acting = regular; intermediate acting = NPH; very rapid acting = lispro, aspart, or glulisine.
Detemir may replace glargine in those regimens using glargine. In any of the regimens using short-acting insulin, very rapid acting insulin may be substituted.

greater than 180, the dose can be increased by 4 U every 3 days. If hypoglycemia occurs, the dose can be reduced by 4 U or 10 percent, whichever is greater. Once the FPG is in target range, testing of blood glucose before each meal should occur. Depending on these results, additional injections of **insulin** are added (Nathan et al, 2009).

As with type 1 diabetes, initial and annual assessments of BP and lipids are also done. If hypertension or hyperlipidemia are found, drugs to treat these conditions are also started early in diabetes management. If glycemic targets are not met with MNT, exercise, weight loss (if appropriate), and **metformin**, then drug therapy is increased by the addition of **insulin** (if not already being used). A **sulfonylurea** may also be added. More than one drug will be necessary for the majority of patients over time (Nathan et al, 2009) and the addition of other drugs is based on the degree and pattern of glycemic control. The ADA/EASD guidelines base the choice of antihyperglycemic drug on the effectiveness of that drug in lowering glucose, extraglycemic effects that may reduce long-term complications, safety profiles, tolerability, ease of use, and expense. Table 33–8, taken from the ADA/EASD consensus document (Nathan et al, 2009), lists the various classes of antihyperglycemic drugs and provides information

Table 33–8 **Summary of Glucose-Lowering Interventions for Type 2 Diabetes**

Intervention	Expected Decrease in HbA_{1c} With Monotherapy (%)	Advantages	Disadvantages
Tier 1: Well-validated core			
Step 1: Initial therapy			
Lifestyle to decrease weight and increase activity	1.0–2.0	Broad benefits	Insufficient for most within first year.
Metformin	1.0–2.0	Weight neutral	GI side effects, contraindicated with renal insufficiency.
Step 2: Additional therapy			
Insulin	1.5–3.5	No dose limit; rapidly effective; improved lipid profile	1 to 4 injections daily; monitoring; weight gain; hypoglycemia; analogues are expensive.
Sulfonylurea	1.0–2.0	Rapidly effective	Weight gain; hypoglycemia (especially with glyburide or chlorpropamide).

Table 33–8 **Summary of Glucose-Lowering Interventions for Type 2 Diabetes—cont'd**

Intervention	Expected Decrease in HbA_{1c} With Monotherapy (%)	Advantages	Disadvantages
Tier 2: Less well-validated			
TDZs (pioglitazone only)	0.5–1.4	Improved lipid profile; potential decrease in MI	Fluid retention; CHF; weight gain; bone fractures; expensive (rosiglitazone not recommended due to potential increase in cardiovascular events)
GLP-1 agonist	0.5–1.0	Weight loss	Two injections daily, frequent GI side effects, long-term safety not established, expensive.
Other therapy			
Alpha-glucosidase inhibitor	0.5–0.8	Weight neutral	Frequent GI side effects; 3 X/d dosing; expensive
Glinide	0.5–1.5*	Rapidly effective	Weight gain; 3 X/d dosing; hypoglycemia; expensive
Pramlintide	0.5–1.0	Weight loss	3 injections daily; frequent side effect; long-term safety not established; expensive
Gliptins (DPP-4 inhibitors)	0.5–0.8	Weight neutral	Long-term safety not established; expensive

*Repaglinide more effective in lowering HbA_{1c} than nateglinide.

Source: Table is adapted from Nathan et al. (2009). Medical management of hyperglycemia in type 2 diabetes: A consensus algorithm for the initiation and adjustment of therapy. *Diabetes Care, 32*(1), 193-203.

about these variables. Monitoring with HbA_{1c} is similar for both types of diabetes. Figure 33–3 shows the algorithm for management of type 2 diabetes. The algorithm emphasizes the following:

- Achievement and maintenance of near normal glucose levels (HbA_{1c} less than 7%)
- Initial therapy with lifestyle interventions and **metformin**
- Rapid addition of drugs and transition to new regimens when target glycemic goals are not achieved or sustained
- Early addition of **insulin** therapy in patients who do not meet target goals. (Nathan et al, 2009)

The guidelines for both BP and lipid control and the use of **aspirin** or another **antiplatelet** drug are not included in these algorithms, but will be discussed in the Complications section. Antiplatelet therapy is recommended in the American Diabetes Association "Standards of Medical Care in Diabetes" (American Diabetes Association, 2009a). Tobacco cessation is discussed in the Lifestyle Modifications section. All of these should be started at the initial assessment.

Initial Assessment

Initial visits for patients with diabetes, regardless of type, are complex. The visits include an extensive history about symptoms; eating habits; physical activity; prior or current infection; symptoms of chronic complications associated with diabetes; current drugs being taken, including over-the-counter (OTC) drugs, and alternative therapies that might affect glucose levels; family history of diabetes, cardiovascular disease, cerebrovascular disease, or dyslipidemia; gestational history, especially related to delivery of an infant weighing more than 9 pounds, toxemia, stillbirth, or history of GDM; and **alcohol** or drug use. Especially critical is assessment of risk factors for cardiovascular disease including smoking, hypertension, or dyslipidemia. **Aspirin** use should be discussed. After a thorough physical examination, including looking at the patient's feet, laboratory data are collected. Appropriate laboratory data are discussed in the Monitoring section. The results of this assessment will determine whether intensive or conventional therapy for glycemic control is better and whether treatment or referral for complications should be started early.

Setting a Glycemic Target

Many studies have shown that treatment regimens that reduce average HbA_{1c} to less than 7 percent are associated with fewer long-term microvascular and neuropathic complications, even at the risk for more episodes of hypoglycemia (American Diabetes Association, 2009a). Some clinical trials suggest a small benefit in microvascular outcomes with a HbA_{1c} score below 7 percent. For selected patients, this lower goal can be suggested if it can be achieved without significant hypoglycemia or other adverse effects of treatment. Such patients might include

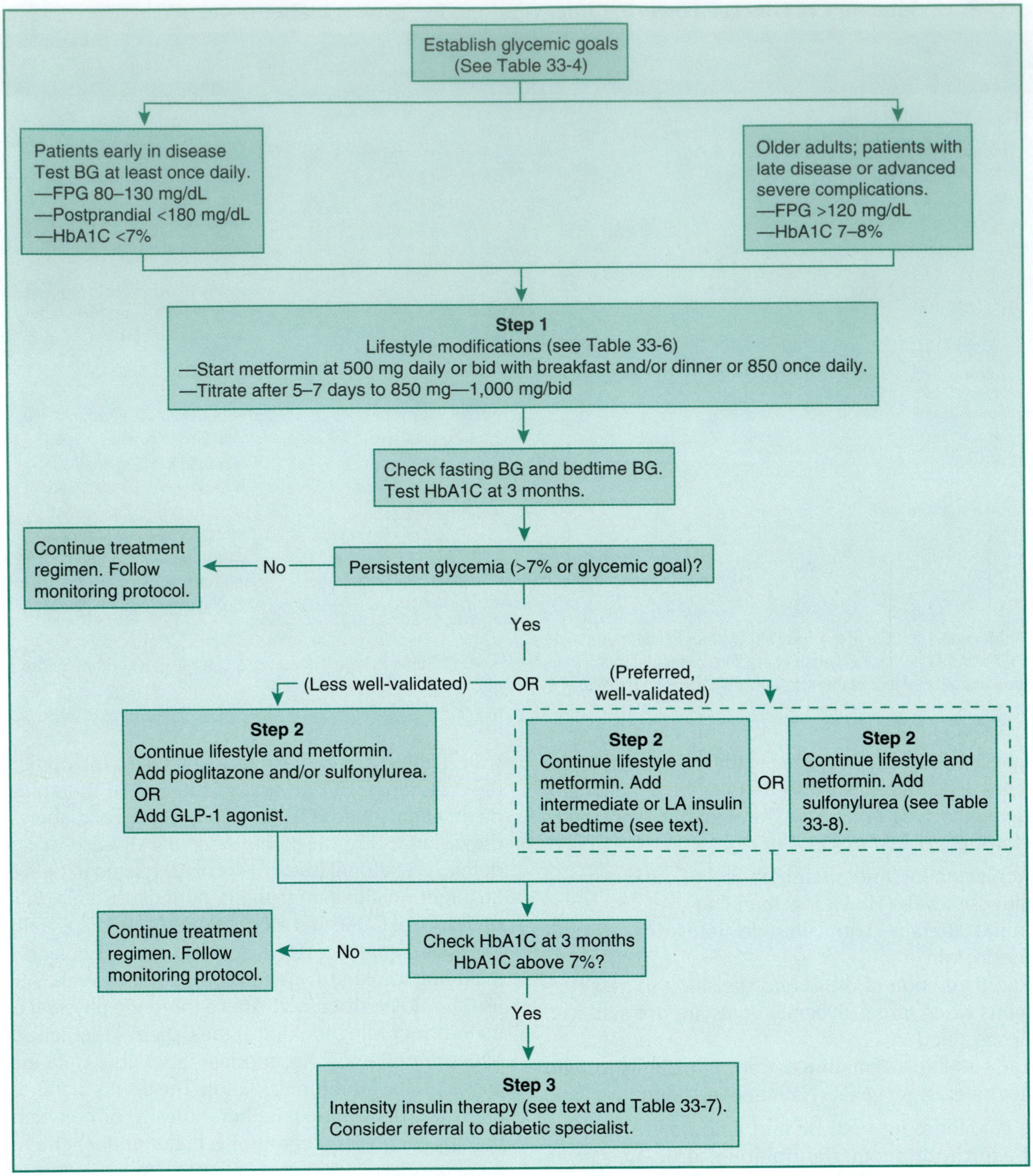

Figure 33–3. Treatment algorithm for type 2 diabetes.

those with short-term duration of diabetes, long life expectancy, and no significant cardiovascular disease (CVD) (American Diabetes Association, 2009a). Several recent studies looking at macrovascular complications (ACCORD, ADVANCE, VDAT) have actually shown increased CVD mortality in patients who were on the intensive control arm of the study in which the HbA_{1c} target approached 6 percent (Abraira, Duckworth, & Moritz, 2008; Action to Control Cardiovascular Risk in Diabetes Study Group [ACCORD] 2008; ADVANCE Collaborative Group, 2008; Duckworth, 2008). Because all three trials were carried out with patients with established diabetes and either known CVD or risk factors suggesting the presence of atherosclerosis, it may be that glycemic targets in the 6.4 to 6.9 percent range play a greater role before macrovascular disease is well developed and minimal or no role when it is advanced. It should be noted that the ADVANCE trial did show evidence of benefits on microvascular and neuropathic complications. Glycemic targets recommended by the American Diabetes Association and key concepts in setting these goals are shown in Table 33–4. Table 33–5 shows the correlation between HbA_{1c} levels and mean plasma glucose levels. Less stringent glycemic targets are recommended for patients with long-standing diabetes and/or advanced macrovascular and microvascular complications; who are older adults (65 years or older) in whom hypoglycemic awareness may be reduced (Bremer, Jauch-Chara, Hallschmld, Schmid, & Schultes, 2009); who are young children (under 13 years); with extensive comorbid conditions; those with severe or frequent hypoglycemia; and with limited life expectancies (5 to 15 years) (American Diabetes Association, 2009a). The VA/DoD Diabetes Guideline Development Group (Pogach et al, 2004) agrees with the importance of individualizing glycemic targets and adds to the list for whom intensive therapy may not be appropriate patients with moderate microvascular disease and type 1 diabetics who have autonomic neuropathy in which the risk of hypoglycemic unawareness is enhanced.

Lifestyle Modifications

The incidence of diabetes and the incidence of obesity in the United States are increasing at approximately the same rate. This increased incidence of obesity is thought to be a primary culprit in the diabetes epidemic. Evidence from the Diabetes Prevention Program Research (2002, 2003) found that even modest lifestyle changes; eating less fat, losing 7 percent of body weight, and exercising 150 minutes weekly, cut the incidence of diabetes dramatically (Daly, Warshaw, Pastors, Franz, & Arnold, 2003; Whittemore, Bak, Melkus, & Grey, 2003). Two studies of lifestyle modification have shown persistent reduction in the rate of conversion of pre-diabetes to type 2 diabetes in follow-up at 3 and 14 years post intervention (Li et al, 2008; Lindstrom et al, 2006).

Patients with pre-diabetes or diabetes should have individualized MNT. MNT has always been an integral part of diabetes management and diabetes self-management education and the results of this study make it even more central to the ability to achieve glycemic goals and to reduce hypertension and dyslipidemia. In overweight and obese **insulin**-resistant patients, even modest weight loss has been shown to reduce **insulin** resistance. Goals of MNT include the following:

- Attain and maintain recommended metabolic outcomes, including glucose and HbA_{1c} level; low-density lipoprotein (LDL) cholesterol, HDL cholesterol, and triglyceride levels; BP; and body weight (see Chaps. 39 and 40 for appropriate goals).
- Modify nutrient intake as appropriate for the prevention and treatment of obesity, dyslipidemia (see Chap. 39), cardiovascular disease (see Chap. 28), hypertension (see Chap. 40), and nephropathy.
- Improve health through healthy food choices and physical activity. Address individual nutritional needs, taking into consideration personal and cultural preferences and lifestyle while respecting the individual's wishes and willingness to change.
- For youth with type 1 diabetes, provide adequate energy to ensure normal growth and development and integrate **insulin** regimens into usual eating and physical activity patterns.
- For youth with type 2 diabetes, facilitate dietary changes that reduce **insulin** resistance.
- For pregnant and lactating women, provide adequate energy and nutrient needed for optimal outcomes.
- For older adults, provide for the nutritional and psychosocial needs appropriate to their age.
- Patients using **insulin** are encouraged to eat at consistent times synchronized with the action of the **insulin** preparation. Patients on intensive therapy may make adjustments in **short-acting insulin** dosages based on the carbohydrate content of their meals and snacks and for deviations from usual eating patterns.

To attain these goals, consultation with a registered dietician familiar with the components of diabetes MNT is key. Additionally, all members of the team caring for a patient with diabetes should be knowledgeable about MNT and supportive of the patient making lifestyle changes. The American Diabetes Association "Nutrition Principles and Recommendations in Diabetes" (2004e) and the "Standards of Medical Care in Diabetes" (2009a) give detailed information on MNT. Table 33–6 provides a summary of these recommendations. Websites that provide low- or no-cost diabetes nutrition education materials include http://www.niddk.nih.gov; http://www.healthsource.org; http://merchant.diabetes.org or http://www.eatright.org/catalogue. Many of these resources are available in Spanish.

Patients with diabetes should also understand the effect exercise has on glucose uptake by skeletal muscle and the resultant alteration in plasma glucose levels. Regular exercise has been shown to improve glucose control, reduce cardiovascular risk factors, contribute to weight loss, and improve well-being. Exercise may also prevent type 2 diabetes in high-risk individuals (American Diabetes Association, 2009a). Therefore, a regular physical activity program, adapted to the presence of complications, is recommended for all patients with diabetes who are capable of participating. Patients with diabetes should be advised to perform moderate to intensive aerobic activity (50% to 70% of maximum heart rate) at least 150 minutes a week. Patients with type 2 diabetes and older adults should perform resistance training three times a week unless it is contraindicated (American Diabetes Association, 2009a). Resistance exercise improves **insulin** sensitivity to about the same extent as does aerobic exercise. Before beginning an exercise program, patients should be evaluated for macro- and microvascular changes that may be worsened by exercise. A graded exercise test is appropriate only for symptomatic patients and those with cardiovascular disease who are older than 35 years, or older than 25 years with type 2 diabetes of more than 10 years duration, or type 1 diabetes more than 15 years duration; those with any additional risk factor for coronary heart disease (see Chap. 28); or those with microvascular disease, peripheral vascular disease, or autonomic neuropathy. The American Diabetes Association's position statement "Physical Activity/Exercise and Diabetes" (2004f) and the "Standards of Medical Care in Diabetes" (2009a) give detailed information on evaluation of the patient before exercise and on prescriptions for the right type of exercise.

Use of tobacco products is a concern with diabetics. A large body of evidence from epidemiological, case-control, and cohort studies provides convincing documentation of the causal link between cigarette smoking and health risks. Individuals with diabetes are at higher risk for morbidity and premature death associated with the development of macrovascular complications found among smokers.

Smoking is also related to the premature development of microvascular complications in diabetes. Smoking cessation is one of the few safe and cost-effective lifestyle modifications that can be recommended for all patients with diabetes. The American Diabetes Association position statement "Smoking and Diabetes" (2004g) gives specific recommendations regarding diabetes and smoking; Chapter 43 focuses on this topic.

Lifestyle modifications make a difference with type 2 diabetes. Some patients (approximately 10%) achieve glycemic targets with lifestyle modifications alone. Nutritional goals for patients with type 2 diabetes include achieving and maintaining not only glycemic control but also appropriate lipid levels and BP. Calories, protein, total fat, saturated fat and cholesterol, carbohydrates, sweeteners, fiber, sodium, and **alcohol** are all included in specific recommendations. Exercise prescriptions for patients with type 2 diabetes are 50 to 70 percent of maximal heart rate, five times per week. Exercise is not recommended if the patient is in poor glycemic control. Specific recommendations related to nutrition and exercise are found in the American Diabetes Association documents cited above and in the References section.

Drug Therapy

Drug therapy with **insulin** is tier 1 in type 1 diabetes with **metformin** being tier 1 therapy in type 2 diabetes. The choice of drug and the decision of monotherapy versus combination therapy are based on the type of diabetes, the glycemic control desired, patient variables, and concomitant disease processes.

Type of Diabetes

Type 1 Diabetes

Patients with type 1 diabetes require **insulin.** Combinations of short-acting, intermediate-acting, and long-acting agents may be used. The pattern of administration of **insulin** is based on the patient's blood glucose, dietary, and exercise patterns. Patients in the Diabetes Complications Control Trial (DCCT) study on tight control had three subject groups. Two groups used combinations of short-acting and intermediate-acting **insulins** given three to four times per day. Patients on very tight control used long-acting **insulin** at night with short-acting **insulin** before each meal or more frequently, based on self-monitored glucose measurements. The third group used an **insulin** pump. The development of the **insulin glargine**, discussed in the **insulin** section in type 1 diabetes, has resulted in a regimen involving one injection per day of **insulin glargine** and individualized doses of other **insulins** based on blood glucose readings throughout the day.

As a general rule, when **insulin** is given twice daily, the dose is split with two-thirds given in the morning and one-third given in the evening. For patients on basal bolus regimens who count carbohydrates, the 1,500 and 500 rules, described in the Clinical Pearl box Rules for Fine-Tuning Insulin Doses, are used to determine **insulin** amount and carbohydrate intake.

Another possibility is to calculate the daily dose of **insulin** at 0.3 U/kg and use premixed 70/30 insulin with two-thirds of the dose in the morning and one-third of the dose in the evening. For patients using **insulin glargine,** one way to calculate the daily dose of insulin is at 0.3 U/kg, start bedtime **glargine** at 50 percent of the total dose, and split the remaining 50 percent with short-acting **insulin** before meals. Patients who are intelligent, motivated, and reliable can be taught to regulate their blood sugar with this intensive control. Less capable patients risk hypoglycemic reactions on this regimen and might not be appropriate candidates or might need higher fasting blood sugar targets than more capable patients.

Table 33–6 lists the commonly used **insulin** regimens. **Insulin** is also discussed in more detail in Chapter 21.

Type 2 Diabetes

Patients with type 2 diabetes can have a variety of oral agents tailored to their specific disease process. Lean patients are less likely to be **insulin** resistant and more likely to benefit from a **sulfonylurea.** Obese patients are more likely to benefit from a **metformin** that acts more on glucose utilization and hepatic glucose storage and production. Both of these classes are considered tier 1 therapy and should be used as main agents with others added as adjuncts. Patients with a high risk for hypoglycemia benefit from drugs, such as **metformin** or **pioglitazone,** that are less likely to produce that effect. **Pioglitazone** is a tier 2 drug and is used as a possible alternative therapy between step 2 and step 3 in the treatment algorithm. Patients with high postprandial blood glucose levels may benefit the addition of an **alpha-glucosidase inhibitor** or a **meglitinide,** but these drugs are not part of the usual treatment algorithm and are useful only in selected patients.

At some point in their disease, many patients with type 2 diabetes may require the addition of **insulin.** The 2009 American Diabetes Association algorithm places **insulin** in the tier 1 category as step 2 therapy. Type 2 diabetics can use a variety of **insulin** regimens. **Insulin glargine**, for example, can be initiated at a dose of approximately 0.1 U/kg while simultaneously starting an oral agent. The likely use of **insulin** over time needs to be discussed early in the disease process with all type 2 patients. These drugs are discussed in more detail in Chapter 21.

Age

Children

Approximately 75 percent of all newly diagnosed cases of type 1 diabetes occur in patients younger than age 18 years. Care of these patients requires integration of diabetes management with the growth and development needs of children, adolescents, and their families. Young patients with diabetes are best cared for by a team that can deal with these special needs. Glycemic targets may need to be modified to take into account that children younger than 7 years lack hypoglycemic awareness because they lack the cognitive capacity to recognize and respond to hypoglycemic signals. Tight control also should be undertaken with extreme caution in children 2 to 7 years because hypoglycemia may impair normal brain development, which is not complete until after 7 years. Overly aggressive dietary manipulation can contribute to lack of adherence, especially in adolescents. Schools and day-care settings must be involved in the treatment of the diabetes, often participating in administration of drugs. Treatment regimens must take all of these needs into account.

Children with type 1 diabetes also have a high risk for CVD. The number of children with type 2 diabetes is currently too small to make a statement about their risk, but CVD is a strong risk factor in adults and likely exists for children as well. Management of complications is discussed in the Hyperlipidemia section.

Children may also develop type 2 diabetes. Prevention of conversion from pre-diabetes to diabetes must take highest priority in children and should focus on decreasing the risk, incidence, and consequences of type 2 diabetes, especially in high-risk ethnic groups. Modifiable risks for type 2 diabetes in children that can be addressed with primary prevention include the prevention of obesity and the promotion of breastfeeding. The use of **alcohol, tobacco**, and drugs should be evaluated in all children and adolescents in whom diabetes is newly diagnosed and should be reevaluated at every visit. **Alcohol** may aggravate hypoglycemia caused by **sulfonylureas** or **insulin** and increase the risk of lactic acidosis in patients who use **metformin.** Family support is essential to the child or adolescent with type 2 diabetes. The whole family should be involved in dietary and activity changes, prevention of complications, as well as drug therapy management and self-monitoring of blood glucose.

For children, the goal weight should be the expected BMI for their age. Weight stabilization rather than weight loss is recommended for prepubertal children. Children who are morbidly obese may be referred to a specialist in weight reduction or a multidisciplinary child obesity clinic.

The BP goal is less than the 90th percentile on the basis of height and weight standards. Treatment of hypertension in children is discussed in Chapter 40. Fasting lipid levels are best obtained after the initial metabolic stabilization (1 to 3 months after diagnosis). The lipid goals are LDL less than 100 mg/dL and total cholesterol less than 170 mg/dL. Treatment of children with dyslipidemia is discussed in Chapter 39.

The HbA_{1c} goal is the same as for adults: less than 7 percent. The drug therapy recommended by the American Academy of Pediatrics (Gahagan & Silverstein, 2003) is **metformin** and **insulin.** Liver function tests should be performed before initiation of **oral hypoglycemic** therapy. **Sulfonylureas** are not currently approved for use in children, although studies in the pediatric population with second generation agents are ongoing. Pediatric endocrinologists have used **sulfonylureas** with **metformin,** when monotherapy has been unsuccessful. If multiple drugs are required, referral to a pediatric endocrinologist may be necessary.

Older Adults

Older adults (older than 65 years) are more likely to have type 2 diabetes and use oral agents to treat their disease. They may suffer severe consequences from a hypoglycemic episode, especially patients with significant atherosclerosis who may be vulnerable to permanent injury. Research on changing nutritional needs with aging is limited and virtually none has been done in subjects with diabetes (American Diabetes Association, 2004e), so the needs of older adults are extrapolated from what is known about the general population. The most reliable indicator of poor nutritional status in older adults is involuntary weight gain or loss of more than 10 pounds or 10 percent of body weight in less than 6 months. Weight loss in overweight older adults should be carefully evaluated. In this population, low body weight has been associated with greater morbidity and mortality.

Exercise training can significantly reduce the decline in maximal aerobic capacity that occurs with age, improve risk factors for atherosclerosis, slow the decline in age-related lean body mass, decrease central adiposity, and improve **insulin** sensitivity. All of these are beneficial in the older adult with diabetes.

Glycemic targets for older adults are generally 10 percent higher than those for younger patients. All **sulfonylureas** may produce severe hypoglycemia. **Second generation** drugs are less likely than **first generation** drugs to have this adverse reaction. **Glimepiride (Amaryl)**, a **third generation sulfonylurea,** is least likely to cause this adverse reaction. Glyburide is the most likely to cause hypoglycemia and is not recommended for the elderly. The risk for hypoglycemia with **repaglinide** or **nateglinide** is about the same as with **second generation**

sulfonylureas, but these drugs are not part of the usual algorithm. Drugs that are less likely to produce hypoglycemia include **metformin**, **alpha-glucosidase inhibitors**, and **pioglitazone**. However, **pioglitazone** should not be used in patients with congestive heart failure because of its fluid-retention side effect. It is not tier 2 and not a good choice in older adults. **Metformin** is often contraindicated in older adults because they may have renal insufficiency or heart failure. **Alpha-glucosidase inhibitors**, which are not part of the usual algorithm, have a good safety profile in this population, but are not well tolerated.

Older adults also have some differences in target organ damage. In a study of renal impairment associated with diabetes in older adults (Wasen et al, 2004), the researchers found that diabetes, compared to HTN, was a more powerful determinant of decreased renal function in older adults. They also found that older type 2 diabetics, especially the very old (older than 80 years), show similarities to target organ damage in type 1 diabetes, with microvascular rather than macrovascular profile. This suggests that glycemic control is still a central issue in older adults to prevent complications of diabetes.

Race and Ethnic Group

The American Association of Clinical Endocrinologists (AACE) (Bloomgarden, 2003) evaluated the differences in diabetes presentation and complications across ethnic groups. *Asian* populations, who have low rates of obesity, have high rates of diabetes and cardiovascular disease. The prevalence of diabetes appears to be higher in the migrant population. Despite low obesity rates, increased intra-abdominal fat showed stronger correlation with hypertension and dyslipidemia than did **insulin** sensitivity per se, and was a marker for diabetes risk. The prevalence of cardiovascular disease may be associated with the higher total and LDL cholesterol, higher triglycerides, lower HDL, and higher concentrations of homocysteine and lipoprotein(a) found in persons of South Asian ethnicity. These data suggest that treatment of hypertension and dyslipidemia and the lifestyle modification related to exercise are necessary in this population.

The SEARCH for Diabetes in Youth Study Group (Liu et al, 2009) looked at *Asian* and *Pacific Islanders* less than 20 years of age. This study found that most participants in the study who had type 2 diabetes were obese (*Asian* 71% and *Pacific Islanders* 100%), with a mean BMI greater than 33 kg/m^2. Of those with type 1 diabetes, *Pacific Islanders* were more likely to be obese, with a mean BMI of 26. The incidence of type 2 diabetes in these populations was almost double that of type 1 diabetes. The study group's recommendation is that a stronger public health focus needs to be made for these youths in the area of type 2 diabetes and obesity.

Hispanics in the United States have a high incidence of obesity, hyper-triglyceridemia, low HDL cholesterol, hypertension, and high FPG. Diabetes prevalence increased 39 percent among *Hispanics*, compared to 30 percent among *African Americans*, and 27 percent among whites from 1990 to 1998. Predictors of conversion from pre-diabetes to diabetes in this population are high LDL and triglycerides and low HDL, high BP, and high BMI. Treatment of hypertension and dyslipidemia, and lifestyle modifications related to nutrition are critical in this group. Because **metformin** has been associated with prevention of conversion from pre-diabetes to diabetes, this may be a good drug for this population.

The SEARCH study of *Hispanics* (Lawrence et al, 2009) found type 1 more prevalent than type 2 in *Hispanic* youth. The study group included children 10 to 19 years. Although there was no gender difference in prevalence, the incidence of type 2 diabetes for female subjects was twice that of male subjects. Poor glycemic control, elevated lipids, and a high prevalence of obesity put *Hispanic* youth at high risk for future diabetes-related complications. Lifestyle modifications play a large role in this group. Drugs that foster weight loss such as **metformin** are good choices here.

African Americans have lesser degrees of dyslipidemia, but greater prevalence of diabetes and hypertension than other ethnic groups. Treatment of hypertension is paramount in this ethnic group. Compared to other ethnic populations, *African American* adolescents have had a huge increase in development of type 2 diabetes. African American children have higher insulin secretion both before and during puberty and lower insulin sensitivity during adolescence. If it is extrapolated that *African American* adults may continue this lower insulin sensitivity, then selecting drugs that improve insulin sensitivity to treat type 2 diabetes in *African Americans* of all ages is appropriate. Drugs with this characteristic include **metformin** and **pioglitazone. Metformin** is also a drug of choice related to the increasing prevalence of obesity among *African Americans*, particularly women.

The SEARCH study with *African American* youth (Mayer-Davis et al, 2009) looked at children from infancy to 19 years. This study found that the incidence of type 1 diabetes was high in this group, especially for those older than age 10 years. The study also found that both types of diabetes substantially affect adolescents in this ethnic group. Among adolescents with either type of diabetes, more than 90 percent were overweight or obese and 60 percent of those with type 2 diabetes came from households with an annual income of less than $25,000. Although lifestyle modifications are a major emphasis in this group, cost variables should especially be taken into account when choosing any drug for this population.

Bloomgarden (2003) did not examine the Native American population, but the SEARCH study group looked at *Navaho* youth ages 15 to 19 (Dabelea et al, 2009). Diabetes is common among members of the *Navaho* nation, but the prevalence and incidence of this disease are higher in older members of the nation than they are among the youth. The vast majority of diabetes among the youth is type 2. These young people are likely to have poor glycemic control, a high prevalence of unhealthy behaviors, and evidence of a severely depressed mood. They have more metabolic factors associated with obesity and insulin resistance (abdominal fat, dyslipidemia, and a higher albumin-to-creatinine ratio). Intervention efforts should be targeted at primary prevention and efforts to prevent or delay the development of chronic complications associated with metabolic factors.

Finally, when looking at ethnicity, *non-Hispanic white* youth (Bell et al, 2009) must be considered. The age group studied in this ethnic group was infancy to 19 years. The incidence of type 1 diabetes in this ethnic group is one of the highest in the world. Although type 2 is still relatively rare, rates are seven times higher than those reported in European countries. Forty percent of the subjects in this study had elevated LDL cholesterol and less than 3 percent met current recommendations for the intake of saturated fat. Of those with type 1 diabetes, 18 percent were smokers and 26 percent of those with type 2 were smokers. Lifestyle and cardiometabolic risk factors require attention in this population.

Obesity

Obesity contributes to diabetes by down-regulating **insulin** receptors, and it contributes to many of the complications associated with diabetes. Weight loss alone improves short-term glycemic levels and has the potential to improve long-term metabolic control. **Metformin** is the oral agent most associated with fostering weight loss and is the tier 1 drug choice in step 1 of the treatment algorithm for patients with central obesity. The lack of weight gain associated with **alpha-glucosidase inhibitors** suggests that these drugs might also be helpful as adjunct therapy for patients with diabetes who are obese. **Alpha-glucosidase inhibitors** are listed in the "other therapy" category by the American Diabetes Association. **Sulfonylureas,** which are also tier 1 drug choices but are step 2 in the algorithm, have been associated with weight gain in most studies; weight gain has been reported in some studies with **pioglitazone**, a tier 2 drug choice.

Concomitant disease processes also affect drug choice. Often these disease processes reflect target organ damage from diabetes. The pathophysiological changes associated with the disease process and/or the drugs commonly used to treat it contribute to determining the best drug therapy, especially for patients with type 2 diabetes.

The American Diabetes Association (2009a) makes specific recommendations for screening and management of chronic complications in type 1 diabetes based on concomitant disorders. They are discussed in the sections that follow.

Coronary Artery Disease and Heart Failure

Large epidemiological studies have shown that in patients with diabetes, the higher the glucose, the greater the incidence of CVD. Collectively, these studies suggest that the risk of a CVD event rises 10 to 30 percent for every 1 percent increase in HbA_{1c} (Sowers & Haffner, 2002). The American Diabetes Association (2009a) states that people with diabetes have a 2- to 4-fold increase in the risk of dying from complications of cardiovascular disease. Other studies have shown a reduction in CVD events and significant microvascular disease in type 2 diabetes with improved glycemic control. A meta-analysis of all glycemic intervention studies in patients with type 2 diabetes showed that intensive therapy (HbA_{1c} greater than 7%) with **insulin** reduced macrovascular events by 28 percent. Three recent studies, ACCORD, VADT, and ADVANCE, did not show a benefit for macrovascular events with stricter glycemic control (6.4% to 6.9%) compared with the standard control of 7 percent. Decline in macrovascular events is more likely related to control of BP, lipids, and smoking.

All patients with known CVD should be treated with an **angiotension-converting enzyme (ACE) inhibitor, aspirin**, and **statin** therapy (if not contraindicated) to reduce the risk of cardiovascular events (American Diabetes Association, 2009a). The American Diabetes Association also recommends that patients with a prior myocardial infarction (MI) have **beta blockers** added to their regimen (if not contraindicated) to reduce mortality.

Atherosclerosis occurs earlier in patients with diabetes than it does in those without elevated glucose levels, and platelets from men and women with diabetes are often hypersensitive to platelet aggregation agents. A major mechanism is increased production of thromboxane, a potent vasoconstrictor and platelet aggregant. **Aspirin** blocks the formation of thromboxane by acetylating cyclo-oxygenase and has been used as both primary and secondary prevention for cardiovascular events in both diabetics and nondiabetics. The American Diabetes Association (2009a) recommends the use of **aspirin** therapy (75 to 162 mg/d) as a primary prevention strategy in patients with type 1 or type 2 diabetes at increased cardiovascular risk, including patients who are older than 40 years or who have additional risk factors (see Chap. 28 for discussion of risk factors for CVD). The same dose is to be used as secondary prevention for those patients with a history of CVD. If **aspirin** is contraindicated (e.g., known **aspirin** allergy), **clopidogrel (Plavix)** 75 mg/day should be used as **antiplatelet** therapy. Combination therapy with both of these agents is reasonable for up to 1 year after an acute coronary syndrome. **Aspirin** therapy is not recommended for patients under 30 years because of a lack of evidence of benefit and is contraindicated for patients under 21 years because of the risk for Reye syndrome. **Metformin** also inhibits platelet aggregations and decreases blood viscosity (Bloomgarden, 2003).

Metformin has been associated with improving cardiovascular risk through its action in improving lipid levels. However, patients with congestive heart failure who take **metformin** have an increased frequency of lactic acidosis and the drug is not recommended for patients requiring pharmacological therapy for congestive heart failure. **Insulin** may be required for these patients.

A bold warning appears in all **sulfonylurea** material stating that the administration of **oral hypoglycemic** drugs has been reported to be associated with increased cardiovascular mortality compared with treatment by diet alone or diet plus **insulin.** Although the research that resulted in the warning was for only one drug in this class, the warning has been extended to all. Some recent studies have suggested that this warning may need to be rethought.

Among the oral agents, **sulfonylureas** are the most associated with risk of hypoglycemia, which may be difficult to recognize in patients concurrently taking **beta blockers,** because **beta blockers** mask the signs and symptoms of hypoglycemia, with the exception of diaphoresis. Patients with coronary artery disease, heart failure, or hypertension are commonly treated with **beta blockers.** If **sulfonylureas** must be given concurrently with **beta blockers, glimepiride** is less likely to cause hypoglycemia than other drugs in the class.

Clinical studies have presented conflicting evidence on the ability of **thiazolidinediones** to modify cardiovascular risk. This controversy relates to the use of **rosiglitazone,** which has been removed from the ADA/EASD guidelines. **Pioglitazone** is still shown on the algorithm in the guidelines, but is not recommended for treating patients with diabetes who also have cardiovascular disease or risks for it. No recommendations currently exist for **meglitidines** related to cardiovascular disease.

ACE inhibitors are central to the management of heart failure and hypertension. **ACE inhibitors** and **angiotensin II receptor blockers (ARBs)** decrease atherosclerosis. These drugs also have been shown to significantly reduce the incidence of diabetic nephropathy. They are the drugs of choice for patients with diabetes who also have these cardiovascular disorders. **Calcium channel blockers (CCBs)** in combination with **ACE inhibitors** also are a rational choice in coexisting cardiovascular diseases and diabetes. **CCBs** have limited effects on glucose metabolism, and the **non-dihydropyridine** type has been shown to have some degree of renal protection.

Coronary artery disease is further discussed in Chapter 28, and heart failure is discussed in Chapter 36.

Hyperlipidemia

Patients diagnosed with type 1 diabetes in childhood have a high risk of developing early subclinical and clinical CVD. Adult patients with type 2 diabetes have an increased prevalence of lipid abnormalities. Although evidence is lacking on type 2 diabetes in children, the assumption is that they will also demonstrate these abnormalities.

Having diabetes is now considered equivalent in cardiovascular risk to having established cardiovascular disease and is listed by the National Cholesterol Education Program (NCEP) as an independent risk factor for coronary heart disease (CHD). The NCEP and the American Diabetes Association both recommend aggressive lipid management aimed at lowering LDL cholesterol, raising HDL cholesterol, and lowering triglycerides, which have been shown to reduce macrovascular disease and mortality in patients with diabetes. The target lipid levels recommended by the American Diabetes Association are shown in Table 33–4.

Diabetes, particularly type 2, can cause a lipid abnormality with a high level of very-low-density lipoprotein (VLDL) and a low level of HDL (American Diabetes Association, 2004c, 2009a). This is seen clinically as high triglyceride levels (200 to 400 mg/dL) and low HDL levels (less than 35 mg/dL).

Treatment for both types of diabetes and for both adults and children consists of optimization of glucose control and MNT using a step 2 American Heart Association (AHA) diet aimed at decreasing the amount of saturated fat to 7 percent of total calories and dietary cholesterol to 200 mg/day. Diabetic control by itself seldom normalizes lipid abnormalities, even with tight glycemic control. A significant number of these patients need direct lipid management. Two classes of **antihyperlipidemic** drugs are first-line therapy for patients with diabetes. **HMG-Co-A reductase inhibitors (statins)** have consistently demonstrated the ability to reduce cardiovascular risk and are first-line therapy for adults and for children over the age of 10 years when the main goal is reduction of LDL cholesterol. These drugs have also been shown to improve endothelial function and cause regression of carotid intimal thickening (McCrindle et al, 2007; Wiegman et al, 2004). Their action is less prominent in reduction of VLDL and triglycerides, but they also have this action. Several secondary prevention studies, including the Heart Protection Study, completed in 2003, show that **statins** have the ability to achieve significant reductions in coronary and cerebrovascular events in patients with diabetes. The American Diabetes Association (2009a), NCEP, Institute for Clinical Systems Improvement (ICSI) (2004), and the VA/DoD (Pogach, 2004) all recommend these drugs as first-line therapy for hyperlipidemia. In fact, the AACE (Bloomgarden, 2003) and the American Diabetes Association (2009a) recommend that a **statin** be given regardless of LDL cholesterol level for diabetic patients with overt CVD or patients without CVD who are over the age of 40 and have one or more CVD risk factors. The ICSI recommends that a **statin** be started early in the treatment protocol along with BP control and **aspirin** therapy.

Fibric acid derivatives act more directly on VLDL and triglycerides. Two studies have shown **gemfibrozil (Lopid)** to be effective for this indication. All the groups previously mentioned list them as second-line drugs. Combining these drugs with **statins** to broaden the lipid abnormalities addressed has resulted in increased risk for rhabdomyolysis and so must be used with great caution.

Ezetimibe is a new class of drug called a **cholesterol absorption inhibitor** that has been shown to be safe in combination with a **statin**. Combinations may be needed because in many patients with diabetes and cardiovascular disease, attaining target LDL goals is difficult (Kennedy, MacLean, Littenberg, Ades, & Pinckney, 2005). **Vytorin** is a combination of **simvastatin** of varying doses and **ezetimibe** 10 mg. A 2009 systematic review of this combination, however, found that the drug was no more effective than either drug taken alone (Sharma et al, 2009). This finding provided additional support for the data from the 2008 ENHANCE trial, which did not show a clinical outcome demonstrating efficacy for **Vytorin.** Because large changes in cholesterol fractions are rarely achieved by monotherapy with one drug class, providers should use individual patient response to select drugs to be used to treat hyperlipidemia.

Nicotinic acid (niacin) also effectively lowers triglycerides; however, it is associated with increased uric acid levels, which also occur in some patients with diabetes. **Nicotinic acid (niacin)** may also increase **insulin** resistance. Given in low doses, **nicotinic acid** produces limited deterioration in glucose control and no changes in HbA_{1c} levels. **Colestipol (Colestid)** and **cholestyramine (Questran)** may improve lipid levels, but they may pose problems for patients with diabetic gastropathy. Discussions of **antihyperlipidemic** drugs, including dosing schedules, and lifestyle modifications that reduce lipids are included in Chapters 16 and 39.

Interventions to improve glycemic control usually lower triglycerides levels, but have little effect on HDL levels. **Metformin** has a modestly favorable impact on lipids because of its actions in the liver. In clinical studies, **metformin** alone or in combination with a **sulfonylurea** lowered mean fasting serum triglycerides, total cholesterol, and LDL and had no adverse effect on HDL. Therefore, it is an appropriate oral agent for patients with diabetes who also have lipid abnormalities. The combination of **gemfibrozil** with **metformin** and a NCEP lipid-lowering diet is the most efficacious in both controlling lipid and lowering blood glucose levels. **Thiazolidinediones** may increase HDL and LDL, but the long-term effect of such changes is unknown. **Acarbose (Precose)**, an **alpha-glucosidase inhibitor**, has also shown beneficial effects for patients with hypertriglyceridemias. **Acarbose** acts on the pathogenesis of these disorders, lowering production of endogenous triglycerides.

Chapter 39 presents more information on treatment of hyperlipidemia.

Hypertension

Hypertension (HTN) is a common comorbid condition in patients with diabetes. It affects 20 to 60 percent of people with diabetes, depending on age, obesity, and ethnicity (American Diabetes Association, 2009b). HTN is also a risk factor for CHD and microvascular complications such as retinopathy and nephropathy. In type 1 diabetes, HTN is often a manifestation of diabetic nephropathy. In type 2 diabetes, HTN is often part of a syndrome that includes glucose intolerance, **insulin** resistance, obesity, hyperlipidemia, and coronary artery disease. In both types of diabetes, the presence of HTN is associated with increased cardiovascular risk, especially for stroke and ischemic heart disease. Control of HTN has been demonstrated to reduce the rate of progression of diabetic nephropathy and hypertensive cerebrovascular disease. HTN control is more important than glycemic control in reducing cardiovascular disease risk. Given the importance of HTN in diabetes management, the American Diabetes Association (American Diabetes Association, 2009a) and *The Seventh Report of the Joint National Committee on Prevention, Detection, Evaluation, and Treatment of High Blood Pressure* (JNC-7) made the target BP for diabetics lower than that for the general population at less than 130/80 mm Hg.

Some drugs used to treat HTN also address other complications of diabetes. **ACE inhibitors** have been shown to improve cardiovascular outcomes in high-risk cardiovascular patients even without HTN. In patients with congestive heart failure, **ACE inhibitors** are associated with better outcome than are **ARBs. ARBs** improve cardiovascular outcomes in patients with HTN, diabetes, and end-organ damage. **ACE inhibitors** reduce the risk for diabetic nephropathy through their reduction of intraglomerular pressure and a reduction in glomerulosclerosis. They have a unique, specific, and beneficial effect on the kidneys of both normotensive and hypertensive patients with diabetes.

ARBs (lorastan [Cozaar] and **irbesartan [Avapro])** have been approved for use in treating diabetic nephropathy. Both **ACE inhibitors** and **ARBs** are recommended by the AACE Hypertension Task Force (2006). **Alpha-adrenergic blockers** are recognized to improve **insulin** sensitivity and have a neutral or mildly beneficial effect on the lipid profile. However, the **alpha-blocker** arm of the Antihypertensive and Lipid-Lowering Treatment to Prevent Heart Attack Trial (ALLHAT) was terminated after interim analysis showed that **alpha blockers** were substantially less effective in reducing congestive heart failure than **diuretic** therapy (Wright et al, 2009). **Alpha blockers** do not appear to have a beneficial effect on diabetic nephropathy. The **non-dihydropyridine** CCBs **(diltiazem** and **verapamil)** may reduce microalbuminuria to an extent comparable with **ACEIs**, but the **dihydropyridine** CCBs may increase it (ACCE, 2006).

Other drugs used to treat HTN, however, can have adverse effects on glycemic control. In very low doses, **diuretics** may safely be used for patients with diabetes (ACCE, 2006), but at moderate to high doses they adversely affect glucose metabolism. They may also potentiate orthostatic hypotensive changes in patients with diabetic neuropathy. **Thiazide diuretics** have been shown to increase peripheral **insulin** resistance and hepatic glucose release. Both of these actions interfere with glycemic control. In one study, **Thiazide diuretics** were associated with a 4-fold excess mortality in patients receiving **diuretics** versus those who were not. **Thiazide diuretics** have demonstrated a slowed progression of nephropathy.

Beta blockers may precipitate diabetes among hypertensive obese patients because of their increase in **insulin** resistance. **Beta$_1$ selective blockers**, by contrast, sometimes increase **insulin** levels. Clearly, if this class of drugs must be used for patients with diabetes (e.g., for MI prevention), the choice should be one with **beta$_1$ selectivity**. The new third generation **beta blockers** such as **nebivolol** or drugs that block both alpha and beta receptors such as **carvedilol** may prove beneficial. These agents cause vasodilation and an increase in **insulin** sensitivity (AACE, 2006). The lack of hypoglycemic awareness with this class of drugs has been discussed previously. HTN is discussed in more detail in Chapter 40.

Nephropathy

Diabetic nephropathy (DN) occurs in 20 to 40 percent of patients with diabetes and is the single cause of end-stage renal disease. Microalbuminuria (30 to 300 mg/24 h) has been shown to be the earliest stage of diabetic nephropathy in type 1 diabetics and a marker for development of nephropathy in type 2 diabetes. Microalbuminuria is also a well-established marker for increased cardiovascular disease risk (American Diabetes Association, 2009a). Patients with microalbuminuria are likely to progress to clinical albuminuria and a decreased glomerular filtration rate over a period of years (Remuzzi, Schieppati, & Ruggenenti, 2003). Once albuminuria occurs, the risk for end-stage renal disease is high in patients with type 1 diabetes and significant for those with type 2. HTN may accelerate the decline in glomerular filtration rate and the progression to end-stage renal disease.

For nephropathy, the American Diabetic Association (2009a) recommends annual screening for microalbuminuria with a random spot urine sample for microalbuminuria-to-creatinine ratio that begins once a child is 10 years of age and has had diabetes for 5 years. Adults with type 1 diabetes should have an annual test to assess urine albumin excretion once they have had diabetes for 5 or more years. All type 2 diabetics should have such screening starting at diagnosis.

Urine excretion of albumin is variable, so two of three specimens collected within a 3- to 6-month period should be abnormal before determining that a patient has crossed a diagnostic threshold. Confirmed, persistently elevated microalbuminuria should be treated with an **ACE inhibitor** or **ARB** with a goal of normalized microalbumin secretion. Evidence suggests that diabetic patients with chronic kidney disease may have little or no detectable albuminuria. Serum creatinine should also be measured at least annually in all adults with diabetes regardless of urine albumin excretion (American Diabetic Association, 2009a).

ACE inhibitors, **ARBs**, and **non-dihydropyridine CCBs** reduce the rate of urinary albumin excretion and may give false-negative tests. To diagnose diabetic nephropathy, microalbuminuria should be confirmed by at least two tests over a period of 3 to 6 months. An estimate of glomerular filtration rate (GFR) using the Levey modification of the Cockcroft and Gault equation to stage a patient's renal disease is also recommended. A tool to do this estimation can be found at www.kidney.org/professionals/dogi/gfrcalculator.cfm and at http://www.nkdep.nih.gov. A referral to a physician experienced in the care of diabetic nephropathy should be considered when the GFR has fallen to less than 80 mL/min/1.73m^2. Consultation with a nephrologist is suggested when the GFR falls to less than 30 mL/min/1.73m^2.

To reduce the risk or slow the progression of nephropathy, the American Diabetes Association and other groups have two recommendations: Optimize glucose control and optimize BP control. Intensive diabetic management and maintenance of BP below 130/80 mm Hg have been effective in reducing the rate of progression to end stage.

In patients with type 1 diabetes, with or without HTN, **ACE inhibitors** have been demonstrated to significantly delay the progression of diabetic nephropathy. In patients with type 2 diabetes, HTN, and microalbuminuria, **ACE inhibitors** and **ARBs** have been shown to delay the progression to macroalbuminuria. In patients with type 2 diabetes, HTN, macroalbuminuria, and renal insufficiency, **ARBs** have been shown to delay the progression to nephropathy (ACCE, 2006; American Diabetes Association, 2009a). Blockade of the renin-angiotensin-aldosterone (RAA) system by **ACE inhibitors** is incomplete. Dual blockade of the RAA system by combining an **ACE inhibitor** and an **ARB** has been shown to provide statistically significant reduction in albuminuria and BP. Although it requires additional monitoring for hyperkalemia, the combination is safe (Wade & Gleason, 2004).

CCBs can be considered for patients who are unable to tolerate **ACE inhibitors** or **ARBs**, but a meta-analysis of studies of patients with diabetes who were treated with **dihydropyridine CCBs** (Remuzzi et al, 2003) found that patients had more severe proteinuria and a more rapid decline in the glomerular filtration rate than those treated with other **antihypertensive** agents.

Several studies (Remuzzi et al, 2003) have shown that intensive glucose control with **sulfonylureas** or **insulin** reduced the risk for diabetic nephropathy as well as other microvascular completions in patients with type 2 diabetes. As discussed in the Older Adults section, diabetes itself is more associated with nephropathy in older adults than is HTN and their renal impairment is more a microvascular than a macrovascular problem (Wasen et al, 2004). **Sulfonylureas** are associated with increased risk for hypoglycemia and careful glucose monitoring is required. Short-acting second generation agents such as **glipizide** or **glimepiride** may be preferred in this drug class. **Metformin** shows a similar reduction in risk for renal failure, but patients who already have significant renal disease should not use **metformin** because of the risk of lactic acidosis. **Pioglitazone** may be considered, but the potential risk of fluid retention needs to be considered.

Studies in patients with varying degrees of nephropathy have shown that protein restriction helps slow the progression of albuminuria, GFR decline, and end-stage renal disease (ESRD). Protein restriction should be considered for patients who demonstrate progression of diabetic nephropathy despite optimal glucose and blood pressure control and the use of an **ACE inhibitor** and/or ARB (American Diabetic Association, 2009a).

Neuropathy

There are 2 kinds of diabetic neuropathy—peripheral and autonomic. Diabetic autonomic neuropathy (DAN) is the earliest and most common complication of diabetes. Its onset is often insidious and screening for it may require several tests. These tests are outlined in Meijer and colleagues (2003). Screening for indications of cardiovascular autonomic neuropathy should be instituted at diagnosis of type 2 diabetes and 5 years after the diagnosis of type 1 (American Diabetes Association, 2009a).

Hypothesis concerning etiologies of DAN include metabolic insult to nerve fibers, neurovascular insufficiency, autoimmune damage, and neurohormonal growth factor deficiency (Vinik, Maser, Mitchell, & Freeman, 2003). Hyperglycemic activation of the polyol pathway leading to accumulation of sorbitol and potential changes in the nicotinamide adenine dinucleotide (NAD) to nicotinamide adenine dinucleotide hydride (NADH) ratio may cause direct neuronal damage. Activations of protein kinase C induces vasoconstriction and reduces neuronal blood flow. Increased oxidative stress, with increased free radical production, causes vascular endothelium damage and reduces nitric oxide bioavailability. Immune mechanisms may also be involved. Reduced neurotrophic growth factors, deficiency of free fatty acids, and formation of advanced glycosylation end products also result in reduced neuronal blood flow. In summary, a multifactorial process is probably involved in DAN.

This multifactorial process affects multiple body systems. Major clinical manifestations are shown in Table 33–9. Treatment is based on the organ system affected but the role of tight glycemic control in preventing or delaying the onset of this complication is clear.

Peripheral diabetic neuropathy is also called distal symmetric polyneuropathy (DPN) entities and the condition may result in pain, loss of sensation, and muscle weakness; it is a major risk factor for development of ulceration and lower extremity amputations. All patients should be screened for DPN at diagnosis and at least annually thereafter, using simple tests such as pinprick sensation, vibration perceptions (using a 128-Hz tuning fork), 10-g monofilament pressure sensation, and assessment of ankle reflexes (American Diabetes Association, 2009a). In addition to maintaining HbA_{1c} concentrations less than 7 percent, therapies are also directed at other factors in DPN. Neuropathic pain is often severe and intractable. Treatment is based on trial and error. No one method is superior to another for an individual patient. **Tricyclic antidepressants** have been used for their effect on the intrinsic pain-suppressing pathways. **Nortriptyline (Aven, Pamelor)** and **desipramine (Norpramin)** are more useful when the patient also experiences orthostatic hypotension because they are less likely to exacerbate it. **Gabapentin (Neurontin)**, an **anticonvulsant**, acts by stabilizing neuronal membranes. Therapy is begun at low doses, followed by gradual titration. **Cymbalta (duloxetine)** and **Lyrica (pregabalin)** are both approved for DPN; some patients get a better response than they do with older medications. **Cymbalta** and **Lyrica** are not

On The Horizon

RECOMBINANT HUMAN NERVE GROWTH FACTOR

A new type of drug used to treat the underlying mechanism of diabetic nephropathy (DN) is currently in phase III trials. Recombinant human nerve growth factor shows promise in improving neurological function and preventing the development of DN.

Table 33–9 **Major Clinical Manifestations of Diabetic Autonomic Neuropathy**

Body System	Manifestations
Cardiovascular	Resting tachycardia, exercise intolerance, orthostatic hypotension, silent myocardial ischemia
Gastrointestinal	Esophageal dysmotility, gastroparesis, constipation, diarrhea, fecal incontinence
Genitourinary	Neurogenic bladder, erectile dysfunction, retrograde ejaculation, loss of vaginal lubrication
Metabolic	Hypoglycemia unawareness, hypoglycemic-associated autonomic failure
Skin	Anhidrosis, heat intolerance, dry skin
Pupillary	Pupillomotor function impairment, Argyll Robertson pupil

Source: Adapted from Vinik, A., Maser, R., Mitchell, B., & Freeman, R. (2003). Diabetic autonomic neuropathy. *Diabetes Care, 26*(5), 1554–1555.

available in generic formulations and are thus more expensive. These drugs are discussed in more detail in Chapter 15. **Capsaicin cream** (0.025% to 0.075%), a Substance P inhibitor, is also helpful in reducing DPN pain. It is applied three or four times daily.

Cardiovascular autonomic neuropathy (CAN) is a serious component of DAN, because it can lead to silent myocardial ischemia and sudden death. Vinik and colleagues (2003) recommend the use of **ACE inhibitors** and **aspirin** and other agents to control BP and lipids as central to the management of CAN. **Cardioselective beta blockers** may also modulate the effects of CAN by opposing the sympathetic stimulus to restore the parasympathetic-sympathetic balance.

Autonomic involvement can affect gastrointestinal, and genitourinary function. **Metoclopramide (Reglan)**, a **prokinetic agent**, is the most commonly used drug to treat gastroparesis; however, it has a relatively high incidence of adverse reactions, especially in children and older adults. This increased risk for adverse reactions is significant because gastric emptying problems are more common in older adults. Diet modification (liquids or softer diet) and referral to a dietician can be helpful.

Genitourinary dysfunction includes reduced bladder contraction force, resulting in urinary stasis, increased risk for bladder infections, and impotence. Bladder contraction force can be enhanced by the use of a **cholinergic agonist** such as **bethanechol (Urecholine)**. Erectile dysfunction has been successfully treated with **alpha blockers** that increase vascular blood flow. The **phosphodiesterase type 5 inhibitors sildenafil (Viagra), tadalafil (Cialis)**, and **vardenafil (Levitra)** are being used for treatment of this problem.

Retinopathy

Diabetic retinopathy (DR) is a highly specific vascular complication of both type 1 and type 2 diabetes. After 20 years of diabetes, nearly all patients with type 1 and more than 60 percent of patients with type 2 diabetes have some degree of retinopathy. A recent study (Wong, Molyneaux, Constantino, Twigg, & Yue, 2008) found that the age of onset of type 2 diabetes significantly affected the development of DR, even more than disease duration and degree of hyperglycemia. This finding supports the importance of delaying the development of diabetes or the movement of pre-diabetes to diabetes and the need for the more stringent metabolic targets for younger patients. Adults and children ages 10 years or older with type 1 diabetes should have an initial dilated and comprehensive examination by an ophthalmologist or optometrist within 5 years after the onset of diabetes. Patients with type 2 should have the examination shortly after the diagnosis of diabetes. These examinations should be repeated annually. Women with diabetes who are planning pregnancy should have an eye examination in the first trimester with close follow-up throughout the pregnancy and 1 year postpartum.

DR is the most frequent cause of blindness among adults ages 20 to 74 years. One of the main reasons for screening is the established efficacy of laser photocoagulation surgery in preventing vision loss.

The DCCT study clearly demonstrated that tight glycemic control reduced or prevented the development of retinopathy by 76 percent as compared with conventional therapy and reduced the progression by 54 percent (Fong et al, 2004). The protective effect of glycemic control has been confirmed in patients with type 2 diabetes (UK Prospective Diabetes Study Group, 1998). The UK Prospective Diabetes Study Group also looked at tight BP control and DR. Investigators found that patients assigned to tight control had a 34 percent reduction in progression of retinopathy and 47 percent reduced risk of deterioration in visual acuity with a reduction of as little as 10/5 mmHg in BP. Other studies have looked at the use of **ACE inhibitors**, but concluded that the decrease in DR may have been related to decrease in BP alone. Aside from the appropriate use of **insulin** or **oral antidiabetic** agents to maintain HbA_{1c} at 7 percent or less, or drugs to control HTN, no pharmacological therapies are available to treat this disorder

Combination Therapy

When monotherapy does not achieve glycemic targets, the treatment regimen is stepped up to combination therapy. Most patients will require more than one drug to achieve HbA_{1c} less than 7 percent. Evidence is lacking that switching drugs within a specific class improves glycemic control. A common mistake is to stop one class of drugs and start another. A more rational approach is to add a second drug.

If **metformin** is to be combined with a **sulfonylurea**, the dose of the **sulfonylurea** may need to be reduced, usually by half, because these drugs tend to potentiate each other, and adverse reactions are more likely without dosage adjustments. However, if blood glucose level is high enough, decreasing the dose of the **sulfonylurea** may not be necessary. The same reduction in the **sulfonylurea** dose arises when an **alpha-glucosidase inhibitor** is added to the regimen. Because of their mechanism of action, **alpha-glucosidase inhibitors** alone do not cause hypoglycemia, but they may do so in combination with **sulfonylureas**. Treatment of this hypoglycemia cannot be accomplished with the usual ingestion of sucrose (hard candy or soft drinks), fructose, or starches because they are disaccharides and **alpha-glucosidase inhibitors** delay their absorption. Because these inhibitors have no inhibitory activity against lactase or monosaccharides, milk, lactose, and glucose can be used to treat hypoglycemia.

Pioglitazone and **sulfonylureas** taken together have additive effects on each other's actions, so the initial dose of the **sulfonylurea** does not need to be reduced. Reduction may occur later. Both fasting and postprandial blood glucose levels decrease. To avoid hypoglycemia when **pioglitazone** is added to a treatment regimen, blood glucose levels must be monitored closely. One study showed that as blood glucose levels dropped, weight went up, with gains of 5.8 to 13 lb. Other studies have not replicated this finding, so the use of this combination for obese patients with diabetes is based on the experience of the provider. If **pioglitazone** is started at a low dose, weight gain usually can be minimized.

Meglitinide dosing, when added to **metformin**, has an additive effect. **Metformin** can also be added to **meglitinide** therapy, with no change in dosing of either drug, if control with the **meglitinide** alone is inadequate. It would be unusual for the initial drug to be a **meglitinide**, because this drug is not listed in early steps of the algorithm.

Insulin may also be added to a regimen. When combined with a **sulfonylurea, insulin** is initially given at bedtime and the **sulfonylurea** in the morning (bedtime **insulin**, daytime **sulfonylurea** [BIDS] or suppertime **mixed insulin**, daytime **sulfonylurea** [SMIDS]). This regimen takes advantage of the increased **insulin** secretion produced by the **sulfonylurea**, whereas the bedtime **insulin** suppresses hepatic glucose production during the early morning hours. This combination is especially useful for patients with elevated fasting blood glucose levels.

When **insulin** is added to the treatment regimen, close monitoring of blood glucose levels is critical. Significant drops in blood glucose, with risk of hypoglycemic reactions, have occurred.

Each of these drug combinations is discussed in more detail, including specific dosing schedules, in Chapter 21.

MONITORING

The American Diabetes Association (2009a, 2009b) has recommendations for laboratory evaluation of patients with diabetes at the initial visit and as part of continuing care. These same data are supported by ICSI (2003). Laboratory evaluation at the initial visit and with continuing care (American Diabetes Association, 2009a) include the following:

1. **Fasting plasma glucose.** A random plasma glucose test may be performed in an undiagnosed symptomatic patient for diagnostic purposes. FPG is also used to determine appropriate drug use in type 1 diabetes related to **insulin.** The use of FPG in type 2 diabetes management has both detractors and adherents.
2. **HbA_{1c}.** This test provides baseline data because it will be the test used for ongoing evaluation of glycemic control. Because HbA_{1c} reflects mean glycemia over the preceding 2 to 3 months, it should be measured every 3 months initially and then every 6 months in patients who are meeting treatment goals and who have stable glycemic control. Variability in HbA_{1c} as a measure of long-term fluctuations in glycemia seems to contribute to the development of diabetic complications as much as the short-term glucose fluctuations that were found in the DCCT data (Kilpatrick, Rigby, & Atkin, 2008). See Table 33–4 for glycemic targets.

   Data published in 2008 (Pani et al, 2008), raises the issue of the effect of age on HbA_{1c} levels. Because HbA_{1c} levels are positively associated with age, the researchers suggest further studies to determine whether age-specific diagnosis and treatment criteria might be appropriate.
3. **Fasting lipid profile.** Hyperlipidemias are common in patients with diabetes and contribute significantly to cardiovascular risk. Adult patients should be tested annually for lipid disorders with fasting cholesterol, triglyceride, HDL, and calculated LDL measurements. The targets for management are LDL below 100 mg/dL, HDL above 50 mg/dL for women and more than 40 for men, and triglycerides below 200 mg/dL. LDL less than 70 is recommended for those with a previous cardiovascular (CV) event. Tests resulting in higher values should be repeated for confirmation, and then management should be instituted according to the NCEP guidelines. Adults with low risk profiles may be tested every 2 years.

   Children older than age 2 years should have a lipid profile after the diagnosis of diabetes and when glucose control has been established. If values fall within accepted risk levels, the test should be repeated every 5 years. Tests resulting in abnormal values require institution of therapy according to NCEP guidelines.
4. **Serum creatinine.** This test is given to all adults but to children only if proteinuria is present. Diabetic nephropathy is a frequent complication of diabetes. Early intervention is necessary to prevent the development of end-stage renal disease.
5. **Tests for microalbuminuria.** Spot urine tests are also given annually for microalbuminuria to patients with type 1 diabetes for at least 5 years and to all patients with type 2 diabetes. Microalbuminuria is the earliest indicator of impaired renal function. This test along with the serum creatinine is used to estimate GFR and the stage of chronic kidney disease, if present.
6. **Thyroid function tests.** The presence of thyroid disorders may cloud the diagnosis and complicate the treatment of diabetes. Patients with type 1 diabetes should be screened for thyroid peroxidase and thyroglobin antibodies at diagnosis. Thyroid-stimulating hormone (TSH) concentrations should be measured after metabolic control has been established. If normal, recheck them every 1 or 2 years.
7. **Electrocardiogram in adults.** Cardiovascular disease is a complication of diabetes, and an electrocardiogram serves as a baseline. Taken alone, electrocardiograms are not sufficient to diagnose most cardiac conditions, but they are part of the diagnostic testing for cardiac disorders.

DIABETES MELLITUS

PATIENT EDUCATION

Related to the Overall Treatment Plan/Disease Process

- ☐ Pathophysiology of diabetes and the long-term effects of inadequate management on target organs
- ☐ Role of lifestyle modification, especially dietary therapy, in improving outcomes and keeping the number and cost of required drugs down
- ☐ Importance of adherence to the treatment regimen
- ☐ Need for regular follow-up visits with the primary care provider and other specialists

Specific to the Drug Therapy

- ☐ Reason for taking the drug(s) and the anticipated action of the drug(s) on the disease process
- ☐ Doses and schedules for taking the drugs
- ☐ Possible adverse reactions (especially hypoglycemia, DKA, and HHNK), how to prevent them, and what to do if they occur
- ☐ Interactions between lifestyle modifications and these drugs

Reasons for Taking the Drug(s)

Patient education about specific drugs is provided in Chapter 21. Specific information related to diabetes includes the following: Tight glycemic control and management of hypertension and hyperlipidemia are central to reducing morbidity and mortality from cardiovascular disease, the leading cause of death in the United States, and to preventing retinopathy and end-stage renal disease. The risks of these complications while maintaining the potential for good quality of life with appropriate treatment must be discussed.

Drugs as Part of the Total Treatment Regimen

Expectations should be clear about what the drugs can and cannot do. Dietary and other lifestyle modifications complement drug therapy and are equally important. Diabetes is a chronic condition. Self-management requires incorporation of drugs, diet, exercise, and glucose self-monitoring into the everyday life of the patient with diabetes.

Adherence Issues

Nonadherence to the treatment regimen may result in increased risk for complications and reduced life expectancy. Health-care providers should be aware of potential problems with nonadherence; discuss the importance of adherence at each follow-up visit; and assist patients in removing barriers to adherence such as lack of social support and cost of the treatment regimen. A team approach with the patient as an active partner should be maximized. Ways to deal with nonadherence are discussed in Chapter 6. Patient education booklets are available from the American Diabetes Association, which can be accessed on the Internet at http://www.diabetes.org.

OUTCOME EVALUATION

Outcome evaluation is against glycemic targets and prevention or development of the common complications of diabetes. The American Diabetes Association has published a position statement on the standards of care for patients with diabetes, including outcome evaluation. These standards include joint establishment of treatment goals and glycemic targets with the patient. Because diabetes requires a considerable amount of self-management, treatment goals and glycemic targets should take into account patient characteristics, such as the patient's capacity to understand and carry out the treatment regimen, the risk for severe hypoglycemia, and other factors that may increase risk or decrease benefit (e.g., very young or very old, end-stage renal disease, advanced cardiovascular or cerebrovascular disease, or other concomitant diseases that will materially shorten life expectancy). In addition, children with diabetes require integration of factors associated with growth and development into their treatment regimen.

To provide this standard of care, a team effort is required, especially when children are the patients. Consultation between diabetic specialists, diabetic educators, nutritionists, and the primary-care provider is critical throughout treatment. If this consultation is ongoing, times when treatment requires more input from a specific member of the team (e.g., intercurrent illness, DKA, HHNK, or recurrent hypoglycemia) will be defined by the team, and interactions between patients and their various providers will be seamless.

PATIENT EDUCATION

Patient education related to diabetes includes management of the disease process, counseling about the risk for development of diabetes, prevention of complications, and the role of the patient in self-management. It is not within the scope of this book to discuss all the patient education required. For that information, the reader is referred to the American Diabetes Association's "Clinical Practice Recommendations." The focus of patient education here is the part that is related to pharmacological management.

Because diabetes requires self-management by the patient as an active member of the treatment team, it must take top priority in a patient's consciousness.

To facilitate adherence to the treatment regimen, patient education should focus on understanding the pathophysiology of diabetes and the long-term effects of inadequate management on target organs; the role of lifestyle modification, especially dietary therapy, in improving outcomes and keeping the number and cost of required drugs down; the importance of adherence to the treatment regimen; and the need for regular follow-up visits with the primary care provider and other specialists.

REFERENCES

Abraira, C., Duckworth, W., & Moritz, T. (2008). Glycaemic separation and risk factor control in the Veterans Affairs Diabetes Trial: An interim report. *Diabetes, Obesity and Metabolism, 11*(2), 150–156.

Action to Control Cardiovascular Risk in Diabetes Study Group (ACCORD). (2008). Effects of intensive glucose lowering in type 2 diabetes. *New England Journal of Medicine, 358,* 2545–2559.

ADVANCE Collaborative Group. (2008). Intensive blood glucose control and vascular outcomes in patients with type 2 diabetes. *New England Journal of Medicine, 358,* 2560–2572.

American College of Cardiology (ACC). (2008). Statement on ENHANCE trial. Retrieved September 10, 2009, from http://www.acc.org.enhance.htm

American Association of Clinical Endocrinologists (AACE) Hypertension Task Force. (2006). American Association of Clinical Endocrinologists medical guidelines for clinical practice for the diagnosis and treatment of hypertension. *Endocrine Practice, 12*(2), 193–222.

American Diabetes Association. (2003). Evidence-based nutrition principles and recommendations for the treatment and prevention of diabetes and related complications. *Diabetes Care, 26*(Suppl. 1), S51–S61.

American Diabetes Association. (2004a). Aspirin therapy in diabetes: Position statement. *Diabetes Care, 27*(Suppl. 1), S72–S73.

American Diabetes Association. (2004b). Diabetic retinopathy: Position statement. *Diabetes Care, 27*(1), 226–229.

American Diabetes Association. (2004c). Dyslipidemia management in adults with diabetes: Position statement. *Diabetes Care, 27*(Suppl. 1), S68–S71.

American Diabetes Association. (2004d). Hypertension management in adults with diabetes: Position statement. *Diabetes Care, 27*(Suppl. 1), S65–S67.

American Diabetes Association. (2004e). Nutrition principles and recommendations in diabetes: Position statement. *Diabetes Care, 27*(Suppl. 1), S36–S46.

American Diabetes Association. (2004f). Physical activity/exercise and diabetes: Position statement. *Diabetes Care, 27*(Suppl. 1), S58–S62.

American Diabetes Association. (2004g). Smoking and diabetes: Position statement. *Diabetes Care, 27*(Suppl. 1), S74–S75.

American Diabetes Association. (2009a). Standards of medical care in diabetes—2009. *Diabetes Care, 32*(Suppl. 1), S13–S61.

American Diabetes Association. (2009b). Diagnosis and classification of diabetes mellitus. *Diabetes Care, 32*(Suppl 1), S62–S67.

American Diabetes Association, North American Association for the Study of Obesity and the American Society for Clinical Nutrition. (2004). Weight management through lifestyle modification for the prevention and management of type 2 diabetes: Rationale and strategies. *Diabetes Care, 27*(8), 2067–2073.

Anand, S., Yusuf, S., Vuksan, V., Devanesen, S., Teo, K., Montague, P., et al. (2000). Differences in risk factors, atherosclerosis, and cardiovascular disease between ethnic groups in Canada: The Study of Health Assessment and Risk in Ethnic Groups (SHARE). *Lancet, 356,* 279–284.

Blakau, B., Lange, C., Fezeu, L., Tichet, J., de Lauzon-Guillain, B., Czernichow, S., et al. (2008). Predicting diabetes: Clinical, biological and genetic approaches. Data from the Epidemiological Study on Insulin Resistance Syndrome (DESIR). *Diabetes Care, 31,* 2056–2061.

Bartels, D. (2004). Adherence to oral therapy for type 2 diabetes: Opportunities for enhancing glycemic control. *Journal of the American Academy of Nurse Practitioners, 16*(1), 8–16.

Bell, R., Mayer-Davis, E., Beyer, J., D'Agostino, R., Lawrence, J., Linder, B., et al, the SEARCH for Diabetes in Youth Study Group. (2009). Diabetes in non-Hispanic white youth: Prevalence, incidence and clinical characteristics. The SEARCH for Diabetes in Youth Study. *Diabetes Care, 32*(3), S102–S111.

Bloomgarden, Z. (2003). American Association of Clinical Endocrinologists (AACE). Consensus conference on insulin resistance syndrome. *Diabetes Care, 26*(4), 1297–1303.

Bloomgarden, Z. (2008a). American College of Endocrinology Pre-Diabetes Consensus Conference: Part one. *Diabetes Care, 3*(10), 2062–2069.

Bloomgarden, Z. (2008b). American College of Endocrinology Pre-Diabetes Consensus Conference: Part two. *Diabetes Care, 31*(11), 2222–2229.

Bremer, J., Jauch-Chara, K., Hallschmid, M., Schmid, S., & Schultes, B. (2009). Hypoglycemia unawareness in older compared with middle-aged patients with type 2 diabetes. *Diabetes Care, 32*(8), 1513–1517.

Brown, J., Wessels, H., Chancellor, M., Stamm, W., Stapleton, A., Steers, W., et al. (2005). Urologic complications of diabetes. *Diabetes Care, 28*(1), 177–185.

Chahal, H., & Chowdhury, T. (2007). Gliptins: A new class of oral hypoglycaemic agent. From the Department of Diabetes and Metabolism, the Royal London Hospital, London, UK. Published by Oxford University Press. Retrieved August 18, 2009, from http://qjmed.oxfordjournals.org/cgi/content/full/hcm081v1

Cowie, C., Rust, K., Ford, E., Eberhardt, M., Byrd-Hoyt, D., Li, C., et al. (2009). Full accounting of diabetes and pre-diabetes in the U.S. populations in 1988–1994 and 2005–2006. *Diabetes Care, 32*(2), 287–294.

Craig, K., Donovam, K., Munnery, M., Owens, D., Williams, J., & Phillips, A. (2003). Identification and management of diabetic nephropathy in the diabetes clinic. *Diabetes Care, 26*(6), 1806–1811.

Cryer, P., Davis, S., & Shamoon, H. (2003). Hypoglycemia in diabetes. *Diabetes Care, 26*(6), 1902–1912.

Dabelea, D., DeGroat, J., Sorrelman, C., Glass, M., Percy, C., Avery, C., et al, the SEARCH for Diabetes in Youth Study Group. (2009). Diabetes in Navaho youth. *Diabetes Care, 32*(3), S141–S147.

Daly, A., Warshaw, H., Pastors, J., Franz, M., & Arnold, M. (2003). Diabetes medical nutrition therapy: Practical tips to improve outcomes. *Journal of the American Academy of Nurse Practitioners, 15*(5), 206–211.

Davies, M., Storms, F., Shutler, S., Bianchi-Biscay, M., & Gomis, R., for the AT.LANTUS Study Group. (2005). Improvement of glycemic control in subjects with poorly controlled type 2 diabetes. *Diabetes Care, 28*(6), 1282–1288.

Diabetes Prevention Program Research Group. (2002). Reduction in the incidence of type 2 diabetes with lifestyle intervention or metformin. *New England Journal of Medicine, 346*(6), 393–403.

Diabetes Prevention Program Research Group. (2003). Within-trial cost-effectiveness of lifestyle intervention or metformin for the primary prevention of type 2 diabetes. *Diabetes Care, 26*(9), 2518–2523.

Dillon, E., Janghorbani, M., Angel, J., Casperson, S., Grady, J., Urban, R., et al. (2009). Novel noninvasive breath test method for screening individuals at risk for diabetes. *Diabetes Care, 32*(3), 430–435.

Duckworth, W. (2008, June). *VADT results*. Paper presented at the 68th annual meeting of the American Diabetes Association, San Francisco, CA.

Feig, D., Palda, V., & Lipscombe, L. (2005). Screening for type 2 diabetes mellitus to prevent vascular complications: Updated recommendations from the Canadian Task Force on Preventive Health Care. *Canadian Medical Association Journal, 172*(2), 177–180.

Fong, D., Aiello, L., Ferris, F., and Klein, R. (2004). Diabetic retinopathy. *Diabetes Care,* 27, 2540–2553.

Gahagan, S., & Silverstein, J. (2003). Prevention and treatment of type 2 diabetes in children, with special emphasis on American Indian and Alaska Native children. American Academy of Pediatrics Committee on Native American Child Health. *Pediatrics, 112*(4), e328–e347.

Hathout, E., Thomas, W., El-Shahawy, M., Nahab, F., & Mace, J. (2009). Diabetic autoimmune markers in children and adolescents with type 2 diabetes. *Pediatrics, 107*(6), e102+.

Heart Protection Study Collaborative Group. (2003). MRC/BHF Heart Protection Study of cholesterol-lowering with simvastatin in 5,963 people with diabetes: A randomized placebo-controlled trial. *Lancet, 361,* 2005–2016.

Howard, A., Arnsten, J., & Gourevitch, M. (2004). Effect of alcohol consumption on diabetes mellitus: A systematic review. *Annals of Internal Medicine, 140*(3), 211–219.

Institute for Clinical Systems Improvement (ICSI). (2004). *Management of type 2 diabetes.* Bloomington, MN: Author. Retrieved June 15, 2005, from http://www.guideline.gov/summary/summary.aspx

Kennedy, A., MacLean, C., Littenberg, B., Ades, P., & Pinckney, R. (2005). The challenge of achieving national cholesterol goals in patients with diabetes. *Diabetes Care, 28*(5), 1029–1034.

Kilpatrick, E., Rigby, A., & Atkin, S. (2008). A1C variability and the risk of microvascular complications in type 1 diabetes: Data from the DCCT. *Diabetes Care, 31*(11), 2198–2202.

Klein, S., Sheard, N., Pi-Sunyer, X., Daly, A., Wylie-Rosett, J., Kulkarni, K., et al. (2004). Weight management through lifestyle modification for the prevention and management of type 2 diabetes: Rationale and strategies. *Diabetes Care, 27*(8), 2067–2073.

Lawrence, J., Mayer-Davis, E., Reynolds, K., Beyer, J., Pettit, D., D'Agostino, R., et al, the SEARCH for Diabetes in Youth Study Group. (2009). Diabetes in Hispanic American youth. *Diabetes Care, 32*(3), S123–S132.

Li, G., Zhang, P., Wang, J., Gregg, E., Yang, W., Gong, Q., et al. (2008). The long-term effect of lifestyle interventions to prevent diabetes in Chine DaQing Diabetes Prevention Study: A 20-years follow-up study. *Lancet, 368,* 1783–1789.

Lindstrom, J., Ilanne-Parikka, P., Peltonen, M., Aunola, S., Eriksson, J., Hemio, K., et al. (2006). Sustained reduction in the incidence of type 2 diabetes by lifestyle intervention: Follow-up of the Finnish Diabetes Prevention Study. *Lancet, 368,* 1673–1679.

Liu, L., Yi, J., Beyer, J., Mayer-Davis, E., Dolan, L., Dabelea, D., et al, the SEARCH for Diabetes in Youth Study Group. (2009). Type 1 and type 2 diabetes in Asian and Pacific Islander U.S. youth. *Diabetes Care, 32*(3), S133–S140.

Mayer-Davis, E., Beyer, J., Bell, R., Dabelea, D., D'Agostino, R., Imperatore, G., et al, the SEARCH for Diabetes in Youth Study Group. (2009). Diabetes in African American youth: Prevalence, incidence and clinical characteristics. *Diabetes Care, 32*(3), S112–S122.

McCance, K., & Huether, S. (2006). *Pathophysiology: The biological basis for disease in adults and children* (5th ed.). St. Louis, MO: Mosby.

McCrindle, B., Urbina, E., Dennison, B., Jacobson, M., Steinberger, J., Rocchini, A., et al, American Heart Association Atherosclerosis, Hypertension and Obesity in Diabetes, American Heart Association Council of Cardiovascular Disease in the Young, American Heart Association Council on Cardiovascular Nursing. (2007). Drug therapy of high-risk lipid abnormalities in children and adolescents. *Circulation, 115*(14), 1948–1967.

Meijer, J., Bosma, E., Lefrandt, J., Links, T., Smit, A., Stewart, R., et al. (2003). Clinical diagnosis of diabetic polyneuropathy with the diabetic neuropathy symptom and diabetic neuropathy examination scores. *Diabetes Care, 26*(3), 697–701.

Mortensen, H., Hougaard, P., Swift, P., Hansen, L., Holl, R., Hoey, H., et al, for the Hvidøre Study Group on Childhood Diabetes. (2009). New definition for partial remission period in children and adolescents with type 1 diabetes. *Diabetes Care, 32*(8), 1384–1390.

Nathan, D., Buse, J., Davidson, M., Ferrannini, E., Holman, R., Sherwin, R., et al. (2009). Medical management of hyperglycemia in type 2 diabetes: A consensus algorithm for the initiation and adjustment of therapy. A consensus statement of the American Diabetes Association and the European Association for the Study of Diabetes. *Diabetes Care, 32*(1), 193–203.

Ohkubo, Y., Kishikawa, H., Araki, E., Miyata, T., Isami, S., Motoyoshi, S., et al. (1995). Intensive insulin therapy prevents the progression of diabetes microvascular complications in Japanese patients with non-insulin-dependent diabetes mellitus: A randomized prospective 6-years study. *Diabetes Research and Clinical Practice, 28,* 103–117.

Pani, L., Korenda, L., Meigs, J., Driver, C., Chamany, S., Fox, C., et al. (2008). Effect of aging on A1C levels in individuals without diabetes: Evidence from the Framingham Offspring Study and the National Health and Nutrition Examination Survey 2001–2004. *Diabetes Care, 31*(10), 1991–1996.

Pogach, L., Brietzke, S., Cowan, C., Conlin, P., Walder, D., Sawin, C., for the VA/DoD Diabetes Guideline Development Group. (2004). Development of evidence-based clinical practice guidelines for diabetes. *Diabetes Care, 27*(Suppl. 2), B82–B89.

Porcellati, F., Rossetti, P., Busciantella, N., Marzotti, S., Lucidi, P., Luzio, S., et al. (2007). Comparison of pharmacolinetics and dynamics of the long-acting insulin analogs glargine and detemir at steady state in type 1 diabetes. *Diabetes Care, 30*(10), 2447–2452.

Randriamboavonjy, V., & Fleming, I. (2009). Insulin, insulin resistance, and platelet signaling in diabetes. *Diabetes Care, 32*(4), 528–530.

Reichard, P., Nilsson, B., Rosenqvist, U. (1993). The effect of long-term intensified insulin treatment on the development of microvascular complications of diabetes mellitus. *New England Journal of Medicine, 329,* 304–309.

Remuzzi, G., Schieppati, A., & Ruggenenti, P. (2003). Nephropathy in patients with type 2 diabetes. *New England Journal of Medicine, 346*(15), 1145–1151.

Schmidt, M., Duncan, B., Vigo, A., Pankow, J., Ballantyne, C., Couper, D., et al, for the ARIC Investigators. (2003). Detection of undiagnosed diabetes and other hyperglycemic states: The Atherosclerosis Risk in Communities Study. *Diabetes Care, 26*(5), 1338–1343.

Sharma, M., Ansari, M. T., Abou-Setta, A. M., Soares-Weiser, K., Ooi, T. C., Sears, M., et al. (2009). Systematic review: Comparative effectiveness and harms of combinations of lipid-modifying agents and high-dose statin monotherapy. *Annals of Internal Medicine, 151*(9), 622–630.

Soinio, M., Marniemi, J., Laakso, M., Lehton, S., & Ronnemaa, T. (2004). Elevated plasma homocysteine level is an independent predictor of coronary heart events in patients with type 2 diabetes mellitus. *Annals of Internal Medicine, 140*(2), 94–100.

Sowers, J., & Haffner, S. (2002). Treatment of cardiovascular and renal risk factors in the diabetic hypertensive. *Hypertension, 40*(6), 781. Retrieved November 2003 from http://ahajournal/org/cgi/content/full

UK Prospective Diabetes Study Group. (1998). Effect of intensive blood-glucose control with metformin on complications in overweight patients with type 2 diabetes. *Lancet, 352,* 854–865.

Vinik, A., Maser, R., Mitchell, B., & Freeman, R. (2003). Diabetic autonomic neuropathy. *Diabetes Care, 26*(5), 1553–1579.

Wade, V., & Gleason, B. (2004). Dual blockade of the renin-angiotension system in diabetic nephropathy. *Annals of Pharmacotherapy, 38*(7), 1278–1282.

Wasen, E., Iosaho, R., Mattila, K., Vahlberg, T., Kivela, S., & Irjala, K. (2004). Renal impairment associated with diabetes in the elderly. *Diabetes Care, 27*(11), 2648–2653.

Welschen, L., Bloemendal, E., Nijpels, G., Dekker, J., Heine, R., Stalman, W., et al. (2005). Self-monitoring of blood glucose in patients with type 2 diabetes who are not using insulin. *Diabetes Care, 28*(6), 1510–1517.

Whittemore, R., Bak, P., Melkus, G., & Grey, M. (2003). Promoting lifestyle change in the prevention and management of type 2 diabetes. *Journal of the American Academy of Nurse Practitioners, 15*(8), 341–349.

Wiegman, A., Hutten, B., deGroot, E., Rodenburg, J., Bakker, H., Buller, H., et al. (2004). Efficacy and safety of statin therapy in children with familial hyperlipidemia: A randomized controlled trial. *Journal of the American Medical Association, 292,* 331–337.

Wong, J., Molyneaux, L., Constantino, M., Twigg, S., & Yue, D. (2008). Timing is everything: Age of onset influences long-term retinopathy risk in type 2 diabetes, independent of traditional risk factors. *Diabetes Care, 31*(10), 1985–1990.

Wright, J., Jr., Probstfield, J., Cushman, W., Pressel, S., Cutler, J., Davis, B., et al, for the ALLHAT Collaborative Research Group. (2009). ALLHAT findings revisited in the context of subsequent analyses, other trials, and meta-analyses. *Archives of Internal Medicine, 169*(9), 832–842.

Yeh, G., Eisenberg, D., Kaptchuk, T., & Phillips, R. (2003). Systematic review of herbs and dietary supplements for glycemic control in diabetes. *Diabetes Care, 26*(4), 1277–1294.

CHAPTER 34

GASTROESOPHAGEAL REFLUX AND PEPTIC ULCER DISEASE

Teri Moser Woo

Chapter Outline

Primary care providers see a variety of gastrointestinal disorders, including gastroesophageal reflux disease (GERD) and peptic ulcer disease (PUD). Over the past few years, many of the medications used to treat these two disorders have become available over the counter (OTC), leading to patients' attempting to self-manage a disorder before they decide to seek care from their provider. This chapter discusses the continuum of care for GERD and PUD from simple OTC antacids to chronic acid suppression therapy.

GASTROESOPHAGEAL REFLUX DISEASE

GERD is a common problem in primary care, and is listed as the primary diagnosis for 6,859,000 ambulatory care visits annually, a rate of 2,332 per 100,000 (National Institutes of Health, 2009a). The severity of the disease varies from occasional postprandial discomfort to severe esophageal inflammation, stricture, bleeding, and even esophageal carcinoma. Gastroesophageal reflux is common and is often called acid reflux because of the acid taste in the back of the mouth or "heartburn" for the burning sensation patients feel in their chest (National Digestive Diseases Information Clearing House [NDDICH], 2007). Persistent acid reflux that occurs more than twice a week is considered GERD and can cause damage to the esophagus due to chronic irritation of the esophageal mucosa (NDDICH, 2007).

Evaluation and management of GERD is best carried out using a stepped approach. In most cases, the primary care provider can manage diagnosis and treatment. Ten to 15 percent of patients with GERD require referral to a gastroenterologist. Although the focus of this chapter is drug therapy, lifestyle modification is central to successful management of GERD and is also discussed.

Pathophysiology

GERD results from the reflux of chyme from the stomach into the esophagus. The physiological action of the lower esophageal sphincter (LES) is critical to maintaining a pressure barrier between the stomach and the esophagus. In patients with GERD, the resting tone of the LES tends to be less than normal, permitting transient relaxation of the LES 1 to 2 hours after eating. This relaxation allows gastric contents to regurgitate into the esophagus. Greenberger (2003) reports on a study that found that gastric juice can separate and form layers over ingested gastric contents in a pocket. After a meal, this highly acidic, unbuffered gastric juice can reflux into the distal esophagus for a distance of 1.8 cm. The median pH of this refluxed gastric juice was 1.6, compared to the pH of 4.7 in the stomach. This acidic layer may be a key factor in the high prevalence of disease in the distal esophagus and explain why the acid that is usually neutralized and cleared from the esophagus by peristaltic action within 1 to 3 minutes cannot be overcome. About 1 to 2 hours after eating, a mean LES tone is restored, but the LES is a complicated region of smooth muscle and many factors can contribute to poor functioning of the LES.

The function of the LES is regulated by the interaction of hormonal, neural, and dietary factors. The hormone gastrin increases resting tone, whereas **estrogen, progesterone, glucagon,** secretin, and cholecystokinin all decrease sphincter tone. The vagus nerve and alpha-adrenergic stimulation help to maintain resting tone. **Tobacco, alcohol,** peppermint, chocolate, and foods with high concentrations of fat or carbohydrate all decrease LES tone.

Medications can increase or decrease LES tone. Drugs that increase LES tone include **bethanechol (Urecholine), metoclopramide (Reglan), pentobarbital (Nembutal), histamine,** and **antacids.** Some of these (**metoclopramide,** antacids) are used to treat GERD. **Anticholinergics, theophylline, meperidine (Demerol),** and **calcium channel blockers** are among the drugs that decrease LES tone. Drugs also contribute to LES tone (Table 34–1).

Factors that increase intra-abdominal pressure can also contribute to GERD by affecting the pressure gradient. Vomiting, coughing, and bending all increase intra-abdominal pressure. Increased abdominal pressure during pregnancy may contribute to GERD, but the underlying reflux cause is the increased circulating estrogen and progesterone, which affect LES tone.

Transient relaxation of LES tone is not the only factor in GERD. Decreased secondary peristalsis and defective mucosal resistance to caustic liquids have also been implicated. Disorders that delay gastric emptying increase exposure time to the acid. Such disorders include gastric or duodenal ulcers, which can cause pyloric edema; strictures that narrow the pylorus; and hiatal hernia, which can weaken the LES. These factors are also targets of treatments for GERD.

The severity of the esophagitis that results from GERD depends on the composition of the gastric contents, the length of time they are in contact with the esophageal mucosa, and the epithelial resistance to acid. If the chyme is highly acidic (see above) or contains bile salts and pancreatic enzymes, reflux esophagitis can be severe. Patients with decreased esophageal peristalsis have longer exposure times between the chyme and the esophageal mucosa. Delayed gastric emptying contributes to reflux esophagitis by lengthening the period during which reflux is possible and by increasing the acid content of chyme.

Reflux esophagitis causes an inflammatory response in the esophageal wall, which results in hyperemia, increased capillary permeability, edema, tissue fragility, erosion and ulcerations. Fibrosis and basal cell hyperplasia are common and precancerous lesions (Barrett's esophagus) can be a long-term consequence (McCance & Huether, 2010).

Table 34–1 Foods and Drugs That Influence GERD

Foods and Drugs	Action on LES Tone
Foods	
Chocolate, spearmint, peppermint, decaffeinated coffee, high-fat or high-carbohydrate meals, alcohol	Decrease LES tone
Acidic foods, citrus fruit and juices, caffeine	Increase gastric acid secretion
Fatty foods	Delay gastric emptying
Drugs	
Tobacco	Decreases LES tone and increases gastric acid secretion
Anticholinergics, theophylline, meperidine, calcium channel blockers	Decrease LES tone
Bethanechol, metoclopramide, pentobarbital, histamine, antacids	Increase LES tone

LES = lower esophageal sphincter.

Signs and Symptoms

Most patients complain of burning substernal pain that radiates upward, often aggravated by meals and by lying down and relieved by sitting up. The burning substernal pain can be confused with the chest pain associated with angina or myocardial infarction and cause considerable patient distress. Nocturnal aspiration of reflux contents can cause recurrent pneumonia, bronchospasm, and cough.

Sore throat, hoarseness, and halitosis are associated with reflux into the back of the throat. A reflex salivary hypersecretion is sometimes described, especially in children.

Dysphagia usually suggests long-standing GERD with acute inflammation, stricture, or both. Solid food may stick in the distal esophagus; repeated swallows and significant amounts of liquid may be required to ensure passage into the stomach.

Table 34–2 shows the signs and symptoms of GERD and potential complications. A predominance of heartburn, regurgitation, or both, occurring after meals (particularly large or fatty meals) are highly specific to GERD. Older adults, who may have decreased gastric acidity or decreased pain perception, may not report these symptoms despite significant disease. They are also more likely to self-treat. Infants and children also have slightly different signs and symptoms and they are discussed in the sections about these specific patient populations.

Table 34–2 **Signs and Symptoms of GERD and Potential Complications**

Signs and Symptoms	Common	Unusual	Extra-esophageal	Potential Complication	Suggestive of Cancer (Alarm)
Heartburn	X				
Regurgitation	X				
Dysphagia	X				X
Hypersalivation		X			
Nausea		X			
Painful swallowing		X			X
Asthma			X		
Noncardiac chest pain			X		X
Chronic cough			X		
Dental disease			X		
Hoarseness			X		
Laryngitis			X		
Respiratory symptoms			X		
Abdominal mass				X	
Hematemesis/melena				X	X
Anemia				X	
Weight loss				X	X
Choking					X

Source: Adapted from VHA/Department of Defense. (2003). *Clinical practice guideline for management of adults with gastroesophageal reflux disease in primary care practice.* Washington, DC: Author.

Diagnosis

Signs and symptoms alone are rarely sufficient to diagnose GERD; however, guidelines differ on their recommendations for diagnostic testing. The American Gastroenterological Association (AGA) recommends no routine testing for straightforward GERD (2008). The AGA recommends diagnostic testing if patients do not respond to twice daily **proton pump inhibitors (PPIs)**, or gastric malignancy or misdiagnosis is a concern. The Institute for Clinical Systems Improvement (ICSI, 2006) recommends nonurgent endoscopy for patients 55 years or older with symptoms of uncomplicated dyspepsia and *Helicobacter pylori* testing for all patients without alarm features. The ICSI guidelines indicate "alarm symptoms" of melena, persistent vomiting, dysphagia, hematemesis, anemia, or involuntary weight loss greater than 5 percent that warrant endoscopy. Diagnostic testing is done by a gastroenterology specialist. The treatment protocol presented here assumes appropriate diagnosis of GERD.

Pharmacodynamics

Each of the contributing factors to the development of GERD is a target for pharmacological management. Drugs can be used to increase LES tone, to reduce the amount of acid in the chyme, to improve peristalsis and thereby decrease the time chyme is available to produce reflux, and to decrease the exposure of the mucosa to highly acid material. The classes of drugs with these actions include **antacids**, **histamine$_2$ blockers**, **cytoprotective agents**, **prokinetics**, and **proton pump inhibitors (PPIs)**. Figure 34–1 depicts the site of action of each of these classes of drugs.

Drugs to Improve Lower Esophageal Sphincter Tone

Metoclopramide and **bethanechol** improve LES tone and have a **prokinetic** function, but are not considered for monotherapy in the treatment of GERD. They are most useful in combination with acid suppression for patients with gastroparesis. **Metoclopramide** and **bethanechol** have not demonstrated significant healing of esophageal lesions.

Antacids also serve a dual purpose: They improve LES tone and increase gastric pH. They are usually patient-initiated drug therapy, along with lifestyle modifications.

Drugs to Reduce the Amount of Acid

Two main classes of drugs are used to reduce acid secretion: **histamine$_2$ receptor antagonists (H_2RAs)** and

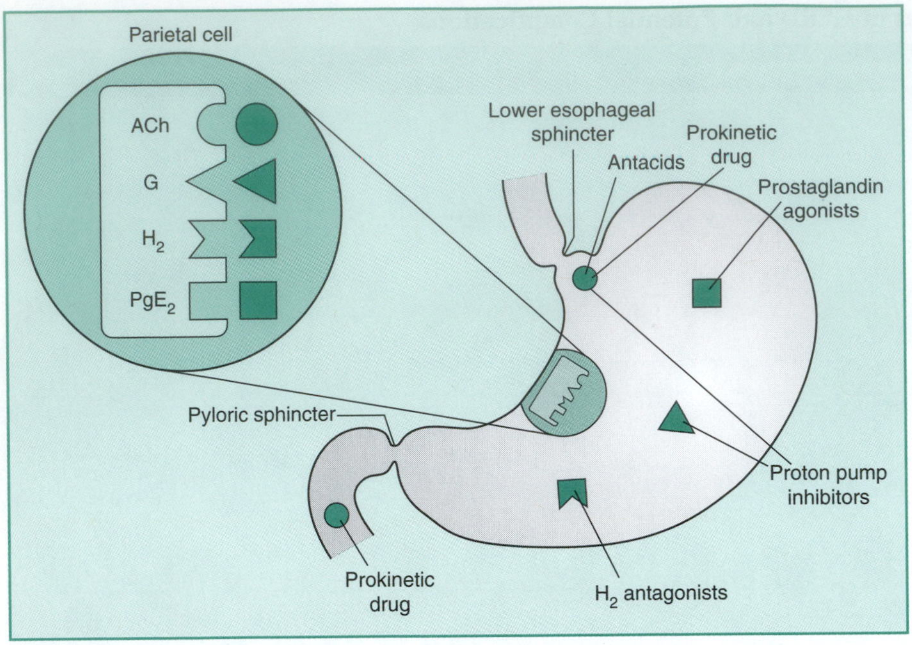

Figure 34–1. Sites of action of drugs used to treat GERD and PUD.

PPIs. H_2RAs act on the parietal cells to decrease the amount of acid produced. In the step-up approach, they are added to **antacid** therapy or used to replace high-dose **antacid** therapy, providing better symptom relief and increasing esophageal healing to about 50 percent. Because most of these drugs are available OTC, many patients may have used these drugs as self-initiated therapy before seeking care. Providers need to determine self-medication for GERD in the initial history. If a step-up approach to therapy is used, H_2RAs are the treatment of choice.

PPIs act one step earlier in the production of acid than do **H_2RAs** and decrease acid secretion by almost 100 percent. In the step-down approach, these are first-line therapy. In the step-up approach, patients with symptoms refractory to lifestyle modification and **histamine$_2$ blocker** therapy and those with erosive esophagitis are candidates for therapy with this class of drugs. **PPIs** improve esophageal healing to about 80 percent.

Studies comparing **PPIs** with **H_2RAs** demonstrated higher global improvement scores for **PPIs** than for **H_2RAs** (ICSI, 2006). However, because of the significant reduction in acid associated with **PPIs**, some guidelines suggest using the lowest dose possible to control symptoms or changing to **H_2RAs** once symptoms have been eliminated in 30 to 60 days (step down). Patients may need some amount of acid suppression to be totally symptom free, even if medications are used intermittently (American Gastroenterological Association [AGA] Institute Medical Position Panel, 2008).

Drugs to Improve Peristalsis

A few patients continue to report symptoms despite reduced acid secretion. These patients may benefit from **prokinetics**, which improve both LES tone and peristalsis. **Metoclopramide** may provide some benefit, but has limited usefulness because of adverse drug reactions.

Drugs to Decrease Mucosal Exposure

Two **cytoprotective** agents are available to decrease the exposure of the gastric mucosa to acid: **sucralfate (Carafate)** and **misoprostol (Cytotec)**. **Sucralfate** acts largely as a Band-Aid to cover sites having erosive damage, but is more often used with ulcers. **Misoprostol** acts by increasing the production of **cytoprotective** mucus. Older adults or those taking multiple drugs may benefit from **sucralfate. Misoprostol** is reserved largely for use when **NSAIDs** are a contributing factor to the increased acid load. These drugs are not mentioned in GERD guidelines, although discontinuance of **NSAIDs** is mentioned.

The pharmacokinetics and pharmacodynamics of each of the categories of drugs are discussed in more detail in Chapter 20.

Goals of Treatment

Therapy for patients with GERD has four goals: (1) Reduce or eliminate the symptoms; (2) heal any esophageal lesions; (3) manage or prevent complications such as stricture, Barrett's esophagus, or esophageal carcinoma; and (4) prevent relapse. Meeting these goals requires a combination of lifestyle modification and drug therapy.

Rational Drug Selection

Algorithm

For most patients, GERD is treated with stepped-approach therapy. The steps are based on symptom relief and degree of esophageal damage. Figure 34–2 presents the step-up

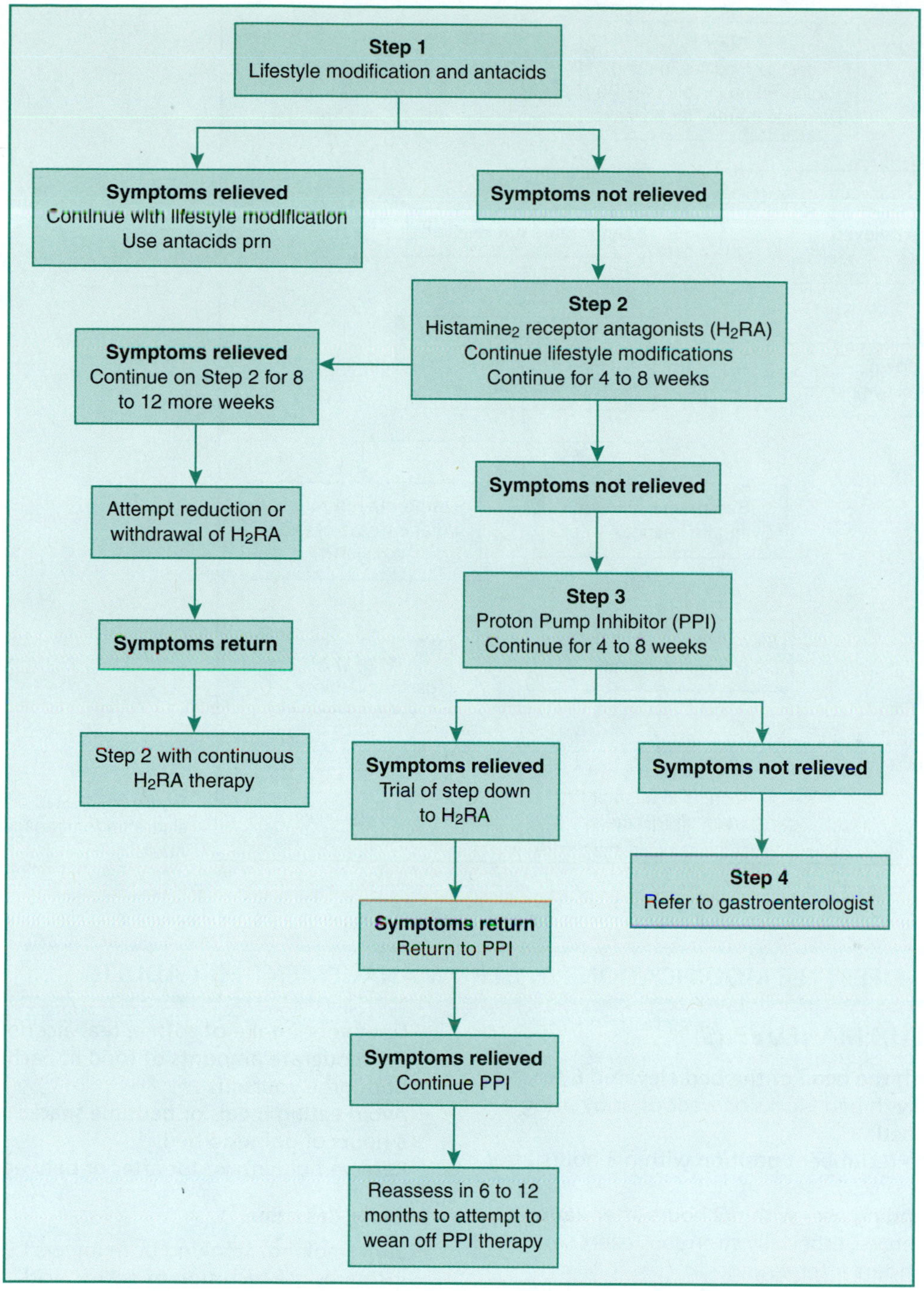

Figure 34–2. Step-up approach algorithm for management of GERD: Adults.

approach and Figure 34–3 presents the step-down approach. Evidence supports both approaches and the provider may select either. The basis for the selection is discussed in lifestyle modifications and drug therapy.

Lifestyle Modifications

Antireflux maneuvers, dietary changes, and cessation of smoking are central to the management of GERD regardless of the step. Antireflux maneuvers reduce back pressure on the LES from intra-abdominal contents. Dietary changes reduce the total volume and acid content of the stomach. Smoking reduces LES tone and increases gastric acid secretion. Box 34–1 lists appropriate lifestyle modifications.

Drug Therapy

Step-Up Approach

Step 1 involves lifestyle modifications and OTC **antacids.** Most patients have tried some step 1 interventions before

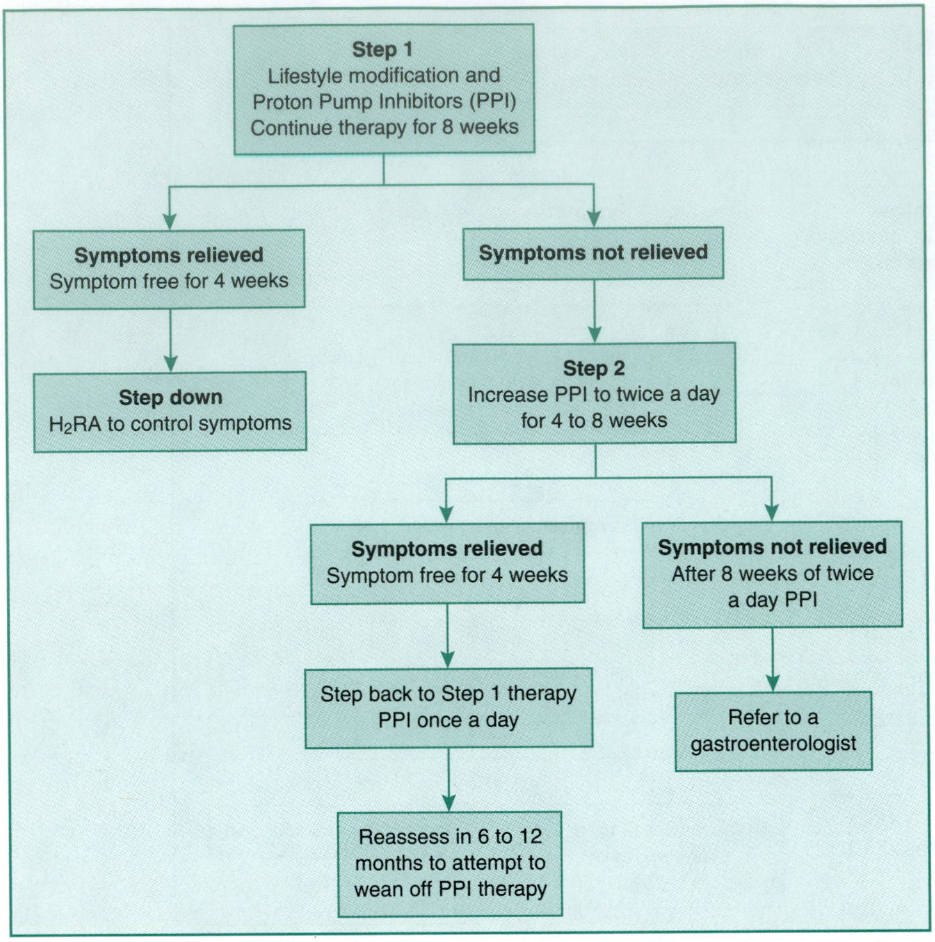

Figure 34–3. Step-down approach algorithm for management of GERD: Adults.

BOX 34–1 LIFESTYLE MODIFICATIONS IN GERD MANAGEMENT FOR ADULTS

ANTIREFLUX MANEUVERS

- Sleep with the head of the bed elevated 6 to 8 inches with bed blocks or wedges or by using a hospital bed.
- Avoid the recumbent position within 3 hours after eating.
- Avoid bending over within 3 hours after eating.
- Avoid exercise, especially strenuous exercise, within 3 hours after eating.
- Attain and maintain appropriate body weight.

Dietary Considerations

- Avoid spicy, acidic, tomato-based, or fatty foods.
- Avoid chocolate, peppermint, onions, and citrus fruits and juices.
- Limit your intake of coffee, tea, alcohol, and colas.
- Eat moderate amounts of food at each meal. Do not gorge yourself.
- Avoid eating meals or bedtime snacks within 3 hours of going to bed.
- Reserve fluid intake for after or between meals.

Smoking Cessation

- Stop smoking. Smoking both lowers LES tone and increases the secretion of gastric acid.
- Smoking cessation is a high priority.

Weight Loss

- Weight loss may improve symptoms

they seek health care. This step alone may be sufficient. If progression to other steps is required, lifestyle modifications are continued throughout the other steps as H_2RAs and PPIs are added. H_2RAs in step 2 are appropriate if no erosive disease is evident.

Step 3 is initiated if symptoms are refractory after 4 to 8 weeks of step 2 therapy. **PPIs** are central to management at this step. They replace the **histamine$_2$ blocker**. Step 3 therapy continues for 4 to 8 weeks. If the response is good, a trial of stepping back down to an H_2RAs is warranted. If symptoms improve, continue with the H_2RAs. If trial of H_2RAs fails, return to the PPI therapy. The patient should be reassessed in 6 to 12 months to determine if he or she can be weaned off therapy. Step 3 is the last phase that is appropriately managed by the primary care provider. Patients who do not respond to PPIs need to be referred to a gastroenterology specialist.

Step 4 requires referral to a gastroenterologist; however, step 3 interventions are continued while the patient is awaiting evaluation. A **prokinetic** agent may be added by the specialist and surgery is considered. The step-up approach is best for patients with mild disease or only occasional symptoms.

Step-Down Approach

In the step-down approach to care, step 1 involves lifestyle modifications and a standard dose of a PPI every morning for 8 weeks (ICSI, 2006). If symptoms are not resolved, step 2 alters the dose of PPI to twice a day for another 4- to 8-week trial period (AGA, 2008). Once the patient is symptom free for 4 weeks, a step down to a lower PPI dose or switch to an H_2RA is tried. The PPI or H_2RA is continued to control symptoms or to move to intermittent therapy when symptoms are relieved. If the patient has no relief after 8 weeks of twice-a-day PPI, the patient warrants a referral to a gastroenterologist. The step-down approach is most appropriate for patients with moderate to severe disease and/or daily symptoms.

Whether the step-up or the step-down approach is chosen, failure to achieve symptom relief after 3 months or the presence of symptoms that suggest complications move the recommendations of all groups to referral for endoscopy. The presence of alarm symptoms suggests endoscopy as part of the initial evaluation.

Patient Variables

Patient variables are also considered in treatment choices. Primary among them is the age of the patient.

Infants and Children

Gastroesophageal reflux (GER) occurs in up to 100 percent of 3-month-old infants, 4 percent of 6-month-olds, and 20 percent of 12-month-olds (Stansbury, 2004). Most (90%–95%) outgrow GER by 12 to 18 months of age. Referral to a pediatric gastroenterologist is suggested if symptoms worsen or do not resolve by that age. Given that most outgrow GER, aggressive management in infants is reserved for the few experiencing concomitant poor weight gain, feeding refusal, arching and crying during feeding, persistent irritability and pain, apnea, and cyanosis suggesting GERD.

In older children, symptoms that suggest GERD include lower chest pain, dysphagia, hematemesis, iron deficiency anemia, wheezing, aspiration or recurrent pneumonia, chronic cough or stridor. The North American Society for Pediatric Gastroenterology, Hepatology, and Nutrition (NASPGHAN) and European Society for Pediatric Gastroenterology, Hepatology, and Nutrition (ESPGHAN) developed an international consensus on the diagnosis and management of GER and GERD and the consensus is used as the guideline for care (Vandenplas et al, 2009).

Diagnosis of GERD in both infants and children is usually done through a thorough history and physical exam with the symptoms being reported (Stansbury, 2004). Any infant with poor weight gain and vomiting should first have a thorough physical exam and be assessed for adequate caloric intake. If caloric intake is adequate, the patient should have the following studies: a complete blood count (CBC), electrolytes, and blood urea nitrogent (BUN). The NASPGHAN/ESPGHAN do not recommend an upper GI series because of low sensitivity and specificity in infants and children (Vandenplas et al, 2009). Esophageal pH monitoring or combined multiple intraluminal impedance (MII) and pH monitoring are the most sensitive and accurate way to diagnose GERD in infants and young children (Vandenplas et al, 2009). Older children or adolescents may be empirically treated with an empirical trial of PPIs for 4 weeks (Vandenplas et al, 2009). No evidence supports empirical treatment of GERD in infants (Vandenplas et al, 2009). Children who present with atypical or extra-esophageal symptoms, do not respond to initial therapy, or have recurrent progressive symptoms should be referred to a gastroenterologist. In children with recurrent vomiting or regurgitation, or difficult or painful swallowing, endoscopy and other invasive tests may be required and referral is appropriate.

Lifestyle modifications are similar to those for adults. Table 34–3 lists the modifications for infants and children.

Infants with GERD

Infants with suspected GERD need consultation with a pediatric gastroenterology specialist because of the difficulty in accurately diagnosing GERD. Empirical medication treatment without studies is not appropriate in infants (Vandenplas et al, 2009). A number of randomized controlled trials in infants have not found consistent improvement in symptoms with either PPIs or H_2RAs (Vandenplas et al, 2009).

Children with GERD

Older children and adolescents need a history and physical examination to confirm the suspicion of GERD. Education regarding disease pathology and lifestyle changes should be implemented. No randomized placebo-controlled trials evaluating lifestyle changes or medications in treating heartburn or GERD in children have been done (Vandenplas et al, 2009). Therefore an approach similar to that used is adults with GERD should be used.

H_2RAs may be prescribed in infants and children with GERD. **Ranitidine (Zantac)**, **cimetidine (Tagamet)**, and **famotidine (Pepcid)** have liquid formulations that make pediatric dosing easier and have been used successfully in children ages 3 months to 16 years.

Table 34–3 **Lifestyle Modifications in GERD Management for Infants and Children**

Antireflux Maneuvers	Dietary Considerations
Infants	
• Keep infant in upright position during feeding and for 30 min after feeding. • Elevated head of crib mattress or bed 30 degrees. Do not use pillow. • Prone position postprandially when infant is awake, but not while asleep.	• Consider commercial antiregurgitation (AR) formula if formula fed. • Do not thicken formulas with rice cereal. • Try 2 wk on hypoallergenic formula. • In breastfed infants, consider cow's milk protein intolerance. A trial of withdrawal of cow's milk and eggs from maternal diet for 2 wk is warranted.
Children	
• Elevate head of bed. • Maintain weight according to guidelines or lose weight if indicated. • Stop smoking (parents or adolescents who smoke)	• Do not eat within 1–3 h of going to bed. • Avoid substances that can cause LES relaxation including caffeine, chocolate, peppermint, garlic, citrus fruits, tomatoes, and alcohol.

LES = lower esophageal sphincter.
Source: Vandenplas et al, 2009.

Alternatively a trial of 2 to 4 weeks of **PPIs** may be started. If the patient does not improve, treatment continues for 8 to 12 weeks. After 12 weeks of therapy, the **PPI** should be discontinued. If symptoms recur, the **PPI** should restarted. If there is no response to the initial 2- to 4-week trial of **PPIs**, the patient should be referred to a gastroenterology specialist (Vandenplas et al, 2009).

The U.S. Food and Drug Administration (FDA) has approved three **PPIs** for use in children: **omeprazole (Prilosec)**, **esomeprazole (Nexium)**, and **lansoprazole (Prevacid)**. Because the long-term effects of their use in children are not known, there is some concern regarding chronic acid suppression. Long-term **PPI** treatment has been associated with increased rates of community-acquired pneumonia, gastroenteritis, and entercolitis (Vandenplas et al, 2009). Long-term therapy with **PPIs** in children warrants consultation with a specialist.

Metoclopramide has adverse reactions in children, including restlessness, insomnia, somnolence, dystonia, and extrapyramidal symptoms. Some of the drug's antidopaminergic adverse reactions do not resolve with drug withdrawal. The new guidelines by NASPGHAN/ESPGHAN do not recommend the use of prokinetics in most children (Vandenplas et al, 2009). Consultation with or referral to a pediatric gastroenterologist is suggested before these drugs are prescribed.

Older Adults

Gastric acid secretion does not decrease with age. However, a subset of this population with long-standing *H. pylori* infection and high expression of interleukin (IL)-1 B may have reduced acid secretion due to atrophic gastritis (Thjodleifsson, 2002). The prevalence of *H. pylori* infection in younger adults is decreasing, but in older adults (older than age 65 years) it ranges from 50 to 70 percent. This has important bearing on acid secretion, because it decreases acid secretion as a result of the production of bacterial products and cytokines, thus enhancing the acid inhibition of **H_2RAs** and **PPIs**. After eradication of *H. pylori*, the acid-reducing efficacy of these drugs is diminished by more than a whole unit when measured on the median 24-hour intragastric pH scale (Haruma et al, 1999). Many early studies of the efficiency of acid-lowering in these two drug classes was done before there was extensive testing for *H. pylori* or the studies included mixed *H. pylori* positive and negative subjects. In addition, acid-related diseases (both GERD and peptic ulcer disease) often present in the older adult population in more severe or unusual forms or with complications, and a high degree of acid inhibition is often indicated (Thjodleifsson, 2002). For this reason, the step-down approach to GERD management is recommended for older adults (see Fig. 34–3).

Subtle differences have emerged between the old and the new **PPIs** that may have little effect on the younger adult, but have significant clinical relevance in the older adult. Studies of the pharmacokinetics of older **PPIs** have demonstrated considerable variation in drug clearance that is reflected in a wide range of efficacy related to acid suppression with standard doses. The bioavailability of **lansoprazole** and **pantoprazole (Protonix)** increases by 50 to 100 percent in older adults, but the plasma clearance of **esomeprazole (Nexium)** is not significantly affected in older adults. **PPIs** are metabolized by cytochrome P450 (CYP450) 2C19 and 3A4, with a greater affinity for 2C19. CYP450 2C19 has two genotypes, resulting in slow metabolizers and extensive metabolizers. The slow metabolizers are more predominant in whites and Asians. **Omeprazole** is the most affected by this genotype and **rabeprazole** is least effected; **esomeprazole** is somewhere in the middle. Given these data, **esomeprazole** and **rabeprazole** provide the most consistent and better acid control in older adults with standard doses than do the other **PPIs** (Thjodliefsson, 2002).

Antacids are generally safe in older adults, but **antacids** with constipation as an adverse reaction may be more problematic for older adults. In addition, many **antacids** have high sodium content, and some older adults are on low- to moderate-sodium diets. Among the H_2RAs, **famotidine (Pepcid)** is generally safe in the older population but should be used with caution in cases of renal insufficiency. **Nizatidine (Axid)** may cause asymptomatic ventricular tachycardia and carries a risk of hepatocellular injury. **Ranitidine (Zantac)** and **cimetidine (Tagamet)** carry risks for confusional states and toxicity in older adults. Because older adults are often taking several prescription and OTC drugs, the increased number of drug interactions associated with **cimetidine** also makes it a less attractive choice.

Among the **prokinetics, metoclopramide** has a risk for central nervous system (CNS) toxicity. In addition, it is contraindicated in congestive heart failure, renal failure, and hypokalemia, all of which are more common in older adults. **Metoclopramide** requires careful thought and monitoring in older adults.

Monitoring

Esophagitis is the cause of 5 to 10 percent of all cases of upper GI bleeding. Monitoring by complete blood count at annual exams is appropriate. The remainder of monitoring is clinical evaluation of symptoms.

Endoscopy to demonstrate the presence of lesions and their healing is the gold standard. It is shown in each algorithm at various steps of therapy. For patients requiring ongoing step 3 or 4 therapy, some specialists recommend endoscopy. Given its cost, others suggest endoscopy every 2 to 3 years because Barrett's esophagus is not reversible.

Long-term use of **PPIs** presents concerns. One concern is the development of precancerous cells due to hypochlorhydria, with enterochromaffin cell–like hyperplasia changes found in chronic **PPI** use (Lodato et al, 2010; Vandenplas et al, 2009). Another concern is an increase in hip fractures in at-risk patients who are on **PPIs** longer than 2 years and on higher doses of **PPIs** (Corley, Kubo, Zhao, & Quesenberry, 2010). Vitamin B_{12} deficiency is also a concern with chronic acid suppression.

Outcome Evaluation

Figures 34–2 and 34–3 show the stepped-approach treatment algorithms for GERD. Outcome evaluation targets relief of symptoms. Evaluation also includes the other goals for therapy: healing of lesions, prevention of complications, and prevention of relapse.

Relapse rates are high for patients with GERD. Lifestyle modifications and some drug therapy are commonly required for life. H_2**RAs** or **PPIs** may be required chronically but at reduced doses. Return of symptoms for a patient who has been pain free and is adherent to the treatment regimen suggests that the provider should increase the dosage of the current drug or move the patient to the next step in the algorithm and arrange for endoscopy evaluation.

Referral to a pediatric specialist is warranted for any infant younger than 2 months who presents with vomiting or other symptoms of GERD. Children and infants older than 2 months who are unresponsive to short-term (2 to 4 wk at each step) empirical treatment or have suspected or demonstrated complications also require referral.

Patients who have mild or typical symptoms and who respond to conservative treatment can be managed by the primary care provider. Patients who do not respond to 4 to 8 weeks of step 2 therapy should have a referral to a gastroenterologist, which means at least consultation with a gastroenterologist. Patients with erosive disease or who do not respond to step 3 therapy require referral to a specialist. These patients are at high risk for Barrett's esophagus, which carries with it a 30-fold greater risk for developing esophageal cancer than the general population.

Patient Education

Patient education should include a discussion of information related to the overall treatment plan as well as that specific to the drug therapy, reasons for the drug being taken, drugs as part of the total treatment regimen, and adherence issues.

PEPTIC ULCER DISEASE

Peptic ulcer disease (PUD) is a common clinical problem estimated to have a lifetime incidence of 12 percent in men and 10 percent in women (Lew, 2009). PUD is listed as the primary diagnosis in 712,000 ambulatory care visits annually and 1,473,000 visits annually have PUD listed as one of the diagnosis (National Institutes of Health, 2009b). The rate of hospital admission for uncomplicated ulcer has decreased significantly, but the incidence has not decreased, making this largely a disease that is treated in the primary care setting. Risk factors for PUD include smoking and habitual use of **NSAIDs** or **alcohol**, but the main culprit is *H. pylori* infection, which has been firmly established as a major cause of PUD. Reduction of stress and other factors that increase gastric acid secretion are still included in disease management.

Peptic ulcers fall into two categories: duodenal ulcers and gastric ulcers. Each has a slightly different pathology and treatment, although they share many aspects of both. They are addressed separately here.

Pathophysiology

PUD is a chronic inflammatory condition of the stomach and duodenum. It is the result of increased acid and

GASTROESOPHAGEAL REFLUX DISEASE

PATIENT EDUCATION

Related to the Overall Treatment Plan/Disease Process

- ☐ Pathophysiology of gastroesophageal reflux and its long-term risks for permanent esophageal damage and cancer of the esophagus
- ☐ Central role of lifestyle modifications in improving prognosis and keeping the number and cost of required drugs down
- ☐ Importance of adherence to the treatment regimen
- ☐ Need for follow-up visits with the primary care provider if the symptoms do not resolve or recur

Specific to the Drug Therapy

- ☐ Reason for the drug(s) being given and the anticipated action of the drug(s) on the disease process
- ☐ Doses and schedules for taking the drug(s)
- ☐ Possible adverse reactions and what to do when they occur
- ☐ Coping mechanisms for complex and costly drug regimens
- ☐ Interaction between lifestyle modifications and these drugs

Reasons for Taking the Drug(s)

Patient education about specific drugs is provided in Chapter 20. Specific information related to GERD: Drugs used to treat GERD are given to reduce symptoms, heal any esophageal ulcers, reduce the risk for permanent esophageal damage or cancer, and prevent relapse of symptoms. Different drugs have different roles with each of these. The expectations should be clear about what the drugs can and cannot do. Drugs alone will not correct the disorder.

Drugs as Part of the Total Treatment Regimen

Lifestyle modification is equally important in disease management. GERD is a chronic condition. Patients with GERD must understand the lifelong nature of the disorder and the need to incorporate the treatment regimen into their everyday lives.

Adherence Issues

Any disease process where lifestyle modifications are central to management is prone to problems with adherence. Health-care providers should be aware of the potential problem of nonadherence, discuss the importance of adherence at each follow-up visit, and assist patients in removing barriers to adherence such as the complexity and cost of the treatment regimen and the presence of adverse reactions.

pepsin secretion; impaired mucosal cytoprotection; use of NSAIDs; *H. pylori;* personal factors such as genetics, smoking, and stress; or a combination of these causes. Definitive diagnosis is via esophagogastroduodenoscopy.

The incidence of gastric ulcers differs from that of duodenal ulcers. Gastric ulcer disease is about one-fourth as common as duodenal ulcer disease. The pathophysiology of the disorders also varies. Table 34–4 compares the incidence, pathophysiology, and signs and symptoms of the two disorders.

Gastric Ulcer Disease

Gastric ulcers tend to develop in the antral region, adjacent to the acid-secreting mucosa of the body. Although the pathogenesis of gastric ulcer disease is unclear, it is generally thought that the underlying defect is a disruption that increases the gastric mucosal barrier's permeability to hydrogen ions. *H. pylori* is seen in 75 to 85 percent of patients with gastric ulcers. Gastric acid secretion may be normal or less than normal. A variety of substances can disrupt this barrier. They are summarized in Box 34–2.

Another suggested contributing factor is increased duodenal gastric reflux of bile across an incompetent pyloric sphincter. An increased concentration of bile salts disrupts the gastric mucosa and decreases the electrical potential across the gastric mucosal membrane. This altered electrical potential permits the diffusion of hydrogen ions into the mucosa, where they disrupt permeability and cellular structure. Once the barrier is broken, the damaged submucosal areas exposed to hydrogen ions release histamine, which stimulates an increase in acid and pepsinogen production, causes local vasodilation, and increases capillary permeability. The pepsinogen produces

Table 34–4 **Comparison of Gastric and Duodenal Ulcer Disease**

Characteristic	Gastric Ulcer	Duodenal Ulcer
Age at onset	50–70	20–50 yr
Gender	Equal in men and women	More common in men
Cancer risk	Increased	Not increased
Pathophysiology		
Parietal cell mass	Normal or decreased	Increased
Acid production	Normal or decreased	Increased
Serum gastrin	Increased	Normal
Serum pepsinogen	Normal	Increased
Associated gastritis	More common	Usually not present
Helicobacter pylori	Present in 60%–80% of cases	Present in 95%–100% of cases
Clinical manifestations: pain	Located in upper abdomen intermittent	Located in upper abdomen intermittent
	Pain>antacid>relief pattern	Pain>antacid or food>relief pattern
	Food>pain pattern	Nocturnal pain common
Clinical course	Chronic ulcer without pattern of exacerbation and remission	Pattern of exacerbation and remission for years*

*This pattern is significantly affected by eradication of *H. pylori.*

BOX 34–2 **SUBSTANCES THAT CAN DISRUPT THE GASTRIC MUCOSAL BARRIER**

Drugs

Alcohol
Aspirin
Caffeine*
Corticosteroids
NSAIDs
Tobacco

Other Causes

H. pylori infection
Bile and pancreatic secretions
Physiological and psychological stress
Salmonella
Spicy, irritating foods*
Staphylococcus organisms
Uremia associated with renal failure

*See discussion in the Lifestyle Modifications section.

mucosal erosion, resulting in the formation of ulcers. The disrupted mucosa becomes edematous and loses plasma proteins. Destruction of small blood vessels results in bleeding.

Pyloric stenosis has also been given as a possible cause of gastric ulcer formation. With pyloric deformity, gastric emptying is poor, resulting in stasis and antral distention. This distention leads to increased gastrin release and gastric acid production.

Chronic gastritis has also been associated with the development of gastric ulcers. It may precipitate ulcer formation by limiting the ability of the mucosa to secrete a protective layer of mucus. Decreased mucosal synthesis of prostaglandin (e.g., NSAIDs) may also create an ulcerogenic environment.

Duodenal Ulcer Disease

Infection with *H. pylori* is the major cause of duodenal ulcers. With the exception of patients taking NSAIDs, 95 to 100 percent of patients with duodenal ulcer are infected with this organism. It is a spiral-shaped bacterium that lives attached to or just above the gastric mucosa. Once *H. pylori* is acquired, colonization continues for life unless the organism is eliminated by antimicrobial treatment or the usually late-in-life development of atrophic gastritis. Essentially everyone who carries the organism in the gastric mucosal layer has evidence of some tissue reaction (e.g., an inflammatory response and chronic active gastritis), yet most colonized patients remain asymptomatic for life. The strain of *H. pylori* with which an individual is colonized (spiral shape, flagella, and specific ability to attach to Lewis B antigens in persons with type O blood) affects risk for disease.

Once attached to the mucosal layer, *H. pylori* releases toxins, proteases, and phospholipase enzymes that promote inflammation and impair the integrity of the mucosal layer. The inflammatory process includes the release of histamine, which acts the same on the duodenal mucosa and on the gastric mucosa. The end result is ulceration. Eradication of *H. pylori* reduces ulcer recurrence (Lew, 2009).

Diagnosis

Diagnosis of ulcerative disease involves radiographic and endoscopic evaluation of the upper GI tract and testing for *H. pylori* colonization. All patients with peptic ulcers should be tested for *H. pylori*, even if they have a history of **NSAID** use. A number of tests can be used, including serological testing, urea breath test, and stool antigen test (Lew, 2009).

Invasive diagnostic procedures are determined in consultation with or by referral to a gastroenterologist. Endoscopy is the gold standard for confirming peptic ulcer disease and to rule out gastric cancer (Lew, 2009). For further discussion of the diagnostic process associated with PUD, the reader is referred to management texts. The treatment protocol presented here assumes appropriate diagnosis of PUD.

Pharmacodynamics

Eradication of *H. pylori* is critical to PUD treatment; therefore, all recommended treatment regimens include a combination of a **PPI** and **antimicrobial** therapy. **Antimicrobial** agents used include **clarithromycin**, **tetracycline**, **amoxicillin**, **levofloxacin**, and **metronidazole**. They are given in triple drug regimen or a quadruple drug regimen that includes **bismuth subsalicylate**. Acid suppression by the **PPI** in conjunction with the **antimicrobial** helps alleviate the ulcer-related symptoms, heals gastric mucosal inflammation, and may enhance the efficacy of the **antimicrobial** agent against *H. pylori* at the mucosal surface. **Antimicrobials** are discussed in more detail in Chapter 24.

Goals of Treatment

Goals of treatment for PUD are (1) to eradicate *H. pylori*, (2) heal any ulcers, (3) manage or prevent complications such as GI bleeding or the development of gastric carcinoma, (4) prevent relapse, and (5) reduce or eliminate symptoms. Meeting these goals requires both lifestyle modification and drug therapy, but lifestyle modification is less important in PUD than it is in GERD.

Rational Drug Selection

Algorithm

The treatment algorithm outlines the steps in treating peptic ulcers that consist of healing the ulcer and preventing ulcer recurrence through eradication of *H. pylori*. Ulcers that are associated with **NSAID** use are discussed in Chapter 25.

As with GERD, step 1 involves lifestyle modifications and OTC **antacids** or **histamine$_2$ blockers**. Most patients have tried some step 1 interventions before they seek health care. This step alone may be sufficient for patients with mild disease and only occasional symptoms, but this step alone is not likely to heal any ulcers. Progression to step 2 is usually required, especially for duodenal ulcers and for those that are a result of *H. pylori* infection. Figure 34–4 shows the stepped algorithm for peptic ulcer disease. See Table 34–5 for diagnostic tests.

Step 2 for patients with uncomplicated gastric ulcers includes testing and treating for *H. pylori* and acid suppressive therapy with **PPIs**. Multiple treatment regimens for *H. pylori* eradication are available, including combining a **PPI** and two antibiotics for 14 days (Lew, 2009). Maintenance therapy with an **antisecretory** agent, usually a **PPI**, at the full healing dose is necessary. Table 34–6 presents the multiple evidence based treatment regimens.

Ulcers complicated by bleeding require endoscopy for diagnosis of the lesion. Healing should also be documented by endoscopy after 12 weeks of **antisecretory** therapy (usually **PPIs**) to document healing. Patients who are taking **NSAIDs** should be switched to a **COX-2 inhibitor** to achieve analgesic and anti-inflammatory effects similar to **NSAIDs**, but with fewer GI complications (Lew, 2009).

Duodenal and gastric ulcers recur in up to 80 percent of patients treated with drugs to reduce gastric acid but not treated for eradication of *H. pylori* infection. By comparison, 6 to 15 percent of patients have recurrent ulcers when their *H. pylori* infection is cured.

Maintenance therapy with an **antisecretory** agent is not generally required after eradication of *H. pylori*. However, it is prudent to prescribe maintenance therapy for certain high-risk groups: smokers; patients older than 60 years; patients with chronic obstructive pulmonary disease, coronary artery disease, or renal failure; patients with a history of bleeding or perforated ulcer; patients with persistent symptoms; and those who must take **NSAIDs** or other ulcerogenic drugs.

Patients with gastric or duodenal ulcers who fail to become symptom free or who develop complications such as GI bleeding while on **antisecretory** therapy require a referral to a gastroenterologist. Surgery is contemplated for gastric ulcer patients.

Lifestyle Modifications

Evidence is lacking that dietary modifications affect the course of PUD. Frequent small meals and decreased consumption of spices, **alcohol**, **caffeine**, and fruit juices have never been demonstrated to affect healing. Dietary changes should be directed at those substances that cause symptoms in each particular patient.

The most important lifestyle modification is smoking cessation. Smoking both increases the risk for gastric and duodenal ulcers and delays their healing.

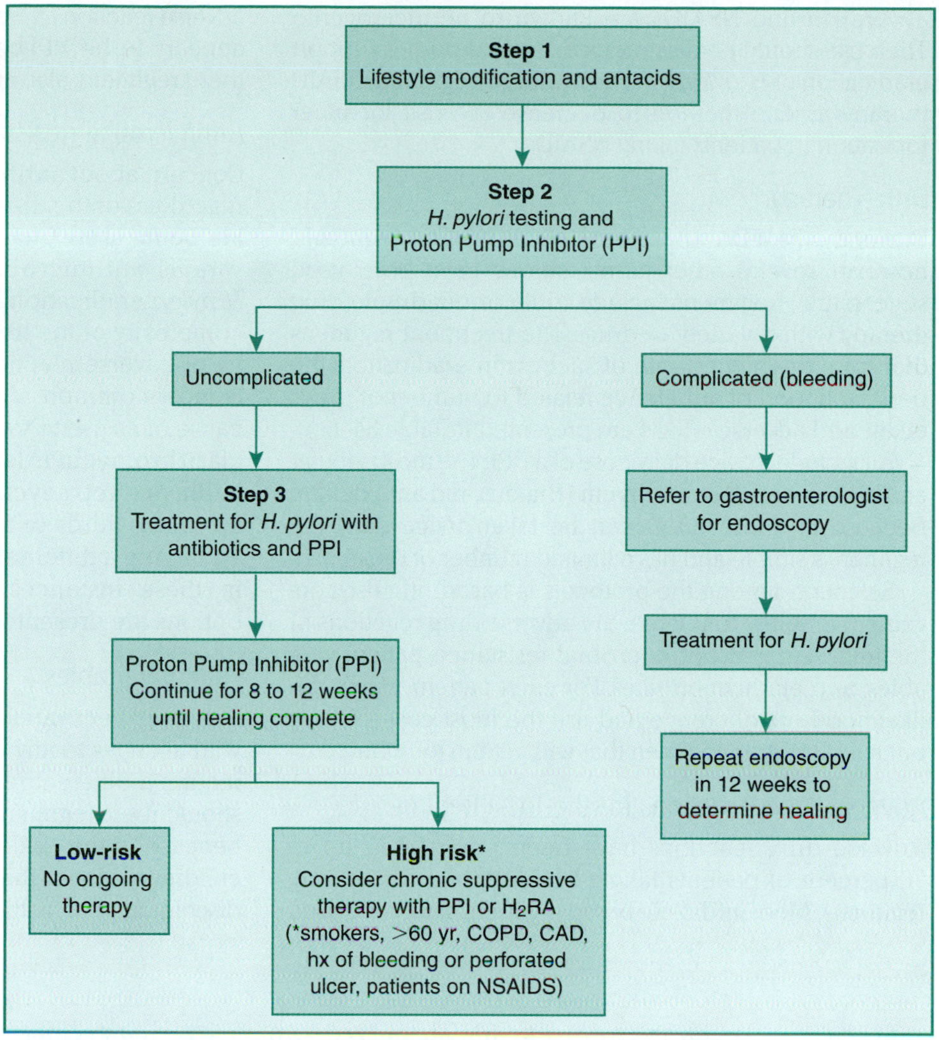

Figure 34–4. Stepped-approach algorithm for peptic ulcer disease.

Table 34–5 Invasive and Noninvasive Diagnostic Tests for *Helicobacter pylori*

Test	Sensitivity	Specificity	Comments
Noninvasive			
Serological ELISA	85%	79%	Detects *H. pylori*, cannot be used to confirm successful cure
Urea breath test	95%–100%	91%–98%	Can be used for screening and confirming cure. PPIs and recent antibiotics can cause false negative
H. pylori stool antigen test	91%–98%	94%–99%	Can be used for initial diagnosis and test of cure
Invasive			
Rapid urease test	93%–97%%	95%–100%	
Culture of biopsy specimen	70%–80%	100%	
Histological evaluation	>95%	95%–98%	

PPI = protein pump inhibitor.

Aspirin and **NSAIDs** are known to be ulcerogenic. Their use should be discouraged. Several studies support eradication of *H. pylori* infection prior to beginning **NSAID** therapy as one method to decrease the risk for ulcer formation in patients taking **NSAIDs**.

Drug Therapy

Currently, the FDA approves eight treatment regimens; however, several other combinations have been used successfully. Regimens include triple or quadruple drug therapy with a variety of drugs. The treatment regimens that have the highest rate of success in eradication, the best likelihood of adherence related to number of drugs taken, and adverse effects are presented in Table 34–6.

All include a twice-daily dose of a **PPI**. The most popular **antibiotics** are **clarithromycin** (**Biaxin**) and **amoxicillin**. Because all these drugs can be taken twice daily, the regimen is simple and has a limited number of drugs.

Selection among the protocols is based on cost, convenience, ability to tolerate the adverse drug reactions of the total regimen, **antimicrobial** resistance, patient variables, and eradication rates. For each patient, assess the likelihood of adherence and use the most cost-effective but simplest drug regimen that will get the job done.

Adverse Drug Reactions for the Total Regimen

Adverse drug reactions have been reported in up to 70 percent of patients taking **bismuth**-based four-drug regimens. **Metronidazole**-based regimens have increased adverse reactions. Overall, the best regimen for tolerability appears to be **PPI**-based three-drug regimens. Happily, these regimens also are highly efficacious.

Antimicrobial Resistance

Concern about **antimicrobial** resistance has increased, regardless of the disease process for which these drugs are being used. Chapter 24 discusses resistance to the various **antimicrobials**. Resistance associated with *H. pylori* eradication has been linked to the length and complexity of the treatment regimen and the tolerability of adverse reactions. Resistance to **metronidazole** is most common and higher in women, probably because of its use to treat genital infections. Resistance to **clarithromycin** is low (10%), as is resistance to **amoxicillin** and **tetracycline**. Acquired resistance occurs in up to two-thirds of treatment failures. Changing drugs and trying a different treatment regimen may be useful in these instances. First- and second-line therapy options are presented in Table 34–6.

Patient Variables

Several patient variables need to be considered. Patients with allergies to any of the drugs in a treatment regimen require a different regimen. Women of childbearing age should use a regimen that does not include **tetracycline** because of the risk for fetal harm. The same is true for children younger than 8 years related to problems with discoloration of teeth. Each of the drugs in these regimens

Table 34–6 **Drug Treatment Protocols for *Helicobacter pylori* Eradication**

	Drug 1	Drug 2	Drug 3	Drug 4	Comments
Triple therapy	Proton pump inhibitor bid	Clarithromycin 500 mg bid or metronidazole 500 mg bid	Amoxicillin 1 g bid	—	Treat for 10–14 d Usual first-line therapy
Triple therapy	Proton pump inhibitor bid	Clarithromycin 500 mg bid	Metronidazole 500 mg bid	—	Treat for 7–14 d Use as first-line therapy in penicillin allergic patients
Quadruple therapy	Proton pump inhibitor bid OR Ranitidine 150 mg bid	Metronidazole 250 mg qid	Tetracycline* 500 mg qid	Bismuth subsalicylate 525 mg qid	Treat for 10–14 d Usually used as second-line therapy in patients who fail first line therapy
Levofloxacin-based triple therapy	Proton pump inhibitor bid	Levofloxacin 250–500 mg bid	Amoxicillin 1 gm bid		Treat for 10–14 d Second-line or rescue therapy

*Children <8 yr should not take tetracycline. Other treatment regimens with dosage adjustments for children are acceptable. Some come with drugs grouped in packets.
Proton pump inhibitors include esomeprazole 40 mg, lansoprazole 30 mg, omeprazole 20 mg, pantoprazole 40 mg, rabeprazole 20 mg.
Source: Lew, 2009.

has potential drug interactions. Other drugs the patient may be taking must be taken into account.

Given all these parameters, the treatment regimen with good to excellent eradication rates, a low to medium adverse reactions profile, likelihood of adherence based on complexity of the regimen and moderate cost, and limited **antimicrobial** resistance appears to be **clarithromycin** plus **amoxicillin** plus a PPI, all taken twice a day for 10 to 14 days.

Monitoring

Monitoring parameters for each of the drugs in these treatment regimens are presented in Chapters 20 and 24. Documentation of ulcer healing by endoscopy 12 weeks after the end of therapy is the gold standard. Cost considerations suggest reserving it for patients who are at high risk for complications, patients with recurrence, and those who will be on long-term therapy. The urea breath test or stool antigen testing can be used to screen symptomatic patients who are suspected of having recurrent ulcers associated with *H. pylori* infection. Note that serological testing for *H. pylori* may be falsely negative if the patient is on PPIs or recently on **antibiotics**. Documentation by endoscopy is optional for low-risk patients.

Outcome Evaluation

Figure 34–4 shows the treatment algorithm for PUD. Outcome evaluation targets eradication of *H. pylori* and relief of symptoms. Evaluation also includes the other goals for therapy: healing of lesions, prevention of complications, and prevention of relapse. Relapse rates are high for patients with PUD but can be significantly reduced with appropriate maintenance therapy or eradication of *H. pylori* infection.

Patients with PUD who remain symptom free without drugs or on maintenance therapy require no more frequent follow-up than with their annual physical examination.

Patients with *H. pylori* infection–associated ulcers that do not respond to the first course of **antimicrobial** therapy should be evaluated for noncompliance. Ask about missed doses, adverse effects of medications, and completion of the therapy prescribed (Lew, 2009). Antibiotic resistance may occur. Culture and sensitivity are not routinely used in PUD treatment. A second course of therapy with a different drug combination for 14 days is recommended (Lew, 2009). If the patient still has symptoms and eradication fails, referral to a gastroenterologist is appropriate. Other causes, such as Zollinger-Ellison syndrome, may be present.

Patient Education

Patient education should include a discussion of information related to the overall treatment plan as well as that specific to the drug therapy, reasons for the drug being taken, drugs as part of the total treatment regimen, and adherence issues.

PEPTIC ULCER DISEASE

PATIENT EDUCATION

Related to the Overall Treatment Plan/Disease Process

- ☐ Understanding the pathophysiology of ulcer formation and its long-term risks for bleeding and cancer of the stomach
- ☐ Role of lifestyle modifications in total treatment regimen
- ☐ Importance of adherence to the treatment regimen, especially in light of antimicrobial resistance
- ☐ Need for follow-up visits with the primary care provider if the symptoms recur or do not resolve

Specific to the Drug Therapy

- ☐ Reason for the drug(s) being given and the anticipated action of the drug(s) on the disease process
- ☐ Doses and schedules for taking the drug(s)
- ☐ Possible adverse reactions and what to do when they occur
- ☐ Coping mechanisms for complex and costly drug regimens
- ☐ Interactions between lifestyle modifications and these drugs

Reasons for Taking the Drug(s)

Patient education about specific drugs is provided in Chapters 20 and 24. Specific information related to PUD includes the following: Drugs used to treat PUD are given to treat *H. pylori,* reduce symptoms, heal any ulcers, reduce the risk for complications, and prevent relapse of symptoms. Different drugs have different roles with each of these.

Continued

PEPTIC ULCER DISEASE—cont'd

PATIENT EDUCATION

Drugs as Part of the Total Treatment Regimen

Lifestyle modification is important in disease management. PUD is often a chronic condition, requiring lifelong maintenance therapy.

Adherence Issues

Any disease process in which lifestyle modifications are required or in which a complex regimen of three or four drugs over a period of weeks is required is likely to have problems with adherence. Health-care providers should be aware of the potential problem of nonadherence, discuss the importance of adherence, and assist patients in removing barriers to adherence, such as the complexity and cost of the treatment regimen and the presence of adverse reactions.

REFERENCES

American Gastroenterological Association (AGA) Institute Medical Position Panel. (2008). American Gastroenterological Association medical position statement on the management of gastroesophageal reflux disease. *Gastroenterology, 135,* 1383–1391.

Corley, D. A., Kubo, A., Zhao, W., & Quesenberry, C. (2010). Proton pump inhibitors and histamine-2 receptor antagonists are associated with hip fractures among at-risk patients. *Gastroenterology, 139*(1), 93–101.

Gold, B., Colletti, R., Abbot, M., Czinn, S., Elitsur, Y., Hassall, E., et al. (2000). *Helicobacter pylori* infection in children: Recommendations for diagnosis and treatment. *Journal of Pediatric Gastroenterology, 31*(5), 490–497.

Greenberger, N. (2003). Update in gastroenterology. *Annals of Internal Medicine, 138*(1), 45–53.

Haruma, K., Mihara, M., Okamoto, E., et al. (1999). Eradication of *Helicobacter pylori* increases gastric acidity in patients with atrophic gastritis of the corpus—evaluation of 24-h pH monitoring. *Alimentary Pharmacology & Therapeutics, 13,* 155–162.

Institute for Clinical Systems Improvement (ICSI). (2006). *Initial management of dyspepsia and GERD.* Bloomington, MN: Institute for Clinical Systems Improvement. Retrieved from http://www.icsi.org

Laine, L., Franz, J., Baker, A., & Neil, G. (1997). A United States multicenter trial of dual and proton pump inhibitor-based triple therapies for *Helicobacter pylori. Alimentary Pharmacologic Therapy, 11,* 913–917.

Lew, E. (2009). Peptic ulcer disease. In N. J. Greenberger (Ed.), *Current diagnosis & treatment gastroenterology, hepatology, & endoscopy* (3rd ed.). New York: McGraw-Hill.

Lodato, F., Azzaroli, F., Turco, L., Mazzella, N., Buonfiglioli, F., Zoli, M., et al. (2010). Adverse effects of proton pump inhibitors. *Best Practices in Research and Clinical Gastroenterology, 24*(2), 193–201.

McCance, K., & Huether, S. (2010). *Pathophysiology: The biological basis for disease in adults and children* (10th ed.). St. Louis, MO: Elsevier Mosby.

National Digestive Diseases Information Clearing House (NDDICH). (2007). *Heartburn, gastroesophageal reflux (GER), and gastroesophageal reflux disease (GERD)* (NIH Publication No. 07–0882). Bethesda, MD: National Institutes of Health. Retrieved from http://digestive.niddk.nih.gov/ddiseases/pubs/gerd/

National Institutes of Health. (2009a). Gastroesophageal reflux disease. In *Burden of digestive diseases in the United States, 2008* (NIH Publication No. 09-6443). Bethesda, MD: National Institutes of Health. Retrieved from http://www2.niddk.nih.gov/AboutNIDDK/ReportsAndStrategicPlanning/

National Institutes of Health. (2009b). Peptic ulcer disease. In *Burden of digestive diseases in the United States, 2008* (NIH Publication No. 09-6443). Bethesda, MD: National Institutes of Health. Retrieved from http://www2 .niddk.nih.gov/AboutNIDDK/ReportsAndStrategicPlanning/

Opekun, A., Abdalla, N., Sutton, F., Hammoud, F., Kuo, G., Torres, E., et al. (2002). Urea breath testing and analysis in the primary care office. *Journal of Family Practice, 51*(12), 1030–1032.

Stansbury, A. (2004). GER and GERD in children. *American Journal for Nurse Practitioners, 8*(3), 37–44.

Thjodleifsson, B. (2002). Treatment of acid-related disease in the elderly with emphasis on the use of proton pump inhibitors. *Drugs and Aging, 19*(12), 911–927.

Vandenplas, Y., Rudolph, C. D., DiLorenzo, C., Hassall, E., Liptak, G., Mazur, L., et al. (2009). Pediatric gastroesophageal reflux clinical practice guidelines: Joint recommendations of the North American Society for Pediatric Gastroenterology, Hepatology, and Nutrition (NASPGHAN) and the European Society for Pediatric Gastroenterology, Hepatology, and Nutrition (ESPGHAN). *Journal of Pediatric Gastroenterology and Nutrition, 49,* 498–547.

CHAPTER 35

HEADACHES

Teri Moser Woo

Chapter Outline

Headaches are a common presenting complaint in primary care, accounting for 18 million outpatient visits per year in the United States. This makes headaches the seventh-leading chief complaint in ambulatory clinics. More than 80 percent of adult Americans report that they experience recurrent headache, with 35 to 50 percent labeling their headache severe enough to disrupt their activities of daily living (Marin, 1998; Smith, 1998). In the United States, 30 million people experience migraine (Gagne et al, 2007). The cost of direct medical care for migraine is $1.25 to $11 billion, and the cost to American employers is $16 to $28 billion annually because of missed work days and impaired work function (Gagne et al, 2007). Successful pharmacological management of headache can improve the quality of life for millions of Americans. The Institute for Clinical Systems Improvement (ICSI) (2009) provides guidelines for treatment of multiple types of headaches, while the US Headache Consortium provides evidence-based guidelines for the treatment of migraine (Matcher et al, 2000). These two evidence-based guidelines are used for treatment recommendations in this chapter.

Headaches affect all age groups, from preverbal children to the older patient. When asked, 20 to 40 percent of school-age children report having had headaches. The onset of migraine usually occurs between the ages of 15 and 25, although younger children may experience migraine. The peak incidence of headache is in young adulthood (25 to 34 years), with the incidence waning as a patient gets older. Onset of headache after age 50 or headaches increasing in frequency or severity should lead to the investigation of underlying neurological disease.

The most common types of headaches can be classified as migraine, tension-type, and chronic daily headache, which may present as a mixed form of tension type and migraine, or transformed migraine. Medication-overuse is also identified as a cause of chronic daily headache. Cluster headaches are rare but severely debilitating. The pharmacological management of these common types of headaches is discussed in this chapter. Pathological headaches, caused by space-occupying lesions, alterations in intracranial pressure, or other pathology, are not discussed here, other than to note when the differential should lead to pathology rather than to common headaches. To assist the provider in diagnosing the correct type of headache, it is helpful to use a headache screening questionnaire that addresses (1) how often the patient is having the headache, (2) how severe the headache is, and (3) how often the patient is taking pain medication or headache relievers (Maizels & Burchette, 2003).

MIGRAINE

Migraine headaches are a complex multifactorial condition, which may be classified in three categories: migraine with aura (classic migraine), migraine without aura (common migraine), and complicated migraine. Classification of migraine, although important for accurate diagnosis, does not affect the pharmacological management. This chapter discusses acute or abortive therapy and preventive therapy, as well as nonpharmacological therapy for treating migraine.

Pathophysiology

There are several theories regarding the pathogenesis of migraine headache. The vascular theory proposes that the aura preceding migraine is caused by vasoconstriction of intracranial vessels, and vasodilation of the affected vessels results in the typical vascular headache pain that throbs in unison with the pulse. The vascular theory has been disputed because not all migraine sufferers have a pulsatile quality to their headache pain.

Considerable evidence associates migraine with changes in serotonin activity that result in release of vasoactive neurotransmitters (substance P, bradykinin, neurokinin A, and calcitonin gene-related peptides). This produces an inflammatory response around the blood vessels of the dura mater and pia mater and is accompanied by dilation of cerebral blood vessels. Specific excitatory serotonin receptors (5-HT_2), when activated, can lead to migraine. Many of the abortive agents used for migraine appear to stimulate inhibitory serotonin receptors (5-HT_1 and 5-HT_{1D}) or block 5-HT_2 receptors.

There is a strong familial component to migraine, with 20 to 60 percent of patients reporting a family history of migraine. Migraine is two to three times more prevalent in women than in men. Women with migraines may have increased headaches around the time of their menstrual periods and if they are taking estrogen-containing medications, such as oral contraceptives. Other known triggers of migraine include **alcohol**, strong light, noxious odors, extreme fatigue, and certain foods. Table 35–1 lists common triggers that may precipitate a migraine headache in patients prone to migraine.

Goals of Treatment

The overall goal of therapy is to minimize the impact of migraine headaches on patients' quality of life, social functioning, and ability to work. A second goal is prevention of migraine by avoiding each patient's identified triggers and prophylaxis for frequent migraine sufferers. Minimizing adverse effects of pharmacotherapy and avoidance of medication overuse/abuse that can lead to medication-overuse headaches should also be goals of both the provider and the patient.

Rational Drug Selection

Pharmacological management of migraine is divided into two major components: acute or abortive therapy and preventive or prophylactic therapy. Most patients with migraine need only abortive therapy for their headaches. If migraine frequency is greater than twice a month and/or severely debilitating or if abortive agents are ineffective, the health-care provider should consider prescribing daily preventive therapy.

Acute Therapy

Acute or abortive therapy is aimed at reversing, aborting, or reducing pain and accompanying symptoms of an attack that is in progress or is anticipated. Acute therapy for migraines can range from simple over-the-counter (OTC) **analgesics** to intramuscular (IM) **dihydroergotamine** that needs to be administered in a clinic or emergency room setting. Oral (PO) therapy may not be effective in patients with associated nausea or vomiting. The stepwise approach to selecting migraine medications for acute treatment is helpful, based on the severity of the pain and associated symptoms. Figure 35–1 is an algorithm that addresses the steps in acute migraine therapy.

The US Headache Consortium, consisting of the American Academy of Family Physicians (AAFP), American Academy of Neurology (AAN), American Headache Society (AHS), American College of Emergency Physicians (ACEP), American College of Physicians (ACP), American Osteopathic Association (AOA), and the National Headache Foundation (NHF), has

Table 35–1 **Common Migraine Triggers**

Factor	Triggers
Environmental factors	Noxious smells and fumes Bright light or glare Tobacco smoke
Foods	Caffeine (coffee, tea, caffeine-containing medications or beverages) Nuts, peanut butter, pea pods, lima or navy beans Alcohol (red wine, beer, liquor) Aged cheese Monosodium glutamate (MSG) (in Chinese food, seasoning salt, processed foods, soups) Chocolate (sweets, foods, drinks) Nitrites and nitrates (processed meats, hot dogs) Onions Avocados Dairy products (ice cream, yogurt, cheese, sour cream, milk, cream) Pickled or smoked foods (pickled herring, smoked fish) Citrus fruits, bananas, figs, raisins Aspartame (in many foods and drinks labeled "sugar free") Sulfites Yeast products (in bread, donuts)
Lifestyle	Hunger/fasting Oversleeping Inadequate sleep Stress Lack of exercise Prolonged sitting in an uncomfortable position Extended computer usage
Hormonal	Menses Menopause Oral contraceptives Hormonal replacement therapy
Medications	Nitroglycerin Oral contraceptives Antihypertensives Theophylline Antibiotics (TMP/SMZ, griseofulvin) Histamine$_2$ blockers (cimetidine, ranitidine) Analgesic or ergotamine overuse Indomethacin

TMP/SMZ = trimethoprim/sulfamethoxazole.

evaluated the evidence regarding the clinical effectiveness of pharmacological treatment of acute attacks and their guidelines are used in this chapter (Matcher et al, 2000). Although this section discusses pharmacological treatment, nonpharmacological therapy—specifically applying ice to the head and/or lying down in a darkened room—must accompany the medication. The patient must be advised not to try to "work through" a migraine by just taking medication.

Simple Analgesics

Simple **analgesics** such as **aspirin** (ASA) and **acetaminophen** (APAP) or **NSAIDs** are the first step in the acute treatment of mild to moderate migraine that is not associated with severe nausea or vomiting. Patients often self-medicate with OTC **analgesics**, relying on advertising messages to choose a medication (Matcher et al, 2000). The health-care provider needs to be aware that most patients have already self-medicated to treat their migraines and that they are often seeking care because their treatment is no longer effective. If the provider decides to begin treatment with an OTC product, educating the patient about the rationale for starting with an OTC product will increase compliance.

Clinical experience and population-based studies have demonstrated the effectiveness of OTC **analgesics** in treating migraine, especially if taken early. The mechanism of action for the various OTC preparations is not completely

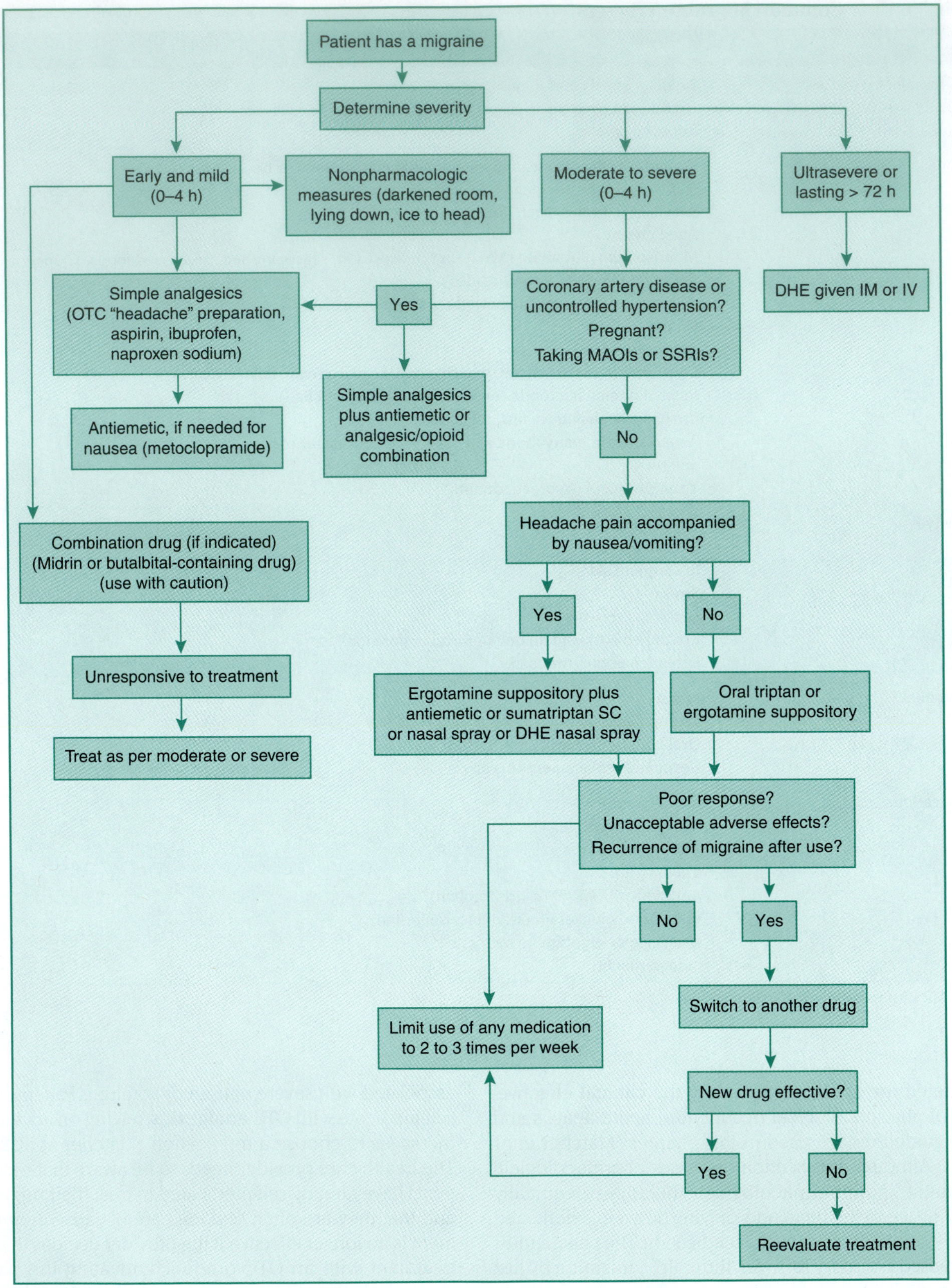

Figure 35–1. Treatment algorithm for acute migraine headache.

understood. ASA is thought to have antiprostaglandin and antiplatelet activity that might deliver relief from migraine attack. There is evidence that ASA may also act centrally and has serotoninergic activity. APAP is thought to act centrally and inhibit prostaglandin synthesis. NSAIDs also inhibit prostaglandin synthesis and have a central analgesic mechanism of action. Their anti-inflammatory and antipyretic activity may also contribute to migraine relief. **Caffeine** is an ingredient in many OTC "headache" preparations (Table 35–2) and plays a role as an analgesic adjuvant when added to ASA or in combination with APAP. The U.S. Food and Drug Administration (FDA) has approved two OTC medications to be labeled specifically for migraine pain: One is a combination of ASA, APAP, and **caffeine (Excedrin Migraine)**, and the other is **ibuprofen in a liquid-filled capsule (Advil Migraine)**.

(Text continues on page 1137)

Table 35–2 Drugs Commonly Used: Headaches

Drug	Initial Dose	Maximum Dose	Strengths Available	Rebound Potential	Comments
			ACUTE THERAPY		
Nonnarcotic Analgesics					
Acetaminophen (OTC: Tylenol)	*Adults:* 650–1,000 mg at onset and every 4–6 h	*Adults:* 4,000 mg/day 2–3 d/wk; 30 dosages/mo	*Tablets:* 160, 325, 500, 650 mg; *Liquid:* 80 mg/0.8 mL 160 mg/5 mL; *Chewable:* 80, 160 mg; *Suppositories:* 80, 120, 325, 650 mg	Yes	Safe in pregnancy, lactation, and in most patients; Not recommended for first-line theory except in pregnant patients; Risk for drug medication-overuse HA
	Children: 10–15 mg/kg/dose	*Children:* 5 doses in 24 h			
Aspirin (OTC: Bayer, Bufferin, Ecotrin)	*Adults:* 650–1,000 mg at onset and every 4–6 h	*Adults:* 4,000 mg/d 2–3 d/wk; 30 dosages/mo	*Tablets:* 325, 500, 650, 975 mg; *Suppositories:* 300, 600 mg	Yes	Contraindicated in pregnancy (Category D); Avoid use within 1 wk of surgery; Risk for medication-overuse HA
	Children: Not recommended				
Ibuprofen (OTC: Motrin IB, Advil, Nuprin; Rx: Motrin)	*Adults:* 200–800 mg at onset, then every 6 h; *Children:* 5–10 mg/kg initially; may repeat every 6–8 h	*Adults:* 2,400 mg/d; *Children:* 40 mg/kg/d	*OTC tablets:* 100, 200 mg; *Rx tablets:* 400, 600, 800 mg; *Suspension:* 100 mg/5 mL; *Chewable:* 50, 100 mg	Unlikely	Contraindicated in third trimester of pregnancy; safe during lactation; Use with caution in kidney disease, ulcer disease, gastritis
Naproxen (Rx: Naprosyn)	*Adults:* 500 mg at onset, then 250 mg every 6–8 h; *Children:* 2.5–5 mg/kg initially and may repeat every 12 h	*Adults:* 1,000 mg/d; *Children:* 15 mg/kg/d	*Tablets:* 250, 375, 500 mg; *Suspension:* 125 mg/mL	Unlikely	Contraindicated in third trimester of pregnancy; safe during lactation; Absorbed more slowly than naproxen sodium; Use with caution in kidney disease, ulcer disease, gastritis

Continued

Table 35–2 **Drugs Commonly Used: Headaches—cont'd**

Drug	Initial Dose	Maximum Dose	Strengths Available	Rebound Potential	Comments
			ACUTE THERAPY		
Nonnarcotic Analgesics					
Naproxen sodium (OTC: Aleve; Rx: Anaprox)	*Adults:* 825 mg at onset, then 200–550 mg in 3–4 h *Children:* Use suspension form of naproxen	*Adults:* 1375 mg/d	*OTC tablets:* 200 mg *Rx tablets:* 275, 550 mg	Unlikely	Contraindicated in third trimester of pregnancy; safe during lactation Naproxen sodium absorbed more quickly than naproxen, reaches peak levels in half the time Use with caution in kidney disease, ulcer disease, gastritis
Ketorolac (Rx: Toradol)	*Adults:* 30–60 mg initially, may repeat 30–60 mg every 6 h *Children:* Not recommended in children <16 yr	*Adults:* 120 mg/d	*Injection:* 15 mg/mL, 30 mg/mL for IM injection	Unlikely, but frequent use should be avoided Contraindicated in pregnancy, lactation, kidney disease, ulcer disease, gastritis	Use for emergency treatment of severe migraine in patients who cannot use other medications
Aspirin/acetaminophen/caffeine combination (OTC: Excedrin, Vanquish)	*Adults:* 2 tablets every 6 h	*Adults:* 8 tablets/d, 2 d/wk	Excedrin: APAP 250 mg, ASA 250 mg, caffeine 65 mg Vanquish: APAP 165 mg, ASA 227 mg, caffeine 33 mg	Yes	Same precautions as for ASA and APAP
Combination Analgesics					
Butalbital compounds (Rx: Fiorinal, Fioricet, Esgic Plus)	*Adults:* 2 tablets at onset, then 1 tablet every 4–6 h *Children:* Not recommended	Adults: 6 tablets per attack 2 d/wk 30 tablets Fioricet:	Fiorinal: Butalbital 50 mg, ASA 325 mg, caffeine 40 mg Butalbital 50 mg, APAP 325 mg, caffeine 40 mg Esgic Plus: Butalbital 50 mg, APAP 500 mg, caffeine 40 mg	Yes	Same as for ASA and APAP Not for first-line therapy Risk for medication-overuse headache, if taken in greater than recommended dosage or more than 2 d/wk
Isometheptene compound (Rx: Midrin, Isocom)	*Adults:* Migraine: 2 capsules at onset, then 1 capsule every h if needed for relief Tension headache: 1 or 2 capsules at onset, followed by one capsule every 4 h *Children:* Not recommended	Migraine: 5 per 12 h, 2 d/wk 20 per mo Tension headache: 8 per 24 h, 2 d/wk 20 per mo	Midrin, Isocom: Isometheptene 65 mg, dichloralphenazone 100 mg, APAP 325 mg	Yes	Adverse interaction with MAOIs Contraindicated in uncontrolled hypertension, CAD, PVD Not considered first-line therapy

Table 35–2 **Drugs Commonly Used: Headaches—cont'd**

Drug	Initial Dose	Maximum Dose	Strengths Available	Rebound Potential	Comments
			ACUTE THERAPY		
Narcotic Analgesics					
Codeine-containing compounds (Rx: Tylenol #3, Empirin #3)	*Adults:* 1 or 2 tablets at onset of attack, then 1 every 4–6 h *Children:* Aspirin-containing preparations contraindicated	*Adults:* 6 tablets per attack, 2 d/wk 10–15 doses/mo	Tylenol #3: APAP 300 mg with codeine 30 mg APAP with codeine liquid: Codeine 12 mg and APAP 120 mg/5 mL Empirin #3: ASA 325 mg with codeine 30 mg	Yes and habit forming Monitor use carefully; if patient is needing more than 15 tablets/mo, reevaluate treatment	Relatively safe during pregnancy Should not be considered first-line therapy Contraindicated in substance-abuse patients Should not be prescribed for chronic daily headache
Meperidine (Rx: Demerol)	*Adults:* Maximum initial dose 150 mg, can repeat 50–100 mg every 3–4 h if needed		*IM injection:* 25 mg/mL, 50 mg/mL, 75 mg/mL, 100 mg/mL	Yes Patients must have someone to drive them home after receiving medication	May be used in pregnancy Use only as "rescue" medication Use sparingly and infrequently when other treatments have been ineffective
Butorphanol (Rx: Stadol NS)	*Adults:* 1 spray to one nostril; may be repeated in 1 h *Children:* Not recommended	*Adults:* 2 sprays (2 mg) per attack, 2 d/wk	Stadol NS: Nasal spray 1 mg/spray	Probably Side effects of orthostasis and sedation	Can be used as a "rescue" medication Effective for nocturnal headaches May be used with caution in pregnancy
Ergot Derivatives					
Ergotamine tablets (Rx: Ergostat, Ergomar)	*Adults:* One tablet sublingual at onset of attack; may repeat every 30 min; max 3 tablets per attack *Children:* Not safe in children	*Adults:* 3 tablets/d, 2 d/wk and 10 mg/wk	Sublingual 2-mg tablets	Yes	Contraindicated in pregnancy (Category X) and lactation Contraindicated in CAD and PVD May cause severe nausea and vomiting
Ergotamine and caffeine combination (Rx: Cafergot, Wigraine)	*Adults:* Tablets: 2 tablets at onset, then 1 tablet every 30 min if needed, up to 6 tablets per attack Suppositories: 1/3–1 suppository at onset; may repeat 1 suppository in 1 h, if needed *Children:* Not recommended	*Adults:* 6 tablets or 2 suppositories per attack, 2 d/wk, 10 mg/wk	Cafergot & Wigraine tablets: Ergotamine 1 mg, caffeine 100 mg Cafergot & Wigraine suppositories: Ergotamine 2 mg, caffeine 100 mg	Yes Suppository form better absorbed	Pregnancy Category X; contraindicated in lactation, CAD, PVD May cause nausea and vomiting May premedicate with an antiemetic

Continued

Table 35–2 **Drugs Commonly Used: Headaches—cont'd**

Drug	Initial Dose	Maximum Dose	Strengths Available	Rebound Potential	Comments
		ACUTE THERAPY			
Ergot Derivatives					
Dihydroergotamine (Rx: DHE 45, Migranal)	*Adults:* Injection: 1 mg IV/IM at onset; may repeat 1-mg dose hourly for total maximum of 3 mg IM or 2 mg IV Intranasal: 1 spray each nostril at onset; may repeat in 15 min *Children:* Not recommended	*Adults:* IM: 3 mg/attack IV: 2 mg/attack IM/IV: 6 mg/wk IM home use: 18 doses/mo Intranasal: 6 sprays/24 h, 8 sprays/wk	DHE 45 injection; 1 mg/mL Migranal 0.5 mg/spray	Unlikely	Contraindicated in pregnancy, lactation, CAD, PVD, and hypertension Premedicate with antiemetic metoclopramide for greater effectiveness
Serotonin Receptor Agonists					
Alomotriptan (Axert)	*Adults ≥18 yr:* 6.25 mg or 12.5 mg once. May repeat × 1 after 2 h *Adolescents age 12–17 yr:* 6.25 mg or 12.5 mg in a single dose may repeat after 2 hours *Children:* Not recommended	2 doses/24 h	6.25-mg tablets 12.5-mg tablets	Likely	Contraindicated in pregnancy ischemic heart disease, CAD, and uncontrolled hypertension None of the triptans can be used within 24 h of ergotamine-containing medications or other triptans Concurrent use of a triptan or use within 2 wk of MAOIs is contraindicated All the triptans interact with SSRIs, causing serotonin syndrome Serious adverse effects rarely reported in adults (stroke, visual loss, and death); have been reported in children after use of SC, oral, and/or nasal sumatriptan Don't use >4 times per mo
Eletriptan (Relpax)	*Adults ≥18 yr:* 20 mg or 40 mg × 1. Reevaluate if no response. May repeat × 1 in 2 h *Children:* Not recommended	Max: 80 mg/d	20-mg tablets 40-mg tablets	Likely	Contraindicated in pregnancy ischemic heart disease, CAD, and uncontrolled hypertension None of the triptans can be used within 24 h of ergotamine-containing medications or other triptans Concurrent use of a triptan or use within 2 wk of MAOIs is contraindicated All the triptans interact with SSRIs, causing serotonin syndrome

Table 35–2 **Drugs Commonly Used: Headaches—cont'd**

Drug	Initial Dose	Maximum Dose	Strengths Available	Rebound Potential	Comments
			ACUTE THERAPY		
Serotonin Receptor Agonists					
Eletriptan (cont'd)					Serious adverse effects rarely reported in adults (stroke, visual loss, and death); have been reported in children after use of SC, oral, and/or nasal sumatriptan Same as sumatriptan Don't use >3 times per mo
Frovatriptan (Frova)	*Adults ≥18 yr:* 2.5 mg with fluids. May repeat × 1 after 2 h *Children:* Not recommended	Max: 7.5 mg/24 h	2.5-mg tablets	Likely	Longer half-life. Slower onset of action, lower rate of migraine recurrence Don't use >4 times per mo
Sumatriptan (Rx: Imitrex, Sumavel DosePro (Sumatriptan Injection)	*Adults ≥18 yr:* Oral: 25–100 mg initially; may be repeated every 2 h for up to 24 h SC injection 6 mg; may repeat × 1 in 1 h Intranasal: 5, 10, or 20 mg; may repeat once after 2 h if needed *Children <18 yr* Not recommended	*Adults:* Oral: 300 mg/d, 4 headaches per mo SC injection: 2 injections/day, 4 headaches per mo Intranasal: 40 mg/day, 4 headaches per mo	*Tablets:* 25, 50 mg *SC Injection:* 6 mg/mL single-dose vial *Nasal spray:* 5 mg/spray, 20 mg/spray	Likely	Contraindicated in pregnancy ischemic heart disease, CAD, and uncontrolled hypertension None of the triptans can be used within 24 h of ergotamine-containing medications or other triptans Concurrent use of a triptan or use within 2 wk of MAOIs is contraindicated All the triptans interact with SSRIs, causing serotonin syndrome Serious adverse effects rarely reported in adults (stroke, visual loss, and death); have been reported in children after use of SC, oral, and/or nasal sumatriptan
Naratriptan (Rx: Amerge)	*Adults:*	*Adults:*	*Tablets:*	Likely	Same contraindications as for sumatriptan
	One 1-mg or 2.5-mg tablet at onset of migraine; may repeat dose in 4 h, if needed	5 mg/24 h, 4 headaches per mo	1 mg, 2.5 mg		
					Longer half-life than other triptans, less likely to cause medication-overuse headache
	Children 12–17 yr:				
	Adult doses are used				

Continued

Table 35–2 **Drugs Commonly Used: Headaches—cont'd**

Drug	Initial Dose	Maximum Dose	Strengths Available	Rebound Potential	Comments
ACUTE THERAPY					
Serotonin Receptor Agonists					
Naratriptan (cont'd)					Interacts with oral contraceptives
	Children <12 yr:				
	Safety has not been established				
Rizatriptan (Rx: Maxalt, Maxalt-MLT)	*Adults* (either form): Take 5–10 mg at onset of migraine; may repeat in 2 h, if needed *Children:* Not recommended in patients <8 yr	*Adults:* 30 mg/24 h, 4 headaches per mo Propranolol patients; use 5 mg dose, up to 3 doses in 24 h	*Maxalt tablets:* 5, 10 mg Maxalt-MLT orally disintegrating tablets: 5, 10 mg	Likely	Same contraindications as for sumatriptan Use with caution in patient concurrently taking propranolol
Zolmitriptan (Rx: Zomig)	*Adults:* 2.5 mg or less initially (may break 2.5-mg tablet in half); repeat if headache returns after 2 h *Children:* Safety not established	*Adults:* 10 mg/24 h, 4 headaches per mo	*Tablets:* 2.5 mg, 5 mg	Likely	Same contraindications as for sumatriptan Use with caution in patients with hepatic dysfunction (<2.5-mg dose) Interacts with oral contraceptives and cimetidine
Antiemetics					
Metoclopramide (Rx: Reglan)	*Adults:* 10 mg either orally or IV either before ergotamine derivative or concurrently with analgesic *Children:* Not recommended	*Adults:* 40 mg/d	*Tablets:* 5 mg, 10 mg *Injection:* 5 mg/mL	N/A	Interacts with cimetidine, digoxin, MAOIs, and cyclosporine Safe in pregnancy Category B
PREVENTIVE THERAPY					
Beta Blockers					
Propranolol (Rx: Inderal)	*Adults:* Start with 60–80 mg/d, and increase every 3–7 d *Children:* 0.5–1 mg/kg/d divided bid and increased every 3–4 d	*Adults:* 240–320 mg/d (monitor blood pressure [BP] and heart rate [HR]: systolic [BP] should be >100 mm Hg and HR >50 bpm) *Children:* 2–4 mg/kg/d	*Tablets:* 10, 20, 40, 60, 80 mg	N/A Pregnancy Category C but safer than some other preventive agents	Contraindicated in CHF, asthma, COPD, PVD, diabetes mellitus, depression, Wolff-Parkinson-White syndrome Start with a trial of 3 mo; as response improves over time, it needs to be tapered slowly (over a week) if discontinued Interacts with many drugs including cimetidine, oral contraceptives, calcium channel blockers

Table 35–2 **Drugs Commonly Used: Headaches—cont'd**

Drug	Initial Dose	Maximum Dose	Strengths Available	Rebound Potential	Comments
			PREVENTIVE THERAPY		
Beta Blockers					
Timolol (Rx: Blocadren)	*Adults:* Start at 20 mg/d; increase slowly *Children:* Not recommended	*Adults:* 60 mg/d	*Tablets:* 5, 10, 20 mg	N/A	Pregnancy Category C Contraindications and drug interactions similar to propranolol
Metoprolol (Rx: Lopressor)	*Adults:* Start at 100 mg/d; increase slowly *Children:* Not recommended	*Adults:* 250 mg/d	*Tablets:* 50, 100 mg	N/A	Pregnancy Category C Contraindications include bradycardia, second- or third-degree heart block, overt heart failure Interacts with many drugs, including calcium channel blockers, digoxin, clonidine, and oral contraceptives
Atenolol (Rx: Tenormin)	*Adults:* 100 mg/d *Children:* Not recommended	*Adults:* 200 mg/d	*Tablets:* 25, 50, 100 mg	N/A	Pregnancy Category D Contraindications include bradycardia, second- or third-degree heart block, overt heart failure Interacts with many drugs, including calcium channel blockers, digoxin, clonidine, and oral contraceptives
Tricyclic Antidepressants					
Amitriptyline (Rx: Elavil)	*Adults:* Start with 10 mg qhs and increase every 2 wk to a total daily dose of 20–50 mg *Children:* Not recommended for children <12 y	*Adults:* 150 mg/d	*Tablets:* 10, 25, 50, 75, 100 mg	N/A	Contraindicated in patients with narrow-angle glaucoma, urinary retention, pregnancy, breastfeeding, concurrent use of MAOIs (within 14 d of each other), and in suicidal patients
Anticonvulsants					
Divalproex (Rx: Depakote)	*Adults:* Initial dose is 125–250 mg bid; may increase 125 mg weekly *Children:* Safety and effectiveness for migraine prevention has not been studied in children <16 yr	*Adults:* 1,000 mg/d	*Tablets:* 125, 250, 500 mg	N/A	Requires baseline assessment of liver function, platelet count, and bleeding time, as hepatic failure and thrombocytopenia are rare adverse effects Monitor LFTs and CBC every 2 wk × 3 Pregnancy Category D

Continued

Table 35–2 **Drugs Commonly Used: Headaches—cont'd**

Drug	Initial Dose	Maximum Dose	Strengths Available	Rebound Potential	Comments
			PREVENTIVE THERAPY		
Anticonvulsants					
Topiramate (Topamax)	*Adults:* Start on 25 mg qhs increase to 25 mg bid in week 2. During week 3 the dose is increased to 25 mg in the morning and 50 mg at night. In week 4 a dose of 50 mg twice a day. 25 mg bid may be effective in some				Not approved in children <12 years
NSAIDs					
Naproxen sodium (OTC: Aleve; Rx: Anaprox)	*Adults:* 550 mg bid	*Adults:* 1,375 mg/d	*OTC tablets:* 200 mg *Rx tablets:* 275, 550 mg	Unlikely	Contraindicated in third trimester of pregnancy; safe during lactation Use with caution in kidney disease, ulcer disease, gastritis
Calcium Channel Blockers					
Verapamil (Rx: Calan, Isoptin)	*Adults:* Start with 40 mg bid and slowly increase *Children:* Not recommended	*Adults:* 480 mg/d	*Tablets:* 40, 80, 120, mg	N/A	Contraindicated in pregnancy (Category C), Parkinson's disease, and depression May be first-line choice in patients with hypertension who cannot take beta blockers
Serotonin Antagonist					
Methysergide (Rx: Sansert)	*Adults:* Start with 2 mg bid; increase slowly *Children:* Not recommended	*Adults:* 8–14 mg/d	*Tablets:* 2 mg	N/A	Most serious side effects is retroperitoneal fibrosis or related conditions with prolonged therapy Patient should have a drug-free period of 3–4 wk after every 6 mo of treatment Contraindicated in pregnancy, CAD, PVD, impaired renal or liver function, and hypertension

APAP = acetaminophen; ASA = acetylsalicylic acid; CAD = coronary artery disease; CBC = complete blood count; CHF = chronic heart failure; COPD = chronic obstructive pulmonary disease; HA = headache; LFTs = liver function tests; MAOIs = monoamine oxidase inhibitors; N/A = information not available; OTC = over the counter; PVD = peripheral vascular disease; SSRIs = selective serotonin reuptake inhibitors.

The dosing of ASA or APAP should be limited to a 1,000-mg dose (10 to 15 mg/kg for children) at the beginning of migraine symptoms or aura, with a maximum of 4,000 mg per day. The US Headache Consortium recommends the combination of **acetaminophen** plus **aspirin** plus **caffeine (Excedrin Migraine)** as a "Group 1 drug with proven pronounced statistical and clinical benefit" (Matcher et al, 2000). APAP has varied results for acute migraine treatment and may not be any better than placebo (Matcher et al, 2000). Medication-overuse headaches are possible if ASA or APAP is used more than 3 days per week.

The **NSAIDs** have been found to diminish the severity and duration of migraine attacks. Although no **NSAID** has been found to be better than another in clinical trials, there is a variable response to the different agents that differs from patient to patient. **Ibuprofen** and **naproxen** are both group 1 drugs with proven clinical efficacy (Matcher et al, 2000). The use of **NSAIDs** can involve trying multiple medications before an effective agent is found. **Naproxen sodium (Anaprox, Aleve)** is often a first choice for migraine, as it is quickly absorbed and well tolerated. The initial starting dose of naproxen sodium is 550 mg, followed by 550 mg twice a day or 275 mg every 6 to 8 hours. The dose of **naproxen sodium** for children is 10 to 20 mg/kg/day divided in twice-daily dosing. Although the majority of **NSAIDs** are given PO, **indomethacin (Indocin)** is also available in suppository form, which may be helpful if the patient is nauseated or vomiting. **Ketorolac (Toradol)** is the only **NSAID** available in an injectable form, which can also be used if the patient is vomiting. Table 35–2 shows the dosing for commonly used **NSAIDs**.

Midrange Analgesics

Midrange **analgesics** are commonly prescribed to treat both migraine and tension-type headaches. Combination products that combine either **butalbital** with ASA or APAP (**Fiorinal** or **Fioricet**) or **isometheptene** with **acetaminophen** and **dichloralphenazone (Midrin)** are effective in treating mild to moderate migraine, although the US Headache Consortium guidelines rate these drugs as group 3 drugs, with inconsistent or conflicting clinical efficacy data (Matcher et al, 2000). These products should be used cautiously because medication-overuse headaches can occur if they are taken in greater-than-recommended dosages or more than 2 days per week. Medication-overuse headaches are discussed later in this chapter.

High-Range Analgesics

High-range **analgesics** include the commonly used **opioids**, which act centrally to treat the pain of migraine. Although **opioids** are controversial in the treatment of migraine, there are patients for whom an **opioid** is the drug of choice. An **opioid** can be prescribed if the patient is pregnant, if vasoconstrictor medications are contraindicated, or if the migraine is not responsive to **ergotamine** or serotonin agonists (discussed later). The **opioids** are group 2 drugs with moderate clinical and statistical benefit (Matcher et al, 2000).

Codeine either alone or in combination with ASA (**Aspirin** with **codeine** #3) or APAP (**Tylenol** with **codeine** #3) is the **opioid** most commonly used to treat migraine. The dose of **codeine** should be 30 to 60 mg, with the lowest effective dose used. **Meperidine (Demerol)** can be given IM if the patient is unable to take oral medications because of nausea and/or vomiting. The maximum initial dose is 150 mg in an adult, and a dose of 50 to 100 mg can be repeated every 3 to 4 hours. Intranasal **butorphanol (Stadol)** can be tried in patients who fail nonopioid therapy or who have contraindications to other migraine medications. The dose of one spray in one nostril has a rapid onset (less than 15 minutes) and can be repeated in 1 hour if needed. Adverse effects include orthostasis and sedation. The patient should limit its use to no more than twice a week. Other **opioids** that are prescribed for migraine include **oxycodone** and **hydrocodone**, even though there is little clinical information to support their effectiveness over newer nonnarcotic agents and their use is not supported by the US Headache Consortium. **Opioids** must be prescribed carefully because of their potential for physical dependence, tolerance, and addiction. Therefore, they should be limited to patients with severe but infrequent headaches or the occasional headache that is unresponsive to nonnarcotic agents.

Ergot Derivatives

Ergot derivatives have been used for many years to treat migraine. **Ergotamine** and **dihydroergotamine** (DHE) act as vasoconstrictors that lead to a decline in the amplitude of pulsation in the extracranial arteries and decreased hyperperfusion of the basilar artery area, without decreasing cerebral hemispheric blood flow. **Ergotamine** controls up to 70 percent of acute migraine attacks, but its adverse effects of nausea and vomiting and its unpredictable oral absorption limit routine use. Pretreatment with an **antiemetic** decreases the nausea and vomiting associated with **ergotamine** use. **Ergotamine** suppositories (**Wigraine, Cafergot**) are better absorbed than PO preparations and can be quite effective if administered at the beginning of migraine symptoms. Misuse of **ergotamine** may lead to medication-overuse headaches, and use should be limited to two doses, twice a week or less (total weekly dose of 10 mg maximum), up to 12 doses per month. Another caution with **ergotamine** is that the vasoconstriction can have serious effects on patients with peripheral vascular disease, coronary heart disease, hypertension, and impaired hepatic or renal function. Exceeding recommended amounts of **ergotamine** can lead to vasospastic adverse effects. **Ergotamine** derivatives are

CLINICAL PEARL

Ergotamine Suppositories

Ergotamine suppositories can provide relief if taken at the beginning of a migraine attack. If a patient has not used **ergotamine** before, instruct the patient to use one-third of a 2-mg suppository initially and repeat in 30 to 60 minutes. Refrigeration makes the suppository easier to slice.

CLINICAL PEARL

Triptans

It is advisable to administer the first dose of any of the **triptans** under direct supervision to monitor for unrecognized coronary disease. The patient should receive the first dose in the clinic (or urgent care center) and be monitored for any adverse cardiovascular effects.

contraindicated in pregnancy because they can produce prolonged uterine contractions that can result in abortion. Thus, all forms of **ergotamine** are Pregnancy Category X. **Ergotamine** is not recommended for children. Most **ergotamine** preparations are group 3 drugs in the US Headache Consortium guidelines, demonstrating conflicting or inconsistent evidence for their use in acute migraine (Matcher et al, 2000).

DHE, although chemically similar to **ergotamine**, does not cause the same peripheral vasoconstrictor effects, making it safer to use and listed as a Group 1 drug by the US Headache Consortium (Matcher et al, 2000). It also causes less nausea than **ergotamine** and does not require pretreatment with an antiemetic. DHE is effective even well into the course of a headache, unlike **ergotamine**, which must be taken at the beginning of migraine symptoms. DHE can be administered IM (D.H.E. 45) or intranasally (**Migranal**). DHE has a longer duration of action than does **sumatriptan**, and so headache recurrence rates are lower. The dosage of DHE 45 is 1 mg (or 1 mL) IM or IV initially and can be repeated at 1-hour intervals to a maximum of 3 mg IM or 2 mg IV. IM DHE can be prescribed for home use if the patient has proper instructions regarding administration. A monthly limit for IM DHE is 18 ampules or 12 headache events. The dose of intranasal DHE is 1 spray (0.5 mg) in each nostril, repeated after 15 minutes, for a dose of 2 mg. Maximum dose is 6 sprays in a 24-hour period and 8 sprays per week. Although intranasal DHE is easier to administer, the patient should be warned that it has a slow onset of action. Precautions for DHE are the same as for **ergotamine**; it is contraindicated in pregnancy, coronary artery disease, peripheral vascular disease, and hypertension. DHE is not recommended for children.

Serotonin Receptor Agonists

Serotonin receptor agonists act selectively as 5-HT_1 receptor agonists, causing vasoconstriction and apparently blocking release of vasoactive substances that lead to migraine. **Sumatriptan (Imitrex)** was the first selective serotonin receptor agonist developed specifically to treat migraine; other agents include **almotriptan** (**Axert**), **naratriptan** (**Amerge**), **rizatriptan** (**Maxalt**), and **zolmitriptan** (**Zomig**). As they differ slightly in pharmacokinetics and individual response, trial of a different **serotonin receptor agonist** is warranted if one is not effective.

Sumatriptan is effective in decreasing the severity of headache in 54 to 80 percent of patients. It is also effective in relieving the nausea, photophobia, and phonophobia that can accompany migraine. **Sumatriptan** should be taken after the aura of migraine passes, as it is found to be effective only after the headache symptoms appear. **Sumatriptan** is available in PO, subcutaneous (SC), and intranasal forms. The dose for PO **sumatriptan** is 25 to 100 mg initially and may be repeated every 2 hours for up to 24 hours (maximum 300 mg in 24 hours). Although an initial dose of 25 mg should be tried with a patient who has never had **sumatriptan**, research has shown that an initial dose of 50 to 100 mg is superior in relieving migraine symptoms (Pfaffenrath, Cunin, Sjonell, & Prendergst, 1998; Carpay, Schoenen, Ahmad, Kinrade, & Boswell, 2004). Carpay et al studied the efficacy and tolerability of fast-disintegrating, rapid release **sumatriptan** and found 51.1 percent of patients who received 50 mg of **sumatriptan** were pain free after 2 hours, whereas 66.2 percent of those who received 100 mg were pain free at 2 hours after dosing. The initial SC dose of **sumatriptan** is 6 mg, and 82 percent of patients report relief in 20 minutes. The dose may be repeated in 1 hour if there is no relief, for a maximum of two 6-mg doses in 24 hours. Intranasal **sumatriptan** has a slower onset than does SC (2 h versus 20 min) and is less effective in relieving headache (62% at 2 h), yet intranasal dosing may be more appealing for children and for patients who fear self-administering injectable medication. After a dose of **sumatriptan**, up to 40 percent of headaches recur within 10 to 14 hours, and a second dose may be necessary. Do not repeat the dose of **sumatriptan** if the patient does not respond to the first dose.

Almotriptan binds with high affinity with 5-HT receptors 1D, 1B, and 1F. **Almotriptan** is rapidly absorbed from the GI tract with a peak of 1 to 3 hours after administration. Two hours after administration of 6.25 mg of **almotriptan**, 55 percent of study subjects reported pain relief from their migraine. When 12.5 mg is administered, 58.5 to 64.9 percent of subjects reported relief (Ortho-McNeil Neurologics, 2009). **Almotriptan** has a mean half-life of 3 to 4 hours and is primarily excreted renally. **Axert** is FDA approved for use in adolescents aged 12 to 17 years.

Naratriptan is similar to **sumatriptan** in its mechanism of action but differs in its pharmacokinetics. **Naratriptan** has a higher PO bioavailability (about 70%) and a longer half-life (6 hours) than does **sumatriptan.** This might lead to a lower rate of headache recurrence, with only 17 to 28 percent of patients reporting recurrence (Mathew, 1997). These differences may lead the practitioner to choose **naratriptan** as the first-line **triptan. Naratriptan** has been studied in adolescents (12 to 17 years), and the reported adverse events do not differ from the adult studies. One factor that may prevent the use of **naratriptan** is that its half-life and plasma levels are increased with concurrent use of **oral contraceptives**, and the dose should be lowered.

Rizatriptan, also a **5-HT$_1$ serotonin receptor agonist**, has oral bioavailability that is better than **sumatriptan** (about 45% versus 15%) but not as good as that of **naratriptan.** Because its half-life is similar to **sumatriptan** (both 2 to 3 hours), cost and PO absorption may be factors when choosing between **rizatriptan** and **sumatriptan. Rizatriptan** is available in PO tablet or PO disintegrating tablet, which may be preferred for some patients with nausea as a major symptom of migraine. One caution with **rizatriptan** is that plasma levels of **rizatriptan** are increased significantly when taken with **propranolol**, and concurrent use should be avoided.

Zolmitriptan has a higher PO bioavailability than do **sumatriptan** and **rizatriptan** (60% in females, 38% in males) and a similar half-life. **Zolmitriptan** is the only **triptan** that interacts with **cimetidine** (doubles the half-life and plasma levels of **zolmitriptan**), and this may be a factor in prescribing. **Zolmitriptan's** half-life and clearance are also affected by **oral contraceptives.**

All **triptans** are contraindicated in patients with coronary artery disease or uncontrolled hypertension because of their potential to constrict coronary artery vessels. The **triptans** are contraindicated in pregnancy. None of the **triptans** can be used if **ergotamine** derivatives have been used in the prior 24 hours because of increased vasospastic reactions; their effects may be additive. The **triptans sumatriptan, zolmitriptan,** and **rizatriptan** interact with **monoamine oxidase inhibitors (MAOIs)**, and should not be used concurrently or within 2 weeks of discontinuing the **MAOI**. All of the **triptans** interact with **selective serotonin reuptake inhibitors (SSRIs)**, causing serotonin syndrome. **Sumatriptan** can be used in children, but consultation with a pediatric neurologist is advisable.

Antiemetics

Antiemetics are an integral part of migraine management. Gastric emptying and oral absorption of medications are decreased in migraine patients, especially those patients with nausea and vomiting as a component of their migraine. A dose of **metoclopramide (Reglan)** is often recommended as part of migraine therapy (ICSI, 2009). Other commonly used **antiemetics** recommended as adjunct therapy by ICSI (2009) are the **phenothiazine antiemetics, perphenazine (Trilafon), prochlorperazine (Compazine)**, and **chlorpromazine (Thorazine).**

Preventive Therapy

Preventive therapy should be considered for any patient who experiences severely incapacitating or frequent severe migraines (more than two per month) and patients who cannot tolerate abortive medications because of either chronic illness (coronary artery disease or hypertension) or the adverse effects of abortive medications. Preventive medication is also recommended if the patient is taking abortive medication more than twice a week. The primary goal of preventive therapy is to use the least amount of medication with the fewest side effects to decrease migraine symptoms. If medication overuse is suspected, it must be treated first before starting the patient on preventive therapy; this topic is covered later in this chapter.

Patients must understand that preventive therapy will not completely eliminate migraine and that a 50 percent reduction in migraine attacks is considered a success. Fewer than 10 percent of patients become headache free with preventive therapy. The patient must also be aware that it may take 4 weeks before preventive therapy begins to be effective and that there is an increase in effectiveness for 3 months. It is common for patients to discontinue preventive therapy after only a couple of weeks and label it as ineffective. Education is the key to success for preventive therapy. Another component to preventive therapy is a headache diary that is initiated prior to preventive therapy and then maintained to determine the frequency, severity, and duration of migraine. This tool enables the provider to assess the effectiveness of preventive therapy. Examples of daily, weekly, and monthly headache diaries can be found at the American Headache Society's Web site (http://www.americanheadachesociety.org).

Because preventive therapy cannot completely eliminate migraines, the patient should also have acute or abortive medications to take for migraine. The provider should recognize interactions between preventive and acute therapies and prescribe accordingly (see Table 35–2). The significance of avoiding migraine triggers, which cannot be overlooked in migraine prevention, is discussed later in the chapter.

Beta Blockers

Beta blockers are one of the first-line choices for migraine preventive therapy (ICSI, 2009), with up to 44 percent reduction in migraine reported. The mechanism of action in migraine prevention is not clear, but it is thought that they may affect the central catecholaminergic system and brain serotonin (5-HT$_2$) receptors. They also block beta receptors in vascular smooth muscle to prevent arterial dilatation. **Propranolol (Inderal)** and **timolol (Blocadren)** are the only **beta blockers** that have been FDA approved for migraine preventive therapy, although **nadolol (Corgard), metoprolol (Lopressor)**, and **atenolol (Tenormin)** have also been shown to be effective.

Propranolol is typically started at a dose of 60 to 80 mg a day and slowly increased every third or fourth day to a maximum of 240 mg per day in adults. Twice-daily dosing has the highest compliance rate. Individual response varies, and the patient should be monitored closely. A pulse below 50 or a systolic blood pressure below 100 mm Hg in the adult suggests that the maximum dosage has been reached. The dose in children is 0.5 to 1 mg/kg a day, divided into two doses and titrated every 3 to 4 days, to a maximum of 2 to 4 mg/kg/day. Pediatric patients should be monitored closely, and consultation with a pediatric neurologist before initiating and during therapy is advisable. A trial of 3 months in both adult and pediatric patients is necessary as the response improves over time. Treatment should be reassessed every 6 months, and it may be discontinued. **Propranolol** needs to be tapered slowly (over a week) to prevent drug withdrawal headache. Adverse effects of **propranolol** include fatigue, lethargy, and depression, and it should not be the first-line drug in depressed patients. It is also not well tolerated by athletes. **Propranolol** is contraindicated in patients with congestive heart failure, asthma, chronic obstructive pulmonary disease, peripheral vascular disease, diabetes mellitus, or Wolff-Parkinson-White syndrome. **Propranolol** is Pregnancy Category C, but it is safer than some of the other preventive agents.

If **propranolol** is not effective or not well tolerated, one of the other **beta blockers** can be tried; failure to respond to one **beta blocker** does not predict response to another. If a patient has asthma or other respiratory disorders, **metoprolol** and **atenolol** may be used because they are cardioselective (see Table 35–2 for dosing of these agents).

Tricyclic Antidepressants

Tricyclic antidepressants, specifically **amitriptyline (Elavil)**, are effective in reducing the frequency, severity, and duration of migraine attacks. **Amitriptyline** modulates neurotransmitters and appears to affect the central serotonin receptor function. Its antimigraine effect is unrelated to its antidepressant effect, and the antimigraine effect can often be achieved at lower doses than are required to treat depression. The patient should be started on 10 mg a day taken before bed and increased every 2 weeks to a total daily dose of 20 to 50 mg. Adverse effects that should be monitored include drowsiness (most common), dry mouth, weight gain, constipation, and orthostatic hypotension. **Amitriptyline** is contraindicated in patients with narrow-angle glaucoma, urinary retention, pregnancy, breastfeeding, and concurrent use of **MAOIs**. Other **tricyclic antidepressants** that may be used include **nortriptyline (Pamelor, Aventyl)**, which causes less drowsiness and anticholinergic effect than does **amitriptyline**.

Antieleptic Drugs

Antieleptic drugs (AEDs) are thought to work on migraines in a similar fashion as their effect on seizures. The AEDs are thought to decrease brain excitability by increasing the threshold for activation of the brainstem areas that are thought to be important for initiating migraine (Carmona & Bruera, 2009). The **AEDs** that are used in migraine include **divalproex (valproate)**, **gabapentin**, and **topiramate** (ICSI, 2009).

Divalproex (Depakote) has FDA labeling as a preventive treatment for migraine. **Divalproex** reduces the number of migraine attacks and also reduces the duration and intensity. It is notably appropriate to use in a patient with coexisting seizure disorder. The initial dose for migraine preventive therapy is 125 to 250 mg twice daily. The dosage can be increased by 125 or 250 mg weekly, to a maximum dose of 1,000 to 1,250 mg per day. Patients who are started on **divalproex** require baseline assessment of liver function, platelet count, and bleeding time, as hepatic failure and thrombocytopenia are rare adverse effects. Clinical monitoring of symptoms for liver failure or bleeding disorders is more indicative of potential problems than routine laboratory monitoring. **Divalproex** serum concentrations should be monitored during therapy if poor compliance, toxicity, or drug reactions are suspected. **Divalproex** is Pregnancy Category D.

Gabapentin has proven efficacy as migraine prophylaxis for some patients and is one of the recommended ICSI migraine prophylaxis drugs (2009). In a controlled clinical trial of **gabapentin** for migraine prophylaxis, 46.4 percent of the **gabapentin** group (2,400 mg/d) had a significant reduction in migraine after four weeks of treatment (Mathew, Rapoport, Saper, Magnus, Klapper, Ramadan, et al, 2001). Patients should be started on **gabapentin** 300 mg daily and titrated up to 2,400 mg per day. A suggested titration is 300 mg daily, titrated up to 900 mg daily at the end of week 1, then titrate up to 1,500 mg per day at the end of week 2. During week 3, the dose is increased to 2,100 mg per day and week 4 the dose increases to 2,400 mg/day (Mathew et al, 2001; ICSI). **Gabapentin** is generally well tolerated, although fatigue, somnolence, and weight gain are known adverse effects.

Topiramate (Topamax) has an FDA indication for migraine prophylaxis. It is rapidly absorbed from the GI tract and has a long duration of action. Migraine patients are started on a dose of 25 mg per day and titrated up in 1-week intervals. During week 1, patients take 25 mg before bed, then 25 mg twice a day in week 2. In week 3, patients take 25 mg in the morning and 50 mg in the evening, then 50 mg twice a day. Dosages of 25 mg of **topiramate** twice daily may be effective (Carmona & Bruera, 2009). **Topiramate** adverse effects include weight loss, somnolence, fatigue, and kidney stones. The AEDs are described in detail in Chapter 15.

NSAIDs

NSAIDs may also be used for migraine preventive therapy. The most commonly used NSAID is **naproxen sodium**, dosed at 550 mg twice a day. **NSAIDs** are particularly effective in treating menstrual migraines if daily dosing is started the week before menses and continued for a week after. In older patients, NSAIDs may pose a higher risk of causing nephrotoxicity or gastrointestinal problems.

Calcium Channel Blockers

Calcium channel blockers are also commonly used for migraine preventive therapy, although their effectiveness has had mixed results, and they should not be a first-line choice. Calcium channel blockers are thought to prevent migraine by inhibiting vasospasm of the cerebral arteries and by preventing cerebral hypoxia during migraine attacks. Verapamil (Calan, Isoptin) is the most commonly used for migraine prevention. Nifedipine and diltiazem are not as effective in controlling migraines and probably should not be prescribed for this use. Calcium channel blockers may be the first-line choice for patients with hypertension who cannot take beta blockers. Dosing of verapamil is shown in Table 35–2. Adverse effects include sedation, weight gain, depression, and extrapyramidal symptoms. Calcium channel blockers are contraindicated in pregnancy, Parkinson's disease, and depression.

Methysergide

Methysergide (Sansert) is an ergot derivative that is a 5-HT_2 receptor agonist that inhibits or blocks the effects of serotonin. Methysergide is not commonly used because of its potential for adverse effects (reported in 30% to 50% of patients). The most serious adverse effect is retroperitoneal fibrosis or related conditions with prolonged therapy. If methysergide is prescribed, the patient should have a drug-free period of 3 to 4 weeks after every 6 months of treatment. Methysergide is contraindicated in pregnancy. Ergot derivatives should be avoided in patients with coronary artery disease, peripheral vascular disease, impaired renal or liver function, or hypertension.

Nonpharmacological Management of Migraine

Nonpharmacological management of migraine includes a variety of interventions and alternative therapies. The first and most important is migraine trigger identification and avoidance. Alternative therapies, including herbs (feverfew and butterbur), vitamins (riboflavin), and coenzyme Q10 are all commonly used in migraine therapy (Taylor, 2009). Nontraditional health care should be addressed; up to 70 percent of patients who seek alternative therapy never discuss it with their health-care provider. Lifestyle issues such as stress and work environment can be modified to decrease migraine attacks or make them more manageable.

Identifying Triggers

Identifying and avoiding triggers can significantly decrease migraines. Many patients identify certain foods, odors, or medications that may cause headache. Table 35–1 lists common migraine triggers. Patients need to be encouraged to use their headache diary to determine if something is a trigger. Common foods like chocolate, yogurt, or the food additive aspartame can trigger a migraine, and patients are often not aware that something is provoking their headaches. Smoking cessation and sleep regulation may also prove helpful in headache prevention.

Alternative Therapies

Alternative therapies that may assist in the treatment of migraine vary considerably. MigraLief is a commonly used herbal supplement containing feverfew, riboflavin, magnesium, and other vitamins that is available OTC. A naturopath may prescribe additional herbal medicine to treat migraines. Other alternative therapies that may be beneficial include acupuncture, aromatherapy, chiropractic manipulation, hypnosis, and reflexology. Patients can try massage therapy, relaxation therapy, and yoga, which all appear to reduce the tension and stress that may lead to migraine. The health-care provider should have access to local health education classes that teach yoga and relaxation classes or a local massage therapist for referral. A simple technique of applying ice to the head can often decrease the severity of pain associated with migraine; patients can be encouraged to try this simple technique as an adjunct to or a substitute for their medication.

Biofeedback

Biofeedback techniques are helpful for many patients. Biofeedback is thought to change vascular dilatation. Although the exact mechanism is unclear, some patients do report improvement in their migraine symptoms. Biofeedback is often combined with other relaxation therapies and may give the patient a feeling of control and mastery over the migraine symptoms.

Monitoring

Patients with migraine headaches should keep a headache diary, especially when a new treatment is begun or if modifications are made in the therapy. The health-care provider can use the diary to determine if the treatment is decreasing the frequency, duration, or severity of the migraine. The diary can also track adverse side effects of the medication prescribed. Overuse of medication can be determined, and an alternative plan developed. Patients should also have their blood pressure monitored for hypertension if they are on a triptan, ergotamine derivative, beta blocker, or calcium channel blocker. Patients on divalproex should have their liver function and complete blood count (CBC) tested every 2 weeks for a total of 6 weeks.

Outcome Evaluation

The goal of migraine treatment is to minimize the impact of migraine headaches on patients' quality of life, social functioning, and ability to work. It is evaluated by discussing with patients how their migraine is affecting their quality of life and by having them record in their headache diary when their headaches adversely affect their quality of life and ability to work. Modification of the treatment plan multiple times until the optimal treatment is found is important in achieving the goal of minimal impact from migraine on quality of life.

Avoidance of patients' identified migraine triggers often decreases the frequency of headache. It is evaluated by having patients record in their headache diaries any headache associated with a specific trigger. If patients are unable to determine if a specific item is a trigger, an elimination diet may be tried. Patients eliminate one item from the common triggers list for 2 weeks and then reintroduce it into their diet. This process may take weeks or months, but the reward of identifying a trigger is worth the perceived inconvenience.

Before beginning preventive therapy for frequent migraine sufferers, patients must be clear that the final goal is to reduce the frequency of migraine by 50 percent and that total elimination of migraine is not a realistic goal. Evaluating the success of preventive therapy by use of the headache diary and by demonstrating a decrease in frequency to patients will assist in clarifying the true success of treatment. It is essential to treat patients for an adequate amount of time (2 to 3 months) before a change in treatment.

Patient Education

Patient education should include a discussion of information related to the overall treatment plan as well as that specific to the drug therapy, reasons for taking the drug, drugs as part of the total treatment regimen, and adherence issues (see the Patient Education box).

Patient education is the key to successful migraine treatment. Patient education related to migraine should focus on the following:

1. An understanding of the diagnosis and nature of migraines.
2. The nonpharmacological measures to prevent and treat migraines, such as trigger identification and avoidance and the use of relaxation, massage, or ice to counter pain.
3. Education about the medication that is prescribed. Specifically, expected side effects, adverse side effects, interactions with other medications, and maximum dosages should be explained. Medication overuse should be addressed at the beginning of treatment.
4. The patient as an integral part of the treatment plan. Therapy is less effective if the patient does not keep a headache diary or uses the medication in a way different from how it was prescribed.
5. Realistic expectations of treatment. The patient will probably not be migraine-free, but the goal is to decrease the severity and frequency of migraines. Acute treatment should provide relief within an hour or two, or a change in therapy may be indicated.
6. Caution the patient about using OTC medications to treat the headache unless they are part of the treatment plan.

HEADACHES

PATIENT EDUCATION

Related to the Overall Treatment Plan/Disease Process

- ☐ Pathophysiology of headache
- ☐ Role of lifestyle modifications
- ☐ Importance of adherence to the treatment regimen
- ☐ Self-monitoring of symptoms and associated symptoms
- ☐ What to do when symptoms and associated symptoms worsen
- ☐ Need for regular follow-up visits with the primary care provider

Specific to the Drug Therapy

- ☐ Reason for taking the drug and its anticipated action in the disease process
- ☐ Doses (including maximum dosage) and schedules for taking the drug
- ☐ Possible adverse effects and what to do if they occur
- ☐ Interactions between other treatment modalities and these drugs
- ☐ Potential for medication-overuse headache

Reasons for Taking the Drug(s)

Patient education about specific drugs is provided in the appropriate chapters. Specific reasons for taking the drug(s) should be discussed on an individual basis, depending on the diagnosis and nature of the headache. Medication overuse should also be discussed at the beginning of treatment.

HEADACHES—cont'd

PATIENT EDUCATION

Drugs as Part of the Total Treatment Regimen

The total treatment regimen includes pharmacological and nonpharmacological measures, as well as the headache diary. A realistic expectation and goals of the individualized treatment plan should be presented.

Adherence Issues

Nonadherence with the treatment regimen may affect functional status. Health-care providers should be aware of the potential problem of nonadherence and discuss the importance of adherence with the patient and family.

Education resources available for both the patient and the provider on the Internet and in print enable better understanding of the pathology and treatment of migraine and other headaches. The patient needs to be directed to reliable information. There are numerous patient-health organizations, pharmaceutical manufacturers, online support groups, and even Web sites that are maintained by private individuals. Box 35–1 provides a short list of the patient-health sites and provider information sites that are considered reliable, comprehensive, and trustworthy and that may be helpful for the health-care provider who cares for patients with headaches.

TENSION-TYPE HEADACHES

Up to 90 percent of all headaches could be classified as tension-type headache. At least 15 percent of patients have experienced their first tension headache by age 10. Tension-type headaches can occur daily and may become persistent and intractable. Like migraine, 75 percent

BOX 35–1 HEADACHE RESOURCES FOR PATIENTS AND HEALTH-CARE PROVIDERS

American Headache Society

http://www.americanheadachesociety.org

The American Headache Society (AHS) is a professional society of health-care providers dedicated to the study and treatment of headache and face pain. Founded in 1959, AHS brings together physicians and other health-care providers from various fields and specialties to share concepts and developments about headache and related conditions.

American Council for Headache Education

http://www.achenet.org

This site is geared for patients and is connected with the American Headache Society. There is patient information on headaches in general, migraines, and prevention and treatment of headaches, as well as a discussion forum for patients. There are specific sections for children and women.

National Headache Foundation

http://www.headaches.org

Nonprofit organization dedicated to educating headache sufferers and health-care professionals about headache causes and treatments.

US Headache Consortium

https://www.americanheadachesociety.org/professional resources/USHeadacheConsortiumGuidelines.asp

The organizations involved in the consortium include the American Academy of Neurology (AAN), the American Headache Society (AHS), the American Academy of Family Physicians (AAFP), the American College of Emergency Physicians (ACEP), American College of Physicians American Society of Internal Medicine (ACP-ASIM), the American Osteopathic Association (AOA), and the National Headache Foundation (NHF).

The consortium completed a landmark evidenced-based review of the literature concerning the diagnosis and treatment of migraine linked from this site.

International Headache Society

http://www.i-h-s.org/

The International Headache Society (IHS) is an international professional organization working with others for the benefit of people affected by headache disorders. The purpose of IHS is to advance headache science, education, and management, and promote headache awareness worldwide. Note: The Web site asks about membership but nonmembers can access all guidelines.

of patients with chronic tension-type headaches are women. Patients may suffer from both tension-type and migraine headaches.

The patient usually describes a band-like pressure that is persistent dull pain. The pain is usually bilateral in location and nonpulsating. The headache may change in intensity and last from 30 minutes to 7 days. Unlike migraine, tension-type headaches are not worsened by physical activity. The patient may have mild nausea or photophobia, but severe nausea, vomiting, and aura are absent. Tension headaches may increase in frequency and severity in times of stress or emotional upheaval. Chronic tension-type headache is diagnosed when the headache is present for more than 15 days per month.

Pathophysiology

The pathology of tension-type headaches is poorly understood. It was thought that muscle contraction was the primary cause of tension headache, and it was previously called muscle contraction headache. The patient may exhibit tenderness of the extracranial soft tissue and of the cervical or masseter muscles. The muscle pain and tenderness in tension headaches may resemble fibromyalgia. Prolonged stress, eyestrain, and sitting for long periods, such as when using a computer, may lead to increased tension headaches. There is little agreement currently about the cause of tension headaches.

Goals of Therapy

The primary goal of tension-type headache treatment is to decrease the frequency and severity of headache and to provide acute relief of headache once it begins. Although total eradication of headaches may not be possible, a combination of relaxation therapy and preventive medication, when necessary, usually decreases the frequency of headache.

Rational Drug Selection

The pharmacological management of tension-type headaches, like migraine, focuses on acute or abortive treatment and preventive therapy. A key distinction between tension headache and migraine treatment is that tension headaches do not respond to **ergotamine** derivatives or **triptans**.

Acute Therapy

Acute therapy in the treatment of tension-type headaches includes a combination of pharmacological and nonpharmacological therapy.

Mild Analgesics

For mild to moderate tension headaches, OTC **analgesics** are quite effective. ASA, **acetaminophen**, or one of the NSAIDs (**ibuprofen** or **naproxen**), taken at the beginning of a tension headache, can be effective in relieving headache pain. The dosing is the same as for migraine. Patients should be cautioned not to use OTC **analgesics** for headache more than two to three times per week because they can cause medication-overuse headache. Patients often self-medicate with OTC products prior to seeking care for their headaches, and therefore a history of what the patient has taken for headache relief and in what amounts is necessary. This history assists the health-care provider in determining if the headache has received adequate amounts of analgesic or if the tension headache is complicated by medication-overuse headache.

Combination Medications

Combination medications are commonly prescribed to treat both migraine and tension-type headaches. Products that combine either **butalbital** with ASA or APAP or **isometheptene** with APAP and **dichloralphenazone** are effective in treating tension headache. These products should be used cautiously because medication-overuse headaches can occur if dosages are higher than recommended or if they are taken more than 2 days per week. The provider should distribute a maximum of 30 tablets of either of these medications per month to make sure the patient is not overusing them.

Preventive Therapy

Preventive therapy should be considered if the patient is having more than one to two headaches per week. Used more than twice a week, the medications used for acute tension headache therapy all have the potential for causing medication-overuse headaches. A trial of preventive medication is likely to be helpful and should be considered early in treatment.

Beta Blockers

Beta blockers can be used for prophylactic treatment of tension headache. The dosing and contraindications are the same as for migraine preventive therapy.

Tricyclic Antidepressants

Tricyclic antidepressants are successful in reducing tension headaches in patients who are depressed and in those who are not. They appear to enhance the endogenous pain-suppressing systems in the brain. **Amitriptyline** and **nortriptyline** are used in the same dosages as for migraine (see Table 35–2). Patients with tension-type headaches may also have depression, and dosing for depression may be successful if a lower dose is not effective.

Nonpharmacological Therapy

Nonpharmacological therapy is central in the preventive treatment of tension-type headaches. Stress management, biofeedback, and regular exercise can help to reduce medication use for tension headaches (ICSI, 2009). Topical heat or cold packs should be applied. Massage therapy and relaxation therapy help to relax the muscle tension that can aggravate tension headaches. Alternative therapies such as acupuncture and herbal medicine prescribed by a naturopath may improve headache symptoms. Referral to a psychologist or psychiatrist may assist in identifying and treating underlying anxiety that may be contributing to the tension headaches.

Monitoring

Monitoring for effectiveness of acute or preventive medication prescribed for tension headache should be done frequently (every 1 to 2 months) at the beginning of treatment. The patient must keep a headache diary to assist in determining if treatment is successful. Once a patient is stable on an acute or preventive medication, the patient can be seen less frequently. The provider should continue to monitor the use of combination drugs (**butalbital** and **isometheptene** compounds) to safeguard against potential medication-overuse headaches developing from overuse.

Outcome Evaluation

Evaluating the success of tension-type headache therapy is achieved by monitoring the patient's headache diary to determine if there is a decrease in the frequency or severity of headaches. If the patient develops new skills, such as stress reduction or relaxation, or begins exercising regularly, these efforts ought to be acknowledged by the health-care provider. As tension-type headaches often last off and on for many years, reevaluation and reworking the treatment regimen may happen multiple times.

Patient Education

Patient education should include a discussion of information related to the overall treatment plan as well as that specific to the drug therapy, reasons for taking the drug, drugs as part of the total treatment plan, and adherence issues. For general patient education information, see the previous Patient Education section.

Patient education information specific to treating tension-type headaches should focus on the following principles:

1. Patients need to know what tension-type headaches are and how they differ from migraines or pathological headaches.
2. Medication education ensures that the acute or preventive medications are taken appropriately. Prevention of medication overuse should be addressed early in the treatment.
3. Nonpharmacological therapies should be encouraged and the patient given local resources available, such as yoga classes, relaxation tapes, and massage therapists.
4. The importance of the patient's participation by keeping a headache diary needs to be stressed. Because most treatment decisions are based on response to therapy, the headache diary is invaluable to the successful management of headaches.

CHRONIC DAILY HEADACHES

Approximately 35 to 45 percent of patients who seek treatment at headache centers suffer from daily or near daily headaches (Mathew, 1997). Use of drugs for acute headache treatment more than nine days a month is associated with increased risk of chronic daily headaches (ICSI, 2009). Chronic daily headaches (CDH) can be classified as chronic tension-type headache, transformed migraine, hemicrania continua, medication-overuse headache, or new daily persistent headache. Chronic tension-type headaches have already been addressed. Medication-overuse is addressed later in this chapter. New persistent daily headache (NPDH) is uncommon, the onset is usually abrupt (patients can often pinpoint the date), and it is usually self-limiting. The cause is thought to be Epstein-Barr virus–induced immune changes. Treatment of NPDH is not discussed in this chapter because little information is available; these patients should be referred to a neurologist for care.

Pathophysiology

The pathology of CDH is often unclear and of mixed origin. There is a clear difference between transformed migraine and hemicrania continua. The boundary between chronic tension-type headache and transformed migraine is less clear and may require a neurology referral for treatment.

The term transformed migraine refers to CDH that starts as episodic migraine headache with onset in adolescence. The initial migraines have the pathogenesis of migraine discussed earlier. In transformed migraine, the overuse of **analgesics** appears to alter platelet membrane transduction, affecting circulating serotonin levels. Other abnormalities in blood biochemistry, such as low intracellular levels of magnesium, may also play a role in transformed migraine (Mendizabal, 1998). There is also a higher incidence of coexisting psychopathology, with a strong association between migraine and depression, anxiety disorders, panic disorders, and neuroticism.

Hemicrania continua, also known as chronic paroxysmal hemicrania, is a rare headache syndrome, and the pathogenesis is unknown. The patient, most often a woman, suffers from multiple (10 to 20) and short-lived (less than 20 minutes) episodes of severe unilateral, excruciating pain in the area of the eye, forehead, and temple.

Goals of Treatment

The first goal of treatment for CDH is to break the pattern of daily headache. The patient is then stabilized on prophylactic or preventive therapy.

Rational Drug Selection

Transformed Migraine

In most patients with transformed migraine, the daily headache cycle can be broken by using repeated doses of IV **DHE**. Approximately 70 to 80 percent of patients respond to **DHE**. The patient is given a test dose of 0.33 mL of **DHE** (1 mg/mL solution) with 5 mg of **metoclopramide** or 10 mg of **prochlorperazine (Compazine)**, followed by 0.5 mL of **DHE** and one of the antinausea medications every 6 hours for 48 to 72 hours. This treatment usually requires inpatient treatment. **DHE** is contraindicated in coronary and peripheral vascular disease.

Alternatives to **DHE** include **chlorpromazine (Thorazine)** and **prochlorperazine**. If the patient has medication overuse headache due to misuse of **analgesics**, **ergots**, or combination medications, the patient has to be detoxified, which is discussed later in this chapter. Treatment of transformed migraine may require consultation with a neurologist.

Preventive pharmacotherapy can be started after the headache cycle is broken. The patient usually responds to migraine-preventive medications such as **propranolol**, **divalproex**, or a **tricyclic antidepressant**. **Amitriptyline** is a good choice if the patient is also depressed. **Fluoxetine (Prozac)** may also be used as a preventive medication; the dose is 40 mg daily. The patient is on preventive medication until the headache days are reduced by 50 percent, and then an additional 3 to 4 weeks, for a total of 6 to 12 weeks.

The patient should also receive alternative therapy to treat CDH. Behavioral counseling, biofeedback therapy, relaxation therapy, physical exercise, and acupuncture are all valid alternative therapies for treatment of CDH.

Hemicrania Continua

Hemicrania continua or chronic paroxysmal hemicrania is a rare disorder that responds completely to **indomethacin** and to nothing else. **Indomethacin (Indocin)** 75 to 150 mg is given daily. Referral to a neurologist is recommended.

Monitoring

Monitoring of patients with CDH who are on preventive therapy requires the patient to keep a diary of headache and medication use. Patients' blood pressure should be monitored if they are on a **beta blocker**, and liver function monitored if on **divalproex**, as per migraine therapy monitoring. Ongoing monitoring of headache is necessary, as 31 percent may have recurrence of headache in spite of preventive medication.

Outcome Evaluation

Patients with CDH are difficult to treat. Treatment success is determined by how effective it has been in breaking the cycle of daily headaches and how effective the preventive treatment is. The patient's headache diary is key in the evaluation of the success of treatment.

Patient Education

Patient education should include a discussion of information related to the overall treatment plan as well as that specific to the drug therapy, reasons for taking the drug, drugs as part of the total treatment plan, and adherence issues. For general patient education information, see the Patient Education box.

Patient education information specific to treating CDH should focus on the following principles:

1. Education about the nature of the disorder, particularly that it is biological in origin, with neurochemical changes producing the headache.
2. Overuse of **analgesics**, leading to medication-overuse headache, must be emphasized.
3. The influence of stress, anxiety, depression, and inability to relax should be discussed, and the patient encouraged to use nonpharmacological therapies to decrease headache.

CLUSTER HEADACHES

Cluster headaches are characterized by intense pain lasting for 15 minutes to 2 hours; they occur in "clusters" of several weeks or months, with the headache subsiding for months at a time, often to recur. The patient can experience one to three attacks a day, usually at the same time of day. They occur most frequently at night, awakening the patient from sleep. Men are affected more than women, with onset in their late twenties. The pain of a cluster headache is unique in that it occurs behind or around one eye, with tearing, conjunctival injection, and drooping of the eyelid common symptoms. There may be nasal congestion, facial flushing, and sweating. The pain is so severe that the patient is unable to lie down or sit still, often pacing the floor in pain.

Pathophysiology

There is no clear etiology for cluster headaches. It is most likely a neuronal disorder originating in the hypothalamus. The clockwork-like timing of cluster headaches suggests that the circadian pacemaker or biological "clock" is dysfunctional.

Goals of Treatment

Relieving the pain of an acute cluster headache and decreasing the length of time of the cluster are the goals of cluster headache management.

Rational Drug Therapy

Most patients with cluster headaches require acute and preventive therapy. The acute attacks are severe and last only a short time; therefore, the intervention must be fast acting. The patient usually requires both acute and preventive medications to manage the headache.

Acute Therapy

Oxygen therapy administered via a 100 percent nonrebreather mask for 15 to 30 minutes often provides immediate relief of cluster headache (ICSI, 2009).

Ergotamine derivatives are also effective for acute cluster headaches, although the PO forms are poorly absorbed. **Ergotamine** suppositories or DHE intranasally or IM has a more rapid onset and is preferred (see Table 35–2 for dosing). **Ergotamine** may also be administered in a 2-mg dose given before bed if nocturnal attacks occur frequently.

Intranasal lidocaine is thought to be effective in treating cluster headache. The patient lies supine, hyperextends the head 45 degrees, and rotates it 30 degrees to the side of the headache. The **lidocaine** nasal solution is then dripped into the nostril on the affected side over 30 seconds. The onset is approximately 5 minutes.

Sumatriptan, if administered SC, may provide relief of acute cluster headaches, although it is not considered a first-line drug. Intranasal **sumatriptan** may also be effective.

Preventive Therapy

Ergotamine administered in a 2-mg dose before bed can prevent nocturnal cluster headaches. **Ergotamine** 1 mg given four times a day may also prevent cluster headaches. **Ergotamine** should be withdrawn every seventh day to prevent ergotism and to determine if the cluster has ceased.

Verapamil can prevent cluster headaches in some patients. **Calcium channel blockers** are thought to prevent cluster headache by inhibiting vasospasm of the cerebral arteries. Dosing of **verapamil** is given in Table 35–2. Cluster headaches appear to need dosing in the high range to achieve headache reduction.

Divalproex can be effective in preventing cluster headaches. The dosing is the same as for migraine prophylaxis (see Table 35–2).

Lithium appears to have some effect on cluster headaches in some patients, and a trial of **lithium** is warranted if the patient does not respond to other preventive medications. The dose for cluster headache prevention is 300 mg daily to a maximum of 300 mg three times a day. The patient needs careful monitoring for adverse effects, including electrocardiogram (ECG), electrolytes, thyroid function, creatinine, and CBC studies.

Nonpharmacological therapies include avoidance of all **alcohol** during the clustering of headaches because **alcohol** often precipitates a headache. Patients often are able to drink **alcohol** between headache clusters without adverse effects. **Tobacco**, stress, anger, and vigorous physical activity should be avoided. The patient needs to maintain a normal sleep pattern, if possible. Cluster headaches do not appear to respond to self-care measures such as massage and relaxation.

Monitoring

Cluster headaches can be severely disabling, and the intense pain and loss of sleep can significantly affect the patient's quality of life. The health-care provider needs to monitor the patient for suicidal thoughts during the headache. The headache diary helps to monitor the effectiveness of acute and preventive medications. A patient treated with **lithium** requires careful monitoring of ECG and chemistries throughout treatment.

Outcome Evaluation

Cluster headaches by definition are self-limiting and will eventually stop, regardless of treatment. The focus of care is to provide measures that shorten or prevent cluster headaches during the cluster. Evaluation of the effectiveness of acute and preventive therapy is accomplished by self-report with a headache diary. Modifications in pharmacological management of cluster headaches should be based on the headache diary.

Patient Education

Patient education should include a discussion of information related to the overall treatment plan as well as that specific to the drug therapy, reasons for taking the drug, drugs as part of the total treatment plan, and adherence issues. For general patient education information, see the Patient Education box.

Patient education information specific to treating cluster headaches should focus on the following principles:

1. Educating the family about cluster headache, particularly the fact that it is a benign condition, in spite of the severe pain experienced during attacks.
2. Self-management of acute medications. The headache is usually brief, and therefore the patient must be able to self-medicate to provide relief. The pain

may be gone by the time the patient can get transportation to a medical clinic.

3. Avoidance of **alcohol** is crucial during clusters of headaches.

MEDICATION-OVERUSE HEADACHES

Drug-rebound or drug-induced headache was reclassified by the International Headache Society as medication-overuse headache in 2008 (Ferrari, Coccia, & Sternieri, 2008). Medication-overuse headache should be considered in any patient who reports daily use of **analgesics**, combination medications such as **butalbital** or **ergotamine** derivatives or one of the **triptans**, with medication overuse reported in one-third of patients with chronic daily headaches (Maizels, 2004). **Caffeine** can also cause withdrawal headache when abruptly discontinued. The headache recurs as the medication wears off, compelling the patient to take another dose of medication, which causes a cycle of medication overuse and rebound. The patient may never have complete relief of pain, leading to a patient concern about serious pathology. A careful history of all the medications, including OTC **analgesics** that the patient takes on a daily basis, can help to determine if drug rebound is the issue or if a patient has CDH. A thorough history and physical examination with negative findings other than medication use is reassuring to the provider, but not always initially to the patient.

The health-care provider needs to be aware of the clinical features of medication-overuse headaches. According to the International Headache Society diagnostic criteria, the following clinical characteristics are found in medication-overuse headache (Silberstein et al, 2005):

1. Headache present on more than 15 days/month, fulfilling criteria 3 and 4 below.
2. Regular overuse for more than 3 months of one or more drugs that can be taken for acute and/or symptomatic treatment of headache.
3. The headache has developed or markedly worsened during medication overuse.
4. Headache resolves or reverts to its previous pattern within 2 months after discontinuation of overused medication.

Other symptoms reported may be worsening of headache as analgesia wears off and the slightest physical or mental exertion brings on the headache (Matthew, 1997). An accurate diagnosis is essential because chronic daily headaches and medication-overuse headache have similar presentation (Silberstein et al, 2005).

Pathophysiology

Dependence on either **ergotamine** or the OTC **analgesics** is thought to have physical and psychological elements. The overuse of simple **analgesics** (ASA or APAP), either alone or in combination with **butalbital** or **caffeine**, has a high potential for causing medication-overuse headache. Although the exact process is unclear, it is thought to suppress or alter the central pain-control mechanism. **Ergotamine** causes a clear pharmacological dependence and subsequent withdrawal. When a patient has analgesic-rebound headache, other headache therapies used for acute or preventive therapy may be resistant to treatment. The patient must be detoxified before preventive therapy can be started.

Goals of Therapy

The goal of treating medication-overuse headache is that the patient will no longer be taking daily doses of **analgesics** or **ergotamine** and will be stabilized on preventive medication. The goal during the withdrawal period should be minimizing the intensity of the withdrawal headache.

Rational Drug Therapy

Treatment of medication-overuse headache involves (1) withdrawal from offending agents, including **caffeine**, (2) transition therapy to support the patient during detoxification, and (3) initiation or adjustment of prophylaxis medication (Maizels, 2004). Anticipating withdrawal from daily or near-daily use of **analgesics**, **butalbital**-containing drugs, **triptans**, or **ergotamine** can make the patient anxious. The provider needs to adequately prepare the patient prior to the detoxification process, as discussed in the Patient Education section. Preventive therapy can be started when the withdrawal process is started or 2 to 3 weeks before or after the withdrawal process. Preventive therapy for migraine and tension-type headache has already been discussed. The advantage of starting preventive therapy either before or after the withdrawal process begins is that the patient may interpret withdrawal symptoms as adverse effects of preventive therapy (Moore & Noble, 1997). The practitioner should consult with a neurologist prior to embarking on detoxification of a patient with medication-overuse headache.

Withdrawal from the simple **analgesics**, ASA and APAP, or **caffeine**-containing medications is usually done on an outpatient basis. The patient stops taking the analgesic and is started on **Midrin** for 1 week and **cyproheptadine (Periactin)**. Another regimen involves a different class of analgesic **(naproxen)**, intranasal DHE, and **antiemetics**.

Butalbital-containing drugs **(Fiorinal, Fioricet)** may need to be tapered slowly because severe problems can develop with abrupt cessation. Serious withdrawal symptoms, such as delirium and seizures, can appear without warning. **Butalbital** use of less than 8 pills (400 mg) per day can be treated on an outpatient basis. Suggested regimens include **Midrin** *plus* **clonazepam (Klonopin)** for 1 week and then taper *or* **phenobarbital** for 1 week *plus* **promethazine (Phenergan)** for 1 to 2 weeks. If the patient is using more than eight pills per day, then inpatient drug detoxification is necessary, using IV DHE, **metoclopramide**, and IV fluids.

Ergotamine overuse can lead to ergotism as well as CDH. If the patient is taking 0.5 to 1 mg of **ergotamine** (either PO or rectally), the patient can be treated as an outpatient. One treatment is to give **naproxen** daily for 1 to 3 weeks *plus* **methylergonovine (Methergine)** *plus* **promethazine** for 1 to 2 weeks (Moore & Noble, 1997). If the patient is taking more than 1 mg per day of **ergotamine**, then inpatient treatment will probably be needed to provide supportive care. The withdrawal headache from **ergotamine** takes up to 72 hours to appear and lasts 72 hours or more.

Some patients may require inpatient management to get their headache under control. Prevention and astute diagnosis are the roles of the primary care provider in the care of medication-overuse headache. Consultation with a headache specialist is warranted to provide optimal evidence-based care for medication-overuse headache.

Monitoring

Monitoring begins with the provider's regulating the number of doses of acute relief medication the patient is allowed to have each month. If OTC analgesic overuse is suspected, then the provider needs to determine the number of doses the patient is taking in a day or a week. During the withdrawal period, the patient's symptoms need to be monitored. If the patient requires IV medication or fluid intervention, the patient may need to be hospitalized. After the patient has been successfully detoxified from the medication, the provider needs to monitor the effectiveness of the preventive medication in preventing headaches. Effective preventive medication decreases the need for acute therapy. Ongoing assessment of **analgesic**, **triptan**, and **ergotamine** use will determine if the patient is overusing again.

Outcome Evaluation

The successful outcome in medication-overuse headache is a patient who is detoxified from the offending medication and is somewhat headache free. The patient may still have an occasional headache and need acute or preventive therapy. Up to 31 percent of patients have recurrence of and often get back into the pattern of overuse of acute therapy medications (Mathew, 1997).

Patient Education

Patient education should include a discussion of information related to the overall treatment plan as well as that specific to the drug therapy, reasons for taking the drug, drugs as part of the total treatment plan, and adherence issues. Patients may have an exacerbation of headache in the first 2 weeks after withdrawal and it may take 4 to 12 weeks after withdrawal for the patient to show improvement (Maizels, 2004). Educating the patient about what to expect during the withdrawal process will reduce anxiety during the process. For general patient education information, see the Patient Education box.

When discussing medication-overuse headache with the patient, the provider must be careful to avoid terms such as "drug abuse." Patients with medication overuse headache began with a primary headache disorder and fell into a pattern of overuse, and to label them as "abusers" can be devastating. Before and during the detoxification period, the provider should explain the plan of care and establish a patient's trust. The patient is about to embark on a process that will surely cause moderate to severe headache, a state that the patient has been trying to avoid.

The following principles regarding medication-overuse headache and the withdrawal process need to be discussed with the patient:

1. A clear description of medication-overuse headache and how it develops should be given to the patient.
2. After stopping the medication, the headache will get worse within 24 hours (72 hours for **ergotamine**) and may last from days to weeks.
3. Patients must be assured that interventions will be taken to make them comfortable and to decrease the severity of headache, including hospitalization, if needed.
4. It may take 1 to 3 months for the patient to have a normal response to acute therapy.

On The Horizon — MIGRAINE MEDICATIONS

A number of drugs are being studied for migraine prevention and chronic daily headache. **Botulism toxin type A (BTX)** injection is a neurotoxin that is undergoing study for effectiveness in treating chronic tension headaches or migraine. **BTX** is injected either in a fixed site or follow-the-pain pattern. A placebo-controlled randomized controlled trial (RCT) trial of 1,300 patients with chronic migraine demonstrated decreased headache and decreased **triptan** use (Lovell & Marmura, 2010).

Zonisamide (Zonegran) is an AED that is being studied to prevent chronic migraine. In a small study (*N* = 33), migraines decreased from 20.7 to 18.0 per month on patients treated with an average of 337.9 mg daily.

Memantine (Namenda) is a noncompetitive antagonist at glutamatergic *N*-methyl-D-aspartate (NMDA) receptors. It is a new class of Alzheimer's medication that is being studied for pain disorders including migraine.

A number of new drugs for acute migraine attacks are in the pipeline, for example, a new **sumatriptan** formula, in which the **Zelrix** patch combines **sumatriptan** with NuPathe's proprietary SmartRelief™ transdermal technology. An inhaled form of dihydroergotamine **(DHE),** labeled **MAP004** is in clinical trials and may be as effective as IV **DHE**.

Source: Lovell & Marmura, 2010.

REFERENCES

American Headache Society. (2007). Information for patients: Types of headaches. Retrieved May 20, 2010, from http://www.achenet.org/education/patients/TypesofHeadaches.asp

Carmona, S., & Bruera, O. (2009). Prophylactic treatment of migraine and migraine clinical variants with topiramate: An update. *Therapeutic and Clinical Risk Management, 5,* 661–669.

Carpay, J., Schoenen, J., Kinrade, F., & Boswell, D. (2004). Efficacy and tolerability of sumatriptan tablets in a fast-disintegrating, rapid-release formulation for the acute treatment of migraine: Results of a multicenter, randomized, placebo-controlled study. *Clinical Therapeutics, 26*(2), 214–223.

Ferrari, A., Coccia, C., & Sternieri, E. (2008). Past, present and future prospects of medication-overuse headache classification. *Headache, 48,* 1096–1102.

Gagne, J. J., Leas, B., Lofland, J. H., Goldfarb, N., Freitag, F., & Silberstein, S. (2007). Quality of care measures for migraine: A comprehensive review. *Disease Management, 10*(3), 138–146.

Institute for Clinical Systems Improvement (ICSI). (2009). *Health care guideline: Diagnosis and treatment of headache* (9th ed.). ICSI; Bloomington, MN. Retrieved from http://www.icsi.org/headache/headache__diagnosis_and_treatment_of_2609.html

Lovell, B. V., & Marmura, M. J. (2010). New therapeutic developments in chronic migraine. *Current Opinion in Neurology, 23,* 254–258

Maizels, M. (2004). The patient with daily headaches. *American Family Physician, 70*(12), 2299–2306.

Maizels, M., & Burchette, R. (2003). Rapid and sensitive paradigm for screening patients with headache in primary care settings. *Headache: The Journal of Head & Face Pain, 43*(5), 441–450.

Mannix, L. K., Frame, J. R., & Solomon, G. D. (1997). Alcohol, smoking and caffeine use among headache patients. *Headache, 37,* 572–576.

Marin, P. A. (1998). Pharmacology update: Pharmacologic management of migraine. *Journal of the American Academy of Nurse Practitioners, 10*(9), 407–412.

Matcher, D. B., Young, W. B., Rosenberg, J. H., Pietrzak, M. P., Silberstein, S. D., Lipton, R. B., et al, & US Headache Consortium. (2000). Evidence-based guidelines for migraine headache in the primary care setting: Pharmacological management of acute attacks. Retrieved May 19, 2010, from http://www.aan.com/professionals/practice/pdfs/gl0087.pdf

Mathew, N. T. (1997). Transformed migraine, analgesic rebound and other chronic daily headaches. *Neurologic Clinics, 15*(1), 167–186.

Mathew, N. T., Rapoport, A., Saper, J., Magnus, L., Klapper, J., Ramadan, N., et al. (2001). Efficacy of gabapentin in migraine prophylaxis. *Headache, 41,* 119–128.

Mendizabal, J. E. (1998). The clinical challenge of chronic daily headaches. *Patient Care Nurse Practitioner, 1*(5), 41–46.

Moore, K. L., & Noble, S. L. (1997). Drug treatment of migraine: Part I. Acute therapy and drug-rebound headache. *American Family Physician, 56*(8), 2039–2048.

Noble, S. L., & Moore, K. L. (1997). Drug treatment of migraine: Part II. Preventive therapy. *American Family Physician, 56*(9), 2279–2286.

Ortho-McNeil Neurologics. (2009). Axert. Retrieved from http://www.axert.com

Pfaffenrath, V., Cunin, G., Sjonell, G., & Prendergast, S. (1998). Efficacy and safety of sumatriptan tablets (25 mg, 50 mg and 100 mg) in the acute treatment of migraine: Defining the optimum doses of oral sumatriptan. *Headache, 38,* 184–190.

Silberstein, S. D., Olesen, J., Bousser, M.-G., Diener, H.-C., Dodick, D., First, M., et al, on behalf of the International Headache Society. (2005). The International Classification of Headache Disorders, 2nd Edition (ICHD-II)—revision of criteria for 8.2 *Medication-overuse headache. Cephalalgia, 25,* 460–465.

Smith, C. M. (1998). Differential diagnosis of headache. *Journal of the American Academy of Nurse Practitioners, 10*(11), 519–524.

Taylor, F. R. (2009). Headache prevention with complementary and alternative medicine. *Headache, 49*(6), 966–968.

CHAPTER 36

HEART FAILURE

Anita Lee Wynne and Sharon Maxey

Chapter Outline

Heart failure (HF) is a major health problem that the American College of Cardiology (ACC) and the American Heart Association (AHA) (Hunt et al, 2005) estimate affects more than 5 million Americans annually, is the underlying reason for 12 to 15 million office visits and 6.5 million hospital visits annually, and causes the deaths of 300,000 people each year. Despite aggressive investigation into treatment options, until very recently the 5-year mortality rate was 50 percent. Of particular importance in its management is the design of a treatment program targeted at the patient's underlying pathophysiology. Such a carefully designed program maximizes outcomes and prevents such treatment complications as prerenal azotemia and dehydration. Because multidrug regimens are often necessary, patient education is essential to limit complications and hospitalizations that result from poor adherence to the treatment regimen.

PATHOPHYSIOLOGY

HF is a complex clinical syndrome that can result from any structural or functional cardiac disorder that results in a cardiac output that is inadequate to satisfy the oxygen demands of the body. In HF several abnormalities occur. Coronary artery disease (CAD) is the underlying cause in about two-thirds of patients with left ventricular dysfunction. Left ventricular dysfunction (systolic heart failure) begins with some injury to the myocardium and is usually a progressive process, even in the absence of additional myocardial insults. The principal mechanism relates to remodeling, which occurs as a homeostatic mechanism to decrease wall stress through increases in wall thickness. The cells generated during remodeling are often abnormal and include a proliferation of connective tissue cells as well. These cells use energy inefficiently and have little contractile ability. The ultimate result is a change in the structure of the left ventricle in which the chamber dilates, hypertrophies, and becomes more spherical. This process generally precedes the development of symptoms, but continues after their appearance and may contribute to the worsening of symptoms despite treatment. One of the advantages of the use of **angiotensin-converting enzyme (ACE) inhibitors** is their action in reducing remodeling. As the left ventricle hypertrophies, the sarcomeres of the muscle cells lengthen so that limited numbers of cross-bridges can form and function appropriately, and contractile force degenerates. Contractility of heart muscle is a function of the interaction of calcium with the actin-troponin-tropomyosin system. Activator calcium released from the sarcoplasmic reticulum facilitates the interaction of actin with myosin to create the cross-bridging that produces contraction. The amount of calcium released depends on the amount in stores and the amount that enters the cell during the plateau phase of the action potential. The reduced force at systole causes the ventricles to supply inadequate blood volume to the body, and blood pressure (BP) drops, even though the ventricle is very full and overstretched. This triggers counter-regulatory mechanisms in the rest of the body, activating the sympathetic nervous system (SNS) and the renin-angiotensin-aldosterone (R-A-A) system (Fig. 36–1). The SNS increases heart rate, tries to increase contractile force, and increases venous tone. A major role of **beta blockers** in HF treatment relates to reducing the SNS activation. The R-A-A system triggers the retention of sodium and water to increase blood volume and venous return (increased afterload). Initially, this brings more venous return to the heart and increases the amount of blood available to the body. In the long term, these adaptive mechanisms actually create more failure. The ventricle that is already full and stretched is required to deal with more volume (increased preload). **Diuretics**, another cornerstone of pharmacological therapy, assist by reducing increased extracellular fluid volume. The pathology of HF is further compounded by the denial of adequate oxygen as the increased heart rate shortens the diastolic filling time and the coronary arteries have less time to fill. The heart demands more oxygen supply and has less.

Types of Heart Failure

Three main forms of HF can occur. Systolic dysfunction typically occurs acutely and often follows a myocardial infarction (MI). Other potential causes include nonischemic cardiomyopathy, use of alcohol and other drugs that depress the myocardium, and conditions that lead to volume overload. The problem is inadequate force generated to eject blood from the ventricles, resulting in decreased cardiac output and ejection fractions of less than 45 percent. Sixty to 80 percent of patients with HF have this form.

Diastolic dysfunction results from inadequate relaxation and loss of muscle fiber elasticity, resulting in a slower filling rate and elevated diastolic pressures. Although cardiac output is reduced, ejection fractions may remain within normal limits. Potential causes include valvular dysfunction, hypertrophic and ischemic cardiomyopathy, uncontrolled hypertension, and hypothyroidism. Many of the changes that occur in the cardiovascular system as a result of aging have a greater impact of diastolic function than systolic function. HF with preserved systolic function is primarily a disease of

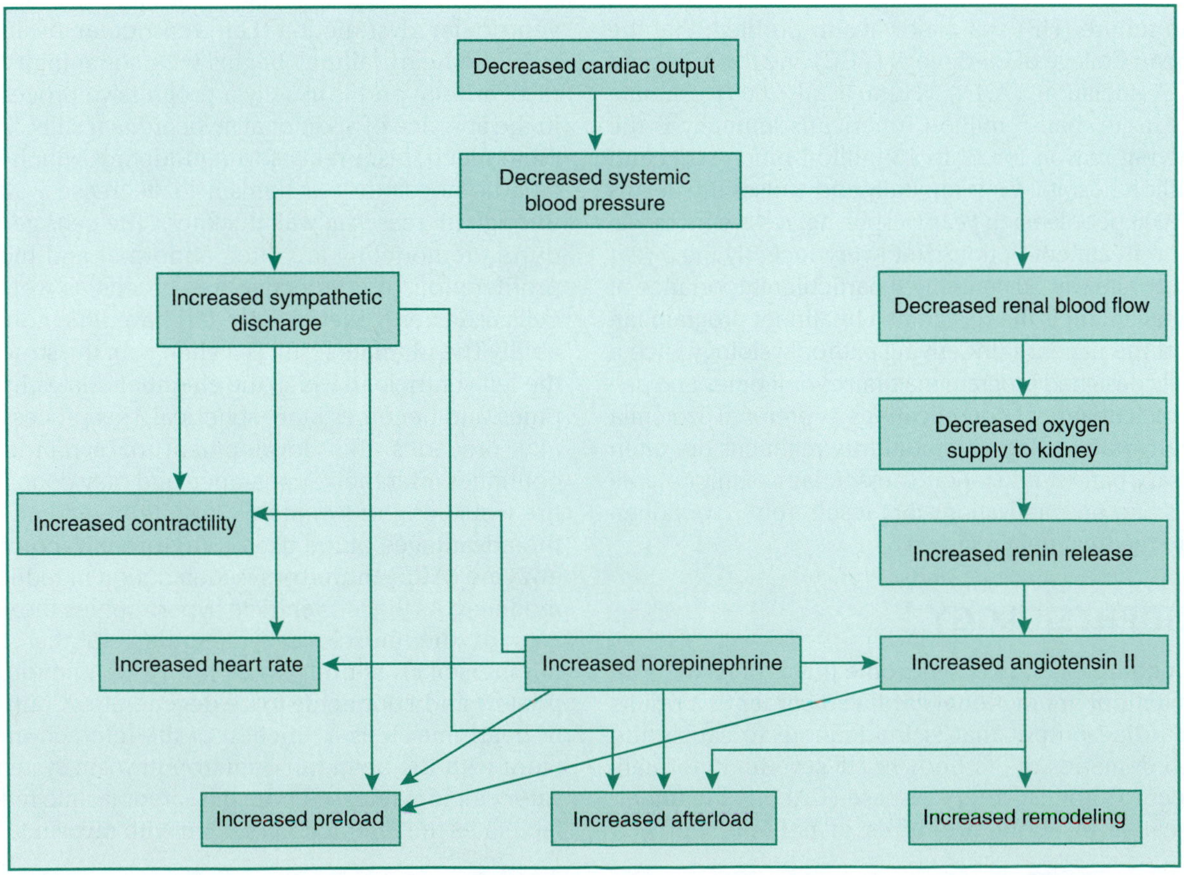

Figure 36–1. Compensatory responses in heart failure.

elderly women (greater than 75 years), most of whom have hypertension. Up to 40 percent of patients with HF have this form, however, the percent increases to 70 percent of HF cases after 80 years (Torosoff & Philbin, 2003). Diastolic dysfunction is also most common in African Americans (Thomas-Kvidera, 2005).

Coronary artery disease (CAD) and atherosclerosis are significant contributing factors for combined systolic-diastolic dysfunction. Framingham data suggest that 76 percent of patients with HF have hypertension or CAD alone or in combination as the cause. Treatment of these underlying disorders often improves the performance of the heart muscle.

"High-output" failure is a fairly rare form that takes place when the demands of the body are so great that even increased cardiac output is insufficient. Causative factors include hyperthyroidism, anemia, and arteriovenous shunts. Treatment for this form is directed at the underlying pathology and is not discussed here.

Classifications of Heart Failure

The New York Heart Association (NYHA) has classified HF based on the severity of symptoms. This functional classification reflects the amount of activity needed to produce symptoms. It is fairly subjective in nature and treatments used do not differ significantly across the classes. In addition, this system does not deal with patients who are asymptomatic or at high risk for the development of HF. The ACC/AHA committee that devised their guidelines sought to develop a staging system that would objectively identify patients throughout the course of their disease and would be linked to treatments that were uniquely appropriate for each stage of their illness. In addition, this classification scheme recognizes that HF, like hypertension (HTN) and CAD, has established risk factors; that evolution of the disorder has asymptomatic as well as symptomatic phases; and that treatment prescribed at each stage can reduce the morbidity and mortality of HF.

Table 36–1 compares these two classifications.

Symptoms of Heart Failure

Symptoms have been described as depending on whether the left or the right ventricle is affected. Lung-focused symptoms (often referred to as "congestion") are associated with left-sided failure, and body-focused symptoms, such as edema, are associated with right-sided failure. With the exception of cor pulmonale, which is clearly right sided in nature, progression of the disease usually involves both ventricles, and the terminology of left-sided versus right-sided failure is less useful clinically. In older adults, the peripheral edema thought to be associated with right-sided HF is actually more often related to venous insufficiency. Peripheral venous disease should be considered as a causative or contributing factor to symptoms in older adults. Regardless of which ventricle is more involved, patients with HF may have a number of symptoms, the most common being breathlessness, fatigue, exercise intolerance, and weight gain secondary to fluid retention. None of these symptoms is specific to HF and several other disorders may present with similar symptoms. Therefore, symptoms alone cannot be relied upon to make the diagnosis, which depends upon good history taking and physical examination, supplemented by diagnostic tests. Diagnostic evaluation will be presented later. The clinical course of the disease depends in large part on the point at which the patient is diagnosed and treatment is started, the appropriate targeting of that treatment, and the underlying pathology.

PHARMACODYNAMICS

Only a small number of HF cases are attributable to specific disorders that can be treated with or improved by

Table 36–1 **Comparison of Classification Systems for Heart Failure (HF)**

New York Heart Association	American College of Cardiology/American Heart Association
Class I. No limitations. Ordinary physical activity does not cause fatigue, breathlessness, or palpitation. (Asymptomatic left ventricular dysfunction is included in this category.)	**Stage A.** Patient at high risk for developing HF but without structural heart disease
Class II. Slight limitations of physical activity. Comfortable at rest, but ordinary physical activity results in fatigue, palpitation, breathlessness, or angina pectoris (symptomatically "mild" HF).	**Stage B.** Patient with a structural disorder of the heart, but who has never developed symptoms of HF
Class III. Marked limitations of physical activity. Although patient is comfortable at rest, less than ordinary physical activity will lead to symptoms (symptomatically "moderate" HF).	**Stage C.** Patient with past or current symptoms of HF associated with underlying structural disease
Class IV. Inability to carry on any physical activity without discomfort. Symptoms of congestive HF are present even at rest. With any physical activity, increased discomfort is experienced (symptomatically "severe" HF).	**Stage D.** Patient with end-stage disease who requires specialized treatment strategies such as mechanical circulatory support, continuous inotropic infusions, cardiac transplantation, or hospice care

surgery. The mainstay of HF therapy is lifestyle management and drug treatment targeted to altering the physiological mechanisms that create or arise from HF. Four main categories of drugs are used to treat HF, whether it is systolic or diastolic in nature. **Diuretics** reduce preload by decreasing extracellular fluid volume and can be used to decrease hypertension that increases afterload. **Angiotensin-converting enzyme (ACE) inhibitors** act on the R-A-A system to decrease preload and afterload. They also affect heart tissue remodeling so that fewer abnormal myocardial cells are generated. **Digoxin**, a **cardiac glycoside**, improves myocardial contractility and cardiac output. **Beta-adrenergic blockers** affect the SNS counterregulatory mechanism of HF. **Aldosterone antagonists** augment the actions of **ACE inhibitors** on the R-A-A system. Three other classes of drugs are used in special circumstances. **Nitrates** improve systolic and diastolic ventricular function by improving oxygen transport to the myocardium for patients with HF who also have angina. **Anticoagulants** are used for patients with HF who also have chronic atrial fibrillation. **Antiplatelets** are used to prevent MI and death in patients with HF who have underlying CAD.

GOALS OF TREATMENT

There are three goals of therapy used to determine treatment options: improvement of symptoms, reduction in morbidity, and reduction in mortality. Specific drug therapies have research support documenting their efficacy in attaining one or more of these goals. Physiological goals are to decrease overload (preload and/or afterload), improve contractility, and decrease heart rate. Rational drug selection can be based on these goals, on the mechanism behind the dysfunction, and on the symptom severity of the disease process.

RATIONAL DRUG SELECTION

Guidelines

Although the ACC/AHA classification system is intended to complement, not replace the NYHA classification, the ACC/AHA guidelines will be the main source of recommendations throughout this chapter. It should be noted that these guidelines are not inconsistent with those produced by the National Collaborating Centre for Chronic Conditions (NCCCC, 2003), the Veterans Health Administration, Department of Veterans Affairs (2003), or the Institute for Clinical Systems Improvement (ICSI, 2004). These latter guidelines are used where noted. These clinical practice guidelines describe the management of patients with both left-ventricular (systolic) dysfunction and diastolic dysfunction and include steps in accurate diagnosis, pharmacological and nonpharmacological therapies, counseling, and patient education. Figure 36–2 depicts the stages in the evolution of HF and the recommended therapy at each stage. All recommendations also follow the same evidence-based format of the previous ACC/AHA guidelines (Hunt et al, 2005), which are:

Class I. Conditions for which there is evidence for and/or general agreement that the procedure or treatment is useful and effective.

Class II. Conditions for which there is conflicting evidence and/or a divergence of opinion about the usefulness/efficacy of a procedure or treatment.

Class IIa. The weight of evidence or opinion is in favor of the procedure or treatment.

Class IIb. Usefulness/efficacy is less well established by evidence or opinion.

Class III. Conditions for which there is evidence and/or general agreement that the procedure or treatment is not useful/effective and in some cases can be harmful. Class III interventions will be mentioned in this chapter only when they may be harmful and are to be avoided.

Diagnosis of Heart Failure

A complete history and physical examination are always important in the diagnosis of any disorder. Specific diagnostic test useful in evaluation of HF including the following:

1. Two-dimensional echocardiograms coupled with Doppler flow studies. This is probably the single most useful diagnostic tool because it facilitates identification of any structural abnormalities. Confirmation by echocardiography of HF diagnosis and/or cardiac dysfunction is mandatory and should be performed shortly after suspicion of HF diagnosis. Echocardiography is the most practical measurement of ventricular dysfunction and can be used to distinguish between systolic dysfunction and preserved systolic function where the ejection fraction is normal (left ventricular ejection fraction [LVEF] greater than 45% to 50%) (Dickstein et al, 2008; Heart Failure Society of America [HFSA], 2006; Hunt et al, 2005; National Heart foundation of Australia/Cardiac Society of Australia and New Zealand [NHFA/CSANZ], 2006; Scottish Intercollegiate Guidelines Network [SIGN], 2007). These patients generally have HF related to diastolic dysfunction.
2. Chest x-rays may show cephalization of the vascular supply and 12-lead ECGs may show left-ventricular hypertrophy and axis deviation (HFSA, 2006; NHFA/CSANZ, 2006; SIGN, 2007). Although both provide baseline information, because they are insensitive and nonspecific neither alone should form the primary basis for determining the specific cause of HF.
3. Complete blood count, urinalysis, serum electrolytes (including calcium and magnesium), blood urea nitrogen (BUN), serum creatinine, blood glucose, liver

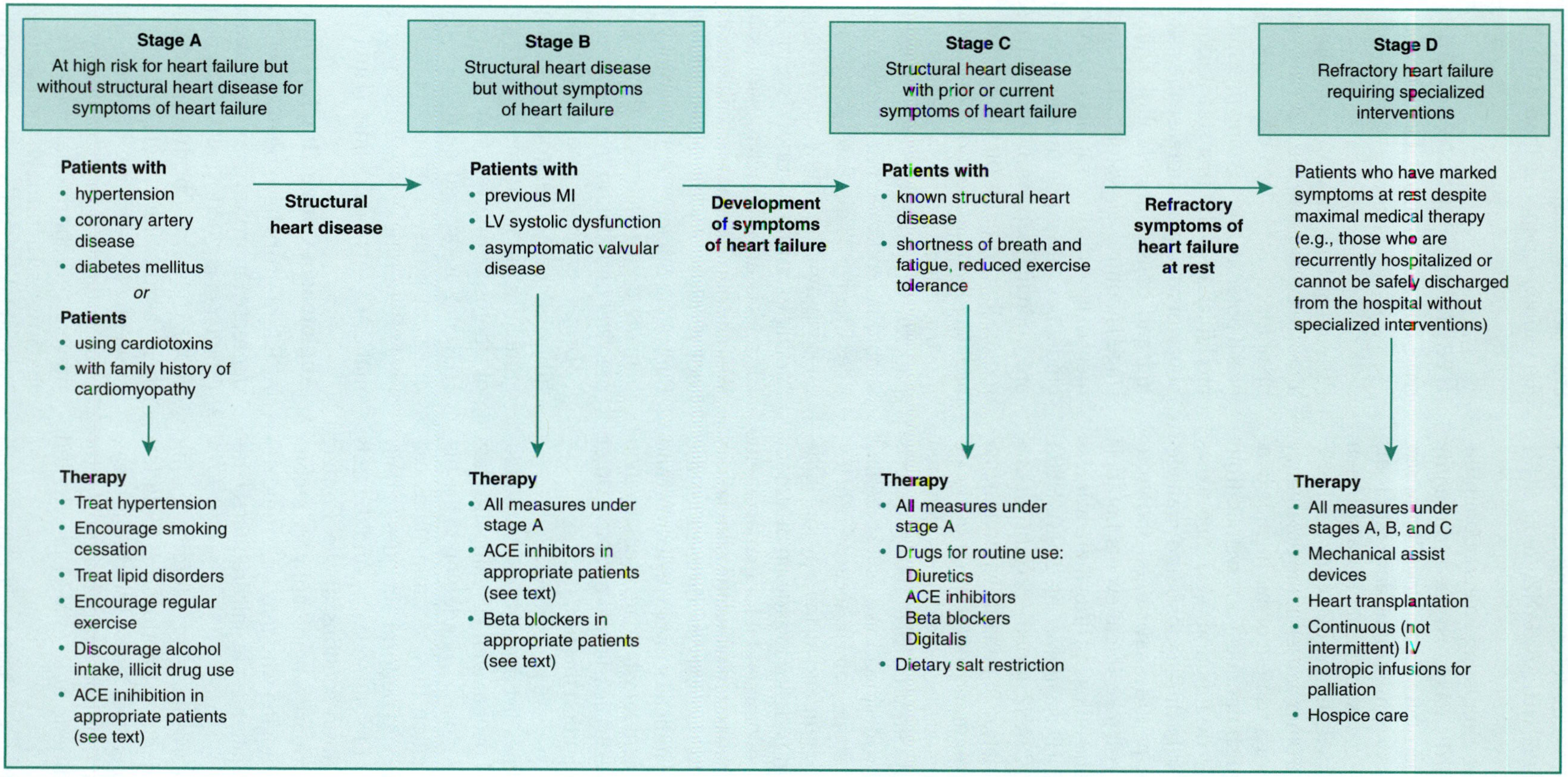

Figure 36–2. Stages in the evolution of HF and recommended therapy by stage.

function studies, and thyroid-stimulating hormone are useful in determining possible treatable underlying causes of HF and in determining end-organ damage (HFSA, 2006; NHFA/CSANZ, 2006; SIGN, 2007)

4. The measurement of circulating levels of brain natriuretic peptide (BNP) has been used to identify patients with elevated left ventricular filling pressures who are likely to exhibit signs and symptoms of HF. The peptide measurement has also been used as an aid in differentiating dyspnea due to HF from dyspnea due to other causes in the emergency setting. Although the assessment of this peptide cannot reliably distinguish patients with systolic from those with diastolic dysfunction, evidence exists supporting its use in both diagnosis and management. Levels of the peptide have been shown to identify patients at risk for clinical events, but their role in monitoring and adjusting drug therapy is less clearly established (Dickstein et al, 2008). HFSA (2006) and NHFA/CSANZ (2006) do not recommend BNP determination in patients without symptoms. They do recommend determination in all symptomatic patients suspected of having HF when the diagnosis is not certain. SIGN (2007) suggests BNP evaluation for widespread use as a screening tool in patients with suspected HF. Because BNP levels tend to fall after commencing therapy for HF, the sensitivity is lower in patients already on treatment, and SIGN does not recommend it for management.
5. Troponin I or T may be tested when the clinical picture suggests an acute coronary syndrome. Increase in cardiac troponins indicates myocyte necrosis and may identify the patient for whom revascularization should be considered (Dickstein et al, 2008). Other guidelines do not mention this test.

The ACC/AHA guidelines list specific recommendations for the evaluation of patient with HF using the class system discussed above. For class I, in addition to the history and physical examination, they recommend assessment of the patient's ability to perform activities of daily living (ADLs), assessment of volume status, and the tests mentioned in the first three sections above. Cardiac catheterization with coronary angiography is recommended for patients with angina who may be candidates for revascularization. The latter test usually requires referral to a specialist.

For class IIa, noninvasive imaging, exercise testing, and measurement of ejection fraction are included. Screening for hemochromatosis is also listed, as is measurement of antinuclear antibody, rheumatoid factor, and urinary vanillylmandelic acid (VMA) in selected patients.

The NCCCC (2003) agrees with the ACC/AHA guidelines for diagnosis but gives more weight to the natiuretic peptides and adds lipid panels to the tests. The ICSI (2004) and the Veterans Health Administration, Department of Veteran's Affairs (2003) also include lipid panels, if not evaluated in the last 5 years, but are less enthusiastic about the natiuretic peptides than is the NCCCC.

Treatment Recommendations Based on Stage of Heart Failure

Stage A

Patients at high risk for developing HF are addressed almost exclusively in the ACC/AHA guidelines. Initial treatment for HF is focused on reversing underlying pathologies if possible and treating precipitating factors. Lifestyle modification is the first step and includes avoidance of behaviors that may increase the risk for HF, such as smoking, and consuming alcohol. Equally important at this stage is control of systolic and diastolic HTN and treatment of lipid disorders in accordance with recommended guidelines. The guidelines for these latter two disorders are found in Chapters 39 and 40. These modifications can reduce the demands on the heart, decrease the risk for or facilitate the treatment of hypertension and CAD, and remove a drug that directly depresses the myocardium. For patients with diabetes mellitus, blood glucose levels should be controlled in accordance with current guidelines. Chapter 33 discusses the guidelines for this disorder. Lifestyle modification (e.g., stopping smoking, not consuming excessive alcohol) is appropriate in all stages of HF and is an adjunct to successful drug therapy. The Web site http://www.heartfailurematters.org is an Internet tool provided by the Heart Failure Association of the European Society of Cardiology (ESC) that permits patients, their relatives, and caregivers to obtain useful, practical information in a user-friendly format.

Drug therapy is also instituted in stage A. **ACE inhibitors**, the cornerstone of therapy for HF in all the guidelines, are recommended for patients with a history of atherosclerotic vascular disease, diabetes mellitus, or HTN and associated cardiovascular risk factors. These drugs can be useful in preventing HF in these high-risk patients. **Beta blockers** are also recommended for stage A in the ACC/AHA guidelines (Hunt et al, 2005).

Angiotensin-Converting Enzyme Inhibitors

ACE inhibitors have been shown to improve symptoms, decrease morbidity, and increases life expectancy (Flather et al, 2000; Neal, MacMahon, Chapman, & Blood, 2000). They affect both preload and afterload through their vasodilating effects, decrease the incidence of remodeling by reducing the local generation and action of angiotensin II in heart muscle (Mancini, 2000), and prevent neurohormonal counterregulatory mechanisms that worsen HF through their action on the R-A-A system. Patients taking **ACE inhibitors** show moderate increases in ejection fraction, decreased left ventricular end-diastolic filling pressures, and improved myocardial energy metabolism. Because they are the only drugs that address all of the pathological mechanisms that produce HF, they are appropriate for all subsets of patients unless these patients are pregnant or have bilateral renal artery stenosis, serum potassium levels above 5.5 mEq, or a history of angioedema. They are also useful for preventing the development of HF in patients with ventricular dysfunction but no overt symptoms (stage B). A significant reduction in the development of symptomatic HF and death from any cause has been demonstrated in these patients. As monotherapy or in combination with **beta blockers, ACE inhibitors** are superior to all other drugs and drug combinations used to treat heart failure. The NCCCC (2003) recommends that "all patients with HF due to left ventricular systolic dysfunction should be considered for treatment with an **ACE inhibitor**" (p. 39) and that such therapy should be started before other drug classes are tried.

Although these drugs are most effective with systolic dysfunction, it is often difficult to ascertain if the patient has systolic or diastolic dysfunction at the time of the initial examination. However, 90 percent of patients with HF have some left ventricular dysfunction (LVD). **ACE inhibitors** are the drugs of choice for LVD and create few ill effects for patients with diastolic dysfunction, even though they are less efficacious with diastolic dysfunction. These drugs are safe to start before it is clear which of the two types of dysfunction exists.

Therapy should be started immediately. There is no need to wait until the disease has progressed. **ACE inhibitors** are commonly used as primary therapy, with other drugs added if symptoms persist or if volume overload develops at a later time. This is consistent with the all of the above guidelines. Start with a low dose to prevent risks of hypotension and hypoperfusion, especially of the kidneys. Beginning with 6.25 mg **captopril (Capoten)**, the only **short-acting ACE inhibitor**, permits discontinuance with rapid clearance of the drug should a renal problem occur. Gradually increase **ACE inhibitor therapy** to improve exercise tolerance and relieve symptoms, while monitoring BP and renal function. BP monitoring is critical not only to assure renal perfusion but also to prevent dizziness and falls. Many patients with heart failure are older adults at high risk for falls with even a limited decrease in cerebral perfusion. Renal function must also be closely watched with BUN, creatinine, and urinalysis. Any deterioration in renal function may require dosage reductions. Because **ACE inhibitors** alter **aldosterone** function, potassium levels may rise. Regular monitoring of serum electrolytes is important. Use of **potassium-wasting diuretics** as concurrent therapy may be helpful. **Potassium-sparing diuretics** are not used.

Debate continues on the choice of the best **ACE inhibitor** for long-term therapy. In randomized, controlled studies, both short-acting and long-acting formulations were equally effective. The long-acting formulations demonstrate some greater risk of prolonged hypotension and impairment of renal function, but only at high doses. However, long-acting forms provide a higher affinity for the ACE receptors and more stable drug levels. They also provide a less complex treatment regimen that is more likely to result in adherence because all **ACE inhibitors** except **captopril** have once-daily dosing. The dosing schedule for different **ACE inhibitors** and the process for changing to a long-acting form is discussed in Chapter 16.

A dry, "tickle" cough occurs in up to 15 percent of patients and is the leading reason patients give for choosing to discontinue therapy. This adverse effect appears to be related to the action of **ACE inhibitors** on the bradykinin system. Because they do not affect this system, **angiotensin II receptor blockers (ARBs)** have actions similar to **ACE inhibitors** but do not produce the cough. **Losartan (Cozaar)** is the only **ARB** officially approved for treatment of HF, especially in older adults. Further trials are underway to determine if other drugs in this class have a similar effect and to support the use of **ARBs** in HF. **ARBs** have not been shown to increase life expectancy compared to **ACE inhibitor** therapy for patients with HF due to systolic dysfunction (Cohn & Tognoni, 2001; Jong, Demers, McKelvie, & Liu, 2002). To date, **ARBs** should be reserved for patients for whom **ACE inhibitors** are indicated, but who are unable to tolerate them; this approach is supported by NCCCC (2003).

Beta Blockers

Unless contraindicated or not tolerated, a **beta blocker** should be given to all patients with a recent or remote history of MI regardless of ejection fraction or presence of HF (Hunt et al, 2005). These drugs improve ventricular function through their action on the HF counterregulatory mechanisms and have cardioprotective properties.

Other class I recommendations for stage A patients include control of ventricular rate in patients with supraventricular tachyarrhythmias, treatment of thyroid disorders, and periodic evaluation for signs and symptoms of HF. Two interesting class III statements are made. Exercise to prevent the development of HF is thought to be ineffective, as is reduction in dietary salt beyond that which is prudent (generally considered to be 2,500 mg/d) for healthy individuals without HTN or fluid retention.

Stage B

Patients with left ventricular dysfunction who have not developed symptoms are classified as stage B. They include patient without symptoms who have had an MI and those with evidence of left ventricular dysfunction. These individuals are at high risk for developing HF, but the likelihood of developing it can be diminished by the use of therapies that reduce the risk of additional injury, the process of remodeling, and the progression of left ventricular dysfunction.

As with stage A, the first drugs of choice are **ACE inhibitors** for these patients as well. **ACE inhibitors** are recommended for all patients with cardiac structural abnormalities who have not yet developed HF (Hunt et al, 2005). The level of evidence to support this recommendation is strong. If the patient has entered the algorithm at stage A, **ACE inhibitors** should be continued. If they enter the algorithm at stage B, **ACE inhibitors** should be started. This is the stage, however, where **beta blockade** is added. **Beta blockers** are recommended for all patients without a history of MI who have a reduced ejection fraction (less than or equal to 40%) with no HF symptoms (Dickstein et al, 2008; Hunt et al, 2005) and for patients with recent MI regardless of ejection fraction.

Beta blockers are also important for MI prophylaxis for patients who develop HF secondary to an acute MI. Care must be taken in prescribing these drugs because they may precipitate acute decompensation. Patients should be clinically stable (e.g., no recent change in **diuretic**) and should be on an optimal dose of **ACE inhibitor** and/or ARB (Dickstein et al, 2008). Very low doses are used, and several months are required to show improvement.

Many large clinical trials (Bonet et al, 2000; Bouzamondo, Hulot, Sanchez, Cucherat, & Lechat, 2001; Brophy, Joseph, & Rouleau, 2001; Dickstein et al, 2008; Packer et al, 2001; Shibata, Flather, & Wang, 2001; Whorlow & Krum, 2000) have shown that some **beta blockers** increase life expectancy in patients with HF due to left ventricular systolic dysfunction, compared with placebo. This effect has been seen in patients in all NYHA functional classes of HF (NCCCC, 2003). The three beta blockers that have the strongest evidence to reduce mortality are **bisoprolol**, **carvedilol**, and **metoprolol succinate** (Hunt et al, 2005). The evidence is strongest for **carvedilol** (which is actually an **alpha$_1$ beta blocker**) and modified release **metoprolol**. There is little evidence of benefits from other **beta blockers**. There is also little evidence to show a clinically significant difference based on selectivity of the **beta blocker** or on those with or without vasodilating properties. There are no randomized clinical trials of **atenolol** in patients with HF. The suggestion by the NCCCC (2003) is that patients who have systolic HF who are not already on a **beta blocker** should be started on one with evidence to support its use (e.g., **cavedilol** or **extended-release metoprolol [metoprolol succinate]**). Although not specifically mentioned in the guidelines, **labetalol (Normodyne)** has the same action as **carvedilol**. **Labetalol** is not recommended, however, for patients with LVEF less than 45 percent. Both can also be used safely with **digoxin** because they do not abolish this drug's **inotropic** action and in combination with **ACE inhibitors** to improve left ventricular function. If the patient developed HF while already on a different **beta blocker** for a concomitant condition such as angina or HTN, the health-care provider has the option to leave them on that drug or change to one of the drugs above. In any case, the "start low and go slow" paradigm should be used with these drugs.

The ICSI (2004) guidelines also recommend **beta blockers** for all NYHA classes of HF and mention the same ones above. The guideline recommends that **carvedilol** be started at 3.125 mg bid and titrated as tolerated up to 25 mg bid maximum with 50 mg bid maximum for patient weighing more than 85 kg. **Metoprolol succinate** can be started at 12.5 mg once daily for two weeks and doubled upward every two weeks as tolerated to a target dose of 200 mg/day. The Veterans Affairs guideline (Veterans Health Administration, Department of Veterans Affairs, 2003) specifies the use of **beta blockers** related to recent MI and also specifically mentions the drugs above. **Beta blockers** are also used for a subset of patients with diastolic dysfunction or cardiomyopathies for whom decreased heart rate could improve cardiac output.

All guidelines suggest that treatment with **digoxin** in stage B patients who are in sinus rhythm is not effective. In addition, the risk for harm is not balanced with any known benefit (Hunt et al, 2005). In the Veterans Affairs guideline (2003) **digoxin** may be used in stage B when the patient has a rapid ventricular response to atrial fibrillation and there is a need to control the rate. The other guidelines would also support its use under these circumstances. **Calcium channel blockers** with negative inotropic effects may be harmful in asymptomatic patients with low LVEF. Other interventions that are useful in selected patients are discussed below.

Stage C

Patients with left ventricular dysfunction with current or prior symptoms of HF are classified as stage C. They are the first stage to have active HF symptoms. All the class I recommendations for stages A and B are also appropriate here. In addition, moderate sodium restriction (1,500 to 2,000 mg/day), along with daily weight monitoring are indicated to facilitate the most effective use of drugs. Physical activity at this stage should be encouraged, except during periods of acute exacerbations because restriction of activity promotes physical deconditioning, which may contribute to the exercise intolerance common with this stage.

Most patients in this stage will require a combination of three to four types of drugs: **ACE inhibitors, beta blockers, cardiac glycosides (digoxin)**, and a **diuretic**. The value of these drugs has been established in numerous large-scale clinical trials and the evidence supporting their use is strong. **ACE inhibitors** and **beta blockers** have already been discussed. **Diuretics** and **digoxin** will be discussed here.

Diuretics

In the presence of fluid overload a **diuretic** is the drug of choice (Dickstein et al, 2008). It should be given until a euvolemic state is achieved and continued to prevent the recurrence of fluid retention. Because of their central role in control of HTN, **diuretics** may be drugs of choice for earlier stages of HF where the goal is control of HTN. This will be discussed later in the section Concomitant Diseases. Even if the patient responds favorably to the **diuretic**, **ACE inhibitors** and **beta blockers** should be initiated or continued after euvolemia has been achieved because **diuretics** cause activation of the R-A-A system and **ACE inhibitors** and **beta blockers** have been shown to improve the long-term prognosis of HF.

Diuretics improve symptoms and reduce morbidity. There is no evidence that they affect mortality. Their main function is to reduce preload associated with volume overload. **Thiazide diuretics** have long been and remain the drugs of choice early in the disease process and for patients with mild disease. However, for stage C patients, **loop diuretics** are more effective. **Potassium-sparing diuretics (aldosterone antagonists)** are too weak to be of benefit as monotherapy. They can be useful as concurrent therapy with **thiazide** or **loop diuretics** to counterbalance the potassium loss common to these latter two groups of drugs. Two drugs in the **aldosterone antagonist class (spironalactone** and **eplerenone)** have shown increased life expectancy and reduced hospitalizations when added to a treatment regimen that included a **loop diuretic** and an **ACE inhibitor** (Pitt et al, 2003). The ACC/AHA guideline recommends **spironalactone** for patients with recurrent class IV symptoms, preserved renal function, and a normal potassium level. The NCCCC guideline (2003) also recommends the drug only for patients who are "severely symptomatic" despite optimal therapy with other drugs. The guideline suggests a starting dose of 12.5 mg once daily and seeking advice from a specialist. For **eplerenone,** the recommended starting dose is 25 mg once daily (Hunt et al, 2005). The doses then may be increased to 50 mg for each of these drugs if needed.

For diastolic HF, **spironalactone** has a definite role. The hormone **aldosterone** contributes to diastolic stiffness by promoting fibrosis. Preliminary studies have shown **aldosterone antagonists** such as **spironalactone** reduce myocardial fibrosis (Weber, 2003), and these agents have a role in the treatment of diastolic HF (Torosoff & Philbin, 2003).

For mild to moderate disease, start therapy with 50 mg **hydrochlorothiazide (HCTZ).** For stage C HF, use a **loop diuretic** such as **furosemide (Lasix)** 20 to 40 mg bid. **Loop diuretics** can cause marked diuresis. Before starting them, discontinue any **thiazide diuretic** currently being used. For **loop diuretics,** divide the daily dose to prevent great diuresis at one time. If the patient does not respond adequately to the divided dose, try giving the entire daily dose in the morning before increasing the dose. The goal with **diuretics** is to give the lowest possible dose that achieves the desired effect. Single daily doses are effective, but during times of increased pathology, oral absorption may be compromised, and the IV route or high doses of oral formulations may be needed. Dosing schedules are given in Chapter 16. Monitor weight gain, changes in exercise tolerance, and electrolytes. **Diuretic** resistance may occur in the presence of decreased renal perfusion or renal stenotic or obstructive pathologies, or with the concurrent administration of **NSAIDs.** If symptoms seem resistant to the standard doses of the **diuretic,** check creatinine clearance. **Thiazide diuretics** cannot be used with creatinine clearances that are lower than 25 mL/minute. **Loop diuretics** can be used with these low creatinine clearances. Patients may also benefit from the addition of **metolazone (Zaroxolyn)** for its synergistic action on diuresis.

Although initiation of **diuretic therapy** is important for patients who have HF with volume overload, it is also important to avoid excessive diuresis, especially for patients who are also on sodium restrictions. Volume depletion can lead to hypotension and prerenal azotemia. For patients concurrently taking **ACE inhibitors**, renal insufficiency can be induced. **Diuretics** may be stopped, if necessary, to allow rehydration before restarting an **ACE inhibitor.** They can be reintroduced after the dose of the **ACE inhibitor** has been stabilized. **ACE inhibitors** augment the effectiveness of **thiazide** and **loop diuretics** because they decrease glomerular filtration fractions and increase the delivery of solute and water to the distal nephron segments that are responsive to the action of these **diuretics.**

Long-term use of **diuretics** can stimulate increased R-A-A activity and sodium retention, which are both counterproductive in treating heart failure. This result is less likely with low doses. In addition to the potential for fluid volume changes, **thiazide** and **loop diuretics** present risks for acid–base and electrolyte disturbances that can be proarrhythmic. Monitoring for these problems is discussed in detail in Chapter 16. The most common electrolyte problem is hypokalemia. Any potassium supplementation must be based on serum levels because not all patients become hypokalemic or require supplementation beyond dietary changes. Potassium supplements must be used cautiously, if at all, for patients concurrently taking **ACE inhibitors,** which cause elevated potassium. Oral potassium supplements should provide chloride as well to prevent diuretic-induced hypokalemic alkalosis. Hypomagnesemia is also common and may impair potassium repletion. **Diuretics** also contribute to abnormal glucose and lipid metabolism. Care must be taken and diagnostic tests frequently monitored when **diuretics** must be used for patients with diabetes or lipid abnormalities.

Cardiac Glycosides

Digitalis was once the only effective drug to treat HF. Its ability to increase contractility by increasing intracellular calcium and inhibiting the sodium-potassium-ATPase pump deals directly with one primary deficit in HF. Unfortunately, clinical research demonstrates that therapy directed at noncardiac targets, such as fluid volume and counterregulatory mechanisms, is more effective in treating HF than are the **inotropes.** Although **digoxin** increases the force of contraction, thereby improving functioning and symptoms and reducing hospitalizations, it has little if any effect on mortality. Although **digoxin** reduces the risk of admission to the hospital for worsening of HF, there are no published data from randomized control trials on the effect of this drug on the signs and symptoms (except for exercise performance) and quality of life of patients with HF (NCCCC, 2003). The development of **ACE inhibitors,** combined with the risks of toxicity and multiple drug interactions associated with the **cardiac glycosides**

(CGs), has moved **digoxin** to a third-line drug except for selected cases and it is recommended for worsening HF due to left ventricular dysfunction despite **ACE inhibitor, beta blocker**, and **diuretic therapy**. Although **beta blockers** would be first-line therapy because they also control HTN and have a role in tachycardia-medicated cardiomyopathy associated with atrial fibriallation, **digoxin** remains a useful drug for HF secondary to atrial fibrillation with a rapid ventricular response because it slows heart rate (Dickstein et al, 2008). **Digoxin** also remains a cornerstone of treatment for HF in patients with severe systolic dysfunction (ejection fractions less than 40% and an audible S_3). In fact, the presence of S_3 is a potent predictor of response to CG **therapy. Digoxin** is less beneficial with ejection fractions of more than 40 percent or in HF secondary to hypertrophic cardiomyopathies. Patients with severe aortic stenosis or poorly compliant, hypertrophied ventricles often require elevated end-diastolic filling pressures to support forward stroke volume. Excessive reduction of preload may markedly decrease cardiac output in these patients, so **diuretics** cannot be used. **Digoxin** is the drug of choice here, although it is not a substitute for valve surgery. **Digoxin** is not useful in HF associated with idiopathic hypertrophic subaortic stenosis, also known as hypertrophic obstructive cardiomyopathy (which it actually worsens), recurrent transient ischemia, or mitral stenosis (unless the patient also has atrial fibrillation). **Digoxin** can also be problematic when treating patients with renal insufficiency. Renal function may decrease during heart failure treatment and the drug may not be adequately excreted, allowing its levels to increase to toxic levels. Digoxin levels should be closely monitored in these patients.

For stable patients, therapy can be started with an oral maintenance dose without resorting to a loading dose. Using a daily dose of 0.25 mg, a therapeutic blood level can be achieved in 5 to 7 days. Check the serum level in 1 week and make any needed adjustments on the basis of clinical response and serum level. Less stable patients require hospitalization for loading doses. Monitor patients on **digoxin** by following heart rate and rhythm, potassium levels, and renal function. Routine monitoring of serum **digoxin** levels is generally overdone. Monitoring should occur in addition to clinical judgment rather than as a substitute for it. Chapter 16 has detailed discussion of the reasons for and process of monitoring associated with the use of **digoxin**, as well as the process of initiating and maintaining **digoxin** therapy.

The decision to begin **digoxin** therapy should not be made lightly. It should be used only when there is clear evidence of chronic systolic dysfunction or one of the disease processes just mentioned. **Digitalis** toxicity occurs in as many as 25 percent of patients, and the mortality rate from this toxicity averages 22 percent. Patients with mild to moderate heart failure often become asymptomatic on optimal doses of **ACE inhibitors** and **diuretics** and do not require **digoxin. Digoxin** should be added for those patients whose symptoms persist despite optimal doses of these two drugs. For patients already on **digoxin**, research evidence supports symptom deterioration when it is suddenly withdrawn. For these patients, **digoxin** should not be withdrawn unless a reversible cause of heart failure has been fully corrected or there is no basis for using the drug in the first place.

Angiotensin II Receptor Blockers

Angiotensin II **receptor blockers (ARBs)** are mentioned as possible drugs to substitute for **ACE inhibitors** in patients who are being treated with **diuretics, beta blockers**, and **digoxin** and who cannot be given an **ACE inhibitor** (Dickstein et al, 2008; Hunt et al, 2005). The use of these drugs is discussed in stage A. It should be noted that the use of an **ARB** before a **beta blocker** in patients who are taking an **ACE inhibitor** is a class III recommendation, meaning it is not effective, and a triple combination of **ACE inhibitor, ARB**, and **beta blocker** should be avoided as it may be harmful.

Calcium Channel Blockers

While the pathology of HF is associated with altered contractility in part associated with calcium movement within the cell, **calcium channel blockers (CCBs)** are listed as a class III "avoid" recommendation in the ACC/AHA guidelines (Hunt et al, 2005). The NCCCC (2003) guidelines state that "**calcium channel blockers** do not improve life expectancy compared with placebo in patients with heart failure who are already receiving an **ACE inhibitor**" (p.50). These same guidelines do acknowledge that **amlodipine, a long-acting dihydropyridine**, is not harmful in terms of adverse events and may be considered for treatment of comorbid HTN and/or angina in patients with HF. It is the only drug in this class that is not to be avoided.

Nitrates

Nitrates are effective for a subset of patients whose primary pathology is increased preload. Their use is discussed related to concomitant conditions. They are also accepted therapy in combination with **hydralazine** when the patient has an intolerance to both an **ACE inhibitor** and an **ARB**. Its use in these patients may reduce the risk of death (Dickstein et al, 2008).

Stage D

Stage D includes patients with refractory end-stage HF. These patients will probably be treated by a specialist and their management is not within the scope of this book.

Cost

The drugs used to treat HF vary in cost from minimal to quite expensive. **Diuretics** are among the least expensive, but they vary from **indapamide (Lozol)** ($25 per month) to **generic HCTZ** ($1.04 per month). The latter is the drug of choice for a variety of reasons, and cost certainly also makes it desirable. None of the **ACE inhibitors** is inexpensive, but several of them are now available as a generic formulation, making them less expensive. Because **digitalis** has been used for so long, it is among the least expensive.

Table 36–2 and the available dosage tables in Chapter 16 include a cost index for many of the drugs commonly used to treat HF.

Additional Patient Variables

Concomitant Diseases

Coronary Artery Disease and the Use of Nitrates

The underlying pathology of HF in the presence of CAD relates to poor oxygenation of the myocardium, which results in angina pectoris. Chapter 28 discusses angina and ischemic heart disease. When these disorders occur with or result in HF, **nitrates** are often added to the treatment regimen. They are relatively selective to epicardial vasculature and improve systolic and diastolic ventricular function by increasing coronary blood flow. The mechanism includes both coronary artery vasodilation and improvement of the uptake of oxygen by the myocardial muscle itself. This mechanism is discussed in some detail in Chapter 16.

They are also effective after MI and for those with CAD as the primary cause of their HF. They reduce symptoms and have some effect on mortality when used in the acute setting. Improvement in mortality in primary care has been demonstrated only when **isosorbide dinitrate** is

Table 36–2 **Drugs Commonly Used: Heart Failure**

Drug	Indication	Initial Dose	Target Dose	Maximum Dose
		Thiazide Diuretics		
Hydrochlorothiazide	Initial therapy for volume overload.	25 mg qd	As needed	50 mg daily
		Loop Diuretics		
	Added therapy when resistant to standard therapy or for decompensation			
Furosemide Bumetanide Torsemide	Furosemide is first choice. Torsemide is best when high doses of furosemide are required	10–40 mg qd 0.5–1 mg qd 5 mg qd	As needed As needed As needed	240 mg daily 10 mg daily 20 mg daily
		ACE Inhibitors		
Captopril Enalapril Lisinopril Quinapril	All subsets of patients. Initial therapy or if symptoms not relieved by diuretic. Drug of choice for patients with diabetes.	6.25 mg tid 2.5 mg bid 5 mg daily 5 mg bid	50 mg tid 10 mg bid 20 mg daily 20 mg bid	100 mg tid 20 mg bid 40 mg daily 20 mg bid
		Angiotensin II Receptor Antagonist		
Losartan Valsartan Candesartan	Patients intolerant to ACE inhibitors	25 mg qd 40 mg qd 4 mg qd	50 mg daily 80 mg qd 32 mg qd	100 daily 320 mg qd
Digoxin	If symptoms unrelieved by ACE inhibitor and diuretic	0.125 mg qd	As needed	As needed
Hydralazine	With isosorbide dinitrate for intolerance to ACE inhibitor	10–25 mg tid	75 mg tid	100 tid
Isosorbide dinitrate	With hydralazine for intolerance to ACE inhibitor	10 mg tid	40 mg tid	80 mg tid
		Beta Blockers		
Labetalol Carvedilol	Patients with diastolic dysfunction or cardiomyopathy in whom reduced heart rate can improve cardiac output.	100 mg bid 3.125 mg bid	400–800 mg 6.25–25 mg bid	1.2 g/d 25 mg bid
		Aldosterone Antagonists		
Eplerenone	Diastolic HF	50 mg qd	50–100 mg qd	50 mg bid
Spironolactone	Diastolic HF	12.5 mg	25 mg qd or 12.5 mg bid	50 mg qd

combined with **hydralazine**, a peripheral vasodilator. This combination is usually reserved for patients who are intolerant of **ACE inhibitors**. Problems with **nitrate** tolerance require special timing of doses, with **nitrate-free** intervals daily. Chapter 16 includes discussion of this problem. The dosage of **isosorbide dinitrate** that produces the most sustained hemodynamic effects and minimizes the development of tolerance appears to be 40 mg every 8 hours. The dosage of **hydralazine** is up to 800 mg every 8 hours to reduce afterload. This is not a long-term management solution and the NCCCC (2003) guideline suggests that it be initiated only by a specialist.

Antiplatelets such as **aspirin** have evidence to support their use in patients with atherosclerotic arterial disease, including CAD. Systematic review evidence (Cohn & Tognoni, 2002) supports **aspirin's** role in reducing the risk of vascular events in these patients. It is recommended by the ACC/AHA and by the ESC group for patients with CAD, although specific evidence for its benefits in patients with HF is lacking (Hunt et al, 2005; Dickstein et al, 2008.). The NCCCC (2003) recommends **aspirin** 75 to 150 mg once daily for patients with a combination of HF and CAD. Some questions have been raised about the possibility that is may reduce some of the benefits of **ACE inhibitors** when taken together (Olson, 2001; Takkouche, Etminan, Caamano, & Rochon, 2002), but the evidence is not robust. It is worth considering this possibility when prescribing both.

Chronic Atrial Fibrillation and the Use of Anticoagulants

Digoxin has already been discussed as the drug of choice for HF patients who have concomitant atrial fibrillation. **Anticoagulants** are also helpful in this situation. Randomized control trials have demonstrated that **warfarin** reduces the risk of stroke in patients with HF and atrial fibrillation (Dickstein et al, 2008; Hunt et al, 2005). No such benefit is shown for patients with HF who are in sinus rhythm (Lip & Gibbs, 2001).

Diabetes and the Use of ACE Inhibitors

Based on data from the Diabetes Complications Control Trial and more recent trials, the American Diabetes Association recommends the use of **ACE inhibitors** as the drugs of choice for the treatment of HTN for persons with diabetes. Their role in HTN is discussed in detail in Chapter 40 and their role in diabetes is discussed in Chapter 33. The same rationale for their use in HTN holds for patients with HF. The ACC/AHA guidelines (Hunt et al, 2005) mention this preference. Because of their demonstrated effect in reducing diabetic nephropathy, **ACE inhibitors** are clearly the drugs of choice to treat HF in patients with diabetes. **ARBs** may also reduce diabetic nephropathy, but this effect has yet to be demonstrated by longitudinal studies.

Patients with diabetes may experience increased glucose levels with **diuretics**. **Thiazide diuretics** in low doses are the least likely to cause this adverse response, followed by **loop diuretics**. **ARBs** are also acceptable drugs for patients with diabetes because of their limited effects on glucose metabolism, lipid profiles, and renal function. **Beta-adrenergic blockers** are generally avoided for patients with diabetes because they have an adverse effect on peripheral blood flow, prolong hypoglycemia, and mask most hypoglycemic symptoms. Recent evidence suggests that these effects may not be as problematic as once thought. The majority of diabetic patients eventually develop coronary disease, with or without heart failure, and **beta blockers** are a first-line drug for cardioprotection. Patients with diabetes who need MI prophylaxis and have concurrent heart failure may be placed on low doses of **beta blockers** and taught to monitor their blood glucose more closely and to recognize diaphoresis as their main indicator of hypoglycemia.

Hypertension and the Early Use of Diuretics

HTN is a common concurrent disorder with heart failure and may contribute to its etiology. Initial therapy for HTN is with **diuretics**, especially for sodium-sensitive patients such as African Americans, older adults, those who are obese, and those with renal insufficiency. The most effective diuretics for both HTN and HF are the **thiazides**. **Loop diuretics** are less effective for HTN but have some use there, and they are helpful for subsets of patients with stage C HF. **ACE inhibitors** are drugs of choice for treating HTN in young and white patients. The dose for treating HTN, however, is double the dose used to treat HF, and the lower dose is required for patients who have both disorders. In patients with low ejection fractions (less than 40 percent), the vasodilating effects of **ACE inhibitors** provide adequate perfusion, even with systolic blood pressure (SBP) at or below 90 mm Hg. Chapter 40 discusses in more detail the drugs helpful in treating HTN. Because a primary goal for all HF patients, including those in stages A and B, is the control of HTN, drugs that assist with both disorders should have preference in rational drug selection.

Hyperlipidemia and the Use of Statins

Hyperlipidemia leading to atherosclerotic changes is also a common concurrent disorder that may contribute to the etiology of HF. Treatment of lipid disorders based on the most current guidelines is a class I recommendations for all HF patients, starting with stage A (Hunt et al, 2005). The Expert Panel on Detection, Evaluation and Treatment of High Blood Cholesterol in Adults (NCEP, 2001) recommends the use of **HMG-Co-A reductase inhibitors (statins)** as first-line therapy when LDL cholesterol-lowering drugs are indicated to achieve treatment goals. **Statins** reduce the frequency of ischemic events (Dickstein et al, 2008) and prolong life expectancy in patients with known CAD (Athryos et al, 2002). The risk of developing HF is also reduced. The benefits of **statins** appear to be universal and not restricted by sex or age, although the ESC guideline (Dickstein et al, 2008) limits their recommendation to the elderly.

Experimental studies suggest that **statins** may improve left ventricular function through mechanisms beyond the prevention of myocardial ischema; however, they may increase the oxidative stress and effects of endotoxin in patients with HF (Krum & McMurray, 2002). The direct effect of **statins** on ventricular function and HF progression has not be specifically studied in a randomized controlled trial. Chapter 39 discusses NCEP recommendations in detail and Chapter 16 discusses the various **statins** and rational drug selection among them.

Diuretics have been associated with transient elevation in lipid levels. This transient problem does not rule them out. **ACE inhibitors**, **ARBs**, **CCBs**, and **digoxin** do not affect lipid levels and may be used for patients with hyperlipidemia. **Beta-adrenergic blockers** increase triglycerides transiently and reduce levels of high-density lipids.

Others

Hyperuricemia can be a problem for patients with gout. **Diuretics** can produce this adverse effect. The least likely to do so are the **thiazides**, followed by the **loop diuretics**. **ACE inhibitors** do not affect uric acid levels directly but can influence renal function, which may indirectly affect uric acid metabolism. **Digoxin** does not affect uric acid metabolism.

Asthma or chronic airway disease may occur with heart failure, especially in older adults. Chronic airway obstruction is the underlying cause of cor pulmonale, right-sided heart failure. Bronchial activity is unchanged by **ACE inhibitors**. In the 10 to 15 percent of patients taking these drugs who experience a cough, **angiotensin II receptor blockers** are an alternative. **Alpha- beta-adrenergic blocker** and **beta-adrenergic blockers** are contraindicated in bronchospastic disorders.

Impaired renal function and electrolyte disturbances also influence drug selection. Because **digoxin** is excreted essentially unchanged by the kidney, renal impairment suggests cautious use and close monitoring of serum drug levels. Renal impairment is also associated with increased potassium levels, and the administration of **potassium-wasting diuretics** often results in decreased potassium levels. Both of these situations increase the risk for **digitalis** toxicity. Dosage adjustments of **digoxin** are required for patients with decreased renal function, especially older adults. Renal clearance is a factor in the choice of **diuretic**, as previously discussed. **Thiazide** and **loop diuretics** may cause hypokalemia. **ACE inhibitors** are contraindicated in bilateral renal artery stenosis, and careful monitoring of renal function is required with their use.

Age

Digoxin has a long history of use in infants and children. **Thiazides** and **loop diuretics** are approved for use with pediatric patients. Both of these drug groups have specific pediatric formulations. Safety has not been established in pediatric patients for **ACE inhibitors**. Older adults have a higher risk for **digitalis** toxicity, and the indications of toxicity are different in children and older adults than they are in most adults. **Digitalis** toxicity is discussed in Chapter 16.

HF is the leading cause of death and hospitalization for adults older than 65 years (Aronow, 2000) and it is the most common Medicare diagnoses related group. A large portion of HF risk in this population is attributable to modifiable risk factors. The Health, Aging and Body Composition study (Kalogeropoulos et al, 2009) researched these factors and suggests that racial differences in risk factors and in hospitalization rate need to be considered in prevention and treatment efforts. **ACE inhibitors** are still the drugs of choice for older adults. Research that includes older adults often excludes patients with serum creatinine levels above 2.0 and older adults often have elevated serum creatinine levels related to the changes associated with aging. Consideration of serum creatinine alone presents some problems. Creatinine clearance may be more accurate in assessing renal function than serum creatinine due to decreased muscle mass in the older adult. The primary reason given in the literature for not reaching goal doses of **ACE inhibitors** in older adults with HF is renal dysfunction, symptomatic hypotension, cough, and hyperkalemia. There are few clinical trials including older adults with HF on goal doses, but several studies indicate that **ACE inhibitors** at target doses would benefit the older adult (Levine, Levine, Bolenbaugh, & Green, 2002).

Older adults are more likely than younger adults to have diastolic dysfunction. **ACE inhibitors** are appropriate for this type of HF, but so are **aldosterone antagonists**. **Eplerenone** has been studied in older adults. No overall identified differences in safety, efficacy, or responses were observed between the older adult and younger subjects.

Pregnancy

ACE inhibitors are contraindicated in pregnancy. **Digoxin** has been used, but blood levels must be monitored closely to avoid toxicity. **Diuretics** decrease plasma volume and may decrease plasma placental perfusion. They are used only when benefits clearly outweigh risks. Jaundice and thrombocytopenia have been seen in neonates after use in the mother. **Beta blockers** are considered safe in the latter part of pregnancy. A general rule of thumb sometimes proposed is that drugs safe to be used in infants are safe for use in pregnancy, but it is important to remember that consideration must be given to the maternal–fetal drug concentration ratio. Some drugs develop much higher levels of concentration in the fetus than they do in the maternal circulation, and the dose that is therapeutic for the mother may be too high for the neonate. It is best to avoid any drug during pregnancy unless the benefits clearly outweigh the risk to the fetus. Pregnant women with HF are probably best treated by a specialist (NCCCC, 2003).

Drug Combinations

Adherence to a treatment regimen is less likely as the regimen becomes more complex. Drug combinations can increase that complexity. They should be reserved for situations in which monotherapy is ineffectual.

Common combinations include **diuretics** and **ACE inhibitors**. When using this combination, withholding or decreasing the dose of the **diuretic** to permit rehydration prior to initiating the **ACE inhibitor** reduces the chances of renal dysfunction and hypotension. The **diuretic** may be reintroduced later with positive effects because the **ACE inhibitor** improves the action of the **diuretic** on the renal tubule. With this combination, monitor BP, potassium, BUN, and creatinine levels, and decrease the **diuretic** dose if BP falls or prerenal azotemia develops.

Diuretics are also commonly used with **digoxin** for patients with systolic dysfunction. The **diuretics** reduce afterload, and **digoxin** improves contractility. Care must be taken with this combination concerning serum potassium levels, as was previously discussed.

For patients who remain symptomatic on a combination of an ACE **inhibitor** and a **diuretic**, **digoxin** may be added. With this combination, fluid status and serum potassium levels must be carefully monitored. For patients with persistent dyspnea after optimal doses of **diuretics**, **ACE inhibitors**, **beta blockers**, and **digoxin**, referral to a specialist is appropriate. The addition of a **vasodilator** to an **ACE inhibitor** may relieve symptoms, particularly for patients with hypertension or evidence of severe mitral regurgitation.

MONITORING

Monitoring to assess effectiveness in treating the pathology includes a variety of tools. NCCCC (2003) recommends the following assessments:

1. Functional capacity, chiefly using the NYHA class, specific quality of life questionnaires, or a maximal exercise test.
2. Assessment of fluid status, chiefly by physical assessment (e.g., daily weights, jugular venous distention, lung crackles, hepatomegaly, peripheral edema, and orthostatic BP).
3. Assessment of cardiac rhythm, chiefly by clinical examination, but a 12-lead ECG may be used if an arrhythmia is suspected. The ACC/AHA guidelines specifically state that Holter monitoring is class III because it is likely not effective.
4. Laboratory assessment, including electrolytes and serum creatinine always. Other tests such as thyroid function, hematology, liver function, and level of anticoagulation may be required depending on the medication prescribed and the comorbidity (p. 63).

Monitoring specific to each drug class is presented in Chapter 16. Serum drug level monitoring is important for **digoxin**. Hypokalemia, which may result from **diuretic therapy**, enhances sensitivity to the toxic effects of **digoxin** and is proarrhythmic in all patients with HF. Hypomagnesemia may impair the effectiveness of **potassium replacement therapy** and should be assessed for patients with refractory hypokalemia. Repeated testing may be useful for patients with a new heart murmur or sudden deterioration, even though they are adherent to the treatment regimen.

OUTCOME EVALUATION

A careful history and physical examination should be the mainstay in determining outcomes and directing therapy. The history includes questions about physical functioning, appetite, mental health, sleep disturbances, sexual functioning, cognitive functioning, and ability to perform the usual ADLs, including occupational and social activities. Specific questions are asked about the presence of weight gain, orthopnea, paroxysmal nocturnal dyspnea, edema, and dyspnea on exertion. The patient should report weight increases greater than 2 lb in any single day, increased pulmonary symptoms, and ankle edema. A worsening of any of these parameters requires evaluation of the treatment regimen and may indicate the need to adjust the therapy, especially **diuretic** dosage.

HF is generally a chronic condition that can be adequately managed in primary care. Consultation or referral to a cardiologist is appropriate when any of the following occurs:

1. Symptoms markedly worsen or the patient becomes excessively hypotensive or experiences syncope.
2. The patient is refractory to standard therapy.
3. There is evidence of renal failure or **digitalis** toxicity.
4. Adequate support is not present in the home to permit the patient to be treated in that situation.
5. Patients who remain symptomatic on a combination of an ACE **inhibitor**, a **beta blocker**, a **diuretic**, and **digoxin** should be seen by a cardiologist at least once. Persistent volume overload despite standard pharmacological management may require more aggressive administration of the current **diuretic**, more potent **diuretics** via the IV route, or a combination of **diuretics**. Additional testing beyond the usual monitoring may demonstrate evidence of concurrent disorders that may be the source of the resistance to therapy. These disorders may be amenable to other therapies. Surgical intervention may be needed, and hospitalization may be appropriate.

The ICSI (2004) also recommends that all patients less than 60 years with class I or II (stage B) HF with either severe left ventricular dysfunction or dilation or significant valvular regurgitation by referred to a cardiologist. These patients may be candidates for heart transplantation or other cardiac surgical procedures.

As with all chronic conditions, lack of adherence to a therapeutic regimen is unfortunately common. Nonadherence with diet and drugs can rapidly and profoundly affect the clinical status of HF patients and increases in

HEART FAILURE

PATIENT EDUCATION

Related to the Overall Treatment Plan and Disease Process

- ☐ Pathophysiology of heart failure, its prognosis, and its long-term effects on other organs of the body besides the heart
- ☐ Role of lifestyle modifications, including dietary and activity modifications, in improving prognosis and keeping the number and cost of required drugs down
- ☐ Importance of adherence to the treatment regimen
- ☐ Self-monitoring of symptoms of worsening failure, including daily weights
- ☐ What to do when symptoms worsen
- ☐ Need for regular follow-up visits with the primary care provider

Specific to the Drug Therapy

- ☐ Reason for the drug being given and its anticipated action in the disease process
- ☐ Doses and schedules for taking the drug
- ☐ Possible adverse effects and what to do it they occur
- ☐ Coping mechanisms for complex and costly drug regimens
- ☐ Interactions between other treatment modalities and these drugs

Reasons for Taking the Drug(s)

Patient education about specific drugs is provided in Chapter 16. Specifically for HF, additional information includes the following: These drugs are given to reduce mortality, reduce symptoms, and improve functional status. Some drugs do all of these **(ACE inhibitors)**; most do only one. The expectations should be clear about what the drugs can and cannot do. HF is a chronic condition that rarely occurs in a short period of time, and it is not likely to be corrected in a short period of time, if at all. Patients with HF must understand the seriousness of this diagnosis, including the 5-year mortality rate of 50 percent and the potential need for surgeries such as heart transplantation. All of this must be done while maintaining hope and emphasizing that good quality of life is possible.

Drugs as Part of the Total Treatment Regimen

The total treatment regimen includes sodium restriction and avoidance of excessive fluid intake. **Diuretics** reduce fluid volume and may interact with dietary restrictions, resulting in orthostatic hypotension. Care should be taken not to reduce fluid volume too quickly, which exacerbates the problem of decreased cardiac output and may lead to hypotension or renal insufficiency. Patients should report symptoms of fluid volume deficit. They should be told to rise slowly from a supine to a standing position to permit the body to redistribute body fluids. Sodium restriction may lead some patients to seek salt substitutes that have a potassium salt as part of their contents. For patients taking **ACE inhibitors,** this can result in excessively high potassium levels. Such salt substitutes should be avoided. Nonsalt herbal seasoning is more appropriate.

Regular aerobic exercise such as walking or cycling may improve functional status and decrease symptoms. Regular, gradually increased exercise may lead to enough improvement, in some cases, to reduce the drugs needed. Timing of exercise with the peak action of drugs is important. Patients are often able to predict the timing of voiding after taking a diuretic or times when other drugs are more likely to produce dizziness. Exercise timing should take these into consideration.

Adherence Issues

Nonadherence with the treatment regimen in HF may reduce life expectancy and certainly affects functional status. Health-care providers should be aware of the potential problem of nonadherence, discuss the importance of adherence at each follow-up visit, and assist patients in removing barriers to adherence (e.g., cost, adverse effects, or complexity of the regimen).

body weight and minor changes in symptoms commonly precede the major clinical episodes that require emergency care or hospitalization. Several factors in the management of heart failure foster this nonadherence. Lifestyle management is central to the treatment regimen for all stages and types of HF, and difficulty in achieving and maintaining lifestyle changes is well documented. Adverse drug reactions and drug costs are also factors. Table 40–9 (Chapter 40) on hypertension details some activities that can improve adherence, and Chapter 6 has additional material to improve positive outcomes.

PATIENT EDUCATION

Patient education should include a discussion of information related to the overall treatment plan as well as lifestyle management (Levitan, Wolk, & Mittleman, 2009), information specific to the drug therapy, reasons for the drug being taken, drugs as part of the total treatment regimen, and adherence issues. Unless contraindicated, all patients should also be encouraged to obtain an **influenza vaccination** every fall. **Pneumococcal immunization** should be provided at diagnosis of HF, if not previously vaccinated. For older adults, if initial vaccination was at 65 years or less, revaccination at 65 years or 5 years after initial immunization, whichever is later, should be done.

REFERENCES

Aronow, W. (2000). Treatment of heart failure in older persons. *Congestive Heart Failure, 9*(3), 142–147.

Athyros, V., Papageorgiou, A., Mercouris, B., Athyrou, V., Symeonidis, A., Basayannis, E., et al. (2002). Treatment with atorvastatin to the National Cholesterol Educational Program goal versus "usual" care in secondary coronary heart disease prevention. The GREek Atorvastatin and Coronary-heart-disease Evaluation (GREACE) study. *Current Medical Research and Opinion, 18*, 220–228.

Bonet, S., Agusit, A., Arnau, J., Vidal, X., Diogene, E., Galve, E., et al. (2000). Beta-adrenergic blocking agents in heart failure: Benefits of vasodilating and non-vasodilating agents according to patients' characteristics: A meta-analysis of clinical trials. *Archives of Internal Medicine, 160*, 621–627.

Bouzamondo, A., Hulot, J., Sanchez, P., Cucherat, M., & Lechat, P. (2001). Beta-blocker treatment in heart failure. *Fundamental and Clinical Pharmacology, 15*, 95–109.

Brophy, J., Joseph, L., & Rouleau, J. (2001). Beta-blockers in congestive heart failure: A Bayesian meta-analysis. *Annals of Internal Medicine, 134*, 550–560.

Cohn, J., & Tognoni, G. (2001). A randomized trial of the angiotensin-receptor blocker valsartan in chronic heart failure. *New England Journal of Medicine, 345*, 1667–1675.

Cohn, J., & Tognoni, G. (2002). Collaborative meta-analysis of randomized trials of antiplatelet therapy for prevention of death, myocardial infarction, and stroke in high-risk patients. *British Medical Journal, 324*, 71–86.

Dickstein, K., Cohen-Solal, A., Filippatos, G., McMurray, J., Ponikowski, P., Poole-Wilson, P. et al. (2008). ESC guidelines for the diagnosis and treatment of acute and chronic heart failure 2008: The Task Force[trunc]. *European Heart Journal, 29*(19), 2388–2442.

Flather, M., Yusuf, S., Kober, L., Pffeffer, M., Hall, A., Murray, G., et al. (2000). Long-term ACE-inhibitor therapy in patients with heart failure or left-ventricular dysfunction: A systematic overview of data from individual patients. ACE-Inhibitor Myocardial Infarction Collaborative Group. *Lancet, 355*, 1575–1581.

Gambassi, G., Froman, D., Lapane, K., Mor, V., Sgadari, A., Lipsitz, L., et al. (2000). Management of heart failure among very older persons living in long-term care: Has the voice of trial spread? *American Heart Journal, 19*, 85–93.

Heart Failure Society of America (HFSA). (2006). Evaluation of patients for ventricular dysfunction and heart failure: HFSA 2006 comprehensive heart failure practice guideline. *Journal of Cardiac Failure, 12*(1), e16–e25.

Hunt, S., Abraham, W., Chin, M., Feldman, A., Francis, G., Ganiats, T., et al. (2005). ACC/AHA 2005 guideline update for the diagnosis and management of chronic heart failure in the adult. A report of the American College of Cardiology/American Heart Association Task Force on Practice Guidelines (Writing Committee to update the 2001 Guidelines for the evaluation and management of heart failure). Bethesda, MD: American College of Cardiology Foundation. 82 pp. Retrieved June 6, 2009, from http://www.guideline.gov/summary/summary.aspx

Institute for Clinical Systems Improvement (ICSI). (2004). Heart failure in adults. *Institute for Clinical Systems Improvement.* Retrieved May 25, 2004, from http://www.guideline.gov/summary/summary.aspx

Jong, P., Demers, C., McKelvie, R., & Liu, P. (2002). Angiotensin receptor blockers in heart failure: Meta-analysis of randomized controlled trials. *Journal of the American College of Cardiology, 39*, 463–470.

Kalogeropoulos, A., Georgiopoulous, V., Kritchevsky, S., Psaty, B., Smith, N., Newman, A., et al. (2009). Epidemiology of incident heart failure in a contemporary elderly cohort. *Archives of Internal Medicine, 169*(7), 708–715.

Krum, H., & McMurray, J. (2002). Statins and chronic heart failure: Do we need a large-scale outcome trial? *Journal of the American College of Cardiology, 39*, 1567–1573.

Levine, T., Levine, A., Bolenbaugh, J., & Green, P. (2002). Reversal of heart failure remodeling with age. *American Journal of Geriatric Cardiology, 11*(5), 299–304.

Levitan, E., Wolk, A., & Mittleman, M. (2009). Consistency with the DASH diet and incidence of heart failure. *Archives of Internal Medicine, 169*(9), 851–857.

Lip, G., & Gibbs, C. (2001). Antiplatelet agents versus control or anticoagulation for heart failure in sinus rhythm. *Cochrane Database Systematic Review*, CD003333.

Mancini, G. (2000). Long-term use of angiotensin-converting enzyme inhibitors to modify endothelial dysfunction: A review of clinical investigations. *Clinical and Investigative Medicine, 23*, 144–161.

National Cholesterol Education Program (NCEP). (2001). *Third Report of the Expert Panel on Detection, Evaluation, and Treatment of High Blood Cholesterol in Adults* (Adult Treatment Panel III). Rockville, MD: National Institutes of Health, National Heart, Lung and Blood Institute.

National Collaborating Centre for Chronic Conditions (NCCCC). (2003). *Chronic heart failure: National clinical guideline for diagnosis and management in primary and secondary care.* Wiltshire, England: Sarum ColourView Group.

National Heart Foundation of Australia./Cardiac Society of Australia and New Zealand (NHFA/CSANZ). (2006). Guidelines for the prevention, detection and management of chronic heart failure in Australia, 2006. Sydney, Australia: National Heart Foundation of Australia. 79 pp. Retrieved June 5, 2009, from http://www.guideline.gov/Compare/comparison.aspx

Naylor, L., Howe, L., Eggert, J., & Heifferon, B. (2004). CHF in the elderly: Using ACEIs appropriately. *Nurse Practitioner, 29*(7), 46–52.

Neal, B., MacMahon, S., Chapman, N., & Blood, P. (2000). Effects of ACE inhibitors, calcium antagonists, and other blood-pressure-lowering drugs: Results of prospectively designed overviews of randomized trials. Blood Pressure Lowering Treatment Trials Collaboration. *Lancet, 356*, 1955–1964.

Olson, K. (2001). Combined aspirin/ACE inhibitor treatment for CHF. *Annals of Pharmacotherapy, 35*, 1653–1658.

Packer, M., Coats, A., Fowler, M., Jatus, H., Krum, H., Mohacsi, P., et al. (2001). Effect of carvedilol on survival in severe chronic heart failure. *New England Journal of Medicine, 344,* 1651–1658.

Pitt, B., Remmer, A., Zannad, F., Neaton, J., Martinez, F., Roniker, B., et al. (2003). Eplerenone, a selective aldosterone blocker, in patients with left ventricular dysfunction after myocardial infarction. *New England Journal of Medicine, 348,* 1309–1321.

Scottish Intercollegiate Guidelines Network (SIGN). (2007). Management of chronic heart failure: A national clinical guideline. Edinburgh, Scotland: Scottish Intercollegiate Guidelines Network (SIGN). 53 pp. Retrieved on June 5, 2009 from http://guideline.gov/Compare/comparison.aspx

Shibata, M., Flather, M., & Wang, D. (2001). Systematic review of the impact of beta blockers on mortality and hospital admissions in heart failure. *European Journal of Heart Failure, 3,* 351–357.

Takkouche, B., Etminan, M., Caamano, F., & Rochon, P. (2002). Interaction between aspirin and ACE inhibitors: Resolving discrepancies using meta-analysis. *Drug Safety, 25,* 373–378.

Thomas-Kvidera, D. (2005). Heart failure from diastolic dysfunction related to hypertension: Guidelines for management. *Journal of the American Academy of Nurse Practitioner, 17*(5), 168–175.

Torosoff, M., & Philbin, E. (2003). Improving outcomes in diastolic heart failure. *Postgraduate Medicine, 111*(3), 51–58.

Veterans Health Administration, Department of Veterans Affairs. (2003). The pharmacological management of chronic heart failure. Washington, DC: Veterans Health Administration, Department of Veterans Affairs. Retrieved May 25, 2005, from http://www.guideline.gov/summary/summary.aspx

Weber, M. (2003). Angiotensin receptor blockers might have a role in treating diastolic heart failure. *Cardiovascular Reviews and Reports, 25*(10), 536–538.

Whorlow, S., & Krum, H. (2000). Meta-analysis of effect of beta-blocker therapy on mortality in patients with New York Heart Association class IV chronic congestive heart failure. *American Journal of Cardiology, 86,* 886–889.

CHAPTER 37

HUMAN IMMUNODEFICIENCY VIRUS DISEASE AND ACQUIRED IMMUNODEFICIENCY SYNDROME

James Raper and Gina Dobbs

Chapter Outline

Since the discovery of human immunodeficiency virus (HIV) in 1981, we have learned a great deal about HIV-associated epidemiology, natural history, pathogenesis, therapy, and immunological host response. However, HIV disease and its sequel, acquired immunodeficiency syndrome (AIDS), remain a global health problem of unprecedented dimensions. HIV has already caused an estimated 25 million deaths worldwide and has generated profound demographic changes in the most heavily affected countries (UNAIDS, 2008). On a global scale, the HIV epidemic has stabilized, although with unacceptably high levels of new HIV infections and AIDS deaths. Globally, an estimated 33 million people were living with HIV in 2007. The annual number of new HIV infections declined from an estimated 3.0 million in 2001 to 2.7 million in 2007. Overall, 2.0 million people died due to AIDS in 2007, compared with an estimated 1.7 million in 2001.

While the percentage of people living with HIV has stabilized since 2000, the overall number of people living with HIV has steadily increased as new infections occur each year, HIV treatments extend life, and new infections still outnumber AIDS deaths. Women account for half of the cases of HIV worldwide, and nearly 60 percent of HIV infections in sub-Saharan Africa. Over the past 10 years, the proportion of women with HIV has remained stable globally, but has increased in many regions. Young people aged 15 to 24 years account for an estimated

45 percent of new HIV infections worldwide. An estimated 370,000 children younger than 15 years became infected with HIV in 2007. Globally, the number of children younger than 15 years living with HIV increased from 1.6 million in 2001 to 2.0 million in 2007. Almost 90 percent live in sub-Saharan Africa (UNAIDS, 2008). In the United States and dependent areas, the cumulative estimated number of diagnoses of AIDS through 2007 was 1,051,875 (Centers for Disease Control and Prevention [CDC], 2007). The cumulative estimated number of deaths of persons with AIDS in the United States and dependent areas was 583,298, including 557,902 adults and adolescents, and 4,891 children under age 13 years (CDC, 2007).

Thanks to increasingly effective **antiretroviral therapy (ART)**, the natural history of HIV disease has been favorably altered. A developing list of potent medications, used in combination therapy, has slowed the progression of HIV disease and has dramatically reduced the death rates for people living with HIV. According to the most recent estimates, there were 571,378 persons (549,196 adults and adolescents, and 2,736 children under age 13 years) living with HIV/AIDS in 34 reporting states (CDC, 2007).

PATHOPHYSIOLOGY

HIV induces defects in host cell–mediated and humoral responses, making the person susceptible to opportunistic infections and certain neoplasms. It is essential to understand the complex pathogenesis of HIV in order to appreciate the impact of HIV on the immune system and the development of interventions to prevent viral replication and advance immunological recovery.

AIDS is a clinical syndrome characterized by progressive immune system suppression, resulting in the development of opportunistic diseases. It is caused by chronic HIV infection. The first reported cases were described in 1981, the causative agent of AIDS was identified as HIV in late 1983, a serological test for HIV infection was available in 1985, and the first therapy was licensed in 1987 (Bennett, 2003). HIV is a member of a family of viruses known as retroviruses, so named because they are able to create DNA copies of their RNA genome, thus reversing (retro) the usual flow of genetic information. HIV is a lentivirus, a type of virus that characteristically produces diseases with a long incubation period leading to cancer, severe immune suppression, or both. The basic pathology in AIDS is a loss of CD4-positive T lymphocytes, cells critical to maintaining cell-mediated immune function. This damage results in progressively severe immune dysfunction.

HIV-1

HIV is a retrovirus that can be divided into two serotypes, HIV-1 and HIV-2; HIV-1 is predominantly responsible for HIV infection worldwide. Retroviruses are RNA-containing viruses that require the formation of proviral DNA within the host to complete their life cycle and infect other cells (Colagreco, 2003). The HIV-1 virus, like other retroviruses, is covered by a lipid bilayer derived from host-cell membranes. Viral glycoproteins are incorporated into the bilayer, as well as host adhesion molecules that may be involved in attachment to target cells (Kilby & Eron, 2003). The early characterization of HIV-1 centered on the CD4 T lymphocytes as the primary target of the HIV virus, the helper cells that are responsible for cell-mediated immune reaction (Ansari & Etzel, 2000; Kilby & Eron, 2003). The infectivity of HIV requires the surface glycoprotein (gp120) and the transmembrane glycoprotein subunit (gp41) of gp160, a viral precursor protein that binds to the CD4 receptor. The presence of a chemokine coreceptor, CCR5, also is required for cell entry (Colagreco, 2003). Following uncoating, the viral RNA is transcribed by the reverse transcriptase enzyme into proviral DNA. The integrase enzyme then integrates the proviral DNA into the host nucleus. The integrated viral genes may remain inactive or become transcribed back into genomic RNA and messenger RNA, which are then translated into viral proteins. Late stages of viral processing involve cleavage of viral proteins by the protease enzyme into new HIV particles, followed by assembly and the release of new infectious virions to infect other cells (Colagreco, 2003).

Viral replication is a dynamic process, involving continuous rounds of de novo virus infection and replication in infected host cells with rapid turnover of both free virus and virus-producing cells (Kilby & Eron, 2003). One billion to 10 billion virions are produced daily. One of the difficulties in eradicating the virus is the existence of an HIV reservoir of latently infected memory CD4 T cells carrying integrated provirus. Those reservoirs of replication-competent virus can persist in resting CD4 T cells of patients that are receiving **ART**. Low-level, ongoing replication of HIV may occur despite suppression of HIV virus with potent combination **ART**. (Kilby & Eron, 2003). To date, complete restoration of immune function has not been possible with **ART**, although partial restoration of pathogen-specific immunity to recall antigens is possible. **ART** can increase the number of circulating CD4 T cells, which is associated with prolonged survival and a diminished rate of common opportunistic infections.

Following initial HIV infection, immediate widespread dissemination of the virus to other lymphatic systems and organs occurs (Ansari & Etzel, 2000). Infectivity is high during primary infection, with high plasma viremia detected in blood and the presence of virus in sexual organs and secretions. During acute infection, the immunological host response involves potent, cytotoxic CD8 T lymphocytes, which limits viral replication and reduces symptomology as plasma viremia declines. In adults, a new steady state plasma HIV RNA "viral setpoint" is established approximately 6 months or longer after the initial infection that can remain stable for months or years before progression to AIDS. The time course of progression to AIDS varies in adults, with average durations of 10 to 11 years reported in the absence of antiretroviral therapy (Ansari & Etzel, 2000).

HIV-2

Although HIV-1 is found around the world, the prevalence of HIV-2 is highest in West Africa. HIV-2 is a zoonosis disease believed to have first infected humans as early as the 1940s by jumping from sooty mangabeys to humans as a result of bush meat hunting and slaughtering. HIV-2 has a lower transmission rate and a less pathogenic course. HIV-2 is common in the following countries: Angola, Benin, Burkina Faso, Cape Verde, Cote d'Ivoire (Ivory Coast), Gambia, Ghana, Guinea, Guinea-Bissau, Liberia, Mali, Mauritania, Mozambique, Niger, Nigeria, Sao Tome, Senegal, Sierra Leone, and Togo.

Transmission

Three principal means of HIV transmission have been identified: blood, sexual contact, and mother-to-child (vertical) transmission (Kirton, 2003). The frequency of transmission is influenced by the amount of infectious virus present in the body fluid and the extent of contact an individual has with body fluids.

Stages—Natural History of HIV

The natural history of HIV disease progresses through several stages. After viral transmission, a symptomatic primary HIV infection, often called acute retroviral syndrome, occurs in 50 to 90 percent of the people infected. The onset of symptoms is usually 2 to 4 weeks following infection, but the incubation may be as long as several months in rare cases. Typically, a flulike viral syndrome develops, with fever, lymphadenopathy, pharyngitis, rash, and myalgias or arthralgias (Freeman & Winland-Brown, 2001). Diarrhea, headaches, and nausea and vomiting are also common.

At this stage, serological tests are not helpful because seroconversion to a positive HIV antibody test usually occurs at 4 to 12 weeks after exposure and infection. Therefore, diagnosis of acute retroviral syndrome must be confirmed by tests for HIV mRNA (viral load). Generally, 95 percent or more of patients seroconvert within 6 months after HIV transmission. The period from infection to 6 months following HIV transmission is known as early HIV disease. At around 6 months after infection, HIV establishes a "set point," representing a stable balance between immune suppression of the virus and ongoing viral replication. In any individual patient, this steady state set point seems to be relatively stable over a period of years in the absence of ART. One possible effect of early therapy is to alter this set point to a level associated with longer survival. The next stage is asymptomatic infection. During this period, the patient is clinically asymptomatic and generally has no abnormal findings on physical examination except enlarged lymph nodes (Freeman & Winland-Brown, 2001). Symptomatic HIV infection is marked by the development of common infections and other conditions that are more severe and persistent in the presence of HIV infections but by themselves do not define AIDS. Examples of the conditions include thrush, oral hairy leukoplakia, peripheral neuropathy, cervical dysplasia, constitutional symptoms, and recurrent herpes zoster. Advanced HIV disease is the development of AIDS as defined by the 1993 CDC case definition (CDC, 1992). This definition includes a list of conditions indicative of severe immunosuppression, as well as the inclusion of all patients with a CD4 count below 200 cells/mm^3.

Viral Structure and Genetic Material

HIV particles appear spherical and their genetic material is enclosed in a special protein shell known as a capsis. HIV also has an outer layer known as an envelope, which is picked up from the host cell membrane as HIV buds out of the cell. Projecting out from the envelope are numerous spikes or knobs that originate from the virus. Each spike consists of three or four molecules of a protein called gp120, which is linked to another protein called gp41; together, the proteins are called gp41. The knobs bind to receptors on cells of the immune system that carry a marker known as the CD4 molecule.

HIV Life Cycle

Entry

HIV can replicate only inside human cells. The process typically begins when a virus particle bumps into a cell that carries on its surface a special protein called CD4. The spikes on the surface of the virus particle stick to the CD4 and allow the viral envelope to fuse with the cell membrane. The contents of the HIV particle are then released into the cell, leaving the envelope behind.

Reverse Transcription and Integration

Once inside the cell, the HIV enzyme reverse transcriptase converts the viral RNA into DNA, which is compatible with human genetic material. This DNA is transported to the cell's nucleus, where it is spliced into the human DNA by the HIV enzyme integrase. Once integrated, the HIV DNA is known as provirus.

Transcription and Translation

HIV provirus may lie dormant within a cell for a long time. But when the cell becomes activated, it treats HIV genes in much the same way as human genes. First, using human enzymes, it converts them into messenger RNA. Then the messenger RNA is transported outside the nucleus, and is used as a blueprint for producing new HIV proteins and enzymes.

Assembly, Budding, and Maturation

Among the strands of messenger RNA produced by the cell are complete copies of HIV genetic material. These gather together with newly made HIV proteins and enzymes to form new viral particles, which are then released from the cell. The enzyme protease plays a vital role at this stage of the HIV life cycle by chopping up long strands of protein into smaller pieces, which are used to construct mature viral cores. The newly matured HIV particles are ready to infect another cell and begin the replication process all over again. In this way the virus quickly spreads through the human body. And once a person is infected, that person can pass HIV on to others in bodily fluids.

GOALS OF TREATMENT

Goals of treatment with **ART** medication are listed in Box 37–1. The most important goals are to (1) achieve maximal suppression of plasma viral load for as long as possible, (2) delay the development of medication resistance, (3) preserve CD4 T-cell numbers, and (4) confer substantial clinical benefits. These goals are achieved by reducing HIV-related morbidity and mortality, improving quality of life, and restoring and preserving immunological function in persons infected with HIV (Moyle et al, 2008).

Unfortunately, complete eradication of HIV infection is not possible with the available **antiretroviral** medications because latently infected CD4 T-cells that are established during the earliest stages of acute HIV infection (Chun et al, 1998) persist with a long half-life in spite of prolonged suppression of HIV plasma viremia (Chun et al, 1997; Finzi et al, 1997, 1999; Wong et al, 1997).

Providers who follow approved treatment guidelines and strategies recognize substantial reductions in HIV-related morbidity and mortality (Mocroft et al, 1998; Mofenson et al, 1999; Palella et al, 1998; Vittinghoff et al, 1999) and reduced vertical transmission from infected mother to infant (Garcia et al, 1999). Higher HIV plasma viral loads are associated with more rapid disease progression (Mellors et al, 1996), whereas other factors, such as heightened T-cell activation with cellular turnover and expression of immune activation markers, probably contribute as well to clinical disease progression and the rate of CD4 T-cell decline (Rodriguez et al, 2006).

The goal of maximal viral suppression with initial ART may be difficult in some patients who have preexisting medication resistance. Unfortunately, about one of every six new HIV cases diagnosed in 2007 involved virus with ARV drug-resistance mutations (CDC, 2010). To be successful, **ART** regimens need to contain at least two, and preferably three, active medicines from multiple medication classes. If maximal initial suppression below the level of HIV detection (less than 50 copies/mL) is not achieved or is lost, it is important to change medication regimens to include at least two active medicines to achieve the maximal suppression goal. If it is not possible to achieve the HIV RNA less than 50 copies/mL goal in a clinically and immunologically stable patient, a time period of persistent detectable viremia may be acceptable while waiting for the availability of new medicine.

In general, viral load reduction to less than 50 copies/mL in most treatment-naïve patients occurs within the first 12 to 24 weeks of therapy. Predictors of virological success are presented in Box 37–2. Virological suppression is always observed. Viral suppression rates in clinical practice may be lower than the 80 to 90 percent seen in clinical trials. However, the use of current easier-to-take, coformulated, and potent ART regimens probably decrease the differences in outcomes between clinical trials and clinical practice (Moore, Keruly, Gebo, & Lucas, 2005). To achieve treatment goals, clinicians and patients must work together to define priorities, investigate options, and mutually determine the best treatment plan.

BOX 37–1 HIV TREATMENT GOALS

- Improve quality of life
- Obtain maximal and durable suppression of HIV
- Prevent vertical HIV transmission
- Prolong survival
- Reduce HIV-related morbidity
- Reduce transmissibility of HIV
- Restore and preserve immunological function

BOX 37–2 PREDICTORS OF ART VIROLOGICAL SUCCESS

- High-level patient adherence to ART regimen
- High potency of antiretroviral medication regimen
- Higher baseline CD4 T-cell count
- Low baseline HIV plasma viral RNA level
- Rapid (i.e., equal to or greater than 1 $\log_{10}$ in 1 to 4 mo) reduction of viral RNA level in response to ART

Rationale for ART Medication Selection

The clinical management of HIV is complex. Practical strategies must be identified so that virological suppression can be attained with therapy plans that patients can adhere to consistently. The treatment of HIV disease is a dynamic, rapidly changing arena, as newer drugs are developed and different combinations evaluated. Selecting the initial combination **ART** regimen is extremely important. Today, there are more than 20 U.S. Food and Drug Administration (FDA) approved **antiretroviral medicines** from six mechanistic classes from which to design combination **ART** regimens. HIV medications are always used in combination to reduce the amount of HIV in the blood (plasma viral load) by helping to block or "inhibit" certain steps during the HIV replication process.

Principles of Therapy

The U.S. Public Health Service has identified certain principles of therapy of HIV infection (CDC, 1998; Panel on Antiretroviral Guidelines for Adults and Adolescent, 2011).

First, ongoing HIV replication leads to immune system damage and progression to AIDS. HIV infection is always harmful, and long-term survival free of clinically significant immune dysfunction is unusual. The extent of HIV replication and its rate of CD4 T-cell destruction are indicated by plasma HIV RNA levels. The extent of HIV-induced immune damage that has already occurred is indicated by the CD4 T-cell counts. Therefore, plasma HIV RNA and CD4 T-cell levels must be regularly measured (every 3 to 6 months) to determine the risk for disease progression in an HIV-infected person and to identify when to initiate or modify antiretroviral treatment regimens (Panel on Antiretroviral Guidelines for Adults and Adolescents, 2011). Treatment decisions should be individualized based on the risk of disease progression as indicated by plasma HIV RNA levels and CD4 measurements. The goal of therapy should be the maximum achievable suppression of HIV replication. The use of potent combination ART to suppress HIV replication to below the levels of detection of sensitive viral-load assays limits the potential for selection of ART-resistant HIV variants.

The most effective way to achieve sustained suppression of HIV replication is the concomitant initiation of combinations of effective anti-HIV medications that are not cross resistant with ART agents. Because there is a finite number of available and effective ART drugs and cross-resistance between specific drugs has been shown, it is critical that every ART drug used in combination therapy be used according to optimal schedules and dosages.

These dosing principles should be applied to HIV-infected children, adolescents, and adults. However, the treatment of HIV-infected children involves unique pharmacological, virological, and immunological considerations (Panel on Antiretroviral Guidelines for Adults and Adolescents, 2009). Women should receive optimal ART even if they are pregnant. In fact, ART of the pregnant woman with **zidovudine** alone or with standard three-drug combinations has dramatically reduced the rates of vertical transmission from mother to child (Panel on Antiretroviral Guidelines for Adults and Adolescents, 2009). Treatment of acute HIV infection should be considered optional at this time (Panel on Antiretroviral Guidelines for Adults and Adolescents, 2009).

INITIATING ART MEDICATIONS

The most current recommendations (Panel on Antiretroviral Guidelines for Adults and Adolescents, 2011) suggest earlier initiation of ART. Specific recommendations state the following:

- ART should be initiated in all patients with a history of an AIDS-defining illness or with CD4 count of less than 350 cells/mm^3.
- ART should be initiated, regardless of CD4 count, HIV-associated nephropathy, and hepatitis B virus (HBV) coinfection when treatment of HBV is indicated.
- A combination **antiretroviral** (ARV) drug regimen is recommended for pregnant women who do not meet criteria for treatment with the goal to prevent perinatal transmission.
- ART is recommended for patients with CD4 counts between 350 and 500 cells/mm^3. (The panel of experts was divided on the strength of this recommendation: 55% of panel members were for strong recommendation and 45% for moderate recommendation.)
- For patients with CD4 counts greater than 500 cells/mm^3, 50 percent of panel members favor starting **antiretroviral** therapy; the other 50 percent of members view treatment as optional in that setting.

However, the potential benefits of early intervention must be weighed against the risks of early therapy. One major factor is nonadherence for patients who are not yet ready to commit to a complex drug regimen and potential adverse effects that may decrease their quality of life. Therefore, the clinician and the patient need to have an in-depth discussion of the potential toxicities and the complexities of the ART regimen. Box 37–3 presents these risks and benefits.

BOX 37–3 POTENTIAL BENEFITS AND RISKS OF ART

Potential Benefits of Early Therapy

- Maintenance of a higher CD4 T-cell count and prevention of potentially irreversible damage to the immune system
- Decreased risk for HIV-associated complications that can sometimes occur at CD4 counts more than 350 cells/μL, including tuberculosis, non-Hodgkin lymphoma, Kaposi's sarcoma, peripheral neuropathy, HPV-associated malignancies, and HIV-associated cognitive impairment
- Decreased risk of nonopportunistic medical conditions, including cardiovascular disease, renal disease, liver disease, and non–AIDS associated malignancies and infections
- Decreased risk of HIV transmission to others, which will have positive public health implications

Potential Risks of Early Therapy

- Treatment-related side effects and toxicities
- Viral resistance to medications because of incomplete viral suppression, resulting in loss of future treatment options
- Less time for the patient to learn about HIV and its treatment and less time to prepare for the need for adherence to ART
- Increased total time exposed to medication, with greater chance of treatment fatigue
- Premature use of ART before the development of more effective, less toxic, and/or better studied combinations of antiretroviral medications
- Transmission of medication-resistant virus in patients who do not maintain full viral suppression

Patients initiating **antiretroviral therapy** should be willing and able to commit to lifelong treatment and should understand the benefits and risks of therapy and the importance of adherence. Patients may choose to postpone therapy, and providers may elect to defer therapy, based on clinical and/or psychosocial factors on a case-by-case basis. The recommended treatment for HIV infection is a combination of three or more medications from two different classes (see Table 37–1). The six different mechanistic classes or "families" of HIV **antiretroviral** medications include **nucleoside reverse transcriptase inhibitors** (NRTIs), also called "nukes"; **nonnucleoside reverse transcriptase inhibitors** (NNRTIs), also called "nonnukes"; **protease inhibitors** (PIs); **fusion inhibitors** (FIs), also called "entry inhibitors"; **integrase strand transfer inhibitor** (INSTIs); and **CCR5 antagonists.** Each class of HIV medications inhibits HIV replication in a different way. The primary difference among the classes is the stage of HIV life cycle that the medications target.

The main mechanism of action of **NRTIs** is the inhibition of replication of retroviruses, including HIV, by interfering with viral RNA-directed DNA polymerase (reverse transcriptase). **NNRTIs** also inhibit replication of HIV by

Table 37–1 ART Medications and Treatment Strategies, Naïve Patients

• NNRTI + 2 NRTIs; or • PI (preferably boosted with ritonavir) + 2 NRTIs; or • INSTI + 2 NRTIs.	
Preferred regimens are those with optimal and durable efficacy, favorable tolerability and toxicity profile, and ease of use. The preferred regimens for nonpregnant patients are arranged by order of FDA approval of components other than nucleosides, thus, by duration of clinical experience.	
NNRTI-Based Regimen	**Comments**
• Efavirenz/emtricitabine/tenofovir	Efavirenz should not be used during the first trimester of pregnancy or in women trying to conceive or not using effective and consistent contraception.
PI-Based Regimens (in alphabetical order)	Atazanavir/r should not be used in patients who require >20 mg omeprazole equivalent/d.
• Atazanavir/r + emtricitabine/tenofovir	
• Darunavir/r (once daily) + emtricitabine/tenofovir	
INSTI-Based Regimen	
• Raltegravir + tenofovir/emtricitabine	
Preferred Regimen† for Pregnant Women	
• Lopinavir/r (twice daily) + zidovudine/lamivudine	
Alternative regimens are those that are effective and tolerable but have potential disadvantages compared with preferred regimens. An alternative regimen may be the preferred regimen for some patients.	
NNRTI-Based Regimens (in alphabetical order)	**Comments**
• Efavirenz + (abacavir or zidovudine)/lamivudine	Nevirapine:
• Nevirapine + zidovudine/lamivudine	• Should not be used in patients with moderate to severe hepatic impairment (Child-Pugh B or C)
PI-Based Regimens (in alphabetical order)	• Should not be used in women with pre-ARV CD4 >250 cells/mm^3 or men with pre-ARV CD4 >400 cells/mm^3
• Atazanavir/r + (abacavir or zidovudine)/lamivudine	Abacavir:
• Fosamprenavir/r (once or twice daily) + either [(abacavir or zidovudine)/lamivudine*] or tenofovir/emtricitabine	• Should not be used in patients who test positive for HLA B*5701
• Lopinavir/r (once or twice daily) + either [(abacavir or zidovudine)/lamivudine*] or tenofovir/emtricitabine	• Use with caution in patients with high risk of cardiovascular disease or with pretreatment HIV-RNA >100,000 copies/mL
• Saquinavir/r + tenofovir/emtricitabine	Once-daily lopinavir/r is not recommended in pregnant women.
Acceptable regimens are those that may be selected for some patients but are less satisfactory than preferred or alternative regimens.	
NNRTI-Based Regimen	**Comments**
• Efavirenz + didanosine + (lamivudine or emtricitabine)	Efavirenz + didanosine + emtricitabine or lamivudine has only been studied in small clinical trials.
PI-Based Regimen	Atazanavir/r is generally referred over atazanavir. Unboosted atazanavir may be used when ritonavir boosting is not possible.
• Atazanavir + (abacavir or zidovudine)/lamivudine	

*Lamivudine may substitute for emtricitabine or vice versa.

†For more detailed recommendations on antiretroviral use in an HIV-infected pregnant woman, refer to "Recommendations for Use of Antiretroviral Drugs in Pregnant HIV-Infected Women for Maternal Health and Interventions to Reduce Perinatal HIV Transmission in the United States," at http://aidsinfo.nih.gov/guidelines.

FIs = fusion inhibitors; INSTIs = integrase strand transfer inhibitor; NNRTIs = nonnucleoside reverse transcriptase inhibitors; NRTIs = nucleoside reverse transcriptase inhibitors; PI = protease inhibitors.

acting as a specific, noncompetitive, reverse transcriptase inhibitor and by disrupting the catalytic site of the enzyme. **PIs** are selective and competitive inhibitors of HIV protease. **PIs** play an essential role in preventing cleavage of protein precursors essential for HIV maturation, infection of new cells, and replication. **FIs** work by blocking an important step in the process of HIV entry into CD4 cells known as fusion. By blocking fusion, **FIs** may prevent HIV from entering and infecting CD4 cells. **Integrase inhibitors (IIs)** work by blocking the integrase enzyme that HIV needs to make more virus. **CCR5 antagonists** work by blocking a molecule called CCR5 that is found on the surface of CD4 cells so HIV cannot enter.

The most extensively studied combination **ART** regimens for treatment-naïve patients include either (1) one **NNRTI** with two **NRTIs** or (2) one **PI** (with or without ritonavir boosting) with two **NRTIs**. The potent inhibitory effect of **ritonavir** on metabolism of the cytochrome P450 (CYP450) 3A4 isoenzyme allows the addition of low-dose **ritonavir** to other **PIs** (except nelfinavir) as a pharmacokinetic booster to increase medication levels and prolong plasma half-lives of the active **PIs**. This "boosting" allows for reduced dosing frequency and/or pill burden, which may improve overall adherence to the **ART** regimen. The increased trough concentration (C_{min}) may improve the antiretroviral activity of the active **PIs**, which can be beneficial when the patient harbors HIV-resistant strains to **PIs** (Dragsted et al, 2003, 2005; Shulman et al, 2002). The potential for increased risk of hyperlipidemia and drug–drug interactions is the major drawback associated with **ritonavir** boosting.

Both **NNRTI**- and **PI**-based regimens result in suppression of HIV RNA levels and CD4 T-cell increases in a large majority of patients (Gallant et al, 2004; Gulick et al, 2006; Riddler et al, 2006; Squires et al, 2004; Staszewski et al, 1999). A list of several preferred and alternative **ART** regimens is available from which to choose (Table 37–1). **ART** regimens vary in efficacy, pill burden, and potential side effects. A patient-specific individualized regimen that maximizes adherence may be more successful in achieving full viral suppression. Many patient-specific characteristics are considered in the selection of **ART** regimen. These characteristics include the following:

- Comorbid conditions (e.g., cardiovascular disease, chemical dependency, liver disease, psychiatric disease, pregnancy, renal diseases, or tuberculosis)
- Convenience (e.g., pill burden, dosing frequency, and food and fluid considerations)
- Gender and pretreatment CD4 T-cell count if considering **nevirapine**
- Genotypic drug resistance testing
- HLA B*5701 testing if considering abacavir
- Patient adherence potential
- Potential adverse drug effects
- Potential drug interactions with other medications
- Pregnancy potential

Medications Used to Treat HIV

There are currently six different mechanistic classes or "families" of HIV antiretroviral medications that include **nucleoside reverse transcriptase inhibitors (NRTIs)**, **nonnucleoside reverse transcriptase inhibitors (NNRTIs)**, **protease inhibitors (PIs)**, **fusion inhibitors (FIs)**, **integrase strand transfer inhibitor (INSTIs)**, and **CCR5 antagonists**. The characteristics of FDA-approved **ART** medications are presented in Table 37–2 and the mechanistic classes are discussed in the following section.

Reverse Transcriptase Inhibitors

Reverse transcriptase inhibitors come in several forms. We will discuss **nucleoside** and **nucleotide** in this section and **non-nucleoside reverse transcriptase inhibitors** in the following section. **Nucleoside** and **nucleotide analogue reverse transcriptase inhibitors** (**NRTIs** and **NtRTIs**) are a class of antiretroviral medicines that inhibit the activity of reverse transcriptase, a viral DNA polymerase enzyme that retroviruses need to reproduce. This class of antiviral medicine was the first to be used to treat HIV and remains a backbone for most ART regimens. Available HIV **NRTIs** include **abacavir**, **didanosine**, **emtricitabine**, **lamivudine**, **stavudine**, **tenofovir**, and **zidovudine**. The only HIV **NtRTI** is **tenofovir**.

Nucleoside Reverse Transcriptase Inhibitors

In order for **NRTIs** to work, they must undergo chemical changes (phosphorylation) to become active in the body. **Nucleotide analogues** bypass this step. Thus, **NtRTIs** are already chemically activated. When HIV infects a cell, reverse transcriptase copies the HIV single-stranded RNA genome into a double-stranded HIV DNA. The HIV DNA is then integrated into the host chromosomal DNA, which allows host cellular processes such as transcription and translation (supra) to reproduce HIV. **NRTIs/NtRTIs** block the function of reverse transcriptase and prevent completion of synthesis of the double-stranded HIV DNA, thereby preventing HIV from reproducing. Whereas **NRTIs/NtRTIs** are analogues of the naturally occurring deoxynucleotides needed to synthesize the viral DNA, their mode of action is to compete with the natural deoxynucleotides for incorporation into the growing viral DNA chain. However, unlike the natural deoxynucleotides substrates, **NRTIs/NtRTIs** lack a 3'-hydroxyl group on the deoxyribose moiety. Thus, following incorporation of an **NRTI/NtRTI**, the next incoming deoxynucleotide cannot form the next 5'-3' phosphodiester bond needed to extend the DNA chain. So, when an **NRTI/NtRTI** is incorporated, viral DNA synthesis is prevented, a process known as chain termination. All **NRTIs/NtRTIs** are competitive substrate inhibitors.

Most **NRITs/NtRTIs** are eliminated via the kidneys so as to require renal adjustment when creatinine clearance

Table 37–2 **Antiretroviral Agent Characteristics**

Drug Name	Form	Usual Adult Dose	Food Effects	Renal Failure Dosing: CrCl 30–59 mL/min	Renal Failure Dosing: CrCl 10–29 mL/min	Renal Failure Dosing: CrCl <10 or dialysis	Liver Failure Dosing	Toxicity
Nucleoside Reverse Transcriptase Inhibitors (NRTIs)								
Abacavir (Ziagen)	300-mg tab; (see also Trizivir); 20 mg/mL po soln.	300 mg bid	No effect	Standard			Usual	Hypersensitivity: fever, rash, GI sx, dyspnea‡, #
Combivir	Zidovudine 300 mg + Lamivudine 150 mg (tab)	1 bid	No effect	Fixed formulation not recommended			Usual	Zidovudine side effects‡
Didanosine (Videx EC)*	125-, 200-, 250-, and 400-mg EC caps†	— / >60 kg / <60 kg EC caps with tenofovir / 400 mg qd / 250 mg qd 250 mg/d / 200 mg/d	½ h before or 2 h after meal Separate dosing of ATV, TPV/r	>60 kg 200 mg/d <60 kg 125 mg/d	>60 kg 125 mg/d <60 kg 100 mg/d	>60 kg 125 mg/d <60 kg 75 mg/d‖	Usual	Pancreatitis, peripheral neuropathy, GI intolerance‡
Emtricitabine (Emtriva)	200-mg cap	200 mg qd	No effect	200 mg q72h	200 mg q96h		Usual	Minimal‡ HBV flare§§
Lamivudine (Epivir)	150, 300 mg tab (see also: Combivir & Trizivir); 10 mg/mL PO soln.	150 mg bid or 300 mg qd	No effect	150 mg x 1 then 100 mg/d	150 mg x 1 then 25–50 mg/kg/d		Usual	Minimal‡ HBV flare§§
Epzicom	Lamivudine 300 mg + Abacavir 600 mg	1 qd	No effect	Fixed formulation not recommended in renal failure			Usual	Abaca hypersensitivity HBV flare§§
Stavudine (Zerit)*	15-, 20-, 30-, 40-mg cap; 1 mg/mL po soln.	Wt >60 kg: 40 mg bid Wt <60 kg: 30 mg bid	No effect	>60 kg 20 mg q12h <60 kg 15 mg q 12 h	>60 kg 20 mg q12h <60 kg 15 mg q24h	>60 kg 20 mg q24h <60 kg 20 mg q24h‖	Usual	Peripheral neuropathy, pancreatitis, lipoatrophy, ascending paresis (rare) ‡

Tenofovir (Viread)	300-mg tab (see also: Truvada)	300 mg qd	Take with meal	300 mg q48h	300 mg 2 d/wk	300 mg q7d[‖]	Usual	Minimal. Renal toxicity (rare) ‡ HBV flare§§
Trizivir (TZV)	Zidovudine 300 mg + Lamivudine 150 mg + Abacavir 300 mg (tab)	1 bid	No effect	Fixed formulation not recommended in renal failure			Usual	Hypersensitivity-reaction (abacavir), bone marrow suppression (zidovudine), GI intolerance (Zidovudine) ‡ HBV flar[10]
Truvada	Tenofovir 300 mg + Emtricitabine 200 mg	1 qd	No effect	Fixed formulation not recommended in renal failure			Usual	Minimal. Renal toxicity, HBV flare§§
Zidovudine (Retrovir)	100 cap, 300-mg tab; (see also Combivir & Trizivir) 10 mg/mL IV soln. 10 mg/mL PO soln.	300 mg bid 200 mg tid	No effect	300 mg bid	300 mg qd	100 mg tid	Usual	Peripheral neuropathy, stomatitis[3]
Protease Inhibitors (PIs)								
Atazanavir (Reyataz)	100-, 150-, and 200-mg capsules	400 mg qd; ATV 300 mg/ritonavir 100 mg qd. Boosting is often preferred and is required if ATV is combined with tenofovir or EFV	Take with food. Avoid concurrent buffered ddI, antacids.	Standard			CPS 7–9: 300 mg qd CPS >9: Avoid	Benign increase in indirect bilirubin, GI intolerance, transaminitis, prolongation of QTc (caution with conduction defects or drugs that do this) ‡‡
Fosamprenavir† (Lexiva)	700-mg tabs	1,400 mg bid or 700 mg/ritonavir 100 mg bid or 1,400 mg/ritonavir 200 mg qd	No effect	Standard			CPS 5–8: 700 mg bid CPS >9: Avoid	Rash, GI intolerance, transaminitis, headache, hepatitis [9]
Indinavir (Crixivan)	200-, 333-, 400-mg caps	800 mg q8h; separate buffered Didanosine ≥1 hr IDV 400 mg/ritonavir 400 mg bid or§ IDV 800 mg/ritonavir 100–200 mg bid§	1 h before or 2 h after meal unless with ritonavir	Standard			600 mg q8h	GI intolerance nephrolithiasis, transaminitis, benign increase in indirect bilirubin [9]

continued

Table 37–2 **Antiretroviral Agent Characteristics—cont'd**

Drug Name	Form	Usual Adult Dose	Food Effects	Renal Failure Dosing: CrCl 30–59 mL/min	Renal Failure Dosing: CrCl 10–29 mL/min	Renal Failure Dosing: CrCl <10 or dialysis	Liver Failure Dosing	Toxicity
Lopinavir/ Ritonavir (Kaletra)	200/50-mg tabs; LPV 80 mg + ritonavir 20 mg/mL po soln [2]	400 mg LPV + 100 mg ritonavir (2 tabs) bid soln: 5 mL bid	No effect	Standard			7	Transaminitis, GI intolerance (esp. diarrhea), asthenia [9]
Nelfinavir (Viracept)	250-, 625-mg tabs 50 mg/g powder	1,250 mg bid or 750 mg tid	Take with high-fat meal	Standard			7	GI intolerance, diarrhea, transaminitis [9]
Ritonavir (Norvir)	100 mg caps 600 mg/7.5 mL PO soln	600 mg q12h§; separate didanosine ≥2 h	Food improves GI tolerance	Standard			7	GI intolerance, paresthesia, transaminitis, taste perversion [9]
Saquinavir† (Invirase)	200 mg caps 500 mg tabs	SQV 1,000 mg bid + ritonavir 100 bid[2] SQV 2,000 mg qd + ritonavir 100 mg qd [2]	Take within 2 h of meal	Standard			7	GI intolerance, transaminitis‡‡
Tipranavir (Aptivus)	250-mg caps	500 mg bid with ritonavir 200 mg bid	Take TPV and ritonavir with food	Standard			CPS B or C: Avoid	Hepatotoxicity - monitor ALT, skin rash, GI intolerance, multiple drug interactions
Non-Nucleoside Reverse Transcriptase Inhibitors (NNRTIs)								
Delavirdine (Rescriptor)	100-, 200-mg tabs	400 mg tid	No effect	Standard			7	Rash
Efavirenz†† (Sustiva)	50-, 100-, 200-mg caps, 600-mg tabs	600 mg hs	Avoid high-fat meal	Standard			7	CNS x 2–3 wk, rash, hepatitis, false + cannabinoid test
Nevirapine (Viramune)	200 mg tabs 50 mg/5 mL PO susp.	200 mg qd x 14 d, then 200 mg bid	No effect	Standard		Standard; give postdialysis	Avoid	Rash, hepatitis; hepatic necrosis esp women with CD4 >250 in first 6 wk

Fusion Inhibitors (FIs)						
Enfuvirtide (Fuzeon, T-20)	90 mg single-use vials to be reconstituted with 1.1 mL H20	90 mg (1 mL) SQ q12h into upper arm, anterior or abdomen (rotate sites).	N/A	Standard	Usual dose	Site reactions

CPS = Child-Pugh score

* The combination of didanosine and stavudine can result in toxicities and the combination should not be used in pregnant women. Efavirenz should be avoided in first trimester of pregnancy and used with caution in women with reproductive potential. Avoid APV liquid in pregnancy.

† The following are no longer available: buffered didanosine, lopinavir/r 133/33 mg cap, amprenavir, or Fortovase.

‡ Class adverse reaction: lactic acidosis with steatosis. Most common with stavudine, ddl, and zidovudine.

§ Various dosing recommendations when using dual PI, PI plus NRTI, or dual PI plus NNRTI.

‖ Give postdialysis.

Registry for hypersensitivity 1-800-270-0425

** More frequent monitoring required. Drug change or dose change could be considered on a case-by-case basis noting the risk of resistance with underdosing.

†† Efavirenz should be avoided in first trimester of pregnancy and used with caution in women with reproductive potential. Avoid APV liquid in pregnancy.

‡‡ Class adverse effects include lipodystrophy with hyperglycemia, fat redistribution, hyperlipidemia, and possible increased bleeding with hemophilia. ATV does not cause hyperlipidemia. All PIs may cause elevated transaminases.

§§ Lamivudine, emtricitabine, and tenofovir; risk of flare of chronic HBV if discontinued.

Source: Adapted from Health Resources and Services Administration. (2006, February). *Tools for grantees: A pocket guide to adult HIV/AIDS treatment.* Retrieved from http://hab.hrsa.gov/tools/HIVpocketguide/PktGDrugTables.htm#DrugTable2; Panel on Antiretroviral Guidelines for Adults and Adolescents. (2011). *Guidelines for the use of antiretroviral agents in HIV-1-infected adults and adolescents.* Department of Health and Human Services. January 10, 2011; 1–166.

is less than 50 mL/minute. **Abacavir** is eliminated by a complex mechanism in the liver. Therefore, it does not require renal function adjustment. However, the half-life of **abacavir** is increased in mild hepatic impairment and must be dose adjusted for Child-Pugh class A and it is contraindicated for classes B and C. Common side effects of the **NRTI/NtRTI** class include anemia, bone marrow suppression, flatulence, headache, myopathy, nausea, rash, renal issues, and vomiting.

Symptomatic and life threatening lactic acidosis may occur with **NRTIs**. Lactic acidosis occurs more commonly in patients with hepatomegaly and hepatic steatosis. **Abacavir** is contraindicated in HLA B*5701 positive patients. Genetic screening for B*5701 effectively predicts the high probability of **abacavir**-associated hypersensitivity reaction, a multisystem syndrome that produces a constellation of symptoms that may include rash, fever, respiratory symptoms, or gastrointestinal symptoms. **Abacavir**-associated hypersensitive reaction can be fatal if **abacavir** is continued or is rechallenged. **Didanosine** and **stavudine** are associated with peripheral neuropathy and pancreatitis. **Tenofovir** is associated with a variety of side effects including decreased bone mineral density, increased biochemical markers of bone metabolism, acute renal failure, acute tubular necrosis, decreased urine volume, Fanconi syndrome, impairment, increased creatinine, interstitial nephritis (including acute cases), nephritis, nephrogenic diabetes insipidus, new onset or worsening renal, proximal renal tubulopathy, renal failure, and renal insufficiency.

NRTI/NtRTIs are sometimes prescribed in fix-dose (fd) combination formulations with other **NRTI/NtRTIs** and other **antiretrovirals** agents to decrease pill burden and simplify ART regimens. **Emtricitabine, lamivudine**, and **tenofovir** are also active against hepatitis B virus.

Nonnucleoside Reverse Transcriptase Inhibitors

Nonnucleoside reverse transcriptase inhibitors (NNRTIs), also known as non-nucleosides or nonnukes, attach themselves to reverse transcriptase and prevent the enzyme from converting RNA to DNA. As a result, HIV's genetic material cannot be incorporated into the healthy genetic material of the cell, and prevents the cell from producing new virus. The pharmacokinetics of **NNRTIs** are complex. Although possessing a common mechanism of action, the approved **NNRTIs, delavirdine, efavirenz, etravirine**, and **nevirapine**, differ in structural and pharmacokinetic characteristics. Each undergoes biotransformation by the CYPP450 enzyme system. This makes them prone to clinically significant drug interactions when combined with other **ARTs**. **NNRTIs** interact with other concurrent medications and complementary/alternative medicines, acting as either inducers or inhibitors of drug-metabolizing CYP450 enzymes. These drug interactions become an important consideration in the clinical use when designing combination regimens, as recommended by current guidelines. Common side effects of the NNRTI class include: difficulty sleeping, dizziness, drowsiness, fatigue, headache, liver problems (which can be severe and life threatening), nausea, vomiting, diarrhea, rash (which can be severe), and vivid dreams.

Protease Inhibitors

Protease inhibitors (PIs) are a class of medications used to treat or prevent viral infection such as HIV and hepatitis C. **HIV-PIs** prevent viral replication by inhibiting the enzyme activity of HIV-1 protease in the CD4 cell that cleaves nascent proteins for final assembly of new virions. All **PIs** have a similar mechanism of action and do not depend on intracellular conversion to be active in the host cell. Available **PIs** include **atazanavir, fosamprenavir, indinavir, lopinavir/ritonavir, nelfinavir, ritonavir, saquinavir**, and **tipranavir**. Like **NNRTIs, PIs** are metabolized by CYP450 enzymes. This makes **PIs** subject to drug interactions with other medicines that use the CYP450 pathway. **Ritonavir** is a very potent CYP450 inhibitor of other **PIs** (except **nelfinavir**) and therefore is commonly paired in low doses to pharmacokinetically intensify the half-life of other **PIs** in a prescribing practice known as **ritonavir** boosting. Drug interactions with boosted and non-boosted **PIs** must be considered when devising an effective, well tolerated **ART** regimen. **PIs** are eliminated in the feces and do not require renal dosing adjustment. Common side effects of the **PI** class include: bleeding problems, diarrhea, gastrointestinal disturbance, hyperglycemia, hyperlipidemia, lipodystrophy, and liver problems that can be severe.

Integrase Strand Transfer Inhibitors

Integrase strand transfer inhibitors (INSTIs) prevent insertion of HIV DNA into the human DNA genome, thereby blocking the ability of HIV to replicate. Integrase is an enzyme that allows HIV genetic material to integrate into the DNA of human CD4 cells, making it possible for the infected cell to make new copies of HIV. By interfering with integrase, **INSTIs** prevent HIV genetic material from integrating into the CD4 cell, thus stopping viral replication. The stage in which HIV genetic material is integrated into human DNA is not fully understood. For that reason, developing an effective **integrase inhibitor** was not easy and many **INSTIs** failed very early in clinical trials. However, **raltegravir** was approved by the FDA in 2007. It acts at the final phase of integration when the viral strand is transferred into the host cell. **Raltegravir** should be used with caution when administered with strong inducers of uridine diphosphate glucuronosyltransferase (UGT1A1), including **rifampin**. These inducers of UGT1A1 may reduce plasma concentrations of **raltegravir**. Similar to **rifampin, ritonavir-boosted tipranavir** reduces plasma concentrations of **raltegravir**. The most common side effects related to **raltegravir** are creatinine kinase elevations, diarrhea, headache, myopathy, nausea, pyrexia, and rhabdomyolysis.

CCR5 Antagonists

CCR5 antagonists selectively bind to the human chemokine receptor CCR5 present on the cell membrane, preventing the interaction of HIV-1 gp120 and CCR5, which is necessary for CCR5-tropic HIV-1 to enter cells. **Maraviroc** is only one CCR5 antagonist licensed by the FDA. CXCR4-tropic and dual-tropic HIV-1 entry are not inhibited by **maraviroc. Maraviroc** is a selective, slowly reversible, small molecule. **Maraviroc** is a substrate of CYP3A and Pgp; therefore, its pharmacokinetics are modulated by inhibitors and inducers of these enzymes/transporters. The CYP3A/Pgp inhibitors **ketoconazole, lopinavir/ritonavir, ritonavir, darunavir/ritonavir, saquinavir/ritonavir,** and **atazanavir ± ritonavir** all increase the C_{max} and the area under the curve (AUC) of **maraviroc.** The CYP3A inducers **rifampin, etravirine,** and **efavirenz** decreased the C_{max} and AUC of **maraviroc.** The most common adverse events reported with **maraviroc** are cough, dizziness, pyrexia, rash, and upper respiratory tract infections. Additional adverse events include diarrhea, edema, esophageal candidiasis, influenza, parasomnias, rhinitis, sleep disorders, and urinary abnormalities.

Fusion Inhibitors

Fusion inhibitors work by attaching themselves to proteins on the surface of CD4 cells or proteins on the surface of HIV and thereby prevent fusion of HIV-1 with CD4 cells. **Enfuvirtide**, the only FDA-approved entry inhibitor that targets the gp120 or gp41 proteins on HIV's surface, was licensed in 2003. By binding to the first heptad-repeat (HR1) in the gp41 subunit of the viral envelope glycoprotein and preventing the conformational changes required for the fusion of viral and cellular membranes, **enfuvirtide** interferes with the entry of HIV-1 into cells by inhibiting fusion of viral and cellular membranes. **Enfuvirtide** is not an inhibitor of CYP450 enzymes. Co-administration of **enfuvirtide** and other drugs that are inducers or inhibitors of CYP450 is not expected to alter the pharmacokinetics of **enfuvirtide.** Common side effects of **enfuvirtide** include skin itchiness, swelling, and pain at the site of the injection (injection site reactions). Other side effects may include dizziness, fatigue, insomnia, and numbness in feet or legs.

COST CONSIDERATIONS

HIV medicines are very expensive. Medication costs vary widely, depending on the choice of medications; the complexity of the ART regimen; where medications are purchased, neighborhood pharmacy versus mail order; and who is doing the purchasing, government versus individual. For most patients, private insurance providers, Medicare, state Medicaid, drug assistance programs, state AIDS Drug Assistance Programs (ADAPs), or community resources pay most of the cost. Patient co-payments also vary widely by individual prescription insurance plan. Many pharmaceutical manufacturers of HIV drugs have implemented co-pay programs to provide financial assistance to patients who qualify financially and medically. Although HIV medications are very costly, not taking them can be even more costly (Chen et al, 2006). Table 37–3 provides some indication of the expense involved in the treatment of HIV.

AIDS Drug Assistance Program

The national AIDS Drug Assistance Program (ADAP) is a major source of medications for the treatment of HIV disease. The program is funded through part B of the Ryan

Table 37–3 **Brand-Name Antiretroviral Medications, Usual Adult Dosing and Monthly Average Wholesale Price by Mechanistic Class**

Generic Name	Brand Name	Usual Adult Dose	AWP	RTV AWP Price*	Total
Nucleoside and Nucleotide Reverse Transcriptase Inhibitors (N/NTRTIs)					
Abacavir (ABC)	Ziagen	300 mg bid or 600 mg daily	$615		$615
Abacavir/lamivudine (ABC/3TC)	Epzicom	600/300 mg daily	$1,073		$1,073
Abacavir/lamivudine/zidovudine (ABA/AZT/3TC)	Trizivir	300/150/300 mg bid	$1,608		$1,608
Didanosine (ddI)	Videx	400 mg EC daily if >60 kg or 250 mg EC daily if <60 kg	$425 $272		$425 $272
Emtricitabine (FTC)	Emtriva	200 mg daily	$437		$437
Emtricitabine/tenofovir (FTC/TDF)	Truvada	200/300 mg daily	$1,118		$1,118
Lamivudine (3TC)	Epivir	150 mg bid or 300 mg daily	$458		$458
Lamivudine/zidovudine (ZDV/3TC)	Combivir	300/150 mg bid	$993		$993

continued

Table 37–3 **Brand-Name Antiretroviral Medications, Usual Adult Dosing and Monthly Average Wholesale Price by Mechanistic Class—cont'd**

Generic Name	Brand Name	Usual Adult Dose	AWP	RTV AWP Price*	Total
Stavudine (d4T)	Zerit	40 mg bid if >60 kg or 30 mg bid if <60 kg	$456 $448		$456 $448
Tenofovir (TDF)	Viread	300 mg daily	$772		$772
Zidovudine (ZDV)	Retrovir	300 mg bid	$535		$535
Non-Nucleoside Reverse Transcriptase Inhibitors (NNRTIs)					
Efavirenz (EFV)	Sustiva	600 mg daily at bedtime	$638		$638
Etravirine (ETV)	Intelence	200 mg bid with a meal	$877		$877
Nevirapine (NVP)	Viramune	200 mg bid; dose is initiated at 200 mg daily for 14 d to reduce rash risk	$547		$547
Protease Inhibitors (PIs)					
Atazanavir (ATV)	Reyataz	400 mg daily (2 caps daily) or 300 mg daily + 100 mg RTV daily	$1,087 $1,077	 $309	$1,087 $1,386
Darunavir (DRV)	Prezista	600 mg bid + 100 mg RTV bid or 900 mg daily + 100 mg RTV daily	$1,102	$617	$1,719
		800 mg daily + Ritonavir 100 mg daily	$1,102	$617	$1,719
Fosamprenavir (FPV)	Lexiva	1,400 mg daily + 100 mg Ritonavir daily or	$869	$309	$1,178
Indinavir (IDV)	Crixivan	800 mg q8h or 800 mg bid + 100–200 mg Ritonavir bid	$548 $365	 $1,234	$548 $1,600
Lopinavir/ritonavir (LPVr)	Kaletra	400/100 mg bid (2 tabs bid)	$842		$842
Nelfinavir (NFV)	Viracept	1,250 mg bid (2 bid)	$844		$844
Ritonavir (RTV)	Norvir	100 mg daily 200 mg daily	$309 $617		$309 $617
Saquinavir mesylate (SQV)	Invirase	1,000 mg bid + RTV 100 mg bid	$1,026	$617	$1,644
Tipranavir (TPV)	Aptivus	500 mg bid with RTV 200 mg bid	$1,187	$1,234	$2,422
Fusion Inhibitors (FIs)					
Enfuviritide (T-20)	Fuzeon	90 mg by subcutaneous injection bid	$3,062		$3,062
CCR5 Antagonists					
Maraviroc (MVC)	Selzentry	300 mg bid	$1,101		$1,101
Integrase Strand Transfer Inhibitors (INSTIs)					
Raltegravir (RAL)	Isentress	400 mg bid	$1,075		$1,075

*RTV (Norvir) co-administration "boosting" is required to achieve therapeutic drug levels and thereby adds to the ART cost.

White HIV/AIDS Treatment Modernization Act (formerly known as the Ryan White Comprehensive AIDS Resources Emergency [CARE] Act), which provides grants to states and territories. Program funds may also be used to purchase health insurance for eligible clients and for services that enhance access to, adherence to, and monitoring of drug treatments. Grants are awarded to all 50 states, the District of Columbia, Puerto Rico, Guam, the U.S. Virgin Islands, and the Pacific jurisdictions. Congress mandates funds that must be used for the ADAP, an important distinction because other part B spending decisions are made locally.

Medication Resistance

Antiretroviral medication resistance occurs when HIV replicates while the patient is taking **ART**. The replication may be the result of poor patient adherence to the ART regimen or possible drug–drug or drug–food interactions, abnormal absorption, distribution, metabolism, or excretion of the medicine, resulting in HIV replication and genetic mutational changes. The first sign of HIV resistance to ART is the presence of detectible plasma viral RNA on two separate viral load measurements. Various assays are used to determine the nature of HIV medication resistance. The most commonly used resistance assays are phenotypic and genotypic assays.

Phenotype assays are used to measure sensitivity to various **antiretroviral** agents. The assay reports HIV sensitivity in terms of a ratio above the normal or wild-type IC_{50}. In other words, it is the half maximal (50%) inhibitory concentration (IC) of a medicine (50% IC, or IC_{50}). This information allows a provider to determine the relative extent of resistance. Genotype assays are used to identify the presence of specific resistance mutations of the HIV genes known to be associated with resistance to specific **antiretroviral** agents (see Table 37–4).

Genotype testing identifies viral mutations on the reverse transcriptase (RT), protease (PR), envelope, and integrase genes. Notation of the specific mutations is standardized by identifying the first letter of the usual amino acid, the location on the gene (number), followed by the first letter of the amino acid change related to the mutation. For example, the M184V mutation conveys that on the 184 position of the RT enzyme, the methionine amino acid residue was replaced with a valine amino acid residue. This is one of the most commonly associated

Table 37–4 **Resistance Mutations to Antiretroviral Medicine**

Antiretroviral Medicine		Codon Mutation
Mutation in reverse transcriptase gene associated with resistance to NRTIs Nucleoside reverse transcriptase inhibitors (NRTIs)		
Multi-NRTI Resistance: 69 Insertion Complex (affects all NRTIs)		M41L, A62V, 69, K70R, L210W, T215Y/F, K219O/E
Multi-NRTI Resistance: 151 Insertion Complex (affects all NRTIs)		A62V, V75I, F77L, F116Y, Q151M
Multi-NRTI Resistance: Thymidine Analogue-Associated mutations (TAMS; affects all NRTIs)		M41L, D67N, K70R, L210W, T215Y/F, K219O/E
Abacavir (ABC)		K65R, L74V, Y115F, M184V
Didanosine (ddI)		K65R, L74V
Emtricitabine (FTC)		K65R, M184V
Lamivudine (3TC)		K65R, M184V
Stavudine (d4T)		M41L, K65R, D67N, K70R, L210W, T215Y/F, K219Q/E
Tenofovir (TDF)		K65R, K70E
Zidovudine (ZDV)		M41L, D67N, K60R, L210W, T215Y/F, K219Q/E
Nonnucleoside Reverse Transcriptase Inhibitors (NNRTIs)		
Efavirenz (EFV)		L100I, K101P, K103N, V106M, V108I, Y181C/I, Y188L, G190S/A, P225H
Etravirine (ETV)		V90I, A98G, L100I, K101E/P,V106I, V179D/E/T, Y181C/I/V, G190S/A, M230L
Nevirapine (NVP)		L100I, K101P, K103N, V106M, V108I, Y181C/I, Y188L, G190S/A
Mutation in the Protease Gene Associated With Resistance to Protease Inhibitors (PIs)		
PIs	**Critical**	**Secondary**
Atazanavir (ATV)	I50L, I84V, N88S	L10I/F/V/C, G16E, K20R/M/I/T/V, L24I, V32I, L33I/F/V, E34Q, M36I/L/V, M46I/L, G48V, F53L/Y, I54L/V/M/T/A, D60E, I62V, I64L/M/V, A71V/I/T/L, G73C/S/T/A, V82A/T/F/I, I85V, L90M, I93L/M
Darunavir (DRV)	I47V, I50V, I54M/L, L76V, I84V	V11I, V32I, L33F, I47V, G73S, L89V
Fosamprenavir (FPV)	I50V, I84V	L10F/I/R/V, V32I,M46I/L, I54L/V/M, G73S, L76V, V82A/F/S/T, L90M

continued

Table 37–4 **Resistance Mutations to Antiretroviral Medicine—cont'd**

Antiretroviral Medicine		Codon Mutation
Indinavir/Ritonavir (IDVr)	M46I/L, V82A/F/T, I84V,	L10I/R/V, K20M/R, L24I, V32I, M36I, I54V, A71V/T, G73S/A, L76V, V77I, L90M
Lopinavir/Ritonavir (LPVr)	V32I, I47V/A, L76V, V82A/F/T/S	L10F/I/R/V, K20M/R, L24I, L33F, M46I/L, I50V, F53L, I54V/L/A/M/T/S, L63P, A71V/T, G73S, L76V, I84V, L90M
Nelfinavir (NFV)	D30N, L90M	L10F/I, M36I, M46I/L, A71V/T, V77I, V82A/F/T/S, I84V, N88D/S
Saquinavir (SQV)	G48V, L90M	L10I/R/V, L24I, I54V/L, I62V, A71V/T, G73S, V77I, V82A/F/T/S, I84V
Tipranavir (TPV)	I47V, Q58E, T74P, V82L/T, I84V	L10V, I13V, K20M/R, L33F, F35G, M36I, K43T, M46L, I54A/M/V, H69K, N83D, L90M
Mutations in the Envelope Gene Associated With Resistance to Fusion Inhibitors (FIs) and CCR5 Antagonists		
Enfuviritide (T-20)	G36D, I37V, V38A/M/E, Q39R, Q40H, N42T, N43D	
Maraviroc (MVC)	Activity limited to CCR5 virus only. CXCR4-CCR5 mixed and CXCR4 viruses do not respond.	
Mutations in the Integrase Gene Associated With Resistance to Integrase Inhibitors (IIs)		
Raltegravir (RAL)	Y143R/H/C, Q148H/K/R, N155H	

Adapted from Johnson et al, 2009.

cytosine analogue-resistant mutations to confer high-level resistance to medications such as emtricitabine and lamivudine. Other RT gene mutations, such as M41L, D67N, K70R, L210W, T215Y/F, and K219O/E, are more commonly known as thymidine analogue mutations, or TAMs. The presence of these mutations affects all **NRTIs**. K65R reduces viral sensitivity to **abacavir**, **didanosine**, **emtricitabine**, **lamivudine**, and **tenofovir** while increasing sensitivity to **zidovudine** (Grant et al, 2010). K103N, a major RT mutation, renders cross-resistance to **efavirenz** and **nevirapine**.

PR gene mutations are classified as critical and secondary. When present, PR mutations render HIV resistant to various **PI** agents. As the number of mutations emerges, HIV develops increasingly high-grade resistance whereby mutation can prevent the **PI** from binding to the catalytic site of action, allowing the normal gag-pol protein to be cleaved and form new virus. Like some RT mutations, some PR mutations confer broad, **PI** class cross-resistance to multiple medicines. L90M and I50L are two examples of very significant critical PR cross-resistance mutations.

Medication resistance to most **PIs** requires multiple mutations in the HIV protease and seldom develops following early virological failure, especially when **ritonavir** boosting is used. However, medication resistance to **efavirenz** or **nevirapine** is conferred by a single mutation in reverse transcriptase and develops rapidly following virological failure (Hirsch et al, 2003).

Pretreatment

About one of every six new HIV cases diagnosed in 2007 involved virus with **ARV drug**-resistance mutations (CDC, 2010). The presence of transmitted medication-resistant viruses, particularly those with **nonnucleoside reverse transcriptase inhibitor (NNRTI)** mutations, may be responsible for not achieving the treatment goal of HIV suppression of less than 50 copies/mL (Wheeler, Mahle, & Bodnar, 2007). Therefore, pretreatment HIV genotypic resistance testing should be considered in selecting the best ART regimen.

Although covered by most insurance providers, resistance assays are expensive. Clinicians should be familiar with the important considerations and limitations associated with HIV resistance testing (see Box 37–4) and be able to explain these to the patient. It is critical that, whenever possible, collection of blood for resistance testing should be performed when the patient is taking **ART** or within 4 weeks of stopping antiretroviral medicine. Resistance testing is not recommended when viral load (VL) is less than 1,000 copies/mL.

Virological Failure

Virological failure, defined as the failure to achieve or maintain suppression of viral replication to less than 50 copies/mL, may be categorized as either (1) incomplete virological response (as when two consecutive HIV RNAs are greater than 400 copies/mL after 24 wk or when HIV RNA is greater than 50 copies/mL by 48 wk in a treatment-naïve patient who is initiating **ART**), or (2) virological rebound (when HIV RNA is repeatedly detected at greater than 50 copies/mL after virological suppression). Baseline HIV RNA affects the time course of suppression. Some patients take longer than others to suppress HIV RNA levels. The timing, pattern, and/or slope of HIV RNA decrease may predict ultimate virological response (Weverling et al, 1998). Unfortunately, there is no

BOX 37–4 HIV DRUG RESISTANCE TESTING: EIGHT IMPORTANT CONSIDERATIONS AND LIMITATIONS

1. Biological cutoffs are based on normal distribution of susceptibility to drug for wild-type strain from treatment-naïve patients.
2. Clinical cutoffs are based on data from clinical trials or cohort studies to determine change in susceptibility that results in reduced virological response.
3. Clinical phenotypic cutoff values include diminished versus no response; partial activity may be useful when treatment options are limited. Analysis complicated by prior drug exposure and activity of other drugs in salvage regimen.
4. Consider phenotyping over genotyping when treatment history is complex and/or significant resistance is expected.
5. May detect resistance only in species that make up more than 10 to 20 percent of viral population.
6. Measures susceptibility to individual medicines, not medication combinations.
7. Phenotypic resistance reported as fold change in IC_{50} for the test strain versus reference wild-type strain.
8. Testing should be performed on therapy whenever possible or within 4 weeks of stopping antiretroviral medicines and is not recommended when VL is less than 1,000 copies/mL.

consensus on the optimal time to change ART when virological failure occurs. The more aggressive approach is to change the medication regimen for any repeated detectable viremia after suppression to less than 50 copies/mL in a patient taking ART. Again, an assessment of adherence is essential. Other approaches for when to change ART allow for detectable viremia up to an arbitrary level (e.g., 1,000 to 5,000 copies/mL when resistance testing can more easily be performed). However, ongoing viral replication in the presence of ART promotes the selection of drug resistance mutations (Barbour et al, 2002) and may limit future ART options. Isolated episodes of viremia ("blips," e.g., single levels of 51 to 1,000 copies/mL) may simply represent laboratory variation (Nettles et al, 2005) and are not usually associated with subsequent virological failure. Rebound to higher viral load levels or more frequent episodes of viremia increase the risk of failure (Greub et al, 2002).

Causes of ART Failure

Although ART is highly successful, it is not without failure. Many factors are associated with an increased risk of ART treatment failure (see Box 37–5). Suboptimal adherence and toxicity may account for 28 to 40 percent

BOX 37–5 FACTORS ASSOCIATED WITH ART FAILURE

Patient factors at baseline:

- AIDS diagnosis
- Comorbid conditions (e.g., affective mental health disorders and active substance use)
- Earlier calendar year of starting ART when less-potent regimens or more poorly tolerated antiretroviral medicines were used
- Higher pretreatment HIV RNA level (regimen specific)
- Lower pretreatment or nadir CD4 T-cell count
- Pretreatment drug-resistant virus
- Prior ART failure, with development of drug resistance or cross-resistance
- ART adverse effects and toxicity
- Nonadherence to ART and medical appointments
- Suboptimal pharmacokinetics caused by variable absorption, metabolism, and/or penetration into HIV reservoirs, food or fasting requirements, adverse drug–drug interactions with concomitant medications and foods
- Suboptimal potency of the ART regimen
- Unknown causes

of treatment failures and regimen discontinuations (D'Arminio Monforte et al, 2000). Multiple risk factors for treatment failure can occur simultaneously. Factors not associated with treatment failure include gender, pregnancy, and history of past substance use.

When ART failure occurs, determining the cause(s) is essential. Candid conversation with the patient and his or her family member(s) coupled with investigation of pharmacy records allows the clinician to explore the various risk factors for ART failure. In assessing ART failure, it is important to identify as many contributing factors as possible. Careful identification of the reasons for failure allows the clinician to address patient needs more effectively and reduces the potential for subsequent ART failure.

Other circumstances should be considered when assessing for virological failure and planning for optimal patient outcomes. In some patients with extensive prior treatment and drug resistance (e.g., when new ART that contains at least two fully active agents cannot be identified), viral suppression below 50 copies/mL is difficult to achieve. When maximal virological suppression cannot be achieved, the goals are to preserve immunological function and to prevent clinical progression. Even partial virological suppression of HIV RNA greater than 0.5 $\log_{10}$ copies/mL from baseline is associated with clinical benefits (Murray, Elashoff, Iacono-Connors, Cvetkovich, & Struble, 1999). However, these marginal benefits must be balanced with the ongoing risk for accumulating additional resistance mutations. It is reasonable to maintain a patient on the same regimen, rather than changing the regimen, depending on the stage of HIV disease.

DISCONTINUATION OR INTERRUPTION OF ANTIRETROVIRAL MEDICATIONS

Discontinuation or interruption of ART is associated with HIV viral rebound, immune decompensation, and clinical progression. Similarly, discontinuation of ART regimens containing **emtricitabine**, **lamivudine**, or **tenofovir** in patients with hepatitis B co-infection may experience an exacerbation of hepatitis on ART discontinuation (Bessesen, Ives, Condreay, Lawrence, & Sherman, 1999). Nonetheless, unplanned interruption of ART may become necessary for a number of reasons. Concurrent illness, severe drug toxicity, surgery that precludes oral therapy, and **antiretroviral** medication nonavailability are some of the common reasons patients discontinue ART. Potential risks and benefits of interruption vary according to a number of factors, including the clinical and immunological status of the patient, the reason for the interruption, the type and duration of the interruption, and the presence or absence of resistant HIV at the time of interruption.

Monitoring

Although ART prolongs life and improves quality of life by suppressing HIV replication and decreasing symptoms of uncontrolled HIV, ART is potentially harmful if not periodically monitored. Monitoring is multidimensional in the care of an HIV-infected patient. In addition to monitoring the effectiveness of ART it is standard of care to monitor the following:

- Adherence to medications and medical visits
- Affective mental health problems
- Alterations in metabolism of lipids and glucose
- Cardiovascular risk
- Hepatitis B and C co-infection
- High-risk behaviors
- Immunization status
- Renal and hepatic function
- Sexually transmitted infections
- Somatic signs and symptoms
- Tobacco, alcohol, and substance use

Plasma HIV RNA by PCR or "viral load" measures the effectiveness of ART to control viral replication. Sequential measurement of the CD4 count is performed to determine the degree of immune system reconstitution. When available, a viral load test is performed shortly after ART is started. If the treatment is working effectively, the viral load will drop to below the level of detection—less than 50 copies/mL. Ideally this occurs within 24 weeks of initiating ART, but for some patients it can take 6 months. Viral load tests are performed every few months. As there can be some variability in viral load test results, the results are monitored over a period of time. An increase in viral load may be followed by a fall in CD4 count and a greater risk of developing opportunistic infections. If viral load is increasing, it is important to determine the cause. Causes for loss of virological control are usually related to impaired medication adherence, drug interactions, altered medication absorption, and development of drug resistance.

OUTCOME EVALUATION

The patient-lived experience of HIV disease and the medications used to treat it are uniquely individual. Patients present to care at various stages of the disease, frequently challenged by multiple life circumstances that complicate the treatment plan. These challenges include, among others active substance abuse, chronic pain, comorbid medical conditions, domestic violence, lack of child care, lack of health insurance, lack of transportation, mental illness, nonadherence to ART and provider visits, opportunistic infection(s), pregnancy, sexual abuse, stigma, unstable living conditions, and victimization. These challenges require a multidisciplinary team to optimize patient outcomes. Owing to complex social and medical problems, optimal patient outcomes are difficult to achieve. Thus, it is critical to formulate attainable treatment plans that are appropriately adapted the individual patient and his or her living situation. A variety of personal and system barriers can potentially diminish patient resolve and confidence in lifelong treatment with ART. Positive predictors of success entail adherence to ART and routine surveillance for effectiveness of therapy and its potentially harmful events.

Although the path to treatment success is arduous without access to specialty HIV health care and modern ART, and drug toxicities and resistance continue to be formidable challengers, effective, well-tolerated therapies coupled with a pipeline of evolving new medications herald a bright future for those chronically infected with HIV. HIV clinicians have immediate Internet access to current comprehensive treatment guidelines from the U.S. Department of Health and Human Services (DHHS) and the International AIDS Society—USA (IAS-USA).

CONCLUSION

Medical care for HIV-infected persons has grown increasingly complex and is beyond the scope of this book chapter. However, a multiplicity of available resources exists to assist clinicians in providing high-quality care to their HIV-infected patients. The U.S. Department of Health and Human Services AIDSinfo Web site (http://www.aidsinfo.nih.gov/) is a dependable source of current, up-to-date information for the following:

- Fact sheets on HIV/AIDS-related drug interactions
- HIV treatment guidelines
- Locating resources on HIV/AIDS-related topics
- Preventive and therapeutic HIV vaccine research
- Research studies on investigational drugs, vaccines, and other new or existing treatments for HIV/AIDS

The Health Resources and Services Administration (HRSA) also provides multiple HIV medical care performance measures at ftp://ftp.hrsa.gov/hab/habGrp1PMs08.pdf. These performance measures can be used to help establish and measure the quality of HIV care being rendered. The performance measures include the following:

- ART adherence assessment and counseling
- ART for pregnant women
- Cervical cancer screening
- Frequency of CD4 measurement
- Hepatitis B vaccination
- Hepatitis C screening
- HIV risk counseling
- Lipid screening
- Medical evaluation visits
- Oral examination
- PCP prophylaxis
- Prescription of ART
- Syphilis screening
- TB screening

The following recommendations and treatment guidelines from the Centers for Disease Control and Prevention are also available at http://www.cdc.gov/hiv/resources/guidelines/index.htm:

- *A Guide to Primary Care for People With HIV/AIDS*
- *A Guide to the Clinical Care of Women With HIV*
- *Adults and Adolescent Treatment Guidelines*
- *Appendix: Recommendations to Help Patients Avoid Exposure to or Infection From Opportunistic Pathogens*
- *Co-Infection Guidelines*
- *Guidelines for Prevention and Treatment of Opportunistic Infections in HIV—Infected Adults and Adolescents*
- *Interim Guidance—HIV-Infected Adults and Adolescents: Considerations for Clinicians Regarding Swine-Origin Influenza A (H1N1) Virus*
- *MMWR: Guidelines for the Prevention and Treatment of Opportunistic Infections Among HIV–Exposed and HIV–Infected Children*
- *Pediatric Treatment Guidelines*
- *Perinatal Guidelines*
- *Sexually Transmitted Diseases Treatment Guidelines*
- *Tuberculosis Treatment Guidelines*

HIV DISEASE

PATIENT EDUCATION

Related to the Overall Treatment Plan/Disease Process

- ☐ After diagnosis, patients need to be educated regarding what it means to be HIV positive (they are infected with the HIV virus) versus what AIDS is (their immune system has been affected and they are at risk for life-threatening infections).
- ☐ Patients need education regarding the chronicity of HIV treatment. The clinician may make an analogy of HIV disease to diabetes; diabetics need insulin for the rest of their life and patients with HIV-disease must take their medications daily for the rest of their lives.
- ☐ HIV-infected patients need to be vaccinated with the recommended adult vaccines, including an annual **influenza vaccine.**
- ☐ Symptoms of opportunistic infections should be discussed so that patients receive early treatment.

Specific to the Drug Therapy

- ☐ Highly active antiretroviral therapy (HAART) is a combination of medications and all should be taken together as prescribed to decrease viral load.
- ☐ Adherence to HAART is critical to prevent the development of drug resistance.

Reasons for Taking the Drug(s)

- ☐ Prevention of serious complications from AIDS.
- ☐ Prevention of transmission of infection to the uninfected (public health issue).

Drugs as Part of the Total Treatment Regimen

- ☐ Importance of seeking treatment when symptoms appear.
- ☐ Patients need routine preventive care including lipid monitoring, cardiovascular health screening, cervical cancer screening, STI screening, and immunizations.

Adherence Issues

- ☐ Importance of following the HAART treatment regimen instructions to prevent resistance and to keep viral loads low.
- ☐ Importance of contacting the health-care provider if side effects or rash appears.
- ☐ The potential for drug interactions.

On The Horizon

FIVE DRUGS FOR THE FUTURE

New HIV-drug development continues.

A new drug nearing approval for treatment-naïve individuals is the following:

Rilpivirine (TMC 278): a new NNRTI that will most likely be a big competitor to Atripla® if studies show it works in a once-daily fixed dose combination with fd(etravirine/tenofovir).

The latest drugs nearing approval for HIV-treatment-experienced persons include the following:

Bevirimat: a maturation inhibitor that may require a resistance test and will be useful in only 60 percent of the population because of naturally occurring mutations in HIV's *gag* gene.

Elvitegravir: in late phase III studies is a new integrase inhibitor that must be boosted and thus be combined in a fixed-dose "quad" pill with a new booster agent and fd (etravirine/tenofovir).

GSK-572: a second generation integrase inhibitor showing powerful suppression of 2.5 logs with only a 50-mg dose in an early 10-day monotherapy study, reported at the 2009 International Aids Society meeting in Cape Town, South Africa. So far it appears not to be cross resistant to the other integrase inhibitors. The drug may be coformulated in a once-daily pill with abacavir and lamivudine.

Vicriviroc: another CCR5 antagonist, useful only against CCR5-sensitive virus.

REFERENCES

Ansari, A. F., & Etzel, J.V. (2000). Immune-based therapies for the management of HIV infection: Highly active antiretroviral therapy and beyond. *Journal of Pharmacy Practice, 13,* 515–532.

Barbour, J. D., Wrin, T., Grant, R. M., Martin, J. N., Segal, M. R., Petropoulos, C. J., et al. (2002). Evolution of phenotypic drug susceptibility and viral replication capacity during long-term virologic failure of protease inhibitor therapy in human immunodeficiency virus-infected adults. *Journal of Virology, 76,* 11104–11112.

Bennett, J. A. (2003). Historical overview of the HIV pandemic. In C. Kirton (Ed.), *ANAC's core curriculum for HIV/AIDS nursing* (2nd ed., pp. 22–29). Thousand Oaks, CA: Sage.

Bessesen, M., Ives, D., Condreay, L., Lawrence, S., & Sherman, K. E. (1999). Chronic active hepatitis B exacerbations in human immunodeficiency virus-infected patients following development of resistance to or withdrawal of lamivudine. *Clinical Infectious Diseases, 28,* 1032–1035.

Centers for Disease Control and Prevention (CDC). (1992). 1993 revised classification system for HIV infection and expanded surveillance case definition for AIDS among adolescents and adults. *MMWR Recommendations and Reports, 41*(RR-17). Retrieved January 10, 2011, from http://www.cdc.gov/mmwr/preview/mmwrhtml/00018871.htm

Centers for Disease Control and Prevention (CDC). (1998). Report of the NIH Panel to define principles of therapy of HIV infection and guidelines for the use of antiretroviral agents in HIV-infected adults and adolescents. *MMWR, 47*(RR-5), 1–82.

Centers for Disease Control and Prevention (CDC). (2007). *HIV/AIDS surveillance report: Cases of HIV infection and AIDS in the United States and dependent areas.* Retrieved from http://www.cdc.gov/hiv/topics/surveillance/basic.htm#hivest

Centers for Disease Control and Prevention (CDC). (2010). Media release at the 17th Conference on Retroviruses and Opportunistic Infections (CROI), San Francisco. Retrieved from http://www.cdc.gov/media/pressrel/2010/r100217.htm

Chen, R. Y., Accortt, N. A., Westfall, A. O., Mugavero, M. J., Raper, J. L., Cloud, G. A., et al. (2006). Distribution of health care expenditures in HIV-infected patients. *Clinical Infectious Diseases, 42*(7), 1003–1010.

Chun, T. W., Engel, D., Berrey, M. M., Shea, T., Corey, L., & Fauci, A. S. (1998). Early establishment of a pool of latently infected, resting CD4(+) T cells during primary HIV-1 infection. *Proceedings of the National Academy of Sciences USA, 95,* 8869–8873.

Chun, T. W., Stuyver, L., Mizell, S. B., Ehler, L. A., Mican, J. A., & Baseler, M. (1997). Presence of an inducible HIV-1 latent reservoir during highly active antiretroviral therapy. *Proceedings of the National Academy of Sciences USA, 94,* 13193–13197.

Colagreco, J. P. (2003). Pathophysiology of HIV infection. In C. Kirton (Ed.). *ANAC's core curriculum for HIV/AIDS nursing* (2nd. ed., pp. 22–29). Thousand Oaks, CA: Sage.

D'Arminio Monforte, A., Lepri, A. C., Rezza, G., Pezzotti, P., Antinori, A., Phillips, A. N., et al. (2000). Insights into the reasons for discontinuation of the first highly active antiretroviral therapy (HAART) regimen in a cohort of antiretroviral naïve patients. I.CO.N.A. Study Group. Italian Cohort of Antiretroviral-Naïve Patients. *AIDS, 14,* 499–507.

Dragsted, U. B., Gerstoft, J., Pedersen, C., Peters, B., Duran, A., Obel, N., et al. (2003). Randomized trial to evaluate indinavir/ritonavir versus saquinavir/ritonavir in human immunodeficiency virus type 1-infected patients: the MaxCmin1 Trial. *Journal of Infectious Disease, 188,* 635–642.

Dragsted, U. B., Gerstoft, J., Youle, M., Fox, Z., Losso, M., Benetucci, J., et al. (2005). A randomized trial to evaluate lopinavir/ritonavir versus saquinavir/ritonavir in HIV-1-infected patients: the MaxCmin2 trial. *Antiviral Therapy, 10,* 735–743.

Finzi, D., Blankson, J., Siciliano, J. D., Margolick, J. B., Chadwick, K., & Pierson, T. (1999). Latent infection of CD4+ T cells provides a mechanism for lifelong persistence of HIV-1, even in patients on effective combination therapy. *Nature Medicine, 5,* 512–517.

Finzi, D., Hermankova, M., Pierson, T., Carruth, L. M., Buck, C., Chaissond R. E., et al. (1997). Identification of a reservoir for HIV-1 in patients on highly active antiretroviral therapy. *Science, 278,* 1295–1300.

Freeman, E., & Winland-Brown, J. E. (2001). Hematologic and immune problems. In L. M. Dunphy & J. E. Winland-Brown (Eds.), *Primary care: The art and science of advanced practice nursing* (pp. 959–1024). Philadelphia: F.A. Davis.

Gallant, J. E., Staszewski, S., Pozniak, A. L., DeJesus, E., Suleiman, J. M., Miller, M. D., et al. (2004). Efficacy and safety of tenofovir DF vs. stavudine in combination therapy in antiretroviral-naïve patients: A 3-year randomized trial. *Journal of the American Medical Association, 292,* 191–201.

Garcia, P. M., Kalish, L. A., Pitt, J., Minkoff, H., Quinn, T. C., Burchett, S. K., et al. (1999). Maternal levels of plasma human immunodeficiency virus type 1 RNA and the risk of perinatal transmission. Women and Infants Transmission Study Group. *New England Journal of Medicine, 341,* 394–402.

Grant, P. M., Taylor, J., Nevins, A. B., Calvez, V., Marcelin, A. G., Wirden, M., et al. (2010). International cohort analysis of the antiviral activities of zidovudine and tenofovir in the presence of the K65R mutation in reverse transcriptase. *Antimicrobial Agents and Chemotherapy, 54*(4), 1520–1525.

Greub, G., Cozzi-Lepri, A., Ledergerber, B., Staszewski, S., Perrin, L., Miller, V., et al. (2002). Intermittent and sustained low-level HIV viral rebound in patients receiving potent antiretroviral therapy. *AIDS, 16,* 1967–1069.

Gulick, R. M., Ribaudo, H. J., Shikuma, C. M., Lalama, C., Schackman, B. R., Meyer, W. A., III, et al. (2006). Three- vs. four-drug antiretroviral regimens for the initial treatment of HIV-1 infection: A randomized controlled trial. *Journal of the American Medical Association, 296,* 769–781.

Health Resources and Services Administration. (2006, February). *Tools for grantees: A pocket guide to adult HIV/AIDS treatment.* Retrieved fromhttp://hab.hrsa.gov/tools/HIVpocketguide/PktGDrugTables.htm#DrugTable2

Hirsch, M. S., Brun-Vezinet, F., Clotet, B., Conway, B., Kuritzkes, D. R., D'Aquila, R. T., et al. (2003). Antiretroviral drug resistance testing in adults infected with human immunodeficiency virus type 1: 2003 recommendations of an International AIDS Society-USA Panel. *Clinical Infectious Diseases, 37*(1), 113–128.

Kilby, J. M., & Eron, J. J. (2003). Novel therapies based on mechanisms of HIV-1 cell entry. *New England Journal of Medicine, 22,* 2228–2238.

Kirton, C. (Ed.). (2003). *ANAC's core curriculum for HIV/AIDS nursing* (2nd ed.). Thousand Oaks, CA: Sage.

Mellors, J. W., Rinaldo, C. R., Jr., Gupta, P., White, R. M., Todd, J. A., & Kingsley, L. A. (1996). Prognosis in HIV-1 infection predicted by the quantity of virus in plasma. *Science, 272,* 1167–1170.

Mocroft, A., Vella, S., Benfield, T. L., Chiesi, A., Miller, V., & Gargalianos, P. (1998). Changing patterns of mortality across Europe in patients infected with HIV-1. EuroSIDA Study Group. *Lancet, 352,* 1725–1730.

Mofenson, L. M., Lambert, J. S., Stiehm, E. R., Bethel, J., Meyer, W. A., & Whitehouse, J. (1999). Risk factors for perinatal transmission of human immunodeficiency virus type 1 in women treated with zidovudine. Pediatric AIDS Clinical Trials Group Study 185 Team. *New England Journal of Medicine, 341,* 385–393.

Moore, R. D., Keruly, J. C., Gebo, K. A., & Lucas, G. M. (2005). An improvement in virologic response to highly active antiretroviral therapy in clinical practice from 1996 through 2002. *Journal of Acquired Immune Deficiency Syndrome, 39,* 195–198.

Moyle, G., Gatell, J., Perno, C. F., Ratanasuwan, W., Schechter, M., & Tsoukas, C. (2008). Potential for new antiretrovirals to address unmet needs in the management of HIV-1 infection. *AIDS Patient Care STDS, 22,* 459–471.

Murray, J. S., Elashoff, M. R., Iacono-Connors, L. C., Cvetkovich, T. A., & Struble, K. A. (1999). The use of plasma HIV RNA as a study endpoint in efficacy trials of antiretroviral drugs. *AIDS, 13,* 797–804.

Nettles, R. E., Kieffer, T. L., Kwon, P., Monie, D., Han, Y., Parsons, T., et al. (2005). Intermittent HIV-1 viremia (blips) and drug resistance in patients receiving HAART. *Journal of the American Medical Association, 293,* 817–829.

Palella, F. J., Delaney, K. M., Moorman, A. C., Loveless, M. O., Fuhrer, J., & Satten, G. A. (1998). Declining morbidity and mortality among patients with advanced human immunodeficiency virus infection. HIV Outpatient Study Investigators. *New England Journal of Medicine, 338,* 853–860.

Panel on Antiretroviral Guidelines for Adults and Adolescents. (2009, December). *Guidelines for the use of antiretroviral agents in HIV-1-infected adults and adolescents.* Department of Health and Human Services. Retrieved May 23, 2010, from http://www.aidsinfo.nih.gov/ContentFiles/AdultandAdolescentGL.pdf

Panel on Antiretroviral Guidelines for Adults and Adolescents. (2011). *Guidelines for the use of antiretroviral agents in HIV-1-infected adults and adolescents.* Department of Health and Human Services. January 10, 2011; 1–166. Retrieved January 10, 2011, from http://www.aidsinfo.nih.gov/ContentFiles/AdultandAdolescentGL.pdf

Perinatal HIV Guidelines Working Group. (2009, April). *Public Health Service Task Force recommendations for use of antiretroviral drugs in pregnant HIV-infected women for maternal health and interventions to reduce perinatal HIV transmission in the United States.* Retrieved from http://aidsinfo.nih.gov/ContentFiles/PerinatalGL.pdf

Riddler, S. A., Haubrich, R., DiRienzo, A. G., Peeples, L., Powderly, W. G., Klingman, K. L., et al. (2006, August). A prospective, randomized, phase III trial of NRTI-, PI-, and NNRTI-sparing regimens for initial treatment of HIV-1 infection—ACTG 5142 [Abstract THLB0204]. XVI International AIDS Conference, Toronto, Canada.

Rodriguez, B., Sethi, A. K., Cheruvu, V. K., Mackay, W., Bosch, R. J., Kitahata, M., et al. (2006). Predictive value of plasma HIV RNA level on rate of CD4 T-cell decline in untreated HIV infection. *Journal of the American Medical Association, 296,* 1498–1506.

Shulman, N., Zolopa, A., Havlir, D., Hsu, A., Renz, C., Boller, S., et al. (2002). Virtual inhibitory quotient predicts response to ritonavir boosting of indinavir-based therapy in human immunodeficiency virus-infected patients with ongoing viremia. *Antimicrobial Agents & Chemotherapy, 46,* 3907–3916.

Squires, K., Lazzarin, A., Gatell, J. M., Powderly, W. G., Pokrovskiy, V., Delfraissy, J. F., et al. (2004). Comparison of once-daily atazanavir with efavirenz, each in combination with fixed-dose zidovudine and lamivudine, as initial therapy for patients infected with HIV. *Journal of Acquired Immune Deficiency Syndrome, 36,* 1011–1019.

Staszewski, S., Morales-Ramirez, J., Tashima, K. T., Rachlis, A., Skiest, D., Stanford, J., et al. (1999). Efavirenz plus zidovudine and lamivudine, efavirenz plus indinavir, and indinavir plus zidovudine and lamivudine in the treatment of HIV-1 infection in adults. *New England Journal of Medicine, 341,* 1865–1873.

UNAIDS. (2008). *2008 report on the global AIDS epidemic.* UNAIDS, the Joint United Nations Programme on HIV/AIDS. Geneva, Switzerland Retrieved from http://data.unaids.org/pub/GlobalReport/2008/jc1510_2008_global_report_pp29_62_en.pdf

Vittinghoff, E., Scheer, S., O'Malley, P., Colfax, G., Holmberg, S. D., & Buchbinder, S. P. (1999). Combination antiretroviral therapy and recent declines in AIDS incidence and mortality. *Journal of Infectious Diseases, 179,* 717–720.

Weverling, G. J., Lange, J. M., Jurriaans, S., Prins, J. M., Lukashov, V. V., Notermans, D. W., et al. (1998). Alternative multidrug regimen provides improved suppression of HIV-1 replication over triple therapy. *AIDS, 12,* F117–122.

Wheeler, W., Mahle, K., & Bodnar, U. (2007, February). *Antiretroviral drug-resistance mutations and subtypes in drug-naive persons newly diagnosed with HIV-1 infection.* Poster session presented at the annual meeting of the Conference on Retroviruses and Opportunistic Infections, Los Angeles, CA.

Wong, J. K., Hezareh, M., Günthard, H. F., Havlir, D. V., Ignacio, C. C., & Spina, C. A. (1997). Recovery of replication-competent HIV despite prolonged suppression of plasma viremia. *Science, 278,* 1291–1295.

CHAPTER 38

HORMONE REPLACEMENT THERAPY AND OSTEOPOROSIS

Anita Lee Wynne and Taynin Kopanos

Chapter Outline

HORMONE REPLACEMENT THERAPY

Hormone replacement therapy (HRT) may be instituted any time there is loss of the body's ability to produce **estrogen** and **progestin.** This would include surgical removal of the ovaries as well as menopause. Until recently, research evidence about the use of HRT has been largely based in observational studies. Such studies have value in raising questions about a given therapy, but they may be flawed because they cannot control for the many variables that can contribute to the findings in a study. For this reason, the discussion and recommendations in this chapter will be based on randomized, placebo-controlled trials where they have been done. Several studies meet this criterion: Heart and Estrogen-progestin Replacement Study (HERS I and HERS II); Estrogen Replacement and Atherosclerosis Trial (ERA); Women's Health Initiative (WHI); Women's Health, Osteoporosis, Progestin, Estrogen Study (HOPE); and Postmenopausal Estrogen/Progestin Interventions Trial (PEPI). The references for each of these trials is found in the References for this chapter and their acronyms will be used throughout this chapter to refer to each study.

Some of these trials such as PEPI (Writing Group of the PEPI Trial, 1996) focused on specific benefits to bone mineral density and prevention of cardiovascular events thought to accrue with the use of HRT. Others looked specifically at cardiovascular effects (Hulley et al, 1998; Hulley et al, 2002). Shumaker and colleagues, (2003) considered the possibility of reduced dementia and cognitive impairment. Wassertheil-Smoller, et al (2003) sought help in the prevention of strokes. Some studies looked at **estrogen replacement therapy** (ERT) without the use of a **progestin** (Garnero, Stevens, Ayers, & Phelps, 2002; Marx et al, 2004; Stevens, Roy, & Phelps, 2002). The Women's Health Initiative, which was started in 1991 and planned a longitudinal study of participants over 15 years, took the broadest look at all the purported health benefits of HRT (Writing Group for the Women's Health Initiative [WHI] Investigators, 2002) and ERT. The HRT arm of the study was stopped in 2002 due to a negative risk to benefit ratio showing an increased incidence of heart disease, stroke, thomboembolic events, and breast cancer among women taking HRT agents. The ERT arm was also stopped early in 2004 because of increased risk of stroke in women taking estrogen only. Age-cohort analysis of the WHI data suggests that the timing of initiation of ERT/HRT may play a role in coronary heart disease (CHD) risks. Women who initiate ERT/HRT at the time of menopause appear to be at less risk to develop CHD related to ERT/HRT use. Data from the HOPE study suggest that lower doses of hormones may be adequate to control the symptoms of menopause and not significantly raise the risk of CHD.

General recommendations from the American Academy of Obstetricians and Gynecologists, the American Society of Reproductive Medicine, the National Association of Nurse Practitioners in Women's Health, the North American Menopause Society, and the U.S. Preventative Services Task Force, along with the U.S. Food and Drug Administration (FDA) support the use of ERT/HRT for the treatment of moderate to severe menopausal symptoms. The use of ERT/HRT to treat and prevent other chronic illness, with the exception of osteoporosis, is no longer encouraged—and the suggestion to consider alternative osteoporosis treatments for women that are not also experiencing menopausal symptoms has been made. Current use guidelines for ERT/HRT proposes utilizing the lowest does of hormones for the shortest duration possible. The WHI results indicate that replacement therapy for up to 5 years is reasonably safe.

Although no single study or series of studies will address all the concerns about the best way to use a given therapy, this chapter will base recommendations on the generally agreed on benefits and risks of HRT and ERT. It is important to note that herbal and dietary approaches to relieve menopausal symptoms have also been tried and sometimes researched. Where there is evidence related to these other approaches, they will be discussed. Additional discussion of hormone therapy related to menopause can be found in Chapter 22.

Pathophysiology

Between the ages of 42 and 56, most women experience a decline in ovarian hormone function, with the resultant natural cessation of menses. At menarche, the ovary starts production of three **steroids: estrogen, progestin,** and **androgen.** These three steroids have a dramatic effect on the brain, hypothalamus, pituitary, and the ovary itself. Sex hormones play an important role in the dynamic process of the formation and remodeling of neuronal circuits and neurotransmitters. The target organs of ovarian steroids are the uterine epithelium, the uterine tubes, the breasts, and the vagina. However, these hormones also play other important roles in the body.

Physiological Effects of Estrogen

Effects of **estrogen** on the reproductive system include maturation of reproductive organs; development of secondary sexual characteristics; regulation of menstrual cycle; and endometrial regeneration postmenstruation. **Estrogen** also effects closure of long bones after the pubertal growth spurt; maintains bone density by decreasing rate of bone resorption through antagonizing the effects of **parathyroid hormone** (PTH); maintains normal structure of skin and blood vessels through its actions on the endothelial cells in the arterial walls, including the induction of nitric oxide to facilitate vasodilation and oxygen uptake by cells; alters plasma lipids (increased high-density lipoprotein [HDL], slight reduction in low-density lipoprotein [LDL], reduced total cholesterol, increased triglycerides) through its action in the liver; reduces motility of the bowel through its modulation of sympathetic nervous system control over smooth muscle; alters production and activity of selected proteins resulting in higher levels of thyroxine-binding globulin, sex-hormone binding globulin, transferrin, and renin substrate; enhances coagulability of blood by increasing the production of fibrinogen; and facilitates loss of intravascular fluid into extracellular space by its action on the **renin-angiotensin-aldosterone** cycle (retention of sodium and water by the kidney) resulting in edema and decreased extracellular fluid (ECF) volume. In the brain, **estrogen** maintains stability of the thermoregulatory center. Decline in this function results in acute activation of the sympathetic nervous system and vasomotor instability, causing hot flushes.

Knowledge of the actions of **estrogen** on areas of the body beyond the reproductive organs combined with the epidemiological evidence of increased incidence of cardiac and related disorders postmenopause, leads to the assumption that the lack of **endogenous estrogen** might be a major contributing factor to this increased incidence. From that conclusion, it was logical to assume that the administration of **exogenous estrogen** would prevent this problem. Although this assumption was supported with some early observational studies, subsequent randomized controlled trials (RCTs) found some flaws in this assumption, and even found that use of replacement hormones increased the cardiovascular risk among some women. The HERS studies found that neither **ERT** nor **HRT** increased nor decreased the incidence of CHD. The WHI study was halted early due to findings of statistically significant increase incidence of CHD, stroke, thromboembolic events and breast cancer in women taking **HRT**, and an increase incidence of stroke in women taking **ERT**. These results challenged the traditional use of **ERT** and **HRT** and raised significant clinical questions in the pharmacologic management of postmenopausal women. As a result, the use of **ERT** and **HRT** to prevent cardiovascular disease is no longer recommended.

Assumptions about the possibility of prevention in other areas such as bone mineral density have been shown valid in several studies. From PEPI through the WHI, studies looking at bone density and estrogen use consistently support the role of **estrogen** in the prevention of bone loss. Even relatively low doses of **estrogen** appear to have a beneficial effect on bone. The use of **estrogen** to prevent osteoporosis is discussed in detail below.

Physiological Effects of Progestin

Effects of **progestin** on the reproductive organs include thickening of the endometrium and increasing its complexity in preparation for pregnancy; thickening of cervical mucus; thinning the vaginal mucosa; and relaxation of smooth muscles of the uterus and fallopian tubes. During pregnancy, **progestin** maintains the thickened endometrium, relaxes myometrial muscles, thickens the myometrium for labor, is responsible for placental development, and prevents lactation until the fetus is born. In the absence of pregnancy, the reduced production of **estrogen** and **progestin** by the corpus luteum results in the shedding of endometrium to produce menstruation. **Progestin** is also responsible for alveolobular development of the secretory apparatus of the breast. **Progestin** also has actions outside the reproductive system. It stimulates lipoprotein activity and seems to favor fat deposition; increases basal insulin levels and insulin response to glucose; promotes glycogen storage in the liver; promotes ketogenesis; competes with **aldosterone** in the renal tubule to decrease Na+ resorption; increases body temperature; and increases ventilatory response to CO_2 resulting in a measurable decrease in $PaCO_2$. The latter occurs only during pregnancy.

Thickening of the endometrium related to **estrogen** stimulation is thought to increase the risk for endometrial cancer and studies have supported a direct correlation between ERT use and an increased incidence of endometrial cancer (Thorneycroft, 2004). To prevent this occurrence, **progestins** have been added to HRT as a way to oppose the effects of estrogen on the endometrium and prevent endometrial hyperplasia. Additional studies indicated that endometrial **estrogen**-related cancer risk is also correlated with estrogen dose and length of exposure. These data, combined with the results of the HRT arm of the WHI, have raised concerns about whether the traditional combination **estrogen-progestin therapy** in a continuous mode is appropriate, and are leading factors that contributed to the recommendations to use the lowest dose for the shortest duration possible, and limit treatment to less than 5 years.

Physiological Effects of Androgens

In the female, small amounts of **androgens** are produced in the ovary and the adrenal gland. Some are precursors to **estrogen (androstenedione)**, serving as an alternate route to **estrogen** production. At puberty, **androgens** contribute to the skeletal growth spurt, growth of pubic and axillary hair, activate sebaceous glands (acne), and play a role in libido. Administration of exogenous **androgens** during menopause is often related to the role they play in skeletal growth and libido.

Menopausal Changes in Hormones

Perimenopause is the transitional period between reproductive and nonreproductive years. During this time approximately 90 percent of women experience extreme variability in frequency and quality of menstrual flow (McCance & Huether, 2006). Commonly, women experience a short cycle with a shortened follicular phase, ovulation, and insufficient luteal phase; followed by a long cycle with extended follicular phase, anovulation, and high **estradiol levels** in the premenstrual phase; followed by a short follicular phase and anovulation cycle. Perimenopausal cycles are correlated with elevated and irregular follicle-stimulating hormone (FSH), decreased inhibin, normal luteinizing hormone (LH), and slightly elevated **estradiol levels**. All of these are associated with reduced follicular genesis. The perimenopausal period may last for up to 10 years in some women, during which time hormone levels continue to fluctuate. Menopause is a period of time in which no menses occur for 12 consecutive months when **estrogen** and **progestin** are low, despite FSH and LH levels that are increased due to lost ovary function. If left intact, the postmenopausal ovary continues to produce androgens. These **androgens**, as well as those from the adrenal gland, are then converted in fatty tissues into less potent **estrogens: estrone** and **estriol**. This peripheral conversion of **androgens** may vary greatly. This variation in peripheral conversion attributes to the spectrum of menopausal symptoms encountered in practice—some women pass through menopause with limited symptoms, whereas others experience severe vasomotor and vaginal symptoms.

These altered levels of hormones result in the symptoms common to the perimenopausal and postmenopausal period. Vasomotor symptoms, which typically begin during the perimenopausal transition, are actually caused by rapid changes in **estrogen** levels rather than low levels, and tend to abate gradually over time for postmenopausal women. ERT/HRT are effective treatments for these symptoms, and data still support the use of both of these replacement therapies for this indication. Breast tissue involutes, yielding a moderate decrease in mammary tissue during perimenopause, and there is significant reduction in glandular breast tissue with associated decrease in fat deposits and connective tissue. Administration of **exogenous estrogen** (ERT) and **HRT** have been associated with increased risk for breast cancer. The data regarding the relative risk of breast cancer among ERT/HRT users have been inconsistent, and will be discussed later. For women at increased risk of breast cancer, ERT/HRT is contraindicated.

The urogenital tract also undergoes changes. The uterus atrophies and decreases in size. The vagina narrows, shortens, and loses some of its elasticity. Vaginal walls lose their ability to lubricate quickly. Intercourse may become painful. The vaginal pH increases, contributing to a higher incidence of vaginitis. The vaginal epithelium also atrophies, resulting in vaginal irritation, burning, itching, white discharge, and vaginal bleeding. Urethral tone declines, associated with an increased the risk for urinary frequency, urgency, and incontinence. Topical **estrogen** has been effective in helping to relieve these symptoms.

Other postmenopausal changes also occur outside the reproductive system. Bone mineral density is reduced, cardiovascular disorders increase, and the risk for various cancers increases. Some of these increased risks can be associated with normal aging (see Chap. 51), which makes it difficult to directly correlate them with loss of female hormones. In the past, ERT and HRT have been used in an attempt to prevent these disorders. However, large-scale studies have questioned the efficacy and safety of some of these uses.

Pharmacodynamics

Estrogens

Estrogen occurs naturally in the body in three forms: **estradiol, estrone,** and **estriol. Estradiol** is the most potent and plentiful and is principally produced by the ovaries. **Androgens** are converted to **estrone** in ovarian and peripheral adipose tissue and **estriol** is the principle metabolite of **estrone** and **estradiol.** Most all of the **estrogens** prescribed for ERT are **estradiol,** although there are formulations of **estrone** as well as combinations of **estradiaol** and **estrone.**

Estradiol formulations are available as conjugated **equine estrogen,** which is marketed as **Premarin,** and as **esterified estrogen (Menest).** Both are taken orally. **Premarin** 0.625 mg, the most commonly prescribed dose, was the **estrogen** used in the WHI. **Estradiol** is also available in oral, injectable/depo, transdermal, and topical formulations. Chapter 22 discusses all these formulations. Oral drugs are subject to extensive metabolizing through the liver and this may explain some of their effects on lipids and coagulation factors. In contrast, the topical and transdermal formulations are not subject to first-pass metabolism, but continue to have associated changes in coagulation and mild changes in lipids.

Estrone formulations include synthetic **conjugated estrogen-A (Cenestin)** and **synthetic conjugated estrogen-B (Enjuvia).** Both of these forms derive their **estrogen** from plant sources. Plant-derived **estrogens** have not been shown to have reduced adverse effects over other estrogen sources.

Progestins

Medroxyprogesterone (MPA) is the primary **exogenous progestin** prescribed, either alone or in combination with **estrogens.** It is a synthetic hormone manufactured and branded as **Provera.** It was the drug used in combination with **estrogen (Prempro)** in the WHI. **Norethindrone (Aygestin)** is another frequently used **progestin.** Their actions are similar to those of the body's own **progesterone** and they are taken orally. Two bioidentical "natural" hormones have FDA approval: **micronized progesterone (Prometrium),** which is taken orally, and **Prochieve** (also sold under the brand name **Crinone**), which is a bioadhesive vaginal gel. Use of the latter for hormone replacement is off-labeled; it has been approved for use in infertility and secondary amenorrhea. Like synthetic **progestins,** bioidentical hormones are manufactured in the laboratory.

Goals of Treatment

The aim of **ERT** and **HRT** is to provide relief from symptoms associated with menopause. Under this general umbrella, are the goals to

- prevent or reduce vasomotor symptoms
- prevent or reduce vaginal atrophy associated with estrogen decline
- reduce the risk for osteoporosis
- ensure that the benefits of **ERT/HRT** outweigh the risk associated with treatment by providing comprehensive pretreatment evaluation of contraindications and risk, and assisting women in making informed decisions about therapy

Treatment of menopausal symptoms and reduction of postmenopausal bone loss with hormone therapy, both by prescription medications or herb supplements, has risks that require careful selection and screening of patients. Each woman should be assessed for the presence and severity of vasomotor and vaginal symptoms and screened for contraindications to therapy and predisposing diseases/risks that would increase the likelihood of an adverse event(s). Patient education requires comprehensive discussion of the current risk and benefits of therapy, the current indications for therapy (as these indications have changed), review of practice recommendations regarding lowest effective dose for the shortest duration of time, and requirements for interval screening and follow-up while on therapy. Clinicians should be prepared to discuss details of the WHI, HOPE, PEPI, and WHIMS (Women's Health Initiative Memory Study) findings with women, as well as critically appraise an individual's risk for adverse events. A full review of the range of treatment options available, including the option for herbal therapies and the option not to engage in therapy, is critical in the management of women in the perimenopausal to postmenopausal years. The use of **ERT/HRT** is an intensely personal, emotional decision for many women since the release of the WHI findings. Clinicians are required to stay current with new research findings and national recommendations when prescribing **ERT/HRT.** It is no longer acceptable to automatically put all perimenopausal and postmenopausal women on essentially the same drug at essentially the same dose. Individualizing treatment options around patient preference, risk/benefit profiles, and research findings will continue to shape the clinical practice of **ERT/HRT.**

Clinicians need to assist patients in making rational decisions about the use of medication therapy in menopause. To assist both the prescriber and the patient in making informed choices, the following questions should be considered: What are the personal benefits of using ERT or HRT? How severe are the symptoms—and what are the key symptoms that need to be treated? What are the risks specific to this individual patient's situation? What health history, lifestyle, or family genetic factors could influence the safety of ERT/HRT therapy? Does the patient wish to investigate pharmaceutical options at this time? What alternative options—such as sleep aids, bisphosphonates, antidepressants, herbal preparations, or lifestyle changes—would be appropriate alternatives to ERT/HRT?

For women who elect to use ERT/HRT, annual risks, benefit assessments, and quality of life issues need to be considered each year when prescriptions are renewed for perimenopausal and postmenopausal hormonal therapy. In addition, nonpharmacological behaviors such as weight loss, smoking cessation, reduced alcohol intake, regular exercise, and healthy dietary habits need to be encouraged at all office visits.

Rational Drug Selection

General consensus recommendations from the leading national organizations of clinicians who care for women, along with those of the U.S. Preventative Services Task Force and FDA, were presented earlier in this chapter. The consensus supports the use of ERT/HRT for the treatment of moderate to severe menopausal symptoms using the lowest does of hormones for the shortest duration possible.

ERT/HRT had been used to treat conditions other than symptomatic management of menopausal symptoms. Recent research has called into question several of these indications and has overturned many of the previous reasons to prescribe these agents in menopausal women. As these additional reasons had been factors in medication selection in the past, the nonvasomotor and nonvaginal reasons for initiating ERT/HRT are briefly explored below.

1. **Cardiac disease.** HRT should not be used to prevent CHD and care should be used in prescribing it to women who have cardiac risk factors. For women with CHD risk factors, the use of **statins** and other **lipid-lowering therapies** are appropriate and these drugs are discussed in Chapters 16 (Drugs Affecting the Cardiovascular and Renal Systems), 39 (Hyperlipidemia), and 40 (Hypertension).
2. **Breast Cancer.** Data regarding the effects of HRT and ERT on breast cancer are inconsistent and controversial. Equally powerful studies reported by Thorneycroft (2004) varied from both causing increased risk to neither causing increased risk. Some evidence suggests that a **progestin receptor** may be involved in invasive breast cancer (Brucker, 2002), which would support more risk for HRT. The **estrogen** and **progesterone** sub-studies of the WHI (Chlebowski et al, 2003) reported an increased risk of invasive breast cancer. No evidence exists that ERT or HRT directly initiates a neoplastic process, but they may be promoters, increasing the rate of division of neoplastic cells. Based on all the available data, it seems prudent to carefully monitor all women on ERT/HRT for breast cancer through monthly breast self-exam, annual office evaluation, and mammography. The use of ERT/HRT is contraindicated in women with a history of breast or gynecological cancers and those with first-degree family members with breast cancer. Duration of therapy also seems to be a factor in breast cancer risk. Women with extended use, especially therapy continued beyond 7 years, seems to increase risk (Thorneycroft, 2004).
3. **Colon Cancer.** HRT and ERT have both been shown to decrease the risk for colon cancer. This has been supported in all studies that specifically looked at this variable. The decrease appears to be approximately 40 percent and the WHI showed a statistically significant reduction. Women with a family/genetic history of colon cancer would benefit from this therapy. However, both clinicians and patients should be aware that ERT/HRT do not have an exclusive indication for use based on this indication alone.
4. **Osteoporosis.** HRT and ERT have both consistently demonstrated to decrease the risk for osteoporosis and hip fracture. Estrogen-containing therapies continue to be indicated for the prevention and treatment of osteoporosis in postmenopausal women with menopausal symptoms and risk for bone loss. HRT is not used solely for the prevention or treatment of osteoporosis. Recent national recommendations suggest that clinicians consider alternative therapies to hormone therapy in women without concurrent vasomotor menopausal symptoms because of the risks associated with hormonal treatments and the excellent track record for sustained bone density achieved with other osteoporosis agents. Osteoporosis and its treatment are discussed later in this chapter.
5. **Vasomotor and vaginal atrophy.** HRT and ERT continue to demonstrate decreased severity of the uncomfortable menopausal symptoms of vasomotor instability (hot flushes) and vaginal dryness. These agents have maintained clinical indication for the use of treating these symptoms.
6. **Cognitive Performance, Sleep Disturbance and Skin Changes.** Data on the effects of HRT or ERT on cognitive changes associate with Alzheimer's disease, on insomnia, and on skin changes such as wrinkles are inconsistent. The Women's Health Initiative Memory Study (WHIMS), a substudy of WHI (Chlebowski et al, 2003) reported an increased risk of developing probable dementia in postmenopausal women 65 years of age or older during 5.2 years of treatment with daily **conjugated estrogen** 0.625 mg alone and during 4 years of treatment

with daily **conjugated estrogen** 0.625 mg combined with **MPA** 2.5 mg, relative to placebo. It is unknown whether this finding applies to younger postmenopausal women. Further study is needed to support the use of hormonal therapies for these indications.

In general, the following recommendations concerning HRT or ERT can be made:

1. Use the lowest dose that relieves the symptoms for the shortest time frame. The optimal time frame appears to be up to 5 years.
2. Individualize the choice of drug and dose based on the woman's risk profile.
3. Monitor women at least annually for changes in risk profile, development of adverse effects, and continued need for therapy.

Estrogen Therapy

Relief of Perimenopausal and Postmenopausal Symptoms

Relief of menopausal symptoms can be dramatic after the initiation of **hormonal therapy**. Women may report feeling more in control of their bodily functions, exhibit improved emotional stability, and reestablish sleep patterns. Dyspareunia and vaginal irritation due to vaginal atrophy improve. Urogenital tissue response to **estrogen** treatment often relieves urinary urgency. A small percentage of women using **ERT/HRT** report headaches, fluid retention, breast tenderness, and change or resumption of erratic menses.

The various formulations of **estrogen** are discussed above and in Chapter 22. For women who have no objections to **estrogens** from animal sources, **conjugated equine estrogen (Premarin)** is available in doses from 0.3 mg to 1.25 mg. Suppression of hot flushes has been shown to be best at 0.625 mg, followed by 0.45 mg and 0.3 mg/day (Liu, 2004). Studies reported by Liu indicate that vasomotor symptoms begin to decrease by week 2 of therapy and reach maximal effect by week 8 of therapy. Dosage increases should not occur, however, until at least a 6- to 8-week interval to give the drug time to reach maximal effect at that dose.

Micronized estradiol (Estrace, Gynodiol) is the only bioidentical **estrogen-alone** product that is available in pill form. It is available in 0.5 mg to 2 mg. Suppression is found at 1-mg and 2-mg doses. The typical regimen is 1 mg taken daily. The lower dose (0.5 mg) has been used for osteoporosis prevention and is less useful for vasomotor symptom relief. Because of the risks associated with hormone therapy, alternative agents considered if osteoporosis is the primary goal of therapy.

For women who prefer **estrogens** derived from plant sources, **estrone-based drugs** are available. **Conjugated-synthetic estrogen-A (Cenestin)** is available in doses from 0.3 mg to 1.25 mg. Patients should be started with **Cenestin** 0.45 mg daily. Subsequent dosage adjustment may be made based on the individual patient response. This dose should be reassessed periodically by the health-care provider. The lowest effective dose of **Cenestin** for the treatment of moderate to severe vasomotor symptoms has not been determined. Studies reported by Liu (2004) found that the majority (77%) of women randomized to **Cenestin** required a total daily dose of 1.25 mg to relieve vasomotor symptoms, whereas the remaining 23 percent required 0.625 mg or less. By week 8, the vasomotor symptoms were significantly decreased. **Conjugated-synthetic estrogen-B (Enjuvia)** is available in doses of 0.625 mg to 1.25 mg, with the lower dose producing relief in many women. **Estropipate (Ogen, Ortho-EST)** is also derived from plant sources and available in 0.75 mg to 6 mg tablets. Following the rule to use the lowest dose to control symptoms, the dosing regimen should start at 0.75 mg.

Several **ERT/HRT** formulations are available in transdermal delivery systems for the indication of managing vasomotor and urogenital menopausal symptoms. The major advantage of this formulation is its once- or twice-weekly application. A potential disadvantage is the incidence of skin irritation (20% to 40%) in users of a patch delivery system (Wysocki & Alexander, 2005). **Menostar** is a transdermal patch that delivers a very low dose (0.014 mg) of **estradiol.** It is indicated only for osteoporosis prevention in women without a uterus, or in combination with a progestin periodically (every 6 to 12 months) during therapy to prevent endometrial hyperplasia.

Complementary and Alternative Therapies

Phytoestrogens and herbals therapies abound for relief of peri- and postmenopausal symptoms. Cherrington and colleagues (2003) and Wysocki and Thorneycroft (2005) report a high level of use of complementary and alternative medicine (CAM) therapies across ethnicities and cultures. The data supporting these treatments for symptom relief are sparse, ambiguous, and largely anecdotal (Langer, 2005). Herbals therapies have long been popular in Germany and in 1978 the German Federal Health Agency established an expert panel, Commission E, to evaluate the safety and efficacy of several hundred herbs. The National Center for Complementary and Alternative Medicine was established in the National Institutes of Health in 1991. Findings from both organizations are routinely published and available for both consumers and clinicians.

Phytoestrogens

Phytoestrogens are plant compounds that are functionally or structurally related to **endogenous estrogens** and their active metabolites. They may be agonistic, partially agonistic, or antagonistic with **estrogen receptors**. **Isoflavones** are **phytoestrogens** that are found largely in soy and red clover. Studies reported by Wysocki and Thorneycroft (2005) have been inconsistent in demonstrating efficacy of soy-based or red clover–based

BOX 38–1 **HORMONE REPLACEMENT THERAPY**

Related to the Overall Treatment Plan/Disease Process

- ☐ Pathophysiology of the changes that take place in the female physiology at menopause that make a woman vulnerable to atrophy of the genital organs, vasomotor instability, and emotional lability, and when lower estrogen levels cause undesirable lipid patterns
- ☐ Role of lifestyle modifications and the various treatment protocols and medications available
- ☐ Importance of adherence to the treatment regimen
- ☐ Need for regular follow-up visits with the primary care provider, including annual screening tests such as mammography

Specific to the Drug Therapy

- ☐ Reasons for the drug's being given
- ☐ Doses and schedules for taking the drug
- ☐ Possible adverse effects and what to do if they occur, especially if uterine bleeding occurs
- ☐ Interactions between other treatment modalities and these drugs

Reasons for Taking the Drug(s)

Additional information includes the following: Quality-of-life issues such as relief of hot flushes; target organ atrophy prevention; treatment of osteoporosis; prevention of early heart disease, which may be more successful, especially in families who have a hereditary tendency for cardiac disease; and the preliminary data on retention of cognition, which seems promising.

Drugs as Part of the Total Treatment Regimen

The total treatment regimen includes the following: Therapy with alternative herbs and healthier lifestyle, which may relieve symptoms but have not proved to bestow reduced morbidity, as has drug therapy; hormonal therapy is indicated for vaginal atrophy and bladder outlet syndrome; and referral to an appropriate specialist to provide the appropriate care when adverse effects occur as a result of estrogen therapy.

Adherence Issues

Nonadherence to the treatment regimen may be a result of various causes. Concerns about the WHI results should be discussed with correction of any inaccurate interpretations of media messages. Nonadherence due to the possible risk of cancer should be discussed, and the absolute risk of cancer rather than relative risk of cancer should be calculated annually. The possibility of minor discomforts, such as breast tenderness, bloating, fluid retention, and the need for follow-up visits, should be discussed prior to therapy. If irregular or unexpected bleeding occurs, patients should be advised to contact their health-care provider for modifications to the treatment regimen rather than stop therapy on their own.

products in improving hot flashes and other menopausal symptoms. Archer (2004) reports that black cohosh, red clover **isoflavone**, gingko biloba, and evening primrose oil have shown no increased efficacy in treating hot flushes in placebo-controlled trials. Wysocki and Thorneycroft (2005) also report that evening primrose oil has not been shown to be effective in limited trials. Most **bioidentical estrogens** are derived from soy, and Wysocki and Alexander (2005) report that to achieve beneficial effects, significantly higher doses than the body produces on its own must be taken. Langer (2005) also warns that these products are not regulated, and cautions that women who are consuming amounts sufficient to achieve effective symptom relief from a **phytoestrogen** may also experience significant **estrogenic stimulation** of the endometrium and breast and be at similar risk for adverse events as are those women who use pharmaceutical agents. FDA-approved **bioidentical hormones** are mentioned above.

Botanicals/Herbals

Plants are used therapeutically in the form of herbs, oils, pills, teas, and tinctures. They may be classified as dietary supplements. The herbal preparations approved for treatment of menopausal symptoms by the German Commission E include black cohosh root and chaste tree fruit. Liu and colleagues (2001) evaluated eight botanicals for **estrogenic activity.** They found that red clover, hops, and chasteberry had significant binding affinities with **estrogen receptors.** Dong quai and licorice had weak binding. Asian ginseng, North American ginseng, and black cohosh displayed no binding to **estrogen receptors.** Langer (2005) reports that black cohosh failed to relieve vasomotor symptoms in a recent small clinical trial. In a study by the National Center for Complementary and Alternative Medicine at the National Institutes of Health, black cohosh failed to show that it reduces the frequency and severity of hot flashes and night sweats in menopausal and perimenopausal participants. Chasteberry contains hormone-like substances with **antiandrogenic effects.** It also has significant binding affinities for both **estrogen-receptor alpha** and **estrogen-receptor beta.** Studies regarding the efficacy of chasteberry have shown symptom reduction; however, questions regarding study design limit the ability to draw clinical conclusions.

For further information on these hormones and herbal remedies, the reader is referred to Chapter 10, the German

Commission E, and the National Center for Complementary and Alternative Medicine.

Non-hormonal Medications

Several non-hormonal medications have demonstrated benefit in reducing menopausal symptoms. **Selective serotonin reuptake inhibitors (SSRIs)** (discussed in Chap. 15) and **clonidine** (Chap. 14) have some demonstrated relief of vasomotor symptoms and sleep disturbance (Langer, 2005). The North American Menopause Society (NAMS, 2006) has published a comprehensive review of alternative treatments for vasomotor symptoms.

Prevention and Management of Vulvovaginal Atrophy and Dryness

In addition to the vasomotor symptoms associated with menopause, the decline in **estrogen** causes the vaginal mucosa and vulvar skin to become thin and atrophic. The result is discomfort, itching, dyspareunia, and increased cases of vaginitis. Low-dose (0.3 to 0.625 mg) oral ERT with **estrogen** from both plant and animal sources has been shown to decrease vaginal pH, thus reducing vaginal infections. It also thickens and revascularizes the vaginal epithelium, increases the number of superficial cells, and reverses vaginal atrophy (Liu, 2004). Vaginal application of **estrogen** also produces these positive effects and improvement in symptoms can be seen in as few as 2 weeks of treatment. Low-dose vaginal **estrogens** (in ring or cream form) have a less stimulating effect on the endometrial tissue and, therefore, a reduced risk for endometrial hyperplasia compared to the oral forms. **Estrace** is a bioidentical vaginal cream approved for the treatment of vaginal and urinary symptoms. The usual doses for all the creams include nightly application. Topical application using vaginal rings and vaginal tablets may be preferred to creams in some patients because of the ease of use and a perception that these options are less "messy" than the creams. The total amount of **estrogen** to which the body is exposed is less with the topical formulations, which may be a consideration for women who have risk factor concerns with ERT. Studies reported by Thorneycroft (2004) found no evidence of increased risk of CHD, breast cancer, or endometrial cancer with the use of vaginal ERT. There was a slight increase in endometrial hyperplasia and it might be prudent to periodically withdraw patients treated with vaginal ERT.

Reduced Risk for Colon Cancer

Colorectal cancer is the third most common cancer in women in the United States and the third most common cause of cancer death in women (Thorneycroft, 2004). Since this cancer is also associated with aging, it clearly is a cancer to be considered with menopause. Reduction in colon and rectal cancers are correlated with both postmenopausal ERT and HRT use and the doses that help with vasomotor symptoms also provide that benefit.

Increased Risk for Endometrial Cancer

There is a clear and consistent increased risk for endometrial cancer in women with a uterus who are treated with unopposed ERT. To help decrease this risk, progestin has been added to hormone treatment options for women with an intact uterus to help prevent endometrial hyperplasia and cancer. The use of unopposed estrogen in a woman with a uterus in contraindicated. Further discussion occurs in **progestin** section below.

Risk for CHD

The first indications that assumptions about ERT/HRT and improved cardiovascular health might not be true happened years before the WHI. The PEPI study, conducted in 1995 (Writing Group of the PEPI Trial, 1996), started to question this hypothesis. Although the drugs tested (**estrogen alone, estrogen with MPA,** and **estrogen with micronized progestin**) increased HDL, lowered LDL and fibrinogen levels, and had no adverse effect on blood pressure, these apparently positive CHD risk factors did not translate into decreased CHD events. The ERA (**estrogen** replacement and atherosclerosis) studies (Herrington et al, 2000; Hodis et al, 2001; Hodis et al, 2003) contributed to the same conclusion. The Heart and Estrogen/Progestin Replacement Study (HERS) was the first large randomized trial that looked at reduction in mortality by using menopausal estrogens. Women with CHD had higher adverse events and incidence of death during therapy. Those women without cardiovascular disease showed modest benefit, but not until the fourth and fifth years of therapy. The definitive study was the WHI, which stopped the **HRT** arm of its study earlier than planned based on an increased risk for CHD versus possible benefits of **HRT**. The **ERT** arm, which includes women who do not have a uterus, failed to show statistically significant benefits in prevention of CHD. It is worth noting that the **ERT** arm of the study was subsequently halted early because of increased incidence of stroke.

The age and years postmenopause of women in the WHI study has raised the possibility that the adverse cardiovascular findings may be related to the length of time that the normal hormone balance had been interrupted prior to initiating of hormone therapy and the vascular capacity to respond. Meta-analysis of age-adjusted cohorts and other studies suggest that the risk of CHD might be substantially less than in women who initiate **ERT/HRT** early in perimenopause and menopause (Archer, 2004; Langer, 2005). **Progestin** has been shown to block **estrogen receptors**, which might interfere with nitric oxide production in the endothelial cells and diminish the beneficial effects of **estrogen**. Questions remain as to the reasons that **HRT** is associated with increased risk over **ERT** alone. These questions need to be answered by further research.

ERT has yet to demonstrate increased CHD risk, but it is important to note that oral **estrogens** are associated with increased levels of C-reactive protein (CRP), a factor associated with increased CHD risk in women (Langer, 2005).

Increased Stroke and Thromboembolic Event Risk

Increased risk for thromboembolic events has been a long-standing concern related to **hormone replacement**, whether **estrogen** alone or in combination with **progestins**. The WHI found significantly increased risk for stroke in postmenopausal women for both ERT and HRT. For HRT the risk was apparent in each decade of age, but for ERT the risk appeared to emerge after age 60 (Langer, 2005). The risk for venous thromboembolic disease, including pulmonary embolism, was doubled in women in the HRT arm, with no difference based on age. There was a nonsignificant increase by about one-third with ERT alone (Anderson et al, 2004). The risk of a thromboembolic event is greatest in the first year after initiating therapy.

Progestin Therapy

Progestin therapy alone is used for contraception (see Chap. 31) or in younger women with menorrhagia. It is used in the perimenopausal and postmenopausal period in combination with **estrogen** to prevent endometrial hyperplasia that increases the risk for endometrial cancer. This combination therapy is discussed below.

Combination Therapy With Estrogen and Progestins

Although HRT is as effective as ERT in preventing the uncomfortable symptoms sometimes associated with menopause, reducing the risk of colon cancer, and reducing the risk for osteoporosis and hip fracture, it is not more effective in these areas. The risks associated with HRT are discussed in the ERT section above. Given the studies that indicate a role in increased risk for CHD, it is prudent to avoid HRT, especially in women with CHD risk factors. For this reason, the only specific indication discussed for combination therapy will be the prevention of endometrial hyperplasia and cancer in a menopausal woman with an intact uterus who are using hormone therapy.

Decreased Risk for Endometrial Cancer

Combinations of **estrogen** and **progestin** are used when the uterus is intact. Research has consistently demonstrated the risk for endometrial cancer in direct correlation with unopposed ERT in women who have an intact uterus (Thorneycroft, 2004). The risk also increases substantially the longer the ERT is used and persists for 5 or more years after ERT has been discontinued. Although this effect appears to be dose related, with higher hyperplasia associated with higher **estrogen** doses, the risk remains for all dose levels of ERT. To prevent this increased incidence of hyperplasia and cancer, **progestin**, which reduces the buildup of endometrial tissue, is added to the treatment regimen.

There are several combinations therapies for use in menopause. The following regimens have been prescribed and all provide effective prevention of endometrial cancer:

1. **Estrogen** (0.625 mg) plus **medroxyprogesterone acetate (MPA)** 2.5 mg daily **(Prempro)**
2. **Estrogen** (0.625 mg) plus **micronized progesterone** 100 mg daily
3. **Estrogen** (0.625 mg) daily plus **MPA** 10 mg for 10 to 12 days
4. **Estrogen** (0.625 mg) daily plus **MPA** 5 mg for 14 days **(Premphase)**
5. **Estrogen** (0.625 mg) daily plus **micronized progesterone** 200 mg for 12 days (PEPI)
6. **Estrogen** (0.625 mg) for days 1 to 25 plus **MPA** days 16 to 25 (the first regimen used, which has the disadvantage of more hot flushes)
7. **Estrogen** (0.625 mg) plus **progestin** Monday through Friday (may experience more hot flashes)

Continuous Versus Cyclical (Sequential) Patterns

The most common reason women give for discontinuing HRT is irregular and unpredictable vaginal bleeding. Continuous regimens (1 and 2 above) eliminate monthly withdrawal bleeding, but they are associated with a higher rate of breakthrough bleeding, especially during the first 6 months of therapy. This is most likely to occur in women who have recently become postmenopausal because endogenous production of **estrogen** is more labile from cycle to cycle in these women. Because currently available data suggest that the best profile for a positive risk/benefit ratio for all indications for ERT/HRT accrue when therapy is started near the time of menopause onset, this unwanted side effect may create a problem for many women.

To deal with breakthrough bleeding issues, cyclical or sequential therapy was introduced. These regimens (3 through 7 above) are preferred until **endogenous hormone** production stabilizes, typically 2 to 3 years after menopause. Differences in potency of various **progestins** result in differences in rates of bleeding. The PEPI study tested **MPA** and **micronized progestin** side by side and found that the **micronized progestin** was associated with less bleeding during the first 6 months than either the continuous or cyclical **MPA** (Lindenfeld & Langer, 2002). With any formulation of **progestin**, breakthrough bleeding decreases substantially after the first 6 months and both drugs produced effective protection from endometrial cancer.

Different types of **progestin** not only have differing effects on the endometrium, they also have differing effects on **estrogen**-associated benefits to lipids. **Norethindrone acetate** has been shown to reverse these benefits on HDL cholesterol while still offering effective endometrial protection. **MPA** and **micronized progestin** do not attenuate the effects of **estrogen** on lipid levels.

Norgestimate improves HDL to a level intermediate between MPA and **micronized progestin**, while also providing good endometrial protection (Langer, 2005).

When initiating therapy for any age group, begin with low doses (0.3 mg) of **conjugated estrogens** every other day for 2 months. Next, increase the **estrogens** to daily use for another 2 months. **Progestin** must be included in the treatment regimens above if the patient has a uterus. If symptoms such as bleeding or breast pain do not occur, increase the **estrogen** to 0.625 mg daily if vasomotor symptoms or vaginal atrophy have not resolved. Some women may need only the lower **estrogen** dosages as long as they have adequate diet. Use of formulations other than oral may reduce the need for the addition of **progestin** due to reduced cancer risk. This reduced risk for different **estrogen** formulations is discussed in the **estrogen therapy** section.

Testosterone Therapy

When traditional HRT/ERT is not successful in suppressing hot flashes and improving sex drive, **estrogen** in combination with **testosterone** has been used empirically.

Peripheral conversion of androgens may augment ERT and reduce hot flushes. Masculinizing adverse effects such as lower voice and increased facial and body hair can occur when **testosterone** is used alone. These adverse effects may not regress after **testosterone** is withdrawn. Traditionally, **testosterone** has been used topically (2%) in **aquaphor** or **petrolatum** for vulvar "dystrophies." See Chapter 44 for newer treatments for vulvovaginitis.

Available formulations are the following:

1. **Esterified estrogen** 0.625 mg plus **testosterone** 1.25 mg
2. **Esterified estrogen** 1.25 mg plus **testosterone** 2.5 mg (this higher **estrogen** is used in postoophorectomy patients under 49 years of age)
3. **Conjugated estrogens** 0.625 mg plus **testosterone** 5 mg
4. **Conjugated estrogens** 1.25 mg plus **testosterone** 10 mg

Figure 38–1 presents a treatment algorithm for HRT/ERT.

Monitoring

Women taking **hormonal therapy** for menopausal symptoms have similar adverse effects and precautions no matter what the **estrogen** source and the route of administration. Annual complete history, physical examination, and mammogram are needed to evaluate for changes in risk profiles that may indicate a need to alter treatments and screen for early adverse effects of therapy. Liver function tests need to be done at baseline, along with a lipid profile, and repeated annually if abnormal. All women older than 45 years need to be screened for adult-onset diabetes mellitus. Most authorities agree that abnormal bleeding and all postmenopausal bleeding require uterine sampling.

Outcome Evaluation

Women may present for treatment complaining of heavy menses. When the bleeding problem is serious enough to cause a drop of 2 g of hemoglobin within one menstrual cycle, management usually requires specialty care. The patient may need a dilation and curettage. It is not uncommon for fibroids and hyperplasia to cause this degree of bleeding. Both conditions may require referral and surgery.

Postmenopausal bleeding—that is, bleeding of any degree after 12 or more months of amenorrhea—needs an evaluation that includes history, physical, pelvic examination, mammogram, pelvic ultrasound, and endometrial biopsy. Laboratory tests are necessary to rule out bleeding disorders and endocrine disease. If all of the work-up demonstrates no disease, then referral for specialty consultation is indicated.

Frequently, older women present with symptoms of urinary incontinence or chronic bladder infections. If there is blood and the culture is negative (even as few as 8–10 RBCs per high-powered field), the patient will need a urological evaluation. Because older women who have not been on ERT/HRT have cervical atrophy, performing an endometrial biopsy in the office is too painful. Other areas of concern in the older woman are pigmented vulvar lesions, ulcerations, and thickened white patches, all of which require biopsies to rule out cancer.

Patient Education

Patient education should include a discussion of information related to the overall treatment plan as well as that specific to the drug therapy, reasons for taking the drug, drugs as part of the total treatment regimen, and adherence issues. Media attention to the WHI has led to some misinformation about ERT/HRT and patients may present to the clinic very fearful about beginning this therapy or wondering if they should stop therapy, even when they have been on such therapy for years without incident. Providers need to inform patients that **hormonal therapy** has a role postmenopause, but that role is limited and therapy should be undertaken based on symptoms and risk assessment.

OSTEOPOROSIS

According to the Surgeon General's Report on Bone Health and Osteoporosis (U.S. Department of Health and Human Services [USDHHS], 2004), an estimated 1.5 million individuals suffer a bone disease–related fracture annually. A white woman older than 50 years has more than a 40 percent chance of having such a fracture during the

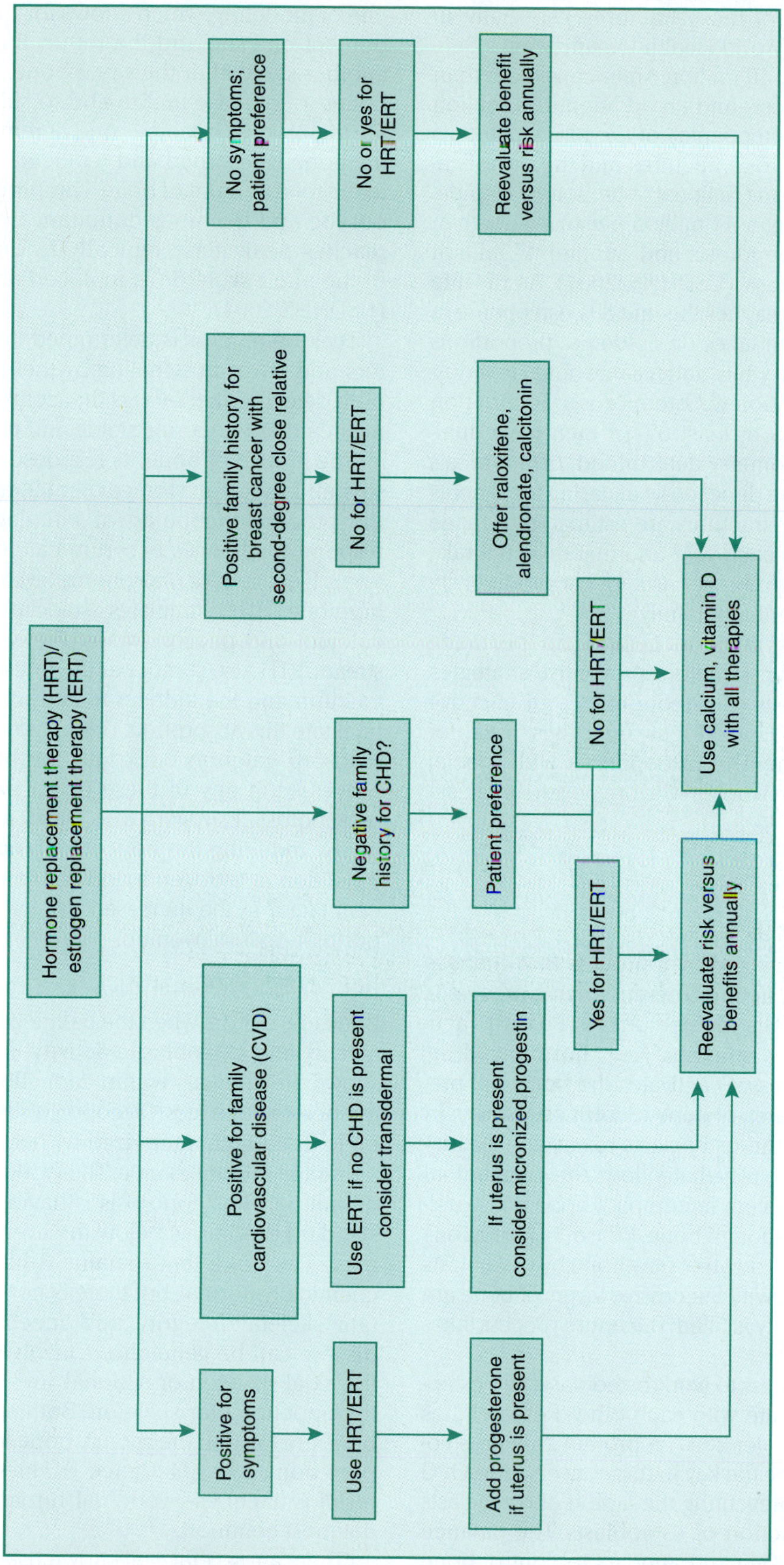

Figure 38–1. Treatment algorithm: Hormone replacement therapy/estrogen replacement therapy.

rest of her life. The lifetime risk for men and nonwhite women is less, but it is still substantial and rising in groups such as Hispanic women. Osteoporosis is the most important underlying cause of these fractures, especially in older adults. Using the World Health Organization's definition, there are roughly 10 million Americans older than 50 years with osteoporosis and an additional 34 million with low bone mass (osteopenia) of the hip, which puts them at risk for osteoporosis, fractures, and the complications associated with them (National Osteoporosis Foundation, 2005). By 2020, roughly 14 million persons older than 50 years will have osteoporosis and another 47 million will have low bone mass (USDHHS, 2004). As the life expectancy of women reaches the mid-80s, osteopenia in perimenopausal women takes on epidemic proportions (50%) especially among white and Asian women in industrial societies (International Osteoporosis Foundation [IOF], 2009). By age 65, at least 6% of men have dual-energy x-ray absorptiometry-determined osteoporosis (Qaseem et al, 2008). The direct costs of caring for patients who have osteoporotic fractures are estimated to range from $12 to $18 billion each year and that does not take into consideration the indirect costs in lost productivity and wages for the patient and family.

Real improvements in bone health can be made through assessment of risk factors, preventive strategies, accurate early diagnosis of osteoporosis, and effective treatment. This section will focus on drugs used for prevention and treatment of osteoporosis with special emphasis on their use in women who are postmenopausal.

Pathophysiology

Normal Bone Physiology

The bony skeleton is created by a process that changes throughout a person's lifetime. The underlying process is *remodeling,* which occurs in three phases. Phase 1 (activation) occurs when a stimulus (e.g., hormone, drug, vitamin, or physical stressor) activates the bone cell precursors in a localized area of bone to form osteoclasts. In phase 2 (resorption), the osteoclasts excavate (resorb) bone, leaving behind a cavity that follows the longitudinal axis of the haversian system in compact bone and parallels the trabeculae in spongy bone. Phase 3 (formation) then results in the laying down of new bone by osteoblasts lining the walls of the cavity. Successive layers of bone are laid down until the cavity is filled. The entire process takes about 3 to 4 months.

In order for this process to work, osteoblasts and osteoclasts must communicate with each other. Research has shown (Kong & Penninger, 2000) a protein called osteoprotegrin (OPG) may be the key in this conversation. OPG binds to OPG-ligand, preventing the action of osteoclasts and stimulating the action of osteoblasts. The balance between OPG and OPG-ligand appears to control bone resorption and growth. The development of drugs to affect the balance between these two may help to treat disease associated with bone loss in the future.

During childhood and adolescence, the process is one of modeling, which allows for the formation of new bone at one site and the removal of older bone from another site within the same bone. This process allows bones to increase in size and to shift in space. Later in life the process becomes one of remodeling when existing bone is resorbed and replaced without an increase in the total amount of bone. This process occurs throughout life and becomes dominant by the time the bone reaches peak mass, typically in one's early 20s. Most of the adult skeleton is replaced about every 10 years (USDHHS, 2004).

Peak bone mass is determined largely by genetic factors, and errors in signaling by these genes can result in birth defects. Other factors that contribute to bone health include diet, endocrine status, and physical activity

The growth of bone, its response to mechanical stressors, and its role in storage of minerals are dependent on the proper functioning of circulating hormones that respond to changes in serum calcium and phosphorus levels. If calcium or phosphorus levels are low, parathyroid hormone (PTH) stimulates osteoclasts to resorb bone, and calcium and phosphorus are released into the bloodstream. PTH also stimulates the intestines to absorb more **calcium** and the kidneys to activate more **vitamin D** to facilitate this absorption. The kidney is also stimulated to reabsorb **calcium** back into the bloodstream. Disease processes in any of these organ systems can produce osteoporosis. Estrogens also play a role in bone remodeling by reducing the bone-resorbing action of PTH. The reduction in estrogen found with menopause is a significant factor in the increased risk for osteoporosis seen in postmenopausal women.

Bone Loss (Osteoporosis)

Bone loss occurs when the balance between osteoclastic activity and osteoblastic activity is altered. Figure 38–2 shows the changes within cancellous bone as a consequence of bone loss. Osteoporosis is a generalized metabolic disease characterized by decreased bone mass as a result of this imbalance. The World Health Organization definition of osteoporosis is having a bone density 2.5 standard deviations below the average adult peak bone mass. The bone that remains is histologically and biochemically normal, but there is not enough of it to maintain skeletal integrity and mechanical support. The disease can be generalized, involving major portions of the axial skeleton or regional, involving one segment of the appendicular skeleton. Both spongy and compact bone are lost, but the spongy bone loss exceeds the compact bone loss (McCance & Huether, 2006). The end result is fractures—vertebral, hip, and wrist fractures are the most common.

There are several well-known risk factors for osteoporosis such as family history, slight build, fair complexion

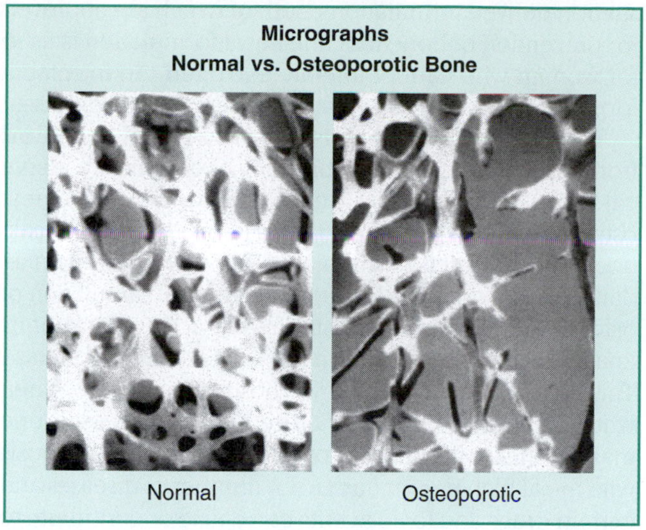

Figure 38–2. Micrographs of normal and osteoporotic bone.

(Scandinavian), age, diets low in **calcium** and **vitamin D**, and minimal sun exposure. Table 38–1 shows these and other risk factors including those for fractures secondary to osteoporosis. There are also a wide variety of diseases and certain drugs and toxic agents that can cause or contribute to development of osteoporosis. Factors associated with increased risk for osteoporosis in men (University of Texas, 2008) include (but are not limited to) the following:

- being older 70 years of age
- **glucocorticoid** use of 5 mg or greater for 3 months or longer
- **anticonvulsants** including **phenobarbital**, **phenytoin**, and **carbamazapine**
- long-term **proton pump inhibitor** use for more than 1 year
- body weight less than 70 kg or weight loss more than 10 percent compared with usual young adult or adult weight in recent years
- heavy tobacco use or consuming more than 14 drinks of **alcohol** per week
- sedentary lifestyle
- deficits in **vitamin D** or **calcium** intake

For women, the same are true with the following exceptions or additions: the age is greater than 62, the body weight is less than 57.7 kg or body mass index (BMI) less than 21 kg/m^2, and there is a history of hip fracture in a parent or a personal history of fracture after menopause (Qaseem et al, 2008). These and other risk factors are shown in Table 38–1.

Ethnic Differences

The bone density of various ethnic groups varies as does their risk for osteoporosis. The National Institute of Arthritis and Musculoskeletal and Skin Diseases (2005a) published some data about these differences. Tools are available to assess osteopenia and osteoporosis risk at http://www.shef.ac.uk/FRAX.

Table 38–1 **Risk Factors for Osteoporosis and Resultant Fractures**

Risk Factors for Osteoporosis
• Thin, small-boned frame
• Estrogen deficiency <45 yr
• Advanced age (62 in women, >70 in men)
• Diet low in calcium and vitamin D
• White and Asian ancestry (African American and Hispanic women are at lower but significant risk)
• Cigarette smoking
• Alcohol intake >2 drinks per day
• Limited physical activity/sedentary lifestyle
Risk Factors for Fracture Secondary to Osteoporosis
• Personal history of fracture as an adult
• History of fragility fracture in a first-degree relative
• Low body weight (57.7 kg for women, 70 kg for men)
• *Weight loss of >10% in recent years*
• *Height loss of ≥1.5 in.*
• Use of oral corticosteroid therapy for >3 mo
• Hormone deprivation therapy used for >1 year as treatment for prostate cancer
• Impaired vision
• Dementia
• Recent falls

Source: Adapted from *Osteoporosis and Asian American Women*, *Osteoporosis and African American Women*, and *Osteoporosis and Hispanic Women* (all from NIAMS documents, 2005); National Osteoporosis Foundation, 2005, *Physician's Guide;* "Bone Health," 2009, in "Menopause and Osteoporosis"; Qaseem et al, 2008; and University of Texas, 2008.

African American Women

Although African American women tend to have higher bone mineral density than white women throughout life, they are still at significant risk for osteoporosis, and the misperception that it does not occur in this population can delay prevention and treatment. As African American women age, their risk for hip fracture doubles approximately every 7 years and they are more likely to die from the hip fracture than are white women. Diseases prevalent in this population, such as sickle cell disease and lupus, can increase the risk for developing osteoporosis. Most African American women consume 50 percent less **calcium** than the Recommended Dietary Allowance (RDA), placing them at risk related to poor **calcium** intake. This is compounded by the fact that 75 percent of all African Americans are lactose intolerant, so they avoid milk and other dairy products that are excellent sources of **calcium**.

Asian American Women

Studies show that Asian Americans share many of the risk factors that apply to white women and are at high risk for developing osteoporosis. Compared to white women, Asian American women tend to consume less **calcium**, in part because 90 percent of Asian Americans are lactose intolerant. Although they generally have lower hip fracture rates than do white women, the prevalence of vertebral fracture is as high.

Hispanic American Women

The prevalence of osteoporosis in Hispanic American women is similar to that of white women. Ten percent of Hispanic American women 50 years and older are estimated to have osteoporosis, and 49 percent are estimated to have bone mass that is low, but not low enough for a diagnosis of osteoporosis. The incidence of hip fracture in this population is on the rise. In addition, this population also consumes less **calcium**, probably also related to lactose intolerance. Finally, Hispanic American women are twice as likely to develop diabetes as are white women, which may increase their risk for osteoporosis.

Pharmacodynamics

Estrogen therapy has long been the gold standard for both prevention and treatment of osteoporosis; however, the results of the Women's Health Initiative called into question the use of **estrogen** for the sole indication of osteoporosis prevention and treatment due to the risks for cardiovascular adverse responses. These risks are discussed earlier under **hormonal replacement therapy**. **Estrogens** prevent osteoporosis by reducing the bone-resorbing action of PTH. **Estrogen** receptors have been found in bone, which validates the hypothesis that **estrogen** may have direct effects on bone remodeling. Chapter 22 provides more detailed discussion on this drug including its dosing.

Raloxifene (Evista) is a **selective estrogen receptor modulator** (SERM) approved for preventing and treating postmenopausal osteoporosis. Because it selectively activates certain **estrogen** pathways in bone and has **anti-estrogen** effects on the uterus and breast, **raloxifene** reduces the resorption of bone with less risk for cardiovascular effects. **Raloxifene** also reduces the risk of cancers of the uterus and breast found with the administration of **estrogen**. This drug also has positive effects on lipid metabolism by decreasing total and LDL cholesterol levels. It does not affect other lipid fractions. **SERMs** are associated with hot flashes, and some perimenopausal and menopausal women discontinue therapy because of this adverse effect. Chapter 22 discusses this drug in more detail.

Bisphosphonates also reduce bone resorption by adhering tightly to bone and inhibiting osteoclastic activity. Although no drug is free of adverse effects, **bisphosphonate** adverse effects are largely gastrointestinal (GI) in nature and not associated with the same life-threatening consequences seen with **estrogen**. They are listed by all guidelines as first-line therapy.

Bisphosphonates are discussed further in Chapter 21.

Calcitonin balances parathyroid hormone by shutting down osteoclastic activity and increasing osteoblastic activity in the presence of hypercalcemia. Low serum calcium levels increase the secretion of endogenous **calcitonin**, with a resulting small decrease in serum calcium. Single injections of **calcitonin** transiently inhibit bone resorption and osteoclasts. It is available in human and salmon-derived formulations, both of which are approved for prevention of bone loss. The nasal formulation is used for women who cannot tolerate **estrogen**. An injectable form is used to treat moderate to severe Paget's disease.

Teriparatide (Forteo) is a **synthetic PTH** derived from recombinant DNA technology. Its actions are identical to that of **human PTH**. Unlike other drugs used to treat osteoporosis in which the action is to prevent bone breakdown, this drug acts to stimulate bone formation. In once-daily doses, it does this through preferential stimulation of osteoblastic activity over osteoclastic activity. Most of its anabolic effects occur within the first 6 months of therapy. This drug is recommended for postmenopausal women who are at high risk for fracture and to increase bone mass in men with primary or hypogonadal osteoporosis who are at high risk for fracture. A number of diseases and certain drugs and toxic agents can cause or contribute to development of osteoporosis (Table 38–2).

Calcium and **vitamin D** are also critical to bone formation and are recommended as complementary agents in the prevention and treatment of osteoporosis (Hodgson et al, 2003; Institute for Clinical Systems Improvement [ISCI], 2008; Kaiser Permanente Care Management Institute, 2008; National Institute for Health and Clinical Excellence [NICE], 2008a; Qaseem et al, 2008; Reid et al, 2009; Scottish Intercollegiate Guidelines Network [SIGN], 2004). Of the 600 to 1,000 mg of **calcium** consumed daily, only 100 to 250 mg are absorbed from the gut. In the steady state, renal excretion of **calcium** and phosphate balances intestinal absorption. The movement of **calcium** and phosphate across the intestinal lining is closely regulated. Intestinal diseases can disrupt this balance. Hormonal regulation of **calcium**, mentioned earlier, greatly affects **calcium** metabolism. Ions such as sodium and fluoride also have an impact on **calcium** balance. Inadequate **vitamin D** can produce a decrease in **calcium** absorption from the intestine and an increase in parathyroid hormone both of which may lead to bone loss and fractures. Amounts of **vitamin D** for optimal bone health are 30 to 100 ng/mL. Deficiency occurs when the amount is less than 20 ng/mL. Drugs taken for other diseases, such as **thiazides** for hypertension, also affect **calcium** metabolism.

Goals of Treatment

The goal of treatment for osteoporosis is that the pharmacological therapy be inexpensive, safe, and effective. Nonpharmacological therapy (and prevention) includes an appropriate exercise program.

The best treatment for osteoporosis is prevention. Developing a healthy lifestyle while building bone mass is the most cost-effective strategy. Excessive dieting and exercise or fad diets that are deficient in essential nutrients contribute to reduced bone mass. **Calcium** is the least expensive drug used in osteoporosis therapy. Generic **calcium carbonate** (**Tums**) costs pennies a day and contains the most elemental calcium per dose. It should be

Table 38–2 **Medical Conditions and Drugs That Increase the Risk for Development of Osteoporosis**

Medical Conditions		
AIDS/HIV	Hemophilia	Parathyroid tumor
Amyloidosis	Inflammatory bowel disease	Pernicious anemia
Ankylosing spondylitis	Type 1 diabetes mellitus	Rheumatoid arthritis
COPD	Lymphoma and leukemia	Severe liver disease
Congenital porphyria	Malabsorption syndromes	Sprue
Cushing's syndrome	Mastocytosis	Stroke (CVA)
Eating disorders	Multiple myeloma	Thalassemia
Gastrectomy	Multiple sclerosis	Thyrotoxicosis
Hemochromatosis	Hyperparathyroidism	Hypogonadism
Drugs		
Aluminum and ***excess use of antacids***	Gonadotropin-release hormones	Progesterone (long acting)
Anticonvulsants (phenobarbital; phenytoin; carbamazepine)	Immunosuppressants	***Aggressive treatment of hypothyroidism with thyroxine***
Cytotoxic drugs	Lithium	Tamoxifen
Glucocorticosteroids equivalent to 5 mg of prednisone or greater for at least 3 months	Long-term heparin use	Total parenteral nutrition
Warfarin use for >1 year	***Selective serotonin reuptake inhibitors***	***Proton pump inhibitors used >1 year***

COPD = chronic obstructive pulmonary disease; CVA = cerebrovascular accident.

Source: Adapted from *Osteoporosis and Asian American Women, Osteoporosis and African American Women,* and *Osteoporosis and Hispanic Women* (all from NIAMS documents, 2005); National Osteoporosis Foundation, 2005, *Physician's Guide;* "Bone Health," 2009, in "Menopause and Osteoporosis"; Qaseem et al, 2008; and University of Texas, 2008.

taken with food to enhance absorption because acid is needed for maximal absorption. **Calcium citrate** contains less elemental calcium, but is better absorbed and may be preferred by patients with reduced gastric acid production (e.g., older adults) or high gastric pH such as those on **proton pump inhibitors** or **histamine$_2$ (H_2) blockers** because it does not require acid for absorption (Kaiser, 2008). **Calcium** formulations are also available with **vitamin D** to improve the uptake of the calcium.

Research indicates that postmenopausal women need some additional drug therapy besides a healthy lifestyle to prevent and treat osteoporosis. Newer drugs such as **calcitonin, bisphosphonates, raloxifene,** and **teriparatide** have not had as wide usage as **estrogen,** but they are recommended at this time for women who have contraindications to **HRT** and for men as well.

Prevention of osteoporosis includes a low-impact aerobic exercise program; however, excessive exercise is not good because stress fractures may result. For treatment of osteoporosis, weight-bearing activity such brisk walking (20 min, 3–4 times/wk) is ideal. Resistance training (lifting weights or using strength-training machines) is a slow process, so programs should start low and work up over a period of months.

Rational Drug Selection

Estrogen Therapy

Studies have shown that there is a direct correlation between rate of bone loss in menopausal women and **estradiol levels** (Fitzpatrick, 2004). Bone resorption has also been shown to be highest in the first postmenopausal year. Women in the immediate postmenopausal years are the ones who are most in need of protection from osteoporosis.

A head-to-head trial comparing the effects of **alendronate** alone, **conjugated equine estrogen** alone, and a combination of the two, found that while both the **alendronate** and **estrogen** alone significantly increased bone mineral density (BMD), the combination was better than either alone (Greenspan et al, 2002). This study also looked at stopping therapy after 2 years by switching women who had been on the drugs to placebo. Those on **alendronate** alone who were switched to placebo had no change in BMD. However, the women initially on **estrogen** who were switched to placebo had a significant decrease in BMD, almost to baseline levels, within 1 year. The same could result in women who react to the WHI study data and stop taking **estrogen.** The WHI raised concerns about the risk for coronary events, stroke, pulmonary emboli, and breast cancer in women who took a combination of **estrogen** and **progesterone.** It is important to note, however, that the number of hip and vertebral fractures was lower at a statistically significant rate for women taking the combination and for women taking **estrogen** alone. Another trial reported by Fitzpatrick (2004), however, found that the addition of **progestin** to **estrogen therapy** did not produce a significant difference in BMD improvement. Findings from the WHI about risks associated with both HRT and ERT alone have led national associations of clinicians that specialize in women's health, the U.S Preventative Services Task Force, and the FDA to recommend that estrogen products not be considered first-line therapy for the prevention and treatment of osteoporosis unless a woman is also experiencing vasomotor or vaginal atrophy menopausal symptoms (details discussed in menopausal sections above). When ERT alone is chosen, low-dose therapy has been shown to produce a positive effect on BMD, even though the dose-related response is less. Lower doses also produce less risk for endometrial hyperplasia in women with an intact uterus; however unopposed estrogen in these women is contraindicated. Endometrial biopsy results from the HOPE trial (Liu, 2004) indicate that there was a 3.17 percent incidence of hyperplasia in the 0.3 mg (**Premarin**) group versus 27.27 percent hyperplasia in the 0.625 mg group at 2 years.

Balancing these risks and the availability of other drugs to prevent and treat osteoporosis should be discussed with women, who can then make an intelligent decision about whether or not to use **estrogen.** Prescribing information is presented earlier in this chapter. Dosing is the same for osteoporosis as recommended for HRT/ERT. Long-term efficacy of taking **estrogen** in lower doses for prevention of osteoporosis remains unknown at this time.

Calcium Therapy

All the guidelines used in this chapter suggest supplementation with **calcium** and **vitamin D** both for prevention of osteoporosis and as part of the treatment protocol. Kaiser (2008) suggests screening for **vitamin D** deficiency and supplementation with **vitamin D** to an acceptable level of greater than 30 ng/ml before initiating **bisphosphonate** therapy.

A major goal of the use of **calcium** and **vitamin D** is prevention of osteoporosis. Bone build-up is largely complete by the time one is a young adult. To assure a sufficient degree of bone density in adulthood, active promotion of adequate levels of **calcium** and **vitamin D** should begin with children and adolescents.

The typical American diet provides 600 to 1,000 mg **calcium** daily. The best **calcium** sources are dairy products and certain vegetables such as broccoli. Whole milk is not recommended for infants until 12 months of age, but yogurt and cheese can be introduced in the infant diet after 6 months of age (Greer & Krebs, 2006). Yogurt has more than 400 mg per 8-oz serving and broccoli has 150 mg. The average absorption of **calcium** from dietary sources is only 10 to 12 percent and **vitamin D** is necessary for optimal absorption. **Calcium** supplementation, up to 1,200 mg, is frequently necessary during childhood growth, pregnancy, and lactation. In women older than 65 years, a high **calcium** intake (500–1,200 mg/d) combined with **vitamin D** (700–800 IU/d) has been shown to reduce the incidence of nonvertebral fractures. The Institute of Medicine of the National Academy of Sciences recommends a daily **calcium** intake for adults aged 19 to 50 years of 1,000 mg/day and 1,200 mg/day for adults older than 50 years. The RDA for **vitamin D** is 200 IU/day for adults younger than 50 years, 400 IU/day for those 51 to 70 years, and 600 IU/day after age 70. For adults who do not get enough sun exposure, the intake may need to be 800 to 1,000 IU/day. Table 38–3 shows the recommended dietary calcium intake in the United States by age. **Calcium** as a part of a daily diet is found in plentiful and inexpensive sources. **Calcium** supplementation is also economical. Table 38–4 presents information on available **calcium** preparations.

When increased demand after menopause exceeds the typical dietary intake (1,500 mg), **calcium** alone as a supplement is not enough to prevent or treat osteoporosis. Patients need pharmacotherapy, used in conjunction with **vitamin D**, exercise, and avoidance of certain lifestyle behaviors.

Some patients complain of constipation with **calcium** in combination with carbonate, and other formulations need to be substituted. The presence of milk allergy and lactose intolerance can also greatly affect the amount of **calcium** in the diet and make supplementation mandatory.

Calcium is always ingested in combination with other ions. Depending on which ion, the dose may need to be given away from mealtimes to avoid reduced absorption.

Table 38–3 **Recommendations for Adequate Dietary Calcium Intake in the United States**

Age	Calcium Intake (mg/d)
0–6 months	210
7–12 months	270
1–3 years	500
4–8 years	800
9–18 years	1,300
19–50 years	1,000
50 to >70 years	1,200

Based on the Food and Nutrition Board of the National Academy of Sciences recommendations. The American Academy of Pediatrics recommends the use of these guidelines.

Table 38–4 **Calcium Preparations**

Drug	Active Calcium	How Supplied
Calcium acetate	25%	1,000 mg in 180 and 1,000 tablets per bottle (250 mg calcium)
Calcium carbonate	40%	650 mg in 1,000 tablets per bottle (260 mg calcium)
Calcium citrate	21%	950 and 2,376 mg in 100 and 300 tablets per bottle (200 mg and 500 mg calcium)
Calcium glubionate	6.5%	1.8 g per 5 mL in 480 mL with sweetener choices of saccharin, sorbitol, or sucrose (115 mg calcium)
Calcium gluconate	9.3%	500-mg, 650-mg, 975-mg, and 1-g tablets in 500 and 1,000 tablets per bottle (45, 58.5, 87.75, and 90 mg of calcium)
Calcium lactate	13%	325 mg and 650 mg in 1,000 tablets per bottle (42.5 mg and 84.5 mg of calcium)
Tricalcium phosphate	39%	1565.2 mg in 60 tablets per bottle (600 mg calcium)

Source: Wolters Kluwer Health, 2009, *Drug facts and comparisons*. St. Louis, MO: Wolters Kluwer Health, Inc.

Most **calcium** supplements in combination are only 40 to 50 percent active, so the practitioner needs to calculate the number of tablets depending on the size of tablet. A 600-mg **Tums** tablet has 240 mg of active **calcium**, and six **Tums** tablets fulfill the requirements for a postmenopausal woman.

Bisphosphonate Therapy

Indications

Primary and Secondary Prevention

NICE (2008a) recommends **alendronate (Fosamax)** for *primary prevention* in women over 70 years who have an independent risk factor for fracture and for women over 75 years with 2 or more risk factors. Women who are over 65 years and who are confirmed to have osteoporosis have this drug recommended by NICE, Kaiser (2008), and the Canadian Consensus Conference (Reid et al, 2009). This drug has also been studied in men. Whereas the NICE group and Kaiser recommend other **bisphosphonates** as alternative treatments, the Canadian Consensus Conference lists **risedronate (Actonel)** at the same level of recommendation as **alendronate. Risedronate** has also been studied in men. Kaiser also recommends **ibandronate (Boniva)** as second-line therapy in *primary prevention* for postmenopausal women over 65 years of age with prior vertebral fractures. The latter drug is not mentioned in other guidelines. The American College of Physicians (Qaseem et al, 2008) also recommends that providers consider drug therapy for men and women who are at risk for developing osteoporosis, but does not specifically state which drugs to use. The NICE (2008b) guidelines also discuss *secondary prevention*. They recommend the same drugs in the same order for this purpose, but limit this recommendation to postmenopausal women who have osteoporosis and have sustained a clinically apparent osteoporotic fragility fracture.

Patients may present with osteopenia, a precursor to osteoporosis. If the patient has other risk factors for osteoporosis and is found to be osteopenic (bone density of 1 to 2.5 standard deviations below the average adult peak bone mass) aggressive treatment with a **bisphosphonate** may be indicated for prevention of osteoporosis.

Treatment of Postmenopausal Women

Among the **bisphosphonates, alendronate (Fosamax), risendronate (Actonel)**, and **ibandronate (Boniva)** are all approved for preventing and treating postmenopausal osteoporosis. All the guidelines recommend **bisphosphonates** as first line therapy for the treatment of osteoporosis ("Bone Health," 2009; Brown et al, 2006; Kaiser, 2008; NICE, 2008b; North American Menopause Society [NAMS], 2006; Qaseem et al, 2008). The best trials have been done with **alendronate** and **risendronate** (ISCI, 2008) for their use with postmenopausal women and all the guidelines give their strongest recommendations to these two drugs. Studies have been done in large numbers of postmenopausal women with low bone mineral density for whom **alendronate** was the treatment in varying lengths of time from 2 to 10 years. In each study, the number of symptomatic fractures was reduced, but in only one study in which the women also had at least one previous vertebral fracture was the difference statistically significant. **Risendronate** had a similar result in research; use for prevention in women without osteoporosis was not helpful in preventing fractures at a statistically significant level, but it was helpful at this level for women who had demonstrated osteoporosis. **Ibandronate** studied in osteoporotic women or those at high risk showed a reduced rate of fractures. Kaiser (2008) and The American College of Physicians (Qaseem et al, 2008) includes this drug in its guidelines, but it has been shown only to prevent vertebral fractures, whereas **alendronate** and **risendronate** have demonstrated the ability to reduce both hip and vertebral fractures.

Dosage schedules vary among guidelines (ICSI, 2008; Kaiser, 2008; Michigan Quality Improvement Consortium, 2003; SIGN, 2004).

Treatment of Men

Kaiser (2008) guidelines also specifically mention treatment for men who are age 70 or older and who are diagnosed with osteoporosis or have a high risk for hip fracture. **Alendronate** is the drug it recommends as first-line therapy and it is approved for treating osteoporosis in men. The American College of Physicians' guideline makes its recommendations for both men and women.

Treatment of Men and Women Taking Corticosteroid Therapy

Both **alendronate** and **risendronate** are approved for use by men and women with **glucorticoid**-induced osteoporosis (Hodgson et al, 2003) and they are recommended as first-line therapy (Drug Facts and Comparisons, 2009; Hodgson et al, 2003; ICSI, 2008; Kaiser, 2008). The **corticosteroid** dose mentioned is equivalent to 5 mg/day of **prednisone** for a duration of 3 or more months. Chapter 21 provides more information on these drugs including their dosing.

Cost Versus Dosing Schedule

Alendronate cost is approximately $82 per month for four once-weekly tablets in a generic formulation with the brand name (**Fosamax**) being only a few dollars more expensive; **risendronate** is approximately $101 for the same monthly supply of four once-weekly tablets that are available in brand name (**Actonel**) only. **Ibandronate** is taken once monthly and costs about $109 for a 1-month supply because it is only available in brand name formulation (**Boniva**). Because the cost is approximately the same for all three drugs, the convenience of once-monthly dosing favors **ibandronate**. However, the cost and convenience of **bisphosphonates** should also be compared with $32 per month for **estrogen** and **estrogen-progestin therapies**, which require daily dosing. Patients with a history of GI bleeding, peptic ulcer disease, and gastroesophageal reflux disease (GERD) may not be the best candidates for **alendronate** because of the esophageal irritation common with this drug.

Adequate supplementation with **calcium** and **vitamin D** is necessary before initiating therapy and some newer formulations have either **vitamin D** or **calcium** included. No dosage adjustment is necessary as long as renal function remains between 35 and 60 mL/minute. At this time, **bisphosphonates** cannot be used with **estrogen**.

Calcitonin Therapy

When given by the intranasal route, **calcitonin** increases spinal bone mass in postmenopausal women with established osteoporosis. **Calcitonin** cannot prevent bone loss in the early postmenopausal woman. A 5-year study in 1,200 women with osteoporosis found statistically significant reduction in vertebral fractures with doses of 200 IU/day or 400 IU/day of the nasal spray. Interestingly, the statistical difference disappeared at the 400-IU/day dose, suggesting the lower dose is more effective. This drug is indicated only for women over 65 or at least years beyond menopause who have severe case of the disease and a history of prior vertebral fracture ("Bone Health," 2009; Kaiser, 2008; NAMS, 2006). It is not approved for prevention of bone loss. **Calcitonin** also has an unexplained analgesic effect on osteoporotic fracture pain.

Currently, this therapy has been shown to be more effective in spinal fractures, rather than in hip and wrist fractures. Use the nasal route of administration for patients with established bone loss. Rhinitis and nasal irritation are the commonest complaints. Examine the nasal mucosa carefully.

Calcitonin should be refrigerated before opening and then kept at room temperature once opened. Dosing with **calcitonin** 200 IU intranasally requires alternating nostrils every other day to reduce mucosal irritation. Other adverse effects are fatigue and flu-like symptoms.

Calcitonin therapy is more costly per month than any of the therapies previously discussed and has a limited fracture prevention efficacy, but has its place for bone pain relief in acute vertebral compression fractures secondary to osteoporosis.

Selective Estrogen Receptor Modulators

Indication

Raloxifene (**Evista**) is currently the only **selective estrogen receptor modulator (SERM)** approved to treat osteoporosis. In one study of 7,705 postmenopausal women with established osteoporosis, vertebral fracture had a statistically significant reduction in patients taking 60 mg to 120 mg of **raloxifene** at the 3-year mark, but at 8 years this difference disappeared. There was, however, a marked reduction in the incidence of invasive breast cancer in women taking this drug for 8 years. Another study of 1,035 postmenopausal women taking **raloxifene** versus placebo had a lower risk for cardiovascular events, most likely secondary to lowered serum LDL. This drug is an improvement over **tamoxifen** and may well prove to be a breast cancer antagonist after further clinical trials. It is indicated for prevention and treatment of osteoporosis in women who do not want to or are unable to take estrogen therapy. It shares with **estrogen** the precaution to avoid use in women who have previously had deep vein thrombus or embolism. It cannot be used in combination with **estrogen** because the receptors affected are different in the presence of **estrogen**.

Professional guidelines differ on the appropriate use of **raloxifene**. NICE (2008a, 2008b) does not recommend this drug for *primary prevention* of osteoporotic fragility fracture in postmenopausal women, but does list it as a second-line drug for secondary therapy. Kaiser (2008) also places it as second-line therapy for women without thrombotic risk who are at increased risk for breast cancer because of its **estrogen-like** effects on bone and **anti-estrogen** effects on the uterus and breast. The Canadian Consensus Conference on Osteoporosis ("Bone Health," 2009; Brown et al, 2006) suggests it as second line therapy to decrease the risk for vertebral fractures. The American College of Physicians' guideline (Qaseem et al, 2008) mentions **raloxifene** to prevent vertebral fractures and NAMS (2006) suggests it be considered for postmenopausal women with low bone mass or younger postmenopausal women with osteoporosis who are at greater risk for fractures of the spine rather than the hip.

Adverse Reactions

When compared with **estrogen** and **progesterone**, **raloxifene**'s adverse reactions were in the areas of more hot flushes, genital and urinary infection, and chest pain. HRT, by contrast, demonstrated more vaginal bleeding, breast pain, and flatulence.

A previous history of venous thromboembolic events such as deep vein thrombosis, pulmonary embolism, and retinal artery embolism is a contraindication for use. Patients with multiple risk factors for osteoporosis should receive BDM assessments to evaluate their need for this drug.

Patients need to be warned that the drug should be discontinued 72 hours prior to prolonged bedrest and to avoid inactivity while traveling by car or plane. Women need to know that this medication will not stop hot flashes; in fact, it could trigger hot flushes at the beginning of therapy.

Cost and Dosing Schedule

The dose of **raloxifene** is 60 mg daily without regard to meals. The cost for a 1-month supply is $84, which is more costly by a small amount than the **bisphosphonates** and over twice the cost of **estrogen**. It must be taken daily. Make sure patients consume or supplement 1,500 mg of **calcium** and 800 IU of **vitamin D** daily.

Raloxifene is discussed in more detail in Chapter 22.

Human Parathyroid Hormone

Teriparatide (Forteo) is the only drug in this class and it has limited indications. It is reserved for women at high risk of fracture, including those with very low bone mineral density with a previous vertebral fracture and who are unable to take a **bisphosphonate** or have had an unsatisfactory response to other therapies (NAMS, 2006; NICE, 2008). Kaiser (2008) recommends it be used only after evaluation by a specialist. A prospective, placebo-controlled trial in a large number of women with postmenopausal osteoporosis whose average age was 70 years found a statistically significant decrease in the incidence of vertebral fracture. The doses used in this study were 20 mcg to 40 mcg once daily for 21 months. The safety and efficacy of this drug have not been evaluated beyond 2 years of treatment. Because it is relatively new, is costly ($202 per injection, given once daily), and has not had safety and efficacy demonstrated long term, it is a third-line drug in treating osteoporosis except for its very limited indications.

Combination Therapy

Additive effects on bone mineral density have been found with **alendronate** plus **raloxifene** combinations. Evidence that this will reduce fractures is still not established and there is some concern that this combination of two different reabsorptive agents could suppress bone turnover to the point that fracture might actually be increased.

Two randomized trials with **teriparatide** and **alendronate** failed to show an additive effect on bone mineral density. One other study found that injecting **teriparatide** intermittently (3 months on, 3 months off) increased bone mineral density more than the **alendronate** alone. The effect on fracture reduction remains to be proven.

One 6-month, randomized, placebo-controlled trial reported on the American College of Rheumatology's Web site (http://www.rheumatology.org/press/2004) used a combination of **teriparatide** plus **raloxifene** versus **teriparatide** plus placebo. This study concluded that concomitant therapy with **teriparatide** and **raloxifene** increased bone formation to a similar degree as **teriparatide** therapy alone, reduced the degree of bone resorption seen with **teriparatide** alone but to a lesser degree, and significantly increased total hip BMD.

Summary

Estrogen is effective in preventing fractures but has cardiovascular and cancer risks. **Raloxifene** is also effective in preventing fractures, has less cardiovascular risk, and actually reduces the risk for breast cancer. It still carries the thromboembolic risks. Both of these require daily dosing. **Bisphosphonates** are effective in preventing fractures, are relatively safe, and have once-weekly or once-monthly dosing. They are listed as first-line therapy in all the guidelines. **Calcitonin** and **PTH** have specific indications and carry cost issues. Their use is limited by these variables. **Calcium**, especially when combined with **vitamin D**, is central to prevention of osteoporosis and the resultant fractures. It is inexpensive and should be used even if other drugs are chosen. Finally, low-impact weight-bearing exercise is critical to prevention of osteoporosis. Figure 38–3 depicts an algorithm for the prevention of osteoporosis in patients without the disease and Figure 38–4 presents a treatment algorithm for osteoporosis.

Monitoring

Before beginning treatment for osteoporosis, rule out common treatable disorders that can also cause low bone density. These include hyperparathyroidism, **vitamin D** deficiency, hyperthyroidism, and renal disease. Tests for these disorders are serum calcium and albumin, 25-hydroxy vitamin D, TSH, and serum creatinine levels, respectively. Serum creatinine levels are drawn prior to initiating therapy (Jamal, Leiter, Bayoumi, Bauer, & Cummings, 2004).

Measurement of bone mineral density is the most accurate predictor of fracture risk and efficacy of these drugs. Each 10 percent change below peak bone mass is associated with a doubling of the fracture risk for patients with osteoporosis. Dual energy x-ray absorptiometry (DEXA) is the gold standard by which bone mineral density and therapy are monitored, but it is expensive. Initial evaluation with DEXA can also suggest when a disease process other

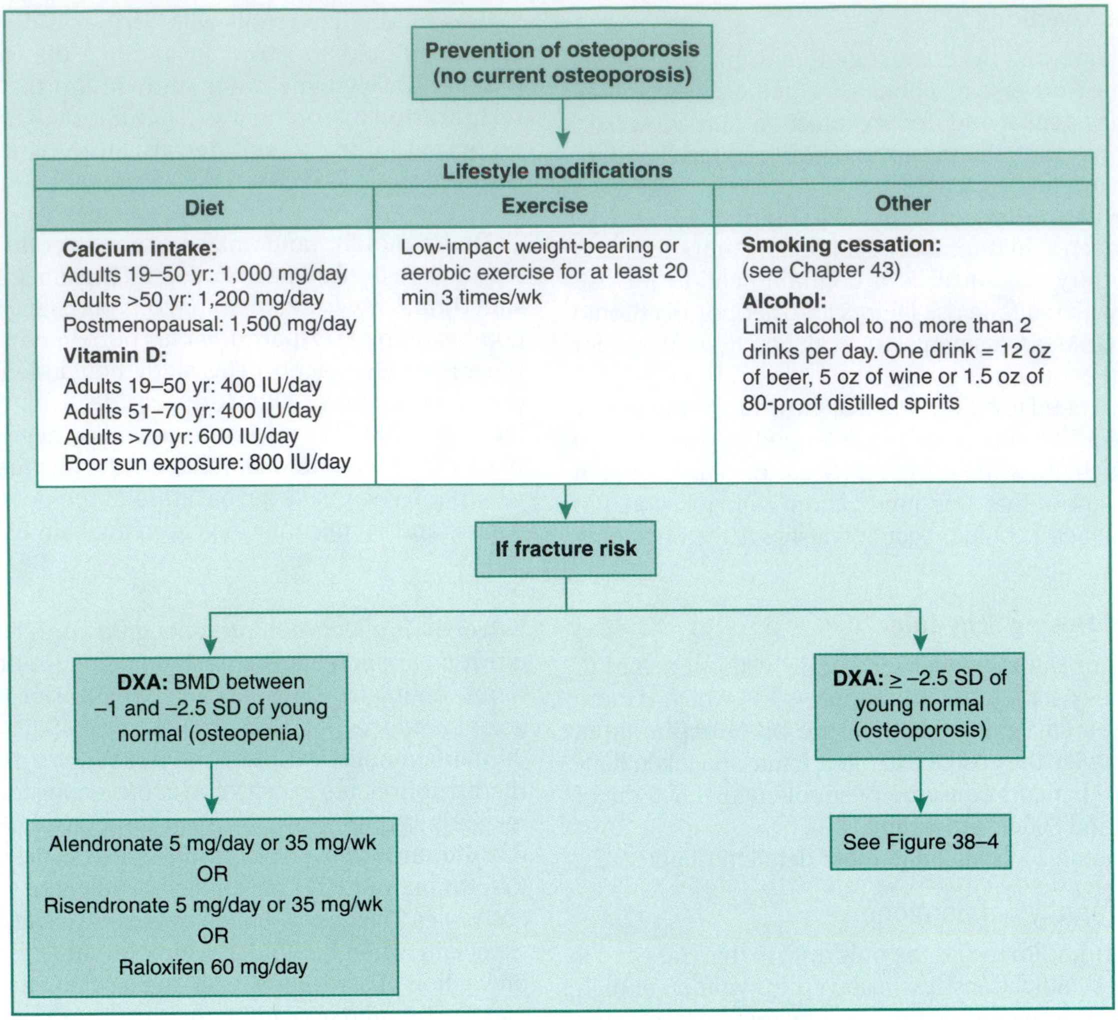

Figure 38–3. Prevention of osteoporosis in patients without the disease.

than aging is the probable cause of the bone loss. Once therapy has been established, DEXA is repeated 1 year later to determine progress. Whether to repeat DEXA at later dates is controversial. According to the American Association of Clinical Endocrinologist (AACE) (Hodgson et al, 2003), DEXA should be used for the following:

1. Women who are **estrogen** deficient, to make decisions about therapy
2. Women who have vertebral abnormalities or osteopenia detected on x-ray, to confirm the diagnosis
3. Patients who are being treated for osteoporosis, to monitor for treatment efficacy
4. Patients receiving long-term **glucocorticoid therapy**, to guide therapy to preserve bone mass
5. Patients with asymptomatic primary hyperthyroidism or other diseases associated with high risk for osteoporosis, to make therapy decisions.
6. All women 40 years and older who have sustained a fracture
7. All women older than 65 years

ICSI (2008) adds the following risk factors:

1. Body weight less than 127 lb or BMI less than or equal to 20
2. Current smoker
3. Surgical menopause before 40 years
4. On **hormone replacement** for more than 10 to 15 years
5. Premenopausal women with amenorrhea for more than 1 year
6. Anyone with severe loss of mobility (unable to ambulate outside one's dwelling without a wheelchair) for more than 1 year

Other articles in the reference list (National Osteoporosis Foundation, 2005; Siminoski et al, 2005; USDHHS, 2004) discuss the use of bone density measurement.

Table 38–5 lists methods for bone density measurements.

Estrogen

Estrogen requires the same monitoring when prescribed for osteoporosis as it does when it is used for ERT/HRT. Obtain annual renal function tests on all patients older

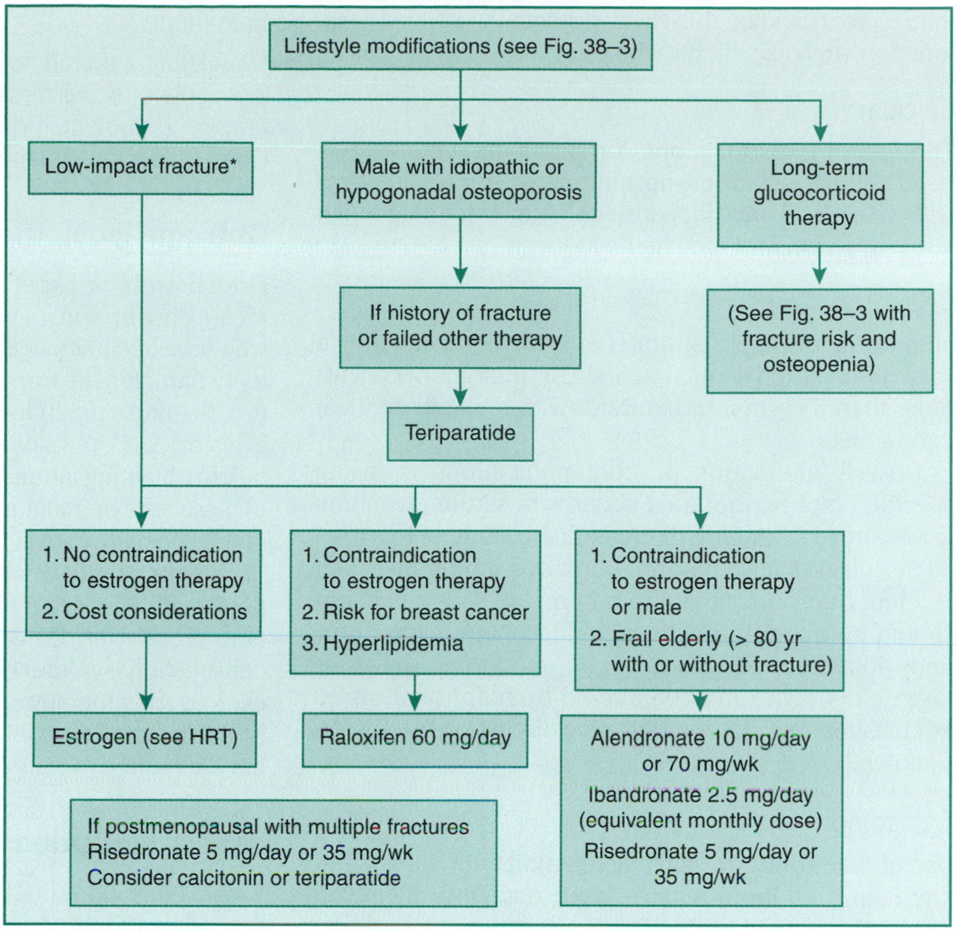

Figure 38–4. Treatment algorithm: Osteoporosis. (Adapted from *Osteoporosis and African American Women; Osteoporosis and Asian American Women; Osteoporosis and Hispanic Women* [all from NIAMS documents, 2005]; and National Osteoporosis Foundation, 2004, *Physician's Guide*.)

Table 38–5 Methods for Bone Density Measurements

Test	Sites Measured	Approximate Cost	Comments
Dual energy x-ray absorptiometry (DEXA)	Spine, hip, total body	$150–$200	Limitations: misdiagnoses low bone mass in patients with arthritis Available: yes, but not in all cities
Peripheral dual energy x-ray absorptiometry (P-DEXA)	Wrist, finger	$50	Limitations: in older adults who tend to have arthritis in these sites (see above). Omits several areas (vertebra and hip) that are common sites of osteoporosis in this age group. Available: yes
Quantitative computed tomography (QCT)	Spine	$100–$150	Limitations: machine must be recalibrated between uses Available: yes
Peripheral QCT (pQCT)	Forearm, wrist	$40–$60	Limitations: better for younger patients needing multiple sites Available: yes
Radiographic absorptiometry (RA)	Hand	$60	Limitations: requires normal baseline; not available for patients with arthritis who have no baseline Available: yes
Single photon absorptiometry (SXA)	Wrist	$50	Limitations: older adults (same as peripheral above) Available: yes
Single energy x-ray absorptiometry (SXA)	Wrist, heel	$35–$120	Limitations: older adults (same as peripheral above) Available: yes
Ultrasound	Heel, tibia, finger	$30–$50	Limitations: new, younger, no x-ray Available: yes
Peripheral instant x-ray imaging (PIXI)	Wrist, heel	$50	Limitations: older adult or young Available: European approval only

than 65 years and on those with potentially reduced renal function, such as patients with diabetes.

Calcium

The use of **calcium** alone for supplementation rarely needs blood test follow-up, but treatment of conditions with **vitamin D** and high-dose **calcium** can induce high levels in serum and then in the kidneys.

Bisphosphonates

Monitoring of **bisphosphonates** is aimed at electrolyte measurement, renal function, and GI symptoms of patients older than 65 years, and of those with multiple medical conditions.

Dosage alterations or contraindications to using specific **bisphosphonates** occur with serum creatinine levels above 2.5 mg/dL or creatinine clearance less than 30 ml/min. Because **bisphosphonates** inhibit intestinal calcium transport, careful monitoring of serum calcium should be done during therapy. Phosphate, magnesium, and potassium should also be monitored because these electrolytes may be altered by **bisphosphonate** administration. Further monitoring discussion is found in Chapter 21.

Calcitonin

Use of **calcitonin** presents the possibility of allergy and circulating antibodies have been detected after 2 to 18 months of therapy. The drug is given intranasally, and a nasal examination should be performed prior to initiation of treatment, and periodically during treatment to look for damage to the nasal mucosa.

Raloxifene

Evaluation of therapy with **raloxifene** can be done every 2 years with bone densitometers, but beneficial effects may be demonstrated as early as 1 year after therapy. Other monitoring is similar to that of **estrogen**.

Outcome Evaluation

Osteoporosis is expected to begin 2 to 5 years after menopause in women not using ERT/HRT. Assess patients who have had fractures, unusual bone pain, high-risk physical characteristics, or a history of **systemic cortisone** use. The nurse practitioner can begin this evaluation with a history and physical examination and then consult before obtaining laboratory tests or imaging studies. If any of these tests or imaging studies indicate pathology, referral for specialty care is indicated.

Patients who have other medical conditions and multiple medications to manage are candidates for consultation or referral. Consider referral if more than one consultation is made with the specialist over medication choices. After therapy is established and the patient is not having adverse drug effects, most primary care providers handle routine monitoring.

Patient Education

Patient education should include a discussion of information related to the overall treatment plan as well as that specific to the drug therapy, reasons for taking the drug, drugs as part of the total treatment regimen, and adherence issues.

OSTEOPOROSIS

PATIENT EDUCATION

Related to the Overall Treatment Plan/Disease Process

- ☐ Pathophysiology of the dynamic relationship between the osteoclasts and osteoblasts in the process of bone metabolism to help the patient understand how the lack of estrogen begins a cascade of events ending with the increased risk of osteoporosis in the early years after cessation of menses. For men, discussion of the role of other factors is important.
- ☐ The role of excessive intake of alcohol, nicotine, and caffeine and low intake of **calcium** and **vitamin D** as modifiable risks for osteoporosis and how nondrug treatments such as diets high in **calcium** and **vitamin D,** exercise, and avoidance of the high-risk lifestyles can help to prevent osteoporosis.
- ☐ An understanding of how knowledge of family history, ethnicity, and genetic characteristics help to identify patients with nonmodifiable risk factors for osteoporosis.
- ☐ Importance of adherence to the treatment regimen
- ☐ Importance of supplementing the diet with additional calcium (up to 1,500 mg) and **vitamin D** (800 mg) to the osteoporosis therapy
- ☐ Self-monitoring of symptoms
- ☐ What to do when symptoms worsen
- ☐ Need for regular follow-up visits with the primary care provider and for screening tests such as BMDs every 2 years.

OSTEOPOROSIS—cont'd

PATIENT EDUCATION

Specific to the Drug Therapy

- ☐ Reason for the drug(s) to be taken and anticipated action in the disease process
- ☐ Doses and schedules for taking the drug(s)
- ☐ Possible adverse effects and what to do if they occur
- ☐ Interactions between other treatment modalities and these drugs

Reasons for Taking the Drug(s)

Patient education specifically for osteoporosis should include the following: that prevention of osteoporosis is more successful than having to treat it later, especially in those who have a hereditary tendency for bone loss disease; treatment of fractures is far more expensive than drug therapy; and postmenopausal fractures are associated with early loss of independent living and reduced life expectancy.

Drugs as Part of the Total Treatment Regimen

The total treatment regimen includes lifestyle modification: healthy diet, dietary supplements, and exercise. However, these lifestyle modifications may not be enough, especially in older patients. Some form of drug therapy is usually necessary. A variety of therapies are available, and selection of estrogen versus nonestrogen therapy is possible with the same results for prevention and treatment of spine, hip, and wrist fractures associated with osteoporosis.

Adherence Issues

Adherence issues include the following:

- ☐ Media reports about disease and drug therapies have an increasing impact on patients and primary care practices.
- ☐ Membership in health maintenance organizations may affect the choice of drugs patients will receive.
- ☐ Patients' fears or issues about drug therapy may not be based on facts.
- ☐ Drug therapy educational handouts should be available to patients and their families.
- ☐ Monitoring appointments is problematic if patients are homebound or transportation is difficult.

REFERENCES

American College of Rheumatology. (2004). Concomitant teriparatide plus raloxifene for the treatment of postmenopausal osteoporosis: Results from a randomized placebo-controlled trial. Retrieved October 28, 2005, from http://www.rheumatology.org/press/2004

Anderson, G., Judd, H., Kaunitz, A., Barad, D., Beresford, S., Pettinger, M., et al. (2003). Effects of estrogen plus progestin on gynecologic cancers and associated diagnostic procedures: The Women's Health Initiative Randomized Trial. *Journal of the American Medical Association, 290*(13), 1739–1748.

Anderson, G., Limacher, M., Assaf, A., Bassford, T., Beresford, S., Black, H., et al. (2004). Effects of conjugated equine estrogen in postmenopausal women with hysterectomy: The Women's Health Initiative randomized trial. *Journal of the American Medical Association, 291,* 1701–1712.

Archer, D. (2004). Hormonal therapy and the postmenopausal woman: Current clinical challenges. *Portraits and Passages: Women's Health Through the Prime of Life.* CE # 04-17.

Barrett-Conner, E., Grady, D., & Stefanick, M. (2005). The rise and fall of menopausal hormone therapy. *Annual Review of Public Health, 26,* 115–140.

Blumenthal, M. (Ed.). (1998). The complete German Commission E monographs. In *Therapeutic guide to herbal medicines.* Austin, TX: American Botanical Council.

Bone health. (2009). (Update of Brown et al, 2006). In: Menopause and osteoporosis: Update 2009. *Journal of Obstetrics and Gynaecology, 31*(Suppl. 1), 34–41.

Boyack, M., Lookinland, S., & Chasson, S. (2002). Efficacy of raloxifene for treatment of menopause: A systematic review. *Journal of the American Academy of Nurse Practitioners, 14*(4), 150–165.

Brown, J., Fortier, M., Frame, H., Lalonde, A., Papaioannou, A., Senikas, V., et al. (2006). Canadian Consensus Conference on osteoporosis. *Journal of Obstetrics and Gynaecology, 28*(2)(Suppl. 1), 95–112.

Brucker, M. (2002). What's a woman to do? *AWHONN Lifelines, 6*(5), 408–417.

Cherrington, A., Lewis, C., McCreath, H., Herman, C., Richter, D., & Byrd, T. (2003). Association of complementary and alternative medicine use, demographic factors, and perimenopausal symptoms in a multiethnic sample of women: The ENDOW Study. *Family and Community Health, 26*(1), 74–83.

Chlebowski, R., Hendrix, S., Langer, R., Stefanick, M., Gass, M., Lane, D., et al. (2003). Influence of estrogen plus progestin on breast cancer and mammography in healthy postmenopausal women: The Women's Health Initiative Randomized Trial. *Journal of the American Medical Association, 289*(24), 3243–3253.

Fitzpartick, L. (2004). Estrogen and bone health. *The Female Patient, 29*(Suppl.), 4–9.

Garnero, P., Stevens, R., Ayres, S., & Phelps, K. (2002). Short-term effects of new synthetic conjugated estrogens on biochemical markers of bone turnover. *Journal of Clinical Pharmacology, 42,* 290–296.

Greenspan, S., Emkey, R., Bone, H., Weiss, S., Bell, N., Downs, R., et al. (2002). Significant differential effects of alendronate, estrogen or combination therapy on the rate of bone loss after discontinuation of treatment of postmenopausal osteoporosis: A randomized, double-blind, placebo-controlled trial. *Archives of Internal Medicine, 137*(11), 875–883.

Greer, F., & Krebs, N. (2006). Optimizing bone health and calcium intakes of infants, children and adolescents. *Pediatrics, 117*(2), 578–585.

Herrington, D., Reboussin, D., Brosnihan, K., Sharp, P., Shumaker, S., Snyder, T., et al. (2000). Effects of estrogen replacement on the progression of coronary artery atherosclerosis (ERA). *New England Journal of Medicine, 343*(8), 522–529.

Hodgson, S., Watts, N., Bilezikian, J., Clarke, B., Gray, T., Harris, D., et al. (2003). American Association of Clinical Endocrinologists medical guidelines for clinical practice for the prevention and treatment of postmenopausal osteoporosis: 2001 edition with selected updates for 2003. *Endocrinology Practice, 9*(6), 544–564.

Hodis, H., Mack, W., Azen, S., Lobo, R. A., Shoupe, D., Maher, P. R., et al. (2003). Hormone therapy and the progression of coronary artery atherosclerosis in postmenopausal women. *New England Journal of Medicine, 349*(6), 535–545.

Hodis, H., Mack, W., Lobo, E., Shoupe, D., Sevanian, A., Maher, P. R., et al. (2001). Estrogen in the prevention of atherosclerosis. A randomized, double-blind, placebo-controlled trial. *Annals of Internal Medicine, 135*(11), 939–953.

Hulley, S., Furberg, C., Barrett-Conner, E., Cauley, J., Grady, D., Haskell, W., et al, for the HERS Research Group. (2002). Noncardiovascular disease outcomes during 6.8 years of hormone therapy: Heart and estrogen/progestin replacement study follow-up (HERS II). *Journal of the American Medical Association, 288*(1), 58–66.

Hulley, S., Grady, D., Bush, T., Furberg, C., Herrington, D., Riggs, B., et al. (1998). Randomized trial of estrogen plus progestin for secondary prevention of coronary heart disease in postmenopausal women. *Journal of the American Medical Association, 280*(7), 605–613.

Institute for Clinical Systems Improvement (ICSI). (2008). *Diagnosis and treatment of osteoporosis.* Bloomington, MN: Author. Retrieved August 3, 2009, from http://www.ICSI.org/osteoporosis

International Osteoporosis Foundation (IOF). (2009). Facts and statistics about osteoporosis and its impact. *Progress in Osteoporosis, 10*(3). Retrieved August 3, 2009, from http://www.iofbonehealth.org

Jamal, S., Leiter, R., Bayoumi, A., Bauer, D., & Cummings, S. (2004, August). Clinical utility of laboratory testing in women with osteoporosis. *Osteoporosis International.* Retrieved October 25, 2005, from http://www.osteoporosis.ca/english/For%20Health%20Professionals/Research

Kaiser Permanente Care Management Institute. (2008). Osteoporosis/fracture prevention clinical practice guidelines. Oakland, CA: Kaiser Permanente Care Management Institute. Retrieved October 11, 2009, from http://www.guideline.gov/summary/summary.aspx

Kern, L., Powe, N., Levine, M., Fitzpatrick, A., Harris, T., Robbins, J., et al. (2005). Association between screening for osteoporosis and the incidence of hip fracture. *Annals of Internal Medicine, 142*(3), 173–181.

Kligler, B. (2003). Black cohosh. *American Family Physician, 68,* 114–119.

Kong, Y., & Penninger, J. (2000). Molecular control of bone remodeling and osteoporosis. *Experimental Gerontology, 35*(8), 947.

Langer, R. (2005). Postmenopausal hormone therapy. *CME Bulletin of the American Academy of Family Physicians, 4*(1), 1–10.

Lindenfeld, E., & Langer, R. (2002). Bleeding patterns of hormone replacement therapies in the postmenopausal estrogen and progestin interventions trial. *Obstetrics and Gynecology, 100,* 853–863.

Liu, J. (2004). Use of conjugated estrogens after the Women's Health Initiative. *The Female Patient, 29,* 8–13.

Liu, J., Burdette, J., Xu, H., Gu, C., vanBreemen, R., Bhat, K., et al. (2001). Evaluation of estrogenic activity of plant extracts for the potential treatment of menopausal symptoms. *Journal of Agricultural and Food Chemistry, 49,* 2472–2479.

Marx, P., Schade, G., Wilbourn, S., Blank, S., Moyer, D., & Nett, R. (2004). Low dose (0.3 mg) synthetic conjugated estrogens A is effective for managing atrophic vaginitis. *Maturitas, 47*(1), 47–55.

McCance, K. L., & Huether, S. E. (2006). *Pathophysiology: The biologic basis for disease in adults and children* (5th ed.). St Louis, MO: Elsevier.

Michigan Quality Improvement Consortium. (2003). *Management of osteoporosis.* Southfield, MI: Author. Retrieved July 11, 2005, from http://www.guideline.gov/summary/summary.aspx

National Institute for Health and Clinical Excellence (NICE). (2008a). Alendronate, etidronate, risedronate, raloxifene and strontium ranelate for the primary prevention of osteoporotic fragility fractures in postmenopausal women. London, England: National Institute for Health and Clinical Excellence (NICE). Retrieved October 11, 2009, from http://www.guideline.gov/summary/summary.aspx

National Institute for Health and Clinical Excellence (NICE). (2008b). Alendronate, etidronate, risedronate, raloxifene, strontium ranelate and teriparatide for the secondary prevention of osteoporotic fragility fractures in postmenopausal women. London, England: National Institute for Health and Clinical Excellence (NICE). Retrieved October 11, 2009, from http://www.guideline.gov/summary/summary.aspx

National Institute of Arthritis and Musculoskeletal and Skin Diseases (NIAMSD). (2005a). *Osteoporosis and African American women.* Retrieved October 25, 2005, from http://www.niams.nih.gov/bone/hi/osteoporosis

National Institute of Arthritis and Musculoskeletal and Skin Diseases (NIAMSD). (2005b). *Osteoporosis and Asian American women.* Retrieved October 25, 2005, from http://www.niams.nih.gov/bone/hi/osteoporosis

National Institute of Arthritis and Musculoskeletal and Skin Diseases (NIAMSD). (2005c). *Osteoporosis and Hispanic women.* Retrieved October 25, 2005, from http://www.niams.nih.gov/bone/hi/osteoporosis

National Osteoporosis Foundation. (2005). Physician's guide to prevention and treatment of osteoporosis. Retrieved October 25, 2005, from http://www.nof/org/physguide/inside. Updated September 2005.

North American Menopause Society (NAMS). (2006). Management of osteoporosis in postmenopausal women: 2006 position statement of the North American Menopause Society. *Menopause, 13*(3), 340–367.

Qaseem, A., Snow, V., Shekelle, P., Hopkins, R., Jr., Forciea, M., Owens, D., the Clinical Efficacy Assessment Subcommittee of the American College of Physicians. (2008). Screening for osteoporosis in men: A clinical practice guideline from the American College of Physicians. *Annals of Internal Medicine, 148*(9), 680–684.

Reid, R. L., Blake, J., Abramson, B., Khan, A., Senikas, V., & Fortier, M. (2009). SOGC Clinical Practice Guideline: Menopause and osteoporosis update 2009. *Journal of Obstetrics and Gynecology Canada, 31*(1), S34–S41.

Rossouw, J., Anderson, G., Prentice, R., Lacroix, A., Kooperberg, C., Stefanick, M., et al. (2002). Risks and benefits of estrogen plus progestin in healthy postmenopausal women: Principal results from the Women's Health Initiative Randomized Controlled Trial. *Journal of the American Medical Association, 288*(3), 321–333.

Sarrel, P. (2004, February). Vasomotor and vascular consideration. *The Female Patient* (Suppl.), 10–80.

Scottish Intercollegiate Guidelines Network (SIGN). (2004). *Management of osteoporosis: A national guideline.* Edinburgh, Scotland: Scottish Intercollegiate Guidelines Network. Retrieved August 3, 2009, from http://www.sing.ac.uk/guidelines

Shumaker, S., Legault, C. Rapp, S., Thal, L., Wallace, R., Ockene, J., et al. (2003). Estrogen plus progestin and the incidence of dementia and mild cognitive impairment in postmenopausal women. *Journal of the American Medical Association, 289*(20), 2651–2662.

Siminoski, K., Leslie, W., Frame, H., Hodsman, A., Josse, R., Khan, A., et al. (2005). Recommendations for bone mineral density reporting in Canada. *Canadian Association of Radiologists Journal, 56*(3), 178–188. Retrieved October 25, 2005, from http://www.osteoporosis.ca/english/For%20Health%20Professionals/Research

Simon, J. (2002). *Hormone replacement therapy: Focus on the menopausal patient.* Clifton, NJ: Continuing Medical Education: Ithaca Center for Postgraduate Medical.

Stevens, R., Roy, P., & Phelps, K. (2002). Evaluation of single- and multiple-dose pharmacokinetics of synthetic conjugated estrogens, A (Cenestin) tablets: A slow-release estrogen replacement product. *Journal of Clinical Pharmacology, 42,* 332–341.

Thorneycroft, I. (2004, February). Unopposed estrogen and cancer. *The Female Patient* (Suppl.), 19–26.

Tice, J., Ettinger, B., Ensrud, K., Wallace, R., Blackwell, T., & Cummings, S. (2003). Phytoestrogen supplements for the treatment of hot flashes:

The Isosflavone Clover Extract (ICE) study: A randomized controlled trial. *Journal of the American Medical Association, 290*, 207–214.

University of Texas, School of Nursing, Family Nurse Practitioner Program. (2008). Risk factor assessment for osteoporosis and/or increased fracture risk in men. Austin, TX: University of Texas, School of Nursing. Retrieved October 11, 2009, from http://www.guideline.gov/summary/summary.aspx

U.S. Department of Health and Human Services (USDHHS). (2004). *Bone health and osteoporosis: A report of the Surgeon General.* Rockville, MD: U.S. Department of Health and Human Services, Office of the Surgeon General. Available at http://www.surgeongeneral.gov/library

Wassertheil-Smoller, S., Hendrix, S. L., Limacher, M., Heiss, G., Kooperberg, C., Baird, A., et al. (2003). Effect of estrogen plus progestin on stroke in postmenopausal women: The Women's Health Initiative: A randomized trial. *JAMA, 289*(20), 2673–2684.

Wolters Kluwer Health. (2009). *Drug facts and comparisons*. St. Louis, MO: Wolters Kluwer Health.

Writing Group for the Women's Health Initiative (WHI) Investigators. (2002). Risks and benefits of estrogen plus progestin in healthy postmenopausal women. *Journal of the American Medical Association, 288*(3), 321–323.

Writing Group of the PEPI Trial. (1996). Effects of hormonal therapy on bone mineral density: Results from the post-menopausal estrogen/progestin interventions (PEPI). *Journal of the American Medical Association, 276*(17), 1394–1396.

Wysocki, S., & Alexander, I. (2005). Bioidentical hormones for menopause therapy: An overview. *Women's Health Care: A Practical Journal for Nurse Practitioners, 4*(2), 9–17.

Wysocki, S., & Thorneycroft, I. (2005). Use of complementary and alternative medicine by menopausal women. *The Forum: A Working Group for Women's Health Care, 3*(3), 18–25.

CHAPTER 39

HYPERLIPIDEMIA

Marylou Robinson and Anita Lee Wynne

Chapter Outline

Cardiovascular diseases are the major cause of death in the United States. Almost 500,000 people die each year from heart attacks, most commonly related to coronary artery disease (CAD). Atherosclerosis, the major cause of CAD, is characterized by deposits of cholesterol and lipoproteins in artery walls. Three major classes of lipoproteins are found in the serum of fasting individuals: low-density lipoproteins (LDL), high-density lipoproteins (HDL), and very-low-density lipoproteins (VLDL). Elevated serum lipoprotein levels are one of the four best-established major risk factors for CAD. More specifically, the risk for CAD is associated with serum cholesterol levels above 200 mg/dL, fasting triglyceride levels above 150 mg/dL, and LDL levels above 100 mg/dL. Lifestyle and pharmacological therapies are directed toward bringing elevated levels of these lipoproteins down to specified levels associated with reduced cardiovascular disease risk. In the Framingham study, a 10 percent decrease in serum cholesterol level was associated with a 2 percent decrease in the incidence of CAD morbidity and mortality. Other studies have confirmed, in men and women who were initially free of coronary heart disease (CHD), a direct relationship between levels of LDL cholesterol and the rate of new-onset CHD. The lifetime risk for developing CHD is 49 percent for men and 32 percent for women (National Cholesterol Education Program [NCEP], 2001). Trials with **HMG-CoA reductase inhibitors (statins)** indicate that a 1 percent decrease in LDL cholesterol reduces the risk of CAD by about 1 percent (NCEP, 2001). Drugs that affect lipid levels differentially affect LDLs, HDLs, VLDLs, and triglyceride levels. In treatment, pharmacotherapy is based on how a drug affects specific lipoprotein levels.

This chapter focuses on the relationship between hyperlipidemia and atherosclerosis. The management of hyperlipidemia is based on the NCEP guidelines and the 2004 amendments (Grundy et al, 2004). Chapter 16 provides specific information for drugs used to lower plasma lipid levels.

PATHOPHYSIOLOGY

Serum fat and cholesterol are carried in the circulation in complexes of lipids and proteins called lipoproteins. Fat is transported as triglycerides and phospholipids, and cholesterol is transported in free and esterified forms. Most of the cholesterol in plasma is carried in LDLs. High concentrations of LDLs are associated with an increased risk of CAD. Serum lipoproteins are formed via two pathways: dietary, or exogenous, and liver synthesis, or endogenous.

Exogenous Pathway

After a meal, fat and cholesterol are absorbed by the intestinal cells, esterified into triglycerides and cholesterol, and then packaged into chylomicrons, which are transported via the lymphatic system to the thoracic duct and enter the venous circulation. Activated endothelial lipoprotein lipase then hydrolyzes the triglycerides into free fatty acids and glycerol, which are removed from the circulation for use by fat and muscle cells. Surface cholesterol is transferred to HDLs. The chylomicrons shrink during this process and become remnants that are removed from the circulation by apolipoprotein (apo) E after it binds to a liver receptor. Antihyperlipidemic pharmacotherapy focuses on the pathway in which fats are absorbed, transported, and metabolized. Medications that affect the absorption of fat and cholesterol in the intestine are classified as **bile acid-binding resins** and medications that increase lipolysis of triglycerides are classified as **fibric acid derivatives.** Lifestyle modifications also affect the absorption, transport, and metabolism of fats through this pathway.

Endogenous Pathway

VLDLs are synthesized and secreted by the liver into the circulation and contain triglycerides and some cholesterol. VLDL is hydrolyzed to free fatty acids and glycerol by lipoprotein lipase in the capillary endothelium. Fat and muscle cells absorb the fatty acid and glycerol. About 50 percent of the VLDL remnants are taken up by apo B and E receptors in the liver, and the other 50 percent stays in the circulation and becomes intermediate-density lipoproteins (IDLs). IDLs are then enriched with cholesterol by hepatic triglyceride lipase to become LDLs, which carry about 75 percent of the circulating cholesterol. LDLs circulate for 2 to 3 days and are removed for use by all types of tissue.

LDL receptors in the liver are down-regulated by the presence of LDL; therefore, one mechanism for lowering LDLs is pharmacotherapy that increases the number of LDL receptors in the liver (**bile acid-binding resins, statins**). Drugs that inhibit VLDL synthesis in the liver (**niacin, fibric acid derivatives**) also reduce LDLs via the endogenous pathway.

Atherogenesis

There are four main types of lipoproteins: VLDLs, IDLs, LDLs, and HDLs. The lipoproteins that contain apo B100 have been identified as the vehicles that facilitate transport of cholesterol into the arterial wall, leading to atherogenesis. LDLs, which make up 60 to 70 percent of the total serum cholesterol, are the major culprit in this process. LDL levels are increased in individuals who consume large amounts of saturated fats and/or cholesterol, who have defects in the hepatic LDL receptor (familial hypercholesterolemia), or who have a polygenic form of increased LDLs. The relationship of elevated LDL cholesterol to the development of CAD is a multistep process beginning relatively early in life (McCrindle et al, 2007). When serum LDL levels exceed a threshold of 100 mg/dL, they cross the arterial wall and become embedded in the arterial lumen. In the arterial lumen, LDLs undergo oxidation, are taken up by macrophages, and form a plaque known as a fatty streak. Atherosclerotic plaques are made up of foam cells, which are transformed macrophages and smooth muscle cells filled with cholesterol. Glycation of lipoproteins in poorly controlled diabetes contributes to foam cell generation. Arterial hypertension also accelerates this process.

The second step of atherogenesis involves the formation of scar tissue over the fatty plaque in the arterial wall. This formation is called a fibrous plaque. Over time, fibrous plaques become unstable and are prone to rupture, causing potentially life-threatening luminal thromboses. Plaque rupture or erosion is responsible for most acute coronary events (e.g., myocardial infarction, unstable angina, and coronary death). Elevated LDL cholesterol provides fatty substrate for plaque formation and the larger the plaque, the more unstable it will be.

HDLs, which make up 20 to 30 percent of total serum cholesterol, are thought to function as acceptors of free cholesterol as it passively diffuses from cells. This reverse transport is the mechanism by which cholesterol may be removed from atherosclerotic plaques. Figure 39–1 shows the relationship of lipid metabolism to atherosclerotic plaque formation. Apo A-I and A-II are the major apos in HDL. The level of apos and HDLs are inversely related to CAD. As serum HDL and apo levels increase, atherogenesis and CAD decrease.

Although LDLs are most commonly the lipoprotein toward which therapy is directed, the ratio of total cholesterol to HDL is actually the most powerful predictor of atherosclerotic CAD risk. Strong epidemiological evidence links low levels of HDL cholesterol to increased coronary morbidity and mortality, and low levels are consistently shown to be an independent risk factor for CHD (NCEP, 2001). The antioxidant and anti-inflammatory properties of HDL also inhibit atherogenesis. Factors that contribute to low HDL are shown in Table 39–1. Each of these factors can be targets of therapy. Drugs that raise HDL levels include **nicotinic acid (niacin)**, **fibrates**, and **statins**.

VLDLs are triglyceride-rich lipoproteins that contain 10 to 15 percent of the total serum cholesterol. The major apolipoproteins (apo) of VLDL are apo B100; apo C I, II and III; and apo E. VLDLs are produced by the liver and are precursors of LDL. Some forms of VLDL, particularly VLDL remnants, appear to promote atherosclerosis similarly to LDL. VLDL + LDL cholesterol is called non-HDL cholesterol. The non-HDL number can be calculated by taking the total cholesterol (TC) and subtracting the HDL. Non-HDL cholesterol includes all lipoproteins that contain apo B, the most important apolipoprotein in the generation of atherosclerotic plaques. Individuals with high triglycerides (200 to 499 mg/dL), present as having most of their cholesterol in these small VLDL remnants. Although LDL receives primary attention for clinical

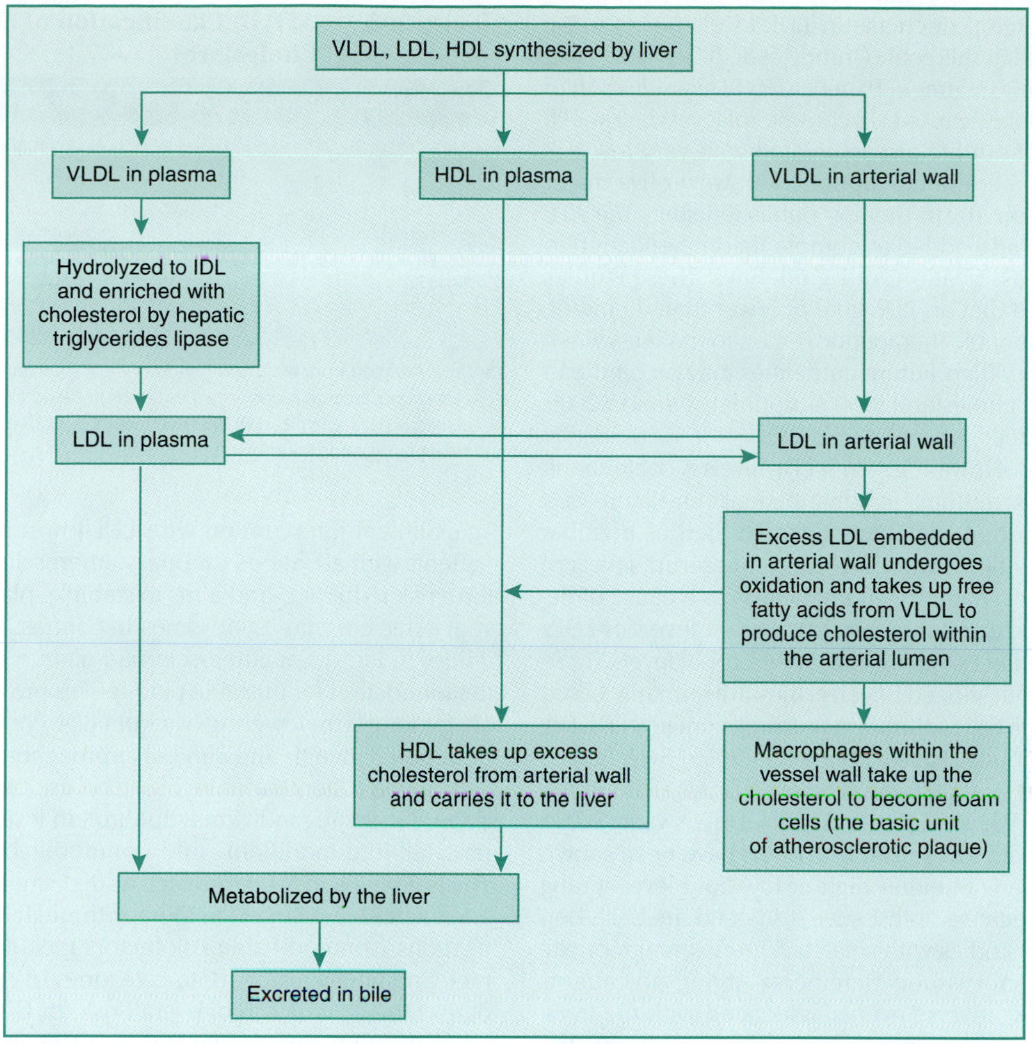

Figure 39–1. Relationship of lipid metabolism to atherosclerotic plaque formation. Excess LDL embedded in the arterial wall undergoes oxidation and takes up free fatty acids from VLDL to produce cholesterol within the arterial lumen. If the excess cholesterol is not taken up by HDL and carried to the liver, macrophages within the vessel wall create atherosclerotic plaque from this excess cholesterol.

Table 39–1 **Factors That Contribute to Low HDL Cholesterol Levels**

Cigarette smoking
Drugs: beta blockers, anabolic steroids, progestational agents
Elevated serum triglycerides
Genetic factors (approximately 50% of cases)
Overweight and obesity (probably most important)
Physical inactivity
Type 2 diabetes mellitus
Very high carbohydrate intake (>60% of total energy intake)

Source: Adapted from the *Third Report of the Expert Panel on Detection, Evaluation and Treatment of High Blood Cholesterol in Adults,* 2001. Rockville, MD: National Institutes of Health, National Heart, Lung, and Blood Institute.

management, growing evidence indicates that both non-HDL (NCEP, 2001) and HDL play important roles in atherogenesis and are correlated with coronary mortality. This correlation is especially true for diabetics (Peters, 2008). For this reason, the latest NCEP guideline gives consideration to VLDL and HDL in the overall management of patients at risk for CAD.

Elevated triglycerides (TG) are now recognized as an independent risk factor for CHD. Because TGs are closely linked with metabolic syndrome and diabetes, they are discussed under concomitant diseases. The NCEP guideline (2001) recommends that triglyceride levels be considered in the treatment protocol when TG levels exceed 150 mg/dL. Pharmacotherapy is first focused on LDL levels. If the medications do not subsequently reduce TG, then pharmacotherapy to address TGs should be considered.

GOALS OF TREATMENT

The positive relationship between elevated cholesterol levels, atherosclerosis, and CAD is well established. The therapeutic goal for the management of hyperlipidemia is to reduce morbidity and mortality from CAD by reducing atherogenesis. Current literature suggests that at least a 30 to 40 percent decrease in LDL levels needs to be achieved to reach this goal (Grundy et al, 2004). Table 39–2 shows the Adult Treatment Panel (ATP) III classification of LDL cholesterol. Because LDL cholesterol levels below 100 mg/dL throughout life are associated with very low risk for CAD, they are termed "optimal." However, five major clinical trials on **statin** therapy published since the ATP III guidelines have added a footnote recommendation to the ATP III classification and guidelines. These studies have indicated that an LDL goal of lower than 70 mg/dL may be a reasonable therapeutic option for patients when CHD risk is very high. Future guidelines may recommend this lower LDL cholesterol level as optimal (Cannon, 2005; Grundy et al, 2004; Nissen et al, 2004).

The degree of lowering serum LDL levels is contentious. Neurological symptoms in some patients and increased cancer risk in diabetics have been studied as possible problems in patients who have very low serum levels of LDLs. Very low LDL has been implicated as a cause of depression, anxiety, and memory loss. Serum levels of LDLs may have an effect on neurological serotonin levels. These concerns are questioned because they are primarily based on case reports with naturally occurring extra low LDL levels, not drug induced states (Zhang et al, 2005). Switching to another **statin** may clear the problem if drugs are found to be the cause (Wagstaff, Mitton, Arvik, & Doraiswamy, 2003). Cancer risks with low serum LDL levels have been shown to be the same with either high or low lipid levels (Yang et al, 2008). Because both issues discussed are based on design-flawed studies with small test groups, major organizations have not issued statements urging precaution. Because many adverse events associated with the treatment of hyperlipidemia have not been established, the reporting of any suspected adverse event is important.

Atherogenesis can occur even when serum LDL cholesterol levels are 100 to 129 mg/dL. Atherogenesis proceeds at a significant rate when levels are 130 to 159 mg/dL; such levels are termed "borderline high." Markedly accelerated atherogenesis occurs at levels of 160 to 189 mg/dL (high) and over 190 mg/dL (very high). Confirmed by log-linear data, a clear increased risk of CHD exists in populations who have higher serum LDL levels (NCEP, 2001). Unfortunately, an independent relationship between LDL reduction and actual percentage of risk reduction is unclear. Data that specify how much a reduction in serum level LDLs decreases how much risk of CHD are not available. Early clinical benefits of **statin** therapy are now recognized to be lipid-independent, but likely related to the reduction of vessel endothelial inflammation (pleiotrophy) (Arnaud, Braunersreuther, & Mach, 2005).

Atherosclerosis can be identified on gross pathological examination of coronary arteries in adolescence and early adulthood (McCrindle, 2007). The cholesterol level in young adulthood predicts the development of CAD later in life. Prospective studies with long-term follow-up have found that elevated serum cholesterol in early adulthood predicted an increased incidence of CAD in middle age. Clinical intervention with LDL-lowering therapy in patients with advanced coronary atherosclerosis is short-term risk reduction and aims to stabilize plaque and prevent acute coronary syndromes. In contrast, LDL-lowering earlier in life slows atherosclerotic plaque development, the foundation for unstable plaque. This provides a rationale for long-term lowering of serum LDL cholesterol using both public health and clinical approaches.

Table 39–2 **ATP III Classification of LDL Cholesterol**

LDL Cholesterol Level (mg/dL)	Category
<100	Optimal
100–129	Near or above optimal
130–159	Borderline to high
160–189	High
>190	Very high

Source: Adapted from the *Third Report of the Expert Panel on Detection, Evaluation and Treatment of High Blood Cholesterol in Adults*, 2001. Rockville, MD: National Institutes of Health, National Heart, Lung, and Blood Institute.

Multiple patient variables based on risk profiles are considered in setting individual lipoprotein level goals. These risks fall into modifiable and nonmodifiable categories. The modifiable risk factors such as diet, smoking behavior, and exercise are targets of therapy through lifestyle modifications. Nonmodifiable risk factors include age, gender, race, and family history. Both categories of risk factors are part of the calculation of overall risk for CAD. Table 39–3 presents the major risk factors for CAD exclusive of the serum LDL cholesterol levels mentioned previously

The patient's CAD risk level is the primary factor that determines the type and intensity of cholesterol-lowering therapy implemented. Those at high risk for CAD should receive more aggressive therapy and have goals of lower target cholesterol and LDL levels than those with less risk. For individuals free of CAD risk, total cholesterol levels below 200 mg/dL and HDL levels above 40 mg/dL are considered acceptable. For those with existing CAD, total cholesterol levels are less important, and the goal becomes reducing LDL levels to below 100 mg/dL and raising HDL levels above 60 mg/dL. Table 39–4 presents the treatment goals for LDL cholesterol levels based on the presence or absence of CAD and risk factors. The *Third Report of the Expert Panel on Detection, Evaluation, and Treatment of High Blood Cholesterol in Adults* (NCEP, 2001) presents algorithms for treatment based on risk stratification with considerations for special populations. The discussion in this chapter is taken from or consistent with those algorithms.

Five factors are considered contributory to low risk and negative risk for CHD: not smoking, normal BP, normal weight, normal glucose metabolism, and low cholesterol levels. Public education programs of the 1980s and 1990s

Table 39–3 **Major Risk Factors for Coronary Heart Disease (CHD) (Exclusive of LDL Cholesterol)**

Risk Factor	Positive Risk	Negative Risk
Age	Male: ≥45	Male: <45
	Female: ≥55	Female: <55
Family history	Premature CHD (MI or sudden death before 55 yr in father or other male first-degree relative or before 65 yr in mother or female first-degree relative)	No family history of CHD
Cigarette smoking	Current smoking (any cigarette smoking in past month)	Nonsmoker
Hypertension	BP ≥140/90 mm Hg or on antihypertensive medication	Normotensive
HDL cholesterol	HDL ≤40 mg/dL	HDL ≥60 mg/dL
Diabetes mellitus	Presence, especially if poorly controlled	Absence

BP = blood pressure; HDL = high-density lipoprotein; MI = myocardial infarction.
Source: Adapted from the *Third Report of the Expert Panel on Detection, Evaluation and Treatment of High Blood Cholesterol in Adults,* 2001. Rockville, MD: National Institutes of Health, National Heart, Lung, and Blood Institute.

Table 39–4 **ATP III Low-Density Lipoprotein Goals**

LDL Cholesterol Patient Category	Goal (mg/dL)
Coronary heart disease (CHD) or CHD risk equivalent	<100
Multiple (two or more) risk factors	<130
Fewer than two risk factors	<160

LDL cholesterol goal for multiple-risk-factor patients with a 10-year risk higher than 20% is less than 100 mg/dL.
Source: Adapted from the *Third Report of the Expert Panel on Detection, Evaluation and Treatment of High Blood Cholesterol in Adults,* 2001. Rockville, MD: National Institutes of Health, National Heart, Lung, and Blood Institute.

contributed to measurable decreases in cardiac disease rates in the United States. This progress is waning with the advent of the obesity epidemic. Currently, the only positive trend is that a lower percentage of the population smokes than did in the 1970s (Ford, Li, Zhao, Peason, & Capewell, 2009). Currently, only 7.5 percent of patients are able to achieve the five low-risk factors, a percentage that has dropped from the 10.5 percent of adults studied in 1994 (Ford et al, 2009). In addition to encouraging patients not to smoke, practitioners need to place emphasis on helping patients achieve optimal weight, BP, glucose metabolism, and cholesterol levels.

RATIONAL DRUG SELECTION

Hyperlipidemia presents a problem in therapeutic management because patients are usually asymptomatic until damage to the cardiovascular system occurs. Central aspects of treatment are lifestyle modifications, especially dietary, which include the reduction of elements that are often perceived as "making food taste good." Finally, patients often want a prescription for a drug that will "cure" the problem, which currently is not a realistic treatment option. The drugs that are prescribed for hyperlipidemia are considered after lifestyle management has failed because the medications available can potentially produce serious adverse events. For effective management of hyperlipidemia, the treatment protocol must be palatable, low cost, and have the fewest possible side effects. The factors to consider before developing a treatment plan are the presence or the absence of CAD, any associated risk factors, and specific patient variables.

Risk Stratification

A gradient potential of CHD risk, along with other CHD risk factors, has been delineated by the NCEP expert panel. Table 39–3 presents the CHD risk factors delineated by the NCEP expert panel. The 2001 NCEP guideline was the first time diabetes was raised to an independent CHD risk equivalent, and where persons with metabolic syndrome were identified as candidates for intensive therapy. Age, gender, diabetes, and the metabolic syndrome are discussed later in a section about additional patient variables. Additional CHD risk equivalents identified by NCEP (2001) included symptomatic carotid artery disease, peripheral arterial disease with an ankle/brachial index less than 0.9, abdominal aortic aneurysm and a 10-year risk of myocardial infarction/coronary heart disease (MI/CHD) death more than 20 percent based on the Framingham algorithm. The reader is referred to the NCEP (2001) document for specific discussion about these risk equivalents.

CHD tends to cluster in families. A positive family history of clinical CHD or sudden death in first-degree male relatives before age 55 or first-degree female relatives before age 65 is an important risk factor. The family history should include relatives with the presence or absence of high cholesterol levels, nonlipid risk factors, and the age of onset of each risk factor. This information provides data to assess for inherited lipoprotein disorders.

The NCEP (2001) guideline is the first to address directly race as a risk factor for CHD. Although no separate treatment algorithm for lipid management based on race is recommended, differences in risk factors and genetic constitution may result in the need for special attention to certain portions of the treatment algorithm. These features are discussed under specific patient variables below.

High Risk: CHD or CHD Risk Equivalent

Patients at high risk are those with clinical evidence of CHD or with CHD risk equivalents. Literature suggests that having coronary disease substantially increases future risk of another coronary event; this risk increases even more in the presence of elevated cholesterol levels. In women with existing CHD, the rates of new coronary events are similar to those of men. In older adults, new events occur with higher frequency than in younger adults with similar cardiac histories (NCEP, 2001). The benefits of lipid lowering in patients with CHD, have been repeatedly demonstrated in clinical studies. Patients without CHD but who have CHD risk equivalents, such as angina, claudication, stroke, TIA, electrocardiogram (ECG) abnormalities, stable angina, or previous coronary revascularization procedures (Knatterud et al, 2000), have similar risk rates to those of patients who have existing CHD.

The NCEP (2001) report cites multiple studies that support placing patients with diabetes in this high-risk category. The absolute risk for first major coronary events for patients with type 2 diabetes approximates that for nondiabetic patients with clinical CHD (Haffner, Lehto, Ronnemaa, Pyorala, & Laasko, 1998; Malmberg et al, 2000). The benefit of lowering LDL cholesterol in patients with type 2 diabetes is well supported. Type 2 diabetics are in this high-risk category because they have an increased MI case fatality rate. In one study, death occurred in 45 percent of men with diabetes and 35 percent of women with diabetes, compared to 38 percent for men and 25 percent for women without diabetes (Miettinen et al, 1998).

The cost effectiveness of treating this high-risk group is discussed extensively in the NCEP (2001) guideline, which states that "at current retail drug prices, **LDL-lowering drug therapy** is highly cost effective in patients with established CHD" (p. II-61). **LDL-lowering drug therapy** is also cost effective for primary prevention in patients with CHD risk equivalents.

Moderate Risk: Two or More Risk Factors

At moderate risk are those patients with two or more CHD risk factors but no clinical evidence of current CHD. NCEP (2001) divides this group into three subcategories of risk depending on 10-year CHD risk as determined by the Framingham Heart Study risk assessment tool: higher than 20 percent, 10 to 20 percent, and less than 10 percent risk. The Framingham tool includes consideration of age, HDL level, systolic blood pressure (BP), total cholesterol, and smoking with different scoring for men and women. Points assigned to each risk factor are added together to determine the total risk score, which corresponds to the patient's 10-year CHD risk. The intensity of lipid-lowering therapy within each category is adjusted according to the 10-year risk and serum LDL cholesterol level. More recent concerns about the validity of the scoring for women are discussed in the section regarding women and hyperlipidemia.

Lower Risk: Zero or One Risk Factor

It should be noted that the lower risk group still has cardiac event risk, although the risk is lower than groups deemed to have high risk. Data from multiple research trials support that lowering LDL cholesterol to target levels is important even for those without CHD, especially in patients with elevated serum LDL cholesterol levels. The Scandinavian Simvastatin Survival Study Group (1994) found that the group without CHD who had high cholesterol had an absolute risk of about 56 percent per decade and those with low HDL in the VA-HIT trial had an absolute risk of about 43 percent per decade (Rubins et al, 1999). Subsequent trials have supported these data. Given that clinical trial participants are likely to be healthier than the general population, and that event rates likely will increase as the patient ages, an event rate of 20 percent per decade presents a minimum estimate of absolute annual risk for those with elevated cholesterol levels.

Patients at low risk for CAD are those with LDL cholesterol levels below 100 mg/dL, HDL cholesterol levels above 60 mg/dL, total cholesterol-to-HDL ratio below 4.5, VLDL cholesterol levels 50 to 100 mg/dL, or fasting triglycerides of 150 to 200 mg/dL, no clinical evidence of CAD, and fewer than two CAD risk factors. These optimal numbers reflect zero risk factors, but do not provide a true "zero risk" for anyone.

Treatment Algorithms

Lifestyle Modifications

Lifestyle modifications are the core of treatment for hyperlipidemia. Lifestyle changes include reduced intake of saturated fats and cholesterol, consuming therapeutic dietary options for lowering LDLs (**plant stanols/sterols** and increased viscous fiber), weight reduction, and increased regular physical activity. NCEP (2001) advocates a two-pronged approach for reducing CHD risk: the population approach and the clinical approach. These two approaches are discussed extensively in the NCEP report. The focus of the population approach includes working with the media so that information from health-care providers is valued and considered credible. Further population-based foci includes promoting U.S. Dietary Guidelines using pamphlets/handouts; promoting regular physical activity, up to 30 minutes on most days of the week; ensuring that weight, height, and waist circumference are measured at every office visit; providing access to body mass index (BMI) tables in the waiting and exam rooms; ensuring that all adults 20 years and older have their blood cholesterol measured and their results explained; ensuring that all adults have their BP measured and their results explained in keeping with the Seventh Report of the Joint National Committee (JNC-7) guidelines (National High Blood Pressure Education Program

[NHBPEP], 2003); making antismoking literature available; and asking all patients about their smoking habits at every office visit. Government-sponsored Web sites for public information are listed in Table 39–5.

Clinical approaches have similar foci as the population-based approach but are directed at specific patients. Clinicians should promote targeted changes in individual lifestyle to produce significant reductions in a patient's risk. These include promoting regular physical activity based on the patient's cardiac status, age, and other factors; teaching about weight management, including 10 percent weight-loss goals for patients who are overweight (Mente, deKoning, Shannon, & Anand, 2009); following NCEP guidelines for diagnosing and treating lipid disorders; following JNC-7 guidelines for diagnosing and treating hypertension (HTN) (NHBPEP, 2003); following the "treating tobacco use and dependence" guideline (U.S. Department of Health and Human Services, 2000); and promoting the Therapeutic Lifestyle Change (TLC) diet using individualized diet counseling and reinforcement of dietary principles during follow-up visits.

The general aim of dietary therapy is to lower cholesterol to target levels while still maintaining a nutritionally adequate eating pattern. Research has demonstrated the benefits of eating a heart-healthy and blood-glucose reducing diet extends across all ethnic groups (Nettelton, Polak, Tracy, Burke, & Jacobs, 2009). Essential components of the TLC diet are the following:

- saturated fats less than 7 percent of total calories
- dietary cholesterol less than 200 mg/day
- **plant stanols/sterols** 2 g/day; **plant sterols** block cholesterol absorption
- increased viscous (soluble) fiber to 10 to 25 g/day; viscous fibers increase bile acid loses
- total calories adjusted to maintain desirable body weight and prevent weight gain

One group of authors note that a combination of plant **sterols** and viscous fiber "is the dietary equivalent of combining a **bile acid-binding resin** and a **statin** (Jenkins, Kendall, & Marchie, 2005).

Table 39–5 **Government-Sponsored Web Sites for Public Information**

Health Approach	Web Site
Diet	*www.nhbli.nih.gov/chd* *www.nhbli.nih.gov/subsites/index.htm (click on Healthy Weight)* *www.nhbli.nih.gov/hbp* *www.nutrition.gov*
Physical activity	*www.fitness.gov*
Cholesterol	*www.nhbli.nih.gov/chd*
Blood pressure	*www.nhbli.nih.gov/hbp*
Smoking cessation	*www.cdc.gov/tobacco/sgr_tobacco_use.htm*

Macronutrient recommendations are the following:

- polyunsaturated fat up to 10 percent of total calories
- monounsaturated fats (olive oil, canola oil, and high-oleic forms of sunflower seed and safflower oils) up to 20 percent of total calories
- total fat 25 percent to 35 percent of total calories
- carbohydrates less than 50 percent to 60 percent of total calories with preference for complex carbohydrates, including whole grains, fruits, and vegetables
- dietary fiber 20 to 30 g/day
- protein approximately 15 percent of total calories

Although not specifically mentioned in the macronutrient recommendations, **alcohol** ingestion is related to CHD. Observational studies consistently show a J-shaped relationship between **alcohol** consumption and total mortality. Case-control, cohort, and ecological studies indicate lower risk for CHD at low to moderate **alcohol** intake. A moderate amount of **alcohol** is no more than 1 ounce of **ethanol** (e.g., 24 oz beer, 10 oz wine, or 2 oz whiskey) for men. Women and lighter-weight people should consume no more than half this amount. There are cardiovascular benefits related to rational **alcohol** intake in men older than 45 years and women older than 55 years. The beneficial mechanism associated moderate **alcohol** use is unknown but may be related to an increase in HDL cholesterol and apo A1, and modest improvement in hemostatic factors (NCEP, 2001).

The dangers of overconsumption of **alcohol** are well known. Patients with levels of **alcohol** consumption in excess of the moderate amount shown in the previous paragraph present with adverse effects that include HTN, arrhythmia, and myocardial dysfunction. **Alcohol** excess also promotes acute pancreatitis and liver dysfunction. Because up to 10 percent of adults in the United States misuse **alcohol**, care should be taken about advice given related to **alcohol** intake with the advantages and disadvantages clearly delineated.

Dietary sodium, potassium, and calcium are also not mentioned in the macronutrient recommendations. Recommendations about these minerals are found in Chapter 9. Many patients with hyperlipidemia also have HTN. The NCEP guideline supports the JNC-7 recommendations about salt, potassium, and calcium intake for persons undergoing cholesterol management. Lifestyle modifications take time and are part of the treatment regimen whether the patient is being treated with medications or not. Modifications involve active assistance from the health-care team. Figure 39–2 shows the steps in achieving therapeutic lifestyle changes. If the LDL cholesterol goal has not been achieved after 3 months of TLC, a decision must be made as to whether to consider adding drug therapy.

Drug Therapy

CHD and CHD Risk Equivalents

For patients with CHD and CHD risk equivalents, the type and intensity of **LDL-lowering drug therapy** is determined by baseline LDL levels. Figure 39–3 shows

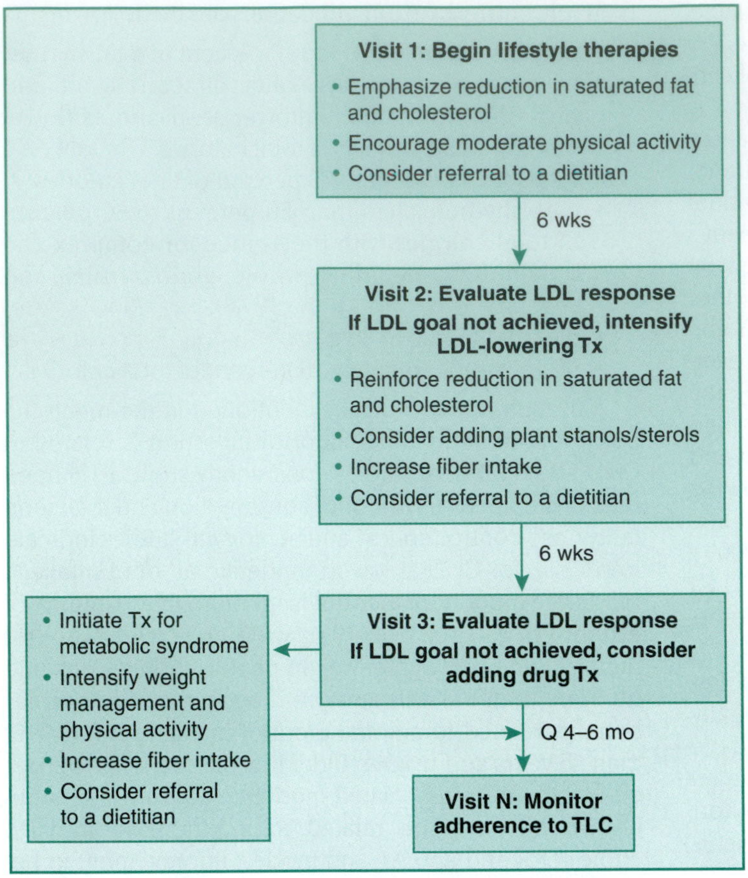

Figure 39–2. Model of steps in Therapeutic Lifestyle Changes (TLC).

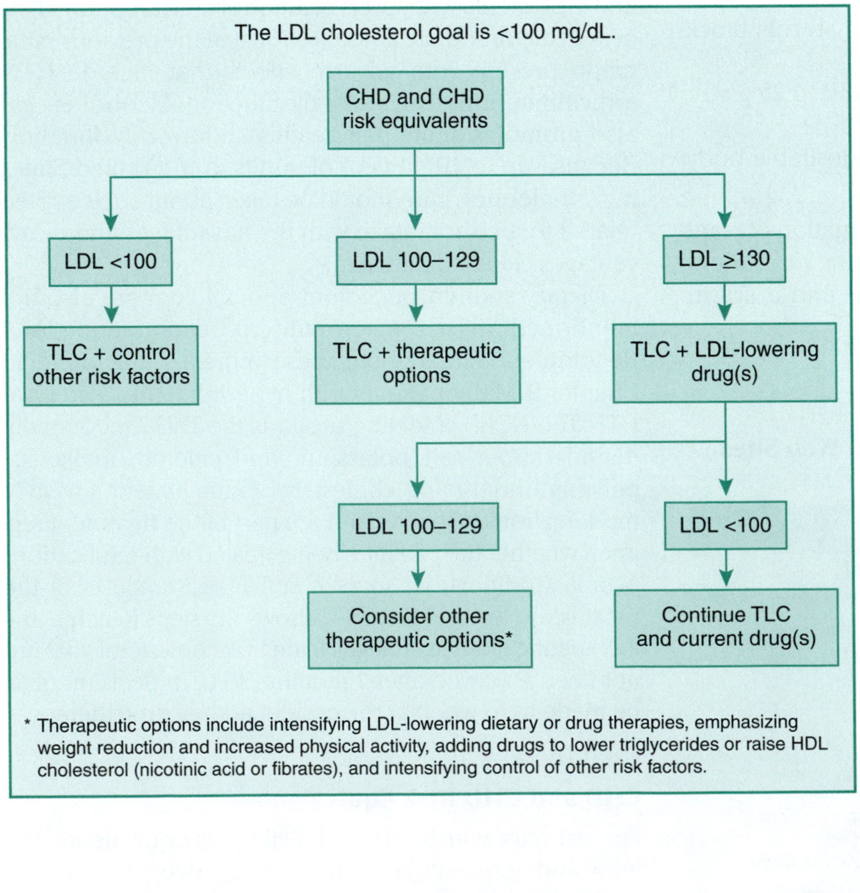

Figure 39–3. Therapeutic approaches for patients with CHD or CHD risk equivalents.

the therapeutic approach for this group of patients. Table 39–6 depicts the level at which TLC and LDL-lowering drugs are initiated.

Persons with a baseline LDL cholesterol at or above 130 mg/dL generally will require **LDL-lowering drugs** to achieve LDL cholesterol levels below 100 mg/dL, so drug therapy (usually with a **statin**) is initiated simultaneously with TLC. If future guidelines recommend that the target LDL cholesterol for very high-risk patients be 70 mg/dL (Cannon, 2005; Grundy et al, 2004; Nissen et al, 2004), the use of drugs for this population will become even more central to their therapy. If the LDL cholesterol level falls into the range of 100 to 129 mg/dL after the initial therapeutic choice, LDL-lowering therapy can be intensified with added dietary therapy or with more *aggressive* drug therapy. If after treatment with the first line therapeutic choice, the patient is near 100-mg/dL, the LDL-lowering therapy can be left unchanged to give the patient more time to achieve a below-100 mg/dL goal. In cases where the patient has metabolic syndrome, dietary therapy is intensified early in the program, with an increased effort to lose excess weight and increase physical activity. If the patient also has elevated triglycerides or low HDL, a **lipid-lowering** agent that focuses on those areas (e.g., **nicotinic acid** or **fibric acid**) may be added as combination therapy.

Patients with a baseline LDL cholesterol of 100 to 129 mg/dL have several possible treatment options. Inclusions of **stanols/sterols** and increased **viscous fiber** in the diet can help achieve serum LDL goals. If LDL cholesterol levels remain above 100 mg/dL after 3 months of maximal dietary therapy, a LDL-lowering drug may be needed. For patients who also have elevated triglycerides or low serum HDL levels, the same recommendation concerning drug selection is used. If the LDL cholesterol goal is near the goal with diet alone, initiation of pharmacotherapy is at the discretion of the provider.

If the baseline LDL cholesterol is below 100 mg/dL, no LDL-lowering therapy is currently recommended. Emphasis is placed on controlling other risk factors. The TLC diet is recommended to help maintain lower serum levels of LDL.

Multiple (2+) Risk Factors

NCEP (2001) distinguishes three risk categories within the multiple risk factor category depending on the Framingham 10-year CHD risk calculation. Intensity of therapy is adjusted based on 10-year CHD risk and serum LDL cholesterol level. Figures 39–4 and 39–5 show the therapeutic approach for this group of patients. Future NCEP guidelines may recommend that the *serum level LDL* goal for this population be reduced to below 100 mg/dL (Grundy et al, 2004). Table 39–7 depicts the level at which TLC and LDL-lowering drugs are currently initiated.

Patients with multiple risk factors and a 10-year risk of more than 20 percent have the same degree of risk as those with CHD or CHD risk equivalents. They are treated with the same protocol as that category. For this reason they are not separately described in Table 39–7.

The LDL cholesterol goal for patients with multiple risk factors and a 10-year CHD risk between 10 to 20 percent is below 130 mg/dL. The therapeutic aim is to reduce short-term risk for CHD. These patients are started on a 3-month trial of TLC, augmented by **plant stanols/sterols** and increased **viscous fiber** in the diet. If the LDL remains above the target after 3 months, drug therapy is considered. If the LDL is at or below target, then the current TLC regimen continues.

Multiple risk factors, and a 10-year CHD risk of less than 10 percent has the same treatment target and approach as for patients with serum LDLs lower than 130 mg/dL. If the baseline serum LDL cholesterol is at or above 130 mg/dL, TLC therapy is initiated. After 3 months of TLC therapy, a lipid panel is performed. If the LDL is at or below 160 mg/dL, the patient remains on TLC therapy with options for intensifying the therapy. If the LDL cholesterol is above 160 mg/dL, drug therapy is considered.

Zero or One Risk Factor

Individuals in the group with zero or one risk factor usually have a 10-year CHD risk of less than 10 percent. The goal for this group is LDL cholesterol levels lower than 160 mg/dL. The primary goal is to reduce long-term risk

Table 39–6 Therapeutic Approaches to Initiation of TLC and Drug Therapy for Persons With Coronary Heart Disease (CHD) or CHD Risk Equivalents

LDL Cholesterol Level	LDL Level to Initiate Therapeutic Lifestyle Changes	LDL Level to Initiate LDL-Lowering Drugs
≥130 mg/dL	≥100 mg/dL	Start drug therapy, simultaneously with dietary therapy
100–129 mg/dL	≥100 mg/dL	Consider drug options*
<100 mg/dL	TLC and emphasize weight control and physical activity	LDL-lowering drugs not required**

LDL = low-density lipoprotein; TLC = therapeutic lifestyle change.

*The LDL cholesterol goal is <100 mg/dL for all groups.

**Some authorities recommend use of LDL-lowering drugs in this category if an LDL cholesterol <100 mg/dL cannot be achieved by TLC. Others prefer the use of drugs that primarily modify other lipoprotein fractions (e.g., nicotinic acid plus fibrate).

Source: Adapted from the *Third Report of the Expert Panel on Detection, Evaluation and Treatment of High Blood Cholesterol in Adults, 2001.* Rockville, MD: National Institutes of Health, National Heart, Lung, and Blood Institute.

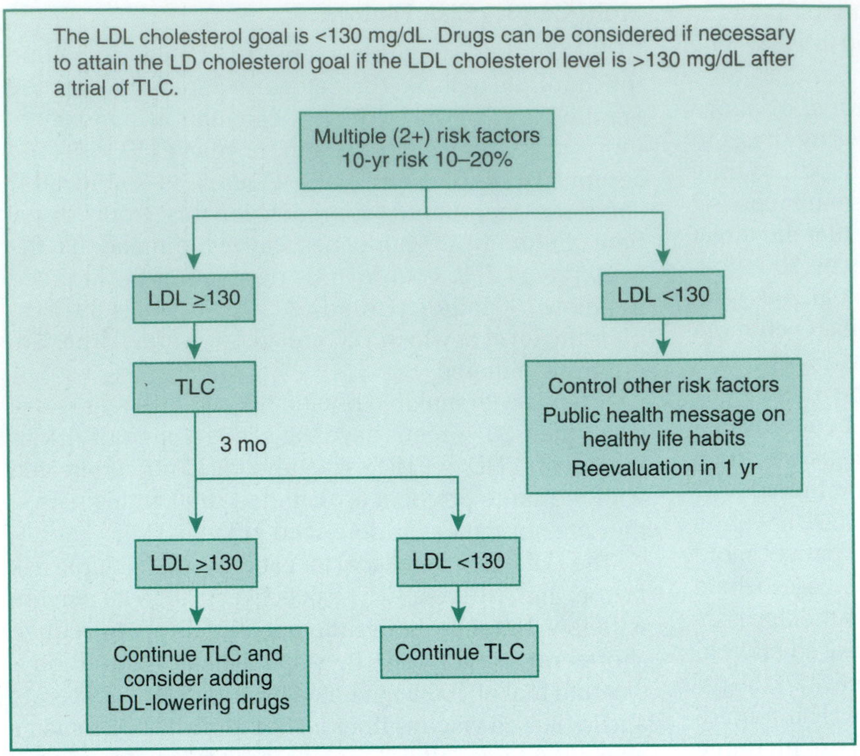

Figure 39–4. Therapeutic approaches for patients with multiple risk factors and 10-year CHD risk 10% to 20%.

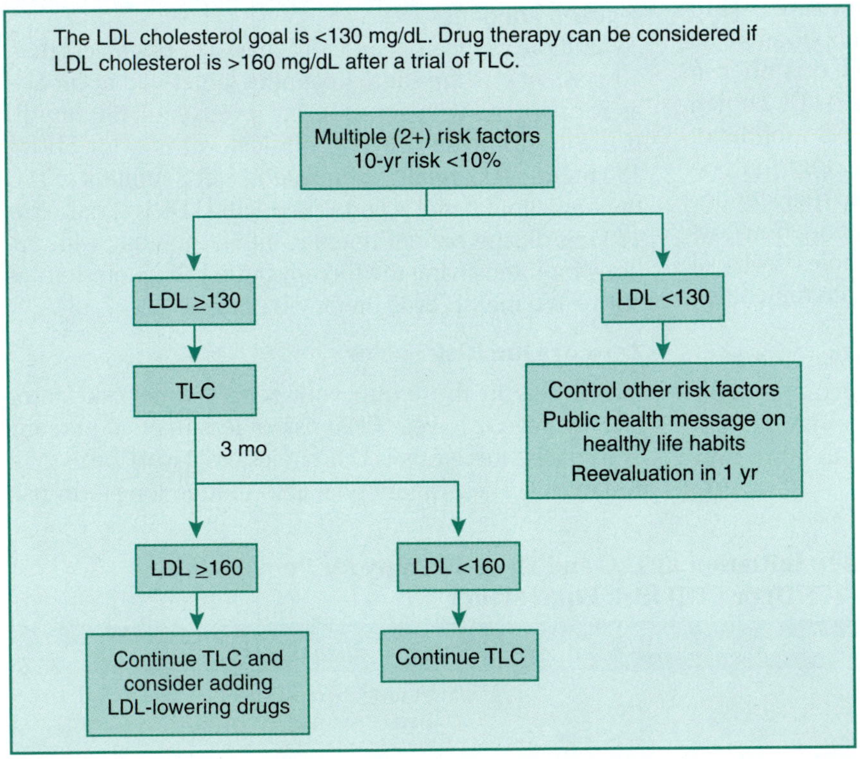

Figure 39–5. Therapeutic approaches for patients with multiple risk factors and 10-year CHD risk less than 10%.

for CHD. Figure 39–6 shows the treatment approach for this group. When baseline LDL cholesterol level is at or above 160 mg/dL, TLC is initiated and continued for 3 months. After 6 weeks, the LDL panel is redrawn and dietary enhancers of LDL lowering (e.g., **plant stanols/sterols** and **viscous fiber**) are increased if needed to achieve the LDL goal. After 3 months, another LDL panel is drawn. If LDL cholesterol is lower than 160 mg/dL, TLC therapy is continued. For LDL cholesterol of 160 to 189 mg/dL, drug therapy is optional. The presence of a severe risk factor, such as smoking, poorly controlled HTN, or very low HDL, suggests beginning drug therapy. If the LDL cholesterol is at or above 190 mg/dL despite TLC therapy, drug therapy is the more likely treatment option. Some patients may

Table 39–7 **Therapeutic Approaches to Initiation of TLC and Drug Therapy for Persons With Multiple (2+) Risk Factors**

10-Year Risk	LDL Goal	LDL Level to Initiate TLC	LDL Level to Consider Drug Therapy
>20%	<100 mg/dL	≥100 mg/dL	See coronary heart disease (CHD) and CHD risk equivalent
10–20%	<130 mg/dL	≥130 mg/dL	≥130 mg/dL
<10%	<130 mg/dL	≥130 mg/dL	≥160 mg/dL

TLC = therapeutic lifestyle change.
Source: Adapted from the *Third Report of the National Cholesterol Education Program Expert Panel on Detection, Evaluation and Treatment of High Blood Cholesterol in Adults,* 2001. Rockville, MD: National Institutes of Health, National Heart, Lung, and Blood Institute.

present with very high LDL cholesterol levels (e.g., greater than 220 mg/dL). These individuals usually have a genetic form of hyperlipidemia that cannot be treated adequately with TLC alone (Table 39–8).

Drug Therapy

The choice of the pharmacotherapy in patients with genetic lipid disorders is based largely on the specific elevated lipoprotein involved. Detailed discussion of each drug class is provided in Chapter 16. In general, LDL cholesterol is the primary target for treatment in hyperlipidemia.

1. **Statins** allow most high-risk patients to attain serum LDL goals. Patients treated with a **statin** may also see a modest decrease in serum triglycerides and an increase in serum HDL. Recent long-term studies have shown **statins** to be safe, to be effective, and to reduce the risk of CHD when used alone or in combination with other agents. Results from the Heart Protection Study Collaboration Group (2002) show that treatment with a **statin** in patients with serum LDL cholesterol levels below 100 mg/dL at baseline reduced the rate of myocardial infarction, stroke, and revascularization by 25 percent.

Statins have ancillary effects beyond their LDL cholesterol-lowering properties. They are especially useful for maximal lowering of LDL levels in secondary prevention and in severe forms of hypercholesterolemia. Many trials have shown **statins** to be

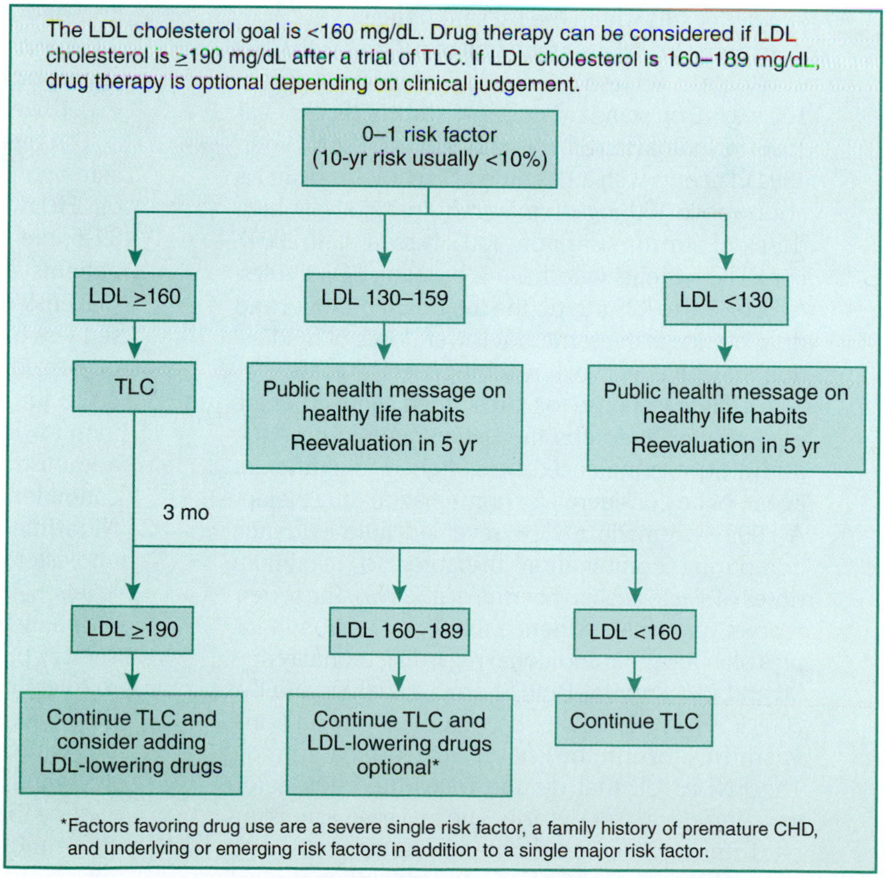

Figure 39–6. Therapeutic approaches for patients with 0 or 1 risk factor.

Table 39–8 **Therapeutic Approaches to Initiation of TLC and Drug Therapy for Persons With 0 or 1 Risk Factor**

LDL Goal	LDL Level to Initiate TLC	LDL Level to Consider Drug Therapy (After TLC)
<160 mg/dL	≥160 mg/dL	≥190 mg/dL Drug therapy optional at 160–189 mg/dL

TLC = therapeutic lifestyle change.
Most persons with 0 or 1 risk factor have a 10-year risk for CHD of <10%.
Source: Adapted from the *Third Report of the Expert Panel on Detection, Evaluation and Treatment of High Blood Cholesterol in Adults,* 2001. Rockville, MD: National Institutes of Health, National Heart, Lung, and Blood Institute.

beneficial in middle-aged men and women, in older patients, and in those patients who are candidates for primary and secondary prevention treatment. For patients with CHD or CHD risk equivalents, this class of drugs should be considered as the first line of drug treatment. The starting dose will depend on the patient's baseline serum LDL cholesterol level with the goal of a serum LDL cholesterol below 100 mg/dL. Most compendiums list LDL-lowering agents according to their impact on serum LDL levels. From greatest impact on serum LDL levels to lowest impact, the drugs are as follows: **rosuvastatin, atorvastatin, simvastatin, lovastatin, pravastin,** and **fluvastatin.** The newest **statin, pitivastatin,** has an LDL-lowering effect that falls within the list's midrange.

In many trials, fewer than half of patients with CHD were able to achieve a serum LDL cholesterol goal of 100 mg/dL on standard doses of **statins** (Sacks et al, 1996; Scandinavian Simvastatin Survival Study Group, 1994). Patients with a baseline LDL cholesterol that is at or above 130 mg/dL may require relatively high doses of **statins** (Cannon, 2005; Nissen et al, 2004). For CHD patients who have a baseline LDL cholesterol of 100 to 129 mg/dL, the treatment protocol and drug choice is the same, but lower doses of medication may be effective in reaching therapy goals

If patient response to a prescribed agent is not adequate after 3 months, the patient should have the **statin** dosage increased, be switched to a different agent, or be considered for combination drug therapy. A 2009 systematic review revealed little evidence comparing combination therapies to maximum doses of single agents (Sharma et al, 2009). The review reports very weak evidence that combination therapies offer anything additional regarding mortality and MI and CVA survival. Both Sharma's analysis and the 2008 ENHANCE trial reports regarding **Vytorin (simvastatin + ezetimibe)** have created great turmoil. The ENHANCE trial demonstrates the cholesterol-lowering efficacy of **Vytorin.** The trial used a nonstandard imaging outcome criterion as its method to prove efficacy, instead of using comparative clinical outcome criteria to determine efficacy (American College of Cardiology [ACC], 2008). Neither report should alter reasonable judgment concerning the use of drug combinations. Medications used in combination therapy all have individually established data confirming that they are helpful in cholesterol reduction. Providers must use individual patient response rates to guide selection of drug therapy. The STELLAR trial results on monotherapy tempered the expectation that massive changes in cholesterol levels would result as dosages of drugs were increased. Typically, only a 6 percent reduction in TC is expected when the dosage of a **statin** is increased (Jones et al, 2003). Another issue to consider in treating patients with increased lipid levels is that monotherapy does not always address all sources of dyslipidemia.

Combination drug therapy (e.g., **statins + bile acid-binding resin** or **nicotinic acid** or **ezetimibe)** should be used if **statin** treatment alone does not sufficiently meet therapeutic goals. Combination drug therapy is helpful in patients who also present with elevated triglycerides and elevated LDLs. Combinations of **statins** with low-dose **niacin** are the most efficacious and practical combination for the treatment of combined familial hyperlipidemia. For treating this disorder, **statins** provide a synergistic action with **bile acid-binding resins** to accomplish more effective lowering of lipid levels. To ensure maximal absorption, the **statin** should be given at least 1 hour before or 4 hours after the administration of the **bile acid-binding resin.** Combination therapy can be achieved by ordering two separate agents or by ordering more convenient, but more expensive, single dosage formulations.

Patients with multiple risk factors or those with zero or one risk factor but without a personal history of CHD may require drug therapy (see Figures 39–4, 39–5, and 39–6). Pharmacotherapy choices for those patients are the same as for patients with CHD or CHD risk equivalent factors, although they are chosen less often or started later in therapy. **Statins** are discussed earlier. The remaining drug classes indicated for lowering serum lipid levels are discussed in following sections. Specifics profiling the dosing, administration, adverse reactions, and patient education for those agents are found in Chapter 16.

2. **Nicotinic acid (niacin)** is effective in lowering total cholesterol and triglyceride levels and raising HDL levels. Evidence indicates that **niacin** reduces total mortality in secondary prevention trials. Side effects such as nausea and flushing are difficult for patients to tolerate and may increase the likelihood of nonadherence. By combining a low-dose **niacin** product with a **bile acid-binding resin,** patients can accomplish effective lowering of VLDL and LDL and reduce the side effects of the niacin. **Slow-release nicotinic acid (Niaspan)** has been studied as another way to reduce the side effects of **niacin** while

still getting therapeutic blood levels of **nicotinic acid**. Based on these studies, a 2 g/day dose is advantageous in reducing lipid levels without causing significant side effects. **Nicotinic acid** is best for treating patients who have elevated total cholesterol and triglycerides, low HDL levels, or both. Because **nicotinic acid** is a vitamin and sold over the counter (OTC), the U.S. Food and Drug Administration (FDA) has issued a statement on using OTC products as a substitute for prescribed cholesterol-lowering drugs, including **nicotinic acid**. The FDA concluded that the nature of hypercholesterolemia and its potential sequelae are such that OTC use of these drugs is not a safe and effective means for treating this condition.

3. **Bile acid-binding resins** have a strong record of efficacy and safety and are most useful for patients with moderately elevated LDL levels and a low CHD risk profile who are unable to reduce their LDL by diet alone. Many young adult men and premenopausal women fit the profile appropriate for treatment with a **bile acid-binding resin** drug. **Bile acid-binding resins** are often used as monotherapy for women who are pregnant or may become pregnant. Low doses of **bile acid-binding resins** can be effective for patients who are close to their target LDL but still need a little extra help. Patients with combined familial hyperlipidemia who find **nicotinic acid** products not tolerable may benefit from a combination treatment that includes a **bile acid-binding resin** and **fibric acid derivative**. **Fibric acid derivatives** do have a significant GI side effect profile and may not be an option for some patients. **Fibric acid derivatives** are contraindicated in patients with elevated serum triglycerides.
4. **Fibric acid derivatives** are effective **triglyceride-lowering drugs** that may modestly lower LDL and raise HDL for some patients. Elevated triglycerides are an independent risk factor for CHD. Because these drugs usually do not produce substantial reductions in LDL cholesterol, they are not appropriate for effective lowering of LDL levels as a primary LDL-lowering agent. They are valuable for patients with very high triglyceride levels, for diabetic patients with elevated triglycerides, and for patients with familial dysbetalipoproteinemia.
5. Drug combinations are commonly used for patients with more than one lipoprotein abnormality. For patients with elevated LDL and triglycerides below 200 mg/dL, the main goal of treatment is to lower LDL levels as hypertriglyceridemia does not carry the same risk for CAD as elevated LDL cholesterol levels. Combinations of **statins** with low-dose **nicotinic acid** are used for patients at high risk for CAD. Combining the powerful LDL-lowering action of the **statins** with the triglyceride-lowering and HDL-raising properties of **nicotinic acid** offers the potential to correct most forms of complex dyslipidemias. The relatively low cost of **nicotinic acid** also makes it an attractive product to use in treatment combinations. **Bile acid-binding resins** combined with low-dose **nicotinic acid** are best for young adults and patients without a high CAD risk. For patients with severe polygenic or familial hyperlipidemias, a **statin** drug combined with a **bile acid-binding resin** may be the most effective treatment option, reducing LDL cholesterol by as much as 70 percent (NCEP, 2001, p. VI-20). If a patient has a triglyceride level of 200 to 400 mg/dL, **nicotinic acid** combined with **fibric acid derivatives** may be effective. The **fibric acid/nicotinic acid** combination is also a good treatment option for atherogenic dyslipidemia.

   The combination of **statins** and **fibrates** carry an increased risk of myopathy. Treatment with this combination should be undertaken carefully and frequent patient monitoring for symptoms of myopathy are necessary. Any reported myopathy symptoms should be followed up with creatinine kinase (CK) testing and the agent should be discontinued if the CK is greater than 10 times the upper limit of normal.
6. Alternative treatments also have a role in managing elevated lipids. **Omega-3 fatty acids** have a place in treating very high triglyceride levels (greater than 500 mg/dL) in adult patients. **Omega-3 fatty acid** treatment results in HDL levels that are typically unaffected and LDL levels that may actually rise. **Omacor** is a prescription formulation that is a more concentrated and quality controlled source of both the eicosapentanoic acid (EPA) and docosahexaenoic acids (DHA) than those found in OTC supplements. **Omacor** has the same "fish burp" side effect as its OTC counterparts, but may be more tolerable to patients because of its twice-a-day dosing schedule. Concerns about mercury content that surround OTC fish oil products are lessened because **Omacor** is regulated like a drug and not a nutritional product. **Red yeast rice**, an alternative therapy for hyperlipidema, appears to mimic **statin** medications. The FDA has issued warnings about some formulations of this product that contain the prescription drug **lovastatin**. Manufacturers claim the yeast growing on their product is the naturally occurring chemical on which **lovastatin** is based. The unregulated production and packaging of these products makes them unsuitable as a substitute for prescription drug therapy, especially in the era of options that include less expensive generic drug formulations.

Additional Patient Variables

Children and Adolescents

Atherosclerosis can begin in childhood, and fatty streaks have been seen in children as young as 10 years old (McCrindle et al, 2007). Up to 25 percent of children and adolescents have cholesterol levels above 200 mg/dL.

Genetic disorders of lipid metabolism occur in 0.5 to 1 percent of the population. Children with such genetic disorders often have total cholesterol levels 1.5 to 3 times higher than normal. Approximately 80 percent of these children will experience symptomatic CAD at an age younger than 20 years. Most cases of elevated cholesterol are related to the same environmental factors that result in adult hyperlipidemia. Treatment of hyperlipidemia in children closely mirrors the regimens used in adults.

Optimal cholesterol levels in children are lower than in adults (McCrindle et al, 2007) because longer duration of elevated lipid levels theoretically translates into longer-term opportunity for vascular wall changes. Total cholesterol should be below 170 mg/dL (LDL less than 100 mg/dL). Borderline cholesterol levels are 170 to 199 mg/dL, and high cholesterol levels are 200 mg/dL or above. Figure 39–7 shows the treatment algorithm for children.

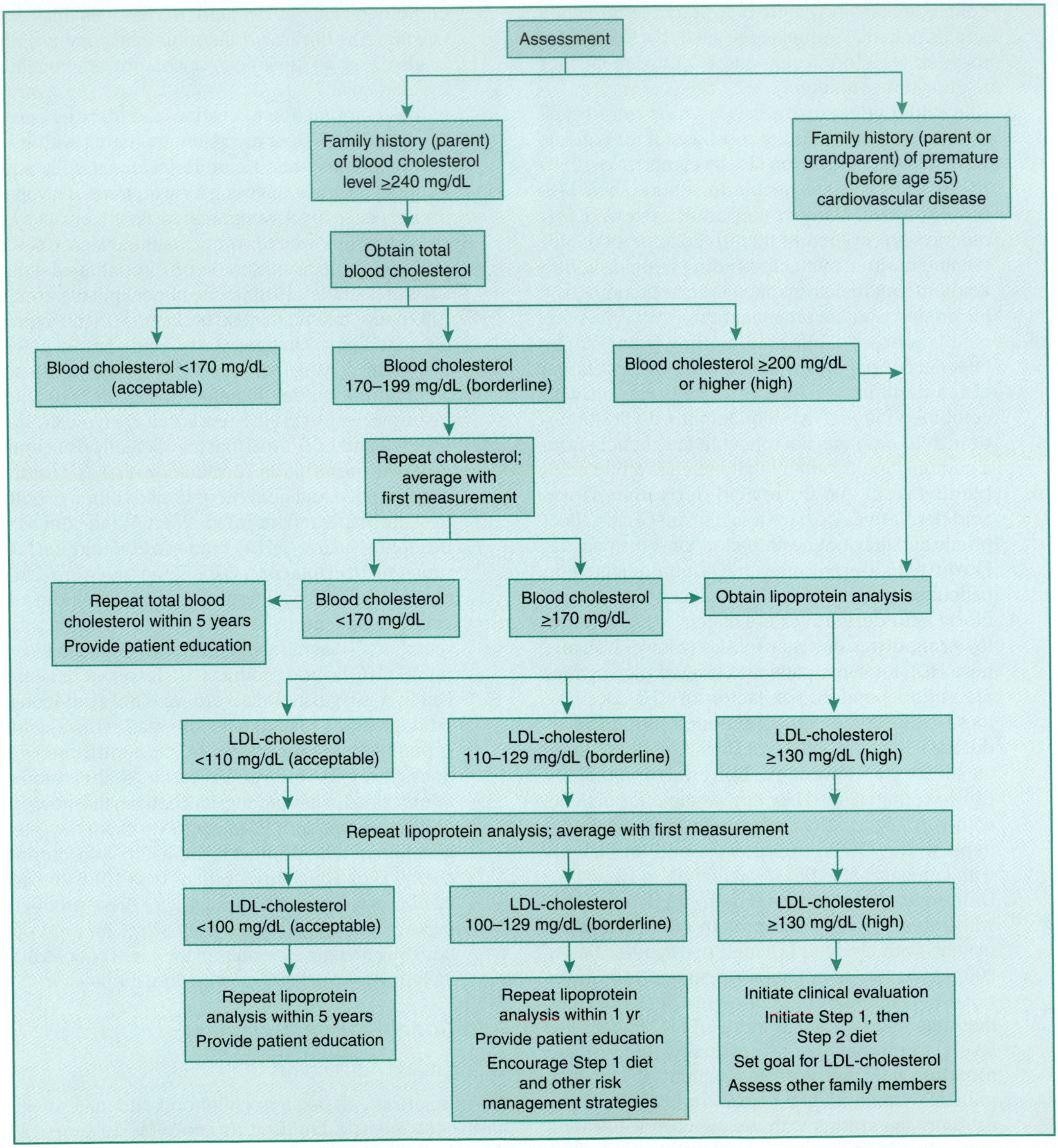

Figure 39–7. Management of blood cholesterol in children.

In children, as with adults, the goal is primary prevention. Lifestyle modifications include aerobic exercise; weight control; and a diet that includes control of salt intake, saturated fat, and cholesterol. In infants, the diet should include breastfeeding and late introduction of solid foods. The use of whole milk until age 1 to provide required fatty acids for neurological development is still recommended; however, children should be switched to 2 percent milk and transitioned to skim milk by age 2 (Daniels & Greer, 2008). Framingham scores do not exist for children; the scores start at age 20 years.

Reduction in CHD risk factors, such as passive smoking; sedentary lifestyle and excessive weight; and appropriate management of hypertension, obesity, and diabetes are all essential in childhood dyslipidemias, just as they are for adults. Attention to individual smoking habits should be implemented by age 10. TLC changes should be initiated as first line of treatment, and maintained for at least a 6-month trial, before pharmacotherapy is considered, except in cases of distinct high risk.

High-risk children include those with familial dyslipidemia syndromes, those with type I diabetes, chronic renal disease, cancer and transplant survivors, and those who have documented coronary vessel issues post Kawasaki disease. A new emphasis is now placed on obese children who develop type II diabetes, as they may exhibit characteristics of metabolic syndrome.

The population approach for therapy includes attention to school lunch programs and alerting parents and children to the dangers of junk food. Providers can take strong stands on increasing emphasis on physical activities during school. Individual focus prevention should include encouragement of after school engagement in active-motion events including sports, dance and general play for at least 60 minutes a day (Gidding et al, 2009). Parents should place limits on sedentary entertainment such as computer games. Studies are underway evaluating the impact of active interactive electronic programs such as Wii games.

Dietary suggestions for children mirror those of adults: saturated fats less than 10 percent of all food stuffs and all fat intakes less than 30 percent (Daniels & Greer, 2008; Gidding et al, 2009). **Fiber, plant stanols,** and **omega-3 fatty acid sources** are all helpful supplements.

When drug therapy is considered, consultation with a pediatrician experienced in lipid disorders is advised. Among the available **antihyperlipidemics, nicotinic acid** has established doses for children and has a history of established safety in children younger than 18 years. **Statins** are useful in children with heterozygous or homozygous familial hyperlipidemia with LDLs greater than 500 mg/dL. Long-term use has not revealed any adverse impact on development, but the population taking medications is very limited. Drug therapy is usually not initiated until patients are at least 8 years old. Positive impact on carotid intima media thickness and mortality mirrors that found in adults.

Guidelines recommend using drugs only for children with high lipid levels and high-risk markers for CAD. Very few children should have to take medications after TLC interventions are implemented. Goals for treatment and lipid lowering impact are similar to those for adults. Monitoring protocols are also the same. Age of initiation of pharmacotherapy for males is age 10 years and for females at the onset of menses. Tanner scales measure levels of maturation in children and the general guide for initiating drug therapy is a Tanner II level of maturation (Daniels & Greer, 2008). Pubescent adolescent females should follow the treatment guidelines for women of childbearing age as discussed later in this chapter. Treatment should consider use of **contraception** because of the potential teratogenic properties of lipid agents. Limited studies have not demonstrated alterations in continued maturation, menstrual cycles, or hormone levels in girls who have taken **statins** for familial dyslipidemias; however, studies were only 1 to 2 years in duration and did not monitor long-term effects.

Current drug monographs should be referenced for approved pediatric dosages. As in adults, drug interactions do occur. Combination therapy with the exception of a **statin** with **estimibe** is generally not prescribed. **Fibric acid medications** are recommended for elevated triglyceride levels, but clinical data concerning their use in pediatric populations are limited. **Bile acid sequestrants** may be a more suitable alternative for prepubescent children.

Specific interventions for children with HTN, obesity, diabetes, and insulin resistance are outside the scope of this chapter. Dyslipidemic responses are associated with HTN above the 95th percentile for age and gender, BMI greater than the 85th percentile and HgA_{1c} levels above 7.0. Readers are referred to those topical headers in other areas of the text.

Middle-Aged Men

Men 35 to 65 years old are at increasing risk for CHD. Up to one-third of all new CHD deaths occur in this age group and most of the excessive risk can be attributed to hyperlipidemia, HTN, and cigarette smoking. Men are also predisposed to abdominal obesity, which increases their risk for metabolic syndrome (NCEP, 2001).

Special attention for cholesterol management in middle-aged men includes consideration of the following:

- Strong evidence of risk reduction from LDL lowering with **statin** therapy for those with CHD or CHD risk equivalents exists. Combination of **statin** and **bile acid-binding resin** is also very useful.
- **Fibrates** or **nicotinic acid** may be used as second-line therapy for lipid lowering in men with low HDL and atherogenic dyslipidemia.
- High prevalence of metabolic syndrome requires intensive TLC.
- Lipid-lowering drugs may be used when LDL is greater than 160 mg/dL or remains at 130 to 159 after TLC.

- The same standards apply to men with multiple risk factors, with the exception of optional drug therapy for those with 10-year risk less than 10 percent.
- Factors favoring drug therapy include higher end of age range, obesity, cigarette smoking, positive family history, and very low serum levels of HDL.

Women

Elevated cholesterol levels confer CHD risk in women as well as in men, but the correlation to CHD is lower for women before age 55. Until that age, women are at lower risk for CHD than their male counterparts, in part because of their higher estrogen levels. After age 55, the most common cause of death in both men and women is cardiovascular disease (NCEP, 2001). Cholesterol levels tend to be higher in women than they are in men, in older groups. Women younger than 45 years are discussed in the Younger Adults section, and women older than 75 years are discussed in the Older Adults section. This section refers to women in the 45- to 75-year age range.

Based on Framingham scoring, only after age 75 do the CHD rates for women approximate those of men. The reason for this disparity is not fully understood. The patterns of risk factors often differ between men and women. BP, LDL cholesterol, and triglycerides rise at an earlier age in adult men than they do in women. At puberty, HDL cholesterol levels decrease in males, but not in females. Because a 10 mg/dL difference in HDL cholesterol may account for a 20 to 30 percent difference in CHD rates, this difference over the adult life span could account for a large portion of the gender disparity.

Although the presence of **bioidentical** and **conjugated equine estrogen** is postulated to raise HDL levels, the results of the Women's Health Initiative study have raised serious questions about supplemental or replacement **estrogen** in combination with **medroxyprogesterone acetate (MPA)**; therefore, **HRT** is no longer recommended for raising HDL (Rossouw et al, 2002). The increased risk of embolism, caused by **estrogen** replacement therapy, causes increased risks to patients in this age group (Grady et al, 2000).

Women's CV health risks are generally underappreciated by both providers and patients, although a significant public health outreach to educate both populations has shown some gains toward clinical treatment parity with men (Ridker, Buring, Rifai, & Cook, 2007). Parity, however, has not been reached. Some researchers have questioned the validity of Framingham scores because the population of women included in the analysis was mostly under age 50. Data were also gathered without much consideration to ethnicity and metabolic syndrome, which has greater and earlier impact on CAD in women (Gleeson & Crabbe, 2009).

The past decade of research has strengthened the addition of novel markers to gain a better appreciation of CHD risk in women. It is anticipated that future NCEP guideline updates may include these markers for both gender risk stratification. The Reynolds Risk Score (Ridker et al, 2007) is one tool used that incorporates novel markers such as C-reactive protein, but has not been validated extensively in diverse populations (Gleeson & Crabbe, 2009). Other novel markers such as homocysteine, coronary artery calcification, and functional capacity tests (including cardiac recovery profiles after exercise) are touted as providing a more refined evaluation of actual risk in women. Because these indications do not yet have a strong evidence base to differentiate care for men and women in published guidelines, some providers are taking the Framingham scores and providing an option to women with strong family histories of early CVD to more aggressively intervene than the current guidelines suggest (Ridker et al, 2007). Those with higher C-reactive protein levels should be included in the more aggressive treatment plans (Cushman et al, 2009).

Special attention for cholesterol management in women 45 to 75 years include consideration of the following:

- For women with CHD or CHD risk equivalents (including diabetes), **statins** are as useful in CHD risk reduction via LDL lowering as they are for men. All secondary prevention trials with these drugs have included women.
- Control of risk factors by **antihypertensive drugs** and **beta blockers** is indicated. Evidence for use of **aspirin** has come under scrutiny for women, but those with high risk are still encouraged to take it if the individualized adverse risk of taking aspirin is lower than the potential benefit.
- For women with multiple risk factors, clinical trials of LDL lowering are generally lacking, and rationale for drug use is extrapolated from benefits for men.
- For women with multiple risk factors, consider LDL-lowering drugs when LDL is at or above 160 mg/dL after TLC. They may also be used when the LDL is 130 to 159 mg/dL and for those requiring more aggressive therapy.
- **LDL-lowering drugs** are generally not indicated for women with multiple risk factors who have a 10-year CHD risk less than 10 percent or for those with zero or one risk factor. Novel cardiac markers may help determine if individual indications exist.
- **HRT** is not recommended for LDL lowering for women in any category.

Older Adults

Most new CHD events and most coronary deaths occur in older adults (men older than 65 years, women older than 75 years) because they have accumulated more coronary atherosclerosis than have younger age groups. Lowering CAD risk by reducing total cholesterol, and specifically LDL levels, is critical in this population. Angiographic studies have shown that even advanced coronary atherosclerosis may respond to reductions in cholesterol. Framingham risk scores are less robust for predicting risk in older adults and measurements of atherosclerosis.

Considering CHD is more prevalent in the older population, more individuals will benefit from risk reduction than in other age groups. Other factors such as concomitant chronic diseases (e.g., congestive heart failure, dementia, advanced cerebrovascular disease, or active malignancy), social circumstances, chronological and functional age, and polypharmacy should be taken into account. Financial considerations must be considered, but in an era of Medicare drug plans and low-cost generics, these considerations have decreased in importance. Older adults who are otherwise healthy should have cholesterol-lowering therapy if they present with elevated lipid levels.

How aggressive the therapy is depends, as it does in younger adults, on the degree of CAD risk. Like younger people, the CHD risk reduction occurs in 6 to 12 months, even in those with long-standing disease. No statistically significant differences in side effect profiles have been noted in elders enrolled in studies.

The same algorithm based on CAD risk is used in elders; however, older adults are less likely to achieve the LDL goal with diet therapy alone and are more likely to require some drug therapy. **Statins** are the first-line of drug treatment used in this age group. **Statins** are well tolerated in this population, with only minor diarrhea and occasional sleep pattern disturbances commonly reported as side effects. Most **statins** can be taken once daily and do not add much complexity to already existing treatment regimens. **Niacin** is also effective, but side effects are not well tolerated. **Niacin** may trigger hypotension that can be dangerous, especially in older adults who may also be on other drugs that can produce orthostatic changes in their blood pressure. **Bile acid-binding resins** have risks for impaction and constipation and are not a good choice for older people. Special attention for cholesterol management in older adults include consideration of the following:

- Older adults respond similarly to risk reduction as do middle-aged adults. Guidelines for use of **LDL-lowering drugs** are, therefore, similar for both groups in the presence of CHD or CHD risk equivalents.
- Prevalence of diabetes, a CHD risk equivalent, is markedly increased in the older population.
- For adults with multiple risk factors, risk assessment by standard risk factors is less reliable, but **LDL-lowering drugs** can be considered when LDL is equal to 130 mg/dL for adults with 10-year CHD risks between 10 and 20 percent.
- Drugs are less likely to be used for adults with 10-year CHD risks of less than 10 percent or zero or one risk factor. However, drugs may be considered if TLC therapy was not successful in bringing the serum LDL below 160 mg/dL for the less than 10 percent group and below 190 mg/dL for the zero or one risk factor group.
- Emphasis should be given to TLC, especially dietary changes, but drugs are more likely to be needed. Elders with poor appetites and risk of malnutrition are not candidates for strict dietary enforcement.
- Consideration for drug interactions related to polypharmacy is important. Elders may be at higher risk for muscle toxicity when **statins** are mixed with **macrolides. Thiazide diuretics** are associated with increasing hyperlipidemic patterns and might be substituted with another class of drugs. Consideration of **statins** with less cytochrome P450 competition, such as **pitavastatin**, may become more commonly considered if this drug, which was introduced in 2009, achieves greater market penetration.
- Patients with very limited life expectancy due to other diseases probably do not benefit from antihyperlipidemic drug therapy. Strict enforcement of TLC is also unnecessary.

Young Adults

CHD is rare in this age group except for patients with severe risk factors such as familial hypercholesterolemia, heavy cigarette smoking, and diabetes. Unfortunately, CHD is becoming more common as the obesity and metabolic syndrome epidemic grows. Coronary atherosclerosis in its early stage may progress rapidly and the rate of development has been shown to correlate with major risk factors. Long-term predictive studies (NCEP, 2001) have shown that elevated cholesterol found in young adults predicts a higher rate of premature CHD in middle age. For this reason, risk factor control is important in young adults as primary prevention.

NCEP (2001) recommends doing lipid profiles beginning at age 20. Such early testing provides an opportunity to begin the public health approach to primary prevention. In addition, all young adults have the right to be informed if they at risk for premature CHD, so that they can consider actions to prevent or postpone its occurrence. Finally, patients with cholesterol levels in the upper quartile of the population are clearly at high long-term risk and TLC intervention should be begun at the earliest possible age. Most young adults with very high LDL cholesterol (greater than 190 mg/dL) are possible candidates for cholesterol-lowering drugs; however, prudence should be exercised in prescribing cholesterol-lowering drugs to this age group. Maximizing TLC and delaying drug therapy is especially important in premenopausal women. Based on the Pregnancy Categories the following recommendations are made:

- **Nicotinic acid** and **fibric acid derivatives** are Pregnancy Category C. Risks and benefits should be carefully weighed before giving these drugs to pregnant women.
- All **statins** are Pregnancy Category X and should not be given to women who have the potential to become pregnant.
- No pregnancy category has been assigned to the **bile acid-binding resins.** Women of childbearing age with elevated cholesterol are best managed with lifestyle modifications. If drug therapy is required, they may be placed on **bile acid-binding resins.** If

this is not effective, they should probably be referred to a lipid specialist.
- All **antihyperlipidemics** should be avoided during breastfeeding.

Special attention for cholesterol management in young adults beyond those listed above for women include consideration of the following:

- CHD is rare in this age group, but persons with heterozygous familial hypercholesterolemia may develop very premature CHD and require intensive **LDL-lowering therapy.** To achieve a level of less than 100 mg/dL usually requires TLC and drugs therapy.
- CHD can also occur in this group for patients with type 1 diabetes or in very heavy cigarette smokers. Clinical judgment is required to determine the LDL goal here.
- Most young adults will not meet the multiple risk factors criteria. Non-LDL risk factors in this age group carry a higher long-term risk and should be the focus of management.
- **LDL-lowering drugs** can be considered when TLC does not bring LDL levels below 160 mg/dL for those with 10-year CHD risks 10 to 20 percent or below 190 mg/dL for those in the lower risk categories.

African Americans

African Americans have the highest overall CHD mortality rates and the highest out-of-hospital coronary death rates of any other ethnic group in the United States, particularly at young ages (Clark et al, 2001). Although the reasons for this excess CHD risk have not be fully elucidated, it can be explained in part by the high prevalence and suboptimal control of coronary risk factors. Current research in HMG-CoA reductase gene variance among ethnic groups shows an interesting, more protective lipid phenotype than other ethnic groups (Chen et al, 2009). Hypertension, left ventricular hypertrophy, diabetes, cigarette smoking, obesity, and physical inactivity are all more prevalent in African Americans than in whites. The predictability of standard risk factors for CHD by the Framingham risk assessment tool appears to be much the same for African Americans as they are for whites, but the risk of death and other serious consequences is disproportionately higher in African Americans. This might be caused by higher C-reactive protein levels (Cushman et al, 2009). Although the ATP III guidelines are generally applicable equally to African Americans and whites, it is important to measure CRP and develop a more aggressive treatment plan if indicated.

Certain differences between African Americans and whites require special attention:

- African American men often have a high normal baseline level of creatinine kinase. CK level should be documented before starting a **statin.**
- Hypertension, a powerful CHD risk factor, is more common in African Americans than whites. If present, left ventricular hypertrophy should be considered in the patient treatment plan as it is a powerful predictor of cardiovascular deaths in African Americans.
- Obesity, especially abdominal obesity, is twice as common in African American women as compared to white women. Metabolic syndrome is a risk factor for CAD.
- Type 2 diabetes, an independent CHD risk factor, is more prevalent in African Americans than whites.
- African Americans with established CHD are at particularly high risk for cardiac death. Nonetheless, the LDL-lowering goals for this group are the same as for whites.
- African Americans are more likely to have multiple risk factors. **LDL-lowering drugs** are warranted when LDL is greater than 130 mg/dL after a TLC trial.

Hispanic Americans

Hispanic Americans are a heterogeneous ethnic group with origins in many different countries. The genetic researchers have found two general haplotypes that affect lipid processing; one was associated with higher risk factors of overall higher TC, TG, and LDL levels with low HDL levels, whereas the other type had much lower risks (Chen et al, 2009). CHD and cardiovascular disease are about 20 percent lower among adult Hispanics than among whites (NCEP, 2001), despite their increased prevalence of diabetes, obesity, lower HDL levels and higher triglyceride levels. While these concomitant conditions may raise their CHD risk score, the Framingham tool has not been validated in this group and probably overestimates the risk (D'Agostino, Grundy, Sullivan, Wilson, for the CHD Risk Prediction Group, 2001). The ATP III panel decided that there was insufficient evidence to justify separate guidelines. There are no special considerations for cholesterol management for Hispanic Americans at this time.

Native Americans (American Indians)

Data from the Indian Health Service indicate that cardiovascular disease rates appear to be increasing in Native Americans. Native Americans were not included in the most recent genetic studies on the metabolism of **statins.** CHD incidence rates among Native American men and women were almost twice as high as those in the biracial Atherosclerosis Risk in Communities Study (Howard et al, 1999). In addition to increased rates of CHD, cardiovascular events in Native Americans appeared more often to be fatal. The significant independent predictors of cardiovascular disease common to both Native American men and women were diabetes, age, LDL levels, albuminuria, and HTN. The increasing incidence of CHD in Native American communities may be related to the increasing prevalence of diabetes in this population. As with the Hispanic population, the Framingham tool appears to overestimate the risk of CHD. Nonetheless, efforts to reduce cholesterol and other CHD risk factors are important because there is a higher incidence of CHD and a higher mortality rate associated with CHD in this population. Despite limited data suggesting some differences, there is no separate algorithm for Native American populations.

Asian and Pacific Islanders

There is limited information on the risks and benefits of lipid management for the reduction of CHD and cardiovascular disease in the Asian and Pacific Islander population. The Honolulu Heart Program is an ongoing prospective study of CHD and stroke in a cohort of Japanese American men living in Hawaii. In this study, CHD and cardiovascular mortality are lower than in the general U.S. population and the Framingham tool appears to overestimate the actual risk. The ATP III panel decided that there should be no separate algorithm for this population. The increased incidence of diabetes in native Hawaiians and Pacific Islanders has not generated a separate algorithm. Some providers question whether alternative BMI charts should be used to determine actual risk levels.

Chinese Americans were included in the recent lipid genetic studies (Chen et al, 2009). Even though this population typically has the lowest BMIs when compared to other racial groups, they have high cardiovascular disease rates. South Asians also have a very high prevalence of coronary disease at younger ages in the absence of standard risk factors. This may be related to the high prevalence of insulin resistance, metabolic syndrome, and diabetes in this population. Efforts to reduce cholesterol and other CHD risk factors in this population appear to be especially important. For these reasons, ATP III recommends that special attention be given to early detection of CHD risk factors in South Asian populations with emphasis focused on metabolic syndrome and diabetes. The treatment algorithm for whites is used in the populations discussed but increased emphasis should be given to intensive TLC implementation.

Concomitant Disease States

Drugs used to treat hyperlipidemia may improve the management of some diseases and worsen others. It is not within the scope of this text to discuss all possible diseases that may coexist with hyperlipidemia, but common diseases that may improve as a result of appropriate drug selection for the treatment of hyperlipidemia are discussed here.

Diabetes Mellitus

Diabetes mellitus is now considered a CHD risk equivalent, so the therapeutic treatment goal for LDL cholesterol levels in diabetic patients, particularly type 2, is less than 100 mg/dL. TLC should be started immediately in all patients presenting with diabetes. Most patients with diabetes will require **LDL-lowering drugs** to achieve target serum LDL levels below 100 mg/dL. If the patient also has high triglycerides, which is common for type 2 diabetics, non-HDL cholesterol becomes a secondary target for therapy. Triglyceride levels at or above 200 mg/dL may require a **fibrate** or low-dose **nicotinic acid** product (less than 3 g/d). In treatment, attention is initially focused on reducing serum LDL levels. After serum LDL levels are in a desirable range, the focus of treatment can change to reducing serum triglyceride levels. **Nicotinic acid** has been shown to have a favorable effect on diabetic dyslipidemia. Unfortunately, nicotinic acid can cause increased insulin resistance. Given in low doses, nicotinic acid produces limited deterioration in glucose control and no changes in glycated hemoglobin levels.

When the baseline serum LDL cholesterol is between 100 and 129 mg/dL, the first line of treatment is intensive TLC, which includes reducing saturated fat and cholesterol in the diet, use of **plant stanols/sterols** and increased **viscous fiber**, weight reduction, increased physical activity, and smoking cessation. Maximal control of nonlipid risk factors such as HTN and hyperglycemia is also the focus of cholesterol management in this population. The drugs of choice for treating HTN in patients with diabetes are **angiotensin-converting enzyme (ACE) inhibitors** or **angiotensin II receptor blockers (ARBs)**.

For all diabetics, **statins** are usually the drugs of choice for lowering serum LDLs. **Statins** are generally well tolerated in this population and have the advantage of lowering VLDL as well. **Bile acid-binding resins** can also be used to lower serum LDLs, but they do not reduce serum VLDL, a lipid fraction commonly elevated in diabetics. Diabetics taking **bile acid-binding resins** should have triglycerides checked regularly, as these medications can elevate serum triglyceride levels.

Additional special attention for lipid management in patients with diabetes include consideration of the following:

- **Fibrates** are well tolerated and do not worsen hyperglycemia, but they are best used in patients with low LDL cholesterol levels and atherogenic dyslipidemia. For type 2 diabetics, generally delay management of atherogenic dyslipidemia until the serum LDL goal is achieved.
- If triglycerides are greater than 200 mg/dL, the non-HDL goal is less than 130 mg/dL.
- Control of nonlipid risk factors is central to management in this population. **Glucophage (metformin)** may help lower hyperglycemia and facilitate weight loss. **Insulin, sulfonylureas, metformin**, and **glitazones** all lower triglycerides. Control of hyperglycemia may eliminate the need for a **fibrate** medication.

Metabolic Syndrome

Patients with metabolic syndrome have an increased risk for coronary disease. Elevated triglycerides present one factor within a set of risk factors in patients who are obese (especially abdominal obesity), sedentary, have low HDL cholesterol, are hypertensive, and have fasting blood glucose levels at or above 110 to 125 mg/dL. Table 39–9

Table 39–9 **ATP III Classification of Triglyceride Levels**

Triglyceride Level (mg/dL)	Category
<150	Normal
150–199	Borderline to high
200–499	High
≥500	Very high

Source: Adapted from the *Third Report of the Expert Panel on Detection, Evaluation and Treatment of High Blood Cholesterol in Adults,* 2001. Rockville, MD: National Institutes of Health, National Heart, Lung, and Blood Institute.

presents the ATP III (NCEP, 2001) triglyceride classifications. The major focus of management for metabolic syndrome is intensive TLC.

Patients with elevated triglycerides typically also have an increase in serum atherogenic VLDL remnants. TLC with the addition of restricting alcohol and avoiding a high-carbohydrate diet form the foundation for triglyceride control in this population. **Statins** are the drugs of choice because they lower both serum LDL and VLDL remnants. In the presence of low serum HDL cholesterol, **nicotinic acid** is an alternative therapy used when the serum LDL cholesterol goal has already been achieved. **Fibrates** can be considered as an alternative option for the treatment of elevated triglycerides.

The Diabetes Prevention Program randomized trial found that both lifestyle modifications and **metformin therapy** were effective in the treatment of metabolic syndrome and reduced the development of metabolic syndrome in participants who had not yet developed the disease (Orchard et al, 2005). The dose of **metformin** used in this trial was 850 mg bid.

Hypothyroidism

Untreated hypothyroidism often presents with symptoms that include hypercholesterolemia. Clinically, patients present with elevated cholesterol, high LDL, and mild VLDL elevation. Every patient found to have elevated cholesterol (LDL greater than 160 mg/dL) should be screened for hypothyroidism. Treatment of the primary problem, hypothyroidism, should be initiated and serum lipid levels should be reevaluated after thyroid levels are normal.

Hypertension

HTN and hyperlipidemia commonly occur together. Patients with concomitant HTN and hypercholesterolemia should have both conditions treated aggressively as these two risk factors act synergistically, greatly increasing CAD risk. Management of HTN is discussed in Chapter 40. Lifestyle modifications are the first approach to treatment of both hypertension and hypercholesterolemia. Dietary Approaches to Stop Hypertension (DASH) has recommended that dietary changes implemented for patients with HTN and hyperlipidemia be the same lowering sodium consumption, recommended for HTN patients, is not problematic for patients with dyslipidemia. Weight control, exercise, and smoking cessation are lifestyle changes that should be stressed to patients with both disorders.

When drug therapy is chosen to treat a disease or condition, consideration must be given to how the medication therapy will affect other health problems that the patient may have. **Diuretics** are now considered first-line therapy for HTN, and some researchers have suggested that all treatment regimens that include more than one drug also include a **diuretic. Thiazide diuretics** are the most commonly prescribed agents for HTN. Higher doses of these drugs can cause modest and often transient increases in serum LDL cholesterol and triglycerides, with little or no adverse effects on HDL cholesterol. The effects of **loop diuretics** are similar to those of **thiazides**, but serum HDL cholesterol levels are generally lower in patients on **furosemide.**

Calcium channel blockers, ACE inhibitors, and **aldosterone antagonists** have little effect on serum lipids. **Beta blockers** without intrinsic sympathomimetic activity (ISA) tend to reduce HDL cholesterol, increase triglycerides, and have variable effects on total serum cholesterol. These effects are minimal, and should not play a role in the selection of a **beta blocker** for treating hypertension. ISA **Beta blockers** combined with **alpha$_1$ beta blockers (labetalol** and **carvedilol)** have no appreciable effect on lipid levels. **Alpha$_1$ blockers** and centrally acting **agonists** provide minimal, beneficial effects on blood lipids by decreasing LDL cholesterol.

Nicotinic acid can cause orthostatic hypotension and should be used with caution in patients who are being treated with **antihypertensives** that have this same side effect. None of the other classes of drugs used to treat hyperlipidemia have a direct effect on blood pressure. **Bile acid-binding resins** may decrease absorption of **antihypertensive medications,** so their administration should be separated by giving the **antihypertensive** 1 hour before or 4 hours after the **bile acid-binding resin. Statins** have no specific interactions with **antihypertensive agents.**

Cost

In today's health-care environment, cost effectiveness of therapy is always an issue. The aggregate cost of CAD in the United States is over $100 billion per year for medication, treatment, and lost wages. Prevention of CAD could greatly reduce this economic burden, and the management of cholesterol levels is one way to prevent CAD. Patients in high-risk categories for CAD related to elevated cholesterol levels have the greatest likelihood of significant benefit from cholesterol reduction. For example, in men 35 to 64 years and women 35 to 54 years with established CAD, intervention with standard doses of **statins** has been estimated to save significant amounts of money otherwise spent on CAD events in untreated patients. In older men and women, the cost/benefit ratios are even better. From a public-health perspective, the cost of cholesterol treatment is clearly justified for older patients. Patients at lower risk for CAD have a less favorable cost/benefit ratio. For this group, the ratio of cost to savings depends on the drug therapy chosen. When evaluating patients on an individual basis, even low-risk patients may benefit from cholesterol reduction therapy. The more recent links between low to moderate lipid levels in middle aged adults to higher risk for development of Alzheimer's disease increases the urgency for earlier and more aggressive treatment of hyperlipidemia beyond just CAD issues (Solomon, Kivipelto, Wolozin, Zhou, & Whitner, 2009).

Obviously, dietary management and reduction of major risk factors, like smoking and limited physical activity, have the best cost/benefit ratio for public health and the individual patient. When drug therapy is chosen, the cost includes laboratory assessment and monitoring as well as the price of the medication. Historically the greatest expense of antihyperlipidemic treatment was drug cost. Today, with the marketing of generic antihyperlipidemic agents, costs associated with the treatment of hyperlipidemia have been reduced significantly. **Nicotinic acid** in its generic form is clearly the least expensive, and even the slow-release form is less expensive than several other **antihyperlipidemic drugs.** Some of the most commonly prescribed **statins** are now available in generic form, but generic equivalents for some drug classifications are limited. Chapter 16 has a detailed discussion of the cost of all of the **antihyperlipidemics.** Many major drug companies offer low-cost or free brand-name medications for those with restricted incomes.

MONITORING

Monitoring for effectiveness of dietary therapy is discussed in the Lifestyle Modifications section. Drug therapy is not usually initiated until a 3-month trial of dietary therapy has been completed. Selection of an agent to treat a lipid disorder is based on a minimum of two lipoprotein levels done 1 to 4 weeks apart during maximum dietary therapy. This provides a baseline for future evaluation of drug efficacy. Baseline lab data (liver function, ALT or AST, and CK) should be gathered before drug treatment begins. Specific diagnostic tests for monitoring each drug class are discussed in Chapter 16.

With good medication compliance, patients should show a lowering of LDL cholesterol within 4 to 6 weeks of initiating therapy. Levels of serum LDL cholesterol should be evaluated 6 to 8 weeks after initiating therapy. **Nicotinic acid** is the exception to this rule. For **nicotinic acid,** repeat measurements should be done when the patient's prescribed dose has been stable for 4 to 6 weeks. For all of these drugs, a second measurement of LDL cholesterol levels is done 6 weeks after the first measurement. A minimum of two measurements is essential for evaluating the efficacy of the drug. For all treatment regimens, if the dose of a drug is increased, or another drug added to the treatment regimen, the patient's laboratory data should be evaluated in another 6 to 8 weeks. An aggressive increase in dosing is recommended for those at highest risk for CAD. After the target LDL cholesterol level is reached, patients should be followed at 8- to 12-week intervals for 1 year. After 1 year of therapy, during which the patient's response to the treatment regimen has been established, and there is no evidence of toxicity, patients should be followed at 4- to 6-month intervals.

Monitoring of HDL and non-HDL levels is a good practice that provides a clear picture of the actual CAD risk status for the patient. Apo levels can be measured, but are expensive. Calculating the non-HDL levels can give an indication of apo levels. Attention to reductions in the C-reactive protein levels are critical in those who have had elevated levels.

OUTCOME EVALUATION

Discontinuation of treatment is quickly followed by a return of the cholesterol to pretreatment levels. Long-term cholesterol control means lifelong adherence to the treatment regimen. Achieving long-term clinical control of high blood cholesterol requires the same interest and attention from the patient and the provider as was given to the initial evaluation and treatment plan. Effective use of follow-up visits and skillful employment of adherence-enhancing techniques are required, including nurturing the patient–provider relationship. The primary care provider can manage hyperlipidemia in most patients. Severe forms of hypercholesterolemia are often the result of a genetic disorder of lipoprotein metabolism. Consultation with a lipid specialist is needed for patients with severe, complex forms of lipid disorders or patients who do not respond to standard therapy. Chapter 6 provides information on how to facilitate drug adherence.

PATIENT EDUCATION

Patient education should include a discussion of the overall treatment plan and the role of medication therapy. Patients who understand the reasons for their drug therapy may show improved compliance with their medication regimens. Tendencies for muscle toxicity appear to run in families. Patients should inquire about **statin** tolerance issues in their older relatives to establish if a potential family risk for myopathies exists. The onset of muscle pain can occur immediately, but frequently does not appear for several months. Reinforcement about reporting myalgias should be addressed with patients at every follow-up appointment.

HYPERLIPIDEMIA

PATIENT EDUCATION

Related to the Overall Treatment Plan and Disease Process

- ☐ Pathophysiology of lipid disorders and their long-term effects on cardiovascular morbidity and mortality
- ☐ Role of lifestyle modification, especially dietary therapy, in improving outcomes and keeping the number and cost of required drugs down
- ☐ Importance of adherence to the treatment regimen
- ☐ Need for regular follow-up visits with the primary care provider

Specific to the Drug Therapy

- ☐ Reason for the drug(s) being given and the anticipated action of the drug(s) on the disease process
- ☐ Doses and schedules for taking the drug(s)
- ☐ Possible adverse reactions, how to prevent them, and what to do if they occur
- ☐ Interaction between lifestyle modifications and the drug(s)

Reasons for Taking the Drug(s)

Patient education about specific drugs is provided in Chapter 16. Specific information related to hyperlipidemia includes the reasons for drug(s) being taken: Antilipidemics are given to reduce morbidity and mortality from the leading cause of death in the United States—cardiovascular disease. Discuss the risk of cardiovascular disease with the patient while maintaining the potential for good quality of life with adequate treatment.

Drugs as Part of the Total Treatment Regimen

The expectations should be clear about what the drugs can and cannot do. Drugs are supplements to dietary and other lifestyle modifications, not substitutes for them. Lipid disorders are chronic conditions. Lifestyle modifications and drug regimens need to be incorporated into patients' everyday lives. Discontinuation of treatment will result in return of lipids to pretreatment levels.

Adherence Issues

Nonadherence to the treatment regimen may increase patients' risk for cardiovascular morbidity and reduce their life expectancy. Health-care providers should be aware of potential problems with nonadherence, discuss the importance of adherence at each follow-up visit, and assist patients in removing barriers to adherence, such as lack of social support and cost of the treatment regimen. Utilization of other health team members, especially the dietitian, should be maximized. Patient education booklets available from the American Heart Association and the National Cholesterol Education Program may supplement dietary instruction.

REFERENCES

Alexander, C., Landsman, P., Teutsch, S., & Haffner, S. (2003). NCEP-defined metabolic syndrome, diabetes and prevalence of coronary heart disease among NHANES III participants age 50 years and older. *Diabetes, 52,* 1210–1214.

American College of Cardiology (ACC). (2008). Statement on ENHANCE trial. Retrieved September 10, 2009, from http://www.acc.org.enhance.htm

Arnaud, C., Braunersreuther, V., & Mach, F. (2005). Toward immunomodulatory and anti-inflammatory properties of statins. *Trends in Cardiovascular Medicine, 15*(6), 202–206.

Cannon C. P. (2005). The IDEAL cholesterol: Lower is better. *Journal of the American Medical Association, 294*(19), 2492–2494.

Chen, Y. C., Chen, Y. D., Li, X., Post, W., Herrington, D., Polak, J. F., et al. (2009). The HMG-CoA reductase gene and lipid and lipoprotein levels: The multi-ethnic study of atherosclerosis. *Lipids, 44*(8), 733–743

Clark, L., Ferdinand, K., Flack, J., Gavin, J., Valantine, H., Watson, K., et al. (2001). Coronary heart disease in African Americans. *Heart Disease, 3,* 97–108.

Cushman, M., McClure, L., Howard, V., Jenny, N., Lakoski, S., & Howard, G. (2009). Implication of increased C-reactive protein for cardiovascular risk stratification in black and white men and women in the U.S. *Clinical Chemistry, 5*(9), 1627–1636.

D'Agostino, R., Grundy, S., Sullivan, L., Wilson, P., for the CHD Risk Prediction Group. (2001). Validation of the Framingham coronary heart disease prediction scores: Results of a multiple ethnic groups investigation. *Journal of the American Medical Association, 286,* 180–187.

Daniels, S., & Greer, F. (2008). Lipid screening and cardiovascular health in childhood. *Pediatrics, 122,* 198–208.

Ford, E., Li, D., Zhao, G., Peason, W., & Capewell, S. (2009). Trends in the prevalence of low risk factor burden for cardiovascular disease among United States adults. *Circulation, 120,* 1181–1188.

Gidding, S., Lichtenstein, A., Faith, M., Karpyn, J., Manella, B., Popkin, J., et al. (2009). Implementing American Heart Association pediatric and adult nutrition guidelines: A scientific statement from the American Heart Association Nutrition Committee of the Council on Nutrition, Physical Activity and Metabolism, Council on Cardiovascular Disease in the Young, Council on Arteriosclerosis, Thrombosis and Vascular Biology, Council on Cardiovascular Nursing, Council on Epidemiology and Prevention and Council for High Blood Pressure Research. *Circulation, 119*(8), 1161–1175.

Gleeson, D., & Crabbe, D. (2009). Emerging concepts in cardiovascular disease risk assessment: Where do women fit in? *Journal of the American Academy of Nurse Practitioners, 21,* 480–487.

Grady, D., Wenger, N., Herrington, D., Khan, S., Furberg, C., Hunninghake, D., et al, for the Heart and Estrogen/Progestin Replacement Study Research Group. (2000). Postmenopausal hormone therapy increases risk for venous thromboembolic disease: The Heart and Estrogen/Progestin Replacement Study. *Archives of Internal Medicine, 132,* 689–696.

Grundy, S., Cleeman, J., Merz, C., Brewer, B., Jr., Clark, L., Hinninghake, D., et al, for the Coordinating Committee of the National Cholesterol Education Program. (2004). Implications of recent clinical trials for the National Cholesterol Education Program Adult Treatment Panel III guidelines. *Circulation, 110,* 227–239.

Haffner, S., Lehto, S., Ronnemaa, T., Pyorala, K., & Laasko, M. (1998). Mortality from coronary heart disease in subjects with type 2 diabetes and in nondiabetic subjects with and without prior myocardial infarction. *New England Journal of Medicine, 339,* 229–234.

Heart Protection Study Collaboration Group. (2002). MRC/BHF Heart Protections Study of cholesterol lowering with simvastatin in 20,536 high-risk individuals: A randomized placebo-controlled trial. *Lancet, 360,* 7–22.

Howard, B., Lee, E., Cowan, L., Devereaux, R., Galloway, J., Go, O., et al. (1999). Rising tide of cardiovascular disease in American Indians: The Strong Heart Study. *Circulation, 99,* 2389–2395.

Jenkins, D., Kendall, C., & Marchie, A. (2005). Diet and cholesterol reduction. *Annals of Internal Medicine, 142,* 793–795.

Jones, P., Davidson, M., Stein, E., Bays, H., McKenney, J., Miller, E., et al. (2003). Comparison of the efficacy and safety of rosuvastatin versus atorvastatin, simvastatin, and pravastatin across doses. (STELLAR trial). *American Journal of Cardiology, 92,* 152–160.

Knatterud, G., Rosenberg, Y., Campeau, L., Geller, N., Hunninghake, D., Forman, S., et al. (2000). Long-term effects on clinical outcomes of aggressive lowering of low-density lipoprotein cholesterol levels and low-dose anticoagulation in the Post Coronary Bypass Graft trial. *Circulation, 102,* 157–165.

Malmberg, K., Yusuf, S., Gerstine, H., Brown, J., Zhao, F., Hunt, D., et al, for the OASIS Registry Investigators. (2002). Impact of diabetes on long-term prognosis in patients with unstable angina and non-Q-wave myocardial infarction: Results of the OASIS (Organization to Assess Strategies for Ischemic Syndromes) Registry. *Circulation, 102,* 1014–1019.

McCrindle, B., Urbina, E., Dennison, B., Jacobson, M., Steinberger, J., Rocchini, A., et al, American Heart Association; Atherosclerosis, Hypertension and Obesity in: American Heart Association Council of Cardiovascular Disease in the Young; American Heart Association Council on Cardiovascular Nursing. (2007). Drug therapy of high-risk lipid abnormalities in children and adolescents. *Circulation, 115*(14), 1948–1967.

Mente, A., deKoning, L., Shannon, H., & Anand, S. (2009). A systematic review of the evidence supporting a causal link between dietary factors and coronary heart disease. *Archives of Internal Medicine, 169*(7), 659–669.

Miettinen, H., Lehto, S., Salomaa, V., Maonen, M., Niemela, M., Haffner, S., et al, for the FINMONICA Myocardial Infarction Register Study Group. (1998). Impact of diabetes on mortality after the first myocardial infarction. *Diabetes Care, 21,* 69–75.

National Cholesterol Education Program (NCEP). (2001). *Third Report of the Expert Panel on Detection, Evaluation, and Treatment of High Blood Cholesterol in Adults* (Adult Treatment Panel III). Rockville, MD: National Institutes of Health, National Heart, Lung and Blood Institute.

National High Blood Pressure Education Program (NHBPEP). (2003). *The Seventh Report of the Joint National Committee on Prevention, Detection, Evaluation, and Treatment of High Blood Pressure* (JNC-7). Rockville, MD: National Institutes of Health, National Heart, Lung and Blood Institute.

Nettleton J. A., Polak, J. F., Tracy, R., Burke, G. L., & Jacobs, D. R., Jr. (2009). Dietary patterns and incident cardiovascular disease in the Multi-Ethnic Study of Atherosclerosis. *American Journal of Clinical Nutrition, 90*(3), 647–654.

Nissen S. E., Tuzcu, E. M., Schoenhagen, P., Brown, B. G., Ganz, P., Vogel, R. A., et al, REVERSAL Investigators. (2004). Effect of intensive compared with moderate lipid-lowering therapy on progression of coronary atherosclerosis: A randomized controlled trial. *Journal of the American Medical Association, 291*(9), 1071–1080.

Orchard, T., Temprosa, M., Goldberg, R., Haffner, S., Ratner, R., Marcovina, S., et al, for the Diabetes Prevention Program Research Group. (2005). The effect of metformin and intensive lifestyle intervention on metabolic syndrome: The Diabetes Prevention Program randomized trial. *Archives of Internal Medicine, 142,* 611–619.

Peters, A. (2008). Clinical relevance of non-HDL cholesterol in patients with diabetes. *Clinical Diabetes, 26,* 3–7.

Ridker, P. M., Buring, J. E., Rifai, N., & Cook, N. R. (2007). Development and validation of improved algorithms for the assessment of global cardiovascular risk in women: The Reynolds Risk Score. *Journal of the American Medical Association, 297*(6), 611–619.

Rossouw, J., Anderson, G., Prentice, R., LaCroix, A., Kooperberg, C., Stefanick, M., et al (Writing Group for the Women's Health Initiative). (2002). Risks and benefits of estrogen plus progestin in healthy postmenopausal women: principle results from the Women's Health Initiative randomized controlled trial. *Journal of the American Medical Association, 288*(3), 321–333.

Rubins, H., Robins, S., Collins, D., Fye, C., Anderson, J., Elam, M., et al, for the Veterans Affairs High-Density Lipoprotein Cholesterol Intervention Trial Study Group. (1999). Gemfibrozil for the secondary prevention of coronary heart disease in men with low levels of high-density lipoprotein cholesterol. *New England Journal of Medicine, 341,* 410–418.

Sacks, F., Tonkin, A., Shepherd, J., Braunwald, E., Cobbe, S., Hawkins, C., et al, for the Prospective Pravastatin Pooling Project Investigators Group. (2000). Effect of pravastatin on coronary disease events in subgroups defined by coronary risk factors: The Prospective Pravastatin Pooling Project. *Circulation, 102,* 1893–1900.

Scandinavian Simvastatin Survival Study Group. (1994). Randomized trial of cholesterol lowering in 4,444 patients with coronary heart disease: The Scandinavian Simvastatin Survival Study (4S). *Lancet, 344,* 1383–1389.

Sharma M., Ansari, M. T., Abou-Setta, A. M., Soares-Weiser, K., Ooi, T. C., Sears, M., et al. (2009). Systematic review: Comparative effectiveness and harms of combinations of lipid-modifying agents and high-dose statin monotherapy. *Annals of Internal Medicine, 151*(9), 622–630.

Solomon, A., Kivipelto, M., Wolozin, B., Zhou, J., & Whitner, R. (2009). Midlife serum cholesterol and increased risk of Alzheimer's and vascular dementia three decades later. *Dementia and Geriatric Cognitive Disorders, 28*(1), 75–80.

U.S. Department of Health and Human Services. (June 2000). *Treating tobacco use and dependence: A systems approach. Clinical Practice Guideline.* Washington, DC: Public Health Service, U.S. Department of Health and Human Services.

Wagstaff, L., Mitton, M., Arvik, B., & Doraiswamy, P. (2003). Statin-associated memory loss: Analysis of 60 case reports and review of the literature. *Pharmacotherapy, 23*(7), 871–880.

Yang, X., So, W., Ko, G. T., Ma, R. C., Kong, A. P., Chow, C. C., et al. (2008). Independent associations between low-density lipoprotein cholesterol and cancer among patients with type 2 diabetes mellitus. *Canadian Medical Association Journal, 179*(5), 427–347.

Zhang, J., McKeown, R. E., Hussey, J. R., Thompson, S. J., Woods, J. R., & Ainsworth, B. E. (2005). Low HDL cholesterol is associated with suicide attempt among young healthy women: The Third National Health and Nutrition Examination Survey. *Journal of Affective Disorders, 89*(1), 25–33.

CHAPTER 40

HYPERTENSION

Anita Lee Wynne and Sharon Maxey

Chapter Outline

Hypertension (HTN) is the most common cardiovascular disease in the United States, and it is also a problem worldwide. According to the *Seventh Report of the Joint National Committee* [JNC-7] *on Prevention, Detection, Evaluation, and Treatment of High Blood Pressure* (National High Blood Pressure Education Program [NHBPEP], 2003), approximately 1 billion individuals worldwide have HTN, and approximately 7.1 million deaths occur each year because of HTN. The World Health Organization (World Health Report, 2002) reports that suboptimal blood pressure (BP) (greater than 115 mm Hg systolic blood pressure [SBP]) is responsible for 62 percent or all cerebrovascular disease and 49 percent of ischemic heart disease. Suboptimal blood pressure is thought to be the number one attributable risk for death throughout the world.

Although the past two decades have seen considerable reduction in deaths from coronary heart disease (CHD) and stroke (CVA), control rates for HTN are still unacceptable. Approximately 30 percent of adults are still unaware of their HTN, 40 percent of individuals who have HTN are not in treatment, and 66 percent of those being treated are not controlled to blood pressures less than 140/90 mm Hg. It is estimated that a reduction of as little as 5 mm Hg of SBP in the general population could result in a 14 percent reduction is CVA mortality, a 9 percent reduction in CHD mortality, and a 7 percent reduction in all-cause mortality in the United States (Whelton et al, 2002). Unfortunately, the declines in deaths rates from CHD and CVA have slowed in the past decade and there is an increasing trend in end-stage renal disease (ESRD). Hypertension is second only to diabetes as the most common cause of ESRD. "Undiagnosed, untreated and uncontrolled hypertension clearly places a substantial strain on the health care delivery system" (NHBPEP, 2003).

PATHOPHYSIOLOGY

Systemic arterial pressure is a function of stroke volume, heart rate, and total peripheral resistance. Alterations in any of these factors result in changes in blood pressure. The major organs involved in regulation of blood pressure are the heart (heart rate [HR] and stroke volume [SV]), the sympathetic nervous system (SNS) (total peripheral resistance [TPR]), and the kidney (extracellular fluid volume and secretion of **renin**). Disease processes that affect stroke volume and heart rate include any that increase extracellular fluid volume, the activity of the SNS, or plasma **norepinephrine** levels and those that produce cardiac rhythm disturbances. Disease processes that affect total peripheral resistance include any that narrow the arteriolar radius or increase blood viscosity. Figure 40–1 shows the relationship of these factors to blood pressure control. In both normotensive and hypertensive patients, blood pressure is maintained by moment-to-moment adjustments in this system.

Factors That Regulate Blood Pressure

Baroreceptors

Change in BP is sensed by baroreceptors located in the carotid arteries and the arch of the aorta. They are sensitive to stretch so that, when stimulated by an increase in BP, they send inhibitory impulses to the sympathetic vasomotor center in the brainstem. Inhibition of efferent nerves in the SNS that innervate cardiac and vascular smooth muscle results in decreased heart rate, decreased force of contraction, and vasodilation of peripheral arterioles. At the same time, increased parasympathetic nervous system (PNS) activity further reduces HR via the vagus nerve. Decreased BP results in a reverse process. This system works well in the maintenance of BP during normal activities; however, in the presence of long-standing HTN, the baroreceptors adapt to the elevated BP levels and "reset" what the body accepts as "normal" BP. Diminished responsiveness to these baroreceptors is one of the most significant cardiovascular effects of aging and a major factor in the lifetime risk of HTN.

Endothelial Factors

In addition to the actions of baroreceptors, vascular endothelium has the ability to produce vasoactive substances and growth factors. Nitric oxide, an endothelium-derived relaxing factor, helps maintain low arterial tone at rest, and inhibits growth of the smooth muscle layer. The vascular endothelium also produces local vasodilators such as prostacyclin and endothelium-derived hyperpolarizing factor. Endothelin, also secreted by the vascular endothelium, is an extremely potent vasoconstrictor and also stimulates vascular smooth muscle growth. Growth of vascular smooth muscle is associated with atherosclerosis and the thickening seen with prolonged exposure to high BP. Endothelial dysfunction may contribute to these changes. Prevention or reversal of endothelial dysfunction may become an important therapeutic area in the future.

Kidneys

The kidneys contribute to BP control by regulation of the renin-angiotensin-aldosterone system. Renin, secreted

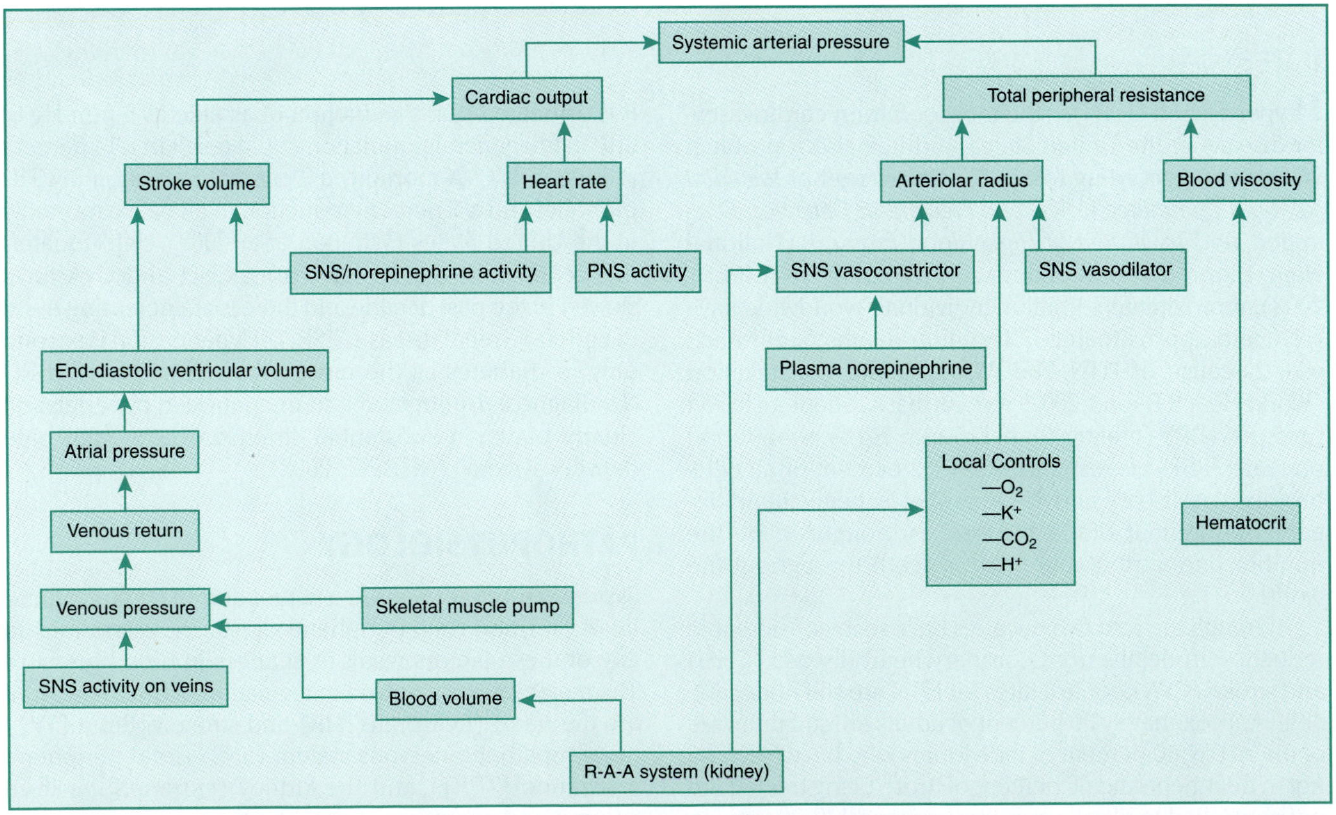

Figure 40–1. Regulation of blood pressure. Systemic arterial pressure is determined by cardiac output and total peripheral resistance. Increases in cardiac output or total peripheral resistance increase systemic arterial pressure, and decreases in these factors decrease systemic arterial pressure. Antihypertensive drugs act at one or more of these anatomical sites of blood pressure control.

by the juxtaglomerular apparatus in the kidney, converts angiotensinogen to angiotensin I. Angiotensin I is then converted by angiotensin-converting-enzyme (ACE) in the lungs to angiotensin II, which effects BP in two different ways. Angiotensin II is a potent vasoconstrictor and increases TPR. In addition, it stimulates the adrenal gland to produce aldosterone, which promotes sodium and water retention, thereby increasing extracellular fluid volume. Recent evidence suggests that angiotensin II also stimulates growth of vascular smooth muscle and may contribute to atherosclerosis and HTN.

Genetic Influences

The level of BP is strongly familial, and recent studies of rare genetic disorders affecting BP have led to the identification of genetic abnormalities associated with several rare forms of HTN. While these studies have been conducted, genetic polymorphisms have been discovered that may harbor genes contributing to primary HTN. To date, none of these genetic abnormalities has been shown, either alone or in joint combination, to be responsible for a clinically significant portion of HTN in the general population; however, research in the area continues (NHBPEP, 2003).

Although 90 to 95 percent of all cases of HTN are primary in nature with no identifiable cause, there are identifiable causes of HTN in which a cure may be effected by appropriate diagnosis and treatment. JNC-7 discusses the laboratory test and diagnostic procedures useful in diagnosing these disorders and common clinical signs and symptoms associated with them. The reader is referred to that document for discussion of secondary HTN. The focus of this chapter is on the diagnosis and management of primary hypertension.

Laboratory Tests and Other Diagnostic Procedures

Confirmation of a diagnosis of HTN is based on BP elevation documented at three different times. Standard measurement techniques including out-of-office or home blood pressure measurements should be used when confirming an initially elevated blood pressure and for all subsequent measures during follow-up and treatment (Institute for Clinical Systems Improvement [ICSI], 2008). Children over 3 years of age who are seen in a medical setting should have their BP measured at least once during every health-care visit. The preferred method for children is auscultation; the correct measurement requires using a cuff that is appropriate to the size of the child's upper arm (NHBPEP Working Group on High Blood Pressure in Children, 2004)

JNC-7 (NHBPEP, 2003) recommends the following laboratory tests before initiating therapy:

1. A 12-lead ECG
2. Urinalysis, including urinary albumin or albumin/creatinine ratio. For those patients with diabetes or renal disease, the latter test of albumin should also be done annually. The presence of albuminuria, including microalbuminuria, even in the setting of normal glomerular filtration rate (gfr), is associated with increased cardiovascular risk
3. Blood glucose and hematocrit
4. Serum potassium
5. Creatinine or the corresponding estimated glomerular filtration rate (gfr). There is a strong relationship between decreased gfr and increases in cardiovascular morbidity and mortality.
6. Serum calcium
7. Lipid profile

Three emerging risk factors—(1) high-sensitivity C-reactive protein (HS-CRP), (2) homocysteine, and (3) elevated heart rate—may also be considered in patients with cardiovascular disease (CVD) but without other risk factors. Analysis of data from the Framingham Heart Study cohort (Ridker, Rifai, Rose, Buring, & Cook, 2002) demonstrated that those with an LDL-C value within the range associated with low CVD risk, but who had an elevated HS-CRP, had a higher risk of CVD compared to those with a low CRP and a high LDL-C. This was especially true in women (Ridker, Hennekens, Buring, & Rifai, 2000). Elevations in homocycteine have also been associated with higher CVD risk, but not as strongly as the HS-CRP (Parsons, Reaveley, Pavitt, & Brown, 2002). Treating elevated homocysteine has not resulted in decreased CVD risk, however.

Target-organ abnormalities are commonly associated with HTN in children and adolescents. Echocardiography is recommended as a primary tool for evaluating these age groups (NHBPEP Working Group on High Blood Pressure in Children and Adolescents, 2004).

Classification of Blood Pressure for Adults

Longitudinal data obtained from the Framingham Heart Study indicate that BP values in the 130 to 139/85 to 89 range are associated with a more than 2-fold increase in relative risk for CVD compared to those with BP below 120/80 (Vasan et al, 2001). Other data suggest increased risk for values as low as 115/80. Based on new data about lifetime risk for hypertension and the increased risk for CVD associated with BP levels previously thought to be normal, the JNC-7 report has reclassified BP levels to include a new term: *prehypertension*. This level of BP ranges from 120 to 130 SBP and/or 80 to 89 diastolic blood pressure (DBP). Individuals in this classification may benefit from early intervention to adopt healthy lifestyles that might reduce BP, decrease the rate of progression to hypertensive levels as the individual ages, or prevent HTN completely.

Another change has been to reduce the total number of classifications from seven to five and to remove risk stratification based on target organ damage from the classification system. This revision combines categories in which the management protocols were very similar and makes the application of the protocols simpler. Table 40–1 shows the BP readings that fall into each of these categories. This classification is based on the average of two or more properly measured, seated BP readings on each of two or more office visits.

PHARMACODYNAMICS

Because primary HTN has no identifiable cause, the treatment necessarily depends on interfering with normal physiological mechanisms that regulate BP. Six classes of drugs lower BP through this interference. **Diuretics** lower BP by depleting the body of sodium and reducing extracellular fluid volume. Agents that act in the renin-angiotensin-aldosterone (R-A-A) system reduce pressure by decreasing sodium and water retention (aldosterone action), by decreasing vasoconstriction (angiotensin direct action), and by increasing vasodilation (bradykinin action). **Adrenergic blockers** and other drugs acting on the SNS lower blood pressure by reducing peripheral vascular resistance, inhibiting cardiac contractility, and increasing venous pooling in capacitance vessels. **Calcium channel blockers** act as **vasodilators** to reduce pressure by relaxing vascular smooth muscle, thereby dilating resistance vessels and increasing the area over which blood must flow and through their negative inotropic activity to reduce cardiac output. Direct **vasodilators** produce the same effect as the **calcium channel blockers** on vascular smooth muscle. Centrally acting agents produce vasodilation mainly through reduction in **norepinephrine.** The latter two classes are used only in specific situations in which other classes are not appropriate. It is unusual that treatment with any one drug class can achieve blood pressure goal and so combinations of two or more drug classes are common. More detailed pharmacokinetics and pharmacodynamics of each of these classes of drugs are discussed in Chapters 14 and 16.

GOALS OF TREATMENT

The positive relationship between hypertension and cardiovascular risk has been long established. "The relationship between BP and risk of CVD events is continuous, consistent, and independent of other risk factors" (Chobanian et al, 2003, p. 1211). The presence of each additional risk factor compounds the risk from HTN. Figure 40–2 shows the 10-year risk for coronary heart disease (CHD) related to the major risk factors of total serum cholesterol, serum high-density lipid (HDL) level, smoking, diabetes, and left ventricular hypertrophy. Easy and rapid calculation of a Framingham CHD risk score using published tables may assist in demonstrating the benefits of treatment to patients. These tables can be accessed on the Web at http://www.nhlbi.nih.gov/. The first goal of HTN management is reduction in cardiovascular risk. Management of other risk factors is essential and should follow the established guidelines for controlling coexisting problems that contribute to cardiovascular risk. A positive relationship has also been shown between HTN and end-organ damage to the eyes, brain, and kidneys. The second goal is prevention of this end-organ damage. To meet these two goals, the following are needed:

1. Prevent the rise of BP with age. The prevalence of HTN increases with advancing age (see the Pathophysiology section above) to the point at which more than 50 percent of adults aged 60 to 69 years and 75 percent of those aged 70 years and older have HTN. The age-related rise in SBP is the primary cause for this increase.

Table 40–1 **JNC-7 Blood Pressure Classifications and Management**

Classification	Systolic BP (mm Hg)	Diastolic BP (mm Hg)	Lifestyle Modification	No Compelling Indication (Drug Therapy)	Compelling Indication (Drug Therapy)
Normal	<120	<80	Encourage	No antihypertensive drug	Drug for compelling indication
Prehypertension	120–139	8–89	Yes	No antihypertensive drug	Drug for compelling indication
Hypertension stage 1	140–159	90–99	Yes	Thiazide-type diuretic for most. May consider ACEI, ARB, BB, CCB, or combination	Drug(s) for compelling indication Other antihypertensive drugs
Hypertension stage 2	≥160	≥100	Yes	Two-drug combinations for most. Usually thiazide-type diuretic and ACEI or ARB, or BB or CCB	Drug(s) for compelling indication Other antihypertensive drugs (ACE, ARB, BB, CCB) as needed

ACEI = angiotinsen-converting enzyme inhibitor; ARB = angiotensin receptor blocker; BB = beta blocker; CCB = calcium channel blocker.
Source: Chobanian, A., Bakris, G., Black, H., Cushman, W., Green, L., Izzo, J., et al, National High Blood Pressure Coordinating Committee. (2003). Seventh Report of the Joint National Committee on Prevention, Detection, Evaluation, and Treatment of High Blood Pressure. *Journal of the American Medical Association, 289,* 2560–2571.

2. Improve control of HTN to below 140/90 mm Hg. Treating HTN to this target is associated with a decreased in cardiovascular disease complications (Hansson et al, 1998). In patients with concurrent HTN and diabetes or renal disease, the BP goal is less than 129/79 mm Hg (American Diabetes Association, 2003; National Kidney Foundation Guideline, 2002).
3. Increase recognition of the importance of controlling isolated systolic hypertension (ISH), as it is the most lethal hypertensive phenotype. Because most persons with HTN, especially those older than 50 years, will achieve control of their DBP once the SBP goal is reached, the primary focus should be on obtaining the SBP goal.
4. Improve recognition of the importance of prehypertension on the development of HTN. Although prehypertension is not a disease category, individuals with SBP between 120 and 139 mm Hg and DBP between 80 and 89 mm Hg have a significantly higher risk for developing HTN, and early recognition of this risk can result in lifestyle modifications that may prevent or delay the development of HTN.
5. Reduce ethnic, socioeconomic, and regional variations in HTN.
6. Improve opportunities for well-tolerated, affordable treatment options, including lifestyle modifications and pharmacological treatment.

Barriers to Goal Achievement

These goals are attainable for a large percentage of patients with HTN with the treatment regimens recommended by the JNC-7. Barriers to achievement of these goals include insufficient health education by health-care providers, lack of reimbursement for health education services, and lack of healthy food choices in many schools, worksites, and restaurants. Another factor is nonadherence to the treatment regimen. Chapter 8 focuses on factors that address these and other barriers to health. This chapter discusses treatment regimens that can enable people to control their BP. The diagnosis and clinical evaluation of HTN are discussed in some detail in the JNC-7 report, and the reader is encouraged to obtain and use that information. Specific recommendations in this chapter are taken from or are consistent with the information in that report.

RATIONAL DRUG SELECTION

Hypertension presents a unique problem in therapeutic management. It is usually a lifelong disease but is asymptomatic until end-organ damage occurs. For this reason, providers often find themselves prescribing lifestyle modifications or drugs that have disturbing adverse reactions to treat a problem that does not make the patient feel ill. For effective management, the choice of treatment should be low in cost, limited in complexity, and with the fewest possible adverse reactions. To achieve this treatment protocol, management is based on classification of HTN, the presence of risk factors, and specific patient variables. For each of these management variables, this chapter discusses lifestyle management, and stepped therapy, including initial monotherapy, stepping up to multiple drugs, and stepping down when possible.

Algorithm for Management of Hypertension

Lifestyle Modifications

Thirty to 65 percent of patients with HTN are obese, a problem frequently compounded by high sodium intake, sedentary lifestyle, and excessive use of alcohol (American Association of Clinical Endocrinologists [AACE] Hypertension Task Force, 2006). Lifestyle modifications directed

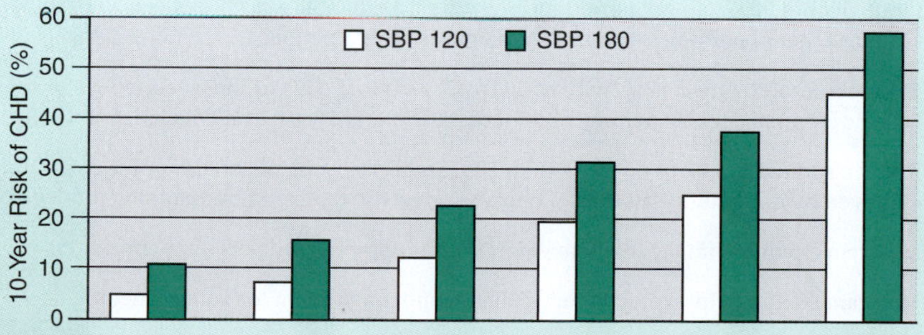

Cholesterol	180	240	240	240	240	240
HDL	50	50	35	35	35	35
Smoking	No	No	No	Yes	Yes	Yes
Diabetes	No	No	No	No	Yes	Yes
LVH	No	No	No	No	No	Yes

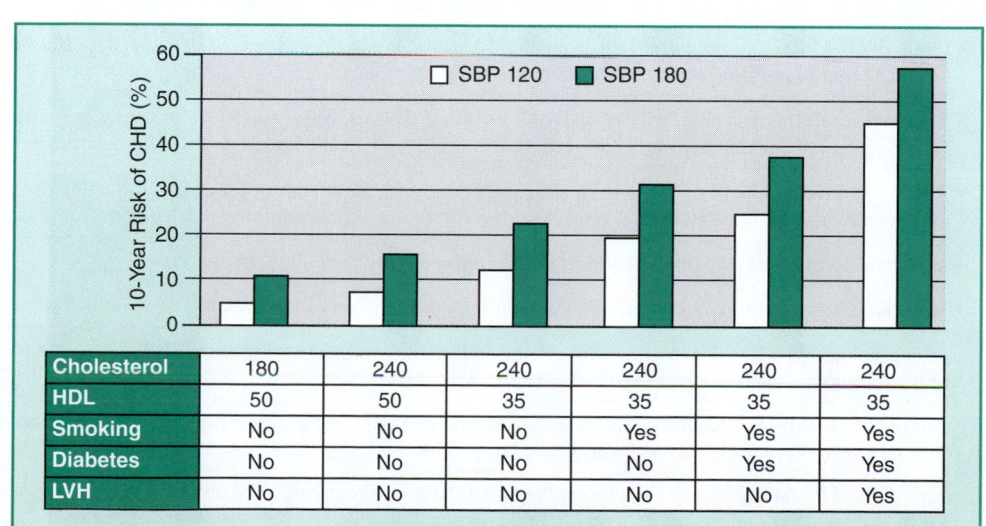

Figure 40–2. Ten-year risk for CHD by SBP and presence of other risk factors. *(Source: Adapted from Anderson, K., Wilson, P., Odell. P., & Kannel, W. [1991]. An updated coronary risk profile: A statement for health professionals.* Circulation, *83, 356–362.)*

at correcting these contributing factors may benefit the patient regardless of the primary course of the HTN and are an important part of first-line therapy. Multiple well-controlled trials have shown that a weight loss of as little as 5 to 10 kg can have a significant beneficial effect on HTN (AACE, 2006).

Treatment of HTN should include lifestyle modifications for all treatment groups, but this is especially true for those with prehypertension. Patients with prehypertension are not candidates for drug therapy based on their level of BP, but should be "firmly and unambiguously advised to practice lifestyle modification in order to reduce their risk for developing hypertension in the future" (Chobanian et al, 2003). Table 40–2 summarizes the lifestyle modifications recommended in JNC-7. Lifestyle modifications reduce BP, prevent or delay the onset of HTN, improve the efficacy of any drug therapy, and decrease cardiovascular risk. Combining two or more lifestyle modifications can achieve better results than one alone.

Stepped Therapy

Patients with all stages of HTN and those with prehypertension who are not able to achieve a BP below 140/90 mm Hg (less than 130/80 mm Hg for those with diabetes or chronic renal disease) require drug therapy. Once the decision is made to begin drug therapy, initial drug choices are based on the presence or absence of compelling indications from concurrent disease processes. Figure 40–3 shows the treatment protocol for hypertension management based on JNC-7 recommendations.

As a general rule, the following steps can lead to achieving the goal level of BP:

1. Set an appropriate minimum therapeutic BP goal based on individual patients and their compelling indications.
2. Be patient and work on attaining the BP goal over many weeks to months. Moving to lower BP quickly is more likely to produce side effects to the drugs that lead to nonadherence. There is no evidence that faster is better.
3. Titrate BP medications no more often than every 4 to 6 weeks. The body needs time to demonstrate full response to the drug.
4. Do not automatically assume symptoms reported by patients are caused by the drug. What may appear to be adverse responses may have other reasons for occurrence. Assigning all symptoms to drug effects may result in changing a drug that is actually working well. Antihypertensive drugs alleviate more adverse responses than they cause.
5. Plan at the beginning of therapy for the use of more than one drug. A single drug is not likely to provide BP control to goal level if the patient is more than 15/10 mm Hg higher than the goal. Explaining to the patient early in treatment the likelihood of more than one drug decreases the risk for nonadherence.
6. Do not ignore ISH in the elderly. Treat to goal SBP in older adults even if DBP is normal, but go more slowly.
7. Extracellular fluid volume must be controlled during any antihypertensive drug therapy in order to achieve BP goals. Include a **diuretic** in any treatment regimen that includes more than one agent.

(Adapted from: Advanstar Medical Economics Healthcare Communications [2004] Reducing cardiovascular risk factors, *Patient Care for the Nurse Practitioner: A CE Activity.* Sponsored by Pfizer Inc.)

Initial Drug Therapy

For most patients, the lowest dose of the initial drug should be used to prevent adverse reactions and too much or too

Table 40–2 **Lifestyle Modifications**

• Lose weight. Loss of as little as 10 lb may significantly reduce blood pressure.
• Limit alcohol intake to no more than 1 oz (30 mL) ethanol (e.g., 24 oz beer, 10 oz wine, 2 oz 100-proof whiskey) per day or 0.5 oz (15 mL) ethanol per day for women and lighter-weight people.
• Increase aerobic physical activity to 30 to 45 min most days of the week. Obese or low-activity patients may need to start with as little as 3 min of activity per day and increase the activity by 1 min each day until the desired 30 to 45 min is achieved.
• Reduce sodium intake to no more than 100 mmol (2,400 mg of sodium or 6 g of sodium chloride) per day. This can often be achieved by not adding salt during cooking or on the table and by watching hidden sources of salt such as canned foods.
• Maintain adequate intake of dietary potassium (approximately 90 mmol per day).
• Maintain adequate intake of dietary calcium and magnesium for general health.
• Stop smoking. The low doses of nicotine found in nicotine replacement therapy (NRT) do not significantly affect blood pressure, and NRT may be used as needed to aid in smoking cessation.
• Adopt the Dietary Approaches to Stop Hypertension (DASH) diet, which is high in fruits, vegetables, and low-fat dairy products as well as low in dietary cholesterol, saturated fat, and total fat.

Source: Adapted from the National High Blood Pressure Education Program. (2003). *Seventh Report of the Joint National Committee on Prevention, Detection, Evaluation, and Treatment of High Blood Pressure.* Rockville, MD: National Institutes of Health, National Heart, Lung and Blood Institute.

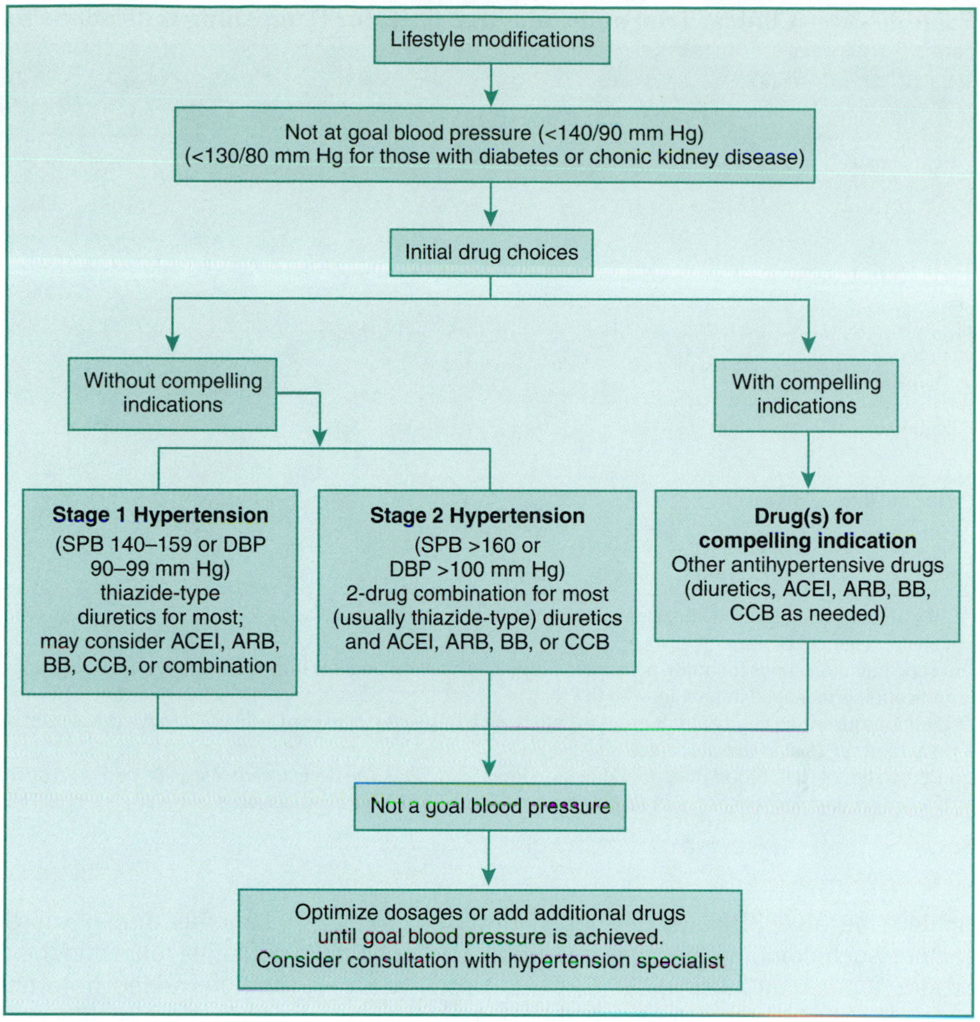

Figure 40–3. Algorithm for Treatment of Hypertension. *(Source: Chobanian, A., Bakris, G., Black, H., et al, National High Blood Pressure Coordinating Committee. [2003]. Seventh Report of the Joint National Committee on Prevention, Detection, Evaluation, and Treatment of High Blood Pressure.* Journal of the American Medical Association, *289, 2560–2571.)*

abrupt a reduction in blood pressure. The dose is then slowly titrated upward, based on patient response. If BP remains uncontrolled after 1 to 2 months, the next dosage level should be prescribed. The ideal drug should provide 24 hours of efficacy with at least 50 percent of the peak effect remaining at the end of the 24 hours. Long-acting formulations are preferred over short acting because (1) adherence is better with once-daily dosing; (2) for many agents, fewer tablets mean lower cost; (3) control of hypertension is smoother; and (4) the risk of sudden death, heart attack, and stroke because of abrupt changes in blood pressure is lessened.

When the decision is made to begin drug therapy and there are no clear indications for another type of drug, a **thiazide-type diuretic** should be chosen because in randomized controlled trials (RCT) comparing **diuretics** with other classes of **antihypertensive** drugs, **diuretics** have been unsurpassed in preventing cardiovascular complications of HTN (ALLHAT Officers and Coordinators, 2002; Wright et al, 2009). Chapter 16 discusses specific **diuretics** and their appropriate use and dosing. In general, the lowest dose that achieves the target BP is best, because higher doses are more likely to produce more potassium loss without significant improvement in BP control. The choice of **diuretic** should be based on level of kidney function. For estimated glomerular filtration rates (EGFR) higher than the mid 40 mL/minute range, a **thiazide diuretic** should be used, as **loop diuretics** are not as effective as **thiazides** in this setting. For EGFRs that are lower than the mid 40 mL/minute range, **loop diuretics**, sometimes in combination with **metolazone**, are more appropriate and are most effective when dosed twice daily.

There are compelling indications for specific other agents, also based on RCTs. Table 40–3 depicts the drug choices appropriate for compelling indications. **Angiotensin-converting enzyme (ACE) inhibitors**, for example, are drugs of choice in diabetes mellitus, heart failure, and myocardial infarction (MI). Other concomitant diseases that may affect the choice of drugs are discussed later.

Monotherapy is acceptable when it controls HTN because adherence is likely to be better, cost is lower, and adverse reactions are apt to be fewer. However, most hypertensive patients will require two or more drugs. Adding a second drug from a different class should be initiated when monotherapy in adequate doses does not

Table 40–3 **Clinical Trial and Guideline Basis for Compelling Indications for Individual Drug Classes**

	RECOMMENDED DRUGS						
Compelling Indication*	**Diuretic**	**BB**	**ACEI**	**ARB**	**CCB**	**Aldo ANT**	**Clinical Trial Basis†**
Heart failure	•	•	•	•		•	ACC/AHA Heart Failure Guideline, MERIT-HF, COPERNICUS, CIBIS, SOLVD, AIRE, TRACE, ValHEFT, RALES, CHARM
Post–myocardial infarction		•	•			•	ACC/AHA Post-MI Guideline, BHAT, SAVE, Capricom, EPHESUS
High risk of coronary disease	•	•	•		•		ALLHAT, HOPE, ANBP2, LIFE, CONVINCE, EUROPA, INVEST
Diabetes	•	•	•	•	•		NKF-ADA Guideline, UKPDS, ALLHAT
Chronic kidney disease			•	•			NKF Guideline, Captopril Trial, RENAAL, IDNT, REIN, AASK
Recurrent stroke prevention	•		•				PROGRESS

ACEI = angiotensin-converting enzyme inhibitor; Aldo ANT = aldosterone antagonist; ARB = angiotensin receptor blocker; BB = beta blocker; CCB = calcium channel blocker.

*Compelling indications for antihypertensive drugs are based on benefits from outcome studies or existing clinical guidelines; the compelling indication is managed in parallel with the BP.

†Conditions for which clinical trials demonstrate benefit of specific classes of antihypertensive drugs used as part of an antihypertensive regimen to achieve BP goal to test outcomes.

Source: National High Blood Pressure Education Program. (2003). *The Seventeenth Report of the Joint National Committee on Prevention, Detections, Evaluation, and Treatment of High Blood Pressure*. Rockville, MD: National Institutes of Health, National Heart, Lung and Blood Institute.

achieve the target BP. Newly developed formulations that include such combinations may permit the best of both worlds; the patient takes just one pill or capsule yet receives the benefit of two drugs, and the combination may cost less than the individual components prescribed separately. The downside is that fixed-dose ratios prevent customization of the regimen.

Some **antihypertensive drugs** are not well suited for monotherapy because they cause troublesome adverse reactions in almost all patients who take them. These drugs include **direct-acting smooth-muscle vasodilators, central alpha$_2$ agonists**, and **peripheral-adrenergic antagonists**. These drugs can be used effectively when combined with other drugs that address these adverse reactions.

When the patient's BP is more than 20 mm Hg above the systolic goal or 10 mm Hg above the diastolic goal, consideration should be given to initial therapy with two drugs, either as separate prescriptions or in fixed-dose combinations. Beginning therapy with more than one drug increases the chances of achieving target BP more rapidly and may produce more BP lowering at lower doses, resulting in fewer adverse responses. Older adults, those at risk for orthostatic hypotension (OH), and diabetics with autonomic dysfunction should have initial multidrug therapy begun with caution.

Stepping Up to Multiple Drugs

If the initial monotherapy drug choice is inadequate at that drug's full dose, two options are considered: addition of another drug or substitution by a different drug. If the patient is tolerating the first choice well, a second drug may be added from another class. The choice of the second drug is influenced by how it might affect the adverse reaction profile of the first drug or by how well these drugs have been shown to work together in clinical studies. An adequate dose of **hydralazine** results in compensatory tachycardia and salt and water retention. The addition of a **beta-adrenergic blocker** prevents the tachycardia, and the addition of a **diuretic** prevents salt and water retention. An **ACE inhibitor** and a **nondihydropyridine calcium channel blocker** may reduce proteinuria in a patient with diabetes better than either drug alone.

If a **diuretic** was not chosen as the first drug, it is usually indicated as the second-step drug because its addition will enhance the effects of most other agents. If the patient is having significant adverse reactions or no response from the initial drug, an agent from another class is substituted. For example, a persistent cough may be annoying enough that a patient will not continue to take an **ACE inhibitor.** Because they do not affect the kallikrein system, **angiotensin II receptor blockers (ARBs)** do not produce this cough, nor do they have the problem with angioedema that is a contraindication to the use of an **ACE inhibitor.** Because the hemodynamic effects are similar, an ARB may be substituted for the **ACE inhibitor.** Documentation of equal long-term cardiac and renal protection for patients with systolic dysfunction and diabetic nephropathy has now been demonstrated for some ARBs;

however, and to date, **ARBs** should be reserved for patients for whom **ACE inhibitors** are indicated but who are unable to tolerate them.

Stepping Down

Although HTN is generally accepted to be a lifelong disease, after it has been controlled effectively for at least 1 year, a decrease in the dosage and number of **antihypertensive drugs** should be considered. The reduction should be deliberate, slow, and progressive and accompanied by vigilant BP monitoring. Step-down therapy is often successful for patients who also are making lifestyle modifications. Any patient whose drugs have been discontinued should have regularly scheduled follow-up visits because BP usually rises again to hypertensive levels within months to years after the drugs have been stopped. This return of HTN is especially common in the absence of continued improvements in lifestyle. If adherence to lifestyle modifications is not likely, maintaining a low-dose **antihypertensive drug** may be preferable to complete discontinuance of all drugs.

Patient Variables

The prevalence of hypertension varies with age, race, education, and many other variables. The patient variables that affect the clinical use and dosing of **antihypertensive medications** include age, gender, race, and concomitant diseases and therapies.

Children and Adolescents

Definitions of hypertension in children and adolescents (age 1 year to 17 years) take into account age and height by sex. Blood pressure in the 90th to less than 95th percentile or if the blood pressure exceeds 120/90 (even if less than 90th percentile) is considered prehypertension in children. Blood pressure in the 95th to 99th percentile is considered hypertension stage 1 and greater than 99th percentile plus 5 mm HG is considered hypertension stage 2 (NHBPEP Working Group on High Blood Pressure in Children and Adolescents, 2004). Table 40–4 shows the values consistent with a diagnosis of hypertension for girls and boys based on age and height. An identifiable cause for the hypertension is more likely in younger children than it is in adults, and such causes should always be sought. Chronic HTN is becoming more common in adolescence and is generally associated with obesity, sedentary lifestyle and a positive family history of HTN and other CVDs. Like adults, children with HTN develop end-organ damage and appropriate assessment for this damage should occur.

Lifestyle modifications, especially weight management and increased physical activity, are initially used, with drug therapy reserved for higher levels of BP or for inadequate response to lifestyle modifications. Adolescents with BP below the 95th percentile should adopt healthy lifestyles similar to those of adults combating prehypertension. Although the choice of drugs is similar to that for adults, dosages should be smaller and adjusted very carefully in children. The U.S. Food and Drug Administration (FDA) recently published new guidelines for pediatric labeling including dosages; this information is published on the Internet at http://www.fda.gov/. The document includes several classes of **antihypertensive** drugs. The clinical use and dosing sections for these drugs, including the new FDA labeling for children's doses are in Chapters 14 and 16. **ACE inhibitors** and **ARBs** should not be prescribed for pregnant or sexually active girls because of their teratogenic effects.

According to the *Seventh Report of the Joint National Committee on the Prevention, Detection, Evaluation, and Treatment of High Blood Pressure* (NHBPEP, 2003), uncomplicated HTN alone is not sufficient reason to restrict asymptomatic children from participating in physical activities because exercise may actually lower blood pressure and prevent HTN. Detailed recommendations regarding HTN in children and adolescents can be found in the Fourth Report of on the Diagnosis, Evaluation, and Treatment of High Blood Pressure in Children and Adolescents (2004) by the National High Blood Pressure Education Program (NHBPEP).

Older Adults

The number of Americans aged 65 and older has increased from 24.2 million to 32.6 million from 1980 to 2000

Table 40–4 **Blood Pressure Readings Consistent With Hypertension in Children and Adolescents (mm Hg)**

Age (Years)	Girls (50th Percentile for Height)	Girls (75th Percentile for Height)	Boys (50th Percentile for Height)	Boys (75th Percentile for Height)
1	104/58	104/58	105/59	102/57
6	115/75	111/73	112/73	114/74
12	123/80	124/81	123/81	125/82
17	129/84	130/85	136/87	138/88

Source: Adapted from the Report by the NHBPEP Working Group on Hypertension Control in Children and Adolescents. From the National High Blood Pressure Education Program, (2003). *Seventh Report of the Joint National Committee on Prevention, Detection, Evaluation, and Treatment of High Blood Pressure*. Rockville, MD: National Institutes of Health, National Heart, Lung and Blood Institute.

and is expected to continue to rise (U.S. Census Bureau, 2002). Hypertension is very common in older adults, occurring in 60 to 71 percent of the population older than 60 years. Among older adults, SBP increases almost linearly with age and is a better predictor of coronary heart disease (CHD), cardiovascular disease (CVD), heart failure, end-stage renal disease (ESRD), and all-cause mortality than is DBP, which increases until about age 55 and then declines. An even better predictor is pulse pressure (SBP minus DBP), which indicates reduced vascular compliance in large arteries. Evidence of this increased risk has led to recognition of the importance of treating isolated systolic hypertension (ISH) in older adults rather than accepting increased blood pressure as a "normal" part of aging. Currently, BP control rates (less than 140/90 mm Hg) are only about 20 percent in older adults with HTN, largely related to poor control of SBP. Benefits of treatment in this age group have been consistently demonstrated in large RCTs (Staessen et al, 1997; Staessen et al, 2000; Systolic Hypertension in the Elderly Cooperative Research Group, 1991). Analysis of multiple treatment trials indicates that the choice of initial agent is less important than the degree of BP reduction achieved (Neal, MacMahon, & Chapman, 2000).

As in younger patients, therapy should begin with lifestyle modifications. Older adults respond especially well to reduced salt intake and weight loss because they are prone to sodium retention and volume excess. In the Trial of Nonpharmacologic Interventions in the Elderly (TONE), reducing sodium to 2000 mg/day reduced BP over 30 months, and about 40 percent of those on the low-salt diet were able to discontinue their **antihypertensive** drugs (Appel et al, 2001). If lifestyle modifications do not achieve the BP goal, drug therapy should begin. In general, the initial dose should be about half that used in younger patients. Use of specific drugs is similar to that recommended in the general algorithm and for individuals with compelling reasons. **Thiazide diuretics** and **beta-adrenergic blockers** in combination with **diuretics** are recommended because they have been shown in RCTs to reduce morbidity and mortality and because they are less expensive for patients who are often on fixed incomes. While considering the comments on orthostatic hypotension below, **diuretics** are still the drugs of choice. **Thiazide diuretics** are particularly useful for ISH because of their greater effects on SBP than on DBP. Morbidity and mortality are both improved in older adults when SBP is reduced, while DBP is held stable at between 85 and 90 mm Hg. It is important to monitor potassium levels with the drugs, especially if the patient is also on digitalis. Even mild hypokalemia may be problematic for older adults with coronary artery disease (CAD). Drug combinations that include both a **thiazide diuretic** and a **potassium-sparing diuretic** are useful for patients who have repeated episodes of hypokalemia.

The BP goal for older adults is the same as it is for younger patients, below 140/90 mm Hg. Any reduction in BP has some benefit, and the closer to the ideal goal, the better. Additional recommendations can be found in the report by the NHBPEP Working Group on Hypertension in the Elderly that is discussed in the JNC-7 document. Special considerations should be given to problems with OH and cognitive dysfunction related to older adults.

Orthostatic Hypotension (OH)

Measurement of BP in older adults requires consideration of the possibility of pseudohypertension caused by excessive vascular stiffness. In addition, older adults are more likely to experience orthostatic changes, and their BP should always be measured standing as well as in the lying position. OH is associated with an increase in age-adjusted mortality and there is a strong correlation between OH and premature death as well as increased numbers of falls and fractures. Severe volume depletion, baroreflex dysfunction, and autonomic insufficiency are common causes in older adults. Certain vasodilator **antihypertensives** (e.g., **alpha blockers** and **alpha beta blockers**) as well as **diuretics** and **nitrates** may exacerbate this problem. Health-care providers should be alert to potential OH symptoms and adjust drug therapy accordingly.

Cognitive Dysfunction and Dementia

Cognitive impairment and dementia occur more commonly in people with HTN. Reduced progression of cognitive impairment may occur with effective treatment of the HTN. Narrowing and sclerosis of small penetrating arteries in the subcortical regions of the brain are often found on autopsy of patients with chronic HTN. These changes may contribute to hypoperfusion, loss of autoregulation, compromise of the blood–brain barrier and white matter demyelination, microinfarction, and cognitive decline. In the SystEUR trial (Forette et al, 1998), **calcium channel blocker** therapy was superior to placebo in slowing the decline of cognitive function, but there was no comparative data with other drug classes. It does appear that **central alpha$_2$ agonists** make cognitive dysfunction worse and so should be avoided or, if there is a compelling reason for their use, used with extreme caution.

Women

Although there are no demonstrated clinical differences between men and women related to BP outcomes or responses to therapy, women do have some unique variables related to hypertension: sexual dimorphism of BP and HTN prevalence, menopause, use of oral contraceptives and hormone replacements, and pregnancy.

Sexual Dimorphism and HTN Prevalence

Women have lower SBP levels than men during early adulthood, but the opposite is true after the sixth decade (Rosenthal & Oparil, 2000). The prevalence of HTN in women follows this dimorphism. The highest prevalence of HTN occurs in elderly black women, with the rate being more than 75 percent in black women older than 75 years.

Menopause

The effect of menopause on BP is controversial. Longitudinal studies have not shown a rise in BP, whereas cross-sectional studies have found significantly higher SBP and DBP in postmenopausal women versus premenopausal women. When there is a rise, it is often attributed to **estrogen** withdrawal, overproduction of pituitary hormones, weight gain, or a combination of these or other undefined neurohormonal influence. Studies of **hormone replacement therapy (HRT)** in postmenopausal women have been inconsistent in findings about changes in BP. Overall, HRT-related change in BP is mainly modest and JNC-7 states that it "should not preclude hormone use in normotensive or hypertensive women" (Chobanian et al, 2003).

Oral Contraceptives

Women taking **oral contraceptives** have a small but detectable increase in both SBP and DBP, but these are usually within the normal range. Relative risk for HTN is significantly increased (RR = 1.8) in current users compared to those who have never used **oral contraceptives**. A strong correlation has also been found in HTN risk for women who smoke and take **oral contraceptives**. Women older than 35 years who smoke should be discouraged from using **oral contraceptives** and highly encouraged to stop smoking. If HTN develops in women taking **oral contraceptives**, then the drugs should be discontinued. Blood pressure usually returns to normal in a few months. If HTN continues, therapy for HTN should be begun. **Oral contraceptives** are often prescribed on a yearly basis, but a more prudent approach may be to prescribe them semiannually so that BP can be checked every 6 months.

Pregnancy

Hypertensive disorders in pregnancy are a major cause of maternal, fetal, and neonatal morbidity and mortality. Hypertension during pregnancy is classified into five categories:

1. **Chronic hypertension.** Hypertension that is present and observable before pregnancy or diagnosed before the 20th week of pregnancy. The goal of management for chronic HTN in pregnant women is to minimize short-term risks while avoiding therapy that compromises the fetus. Women in stage 1 HTN are considered at low risk for cardiovascular complications during pregnancy and are best managed by lifestyle modifications only, although aerobic exercise should be limited, and weight reduction should not be attempted, even in obese pregnant women. A meta-analysis of 45 RCTs of treatment with a variety of antihypertensives in stage1 and stage 2 HTN in pregnancy showed a direct relationship between treatment-induced drops in mean arterial pressure and the proportion of small-for-gestational-age infants (von Dadelszen et al, 2000). It appears judicious to carefully consider whether to continue **antihypertensive drugs** during pregnancy unless the pregnant woman has target organ damage or requires multiple **antihypertensive drugs** to control BP. In all cases, treatment should be reinstituted if the BP reaches 150 to 160 systolic or 100 to 110 diastolic. Drug selection is then based on the safety of the fetus. Table 40–5 summarizes the treatment options. **Methyldopa** has been studied the most and is recommended for women whose chronic hypertension is first diagnosed in pregnancy. **Beta-adrenergic blockers** are equally effective and are safe during the second and third trimesters, but their use in the first trimester has been associated with growth retardation in the fetus. **Labetalol** is equally effective as **methyldopa** and has fewer side effects. If the hypertension is diagnosed before the pregnancy, **diuretics** and many other **antihypertensives** may be continued. Chapters 14 and 16 delineate safety issues in pregnancy for various drugs used to treat hypertension. **ACE inhibitors** and **ARBs** should never be used in pregnancy because of their teratogenic effects.
2. **Preeclampsia.** Preeclampsia is a pregnancy-specific condition. It involves HTN and proteinuria (greater than 300 mg/24 h) after 20 weeks' gestation. Preeclampsia rarely disappears on its own and usually worsens with time. It may be superimposed on existing chronic hypertension. Because of the risk for development of eclampsia, treatment includes bedrest (although strict bedrest is not recommended) (Magee, Helewa, Moutquin, & von Dadelszen, 2008), control of BP, seizure prophylaxis, and timely delivery. **Antihypertensive therapy** is prescribed only for maternal safety because it does not improve perinatal outcomes and may adversely affect utero-placental blood flow. Drug selection depends on time of delivery. If delivery is more than 48 hours away, **methyldopa, labetalol,** or **calcium channel blockers** are acceptable. If delivery is imminent, **parenteral agents** such as **hydralazine** or **labetalol** may be used.
3. **Chronic HTN with superimposed preeclampsia.** This classification is treated as in number 1.
4. **Gestational HTN.** This classification involves HTN without proteinuria occurring after 20 weeks gestation. It is a temporary diagnosis and requires careful monitoring as it may evolve into preeclampsia. Some bedrest may be useful, but there is insufficient evidence to make a recommendation about the usefulness of salt restriction (Magee, et al, 2008).
5. **Transient HTN.** This is a retrospective diagnosis and BP is normal by 12 week postpartum. It may be predictive of future primary HTN (NHBPEP, 2000).

Table 40–5 **Antihypertensives Recommended in Pregnancy**

The report of the NHBPEP Working Group on High Blood Pressure in Pregnancy permits continuation of drug therapy in women with chronic hypertension (except for angiotensin-converting enzyme [ACE] inhibitors). In addition, angiotensin II receptor blockers should not be used during pregnancy. In women with chronic hypertension with diastolic levels of 100 mm Hg or greater (lower when end-organ damage or underlying renal disease is present) and in women with acute hypertension when levels are 150 mm Hg or greater, the following drugs are recommended:

Recommended Drug	Comments
Alpha beta blockers	Labetalol (C) is equally effective as methyldopa but has fewer adverse responses.
Beta blockers	Atenolol (C) and metoprolol (C) appear to be safe and effective in late pregnancy; labetalol (C) also appears to be effective.
Calcium antagonists	Potential synergism with magnesium sulfate may lead to precipitous hypotension (C).
Central alpha agonists	Methyldopa (C) is the recommended drug of choice
Direct vasodilators	Hydralazine (C) is the parenteral drug of choice, based on its long history of safety and efficacy.
Diuretics	Diuretics (C) are recommended for chronic hypertension if prescribed before gestation or if patients appear to be salt-sensitive; they are not recommended in preeclampsia.

ACE inhibitors (D) and angiotensin II receptor blockers (D) may result in fetal abnormalities including death; these drugs should not be used in pregnancy.

Pregnancy Category C = adverse effects in animals; no controlled trials in humans; use it risk appears justified. Pregnancy Category D = positive evidence of fetal risk.

Source: From the National High Blood Pressure Education Program, (2003). *Seventh Report of the Joint National Committee on Prevention, Detection, Evaluation, and Treatment of High Blood Pressure.* Rockville, MD: National Institutes of Health. National Heart, Lung and Blood Institute.

Racial and Ethnic Minorities

The prevalence of HTN and the degree of control to target BP among different racial and ethnic groups varies (Hajjar & Kotchen, 2003). Native Americans have the same or slightly higher prevalence rates than does the white population. Hispanics have the same to slightly lower prevalence rates, despite their increased incidence of obesity and type 2 diabetes mellitus. Asians have about the same prevalence and appear to be more responsive to antihypertensive drugs than whites. The prevalence of hypertension in African Americans is among the highest in the world and an estimated 30 percent of all deaths in this population are attributable to HTN. Hypertension develops at younger ages than it does in whites, and the average BP is much higher than it is in the whites. They also have a higher rate of severe hypertension and more end-organ damage from their hypertension. Their stroke rate is 80 percent higher, their heart disease mortality is 50 percent higher, and their hypertension-related ESRD is 320 percent higher than that of the general population. The comorbidity of type 2 diabetes and HTN is particularly true in African Americans, among whom up to 14 percent of adults may have both disorders (AACE, 2006). This has led the International Society on Hypertension in Blacks to publish a consensus statement dealing with these issues (Douglas et al, 2003).

The underlying pathology associated with hypertension in African Americans is thought to be salt sensitivity. In general, this population has low **renin** activity, and so the R-A-A system is thought not to play a major role. This increased sensitivity to salt, along with the high prevalence in this population of obesity, cigarette smoking, and type 2 diabetes mellitus, means that lifestyle modifications are especially efficacious. Salt intake should be reduced to less than 6 g per day, and weight should be reduced, if necessary, to approach ideal body weight. If these modifications do not result in achievement of the BP goal, **diuretics** have been proved in RCTs to reduce morbidity and mortality and are the first agents of choice unless there are compelling reasons to choose another drug class. **Calcium channel blockers** are also effective in this population. Monotherapy with **ACE inhibitors** is less effective because of the low **renin** activity. In the presence of diabetes mellitus, however, **ACE inhibitors** should be used. Monotherapy with **beta-adrenergic blockers** is also less effective but may be used for post-MI patients. The interracial differences in BP-lowering observed with any drug class are abolished when the drugs is combined with a **diuretic.** Despite noted differences in BP response at the population level, race alone is a poor predictor of BP response to any particular class of drugs if they are given in adequate doses and with sufficient time to work.

The high prevalence of stage 2 hypertension in the African American population means that they frequently require multidrug therapy, which may result in a higher prevalence of adverse responses. For the proportion of African Americans who do not trust the white-dominated medical system, these adverse effects—related to drugs that treat a disease that exists for them only because a medical device (the blood pressure cuff) tells them they have it—increase their distrust, especially when these adverse responses include personal problems such as impotence. All possible steps should be taken to deal with adherence issues in this population, with consideration for cultural ramifications.

Racial differences in adverse responses to antihypertensive drugs may occur even in monotherapy. African Americans and Asians, for example, have a 3- to 4-fold higher risk of angioedema (ALLHAT, 2002; Brown, Ray, Snowden, & Griffin, 1996; Wright, 2009) and more cough has been attributed to **ACE inhibitors** than it has in whites (Elliot, 1996). Unfortunately, insufficient numbers of Mexican Americans and other Hispanic Americans, Native Americans, or Asian/Pacific Islanders have been included in most of the major clinical trials to make strong recommendations about their responses to individual **antihypertensives.**

Adherence to dietary recommendations also may vary by ethnicity. In a study of nearly 6,000 adults aged 45 to 84 years, there was a significant variation in Dietary Approaches to Stop Hypertension (DASH) goal attainment among ethnic groups (Gao et al, 2009). Chinese Americans were more likely to meet cholesterol goals, but less likely to meet magnesium and potassium goals. African Americans and Hispanics had problems with calcium intake and had less goal attainment related to saturated fat and magnesium.

Concomitant Diseases and Therapies

Antihypertensive drugs may improve the management of some diseases and worsen that of others (Table 40–6). Selection of an **antihypertensive** that also treats a concomitant disease can simplify the overall therapeutic regimen, reduce cost, and increase the likelihood of adherence. It is not within the scope of this book to discuss all possible diseases that may coexist with HTN, but the most common diseases that benefit from appropriate selection of an antihypertensive are discussed here.

Cerebrovascular Disease

The risk of complications of cerebrovascular disease, including CVA and dementia, increases as a function of BP levels. Most ischemic strokes occur in individuals with prehypertension or stage 1 HTN. No specific drug has been proven to be clinically superior to all others for stroke prevention. Management of BP during an acute stroke remains controversial. BP elevated in the immediate poststroke period is thought by some to be a compensatory physiological response to improve cerebral perfusion. It is, therefore, common practice to initially withhold therapy until the patient is stable, and then treatment is instituted with a goal to reduce BP gradually. Specific guidelines are

Table 40–6 **Drug Choice Based on Concomitant Disease States**

Disease State	Drug Choice
Compelling Indications Unless Contraindicated	
Diabetes mellitus (type 1) with proteinuria	ACE inhibitors
Heart failure	ACE inhibitors Diuretics
Isolated systolic hypertension (older adults)	Diuretics (preferred) CA (long-acting DHP)
Myocardial infarction	Beta blockers (non-ISA) ACE inhibitors (with systolic dysfunction)
May Have Favorable Effects on Comorbid Conditions	
Angina	Beta blockers CA
Atrial tachycardia and fibrillation CA (non-DHP)	Beta blockers CA (non-DHP)
Cyclosporine-induced hypertension (caution with the dose of cyclosporine)	CA
Diabetes mellitus (types 1 and 2) with proteinuria	ACE inhibitors (preferred) CA
Diabetes mellitus (type 2)	Diuretics (low dose)
Dyslipidemia	Alpha blockers
Essential tremor	Beta blockers (non-CS)
Heart failure	Carvedilol Losartan potassium

Continued

Table 40–6 **Drug Choice Based on Concomitant Disease States—cont'd**

Disease State	Drug Choice
Hyperthyroidism	Beta blockers
Migraine	Beta blockers (non-CS) CA (non-DHP)
Myocardial infarction	Diltiazem hydrochloride Verapamil hydrochloride
Osteoporosis	Thiazides
Preoperative hypertension	Beta blockers
Prostatism (BPH)	Alpha blockers
Renal insufficiency (caution in renovascular hypertension and creatinine 265.2 mmol/L or higher [3 mg/dL])	ACE inhibitors
May Have Unfavorable Effects on Comorbid Conditions (May Be Used With Special Monitoring Unless Contraindicated)	
Bronchospastic disease	Beta blockers
Depression	Beta blockers Central alpha agonists Reserpine (contraindicated)
Diabetes mellitus (types 1 and 2)	Beta blockers Diuretics (high dose)
Dyslipidemia	Beta blockers (non-ISA) Diuretics (high dose)
Gout	Diuretics
Heart block (second and third degree)	Beta blockers (contraindicated) CA (non-DHP) (contraindicated)
Heart failure	Beta blockers (except carvedilol) CA (except amlodipine besylate, felodipine)
Liver disease	Labetalol hydrochloride Methyldopa (contraindicated)
Peripheral vascular disease	Beta blockers
Pregnancy	ACE inhibitors (contraindicated) Angiotensin II receptor blockers (contraindicated)
Renal insufficiency	Potassium-sparing agents
Renovascular disease	ACE inhibitors Angiotensin II receptor blockers

ACE = angiotensin-converting enzyme; CA = calcium channel blockers; CS = cardiac specific; DHP = dihydropyridine; non-ISA = nonintrinsic sympathomimetic action.

Source: From the National High Blood Pressure Education Program. (1997). *The Sixth Report of the Joint National Committee on Prevention, Detection, Evaluation, and Treatment of High Blood Pressure* (NIH Publ. No. 98–4080). Rockville, MD: National Institutes of Health, National Heart, Lung and Blood Institute.

provided by the American Stroke Association (Adams et al, 2003).

Coronary Artery Disease

Coexisting CAD and hypertension place patients at especially high risk for cardiovascular morbidity and mortality. Antihypertensive therapy is essential, and its benefits well established. Blood pressure should be reduced to a goal of 140/90 mm Hg, with lower BP desirable in patients with angina. Excessively rapid lowering of BP, however, may result in reflex tachycardia and sympathetic stimulation and should be avoided. Lowering DBP below 55 to 60 mm Hg also present problems and has been associated with increased cardiovascular events, including MI (Systolic Hypertension in the Elderly, 1991; University of Michigan Health System, 2009). Antihypertensive drugs that have reflex tachycardia and sympathetic stimulation as adverse reactions (**alpha-adrenergic blockers**, **nitrates**, and peripheral vasodilators) should also be avoided. Long-acting calcium channel blockers and beta-adrenergic blockers are especially helpful to patients with concomitant angina. Short-acting calcium channel blockers should not be used. After MI, beta-adrenergic blockers with intrinsic sympathomimetic activity are the drugs of choice because they reduce the risk of subsequent MI or sudden cardiac death. ACE inhibitors and ARBs are also useful after MI, especially with concomitant left ventricular (LV) dysfunction, to prevent heart failure and mortality.

Stable Angina and Silent Ischemia

Therapy in these disorders is directed toward preventing MI and death and reducing symptoms of angina and occurrence of ischemia. Unless contraindicated, drug therapy should begin with a beta-adrenergic blocker. Beta-adrenergic blockers reduce symptoms, improve mortality, and reduce cardiac output and heart rate, which decreases myocardial oxygen demand. If angina and BP are not controlled by beta-adrenergic blockers alone, or if these drugs are contraindicated, a long-acting calcium channel blocker may be used. These drugs decrease total peripheral resistance, which leads to reduction in BP and wall tension. Nondihydropyridine calcium channel blockers also decrease heart rate, but when combined with a beta-adrenergic blocker they may produce severe bradycardia or high degrees of heart block. Therefore, dihydropyridine calcium channel blockers are preferred for combination therapy with a beta-adrenergic blocker. If angina is still not controlled, a nitrate can be added. Chapter 28 further discusses the management protocol for angina.

Left Ventricular Hypertrophy

Left ventricular hypertrophy (LVH) is a cardiac adaptation to the increased afterload generated by persistent hypertension. LVH is a major independent risk factor for sudden cardiac death, MI, stroke, and other cardiovascular events. In addition to lifestyle modification with salt reduction and weight loss, antihypertensive drugs (except direct vasodilators such as hydralazine and minoxidil) are capable of reducing left ventricular mass and wall thickness and reducing cardiovascular risks. ACE inhibitors have been demonstrated to be the most effective in reducing LV mass in patients with LV hypertrophy, beta-adrenergic blockers had the least reduction in mass and intermediate effects occurred with diuretics and calcium channel blockers. The LIFE study demonstrated a reduction for the ARB losartan (Cozaar) similar to that of ACE inhibitors (Dahlof et al, 2002). Reduction of LV mass is associated with lower overall CVD risk. The combination of an ACE inhibitor and a diuretic has proved to be most effective in regressing LVH and reducing cardiovascular risks.

Heart Failure

Hypertension is the major cause of left ventricular failure in the United States. Control of BP with lifestyle modifications and drug therapy improves myocardial function and reduces the risk for heart failure and cardiovascular mortality. HTN precedes the development of heart failure in approximately 90 percent of patients and this is most important in African Americans and older adults. CAD is the cause of heart failure in approximately two-thirds of heart failure patients. A variety of neurohormonal systems, especially the R-A-A and SNS are activated by the LV dysfunction seen in heart failure. Such activation may lead to abnormal ventricular remodeling, further LV enlargement, and reduced cardiac contractility. This progression can be significantly reduced by effective therapy with ACE inhibitors alone or in conjunction with diuretics and beta-adrenergic blockers. Heart failure is a compelling indication for the use of ACE inhibitors. When ACE inhibitors are not well tolerated, the LIFE study (Dahlof et al, 2002) demonstrated that the ARB losartan (Cozaar) was equally effective alone or in the same combinations. The alpha and beta-adrenergic blocker carvedilol (Coreg) has also been shown to be beneficial when combined with an ACE inhibitor, but carvedilol is quite expensive. The dihydropyridines amlodipine (Norvasc) and felodipine (Plendil) have been demonstrated to be safe for treating angina and hypertension in patients with advanced left ventricular dysfunction when they are used in addition to ACE inhibitors, diuretics, or beta-adrenergic blockers, but other calcium channel blockers are not recommended for these patients. Aldosterone antagonists in low doses (12.5 to 25 mg daily) may provide additional benefits for patient with severe LV dysfunction. Chapter 36 discusses the treatment of heart failure in more detail.

Renal Parenchymal Disease

Hypertension may result from any form of renal disease that reduces the number of functioning nephrons, leading to salt and water retention and then to increased extracellular fluid (ECF) volume. Evaluation of renal function in hypertensive patients should include serum creatinine levels (even small elevations reflect large losses in glomerular filtration rate) and urinalysis to detect proteinuria or hematuria. Reversible causes of renal failure should always be sought and treated. Blood pressure goals for patients with proteinuria in excess of 1 g/24 hours should be 125/75 mm Hg or less, with whatever antihypertensive therapy is necessary. Sodium restriction is recommended to a level lower than that recommended for uncomplicated hypertension, and dietary restriction of potassium and phosphorus is recommended when creatinine clearance is below 30 mL/minute.

All classes of antihypertensive drugs are effective, and multiple drugs may be needed. ACE inhibitors have been the most effective in patients with diabetic nephropathy, proteinuria of 1 g or more per 24 hours, and renal insufficiency. ACE inhibitors are the drug class of choice to control HTN and slow progression of renal failure for all patients who have HTN and renal insufficiency unless they are specifically contraindicated (see below).

In patients with serum creatinine levels of 3 mg/dL or more, **ACE inhibitors** should be used with caution. Chapter 16 provides more detailed discussion of this treatment protocol. **Thiazide diuretics** are not effective with renal insufficiency manifested by serum creatinine levels 2.5 mg/dL or more, and **loop diuretics** such as **furosemide (Lasix)** are needed, often at relatively large doses. **Potassium-sparing diuretics** should be avoided in renal insufficiency. Chapter 16 also discusses the use of **diuretics** in more detail.

Renovascular Disease

Clinical clues to renovascular disease include (1) onset of HTN before age 30 or recent onset of severe HTN after age 55; (2) an abdominal bruit, particularly if it continues into diastole and is lateralized; (3) accelerated or resistant HTN; (4) recurrent (flash) pulmonary edema; (5) renal failure of uncertain etiology; (6) coexisting diffuse atherosclerotic vascular disease, especially in heavy smokers; and (7) acute renal failure precipitated by **antihypertensive therapy**, especially with **ACE inhibitors** or **ARBs** (Pohl, 1999). Patients with renovascular disease may require surgical interventions to stabilize their BP and no specific **antihypertensive medications** are recommended.

Diabetes Mellitus

HTN is disproportionately increased in diabetics and persons with HTN are 2.5 times more likely to develop diabetes within 5 years (Gress, Nieto, Shahar, Wofford, & Brancati, 2000; Sowers & Bakris, 2000). Coexistence of HTN and diabetes is especially concerning because both have strong links to CVD, CVA, progression to renal disease, and diabetic retinopathy. Studies (Adler et al, 2000; Dahlof et al, 2002; Heart Outcomes Prevention Evaluation Study Investigators, 2000) have shown that a reduction of as little as 10 mm Hg in SBP was associated with average reductions in diabetes-related mortality by 15 percent; MI by 11 percent; and retinopathy and nephropathy by 13 percent. The rate of decline in diabetic nephropathy has been reported to be a continuous function of arterial pressure down to approximately 124 to 130 mm Hg SBP and 70 to 75 mm Hg DBP (Nelson et al, 1996). **Antihypertensive drug therapy** should be initiated, along with lifestyle modifications (especially weight loss), to reach a blood pressure goal of below 129/79 mm Hg for all patients with diabetes mellitus (Chobanian et al, 2003; American Diabetes Association, 2009). **ACE inhibitors**, **ARBs**, **beta-adrenergic blockers**, **calcium channel blockers**, and **diuretics** in low doses are preferred because of their lower effects on glucose metabolism, lipid profiles, and renal function. Of this group, **ACE inhibitors** are considered best because of their demonstrated reduction in risk for diabetic nephropathy (AACE, 2006). They work well alone but are more effective when combined with a **thiazide diuretic**. **Thiazide diuretics**, however, can worsen blood glucose control in some patients and can increase the likelihood of developing diabetes in **insulin**-resistant patients (AACE, 2006). These drugs should be used at the lowest effective dosage in conjunction with adequate **potassium** replacement or the addition of a **potassium-sparing agent**. If **ACE inhibitors** are not well tolerated, **ARBs** may be considered. **Beta-adrenergic blockers** are beneficial as part of multidrug therapy, but their value as monotherapy is less clear. The new third generation **beta blockers** such as **nebivolol** or drugs that block both alpha and beta receptors such as **carvedilol** may prove to be beneficial. These agents cause vasodilation and an increase in insulin sensitivity (AACE, 2006). Other **beta-adrenergic blockers** have an adverse effect on peripheral blood flow, prolong hypoglycemia, and mask most hypoglycemic symptoms. If there is a compelling reason for a patient with diabetes to use them, they should be combined with a **diuretic**. The patient should be taught that **beta-adrenergic blockers** do not mask diaphoresis as a symptom of hypoglycemia; this symptom should be carefully watched for and lead to immediate blood glucose monitoring. Chapter 16 discusses this treatment protocol in more detail. **Calcium channel blockers** have also been shown to have some degree of renal protection and are most helpful as part of multidrug therapy. The nondihydropyridine **calcium channel blockers (diltiazem** and **verapamil)** may reduce microalbuminuria to an extent comparable with **ACEIs**, but the dihydropyridine **calcium channel blockers** may increase it (ACCE, 2006). Most diabetics will require two or more drugs to achieve BP control.

Metabolic Syndrome

Metabolic syndrome is a constellation of cardiovascular risk factors related to HTN, abdominal obesity, dyslipidemia, and insulin resistance (National Cholesterol Education Program, 2002). The prevalence of this syndrome is highly age dependent with 7 percent of adults 20 to 29 years demonstrating it, whereas 40 percent or more of Americans older than 60 years demonstrate it. The risk for fatal CHD is increased 4-fold and for CVD is increased 2-fold for individuals with this syndrome, even after adjustment for age. Patients with this syndrome also have a 5- to 9-fold increased risk for developing diabetes. The cornerstone of clinical management of metabolic syndrome in adults is lifestyle modification and most patients with this syndrome fall into prehypertension or stage 1 hypertension categories. If BP exceeds 140/90 mm Hg, drug therapy is indicated based on the general hypertension treatment algorithm.

Dyslipidemia

Lifestyle modifications are the first approach to treatment of both dyslipidemia and HTN. Emphasis is placed on control of weight; reduced intake of sodium, saturated fat, cholesterol, and **alcohol**; and increased physical activity. When drug therapy is chosen, drug effects on lipid metabolism are the primary consideration. **Alpha-adrenergic blockers** may decrease serum cholesterol to a limited degree and increase HDL. **ACE inhibitors**, **ARBs**, **calcium channel blockers**, and **central adrenergic agonists** have neutral effects on lipids. **Beta-adrenergic blockers** increase triglycerides transiently and reduce levels of HDLs. They are chosen mainly for patients with previous MIs who need their protective effects against sudden cardiac death and recurrent MI. In high doses, **thiazide** and **loop diuretics** can cause at least short-term increases in levels of cholesterol, triglycerides, and low-density lipids (LDLs). Dietary modifications can reduce these effects. Low doses of **thiazide diuretics** do not produce these effects and can be safely used. The Systolic Hypertension in the Elderly Program was conducted in the 1980s with the final results published in 1991 (Hulley et al, 1985; Systolic Hypertension in the Elderly Cooperative Research Group, 1991; Perry, Jr., 2010). Follow up studies were conducted 14 years later in 2008 (Vagaonescu et al, 2008). Each of these studies investigated the use of **chlorthalidone**, a **diuretic**, as initial monotherapy or in combination to treat systolic hypertension in a population 60 years of age or older. The risks for cerebrovascular and coronary events were reduced equally in persons with normal lipid levels and those with elevated lipid levels.

Lowering lipid levels also reduces cardiovascular risks that are shared in common with HTN. Selection of appropriate **cholesterol-lowering drugs** is discussed in the guidelines from the National Cholesterol Education Program (2002) and in Chapter 39.

Bronchial Asthma or Chronic Airway Diseases

Hypertension is relatively common in acute asthma and may be related to treatment with **beta agonists** or **systemic corticosteroids.** Bronchial reactivity is unchanged by **ACE inhibitors**, which are safe for most patients with asthma. If the patient is one of the 10 to 15 percent who experience the adverse effect of a cough, ARBs are an alternative. **Beta-adrenergic blockers** and **alpha- and beta-adrenergic blockers** may exacerbate asthma and should not be used unless there are compelling reasons for doing so. The topical ophthalmic **beta-adrenergic blockers** such as **timolol** (Timoptic) may also worsen asthma.

Many over-the-counter (OTC) drugs used as **decongestants** and cold and asthma remedies contain a sympathomimetic drug that can raise blood pressure. They are generally safe when taken in limited doses by patients who are on **antihypertensive** therapy. **Cromolyn sodium, ipratropium bromide,** or **corticosteroids** by inhalation can be used safely for nasal congestion by patients with hypertension.

Cost

The cost of **antihypertensive** drug therapy should be considered in drug selection, especially for patients who require multiple drugs (Table 40–7). In most cases, generic formulations are acceptable and cheaper than brand-name counterparts. Nongeneric newer agents are usually more expensive. If the newer agent is equally effective and there are no compelling reasons for its use, cost should be a major factor in choosing the initial therapy. If the newer agent is more effective or there is a compelling reason for its use, cost should be a secondary consideration. Using combinations can also reduce drug cost. Table 40–8 lists some of the more common drugs found in combination tablets.

Table 40–7 Selected Antihypertensive Drugs and Their Cost

Drug	Dosage (mg/d)	Cost*
ACE Inhibitors		$6 for all strengths in generic
Benazepril	10–40	$20 for 10 and 20 mg for brand
Captopril	12.5–150	$4 (generic) $97 (brand)
Enalapril	2.5–40	$6 (generic) $54–119 (brand)
Lisinopril	5–40	$6 (generic) $40 (brand)
Alpha-Adrenergic Blockers		
Prazosin	1–20	$10 for 1 mg, 2 mg; $20 for 5 mg
Terazosin	1–20	$13
Angiotensin II Receptor Antagonist		
Losartan	25–100	$60 (Cozaar brand)
Beta-Adrenergic Blockers		
Atenolol	25–100	$5 (generic)
Metoprolol	50–200	$6 (generic)
Propranolol	40–240	$4 (generic)
Propranolol extended-release	80–240	$30 (generic)
Calcium Channel Blockers		
Amlodipine	2.5–10	$13–17 (generic) $46 (Norvasc brand)
Diltiazem CD	120–360	$42
Diltiazem SR	120–360	$36
Diuretics		
Furosemide	20–320	$5 (generic)
Hydrochlorothiazide	12.5–50	$5 (generic)
Indapamide	2.5–5	$3 (generic) $59 brand
Spironolactone	25–100	$9 (generic)
Triamterine	50–150	$9.77 (generic) $92 (brand)

*Cost in 2010 dollars for 30-day prescription.

Table 40–8 **Common Combinations of Antihypertensive Drugs**

Combination*	Fixed-Dose Combination (mg)†	Brand Name
ACEIs and CCBs	Amlodipine/benazepril hydrochloride (2.5/10, 5/10, 10/20) Enalapril maleate/felodipine (5/5) Trandolapril/verapamil (2/180, 1/240, 2/240, 4/240)	Lotrel Lexxel Tarka
ACEIs and diuretics	Benazepril/hydrochlorothiazide (5/6.25, 10/12.4, 20/12.5, 20/25) Captopril/hydrochlorothiazide (25/15, 25/25, 50/15, 50/25) Enalapril maleate/hydrochlorothiazide (5/12.5, 10/25) Lisinopril/hydrochlorothiazide (10/12.5, 20/12.5, 20/25) Moexipril HCL/hydrochlorothiazide (7.5/12.5, 15/25) Quinapril HCL/hydrochlorothiazide (10/12.5, 20/12.5, 20/25)	Lotensin HCT Capozide Vaseretic Prinzide Uniretic Accuretic
ARBs and diuretics	Candesartan cilexetil/hydrochlorothiazide (16/12.5, 32/12.5) Eprosartan mesylate/hydrochlorothiazide (600/12.5, 600/25) Irbesartan/hydrochlorothiazide (150/12.5, 300/12.5) Losartan potassium/hydrochlorothiazide (50/12.5, 100/25) Telmisartan/hydrochlorothiazide (40/12.5, 80/12.5) Valsartan/hydrochlorothiazide (80/12.5, 160/12.5)	Atacand HCT Teveten/HCT Avalide Hyzaar Micardis/HCT Diovan/HCT
BBs and diuretics	Atenolol/chlorthalidone (50/25, 100/25) Bisoprolol fumarate/hydrochlorothiazide (2.5/6.25, 5/6.25, 10/6.25) Propranolol LA/hydrochlorothiazide (40/25, 80/25) Metoprolol tartrate/hydrochlorothiazide (50/25, 100/25) Nadolol/bendrofluthiazide (40/5, 80/5) Timolol maleate/hydrochlorothiazide (10/25)	Tenoretic Ziac Inderide Lopressor HCT Corzide Timolide
Centrally acting drug and diuretic	Methyldopa/hydrochlorothiazide (250/15, 250/25, 500/30, 500/50) Reserpine/chlorothiazide (0.125/250, 0.25/500) Reserpine/hydrochlorothiazide (0.125/25, 0.125/50)	Aldoril Diupres Hydropres
Diuretic and diuretic	Amiloride HCl/hydrochlorothiazide (5/50) Spironolactone/hydrochlorothiazide (25/25, 50/50) Triamterene/hydrochlorothiazide (37.5/25, 50/25, 75/50)	Moduretic Aldactone Dyazide, Maxzide

*Drug abbreviations: ACE = angiotensin-converting enzyme inhibitor; ARB = angiotensin receptor blocker; BB = beta blocker; CCB = calcium channel blocker.

†Some drug combinations are available in multiple fixed doses. Each drug dose is reported in milligrams.

Source: Chobanian, A., Bakris, G., Black, H., Cushman, W., Green, L., Izzo, J., et al, National High Blood Pressure Coordinating Committee. (2003). Seventh Report of the Joint National Committee on Prevention, Detection, Evaluation, and Treatment of High Blood Pressure. *Journal of the American Medical Association, 289,* 2560–2571.

Shopping at different sources to check prices is often worthwhile. Some drugs have the same cost for a higher-dose as a lower-dose tablet, and the tablet can be divided to reduce cost. These cost-saving measures are discussed in more detail in Chapters 14 and 16.

Treatment costs include not only the price of the drug but also the price of any routine or special laboratory tests, supplemental therapies, clinic visits, and time lost from work for clinic visits. Maintaining contact with a patient and regularly checking BP are important factors in adherence, but they can also add cost. Teaching the patient how to do home BP monitoring and use of telecommunication or e-mail to maintain contact can reduce these costs.

In an era of managed care, the cost of treating HTN is always under scrutiny. Managed-care agencies can be reminded, however, that the cost of HTN management that results in good control is lower than the cost that may be avoided by reducing hypertension-associated heart disease, stroke, and renal failure, which may result in expensive hospitalizations. RCTs have shown that these reductions occur in a relatively short period of time and are sustained for years.

MONITORING

The single-most important monitoring parameter is BP measurement. Equipment used to monitor BP should be regularly inspected and validated. The operator should be trained and regularly retrained in the appropriate technique and the patient must be properly prepared and positioned. **Caffeine**, exercise, and smoking should be avoided for at least 30 minutes prior to measurement. The person should be seated in a chair (not on the examination table) for at least 5 minutes with feet on the floor and arm supported at heart level. An appropriately sized cuff (cuff bladder encircling at least 80% of the arm) should be used. At least two measurements are taken and the average recorded. The health-care provider should provide to patients verbally and in writing their specific BP numbers and the BP goal of their treatment.

Home or clinic blood pressure measurement in the early morning before the patient has taken the **antihypertensive drug(s)** provides data about the adequacy of management related to the increase in blood pressure after arising. Measurement in the late afternoon or evening helps to monitor control across the day. Because the stress of a clinic visit may result in higher blood pressure readings in the clinic, blood pressure goals based on home monitoring are usually lower than those based on clinic monitoring.

OUTCOME EVALUATION

Evaluation of hypertensive patients has three objectives: (1) to assess lifestyle and identify other cardiovascular risk factors or concomitant disorder that may affect prognosis and guide treatment, (2) to reveal identifiable causes of HTN, and (3) to assess the presence or absence of target organ damage and CVD. Figure 40–2 shows the treatment protocol for HTN management. Evaluation against specific BP goals occurs throughout the protocol. The main indications for substitution of a drug from a different class are no response and troublesome adverse reactions to initial drug therapy. Specific drugs to substitute were previously discussed. When this substitution does not result in achievement of the target BP, drugs from other classes are continually added until the goal is reached.

When standard therapy is not successful in achieving goal BP (refractory hypertension), when a secondary cause of the hypertension is suspected, when the patient has complex concomitant conditions, or when renal failure worsens even with adequate control, referral to a HTN specialist is appropriate. Referral to a physician for immediate hospitalization is indicated with evidence of malignant hypertension (greater than 130 mm Hg diastolic reading, retinal hemorrhages, bulging disks, mental status changes, or new-onset heart failure).

Laboratory data and other monitoring parameters related to specific drugs are discussed in Chapters 14 and 16 for each drug class. Annual evaluations for target organ damage should include a 12-lead electrocardiogram (ECG), urinalysis, complete blood count (CBC), blood chemistry (potassium, sodium, creatinine, fasting glucose, total cholesterol), and HDL levels. Optional tests include creatinine clearance, 24-hour urine protein, LDL levels, thyroid-stimulating hormone levels, and limited echocardiography. For patients with diabetes, microalbuminuria and glycosylated hemoglobin studies are essential. Physical examination includes funduscopic examination, neurological examination, and assessment of heart and lung sounds, peripheral pulses, and bruits.

Adherence Issues

Lack of adherence to a therapeutic regimen to control BP is unfortunately very common. Several factors in HTN management foster this nonadherence. Lifestyle modification is a foundation of HTN management, and difficulty in achieving and maintaining lifestyle changes is well documented. Adverse drug reactions and drug costs are also factors in nonadherence. Sexual dysfunction, fatigue, and depression are common adverse reactions to several classes of **antihypertensive drugs.** A systematic team approach that uses health professionals and community resources can assist in providing the necessary education, support, and follow-up to improve adherence. The ultimate improvement in adherence is related to the patients having a positive experience with, and trust in, their healthcare provider. Better communication improves outcomes and empathy builds trust. Table 40–9 details some activities that can improve adherence. Chapter 6 has additional material on improving positive outcomes.

PATIENT EDUCATION

Patient education should include a discussion of information related to the overall treatment plan as well as that specific to the drug therapy, reasons for the drug's being taken, drugs as part of the total treatment regimen, and adherence issues.

Table 40–9 **Factors to Improve Adherence to Therapy**

• Be aware of signs of patient nonadherence to antihypertensive therapy and monitor for them.
• Establish the goal of therapy jointly with the patient: to reduce blood pressure to nonhypertensive levels with minimal or no adverse effects.
• Educate patients about the disease and involve them and their families in its treatment; have them measure blood pressure at home.
• Maintain regular contact with patients; consider telecommunication.
• Keep treatment regimen as inexpensive and simple as possible.
• Encourage lifestyle modifications and provide support for them.
• Integrate drug regimen into routine activities of daily living.
• Prescribe drugs according to pharmacological principles, favoring long-acting formulations.
• Be willing to stop unsuccessful therapy and try a different approach.

Continued

Table 40–9 **Factors to Improve Adherence to Therapy—cont'd**

• Anticipate adverse reactions and adjust therapy to prevent, minimize, or ameliorate them.
• Continue to add effective and tolerated drugs, stepwise, in sufficient doses to achieve the goals of therapy while reducing the likelihood of adverse reactions.
• Encourage a positive attitude about achieving therapeutic goals.
• Use nurse case management and a team approach.

Source: Adapted from the National High Blood Pressure Education Program. (2003). *Seventh Report of the Joint National Committee on Prevention, Detection, Evaluation, and Treatment of High Blood Pressure.* Rockville, MD: National Institutes of Health, National Heart, Lung and Blood Institute.

HYPERTENSION

PATIENT EDUCATION

Related to the Overall Treatment Plan and Disease Process

- ☐ Pathophysiology of hypertension and its long-term effects on target organs
- ☐ Role of lifestyle modifications in improving prognosis and keeping the number and cost of required drugs down
- ☐ Importance of adherence to the treatment regimen
- ☐ Self-monitoring of blood pressure
- ☐ Indications of target organ damage
- ☐ Need for regular follow-up visits with the primary care provider

Specific to the Drug Therapy

- ☐ Reason for taking the drug(s) and the anticipated action of the drug(s) on the disease process
- ☐ Doses and schedules for taking the drug(s)
- ☐ Possible adverse reactions and what to do when they occur
- ☐ Coping mechanisms for complex and costly drug regimens
- ☐ Interaction between lifestyle modifications and these drugs

Reasons for Taking the Drug(s)

Patient education about specific drugs is provided in Chapters 14 and 16. Specific information related to hypertension includes the reasons for taking the drug(s): Antihypertensive drugs are given to reduce mortality and decrease target organ damage. Some drugs do both; most do one or the other. The expectations should be clear about what the drugs can and cannot do. Hypertension is a chronic condition that rarely develops in a short space of time and is not likely to be corrected in a short space of time, if at all. Patients with hypertension must understand the lifelong nature of the disorder and the need to incorporate the treatment regimen into their everyday lives. The risk of target organ damage must be discussed, but hope must be maintained, and the potential for good quality of life with adequate treatment must be emphasized.

Drugs as Part of the Total Treatment Regimen

The total treatment regimen includes salt reduction and avoidance of excessive fluid intake. **Diuretics** reduce fluid volume and may interact with dietary sodium reduction, resulting in OH. Care should be taken not to reduce salt and fluid too quickly. Patients should be taught to report signs and symptoms of fluid volume deficit. Sodium reduction may lead some patients to seek salt substitutes that have potassium as part of their contents. For patients taking **ACE inhibitors** or **ARBs,** this choice can result in excessively high potassium levels. Such salt substitutes should be avoided. Nonsalt herbal seasoning is more appropriate.

Vasodilators can produce OH. Tell patients to rise slowly from a supine position to permit the body to redistribute body fluids.

Regular aerobic exercise such as walking or cycling can improve blood pressure control. Gradually increased, regular exercise may lead to improvement in blood pressure level and reduce the drug(s) needed.

Adherence Issues

Nonadherence with the treatment regimen may reduce life expectancy and affect the functioning of target organs. Health-care providers should be aware of the potential problem of nonadherence, discuss the importance of adherence at each follow-up visit, and assist patients in removing barriers to adherence, such as the complexity and cost of the treatment regimen and the presence of adverse reactions.

REFERENCES

Adams, H., Jr., Adams, R., Brott, T., del Zoppo, G., Furlan, A., Goldstein, L., et al. (2003). Guidelines for the early management of patients with ischemic stroke: A scientific statement from the Stroke Council of the American Stroke Association. *Stroke, 34,* 1056–1083.

Adler, A., Stratton, I., Neil, H., Yudkin, J., Matthews, D., Cull, C., et al. (2000). Association of systolic blood pressure with macrovascular and microvascular complications of type 2 diabetes (UKPDS 36): Prospective observational study. *British Medical Journal, 321,* 412–419.

ALLHAT Officers and Coordinators for the ALLHAT Collaborative Research Group. (2002). Major outcomes in high-risk hypertensive patients randomized to angiotensin-converting enzyme inhibitor or calcium channel blocker vs diuretic: The Antihypertensive and Lipid-Lowering Treatment to Prevent Heart Attack (ALLHAT). *Journal of the American Medical Association, 288,* 2981–2997.

American Association of Clinical Endocrinologists (AACE) Hypertension Task Force. (2006). American Association of Clinical Endocrinologists medical guidelines for clinical practice for the diagnosis and treatment of hypertension. *Endocrine Practice, 12*(2), 193–222.

American Diabetes Association. (2003). Treatment of hypertension in adults with diabetes. *Diabetes Care, 26,* 80–S82.

American Diabetes Association. (2009). Standards of medical care in diabetes-2009. *Diabetes Care, 32* (Suppl. 1) S13–S61.

Appel, I., Espeland, M., Easter, L., Wilson, A., Folmar, S., & Lacy, C. (2001). Effects of reduced sodium intake on hypertension control in older individuals: Results from the Trial of Nonpharmacologic Interventions in the Elderly (TONE). *Archives of Internal Medicine, 161,* 685–693.

Brown, N., Ray, W., Snowden, M., & Griffin, M. (1996). Black Americans have an increased rate of angiotensin converting enzyme inhibitor-associated angioedema. *Clinical Pharmacology Therapy, 60,* 8–13.

Chobanian, A., Bakris, G., Black, H., Cushman, W., Green, L., Izzo, J., et al, National High Blood Pressure Coordinating Committee. (2003). Seventh Report of the Joint National Committee on Prevention, Detection, Evaluation, and Treatment of High Blood Pressure. *Journal of the American Medical Association, 289,* 2560–2571.

Dahlof, B., Devereux, R., Kjeldsen, S., Julius, S., Beevers, G., Faire, U., et al. (2002). Cardiovascular morbidity and mortality in the Losartan Intervention For Endpoint reduction in hypertension study (LIFE): A randomized trial against atenolol. *Lancet, 359,* 995–1003.

Douglas, J., Bakris, G., Epstein, M., Ferdinand, K., Ferrario, C., Flack, J., et al. (2003). Management of high blood pressure in African Americans: Consensus statement of the Hypertension in African Americans Working Group of the International Society on Hypertension in Blacks. *Archives of Internal Medicine, 163*(5), 525–541.

Elliot, W. (1996). Higher incidence of discontinuance of angiotensin converting enzyme inhibitors due to cough in black subjects. *Clinical Pharmacology Therapy, 60,* 582–588.

Forette, F., Seux, M., Staessen, J., Thijs, L., Birkenhager, W., Barbarskiene, M., et al. (1998). Prevention of dementia in randomized double-blind placebo-controlled Systolic Hypertension in Europe (Syst-EUR) trial. *Lancet, 352,* 1347–1351.

Gao, S., Fitzpatrick, A., Psaty, B., Jiang, R., Post, W., Cutler, J., et al. (2009). Suboptimal nutritional intake for hypertension control in 4 ethnic groups. *Archives of Internal Medicine, 169*(7), 702–707.

Gress, T., Nieto, F., Shahar, E., Wofford, M., & Brancati, F. (2000). Hypertension and antihypertensive therapy as risk factors for type 2 diabetes mellitus. Atherosclerosis risk in communities study. *New England Journal of Medicine, 342,* 905–912.

Hajjar, I., & Kotchen, T. (2003). Trends in prevalence, awareness, treatment and control of hypertension in the United States 1988–2000. *Journal of the American Medical Association, 290,* 199–206.

Hansson, L., Zanchetti, A., Carruthers, S., Dahlof, B., Elmfeldt, D., Julius, S., et al. (1998). Effects of intensive blood-pressure lowering and low-dose aspirin in patients with hypertension: Principal results of the Hypertension Optimal Treatment (HOT) randomized trial. *Lancet, 351,* 1755–1762.

Heart Outcomes Prevention Evaluation Study Investigators. (2000). Effects of an angiotensin-converting-enzyme inhibitor, ramipril, on cardiovascular events in high-risk patients. *New England Journal of Medicine, 342,* 145–153.

Hulley, S., Furberg, C., Gurland, B., McDonald, R., Perry, H., Schnaper, H., et al. (1985). Systolic Hypertension in the Elderly Program (SHEP): Antihypertensive efficacy of chlorthalidone. *American Journal of Cardiology, 56*(15), 913–920.

Institute for Clinical Symptoms Improvement (ICSI). (2008, October). Hypertension diagnosis and treatment. 59 pp. Retrieved June 16, 2009, from http://www.guideline.gov/

Magee, L., Helewa, M., Moutquin, J., & von Dadelszen, P. (2008). Treatment of the hypertensive disorders of pregnancy. In: Diagnosis, evaluation and management of the hypertensive disorders of pregnancy. *Journal of Obstetrics and Gynaecology of Canada, 30*(3 Suppl. 1), 24–36.

National Cholesterol Education Program. (2002). Third report of the Expert Panel on Detection, Evaluation, and Treatment of High Blood Cholesterol in Adults (Adult Treatment Panel III): Final report. *Circulation, 106,* 3143–3421. Retrieved March 8, 2011 at http://www.nhlbi.nih.gov/guidelines/cholesterol

National Health and Nutrition Examination Survey. Available from National Center for Health Statistics Web site of the CDC, http://www.cdc.gov/nchs/nhanes.htm (accessed March 8, 2011).

National High Blood Pressure Education Program (NHBPEP). (2000). Report of the National High Blood Pressure Education Program Working Groups on High Blood Pressure in Pregnancy. *American Journal of Obstetrics and Gynecology, 183,* S1–S22.

National High Blood Pressure Education Program (NHBPEP). (2003). *Seventh Report of the Joint National Committee on Prevention, Detection, Evaluation, and Treatment of High Blood Pressure* (JNC-7). Rockville, MD: National Institutes of Health, National Heart, Lung and Blood Institute.

National High Blood Pressure Education Program (NHBPEP). (2004). The fourth report on the diagnosis, evaluation, and treatment of high blood pressure in children and adolescents. *Pediatrics, 114*(Suppl. 2), 555–576.

National Kidney Foundation Guideline. (2002). Kidney Disease Outcome Quality Initiative clinical practice guidelines for chronic kidney disease: Evaluation, classifications, and stratification. *American Journal of Kidney Disease, 39,* S1–S246.

Neal, B., MacMahon, S., & Chapman, N. (2000). Effects of ACE inhibitors, calcium antagonists, and other blood-pressure-lowering drugs: Results of prospectively designed overviews of randomized trials. *Lancet, 356,* 1955–1964.

Nelson, R., Bennett, P., Beck, G., Tan, M., Knowler, W., Mitch, W., et al. (1996). Development and progression of renal disease in Pima Indians with non-insulin-dependent diabetes mellitus. *New England Journal of Medicine, 335,* 1636–1642.

Parsons, D., Reaveley, D., Pavitt, D., & Brown, E. (2002). Relationship of renal function to homocysteine and lipoprotein(a) levels: The frequency of the combination of both risk factors in chronic renal impairment. *American Journal of Kidney Disease, 40,* 916–923.

Perry, Jr., H. (2010). SHEP: Systolic Hypertension in the Elderly Program. *The Internet Stroke Center.* Washington University in St. Louis: School of Medicine. Retrieved October 3, 2010 at http://www.strokecenter.org/trials/TrialDetail.aspx?tid=338.

Pohl, M. (1999). Renovascular hypertension and ischemic nephropathy. In C. Wilcox (Ed.), *Atlas of diseases of the kidney.* Philadelphia: Current Medicine.

Ridker, P., Hennekens, C., Buring, J., & Rifai, N. (2000). C-reactive protein and other markers of inflammation in the prediction of cardiovascular disease in women. *New England Journal of Medicine, 342,* 836–843.

Ridker, P., Rifai, N., Rose, L., Buring, J., & Cook, N. (2002). Comparison of C-reactive protein and low-density lipoprotein cholesterol levels in the prediction of first cardiovascular events. *New England Journal of Medicine, 347,* 1557–1565.

Rosenthal, T., & Oparil, S. (2000). Hypertension in women. *Journal of Human Hypertension, 14,* 691–704.

Sowers, J., & Bakris, G. (2000). Antihypertensive therapy and the risk of type 2 diabetes mellitus. *New England Journal of Medicine, 342,* 969–970.

Staessen, J., Fagard, R., Thijs, L., Celis, H., Arabidzem, C., Birkenhager, W., et al. (1997). Randomized double-blind comparison of placebo and active treatment for older patients with isolated systolic hypertension. The Systolic Hypertension in Europe (Syst-EUR) Trial. *Lancet, 350,* 757–764.

Staessen, J., Gasowski, J., Wang, J., Thijs, L., Den Hond, E., Boissel, J., et al (2000). Risks of untreated and treated isolated systolic hypertension in the elderly: Meta-analysis of outcome trials. *Lancet, 355,* 865–872.

Systolic Hypertension in the Elderly Cooperative Research Group. (1991). Prevention of stroke by antihypertensive drug treatment in older persons with isolated systolic hypertension. *Journal of the American Medical Association, 265,* 3255–3264.

University of Michigan Health System. (2009, February). UMHS hypertension guideline. Retrieved June 6, 2009, from http://www.guideline.gov/

U.S. Census Bureau. (2002). Persons 65 years old and over characteristics by sex: 1980–2000. *Statistical abstracts of the United States: 2002* (p. 43). Washington, DC: U.S. Census Bureau.

Vagaonescu, T., Wilson, A., & Kostis, J. (2008). Atrial fibrillation and isolated systolic hypertension: The Systolic Hypertension in the Elderly Program and Systolic Hypertension in the Elderly Program Extension Study. *Hypertension, 51,* 1552–1556.

Vasan, R., Larson, M., Leip, E., Evans, J., O'Donnell, C., Kannel, W., et al. (2001). Impact of high-normal blood pressure on the risk of cardiovascular disease. *New England Journal of Medicine, 345,* 1291–1297.

von Dadelszen, P., Ornstein, M., Bull, S., Logan, A., Koren, G., & Magee, L. (2000). Fall in mean arterial pressure and fetal growth restriction in pregnancy hypertension: A meta-analysis. *Lancet, 355,* 87–92.

Weir, M., Chrysant, S., McCarron, D., Canossa-Terris, M., Cohen, J., Gunter, P., et al. (1998). Influence of race and dietary salt on the antihypertensive efficacy of an angiotensin-converting enzyme inhibitor or a calcium channel antagonist in salt-sensitive hypertensives. *Hypertension, 31,* 1088–1096.

Whelton, P., He, J., Appel, L., Cutler, J., Havas, S., Kotchen, T., et al. (2002). Primary prevention of hypertension: Clinical and public health advisory from the National High Blood Pressure Education Program. *Journal of the American Medical Association, 288,* 1882–1888.

World Health Report. (2002). *Reducing risks, promoting healthy life.* Geneva, Switzerland: World Health Organization.

Wright, J., Jr., Probstfield, J., Cushman, W., Pressel, S., Cutler, J., Davis, B., et al, for the ALLHAT Collaborative Research Group. (2009). ALLHAT findings revisited in the context of subsequent analyses, other trials, and meta-analyses. *Archives of Internal Medicine, 169*(9), 832–842.

CHAPTER 41

HYPERTHYROIDISM AND HYPOTHYROIDISM

Marylou Robinson

Chapter Outline

Thyroid disorders are among the most common disease processes seen in primary care. About 5 percent of U.S. adults have thyroid disease or take thyroid drugs. Untreated thyroid disease can result in long-term complications in every body system, especially the cardiovascular system. Most thyroid disorders involve thyroid gland malfunction, but secondary hypothyroid or hyperthyroid issues can stem from pituitary axis interruptions.

Hyperthyroidism is seen in 2 percent of women and in one-tenth as many men. It is most common from age 20 to 40. In children and older adults, hyperthyroidism can produce cardiomegaly and heart failure. Elders are also at risk for osteoporosis. In adolescents, hyperthyroidism can interfere with normal growth because of alterations in basic metabolism. Untreated hyperthyroidism in pregnancy increases the risk for first-trimester spontaneous abortion, stillbirths, and neonatal mortality.

Hypothyroidism also is more common in women, with a prevalence of 6 per 1,000. Prevalence increases with aging. Approximately 5 percent of older adults of both genders manifest evidence of hypothyroidism. In children, hypothyroidism can result in decreased mental and physical growth. In adults, it increases the risk for heart disease related to altered lipoprotein metabolism.

Treatment for these two disorders includes lifestyle management and drug therapy. Pharmacological management includes **thyroid hormones** to treat hypothyroid conditions and **antithyroid agents** such as **propylthiouracil (PTU), methimazole (Tapazole),** and **radioactive iodine** (I^{131}) or strong **iodine solutions** for hyperthyroid states. These drugs are discussed in detail in Chapter 21. Symptom management may also include other drugs, such as **beta blockers,** which are discussed in Chapter 14. This chapter discusses the management of hyperthyroidism and hypothyroidism that is usually done by primary care providers and provides only an overview of specialty-based directives and activities.

THYROID HORMONE SYNTHESIS

The synthesis of thyroid hormones is dependent on the functioning of the hypothalamic-pituitary-thyroid axis. The secretion of thyrotropin-releasing hormone (TRH) by the hypothalamus in response to cold, stress, and decreased levels of thyroxine (T4) stimulates the synthesis of thyroid-stimulating hormone (TSH) by the anterior pituitary. TSH, in turn, stimulates the thyroid gland to produce of thyroid hormones. Thyroid hormones (T4 and triiodothyronine [T3]) are synthesized from iodine and tyrosine molecules by follicular cells in the thyroid gland.

Dietary iodine of about 100 to 150 mcg/day is required for normal thyroid hormone production. In the United States, adequate iodine is found in foodstuffs and in iodized salt. In the past 20 years, there has been a reduction of typical intake with the healthy eating movement away from eggs and salty foods. Food manufacturers also switched to more noniodized salt in frozen meals and bread products. Per the National Health and Nutrition Examination Survey [NHANES] 2003–2004, U.S. average consumption is still adequate (Caldwell, Miller, Wang, Jain, & Jones, 2008).

Dietary iodine absorbed from the gastrointestinal (GI) tract is carried in the blood as iodide. When it reaches the thyroid gland, it is actively taken up by the iodide pump, located at the base of the thyroid follicles. The iodide pump is controlled by the serum iodide concentration: Low concentration increases pump activity and high concentration inhibits pump activity. The iodide is then oxidized within seconds by the thyroid peroixdase enzyme and binds to tyrosine residues in thyroglobin to form monoiodotyrosine and diiodotyrosine. The coupling of these two iodides forms T4 or T3, which is then stored in the thyroglobin.

The thyroid gland mainly produces T4. About 20 percent of T3 is synthesized and released from the thyroid gland. The remainder is converted from T4 to T3 peripherally when additional thyroid hormone is needed. Conversion of T4 to T3 is stimulated by cold temperatures and stress. Conversion is inhibited by acute and chronic illness, starvation, and some drugs (see Table 41–1). Practitioners must, therefore, consider the role of medications, stress, and other disease states when evaluating patients with newly diagnosed thyroid imbalances. T4 and T3 in plasma are reversibly bound to protein, mainly thyroxine-binding globulin. Only a small portion (0.04% of total T4 and 0.4% of total T3) exists in a free form; however, only this free form is clinically active. The amount of active thyroid hormone in the plasma produces a feedback loop that inhibits or further stimulates TRH and TSH secretion to decrease or increase thyroid hormone production. This mechanism is depicted in Chapter 21.

Table 41–1 **Drug Effects on Thyroid Function**

Drug	Effect on Thyroid Function
Amiodarone	• Releases iodine as drug is metabolized • Inhibits peripheral conversion of T4 to T3 • Can produce thyrotoxicosis
Carbamazepine	Increases metabolism of T4, resulting in decreased total T4
Estrogen	Increases thyroid-binding globulin levels
Glucocorticoids	Impair basal and TRH-stimulated TSH concentration
Levodopa	Chronic administration displaces thyroid hormone from thyroid-binding globulin, resulting in suppressed TSH response
Lithium	Blocks iodine uptake by thyroid gland, resulting in decreased hormone production
Phenytoin	• Decreases TSH response to TRH by 50% • Enhances cellular uptake and metabolism of T4, resulting in decreased total T4
Propranolol	Inhibits peripheral conversion of T4 to T3
Salicylates (in doses >4 g/d)	Suppress TSH response by inhibiting binding of T4 and T3 to thyroid-binding globulin
Theophylline	Beta-adrenergic stimulation of hypothalamus results in increased TSH response

TRH = thyroid-releasing hormone; TSH = thyroid-stimulating hormone.

THYROID FUNCTION TESTS

Several tests can be used to evaluate thyroid function. These tests and their normal values are listed in Table 41–2. The most commonly used tests in primary care are TSH and free T4 values. Serum TSH measurement is the single most reliable test to diagnose all common forms of hypothyroidism and hyperthyroidism. The sensitive or ultrasensitive forms of the TSH test should be used to avoid missing subclinical conditions. Subclinical conditions exist when TSH is normal, but free thyroxine (FT4) and free triiodothyronine (FT3) are abnormal (see the sections Subclinical Hyperthyroidism and Subclinical Hypothyroidism).

Altered serum TSH confirms the diagnosis in all patients with primary hypo- or hyperthyroidism, but it will not reliably identify all hypothyroid patients with secondary (central) disturbances wherein TSH values may be atypically low, normal, or elevated. When pituitary or hypothalamic disease is suspected as the cause of hypothyroidism, FT4 concentrations should be measured in addition to TSH. When less-sensitive TSH tests are the only ones available, FT4 and FT3 measurement can give addition information to validate the TSH (American Association of Clinical Endocrinologists [AACE], 2006).

Abnormal results from other commonly obtained laboratory tests may also suggest hypo- or hyperthyroidism.

Table 41–2 **Thyroid Function Tests**

Test	Normal Value	Values in Hyperthyroidism	Values in Hypothyroidism
Free thyroxine index (FT4I)	1.3–4.2	High	Low
Free triiodothyronin index (FT3I)	22–56	High	Normal or low
Free T4 (FT4)	0.7–1.86 ng/dL (9–24 pmol/L)	High	Low
Free T3 (FT3)	0.2–0.52 ng/dL (3–8 pmol/L)	High	Low
Thyrotropin-stimulating hormone (TSH)	0.3–5 microUnits/mL	Low	High
Thyrotropin-releasing hormone (TRH)	>6 microUnits/mL in serum TSH 45 min after injection; blunted TSH response (<2 microUnits/mL) in patients >40 yr	No response	Exaggerated rise

Hypercholesterolemia, hyponatremia, anemia, elevated creatinine kinase and lactate dehydrogenase, and hyperprolactinemia all suggest hypothyroidism. Hypercalcemia, elevated alkaline phosphatase, and elevated hepatocellular enzymes suggest hyperthyroidism. These laboratory findings justify thyroid function tests, especially if they are sustained for 2 weeks or more, occur in combination, or occur in patients with increased risk for thyroid disease (AACE, 2006).

Thyroid abnormalities can present with the development of enlarging thyroid tissues called goiters. This tissue growth may be euthyroid (normal functioning), it may be collections of subfunctioning tissue, or it may be focal cellular growths (nodules) that may produce excess amounts of thyroid hormone. The trigger for excess growth may be autoimmune processes or abnormal cellular disturbances. Goiter size or presence of palpable nodules does not correlate with underlying function. Moreover, abnormalities can exist without goiter presence. Generally, the work-up for a goiter will include serum thyroid antibody screens and a baseline ultrasound. Calling the endocrinology team and requesting which exact tests are required before the initial consultation will usually speed diagnosis and preclude unnecessary repetition of laboratory tests.

Suspicion of cancer or to determine whether nodules are "hot" or "cold" in terms of production of excess hormone, is confirmed with thyroid scanning. The radioisotope I^{123} dose and residual radiation levels used for these tests does not trigger the same precautions linked with I^{131} used to treat hyperthyroidism . In cases that are not urgent, individuals previously on **levothyroxine** are switched to **liothyronine** to deplete the organ of hormone for 2 to 6 weeks prior to the scan. Ideally, the person stops all hormones for the last 2 weeks in order to facilitate the iodine uptake capacity of the thyroid. A synthetic hormone **thyrotropin alpha (Thyrogen)** can be given to preclude hypothyroid-like symptoms of hormone withdrawal. The **Thyrogen** does not interfere with iodine uptake, but might cause false negative results in some individuals compared to the earlier standard practice of inducing a short-term hypothyroid state (New York Thyroid Center, 2007). Timing of scans and dosing of medications should be coordinated with the endocrinology team.

SCREENING

The U.S. Preventive Services Task Force (2004) found that the evidence is insufficient to recommend for or against routine screening for thyroid disease in adults. Testing can detect subclinical thyroid disease in people without symptoms of thyroid dysfunction, but the evidence is poor that treating these individuals changes their health status. Screening high-risk groups such as postpartum women, people with Down syndrome, and older adults is more likely to find subclinical disease, but the progression of subclinical thyroid disease to overt disease in patients without a history of prior thyroid issues is not clearly established.

Subclinical hypothyroidism is associated with poor obstetrical outcomes and poor cognitive development in children; nonetheless, the American College of Obstetricians and Gynecologists (ACOG, 2007) states that performance of thyroid function tests in asymptomatic pregnant women with mildly enlarged thyroid glands is also not warranted. Conversely, the American Association of Clinical Endocrinologists (AACE, 2006) recommends TSH measurement in women of childbearing age before pregnancy or during the first trimester. The literature agrees that no thyroid function tests should be performed unless disease is suspected by the presence of symptoms or suspicion of undiagnosed disease to include the aging, those with new cardiovascular issues and extreme fatigue.

In summary, the recommendations are conflicting, as are the data, about whether screening does any long-term good. The consensus seems to be that patients with symptoms that might be caused by thyroid dysfunction probably should be screened. Asymptomatic patients probably should not be screened unless they fall into specific risk groups.

HYPERTHYROIDISM

Pathophysiology

Thyrotoxicosis, or hyperthyroidism, occurs when the feedback loop fails and excessive levels of thyroid hormone are circulating. Extreme thyrotoxicosis is called thyroid storm, a life-threatening condition beyond the scope of this text. The cause of excessive secretion may be a hyperfunctioning thyroid nodule, toxic diffuse goiter (Graves' disease), anterior pituitary disorders, toxic multinodular goiter (Plummer's disease), or iodine- induced disease, including **amiodarone** therapy (AACE, 2006). Identifiable risk factors for hyperthyroid dysfunction include diabetes mellitus, pernicious anemia, primary adrenal insufficiency, vitiligo, leukotrichia (prematurely gray hair), and drugs or other compounds that contain iodine or affect iodine metabolism. Viruses and pregnancy are two of many conditions that can trigger thyroiditis.

By far, the most common hyperthyroid etiology (60% to 90% of all cases) is Graves' disease. Graves' disease is an autoimmune disorder characterized by generation of abnormal immunoglobulin G (IgG) autoantibodies to thyroid peroxidase and thyroglobin. The antibodies bind to the TSH receptors, activating excessive glandular growth and hormone production. Normally, any hyperfunction of the thyroid gland would lead to suppression of TSH and TRH; however, in autoimmune conditions, the feedback system is altered.

The hyperfunction of the thyroid gland with Graves' disease results in a dramatic increase in iodine uptake and subsequent systemic metabolism. The thyroid gland becomes more vascular and enlarges, forming a goiter. A disproportionate increase in T3 production is a hallmark of longer-term overstimulation of the gland. The overproduction leads to a decreased concentration of thyroid-binding globulin and increased circulating levels of free hormone. These hormone levels are responsible for the many thyrotoxic symptoms.

The clinical features of hyperthyroidism are attributable to metabolic effects of increased circulating levels of thyroid hormone. Typical effects include heat intolerance and heightened sensitivity to sympathetic nervous system stimulation. Table 41–3 shows the most common systemic effects of hyperthyroidism. Treatment goals are to diminish negative cardiovascular effects while returning the patient to a euthyroid state.

Table 41–3 **Systemic Effects of Hyperthyroidism**

Body System	Clinical Manifestation	Underlying Mechanism
Cardiovascular	Increased cardiac output, decreased peripheral vascular resistance, tachycardia at rest, arrhythmias	Increased metabolism and need to dissipate heat
Respiratory	Dyspnea and reduced vital capacity	Weakness of respiratory muscles
Gastrointestinal	• Increased appetite with concurrent weight loss	Increased utilization of carbohydrates, proteins, and fats to support rapid metabolism
	• Diarrhea, nausea, vomiting, abdominal pain	Increased peristalsis and cholesterol conversion salts
	• Decreased serum lipid levels	Malabsorption of fat, fat stores depleted for energy, increased excretion of cholesterol in feces
	• Decreased tissue stores of glucose, protein, and vitamins	Increased glucose utilization, use of protein as energy source, and impaired conversion of B vitamins to their coenzymes, causing an increased need for water- and fat-soluble vitamins
Integumentary	• Excessive sweating, flushing, warm skin	Need to dissipate heat
	• Temporary hair loss; hair fine, soft, and straight; nails grow away from nail beds	Hyperdynamic circulatory state
Reproductive	Oligomenorrhea or amenorrhea in women; impotence or decreased libido in men	Hypothalamic or pituitary disturbances; increased production of sex hormone–binding globulin
Neurological	• Restlessness, short attention span, fatigue, insomnia, emotional lability	Alteration in cerebral metabolism
	• Ocular manifestations, including decreased blinking and fine tremor of the lid	Hyperactivity of sympathetic nervous system

Table 41–3 **Systemic Effects of Hyperthyroidism—cont'd**

Body System	Clinical Manifestation	Underlying Mechanism
Musculoskeletal	• Hypercalcemia	Excessive bone resorption
	• Loss of muscle mass	Excessive protein catabolism
Endocrine	• Enlarged gland; systolic or continuous bruit of thyroid gland	Hyperactivity of the gland and increased circulation to support that hyperactivity
	• Diminished sensitivity to exogenous insulin	Increased insulin degradation

Many patients with Graves' disease experience ocular symptoms. These symptoms include functional abnormalities (e.g., lid lag with upward or downward gaze) related to hyperactivity of the sympathetic nervous system (McCance & Huether, 2006). Other changes involve orbital and periorbital edema and altered fat deposition. More than half of Graves' disease patients develop the characteristic wide-eyed stare with protrusion of the globe (exophthalmus). These ocular concerns can exist in tandem. The provider must recognize that the absence of classic exophthalmus does not negate the need for ophthalmological consultation. Occular changes can result in damage to the cornea, the retina, and/or the optic nerve, any of which may lead to blindness (McCance & Huether, 2006). A small number of patients with Graves' disease experience pretibial myxedema (Graves' dermopathy), characterized by subcutaneous swelling of the anterior portions of the legs, and occasionally in the hands, with bumpy, erythematous skin. This puts skin integrity at risk. Note that this form of myxedema is not synonymous with myxedema coma from profound hypothyroidism.

Pharmacodynamics

Antithyroid drugs reduce the production of thyroid hormones. **Propylthiouracil (PTU)** and **methimazole** inhibit the synthesis of new thyroid hormone by the thyroid gland, but do not inactivate existing or stored hormone. **PTU** also inhibits the peripheral conversion of T4 to T3. Neither of these drugs treats the underlying pathophysiology of hyperthyroidism. Resumption of hormone synthesis occurs quickly after drugs are withdrawn, because iodine is no longer blocked from use.

A treatment typically requires 6 to 12 months for total reversal of hyperthyroid symptoms. Dosing schedules for these two drugs are provided in Chapter 21. Some authorities advocate high-dose therapy; others favor low doses. Relapse rates appear to be higher in those taking lower doses. Higher doses increase the probabilities for development of post-treatment hypothyroidism. This sequela may not surface for several years.

Trials have shown no clinical outcome differences when **methimazole** is compared with PTU; however, the most recent concerns of hepatic toxicity with PTU have resulted in a withdrawal of the indication for use in children and for those with hepatic issues (U.S. Food and Drug Administration, 2009, 2010). **Methimazole** should be preferentially used in almost all cases. Adherence is significantly better for patients on **methimazole,** owing to its once-daily dosing schedule. Both drugs are relatively inexpensive.

Beta blockers address the symptoms of hyperthyroidism by decreasing the response to sympathetic stimulation and are used as adjunct therapy to control uncomfortable or unhealthy tachycardia. Low doses are all that are typically needed, with early onset symptom management evident. The most commonly prescribed drugs in this class are **propranolol,** because of its short half-life, and **atenolol,** because of its once-daily dosing. Patients with unstable hypoglycemia and severe reactive airways dependent on rescue inhalers may do better on the **cardioselective beta blockers** such as **atenolol.** The drugs are gradually withdrawn as the patient becomes euthyroid.

Iodides block peripheral conversion of T4 to T3 and inhibit hormone release. **Potassium iodine** was the earliest of the **iodides** to be used for this purpose. It is mainly used for preoperative preparation before thyroid surgery. Not only are the levels of circulating hormone reduced, but the vascularity of the tissue is also lessened. Dilution in fruit juices can make them more palatable and protect the teeth from discoloration.

Goals of Treatment

The goal of therapy for patients with hyperthyroidism is correction of the hypermetabolic state, with a minimum of adverse reactions and with the smallest incidence of resultant hypothyroidism. This means symptom relief and normalization of TSH and FT4 levels. **Beta blockers** can reduce symptomatic effects in the short term, but definitive therapy usually requires at least the addition of an **antithyroid agent** or surgery.

Rational Drug Selection

Three main avenues of treatment are used for patients with hyperthyroidism: (1) **antithyroid drugs,** (2) **radioactive** iodine, and (3) surgery. Radioactive iodine and the antithyroid drugs are also discussed in Chapter 21. Iodides are sometimes useful as supplemental suppressive drugs or for individuals who refuse I^{131} or cannot tolerate surgery. Presurgical use of iodides is indicated for those with cardiovascular compromise or for the elderly. Such use also decreases the immediate postoperative spike in hyperthyroid symptomatology experienced by many.

Lifestyle Management

Lifestyle management is primarily diet related. The thyroid gland requires adequate amounts of iodine to produce thyroid hormones. Patients should be taught how to recognize iodine sources in their diets. These include iodized salt; seafood products, especially shellfish; and seaweed. Vitamin supplements that have minerals and many over-the-counter (OTC) cold medications, especially cough syrups, should be screened for iodine on the labels.

The potential for nutritional deficits is the major concern, related to the hypermetabolic state. A high-calorie (4,000 to 5,000 kcal/d) diet may be necessary to satisfy hunger and prevent tissue breakdown. To provide this number of calories, six meals a day may be required, as well as snacks that are high in protein; carbohydrates; minerals; and vitamins, particularly vitamins A and B_6 and ascorbic acid. Caffeinated fluids and highly seasoned food should be avoided because they augment the tachycardiac and hot flushing symptoms of hyperthyroidism.

Other lifestyle concerns include providing adequate rest and avoiding external sources of stress, including work, domestic issues, and undo worry. Circulating catecholamines have more intensive cardiovascular effects in the presence of excessive thyroid hormone. Risks for triggering angina and dysrhythmias are heightened. Insomnia is made worse by any heat intolerance or sweating. Relaxation therapy and yoga are potential helpful interventions. Climate control, especially during hot weather, can reduce the burden of feeling hot.

Drug Therapy

Choices in drug therapy are based on patient variables (severity of the disease, duration of the disease, age of the patient, pregnancy, and the likelihood of patient adherence to the treatment regimen) and on drug-related variables (cost and adverse reactions). Figure 41–1 depicts some drug choices based on these variables.

Patient Variables

Severity of Disease

Antithyroid drugs are prescribed with the intent of achieving spontaneous remission of the disease. Patients most likely to achieve remission are those with mild disease and small goiters (AACE, 2006). Methimazole is the initial drug of choice because of the hepatic risks of PTU (U.S. Food and Drug Administration, 2010). Because these drugs do not inhibit the action of existing or stored thyroid hormone, clinical response typically takes 4 to 8 weeks with either drug. PTU is available in 50-mg tablets, and the dose varies from 150 to 300 mg daily. Because of its short half-life, the dose is divided and taken three times daily. Methimazole comes in 5- and 10-mg tablets. Dosing is usually started at 15 mg daily. Its longer half-life means that once-daily dosing may be tried.

Beta blockers may be added temporarily to reduce symptoms while the patient is awaiting clinical response to the antithyroid drugs. Some patients with long-standing hyperthyroidism may be relatively resistant to the effects of beta blockers, so larger and more frequent doses may be necessary. Propranolol is the drug most widely used, with the usual starting dose at 80 to 160 mg/day. Larger doses (360 to 480 mg/day) are sometimes necessary. Adequate doses of these drugs are determined by measuring resting and exercising heart rates and degree of symptom relief. These drugs can be tapered and discontinued once the patient is no longer hyperthyroid.

In severe thyrotoxic states, adjuvant treatment with iodides may be needed. Excess iodine limits the activity of thyroid peroxidase, thus decreasing iodide oxidation and rapidly blocking the release of T3 and T4 from the thyroid. Patients with Graves' disease are more sensitive to the inhibitory effects of iodine than are healthy individuals. The inhibitory effects of iodides, however, are short term in some individuals. Potassium iodide is given orally as Lugol's solution (8 mg/drops [gtt]) or as saturated solution of potassium iodide (SSKI; 35 to 50 mg/gtt). The dose of Lugol's solution is 3 to 5 drops and for SSKI it is 1 drop, both given tid.

Duration of Disease

Beta blockers provide excellent symptomatic relief for transient disorders (e.g., thyroiditis) because spontaneous remission is the rule. Aspirin, NSAIDs, and corticosteroids may also be used in subacute thyroiditis to control inflammatory symptoms. These drugs are equally useful for postpartum thyroiditis, where they are given for 3 months. Dosage is based on symptom relief.

Graves' disease requires longer duration dosing. Endocrinologists do not agree on the best treatment for Graves' disease, except in the case of older adults and cardiac patients, for whom radioactive iodine is the treatment of choice. For younger or middle-aged patients, an initial 1-year trial of antithyroid drugs is considered a reasonable starting point for treatment. Both drugs are equally useful. PTU's peripheral activity involving conversion of bound and free hormone is not clinically significant except at high doses, at which it is especially useful for severe hyperthyroidism and thyroid storm. PTU is initiated at 300 mg daily in three equally divided doses given 8 hours apart. Patients with severe disease may require 400 mg daily. Maintenance doses are 100 to 150 mg daily.

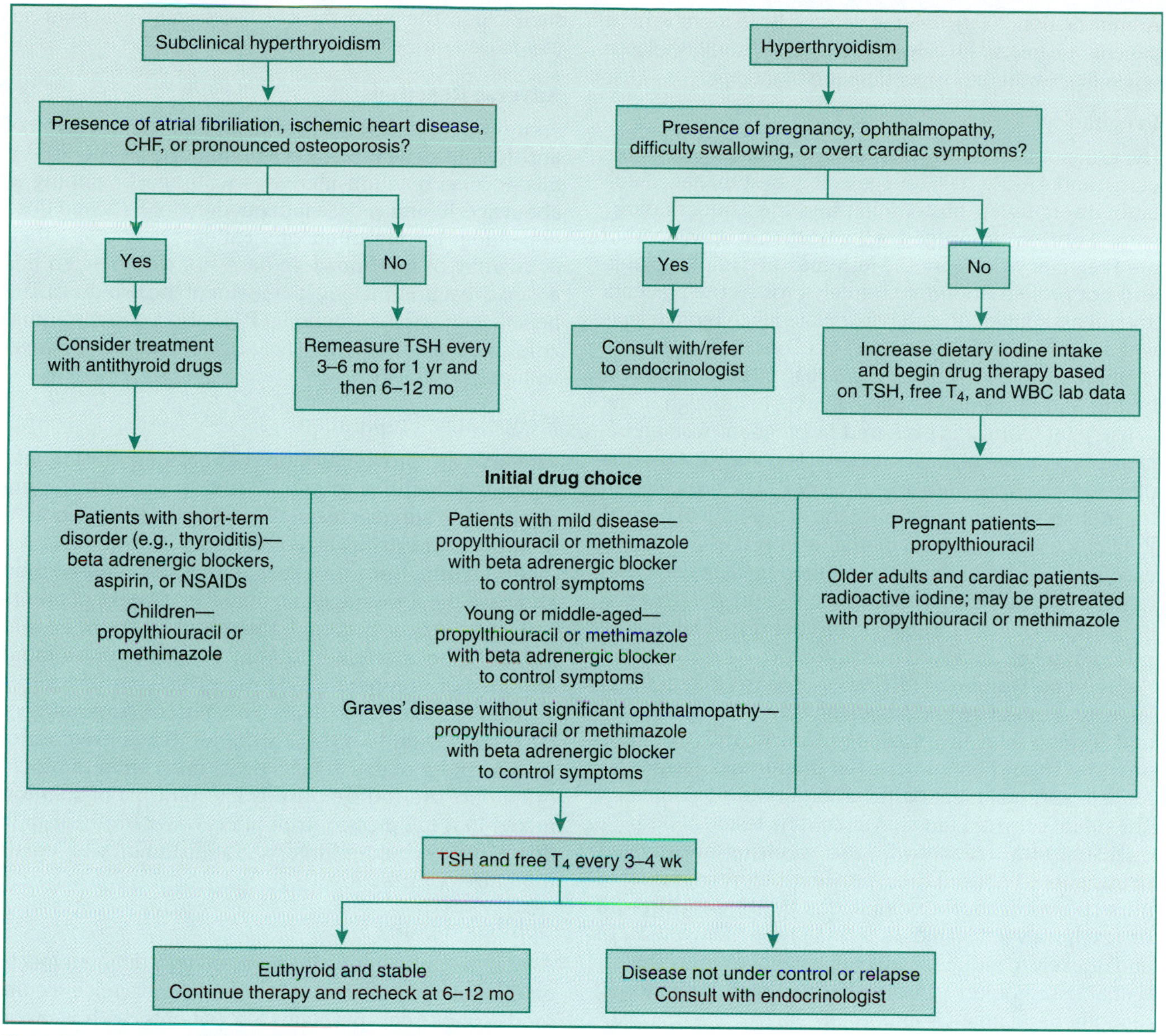

Figure 41–1. Drug therapy algorithm: Hyperthyroidism.

Methimazole is commonly initiated at 20 to 30 mg daily. One advantage to **methimazole** is that doses may be divided and given every 8 hours, or once-daily dosing may be tried. Once-daily dosing reduces the complexity of the treatment regimen. Once control of symptoms and appropriate levels of thyroid hormone production are achieved, the doses of both drugs can be tapered to the lowest amount needed to maintain a euthyroid state. Treatment is continued for 12 to 24 months and then stopped to see if a relapse occurs. Relapse is more common for patients treated less than 12 months. Patients who fail to achieve control of symptoms with **antithyroid drugs**, who are unable to tolerate the therapy, or who experience a relapse after completion of therapy are candidates for **radioactive iodine** or surgery.

The Graves' treatment regimen often includes supplementation with **beta blockers** for symptom relief. **Atenolol** offers the advantages of fewer adverse reactions, based on its $beta_1$ selectivity, and once-daily dosing for patients who are less adherent if the regimen is too complex. **Propranolol** offers the advantage of peripheral blockage of conversion of T4 to T3.

Age of Patient

Older adults are preferentially treated with **radioactive iodine** because of less tolerance for persistent cardiovascular stress. They may be pretreated with **antithyroid drugs** to bring them closer to euthyroid status before **radioactive iodine** therapy is initiated. Some endocrinologists prefer **antithyroid drug** therapy in childhood Graves' disease (AACE, 2006), waiting until adolescence for I^{131} therapy. PTU related hepatic toxicity has triggered the U.S. Food and Drug Administration's (FDA) 2009 recommendation that only **methimazole** be used in pediatrics (U.S. Food and Drug

Administration, 2009). Treatment lasts 6 to 18 months; most patients are treated for at least 1 year. As with adults, relapse is less likely with the longer duration of therapy.

Pregnancy

Hyperthyroidism during pregnancy presents special concerns, and AACE (2006) suggests it is best managed collaboratively by an obstetrician and the endocrinology team. **Antithyroid drugs** are the treatment of choice, but are Pregnancy Category D. **Methimazole** is lipid soluble and not protein bound, so it freely crosses the placenta and breast epithelium and is associated with birth defects when used in the first trimester (U.S. Food & Drug Administration, 2010). **PTU**, conversely, is 80 to 90 percent protein bound and ionized at physiological pH. Although it can cause fetal harm, it is preferred in pregnant women because its pharmacokinetics makes it less likely to cross the placenta. The lowest possible dose of **PTU** is used to keep the mother's thyroid function at the upper limit of normal. Pregnancy itself has an ameliorating effect on Graves' disease, so the dose of the drug required usually decreases as the pregnancy progresses. In some cases, the drug can be withdrawn 2 to 3 weeks before delivery if laboratory values indicate improved functioning.

Pregnant women with Graves' disease may transfer large amounts of thyroid-stimulating antibody to the fetus and induce fetal thyrotoxicosis. The infant's pediatric provider should be informed of the mother's hyperthyroidism and treatment of this disorder during pregnancy. The infant's thyroid function should be tested at birth.

Postpartum patients who are receiving **antithyroid drugs** should consult their provider before choosing to nurse their infants. Breast milk can transfer **antithyroid drugs**; however, the amount is small, especially with **PTU**, and unlikely to induce significant hypothyroidism. The potential risk should be discussed, and careful monitoring of mother and infant is important.

Adherence

Drug treatment is effective only if the drugs are taken as prescribed. Adherence to a treatment regimen is less likely if it is complex or leads to significant adverse reactions. **Antithyroid drugs** have limited overt adverse reactions but may need to be taken three times daily, making the treatment regimen complex. This complexity is especially problematic if the treatment regimen also involves a **beta blocker** that has significant adverse reactions and must also be taken three times daily but on a different schedule. To facilitate adherence, both **methimazole** and **atenolol** can be given once daily, and both have fewer adverse reactions than other drugs in their classes. Other factors that influence adherence are discussed in Chapter 6.

Drug-Related Variables

Cost

Costs based on the adjusted whole price are outlined in Chapter 21 tables. The actual retail price can vary significantly. The prices must be assessed at local pharmacies to determine true expense.

Adverse Reactions

A rare (0.3% to 0.6%) but potentially fatal complication of **antithyroid drug** therapy is agranulocytosis. The risk for this adverse reaction increases with age, beginning at about age 40, and is dose independent for **PTU** and dose dependent for **methimazole**. Patients taking less than 30 mg/day of **methimazole** have not experienced this adverse reaction, making it the safer of the two drugs. The hepatic concerns surrounding **PTU** also make **methimazole** a safer alternative for all age groups, especially those with polypharmacy.

Preoperative Preparation

Primary care providers should coordinate dosing and tapering schedules of any thyroid drugs with the endocrine and surgical teams. Preoperative administration of **antithyroid drugs** is required to avoid precipitating thyroid storm. **Beta blockers** may also be prescribed and have the advantage that only 1 to 2 weeks of preoperative therapy is required. The addition of **potassium iodide** to **beta blocker** therapy produces more rapid and greater preoperative control. This combination is especially useful for patients who must undergo surgery fairly quickly and for those who fail to achieve control (resting pulse of less than 90 beats/min) on **beta blockers** alone. The **iodide** dose is 2 to 6 drops of solution mixed in a full glass of fruit juice, water, broth, or milk tid for 10 days before surgery. Administration with meals minimizes GI irritation.

Ophthalmopathy

Although ophthalmopathy is caused by a different mechanism from that which causes hyperthyroidism, it is a common concurrent problem for patients with Graves' disease. Approximately 20 percent of patients with eye involvement that predates the treatment of their hyperthyroidism experience an exacerbation after treatment is initiated. Successful treatment of hyperthyroidism does not necessarily improve eye conditions, but treatment-induced hypothyroidism increases the risk for worsening the eye disorders. **Radioactive iodine** has the highest risk for post-treatment hypothyroidism, with up to 50 percent of patients becoming hypothyroid. **Antithyroid drugs** are much less likely to result in post-treatment hypothyroidism and are often chosen in preference to other therapies for patients with ophthalmopathy. Patients are also advised to wear sunglasses, use artificial tears, and elevate the head of their bed and use corneal protectors for severe exophthalmus when sleeping. Bedtime **diuretics** may also be prescribed (AACE, 2006). AACE recommends consultation with an ophthalmologist experienced in the treatment of orbital disease in the management of these cases, because extensive testing, including orbital ultrasonography, CT scanning, or MRI imaging, may be necessary, and treatment may include **corticosteroids**, retro-orbital irradiation, or surgical intervention.

Monitoring

Monitoring therapy includes attention to clinical status and thyroid function test results. Clinical status is assessed by watching weight, degree of heat tolerance, appetite, anxiety level, energy level, resting heart rate, and skin texture and temperature. For patients with ophthalmopathy, assessment also includes changes in visual acuity, increasing corneal dryness, and adherence to suggestions such as sunglass use. Scheduling of ophthalmic appointments should be done frequently to monitor for complications that can include cataract development, corneal scarring, and retinal detachments.

The same tests that are used to diagnose hyperthyroidism are used to monitor the effectiveness of treatment. The amount of circulating thyroid hormone is monitored by changes in TSH and free T4. TSH is the best outcome measure because the goal is normalization of TSH. It also provides the earliest evidence of overtreatment or development of hypothyroidism.

Initially, patients are seen every 3 to 4 weeks, and TSH and free T4 levels are drawn at these times until the patients are euthyroid. Once a patient is stable and euthyroid, the frequency of visits, decreases, and thyroid testing and clinical evaluation are done at 3 months, at 6 months, and then annually, based on symptom relief (AACE, 2006).

Pregnant patients are usually monitored each visit because the progression of pregnancy is associated with altered thyroid hormone production, and dosage adjustments are commonly required. Pregnant patients with Graves' disease may have thyroid-stimulating antibodies in their circulation that can cross the placenta and affect the fetus. Measurement of maternal thyroid-stimulating antibody may be useful to assess potential fetal risk (AACE, 2006; ACOG, 2008).

Close monitoring of white blood cell (WBC) counts is important during the first 4 months of therapy, especially in those over age 40. Mild leukopenia is common, occurring in up to 10 percent of patients. Although it does not require discontinuance of the drug, leukocyte counts below 1,500 mm^3 are indications for stopping therapy. Agranulocytosis, a rare but potentially fatal adverse reaction, usually occurs within 2 months and rarely beyond 4 months after initiation of therapy with **antithyroid drugs**. Onset is rapid, so it is prudent, to obtain a baseline WBC count before initiating therapy.

Special monitoring for I^{131} patients is not indicated. Half of the dose is gone in a week. After 2 months only 1 percent remains in the body. Because one-third of patients have hyperthyroid symptoms return, assessments are necessary to monitor for return of hyperthyroid symptoms. Long-term effects do not appear to include localized, or distant, cancers related to the radioactive exposure.

Outcome Evaluation

Figure 41–1 shows the drug treatment protocol for hyperthyroidism. Evaluation is based on reduction of clinical symptoms and normalization of TSH and free T4 levels. The main indications for substituting surgery or **radioactive iodine** for **antithyroid drugs** are a patient's failure to achieve control of symptoms with **antithyroid drugs**, a patient's inability to tolerate the therapy, and relapse after completion of therapy. Having persistently high antibody titers after discontinuation of an **antithyroid drug** is predictive of relapse.

Consultation with or referral to the endocrinology team is appropriate when:

1. A patient who requires surgery or **radioactive iodine** therapy. These patients may require hospitalization and coordination with the surgeon.
2. Hyperthyroidism occurs during pregnancy or when those on antithyroid drugs become pregnant. Lactating women are also best managed with at least consultation with the endocrinology team.
3. Patients with severe ophthalmopathy require consultation or referral, depending on the degree of symptoms. Visual impairment may require hospitalization and very high-dose corticosteroid therapy or surgical decompression.
4. Referral is also considered when the patient has an obstruction to swallowing or desires cosmetic improvement post-treatment that may require surgery.
5. Prompt hospital admission is needed if heart failure, rapid atrial fibrillation, or angina develops.

Patient Education

Patient education should include discussion of information related to the overall treatment plan, as well as that specific to the drug therapy, reasons for taking the drug, drugs as part of the total treatment regimen, and adherence issues.

Patients receiving I^{131} should be instructed on dietary sources of iodine and to check for OTC sources of iodine such as multivitamins with minerals and cough syrups. Reduced levels of iodine before scans and treatments facilitate better **radioactive iodine** uptake. The following recommendations come from the American Thyroid Association (2005). Patients should delay return to work for a day and limit use of public transportation for 1 day to reduce exposure of radiation to others. In the home and at work, individuals are instructed to keep others at arm's length—distance of about 3 feet—for the next 2 to 3 days. Forcing fluids to help excrete the ions and flushing toilets twice to reduce residual elements in the reservoir also is suggested for 2 to 3 days. Eating utensils should not be shared, with a recommendation for disposable plates and utensils, the use of which will preclude the need to wash dishes separately. Sleeping alone and avoiding close personal contact, especially with infants and pregnant women, extends for 5 to 11 days. Saliva, vaginal secretions, tears, and sweat are possible sources of contamination during that period. Those patients receiving very high doses for cancer treatment are given a wallet card to carry in the highly unlikely chance of radiation detection alarms found at some worksite and federal buildings.

HYPERTHYROIDISM

PATIENT EDUCATION

Related to the Overall Treatment Plan and Disease Process

Understanding the pathophysiology of hyperthyroidism and its prognosis.
Role of iodine intake in thyroid hormone production.
Importance of adherence to the treatment regimen.
Need to take the drug for at least 1 year.
Indications of relapse or complications that need to be reported.
Importance of discussing pregnancy or the potential for pregnancy with the primary care provider.
Need for regular follow-up visits with the primary care provider.

Specific to the Drug Therapy

Discussion of the reasons for taking the drug(s) and the anticipated action of the drug(s) on the disease process. It is especially important to inform the patient that **antithyroid drugs** take 4 to 8 weeks to have a noticeable effect.
Doses and schedules for taking the drug(s).
Possible adverse reactions and what to do when they occur.
Patient education specific to **antithyroid drugs** is provided in Chapter 21.
Patient education specific to **beta-adrenergic blockers** is provided in Chapter 14.

SUBCLINICAL HYPERTHYROIDISM

Subclinical hyperthyroidism is characterized by a serum TSH level less than 0.1 microUnits/mL and a normal FT4 and FT3. Exogenous TSH suppression or endogenous production of thyroid hormones appears to be sufficient in this disorder to keep FT4 and FT3 levels normal, but to suppress pituitary TSH production and secretion. Studies report a prevalence of less than 2 percent in the adult and older adult population (AACE, 2006). The clinical significance is the potential for progression to overt hyperthyroidism, exacerbation of any concurrent cardiac problems, and decrease in bone mineral density if it is more than a transient situation. How often these "potential" problems occur is a matter of debate, and different professional groups differ on their views of whether to screen for and/or treat this disorder. According to AACE (2006), patients with subclinical hyperthyroidism attributable to nodular thyroid disease warrant treatment because there is a high rate of conversion to clinical disease. Postmenopausal women, who are already at risk for osteoporosis, may also warrant treatment. In older adults, the relative risk for atrial fibrillation increases 3-fold for those with subclinical hyperthyroidism, so treatment is prudent. However, in most patients, no treatment is necessary (AACE, 2006).

Patients with subclinical hyperthyroidism should have periodic clinical and laboratory assessment to determine individual therapeutic options. Because persistent rather than transient hormonal abnormalities are more often associated with clinical problems that suggest treatment, assessment of TSH levels along with FT4 and FT3 at 2- to 4-month intervals appears appropriate. If sustained TSH suppression (less than 0.1 microUnits/mL) is established, then treatment is probably appropriate.

HYPOTHYROIDISM

Pathophysiology

The underlying mechanisms that cause hypothyroidism can be primary or secondary. Primary disorders include the following:

- Defective hormone synthesis resulting from autoimmune thyroiditis, endemic iodine deficiency, or **antithyroid drugs** that were used to treat hyperthyroidism
- Congenital defects or loss of tissue after treatment for hyperthyroidism

Secondary causes of hypothyroidism, which are less common, include conditions that cause either pituitary or hypothalamic failure. In secondary disorders, the TSH response is inadequate, so that the gland is normal or reduced in size, and both T3 and T4 synthesis is equally reduced.

Primary hypothyroidism is based on the hypothalamic-pituitary-thyroid gland feedback system and occurs when the hypothalamus responds to a decreased thyroid hormone level with an increase in TRH, resulting in increased TSH secretion, which in turn stimulates thyroid gland enlargement, goiter formation, and preferential synthesis of T3 over T4. Of all patients with hypothyroidism, 95 percent have primary thyroid disease.

Primary Disease

Hashimoto's thyroiditis is an immune-mediated disorder in which all components of the thyroid gland are injured, but especially the TSH receptors. Antibodies generated to attack glandular antigens impair TSH response, hormone synthesis, and hormone release. Most patients with this disorder have mild disease and may remain euthyroid. Approximately 70 percent go on to develop permanent hypothyroidism.

A common variant of this disorder is postpartum thyroiditis with hypothyroid characteristics, which may affect up to 7 percent of postpartum women. Antibody production in this disorder peaks in 3 to 4 months after delivery and then declines. Symptoms resolve spontaneously in 95 percent of patients, and most return to euthyroid states.

Subacute thyroiditis is a nonbacterial inflammation of the thyroid often preceded by a viral infection. It is accompanied by fever, tenderness, and enlargement of the gland. Elevated levels of thyroid hormone are due to the release of stored thyroglobin related to the inflammatory process. Symptoms last 2 to 4 months. Anti-inflammatory agents such as **NSAIDs** may be used to address the inflammation, and **beta blockers** may be used to reduce symptoms. **Thyroid hormone replacements** may also be used temporarily. There is usually spontaneous remission of the disorder, but it can become chronic.

Congenital hypothyroidism occurs in infants as a result of absent thyroid tissue (thyroid dysgenesis) and hereditary defects in thyroid hormone synthesis. It is more common in female infants. Because thyroid hormone is essential for embryonic growth, especially of brain tissue, an infant with no T4 during fetal life will be mentally retarded. This condition can largely be reversed with administration of T4 immediately after birth. Capillary blood screening of all infants in the United States and Canada before discharge from the hospital or birthing center tests for this disorder. Infants suspected of the disorder are referred immediately to a pediatric endocrinologist.

Endemic iodine deficiency has not been a problem in the United States since the early 1900s. The addition of iodine to table salt has largely eliminated this form of hypothyroidism.

Secondary Disease

Secondary hypothyroidism most commonly is a result of a pituitary disorder. The net result is inadequate TSH production, and the thyroid gland does not produce either thyroid hormone. Common disorders of the pituitary that are associated with secondary hypothyroidism include Cushing's syndrome, acromegaly, and pituitary adenomas.

Other secondary causes of hypothyroidism include the administration of drugs that reduce thyroid hormone production (see Table 41–1) and treatment or overtreatment of hyperthyroidism.

Regardless of the etiology of hypothyroidism, the clinical features are attributable to the metabolic effects

Table 41–4 **Systemic Effects of Hypothyroidism**

Body System	Clinical Manifestation	Underlying Mechanism
Cardiovascular	Reduced stroke volume and heart rate (reduced cardiac output); increased peripheral vascular resistance to maintain blood pressure; decreased blood flow to tissue; sinus bradycardia; ECG changes	Decreased metabolic demands and loss of regulatory and rate-setting effects of thyroid hormone
Hematologic	Decreased red blood cell mass (normocytic/normochromic anemia); macrocytic anemia associated with B_{12} deficiency and inadequate folate or iron absorption	Decreased basal metabolic rate and oxygen requirements, decreased production of erythropoietin. Possible association between thyroid hormone and hematologic response to B_{12}
Respiratory	Dyspnea, hypoventilation, CO_2 retention	Myxedematous changes in respiratory muscles
Gastrointestinal	Decreased appetite, constipation, weight gain, fluid retention; decreased protein metabolism (lightly positive nitrogen balance); decreased glucose absorption; elevated serum lipid levels	Decreased metabolic demand; reduced peristaltic activity; increased capillary permeability to proteins; depressed insulin degradation; depressed lipid synthesis and degradation
Renal	Increased total body water; reduced erythropoietin production; dilutional hyponatremia	Reduced blood flow and glomerular filtration rate, leading to decreased excretion of water
Integumentary	Dry, flaky skin; dry, brittle hair; reduced growth of nails and hair; slow wound healing; myxedema; cool skin	Reduced sweat and sebaceous gland secretion; increased hyaluronic acid binds water and causes a puffy appearance; decreased circulation to skin; reduced tissue regeneration

Continued

Table 41–4 **Systemic Effects of Hypothyroidism—cont'd**

Body System	Clinical Manifestation	Underlying Mechanism
Reproductive	Anovulation, decreased libido, high incidence of spontaneous abortion in women; decreased libido and oligospermia in men	Increased estriol formation in women, decreased androgen secretion in men, decreased levels of sex hormone–binding globulin in both genders
Neurologic	Confusion, slow speech and thinking; memory loss; hearing loss; night blindness; slow; clumsy movements; cerebellar ataxia	Decreased cerebral blood flow, resulting in cerebral hypoxia
Musculoskeletal	Muscle and joint aching and stiffness; reduced deep tendon reflexes; increased bone density	Decreased innervation of muscles; decreased bone formation and resorption
Endocrine	Increased TSH production; decreased cortisol turnover rate but normal serum cortisol levels	Impaired thyroid hormone synthesis; decreased deactivation of cortisol

ECG = electrocardiogram; TSH = thyroid-stimulating hormone.

of decreased circulating levels of thyroid hormone. These effects include decreased energy metabolism and heat production. The patient develops a low basal metabolic rate, cold intolerance, lethargy, and a slightly lowered body temperature. Table 41–4 shows the most common systemic effects of hypothyroidism.

Long-standing undertreated hypothyroidism often results in myxedema, a condition similar to the pretibial myxedema seen in Graves' disease. It is a result of connective tissues being separated by an increased amount of protein and mucopolysaccharides. These protein-mucopolysaccharide complexes bind water, producing pitting, boggy edema, especially around the eyes, hands, and feet and in the supraclavicular fossae. They also produce thickening of the tongue and the laryngeal and pharyngeal membrane, resulting in thick, slurred speech and hoarseness. Myxedema coma can occur, which is a medical emergency, signaling severe hypothyroidism. Signs and symptoms include hypoventilation, hypotension, hypoglycemia, and lactic acidosis. Older adults with vascular disease and untreated hypothyroidism are especially at risk.

Pharmacodynamics

For patients who are clinically hypothyroid, replacement therapy with thyroid hormones is indicated. Administration of **synthetic thyroid hormones (levothyroxine** [T4], **liothyronine** [T3], and **liotrix** [a 4:1 **mixture of T4 and** T3]) produces the same effects on body tissues as the body's own thyroid hormones, including the negative feedback required to reduce further secretion of TSH. Dosing schedules for these drugs are provided in Chapter 21. These drugs are inexpensive and relatively free of adverse reactions, but there are conditions (discussed below) in which they are contraindicated or to be used with caution.

Goals of Treatment

The goal of therapy for patients with hypothyroidism is correction of the hypometabolic state with a minimum of adverse reactions. Adequate replacement should result in resolution of fatigue, loss of excess weight, improved functioning of all body systems, and prevention of complications, especially cardiovascular and neurological ones. This means normalization of TSH and FT4 levels.

Rational Drug Selection

Thyroid hormones were originally ground-up thyroid glands of animals, and such preparations are still available today. Because the pharmacokinetics of such drugs and the concentration of thyroid hormone within them are highly variable, they have been replaced in practice with synthetic formulations. Patients may purchase the "natural" forms in health food stores, and complementary medicine health-care providers may prescribe them. It is important to ask in the history about this possibility. The focus of this chapter is **synthetic thyroid hormones.**

Drug Therapy

Patients develop the symptoms of hypothyroidism slowly and are often quite low in thyroid hormone before they are diagnosed as having the condition. These patients have adapted to this low level of hormone and are very sensitive to the effects of **synthetic thyroid hormone** replacement. Treatment of mild to moderate hypothyroidism should be gradual. With adequate therapy, the first signs of clinical response to therapy are a modest weight loss, an increase in pulse rate, and resolution of constipation. Other symptoms, such as myxedema, cardiovascular problems, and elevated creatine kinase levels, take more time to improve. Most patients feel better in about 2 weeks, and clinical resolution usually occurs in about 3 months. All patients with TSH greater than 10 microUnits/mL. should be treated (AACE, 2006).

All of the synthetic forms of thyroid hormone have been successfully used to treat hypothyroidism. Drug choice is based on patient and drug variables. Figure 41–2 depicts the treatment algorithm based on these variables.

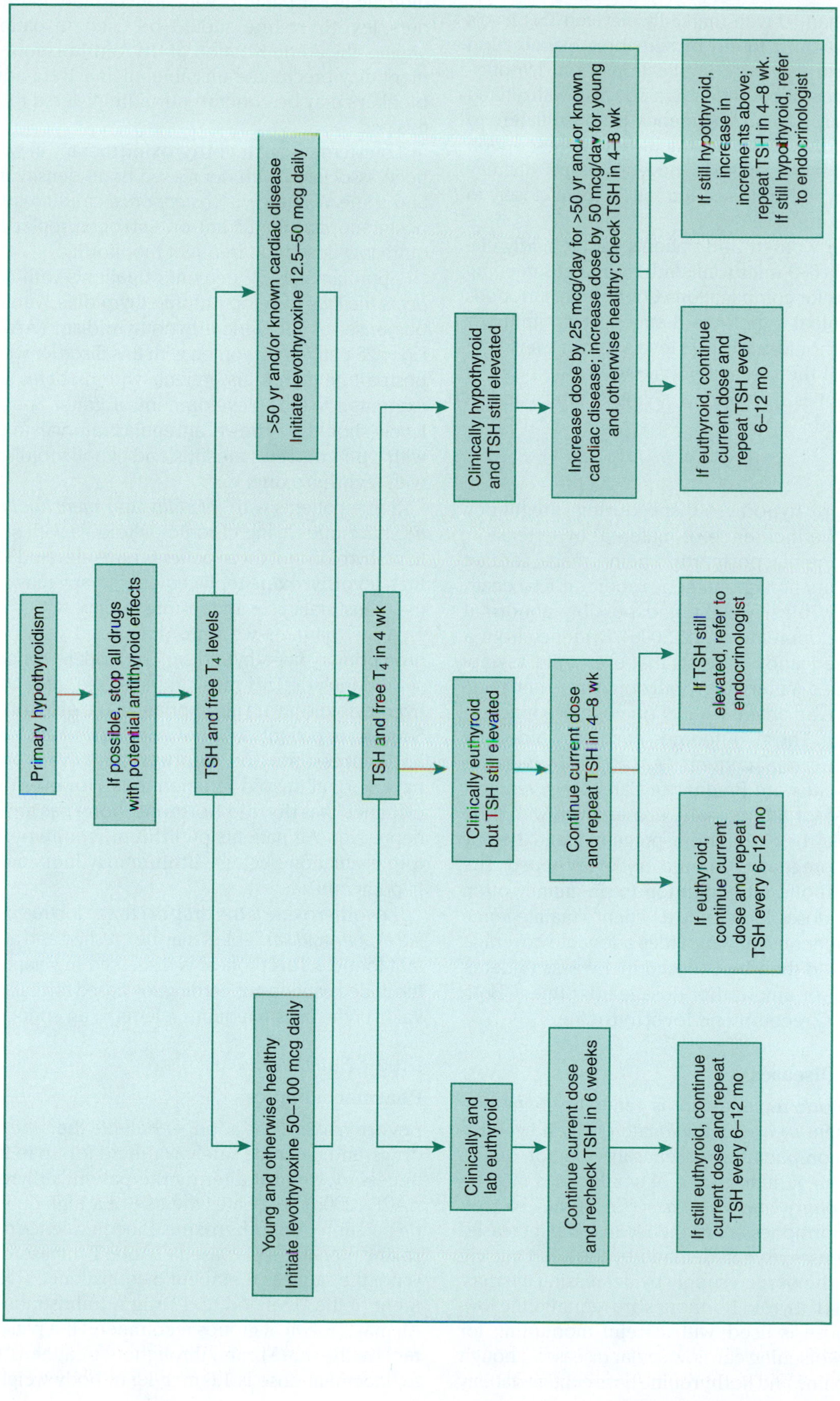

Figure 41–2. Drug therapy algorithm: Hypothyroidism.

Patient Variables

Age and Gender

Women older than 50 with markedly elevated TSH levels (= 10 microUnits/mL) found by screening examination have the highest risk for complications from hypothyroidism, such as cardiac conditions associated with altered lipid metabolism. Research evidence is not sufficient to recommend or discourage treatment, but the best option seems to be to treat patients who have symptoms that may be caused by hypothyroidism and follow them closely to see if symptoms improve.

Men, younger women, and patients with a mildly elevated TSH level (6–9 microUnits/mL) found at screening have a lower risk for complications. Controversy surrounds treating subclinical hypothyroid states. At a minimum, these patients should have TSH levels drawn every 2 to 5 years to see if the disease progresses to the point at which treatment is appropriate. Symptomatic patients should be treated.

Pregnancy

Untreated overt hypothyroidism during pregnancy may increase the incidence of maternal hypertension, preeclampsia, anemia, postpartum hemorrhage, cardiac ventricular dysfunction, spontaneous abortion, fetal death or stillbirth, low birth weight, and possibly abnormal fetal brain development (AACE, 2006). Evidence from a population-based study suggests that even mild, asymptomatic, untreated maternal hypothyroidism during pregnancy may have an adverse effect on cognitive function in the offspring. These outcomes can be avoided by thyroid hormone replacement (AACE, 2006). Because **thyroid hormones** are Pregnancy Category A, replacement is advised for all pregnant women even with mild disease. They may be given during pregnancy, and therapy begun before pregnancy should not be stopped. The increased metabolic rate common to pregnancy often requires higher doses. Increasing a patient's maintenance dose by 25 percent usually provides adequate coverage. TSH levels should then be checked in 4 weeks to determine the need for any further dosage adjustment. Both AACE and ACOG recommend **levothyroxine.**

Concomitant Diseases

Thyroid hormone replacement is generally contraindicated after recent *myocardial infarction* (MI). If hypothyroidism is a complicating or causative factor of the cardiac problem, judicious use of small doses may be called for. *Coronary artery disease* (CAD) may worsen when thyroid hormones are given because the increased heart rate increases oxygen demand by the heart muscle and decreases the oxygen supply by decreasing the diastolic filling time. If thyroid hormones are required, the lowest possible dose is used, with careful monitoring for indications of worsening cardiovascular disease. Although both **levothyroxine** and **liothyronine** have content stability, **liothyronine** is three to four times more active than **levothyroxine**, making it more likely to produce cardiotoxicity. For patients with concomitant cardiac disorders, **levothyroxine** should be used. In patients with *angina*, the administration of **thyroid hormone** replacement may precipitate unstable angina. **Beta-adrenergic blockers** may be concurrently administered to decrease this risk.

Long-term use of **levothyroxine** therapy in women has been associated with decreased bone density in the hip and spine. Women with *osteoporosis* and those who are postmenopausal and not on **estrogen** replacement require low doses and frequent monitoring.

Approximately 10 percent of patients with *type 1 diabetes mellitus* develop chronic thyroiditis, with an insidious onset of subclinical hypothyroidism (AACE, 2006). Up to 25 percent of women with this disorder will develop postpartum thyroiditis. Patients with diabetes should be examined for the development of goiter. Sensitive TSH levels should be drawn at regular intervals on patients with type 1 diabetes mellitus, and hypothyroidism treated with **levothyroxine.**

Some patients with *infertility* and *menstrual irregularities* have underlying chronic thyroiditis with subclinical hypothyroidism. If these patients have elevated TSH levels, then **levothyroxine** replacement therapy may normalize the menstrual cycle and restore fertility.

A few patients who are diagnosed with *depression* have primary hypothyroidism. The work-up for depression should include TSH measurement and treatment of any hypothyroidism with appropriate doses of **levothyroxine.** Sometimes patients who have depression are treated with **antidepressants** and **levothyroxine** even though they have normal thyroid function tests. However, there is no evidence that **thyroid hormone** alone has any effect on depression. All patients on **lithium** require periodic thyroid evaluation because **lithium** may induce goiter and hypothyroidism.

Levothyroxine is the drug of choice for treating *congenital hypothyroidism*. Tablets may be crushed and added to infant formula. This process is discussed in Chapter 21 with the added caution concerning soy-based formulas. Congenital hypothyroidism requires referral to an endocrinologist.

Drug-Related Variables

Pharmacokinetics

Levothyroxine has a longer half-life than the other two drugs, and it can be safely withheld for up to 2 weeks, if necessary, without altering the patient's thyroid status. AACE (2006) advocates the use of a high-quality brand preparation of **levothyroxine.** Bioequivalence of **levothyroxine** preparation is based on total T_4 measurement and is not the same as therapeutic equivalence ("Joint Statement of the U.S. Food and Drug Administration," 2004). All major medical groups recommend the patient should receive the same brand throughout treatment. The mean replacement dose is 1.6 mcg/kg of body weight per day.

The initial dose may range from 12.5 mcg/day to a full replacement dose based on the age, weight, and cardiac status of the patient and the severity and duration of the hypothyroidism.

Thyroid hormone absorption can be affected by malabsorptive states and patient age. Because **levothyroxine** has a narrow therapeutic range, small differences in absorption can result in clinical changes. The surge in soy-based products generated concern about absorption issues, which have not come to fruition, except for infants (Messina & Redmond, 2006). Drug interactions also present a problem. Table 21–34 in Chapter 21 lists these drug interactions. Titrations in dosage may initially occur after 4 weeks, but any future titrations should occur at no sooner than 6-week intervals. The TSH level is the most important monitoring variable. Once it is in normal range, the frequency of visits and laboratory studies can be decreased. Although treatment is individualized, the usual follow-up visit is after 6 months and then annually.

Recently, there has been a resurgence of interest in the use of combination **thyroid hormones** to treat hypothyroidism. A meta-analysis concluded that physiological combinations of **levothyroxine** plus **liothyronine** did not offer any objective advantage over **levothyroxine** alone (Groszinski-Glasberg, Fraser, Nashshoni, Weizman, & Leibovici, 2006).

If there is a need to rapidly correct a hypothyroid state, **liothyronine** is preferable because of its rapid onset and dissipation of action. The advantages of rapid onset and dissipation, however, must be weighed against the wide swings in T3 levels and possible cardiotoxicity of **liothyronine**. Dosing schedules for both drugs are shown in Chapter 21.

Cost

Generic forms of all the **thyroid hormones** are less expensive than brand names; however, bioequivalence does not exist between brands and cannot be assumed between generic forms. A cost index is provided in Chapter 21.

Monitoring

Levothyroxine is the easiest to monitor with standard TSH and free T4 laboratory measurements of thyroid function. Monitoring **liothyronine** therapy is more difficult, and it is best used for TSH suppression. **Liotrix** offers no clear benefit over either of these other drugs on any of these parameters.

Monitoring thyroid replacement therapy has three parameters: clinical symptoms, TSH, and free T4. Despite some controversy, clinical symptoms alone are generally not an effective monitoring parameter because they do not correlate well with laboratory findings. They are important in conjunction with laboratory data.

The most accurate monitoring parameter is a sensitive TSH test because it correlates most closely with physiological measurements of **thyroid hormone** effects. TSH is evaluated for diagnosis, at initiation of therapy, and every 4 to 8 weeks after therapy has begun until the patient achieves stable euthyroid status. Normalized and stable TSH levels often take 6 to 12 months to achieve. TSH is also repeated 6 to 8 weeks after any dosage adjustment because it takes approximately this amount of time for the new dosage to stabilize, especially with the long half-life of **levothyroxine**. Once the patient is euthyroid and stable, TSH monitoring occurs every 12 months, depending on symptoms and stability.

Controversy exists as to where the cutoff range of TSH is at which treatment should initially begin. Providers should be attuned to the fact that the diagnostic cut point for hypothyroid disease and the therapeutic range for treatment differ in practice. The current practice is that the TSH should remain between 0.3-3.0 microunits/mL during therapy, preferably between 1.0 and 2.0. If the TSH level falls below the lower limit of normal or becomes undetectable, the dose of **thyroid hormone** used for replacement is excessive. Measurement of free T4 can help to determine how excessive the dose is. FT4 may correlate poorly with physiological status during the initial therapy period. It is more reliable once the patient is stable (e.g., after 12 months).

During pregnancy, elevated estrogen increases thyroid-binding globulin levels, which alters total T4 values but not FT4. During pregnancy, both TSH and FT4 levels are evaluated to determine appropriate replacement dosage. Tests are done at 8 weeks and 6 months of gestation. The goal is to normalize TSH and maintain FT4 at the upper limits of normal. Women with hypothyroidism who become pregnant may have their thyroid function change. In general, the dosage of **thyroid hormone** may need to be increased and these patients should have their serum TSH level evaluated every 6 weeks during pregnancy to ensure that the dose of **levothyroxine** is appropriate. Primary care providers should consult with an endocrinologist for management of pregnant patients.

Anemia is a frequent concomitant disease with hypothyroidism. A complete blood count (CBC) should be drawn at initiation of therapy. After a thorough work-up of any anemia to assess for other possible causes (e.g., iron deficiency, blood loss, vitamin B_{12} or folic acid deficiency), hypothyroidism should be treated with standard **thyroid hormone** replacement. Management of anemia, including monitoring parameters, is discussed in Chapter 27.

Other common concomitant disorders with hypothyroidism that require monitoring include hypercholesterolemia and hypertension. Management of these disorders, including monitoring parameters, is discussed in Chapters 39 and 40.

Outcome Evaluation

Figure 41–2 shows the drug treatment protocol for hypothyroidism. Evaluation is based on reduction of clinical symptoms and normalization of TSH and FT4 levels. Although most health-care providers can diagnose and treat hypothyroidism, certain situations suggest referral to a clinical endocrinologist experienced in the spectrum of thyroid disease. AACE (2006) recommends consultation for the following situations:

- Patients age 18 years or under
- Patients unresponsive to therapy
- Pregnant patients
- Cardiac patients
- Presence of goiter, nodule, or other structural changes in the thyroid gland
- Presence of other endocrine diseases

Additional situations for referral include the following:

- Failure to achieve control of symptoms or normalized TSH within 12 months by standard doses despite patient adherence to the treatment regimen.
- Relapse after a period of stability on a standard dose.
- Pending surgery. Careful anesthesia planning is required because clearance of anesthetics is reduced.
- Lactating women are also best managed with at least consultation with an endocrinologist.

Patient Education

Patient education should discuss the overall treatment plan, as well as information specific to the drug therapy, reasons for taking the drug, drugs as part of the total treatment regimen, and adherence issues.

HYPOTHYROIDISM

PATIENT EDUCATION

Related to the Overall Treatment Plan and Disease Process

Understanding the pathophysiology of hypothyroidism and its prognosis.

Role of iodine intake in thyroid hormone production.

Importance of adherence to the treatment regimen.

Length of time the drug will need to be taken. For those with thyroiditis, this may be less than 12 months. For many with primary hypothyroidism, the treatment will be lifelong. The patient should be informed not to stop taking the drug without first consulting the health-care provider.

Indications of relapse or complications that need to be reported.

Importance of discussing pregnancy or the potential for pregnancy with the primary care provider.

Need to wear a medical identification bracelet stating that patient is taking **thyroid hormone** replacement and to inform any provider who sees him or her that this is the case. This is especially important if this provider prescribes any new drugs for the patient.

Need for regular follow-up visits with the primary care provider, which will include laboratory monitoring of thyroid function to determine the status of the hypothyroidism and any needed dosage adjustments of the drug therapy.

Specific to the Drug Therapy

Discussion of the reasons for taking the drug(s) and the anticipated action of the drug(s) on the disease process. It is especially important to inform the patient that **thyroid hormone** replacement may take 4 to 8 weeks to have a noticeable effect.

Doses and schedules for taking the drug(s).

Possible adverse reactions (e.g., rapid heart rate, cardiac arrhythmias, chest pain, insomnia, diarrhea, or heat intolerance) and what to do when they occur.

Additional patient education specific to thyroid hormones is provided in Chapter 21.

SUBCLINICAL HYPOTHYROIDISM

Subclinical hypothyroidism refers to mildly increased serum TSH levels in the setting of normal FT4 and FT3. It is a common disorder, ranging from 1 to 10 percent of the adult population, with increased frequency in women, older adults, and those with higher dietary iodine intake. Subclinical hypothyroidism is usually asymptomatic and discovered on routine screening of TSH. The most common cause is Hashimoto's disease. Progression to overt hypothyroidism is reported to vary from 3 to 20 percent.

Potential risks for this condition, besides progression to hypothyroidism, include cardiovascular disease, hyperlipidemia, and neuropsychiatric effects. AACE (2006) reports that studies have suggested that treatment will reduce cardiovascular risk factors, improve lipid profile, and minimize behavioral abnormalities. They question the validity of some of these studies. The treatment of this disorder remains controversial. AACE (2006) recommends treatment for selected patients with TSH levels 5 and 10 micro Units/mL who also have goiter or positive thyroid peroxidase antibodies. These patients have the highest rate of conversion to overt hypothyroidism. An initial dose of

levothyroxine 25 to 50 mcg/day can be used, the serum TSH measured in 6 to 8 weeks, and the dose adjusted as needed. As with overt hypothyroidism, the target TSH level should be between 0.3 and 3.0 microUnits/mL. Once this level is achieved, an annual evaluation is sufficient.

REFERENCES

American Association of Clinical Endocrinologists (AACE). (2006). American Association of Clinical Endocrinologists medical guidelines for clinical practice for the evaluation and treatment of hyperthyroidism and hypothyroidism. (Amended version from original *Endocrine Practice 2002, 8*[6], 457–469.) Retrieved August 10, 2009, from http://www.aace.com/pub/pdf/guidelines

American College of Obstetricians and Gynecologists (ACOG). (2007). Routine thyroid screening not recommended for pregnant women [ACOG News release]. Retrieved August 10, 2009 from http://www.acog.org

American College of Obstetricians and Gynecologists (ACOG). (2008). *Thyroid disease in pregnancy.* ACOG Practice Bulletin No. 37. (Bulletin from 2002; reaffirmed 2008.) Retrieved August 10, 2009, from http://www.acog.org

American Thyroid Association. (2005). Radioactive iodine uses for thyroid diseases. Retrieved August 31, 2009, from http://www.thyroid.org/patients/patient-brochures/radioactive.html

Caldwell, K., Miller, G., Wang, R., Jain, R., & Jones, R. (2008). Iodine status of the U.S. population. National Health and Nutrition Examination Survey 2003–2004. *Thyroid, 18*(11), 1207–1214.

Grozinski-Glasberg, S., Fraser, A., Nashshoni, E., Weizman, A., & Leibovici, L. (2006).. Thyroxine-triiodothyronine combination therapy versus thyroxine monotherapy for clinical hypothyroidism: Meta-analysis of randomized controlled trails. *Journal of Clinical Endocrinology & Metabolism, 91*(7), 2592–2599.

Joint statement of the U.S. Food and Drug Administration's decision regarding bioequivalence of levothyroxine sodium. (2004). *Thyroid 2004, 14*, 486.

McCance, K., & Huether, S. (2006). *Pathophysiology: The biological basis for disease in adults and children* (5th ed.). St. Louis, MO: Mosby.

Messina, M., & Redmond, G. (2006). Effects of soy protein and soybean isoflavones on thyroid function in healthy adults and thyroid patients: A review of the relevant literature. *Thyroid, 16*(3), 249–258.

New York Thyroid Center. (2007). Radioactive iodine preparation and precautions. Retrieved August 31, 2009, from http://www.cumc.columbia.edu/dept/thyroid/raiprep.html

U.S. Food & Drug Administration. (2009). Propylthiouracil-induced liver failure. Retrieved June 5, 2009, from http://www.fda.gov/Drugs/DrugSafety/PostmarketDrugSafetyInformationfor PatientsandProviders/ucm162701

U.S. Food & Drug Administration. (2010). FDA Drug Safety Communication: New boxed warning on severe liver injury with propylthiouracil. Retrieved April 21, 2010, from http://www.fda.gov/Drugs/DrugSafety/PostmarketDrugSafetyInformationfor PatientsandProviders/ucm209023.htm

U.S. Preventive Services Task Force. (2004). Screening for thyroid disease: Recommendation statement. *Annals of Internal Medicine, 140*, 125–127.

CHAPTER 42

PNEUMONIA

Teri Moser Woo

Chapter Outline

Pneumonia is a common condition seen in primary care as well as in acute care. A provider may see patients of all ages with pneumonia and therefore needs to be familiar the common pathogens and treatment for each unique population.

ADULT PATIENTS WITH PNEUMONIA

Pneumonia affects more than 5 million people a year in the United States, making it one of the more commonly seen medical problems and the seventh leading cause of death in the United States (Mandell et al, 2007; National Center for Health Statistics, 2009). The incidence rates average 12 per 1,000, increasing with age to more than 30 per 1,000 in patients over age 75. As in most bacterial illnesses, those patients of the extremes of age are most severely affected, with infants and older adults often requiring hospitalization and IV antibiotics.

Pathophysiology

Pneumonia develops when an organism invades the lung parenchyma and the host defenses are depressed. Bacterial pneumonia results when the lung's primary defense mechanisms are altered, either by a viral infection or by immunological problems. Chronically ill patients of all ages are more prone to pneumonia, usually because of their underlying medical problem. There may be other origins of pneumonia besides bacterial organisms, such as viral, fungal, rickettsial, and parasitic organisms; inflammatory processes; and inhalation of toxic substances.

Pneumonia should be considered in any patient who presents with respiratory symptoms such as cough, dyspnea, or sputum production. Fever or abnormal breath sounds, such as crackles, would strengthen the suspicion of pneumonia. Chest radiographs assist in confirming the diagnosis of pneumonia versus other respiratory disorders such as lung abscess or tuberculosis (Mandell et al, 2007).

The predominant organism found in pneumonia depends on the age and health status of the patient. For all ages (except neonates), *Streptococcus pneumoniae* is the most commonly found organism in pneumonia (Mandell et al, 2007). *S. pneumoniae* is identified as the causative organism in 60 to 75 percent of adults with bacterial pneumonia, based on sputum culture. Nontypeable *Haemophilus influenzae* and *Moraxella catarrhalis* are common pathogens in patients with underlying lung disease. *Staphylococcus aureus* has become a common copathogen in influenza-associated pneumonia. *Mycoplasma pneumoniae*, a pathogen difficult to detect on gram stain or culture, is another common cause of pneumonia. Viruses are the cause of pneumonia in many patients; with viruses identified in 18 to 36 percent of pneumonia cases (Mandell et al, 2007). It must be noted that the responsible organism is not identified in up to 50 percent of patients with community-acquired pneumonia (CAP) (American Thoracic Society [ATS], 2001). Table 42–1 lists the common pathological agents for CAP at different ages.

In the past, practitioners attempted to determine the most likely pathogen by the clinical presentation of the patient, using terms like typical and atypical. Typical infections were those caused by *S. pneumoniae, H. influenzae, S. aureus,* or gram-negative bacteria. The presentation of typical pneumonia included fever, chills, yellow or green sputum, pleuritic chest pain, and lobar consolidation on chest x-rays; the presentation of atypical pneumonia included a gradual onset of cough, no or scant sputum, low-grade fever, myalgias, arthralgias, and lack of consolidation on x-rays. It was thought that patients with atypical pneumonia most likely had *M. pneumoniae, Legionella pneumophila,* or a viral infection. In clinical practice, these classifications have little usefulness, as numerous studies have shown that few reliable clinical features distinguish between the different bacterial pathogens (ATS, 2001).

Goals of Treatment

The ultimate goal of treatment for all patients is return to the respiratory status they had before the illness. Initially, patients who are responding to empirical **antibiotic therapy** should show improved clinical condition in 48 to 72 hours. Fever should resolve in 2 to 4 days, and leukocytosis usually resolves by day 4 of treatment (ATS, 2001). The patient's chest x-ray may actually deteriorate, however, and not return to baseline for weeks or months. In previously healthy adults younger than age 50 years, 66 percent of patients with pneumonia return to baseline chest x-rays within 4 weeks. In older patients or those who have previously had respiratory or other chronic illness, only 26 percent of patients have normal chest x-rays by the fourth week of treatment (ATS, 2001). Children may require 6 to 8 weeks for the chest x-ray to return to normal (Kercsmar, 1998). Therefore, a clear chest x-ray may not be the best indicator of successful treatment initially. The best indicator of improvement in clinical status is that the overall clinical manifestations of pneumonia (e.g., fever and increased white blood cell [WBC] count) should improve. Older patients, those with multiple coexisting illnesses, and increased severity of disease will have delayed resolution of clinical signs and symptoms (level II evidence) (ATS, 2001).

Rational Drug Selection

Clinical Guidelines

In 1993, the American Thoracic Society (ATS) issued guidelines for the initial management of adults with CAP that discuss the diagnosis, assessment of severity, and initial antimicrobial therapy; these guidelines were revised and updated in 2001. In 2007, the Infectious Diseases Society of America and the American Thoracic Society published a consensus document on the management of community-acquired pneumonia (Mandell et al, 2007). The original ATS guidelines published in 2001 are similar to those used in Europe and Canada (Woodhead, 1998), and break down the treatment into severely ill and not severely ill patients, patients who require hospitalization, and those who require intensive care unit (ICU) hospitalization (ATS, 2001; Mandell et al, 2007; Riley, Aronsky, & Dean, 2004). These categories include the following:

1. Previously healthy outpatients with no history of cardiopulmonary disease, and no modifying factors such as risk for drug-resistant streptococcal pneumonia (DSRP) (excludes those with HIV).
2. Outpatients with cardiopulmonary disease (congestive heart failure or chronic obstructive pulmonary disease [COPD]), diabetes, liver or renal disease,

Table 42–1 **Community-Acquired Pneumonia: Common Pathogens by Age**

Age	Common Pathogens
Neonates	Coliform bacteria, cytomegalovirus, enterovirus, group B streptococci, herpesvirus, *Mycoplasma hominis, Ureaplasma urealyticum*
Infants 4–16 weeks	Cytomegalovirus, influenza virus, parainfluenza virus, respiratory syncytial virus (RSV), *Chlamydia trachomatis, Haemophilus influenzae, Staphylococcus aureus, Streptococcus pneumoniae, U. urealyticum*
Children up to 5 years	Adenovirus, group A streptococci, influenza virus, RSV, *H. influenzae, S. aureus, S. pneumoniae*
Children over 5 years through adolescence	Influenza virus, varicella, *Chlamydia pneumoniae, H. influenzae, Legionella pneumophila, Mycoplasma pneumoniae, S. pneumoniae*
Adults group I: no cardiopulmonary disease and no modifying factors	Respiratory viruses, *C. pneumoniae, H. influenzae, M. pneumoniae, S. pneumoniae;* other (1%): endemic fungi, *Legionella* spp., *Mycobacterium tuberculosis, S. aureus*
Adults group II: with cardiopulmonary disease and/or modifying factors	Aerobic gram-negative bacilli, respiratory viruses, *H. influenzae, S. aureus, S. pneumoniae* (including DSRP); other (1%): endemic fungi, *Legionella Moraxella catarrhalis, M. tuberculosis, Mycoplasma pneumoniae,* mixed infection

DSRP = drug-resistant streptococcal pneumonia; RSV = respiratory syncytial virus.

alcoholism, malignancies, asplenia, immunosuppression, use of antimicrobials in the past 3 months, and/or modifying factors (risk factors for DSRP [age greater than 65] or gram-negative bacteria).

3. Inpatients not admitted to the ICU who have the following:
   a. Cardiopulmonary disease and/or other modifying factors, such as having recently stayed at a nursing home.
   b. No cardiopulmonary disease, and no other modifying factors.
4. ICU-admitted patients who have the following:
   a. No risks for *Pseudomonas aeruginosa*
   b. Risks for *P. aeruginosa*

Basically, the practitioner needs to take into consideration the comorbidities of patient (cardiopulmonary disease), the severity of the illness at initial presentation, and the treatment setting (outpatient or hospital). In the 1993 ATS guidelines, age was a factor in decision making, but studies have found that age alone has little impact on the bacterial etiology of pneumonia (ATS, 2001). The only exception is that patients over age 65 are at risk for DSRP, which automatically places them in group 2, but age does not affect susceptibility to other organisms. Because most primary care practitioners are in the ambulatory setting, the first two categories, which outline the treatment of the outpatient, are discussed here.

In selecting treatment, the practitioner must also decide whether to treat the patient on an outpatient basis or in a hospital. The presence of any one of the following warrants admission to a hospital: respiratory rate greater than 30, temperature above 101°F, a Pao_2 less than 60 mm Hg, or a $Paco_2$ greater than 50 mm Hg on room air. Age over 65 years, presence of coexisting illnesses such as COPD, diabetes mellitus, and chronic renal failure, congestive heart failure, chronic liver disease, **alcohol** abuse, and malnutrition all increase mortality of pneumonia and should warrant consideration for initial treatment as an inpatient (ATS, 2001). A severity-of-illness scale such as CURB-65 may be used to guide hospital admission decision making. The CURB-65 criteria evaluate confusion, uremia, respiratory rate, low blood pressure, age 65 years or greater; patients with a score of 2 or above require either hospitalization or intensive home health services (Mandell et al, 2007). Even in the absence of any of these complicating factors or findings, the severity of the overall clinical picture may warrant hospitalization.

If the patient can be treated on an outpatient basis, the practitioner, using the ATS guidelines, determines the appropriate treatment based on the modifying factors that increase the risk of infection with specific pathogens. The treatment decision is based on the slightly different organism found in each group. Figure 42–1 is an outpatient treatment algorithm for adults with CAP.

Dosing Regimen

Initial empirical therapy for the previously healthy outpatient with no cardiopulmonary disease, no antibiotics in the past 3 months (no risk for DRSP), and no modifying factors (group 1) is to treat with an **advanced-generation macrolide** (level I evidence), such as **azithromycin** or **clarithromycin**, with **doxycycline** (level III evidence) a second choice if the patient is allergic or intolerant to **macrolides**. **Erythromycin** is the least expensive **macrolide**, whereas the ATS guidelines note that the newer **macrolides** have a lower incidence of gastrointestinal (GI) side effects and require fewer doses, improving the likelihood of patient compliance with therapy (Abramoqicz, 2003; Mandell et al, 2007). **Azithromycin** 500 mg on day 1, followed by 250 mg/day for days 2 to 5 is one choice (about $25 per course of treatment with generic medication), with **clarithromycin** 250 to 500 mg twice a day for 7 to 10 days (about $73 for 10 days of treatment, either strength) also an appropriate choice. **Erythromycin** 500 mg given PO qid for 7 to 10 days is the least expensive (about $17 for 7 days of treatment). Patients may also be prescribed **erythromycin** 333 mg tid (about $16 for 10 days) or 500 mg bid ($15 for 10 days). If patients have GI upset from the **erythromycin** at a dose of 500 mg qid, they may respond to 250 mg of **erythromycin** given qid. The patient should begin to exhibit clinical response in 48 to 72 hours; therefore, unless the patient is deteriorating, treatment should not be altered for 72 hours (level III evidence) (ATS, 2001). Length of treatment with community-acquired pneumonia should be for a minimum of 5 days (level I evidence) and the patient should be afebrile for 48 to 72 hours and vitals signs, including oxygen saturation, within normal limits (Mandell et al, 2007).

Presence of comorbidities, such as chronic heart, lung, liver, or renal disease; diabetes mellitus; alcoholism; malignancies; asplenia; immunosuppressant conditions or use of immunosuppressant drugs; use of antimicrobials within the previous 3 months; or other risk for DRSP infection requires a respiratory **fluoroquinolone** such as **moxifloxacin, gemifloxacin,** or **levofloxacin** (Mandell et al, 2007). An alternative treatment in patients with comorbidities is a **beta lactam** *plus* a **macrolide** (level I evidence). High-dose **amoxicillin** (1 gm tid) or **amoxicillin/clavulanate (Augmentin)** is the preferred choice (Mandell et al, 2007). Alternatives include **cefpodoxime, cefuroxime,** or parenteral **ceftriaxone** followed by oral **cefpodoxime. Doxycycline** may be used as an alternative to the **macrolide** (level II evidence). In regions with a high rate (125%) of infection with high-level (MIC 16 mg/mL) macrolide-resistant *S. pneumoniae,* consider use of a respiratory **fluoroquinolone (levofloxacin, gemifloxacin, or moxifloxacin)** or a **beta lactam** plus a **macrolide** (level III evidence). The patient should begin to demonstrate clinical improvement in 48 to 72 hours and length of treatment is a minimum of 5 days.

If the patient is over age 60 years or has comorbidities, is stable enough for home therapy, but oral intake is not assured, home parenteral therapy is an option. The drugs

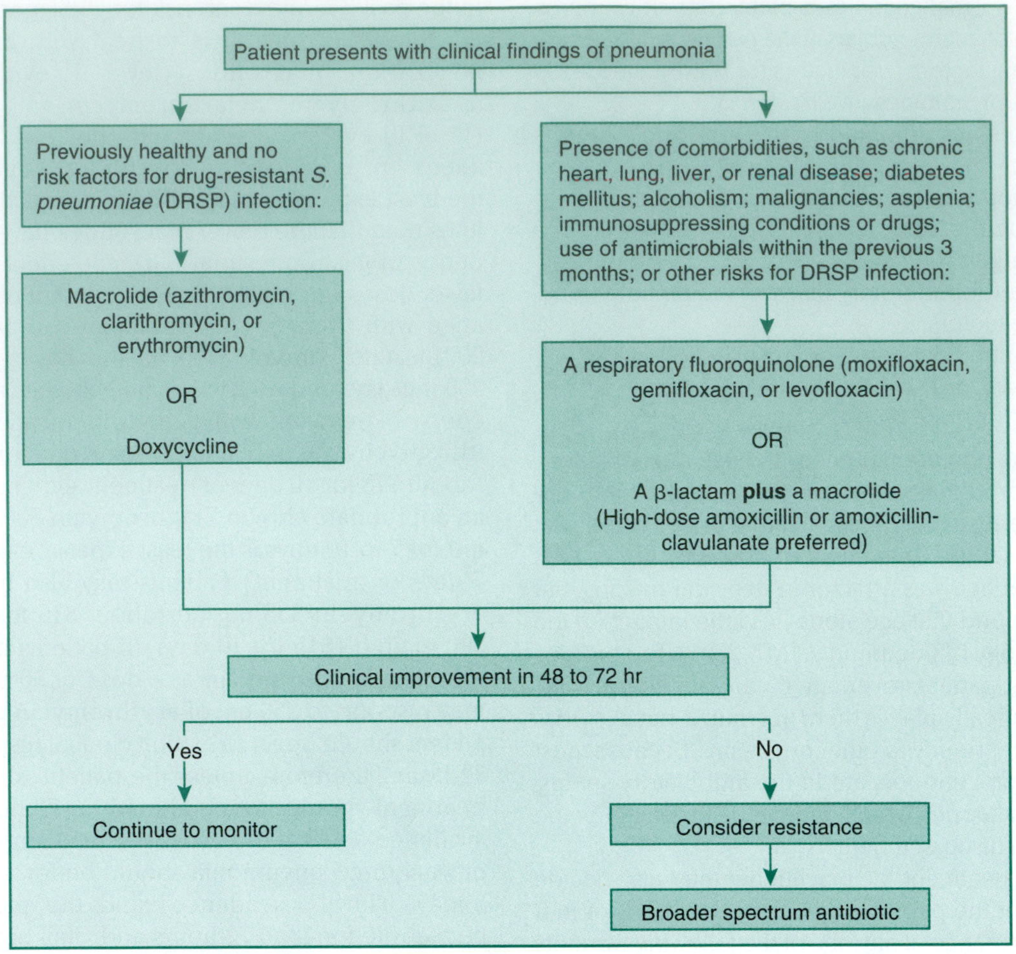

Figure 42–1. Treatment algorithm: Outpatient treatment of adults with community-acquired pneumonia.

of choice for these patients are **ceftriaxone (Rocephin)** 1 g daily via IV or IM or **levofloxacin** 500 mg IV daily. Consider adding a **macrolide** to **ceftriaxone** for coverage against atypical pathogens if indicated. Once clinical response is observed, the patient is switched to oral therapy, as described previously. Although parenteral therapy is expensive, it is still much more cost effective than a hospital stay.

Patient Variables

Patient With Nursing Home–Acquired Pneumonia

Patients with nursing home–acquired pneumonias are classified by the ATS guidelines as group 2 patients, with nursing home residence considered a modifying factor. The ATS document (2001) does identify certain pathogens that need to be considered in residents of long-term care facilities: aerobic gram-negative pathogens, Enterobacteriaceae, *Mycobacterium tuberculosis,* and certain viral agents (adenovirus, respiratory syncytial virus [RSV], and influenza). Anaerobes should be considered if the patient has poor dentition or swallowing disorder (ATS, 2001; Muder, Agahbabian, Loeb, Solot, & Higbee, 2004). These pathogens should be part of the differential for treating a patient who resides in a long-term care facility, yet the ATS recommends that nursing home patients should be initially treated in the same fashion as other group 2 patients. Note the 2007 consensus statement does not directly address nursing home–acquired pneumonia.

Pregnant Patient With Pneumonia

Pregnant women are at a slightly higher risk for infections than are other women because of diminished lymphocyte function and decreased functional residual capacity of the lung during pregnancy (Sheffield & Cunningham, 2009). The prevalence of pneumonia in pregnancy is 0.5 to 1.5 cases per 1,000 pregnancies (Sheffield & Cunningham, 2009). Risk factors that appear to be associated with antepartum pneumonia include anemia, prior lung disease, and illicit drug use. The pathogens found in CAP are also the predominant pathogens in antepartum patients with pneumonia; the main pathogens causing pneumonia are *S. pneumoniae, H. influenzae, M. pneumoniae,* and viruses (Lim, Macfarlane, & Colthorpe, 2003). Viruses such as influenza (both type A and type B), varicella, and measles are associated with significant morbidity for pregnant women with pneumonia (Riley, 1997). During the pandemic H1N1 influenza epidemic of 2009, infected pregnant women were found to be at high risk for hospitalization and severe complications, specifically pneumonia leading to acute respiratory distress syndrome (Centers for Disease Control and Prevention [CDC], 2009; Jamieson et al, 2009; Sheffield & Cunningham, 2009).

A review of the effects of pneumonia on pregnant patients suggests that maternal and fetal morbidity remain a concern. The complications found were maternal death, fetal death, and preterm labor, with preterm labor rates as high as 44 percent in some studies (Riley, 1997; Sheffield & Cunningham, 2009). Pregnant women with pneumonia require treatment with the appropriate antimicrobial/antiviral and consultation with a perinatologist as occult onset of preterm labor may occur (Ramsey & Ramin, 2001). **Antibiotic therapy** for the pregnant patient is similar to treatment of other adults with CAP: The **macrolides erythromycin, azithromycin,** and **clarithromycin** are safe during pregnancy, although **erythromycin** or **azithromycin** is the first choice, as each is Pregnancy Category B, whereas **clarithromycin** is Pregnancy Category C. Sheffield and Cunningham report a 99 percent treatment success rate among previously healthy pregnant women treated with macrolides (2009). **Doxycycline,** a **tetracycline,** is not used during pregnancy because it may cause discoloration of deciduous teeth in neonates. Women with comorbid conditions or recent antibiotics should be treated with a βeta lactam plus a macrolide (Mandell et al, 2007).

Prevention of viral causes of pneumonia is key to the health of the pregnant patient. The patient who has not previously had varicella should receive the **varicella vaccine** prior to planning a pregnancy (**Measles/Mumps/Rubella [MMR]** cannot be given during pregnancy.) The pregnant patient should receive an **influenza vaccine,** including **H1N1 vaccine,** in the fall of the year, and any patient with a chronic medical condition should receive a **pneumococcal vaccine.**

Lifestyle Modifications

Although the mainstay of treatment is **antibiotic therapy,** other measures improve outcome. Adequate hydration enables the patient to liquefy any secretions present. Also, patients who are ill with pneumonia often are anorectic and have decreased fluid intake, so education regarding "pushing" fluids is helpful. Rest is one aspect of therapy that younger, working patients may have a hard time accepting. Encouraging patients to not work for a few days will speed the healing process. Tobacco smoke irritates the lungs and increases the coughing associated with the pneumonia. The patient and other household members should refrain from smoking.

Monitoring

The practitioner needs to monitor the patient's clinical status closely. Early identification of the need for hospitalization will enhance the outcome of the illness. The patient's fever, respiratory status, hydration, and activity tolerance all need to be monitored for early signs of either improvement or deterioration.

Outcome Evaluation

As previously mentioned, the patient needs to be monitored for response to empirical **antibiotic therapy.** The patient should become afebrile in 2 to 4 days. Leukocytosis most often resolves by the fourth day of treatment. Radiographic improvement usually requires more time and is not an indicator of improvement. If the chest x-ray worsens yet the patient shows clinical improvement that is the natural progression of the disease. Up to 15 percent of patients do not respond to appropriate initial empiric antibiotic therapy (Mandell et al, 2007). In severe CAP, if the radiographic findings worsen *and* the clinical picture worsens, then that is a predictor of increased morbidity and mortality (ATS, 2001; Mandell et al, 2007).

If no improvement in clinical status occurs within 72 hours, the practitioner needs to consider that the pathogen is not being treated appropriately. Two possibilities exist. One is that the **antibiotic** chosen is not treating the pathogen. Another consideration is that the pathogen is resistant to the **antibiotic** chosen. In an era of increasing **antibiotic** resistance, the practitioner is always choosing between the narrowest treatment spectrum and the shotgun approach to treatment. There are more powerful oral **antibiotics** available than those the ATS recommends for empirical therapy, but if all practitioners routinely overprescribe them, then resistance will soon develop. Therefore, the prudent practice is to start with the recommendation and save the broader-spectrum antibiotics for true cases of resistance.

Patient Education

Patient education related to pneumonia should focus on the following:

1. The patient should understand that pneumonia might be bacterial, viral, or mycoplasmal and the expected course of improvement for each. The patient should know that the initial clinical picture might not clearly indicate what type of pathogen is causing the pneumonia. The response to treatment will help to clarify the pathogen.
2. The patient should understand the **antibiotic** that is prescribed, including expected adverse reactions, drug interactions, and length of treatment.
3. Lifestyle modifications, such as increased hydration, smoking cessation, and rest, should all be discussed.
4. Symptoms of worsening status should be described and the patient told to notify the practitioner or seek urgent care if symptoms worsen rather than improve. Patients should be told to expect clinical improvement in 48 to 72 hours.

Patient education should also focus on prevention.

CLINICAL PEARL

Immunizations

Pneumococcal vaccine is recommended for specific groups of patients. Pneumococcal conjugate (PCV13) is recommended universally for all infants as part of the routine infant series. All patients with chronic medical conditions who are at high risk for infections should get a **pneumococcal polysaccharide vaccine.** Chronic medical conditions that warrant **pneumococcal** vaccination include chronic lung disease (including asthma); chronic cardiovascular diseases; diabetes mellitus; chronic liver diseases, cirrhosis; chronic alcoholism; functional or anatomic asplenia; immunocompromising conditions (including chronic renal failure or nephrotic syndrome); and cochlear implants and cerebrospinal fluid leaks (CDC, 2010). The **influenza vaccine** previously was advised for patients with chronic medical or respiratory infections (e.g., COPD, asthma); now it is recommended that all persons older than age 6 months be vaccinated annually.

PEDIATRIC PATIENTS WITH PNEUMONIA

Pneumonia in the pediatric patient can cause the infant or child to become quite ill very rapidly. Specific pathogens are more likely at certain ages (Brady, 2009). In children, treatment is determined by the organism most likely to be causing the pneumonia or by positive cultures for a specific organism. Children may be treated on an outpatient basis if their clinical condition is stable. Indications for hospitalization in children beyond early infancy include moderate to severe respiratory distress, failure to respond to oral antibiotics, lobar consolidation in more than one lobe, immunosuppression, empyema, abscess or pneumatocele, or underlying cardiopulmonary disease. This section focuses on the outpatient treatment of pneumonia in children. Neonates (children less than 30 days old) with pneumonia require hospitalization, with few exceptions; therefore, this group is not discussed in this chapter.

Pathophysiology

S. pneumoniae is the most common cause of bacterial pneumonia in children of all ages (Brady, 2009; Cunha, 2004; Kaplan, 2004; Michelow et al, 2004). **Pneumococcal vaccine (PCV7, Prevnar)** has decreased overall prevalence of invasive pneumococcal disease and pneumococcal pneumonia. Su-Ting and Tancredi (2010) reviewed the national Kid's Inpatient Database for 2006 hospital admissions for pneumonia and empyema, and determined the prevalence of *S. pneumoniae* related in-patient pneumonia dropped from 8.9 percent in 1997 to 4.9 percent in 2006. In children, the most common organisms after *S. pneumoniae* vary according to age (see Table 42–1). *S. pneumoniae* is rarely found in neonates, whereas perinatal infection from group B streptococci is often the leading pathogen in this age group. *C. trachomatis,* another perinatal infection, can occur in 5 to 20 percent of 3- to 16-week-old infants whose mother has untreated disease at the time of birth. Viral infections should also be considered, with mixed viral-bacterial pneumonia identified in up to 30 percent of children hospitalized with pneumonia (McCracken, 2000; Michelow et al, 2004). In a recent study of children less than age 5 years with radiologically confirmed community-acquired pneumonia diagnosed in the emergency department, the viral pathogens identified were the following: Respiratory syncytial virus (RSV) accounted for 23.1 percent; human metapneumovirus, 8.3 percent; adenovirus, 3.4 percent; influenza A, 2.9 percent; and parainfluenza, 2.9 percent (Wolf et al, 2010). The clinical findings or age can often differentiate among the pathogens that cause pneumonia in children.

Goals of Treatment

The goals of treatment for pediatric patients with pneumonia are the same as the goals for adults with pneumonia.

Rational Drug Selection

Patient Variables

Infants With Chlamydial Pneumonia

Infants who are 2 to 19 weeks old and who present as afebrile, with a repetitive staccato cough and tachypnea, cervical adenopathy, and rales, are likely to have chlamydial pneumonia (American Academy of Pediatrics [AAP], 2009a). Wheezing is rare. Chest x-ray will show hyperinflation and bilateral diffuse infiltrates. The patient may also have nasal stuffiness and otitis media. Diagnosis is confirmed by detecting chlamydia-specific immunoglobulin M (IgM) in serum (1:32 or greater is diagnostic) (AAP, 2009a).

Drug Therapy

The standard treatment for infants with confirmed chlamydial pneumonia is **erythromycin (EryPed)** 50 mg/kg daily for 14 days or oral **azithromycin (Zithromax)** for 5 days (AAP, 2009a). These infants can usually be treated as outpatients if they are able to eat and maintain hydration. An association between the use of **erythromycin** and hypertropic pyloric stenosis in infants less than 6 weeks of age has been reported. The AAP continues to advise use of **erythromycin** for treatment of diseases caused by *C trachomatis,* and recommends any cases of pyloric stenosis associated with the use of **erythromycin** or **azithromycin** be reported to Medwatch (AAP, 2009a). A diagnosis of *C. trachomatis* infection in an infant should prompt treatment of the mother and her sexual partner(s). See Table 42–2 for drugs commonly used with patients with CAP.

Table 42–2 **Drugs Commonly Used: Community-Acquired Pneumonia**

Drug	Dose	Length of Treatment	Strengths Available	Comments
Amoxicillin (Amoxil, Trimox)	*Adults and children ≥16 yr:* 875 mg q12h or 500 mg q8h *Children:* 80–100 mg/kg/day divided bid or tid	*Adults:* 7–14 days *Children:* 7–14 days	Tablets: 500 mg, 875 mg Capsules: 250 mg, 500 mg Chewable tablets: 125 mg, 200 mg, 250 mg, 400 mg Powder for suspension: 50 mg/mL, 125 mg/5 mL, 200 mg/5 mL, 250 mg/5 mL, 400 mg/ 5 mL	
Amoxicillin/ clavulanate (Augmentin)	*Adults:* 875 mg q12h *Children <3 mo:* 30 mg/kg/day of amoxicillin divided q12h *Children >3 mo:* 80–90 mg/kg/d of amoxicillin divided q12h. Use Augmentin ES-600 formula or combine Augmentin and amoxicillin to equal amoxicillin 80–90 mg/kg/day	10–14 days for all patients	Tablets: 250 mg amoxicillin with 125 mg clavulanate, 500 mg amoxicillin with 125 mg clavulanate, 875 mg amoxicillin with 125 mg clavulanate Chewable tablets: 125 mg amoxicillin with 31.25 mg clavulanate, 200 mg amoxicillin with 28.5 mg clavulanate, 250 mg amoxicillin with 62.5 mg clavulanate, 400 mg amoxicillin with 57 mg clavulanate Suspension: 125 mg amoxicillin with 31.25 mg clavulanate/5 mL, 200 mg amoxicillin with 28.5 mg clavulanate/5 mL, 250 mg amoxicillin with 62.5 mg clavulanate/5 mL, 400 mg amoxicillin with 57 mg clavulanate/ 5 mL, 400 mg amoxicillin with 57 mg clavulanate Augmentin ES-600 600 mg amoxicillin with 42.9 mg clavulanate per 5 mL	Children's dose is based on amoxicillin content. Because of the clavulanate content, two 250-mg tablets are not the same as one 500-mg tablet. Because of the different clavulanate levels in the suspensions, it is not appropriate to dose the 125-mg/5-mL or the 250-mg/5-mL suspensions twice a day Children should not be given the 250-mg tablet until they are >40 kg In children, if combining Augmentin and amoxicillin, do not exceed 6.4 mg/kg/day of clavulanate

Continued

Table 42–2 **Drugs Commonly Used: Community-Acquired Pneumonia—cont'd**

Drug	Dose	Length of Treatment	Strengths Available	Comments
Azithromycin (Zithromax)	*Adults:* 500 mg on day 1, then 250 mg daily for days 2–5 *Children:* day 1, 10 mg/kg, followed by 5 mg/kg on days 2–5	5 days	Capsules: 250 mg Z-pak: 6 250-mg tablets with instructions for daily dosing Suspension: 100 mg/5 mL, 200 mg/5 mL	
Ceftriaxone (Rocephin)	*Adults:* 1–2 g every 12–24 h *Children:* 50 mg/kg/day up to 2 g/d	Based on clinical response, switch to oral therapy when able	Powder for Injection: 250 mg, 500 mg 1 g	Broad spectrum Expensive but less expensive than hospitalization
Erythromycin base (E-Mycin, Ery-Tab)	*Adults:* 250–500 mg q6h *or* 333 mg q8h *or* 500 mg q12h *Children:* 30–50 mg/kg/day divided into tid dosing	*Adults:* 7–14 days *Children:* 10–14 days	Tablets: 250 mg, 333 mg, 500 mg	Should be taken with food to decrease GI upset
Erythromycin estolate (Ilosone)	*Adults:* 250–500 mg q6h *or* 333 mg q8h *or* 500 mg q12h *Children:* 30–50 mg/kg/d divided into tid dosing	*Adults:* 7–14 days *Children:* 10–14 days	Tablets: 500 mg Capsules: 250 mg Suspension: 125 mg/5 mL, 250 mg/5 mL	Should be taken with food to decrease GI upset
Erythromycin ethylsuccinate (E.E.S., EryPed)	*Adults:* 400–800 mg q6h–12h *Children:* 30–50 mg/kg/d divided in q6h *or* q12h dosing	*Adults:* 7–14 days *Children:* 10–14 days	Tablets: 400 mg Chewable tablets: 200 mg Drops: 100 mg/ 2.5 mL Suspension: 200 mg/5 mL, 400 mg/5 mL	Should be taken with food to decrease GI upset
Gatifloxacin (Tequin)	*Adults ≥18 yr:* 400 mg daily	7–14 days	Tablets: 400 mg	Expensive
Levofloxacin (Levaquin)	*Adults:* 500 mg once a day	7–14 days	Tablets: 250 mg, 500 mg Injection: 500 mg	Expensive
Moxifloxacin (Avelox)	*Adults ≥18 yr:* 400 mg once a day	7–14 days	Tablets: 400 mg	Expensive
Ofloxacin (Floxin)	*Adults ≥18 yr:* 400 mg q12h	10 days	Tablets: 400 mg	Expensive
Sparfloxacin (Zagam)	*Adults ≥18 yr:* 400 mg PO day 1 then 200 mg PO daily for 10 days	10 days	200-mg tablets	Expensive

Children With Bacterial Pneumonia

Bacterial pneumonia in children usually occurs as a secondary infection following a viral infection. Primary bacterial pneumonia is less common. The viral infection affects the lung defenses, setting the stage for secondary bacterial infection. Prior to universal PCV7 vaccination, the pathogen was identified as *S. pneumoniae* in 73 percent of bacterial pneumonia, and 24 to 33 percent of all cases of childhood pneumonia (McCracken, 2000; Michelow et al, 2004). The prevalence of *S. pneumoniae* is decreasing, but it remains the leading cause of bacterial pneumonia in children, especially those under age 5 (Su-Ting & Tancredi, 2010). The clinical findings may include the following: fever (usually high), cough, shaking and chills, tachypnea, tachycardia, cyanosis, fine crackles (rales), decreased breath sounds, abdominal pain, and vomiting. Oxygen saturation less than 94 percent may be present. Symptoms can worsen suddenly, and children can become quite ill. Definitive diagnosis of a bacterial infection includes an elevated WBC with a left shift (greater than 15,000) and a chest x-ray that demonstrates lobar consolidation (Cincinnati Children's Hospital Medical Center, 2005). Blood cultures are not routinely necessary. If pneumatoceles are seen on chest x-ray, suspect staphylococcal pneumonia.

Drug Therapy

If *S. pneumoniae* is the suspected organism based on the clinical picture, then high-dose **amoxicillin** (80 to 100 mg/kg daily, divided in three doses) is the drug of choice for 7 to 10 days of outpatient treatment (Cincinnati Children's Hospital Medical Center, 2005; Cunha, 2004; Kaplan, 2004). If highly resistant pneumococci are in the community, the practitioner may choose between IV or IM **ceftriaxone** (50 mg/kg in one daily dose, not to exceed 2 g/d) followed by appropriate oral therapy after 1 or 2 doses of **ceftriaxone** or inpatient treatment using **vancomycin.** Patients who are treated early in the course of the illness usually respond to high-dose **amoxicillin.** *S. pneumonia* may be resistant to macrolides (AAP, 2009c; Cincinnati Children's Hospital Medical Center, 2005). Macrolides are not considered first-line therapy for children under age 5 unless the child has a type I reaction to beta lactams (AAP, 2009c).

If *S. aureus* is the confirmed or highly suspected organism (6.2% prevalence in the Su-ting & Tancredi, 2010, study), the patient may be treated with IM or IV **ceftriaxone** (50 mg/kg in one dose daily) or hospitalized and given **methicillin, nafcillin,** or **oxacillin** (AAP, 2009d). **Vancomycin** would be added to the regimen if methicillin-resistant *S. aureus* (MRSA) is suspected. Patients with *S. aureus* pneumonia are usually quite ill and require hospitalization for at least a few days. They may require a chest tube if there is significant empyema.

Children and Adolescents With Mycoplasma Pneumonia

Mycoplasma pneumonia is the most common type in children over age 5 years. The disease is usually mild. The typical history includes upper respiratory symptoms, fever, dry cough, malaise, sore throat, headache, and possibly chills. Symptoms often last for 3 to 4 weeks (AAP, 2009b). A maculopapular rash may develop in up to 10 percent of children with mycoplasma pneumonia (AAP, 2009b). *M. pneumoniae* may be associated with asthma exacerbation. The patient may have been treated with **amoxicillin** for "bronchitis" without improvement. Chest x-ray reveals bronchovascular markings with areas of atelectasis. Confirmation of *M. pneumoniae* as the pathogen is determined by the presence of *Mycoplasma*-specific IgG or IgM in the serum (Kercsmar, 1998). Polymerase chain reaction (PCR) test for *M. pneumoniae* is the standard, as a culture may take up to 21 days (AAP, 2009b). Serum cold hemagglutinin titers are only positive in 50 percent of children with mycoplasma pneumonia (AAP, 2009b).

Drug Therapy

Mycoplasma pneumonia is usually mild and will resolve without treatment, although observation data indicate children will have a shorter duration of symptoms and fewer relapses if treated with an antimicrobial (AAP, 2009b). The treatment of choice for mycoplasma pneumonia is a macrolide. **Erythromycin** 40 to 50 mg/kg daily is given qid or tid or, for larger children, 333 mg PO tid for 10 days (AAP, 2009b). **Erythromycin** is inexpensive and provides good coverage for other atypical organisms. Another choice is **azithromycin** (10 mg/kg on day 1 and 5 mg/kg on days 2 through 5). **Azithromycin (Zithromax)** is also packaged in a "Z-pak," a 5-day dose pack for older children or children over 50 kg; printed on the package are instructions to take two 250-mg capsules on day 1 and one capsule daily thereafter. **Clarithromycin (Biaxin)** may also be prescribed. Because mycoplasmas lack a cell wall, they inherently are resistant to beta lactam agents.

Monitoring

Patients with bacterial pneumonia need to be monitored closely for clinical improvement or deterioration. If the patient is being treated with the appropriate **antibiotic,** children often show rapid improvement, much faster than adults. Children can also deteriorate rapidly, and any infant or young child who is not hospitalized needs to be seen in the clinic the following day for reassessment. Recommendations are that families receive clear instructions regarding the symptoms of deterioration in respiratory status.

If cultures were drawn, results are usually available in 24 hours, and the practitioner needs to determine (1) if the appropriate **antibiotic** has been chosen and (2) the level of resistance the organism has to the chosen **antibiotic.** If the patient is improving clinically, there is no need for repeat blood counts or cultures. If the patient is not improving or the clinical condition worsens, a repeat chest x-ray can determine if effusions or empyema is developing.

Patients with mycoplasma pneumonia should be monitored for clinical improvement. The cough may last for weeks after the infection is treated. *M. pneumoniae* can spread to the blood, central nervous system, heart, skin, and joints, so monitoring for these complications is prudent. A child with sickle cell disease who contracts mycoplasma pneumonia develops a more severe pulmonary disease than the average child (Brady, 2009).

All children with pneumonia need monitoring of their hydration status. Nutritional intake should also be assessed in infants who may be ill for a few days. The parents' ability to successfully administer medication and their ability to monitor their child's status are essential to the successful outpatient treatment of children with pneumonia.

Outcome Evaluation

Like the adult patient, the child with pneumonia must be monitored for response to the **antibiotic** therapy. The child should become afebrile in 24 to 48 hours. There may be a residual cough for weeks, which should lessen with time. If the child's clinical status fails to improve in 48 to 72 hours, then the treatment plan must be reconsidered. There may be bacterial resistance to the **antibiotic**, or the patient might have mycoplasma pneumonia, which requires a **macrolide antibiotic**.

Patient Education

Patient education when a child has bacterial pneumonia focuses on the following:

1. How to assess the child's respiratory status and signs of respiratory deterioration. Clear instructions, such as "If breathing over __ breaths per minute, call the practitioner," help parents monitor their child at home.
2. A clear plan of where the parents should take a child whose status worsens during the evening or night. Given the variable insurance rules regarding after-hours care, the practitioner needs to explain to parents how to access high-quality pediatric after-hours care in the event of deterioration in the child's status. Not all urgent-care clinics are equipped to handle a child in respiratory distress, and an emergency room is probably the best place for the child to be assessed. Use of the emergency 911 system for respiratory distress should be discussed with families, with clear guidelines given as to what constitutes respiratory distress.
3. How to administer medication appropriately. Make sure the parents have a medicine syringe to accurately administer the oral medications. Some medications must be taken on an empty stomach, and others must be taken with food, and the parents need to be reminded about any special instructions regarding the administration of the **antibiotic**.
4. The parents need to know how to assess hydration and what parameters are expected for urine output. Instructions that clearly define minimum output are the easiest to understand, for example, "Your infant should have a wet diaper every 6 to 8 hours at a minimum."

REFERENCES

Abramoqicz, M. (Ed.). (2003). Drugs for pneumonia. *Treatment Guidelines from the Medical Letter, 1*(13), 83–88.

American Academy of Pediatrics (AAP). (2009a). *Chlamydia trachomatis.* In L. K. Pickering (Ed.), *Red book: 2009 Report of the Committee on Infectious Diseases* (28th ed., pp. 255–259). Elk Grove Village, IL: American Academy of Pediatrics. Retrieved February 13, 2010, from http://aapredbook.aappublications.org/cgi/content/full/2009/1/3.27.3

American Academy of Pediatrics (AAP). (2009b). *Mycoplasma pneumoniae* and other *Mycoplasma* species infections. In L. K. Pickering (Ed.), *Red book: 2009 Report of the Committee on Infectious Diseases* (28th ed., pp. 473–475). Elk Grove Village, IL: American Academy of Pediatrics. Retrieved February 13, 2010, from http://aapredbook.aappublications.org/cgi/content/full/2009/1/3.84

American Academy of Pediatrics (AAP). (2009c). Pneumococcal infections. In L. K. Pickering (Ed.), *Red book: 2009 Report of the Committee on Infectious Diseases* (28th ed., pp. 524–535). Elk Grove Village, IL: American Academy of Pediatrics. Retrieved February 13, 2010, from http://aapredbook.aappublications.org/cgi/content/full/2009/1/3.102

American Academy of Pediatrics (AAP). (2009d). Staphylococcal infections. In L. K. Pickering (Ed.), *Red book: 2009 Report of the Committee on Infectious Diseases* (28th ed., pp. 601–615). Elk Grove Village, IL: American Academy of Pediatrics. Retrieved February 13, 2010, from http://aapredbook.aappublications.org/cgi/content/full/2009/1/3.124

American Thoracic Society (ATS). (2001). Guidelines for the management of adults with community-acquired pneumonia: Diagnosis, assessment of severity, antimicrobial therapy and prevention. *American Journal of Respiratory and Critical Care Medicine, 163,* 1730–1754.

Brady, M. (2009). Respiratory disorders. In C. E. Burns, A. M. Dunn, M. A. Brady, N. B. Starr, & C. Blosser (Eds.), *Pediatric primary care: A handbook for nurse practitioners* (4th ed.). Philadelphia: Saunders.

Centers for Disease Control and Prevention (CDC). (2009) Interim guidance: considerations regarding 2009 H1N1 influenza in intrapartum and postpartum hospital settings. Retrieved from http://www.cdc.gov/h1n1flu/guidance/obstetric.htm

Centers for Disease Control and Prevention (CDC). (2010). Recommended Adult Immunization Schedule—United States, 2010. *Mortality and Morbidity Weekly Report, 59*(1), 1–4.

Cincinnati Children's Hospital Medical Center. (2005). Evidence-based clinical practice guideline of community-acquired pneumonia in children 60 days to 17 years of age. Cincinnati, OH: Cincinnati Children's Hospital Medical Center. Retrieved from http://www.cincinnatichildrens.org/assets/0/78/1067/2709/2777/2793/9199/1633ae60-cbd1-4fbd-bba4-cb687fbb1d42.pdf

Cunha, B. A. (2004). Therapeutic implications of antibacterial resistance in community-acquired respiratory tract infections in children. *Infection, 32*(2), 98–108.

Jamieson, D. J., Honein, M. A., Rasmussen, S. A., Williams, J. L., Swerdlow, D. L., Biggerstaff, M. S., and Novel Influenza A H1N1 Pregnancy Working Group (2009). H1N1 2009 influenza virus infection during pregnancy in the USA. *Lancet, 374,* 451–458.

Johanson, W. G. (1996). Overview of pneumonia. In C. J. Bennett & F. Plum (Eds.), *Cecil textbook of medicine* (20th ed.). Philadelphia: Saunders.

Kaplan, S. L. (2004). Review of antibiotic resistance, antibiotic treatment, and prevention of pneumococcal pneumonia. *Paediatric Respiratory Reviews, 5*(Suppl. A), S153–S158.

Kercsmar, C. M. (1998). The respiratory system. In R. E. Behrman & R. M. Kliegman (Eds.), *Nelson essentials of pediatrics* (3rd ed.). Philadelphia: Saunders.

Lim, W. S., Macfarlane, J. T., & Colthorpe, C. T. (2003). Treatment of community-acquired lower respiratory tract infections during pregnancy. *American Journal of Respiratory Medicine, 2*(3), 221–233.

Mandell, L. A, Wunderink, R. G., Anzueto, A., Bartlett, J. G., Campbell, G. D., Dowell, S. F., et al. (2007). Infectious Diseases Society of America/American Thoracic Society consensus guidelines on the management of community-acquired pneumonia in adults. *Clinical Infectious Disease, 44*(Supp. 2), S27–S72.

Marrus, T. K., & Chan, C. K. (1998). Use of guidelines in treating community-acquired pneumonia. *Chest, 113,* 1689.

McCracken, G. H. (2000). Diagnosis and management of pneumonia in children. *Pediatric Infectious Disease Journal, 19,* 924–928.

Michelow, I. C., Olsen, K., Lozano, J., Rollins, N. K., Duffy, L. B., Zeiger, T., et al. (2004). Epidemiology and clinical characteristics of community-acquired pneumonia in hospitalized children. *Pediatrics, 113,* 701–707.

Muder, R. R., Agahbabian, R. V., Loeb, M. B., Solot, J. A., & Higbee, M. (2004). Nursing home-acquired pneumonia: An emergency department treatment algorithm. *Current Medical Research and Opinion, 20*(8), 1309–1320.

National Center for Health Statistics. (2009). National vital statistics report. *Deaths: Final Data for 2006, 57*(14). Retrieved from http://www.cdc.gov/nchs/data/nvsr/nvsr57/nvsr57_14.pdf

Ramsey, P. S., & Ramin, K. D. (2001). Pneumonia in pregnancy. *Obstetrics and Gynecology Clinics of North America, 28*(3), 553–569.

Riley, L. (1997). Pneumonia and tuberculosis in pregnancy. *Infectious Disease Clinics of North America, 11,* 119.

Riley, P. D., Aronsky, D., & Dean, N. C. (2004). Validation of the 2001 American Thoracic Society criteria for severe community acquired pneumonia. *Critical Care Medicine, 32*(12), 2398–2402.

Sheffield, J. S., & Cunningham, F. G. (2009). Community-acquired pneumonia in pregnancy. *Obstetrics & Gynecology, 114*(4), 915–922.

Su-Ting, T. L., & Tancredi, D. J. (2010). Empyema hospitalizations increase in U.S. children despite pneumococcal conjugate vaccine. *Pediatrics, 125*(1), 26–33.

Wolf, D. G., Greenberg, D., Shemer-Avni, Y., Govon-Lavi, N., Bar-Jiv, J., & Dagan, R. (2010). Association of human metapneumovirus with radiologically diagnosed community-acquired alveolar pneumonia in young children. *Journal of Pediatrics, 156*(1), 115–120.

Woodhead, M. (1998). Community-acquired pneumonia guidelines: An international comparison. *Chest, 113,* 183S.

CHAPTER 43

SMOKING CESSATION

Teri Moser Woo

Chapter Outline

The current rate of adults over age 18 years who smoke cigarettes in the United States is 20.8 percent, representing a steady decline in smoking rates from a high of 41.9 percent in 1965 (National Center for Health Statistics, 2008). Smoking is the leading cause of death in the United States, accounting for more than 438,000 deaths annually (National Cancer Institute, National Institute of Health, 2008). Tobacco use contributes to the development of cancers, cerebrovascular disease, cardiovascular disease, dental disease, gastrointestinal (GI) disorders, and respiratory disease, making it the most preventable health problem in developed countries. Smokers who do not quit by age 35 have a 50 percent chance of dying from a tobacco-related disease. Patients' tobacco use needs to be addressed by all primary care providers, especially those who care for children, as the 2006 National Survey on Drug Use & Health indicated that 12.9 percent of children age 12 and older use tobacco in some form (National Center for Health Statistics, 2008). Secondhand or environmental exposure to tobacco smoke also poses a health hazard to nonsmokers, and the health-care provider plays an important role in educating parents of young children about the effects of secondhand smoke. Education about secondhand smoke should be used as an opportunity to offer tobacco cessation to the smoking family member, thereby decreasing the health risks for the whole family.

A review of the physiological and psychological process of addiction will assist the health-care provider in understanding the rationale for pharmacological intervention. Tobacco smoke contains many different chemicals, many of them known health hazards (ammonia, formaldehyde, carbon monoxide, benzene, arsenic, and lead). The addictive component in tobacco is nicotine. Nicotine has all the components of an addictive substance, similar to those of heroin, in which "addiction is characterized by compulsive drug seeking and use, even in the face of negative health consequences" (National Institute on Drug Abuse, 2006).

The many forms of tobacco include cigarettes, pipes, cigars, smokeless tobacco, and snuff, and patients can be addicted to any of them. The health-care provider needs to assess if the patient is using any form of tobacco and address cessation in the patient's plan of care. Although behavioral modification also plays an important part in quitting, it is discussed only briefly as a component of the treatment plan because this chapter focuses on pharmacological management.

PATHOPHYSIOLOGY

Nicotine is a naturally occurring substance that is soluble in water and lipids. It is readily absorbed from many sites, including the lungs, mucosa, skin, and GI tract.

Nicotine Delivery

Nicotine is absorbed rapidly from tobacco smoke into the pulmonary circulation. It is then transported via the bloodstream to the brain, where it reaches the nicotine cholinergic receptors in 10 to 15 seconds after a puff. The mean time to peak concentration in the bloodstream is 7 to 8 minutes. Each puff contributes to maintaining the nicotine concentration. With each cigarette averaging 10 puffs, the pack-a-day smoker reinforces the blood nicotine level 200 times per day, with each puff providing distinct reinforcement of the habit. Smokeless tobacco is absorbed more slowly from the oral or nasal cavity.

Nicotinic Receptors

The neuronal nicotinic receptors appear to be complex, with the complexity contributing to the different responses to nicotine agonists. Chronic use of nicotine results in an increased number of brain nicotinic receptors, which appears to be an important factor in the development of tolerance of and dependence on nicotine.

Nicotine has both stimulant and depressant effects in the central nervous system (CNS). The stimulant effect is exerted mainly at the cortex, producing increased alertness and cognitive performance. Nicotine activates the nucleus accumbens "reward" system in the limbic system, causing increased extracellular fluid dopamine levels in the region. This increases the "reinforcing" quality of nicotine. IV administration of nicotine activates neurohormonal pathways, releasing acetylcholine, norepinephrine, dopamine, serotonin, vasopressin, beta endorphins, growth hormone, and adrenocorticotropic hormone (ACTH).

Nicotine Withdrawal Syndrome

Nicotine withdrawal syndrome is characterized by craving, nervousness, irritability, impatience, hostility, labile mood, difficulty in concentrating, restlessness, and anxiety. Physical symptoms include decreased heart rate, increased appetite, and weight gain averaging 5 to 6 pounds. Somatic complaints such as myalgia, headache, constipation, and fatigue are common. The urge to smoke is closely related to low blood nicotine levels, which bring on early morning withdrawal symptoms. The smoker may not be smoking to achieve the effects of nicotine but rather to avoid withdrawal symptoms.

GOALS OF TREATMENT

The goal of tobacco cessation treatment is the complete discontinuation of tobacco. It can be achieved either "cold turkey" without pharmacological intervention or by using **nicotine replacement therapy**, which is then gradually reduced over time to zero. If **bupropion (Zyban)** is used, the goal is for the patient to be tobacco free at the end of the 7 to 12 weeks of therapy. Twelve weeks is the recommended treatment length if **varenicline (Chantix)** is prescribed.

RATIONAL DRUG SELECTION

The pharmacological management of tobacco cessation involves three different treatment modalities: **nicotine replacement therapy**, the **antidepressant bupropion**, and the **nicotine receptor partial agonist varenicline**. The combination of **bupropion** and **nicotine replacement** via a **nicotine patch** or **lozenge** may provide higher long-term rates of smoking cessation (Jorenby et al, 1999; Piper et al, 2009; Steinberg et al, 2009). All of the **nicotine replacement therapy** products deliver nicotine to the CNS at a lower dose and slower rate than do tobacco cigarettes, and all the products can double quit rates (Abramowicz, 2003). **Varenicline (Chantix)** has a reported continuous abstinence rate of 43.9 percent after 9 to 12 weeks of therapy (Garrison & Dugan, 2009).

Nicotine Replacement Therapy

Nicotine replacement therapy comes in five different forms: gum, lozenge, transdermal patch, inhaler, and nasal spray. The gum and transdermal patch **Nicotrol**, the transdermal patch **Habitrol**, and the lozenge **Commit** are available over the counter (OTC); the inhaler **(Nicotrol Inhaler)** and the spray **(Nicotrol NS)** are by prescription. Although the patient can self-treat with the OTC products, the health-care provider should educate the patient regarding their proper use to ensure successful treatment. **Nicotine replacement** does not achieve the same peak levels of nicotine as does smoking, but it does achieve a level high enough to suppress nicotine withdrawal symptoms. **Nicotine replacement therapy** is recommended for patients who smoke more than 20 cigarettes per day (one pack), patients who smoke within 30 minutes of awakening in the morning, and patients who have tried to quit previously and have failed because of strong withdrawal symptoms and craving within the 1st week of quitting. Cooper and colleagues (2004) found that patients treated with **nicotine replacement therapy** combined with nonpharmacological interventions (behavioral counseling or telephone intervention contact) reported greatest adherence to treatment.

Nicotine polacrilex gum is Pregnancy Category C, and **transdermal nicotine** is Pregnancy Category D, as nicotine is associated with decreased fetal breathing movements, probably caused by decreased placental perfusion. **Nicotine replacement therapy** is contraindicated immediately after myocardial infarction (MI) in patients with life-threatening arrhythmias and severe or worsening angina pectoris.

Nicotine Gum

Nicotine gum improves smoking cessation rates of 40 to 60 percent compared with controls through 12 months of follow-up. The active ingredient in **nicotine gum (Nicorette)** is **nicotine polacrilex**, a nicotine resin complex. The nicotine is bound to an ion exchange resin that is released only during chewing. The medication is administered when the patient places a piece of gum in his or her mouth and chews slowly five to eight times, until a peppery taste appears. The patient then "parks" the gum in the buccal space. Intermittent chewing and parking the gum over a period of 30 minutes promotes slow buccal absorption. Chewing too quickly causes an excess amount of nicotine to be released into the bloodstream, producing nausea, throat irritation, and hiccoughs. The patient should avoid smoking while chewing **nicotine gum,** as toxicity symptoms may occur (nausea, vomiting, and headache). **Nicotine gum** should not be the first-line choice for patients with temporomandibular joint (TMJ) disease or peptic ulcer disease on account of adverse effects.

Nicotine polacrilex gum takes 30 minutes to reach its peak serum concentration. The patient who is just beginning a tobacco-cessation program should chew one piece of 2- or 4-mg gum per hour. Abstinence rates appear to be higher when the patient chews the gum on a fixed schedule of every hour or every 2 hours. The patient who smokes more than 25 cigarettes per day should be started on the 4-mg dose initially and not exceed the maximum number of pieces per day of gum (30/d of 2 mg, 20/d of 4 mg). Acidic foods (coffee, soft drinks, juice) interfere with the buccal absorption of nicotine from **nicotine polacrilex** and should be avoided for 15 minutes before, during, and 15 minutes after chewing the gum.

After the patient has successfully quit smoking for 6 weeks, a gradual weaning of the gum dosage should begin. Suggestions for a gradual withdrawal of treatment are as follows:

1. Weeks 7 to 9, chew one piece of gum every 2 to 4 hours.
2. Weeks 10 to 12, chew one piece of gum every 4 to 8 hours.
3. After 12 weeks, discontinue nicotine gum and suggest substituting sugarless gum if needed.

Online support for quitting smoking is available from the brand-name drug manufacturer at http://www.nicorette.com, and includes tools for dealing with cravings and lapses.

Nicotine Lozenge

Nicotine polacrilex lozenge (Nicorette Lozenge) is indicated as an adjunct in smoking-cessation therapy. The usual dose is either a 2-mg or 4-mg lozenge, based on how early in the day the smoker smoked the first cigarette. If a smoker has the first cigarette of the day 30 minutes or more after awakening, then the 2-mg lozenge is indicated. The 4-mg lozenge is used if the smoker has the first cigarette within 30 minutes of arising. The lozenge dissolves over 20 to 30 minutes with peak serum levels of nicotine reached in 20 to 30 minutes after the lozenge dissolves in the mouth. The patient should not chew or swallow the lozenge, as there is a significant first-pass metabolism and will decrease bioavailability (Abramowicz, 2003). The patient should use 1 lozenge every 1 to 2 hours for the first 6 weeks, at least 9 lozenges per day with a maximum of 20 lozenges per day. Dosing should taper based on a set schedule similar to that for **nicotine polacrilex gum:**

1. Weeks 1 to 6, one lozenge every 1 to 2 hours.
2. Weeks 7 to 9, one lozenge every 2 to 4 hours.
3. Weeks 10 to 12, one lozenge every 4 to 8 hours.

The patient should not eat or drink for 15 minutes before or while the lozenge is dissolving in the mouth. There may be a tingling sensation in the mouth as the lozenge dissolves. Online quitting support is available at http://www.nicorette.com/.

> **CLINICAL PEARL**
>
> **Nicotine Gum**
> Patients complain about the taste of the **nicotine gum.** Suggest that the patient try the mint-flavored variety, which patients seem to tolerate better.

Nicotine Transdermal System

The **transdermal nicotine system,** or **"patch,"** provides a slow, cutaneous absorption of nicotine over many hours. The patch is applied to clean, nonhairy skin on the upper body or upper arm when the patient wakes up. Peak nicotine levels occur in 2 to 6 hours (brand dependent) and then gradually decrease. Once the patch is removed, nicotine levels in the blood reach a nondetectable level in 10 to 12 hours in nonsmokers. There are different strengths of patches available and patches that are for 16-hour and for 24-hour use, allowing for dose regulation (Table 43–1). The 16-hour patch works well for the light to average smoker but is not effective for early morning withdrawal symptoms. The 24-hour patch provides a steady-state blood level of nicotine, with minimum peaks and troughs, and avoids morning withdrawal symptoms. The disadvantage of the 24-hour patch is that there are more adverse effects, including sleep disruption. Evaluating the patient's smoking habit and determining if early morning withdrawal is an issue will enable the provider to recommend the best **transdermal system** for the patient. **Transdermal nicotine** approximately doubles 6- to 12-month abstinence rates over those produced by placebo interventions.

The **transdermal nicotine system** has the advantage of delivering a steady-state level of nicotine that prevents nicotine withdrawal symptoms while allowing the smoker to work on the behavioral aspects of quitting. Unlike nicotine gum, the patch has the advantage of not reinforcing the oral aspects of smoking. Patients appreciate the ease of administration and once-daily dosing. Weaning off the **transdermal nicotine system** is accomplished by decreasing the dose of the patch on a scheduled basis. Longer duration of use and weaning, rather than abrupt

Table 43–1 **Drugs Commonly Used: Smoking Cessation**

Drug	Strength Available	Dosage	Comments
Nicotine Gum			
Nicotine polacrilex (Nicorette)	2 mg 4 mg	If smoking <20–25 cigarettes/day: chew one 2-mg piece every 1–2 h (at least 9/d), max of 30/d If smoking >20–25 cigarettes/day: chew one 4-mg piece every 1–2 h (at least 9/d), max of 20/d After 6 wk decrease dose to 1 every 2–4 h for 3 wk, then 1 piece every 4–8 h for 3 wk, and then discontinue Alternative: After 6 wk, gradually wean the dose by decreasing one piece of gum/d every 4–7 days	Abstinence rates are higher if gum is chewed on a scheduled basis, rather than prn. Acidic foods and drinks interfere with absorption, so they should be avoided during and for 15 min before and after chewing nicotine gum. The use of nicotine gum for longer than 6 mo is not recommended.
Nicotine Transdermal Patch			
Habitrol (OTC)	21 mg/d 14 mg/d 7 mg/d	If >10 cigarettes/d: 21 mg/d for first 6 wk, 14 mg/d for next 2 wk, and 7 mg/d for final 2 If ≤10 cigarettes/d: 14 mg/d for 6 wk, then 7 mg/d for final 2–4 wk *Length of treatment:* 8–12 wk	24-h patch Apply to clean, nonhairy area on upper body or upper arm upon waking. Rotate application site.
Nicoderm CQ (OTC)	21 mg/d 14 mg/d 7 mg d	21 mg/d for first 6 wk, 14 mg/d for next 2 wk, and 7 mg/d for final 2 wk *Low-dose regimen:** 14 mg/d for 6 wk then 7 mg/d for final 2–4 wk *Length of treatment:* 8–12 wk	24-h patch Apply to clean, nonhairy area on upper body or upper arm upon waking. May remove after 16–24 h.
Nicotrol Step-Down Patch (OTC)	15 mg/6 h 10 mg/16 h 5 mg/16 h	15 mg/16 h for first 6 wk, 10 mg/16 h for 2 wk, then 5 mg/16 h for final 2 wk *Alternative:* Use 15 mg/16 h patch daily for 6 wk, then discontinue *Length of treatment:* 10 wk	16-h patch Apply to clean, nonhairy area on upper body or upper arm upon waking. Remove after 16 h (before bed).
Prostep (OTC)	22 mg/d 11 mg/d	22 mg/d for 4–8 wk, then 11 mg/d for 2–4 wk *Low-dose regimen:** 11 mg/d for 4–8 wk *Length of treatment:* 6–12 wk	24-h patch Apply to clean, nonhairy area on upper body or upper arm upon waking.
Nicotine Nasal Spray			
Nicotrol NS (Rx)	0.5 mg/spray 1 dose = 1 mg, or 1 spray in each nostril	Start with 1–2 doses (2–4 sprays)/h, Max of 5 sprays/h, 40 sprays/d *Length of treatment:* max 3 mo	Can be used ad lib. Advise patient not to sniff, inhale, or swallow the spray.
Nicotine Inhaler			
Nicotrol inhaler (Rx)	10 mg/cartridge (4 mg nicotine delivered)	Patient puffs on mouthpiece frequently and continuously for 20 min. Initially, begins with at least 6 cartridges/d (max 16 cartridges/d) for the first 3–6 wk. Gradually decrease over 12 wk *Length of treatment:* max 6 mo	Provides oral stimulation similar to smoking.
Nicotinic Receptor Partial Agonists			
Varenicline (Chantix)	Strength: 0.5 mg, 1.0 mg	*Patients ≥18 yr:* 0.5 mg po daily for the first 3 d, then 0.5 mg bid days 4–7. On day 8 increase to 1.0 mg bid *Length of treatment:* 12 wk, may continue for another 12 wk	Start 1 wk before quit date. Take on full stomach with a glass of water. Reduce dose if intolerable nausea or other side effects occur. Monitor closely for signs of mood change or suicide ideation.

Table 43–1 **Drugs Commonly Used: Smoking Cessation—cont'd**

Drug	Strength Available	Dosage	Comments
Antidepressant			
Bupropion (Zyban) (Rx)	150-mg tablet	*Patients ≥18 yr:* Begin 150 mg/d 1–2 wk prior to quit date. Increase dose to 150 mg bid (at least 8 h apart) after 3 d *Length of treatment:* 7–12 wk	May be combined with nicotine replacement. Avoid bedtime dosing, which may cause insomnia. Do not use with other forms of bupropion. Monitor closely for signs of mood change or suicide ideation.

*Low-dose therapy is used for patients weighing less than 100 lb, patients with cardiovascular disease, and patients who smoke one-half pack per day or less.
OTC = over the counter.

withdrawal of the **nicotine** patch had the greatest effectiveness in a review of nicotine replacement for smoking cessation (Silagy, Lancaster, Stead, Mant, & Fowler, 2004).

One disadvantage of the **nicotine patch** is that patients report that they are unable to self-regulate the dose if they are exhibiting withdrawal symptoms. This makes the patch less effective for highly dependent smokers, and a highly dependent smoker who is started on a **transdermal nicotine system** should be started on a high-dose, 24-hour system to decrease withdrawal symptoms. The patient *must* refrain from smoking while using the **nicotine patch** because life-threatening dysrhythmias or acute myocardial infarction may occur.

The most common adverse effect of the **nicotine patch** is skin irritation, with 35 to 47 percent of patients reporting some skin irritation during clinical trials. Advising the patient to change the site every day and not to reuse the site within a week can minimize this problem. The amount of skin irritation differs with the brand and dose used, so a change may alleviate the problem. If the patient exhibits symptoms of sleep disturbance or insomnia while using the **transdermal nicotine system**, first determine whether the patient has signs of too high a dose or early morning withdrawal. Delayed onset of sleep is usually associated with too high a dose and early awakening associated with withdrawal symptoms. The provider can either switch the patient from the 24-hour to the 16-hour patch to decrease the dose or, if the patient is already using the 16-hour patch, decrease the dose. If withdrawal is the problem, then increase the patch from a 16-hour to a 24-hour or increase the dose of the patch. The patient needs to be aware that some adjustment of the dose may be necessary to provide effective relief of symptoms with minimum adverse effects. Advise the patient to report any adverse effects so that adjustments can be made.

Other adverse effects observed include symptoms of **nicotine** toxicity (headache, nausea, and vomiting) with higher-dose **patches** and with smoking while using a patch. If symptoms of toxicity occur, remove the **patch** and flush the skin area with water. *Do not use soap,* which increases **nicotine** absorption from the site. **Nicotine** will continue to be delivered into the bloodstream for a number of hours because there is a deposit of **nicotine** under the skin. Patients should report any symptoms of toxicity immediately to their health-care provider. Generic **transdermal nicotine** is available at substantial savings to the patient.

Nicotine Nasal Spray

Nicotine nasal spray (Nicotrol NS) is an inhaled of **nicotine replacement therapy.** The usual dose is one to two sprays in each nostril per hour, not to exceed five sprays per hour and not to exceed 40 doses/day. The advantage to **nicotine nasal spray** is rapid achievement of peak blood levels, with peak levels reached in 4 to 15 minutes after a single 1-mg (two-spray) dose. This speed is advantageous for patients who report severe withdrawal symptoms because the rate of absorption into the bloodstream is similar to that of smoking cigarettes, providing immediate relief of withdrawal symptoms through self-administration. Patients can have a sense of control over their nicotine cravings.

Patients need to be instructed *not to inhale, swallow, or sniff* the spray, unlike many other inhaled medications. The most common adverse effect is nasopharyngeal and ocular mucosa irritation. The use of **nicotine nasal spray**

CLINICAL PEARL

Nicotine Patch
Advise patients to dispose of used **nicotine patches** out of the reach of children or animals. Enough **nicotine** is left in a *used* patch to lead to toxic levels in a child or small animal.

can cause serious arrhythmias and elevated blood pressure and should be avoided immediately after MI because it may cause angina. If the patient is experiencing any cardiac symptoms, then **nicotine nasal spray (Nicotrol NS)** can be abruptly discontinued, an advantage of this delivery system over the longer-acting nicotine products.

With **nicotine nasal spray**, there is potential for abuse, as patients report a "head rush" and the sensation of feeling good, similar to that of cigarette smoking. Careful monitoring of the use of **nicotine spray** and advising patients of the potential for replacing their cigarette addiction with an addiction to the **nicotine spray** can help to avoid this problem. Three months is the recommended maximum length of treatment with **nicotine nasal spray**.

Nicotine Inhaler

The **nicotine (Nicotrol) inhaler** is a unique delivery method of **nicotine replacement therapy** in that the medication stimulates the act of smoking a cigarette. The inhaler consists of two parts, a cartridge containing 10 mg of nicotine (4 mg of delivered drug) and a mouthpiece. The patient puffs continuously on the inhaler for 20 minutes, providing the nicotine equivalent of two cigarettes. The patient should use at least six cartridges per day for 3 to 6 weeks. A maximum of 16 cartridges is used for the first 12 weeks. After 12 weeks the dose is reduced gradually, with a maximum of 6 months of treatment. Adverse effects include coughing, mouth and throat irritation, and dyspepsia.

Antidepressants

Antidepressants are thought to be helpful in smoking cessation because of the relationship between depressed mood and smoking behavior. During tobacco withdrawal, patients often exhibit depressed and anxious moods. Several **antidepressants**, including **bupropion**, **doxepin**, and **nortriptyline**, have been shown to be effective in smoking cessation. This chapter discusses **bupropion (Zyban)**, currently the only **antidepressant** approved by the U.S. Food and Drug Administration (FDA) for smoking cessation.

Bupropion

Bupropion is chemically unrelated to other **antidepressants**, and the mechanism by which it enhances the ability to abstain from smoking is unknown. It is presumed that **bupropion**'s action as a weak inhibitor of neuronal uptake of dopamine and norepinephrine accounts for its ability to assist in smoking cessation. **Bupropion** is started 1 to 2 weeks before the quit-smoking date. The patient begins taking 150 mg daily for 3 days and then increases the dose to 150 mg twice a day at least 8 hours apart, avoiding bedtime dosing. On the quit day, the patient can quit cold turkey or use a **nicotine replacement therapy** along with the **bupropion**. **Bupropion** and the **nicotine patch** are a successful combination, more successful than the **nicotine patch** alone. Therapy continues for 7 to 12 weeks, although treatment may be extended an additional 12 weeks up to 6 months if smoking cessation is successful. If the patient has not made significant progress toward quitting by week 7 of treatment it is unlikely he or she will successfully quit during the attempt and **bupropion (Zyban)** should be discontinued.

Bupropion is contraindicated in patients with seizure disorders, bulimia, and anorexia nervosa and within 14 days of the use of **monoamine oxidase inhibitors (MAOIs)**. **Bupropion** should not be used in patients with a history of stroke, brain tumor, brain surgery, or history of closed head injury (Abramowicz, 2003). Frequency of dosing is reduced in patients with renal failure, as the drug and drug metabolites may accumulate. **Bupropion** should be used with caution in patients with hepatic cirrhosis, with the dose decreased to 150 mg every other day. Although it is Pregnancy Category B, it is not recommended during pregnancy or for use in children under age 18. Nondrug treatments should be tried first in pregnant patients. If used with **nicotine replacement therapy**, the patient should be monitored for hypertension. **Bupropion** is the active ingredient in **Wellbutrin**, used to treat depression. The concurrent use of **bupropion (Zyban)** and **Wellbutrin** is contraindicated. The most frequent adverse effects of **bupropion** are insomnia (40%), dizziness (10%), and dry mouth (10%). Constipation is also a reported adverse effect, and the patient should be advised to increase fiber and fluid intake during treatment.

Bupropion is the active ingredient in the antidepressant **Wellbutrin** and as such received a black box warning regarding increased risk of suicide ideation and suicidality in children, adolescents, and young adults. **Zyban** is not approved for use in children under 18 years of age for smoking cessation. Patients prescribed **Zyban** should be monitored closely for signs of suicide ideation when treatment is started.

Nicotinic Receptor Partial Agonists

Varenicline (Chantix) was approved by the FDA in 2006 as a pharmacological aid to quit smoking. **Varenicline** is a partial agonist/antagonist with affinity and selectivity for alpha(4) beta(2) ($\alpha 4\beta 2$) nicotinic acetylcholine receptors. Its mechanism of action appears to be its action as an agonist on the $\alpha 4\beta 2$ receptors, as well as an antagonist preventing nicotine from binding to the receptors. **Varenicline** is highly selective to the $\alpha 4\beta 2$ and is moderately selective to the 5-HT3 receptor. By preventing binding of nicotine to the nicotinic receptors, there is less dopaminergic reinforcement and reward for smoking, as well as decreased withdrawal symptoms with smoking cessation. The patient experiences reduced cravings and decreased satisfaction with smoking.

To begin smoking cessation therapy with **varenicline (Chantix)**, the patient chooses a quit date and **varenicline** is started 1 week before the scheduled quit date. **Varenicline** reaches steady state in 4 days from the onset of therapy. A titration of **varenicline** up to 1 mg twice a day is required, with the manufacturer suggesting a schedule of 0.5 mg once a day for the first 3 days, then 0.5 mg twice a day on days 4 to 7. The dose may be increased to 1 mg twice a day on day 8 and continue throughout treatment. **Varenicline** is administered after eating with a full glass of water. Treatment should continue for 12 weeks. If the patient has successfully quit smoking, treatment with an additional 12 weeks of therapy is thought to increase the long-term likelihood of abstinence.

Nausea is the most common adverse effect reported when taking **varenicline**, with 16–41 percent of patients reporting nausea compared in double blind trials (Garrison & Dugan, 2009). Patients also report insomnia and headache at higher rates than placebo when taking **varenicline**. The most concerning adverse effect of **varenicline** has been found in post-marketing surveillance related to changes in behavior, agitation, depressed mood, suicidal ideation, and actual suicidal behavior (U.S. Food and Drug Administration, 2008). These concerns prompted a modification of the label highlighting a warning regarding neuropsychiatric symptoms and noting **Chantix** was not studied in patients with preexisting serious psychiatric illness such as schizophrenia, bipolar disorder, and major depressive disorder, therefore safety in these patients has not been established. **Varenicline (Chantix)** is Pregnancy Category C and is not recommended for pregnant or nursing women. **Varenicline** should not be prescribed for children under 18 years of age. Pharmacokinetic properties of **varenicline** in a small study ($N = 16$) of the elderly appears to be similar to younger adults, although as a renally eliminated drug dosing may need to be adjusted in older patients with decreased renal function.

Alpha$_2$ Adrenergic Agonists

Clonidine has been used as a second-line treatment for smoking cessation, although this is not an approved indication by the FDA. **Clonidine** is available in tablets and patch and may be used in patients who refuse or cannot tolerate **nicotine replacement**, **varenicline**, or **bupropion**. The starting dose is 0.1 mg/day, increasing slowly to a maximum of 0.3 mg/day. Side effects are the same as if using **clonidine** for hypertension: dry mouth, sedation, dizziness, and hypotension (Abramowicz, 2003).

Combination Therapy

The Agency for Health Care Policy and Research (AHCPR) has published *Smoking Cessation: Clinical Practice Guidelines* (Fiore et al, 2008), which recommend that the provider consider combining multiple first-line medications (level A evidence) for smoking cessation:

- Long-term (more than 14 weeks) **nicotine** patch plus other **nicotine** replacement therapy (NRT) (gum and spray).
- The **nicotine** patch plus the **nicotine** inhaler.
- The **nicotine** patch plus **bupropion** SR (sustained release).

Steinberg and colleagues (2009) evaluated the use of triple-medication therapy (**nicotine** patch at 21 mg/d, **nicotine** oral inhaler to be used as needed, and **bupropion** 150 mg/d) in medically ill smokers, including those with cardiovascular disease, chronic pulmonary disease, cancer, hypertension, diabetes, and current pulmonary infection. The study found that patients who used a combination of **nicotine** patch, **nicotine** inhaler, and **bupropion** had a 16 percent higher abstinence rate at 6 months than did those who used **nicotine** patch alone (35% vs. 19% [CI 1% to 31%]), with no higher incidence of adverse effects (Steinberg et al, 2009). This study is significant as it addresses the concerns of providers to prescribe smoking cessation medications to patients with chronic illness, as well as validating the use of combination therapies.

Nonpharmacological Treatment of Nicotine Addiction

The AHCPR *Smoking Cessation: Clinical Practice Guidelines* recommend a number of nonpharmacological interventions (Fiore et al, 2008):

1. Smoking-cessation interventions should include either individual or group counseling. There is strong evidence (level A) that a combination of medication and counseling is more effective than is either method alone.
2. Smokers should be offered access to support through a telephone hot line, help line, or online support group, when feasible, as a self-help intervention.
3. Smoking-cessation interventions should include problem solving, skills training, relapse prevention, and stress management to increase cessation success rates.

The provider needs to consider quit rates and cost effectiveness when determining what nonpharmacological smoking cessation therapy to recommend. Higher quit rates are found with more intensive therapies and use of multiple therapies, for example, combining behavioral counseling and individualized computer reports (Lerman, Patterson, & Berrettini, 2005; Ramon & Bruguera, 2009), a combination of counseling and pharmacological therapies, or a combination of pharmacological therapies (Fiore et al, 2008).

Other nonpharmacological therapies include hypnosis, acupuncture, and massage. Self-massage of the ear or hand with circular or stroking motions decreases feelings of anxiety, depressed mood, withdrawal cravings, and craving intensity in smoking patients attempting to quit (Hernandez-Reif, Field, & Hare, 1999). Relaxation and exercise are also central to smoking-cessation therapy to counter the anxiety that is associated with **nicotine** withdrawal and to decrease the amount of weight gained during cessation. The successful treatment of the smoker who desires to quit will include a variety of treatment modalities, both pharmacological and nonpharmacological.

Patient Variables

Pregnant Women

A pregnant woman who smokes places herself and her fetus in danger. Smoking is associated with low birth weight and prematurity, as well as increased perinatal mortality. Smoking cessation during pregnancy is ideal for the developing fetus. Pregnant smokers are advised to quit smoking without the use of **nicotine replacement therapy.** The benefits and risks of **nicotine replacement therapy** have not been studied on pregnant patients, but the risk of smoking is thought to outweigh the short-term risk of low-dose **nicotine replacement.** Therefore, the FDA has classified **nicotine gum** as a Pregnancy Category C medication; the **transdermal patch** and **inhaled** forms continue to be classified as Pregnancy Category D. The manufacturer of **Nicorette gum** continues to recommend that nonpharmacological measures be used first. **Bupropion (Zyban)** and **varenicline (Chantix)** are not recommended during pregnancy.

Children

Children should never receive **nicotine replacement** products, **bupropion,** or **varenicline** for tobacco cessation. Their use is usually experimental, and children are rarely nicotine addicted. Primary education about tobacco use is the appropriate method to be used with children who may be tempted to smoke. Toxic levels of nicotine are reached quickly in children, and all nicotine products should remain out of their reach. Adults should be advised to dispose of used **nicotine patches** in a safe manner, so that children cannot touch or play with the used patch.

Adolescents

Adolescent patients pose a challenge because most adult smokers began as teenage smokers. The American Academy of Pediatrics, in *Guidelines for Adolescent Preventive Services* and *Bright Futures: Guidelines for Health Supervision of Infants, Children, and Adolescents,* recommends screening for tobacco use beginning at the 11- to 14-year-old well child care visit (Hagan, Shaw, & Duncan, 2008). Physically and psychologically, adolescents can be addicted to tobacco (Prokhorov, Pallonen, Fava, Ding, & Niaura, 1996). The peer group norm can lead teens to use tobacco, even when they know it is illegal and a poor choice for them to make. Tobacco-cessation programs in this age group need to be geared toward identifying the teen smoker early and providing support for quitting. The provider who identifies a teen smoker who is ready to quit can choose a variety of options. It is essential for the teen to have a peer support group of other teen nonsmokers. Many schools have drug and alcohol counselors who organize support groups in the school. There has been minimal research in adolescents regarding **nicotine replacement therapy.** Because adolescent smokers report the same nicotine withdrawal and cravings as do adults, a teenager who smokes 20 or more cigarettes per day warrants the trial use of **nicotine replacement. Transdermal nicotine replacement** has been studied in adolescent patients and may be the best choice for treatment.

Buying tobacco products is illegal for adolescents under age 18, although a study of 4078 adolescents found 50 percent of respondents stating they could easily access nicotine replacement products (Klesges, Johnson, Somes, Zbikowski, & Robinson, 2003). Writing a prescription for the product and having the parent purchase the product will allow the patient access to **nicotine replacement therapy** legally. The adolescent needs to have clear directions regarding not smoking while using **nicotine replacement** and the symptoms of nicotine toxicity. Careful education and monitoring of the patient throughout therapy will decrease adverse outcomes.

> **CLINICAL PEARL**
>
> **Constipation and Tobacco Cessation**
> Many patients experience constipation during tobacco cessation as the stimulating effects of nicotine on the GI system are decreased. Increased dietary fiber, increased fluids, and use of a bulk-producing laxative **(Metamucil** or **Citrucel)** will help with this problem.

MONITORING

The patient needs to be monitored closely during all phases of tobacco cessation. As patients begin therapy, they need to be monitored for signs of nicotine withdrawal or, in the case of **nicotine replacement,** nicotine toxicity. The dose of **nicotine replacement** can be adjusted up or down, based on a patient's clinical symptoms. As patients are weaned down on the dose of **nicotine replacement** (every 2 to 3 weeks), they need to be monitored for increasing withdrawal symptoms. After patients are weaned off **nicotine replacement,** they need to be continually assessed as to their abstinence from tobacco. It is not unusual for patients to relapse, and the health-care provider needs to provide support for their repeated attempts to quit.

Patients who are using **varenicline** for tobacco cessation need to be monitored for neuropsychiatric symptoms such as changes in behavior, agitation, depressed mood, suicidal ideation, and suicidal behavior. Patients and family members need to be informed to stop taking **varenicline** and report symptoms to their health-care provider immediately.

Smoking alters the metabolism of several medications, and patients taking them need to be monitored closely and the dosage of their medications adjusted accordingly as they successfully quit. Both smoking and nicotine can increase circulating cortisol and catecholamines. Patients taking **adrenergic agonists (isoproterenol, phenylephrine)** or **adrenergic blockers (beta blockers)** must be monitored closely as they decrease their nicotine dependence. Smoking may reduce the diuretic effects of **furosemide** and reduce cardiac output, and smoking cessation may reverse these actions. **Glutethimide (Doriden)** absorption may be decreased with smoking cessation. First-pass metabolism of **propoxyphene (Darvocet)** may be decreased with smoking cessation. Smoking cessation potentiates **theophylline, insulin, pentazocine, oxazepam, tricyclic antidepressants** (e.g., **imipramine**), **caffeine**, and **acetaminophen.** Careful assessment of medications that the patient is taking prior to beginning a tobacco-cessation program will decrease the adverse effects during cessation.

OUTCOME EVALUATION

The goal of tobacco cessation is for the patient to be tobacco free at the end of treatment. Understanding that nicotine is highly addictive and that there are behavioral patterns ingrained in a smoker's habit can help define successful treatment. The patient who quits smoking cold turkey and is successful over the long term clearly has a positive outcome. The patient who uses **nicotine replacement, bupropion**, or **varenicline** for a number of weeks and then is tobacco free for a long period of time (more than 12 months) also has a positive outcome.

The reality of tobacco-cessation treatment is that many patients relapse. Recognizing that many smokers quit for a while two or three times before successfully achieving long-term cessation will enable the patient and the provider to view any period of abstinence as one step closer to long-term success. By supporting patients during this process and assuring them that they are not failures if they begin smoking again, the health-care provider preserves an environment in which patients can again attempt quitting when they are ready.

PATIENT EDUCATION

Patient education should include a discussion of information related to the overall treatment plan as well as that specific to the drug therapy, reasons for the drug's being taken, drugs as part of the total treatment regimen, and adherence issues.

Patients should be taught that there is a relationship between smoking cessation and development of mouth ulcers, not related to the smoking-cessation medications. Forty percent of quitters develop mouth ulcers in the first 2 weeks after quitting, with most ulcers (60%) resolving by 4 weeks. The more dependent quitters are more likely to report ulcers (McRobbie, Hajek, & Gillison, 2004).

Educational Resources

Many resources pertaining to tobacco cessation are available for providers and patients. The American Lung Association (ALA) has local chapters that can provide posters;

SMOKING CESSATION

PATIENT EDUCATION

Related to the Overall Treatment Plan/Disease Process

- ☐ Education regarding the physical and psychological aspects of tobacco addiction
- ☐ Role of lifestyle modifications
- ☐ Importance of adherence to the treatment regimen
- ☐ Need for regular follow-up visits with the primary care provider

Specific to the Drug Therapy

- ☐ Doses and schedules for taking the drug
- ☐ Possible adverse effects and what to do if they occur
- ☐ Interactions between other treatment modalities and these drugs

Reasons for Taking the Drug(s)

These drugs are given to help a person stop smoking. The medications that are used for smoking cessation need to be used as prescribed; overuse or underuse will increase treatment failure or lead to adverse effects. The patient needs to understand the danger of nicotine toxicity, know the symptoms, and have clear instructions to cease the medication and notify the health-care provider. The patient must not smoke while using a **nicotine replacement. Nicotine replacement** products, even after they are used, can be toxic to children and to pets; therefore, all of the products need to be handled carefully and disposed of properly after use.

SMOKING CESSATION –cont'd

PATIENT EDUCATION

Drugs as Part of the Total Treatment Regimen

The total treatment regimen includes nonpharmacological strategies. Nonpharmacological strategies such as relaxation, acupuncture, massage, exercise, and group therapy should be discussed and patients encouraged to incorporate multiple strategies to help them be successful.

A weight gain of 5 to 8 lb is common during tobacco cessation. Patients need to avoid strict diets during tobacco cessation and increase exercise during cessation treatment. After they have been tobacco free for a few months, they can then work on weight reduction. Encouraging exercise during treatment will decrease the amount of weight gained.

Adherence Issues

Patients should know that having quit before and resumed their habit does not predict that they cannot be successful and that patients often quit for a while and then lapse two or three times before they succeed.

Many patients need external motivation to be successful at tobacco cessation. Identifying each patient's motivation and reminding her or him of it at each visit will assist patients in refocusing their goals when they feel like giving up. Common motivators include the health of their children or spouse and their own health. Pointing out the cost savings of quitting smoking, which can add up to over $250 a month for a pack-a-day smoker in New York City, where cigarettes are $9.00 a pack, can also help patients focus on their goal. Have them place a photo of what they will buy with their savings in a prominent place (the refrigerator or bathroom mirror) as a reminder.

On The Horizon: TOBACCO-CESSATION THERAPIES

The future looks promising for tobacco-cessation therapies. Currently, a sublingual form of **nicotine replacement,** in a 2-mg or 4-mg dose, is available in Europe and Canada. Scientists are also investigating the potential of a vaccine that stimulates antibodies that block nicotine receptors in the brain and will be used to prevent relapse in smokers who quit.

written educational materials to promote tobacco cessation; and materials for the Great American Smokeout, an annual antismoking event. Both the American Cancer Society (ACS) and the American Heart Association (AHA) have local chapters that can also provide educational materials to health-care providers. There are Web sites devoted to tobacco cessation that health-care providers can access. The key AHCPR *Clinical Guidelines* are available at http://www.ahrq.gov/clinic/tobacco. Smoking support information with links to multiple resources is available at the ALA Web site, http://www.lungusa.org. At the RxList Web site, http://www.rxlist.com, the provider can type in a medication and print or e-mail the patient information about the medication. With the abundance of resources available to the health-care provider, patient education should be easily incorporated into the care of the patient.

REFERENCES

Abramowicz, M. (Ed.). (2003). Drugs for tobacco dependence. *Treatment Guidelines from the Medical Letter, 1*(10), 65–68.

Cooper, T. V., DeBon, M. W., Stockton, M., Klesges, R. C., Steenbergh, T. A., Sherrill-Mittleman, M., et al. (2004). Correlates of adherence with transdermal nicotine. *Addictive Behaviors, 29,* 1565–1578.

Cromwell, J., Bartosch, W. J., Fiore, M. C., Hasselblad, V., & Baker, T. (1997). Cost effectiveness of the clinical practice recommendation in the AHCPR guidelines for smoking cessation. *Journal of the American Medical Association, 278,* 1759–1766.

Fiore, M. C., Jaén, C. R., Baker, T. B., Bailey, W. C., Benowitz, N. L., Curry, S. J., et al. (2008). Treating tobacco use and dependence: 2008 update. *Clinical practice guideline.* Rockville, MD: U.S. Department of Health and Human Services, Public Health Service.

Garrison, G. D., & Dugan, S. E. (2009). Varenicline: A first-line treatment option for smoking cessation. *Clinical Therapeutics, 31*(3), 463–491.

Hagan, J. F., Shaw, J. S., & Duncan, P. M. (Eds.). (2008). *Bright futures: Guidelines for health supervision of infants, children, and adolescents* (3rd ed.). Elk Grove Village, IL: American Academy of Pediatrics.

Heishman, S. J., Balfour, D. J. K., Benowitz, N. L., Hatsukami, D. K., Lindstrom, J. M., & Ockene, J. K. (1997). Society for Research on Nicotine and Tobacco: Conference summary. *Addiction, 92*(5), 615–633.

Hernandez-Reif, M., Field, T., & Hare, S. (1999). Smoking cravings are reduced by self-massage. *Preventive Medicine, 28*(1), 28–32.

Hjalmarson, A., Nilsson, F., Sjöström, L., & Wiklund, O. (1997). The nicotine inhaler in smoking cessation. *Archives of Internal Medicine, 157,* 1721–1728.

Hurt, R. D., Offord, K. P., Croghan, I. T., Croghan, G. A., Gomez-Dahl, L. C., Wolter, T. D., et al. (1998). Temporal effects of nicotine nasal spray and gum on nicotine withdrawal symptoms. *Psychopharmacology, 140,* 98–104.

Jimenez-Ruiz, C., Kunze, M., & Fagerstrom, K. O. (1998). Nicotine replacement: A new approach to reducing tobacco-related harm. *European Respiratory Journal, 11,* 473–479.

Jorenby, D. E., Leischow, S. J., Nides, M. A., Rennard, S. I., Johnston, J. A., Hughes, A. R., et al. (1999). A controlled trial of sustained-release bupropion, a nicotine patch, or both for smoking cessation. *New England Journal of Medicine, 340*(9), 685–691.

Klesges, L. M., Johnson, K. C., Somes, G., Zbikoswki, S., & Robinson, L. (2003). Use of nicotine replacement therapy in adolescent smokers and nonsmokers. *Archives of Pediatric and Adolescent Medicine, 157*(6), 517–522.

Krawiec, J. V., & Pohl, J. M. (1998). Smoking cessation and nicotine replacement therapy: A guide for primary care providers. *American Journal for Nurse Practitioners, 2*(1), 15–33.

Lerman, C., Patterson, F., & Berrettini, W. (2005). Treating tobacco dependence: State of the science and new directions. *Journal of Clinical Oncology, 23*(2), 311–323.

McRobbie, H., Hajek, P., & Gillison, F. (2004), The relationship between smoking cessation and mouth ulcers. *Nicotine & Tobacco Research, 6*(4), 655–659.

National Cancer Institute, National Institute of Health. (2008). Tobacco facts. *Tobacco statistics snapshot*. Bethesda, MD: National Institute of Health. Retrieved March 8, 2011, from http://www.cancer.gov/cancertopics/tobacco/statisticssnapshot#0_references

National Center for Health Statistics. (2008). *Health, United States, 2008. With Chartbook on trends in the health of Americans*. Hyattsville, MD: U.S. Department of Health and Human Services. Retrieved March 8, 2011, from http://www.cdc.gov/nchs/data/hus/hus08.pdf#063

National Institute on Drug Abuse. (2006). Tobacco addiction. *National Institute on Drug Abuse: Research report series* (NIH Publication No. 06-4342). Retrieved March 8, 2011, from http://www.nida.nih.gov/ResearchReports/Nicotine/Nicotine.html

Piper, M. E., Smith, S. S., Schlam, T. R., Fiore, M. C., Jorenby, D. E., Fraser, D., et al. (2009). A randomized placebo-controlled clinical trial of 5 smoking cessation pharmacotherapeutics. *Archives of General Psychiatry, 66*(11), 1253–1262.

Prochazka, A. V., Weaver, M. J., Keller, R. T., Fryer, G. E., Licari, P. A., & Lofaso, D. (1998). A randomized trial of nortriptyline for smoking cessation. *Archives of Internal Medicine, 158*, 2035–2039.

Prokhorov, A. V., Pallonen, U. E., Fava, J. L., Ding, L., & Niaura, R. (1996). Measuring nicotine dependence among high-risk adolescent smokers. *Addictive Behaviors, 21*(1), 117–127.

Ramon, J. M., & Bruguera, E. (2009). Real world study to evaluate the effectiveness of varenicline and cognitive-behavioural interventions for smoking cessation. *International Journal of Environmental Research and Public Health, 6*, 1530–1538. doi:10.3390/ijerph6041530

Schneider, N. G., Lunell, E., Olmstead, R. E., & Fagerström, K. (1996). Clinical pharmacokinetics of nasal nicotine delivery: A review and comparison to other nicotine systems. *Clinical Pharmacokinetics, 31*(1), 65–80.

Silagy, C., Lancaster, T., Stead, L., Mant, D., & Fowler, G. (2004). Nicotine replacement therapy for smoking cessation. *Cochrane Database of Systematic Reviews*, 3. Art. No.: CD000146. doi:10.1002/14651858.CD000146.pub2

Steinberg, M. B., Greenhaus, S., Schmelzer, A. C., Bover, M. T., Foulds, J., Hoover, D. R., et al. (2009). Triple-combination pharmacotherapy for medically ill smokers: A randomized trial. *Annals of Internal Medicine, 150*(7), 447–454.

U.S. Food and Drug Administration. (2008). *FDA issues public health advisory on Chantix: Agency requests that manufacturer add new safety warnings for smoking cessation drug.* Bethesda, MD: U.S. Food and Drug Administration. Retrieved March 8, 2011, from http://www.fda.gov/NewsEvents/Newsroom/PressAnnouncements/2008/ucm116849.htm

CHAPTER 44

SEXUALLY TRANSMITTED INFECTIONS AND VAGINITIS

Jacqueline Webb

Chapter Outline

Two common concerns seen by primary care providers are sexually transmitted infections (STIs) and vaginitis. The Centers for Disease Control and Prevention (CDC) national surveillance data indicate there are approximately 19 million new STIs each year, at a cost of $15.9 billion annually (CDC, 2009). Vaginitis is an inflammation of the vagina that may be caused by STIs, or it may be the result of other factors. This chapter discusses the pharmacological management of STIs and vaginitis.

SEXUALLY TRANSMITTED INFECTIONS

Management of STIs requires recognizing vulnerable populations with high rates of sexually transmitted infections and an understanding of drug resistance. In the 1950s and 1960s, **penicillin** was the drug of choice for treatment of most STIs. By 1995, **antibiotic** resistance threatened the ability to control bacterial infections such as syphilis, gonorrhea, and chlamydia. Over growing concerns based on the Gonococcal Isolate Surveillance Project (GISP), by 2006 the CDC no longer recommended the use of **fluoroquinolones** for the treatment of gonococcal infections and associated conditions such as pelvic inflammatory disease (PID) (CDC, 2006).

Populations at Risk

Managing STIs must also take into consideration identifying populations most at risk. Rates of gonorrhea and chlamydia are highest among adolescents. Young women aged 15 to 24 years have the highest rate of chlamydia, with rates more than five times as high as women overall (CDC, 2009). In 2008, the rate of chlamydia among black women was nearly eight times higher than the rate among white women (2,056.9 and 264.4 per 100,000 women, respectively). The chlamydia rate among black men was almost 12 times as high as the rate among white men (928.8 and 79.4 per 100,000 men, respectively) (CDC, 2009). Although research seems to demonstrate that white Americans acquire STIs predominantly through high-risk sexual behaviors, black Americans acquire them through both high- and low-risk behaviors, which contributes to the disparity in STI rates (Aral, Adimora, & Fenton, 2008).

The number of patients requiring services for STIs has increased in proportion to those who are sexually active, and the number of patients with viral infections has increased exponentially. Viral STIs are incurable and produce lifelong periods of exacerbations and remissions. In 2006, the CDC estimated at least 50 million persons in the United States to be infected with genital herpes simplex virus (HSV). Those who have unprotected sexual contact with multiple partners are virtually guaranteed to acquire

HSV-2 (Ribes, Steele, Seabold, & Baker, 2001). In the third National Health and Nutrition Examination Surveys (NHANES III), seropositivity with HSV correlated with a higher lifetime number of sexual partners and with cocaine use, both of which are behavioral risk factors associated with the acquisition of HIV (Armstrong et al, 2001).

STI as Precursor to Cancer

Scientific identification of the viral genotype of HPV (also known as genital warts) has enabled primary care providers to view cancer of the cervix in women and anus in men and women as an STI. Cervical cancer is the second leading cause of female cancer death worldwide, with an estimated 240,000 deaths yearly (World Health Organization [WHO], 2006). Although more than 30 types of HPV can infect the genital tract, genotypes 16, 18, 31, 33, and 35 have been strongly associated with cervical neoplasia, with 16 and 18 the most prevalent (CDC, 2010). Most HPV infections do not cause clinical complications and as many as 91 percent of new infections clear up within 2 years (Gerbeding, 2004). Because most HPV infections are asymptomatic, early diagnosis and treatment of suspicious lesions are essential to prevent the spread of potentially cancerous lesions. In 2009 the American College of Obstetricians and Gynecologists (ACOG) revised its cancer screening guidelines to recommend that the first cervical screening should be at age 21 years and rescreening can be less frequent than previously recommended (American College of Obstetricians and Gynecologists, 2009; Wright et al, 2007). However, risk factors that may indicate the need for more frequent screening include HIV infection; immunosuppression; history of diethylstilbestrol (DES) exposure in utero; and abnormal Pap test results such as cervical intraepithelial neoplasia (CIN) 2, CIN 3, or history of cervical cancer. Although Pap tests are fairly common in the United States, about 17 percent of American women aged 18 to 64 in 2005 had not been tested in the past previous 3 years (Partnership for Prevention, 2007). These are the women who may account for the majority of cervical cancer diagnoses.

Pathophysiology

The pathogenic potential of the viruses and bacteria capable of causing STIs and general discomfort depends on several factors: age of host, sex of patient, number of sexual partners, pregnancy, immune system status, and coexisting infections. These are examples of the numerous factors to be considered when managing STIs. Age of the host is, perhaps, one of the most important factors for the nurse practitioner to consider. Prepubertal, lactating, and postmenopausal women lack the vaginal effects of estrogen (Markusen & Barclay, 2003). This estrogen deficit results in a thin vaginal mucosa and vaginal epithelium. As a result, the vaginal area becomes more susceptible to infection and trauma. In addition to lacking the effects of estrogen, the pH of the vagina can be abnormally high (5.0 to 7.0) for some women and the normally acidogenic flora of the vagina may be replaced by mixed flora, which predisposes to infection. The normally acidic environment of the vagina (pH 3.5 to 4.1) promotes growth of the normal flora and helps prevents growth of infectious or irritative organisms. Although most women grow between three and eight types of bacteria, which are considered part of the "normal flora," lactobacilli and corynebacteria are the most common organisms (Markusen & Barclay, 2003). Treatments such as **antibiotic therapy** or a behavior such as having multiple sex partners triggers a nonphysiological response, and the "normal flora" of the vagina becomes disturbed enough to produce pathological symptoms (bacterial vaginosis). Postmenopausal women may experience vulvovaginal pain as a direct result of decreased estrogen production, which results in a thin, superficial epithelium. Some of the irritative symptoms may be also caused by infection. This reduced layer of epithelial cells can make the woman more vulnerable to infection and trauma (atrophic vaginitis). Infection can be from a woman's own perineal bacterial flora, and trauma can be a result of normal sexual relations. Other common irritants to the vaginal ecosystem are "forgotten" tampons, douches, contraceptive preparations, diabetes mellitus, and even stress.

Sex of the patient is another factor to consider. The overall reported rate of chlamydia infection among women (583.8 cases per 100,000 females) was almost three times the rate among men (211.1 cases per 100,000 males) (CDC, 2009). Research suggests that men are less likely to be tested for sexually transmitted infections (CDC, 2009).

In women, STIs are a common cause of vaginitis. Presenting symptoms often include discharge and vaginal irritation. However, it is important to note that not all vaginitis is infectious and that those infected with an STI are often asymptomatic. The differential diagnosis of vaginal discharge is presented in Table 44–1. Treatments for infectious vaginitis that may be acquired without sexual contact as well as for noninfectious vaginitis are discussed later in this chapter.

Genital contact between people is required for transmission of most STIs, although fomite transmission (such as through vibrators, toilet seats, and bath towels) has occurred with hardier organisms. Women tend to experience more morbidity than men because of the secretions deposited during the sex act. Transmission from one partner to the other can be facilitated or impeded by alterations in vaginal pH, the presence of inflammation caused by spermicides, and the mucosal integrity of either partner. Bacteria and viruses can invade the mucosal lining of the oral, genital, or anal tract. All bodily secretions, especially blood, can transmit infection from human to human.

Goals of Treatment

There are four main goals of STI treatment that primarily address treatment of the infection and prevention of

Table 44–1 **Differential Diagnosis of Vaginal Discharge**

Discharge Appearance	Symptoms	pH	Diagnostic Tests	Microscope Findings	Disease/Syndrome
White, curdy	+ Burn, itch	<4.5	Culture/KOH	Budding yeast hyphae	Moniliasis Candidiasis
Mucopurulent, thick	+ Irritating	Normal	DNA/culture	WBCs > 10/hpf	GC/Chlamydiasis
Thin, white, odor	+ Itch, odor a big issue	>4.5	+Amine/culture-change in vaginal flora	"Clue cells" (coccoid bacteria that obscure epithelial cell borders)	Bacterial vaginosis (BV)
Blood-tinged, purulent	+ Itch, dysuria, foul odor	<4.5	Wet mount = + Trichomonads	Trichomonads >10 WBCs/hpf	Trichomoniasis
Nonspecific, white	+ Pruritus, burn	3.5–4.5	Culture reports change in normal flora	4+ *Lactobacillus*	Cytological
Scanty, may be white or yellow	+ Burn, sore, cracks	>5–7	Culture is negative	Several epithelial cells	Atrophic
White	None	3.8–4.2	Not necessary	1–2+ *Lactobacillus*	Normal

disease spread. There is ample literature to validate that STIs are preventable through safe sexual behavior, therefore the first goal of therapy is to educate patients about high-risk behaviors, especially those patients between ages 15 and 25 years, when the incidence of chlamydia infection is the highest. Prevention of long-term sequelae of unsafe sex is the second goal of therapy. Four complications of STIs are tubal occlusion leading to infertility and ectopic pregnancy, neonatal morbidity and mortality caused by transmission during pregnancy and parturition, genital cancers, and possible exposure to HIV because of its association with other STIs. Only two vaccines are available against viral STIs: **hepatitis B** and HPV. **Hepatitis B vaccine** was introduced in 1982 and the vaccine that protects against four high-risk strains of HPV was introduced in 2006. Identifying patients that have not received these vaccines is an important step that needs careful monitoring in primary care settings. The third goal of therapy is to choose the most specific, cost-effective drug that has the best regimen for adherence, after verifying the diagnosis and assessment of pregnancy. The fourth goal of therapy is to reduce morbidity and provide comfort for those chronic viral and inflammatory conditions that are not curable.

Rational Drug Selection

Guidelines

Treatment for STIs is based on national guidelines recommended by the CDC (2010). Nurse practitioners and other health-care providers play a crucial role in the diagnosis, treatment, and counseling of STIs. The treatment information presented in this chapter is consistent with the CDC's *Sexually Transmitted Diseases Treatment Guidelines*. Specific treatment for STIs are outlined in Table 44–2. The CDC guidelines in their entirety can be accessed from the following Web site: http://www.cdc.gov/STD/treatment/. Chapter 24 has more information about the specific **antibiotics** and **antifungals**. Chapters 25 and 32 discuss drugs used for inflammatory disorders and for conditions of the integumentary system.

Syphilis

Syphilis is a systemic disease caused by *Treponema pallidum* has been present in society for centuries. Syphilis is spread by direct contact of the mucosal tissue to infected lesions. There has been an increase of congenital cases (4-fold) since 1950, which may be a result of illicit drug use. Diagnostic symptoms may present as early as 5 days and as late as 90 days after exposure to the organism. Primary syphilis infection presents with ulcer or chancre at the site of infection. Secondary infection has manifestations that include rash, mucocutaneous lesions, and adenopathy. Not all vaginal "warts" are attributed to HPV disease, as anogenital condylomata lata are a common symptom of secondary syphilis, as well as a generalized papulosquamous eruption. Tertiary infections with syphilis present with cardiac, neurological, ophthalmic, auditory, or gummatous lesions. Neurosyphilis may occur at any stage but is most common in late latent stage. During the late latent phase, the infected patient is not infectious, unless pregnant or through blood transmission. Treatment of latent syphilis is intended to prevent occurrence or progression of late complications. Latent infections lack clinical symptoms and are detected by serological testing. Misdiagnosis or delayed diagnosis is possible because of the low level of suspicion in many family practice settings.

All women should be screened for syphilis early in pregnancy, with many states mandating screening with

Table 44–2 **Drugs Commonly Used: Sexually Transmitted Infections**

Pathogen	First Choice	Alternative Choice
Bacterial Pathogens		
Syphilis, primary and secondary	Benzathine penicillin G *Adults including pregnant women:* 2.4 million units (IM) one dose *Children*: 50,000 units/kg in one dose Maximum dose: 2.5 million units	Pregnant patients allergic to penicillin should be desensitized. Nonpregnant use doxycycline 100 mg bid for 14 days *or* tetracycline 500 mg qid for 14 days.
Syphilis, early latent (tertiary)	Benzathine penicillin G *Adults including pregnant women:* 2.4 million units (IM) one dose *Children:* 50,000 units/kg in one dose Maximum dose: 2.4 million units	
Syphilis, late latent or unknown	3 weekly doses of benzathine penicillin G 2.4 million units (total 7.2 million units) *Children:* 50,000 units/kg IM weekly for three weeks, (total 150,000 units/kg up to adult dose of 7.2 million units)	Pregnant patients 2.4 million units weekly x 3 weeks.
Gonococcal infections: (uncomplicated infections of cervix, urethra, and rectum)	Ceftriaxone 250 mg IM in a single dose *or* cefixime 400 mg PO *plus* treatment for chlamydia if chlamydial infection is not ruled out: azithromycin 1 g PO in one dose *or* doxycycline 100 mg PO bid × 7 d	Spectinomycin 2 g in a single IM dose *or* ceftizoxime 500 mg IM or cefoxitin 2 g IM administered with Probenecid 1 g PO or cefotaxime 500 mg IM
Gonococcal infections (pharynx)	Ceftriaxone 250 mg IM in a single dose plus azithromycin 1 gm in a single dose or doxycycline 100 mg bid for 7 days	
Chlamydia (adults and adolescents)	Azithromycin 1 g PO one dose *or* doxycycline 100 mg bid for 7 d	Erythromycin base 500 mg PO qid for 7 d *or* erythromycin ethylsuccinate 800 qid PO for 7 d *or* ofloxacin 300 PO bid for 7 d *or* levofloxacin 500 mg PO daily for 7 days.
Chlamydia (pregnancy)	Azithromycin 1 g PO single dose *or* amoxicillin 500 mg PO tid for 7 d	Erythromycin base 500 mg PO qid for 7 d *or* erythromycin ethylsuccinate 800 mg PO qid for 7 d *or* erythromycin ethylsuccinate 400 mg. PO qid for 14 d *or* erythromycin base 250 mg PO qid for 14 d.
Chancroid	Azithromycin 1 g PO in one dose *or* ceftriaxone 250 mg (IM) in one dose *or* ciprofloxacin 500 mg PO bid for 3 d *or* erythromycin base 500 mg PO qid for d	Ciprofloxacin is not for patients under age 18 yr and those who are pregnant *or* lactating.
Granuloma inguinale (donovanosis)	Doxycycline 100 mg PO bid for at least 3 wk or until ulcers completely heal	Ciprofloxacin 750 PO bid for 3 wk *or* erythromycin base 500 mg PO qid for 3 wk *or* azithromycin 1 g PO weekly for 3 wk or trimethoprim-sulfamethoxazole one double-strength (DS) tablet PO bid for 3 wk.
Lymphogranuloma venereum	Doxycycline 100 mg PO bid for 21 d	Erythromycin base 500 mg PO qid for 21 d. Do not use doxycycline in pregnant *or* lactating women.
Bacterial vaginosis	Metronidazole 500 mg PO bid for 7 d *or* clindamycin cream 2% 5 g (one applicator) at bedtime for 7 d *or* metronidazole gel 0.75% 5 g (one applicator) at bedtime for 5 d *Pregnant women:* metronidazole 500 mg bid for 7 d *or* metronidazole 250 mg tid for 7 days or clindamycin 300 mg bid for 7 days	Tinidazole 2 gm PO daily for 2 days *or* tinidazole 1 gm PO daily for 5 days *or* clindamycin 300 mg PO bid for 7 days *or* clindamycin ovules 100 mg intravaginally at bedtime for 3 days

Table 44–2 **Drugs Commonly Used: Sexually Transmitted Infections—cont'd**

Viral Pathogens	First Episode	Recurring Episodes
Herpes simplex types 1 and 2	Acyclovir 400 mg PO tid for 7–10 d *or* acyclovir 200 mg PO 5 times for 7–10 d *or* famciclovir 250 mg PO tid for 7–10 d *or* valacyclovir 1 g PO bid for 7–10 d	Treatment for recurrent genital herpes can be administered either episodically to ameliorate or shorten duration of lesions or continuously as suppressive therapy to reduce frequency of recurrences. Episodic therapy: Acyclovir 400 mg PO tid for 5 days or acyclovir 800 mg bid for 5 d or acyclovir 800 mg tid for 2 d or famciclovir 125 mg bid for 5 d or famciclovir 1,000 mg bid for 1 day or valacyclovir 500 mg bid for 3 d or valacyclovir 1.0 g PO once a d for 5 d. Suppression daily is same dosage but given: acyclovir 400 bid; famciclovir 250 mg bid; valacyclovir 500 mg once daily; valacyclovir 1,000 mg once daily.
Human Papillomavirus		
Human papillomavirus (HPV) (cervical)	Provider-applied (nonpregnant): needs specialized training to treat Cervical HPV lesions.	Patient-applied (nonpregnant): needs colposcopy, biopsy prior to treatment. Patient-applied (pregnant): needs specialist management.
Human papillomavirus (HPV) (vaginal)	In the absence of genital warts or cervical SIL, treatment is not recommended for subclinical genital HPV infection. Genital HPV infection frequently goes away on its own, and no therapy has been identified that can eradicate infection (CDC, 2010). <10 genital warts; Provider-applied (nonpregnant): cryotherapy: apply every 2 wk; OK with pregnancy, *or* TCA or BCA 80%–90% Apply every wk; allow tissues to heal between applications; OK with pregnancy, *or* podophyllin resin 10%–25%; apply, dry, wash off by 4 h; treat weekly *or* surgical removal by shave technique, curettage, or electrosurgery; *alternative therapies*: intralesional interferon, not with pregnancy, *or* laser surgery, not with pregnancy	Patient-applied (nonpregnant): Podofilox 0.05% solution or gel bid for 3 d, 4 d off, up to 4 cycles. Imiquimod 5% cr: Apply 3 times/wk at bedtime, wash off in a.m. Duration 8–16 wk. Patient-applied (pregnant): not safe.
Human papillomavirus (HPV) (urethral)	Provider-applied (nonpregnant): cryosurgery *or* podophyllin 10%–25% as above	Patient-applied (nonpregnant): none Patient-applied (pregnant): none
Human papillomavirus (HPV) (anal, outside sphincter)	Provider-applied (nonpregnant): cryosurgery *or* TCA or BCA 80%–90% as above *or* surgical removal	Patient-applied (nonpregnant): none Patient-applied (pregnant): none
Human papillomavirus (HPV) (oral)	Provider-applied (nonpregnant): cryosurgery *or* surgical removal	Patient-applied (nonpregnant): none Patient-applied (pregnant): none
Fungal Pathogen	**Intravaginal**	**Oral**
Candidia albicans	Butoconazole 2% 5 g for 3 d Clotrimazole 1% 5 g for 7–14 d Clotrimazole 100-mg tablet 2 tabs for 3 d Clotrimazole 100-mg tab for 7 d Clotrimazole 500-mg tab given only once Miconazole 2% 5 g for 7 d Miconazole 200-mg supp for 3 d Miconazole 100-mg supp for 7 d Miconazole 1,200-mg suppository for 1 day Nystatin 100,000-unit tab for 14 d Tioconazole 6.5% oint 5 g in one dose Terconazole 0.4% cr 5 g for 7 d Terconazole 0.8% cr 5 g for 3 d Terconazole 80-mg supp for 3 d	Fluconazole 150-mg tablet in one dose. Note: Cream and ointments may weaken condoms and diaphragms.

Continued

Table 44–2 **Drugs Commonly Used: Sexually Transmitted Infections—cont'd**

Pathogen	First Choice	Alternative Choice
Protozoan Pathogen		
Trichomoniasis	Metronidazole 2 g PO in one dose or tinidazole 2 g PO in a single dose	Metronidazole 500 mg PO bid for 7 d.
Ectoparasitic Pathogens		
Pubic lice	Permethrin 1% cream rinse to affected areas, wash off in 10 min *or* pyrethrins with piperonyl butoxide applied to affected areas, wash off in 10 min Permethrin 5% cream: apply to all body, wash off 8–14 h	Alternative regimens: malathion 0.5% lotion applied for 8–12 hr, then wash off *or* ivermectin 250 mcg/kg repeated in 2 wk Pregnant/lactating women: can be treated with either permethrin or pyrethrins with piperonyl butoxide.
Scabies	Permethrin cream 5% applied to all areas of body from neck down and washed off 8–14 h after application *or* Ivermectin 200 mcg/kg orally, repeated in 2 wk	Lindane 1% lotion or 30 g cream apply to all body, wash off after 8 h Note: Lindane is not recommended as first-line therapy because of toxicity. Only use if pt. cannot tolerate other therapies. Lindane should *not* be used immediately after a bath or shower, or in persons with dermatitis, women who are pregnant/lactating and children <2 yr.

BCA = bichloroacetic acid; TCA = trichloroacetic acid.
Source: Adapted from *Sexually transmitted diseases treatment guidelines (2010)*. Atlanta, GA: Centers for Disease Control and Prevention.

the first prenatal visit (CDC, 2010). In communities and populations with high prevalence of syphilis, patients are screened at 28 to 32 weeks' gestation and at delivery to avoid possible neonatal transmission (CDC, 2010). The high-risk category for repeated screening is described as a person who has a history of multiple sex partners, a history of current or recent STIs, or a user of street drugs (Hatcher, Trussell, & Kowal, 2008).

Parenteral Penicillin G (rather than **oral penicillin**) has been used effectively for more than 50 years and is the preferred drug for the treatment of all stages of syphilis; dosing is found in Table 44–2. Patients who are **penicillin** allergic may be treated with 14 days of **doxycycline** or **tetracycline** (see Table 44–2). **Doxycycline** causes less gastrointestinal upset, so may have better compliance than **tetracycline** (CDC, 2010). **Parenteral penicillin G** is the only therapy with documented efficacy for syphilis during pregnancy, with dosing the same as for non-pregnant patients (CDC, 2010). Pregnant women with syphilis in any stage who report **penicillin** allergy should be desensitized and treated with **penicillin.**

Gonorrhea

First isolated in 1879, the gram-negative intracellular diplococcus *Neisseria gonorrhoeae* can be transmitted through the urethra, rectum, pharynx, vagina, or eye. In the United States, an estimated 700,000 new *N. gonorrhoeae* infections occur each year (CDC, 2010). Men tend to become symptomatic when infected. Many infected women have no symptoms until complications, such as pelvic inflammatory disease (PID), have occurred (CDC, 2010). The incubation period can be 2 days to 2 weeks. Patients infected with gonorrhea are often co-infected with chlamydia. This finding led to the recommendation that patients being treated for gonorrhea also need treatment for chlamydia (CDC, 2010).

Complications of gonococcal infection include PID, tubal scarring, infertility, ectopic pregnancy, salpingitis, or disseminated gonococcal (GC) infection. Disseminated GC infection is characterized by pustular dermatitis, asymmetrical arthralgia, tenosynovitis, or septic arthritis. An infected pregnant woman is at risk for endometritis after procedures such as therapeutic abortions, chorionic villus sampling, or dilation and curettage. Between 30 and 50 percent of newborns of women with GC cervicitis develop GC conjunctivitis. Drug resistance has had a significant impact on the treatment of gonorrhea. Previous CDC guidelines recommended a **fluoroquinolone (ciprofloxacin)** for treatment of gonorrhea. Over the past 10 years the prevalence of **fluoroquinolone** resistance in *N. gonorrhoeae* has been increasing and as of 2007, the CDC no longer recommends the use of **fluoroquinolones** for the treatment of *N. gonorrhoeae* infections. Only one class of drugs, the **cephalosporins,** continues to be recommended for the treatment of gonorrhea (CDC, 2007a; CDC, 2010). For the treatment of uncomplicated urogenital and anorectal gonorrhea, the CDC now recommends a single intramuscular dose of **ceftriaxone** 250 mg or a single oral dose of **cefixime** 400 mg. For persons with severe **cephalosporin** allergies, providers should consult with an infectious disease specialist (CDC, 2010).

Pregnant patients are treated with **ceftriaxone** 250 mg IM or **cefixime** 400 mg orally. Pregnant patients may also be treated with **azithromycin** 2 grams if they cannot tolerate **cephalosporins** (CDC, 2010).

Patients infected with *N. gonorrhoeae* infections frequently are co-infected with *Clamydia trachomatis* infections. This co-infection has led the CDC to recommend that patients treated for gonococcal infection also be treated routinely with a regimen effective against *C. trachomatis* infections (CDC, 2010). The recommended dual treatment is **ceftriaxone** or **cefixime** *plus* **azithromycin** 1 gm orally in a single dose or **doxycycline** 100 mg orally twice daily for 7 days.

Sexual partners require treatment. To prevent re-infection patients and their partners should abstain from intercourse until therapy is completed.

Women have a high rate of re-infection in the six months after treatment. The CDC recommends repeat screening of all women 3 to 6 months after treatment regardless of whether their sex partner is treated (CDC, 2010).

Chlamydia

C. trachomatis is a silent disease that causes serious sequelae such as PID, ectopic pregnancy, and infertility. Some women who have uncomplicated cervical infection already have subclinical upper reproductive tract infections. Asymptomatic infection is common among both men and women. Chlamydial genital infections occur frequently among sexually active adolescents and young adults. All sexually active women age 25 years or younger should be screened for chlamydia infection at least annually, even if symptoms are not present. Older women who have a new or multiple sex partner should also be screened. Screening can be completed via urine testing or by endocervix or vaginal swab.

The CDC recommended treatment for chlamydia infection is **azithromycin** 1 gram orally in a single dose or **doxycycline** 100 mg twice a day for 7 days (CDC, 2010). Either treatment is efficacious, although the single-dose **azithromycin** may have a higher compliance rate (CDC, 2010). Pregnant women are treated with either **azithromycin** or **amoxicillin** (see Table 44–2). Alternative therapy with **erythromycin** is recommended for pregnant women, but adverse reactions and reduced effectiveness make it less desirable for nonpregnant women.

Except in pregnant women, a test of cure (repeat testing 3 to 4 wk after completing therapy) is not recommended for persons treated with the recommended or alternative regimens, unless therapeutic compliance is in question (CDC, 2010). Pregnant women should have follow up testing after treatment and should be retested 3 months after treatment (CDC, 2010). The majority of post-treatment infections result from reinfection. To minimize transmission, persons being treated for chlamydia should be instructed to abstain from sexual intercourse for 7 days after single-dose therapy or until completion of a 7-day regimen. Treatment of sex partners will also minimize the risk of reinfection.

Co-infection with *C. trachomatis* often occurs in patients with gonorrhea infections, as noted previously. Therefore, dual therapy for gonorrhea and chlamydial infections is the accepted treatment standard.

All sexual partners in the past 60 days should be referred for testing and treatment. The most recent partner, even if more than 60 days should be evaluated. Expedited partner therapy is recommended to decrease reinfection (CDC, 2010).

Chancroid

Chancroid, caused by *Haemophilus ducreyi,* is endemic in some areas of the United States and is common in many of the world's poorest regions such as areas of Africa, Asia and the Caribbean (WHO, 2010). Co-infection with HIV and, to a lesser extent, with syphilis and HSV can occur. Diagnosis is difficult because of the lack of available and sensitive testing media. As a result, treatment is initiated when these criteria are satisfied: (1) one or more painful ulcers, (2) negative tests for syphilis and HSV, and (3) the appearance of ulcers with suppurative inguinal adenopathy.

Chancroid usually starts as a small papule that rapidly becomes pustular and then it eventually ulcerates. The ulcer enlarges and begins to develop ragged and uneven borders, and is surrounded by an erythematous rim. Unlike syphilis, chancroid lesions are tender. Treatment recommendations include **azithromycin** 1 g orally in a single dose or **ceftriaxone** 250 mg intramuscularly (IM) or **ciprofloxacin** 500 mg orally twice a day for 3 days or **erythromycin** 500 mg orally three times a day for 7 days (CDC, 2010). Pregnant women are treated with **azithromycin**, **ceftriaxone**, or **erythromycin**. **Ciprofloxacin** should not be prescribed to pregnant women.

Patients are re-examined 3 to 7 days after therapy is started (CDC, 2010). Ulcers usually improve symptomatically after 3 days. Ulcers may take up to 2 weeks to heal. Although treatment is successful, there still may be significant scarring. Poor response to treatment may indicate the patient is co-infected with another STI, has HIV or the pathogen is resistant. Healing may be slower for uncircumcised men with ulcers under their foreskin.

In those men who are uncircumcised or have HIV disease, response to treatment may not be as good, therefore patients should have HIV testing at the time of chancroid diagnosis (CDC, 2010). Follow-up is recommended because lack of response may indicate presence of HIV disease owing to the fact that chancroid is a cofactor for HIV transmission. Patients should be retested for syphilis and HIV at 3-month intervals after the diagnosis of chancroid, if the initial test results were negative (CDC, 2010). If the lymphadenopathy is fluctuant, incision and drainage may be necessary to enhance healing.

Treatment of sexual partners should be examined and treated if they have had sexual contact with the patient in the 10 days preceding diagnosis.

Granuloma Inguinale (Donovanosis)

Granuloma inguinale is a genital ulcerative disease caused by the intracellular gram-negative bacterium

Klebsiella granulomatis (formerly known as *Calymmatobacterium granulomatis*). This infection results in ulcers that are painless and without lymphadenopathy. Granuloma inquinale usually affects the skin and mucous membranes in the genital region and results in nodular lesions that progress to large beefy lesions that are difficult to heal and bleed easily on contact. The ulcers progressively expand and are locally destructive. The mode of transmission of granuloma inguinale primarily occurs through sexual contact; however, it may have low infectious capabilities because repeated exposure is necessary for clinical infection to occur. Additionally, granuloma inguinale may also be obtained through the fecal route or by passage through an infected birth canal (CDC, 2006). Most infections are endemic in tropical and developing areas of India, Papua New Guinea, central Australia, and southern Africa. The recommended antibiotic treatment for granuloma inguinale is **doxycycline** 100 mg twice a day for 3 weeks (CDC, 2010). Alternatives include **ciprofloxacin** (750 twice a day for 3 weeks), **erythromycin** (500 qid for 3 weeks), **azithromycin** (1 gram weekly for 3 weeks) or **trimethoprim/sulfmethoxazole** (one DS twice a day for 3 weeks). Treatment is long, a minimum of 3 weeks or until all lesions have completely healed (CDC, 2010). Relapse is common within 6 to 18 months despite the best therapy. Although treatment stops progression of lesions, prolonged therapy may be required to permit granulation and re-epithelialization of the ulcers. Sex partners should have clinical signs and symptoms prior to initiation of therapy.

Lymphogranuloma Venereum

Lymphogranuloma venereum (LGV), caused by *C. trachomatis* serovars L1, L2, or L3, rarely occurs in the United States. However, LGV infection manifestations share characteristics with chancroid, such as unilateral tender lymphadenopathy and self-limited genital ulcers. Homosexual men may present with proctocolitis and women with perianal inflammation, with the complication being strictures or fistulas. LGV can become an invasive systemic infection, and if it is not treated early, LGV proctocolitis may lead to chronic, colorectal fistulas and strictures. The diagnosis is made serologically and the recommended treatment is **doxycycline** 100 mg twice a day for 21 days; an alternative treatment is **erythromycin base** 500 mg four times a day for 21 days (CDC, 2010). Pregnant women are treated with **erythromycin**. Local lesions (buboes) may require incision and drainage. Patients may need further testing to rule out the high rate of coexisting STIs.

Sexual partners who had contact with the patient in the past 60 days should be examined and treated (CDC, 2010).

Bacterial Vaginosis

Bacterial vaginosis (BV), the most prevalent of vaginal infections, is caused by a replacement of the normal vaginal flora by an overgrowth of organisms such as *Prevotella* spp., *Mobiluncus* spp., *Gardnerella vaginalis*, or *Mycoplasma hominis*. Although BV is not considered an STI, women who have never been sexually active are rarely affected. BV is associated with having multiple sex partners, douching, and lack of vaginal lactobacilli. BV has caused endometritis and PID after invasive procedures such as endometrial biopsy, intrauterine device insertion, cesarean delivery, hysterectomy, and therapeutic abortion.

BV can be diagnosed by the use of clinical or Gram's stain criteria and must include three of the four following signs and symptoms: (1) a homogeneous, white, noninflammatory discharge that smoothly coats the vaginal walls, (2) vaginal pH of more than 4.5, (3) positive whiff test (fishy odor) with 10 percent potassium hydroxide (KOH), or (4) the presence of "clue cells" (vaginal epithelial cell peppered with coccoid bacteria) under high-power microscopy.

All symptomatic women should be treated. The recommended **metronidazole** regimens are equally effective. **Metronidazole** 500 mg orally twice a day for 7 days; **metronidazole** gel, 0.75 percent, one full applicator (5 g) intravaginally, once a day for 5 days; or **clindamycin** cream, 2 percent, one full applicator (5 g) intravaginally at bedtime for 7 days are the current CDC (2010) recommendations. **Metronidazole** 2 g single-dose therapy has the lowest efficacy for BV and is no longer a recommended or alternative regimen (CDC, 2006). Vaginal **clindamycin cream** is less effective than the **metronidazole** regimen, but it provides an option for women allergic to **azoles**. When mixed with alcohol, **metronidazole** has produced **disulfiram**-like reactions. Alcohol should not be consumed during or for at least 1 day following completion of **metronidazole** therapy (American Society of Health-System Pharmacists, 2010; CDC, 2010). **Clindamycin cream** is oil based and may weaken latex condoms and diaphragms. Owing to the fact that treatment of the sex partner has not been shown to be effective in preventing reoccurring infections, routine treatment of sexual contacts is not recommended.

BV during pregnancy is associated with premature rupture of membranes, preterm labor, preterm birth, and postpartum endometriosis. For this reason, pregnant women should be screened for BV once the diagnosis of pregnancy is made. Current data do not support the use of topical agents to treat BV during pregnancy. There has been evidence to show adverse events after the use of **clindamycin cream**. For this reason, treatment of BV in the pregnant woman should be oral, rather than topical, with a medication that is safe during pregnancy. **Metronidazole** 500 mg orally twice a day for 7 days or **metronidazole** 250 mg three times a day for 7 days may be used or **clindamycin** 300 mg twice daily for 7 days can be prescribed for pregnant women (CDC, 2010).

Vulvovaginal Candidiasis

Vulvovaginal candidiasis (VVC) may be caused by several yeast species, although *Candida albicans* is the most common. It is estimated that 75 percent of women will have at least one episode of VVC, and 40 to 45 percent will have two or more episodes (CDC, 2010). For many women, a recent history of **antibiotic** use is often the cause. The patient with chronic recurrent disease is often diabetic. Women who closely control their blood sugar have fewer reported infections. Although this disease is often diagnosed when women are checked for STIs, it is not necessarily passed sexually. Sexual partners may be treated simultaneously if they are symptomatic with *Candida*. The diagnosis for VVC can be made in a woman by wet preparation (saline, 10% KOH), Gram's stain, or culture.

The **azoles** as a drug class are the most effective treatment. In 90 percent of infections, a single oral dose of **fluconazole** provides a cure. The recommended creams and suppositories for the treatment of VVC are oil based and may weaken latex condoms and diaphragms. Self-medication with over-the-counter (OTC) preparations is advised only for women who have been previously diagnosed with VVC and who have a recurrence of the same symptoms. VVC often occurs during pregnancy. Only **topical azole therapies**, applied for 7 days, are recommended for use among pregnant women.

Azoles do stimulate the cytochrome P450 (CYP450) enzyme system in the liver and have potential drug interactions with **calcium channel antagonists**, **cisapride**, **warfarin**, **oral hypoglycemic agents**, **phenytoin**, **protease inhibitors**, **theophylline**, and **rifampin**.

An alternative treatment for vaginal *Candida* is to use **fluconazole** 150 mg oral tablet, one tablet in a single dose (CDC, 2010). Severe vulvovaginitis, characterized by extensive vulvar erythema, edema, excoriation, and fissure formation may not clear with standard short therapy. The CDC (2010) recommends two doses of **fluconazole** 150 mg, with the second dose 72 hours after initial dose or 7 to 14 days of a topical **azole**. Recurrent vulvovaginal candidiasis may be treated with oral **fluconazole** (100 mg, 150 mg, or 200 mg) weekly for 6 months (CDC, 2010).

Herpes Simplex Virus Type 1 and Herpes Simplex Virus Type 2

Genital herpes is recurrent and incurable. Two serotypes of HSV have been identified: HSV-1 and HSV-2. Most recurrences are a result of HSV-2. At present, approximately 50 million people have genital HSV infection. Most persons infected with HSV-2 have not been diagnosed and shed the virus in the genital tract without obvious symptoms (CDC, 2010).

Medications are up to 75 percent effective for symptom relief and speed of healing ulcers. Restoring and preserving quality of life is important in the patient with genital herpes. Suppressive therapy is recommended for patients experiencing six or more outbreaks each year. Most patients experience fewer episodes after 1 year of suppressive therapy. However, suppressive treatment can be effective in patients with less frequent attacks. Suppressive **antiviral therapy** reduces but does not eliminate subclinical viral shedding. Systemic medication with **acyclovir**, **famciclovir**, and **valacyclovir** are the mainstay of treatment for genital herpes. **Topical antiviral therapy** is not recommended. **Antiviral therapy** for recurrent genital herpes can be administered episodically or continuously as suppressive therapy. **Episodic therapy** is effective in shortening the duration of outbreaks if started within the first 24 hours of lesion outbreaks or during the prodromal phase (burning, itching, and tingling) that often precedes outbreaks. In order for the **antiviral treatment** to be effective, the provider should supply the patient receiving episodic treatment for HSV with a prescription to self-medicate immediately when symptoms begin. Consider reassessing the need for suppressive therapy annually by temporarily discontinuing the drug to see if outbreaks occur.

Patients with HIV infection or who are immunocompromised because of other causes may have prolonged or severe, painful episodes of genital, perianal, or oral herpes. Drug choices and dosing for HSV in the HIV patient is the same as for those with a first episode (or initial outbreak). Episodic or suppressive therapy with oral **antiviral agents** is beneficial.

Perinatal transmission of HSV is low (less than 1 percent) in women who have a history of genital HSV, but because recurrent herpes is common in pregnant women there is concern for transmission to the neonate at birth (CDC, 2010). The safety of **acyclovir**, **valacyclovir**, and **famciclovir** in pregnant women has not been well established. However, **acyclovir** can be administered orally to pregnant women with first episode genital herpes or severe recurrent herpes (CDC, 2010). Perinatal transmission of HSV is 30 percent to 50 percent if women are infected near delivery and can be life threatening, therefore protected sex is necessary if sex partners are infected (CDC, 2010). Cesarean delivery does not ensure protection from HSV-2 infection. Pregnant women with HSV require careful management by a obstetrical specialist during pregnancy and delivery.

Human Papillomavirus

According to the CDC, by the age of 50 more than 80 percent of American women will have contracted at least one strain of genital HPV. Both men and women can be carriers of HPV (CDC, 2010). Most HPV infections are asymptomatic or not visible. Reports indicate that more than 40 viral types are currently transmitted. Types 6 and 11 are associated with visible "warts" and are associated with conjunctival, nasal, oral, and laryngeal lesions. Patients with visible warts may be infected with several types simultaneously. Other types (16, 18, 31, 33, and 35) are associated with cervical neoplasia and detected through the Pap smear process (CDC, 2006). Lesions may be penile, scrotal, cervical, vaginal, urethral, oral, or perianal. HPV type 6 or 11 are commonly found before, or at the time of, detection of genital warts; however, the use of HPV testing for genital wart diagnosis is not recommended.

Genital warts are usually flat, papular, or pedunculated growths on the genital mucosa. Diagnosis of genital warts is made by visual inspection and may be confirmed by biopsy, although biopsy is needed only under certain circumstances (for example, if the diagnosis is uncertain; the lesions do not respond to standard therapy; the disease worsens during therapy; the patient is immunocompromised; or warts are pigmented, indurated, fixed, bleeding, or ulcerated). No data support the use of HPV nucleic acid tests in the routine diagnosis or management of visible genital warts (CDC, 2006).

The application of 3 to 5 percent **acetic acid** usually turns HPV-infected genital mucosal tissue to a whitish color. However, **acetic acid** application is not a specific test for HPV infection, and the specificity and sensitivity of this procedure for screening have not been defined. Therefore, the routine use of this procedure for screening to detect HPV infection is not recommended (CDC, 2006). However, those clinicians who are experienced in the management of genital warts have determined that this test is useful for identifying flat genital warts.

In addition to the external genitalia (that is, penis, vulva, scrotum, perineum, and perianal skin), genital warts can occur on the uterine cervix and in the vagina, urethra, anus, and mouth. Intra-anal warts are observed predominantly in patients who have had receptive anal intercourse; these warts are distinct from perianal warts, which can occur in men and women who do not have a history of anal sex. In addition to the genital area, genital warts are usually asymptomatic, but depending on the size and anatomical location, genital warts can be painful, friable, or pruritic.

HPV types 16, 18, 31, 33, and 35 are found occasionally in visible genital warts and have been associated with external genital squamous intraepithelial neoplasia. These HPV types also have been associated with vaginal, anal, and cervical intra-epithelial neoplasia (CIN). They have also been associated with anogenital and some head and neck squamous cell carcinomas. Patients who have visible genital warts are frequently infected simultaneously with multiple HPV types (CDC, 2006). Management of HPV involves removing warts if the patient is symptomatic due to location, size, and number of warts and monitoring for the development of cancer cells especially in patients with abnormal Pap test results.

The primary goal of treating visible genital warts is the removal of the warts. In the majority of patients, treatment can induce wart-free periods. If left untreated, visible genital warts might resolve on their own, remain unchanged, or increase in size or number. Treatment possibly reduces, but does not eliminate, HPV infection. So far existing data indicate that currently available therapies for genital warts might reduce, but probably do not eradicate, HPV infections. No evidence indicates that the presence of genital warts or their treatment is associated with the development of cervical cancer (CDC, 2006).

The patient's symptoms, number of warts, where the warts are on the body, and size of warts are some of the factors that need to be considered in selecting a treatment modality. Other factors include cost of treatment, patient preference, the experience of the provider, and access to wart morphology. In general, warts located on moist surfaces or areas such as the armpits, underneath pendulous breasts, groin, creases of the neck, or skinfolds respond better to topical treatment than do warts on skin surfaces that are drier. The majority of patients will need more than one treatment and most respond within 3 months of therapy. Treatment regimens are classified into patient-applied and provider-applied modalities.

For external genital warts the CDC (2010) recommends patient-applied therapy to include **podofilox** 0.5 percent solution or gel or **imiquimod** 5 percent cream. These therapies need to be applied several times a week. Provider-applied management includes cryotherapy with **liquid nitrogen** or **cryoprobe** or **podophyllin resin** 10 to 25 percent in a compound tincture of benzoin or **trichloroacetic acid (TCA)** or **bichloroacetic acid (BCA)** 80 to 90 percent. An alternative provider-applied management includes the use of intralesional interferon or laser surgery. Surgical referral should be considered by the nurse practitioner when the size, number of warts, ineffective response to topical treatments, and location of warts make it difficult to treat effectively. **Imiquimod**, **podophyllin**, and **podofilox** should not be used during pregnancy. Because genital warts can proliferate and become friable during pregnancy many specialist recommend their removal during pregnancy.

There is no evidence to suggest that one treatment is superior to another. Only trained nurse practitioners should administer cryotherapy. Treatment regimens should be changed if warts do not resolve in three to six treatments. Treatment of these lesions may result in chronic pain syndromes of the vulva, but these are extremely rare. In the absence of genital warts or cervical squamous intraepithelial lesion (SIL) the CDC does not recommend treatment for subclinical genital HPV infection.

Currently in the United States, two vaccines to prevent HPV infection are currently on the market: **Gardasil** and **Cervarix**. Both vaccines protect against two of the HPV types (HPV-16 and HPV-18) that can cause cervical cancer and some other genital cancers; **Gardasil** also protects against HPV-6 and HPV-11, two of the HPV types that cause genital warts. **Gardasil** has been shown to also be effective in preventing genital warts in males, and use for men and boys was approved by the U.S. Food and Drug Administration (FDA) in October 2009.

Trichomoniasis

Trichomonas spp. are protozoa, and protozoan infections require a different therapeutic approach. Infection with these organisms requires treatment of sex partners. Men are rarely symptomatic but may harbor *Trichomonas* in the prostate gland for years if left untreated. Many women have a malodorous, yellow green vaginal discharge with vulvar irritation. However, some women have minimal discharge and may be asymptomatic. The availability of rapid testing has increased the sensitivity and specificity significantly compared to the use of microscopy which requires provider experience and immediate evaluation of wet prepared slides to capture the classic *Trichomonas* movement. The diagnosis is therefore often missed because wet mounts must be viewed quickly. Urine sediment microscopy may frequently demonstrate this organism fortuitously.

The treatment regimen for trichomoniasis includes **metronidazole** 2 grams orally in one dose or **tinidazole** 2 grams orally in a single dose (CDC, 2010). Patients may also be treated with **metronidazole** 500 mg twice a day for 7 days. Patients need to be advised to avoid consuming alcohol during treatment with **metronidazole** it may elicit a **disulfiram** reaction. Topical **metronidazole** or **clindamycin** are no longer recommended in the treatment of trichomoniasis due to poor efficacy (less than 50 percent cure) compared with oral treatment (CDC, 2010). Rescreening for *T. vaginalis* 3 months after treatment may be considered in sexually active women, due to a high (17 percent) reinfection rate (CDC, 2010).

Pregnant women who are infected with vaginal trichomoniasis are at risk of preterm labor, premature rupture of membranes and low birth weight (CDC, 2010). Treatment for symptomatic women or asymptomatic women after 37 weeks gestation is **metronidazole** 2 grams in a single dose, regardless of stage of pregnancy (CDC, 2010). The safety of **tinidazole** in pregnancy has not been well evaluated. Pregnant women should be followed up in 1 month.

Sexual partners should be treated for trichomoniasis and patients should be instructed to abstain from intercourse until both partners are treated an asymptomatic (CDC, 2010).

Pediculosis Pubis (Genital Lice)

Pediculosis pubis (i.e., genital lice), commonly called crabs, is an ectoparasitic infection that is treated differently based on where the lice are found (e.g., scalp, body, or the pubic area). Pubic lice are sexually transmitted. The organism is genetically programmed to attach to hair of different diameters. Considerable resistance to medication for treatment of head lice has been seen, but pediculosis is still eradicated by the methods listed in Table 44–2. Decontamination of household and personal items with hot washing or dry-cleaning is usually adequate. Pubic lice cannot live away from the body for more than 72 hours, and fumigating the home is not necessary if the previous methods are observed.

Pubic lice may be treated with **pyrethrins**, which are **permethrin** 1 percent, **pyrethrin** lotion, or shampoo. Advise the patient to thoroughly saturate hair with lice medication. Leave medication on for 10 minutes then thoroughly rinse off medication with water. Dry off with a clean towel. (CDC, Division of Parasitic Diseases, 2008a). Reapply in 7 days if there is evidence of live lice.

Resistance to pediculicides is becoming more frequent and widespread. Pubic lice may also be treated with an application of **lindane** 1 percent cream, lotion, or shampoo. A thin layer of cream or lotion is applied to the hair and skin surrounding the pubic area and left on for 12 hours. If **lindane** shampoo is used, the shampoo is massaged into dry pubic hair and left on for 5 to 10 minutes. If axillary or thigh hair is also infested, then use the cream or lotion. Reapply in 7 days if there is evidence of live lice. **Malathion** 0.5 percent lotion is an option for treatment and is applied for 8 to 12 hours and then washed off; it may be used when treatment failure is believed to have occurred because of resistance (CDC, 2006; Chosidow, 2000). Further discussion of the treatment of body lice is discussed in Chapter 32.

Scabies

Sarcoptes scabiei is the parasite involved in scabies. The most common predominant symptom is pruritus. After a person is infested with scabies for the first time, sensitization can take up to several weeks to develop. Pruritus can then occur within 24 hours following a subsequent infestation. Scabies is passed sexually in adults, but adults and particularly children may become infected by sleeping on infected sheets in motels and hotels.

Permethrin 5 percent cream (**Elimite, Acticin**) is the drug of choice for the treatment of scabies, especially in pregnant women or young children. The cream is massaged into the skin from the neck to the soles of feet. It should be left on for 8 to 14 hours and then washed off in the shower. **Lindane** 1 percent is recommended only as an alternative regimen. **Lindane** should not be used immediately after bathing or by people with extensive dermatitis. **Lindane** is contraindicated in pregnant and lactating women and in children less than 2 years of age.

In patients who are immunocompromised or who have refractory scabies, **ivermectin** 200 mcg/kg orally may be used. The **ivermectin** may need to be repeated in 2 weeks. **Ivermectin** is not active against nits.

Bedding and clothing should be decontaminated or removed from body contact for at least 72 hours. Patient education is important when treating ectoparasitic infections. The rash and pruritus of scabies can persist for up to 2 weeks after treatment. Sexual contacts, and family members may be in the incubation period (4 wk), and so all family members and close contacts need simultaneous treatment to prevent recurrence. Reinfection from family members or fomites might occur in the absence of appropriate contact treatment and decontamination of bedding and clothing. The treatment of scabies is discussed in depth in Chapter 32.

Special Treatment Situations

Certain treatment situations warrant special consideration, including PID, sexual assault, and men who have sex with men. Delay in treatment of PID or treatment with the wrong **antibiotic** can result in continued spread of the organism. A woman who presents for care with signs of PID needs treatment as though she has all types of infection, including gonorrhea, *Chlamydia,* and BV. The sexual assault victim needs urgent evaluation, with testing, prophylactic antibiotics, and emergency contraception offered. Men who have sex with men also present a special treatment challenge and are described in more detail below. Box 44–1 reviews the **antibiotic** choices for these special treatment situations.

Pregnancy

All pregnant women and their sexual partners should be asked about STIs, counseled about the possibility of perinatal infection, and ensured access to treatment. A pregnant woman with an STI requiring **antibiotic** treatment may present as a treatment challenge for the nurse practitioner. **Ciprofloxacin, ofloxacin,** and **doxycycline** are also contraindicated in pregnancy.

Children

STIs in children, if acquired after the neonatal period, should raise the index of suspicion about the possibility of child abuse. Nurse practitioners or other health providers must perform extensive evaluation and referral to a child abuse specialist in order to effectively evaluate and treat this population.

The use of **fluoroquinolones** in children younger than 18 years is controversial. Therapy with this particular class of drugs has caused articular cartilage damage in some studies utilizing young animals. Owing to the fact that no joint damage attributable to **quinolone** therapy has been observed in children treated with prolonged **ciprofloxacin**, the CDC (2006) recommendations include treating children weighing more than 45 kg with any regimen recommended for adults.

Adolescents

According to the CDC (2010), the reported rates of chlamydia and gonorrhea are highest among females aged 15 to 19 years. This population of young adults also has the highest risk for acquiring HPV. Reasons cited for these risks include (1) engaging in frequent unprotected intercourse, (2) being biologically more susceptible to infection, (3) having partnerships of limited duration, and

BOX 44–1 SITUATIONS REQUIRING SPECIAL TREATMENT

Sexual Assault

PREGNANT

Patient needs specialty consultation; may need hospitalization.

NONPREGNANT

For nonpregnant prophylaxis management, the examination should include the following:

- STI testing: *Neisseria gonorrhoeae, Chlamydia trachomatis,* trichomoniasis, HIV, hepatitis B, and syphilis
- **Hepatitis B** vaccine (if not already immunized and empiric treatment) and
- **Ceftriaxone** 125 mg (IM) in 1 dose and
- **Metronidazole** 2 g PO in 1 dose and
- **Azithromycin** 1 g PO in 1 dose or
- **Doxycycline** 100 mg PO bid for 7 days

Emergency contraception should be offered.

Pelvic Inflammatory Disease (PID)

PREGNANT

Patient needs specialty consultation; may need hospitalization.

NONPREGNANT

Recommended oral treatment for women with mild-to-moderately severe acute PID includes the following:

- **Ceftriaxone** 250 mg IM as single dose plus **doxycycline** 100 mg PO bid for 14 days with or without **metronidazole** 500 mg PO bid for 14 days

  or
- **Cefoxitin** 2 g IM in a single dose and **probenecid** 1 g PO as single dose *plus* **doxycycline** 100 mg PO bid for 14 days with or without **metronidazole** 500 mg PO bid for 14 days

  or
- Other parenteral third generation **cephalosporin** (e.g., **ceftizoxine** or **cefotaxine**) *plus* **doxycycline** 100 mg PO bid for 14 days with or without **metronidazole** 500 mg PO bid for 14 days

Men Who Have Sex With Men

GONORRHEA

- **Ceftriaxone** 250 mg (IM) in 1 dose *or*
- **Cefixime** 400 mg PO in 1 dose *plus* treatment for chlamydia if chlamydial infection is not ruled out. Alternative regimens:
- Spectinomycin 2 g (IM) in 1 dose

CHLAMYDIA

- **Azithromycin** 1 g PO in 1 dose *or*
- **Doxycycline** 100 mg PO bid for 7 days

For the most up-to-date STI prescribing guidelines, go to the Centers for Disease Control and Prevention Guidelines Web site, http://www. cdc.gov/std/.

(4) difficulty gaining access to care. Adolescents in most states can consent to the confidential diagnosis and treatment of STIs. In these states, nurse practitioners need to be aware that medical care for STIs can be provided to adolescents without parental consent or knowledge.

Pelvic Inflammatory Disease

Delay in treatment of STIs and other diseases (bacterial vaginosis) can result in PID and infertility. Organisms that cause PID can be sexually transmitted *(N. gonorrhoeae* and *Chlamydia)*, part of the normal flora *(G. vaginalis* and *Haemophilus influenzae)*, or atypical agents (cytomegalovirus and *Mycoplasma hominis*).

PID is difficult to diagnose owing to (1) the wide variation in signs and symptoms and (2) the fact that more than one organism may be involved. Empirical treatment of PID should be initiated if the following minimum criteria are met and no other cause for the symptoms (e.g., appendicitis) can be found: (1) uterine/adnexal tenderness or (2) cervical motion tenderness. Additional criteria that support the diagnosis of PID include (1) oral temperature higher than 38.3°C, (2) abnormal cervical or vaginal mucopurulent discharge, (3) presence of white blood cells upon saline microscopy examination, (4) elevated erythrocyte sedimentation rate, (5) elevated C-reactive protein, and (6) laboratory documented cervical infection with gonorrhea or chlamydia.

Treatment for PID is a multidrug regimen and must provide empirical, broad-spectrum coverage of the most likely pathogens. The nurse practitioner who suspects PID must begin treatment as soon as possible. Prevention of long-term complications has been linked directly with immediate administration of appropriate **antibiotics**. A woman who presents for care with signs and symptoms suggestive of PID needs to be treated as if she has all types of infection. When tubo-ovarian abscess is present, the use of **clindamycin** or **metronidazole** with **doxycycline** for continued treatment, rather than **doxycycline** alone, provides more effective anaerobic coverage.

A woman may need IV **antibiotics** and/or hospitalization if her temperature is high and/or if she cannot tolerate oral drugs. The transition from IV therapy to oral therapy can usually be initiated within 24 hours of clinical improvement. Consider changing patients who fail to respond to oral therapy within 72 hours to parenteral therapy. The PID patient should show substantial clinical improvement within 3 days after initiation of therapy. Patients who do not improve within this time period usually require hospitalization, additional diagnostic testing, and surgical intervention. All pregnant women with PID should be hospitalized and treated with parenteral antibiotics.

Sexual Assault

Trichomoniasis, bacterial vaginosis, gonorrhea, and chlamydial infection are the most frequently diagnosed infections among women who have been sexually assaulted. Routine prophylaxis for STIs after a sexual assault is recommended. HBV infection might be prevented by post-exposure administration of hepatitis B immune globulin and hepatitis B vaccine.

Sexual assault victims should be evaluated for ingestion of date rape drugs. The date rape drug **Rohypnol (flunitrazepam)** is available illegally in the United States. This drug has been associated with an increased incidence of adolescent date rape (American Academy of Pediatrics [AAP], 2009. **Flunitrazepam**, a very rapid onset **benzodiazepine** with amnesic properties, is a tasteless drug that can go undetected if added to any drink (Kosten, 2009). The tasteless properties of these drugs make the victim incapable of protecting him- or herself. Owing to the amnesic properties, the sexual assault victim is unable to remember the events of the incident after the drug effects have worn off. These drugs, in the amounts most commonly used, produce intoxication and can produce fatalities if used with other respiratory depressants (such as large amounts of **alcohol** or **opioids**).

Men Who Have Sex With Men

The CDC (2007) recommendations include frequent STI screening (at 3- to 6-mo intervals) for high-risk males. Vaccinations against hepatitis A and B are recommended for all men who have sex with men (MSM) in whom previous infection or immunization cannot be documented. Men should be offered the HPV4 vaccine, regardless of their sexual orientation. Owing to the increased incidence of **fluoroquinolone**-resistant *N. gonorrhoeae* (QRNG) in Asia, the Pacific Islands (including Hawaii), and California, **fluoroquinolones** are no longer recommended for treating proven or suspected GC infections in men who have sex with men in the United States (CDC, 2007a).

Cefixime 400-mg dose is the only CDC-recommended oral agent for the treatment of gonorrhea. A single IM dose of **ceftriaxone** 250 mg is recommended for uncomplicated urogenital and anorectal gonorrhea. Alternative parenteral single-dose regimens for urogenital and anorectal gonorrhea may also include **ceftizoxime** 500 mg, **cefoxitin** 2 g with **probenecid** 1 g orally, or **cefotaxime** 500 mg. For persons with **penicillin** or **cephalosporin** allergies, a single IM dose of **spectinomycin** 2 g is a recommended alternative (CDC, 2007a).

The same STI treatment principles applied to heterosexuals are relevant to men having sex with men. If the nurse practitioner treats for gonorrhea, then treatment for possible co-infection with chlamydia should be prescribed. The reverse statement is also true.

Hepatitis

Serological testing is necessary for all suspected cases of hepatitis. In the United States almost half of all reported hepatitis A cases have no specific risk factors identified. However, among adults with identified risk factors, the majority of cases are among MSM, persons who use illegal drugs, and international travelers (CDC, 2006). Only about 1.8 percent of patients die from liver disease as a result of hepatitis A, but there is considerable morbidity, well worth the cost and inconvenience of two vaccine injections. Currently two products are available for the prevention of hepatitis A (HAV) infection: hepatitis A vaccine and immune globulin (Ig) for IM administration. No specific treatment therapy is available for persons with acute hepatitis A or B; treatment is supportive.

Chronic infections of hepatitis B occur in 1 to 6 percent of infected adults; however, they occur in 90 percent of infected newborns. The risk for premature death from either cirrhosis or hepatocellular carcinoma among persons infected with hepatitis B is between 15 and 25 percent (CDC, 2006). Hepatitis B virus (HBV) is passed through vertical transmission. Sexual transmission among adults accounts for most HBV infections in the United States. Prevention aimed at several groups is necessary. Prevention strategies include screening all pregnant women, vaccinating all newborns, vaccinating older children at high risk (e.g., Alaskan Natives, Pacific Islanders) and residents in households with first generation immigrants from countries that have high levels of endemic disease, vaccinating children aged 11 and 12 who do not fit into the preceding categories, and vaccinating teens and adults at high risk (sexual behaviors confer increased risk). Hepatitis A and B are the only **vaccines** available for preventable hepatitis diseases. There is no vaccine for hepatitis C.

Two products have been approved for hepatitis B prevention: **hepatitis B immune globulin (HBIG)** and **hepatitis B vaccine**. **HBIG** provides 3 to 6 months of temporary protection from hepatitis B infection. There are two monovalent **hepatitis B vaccines** for use in adolescents and adults: **Recombivax HB** and **Engerix-B**. There is also a combination vaccine of hepatitis A and B for use in adults, **Twinrix**. See Chapter 19 or http://www.cdc.gov/vaccines for more information.

Hepatitis C virus (HCV) is the most common chronic bloodborne infection in the United States. HCV transmission occurs by direct percutaneous exposure to infected blood, as well as by occupational, perinatal, and sexual exposure. Sexual transmission of HCV accounts for up to 15 to 20 percent of HCV infections (CDC, 2007a). Furthermore, coinfection with HIV increases the risk for sexual transmission of HCV. Newly infected persons with HCV commonly are either asymptomatic or have a mild clinical illness and may not seek medical care. HCV RNA can be detected within 1 to 3 weeks of exposure. Chronic HCV infections develop in 60 to 85 percent of HCV- infected persons. Of these, 60 to 70 percent have evidence of active liver disease. No vaccine is available for HCV, and prophylaxis with immune globulin is not effective in preventing HCV infection after exposure (CDC, 2006).

Human Immunodeficiency Virus

The immunosuppressive pathology of HIV predisposes some infected individuals to STIs. HIV affects the immune system, which in turn has an impact on diagnostic testing and evaluation of some of these infections. In addition, those infected with HIV often have a suboptimal response to treatment or present as treatment failures when infected with an STI. As a result, HIV-infected patients who have concurrent STI infections may require longer, more aggressive courses of therapy. When included as part of the treatment recommendations, nurse practitioners should consider prescribing **suppressive therapy** (HSV **vaccine**) sooner rather than later. Treatment of HIV infection is covered in Chapter 37.

Penicillin Allergy

Individuals infected with an STI, but who have an allergy to **penicillin**, also present as a treatment challenge. There are no CDC recommendations or proven alternatives to **penicillin** for the treatment of neurosyphilis, congenital syphilis, or syphilis in pregnant women. **Penicillin** is also the treatment of choice in HIV-infected patients. However, the administration of **penicillin** to those allergic to the drug can cause severe, immediate anaphylaxis, which can be fatal. As a general rule, **penicillin** should never be used in **penicillin**-allergic patients. Those patients needing **penicillin** should be referred to allergy specialists who can safely perform allergy skin testing and acute desensitization to eliminate anaphylactic sensitivity.

Monitoring

Drug sensitivity, patient intolerance, and noncompliance with drugs requiring multiple daily doses frequently necessitate use of alternate drugs. Although treatments for most STIs are quite effective, follow-up is necessary. Viral STIs present a challenge for most health care providers. Patient education, appropriate viral testing, and evaluation of possible concurrent infections are necessary components of any management. It is important to be sure that all sexual partners have been treated and that the organism in question has either been eradicated or brought under control. Asymptomatic partners may be resistant to treatment and may require education and assistance from the local health department. Laboratories are required by law to report most STIs to the state, so patients need to know that they will be contacted for verification of treatment.

Outcome Evaluation

Infection in the genital tract with *Chlamydia* or gonorrhea, if not treated in a timely manner, may ascend and invade the fallopian tubes, thus causing life-threatening PID and sepsis. A pregnant patient with an untreated STI may spontaneously abort and hemorrhage. Sepsis and bleeding require hospitalization and parenteral therapy. Consultation and referral to a gynecologist must be completed swiftly to prevent further complications. The specialist, in turn, will need information that only the nurse practitioner may possess: the patient's full past medical history, laboratory findings, previous treatments, and drug allergies.

On The Horizon

TREATMENT OF SEXUALLY TRANSMITTED INFECTIONS

Clinical development and trials are in progress for vaccines against a number of STIs, including HIV and HSV. Numerous **antiviral agents** have been investigated for the treatment of chronic HBV infections. Studies indicate that current monotherapy with conventional interferon-alpha, **lamivudine,** and **adefovir dipivoxil** may not be best practice. In addition, conventional **interferon-alpha** needs to be administered subcutaneously daily or thrice weekly and is associated with frequent adverse events. Although nucleoside–nucleotide analogues such as **lamivudine** and **adefovir dipivoxil** are well tolerated, 1-year therapy with either **lamivudine** or **adefovir dipivoxil** results in low hepatitis B e antigen (HBeAg) seroconversion rates. **Pegylated interferon alpha-2a**, an immunomodulatory agent, is a new drug that has just completed phase III clinical trials for the treatment of both HBeAg positive and HBeAg negative chronic HBV infection. The advantage of pegylated **interferon alpha-2a** in achieving sustained virological response over nucleoside–nucleotide analogues is becoming more apparent in the HBeAg negative group. In both of these phase III studies, sustained off-treatment responses appear to have better results in the use of **lamivudine.** These recent data put **pegylated interferon alpha-2a** as the first choice of anti-HBV therapy, especially in young and motivated patients with chronic HBV infection (Lai, Hui, Leung, & Lau, 2006).

Patient Education

Patient education should include a discussion of information related to the overall treatment plan as well as that specific to the drug therapy, reasons for taking the drug, drugs as part of the total treatment regimen, and potential compliance issues. Partner education is also important to consider. Assessment of the barriers to drug adherence need to be explored and discussed with the patient.

VAGINITIS

Treatment of female genital complaints across a woman's lifespan is common in primary care practice. The three diseases most frequently associated with vaginal discharge are trichomoniasis, bacterial vaginosis, and candidiasis. *C. trachomatis* and *N. gonorrhoeae* are less frequent causative organisms. Because of embarrassment, many patients, both old and young, try to get treatment over the phone. Diagnosing vaginal discharge and vulvar conditions requires examination of the area affected and microscopic examination of vaginal secretions. Not all practitioners are adept at microscopy, but in this area, the diagnosis may be elusive without prompt examination of vaginal discharge. This chapter earlier discussed the most common STIs and their treatment. Vaginal infections can be sexually transmitted, but some may also be acquired

SEXUALLY TRANSMITTED DISEASES

PATIENT EDUCATION

Related to the Overall Treatment Plan/Disease Process

- ☐ Importance of routine Pap smears in women and testicular self-examinations (TSE) in men.
- ☐ Prevention of high-risk sexual behaviors.
- ☐ Avoidance of sexual intercourse until the organism is either eradicated (bacterial) or under control (viral).
- ☐ Include immunization against selected STDs as part of treatment regimen.

Specific to the Drug Therapy

- ☐ Many OTC products are available to treat symptoms (see Table 42–2).
- ☐ Douching is no longer recommended because of the potential for pelvic infection and destroying the normal flora of *Lactobacillus.*
- ☐ BV must be diagnosed and treated on the same day in patients suspected of being pregnant (BV may cause preterm labor).
- ☐ Importance of assessment of pregnancy status *before* prescribing.
- ☐ Choosing an agent that has daily or twice-daily dosing increases patient compliance with treatment.

Reasons for Taking the Drug(s)

- ☐ Prevention of serious complications such as PID and infertility.
- ☐ Prevention of transmission of infection to the uninfected (public health issue).
- ☐ Prevention of dyspareunia, which affects normal sexual relations.

Drugs as Part of the Total Treatment Regimen

- ☐ Importance of seeking treatment when symptoms appear.
- ☐ Importance of culturing asymptomatic young persons (aged 15 to 24) every 6 months.

Continued

SEXUALLY TRANSMITTED DISEASES—cont'd

PATIENT EDUCATION

Adherence Issues

Importance of following the labeled instructions to totally eradicate the infection.

- ☐ Importance of finishing the full course of **antibiotics.**
- ☐ Importance of contacting the health-care provider if side effects or rash appears.
- ☐ The potential for drug interactions (the **macrolides** with **antifungal, systemic antifungals,** and **birth control pills).**

without sexual contact: VVC, some types of bacterial vaginosis, cytolytic vaginosis, atrophic vaginitis with secondary bacterial infection, and some types of streptococcal infections. *Staphylococcus aureus,* found in toxic shock syndrome, is associated with foreign bodies (tampons) inadvertently left during menses. Treatment of vulvovaginal infections is discussed separately from those vulvovaginal conditions that present with vaginal burning, pruritus, and dyspareunia, yet are not infectious.

Pathophysiology

Normal vaginal discharge contains desquamated vaginal epithelial cells, cervical secretions, lactic acid, and bacteria that are both anaerobic and aerobic. Vaginal microflora, predominantly *Lactobacillus,* appear under the microscope as unclumped, rod-like organisms. Hormones, age influence, and infections may alter the delicate balance. The most common infections are due to bacteria, yeast, and parasites.

Conditions not covered earlier in the chapter are discussed here.

Cytolytic Vaginosis

In cytolytic vaginosis, an overgrowth of *Lactobacillus* occurs late in the menstrual cycle. It is frequently treated as a chronic yeast infection. Diagnosis is made by absence of *Trichomonas,* hyphae, clue cells, and white blood cells under microscopy. The pH may be as low as 3.5, and treatment is aimed at raising the pH rather than eradicating all bacteria. Treatments that involve douching of medications are discouraged. Instead, patients are encouraged to make vaginal suppositories from clear gelatin capsules (size 0) filled with sodium bicarbonate (baking soda) and dose twice weekly in the last week of the menstrual cycle.

Atrophic Vaginitis

Atrophic vaginitis with secondary infection occurs owing to estrogen deficiency. As a result, the thinned vaginal epithelium has reduced defenses against common perineal bacteria. Culturing is necessary, as well as microscopy. See Table 44–2 for treatment once the infecting organism is diagnosed and Table 44–3 for treatment of the underlying atrophic conditions.

Toxic Shock Syndrome

S. aureus associated with toxic shock syndrome (TSS) can be life threatening. This patient requires immediate referral for hospitalization. *S. aureus* commonly colonizes skin and mucous membranes in humans. TSS has been associated with use of tampons and intravaginal contraceptive devices in women and occurs as a complication of skin abscesses or surgery. Risk groups include menstruating women, women using barrier contraceptive devices, persons who have undergone nasal surgery, and persons with postoperative staphylococcal wound infections (CDC, 2007b). Some women harbor *S. aureus* in their normal vaginal secretions but experience no symptoms until using tampons sets up an anaerobic climate. Criteria for making this diagnosis and treatment are based on CDC guidelines and include four of the following five diagnostic criteria: fever of 38.9°C (102°F) or higher, presence of a diffuse macular erythroderma, desquamation 1 to 2 weeks after onset of illness (palms and soles), hypotension (orthostatic changes of 15 mm Hg diastolic pressure or syncope), and involvement of three or more organ systems (GI, muscular, mucous membrane, renal, hepatic, hematological, and central nervous system [CNS]) (CDC, 2007b).

Noninfectious Vaginal Conditions

Noninfectious vaginal conditions may result from the following:

1. Normal cyclical hormonal changes, which occur at midcycle under high estrogen levels, and premenses, which is under progestin dominance. The changes in amount of vaginal secretions may concern some women, and microscopy may be necessary to reassure the patient and to rule out pathological organisms.
2. Irritant or allergic products, such as those found in hygiene and **contraceptive** products (e.g., **spermicides** and latex).
3. Atrophic conditions, such as those associated with the postpartum period and breastfeeding and those associated with postmenopausal vaginal atrophy.

Other Conditions

Less common and more worrisome are inflammatory, collagen, and epidermal sclerosing conditions, which are

Table 44–3 **Treatment for Noninfectious Vulvovaginal Conditions**

Condition	Drug Used	Nondrug Treatment
Chemical or other irritants spermicidals, douching solutions	Systemic steroid burst Medrol Dosepak	Avoid products with color and fragrance. Always use sanitary pads. Treat urinary incontinence with hygiene and disposable pads. Referral to urology for surgical correction.
Allergic, hypersensitivity, contact dermatitis, lichen simplex, foreign body	Steroid burst if severe reaction occurs Topical preferred over systemic	Avoidance and education about use of excessive hygiene measures. Use of Crisco (vegetable shortening) and avoidance of detergents in older women.
Traumatic vaginitis (may be factitious)	Treat with short-term (2–4 wk) clobetasol 0.05% tid. May add hydroxyzine (Atarax) 10 mg prn	Education and counseling about breaking the scratch-itch cycle.
Postpuerperal atrophic vaginitis	Vaginal application of conjugated or synthetic estrogen 1 g twice weekly	Water-soluble vaginal lubricant during intercourse—over a dozen effective lubricant choices.
Desquamative inflammatory vaginitis (steroid responsive)	If short course is helpful, consult about length of therapy; need tissue diagnosis	Avoid harsh scrubbing, soaps, and other over-the-counter vaginal products.
Erosive lichen planus	Steroids are usually necessary; need tissue diagnosis and consult or refer	Avoid excessive hygiene measures; there are "vulvar" specialists in gynecology.
Collagen vascular disease, Behçet's and pemphigus syndromes	Refer aggressive and painful lesions for diagnosis and treatment May use low-dose (25–50 mg) tricyclic antidepressants for pain control	Support groups may be helpful for some patients.
Hormonal Changes (normal responses)		
1 Midcycle	None	If culture and microscopy clear, then educate and reassure patient.
2 After intercourse	None	If culture and microscopy are clear, then educate and reassure.
3 Atrophic	If culture and microscopy are clear, then vaginal estrogen or Estratest hs (in 2 dosages 1.25 mg or 0.625 mg [conjugated estrogen] with 2.5 mg or 1.25 [methyltestosterone])	May require 3–6 mo of therapy for full therapeutic benefit.
Epithelial disorders (previously called dystrophies), lichen sclerosus (white lesions)	Clobetasol ointment 0.05% bid for 4 wk, then once daily for 4 wk, then twice per wk for maintenance	Support group may be helpful for some patients.

Sources: Advisor Forum. (2010). Treating vaginal dryness without causing recurrent DVT. *Clinical Advisor for Nurse Practitioners, 13*(1), 41; Centers for Disease Control and Prevention (CDC). (2007).
Doseck, J., & Stern, L. (2009). Treatment options for bacterial vaginosis. *Clinical Advisor for Nurse Practitioners, 12*(11); Levin, S., & O'Connell, C. B. (2010). Topical estrogens for postmenopausal women. *Clinical Advisor for Nurse Practitioners, 13*(2); Thompson, I. M., Teichman, J. M., Elston, D. M., & Sea, J. (2010). Noninfectious penile lesions. *Journal of the American Academy of Family Physicians, 81*(2).

commonly diagnosed in older women: inflammatory conditions related to trauma from excessive washing, wiping, and scratching; inflammatory conditions reflecting collagen-vascular disease; and inflammatory conditions associated with white or pigmented lesions that may be dysplastic or cancers.

Goals of Treatment

The goals of treatment are to treat the infection or inflammation, prevent reinfection, and prevent complications of the infection or inflammation. The infection cannot be treated without an accurate diagnosis. Patients often call the office numerous times for prescriptions for yeast infections, yet frequently they do not have monilial vaginitis. This telephone diagnosis has a 50-50 chance of being correct. Patients end up spending money on medications that probably will not help their symptoms. In addition, prescribing an ineffective **antibiotic** exposes the patient to potential side effects, adverse effects, and drug–drug interactions. For patients aged 15 to 24, there is a good chance the problem is *Chlamydia,* but for patients age 50 to 70, vaginal symptoms are more often related to atrophy of the genital tissues, vulvar presentation of collagen-vascular disease, or cancer.

Reinfection occurs when the etiology of the vaginal irritation is not known. If lack of estrogen is making the vaginal tissues thin and vulnerable to bleeding, then treatment with an **antibiotic** alone allows the infection to recur. Treatment with **vaginal estrogen** or the **vaginal ring** thickens the vaginal epithelium and permits natural defenses (intact mucous membranes) to prevail.

Complications of the infection can occur when symptoms of itching and irritation go untreated and the affected tissues thicken and lose elasticity (lichenification). When vulvar tissues become inflamed and heal, they often shrink in size so that the vagina will not allow sexual penetration. Early and aggressive treatment of conditions such as lichen sclerosus delays permanent hardening of the epidermis and dermal layers of the vulva.

Rational Drug Selection

Guidelines

Treatment of STI infections is dictated by the CDC guidelines, but treatment for nuisance infections may vary according to severity of patient symptoms or health-care provider preference. Many women prefer the convenience of taking one pill (one dose that lasts 1 wk) for yeast infection, but some authorities fear emergence of resistance of *C. albicans* with chronic oral medication (Sinofsky, 1999), although recent studies are not showing a resistance when used for 6 months or less (Sobel, 2005). The concept of keeping treatments specific is encouraged throughout medicine. Choice of a specific drug instead of a broad-spectrum drug reduces the problem of developing resistant organisms.

Cost

Many fungal infections are easily eradicated with **topical antifungals** such as **miconazole,** which is available OTC. Maximizing the use of OTC agents is a more cost-effective approach for the patient, especially for those without insurance, to cover the cost of a written prescription.

Patient Variables

For most patients, wait to treat *Trichomonas* vaginal infections until after the first 12 weeks of pregnancy. Nevertheless, pregnant women need to have bacterial vaginosis treated early because preterm labor is possible with this seemingly minor infection. The presence of other medical conditions, such as diabetes, use of **progestin-containing contraceptives,** and tissue immunity factors, contribute to chronic monilial vaginitis.

Drug Variables

Many vulvovaginal conditions can be treated topically with as much efficacy as oral medication. Use of **intravaginal antibiotics** and **antifungals** does not affect the absorption of **oral contraceptives** or other medications that patients may be taking. **Topical steroids** can be used for longer periods without suppressing the adrenal gland and reducing total body immunity.

Monitoring

Episodic vaginal irritations that require topical treatment do not need to be monitored, but when patients become chronically infected or require oral medications, then pelvic examination and microscopy of vaginal discharge must be scheduled.

Outcome Evaluation

When a patient has a dermal condition that the practitioner has not seen before, a consultation is required. Consultation is also necessary when pigmented or white lesions are seen during examination. If patients remember that they were born with pigmented lesions (birthmarks), then biopsy is generally not necessary.

When patients do not respond to initial or follow-up treatments, consider referral. If the provider is not adept or comfortable with vulvar biopsies, then referral for specialty care is necessary. When conditions of the vulva appear in the very young (patients aged 1 to 12), in the older adult (patients age 60 or older), or in the pregnant patient, referral is recommended.

Patient Education

Patient education should include a discussion of information related to the overall treatment plan as well as that specific to the drug therapy, reasons for taking the drug, drugs as part of the total treatment regimen, and adherence issues.

VAGINITIS

PATIENT EDUCATION

Related to the Overall Treatment Plan/Disease Process

- ☐ Knowledge of many causes of vaginal irritation, ranging from allergy to inflammatory conditions associated with local and systemic disease.
- ☐ Knowledge of the physiological changes in vaginal epithelium from age 12 to 50.
- ☐ Hygiene issues such as types of clothing for underwear, wiping correctly, and emptying bladder before and after intercourse.

VAGINITIS—cont'd

PATIENT EDUCATION

Specific to the Drug Therapy

- ☐ Many OTC products that were previously under prescriptive authority are available to treat symptoms and are still efficacious.
- ☐ Douching is no longer recommended because of the potential for pelvic infection and its destruction of the normal flora of *Lactobacillus.*

Reasons for Taking the Drug(s)

- ☐ Prevention of dyspareunia, which affects normal sexual relations.
- ☐ Control of miserable chronic conditions like lichen sclerosus.

Drugs as Part of the Total Treatment Regimen

- ☐ Importance of seeking treatment when symptoms first appear to obtain the correct diagnosis.
- ☐ Drug treatment early may prevent long-term morbidity (atrophy, sclerosis, and cancers).

Adherence Issues

- ☐ Importance of following the labeled instructions to totally eradicate the infection.
- ☐ Importance of contacting the health-care provider if side effects or rash appears.
- ☐ Potential for drug interactions (the **macrolides with antifungal, systemic antifungals,** and **birth control pills).**

REFERENCES

American Academy of Pediatrics (AAP). (2009). *Red book: Report of the Committee on Infectious Disease* (28th ed.). Elk Grove Village, IL: American Academy of Pediatrics.

American College of Obstetricians and Gynecologists (2009). New ACOG cervical cancer screening recommendations. Retrieved from http://www.acog.org/departments/dept_notice.cfm?recno=20&bulletin=5021

American Society of Health-System Pharmacists. (2010). *AHFS drug information.* Bethesda, MD: Author.

Aral, S. O., Adimora, A. A., & Fenton, K. A. (2008). Understanding and responding to disparities in HIV and other sexually transmitted infections in African Americans. *Lancet, 372*(9635), 337–340.

Armstrong, G. L., Schillinger, J., Markowitz, L., Nahmias, A. J., Johnson, R. E., McQuillan, G. M., et al. (2001). Incidence of herpes simplex virus type 2 infection in the United States. *American Journal of Epidemiology, 153*(9), 912–920.

Banikarim, C., & Chacko, M. (2005). Pelvic inflammatory disease in adolescents. *Seminars in Pediatric Infectious Diseases, 16*(3), 175–180.

Beeching, N. J. (2005). Tetanus in injecting drug users. *British Medical Journal, 330*(7488), 208–209.

Centers for Disease Control and Prevention (CDC). (2006). Sexually transmitted diseases treatment guidelines. *Morbidity and Mortality Weekly Report, 55*(RR-11), 1–94.

Centers for Disease Control and Prevention (CDC). (2007a). Update to CDC's Sexually Transmitted Diseases Treatment Guidelines, 2006: Fluoroquinolones no longer recommended for treatment of gonococcal infections. *Morbidity and Mortality Weekly Report, 56*(14), 332–336.

Centers for Disease Control and Prevention (CDC). (2007b). Toxic-shock syndrome: 1997 case definition. (Updated July 26, 2007.) Retrieved from http://www.cdc.gov/ncphi/od/ai/casedef/toxicsscurrent.htm

Centers for Disease Control and Prevention, Division of Parasitic Diseases. (2008a). Pubic lice infestation. Retrieved from http://www.cdc.gov/lice/pubic/index.html

Centers for Disease Control and Prevention, Division of Parasitic Diseases (CDC). (2008b). Scabies. Retrieved from http://www.cdc.gov/scabies/treatment.html

Centers for Disease Control and Prevention (CDC). (2009). *Trends in reportable sexually transmitted diseases in the United States, 2008: National surveillance data for chlamydia, gonorrhea, and syphilis.* Atlanta, GA: Centers for Disease Control and Prevention. Retrieved from http://www.cdc.gov/STD/stats08/trends.htm

Centers for Disease Control and Prevention (CDC, 2010). Sexually transmitted treatment guidelines, 2010. *Morbidity and Mortality Weekly Report, 59*(RR-12), 1–116.

Chosidow, O. (2000). Scabies and pediculosis. *Lancet,* 355, 819–826.

Farage, M. (2005). Vulvar susceptibility to contact irritants and allergens: A review. *Archives of Gynecology and Obstetrics, 272*(2), 167–172.

Forhan, S., Gottlieb, S., Sternberg, M., Xu, F., Deblina Datta, S., McQuillan, G., et al. (2009). Prevalence of sexually transmitted infections among female adolescents aged 14 to 19 in the United States. *Pediatrics, 124*(6), 1505–1512. doi:10.1542/peds.2009-0674

Gerberding, J. L. (2004). *Report to Congress: Prevention of genital human papillomavirus infection* (p. 10). Atlanta, GA: Centers for Disease Control and Prevention.

Goroll, A., May, L., & Mulley, A. (2010). *Primary care medicine* (6th ed.). Philadelphia: Lippincott.

Hatcher, R., Trussell, J., & Kowal, D. (2008). *Contraceptive technology* (19th ed.). New York: Ardent Media.

Harper, D. (2009). Clinical diagnosis of vaginitis was moderately accurate in symptomatic women. *Evidence-Based Medicine, 14*(3), 88.

Janos, M., & White, G. (1997). The vestibulitis syndrome. *Journal of Reproductive Medicine, 42*(3), 145–152.

Judlin, P. (2010). Current concepts in managing pelvic inflammatory disease. *Current Infectious Diseases, 23*(1), 83–87

Kaufman, M. (2008). Care of the adolescent sexual assault victim. *Pediatrics, 122,* 462–470.

Kastrup, E. (Ed.). (2010). *Drug facts and comparisons.* St. Louis, MO: Wolters Kluwer.

Katzung, B. (2009). *Basic and clinical pharmacology* (11th ed.). Norwalk, CT: Appleton & Lange.

Kim, J., Wright, T., & Goldie, S. (2002). Cost-effectiveness of alternative triage strategies for atypical squamous cells of undetermined significance. *Journal of the American Medical Association, 287*(18), 2382–2390.

Kisa, S., & Taskin, L. (2009). Validity of the symptomatic approach used by nurses in diagnosing vaginal infections. *Journal of Clinical Nursing, 18*(7), 1059–1068.

Kosten, T. R. (2009). Drugs of abuse. In B. G. Katzung (Ed.), *Basic & clinical pharmacology* (11th ed.). San Francisco: McGraw-Hill.

Kusseling, F., Shaperio, M., Greenberg, J., & Wenger, N. (1996). Understanding why heterosexual adults do not practice safer sex: A comparison of two samples. *AIDS Education and Prevention, 8*(3), 247–257.

Lai, L., Hui, C., Leung, N., & Lau, G. K. (2006). Pegylated interferon alpha-2a (40kDa) in the treatment of chronic hepatitis B. *Internation Journal of Nanomedicine, 1*(3), 255–262.

Lawrence, L., Chee-Kin, H., Nancy, L., George, L. K., Lai, L., Hui, C., et al. (2006). Pegylated interferon alpha-2a, (40 dDa) in the treatment of chronic hepatitis B. *International Journal of Nanomedicine, 1*(3), 255–262.

Markusen, T. E., & Barclay, D. L. (2003). Benign disorders of the vulva and vagina. In A. H. DeCherney & L. Nathan (Eds.), *Current obstetric & gynecologic diagnosis & treatment.* San Francisco: McGraw-Hill.

Montgomery, K., & Bloch, J. (2010). The human papillomavirus in women over 40: Implications for practice and recommendations for screening. *Journal of the American Academy of Nurse Practitioners, 22*(2), 92–100.

Neill, S. M., Tatnall, F. M., & Cox, N. H. (2002). Guidelines for the management of lichen sclerosus. *British Journal of Dermatology, 147,* 640–649.

Nunez, J. T., Delgado, G., Pino, G., Giron, H., & Bolet, B. (2002). Smoking as a risk factor for preinvasive female and invasive cervical lesions in female sex workers in Venezuela. *International Journal of Gynecology Obstetrics, 79*(1), 7–60.

O'Keefe, R., Scurry, J., Dennerstein, G., Sfameni, S., & Brenan, J. (1995). Audit of 114 non-neoplastic vulvar biopsies. *British Journal of Obstetrics and Gynaecology, 102,* 780–786.

Paavonen, J. (2006). Update vulvodynia: A therapeutic challenge. *Women's Health, 2*(2), 289–296. doi:10.2217/17455057.2.2.289

Partnership for Prevention. (2007). *Preventive care: A national profile on use, disparities and health benefits.* Washington, DC: Partnership for Prevention.

Ribes, J. A., Steele, A. D., Seabold, J. P., & Baker, D. J. (2001). Six-year study of the incidence of herpes in genital and nongenital cultures in a central Kentucky medical center patient population. *Journal of Clinical Microbiology, 39*(9), 3321–3325. doi:10.1128/JCM.39.9.3321-3325.2001

Rodriquez, M., Schiff, E., & Tzakis, A. (1998). Hepatitis A: Potentially serious disease. *Annals of Internal Medicine, 129*(6), 506.

Secor, R. (1997). Vaginal microscopy: Refining the nurse practitioner's technique. *Clinical Excellence for Nurse Practitioners, 1*(1), 29–34.

Setterfield, J. F., Neill, S., Shirlaw, P. J., Theron, J., Vaughan, R., Escudier, M., et al. (2006). The vulvovaginal gingival syndrome: A severe subgroup of lichen planus with characteristic clinical features and a novel association with the class II HLA DQB1*0201 allele. *Journal of American Academy of Dermatology, 55*(1), 98–113.

Sinofsky, F. (1999). Vulvovaginal candidiasis: Topical versus oral therapy. *The Female Patient, 24*(5), 35–39.

Sobel, D. J. (2005). Genital candidiasis. *Medicine,* 33, 62–65.

Smith, Y. R., & Quint, E. H. (2001). Clobetasol propionate in the treatment of premenarchal vulval lichen sclerosus. *Obstetrics & Gynecology, 98*(4), 588–591

Tyring, S., Diaz-Mitoma, F., Shafran, F. S., Locke, L., Sacks, S., & Young, C. (2003). Oral famciclovir for the suppression of recurrent genital herpes: The combined data from two randomized controlled trials. *Journal of Cutaneous Medicine and Surgery, 7*(6), 449–454.

U.S. Preventive Services Task Force. (2002). *Guide to clinical preventive services* (3rd ed.). Baltimore: Williams & Wilkins.

Wallace, L., Scoular, A., Hart, A. G., Reid, M., Wilson, P., & Goldberg, P. D. (2008). What is the excess risk of infertility in women after genital chlamydia infection? A systematic review of the evidence. *Sexually Transmitted Infections, 84,* 171–175.

Wendel, G., Stark, B., Jamison, R., Molina, R., & Sullivan, T. (1985). Penicillin allergy and desensitization in serious infections in pregnancy. *New England Journal of Medicine, 312,* 1229–1232.

Winer, R. L., Lee, S. K., Hughes, J. P., Adam, D. E., Kiviat, N. B., & Koutsky, L. A. (2003). Genital human papillomavirus infection: Rates and risk factors in a cohort of female university students. *American Journal of Epidemiology, 157,* 218–226. [Erratum, *American Journal of Epidemiology,* 2003, *157,* 858.]

World Health Organization (WHO). (2006). Viral cancers: Human papillomavirus. *Initiative for Vaccine Research (IVR).* Retrieved from http://www.who.int/vaccine_research/diseases/viral_cancers/en/

Wright, T. C., Massad, L. S., Dunton, C. J., Spitzer, M., Wilkinson, E. J., Solomon, D. (2007). 2006 consensus guidelines for the management of women with abnormal cancer screening tests. *American Journal of Obstetrics & Gynecology, 197*(4), 346–355.

Zhao, C., Florea, A., & Austin, R. (2010). Clinical utility of adjunctive high-risk human papillomavirus DNA testing in women with Papanicolaou test findings of atypical glandular cells. *Archives of Pathology & Laboratory Medicine, 134*(1), 103–108.

CHAPTER 45

TUBERCULOSIS

Teri Moser Woo

Chapter Outline

Tuberculosis (TB) presents a serious threat to global health, with over 2 billion infected people and 1.77 million deaths worldwide in 2008 (World Health Organization [WHO], 2009a). Nearly one-third of the world population is infected with *Mycobacterium tuberculosis*. In 1993, the World Health Organization (WHO) declared a global emergency concerning TB, the number one infectious disease killer worldwide.

Between 1993 and 2003, TB incidence in the United States decreased significantly (44%), most likely because of increased attention and funding for TB prevention programs (Centers for Disease Control and Prevention [CDC], 2005). Yet TB continues to present a significant health problem; in 2007 alone, 13,299 TB cases were reported to the Centers for Disease Control and Prevention (CDC) from all 50 states and the District of Columbia (DC) (CDC, 2008). This is a striking number of new cases for a disease that is preventable and curable.

In the United States, federal funding for TB programs decreased in the 1970s, with states and the federal government spending less money on TB prevention. Because of decreased funding and the growing worldwide HIV epidemic, the emergence of drug-resistant TB has been inevitable. Drug-resistant TB has been increasing worldwide since the mid-1980s. In response to this growing issue, in1993 the U.S. Congress increased funding for TB, and the CDC established three National Model TB Centers (in San Francisco, Newark, and New York City) and a National Tuberculosis Surveillance Network. Surveillance indicates cases of multidrug-resistant (resistance to at least **isoniazid** and **rifampin**) TB decreased from 2.5 percent of TB cases in 2006 to 1.1 percent in 2007 and extensively drug-resistant (XDR) TB (resistance to **isoniazid** and **rifampin** plus resistance to any **fluoroquinolone** and at least one of three injectable second-line anti-TB drugs [i.e., **amikacin, kanamycin,** or **capreomycin**]) from four cases in 2006 to two cases in 2007 (CDC, 2008).

Acquired resistance to TB medications stems from inadequate or inappropriate prescribed treatment regimens or from patient noncompliance. In a recent study of TB rates in Asian/Pacific Islanders and non-Hispanic whites in the United States between 1993 and 2006, the rate of TB resistance to **isoniazid** was 8.6 percent; resistance to multiple drugs was 1.2 percent, and extensively resistant TB was 1.9 percent (Managan et al, 2009). In Canada 9.5 percent of TB isolates were resistant to at least one first-line anti-tuberculosis drug in 2009, predominately (85 percent) INH, and 1.4 percent of isolates were resistant to multiple drugs (Public Health Agency of Canada, 2010). The problem of multidrug-resistant (MDR) TB is worldwide, with 60 percent of MDR TB occurring in China, India, the Russian Federation, and South Africa (WHO, 2009b). WHO is concerned with MDR TB and has partnered with the International Union Against Tuberculosis and Lung Disease (IUATLD), and the Gates Foundation to develop a Call to Action including a goal of universal access to MDR/XDR-TB diagnosis and treatment by 2015 (WHO, 2009b).

Both the diagnosis and treatment of TB have become complex. Diagnostic criteria depend not only on the results of testing, but also on the patient's immigration and immune status. Multidrug regimens that vary according to the patient's risk factors require the practitioner to be familiar with a wide variety of treatment regimens. Compliance with long treatment courses is an issue in the treatment of TB. Noncompliance leads to the emergence of drug-resistant TB. This chapter addresses the treatment of TB and strategies to increase compliance with the treatment regimen, as well as the drug regimen used for TB prevention.

PATHOPHYSIOLOGY

TB is an infectious disease caused by *M. tuberculosis*, an organism that is inhaled into the alveolus, where it is ingested by the pulmonary macrophage. The bacilli multiply and spread to local pulmonary areas and to extrathoracic organs via the lymphatic system. The infected macrophage releases a substance that attracts T lymphocytes. The infected macrophage presents antigens from the phagocytosed bacilli to the lymphocytes, producing a series of committed immune effector cells. This causes a delayed hypersensitivity and, combined with the newly activated macrophages, leads to intracellular killing of the bacilli and granuloma formation.

M. tuberculosis and most of the other mycobacteria grow quite slowly, with a doubling time of 18 hours. Thus, skin test reactivity does not occur until 4 to 6 weeks after infection, with longer intervals noted. Colonies on culture media do not appear for 3 to 5 weeks, creating delays in culture confirmation and drug susceptibility testing.

Infection is spread almost exclusively by aerosolization of contaminated lung secretions. This organism primarily affects the pulmonary tissue, although extrapulmonary TB is not uncommon, especially in immunocompromised patients. Patients with cavitary lung disease cough frequently and, therefore, are particularly infectious. The aerosolized droplets can remain suspended in room air for many hours. The skin and respiratory mucous membranes of a healthy normally exposed person are resistant to invasion. The problem occurs with heavy or prolonged exposure to an infected or immunocompromised person. The very young and the very old or debilitated are also more susceptible because of decreased host defenses.

Pulmonary TB presents with the classic symptoms of TB: cough with productive, purulent secretions, often with blood streaks. Other symptoms include wide temperature variations, malaise, fatigue, wasting, chest pain, and dyspnea. Sweating, including night sweats, is common.

Extrapulmonary TB presents with a more problematic set of symptoms, often mimicking other diseases. Lymphatic TB may present initially as unilateral, painless cervical lymphadenopathy. TB bacilli can also settle in the genitourinary tract, bones or joints, meninges, gastrointestinal (GI) tract, and pericardium. When these extrapulmonary sites are infected, the symptoms are often vague and difficult to define. The suspicion of TB and intradermal testing as part of a work-up for other diseases may lead to a quicker diagnosis. Also of concern is that the tuberculin skin test can be negative 20 to 25 percent of the time. Appropriate biopsy and culture of affected tissues or cerebrospinal fluid—which usually require consultation with a specialist in infectious diseases—increase the likelihood of an accurate diagnosis.

GOALS OF TREATMENT

The initial goal of treatment in TB is an accurate diagnosis. This requires a practitioner who understands the current guidelines for screening and puts TB high on the differential list for any pulmonary or other illness with vague presenting symptoms. A second goal is the patient's completion of the recommended therapy, as failure to complete therapy can lead to drug-resistant TB. Finally, the effectiveness of treatment must be evaluated. Effective treatment of TB is not only intended to treat the sick patient, but also to prevent the transmission of *M. tuberculosis* to the public.

Patients who have positive sputum cultures at the beginning of treatment should have monthly cultures, and the culture should convert to negative. A final chest x-ray is needed for documentation of baseline for future films, but the x-ray is not as important as the sputum examination (American Thoracic Society [ATS], 2003). In patients with radiographic abnormalities consistent with TB, an effort should be made to establish a diagnosis via sputum culture. The CDC recommends that three sputum specimens should be obtained if pulmonary involvement is suspected (CDC, 2003a). Bronchoscopy may be necessary to obtain an accurate diagnosis. If presumptive treatment is the only option, the key indicators for response to therapy are the chest x-ray findings. Improvement should be noted within the first 3 months of therapy. If there is no improvement, then either resistance or inaccurate diagnosis must be considered. The CDC recommends that all patients with TB have testing for HIV infection at the time treatment is initiated, if not earlier (CDC, 2003a).

RATIONAL DRUG SELECTION

Risk Stratification

Although anyone may become infected with TB, some populations are identified as being at greater risk: children up to age 4 years, the infirm elderly, and immunocompromised patients, including those with HIV infection or AIDS and organ transplant recipients. Foreign-born people are also at higher risk, accounting for over half of U.S. TB cases (Cain et al, 2007) and 66 percent of Canadian cases (Public Health Agency of Canada, 2007). The top five countries of origin for foreign-born TB cases from 2001 to 2007 were Mexico, Philippines, India, Vietnam, and China (CDC, 2008). Canadian statistics reflect the immigration patterns of the country with the world regions of Western Pacific, Southeast Asia, and Africa accounting for the highest prevalence of foreign-born TB cases (Public Health Agency of Canada, 2007). In the United States and Canada, certain populations are identified as being at higher risk, specifically medically underserved, low-income populations, including high-risk racial or ethnic minority populations, people who are homeless, blacks, Hispanics, and Native Americans/Canadian aboriginal peoples. Nonwhite patients have a peak incidence of TB between ages 25 and 44, significantly younger than that of whites, which is over age 70. Residents of long-term-care facilities (nursing homes, prisons, and mental institutions) are also at higher risk.

Screening

Targeted screening for TB is usually based on the patient's presenting with an identified risk factor. In some areas of the country, routine TB testing is part of all health maintenance visits because of an increased incidence of TB in the area. Many pediatric health-care providers routinely screen all 12-month-old infants. Patients identified as being at risk are those with compromised immune systems (e.g., HIV positive or undergoing immunosuppressive therapy or prolonged adrenocorticosteroid therapy), close contacts of patients with newly diagnosed infectious TB, injection drug users known to be HIV seronegative, foreign-born persons from high-prevalence countries, medically underserved low-income populations, and residents and staff of long-term-care facilities or prisons. All health-care providers should be screened routinely.

Two screening methods for TB may be used, the tuberculin skin test (TST) or the QuantiFERON-TB Gold test. The most commonly used screening test is an intradermal injection of TB protein antigens (such as **purified protein derivative [PPD]**). In 48 to 72 hours, an induration response is considered positive, based on the population being tested. The CDC in the United States and the Ontario Lung Association in Canada (2009) have slightly different criteria for positive tuberculin skin test results. The CDC (2007) states that for adults and children with HIV infection, close contacts of people with infectious TB, and patients with fibrotic lesions on chest x-ray (especially in upper lung regions), an induration of 5 mm or more is considered positive. A reaction of 10 mm or more is considered positive for other high-risk adults and children, including infants and children under age 4. For people not considered at risk for TB infection, a reaction of 15 mm or more is considered positive. The Canadian criteria for a positive skin test are the following: An induration 0 to 5 mm in diameter is considered positive in HIV infection with immune suppression and the expected likelihood of TB infection is high; 5- to 9-mm induration is considered positive in patients with HIV infection, close contacts of contagious case children suspected of having TB, abnormal chest x-ray with fibronodular disease, or immune suppression; and greater than 10-mm induration is positive in all other cases (Ontario Lung Association, 2009).

In 2005 the U.S. Food and Drug Administration (FDA) approved QuantiFERON-TB Gold as an aid in diagnosing *M. tuberculosis* infection, both latent and active TB disease (Mazurek et al, 2005). Health Canada approved QuantiFERON-TB in 2006. The QuantiFERON-TB Gold (QFT-G) is an enzyme-linked immunoassay (ELISA) test that tests for the proteins present in *M. tuberculosis* that are absent from bacille Calmette-Guérin (BCG) vaccines (Mazurek et al, 2005). A positive QFT-G should be treated in the same manner as a positive TST: The patient needs a medical evaluation, including a chest x-ray, to rule out latent versus active TB infection.

Drug Therapy for Infectious Tuberculosis

Treatment of infectious TB requires the practitioner to apply three basic principles, as recommended by the American Thoracic Society, CDC, and the Infectious Diseases Society of America (CDC, 2003b):

1. Treatment regimens must contain multiple drugs to which the organisms are susceptible.
2. The drugs must be taken regularly.
3. Drug therapy must continue for a sufficient period of time.

Another fundamental principle of managing TB patients is never add a single drug to a failing treatment regimen (ATS, 2003).

Many combinations of drugs and frequencies of administration are possible, but the initial phase of treatment is critical to prevent drug resistance and improve outcomes. Treatment for TB has two phases: the first phase or initiation phase (bactericidal or intensive phase), which lasts for 2 months, and the continuation phase (sterilizing phase), which lasts for 4 to 7 months (Blumberg, Leonard, & Jasmer, 2005). This chapter discusses the treatment regimens that may be used. As newer medications are approved, these regimens may change, but the basic principles remain (Table 45–1).

Table 45–1 **Drug Regimens for Culture-Positive Pulmonary Tuberculosis Caused by Drug-Susceptible Organisms**

Initial Phase			Continuation Phase				Rating (Evidence)	
Regimen	*Drugs*	*Interval and Doses‡ (Minimal Duration)*	*Regimen*	*Drugs*	*Interval and Doses‡ (Minimal D uration)*	*Range of Total Doses (Minimal Duration)*	*HIV-*	*HIV+*
1	INH RIF PZA	7 d/wk for 56 doses (8 wk) or 5 d/wk for 40 doses (8 wk)¶	1a	INF/RIF	7 d/wk for 126 doses (18 wk) or 5 d/wk for 90 doses (18 wk)¶	182–130 (26 wk)	A (I)	A (II)
	EMB		1b	INH/RIF	Twice weekly for 36 doses (18 wk)	92–76 (26 wk)	A (I)	A (II)*
			1c**	INH/RPT	Once weekly for 18 doses (18 wk)	74–58 (26 wk)	B (I)	E (I)
2	INH	7 d/wk for 14 doses (2 wk). Then twice weekly for 12 doses (6 wk) or 5 d/wk for 10 doses (2 wk).¶ Then twice weekly for 12 doses (6 wk)	2a	INH/RIF	Twice weekly for 36 doses (18 wk)	62–58 (26 wk)	A (II)	B (II)*
	RIF PZA EMB		2b**	INH/RPT	Once weekly for 18 doses (18 wk)	44–40 (26 wk)	B (I)	E (I)
3	INH RIF PZA EMB	Three times weekly for 24 doses (8 wk)	3a	INH/RIF	Three times weekly for 54 doses (18 wk)	78 (26 wk)	B (I)	B (II)
4	INH RIF	7 d/wk for 56 doses (8 wk) or 5 days/wk for 40 doses (8 wk)¶	4a	INH/RIF	7 d/wk for 217 doses (31 wk) or 5 d/wk for 155 doses (31 wk)¶	273–195 (39 wk)	C (I)	C (II)
	EMB		4b	INH/RIF	Twice weekly for 62 doses (31 wk)	118–102 (39 wk)	C (I)	C (II)

EMB = ethambutol; INH = isoniazid; PZA = pyrazinamide; RIF = rifampin; RPT = rifapentine.

*Definitions of evidence ratings: A = preferred; B = acceptable alternative; C = offer when A and B cannot be given; E = should never be given.

†Definition of evidence ratings: I = randomized clinical trial; II = data from clinical trials that were not randomized or were conducted in other populations; III = expert opinion.

‡When DOT is used, drugs may be given 5 d/wk and the necessary number of doses adjusted accordingly. Although no studies compare five with seven doses, extensive experience indicates this would be an effective practice.

§Patients with cavitation on initial chest radiograph and positive cultures at completion of 2 months of therapy should receive a 7 month's (31 weeks either 217 doses [daily] or 62 doses [twice weekly]) continuation phase.

¶Five-day-a-week administration is always given by DOT. Rating for 5 d/wk regimens is A III.

#Not recommended for HIV-infected patients with CD4+ cell counts <100 cells/mcL.

**Options 1c and 2b should be used only in HIV-negative patients who have negative sputum smears at the time of completion of 2 months of therapy and who do not have cavitation on initial chest radiograph (see text). For patients started on this regimen and found to have a positive culture from the 2-month specimen, treatment should be extended an extra 3 months.

Source: Centers for Disease Control and Prevention. (2003). Treatment of tuberculosis, American Thoracic Society, CDC, and Infections Diseases Society of America. *Morbidity and Mortality Weekly Report, 52*(RR-11)

There are several new combination drugs available to treat TB. Combination tablets offer ease of dosing with one tablet, but may be more expensive than single ingredient tablets. **Rifater** tablets contain 120 mg **rifampin**, 50 mg **isoniazid**, and 300 mg **pyrazinamide** and cost $195.43 for 60 tablets (http://www.drugstore.com). **Rifamate** or **IsonaRif** capsules contain 300 mg **rifampin** and 150 mg **isoniazid** and cost $243.83 for 60 capsules, which is a 30-day supply for adults (http://www.drugstore.com). In comparison, **rifampin** 300 mg capsule is $129.98 for 60 capsules (http://www.drugstore.com) and **isoniazid** 300 mg tablets are $13.99 for 30 tablets (http://www.drugstore.com), for a total of $143.97 for a 30-day supply. The $100 difference in cost is significant for clients who must pay all or a large part of their drug costs. The ATS (2003) guidelines note that no evidence supports combination medications over single-ingredient drugs, although the combination drugs may be preferable if directly observed therapy (DOT) is not used.

Six-Month Regimen

A 6-month regimen is recommended for patients who adhere to treatment and have fully susceptible organisms. This regimen consists of 2 months of four-drug therapy administered daily: **isoniazid** (INH), **rifampin** (RIF), **pyrazinamide** (PZA), and **ethambutol** (EMB), followed by 4 months of INH and RIF. Alternative regimens for the first 2 months of therapy include the same four drugs (INH, RIF, PZA, and EMB) given (regimen 2) daily for 2 weeks followed by two times weekly for 6 weeks; or (regimen 3) three times a week for 8 weeks (CDC, 2003a). This four-drug therapy is effective even when the infecting organism is resistant to INH. Dosing for the continuation phase (after the initial 2 mo) should consist of INH and RIF (regimen 1) daily, (regimen 2) twice weekly, (regimen 3) three times weekly for 4 months (CDC, 2003a). **Streptomycin** is substituted for EMB in children too young to be monitored for visual acuity.

This 6-month treatment can be used in patients who have HIV infection and patients who are not infected with HIV. Patients who have HIV infection should be monitored for treatment response, and their therapy should be prolonged if suboptimal response is found. The continuation phase of treatment should be followed for an additional 3 months for patients who have cavitation on the initial or follow-up chest radiograph and are still culture positive after the initial 2 months of treatment (CDC, 2003a).

Nine-Month Regimen

A 9-month regimen of INH and RIF may be used for patients who cannot take PZA or who have isolates resistant to PZA. EMB (**streptomycin** in young children) should also be included in the treatment protocol for the first 2 months, followed by INH and RIF given either daily or twice weekly for 7 months (CDC, 2003a). Dosages for the drugs commonly used for treatment and prevention are shown in Table 45–2.

Table 45–2 **Drugs Commonly Used: Tuberculosis**

Drug	Preparation	Adults/ Children†	Doses* Daily	1 ×/wk	2 ×/wk	3 ×/wk
FIRST-LINE DRUGS						
Isoniazid (INH)	Tablets (50 mg, 100 mg, 300 mg); elixir (50 mg/5 mL); aqueous solution (100 mg/mL) for IV or IM injection	*Adults* (max)	5 mg/kg (300 mg)	15 mg/kg (900 mg)	15 mg/kg (900 mg)	15 mg/kg (900 mg)
		Children (max)	10–15 mg/kg (300 mg)	—	20–30 mg/kg (900 mg)	—
Rifampin (RIF)	Capsule (150 mg, 300 mg); powder may be suspended for oral administration; aqueous solution for IV injection	*Adults* ‡ (max)	10 mg/kg (600 mg)	—	10 mg/kg (600 mg)	10 mg/kg (600 mg)
		Children (max)	10–20 mg/kg (600 mg)	—	10–20 mg/kg (600 mg)	—

Continued

Table 45–2 **Drugs Commonly Used: Tuberculosis—cont'd**

Drug	Preparation	Adults/ Children†	Doses* Daily	1 ×/wk	2 ×/wk	3 ×/wk
FIRST-LINE DRUGS						
Rifabutin	Capsule (150 mg)	*Adults* ‡ (max)	5 mg/kg (300 mg)	—	5 mg/kg (300 mg)	5 mg/kg (300 mg)
		Children	Appropriate dosing for children is unknown	Appropriate dosing for children is unknown	Appropriate dosing for children is unknown	Appropriate dosing for children is unknown
Rifapentine	Tablet (150 mg, film coated)	*Adults*	—	10 mg/kg (continuation phase) (600 mg)	—	—
		Children	Not approved for use in children	Not approved for use in children	Not approved for use in children	Not approved for use in children
Pyrazinamide (PZA)	Tablet (500 mg, scored)	*Adults* :				
		Wt: 40–55 kg	1,000 mg	—	2,000 mg	1,500 mg
		Wt: 56–75 kg	1,500 mg	—	3,000 mg	2,500 mg
		Wt: 76–90 kg	2,000 mg	—	4,000 mg	3,000 mg
		Children (max)	15–30 mg/kg (2.0 g)	—	50 mg/kg (2 g)	—
Ethambutol (EMB)	Tablet (100 mg, 400 mg)	*Adults*				
		Wt: 40–55 kg	800 mg	—	1,600 mg	1,200 mg
		Wt: 56–75 kg	1,200 mg	—	2,800 mg	2,000 mg
		Wt: 76–90 kg	1,600 mg	—	4,000 mg	2,400 mg
		Children§ (max)	15–20 mg/kg daily (1.0 g)	—	50 mg/kg (2.5 g)	—
SECOND-LINE DRUGS						
Cycloserine	Capsule (250 mg)	*Adults* (max)	10–15 mg/kg/d (1.0 g in 2 doses), usually 500–750 mg/d in 2 doses¶	No data to support intermittent administration	No data to support intermittent administration	No data to support intermittent administration
		Children (max)	10–15 mg/kg/d (1.0 g/d)	—	—	—
Ethionamide	Tablet (250 mg)	*Adults** (max)	15–20 mg/kg/d (1.0 g/day), usually 500–750 mg/d in a single daily dose or 2 divided doses*	No data to support intermittent administration	No data to support intermittent administration	No data to support intermittent administration
		Children (max)	15–20 mg/kg/d (1.0 g/d)	No data to support intermittent administration	No data to support intermittent administration	No data to support intermittent administration

Table 45–2 **Drugs Commonly Used: Tuberculosis—cont'd**

Drug	Preparation	Adults/ Children†	Doses* Daily	1 ×/wk	2 ×/wk	3 ×/wk
SECOND-LINE DRUGS						
Moxifloxacin	Tablets (400 mg): aqueous solution (400 mg/ 250 mL) for IV injection	*Adults*	400 mg daily	No data to support intermittent administration	No data to support intermittent administration	No data to support intermittent administration
		Children	‡‡	‡‡	‡‡	‡‡
Gatifloxacin	Tablets (400 mg); aqueous solution (200 mg/ 20 mL; 400 mg/ 40 mL) for IV injection	*Adults*	400 mg daily	No data to support intermittent administration	No data to support intermittent administration	No data to support intermittent administration
		Children	§§	‡‡	‡‡	‡‡

*Dose per weight is based on ideal body weight. Children weighing more than 40 kg should be dosed as adults.

†For purposes of this document, adult dosing begins at age 15 years.

‡Dose may need to be adjusted when there is concomitant use or protease inhibitors or non-nucleoside reverse transcriptase inhibitors.

§The drug can likely be used safely in older children but should be used with caution in children less than 5 years of age, in whom visual acuity cannot be monitored. In younger children, EMB at the dose of 15 mg/kg per day can be used if there is suspected or proven resistance to INH of RIF.

¶Note: Although this is the dose recommended generally, most clinicians with experience using cycloserine indicate that few patients can tolerate this amount. Serum concentration measurements are often useful in determining the optimal dose for a given patient.

#The single daily dose can be given at bedtime or with the main meal.

**Dose: 15 mg/kg per day (1 g) and 10 mg/kg in persons more than 59 years of age (750 mg). Usual dose: 750–1,000 mg administered IM or IV, given as a single dose 5–7 d/wk and reduced to two or three times per week after the first 2–4 months or after culture conversion, depending on the efficacy of the other drugs in the regimen.

††The long-term (more than several weeks) use of levofloxacin in children and adolescents has not been approved because of concerns about effects on bone and cartilage growth. However, most experts agree that the drug should be considered for children with tuberculosis caused by organisms resistant to both INH and RIF. The optimal dose is not known.

‡‡The long-term (more than several weeks) use of moxifloxacin in children and adolescents has not been approved because of concerns about effects on bone and cartilage growth. The optimal dose is not known.

§§The long-term (more than several weeks) use of gatifloxacin in children and adolescents has not been approved because of concerns about effects on bone and cartilage growth. The optimal dose is not known.

Source: Centers for Disease Control and Prevention. (2003). Treatment of tuberculosis, American Thoracic Society, CDC, and Infections Diseases Society of America. *Morbidity and Mortality Weekly Report, 52*(RR-11).

Drug Therapy for Drug-Resistant Tuberculosis

Drug-resistant TB has been increasing worldwide for the past 20 years. Microbial resistance to **anti-TB drugs** may be either primary or acquired. Primary resistance occurs in the patient who has never been treated for TB. Risk factors for primary resistance include exposure to a patient who has drug-resistant TB, immigration from a country with a high prevalence of drug-resistant TB, and a greater than 4 percent incidence of resistant TB in the community. Acquired or secondary resistance occurs in a patient who has been previously treated for TB. Poorly or inadequately treated TB is the leading cause of secondary resistance, with global prevalence of MDR TB reported in 20 percent of cases worldwide (LoBue, Sizemore, & Castro, 2009). Extensively resistant TB (resistant to multiple second-line drugs) is found in 4 percent of MDR TB in the United States (LoBue et al, 2009). Extensively resistant TB is resistant both to **isoniazid** and **rifampin**, and to any **fluoroquinolone** drug and at least one of three second-line injectable drugs (**amikacin**, **kanamycin**, or **capreomycin**). Drug resistance can be proved only by susceptibility testing.

For treatment of drug- or multidrug-resistant TB, the administration of at least two drugs to which susceptibility has been demonstrated is recommended. For isolated INH resistance, the 6-month, four-drug (INH, RIF, EMB, PZA) protocol is recommended (ATS, 2003).

If INH resistance is documented in a patient on a 9-month regimen (without PZA), then INH should be discontinued. If EMB was included in the initial regimen, then treatment with RIF and EMB should continue for a minimum of 12 months. If the initial treatment did not include EMB, then drug susceptibility should be repeated. INH needs to be discontinued, and two new drugs should be added. The regimen may need to be adjusted when drug susceptibility tests results are available.

If a patient is resistant to multiple first-line drugs (INH, RIF, EMB, PZA), then at least three new drugs that the organism is susceptible to should be administered. These second-line drugs include **capreomycin (Capastat)**, **cycloserine (Seromycin)**, **EMBionamide (Trecator)**, **kanamycin (Kantrex)**, **para-aminosalicylic acid (Sodium P.A.S.)**, **levofloxacin (Levaquin)**, and **moxifloxacin (Avelox)** (see Table 45–2). This regimen should be followed until sputum cultures are clear; then the patient should have 12 months of two-drug therapy. Often, 24 months of therapy are given to patients who have TB that is resistant to multiple first-line drugs. Patients with resistant TB should have their medications administered via DOT (Box 45–1).

Second-line treatment usually requires injectable medications, which complicates the treatment regimen. **Fluoroquinolones** such as **levofloxacin**, **moxifloxacin**, and **gatifloxacin** are all active against *M. tuberculosis*. Based on the evidence so far, **levofloxacin** is the preferred **oral fluoroquinolone** for treating drug-resistant TB or when first-line agents cannot be used because of intolerance (CDC, 2003b). Patients with extensively resistant TB require broader coverage including parenteral **cycloserine (Seromycin)** and a **fluoroquinolone**. In a recent study of 48 patients with extensively resistant disease, patients were prescribed an average of 5.3±1.3 **antimycobacterial agents** for which either susceptibility had been documented or the duration of prior exposure had not exceeded 1 month and susceptibility had not been tested, leading to a 60 percent cure rate (Mitnick et al, 2008). Any patient whose TB demonstrates resistance must be seen by an infectious disease specialist who treats patients with TB. Inadequate treatment is one of the leading causes of secondary resistant TB.

BOX 45–1 DIRECTLY OBSERVED THERAPY

Directly observed therapy (DOT) reduces the risk of developing drug resistance. In DOT, the patient is required to take all of the medication in front of a health-care or other service provider. The Centers for Disease Control and Prevention (CDC), the American Thoracic Society (ATS), and the World Health Organization (WHO) recommend the widespread or universal use of DOT in the treatment of TB. DOT has been demonstrated to ensure the highest degree of compliance with the medication regimen. Compliance with DOT can be increased in many ways including convenient clinic times and locations and incentives such as food, clothing, bus or carfare money, and gifts.

Algorithm

Treatment of TB begins with an accurate diagnosis. Once a screening test for TB is considered positive, treatment begins, even if a definitive diagnosis of TB has not been made. Therapy may be altered, based on the patient's risk factors or on the sensitivity of the organisms to the medications being used. DOT should be considered at any point of therapy based on patient history and local drug-resistance pattern. A treatment algorithm is presented in Figure 45–1.

Extrapulmonary Tuberculosis

Extrapulmonary TB is often difficult to diagnose. Once a bacteriological examination has determined a diagnosis of TB, the treatment is basically the same as for pulmonary TB. Although little research has been done regarding the effectiveness of shortened treatment for extrapulmonary TB, the ATS guidelines recommend 6 to 9 months of therapy as probably effective (2003). Infants and children with miliary TB, bone or joint TB, and TB meningitis should receive 12 months of therapy.

Response to treatment is more difficult to monitor in patients with extrapulmonary TB than in those with pulmonary TB and must often be determined based on clinical and radiographic improvement. Bacteriological evaluation of extrapulmonary sites often requires invasive procedures to evaluate treatment. Referral to an infectious disease specialist is usually necessary to ensure optimal treatment.

Patient Variables

Pregnancy and Lactation

TB infection during pregnancy presents in the same manner as does TB in nonpregnant patients. The clinical symptoms include cough, weight loss, fever, malaise and fatigue, and hemoptysis. Eighty-five percent of patients have upper lobe disease; extrapulmonary TB is rare in pregnant patients. TB screening during pregnancy is recommended for all patients. Positive results are the same as for nonpregnant patients. Patients who have active untreated TB at the time of delivery need to be placed in respiratory isolation and separated from their infants. Therefore, it is best to treat TB prior to delivery.

The initial treatment regimen for pregnant women is INH and RIF. EMB should be included unless INH resistance is unlikely. The length of therapy is 6 months. **Pyridoxine (vitamin B_6)** 25 mg/day should be added to the regimen in pregnant or lactating patients to decrease the incidence of peripheral neuropathy associated with INH (ATS, 2003).

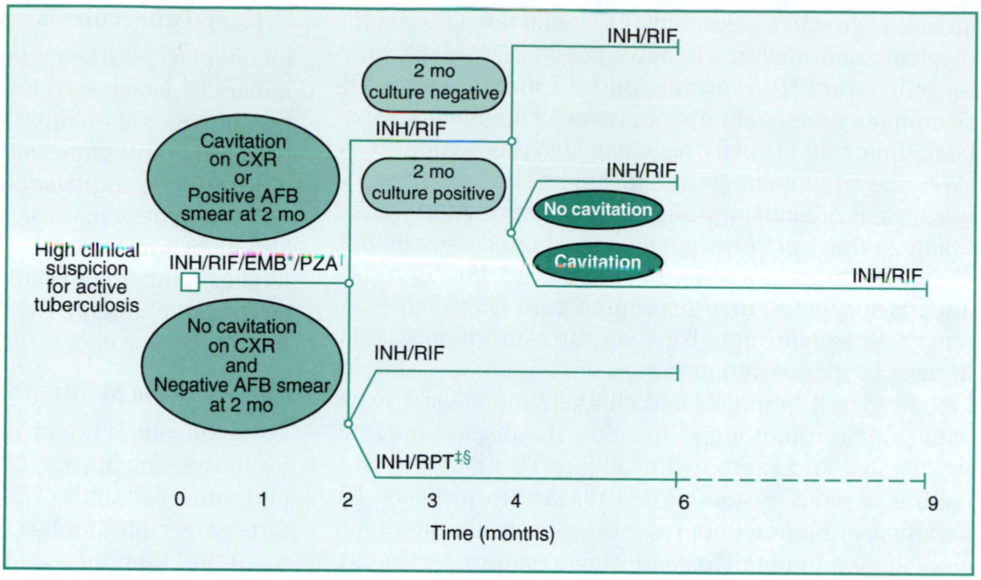

Patients in whom tuberculosis is proved or strongly suspected should have treatment initiated with isoniazid, rifampin, pyrazinamide, and ethambutol for the initial 2 months. A repeat smear and culture should be performed when 2 months of treatment have been completed. If cavities were seen on the initial chest radiograph or the acid-fast smear is positive at completion of 2 months of treatment, the continuation phase of treatment should consist of isoniazid and rifampin daily or twice weekly for 4 months to complete a total of 6 months of treatment. If cavitation was present on the initial chest radiograph and the culture at the time of completion of 2 months of therapy is positive, the continuation phase should be lengthened to 7 months (total of 9 months of treatment). If the patient has HIV infection and the CD4⁺ cell count is <100/μL, the continuation phase should consist of daily or 3 times weekly isoniazid and rifampin. In HIV-uninfected patients having no cavitation on chest radiograph and negative acid-fast smears at completion of 2 months of treatment, the continuation phase may consist of either once weekly isoniazid and rifapentine, or daily or twice weekly isoniazid and rifampin, to complete a total of 6 months (bottom). Patients receiving isoniazid and rifapentine, and whose 2-month cultures are positive, should have treatment extended by an additional 3 months (total of 9 months).

*EMB may be discontinued when results of drug susceptibility testing indicate no drug resistance.

†PZA may be discontinued after it has been taken for 2 months (56 doses).

‡RPT should not be used in HIV-infected patients with tuberculosis or in patients with extrapulmonary tuberculosis.

§Therapy should be extended to 9 months if 2-month culture is positive.

CXR = chest radiograph; EMB = ethambutol; INH = isoniazid; PZA = pyrazinamide; RIF = rifampin; RPT = rifapen - tine.

Figure 45–1. Treatment algorithm for TB.

Source: American Thoracic Society, CDC, and Infectious Diseases Society of America (2003). Treatment of Tuberculosis. MMWR, 52 (RR11), 1–77.

Pregnant patients have a 2.5-fold higher risk of INH-induced hepatitis than other patients (Riley, 1997). RIF may also be associated with maternal hepatitis. Monthly monitoring of liver function tests will detect any change in liver function indicating hepatitis.

INH, RIF, and EMB all cross the placenta, but these drugs have not been demonstrated to have teratogenic effects (ATS, 2003). **Streptomycin** and other **aminoglycosides** are contraindicated because of harmful effects on the fetus, including congenital deafness and altered ear development. **Streptomycin** is Pregnancy Category D.

PZA is recommended for routine use in pregnant women by WHO, but the drug has not been used routinely in the United States because of lack of safety studies. Some U.S. public health officials are using PZA in pregnant women without reported adverse effects (CDC, 2003a). If PZA is not included in the initial treatment regimen, then 9 months of therapy needs to be considered.

Breastfeeding is not contraindicated during treatment. Small amounts of INH and RIF are excreted into breast milk, but these amounts are well below the therapeutic dose. EMB and PZA are both excreted in very small amounts as well. The risk of toxic reactions in the infant may be further minimized if the mother breastfeeds just prior to taking a dose of TB medication. Breastfeeding does not provide effective treatment for active or latent TB infection in a nursing infant; therefore, newborns should be evaluated for congenital TB (ATS, 2003; Public Health Agency of Canada, 2009). **Pyridoxine (vitamin B_6)** 25 mg/day is recommended in lactating women taking INH (ATS, 2003).

Pediatric Patients

Primary Pulmonary Tuberculosis

Children pose challenges in the treatment of TB because older infants and children may present with a positive screening test and are asymptomatic, yet may have primary pulmonary TB. A chest x-ray may be normal or demonstrate minimum abnormalities (infiltrates with hilar adenopathy). WHO published guidelines for diagnosis of TB in children, which include the following: (1) careful history, including TB contacts; (2) clinical examination, including growth assessment; (2) TB skin test; (3) bacteriological confirmation whenever possible; (4) chest x-ray for pulmonary TB or evaluation for extrapulmonary TB (lymph node biopsy, lumbar puncture if meningitis is suspected, etc); and (5) HIV testing in high prevalence areas (WHO, 2006). Obtaining sputum cultures for confirmatory diagnosis is difficult in young children; use of drug susceptibility testing from presumed source case can guide the choice of drugs in children (CDC, 2003a). If drug resistance is suspected or if no source case is available, attempts to isolate organisms via three morning gastric lavages, bronchoalveolar lavage, or tissue biopsy should be considered. In infants and children under age 3 years with primary pulmonary infection, the disease may be progressive and merge with miliary TB or progressive central nervous system (CNS) disease to produce TB meningitis. Children under age 13 years usually have paucibacillary pulmonary disease (low organism numbers), and cavitating disease is rare (less than 6% of cases) (WHO, 2006). Primary infection in older children and adolescents presents with an upper lobe infiltrate and cavitation without calcification. Progressive disease does occur in immunocompromised children of all ages.

Progressive Pulmonary Tuberculosis

Progressive pulmonary TB in children occurs when the primary infection is not contained and produces bronchopneumonia or when the lesions involve a whole lobe (usually middle or lower) and cavitation develops. Weight loss, fever, night sweats, malaise, hemoptysis, and productive cough are common symptoms.

Miliary Tuberculosis

Infants and children under age 3 years frequently develop miliary TB, which is widespread dissemination with infection of multiple organs. The lesions are the size of millet seeds, thus the name *miliary* TB. The infant or child is quite ill, often with a sudden onset, and may have a high fever, weakness, malaise, anorexia, hepatosplenomegaly, and night sweats. A chest x-ray reveals diffuse miliary infiltrates. A tuberculin skin test (PPD) may be nonreactive as a result of anergy. The child may need a liver or bone marrow biopsy to determine an accurate diagnosis.

Tuberculosis Meningitis

TB meningitis is the most serious complication of TB. It usually occurs in young children (younger than 5 years) and within 6 months of primary infection. The disease has three stages: prodromal (lasts 1 wk), neurological involvement, and then increasing neurological involvement resulting from increasing intracranial pressure. The skin test (PPD) is positive in two-thirds of cases, but anergy may be present in very ill patients.

Drug Therapy

Drug therapy for pediatric patients depends on the infection or disease category, as noted in Table 45–3. The standard **anti-TB drugs** INH and RIF are used for asymptomatic infection and for 6 to 9 months. Multidrug regimens, as noted in Table 45–3, are used for progressive disease. EMB may be used in pediatric patients if risk of drug-resistant organisms is present (ATS, 2003). DOT should be used for all children with TB (ATS, 2003). If

Table 45–3 Treatment of Tuberculosis in Infants, Children, and Adolescents

Disease Category	Drug Therapy	Comments
Asymptomatic infection (positive skin test only)	*9-mo regimen:* INH-susceptible: INH daily	Twice-weekly therapy may be used if daily therapy is not feasible.
	INH-resistant: RIF daily	Children who with INH resistant TB should be treated for 12 mo.
Pulmonary disease	*6-mo regimen:* INH, RIF, and PZA daily for first 2 mo, followed by 4 mo. of INH and RIF daily *or* INH, RIF, and PZA daily for 2 mo., followed by 4 mo. of INH and RIF twice weekly *9-mo regimen:* 9 mo of INH and RIF daily *or* 1 mo of INH and RIF daily, followed by 8 mo of INH and RIF twice weekly	If drug resistance is a concern, then a 4-drug regimen is used (INH, RIF, PZA, and ETH or streptomycin) for the first 2 mo.
Extrapulmonary TB (meningitis, miliary, bone, and joint)	*12-mo regimen:* INH, RIF, PZA, and streptomycin daily for 2 mo, followed by 10 mo of INH and RIF daily or INH, RIF, PYZ, and streptomycin daily, followed by INH and RIF twice weekly	4-drug therapy is used for the first 2 mo of treatment, until drug susceptibility is known.
Extrapulmonary TB (other than meningitis, miliary, bone, or joint)	Same as for pulmonary disease	

ETH = ethionamide; INH = isoniazid; PZA = pyrazinamide; RIF = rifabutin.
DOT (directly observed therapy) should be used for all children with tuberculosis. Parents should not be relied on to administer medications (CDC, 2003a).

children are not able to swallow pills, administrating medications requires crushing the pills, and tolerance must be monitored. Parents should not be relied on to correctly administer TB treatment.

Adverse Reactions

RIF and **INH** can be administered to children safely, with minimal adverse reactions. Patients should be monitored for liver function alterations, especially if the patient presents with a flu-like illness. Pyridoxine deficiency associated with **INH** can be prevented in infants, children, and adolescents with 25 mg/day of **vitamin B_6** supplementation (ATS, 2003; Public Health Authority of Canada, 2009). **EMB** is an effective drug, but its main limitation is ocular toxicity, which causes optic neuritis, leading to blurred vision, color blindness, and visual field constriction. Although the visual changes associated with **EMB** are reversible, it should not be prescribed to children under age 6 years whose visual changes cannot be accurately monitored. **Streptomycin** can be used in children in place of **EMB**, but it is used for only a short time (12 weeks or less), and patients should be monitored for ototoxicity and nephrotoxicity. **PZA** is used in multidrug therapy in children and has few adverse reactions.

Newborn Infants

Management of the newborn infant whose mother (or other household contact) has TB is based on individual considerations. Infants born to mothers with active disease are at high risk for TB in the first year of life (CDC, 2003a). Unfortunately, in infants, the skin test may not be positive until age 6 months.

If the mother has a positive **PPD** but no evidence of active disease, then the family and household contacts must be investigated. If no evidence of active disease is found in the mother or extended family, the infant needs to have a **Mantoux** (**5 TU PPD**) skin test at 4 to 6 weeks of age and at 3 to 4 months of age. If the TB status of household contacts cannot be evaluated, the infant may be started on **INH** (10 mg/kg/d).

If the mother has newly diagnosed TB but is not contagious at delivery, the newborn infant requires a chest x-ray and **Mantoux** test at age 4 to 6 weeks. If these are negative, then the child is monitored at age 3 to 4 months and again at 6 months, with repeat **Mantoux** skin tests. **INH** is started at birth and discontinued at 3 to 4 months (some sources say 6 months) if the **PPD** is negative and the family has no active disease. The infant should receive **INH** even if the initial chest x-ray and **PPD** are negative because cell-mediated immunity of a degree sufficient to mount a significant reaction to skin testing can develop as late as age 6 months in an infant infected at birth. The mother may breastfeed. The infant should be examined carefully at monthly intervals. In cases of poor compliance, maternal positive sputum, or uncertain supervision, the infant may be given **bacille Calmette-Guérin (BCG) vaccine**. BCG does not prevent TB but may decrease the severity of the disease.

If the mother has active disease and is contagious at the time of delivery, the infant and mother should be separated until the mother is no longer contagious. The infant is managed the same as if the maternal disease were not contagious at the time of delivery.

If the mother has hematogenous spread of TB (bone, meningitis, or miliary TB), congenital TB is possible. If the infant is suspected of having congenital TB, **INH** is given for 6 months. If the **PPD** is positive at 6 months, then the **INH** is continued until age 9 months. As for any mother with active disease at delivery, a chest x-ray and Mantoux skin test should be done shortly after birth, and the infant should be monitored closely, with monthly assessments.

The HIV-Positive Patient

Worldwide, 1.37 million patients with TB have HIV infection according to WHO (2009). In the early stages of HIV infection, the clinical manifestations of TB are similar to those of a normal host. As the T-lymphocyte count decreases, changes occur:

1. A steady reduction in the percentage of patients will have a positive TB skin test, decreasing to 10 to 20 percent of patients with advanced AIDS.
2. Extrapulmonary TB increases, with 60 to 80 percent of patients with CD4 counts below 50 demonstrating extrapulmonary infection.
3. Changing patterns of disease are noted on chest x-ray, although 56 percent of HIV/AIDS patients with TB still present with upper lobe disease (Refaie, Chaudry, Alfakir, & Khan, 2010).

The treatment regimen for patients with HIV infection or AIDS as well as TB is the same as it is for uninfected adults (6-mo regimen, with initial 2-month, four-drug [**INH**, **RIF**, **PZA**, and **EMB**] phase followed by 2 mo of **INH** and **RIF**). Two exceptions to this recommendation for the patient who is HIV positive are that (1) once-weekly **RIF** should not be used in any HIV-infected patient; (2) twice-weekly **INH-RIF** or **rifabutin** should not be used for patients with CD4 counts lower than 100/mcL.

Patients with HIV infection or AIDS are usually on multiple drugs besides the **anti-TB medication**; therefore, the patient should be monitored for interactions between the medications. **RIF** is known to alter the liver's metabolism of many drugs, leading to treatment failure or suboptimal response in the patient on multiple medications. A complex drug interaction also takes place between **RIF** and **protease inhibitors** that can create a therapeutic challenge, possibly leading to changes in the **antiretroviral** regimen. All HIV-infected patients who are undergoing treatment with **isoniazid** should be on **pyridoxine** (**vitamin B_6**) 25 to 50 mg daily or 50 to 100 mg twice weekly to reduce the occurrence of **isoniazid**-induced side effects in the central and peripheral nervous system. Providing an optimal outcome to a patient with HIV infection or AIDS with TB will require referral to an infectious disease specialist. Recommendations regarding treating HIV-infected patients with TB change frequently as new **antiretroviral agents** are introduced; providers can find up-to-date information at the CDC's Division of Tuberculosis Elimination site (http://www.cdc.gov/tb/).

MONITORING

Patients with positive pretreatment sputum for *M. tuberculosis* are best monitored by repeat sputum cultures monthly until sputum cultures are negative. After 2 months of treatment with INH and RIF, more than 80 percent of patients who had positive sputum cultures at the beginning of treatment should have converted to negative. Patients should be monitored monthly and should have a sputum smear and culture at the end of the course of treatment. DOT should be considered for all cases of TB.

Radiographic monitoring is not as important as sputum examination during the course of treatment (ATS, 2003). At the completion of treatment, a chest x-ray should be done to provide a baseline for comparison with any future films.

In patients with negative pretreatment sputum yet having radiographic findings consistent with TB, an extensive effort to make a microbiological diagnosis is necessary. These patients most likely need medical evaluation by a pulmonologist. Bronchoscopy to perform biopsies and bronchoalveolar lavage should be considered to confirm the diagnosis of TB. If presumptive treatment is started without sputum cultures, then the chest x-rays should be repeated. Failure to show improvement of the lesions on the chest film after 3 months of therapy strongly suggests a misdiagnosis or a lesion that is an old TB lesion (not currently active).

Adverse Reactions to the Medications

Patients should also be monitored for adverse reactions to the medications used to treat TB by means of a baseline measurement of hepatic enzymes, bilirubin, serum creatinine, a complete blood count (CBC), and platelet count. Patients who are taking PZA require a baseline serum uric acid. A baseline ophthalmology examination for visual acuity and a red green color examination are required for patients on EMB. These baseline tests are used to determine any underlying abnormality that would affect the treatment regimen. Children generally do not require baseline laboratory tests, except visual acuity, unless they have some underlying medical condition that may complicate the treatment regimen.

INH has a black box warning regarding the development of severe and sometimes fatal hepatitis, even after many months of treatment. The risk is age related, with the highest incidence in persons aged 50 to 64 years (23 cases per 1,000). Increased risk for hepatitis is associated with daily alcohol use, chronic liver disease, and IV drug use. Black and Hispanic women, as well as any woman during the postpartum period who takes INH, may have increased risk of developing fatal hepatitis. All patients taking INH should have monthly symptom reviews to screen for hepatitis. Symptoms to screen for include unexplained anorexia, nausea, vomiting, dark urine, icterus, rash, persistent paresthesias of hands or feet, fatigue, weakness, fever longer than 3 days, or abdominal tenderness especially in the right upper quadrant. Liver enzymes should be measured in patients over age 35 years prior to starting INH, and then periodically throughout treatment.

Once treatment is begun, patients are monitored clinically for adverse reactions. They usually do not need routine laboratory tests unless laboratory abnormalities are present prior to beginning therapy. Patients should be told of the symptoms associated with the most common adverse reactions to the medications. They should report all flu-like illness immediately and see their health-care provider at least monthly during treatment. At the monthly visit, the provider should ask specific questions regarding adverse reactions to the medication and follow any positive answer with confirming laboratory tests.

Adult patients treated for TB are at risk for peripheral neuropathy associated with INH therapy; therefore, they also need 25 to 50 mg per day of **pyridoxine (vitamin B_6)** to decrease the likelihood of developing this serious but avoidable adverse reaction.

OUTCOME EVALUATION

Because of the lengthy treatment time for TB and the increased incidence of resistant organisms found with inadequate treatment, health-care providers should include both the actual sputum culture evaluation and the patient's compliance with the medication regimen in judging the success of the treatment. Ideally, the patient will have TB-free sputum within the first 2 months of treatment and a clear sputum culture throughout the rest of the treatment. After treatment, no standard follow-up is required. If a patient is immunosuppressed, reevaluation is suggested 6 months after treatment has been completed. Any relapse is most likely to occur within the first 2 years after treatment.

PATIENT EDUCATION

Extensive patient education is essential to successful TB treatment. Administration should be explained, including the instructions to take isoniazid on an empty stomach because food reduces bioavailability. The patient must also understand the purpose for the long, multidrug treatment regimen and be a partner in the process. Compliance is a major issue in TB treatment; therefore, all teaching should have the underlying theme of taking all medication as scheduled. Research has found that patients who receive health education and counseling have higher compliance rates (Ailinger & Dear, 1998). The lengthy treatment requires that education be repeated and reviewed at the monthly visits. Because patients may be illiterate or understand little English, education should be presented in a variety of media, such as videotapes in a patient's primary language. Peer health counselors may also be helpful in educating patients with TB.

PREVENTION OF TUBERCULOSIS

Most patients infected with the tubercle bacillus never develop active TB. Approximately 90 to 95 percent of those infected are able to mount an immune response that prevents active TB infection (CDC, 2005). The goal of preventive therapy is early identification of patients at risk of developing active TB so that they can be treated with drugs to prevent their conversion to active disease. Patients at risk for developing active TB include those who have been newly exposed to persons with active TB and those who have dormant infections that are at risk for reactivation.

Skin testing with **PPD** or **Mantoux** is a necessary screening test to determine if the patient has been infected. Evaluation of the results of the skin test is based on the likelihood of infection and the risk of active TB if infection has occurred. If the patient is HIV positive or has fibrotic lesions on chest x-ray, a reaction of 5 mm or more is considered positive. A reaction of 10 mm or more is considered positive in other at-risk patients, including infants and children. In patients who are not in any high-risk category or high-risk environment, a result of 15 mm or more is considered positive.

Patients are considered high risk if they have the following medical conditions: diabetes mellitus, prolonged therapy with **adrenocorticosteroids**, **immunosuppressive therapy**, hematological or reticuloendothelial diseases such as leukemia or Hodgkin's disease, injection drug use by a patient known to be HIV seronegative, end-stage renal disease, and any clinical presentation that consists of substantial rapid weight loss or chronic malnutrition. A person who is in a high-incidence group with a skin test reaction of 10 mm or more is a candidate for preventive therapy, even without any of these risk factors. High-incidence groups include foreign-born people from high-prevalence countries; medically underserved, low-income populations; and residents of long-term-care facilities.

Pathophysiology

Most cases of TB in the United States and Canada occur from reactivation of latent infection acquired at an earlier time, months or years before, when the patient's immune system was able to mount a sufficient defense. The patient has no outward sign of ever having been infected by TB. All that remains to identify that the patient was exposed to TB is a positive tuberculin skin test. Reactivation, leading to active infection, occurs in patients who, for whatever reason, cannot muster a sufficient immune response.

Drug Therapy

Drug therapy for TB prevention consists of INH alone. It is given in a single daily dose of 300 mg for adults and 10 to 15 mg/kg for children, not to exceed 300 mg. Or it may be given as a twice-weekly dose of 10 to 15 mg/kg (maximum 900 mg/dose) in adults and 20 to 30 mg/kg (maximum 900 mg/dose) for children (Abramowicz, 2004). DOT is recommended for twice-weekly dosing. For many years, the standard length of preventive therapy has been 12 months. More recently, 6- and 9-month regimens have been used and are effective if the proper number of doses of INH is taken (CDC, 2000) Patients who are HIV positive should receive 12 months of therapy. The American Academy of Pediatrics recommends 9 months of therapy for children. Shortened 2-month therapy that combines RIF and PZB is no longer recommended because of high rates of hospitalization and death from liver injury associated with the treatment (CDC, 2003b).

The INH should be dispensed in monthly allotments, with the patient's compliance monitored at least monthly. For patients who may have questionable adherence, DOT is recommended. If resources prohibit daily DOT, then INH may be given twice a week at the dose of 15 mg/kg, utilizing DOT to monitor adherence.

Prior to beginning drug therapy with INH, evaluate the patient as follows:

1. Exclude active TB by both radiographic and bacteriological tests. All patients with a positive skin test require a chest x-ray to rule out pulmonary TB. If the chest x-ray is consistent with pulmonary TB, then an extensive evaluation to rule out active disease is necessary. Bacteriologic studies of the sputum and comparisons with old x-rays are helpful in gaining a clear clinical picture of when the patient has active disease. Because of the risk of developing INH resistance when only INH is used for active disease, patients with any suspicion of active disease should be started on multidrug therapy until the final diagnosis is clarified.
2. Determine if the patient has a history of adequate TB preventive therapy.
3. Determine if the patient has had prior INH therapy to decide if the patient has had adequate drug therapy.
4. Look for any contraindications to the administration of INH therapy: previous INH-induced hepatitis, history of severe INH reactions, or liver disease of any etiology.
5. Identify patients who require special cautions. They include patients over age 35 years as well as patients with daily alcohol use, previous problems with INH therapy, current chronic liver disease, and injection drug use. Other patients requiring cautions include pregnant women and patients at higher-risk for developing fatal hepatitis (women, particularly black and Hispanic women). Hepatitis risk is also increased in the postpartum period.

Monitoring

Patients receiving preventive TB therapy with INH should be monitored at least monthly. At monthly visits, the health-care provider should carefully assess the patient's compliance and ask the patient about symptoms of adverse effects of INH, specifically liver damage. A standardized form should be used to evaluate the patient for symptoms of liver damage, including unexplained anorexia; nausea; vomiting; dark urine; icterus; rash; persistent paresthesias of the hands and feet; persistent fatigue, weakness, or fever for more than 3 days' duration; and abdominal tenderness. If these or other signs or symptoms occur during preventive therapy, patients should contact their health-care provider immediately.

Of those receiving INH therapy, 10 to 20 percent will have mildly abnormal liver enzymes, which usually resolve even if the INH is continued. Patients over age 35 years have the highest frequency of hepatitis; therefore, a baseline transaminase should be obtained before therapy is begun for such patients, and the study should be repeated monthly during therapy. If values are greater than three to five times normal, then INH should be discontinued (ATS, 1994). Other patients at risk for developing hepatitis are those who have chronic liver disease, injection drug users, and those who use alcohol daily. Monthly liver function tests are not a substitute for monthly clinical evaluations of the patient on preventive therapy.

Outcome Evaluation

The success of preventive TB therapy is determined by the absence of active disease and by whether the patient has been compliant with the prescribed drug treatment. Because patients who are receiving preventive therapy often do not feel ill or have any overt symptoms, compliance with the long treatment regimen is even more difficult than for patients with active TB.

Patient Education

Education for patients receiving preventive TB therapy is similar to education for those receiving treatment for active TB. The key difference is stressing the need for months of treatment to a patient who often has no symptoms and feels well. Education should occur in the patient's primary language and at an appropriate literacy level. Patients must understand that adherence to the treatment regimen is essential, and the health-care team cannot emphasize it enough.

On The Horizon — DRUGS OF THE FUTURE

The current drugs used for standard TB treatment are more than 40 years old, and renewed interest in TB drug research has been spawned by the Global Alliance for TB Drug Developments. Currently at least three drugs are in clinical trials for TB treatment, including **moxifloxacin** in phase III clinical development, **PA-824** and **TMC 207** in phase II development, with an additional 19 drugs in the discovery and preclinical phase (Global Alliance for TB Drug Development, 2009).

TUBERCULOSIS — PATIENT EDUCATION

Related to the Overall Treatment Plan and Disease Process

- ☐ A clear description of the pathophysiology and mode of transmission of TB: Patients need to understand that they can be infectious to their close contacts if they do not receive adequate treatment.
- ☐ A thorough outline of the complete treatment regimen, including an estimated length of time for treatment: Patients need to know up front that they will be receiving months and possibly more than a year of treatment.
- ☐ Importance of adherence to the treatment regimen.
- ☐ Importance of regularly scheduled follow-up appointments.

Specific to the Drug Therapy

- ☐ A written plan of the medication schedule is essential, especially with multidrug regimens.
- ☐ Possible adverse effects of the medications and importance of reporting immediately to the health-care provider any vague, flu-like symptoms.

Reasons for Taking the Drug(s)

- ☐ The drugs are given to prevent or eliminate infection by *M. tuberculosis.*

TUBERCULOSIS—cont'd

PATIENT EDUCATION

Drugs as Part of the Total Treatment Regimen

Tuberculosis medications are a part of the total treatment regimen, which also includes strict pulmonary care.

Adherence Issues

Extensive patient education is essential to successful treatment. The patient must understand the purpose for the long, multidrug treatment regimen and be a partner in the treatment. Adherence is a major issue; therefore, all teaching should have the underlying theme of taking all medication as scheduled. Researchers have found that patients who receive health education and counseling have higher compliance rates (Ailinger & Dear, 1998). The long period of treatment requires education that is repeated and reviewed at the monthly visits. To teach patients who may be illiterate or who understand only minimum English, education should be conducted in a variety of media, such as videos in the patient's primary language. Peer health counselors may also help to educate patients with TB. DOT may enhance compliance with and adherence to therapy.

REFERENCES

Abramowicz, M. (Ed.). (2004). Drugs for tuberculosis. *Treatment Guidelines from the Medical Letter, 2*(28), 83–88.

Ailinger, R. L., & Dear, M. R. (1998). Adherence to tuberculosis preventive therapy among Latino immigrants. *Public Health Nursing, 15*(1), 19–24.

American Thoracic Society (ATS). (2003). American Thoracic Society/Centers for Disease Control and Prevention/Infectious Diseases Society of America: Treatment of tuberculosis. *American Journal of Respiratory and Critical Care Medicine, 167,* 603–662.

Blumberg, H. M., Leonard, M. K., & Jasmer, R. M. (2005). Update on the treatment of tuberculosis and latent tuberculosis infection. *Journal of the American Medical Association, 293*(22), 2776–2784.

Cain, K. P., Haley, C. A., Armstrong, L. R., Garman, K. N., Wells, C. D., Iademarch, M. F., et al. (2007). Tuberculosis among foreign-born persons in the United States: Achieving tuberculosis elimination. *American Journal of Respiratory and Critical Care Medicine, 175,* 75–79.

Centers for Disease Control and Prevention (CDC). (2000). Targeted tuberculin testing and treatment of latent tuberculosis infection. *Morbidity and Mortality Weekly Report, 49*(RR-06), 1–54.

Centers for Disease Control and Prevention (CDC). (2003a). Treatment of tuberculosis, American Thoracic Society, CDC, and Infectious Diseases Society of America. *Morbidity and Mortality Weekly Report, 52*(RR-11), 1–77.

Centers for Disease Control and Prevention (CDC). (2003b). Update: Adverse event data and revised American Thoracic Society/CDC recommendations against the use of rifampin and pyrazinamide for treatment of latent tuberculosis infection—United States, 2003. *Morbidity and Mortality Weekly Report, 52*(31), 735–739.

Centers for Disease Control and Prevention (CDC). (2005). Trends in tuberculosis—United States—2004. *Morbidity and Mortality Weekly Report, 54,* 245–249.

Centers for Disease Control and Prevention (CDC). (2008). *Reported tuberculosis in the United States, 2007.* Atlanta, GA: U.S. Department of Health and Human Services, CDC.

Dasgupta, K., & Menzies, D. (2005). Cost-effectiveness of tuberculosis control strategies among immigrants and refugees. *European Respiratory Journal, 25,* 1107–1116.

Global Alliance for TB Drug Development. (2009). TB drug portfolio. Retrieved March 8, 2011, from http://www.tballiance.org

Haddad, M. B., Wilson, T. W., Ijaz, K., Marks, S. M., & Moore, M. (2005). Tuberculosis and homelessness in the United States, 1994–2003. *Journal of the American Medical Association, 293*(22), 2762–2766.

Hampton, T. (2005). TB drug research picks up the pace. *Journal of the American Medical Association, 293*(22), 2705–2707.

Heymann, J. S., Sell, R., & Brewer, T. F. (1998). The influence of program acceptability on the effectiveness of public health policy: A study of directly observed therapy for tuberculosis. *American Journal of Public Health, 88*(3), 442–445.

LoBue, P., Sizemore, C., & Castro, K. G. (2009). Plan to combat extensively drug-resistant tuberculosis recommendations of the federal Tuberculosis Task Force. *Morbidity and Mortality Weekly Report, 58*(RR03), 1–43.

Manangan, L., Elmore, K., Lewis, B., Pratt, R., Armstrong, L., Davison, J., et al. (2009). Disparities in tuberculosis between Asian/Pacific Islanders and non-Hispanic Whites, United States, 1993–2006. *International Journal of Tuberculosis and Lung Disease, 13*(9), 1077–1085.

Mazurek, G. H., Jereb, J., LoBue, P., Iademarco, M. F., Merchock, B., & Vernon, A. (2005). Guidelines for using QuantiFERON-TB Gold test for detecting *Mycobacterium tuberculosis* infection, United States. *Morbidity and Mortality Weekly Report, 54*(RR-15), 49–55.

Mitnick, C. D., Shin, S. S., Seung, K. J., Rich, M. L., Atwood, S. S., Furin, J. J., et al. (2008). Comprehensive treatment of extensively drug-resistant tuberculosis. *New England Journal of Medicine, 359*(6), 563–74.

Ontario Lung Association. (2009). *Tuberculosis information for health care providers* (4th ed.). Toronto, ON: Lung Association. Retrieved from http://www.on.lung.ca

Ormerod, L. P. (2005). Multidrug-resistant tuberculosis (MDR-TB): Epidemiology, prevention and treatment. *British Medical Bulletin, 73,* 17–24.

Public Health Agency of Canada. (2007). *Tuberculosis in Canada.* Ottawa, ON: Public Health Agency of Canada.

Public Health Agency of Canada (2009). *Tuberculosis: Information for Health Care Providers. 4th Edition.* Ottawa, ON: Public Health Agency of Canada.

Public Health Agency of Canada (2010). *Tuberculosis: Drug resistance in Canada—2009.* Ottawa, ON: Public Health Agency of Canada.

Rafaie, T., Chaudry, F. A., Aflakir, M., & Khan, M. A. (2010). Chest x-ray presentation of pulmonary tuberculosis in patients with HIV/AIDS. American Journal of Respiratory and Critical Care Medicine, 181, A1787.

Rey, E., Pons, G., Crémier, O., Van Zelle-Kervroëdan, F., Pariente-Khayat, A., d'Athis, P., et al. (1998). Isoniazid dose adjustment in a pediatric population. *Therapeutic Drug Monitoring, 20*(1), 50–55.

Riley, L. (1997). Pneumonia and tuberculosis in pregnancy. *Infectious Disease Clinics of North America, 11*(1), 119–133.

World Health Organization (WHO). (2006). Guidance for national tuberculosis programmes on the management of tuberculosis in children. Geneva, Switzerland: World Health Organization. Retrieved March 8, 2011, from http://whqlibdoc.who.int/hq/2006/WHO_HTM_TB_2006.371_eng.pdf

World Health Organization (WHO). (2009a). Tuberculosis [Fact sheet]. Geneva, Switzerland: World Health Organization. Retrieved March 8, 2011, from http://www.who.int/mediacentre/factsheets/fs104/en/index.html

World Health Organization (WHO). (2009b). Health ministers to accelerate efforts against drug-resistant TB. Geneva, Switzerland: World Health Organization. Retrieved March 8, 2011, from http://www.who.int/mediacentre/news/releases/2009/tuberculosis_drug_resistant_20090402/en/

CHAPTER 46

UPPER RESPIRATORY INFECTIONS, OTITIS MEDIA, AND OTITIS EXTERNA

Teri Moser Woo

Chapter Outline

Upper respiratory infections (URIs) are the most common minor acute illnesses seen in primary care. The most common secondary infections seen with viral URIs are sinusitis and, in children, otitis media (OM). Practitioners encounter these illnesses countless times among their patients and should be aware of the pathogens commonly found and the pharmacological and nonpharmacological management of these illnesses. This chapter discusses the pharmacological management of these acute illnesses, as well as the management of otitis externa (OE).

VIRAL UPPER RESPIRATORY INFECTION

Viral URIs, also known as common colds, are the most frequent disease seen in a primary care practice and also the number one cause of absenteeism from work and school. The frequency of viral URIs varies with age, with adults averaging 2.5 colds a year (Fendrick, Monto, Nightengale, & Sarnes, 2003) and children age 1 to 5 averaging 7 or 8 (Friedman & Sexton, 2009). Infants have an average of 6 or 7 colds per year, but being in day care increases their incidence of colds to 9 to 11 in the first year of life. Overall, the common cold accounts for 22 million missed school days and 20 million missed workdays due to caring for an ill child; the total economic cost of the common cold is estimated at $25 billion annually (Bramley, Lerner, & Sames, 2002).

A viral URI usually starts with the symptoms of nasal congestion, rhinorrhea, malaise, and scratchy throat. The nasal discharge typically starts out thin and clear and then thickens and progresses to a green or yellow color. Generalized muscle aches may be present, but fever is usually absent in adults. Young children may have a low-grade fever for 2 or 3 days. Fever in adults or a high fever in children suggests influenza or a secondary infection, such as sinusitis or OM. URI symptoms are irritating but not severe. More severe symptoms should be investigated for secondary infection or other bacterial infection. Most patients are symptom free in 7 to 10 days from the beginning of the illness.

Pathophysiology

The rhinovirus causes approximately 50 percent of all viral URIs (Pappas & Hendley, 2009). There are more than 100 serotypes of rhinovirus (American Academy of Pediatrics [AAP], 2009a); therefore, even though immunity is produced by rhinoviral infections, the patient can quickly become infected with another strain of rhinovirus. The common story heard in the clinic is that the patient has just gotten over a cold and now it has come back. Other viruses found with the common cold include, but are not limited to, adenovirus, respiratory syncytial virus, parainfluenza virus, influenza viral strains and human metapneumovirus (Pappas & Hendley, 2009). These viruses are transmitted between people by airborne droplets or by direct transmission of the virus in secretions via hand contact.

Goals of Treatment

Viral URIs are self-limiting and require no treatment other than symptomatic relief; therefore, the major goal in treating a patient with a viral URI is relieving irritating symptoms, specifically nasal congestion.

Rational Drug Selection

Drug Therapy

Although viral URI (the common cold) is a self-limited disease that requires no treatment, a huge industry touts nonprescription medications for treatment of colds. First, note that **antibiotics** have no place in the treatment of the common cold. Using **antibiotics** for a viral infection increases the likelihood of antimicrobial resistance to secondary bacterial infections that may occur in the upper respiratory tract. **Antihistamines** have not been proved to alter the course of a common cold, yet many over-the-counter (OTC) cold preparations contain some form of **antihistamine**, probably for their "drying" effect.

The mainstay of pharmacological management for a cold is the **decongestant**, either systemic or topical. **Decongestants** cause vasoconstriction of the capillaries in the nasal mucous membranes. This results in shrinkage of the mucous membrane, which promotes drainage and decreases the nasal stuffiness that accompanies a URI. Dosing of common **decongestants** can be found in Table 46–1. **Topical decongestants** (Afrin, Neo-Synephrine) may be helpful for temporary relief of congestion without causing systemic side effects. **Topical decongestants** may be used safely for up to 3 consecutive days. Prolonged use of **topical decongestants** will lead to rebound congestion. **Analgesics** such as **acetaminophen** (Tylenol), **aspirin**, and **ibuprofen** (Motrin) can be given for malaise.

Table 46–1 **Drugs Commonly Used: Viral Upper Respiratory Infections**

Drug	Adult Dose	Pediatric Dose	Strengths Available	Comments
Oral Decongestants				
Pseudoephedrine HCI (Sudafed, Genafed, Pseudo Tabs, Pediacare)	60 mg q4–6h Extended release: 120 mg q12h	*Children 6–12 yr:* 30 mg q4–6h	Tablets: 30 mg, 60 mg	*Adults:* do not exceed 120 mg in 24 h
		**Children 2–5 yr:* 15 mg q4–6h *Infants–2 yr:* 1 mg/kg or 0.1 mL/kg of 7.5 mg/0.8 mL drops	Extended release: 120 mg Liquid: 15 mg/5 mL, 30 mg/5mL Drops: 7.5 mg/0.8 mL Capsules: 60 mg	*Children:* do not exceed 4 doses/d *Not recommended in children under age 4 yr
Pseudoephedrine sulfate (Afrin, Drixoral Non-Drowsy)	120 mg q12h	Not for use in children <12 yr	Extended release: 120 mg	Do not crush or chew
Phenylephrine (Sudafed PE)	*Adults:* 10 mg q4h Maximum of 60 mg/24 h	**Children 2–6 yr:* 2.5–5 mg every 12 h *Children >6 yr:* 5–10 mg q12h	Tablet: 10 mg Chewable tablet: 10 mg Dissolving tablet: 10 mg	*Decongestants are not recommended in children < age 4 yr

Table 46–1 **Drugs Commonly Used: Viral Upper Respiratory Infections—cont'd**

Drug	Adult Dose	Pediatric Dose	Strengths Available	Comments
Topical Decongestants				
Phenylephrine HCl (Neo-Synephrine, Nostril, Sinex, Alconefrin, Rhinall)	2–3 sprays each nostril; repeat q3–4h	*Children 6–12 yr:* 2 sprays each nostril q4h *Children >6 mo:* 1 to 2 drops each nostril q3h	Spray: 0.125%, 0.16%, 0.25%, 0.5%, 1% Drops: 0.25%, 0.5%, 1%	Do not use for longer than 3 d because of rebound congestion; rarely used in young children.
Oxymetazoline HCl (Afrin, 12 Hour Nasal, Dristan Long Lasting, Allerest 12 Hour, Afrin Children's Nose Drops)	2 or 3 sprays or drops of 0.05% solution in each nostril bid or q10–12h	*Children ≥6 yr:* 2 or 3 drops of 0.025% solution in each nostril bid, morning and evening	Solution: 0.05%, 0.025%	Do not use for longer than 3 d because of rebound congestion. Do not use in children <6 yr.

There have been recent concerns about the use of **pseudoephedrine** to manufacture **methamphetamine** and a number of states have decreased access to OTC **pseudoephedrine**. Some states have declared **pseudoephedrine** a prescription medication; Oregon made it a Schedule III drug. In 2006 the Combat Methamphetamine Epidemic Act was incorporated into the USA Patriot Act, requiring special handling of **pseudoephedrine**, **ephedrine**, and **phenylpropanolamine**, all precursors to **methamphetamine**. The law requires precursors to **methamphetamine** to be placed behind the pharmacy counter nationwide to restrict access. Retailers must ask for purchaser identification and limit the amount of drug purchased to a 30-day supply. Providers need to be aware of the changing laws in their state or province of practice and provide a prescription for **pseudoephedrine** as needed. Many manufacturers have begun to create new products that replace the **pseudoephedrine** with **phenylephrine (Sudafed PE)**, a **decongestant** that cannot be used to manufacture **methamphetamine** (see Table 46–1).

The use of cough and cold medications in young children, specifically children under age 5 years, has become an area of significant debate. The safety of cough and cold medications, specifically those containing **decongestants**, has been questioned after a number of reports of deaths of infants taking cold medications (Taverner & Latte, 2007). **Decongestants** have questionable efficacy in children, with a *Cochrane Review* of the use of **decongestants** to treat nasal congestion associated with the common cold found a small (6%) but statistically significant improvement in congestion in adults, but insufficient evidence regarding effectiveness in children (Taverner & Latte, 2007). In October 2007 a U.S. Food and Drug Administration (FDA) panel recommended that all pediatric cough and cold medications be relabeled as not indicated for use in children under age 4 years. This led to a voluntary withdrawal of infant drop formulations of cough and cold medications from the market in October 2007.

Nonpharmacological Therapy

Nonpharmacological therapy or lifestyle management includes increasing fluid intake, using nonmedicated cough drops, using nasal saline spray or drops to decrease the viscosity of nasal secretions, and rest. Patients and parents or other family members need to be reminded that anorexia is often associated with the common cold and that fluids often need to be forced on the ill person to maintain adequate hydration. Infants who are congested often cannot breathe and drink liquids from the bottle or breast at the same time; therefore, their fluid intake may be inadequate. Parents need to be encouraged to suction the infant's nose with a nasal bulb syringe to clear secretions before the infant eats or drinks. Nasal saline spray is also beneficial in thinning secretions at all ages to make blowing or bulbing secretions more effective. Patients can make their own saline solution by adding a quarter tsp salt to 8 oz warm water. If a dropper is not available, patients can use a cotton ball saturated with saline solution to squeeze three or four drops into each nasal passage. Many patients are overcommitted and overworked and must be reminded of the restorative powers of rest. Encouraging patients to take a day or two off from work is much more effective than prescribing an unnecessary **antibiotic**.

Monitoring

The patient with a viral URI should be monitored for signs of secondary bacterial infection. Monitor **decongestant** use in cardiac patients, who may have increased hypertension from the added vasoconstriction caused by **oral decongestants**. Older adults are more likely to have adverse reactions from **decongestants**.

Outcome Evaluation

Secondary bacterial infections may complicate the common cold. The most common complication in adults is sinusitis, which occurs in approximately 0.5 to 2.5 percent of colds (Friedman & Sexton, 2009). In children, sinusitis is a common secondary infection (5% of colds), as is OM, which occurs in about 5 to 10 percent of children with colds (Contopoulos-Ioannidis, Ioannidis, & Lau, 2003). Some children appear more apt to get OM as a secondary infection, possibly because differences in middle ear and eustachian tube anatomy predispose them to ear infections. Adults may not get acute otitis media as often as do children, but 50 to 80 percent of adults will develop eustachian tube dysfunction after a rhinovirus or influenza A URI infection (Friedman & Sexton, 2009; McBride, Doyle, Hayden, & Gwaltney, 1989). This chapter discusses sinusitis and otitis media, common complications of URI. Another complication of viral URIs is exacerbation of asthma symptoms, occurring in 30 to 50 percent of the colds acquired by people with asthma. See Chapter 30 for asthma management.

Patient Education

Patient education for a viral URI is centered on symptomatic treatment and proper dosing of **decongestants.** Parents should be educated about avoiding the use of cough and cold medications in children, especially those age 4 years and younger. Patients need to be assured that most URIs resolve in 7 to 10 days and that very little can be done to shorten the course of the disease. **Antibiotics** are not necessary for viral infections, and education regarding the signs and symptoms of a secondary bacterial infection needs to be provided.

SINUSITIS

Diagnosis of sinusitis is based on clinical symptoms and the course of the illness. Any URI lasting longer than 10 days without improvement is, by definition, sinusitis (American Academy of Allergy, Asthma, and Immunology [AAAAI], 2005; Rosenfeld et al, 2007), with a 60 percent chance that sinus aspiration will identify a bacterial infection (Gwaltney, Scheld, Sande, & Sydnor, 1992). In adults, three symptoms have high specificity and sensitivity for diagnosing acute sinusitis: purulent rhinorrhea, facial pain or pressure, and nasal obstruction (Chan & Kuhn, 2009). Patients may have a headache that worsens when they bend over, and they may have a cough that is worse at night. A sudden worsening of symptoms after improvement is also suggestive of sinusitis (Chan & Kuhn, 2009). Children have subtler symptoms. Because their frontal sinuses are not completely developed until they are 10 years old, children often do not have the classic frontal headache of sinusitis. Children may vomit owing to gagging on mucus. Children have colds more frequently than do adults. Therefore, a careful history of whether the

CLINICAL PEARL

Nutritional or Herbal Therapy

Nutritional or herbal therapy is often thought to decrease symptoms of the common cold. In the 1970s, Linus Pauling first brought forward the idea that **vitamin C** prevents and alleviates episodes of the common cold. Although this has still not been scientifically proved, many patients continue to take **vitamin C** at the first sign of a cold.

Zinc lozenges have also been brought forth as a treatment for the common cold. It is thought that zinc ions inhibit rhinovirus replication in vitro. A systematic review of seven randomized controlled trials (RCTs) (754 patients total) found two of the studies suggested reduced duration and severity of upper respiratory infection (URI) symptoms (Marshall, 2000). Another review of 14 placebo-controlled trials, published from 1966 to 2000, found one well-designed study that found improvement with the use of **zinc nasal gel** (Caruso, Prober, & Gwaltney, 2007). In a more recent RCT, the group of patients took a 13.3-mg **zinc lozenge** every 2 to 3 hours while awake and had a significantly shorter duration of cold symptoms (4.0 days vs. 7.1 days; P is less than 0.0001), shorter duration of cough (2.1 days vs. 5.0 days), and nasal discharge (3.0 vs. 4.5 days) than did the placebo control group (Prasad, Beck, Bao, Snell, & Fitzgerald, 2008). In light of these studies, **zinc lozenges** may decrease URI symptoms in some patients. **Zinc nasal gels (Zicam)** should be avoided after reports of permanent anosmia and an FDA warning to avoid their use.

Another common herbal therapy that patients may be using for their cold symptoms is **echinacea. Echinacea** is widely used in Europe for the prevention and treatment of colds and flu. Its use is increasing in the United States. A number of European studies have demonstrated the immune-enhancing properties of **echinacea,** specifically increasing T-cell activity and interferon. Among European providers, **echinacea** is the leading herbal recommendation for the prevention of colds and flu. **Echinacea** is available in tablet, liquid, and tea bag form. The correct dosage is 900 mg daily divided into two or three doses, or 40 drops of the juice three times a day. Length of therapy should not exceed 8 weeks. There are no reported side effects at the recommended dosages. It appears to be safe during pregnancy and lactation. The only true contraindication is having a progressive systemic disease such as tuberculosis or multiple sclerosis or an autoimmune illness. **Echinacea** is a relative of the daisy; therefore, patients who are allergic to daisies should also avoid any form of **echinacea** (Brown, 1996).

symptoms have actually been prolonged or whether the patient has a new viral URI is essential. Children and adults alike may have puffy eyes and a cough that worsens when they lie down. Radiological studies are of questionable validity because sinus films look the same for a viral URI and a sinus infection. The length of the illness and the severity of symptoms often distinguish the two. Sinus infections can be either acute or chronic. Chronic sinusitis is defined as signs and symptoms consistent with sinusitis that last longer than 12 weeks (Chan & Kuhn, 2009; Rosenfeld et al, 2007).

Pathophysiology

The most common bacterial organisms found in acute sinusitis are *Streptococcus pneumoniae, Haemophilus influenzae, Moraxella catarrhalis,* and more rarely, *Staphylococcus. Staphylococcus,* gram-negative enteric organisms and anaerobic bacteria, are more common in chronic sinusitis. Rarely, the causative organism in chronic sinusitis is fungal, with *Aspergillus* the most common fungus found. Patients who are immunocompromised develop severe infection, even invasive infections with eye, mouth, and brain extensions. Culture of the nasal mucosa is not helpful in determining the causative agent in sinusitis. If the patient is not responding to therapy, sinus aspiration or endoscopic aspiration is the only accurate way to determine the organism involved; both procedures require referral to otolaryngology.

Goals of Treatment

The overall goal for the treatment of sinusitis is absence of infection, demonstrated by the patient's freedom from all symptoms of a sinus infection.

Rational Drug Selection

Given the most likely organisms to be found in both children and adults, the first choice for **antibiotic therapy** in acute sinusitis is **amoxicillin** (AAAAI, 2005; Hwang & Getz, 2009; Rosenfeld et al, 2007). **Amoxicillin** is inexpensive and well tolerated (Table 46–2). For adults, the dose is 500 mg given three times a day, and in children, the daily dose is

Table 46–2 **Drugs Commonly Used: Sinusitis and Otitis Media**

Drug	Dose	Length of Treatment	Strengths Available	Comments
Amoxicillin (Amoxil, Trimox)	*Adults and children >20 kg*: 500 mg q8h *Children:* 80–90 mg/kg/d divided in 3 doses	Sinusitis: 10–14 days or until 7 d after symptom-free (may need 21 d of treatment) Otitis media: 7–10 d	Capsules: 250 mg, 500 mg Chewable tablets: 125 mg, 200 mg, 250 mg, 400 mg Powder for suspension: 50 mg/mL, 125 mg/5 mL, 200 mg/5 mL, 250 mg/5 mL, 400 mg/5 mL	First choice for non–penicillin allergic patients. Higher doses may be used for children who have recently been on antibiotics or in day care, up to 90 mg/kg/d.
Amoxicillin and clavulanate (Augmentin)	*Adults:* 500 mg q12h or 250 mg q8h *Children <3 mo:* 30 mg/kg/d of amoxicillin divided q12h *Children >3 mo, <40 kg:* 25–45 mg/kg/d of amoxicillin divided q12h (use 200 mg/5 mL or 400 mg/5 mL suspension) *or* 20–45 mg/kg/d of amoxicillin if using 125 mg/5 mL or 250/5 mL suspension dosed every 8 hours. Drug-resistance dosing: 80–90 mg/kg/d divided every 12 hours. Use Augmentin ES or a 7:1 bid formulation	10–14 d for all patients	Tablets: 250 mg amoxicillin & 125 mg clavulanate; 500 mg amoxicillin & 125 mg clavulanate; 875 mg amoxicillin & 125 mg clavulanate Chewable tablets: 125 mg amoxicillin & 31.25 mg clavulanate; 200 mg amoxicillin & 28.5 mg clavulanate; 250 mg amoxicillin & 62.5 mg clavulanate; 400 mg amoxicillin & 57 mg clavulanate Suspension: 125 mg amoxicillin & 31.25 mg clavulanate/ 5 mL; 200 mg amoxicillin & 28.5 mg clavulanate/5 mL; 250 mg amoxicillin & 62.5 mg clavulanate/5 mL; 400 mg amoxicillin & 57 mg clavulanate/5 mL; 400 mg amoxicillin & 57 mg	Children's dose is based on amoxicillin content. Because of the clavulanate content, two 250-mg tablets are *not* the same as one 500-mg tablet. Because of the different clavulanate levels in the suspensions, it is not appropriate to dose the 125-mg/5 mL or the 250-mg/5 mL suspensions bid. Children should not be given the 250-mg tablet until they are >40 kg. High-dose amoxicillin/clavulanate requires use of a formula of 600 mg amoxicillin/42.9 mg clavulanate per 5 mL.

Continued

Table 46–2 **Drugs Commonly Used: Sinusitis and Otitis Media—cont'd**

Drug	Dose	Length of Treatment	Strengths Available	Comments
			clavulanate (Augmentin ES = 600) amoxicillin 600 mg/5 mL and 42.9 mg clavulanate/5 mL (Augmentin ES = 600) Amoxicillin 600 mg/5 mL & 42.9 mg clavulanate/ 5 mL	
Azithromycin (Zithromax)	*Children:* 10 mg/kg as 1 single dose on the first day, then 5 mg/kg/d on days 2 through 5; do not exceed adult dose *Adults:* 500 mg single dose the first day, followed by 250 mg daily for days 2 through 5	5 d	Suspension: 100 mg/5 mL, 200 mg/5 mL Capsules: 250 mg Z-pak (six 250-mg tablets with instructions for daily dosing)	Convenient dosing. 5-d course of treatment. Broad spectrum. Use as second-line drug for otitis media in penicillin-allergic patients.
Cefdinir (Omnicef)	*Adults ≥13 yr:* 300 mg q12h or 600 mg q24h *Children:* 14 mg/kg/d in 1 or 2 doses	AOM: 5–10 d Sinusitis: 10 d	Capsules: 300 mg Suspension: 125 mg/5 mL 250 mg/5 mL	Do not use for type 1 Penicillin = allergic patients (urticaria of anaphylaxis). Adjust dosing for renal insufficiency.
Cefpodoxime (Vantin)	*Adults:* 200 mg q12h *Children:* 10 mg/kg/d divided q12h (max dose 400 mg)	5–14 d	Tablets: 100 mg, 200 mg Suspension: 50 mg/5 mL, 100 mg/5 mL	Broad spectrum Very expensive
Cefprozil (Cefzil)	*Adults and children* >12 yr: 500 mg q12h *Children:* 30 mg/kg/d divided into 2 doses 12 h apart	10–14 d	Tablets: 250 mg, 500 mg Suspension: 125 mg/5 mL, 250 mg/5 mL	Broad-spectrum coverage Expensive
Ceftibuten (Cedax)	*Adults:* 400 mg once daily *Children:* 9 mg/kg/d in 1 daily dose	10 d	Tablets: 400 mg Suspension: 90 mg/5 mL, 180 mg/5 mL	Must be given on an empty stomach.
Ceftriaxone (Rocephin)	*Children:* 50 mg/kg given as 1 IM dose (maximum of 1 g/dose)	One dose only	Powder for injection: 250 mg, 500 mg, 1 g	May be used as 1-time dose for otitis media in children. Very expensive compared with amoxicillin. Broad spectrum
Cefuroxime (Ceftin)	*Adults and children >12 yr:* 250 mg or 500 mg q12h *Children:* 30 mg/kg/d given q12h up to 1,000 mg/d	10 d	Tablets: 125 mg, 250 mg, 500 mg Suspension: 125 mg/5 mL Note: Tablets and suspension are *not* bio-equivalent and are *not* substitutable on a mg-for-mg basis	Prolonged half-life in patients with renal failure. Suspension must be given with food. Broad spectrum Expensive

Table 46–2 **Drugs Commonly Used: Sinusitis and Otitis Media—cont'd**

Drug	Dose	Length of Treatment	Strengths Available	Comments
Erythromycin-sulfisoxazole (Pediazole)	*Children:* Dose by erythromycin content: 50/mg/kg/d in 3 divided doses	10–14 d	Suspension: 200 mg erythromycin with 600 mg sulfisoxazole/5 mL	Broad-spectrum activity. Used for treatment of otitis media in penicillin-allergic children. Poor taste.
Trimethoprim (TMP)-sulfamethoxazole (SMZ) (Bactrim, Septra, Cotrim)	*Adults:* 160 mg TMP & 800 mg SMZ q12h	10–14 d for all patients	Tablets: 80 mg TMP & 400 mg SMZ	Do not prescribe in children <2 mo
	Children >2 mo: 8 mg/kg TMP & 40 mg/kg SMZ q12h		Double-strength tablets: 160 mg TMP & 800 mg SMZ Oral suspension: 40 mg TMP & 200 mg SMZ/5 mL	*Dosing tip:* Dose of suspension is 1 mL/kg/d divided in 2 doses

80 to 90 mg/kg per day, divided in three doses. The usual length of treatment is 10 to 14 days; if the patient is responding slowly, treat until the patient is symptom free and then an additional 7 days (AAAAI, 2005; Contopoulos-Ioannidis et al, 2003). The course of treatment may be up to 21 days in acute sinusitis. If the patient is allergic to **penicillin**, **trimethoprim/sulfamethoxazole (Septra)** and **erythromycin** are also acceptable (Hwang & Getz, 2009). Acute sinusitis may also be treated with many of the **cephalosporins**, **azithromycin**, or a **fluoroquinolone**, but use of the narrower spectrum antibiotics **amoxicillin** and **trimethoprim/sulfamethoxazole** are recommended as first line treatment (Rosenfeld et al, 2007). Children who meet criteria for sinusitis should be treated with **amoxicillin** as first-line therapy, although children who are in day care or who have had antibiotics in the past 90 days are at risk for resistance and should be treated with **amoxicillin/clavulanate** (80 to 90 mg/kg/d), **cefdinir** (14 mg/kg/d), **cefuroxime** (30 mg/kg/d) or **cefpodoxime** (10 mg/kg/d) (Wald, 2010). Adults who have a child in day care should be started on high-dose **amoxicillin** (1 g qid) as they are at risk for having a beta-lactamase-producing *S. pneumoniae* (Hwang & Getz, 2009; Rosenfeld et al, 2007).

If the patient is worsening or not improving in 7 days, bacterial resistance needs to be considered. It is important to discern between slow improvement and failure to improve as sinusitis may slowly resolve (Rosenfeld et al, 2007) The drugs of choice for sinusitis that fails to improve after a week of first-line therapy are high-dose **amoxicillin/clavulanate (Augmentin)** or in adults a respiratory **fluoroquinolone (levofloxacin, moxifloxacin, gemifloxacin)** (Rosenfeld et al, 2007). **Fluoroquinolones** should not be prescribed for children or adolescents because of the potential for adverse reactions, which is discussed further in Chapter 24. Children who fail to improve are treated with high-dose **amoxicillin/clavulanate** (80 to 90 mg/kg/d of **amoxicillin** component), **cefdinir** (14 mg/kg/d), **cefuroxime** (30 mg/kg/d), or **cefpodoxime** (10 mg/kg/d) (Wald, 2010). Failure to respond indicates either misdiagnosis of sinusitis or resistance. Although radiological evaluation is not indicated in patients initially diagnosed with sinusitis, failure to improve warrants either plain sinus films or computed tomography (CT) to confirm diagnosis. Consultation with an otolaryngologist may also be warranted to determine the need for sinus aspiration to guide **antimicrobial** choice (Hwang & Getz, 2009; Wald, 2010).

Chronic sinusitis is defined by 12 weeks of symptoms and the documentation of inflammation either by examination or radiographic findings (Rosenfeld et al, 2007). **Amoxicillin/clavulanate** is the drug of choice in chronic sinusitis. Patients with chronic sinusitis may also need a short course of **inhaled** or **oral corticosteroids**, drugs with no proven efficacy in acute sinusitis (Chan & Kuhn, 2009). Hypertonic or isotonic saline washes are a critical part of chronic sinusitis treatment. Patients who fail to respond to **antibiotics** may need referral to an otolaryngologist. Other causes for chronic sinusitis need to be considered, including allergies and immunodeficiency (Rosenfeld et al, 2007). Figure 46–1 provides an algorithm for the treatment of sinusitis.

Monitoring

Patients who are being treated with **antibiotics** for sinusitis need to be monitored for adverse reactions to the **antibiotics** and for their response to treatment. They should begin to respond in 3 to 4 days. If there is no improvement in clinical symptoms, then bacterial resistance must be considered.

Outcome Evaluation

Sinusitis symptoms should resolve after 7 days of treatment. Chronic or recurrent sinusitis requires a referral to

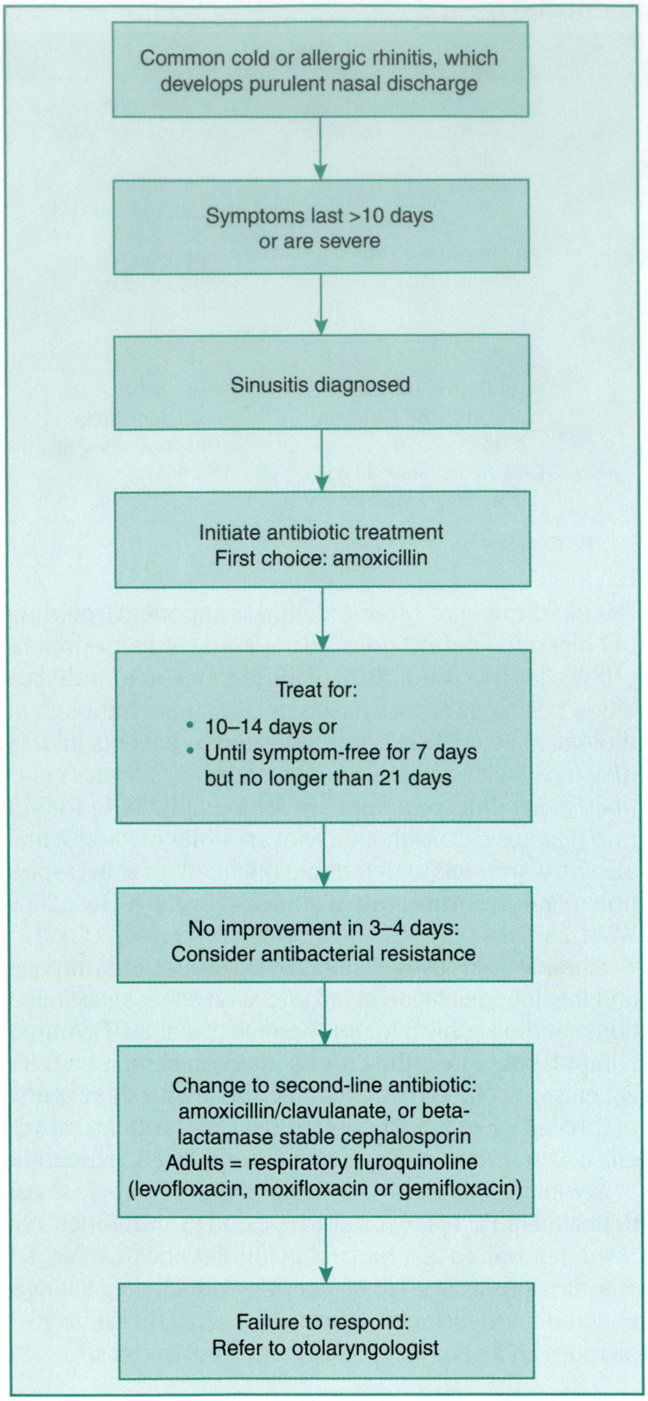

Figure 46–1. Algorithm for treatment of sinusitis.

an otolaryngologist. Often, surgical intervention is needed to provide adequate drainage from the sinuses. Untreated sinusitis can lead to invasive disease such as orbital cellulitis or brain involvement. These are both medical emergencies and fortunately rare, usually seen only in immunocompromised patients. As with viral URIs, acute or chronic sinusitis may exacerbate asthma.

Patient Education

Nonpharmacological management includes **decongestants**, either topical or systemic, to improve nasal obstruction. Patients should be warned against long-term use of **topical decongestants**, but they can be very helpful in providing symptomatic relief during the few days it takes to respond to **antibiotics**. Saline nasal spray or wash prevents crusting of secretions in the nasal cavity, facilitating removal of secretions. Adequate hydration is essential in liquefying secretions. The facial pain and headache associated with sinusitis can be severe, and the patient should be encouraged to take **acetaminophen** or **ibuprofen** for pain. A warm pack to the frontal and maxillary sinuses often provides pain relief. Running a humidifier at night can alleviate the dry mouth caused by mouth breathing during sleep. Breathing in hot steam often helps clear nasal passages, but caution patients about burns.

Sinusitis causes the air passages in the sinuses to become swollen and blocked and to trap air. Therefore, sinusitis poses a hazard to patients who dive because of the changing air pressures in the sinuses, and diving is contraindicated. Patients who are planning to fly or to drive over mountain ranges can use **topical decongestants** prior to the trip to prevent the pain associated with the changing air pressures in the air trapped in the sinuses.

OTITIS MEDIA

The most common reason that children in the United States receive **antibiotics** is for acute otitis media (AOM); an estimated 10.3 million visits annually are coded AOM (Coco, Vernacchio, Horst, & Anderson, 2010). OM may occur at any age, but the most common presentation is in children under age 10 years. In the first year of life, 60 to 80 percent of infants have at least one episode of AOM, and 80 to 90 percent of children have at least one episode of AOM by age to 2 to 3 years (Paradise et al, 1997; Teele, Klein, & Rosner, 1989). The estimated annual cost of OM treatment is more than $5 billion. Every practitioner encounters OM, and those who work with children see OM daily. Defining AOM and otitis media with effusion (OME) would seem to be a simple task, yet there is great diversity in the criteria for diagnosis and management among primary care providers (Altemeier, 1998). Criteria for the diagnosis of AOM and OME, as well as their management, are discussed in this section of the chapter.

The hallmark symptom of OM is ear pain, often unilateral. Patients may also complain of hearing loss in the affected ear. Preverbal children may tug or poke at the affected ear, be irritable, and sleep poorly. Fever often accompanies AOM. Patients may also report tinnitus, dizziness, an unsteady gait, or balance problems. In children, vomiting and diarrhea may be associated with OM.

Diagnosis of AOM requires: (1) a history of acute onset of symptoms; (2) the presence of middle ear effusion; and

(3) signs and symptoms of middle ear inflammation (AAP/AAFP, 2004). OME is fluid in the middle ear without any signs or symptoms of acute illness. Erythema is nonspecific, and AOM should never be diagnosed on the basis of tympanic membrane (TM) color alone, as the TM can redden from crying or a fever. Fluid in the middle ear is assessed by observing white or yellow fluid, seeing air/fluid level, observing air bubbles, or noting decreased TM movement via pneumatic otoscopy. A thin walled bulla is seen with bullous myringitis, a very painful form of AOM.

Pathophysiology

AOM occurs when there is a combination of eustachian tube dysfunction, which blocks the flow of secretions from the middle ear to the pharynx, and negative pressure developing in the middle ear, which causes reflux of bacteria into the middle ear space. This combination results in a middle ear effusion that becomes infected with nasopharyngeal bacteria. A predisposing factor in young children (<5 years) is that they have shorter, more horizontal, and more flaccid eustachian tubes, and bacteria are more easily drawn into the middle ear space. Certain risk factors predispose children to AOM: URIs, Down syndrome, cleft palate, HIV infection, and Eskimo or Native American heritage. Children who are bottle-fed formula have a higher incidence of AOM than do breast-fed infants. Children who live with one or more tobacco smokers have an increased risk of OM, with a 1.4 odds ratio of recurrent AOM if either parent smokes (Adair-Bischoff & Sauve, 1998; Strachan & Cook, 1998). Immunocompromised patients and patients with indwelling nasogastric tubes have an increased incidence of OM, regardless of age.

S. pneumoniae, *H. influenzae*, and *M. catarrhalis* are the most common pathogens found in AOM in both children and adults. *S. pneumoniae* accounts for 25 to 50 percent of AOM, *H. influenzae* for 15 to 30 percent, and *M. catarrhalis* for 3 to 20 percent of pathogens found upon culture of middle ear aspirates (Adderson, 1998; AAP & AAFP, 2004). Some evidence suggests that the microbiology of AOM is changing as a result of routine use of **heptavalent pneumococcal vaccine**; *S. pneumoniae* isolates from middle ear fluid are decreasing from 45 to 30 percent (Casey & Pichichero, 2004), and vaccine specific isolates are decreasing from 70 to 36 percent (Block et al, 2004). The **conjugate Hib vaccine** has not affected AOM caused by *H. influenzae* because approximately 90 percent of *H. influenzae* in AOM is nontypeable. Viruses (respiratory syncytial virus, rhinovirus, coronavirus, adenovirus, and parainfluenza virus) alone or as a copathogen are found in 40 to 75 percent of AOM cases (AAP & AAFP, 2004).

Goals of Treatment

The goal for the treatment of AOM is to clear infection from the middle ear fluid with the use of **antibiotics**. If the **antibiotic** chosen is effective against the pathogen, then the infection clears. Because the treatment of AOM is empiric based on the most commonly found pathogens, at times, a change of **antibiotic** is necessary to treat the infection. The goal remains the same: clearing infection from the middle ear fluid.

Rational Drug Selection

Guidelines

There is much controversy regarding the treatment of OM. In 2004, the AAP and the AAFP issued a joint clinical practice guideline for the diagnosis and treatment of AOM, which provides an evidence-based approach caring for the child aged 2 months to 12 years with uncomplicated AOM.

The AAP & AAFP (2004) recommendations are the following:

1. Diagnosis of AOM includes the following criteria: (a) history of acute onset of signs and symptoms; (b) middle ear effusion (MEE); and (c) signs and symptoms of middle ear inflammation.
2. Pain must be assessed and adequate pain management provided.

3a. Observation for 48 to 72 hours without prescribing an **antibiotic** is an option for children who meet criteria (age 2 years or older with nonsevere illness, or uncertain diagnosis, follow-up assured).

3b. If treating with an **antibiotic**, **amoxicillin** is the first choice for most children. **Amoxicillin** should be dosed at 80 to 90 mg/kg per day. Patients with severe illness (fever of 39°C or higher, moderate to severe otalgia) and those who warrant coverage for beta lactamase–positive *H. influenzae* and *M. catarrhalis*, should be prescribed **amoxicillin/clavulanate** (90 mg/kg/d of **amoxicillin** and 6.4 mg/kg/d of **clavulanate** in two divided doses) as the drug of choice.

4. If patient fails to respond to initial management option (3a or 3b) within 48 to 72 hours, the clinician must reassess the patient to confirm AOM and exclude other causes of illness. If initially managed with observation, then **antibiotics** should be started. If an **antibiotic** was initially prescribed, then the **antibiotic** should be changed.
5. Clinicians should encourage prevention of AOM through the reduction of risk factors such as reconsidering day-care attendance, breastfeeding for the first 6 months of life, avoiding "bottle propping" or supine bottle feeding, reducing pacifier use in the second 6 months of life, and reducing exposure to tobacco smoke.
6. There are no recommendations for complementary or alternative medication (CAM) for the treatment of AOM based on limited evidence.

Figure 46–2 provides an algorithm for treating OM.

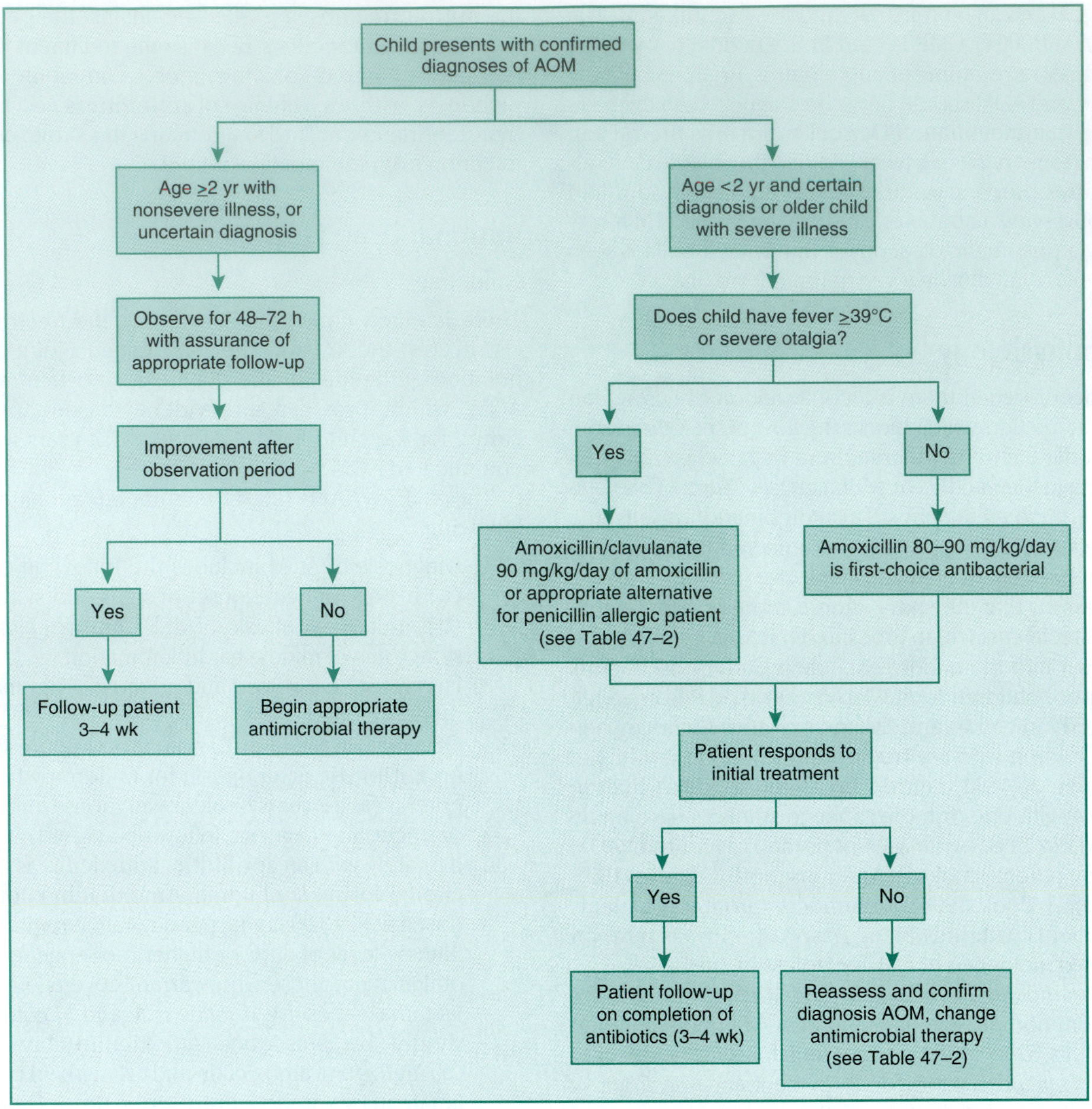

Figure 46–2. Algorithm for treatment of AOM.

Antimicrobial Resistance

The emergence of antimicrobial resistance among respiratory pathogens has caused primary care providers to reevaluate their routine use of **antibiotics** for all illnesses, especially OM. More than 95 percent of *M. catarrhalis* produces beta lactamase, which can be resistant to **amoxicillin** and other **penicillins** (AAP, 2009a). *H. influenzae*, another beta lactamase producer, is 30 to 40 percent resistant to **amoxicillin** (AAP, 2009b). Between 15 and 50 percent of upper respiratory tract isolates of *S. pneumoniae* are not susceptible to penicillin; approximately 50 percent of these are highly resistant to penicillin, and 50 percent are intermediate in resistance (AAP & AAFP, 2004). *S. pneumoniae* is also resistant to the common macrolides erythromycin (35.3% resistance), azithromycin (35.3% resistance), and clarithromycin (35.2% resistance) (Jenkins & Ferrell, 2009). Resistant *S. pneumoniae* is more common among children who are in day care, have recurrent AOM, are younger than 2 years, or have been recently treated with **beta lactamase antibiotics** (AAP & AAFP, 2004). In light of this increasing resistance among common OM pathogens, the provider needs to decide carefully whether an **antibiotic** is necessary and, in the case of treatment failure, consider the possibility of resistant bacterial strains. The common **antibiotics** and their dosages used for OM are listed in Table 46–2.

Dosing Regimen

Amoxicillin remains the first-line drug of choice for AOM in spite of resistance per the AAP and AAFP guidelines for the management of AOM (2004). **Amoxicillin** is dosed at 80 to 90 mg/kg per day, which raises the concentration in the middle ear to be effective against intermediate and resistant strains of *S. pneumoniae*. Conversely, patients who have had repeated episodes of AOM or have been on **antibiotics** in the past 30 days should be treated with beta lactamase–stable **amoxicillin/clavulanate** or **beta lactamase–stable cephalosporin** if **penicillin** allergic. Table 46–3 discusses **antibiotic** treatment options for AOM in patients who have been on **antibiotics** recently.

Length of Treatment

Length of treatment has also been investigated in recent years. In the United States, AOM has traditionally been treated for 10 days with **antibiotics.** There are few controlled studies to support the practice. Compliance and completion of the 10-day regimen have also been an issue. A number of studies have compared outcomes after 5 or 7 days of **antibiotics** versus 10 days. For patients over age 5 years, a shortened 5-day course of treatment is probably adequate (AAP & AAFP, 2004; Paradise, 1997). In an analysis of nine studies comparing shortened therapy with traditional 10-day therapy, Paradise (1997) concluded that short-course **antimicrobial treatment** for AOM is probably not adequate for children under age 5 years, especially children age 2 years or younger. Dowell, Mary, Phillips, Gerber, and Schwartz (1998a) put forth a set of principles for the judicious use of **antimicrobial agents** in the treatment of OM, one of which is that uncomplicated AOM may be treated in patients older than age 2 for 5 to 7 days. The AAP and AAFP guidelines (2004) recommend the length of treatment in children under age 6 years to be 10 days and in children age 6 years and older with moderate disease a 5 to 7 day course of antibiotics. These guidelines have not been updated and remain the standard of care (Klein & Pelton, 2010).

Watchful Waiting (No Antibiotics)

With the guidelines recommending a period of "watchful waiting" for 48 to 72 hours in low-risk patients, providers must have confidence in their decision not to treat with antibiotics. Providers are concerned not only about the prudence of the treatment but also about the acceptance of watchful waiting by parents of children with OM. Since the recommendation for judicious use of **antibiotics** was published by Dowell and colleagues (1998a), there has been a movement to look critically at the appropriate diagnosis of AOM and the universal use of **antibiotics.** Finkelstein and colleagues (2003) examined a large database of pediatric visits for AOM and the prescribing of **antibiotics** and found a 59 percent reduction in the prescribing of **antibiotics,** attributed to a decrease in the diagnosis of AOM. Undoubtedly, the clarification and consistency of the diagnosis of AOM have had an impact on the overall use of **antibiotics** for AOM. Whereas previously **antibiotics** were prescribed for any TM that was not "perfect," the recommendation by Dowell and colleagues (1998a) indicated that **antimicrobials** are not indicated for OME, nor for prophylactic use. The AAP and AAFP guidelines (2004) are even clearer: in order to diagnose AOM, the clinician should confirm a history of acute onset, document signs of MEE, and evaluate for signs and symptoms of middle ear inflammation.

Acceptance of watchful waiting among parents of children with AOM has been evaluated. A *Cochrane Review* of 10 studies examining delayed antibiotics for respiratory infections including AOM indicates delayed antibiotic prescription slightly reduces parent satisfaction compared to immediate antibiotics (87% vs. 92%) (Spurling, Del Mar, Dooley, & Foxlee, 2007). A recent study examining the AAP recommendation of watchful waiting indicates that although antibiotic prescribing in children under age 2 years decreased 21 to 26 percent, parental sick days increased 13 to 14 percent (Meropol, Glick, & Asch, 2008). The increase in parental sick days may be a reason for decreased parental satisfaction with watchful waiting.

Providing a "safety-net" prescription for parents to fill after an initial period of observation or watchful waiting is an option for the treatment of AOM. Initial observation of AOM for 48 to 72 hours has been a recommendation of the Dutch College of General Practitioners for almost 30 years (Culpepper & Froom, 1997). Using these guidelines,

Table 46–3 **Treatment Options for Otitis Media**

Temperature >39°C (102.2°F) and Severe Otalgia	Treatment Failure Initial Treatment	Treatment Failure (Days 3–5)	(Days 10–28)
No	High-dose amoxicillin (80–90 mg/kg/d)	*Amoxicillin & clavulanate	Same as day 3
		Cefuroxime, Cefdinir	
		Cefpodoxime	
		Cefriaxone (IM)	
		Cefixime	
Yes	High-dose amoxicillin/clavulanate (80–90 mg/kg/d)	IM ceftriaxone	IM ceftriaxone × 3 d or tympanocentesis

*High-dose amoxicillin & clavulanate = 80–90 mg/kg/d of the amoxicillin component, with 6.4 mg/kg/d of clavulanate.

Dutch children have outcomes at 2 months similar to those of children from other countries treated with **antibiotics**. Siegel and colleagues (2003) studied the use of a safety-net **antibiotic** prescription in a study of 194 patients in 11 practice sites and found 31 percent filled the **antibiotic** prescription. Of the 69 percent of parents who did not fill the **antibiotic** prescription, 97.4 percent said they were willing to use **pain medication** without **antibiotics** in the future (Siegel et al, 2003). Meropol and colleagues (2008) found that using the watchful waiting approach reduced antibiotic use 67 percent in children aged 2 to 12 years. The pediatric provider needs to educate parents about the rationale for initial observation of AOM and provide adequate pain relief during the observation period to ensure success with this approach.

Pain Relief

Regardless of whether the patient receives **antibiotics**, all children require pain relief for the first 24 to 72 hours of treatment. Adequate dosing of **acetaminophen** (15 mg/kg per dose) or **ibuprofen** (5 to 10 mg/kg per dose) is necessary. It is the provider's responsibility to determine the dose of **analgesic** that ensures adequate pain relief. **Topical analgesia (Auralgan otic solution**, a combination of **antipyrine, benzocaine**, and **u-polycosanol 410 otic solution)** can be applied. In a study of children aged 5 years or older who were being adequately dosed with **acetaminophen** (15 mg/kg), the study patients who received **Auralgan** reported lower ear pain scores than did the control group who received the placebo (olive oil). A number of the study patients reported dramatic and immediate reductions in pain (Hoberman, Paradise, Reynolds, & Urkin, 1997). Some providers stock **Auralgan** in the clinic to provide immediate pain relief for their OM patients. **Auralgan** should never be used before the provider observes an intact TM.

Monitoring

Monitoring the effectiveness of the treatment chosen, either to prescribe **antibiotics** or to provide symptomatic care for the first 2 to 3 days, is essential to the optimal outcome for the patient. Patients may still experience pain with OME, even if the appearance of the TM improves. Patients with persistent symptoms or failure to improve in 48 to 72 hours should be reexamined to determine whether the initial plan (whether antibiotics were prescribed or not) needs to be reevaluated (Klein & Pelton, 2010. If symptoms resolve, patients younger than 2 years of age should be reexamined in 8 to 12 weeks after beginning **antibiotics**, with the understanding that, at 4 weeks, there is a 40 percent chance that fluid is still present in the middle ear and that effusions can last up to 3 months (AAP & AAFP, 2004; Dowell et al, 1998a; Klein & Pelton, 2009; Mason, 1996). Older children (older than 2 years) without language or learning problems can be followed at their next scheduled well child exam, sooner if there are concerns (Klein & Pelton, 2009). If older children have known language or learning problems, they should be examined 8 to 12 weeks after the AOM. **Antibiotics** are not appropriate for the initial treatment of OME, and there is controversy regarding their use at all for this indication, even after 3 months of persistent effusion. Persistent effusion beyond three months is an indication for a referral to otolaryngology.

Outcome Evaluation

The patient should be evaluated 8 to 12 weeks from the beginning of treatment to determine if the infection is completely resolved. The provider may choose to evaluate the patient sooner, with the understanding that some MEE may remain.

Patient Education

Two areas have to be covered in educating patients and families about the use of **antibiotics** for AOM: the proper use of the prescribed **antibiotic** and the predicted course of the infection once **antibiotics** are started. The instructions regarding the **antibiotic** dosage and timing of doses must be clear, and any questions regarding the medication answered. Expected adverse reactions, such as the mild diarrhea that may accompany many of the **antibiotics**, must be discussed. Patients and family members should be aware that the expected course of the ear infection, once **antibiotics** are started, is some symptomatic relief in 24 to 48 hours. Use of **acetaminophen** or **ibuprofen** for pain relief is necessary during this initial period to provide comfort. Parents should be encouraged to give their children a dose of **ibuprofen** or **acetaminophen** just before bedtime because children seem to complain of greater ear pain at night during the healing stages. Patients who are still having significant pain after 48 hours should be reexamined for the possibility of a resistant organism. Bacterial resistance ought to be mentioned, and the patient should be encouraged to complete the course of medication to prevent the development of antibacterial resistance to a partially treated organism.

OTITIS EXTERNA

OE (external OM) is an acute infection that causes an inflammatory reaction in the external auditory canal. It is also known as swimmer's ear.

The patient generally presents with severe ear pain, which may have begun as itching and irritation. The pain is generally unilateral and localized to the ear. Manipulation of the pinna or tragus causes moderate to severe pain, a finding that is usually absent in OM. The TM is normal in OE, but the external auditory canal may be swollen such that the TM is difficult to visualize. Malignant OE is found in patients with diabetes and presents as severe cellulitis due to *Pseudomonas aeruginosa*.

Pathophysiology

Trauma or prolonged exposure to moisture predisposes to infection. The chlorine in swimming pools kills the normal flora in the external ear canal, which allows growth of pathogens. The most common organism found is *P. aeruginosa,* followed by *Staphylococcus aureus.*

Goals of Treatment

The goal of treatment of OE is resolution of the infection, pain control, and prevention of recurrence.

Rational Drug Selection

The medications used in the treatment of OE include combination products (**Cortisporin, Pediotic**) that contain a **corticosteroid (hydrocortisone)** and **antibiotic(s) (neomycin, polymyxin B, ciprofloxacin), antibiotic** alone (**gentamicin, ofloxacin**), and **acid** or **alcohol drops** (Otic Domeboro, Burow's Otic, Vosol, Vosol HC).

The medication of choice is **antibiotic/steroid eardrops**, which combine an **antibiotic(s)** and an anti-inflammatory such as **neomycin sulfate, polymyxin B,** and **hydrocortisone** (Cortisporin Otic, Pediotic); **colistin, neomycin,** and **hydrocortisone** (Coly-Mycin S Otic); or **ciprofloxacin** and **hydrocortisone** (Cipro HC Otic). Eyedrops can be used for external otitis, including **tobramycin** and **dexamethasone** (Tobradex eyedrops), **gentamicin** and **prednisolone** (Pred-G), and **sulfacetamide** and **prednisolone** (Vasocidin solution).

Acid and **alcohol solutions** may also be used. Common products are **Otic Domeboro** and **Burow's Otic**, which contain 2 percent acetic acid in aluminum acetate solution. Another **acid solution, Vosol Otic**, contains 2 percent acetic acid solution and 3 percent propylene glycol. These solutions reduce inflammation and are **antibacterial** and **antifungal**.

Treatment consists of irrigation and **antibiotic eardrops**. The medication of choice is **antibiotic/steroid eardrops**. The routine dosing is three to four drops administered four times a day. Suspension formulations are less ototoxic than solution preparations of eardrops. A cotton wick may be necessary if the ear canal is extremely swollen. For severe cellulitis, parenteral **antistaphylococcal** and **antipseudomonal antibiotics** are necessary. Pain can be severe but patients should have relief with topical therapy, and should only need NSAIDs for pain (Goguen, 2009).

Monitoring

The patient should begin to experience relief from pain in 3 or 4 days. Reevaluation in 1 week determines if the patient is clinically improving. Referral to a dermatologist or otolaryngologist may be necessary if there is no improvement.

Outcome Evaluation

To evaluate the effectiveness of OE treatment, the provider determines if the infection is resolved after treatment with **antibiotic/steroid eardrops**.

Patient Education

Educate the patient to prevent OE by avoiding pooling of water in the ears and by using a mildly acidic solution after swimming. Patients can instill three to four drops of a 1:1 solution of water and white vinegar or 70 percent ethyl alcohol. Commercially available products (**EarSol, Swim-Ear**) can also be used. Earplugs may be helpful for swimmers to avoid developing external otitis.

Explain proper irrigation of debris prior to instillation of eardrops to ensure that the medication contacts the affected area. Swimming should be avoided until external otitis has cleared, ideally for 7 to 10 days (Goguen, 2009). Monitoring for increasing severity is essential to detect cellulitis early in the diabetic patient. The patient may take **ibuprofen** or another **analgesic** for the first 24 to 48 hours of treatment to provide pain relief.

REFERENCES

Adair-Bischoff, C. E., & Sauve, R. S. (1998). Environmental tobacco smoke and middle ear disease in preschool age children. *Archives of Pediatric and Adolescent Medicine, 152,* 127–133.

Adderson, E. E. (1998). Preventing otitis media: Medical approaches. *Pediatric Annals, 27,* 101.

Aitken, M., & Taylor, J. A. (1998). Prevalence of clinical sinusitis in young children followed up by primary care pediatricians. *Archives of Pediatric and Adolescent Medicine, 152*(3), 244–248.

Altemeier, W. A. (1998). A pediatrician's view: Earaches. *Pediatric Annals, 27,* 62–64.

American Academy of Allergy, Asthma, and Immunology (AAAAI); R. G. Slavin, S. L. Spector, & I. L. Bernstein (Eds.). (2005). The diagnosis and management of sinusitis: A practice parameter update. *Journal of Allergy and Clinical Immunology, 116*(6), S13–S47.

American Academy of Pediatrics (AAP) & American Academy of Family Physicians (AAFP). (2004). Clinical Practice Guidelines: Diagnosis and management of acute otitis media. *Pediatrics, 113*(5), 1451–1465.

American Academy of Pediatrics (AAP). (2009a). *Moraxella catarrhalis* infections. In L. K. Pickering (Ed.), *Red book: 2009 Report of the Committee on Infectious Diseases* (28th ed., p. 467). Elk Grove Village, IL: American Academy of Pediatrics. Retrieved from http://aapredbook.aappublications.org/cgi/content/full/2009/1/3.82

American Academy of Pediatrics (AAP). (2009b). *Haemophilus influenzae* infections. In L. K. Pickering (Ed.), *Red book: 2009 Report of the Committee on Infectious Diseases* (28th ed., pp. 314–321). Elk Grove Village, IL: American Academy of Pediatrics. Retrieved from http://aapredbook.aappublications.org/cgi/content/full/2009/1/3.47

Block, S. L., Hedrick, J., Harrison, C. J., Tyler, R., Smith, A., Findlay, R. et al. (2004). Community-wide vaccination with the heptavalent pneumococcal conjugate significantly alters the microbiology of acute otitis media. *Pediatric Infectious Disease Journal, 23*(9), 829–833.

Bramley, T. J., Lerner, D., & Sames, M. (2002). Productivity losses related to the common cold. *Journal of Occupational and Environmental Medicine, 44*(9), 822–829.

Brown, D. J. (1996). *Phytotherapy: Herbal medicine meets clinical science.* Bothell, WA: Bastyr University.

Canafax, D. M., Yuan, Z., Chonmaitree, T., Deka, K., Russlie, H. Q., & Giebink, G. S. (1998). Amoxicillin middle ear fluid penetration and pharmacokinetics in children with acute otitis media. *Pediatric Infectious Disease Journal, 17*(2), 149–155.

Caruso, T. J., Prober, C. G., & Gwaltney, J. M. (2007). Treatment of naturally acquired common colds with zinc: A structured review. *Clinical Infectious Disease, 45*(5), 569–574.

Casey, J. R., & Pichichero, M. E. (2004). Changes in frequency and pathogens causing acute otitis media in 1995–2003. *Pediatric Infectious Diseases Journal, 23,* 824–828.

Chan, Y., & Kuhn, F. A. (2009). An update on the classifications, diagnosis and treatment of rhinosinusitis. *Current Opinion in Otolaryngology & Head and Neck Surgery, 17,* 204–208.

Coco, A., Vernacchio, L., Horst, M., & Anderson, A. (2010). Management of acute otitis media after publication of the 2004 AAP and AAFP clinical practice guideline. *Pediatrics, 125*(2), 214–220.

Conrad, D. A. (1998). Should acute otitis media ever be treated with antibiotics? *Pediatric Annals, 27,* 66.

Contopoulos-Ioannidis, D. G., Ioannidis, J. P. A., & Lau, J. (2003). Acute sinusitis in children: Current treatment strategies. *Pediatric Drugs, 5*(2), 71–80.

Culpepper, L., & Froom, J. (1997). Routine antimicrobial treatment of acute otitis media: Is it necessary? *Journal of the American Medical Association, 278,* 1643.

Dowell, S. F., Butler, J. C., Giebink, G.S., Jacobs, M.R., Jernigan, D., Musher, D. et al. (1999). Acute otitis media. Management and surveillance in an era of pneumococcal resistance: A report from the Drug-Resistant *Streptococcus pneumoniae* Therapeutic Working Group (DRSPTWG). *Pediatric Infectious Disease Journal, 18*(1), 1–9.

Dowell, S. F., Mary, S. M., Phillips, W. R., Gerber, M. A., & Schwartz, B. (1998a). Otitis media: Principles of judicious use of antimicrobial agents. *Pediatrics, 101*(Suppl. 1), 165–169.

Dowell, S. F., Mary, S. M., Phillips, W. R., Gerber, M. A., & Schwartz, B. (1998b). Principles of judicious use of antimicrobial agents for pediatric upper respiratory tract infections. *Pediatrics, 101*(Suppl. 1), 163–165.

Fendrick, A. M., Monto, A. S., Nightengale, B., & Sarnes, M. (2003). The economic burden of non-influenza-related viral respiratory tract infection in the United States. *Archives of Internal Medicine, 163*(4), 487–494.

Finkelstein, J. A., Stille, C., Nordin, J., Davis, R., Raebel, M. A., Roblin, D., et al. (2003). Reduction in antibiotic use among U.S. children, 1996–2000. *Pediatrics, 112*(3), 620–627.

Finkelstein, J. A., Stille, C. J., Rifas-Shiman, S. L., & Goldman, D. (2005). Watchful waiting for an acute otitis media: Are parents and physicians ready? *Pediatrics, 115*(6), 1466–1473.

Friedman, N. D., & Sexton, D. J. (2009). The common cold in adults: Diagnosis and clinical features. *UpToDate Online.* Retrieved from http://www.uptodate.com/online/content/topic.do?topicKey=pc_id/2155&source=preview&selectedTitle=1~150&anchor=H3#H9

Goguen, L. A. (2009). External otitis. *UpToDate Online.* Retrieved from http://www.uptodate.com/online/content/topic.do?topicKey=pc_id/2947&selectedTitle=1%7E150&source=search_result#H14

Gwaltney, J. M., Scheld, W. M., Sande, M. A., & Sydnor, A. (1992). The microbial etiology and antimicrobial therapy of adults with acute community-acquired sinusitis: A fifteen-year experience at the University of Virginia. *Journal of Clinical Immunology, 90*(3 Part 2), 457–461.

Hickey, S. M., & Nelson, J. D. (1997). Mechanisms of antibacterial resistance. *Advances in Pediatrics, 44,* 1.

Hoberman, A., Paradise, J. L., Reynolds, E. A., & Urkin, J. (1997). Efficacy of Auralgan for treating ear pain in children with acute otitis media. *Archives of Pediatric and Adolescent Medicine, 151,* 675.

Hwang, P. H., & Getz, A. (2009). Acute sinusitis and rhinosinusitis in adults. *UpToDate Online.* Retrieved from http://www.uptodate.com/online/content/topic.do?topicKey=pc_id/5943&source=see_link#H15

Jenkins, S. G., & Farrell, D. J. (2009). Increase in pneumococcus macrolide resistance, United States. *Emerging Infectious Diseases, 15*(8), 1260–1264. Retrieved from http://www.cdc.gov/EID/content/15/8/1260.htm

Klein J. O., & Pelton, S. (2009). Otitis media with effusion (serous otitis media) in children. *UpToDate Online.* Retrieved from http://www.uptodate.com/online/content/topic.do?topicKey=pedi_id/12751&selectedTitle=1%7E37&source=search_result

Klein, J. O., & Pelton, S. (2010). Acute otitis media in children: Epidemiology, pathogenesis, clinical manesfestations, and complications. *Up ToDate Online.* Retrieved from http://www.uptodate.com/patients/content/ topic.do?topicKey=~X8HJRL3o3L4fY

Leibovitz, E., Raiz, S., Piglanski, L., Greenberg, D., Yagupsky, P., Fliss, D. M., et al. (1998). Resistance pattern of middle ear fluid isolates in acute otitis media recently treated with antibiotics. *Pediatric Infectious Disease Journal, 17,* 463.

Marshall, I. (2000). Zinc for the common cold. *Cochrane Database,* 2: CD001364.

Mason, W. H. (1996). The management of common infections in ambulatory children. *Pediatric Annals, 25,* 620.

McBride, T. P., Doyle, W. J., Hayden, F. G., & Gwaltney, J. M. (1989). Alterations of the eustachian tube, middle ear, and nose in rhinovirus infection. *Archives in Otolaryngology, Head and Neck Surgery, 115*(9), 1054–1059.

Meropol, S. B., Glick, H. A., & Asch, D. A. (2008). Age inconsistency in the American Academy of Pediatrics guidelines for acute otitis media. *Pediatrics, 121*(4), 657–668.

O'Brien, K. L., Dowell, S. F., Schwartz, B., Marcy, S. M., Phillips, W. R., & Gerber, M. D. (1998). Acute sinusitis: Principles of judicious use of antimicrobial agents. *Pediatrics, 101*(Suppl.), 174.

Pappas, D. E., & Hendley, J. O. (2009). The common cold in children. *Up ToDate Online.* Retrieved from http://www.uptodate.com/online/content/topic.do?topicKey=pedi_id/16291&source=see_link#H2

Paradise, J. L. (1997). Short-course antimicrobial treatment for acute otitis media: Not best for infants and young children. *Journal of the American Medical Association, 278,* 1640.

Paradise, J. L., Rockette, H. E., Colborn, D. K., Bernard, B. S., Smith, C. G., Kurs-Lasky, M., et al. (1997). Otitis media in 2253 Pittsburgh-area infants: Prevalence and risk factors during the first two years of life. *Pediatrics, 99*(3), 318–333.

Prasad, A. S., Beck, F. W., Bao, B., Snell, D., & Fitzgerald, J. T. (2008). Duration and severity of symptoms and levels of plasma interleukin=1 receptor antagonist, soluble tumor necrosis factor receptor, and adhesion molecules in patients with common cold treated with zinc acetate. *Journal of Infectious Disease, 197*(6), 795–802.

Prince, A. (1998). Infectious diseases. In R. E. Behrman & R. M. Kliegman (Eds.), *Nelson essentials of pediatrics* (3rd ed., p. 341). Philadelphia: Saunders.

Rosenfeld, R. M., Andes, D., Bhattacharyya, N., Cheung, D., Eisenberg, S., Ganiats, T. G., & Witsell, D. L. (2007). Clinical practice guideline: Adult sinusitis. *Otolaryngology—Head and Neck Surgery, 137,* S1–S31.

Siegel, R. M., Kiely, M., Bien, J. P., Joseph, E. C., Davis, J. B., Mendel, S. G., et al. (2003). Treatment of otitis media with observation and a safety-net antibiotic prescription. *Pediatrics, 112*(3), 527–531.

Simon, R. P. (1998). Parameningeal infections. In R. E. Behrman & R. M. Kliegman (Eds.), *Nelson essentials of pediatrics* (3rd ed., p. 2080). Philadelphia: Saunders.

Spurling, G. K. P., Del Mar, C., Dooley, L., & Foxlee, R. (2007). Delayed antibiotics for respiratory infections. *Cochrane Database of Systematic Reviews,* 3. Art. No.: CD004417.

Strachan, D. P., & Cook, D. G. (1998). Health effects of passive smoking. *Thorax, 53*(1), 50–56.

Taverner, D., & Latte, J. (2007). Nasal decongestants for the common cold. *Cochrane Database of Systematic Reviews (Online),* 1, Art. No.: CD001953.

Teele, D. W., Klein, J. O., & Rosner, B. (1989). Epidemiology of otitis media during the first seven years of life in children in greater Boston. *Journal of Infectious Diseases, 160*(1), 83–94.

Van Buchem, F., Peeters, M., & van't Hof, M. (1985). Acute otitis media: A new treatment strategy. *British Medical Journal (Clinical Research Edition), 290*(6474), 1033–1037.

Wald, E. R. (2010). Acute bacterial sinusitis in children: Microbiology and treatment. *UpToDate Online.* Retrieved from http://www.uptodate.com/online/content/topic.do?topicKey=pedi_id/21866&selected Title=1%7E150&source=search_result

CHAPTER 47

URINARY TRACT INFECTIONS

Teri Moser Woo

Chapter Outline

Urinary tract infections (UTIs) are responsible for 8.27 million (1.41 million men; 6.86 million women) office visits per year (Litwin & Sagel, 2007). UTIs are more common in women because the short female urethra provides easy access to the bladder for bacteria. The lifetime risk of a woman developing a UTI is 60.4 percent (Foxman, Barlow, D'Arcy, Gillespie, & Sobel, 2000). In a study of self-reported UTI, 10.8 percent of women over age 18 years stated they had a UTI in the past 12 months (Foxman et al, 2000). UTIs also occur in men who have a 13.6 percent lifetime risk, with most UTIs related to urinary tract obstructions such as benign prostatic hypertrophy reflected in the increased incidence of UTI as men age (Griebling, 2007a). UTIs affect 2.6 percent to 3.4 percent of children annually, with a childhood risk of developing a UTI 2 percent for boys and 8 percent for girls (Freedman, 2007). In infant males, circumcision decreases the risk of developing a UTI, with the rate in the first 6 months of life in uncircumcised boys 12 times higher than in circumcised boys (Freedman, 2007). Vesicoureteral reflux, constipation, and dysfunctional voiding all increase the risk for UTI in children (Freedman, 2007).

Most patients with UTIs do not experience long-term complications from these disorders. Those who do usually have a comorbid condition such as vesicoureteral reflux, renal stones, neurogenic bladder, diabetes, or obstruction. This chapter discusses the management of uncomplicated UTIs in otherwise healthy patients who do not have these comorbid conditions and who do not have retention catheters inserted.

PATHOPHYSIOLOGY

A complex interaction between host and microbial factors leads to UTIs. The anatomy and physiology of the genitourinary tract offer protective defenses against UTIs, although certain factors may increase risk for developing a UTI in certain populations. Likewise, behavioral factors may contribute to developing UTIs.

Host Factors

Anatomy and Physiology of the Genitourinary Tract

The bladder has unique intrinsic defenses against infection. Periodic washout, by voiding, of the bacteria that perpetually colonize the urethra is one of the main defense mechanisms. The bladder also deters microbial adherence to the mucosa through the antibacterial properties of the urinary bladder epithelium. Patients who have repeated UTIs appear to have altered bladder epithelial cells that facilitate adherence of bacteria to the mucosa rather than deter it. The low pH and high osmolality of urea and secretions from the uroepithelium and a competent urethral valve that prevents backflow also decrease

UTIs. The longer urethra and prostatic secretions decrease the risk of infection in men.

These defense mechanisms are severely limited if residual urine is regularly present after voiding. Pregnancy increases the risk for UTIs because of pressure on the bladder from the enlarging fetus, increased incidence of residual urine, and changes in estrogen levels. Genetic factors, including expression of HLA-A3 and Lewis blood group Le(a-b-) or Le(a+b-), may put women at higher risk for developing UTIs (Griebling, 2007b). Estrogen deficiency and concomitant decreased acidification of the vagina, with increased vaginal colonization by *Enterobacteriaceae*, also contribute to increased risk in postmenopausal women. Men who develop benign prostatic hypertrophy (BPH) are at increased risk of developing a UTI due to bladder outlet obstruction (Griebling, 2007a). Fecal and urinary incontinence, lack of estrogen, immunocompromised states—including diabetes mellitus and taking **antibiotics** for other infections—have been associated with increased risk in the older adult. Any instrumentation of the urinary tract—including catheter placement or cystoscopy—place patients at risk of developing a UTI (Griebling, 2007a).

Behavioral Factors

Sexually active women are at higher risk than sexually inactive women for developing UTIs. Frequency of sexual intercourse, diaphragm or spermicide use, and failure to void within 10 to 15 minutes of coitus have all been associated with a risk for UTIs in women (Griebling, 2007b; Towers, 2000). Reasons for the increased risk may be urethral trauma, decreased urge to void, and residual urine. Diaphragm or spermicide use also appears to compromise host defense mechanisms to the extent necessary for virulent strains of bacteria to become capable of causing an infection.

Other behavioral factors have been inconsistently associated with UTI and are subject to some controversy. Purposely resisting the urge to void has been associated with UTIs in some studies and not in others. Increased fluid intake has also had an inconsistent association, although it is difficult to find a reason not to suggest adequate fluid intake for a variety of reasons, including increasing bacterial washout through more frequent voiding. Cranberry juice has an "on-again, off-again" history of association with prevention of UTI (Berger, 2005). Little evidence indicates that the direction of wiping after bowel movements, the use of oral contraceptives or tampons, or the habit of taking bubble baths or douching contributes to UTIs.

Microbial Factors

Ability of the Bacteria to Adhere to Epithelial Cells

Escherichia coli is responsible for 85 percent of community-acquired UTIs and 50 percent of hospital-acquired UTIs. This organism is successful in part because it contains fimbriae that allow attachment to host cell receptor sites on the bladder mucosa. Some women are thought to be genetically susceptible to certain strains of *E. coli* attachment. Other organisms that commonly infect the urinary tract include *Klebsiella, Proteus* (more common in men), *Pseudomonas,* and *Staphylococcus saprophyticus.*

Virulence of the Organism

Coliforms cultured from women with recurrent UTIs were more virulent than those cultured from patients with first-time infections or from the fecal flora of patients who had no history of UTIs.

Ability of the Organism to Survive the Urinary Tract Environment

Some bacteria are more tolerant of the low pH of urine. Table 47–1 lists the factors shown by research to be associated with the occurrence of UTIs. It also lists those factors that have been inconsistently related to UTIs or not demonstrated by research to be associated with UTIs.

Inflammatory Reaction to Bacteria

Infection with any organism initiates an inflammatory response and the symptoms of cystitis. The inflammatory edema in the bladder wall stimulates stretch receptors, which discharge with even small volumes of urine, producing the urgency and frequency or urination association with UTIs. Prostaglandins released from the mast cell as part of the inflammatory response produce pain. They also increase vascular permeability, which may be exhibited as hematuria.

Diagnosis of UTI is based on symptoms and laboratory data. Presenting symptoms of UTI vary with age. Table 47–2 shows the various symptoms by age. Symptom presentation is similar for both men and women. All ages often exhibit dark, cloudy, and malodorous urine. Urethral discharge in men is more commonly associated with sexually transmitted infections (STIs) than with UTIs. STIs are discussed in Chapter 44.

Laboratory data for diagnosis include urinalysis (UA) and urine culture and sensitivity. The most common findings from a clean-catch urine specimen are (1) a positive leukocyte esterase or pyuria (usually greater than 5 white blood cells [WBCs] per high-power field), which has a sensitivity range of 90 to 100 percent and a specificity range of 58 to 91 percent; (2) the presence of bacteria, which has a sensitivity of approximately 81 percent and a specificity of approximately 83 percent; (3) and/or a positive dipstick for nitrates. When all are positive, the sensitivity is 99 to 100 percent and the specificity is up to 92 percent. The presence of casts or hematuria suggests an upper UTI. Quantitative urine cultures are the most reliable method for diagnosing UTIs; however, they require trained personnel, are more expensive, and take time to complete, which might lead to postponing treatment of symptomatic patients. Cultures are usually reserved for

Table 47–1 **Factors Associated With Urinary Tract Infections**

Host Factors	Microbial Factors	Inconsistent or Not Associated Factors
	Anatomical and Physiological	
• Periodic washout with voiding* • Bladder epithelial cells that prevent adherence of bacteria* • Acid pH of urine* • Osmolality of urine* • Competent urethral valves to prevant backflow of urine* • Pregnancy • Estrogen deficiency • Residual urine • Lack of circumcision in males • Benign prostate hyperplasia	• Ability of the organism to adhere to epithelial cells • Virulence of the organism • Ability of the organism to survive the urinary tract environment	• Ingestion of cranberry juice* • Purposely resisting the urge to void • Increased fluid intake* • Wiping from front to back after defecation* • Oral contraceptive use • Tampon use • Bubble baths • Douching
	Behavioral	
• Frequent sexual intercourse • Diaphragm use • Spermicide use • Failure to void 10–15 min after coitus • Multiple sexual partners • Anal intercourse • Fecal and urinary incontinence		

*These factors are negatively associated with UTIs and may prevent them.

children and men and for recurrent UTIs in women. Pregnant women should be screened for bacteriuria by urine culture at least once in early pregnancy since this population is at risk for asymptomatic UTI (Institute for Clinical Systems Improvement [ICSI], 2004; Nicolle et al, 2005). Nicolle and colleagues do not recommend screening for or treatment of asymptomatic bacteriuria for premenopausal, nonpregnant women; diabetic women; older persons living in the community; older adults who are institutionalized; or catheterized patients while the catheter is still in place. Older institutionalized adults who exhibit altered mental status from their norm should be screened for UTI, as this symptom may indicate UTI in the absence of other reported symptoms.

PHARMACODYNAMICS

There is a wide range of antimicrobial agents available for treatment of UTIs. They include trimethoprim/sulfamethoxazole (Bactrim, Septra), nitrofurantoin (Furadantin, Macrodantin), fluoroquinolones (ciprofloxacin [Cipro], gatifloxacin [Tequin], levofloxacin [Lavaquin], ofloxacin [Floxin]), cephalosporins (cephalexin [Keflex], cefixime [Suprax]), and penicillins

Table 47–2 **Urinary Tract Infection Symptoms by Age**

Neonate	Failure to thrive, irritability, fever, hypothermia, sepsis, jaundice, vomiting, acidosis
Infant	Failure to thrive, irritability, fever, hypothermia, sepsis, jaundice, vomiting, acidosis, hematuria, urinary frequency, dysuria
Preschool- or school-age child	Abdominal or suprapubic pain, dysuria, frequency, urgency, enuresis, urinary incontinence
Adult	• Dysuria, frequency, urgency, burning on urination, incontinence, urethral pain, suprapubic pain, low back pain, hematuria. • Significant fever is unusual in bladder infections but may occur, along with severe flank pain and costovertebral tenderness, in upper UTIs • Patients with upper UTIs may also demonstrate headache, malaise, nausea, and vomiting • Symptoms are similar for women and men
Older adult	• Same symptoms as adult, but also mental status changes from patient's norm • Urinary incontinence

(amoxicillin [Amoxil], amoxicillin/clavulanate [Augmentin]). The spectrum of antimicrobial activity varies among these agents. Recent studies have shown a slight but generalized decrease in bacterial susceptibility to some of these agents. Each of these is discussed in Chapter 24.

A *Cochrane Review* of the use of cranberries in the treatment of UTI concluded that cranberry products decrease the incidence of symptomatic UTIs over a 12-month period, especially in patients with recurrent UTIs (Jepson & Craig, 2008). Studies indicate that a substrate in cranberries may exert a bacteriostatic effect by inhibiting the adherence of organisms to the mucosal surface of the bladder. Cranberries also change the surface properties of *E. coli*, preventing it from adhering to the bladder wall (Jepson & Craig, 2008). The recommended dose is one 300- to 400-mg cranberry tablet daily or three 8-ounce glasses of unsweetened, pure cranberry juice daily (not cranberry drink) (Jepson & Craig, 2008). A wide variety of cranberry products is available OTC. **Azo-Cranberry** contains 450 mg of natural cranberry concentrate powder; **Nature's Way Cranberry** and **GNC Cranberry** capsules contain 500 mg of cranberry concentrate.

Symptomatic relief is often provided by **urinary analgesics**. The primary ingredient in these products is **phenazopyridine**, an azo dye taken orally that exerts a **topical analgesic** effect on the urinary tract mucosa when it is excreted into the urine. This dye is available under several different brand names. **Azo-Standard**, **Prodium**, **Pyridium**, **Uricalm**, and **Urogesic** all contain **phenazopyridine** 95 mg.

GOALS OF TREATMENT

Eradication of the causative organism is the primary goal of therapy. Relief of symptoms and prevention of recurrent infections are also therapeutic goals.

RATIONAL DRUG SELECTION

The main focus of this section is appropriate selection and use of drugs to treat both upper and lower UTIs.

Algorithm

This chapter does not discuss the testing involved in the diagnosis of UTIs beyond that needed for treatment decisions. The treatment protocol here assumes accurate diagnosis of the UTI by means of the appropriate diagnostic tools, including laboratory data. Once the diagnosis has been made, treatment regimens are determined.

Treatment of UTIs is directed at the three goals of eradication of organisms, relief of symptoms and prevention of recurrence. The infecting organism is eradicated with **antimicrobial therapy**. Treatment for symptom relief often includes **urinary analgesics**. Prevention of recurrence may involve **prophylactic drug therapy** but involves lifestyle management as well.

Drug Therapy

Drug therapy is aimed at eradicating the infecting organism. Appropriate **antimicrobial** selection is based on drug variables—spectrum of activity of the drug, potential adverse drug reactions, patterns of resistance to the **antimicrobial**, and cost—and patient variables—age, gender, pregnancy, and the underlying cause of the UTI.

Drug Variables

Spectrum of Activity

Lower tract UTIs are most commonly caused by gram-negative bacteria (95% of UTIs), with *E. coli* the most prevalent organism (80% of all lower UTIs are caused by *E. coli*) (Wagenlehner, Weidner, & Naber, 2005). Among community-acquired infections, *S. saprophyticus*, *Klebsiella*, and gram-negative enteric bacilli cause almost all the UTIs not caused by *E. coli*. In children, additional organisms include *Klebsiella* in neonates and *Proteus* in boys. All of the antimicrobial agents mentioned have a spectrum of activity that covers these organisms.

Empirical treatment with **trimethoprim/sulfamethoxazole (TMP/SMX, Septra, Bactrim)** is the first-line treatment choice when no complicating factors are present. **TMP/SMX** has fallen out of favor in spite of its being the recommended first-line drug per guidelines, inexpensive, and effective (Griebling, 2007b; Grover et al, 2007). A 3-day treatment is cost effective, increases compliance, and reduces risk of developing *Candida* vaginitis (Thomas & Porter, 2007). The recommended dose for treating uncomplicated UTI in adults is one double-strength tablet bid for 3 days (Hooton, 2011). The dose of **TMP/SMZ** to treat UTIs in children older than 2 months of age is 6 to 12 mg trimethoprim/30 to 60 mg sulfamethoxazole/kg/day in two divided doses (1 mL suspension per kg/d). Children should be treated with a 10-day regimen. Resistance to **TMP/SMZ** is seen in patients who have had antibiotic therapy for any reason in the past 3 months or if they have been hospitalized recently.

An alternative first-line treatment is the **fluoroquinolone ciprofloxacin**. The dose is 250 mg bid for 3 days or **ciprofloxacin extended release (Cipro XR)** 500 mg daily for 3 days. Note that generic **ciprofloxacin** is similar in cost to **TMP/SMZ**, but **Cipro XR** is significantly more expensive ($4 versus $28 for a 3-day supply). Other **fluoroquinolones** that may be used as second-line therapy include **Gatifloxacin** 200 to 400 mg daily and **levofloxacin** 250 mg daily. **Moxifloxacin** and **gemifloxacin** are not approved for use with UTIs because they have poor concentration in the urine. **Fluoroquinolone** resistance has been steadily increasing, with 24.2 percent of *E. coli* resistant to **ciprofloxacin** and 24 percent resistant to **levofloxacin** (Kashanian et al, 2008). Cross-resistance occurs with the **fluoroquinolones**. **Fluoroquinolones** are not prescribed to children or pregnant women because of concern for adverse effects on joints and cartilage in animal studies. The exception is **ciprofloxacin**, which has U.S. Food and Drug Administration (FDA) approval as second-line therapy in complicated UTI or pyelonephritis in children.

Beta-lactam antibiotics such as **amoxicillin** or the **cephalosporins (cephalexin, cefpodoxime, cefixime)** can be prescribed as second-line therapy to patients who are allergic to **sulfa** drugs or the **fluoroquinolones** or as first-line treatment for women who are pregnant. Twenty-five to 70 percent of *E. coli* is resistant to **amoxicillin**; therefore, it should not be used as first-line therapy unless patient factors warrant its use.

Nitrofurantoin is an effective treatment for UTIs, with a low *E. coli* resistance rate of 2.1 percent in a recent study comparing it to **TMP/SMZ**, **ciprofloxacin**, and **levofloxacin** (Kashanian et al, 2008). The adult dose for **nitrofurantoin** is 50 to 100 mg four times a day for 7 to 10 days. The pediatric dose is 5 to 7 mg/kg/day divided every 6 hours for 7 to 10 days. Shortened therapy should not be used. This drug can be used prophylactically in adults and children who have recurrent UTIs more often than three times per year. **Nitrofurantoin** is Pregnancy Category B, but should be avoided in pregnancy near term, in labor, and during lactation when the infant is less than 1 month of age because of a risk for the infant to develop hemolytic anemia.

Any of these treatments generally sterilizes the urine and produces symptom relief in 24 or fewer hours. Patients who are very symptomatic or have severe burning on urination can have **phenazopyridine** 200 mg three times a day added to their treatment regimen for 2 to 3 days as a **urinary analgesic**.

Complicating factors in which short-course (3-day) therapy is not appropriate (ICSI, 2002) include the following:

- Symptoms longer than 7 days' duration
- Shaking chills (rigors)
- Flank pain: midback, severe, new occurring with onset of UTI symptoms
- History of diabetes, pregnancy, immunosuppressed, renal calculi, renal insufficiency, discharge from hospital or nursing home within the past 2 weeks, four or more UTIs in past year, failure of this drug to treat UTI within the past 4 months, or resident of extended-care facility

For patients with complicating factors, longer treatment protocols are needed or referral may be appropriate. Urine culture should be used to guide therapy.

All of the drugs discussed so far may also be used for prophylaxis. The drug of choice for adults for prophylaxis or for recurrent infections (more than three infections in 1 year) is **trimethoprim/sulfamethoxazole** one single-strength tablet daily at bedtime for a minimum of 6 months or a self-administered single dose of two double-strength tablets at symptom onset. For children, the recommended dose of **trimethoprim/sulfamethoxazole** is 2 mg trimethoprim/10 mg sulfamethoxazole per kg as a single bedtime dose (American Academy of Pediatrics, 1999). The **nitrofurantoin** adult dose is 50 to 100 mg at bedtime and children 1 to 2 mg/kg/day in a single dose (Gaylord & Starr, 2009).

Patients with risk factors for STIs, a positive dipstick for leukocyte esterase or hemoglobin, and a negative Gram's stain are likely to have a UTI complicated by *Chlamydia trachomatis*. The recommended drug for these patients is **doxycycline (Doxy-Caps, Vibramycin)** 100 mg bid for 7 days. The alternative drug is **azithromycin (Zithromax)** 1 g in a single dose. **Azithromycin** is the preferred drug if the patient's adherence to the 7-day regimen is questionable.

Upper UTIs (e.g., pyelonephritis) involve the same likely organisms because the infections are most often ascended from a bladder infection; *E. coli* is the identified organism in more than 80 percent of pyelonephritis cases. Failure of a 3-day course of **antimicrobials** generally indicates an upper UTI. Uncomplicated pyelonephritis in adults can usually be treated with an oral **antibiotic** with a 90 percent success rate (Ramakrishnan & Scheid, 2005). A pyelonephritis is uncomplicated if it is caused by a typical pathogen in an immunocompetent person with a normal urinary tract (Ramakrishnan & Scheid, 2005). The ICSI recommends **ciprofloxacin** 500 mg twice a day for 7 to 14 days as the first-line drug for nonpregnant adults (2004). Other **fluoroquinolones (gatifloxacin** 400 mg daily, **levofloxacin** 250 mg daily, or **ofloxacin** 400 mg bid) may also be used. The alternative drugs recommended are **amoxicillin/clavulanate** or an oral **cephalosporin** with the treatment extending for 14 days. Pregnant patients should be treated with **amoxicillin** or **amoxicillin/clavulanate** and followed closely. Patients with acute pyelonephritis who are not acutely ill or in whom oral therapy can be assured (i.e., not vomiting) may benefit from 1 to 2 g **ceftriaxone** IM at the time of diagnosis and switched to oral therapy on day 2 of treatment. Acutely ill patients require initiating parenteral therapy in an inpatient observation unit or hospital admission for IV fluids and parenteral antibiotics.

Potential Adverse Drug Reactions

A significant number of patients have allergies to **sulfonamides** and **penicillins**. Approximately 15 percent of patients allergic to **penicillin** are also allergic to the other class of **beta-lactam drugs, cephalosporins**. Note: Patients with allergies to other substances such as pet dander and pollens are at high risk for drug allergies. Patients allergic to **sulfonamides** and **penicillins** can be treated with **nitrofurantoin** 50 to 100 mg bid.

Amoxicillin and **cephalosporins** have a negative effect on bowel flora and often result in diarrhea. This adverse reaction is much less common with **trimethoprim**, and **nitrofurantoin** does not affect bowel flora. Patients with bowel disease should be given either of the latter two drugs.

The **fluoroquinolones**—including **ciprofloxacin**—that are usually well tolerated have a black box warning regarding the development of tendonitis and tendon rupture, even after therapy has been completed. The risk is greatest in patients over age 60 years, those on corticosteroid therapy, and patients with previous tendon disorders or who exercise strenuously. **Fluoroquinolones** may have central nervous system effects including increased intracranial pressure, dizziness, confusion, tremors, hallucinations, depression, and rarely, suicidal thoughts (Bayer Healthcare Pharmaceuticals, 2009). Patients with a known seizure disorder or a disorder that may predispose them to seizures should not be prescribed **fluoroquinolones**, as the drugs may lower the seizure threshold. **Fluoroquinolones** should not be prescribed for pregnant women because of the risk of joint disorders in the fetus and green discoloration of primary teeth developing in newborns. **Fluoroquinolones** are not the drug of first choice in pediatric patients because of concerns for joint disorders. The only exception is **ciprofloxacin,** which can be prescribed as second-line therapy in complicated UTIs and pyelonephritis in children ages 1 year to 17 years.

Long-term therapy with **nitrofurantoin** has been associated with pulmonary fibrosis and peripheral neuropathy. Short-term therapy has not been associated with this problem. If this drug is chosen for prophylaxis, it should be used for no more than 3 months. **Nitrofurantoin** should not be prescribed to pregnant women at term or during labor because of the risk of hemolytic anemia in the newborn. The drug should also be avoided in lactating women whose infants are less than a month of age for the same reason.

Resistance Patterns

Drug resistance to **antimicrobial therapy** is a major factor in drug selection. In the United States, the resistance of *E. coli* to **trimethoprim/sulfamethoxazole** is approximately 15 to 20 percent and the same level of resistance has recently been reported for **ciprofloxacin** and **levofloxacin** (Griebling, 2007b; Kashanian et al, 2008). Resistance to **fluoroquinolones** among *E. coli* isolates has been increasing; and they should be thoughtfully prescribed. Resistance patterns vary in other countries. Prais and colleagues (2003) report research data from Israel, the United Kingdom, the Netherlands, and South Africa that show a clear difference in resistance patterns. In all of these countries, however, resistance to **trimethoprim/sulfamethoxazole** is lower than to any other drugs. **Nitrofurantoin** resistance was less than 10 percent in all countries studied and only 2 percent in the United States. Prais and colleagues (2003) also found that **cephalexin** was inadequate to resolve UTI in approximately one-third of cases, but 95 percent of the organisms were susceptible to **cefuroxime axetil** and **amoxicillin/clavulanate. Amoxicillin** is no longer recommended for empirical therapy in the United States because up to one-third of the UTI organisms are resistant. Providers should be aware of local resistance patterns in their community. Providers can consult with their reference laboratory regarding the antibiogram pattern of resistance. The resistance patterns seen in inpatients may be different from community patterns of resistance.

Cost

Trimethoprim/sulfamethoxazole is the least expensive of the **antimicrobials**, especially when it can be given for 1 to 3 days. Generic **ciprofloxacin** is comparable in cost with **TMP/SMZ** for a 3-day supply, but be aware that brand-name **Cipro XR** is significantly more expensive than generic **ciprofloxacin. Nitrofurantoin** is also relatively inexpensive, although the brand-name **Macrodantin** that has bid dosing is more expensive. Cost comparisons for the **antimicrobials** are presented in Chapter 24.

Table 47–3 summarizes **antimicrobial** recommendations for upper and lower UTIs. Recommendations are included for adults and children. Figure 47–1 depicts the treatment protocol for management of UTIs in adult women.

Patient Variables

Age

Infants and Children

Signs and symptoms of UTI in infants and very young children are different from those in adults. The likelihood of UTI, especially with fever, increases in these circumstances: a history of crying on urination, foul-smelling urine, altered urination pattern, irritability, vomiting, diarrhea, and failure to thrive. All infants with fever of unknown origin should have a catheterized urine specimen obtained to rule out a UTI. The most accurate diagnosis of a UTI in a non–toilet trained child is made with a catheterized urine sample. Bagged urine samples should not be used to diagnose a UTI (AAP, 1999). The common UTI symptoms of dysuria, urgency, frequency, and hesitancy may be present in preschool-age children, but are difficult to discern in this age group. The older the child is, the more likely he or she is to have the "classic" UTI symptoms of dysuria and frequency.

Febrile UTI is treated aggressively in infants and children, as fever is often an indication of pyelonephritis (Gaylord & Starr, 2009). Infants and children with febrile UTI should receive parenteral antibiotics for the first 24 hours or until afebrile. **Ceftriaxone** 50 to 75 mg/kg divided every 12 to 24 hours IV/IM is often used in children older than 3 months because of the convenience of 24-hour dosing. Other appropriate parenteral antibiotic choices are **cefotaxime, deftazidime, ampicillin,** or **gentamicin** (see Table 47–3 for dosing).

All infants and children with febrile UTI are evaluated daily until afebrile. Complicated febrile UTI in children warrants inpatient treatment with IV antibiotics. Symptoms

Table 47–3 **Drugs Commonly Used: Upper and Lower Urinary Tract Infections**

Indication	Primary Choices	Alternative Choices
	Upper UTIs (Adults)	
Simple, uncomplicated upper UTI Mild to moderately ill	• Ciprofloxacin 500 mg bid for 14 d • Trimethoprim-sulfamethoxazole double-strength 1 tablet bid for 14 d *or* • Ofloxacin 400 mg bid for 14 d If client status warrants: give 1 to 2 g ceftriaxone IV on day 1, switching to one of the oral medications above on day 2	• Amoxicillin-clavulanate 500 mg bid for 14 d • Cefixime 200 mg bid for 14 d
	Lower UTIs	
Simple, uncomplicated lower UTI in adults Symptomatic or asymptomatic and reinfection (single event)	• Trimethoprim-sulfamethoxazole double-strength 1 tablet bid for 3 d *or* • Ciprofloxacin 250 mg bid for 3 d • Ciprofloxacin Extended Release 500 mg daily for 3 d	• Nitrofurantoin 50–100 mg bid for 7 d if resistance to *Escherichia coli* ≥20% • Gatifloxacin 200–400 mg daily for 3 days • Levofloxacin 250 mg daily for 3 d
Simple, uncomplicated lower UTI Serial reinfections (more than 3/yr)	• Trimethoprim-sulfamethoxazole double-strength 1 tablet bid for 3 d with onset of symptoms	• Ciprofloxacin 250 mg bid for 3 d with onset of symptoms
Simple, uncomplicated lower UTI associated with intercourse prophylaxis	• Trimethoprim-sulfamethoxazole double-strength 1 tablet single dose after intercourse	• Ciprofloxacin 250-mg single dose after intercourse
Simple, uncomplicated lower UTI recurrence prophylaxis	• Trimethoprim-sulfamethoxazole double-strength 1 tablet daily at bedtime for at least 6 mo	• Nitrofurantoin 50 mg daily at bedtime for no more than 3 mo
Complicated lower UTI or symptomatic after 3 d of therapy	• Trimethoprim-sulfamethoxazole double-strength 1 tablet bid for 7–14 d • Ciprofloxacin 250 mg bid for 7–14 d	• Nitrofurantoin 100 mg bid for 7–14 d • Ofloxacin 200 mg bid for 7–14 d
	Special Considerations	
Risk factors for STD	• Doxycycline 100 mg bid for 7 d	• Azithromycin 1-g single dose
Pregnancy	• Nitrofurantoin 100 mg bid for 7 d	• Amoxicillin 500 mg tid for 7 d • Cefixime 200 mg bid for 7 d
Afebrile children: >1 month	• Trimethoprim-sulfamethoxazole 6 to 12 mg/kg/d trimethoprim plus 30 to 60 mg/kg/d sulfamethoxazole given in 2 divided doses for 10 d in infants >2 months of age	• Nitrofurantoin 5 to 7 mg/kg/d in 3 or 4 divided doses x 10 d • Amoxicillin 40 mg/kg/d in 2 or 3 divided doses x 10 d if no resistance in the community • Augmentin 40 mg/kg/d of amoxicillin component divided TID x 10 d • Cefixime 8 mg/kg/d • Cephalexin 25 to 50 mg/kg/d in 3 or 4 doses • Cefpodoxime 10 mg/kg/d in 2 divided doses

Febrile UTI in children >1 month of age	• Parenteral antibiotics for first 24 h or until afebrile
	  • Ceftriaxone 50 to 75 mg/kg every 12 to 24 h
	  • Cefotaxime 150 mg/kg/d divided every 6 to 8 h
	  • Ceftazidime 150 mg/kg/d divided every 6–8 h
	• Oral antibiotics are started once the child is afebrile and continued for 10 to 14 d, followed by prophylaxis until radiological work-up is complete
	• Oral antibiotic choices are the same as for afebrile UTI	

Estrogen deficiency/ postmenopausal female	• Vaginal estrogen cream 0.5–2 g intravaginally daily	
Advanced age	• No treatment if asymptomatic	

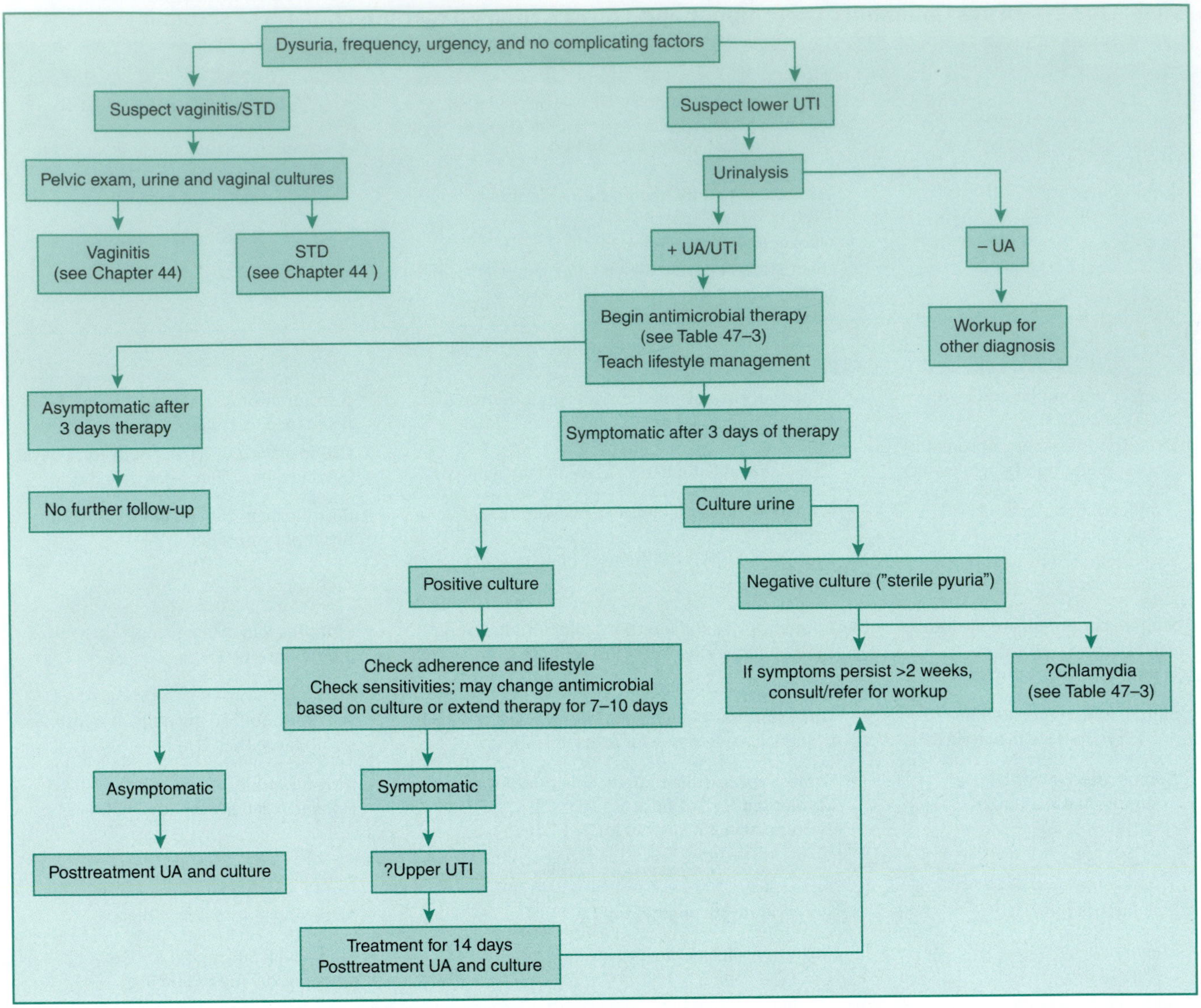

Figure 47–1. Treatment protocol: Urinary tract infections in women.

warranting inpatient treatment include high fever, toxic appearance, persistent vomiting, moderate to severe dehydration, poor compliance (Gaylord & Starr, 2009). In addition, any patient younger than age 6 months who appears toxic should receive initial inpatient treatment for febrile UTI.

The goals for treatment of UTI in infants and children are the same as those for adults, with the exception that a search should be made for anatomical abnormalities of the bladder and kidneys. The American Academy of Pediatrics (1999) and Cincinnati Children's Hospital (2006) guidelines recommend a cystogram and renal ultrasound in the following children with UTI: all males, all females younger than 36 months, and females age 3 to 7 years with a fever of 38.5°C or above. Infants and young children are at higher risk for incurring acute renal injury, because the incidence of vesicoureteral reflux is higher in this age group than it is in older children (American Academy of Pediatrics, 2000; Cincinnati Children's Hospital, 2006). In addition, the risk of renal damage increases as the number of recurrences of UTI increases. Children with documented or suspected vesicoureteral reflux, renal scarring, or structural abnormalities of the urinary tract should be referred to a pediatric urologist. Children with an identified renal or bladder stone should also be referred to a pediatric urologist. Children should be on prophylactic antibiotics until the urological evaluation is complete.

Adolescents with pyelonephritis or a second UTI with documented positive urine cultures and no history of recent sexual activity require at least consultation (Gaylord & Starr, 2009). The American Academy of Pediatrics guidelines for the treatment of febrile UTI have not been updated since 1999. An update is due and is expected in 2011.

Older children (older than age 5) can be treated with the same drugs as adults, whether they are asymptomatic or symptomatic, but the extent of treatment may need to be 7 to 14 days. In a meta-analysis of published randomized, controlled trials in children 0 to 18 years of age comparing long-course (7 to 14 days) with short-course (3 days or less) **antibiotic treatment** of UTI, long-course therapy was associated with fewer treatment failures with concomitant increase in reinfections, even when studies including subjects with evidence of pyelonephritis were excluded from the analysis. Based on this analysis, Keren and Chan (2002) recommend that clinicians continue to treat children with UTI for 7 to 14 days until more accurate methods of distinguishing upper from lower UTIs in children are available.

Consideration should be given to the effect of the agent chosen on bowel flora, which is highly correlated with diarrhea. Younger children are more likely to experience fluid volume deficits secondary to diarrhea. Among the available drugs, **nitrofurantoin** has the least effect on bowel flora and **amoxicillin** has the most effect. The effect of **trimethoprim/sulfamethoxazole** is only slightly more than that of **nitrofurantoin.** Figure 47–2 shows the treatment protocol for management of UTIs in children.

Older Adults

Elderly patients are at increased risk for UTIs and asymptomatic bacteriuria. In 1999, UTI was reported as the admitting or current diagnosis in 7.1 percent of female and 5.6 percent of male nursing home residents (Griebling, 2007a). Asymptomatic bacteriuria may be present in more

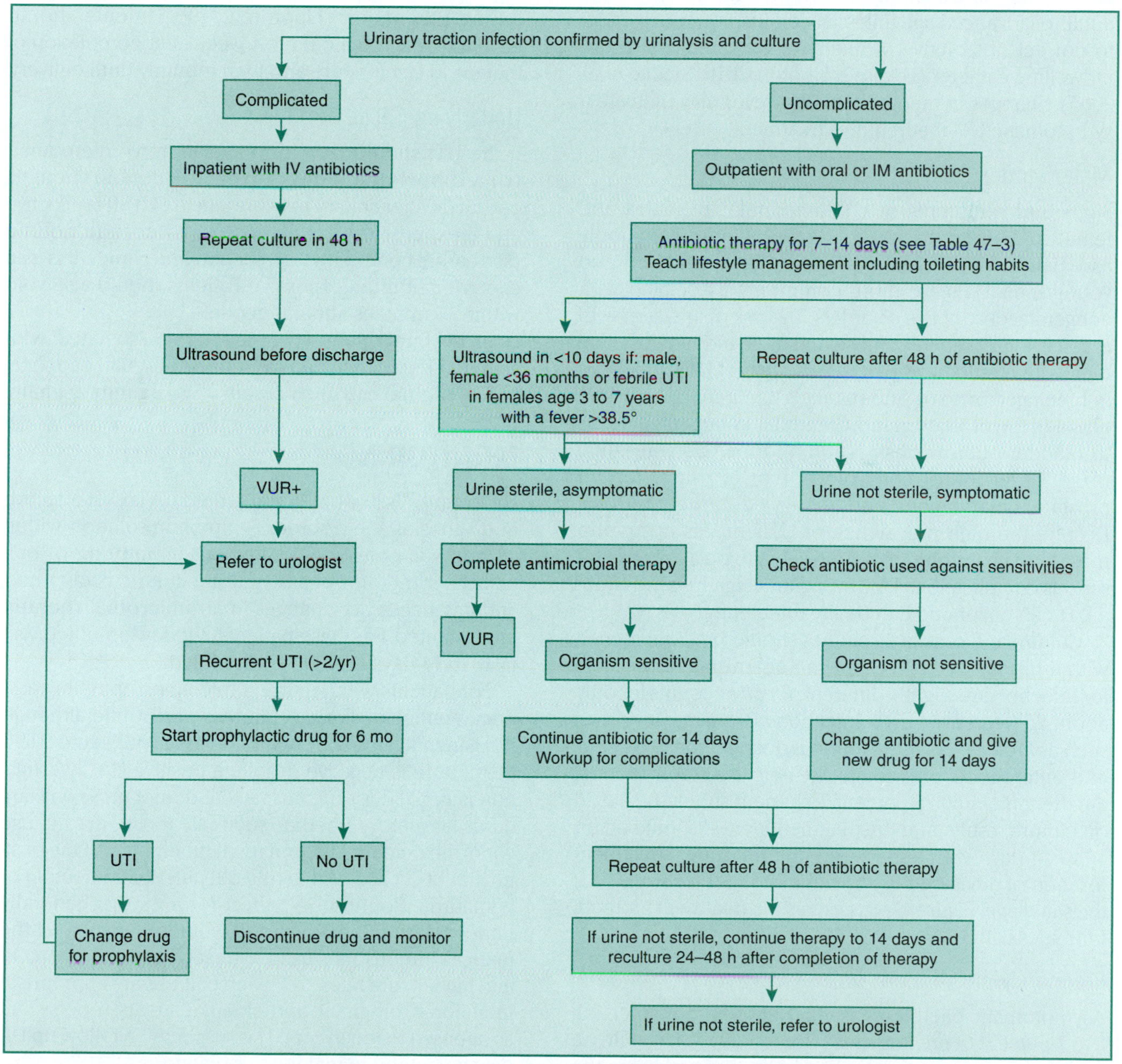

Figure 47–2. Treatment protocol: Urinary tract infections in children.

than 20 percent of women over age 80 years and 6 to 15 percent of men over age 75 years living independently in the community (Fekete & Hooton, 2010). Asymptomatic bacteriuria is defined by the Infectious Diseases Society of America (IDSA) guidelines as two consecutive clean-catch voided urine specimens in women and one clean catch in men with isolation of a single organism in quantitative counts of greater than 10^5 cfu/mL (Fekete & Hooton).

A symptomatic bacteriuria is commonly associated with urinary incontinence, multiple medical illnesses, and impairment of mental status. Treatment with **antimicrobial therapy** is frequently unsuccessful in eradicating the infection and may be associated with the development of more resistant bacteria. Choice of **antimicrobial** should be based on culture and sensitivity tests rather than done empirically. No treatment is indicated in asymptomatic adults of advanced age unless in conjunction with surgery to correct obstructive uropathy or after removal of an indwelling catheter (Fekete & Hooton, 2010; Nicolle et al, 2005). Changes in mental status, however, may indicate a symptomatic UTI that requires treatment.

Male Gender

Signs and symptoms of UTI are similar in males and females. Urethral discharge in men is more commonly associated with STDs than with a UTI. In children and young men, UTIs are more commonly associated with congenital obstructive disorders. The risk of infection with *E. coli* is increased in homosexual men and heterosexual men with a colonized partner. The rate of UTIs increases in men aged 50 to 65 and parallels the increase in hyperplasia of the prostate gland. Glandular enlargement leads to bladder outflow obstruction and increased residual urine. Older adult men (older than 65) have further prostate enlargement and increased urine residuals. Despite the high prevalence of UTIs in this age group, most remain asymptomatic and seem to be at low risk for serious complications. However, gram-negative sepsis from a UTI can occur and can be life threatening.

Culture and sensitivity studies should be done in men with a history of UTI. In men, the organisms responsible for infection are slightly different. *E. coli* accounts for only about 25 percent of their infections. Gram-negative rods such as *Proteus* and *Pseudomonas* account for 50 percent, and enterococci and coagulase-negative staphylococci are the remaining 25 percent. Treatment should be based on culture results, and the treatment period should be for 10 to 14 days, with a follow-up culture drawn. Treatment for men of advanced age is similar to that for women of the same age. Figure 47–3 presents the treatment protocol for males with UTIs.

Pregnancy

Asymptomatic bacteriuria is relatively common, affecting 2 to 7 percent of pregnancies (Hooton, 2010). It should be treated because eradication of bacteriuria reduces the high incidence of symptomatic UTI that commonly occurs later; treatment may reduce the risk for preterm birth. All pregnant women should be screened for bacteriuria by urine culture at least once early in pregnancy, and they should be treated if the results are positive (Hooton, 2010; Nicolle et al, 2005). Periodic screening for recurrent bacteriuria should be done following completion of therapy to ensure clearance of the infection and to monitor for any recurrence. Women who are culture negative at early screening do not require additional screening later in pregnancy. Symptoms of UTI should always result in urine testing and treatment if needed throughout pregnancy.

Nitrofurantoin 100 mg bid for 5 to 7 days, **amoxicillin/clavulanate** 500 mg bid for 3 to 5 days, and third generation **cephalosporins** (**cefpodoxime** 100 mg every 12 hours for 3 to 7 days) are all acceptable during pregnancy (Hooton, 2010). Patients should have a repeat urine culture 1 week after completion of therapy to test for cure and then monthly until delivery.

Underlying Cause

If the UTI should develop in relation to intercourse, **trimethoprim/sulfamethoxazole** (double-strength, one tablet after coitus) may prevent the UTI. It is effective and inexpensive. A single dose of a **fluoroquinolone** (see earlier comments) is a second-line choice. It is also effective but more expensive. Patients should also void within 10 minutes after intercourse.

In postmenopausal women, UTIs associated with estrogen deficiency can be reduced by daily application of **vaginal estrogen cream** 0.5 to 2 g intravaginally.

MONITORING

For lower UTIs in women, a standard UA is cost effective in diagnosing the disorder. Symptom resolution within 48 hours is considered sufficient monitoring of outcome. If symptoms persist, a urine culture is obtained, and any necessary changes in **antimicrobial therapy** are instituted. For these patients, a follow-up office visit in 10 to 14 days should be scheduled.

For patients with recurrent infections, obtaining and documenting one urine culture is worthwhile, although it is generally unnecessary for women with acute UTI. If the culture is negative despite a positive UA, investigation is needed for organisms that do not grow on standard laboratory media, such as those that cause gonorrhea, chlamydia, and renal tuberculosis. One post-treatment UA is useful to rule out persistent infection or hematuria. Routine UA to test for a cure is generally unnecessary in healthy adult women because all the main **antimicrobials** used to treat UTIs have 91 percent and higher cure rates. Follow-up cultures are appropriate in children, pregnant, and elderly patients. If persistent as opposed to recurrent UTI is suspected, a follow-up UA may be helpful in making this diagnosis.

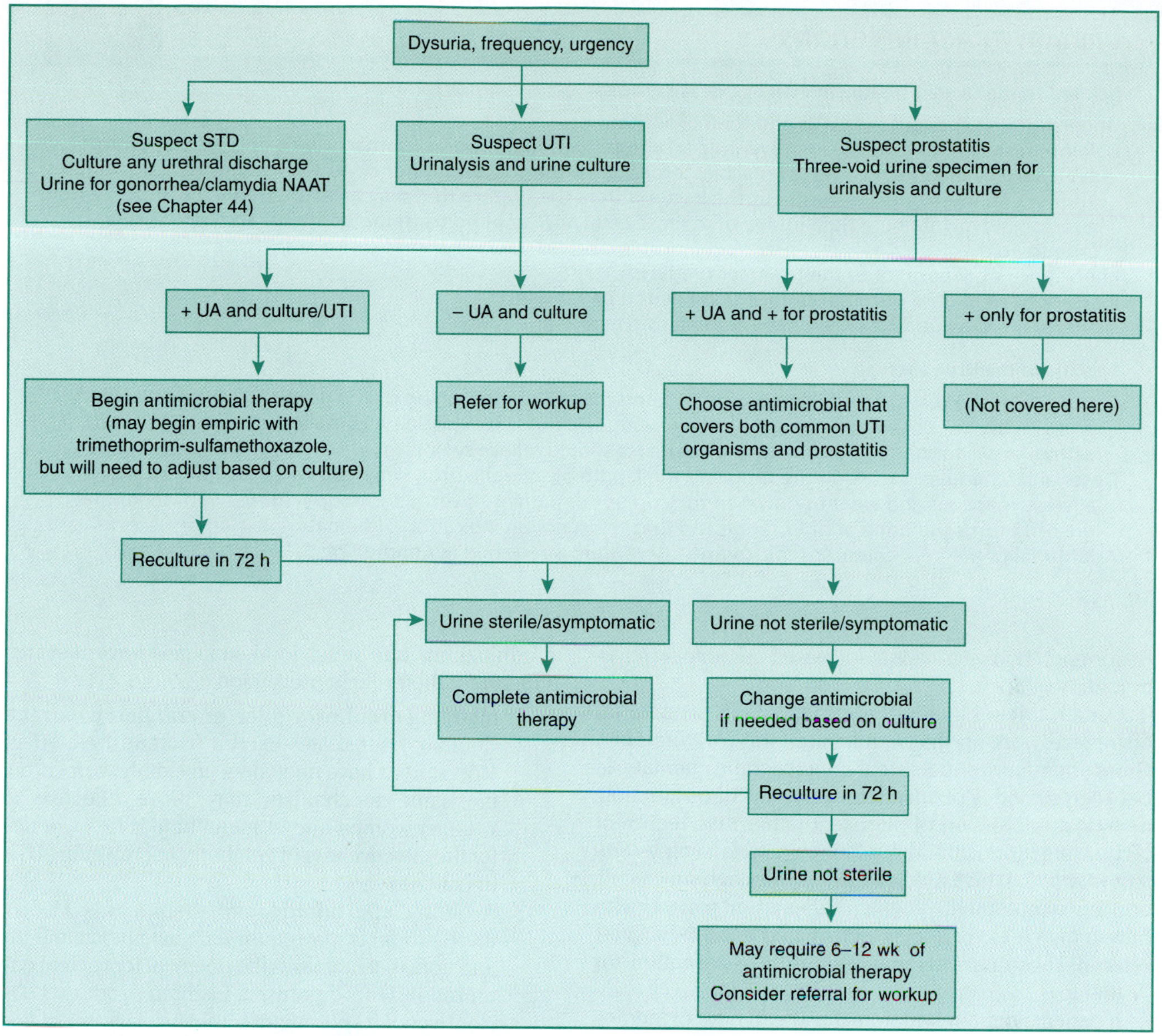

Figure 47–3. Treatment protocol: Urinary tract infections in men.

All children age 5 years and younger need radiological evaluation and appropriate referral to a pediatric urologist. Older children with simple, uncomplicated UTI require urine culture for diagnosis of the offending organism, and a culture after completion of therapy. Failure to produce sterile urine after 14 days of therapy suggests referral.

Pregnant patients with a positive urine culture should have a follow-up urine culture every 2 weeks until delivery and at their postpartum evaluation to validate sterile urine. Reinfections require prophylactic **antimicrobial therapy.** For upper UTIs, an initial telephone assessment of the patient's symptoms and response to therapy is important within 24 hours. A second assessment with an office visit should occur in 2 to 3 days. If symptoms do not resolve or if they worsen, hospitalization may be required. A urine culture should be done 1 to 2 weeks after therapy in pregnant patients, children, patients who remain symptomatic, and those for whom suppression therapy is being considered. Follow-up cultures are optional for all other patients.

OUTCOME EVALUATION

Neonates, infants, and children under age 5 years who present with clinical and laboratory evidence of UTIs should be referred to a pediatric urologist. The cause is likely to be an anatomical obstructive problem, especially in boys. Although adults do not often have long-term complications from UTIs, 10 percent of children with reflux nephropathy go on to develop hypertension with bilateral scarring of the kidney within 10 years. Risk for development of end-stage renal disease after UTI is rare in adults but is 1:500 for children who later develop hypertension.

URINARY TRACT INFECTIONS

PATIENT EDUCATION

Related to the Overall Treatment Plan or Disease Process

Understanding the causes of UTIs and their prognoses.

Role of lifestyle modifications in preventing UTIs, especially ingestion of cranberry juice or cranberry extract; avoidance of diaphragms and spermicides, especially those containing nonoxynol-9; voiding 10 to 15 minutes after sexual intercourse to wash out the bacteria from the urethra that may have entered the bladder during intercourse; maintaining fluid intake of at least 2,000 mL/day of noncaffeinated fluids; and not resisting the urge to void.

Importance of adherence to the treatment regimen.

Indications of relapse or complications that need to be reported.

Need for a follow-up visit only if patient remains symptomatic.

Specific to the Drug Therapy

Discussion of the reasons for taking the drug(s) and the anticipated action of the drug(s) on the disease process. The patient should be asymptomatic within 48 hours for simple, uncomplicated lower UTIs and within 7 days for upper UTIs. **Urinary analgesics** should relieve symptoms within 24 hours.

Doses and schedules for taking the drug and the length of time the drug will need to be taken. Possible adverse reactions and what to do when they occur. For patients given **phenazopyridine,** warn them that the drug turns the urine bright orange and that this is not an indication of hematuria.

Additional patient education specific to **antimicrobials** is provided in Chapter 24.

Recurrent UTI in girls leads to increased risk for new infection in pregnancy.

Certain criteria in adults also suggest the need for an aggressive work-up that requires referral to a urologist. Gross hematuria; persistent microscopic hematuria between episodes of infection; symptoms of obstruction; a clinical impression of persistent rather than recurrent UTI, or infection with urea-splitting bacteria, such as *Proteus mirabilis,* which are associated with staghorn calculi; and any symptomatic pregnant patients and patients who have a high fever or appear dehydrated or septic suggest referral. These patients may require hospitalization for IV therapy.

If patients remain symptomatic after 3 days of therapy for a simple, uncomplicated lower UTI or after completion of 10 to 14 days of therapy for an upper UTI, a culture should be done to determine the causative organism, and a different **antimicrobial** may be needed.

PATIENT EDUCATION

Patient education should include a discussion of information related to the overall treatment plan as well as that specific to the drug therapy, reasons for taking the drug, drugs as part of the total treatment regimen, and adherence issues. Lifestyle changes to prevent UTIs should be addressed, especially with patients who have recurrent UTIs.

Lifestyle Management

Prevention is the key to management of UTIs. Although lifestyle management may not always prevent UTIs, studies confirm several practices that may help to prevent UTIs, especially in women. The following lifestyle modifications and behavioral strategies have research support for their role in prevention:

1. Ingesting **cranberry juice** or **cranberry extract.** Cranberry substrates exert a bacteriostatic effect. Most studies have been done in elderly women, but the same mechanism may prove effective in younger women and in men. There is no evidence for the effectiveness of cranberry in preventing UTIs in children.
2. Avoiding **spermicide** and diaphragms. Use of these products may cause a change in vaginal pH and flora that increases the potential for vaginal colonization with organisms likely to produce UTIs. **Nonoxynol-9 spermicides** are especially associated with increased incidence of bacteriuria. The essential first step to UTIs in women is frequently thought to be the colonization of the vaginal introitus.
3. Voiding 10 to 15 minutes after sexual intercourse. Urination washes out the bacteria from the urethra that may have entered the bladder during intercourse.

Additional measures that have inconsistent support but would not be harmful and are likely to be helpful include the following:

1. Maintaining fluid intake of at least 2,000 mL/day of noncaffeinated fluids. Sufficient fluid is necessary to ensure regular voiding throughout the day. Caffeinated fluids have a mild diuretic effect but are less likely to maintain fluid volume balance.
2. Not resisting the urge to void. "Holding" urine may stretch the bladder and cause small breaks in the bladder mucosal layer that provide entrance for bacteria. Holding also increases the risk for growth of bacteria in residual urine.

3. Avoiding douche products that change the vaginal pH and flora. This practice may decrease the likelihood of vaginal canal colonization.

REFERENCES

American Academy of Pediatrics. (1999). Practice parameter: The diagnosis, treatment, and evaluation of initial urinary tract infections in febrile infants and young children. Committee on Quality Improvement: Subcommittee on Urinary Tract Infections. *Pediatrics, 103*(4), 843–852.

Bayer Healthcare Pharmaceuticals. (2009). Cipro [Manufacturer's label]. Retrieved from http://www.univgraph.com/bayer/inserts/ciprotab.pdf

Berger, R. (2005). Cranberries for preventing urinary tract infections. *Journal of Urology, 173*(6), 1988.

Burns, C., Dunn, A., Brady, M., Barber-Starr, N., & Blosser, C. (2004). *Pediatric primary care: A handbook for nurse practitioners* (3rd ed.). Philadelphia: Saunders.

Cincinnati Children's Hospital. (2006). UTI Guideline Team, Cincinnati Children's Hospital Medical Center: Evidence-based care guideline for medical management of first urinary tract infection in children 12 years of age or less (Guideline 7, pp. 1–23). Retrieved from http://www.cincinnatichildrens.org/svc/dept-div/health-policy/ev-based/uti.htm

Fekete, T., & Hooton, T. M. (2010). Approach to the adult with asymptomatic bacteriuria. *UpToDate.* Last updated April 2010. Retrieved from http://www.uptodate.com/online/content/topic.do?topicKey=uti_infe/6290&selectedTitle=1%7E150&source=search_result

Foxman, B., Barlow, R., D'Arcy, H., Gillespie, B., & Sobel, J. D. (2000). Urinary tract infection: Self-reported incidence and associated costs. *Annals of Epidemiology, 10,* 509–515.

Freedman, A. L. (2007). Urinary tract infection in children. In M. S. Litwin & C. S. Saigal (Eds.), *Urologic diseases in America* (NIH Publication No. 07–5512, pp. 439–457). U.S. Department of Health and Human Services, Public Health Service, National Institutes of Health, National Institute of Diabetes and Digestive and Kidney Diseases. Washington, DC: U.S. Government Printing Office.

Gaylord, N. M., & Starr, N. B. (2009). Genitourinary disorders. In C. E. Burns, A. M. Dunn, M. A. Brady, N. B. Starr, & C. G. Blosser (Eds.), *Pediatric primary care* (pp. 866–905). St. Louis, MO: Saunders.

Griebling, T. L. (2007a). Urinary tract infection in men. In M. S. Litwin & C. S. Saigal (Eds.), *Urologic diseases in America* (NIH Publication No. 07–5512, pp. 621–645). U.S. Department of Health and Human Services, Public Health Service, National Institutes of Health, National Institute of Diabetes and Digestive and Kidney Diseases. Washington, DC: U.S. Government Printing Office.

Griebling, T. L. (2007b). Urinary tract infection in women. In M. S. Litwin & C. S. Saigal (Eds.), *Urologic diseases in America* (NIH Publication No. 07–5512, pp. 588–617). U.S. Department of Health and Human Services, Public Health Service, National Institutes of Health, National Institute of Diabetes and Digestive and Kidney Diseases. Washington, DC: U.S. Government Printing Office.

Grover, M. L., Bracamonte, J. D., Kanodia, A. K., Bryan, M. J., Donahue, S. P., Warner, A., et al. (2007). Assessing adherence to evidence-base guidelines for the diagnosis and management of uncomplicated urinary tract infection. *Mayo Clinic Proceedings, 82*(2), 181–185.

Hooton, T. M. (2010). Urinary tract infections and asymptomatic bacteriuria in pregnancy. *UpToDate*. Last updated July 2010. Retrieved from http://www.uptodate.com/online/content/topic.do?topicKey=uti_infe/7516&source=see_link

Hooton, TM (2011). Acute cystitis in women. UpToDate Online. Retrieved from http://www.uptodate.com/contents/acute-cystitis-in-women?source=preview&anchor=H18&selectedTitle=7~150#H19

Institute for Clinical Systems Improvement (ICSI). (2004). *Uncomplicated urinary tract infection in women.* Bloomington, MN: ICSI.

Jepson, R. G., & Craig, J. C. (2008). Cranberries for preventing urinary tract infections. *Cochrane Database of Systematic Reviews,* (1):CD001321.

Kashanian, J., Hakimian, P., Blute, M., Wong, J., Khanna, H., Wise, G. et al. (2008). Nitrofurantoin: The return of an old friend in the wake of growing resistance. *British Journal of Urology International, 102,* 1634–1637.

Keren, R., & Chan, E. (2002). A meta-analysis of randomized, controlled trials comparing short- and long-course antibiotic therapy for urinary tract infections in children. *Pediatrics, 109*(5), e70.

Litwin, M. S., & Saigal, C. S. (2007). Introduction. In M. S. Litwin & C. S. Saigal (Eds.), *Urologic diseases in America* (NIH Publication No. 07–5512, pp. 588–617). U.S. Department of Health and Human Services, Public Health Service, National Institutes of Health, National Institute of Diabetes and Digestive and Kidney Diseases. Washington, DC: U.S. Government Printing Office.

McCance, K., & Huether, S. (2006). *Pathophysiology: The biological basis for disease in adults and children.* St. Louis, MO: Mosby.

Nicolle, L., Bradley, S., Colgan, R., Rice, J., Schaeffer, A., & Hooton, T. (2005). Infectious Diseases Society of America guideline for the diagnosis and treatment of asymptomatic bacteriuria in adults. *Clinical Infectious Diseases, 40*(5), 643–654.

Prais, D., Straussberg, R., Avitzur, Y., Nussinovitch, M., Harel, L., & Amir, J. (2003). Bacterial susceptibility to oral antibiotics in community acquired urinary tract infection. *Archives of Disease in Childhood, 88,* 215–218.

Ramakrishnan, K., & Scheid, D. C. (2005). Diagnosis and management of acute pyelonephritis in adults. *American Family Physician, 71,* 933–42.

Towers, P. (2000). Urinary tract infections. *Journal of the American Academy of Nurse Practitioners, 12*(4), 149–154.

Wagenlehner, F., Weidner, W., & Naber, K. (2005). Emerging drugs for bacterial urinary tract infections. *Expert Opinion on Emerging Drugs, 10*(2), 275–298.

UNIT IV

Special Drug Treatment Considerations

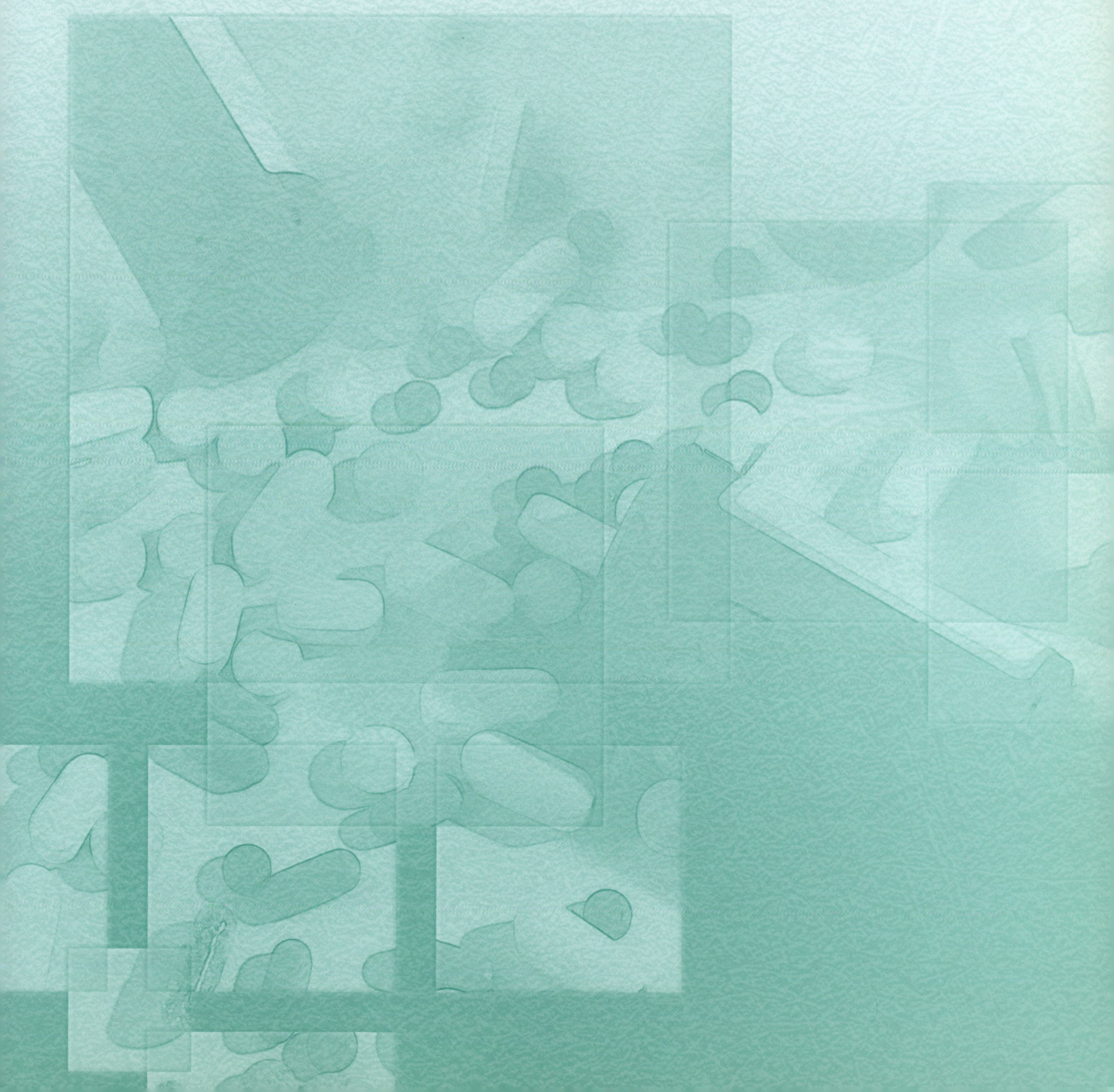

CHAPTER 48

WOMEN AS PATIENTS

Kathleen Bell and Anita Lee Wynne

Chapter Outline

Differences in patterns of health and illness between females and males have been well documented. Women tend to pay more attention to changes in health patterns, seeking health care earlier and more often than men. Even when diagnosed with similar medical conditions (such as cardiac disease or Alzheimer's disease) adult women have very different needs for care than do their male counterparts. Adherence to a prescribed medication regimen may be affected by gender, especially if the adverse effects have a particular impact on females (e.g., hirsutism or risk of thromboembolic disorders). This chapter will discuss treatment of common conditions experienced by women as a special population.

To review growth and development briefly, both sexes progress similarly until puberty, when increases in estrogen and progesterone prepare women for fertility and reproduction. Menopause signals the cessation of reproductive capability for females. During puberty, males respond to the influence of increased androgens, triggering a cascade of changes such as increased height, weight, and muscle mass and the genital changes that accompany the ability to reproduce. Whereas females are born with all of their gamete cells already present, sperm production in males begins at puberty and continues throughout their adult lives until levels of testosterone start to wane, usually in their sixth or seventh decade.

Prescribing for women in their childbearing years requires constant awareness of the possibility of pregnancy in order to avoid exposing the developing fetus to potential teratogens. Sexually active women who use birth control also become pregnant. In the United States, 3 million unintended pregnancies occur annually (Trussell, Vaughn, & Stanford, 1999). Sexual activity (especially if begun early) can lead to lifelong viral infections or silent bacterial infections that scar delicate fallopian tubes and change cervical tissues, contributing to infertility. Early sexual activity in adolescents exposes them to risks of both infection and pregnancy, at a time when their bodies are still growing and their personalities are not yet mature.

Teenage pregnancy is associated with inconsistent prenatal care, smaller infants, and preterm labor. These infants are at high risk for developmental disorders and other medical conditions associated with low birth weight. Neglect and abuse account for two deaths per 1,000 healthy infants born to adolescents 15 years or younger, and the risk from sudden infant death syndrome (SIDS) increases (Moos, 2005).

Breastfeeding is another time when prescribing for women requires special care and knowledge. For information on pharmacokinetics about breastfeeding to assist the practitioner in making safe decisions about prescribing, see Chapter 50. Areas discussed in Chapter 50 include maternal pharmacokinetics, infant suckling pattern, infant pharmacokinetics, variable infant susceptibility to drugs, and milk-to-plasma ratios.

Cultural attitudes, behaviors, and beliefs related to health can affect how a woman responds to and complies with health advice. Caring for women from different cultures requires knowledge of the treatments they will accept, of their personal values and beliefs, and of the customs of their identified cultural group. With the assistance of an interpreter, health-care providers should provide written and verbal instruction to women with language barriers (Olds, London, Ladewig, & Davidson, 2004). Translation alone may not be an issue. The patients may not understand explanations if they lack basic education in their own country. Cultural influences are discussed in detail in Chapter 7.

During the 1980s abuse of children and women was recognized as a significant public health problem. Although boys have also been abused, most abuse has been against girls and women. "Domestic violence against women is a major public health concern. Abuse often increases in frequency and severity over time and leads to significant social, psychological, and medical consequences" (Bohn, Tibben, & Campbell, 2004, p. 561). Intimate partner violence (IPV), which can vary in frequency and severity, is a type of violence that occurs among heterosexual and same-sex couples. IPV is also a serious public health problem (Centers for Disease Control and Prevention [CDC], 2005b). Statistics about IPV vary because of differences in the way different data sources define IPV and collect data. In addition, most IPV incidents are not reported to the police; thus, available data underestimate the true extent of the problem (CDC, 2005a).

Women are at high risk for violence during pregnancy, a complication that can lead to many other problems: miscarriage, placental abruption, low-birth-weight infants, premature labor or birth, substance abuse, late entry to prenatal care, intrauterine fetal death, and sexually transmitted and urinary tract infections (Bohn et al, 2004; Schoening, Greenwood, McNichols, Heermann, & Agrawal, 2004).

The American Nurses Association (ANA), the Association of Women's Health, Obstetrics and Neonatal Nurses (AWHONN), the American College of Obstetricians and Gynecologists (ACOG), and the American Medical Association (AMA) recommend that practitioners screen all patients for IPV at every encounter with the health-care system, regardless of the reason for which health care is being sought. Routinely asking all women about physical and emotional abuse increases a practitioner's opportunity to uncover the underlying causes of women's physical symptoms or depression, conditions that may be related to some form of abuse (Schoening et al, 2004). Women are four times more likely to report abuse if they are simply asked!

In most of the world, the majority of the older population is comprised of women. This demographic phenomenon has been called the feminization of later life (Ginn, Street, & Arber, 2001). Women's life expectancy in developed countries is an average of 7 years longer than that of men, with the gender gap narrowing to 3 years in developing countries (mostly due to high maternal mortality rates) (United Nations Populations Fund, 2008). The feminization of later life carries consequences that include a high incidence of widowhood, living alone, disability, and poverty. Women are more likely to live alone than are their male counterparts, who frequently marry again. In addition, an increase in chronic illness also accompanies women's longer life spans, including cardiovascular disorders, strokes, diabetes, arthritis, and Alzheimer's disease. Management of chronic illnesses in the face of economic concerns in this vulnerable population presents significant challenge for health-care providers.

In the United States, women are the most impoverished subgroup of society. At both ends of the demographic spectrum, single mothers with children and elderly women are the poorest of the poor (U.S. Department of Health and Human Services, Office of the Assistant Secretary for Planning and Evaluation, 2005). Lack of health insurance coverage leads many women not to fill prescriptions or to take or administer medications on an altered schedule. Prescribers must adequately assess a patient's financial status and be aware of the possibility that a woman's noncompliance may be primarily economically driven.

Practitioners often neglect the complex needs of older women, maintaining a symptom-specific focus. By age 65, half of all women have two or more chronic conditions (Agency for Healthcare Research and Quality [AHRQ], 2002). The need for polypharmacy that often results from multiple comorbidities necessitates a more holistic approach to these patients' care.

Although defining disability can be a daunting task because of a multitude of components, practitioners need to be aware that 28.6 million women/girls, or 21.3 percent of all females in the United States, have some type of disability (Disability Statistics Center, 2002). Because of their longer life expectancy, women are more likely than men to be disabled, with the most prevalence among women over age 85. Disability refers to a chronic physical or mental health problem or an impairment that restricts an individual's ability to perform one or more activities (Olds et al, 2004). Various categories of disabilities include developmental (present before the age of 22), neurological, psychiatric, and sensory. Autoimmune diseases are categorized as neurological disabilities, as is Alzheimer's disease (AD). Psychiatric disabilities include depression, anxiety, panic disorders, and phobias. Women have 50 percent higher rates than do men of all of these disabling conditions. Chapters 14 (Autonomic Nervous System Drugs), 29 (Anxiety and Depression), and 51 (Geriatric Patients) discuss these conditions and the drugs to treat them in more detail.

As women age, changes in cognitive functioning—learning, memory, concentration, and planning ability—often occur. Clinically apparent cognitive decline is called dementia (Olds et al, 2004). In the United States, Alzheimer's disease (AD) is the most commonly occurring form of dementia, and in women the prevalence increases about 5 percent every year. Incidence reaches 50 percent in women over age 85 (Naftolin, 2002). **Acetylcholinesterase inhibitors** are the only medications approved by the U.S. Food and Drug Administration (FDA) to treat cognitive dysfunction. Evidence is conflicting about the effect of **estrogen** or **hormone replacement therapy (HRT)** in either prevention or the delay of AD onset in women.

In 1999, the National Institutes of Health (NIH) published "Agenda for Research in Women's Health for the 21st Century" (1999). This document stated that "gaps in knowledge remain regarding the behavior of drugs in women and gender-related pharmacokinetic and pharmacodynamic differences." Since that time research has included more women as subjects, but work needs to continue in this area.

In this chapter, the biological and molecular basis for sex-related differences in pharmacokinetics, pharmacodynamics, drug effects, and safety will be discussed based on the current science.

PHARMACOKINETICS AND PHARMACODYNAMICS IN WOMEN

Pharmacokinetics

Gender differences occur in all phases of pharmacokinetics between men and women. Table 48–1 presents some gender differences in pharmacokinetic properties. Women have longer gastric emptying times, which influence the absorption and bioavailability of some drugs. The volume of distribution (Vd) of drugs is dramatically altered by body composition. The higher percentage of body fat means a larger Vd for **lipophilic agents** (Gandhi, Aweeka, Greenblatt, & Blaschke, 2004; Kleist, 2005). The fat-soluble drug **diazepam (Valium)** has been observed to have a significantly larger Vd in women, and the water-soluble drug **metronidazole (Flagyl)** demonstrates a lower Vd, although increased clearance in women accounts for a lower area under the curve (AUC) for this drug in females. Water-soluble

Table 48–1 **Gender Differences in Pharmacokinetic Parameters**

Pharmacokinetic Parameter	Sex-Based Difference
Absorption and bioavailability	• Gastric emptying time is slower in females, mainly related to the effects of estrogen. Drugs absorbed in the stomach will have longer exposure to absorption sites. • Gastric levels of alcohol dehydrogenase are lower in females. Plasma concentrations are greater in females than males after ingestion of similar amounts of alcohol. • Gastric acid secretion, pH, osmolality, electrolyte concentrations, and levels of bile acids and proteins do not vary significantly between sexes.
Distribution	• Females have lower body weights and BMI than males. • Females have a higher proportion of body fat. Lipophilic drugs are more readily absorbed and have relatively greater volumes of distribution than hydrophilic drugs. • Plasma volume is lower in females. Drugs with high volumes of distribution will be more concentrated in the plasma of females. • Organ blood flow is lower in females. • Estrogen is distributed attached to a serum-binding globulin. Exogenous estrogens increase levels of many serum-binding globulins such as corticosteroid-binding globulin and thyroxine-binding globulin resulting in less free drug.
Metabolism	• Studies have been inconsistent in showing differences in CYP450 substrates; the general trend is toward high rates of metabolism for CYP450 3A4 substrates and lower rates for 1A2 and 2D6 substrates. • Females have lower levels of p-glycoprotein and higher rates of drug clearance for drugs that are substrates of p-glycoprotein.
Excretion	• Gender differences in rates of renal excretion of most drugs are probably more related to simple weight differences. • Drugs that are actively secreted by the kidney may show gender differences, but further study is required to demonstrate this difference.

BMI = body mass index.

fluoroquinolones also have a smaller Vd in women. Both the oral clearance and Vd of **prednisolone** are significantly lower in women (Ghandi et al, 2004). **Tricyclic antidepressants** take longer to reach a steady state in women because of the drugs' lipophilic distribution. As a result, women experience more adverse reactions after the drug saturates all the sites in adipose tissues and more active drug remains in the bloodstream.

Gastric levels of **alcohol** dehydrogenase are lower in women so a greater fraction of ingested **alcohol** would be oxidized in men prior to absorption than in women. This is a significant factor behind why blood **alcohol** levels are disproportionately higher in women after ingestion of similar amounts of **alcohol.**

Gender-based differences in drug metabolism play a larger role in inter-gender pharmacokinetic differences than any of the other parameters. While hepatic blood flow is lower in women, differences in hepatic enzymes seem to be the major factor in variability. The frequency of variant alleles for the CYP450 system has been shown to exist both between races and sexes. Studies have shown that CYP 3A4 activity is 24 percent higher in women (Gandhi et al, 2004) and CYP 1A2 is lower (Davis, 1998). It is acknowledged that some studies demonstrated that the mean amounts of these isoenzymes did not differ (Gandhi et al, 2004), but specific drugs have shown differences. For example, **Erythromycin** is more rapidly cleared in women than it is in men, which is thought to be related to its CYP450 3A4–mediated effect. Orally administered **verapamil (Isoptin, Calan)** clears more quickly in men than it does in women based in part on its CYP 3A4 metabolism. Higher absolute bioavailability of this drug in women may explain the greater pharmacodynamic effects on blood pressure and heart rate in women. The CYP 2D6 isoenzyme is important in the metabolism of many **psychotropic drugs.** One study showed that tardive dyskinesia develops more frequently in female Chinese schizophrenics secondary to increased frequency of a defective CYP 2D6 allele in Chinese women (Gandhi et al, 2004).

Propranolol (Inderal) was one of the earliest drugs to show a clear gender difference in metabolic clearance of a drug. Oral doses of this drug had a significantly higher (63%) rate of clearance in men than it did in women (Kleist, 2005). IV doses demonstrated no differences, indicating that this was a hepatic first-pass metabolism issue. Women might be expected, therefore, to show a significantly greater clinical response to oral doses of this drug than men.

The difference in clearance rates among the **benzodiazepines** can be explained in part by CP450 (oxidative) versus conjugative activity for drug metabolism. Those that undergo oxidative metabolism (**alprazolam, diazepam,** and **midazolam**), which is higher in women, are more rapidly metabolized than those that undergo conjugation (**chlordiazepoxide, temazepam,** and **oxazepam**), which is lower in women. The gender-related difference in CYP 2D6 activity and p-glycoprotein expression may be an important reason for different responses to **antidepressants** such as **serotonin reuptake inhibitors** (Kleist, 2005). Finally, **oral contraceptives** have been demonstrated to significantly inhibit CYP 2C19 activity, which accounts for many drug interactions with other drugs using this substrate.

Studies aimed at showing differences in drug metabolism based on menopausal status have been inconsistent. Conflicting data exist on whether menopausal status or **estrogen** and **progesterone** level in HRT significantly affects drug metabolism and, therefore, no recommendations can be made at this time.

Kleist (2005) reminds us that many of these effects have been subtle and their overall clinical relevance remains to be demonstrated. With the exception of **propranolol** and **verapamil,** in which the differences in outcome have been clearly significant, and **erythromycin,** which appears to be more effective in women, the provider should use these data to alter individual drug regimens cautiously.

Excretion of drugs by the kidney depends on weight, body surface area, age, and gender. Renal clearance of drugs that are not actively secreted or reabsorbed is dependent on the glomerular filtration rate, which is directly proportional to weight and consequently higher (on average) in men. Gender differences in excretion, therefore, are thought to be largely related to weight differences. Drugs that are actively secreted by the kidney may show gender-based differences, but further study in humans is necessary to clearly demonstrate this difference (Gandhi et al, 2004).

Pharmacodynamics

Pharmacodynamic differences in drug response based on gender have not been studied to the same extent as pharmacokinetic differences. Pharmacodynamic differences are demonstrated only when the same plasma concentration of a drug in both males and females yields a different pharmacological outcome. The clinical relevance of gender-related differences in pharmacodynamics appears with greater risk for adverse drug responses (1.5% to 1.7% higher) in women (Rademaker, 2001). However, not all drugs that have pharmacokinetic differences have pharmacodynamic differences.

The pharmacokinetic differences seen in **prednisolone** correlate with increased **cortisol** and T-helper lymphocyte suppression in women. This difference may be mediated by endogenous **estrogen,** because increased sensitivity has been found at higher **estradiol** concentrations, which may translate into clinical differences in postmenopausal women. The pharmacokinetic differences seen in **verapamil** lead to pharmacological effects of greater reductions in blood pressure and heart rate in women.

Gender differences in response to various **analgesics** have been well studied. **Opiates** seem to have a greater **analgesic** effect in women (Gandhi et al, 2004; Kleist,

2005), but this difference is accompanied by an increase in adverse effects, especially nausea and vomiting. These differences in pharmacological response appear to be due to pharmacodynamic differences, including gender differences in drug-receptor affinity, receptor density, or signal transduction pathways (Gandhi et al, 2004). The effects of several **cardiovascular drugs** on women are different from their effects on men. Women aged 15 to 50 years have longer QT intervals, making them more vulnerable to cardiac arrhythmias. **Macrolide antibiotics** cause a woman's heart to repolarize more slowly. Pharmacokinetic differences in females may explain the increased incidence of life-threatening ventricular arrhythmias, which are twice as common in women who are taking **erythromycin** (Kleist, 2005). Women taking oral **anticoagulants (warfarin)** or **thrombolytic agents** (e.g., after myocardial infarction [MI]) have less benefit with respect to mortality, but more bleeding episodes (Kleist, 2005; Gandhi et al, 2004). **Aspirin** is often prescribed for MI and stroke prevention. Randomized trials have shown that although **aspirin** lowers the risk for ischemic stroke in women, it has little effect on their risk for MI; the opposite is true in men (Kleist, 2005). The exact mechanism for this gender-related difference in outcome has yet to be elucidated.

Many **psychotropic drugs** appear to exhibit gender-mediated differences in pharmacodynamics. In general, women show both greater improvement in symptoms and more severe adverse reactions with **antipsychotics** (Gandhi et al, 2004). These effects appear to be related to the **antidopaminergic** actions of **estrogens**, duplicating the major mechanism of action of typical **antipsychotics.** These findings have resulted in a trend toward prescribing lower doses for women. **Tricyclic antidepressants** exhibit both pharmacokinetic and pharmacodynamic differences between genders. Studies have shown that premenopausal women respond better to **selective serotonin reuptake inhibitors (SSRIs)**, and men respond better to **tricyclic antidepressants** (Anderson, 2003; Davis, 1998). Another example is **lithium** and its increased bioavailability because of renal excretion. This pharmacokinetic difference can result in levels of this drug that are higher in women. The narrow therapeutic range for this drug means the risk for toxicity is increased in women. Drug levels drawn early in therapy may prevent toxicity in drugs, such as **lithium**, **digoxin**, and **theophylline**, which have narrow margins of safety.

Infection with HIV and the development of AIDS are increasing in females, as is the use of **antiretroviral drugs.** Multiple studies have shown differences in treatment efficacy, toxicity profile, and drug pharmacokinetics between women and men (Gandhi et al, 2004). Women experience more frequent and severe adverse effects with various **protease inhibitors**, including higher rates of gastrointestinal and neurological adverse effects, with **ritonavir** secondary to higher plasma concentrations of this drug. They also demonstrate higher rates of allergic reactions and nephrolithiasis with **protease inhibitors.** Related problems (neuropathy, pancreatitis, and toxicity-driven regimen changes) also occur more often in women (Gandhi et al, 2004). A few studies have shown increased efficacy of **antiretrovirals** in women compared to men, including slower rates of disease progression and hospital admissions related to HIV disease in women on **highly active antiretroviral therapy (HAART) therapy** (Moore, Sabin, Johnson, & Phillips, 2002). Further discussion of HIV infection and AIDS is found in Chapter 37.

In summary, an increasing number of gender-related differences in pharmacokinetics and pharmacodynamics are emerging. Kleist (2005) warns, however, that these differences generally have not had an impact on drug dosing and most drugs on the market have a wide enough therapeutic index that minor differences usually do not reach clinical significance. Clinical significance can be seen in drugs that have marked gender-specific pharmacokinetic differences and those with narrow therapeutic indices, a steep dose-concentration curve, or both. As more clinical trials include both women and men, more pharmacodynamic and pharmacotherapeutic differences may appear.

FACTORS THAT INFLUENCE MEDICATION ADMINISTRATION

Puberty

Adolescent female athletes may display a combination of symptoms including amenorrhea, disordered eating, and osteoporosis, called the "female athlete triad" (Gibson & Coupey, 2007). This syndrome is a disruption in normal growth and development caused by inadequate nutrition (caloric intake lower than expenditure) and overexercising (strenuous athletic training). These two behaviors lead to suppression of the hypothalamic-pituitary-ovarian axis, which in turn leads to reduced estrogen levels, amenorrhea, and decreased bone mineralization. Incidence of secondary amenorrhea (defined as absence of menses for 6 months in a girl who has had at least one menstrual period) runs between 10 percent and 50 percent in highly trained female athletes. Many young athletes present with primary amenorrhea (absence of menses by age 13 with secondary sex characteristics or absence of menses by age 15 with secondary sex characteristics). **Hormonal therapy** is not successful with this type of hypogonadism; however, other strategies that decrease the risk for osteoporosis should be incorporated into the routine health care of adolescent females in order to promote positive lifetime habits. Strategies include increasing daily **calcium** intake; assessing amount of **vitamin D** exposure, level of physical activity, and choice of contraception; and assessing for primary or secondary amenorrhea.

Persistent low levels of estrogen in adolescents are of concern regarding bone mineralization. Forty percent of bone accrual occurs during adolescence with bone formation continuing up to age 30 years after which a gradual bone loss begins (Moos, 2005), so building bone during this developmental stage is crucial. Because adolescents have not yet reached peak bone mass, interpreting adolescent bone density measurements should be done appropriately with pediatric/adolescent-specific software that calculates Z scores, rather than T scores. Without appropriate intervention, girls with low bone density may never achieve adequate bone mass and run the risk of fractures and osteoporosis. **Bisphosphonates** (used to treat osteopenia in postmenopausal women) are not FDA approved for use in the teen population. Adequate **calcium** intake along with **vitamin D** can help build bone mass. Successful management of the female athlete triad must be multidisciplinary, requiring the support of coaches, family, trainers, nutritionists, physicians, and counselors (Gibson & Coupey, 2007)

As adolescent diets are often not healthy, strategies that decrease the risk for osteoporosis should be incorporated into the routine health care of adolescent females in order to promote lifetime wellness habits. A daily intake of 1,300 mg of **calcium** daily is recommended for females aged 9 through 18 years, an amount that can be obtained by drinking three cups of low-fat or skim milk and consuming 8 ounces of low-fat yogurt. If a young woman consistently is unable to meet the recommended daily amount of **calcium** through diet alone, **calcium carbonate (Tums, Caltrate, or Viactiv)** should be consumed with food to maximize absorption. Because **vitamin D** is required for optimal **calcium** absorption, a daily multivitamin that includes at least 400 IU **vitamin D** should also be taken (Moos, 2005). Adolescents should also be discouraged from smoking, because smoking has been associated with poor uptake of the nutrients needed to build healthy bone.

Another concern related to bone mineral density (BMD) is long-term use of **medroxyprogesterone acetate (Depo-Provera)**, an injectable form of birth control used by approximately 10 percent of adolescents. In 2004, the FDA announced a black box warning for this drug when studies demonstrated an association between long-term **Depo-Provera** use and significant BMD loss. Because adolescent females have yet not reached their peak BMD, prolonged use of **Depo-Provera** may put these girls at increased risk for osteoporosis. Mounting evidence suggests bone mass recovery occurs when the drug is discontinued; however, the long-term impact of this drug on BMD throughout a woman's life remains unknown. The FDA warning indicates that **Depo-Provera** should not be used as a birth control method for longer than two years (Moos, 2005). Treatment of osteoporosis, including nutrition, is discussed in Chapter 38.

Another concern common in adolescent girls and young women is **iron**-deficiency anemia (IDA), a condition often related to heavy menstruation. Oral **iron** supplementation is recommended to replenish **iron** loss during menstruation. Girls going through puberty may also be avoiding red meat, a good source of **iron**, in favor of lower-calorie salads and vegetables. Although green, leafy vegetables contain **iron**, plant sources are not as fully absorbed as the **iron** found in meats. IDA is discussed in more detail in Chapter 27.

Pregnancy

Extraordinary anatomical and physiological changes occur in a woman's body during pregnancy. Her body changes shape and size, and every organ system modifies its function to create a protective and nurturing environment for the developing fetus (Olds et al, 2004). Drug absorption through the lungs, skin, and mucous membranes is increased because of increased cardiac output, which peaks at 20 to 24 weeks' gestation. Increases in cardiac output may be 30 to 50 percent above prepregnancy levels. Plasma volume is 50 percent higher by the third trimester; most of the volume is in the products of conception. Clearance of some drugs is altered by these changes. **Phenytoin** clearance, for example, is increased during the second and third trimesters. Although this drug is potentially teratogenic, the risk of seizure is much more dangerous to the mother and the fetus. **Theophylline** blood levels may rise because of decreased renal clearance (Olds et al, 2004). Other drugs with effects similar to **theophylline** are preferred during pregnancy.

IDA is one of the most common complications of pregnancy and is primarily due to expansion of plasma volume without equivalent expansion of maternal hemoglobin mass. This condition is called physiologic anemia (Olds et al, 2004). IDA puts a pregnant woman at risk for susceptibility to infections, fatigue, and an increased chance of preeclampsia and postpartum hemorrhage. In addition, a pregnant woman with IDA tolerates even minimal blood loss during birth poorly and may experience delayed healing of an episiotomy, laceration, or cesarean birth incision (Olds et al, 2004).

Dietary **iron** is necessary for hemoglobin production, and during pregnancy hemoglobin is vital for transport of oxygen to the growing fetus. Daily **iron** intake of 1,600 mg is necessary during pregnancy with the greatest need for **iron** intake in the last 20 weeks. Stinging nettle *(Urtica dioica)* and chlorophyll are good sources of **iron** for pregnant women who find it difficult to consume adequate amounts of **iron-containing** foods. Stinging nettle can be consumed as a cooked green leafy vegetable, added to soups, or drunk as a tea. The tea is prepared by adding boiling water to two teaspoons of the dried or fresh herb then steeped for several minutes. A woman should drink

CLINICAL PEARL

Prescribing for Adolescents

Become knowledgeable about the laws in your state regarding treatment of sexually transmitted infections, contraception, and medical record confidentiality in minor patients.

two cups of tea per day with cinnamon and honey added to improve the taste (Olds et al, 2004). Table 48–2 lists herbs to avoid in pregnancy.

The physiologic anemia of pregnancy is commonly treated with **ferrous sulfate.** This oral preparation should be taken with **vitamin C** for increased absorption, and should be taken after meals to reduce gastrointestinal irritation. Most prenatal vitamins contain the required 60 to 120 mg of **iron** for pregnancy. Because women with IDA may be asymptomatic, and because not all pregnant women need large quantities of supplemental **iron,** monitoring hemoglobin and hematocrit is necessary. To prevent IDA, an **iron** supplement of 30 mg/day should be initiated at the first prenatal visit, and pregnant women should be advised to eat an **iron**-rich diet (Olds et al, 2004).

Pregnancy may present an opportune time for women to modify unhealthy or high-risk lifestyle behaviors. For example, illicit drug use may be corrected or reduced when patients are motivated by the birth of a child. Although legal, **nicotine** and **alcohol** are harmful to the developing fetus.

The use of **caffeine** during pregnancy remains controversial. At this time, no conclusive evidence links **caffeine** consumption to birth defects or spontaneous abortion (Olds et al, 2004). **Caffeine** is found in beverages such as coffee, teas, colas and some other sodas, in foods such as chocolate, and some over-the-counter (OTC) pain relievers. **Caffeine,** a central nervous system **stimulant,** causes mood swings and diuresis and readily crosses the placenta to the fetus, who is unable to metabolize it effectively. **Caffeine** may cause fetal or newborn cardiac arrhythmias. Some women may choose to avoid **caffeine** intake during pregnancy altogether. Until more information is available, pregnant women should be counseled about sources of **caffeine** and advised to limit their consumption to 150 to 300 mg a day or less (American Pregnancy Association, 2005; Olds et al, 2004).

Smoking has been linked to higher infertility rates in both men and women. Women who smoke have a higher risk for spontaneous abortion, preterm birth, placenta previa, abruptio placentae, and premature rupture of membranes. The risk is directly related to the number of cigarettes smoked, so any decrease in smoking will improve fetal outcomes. Two main ingredients in cigarette smoke affect the fetus: carbon monoxide and **nicotine.** Carbon monoxide competes for oxygen binding sites on fetal hemoglobin and **nicotine** causes vasoconstriction in both the mother and the fetus. The compound effect of these two ingredients is decreased availability and delivery of oxygen to maternal and fetal tissues, including the uterus and placenta.

Alcohol causes decreased folic acid and thiamine absorption. Mothers who drink **alcohol** while pregnant frequently deliver low-birth-weight infants, and they risk their infants' having problems of growth and development associated with fetal alcohol syndrome. To date, no safe level of **alcohol** consumption during pregnancy has been identified; therefore, women should be counseled to abstain from **alcohol** during pregnancy (*Drug Facts and Comparisons,* 2009; Olds et al, 2004).

Complementary and alternative therapies, such as the use of medicinal herbs, are currently being evaluated with randomized methodologies to evaluate their efficacy. Many herbs can be useful for treating pregnancy associated discomforts. Examples include ginger for nausea and vomiting, horse chestnut for varicose veins, and meadowsweet for heartburn (Blumenthal, Goldberg, & Brinckman, 2000; Gottlieb, 2000; Hardy, 2000). Women interested in taking herbs during pregnancy should be advised (1) to avoid most herbs during the first trimester (except up to 1 g of ginger per day), (2) to avoid standardized or highly concentrated extracts, and (3) not to ingest essential oils (Hardy, 2000; Olds et al, 2004). Table 48–2 presents selected herbs that are contraindicated during pregnancy and some that may be beneficial.

Menopause

Menopause, a natural passage in a woman's life, is a time of transition that marks the end of a woman's reproductive abilities. Women experience changes in their reproductive, musculoskeletal, and cardiovascular systems as well as vasomotor and cognitive function changes. Despite the significance of these changes, fewer than 30 percent of women going through menopause have engaged in discussion with their health-care provider about menopausal

Table 48–2 **Use of Selected Herbs During Pregnancy**

Common Name	Comments
	Selected Herbs to Avoid in Pregnancy
Alder buckthorn	Very potent stimulators of bowel peristalsis known to irritate the uterus in sensitive women that may cause premature labor.
Angelica, dong quai	Uterine stimulant or may induce abortion/preterm labor. Dong quai is also an anticoagulant.
Arbor vitae and aloe	Oil-containing plants and essential oils that should not be taken internally during pregnancy.
Autumn crocus	Alkaloid-containing herbs that can be very potent, and are best avoided in pregnancy.
Barberry	Uterine stimulant.
Black cohosh	Uterine stimulant.

Continued

Table 48–2 **Use of Selected Herbs During Pregnancy—cont'd**

Common Name	Comments
	Selected Herbs to Avoid in Pregnancy
Blessed thistle	Powerful laxative; may overstimulate digestion and metabolism, causing fluid and electrolyte imbalances.
Blue cohosh	Uterine stimulant.
Cascara sagrada	Powerful laxative; may overstimulate digestion and metabolism, causing fluid and electrolyte imbalance.
Ephedra	Cardiovascular stimulant.
Feverfew	Uterine stimulant.
Ginseng	Thought to affect the hormonal system.
Goldenseal	Uterine stimulant.
Gotu kola	Potential teratogen.
Juniper	Potential teratogen.
Licorice root	Powerful laxative; may overstimulate digestion and metabolism, causing fluid and electrolyte imbalances.
Mugwort	Uterine stimulant.
Pennyroyal	Uterine stimulant.
Senna	Powerful laxative; may overstimulate digestion and metabolism, causing fluid and electrolyte imbalances.
Yarrow root	Uterine stimulant.
	Selected Herbs That May Be Beneficial in Pregnancy
Chamomile flowers	The safest herbs to use during pregnancy are those considered food or tonic herbs. May be taken in capsule form or used as a tea or infusion for nausea.
Black haw/cramp bark	Uterine relaxant; used for cramping/miscarriage prevention.
Dandelion greens and root	For anemia.
False unicorn root	Uterine tonic; used with black haw/cramp bark to prevent miscarriage.
Ginger root	For nausea.
Jasmine	Essential oils that can be safely used in aromatherapy during pregnancy. Do not ingest or use internally.
Nettle leaf	Allergy prevention.
Peppermint leaf	Used for nausea.
Red raspberry leaf	Uterine relaxant; used for cramping/miscarriage prevention.
Slippery elm bark	Uterine relaxant; used for cramping/miscarriage prevention.

symptoms, risk for chronic disease, or hormone use (Olds et al, 2004; Smith, 2005).

Many options for managing menopausal symptoms are available, such as the use of exercise, relaxation techniques, massage therapy, acupuncture, herbs, or pharmaceuticals such as **HRT** (Smith, 2005). Some women are unable or choose not to take **HRT** and have turned to **phytoestrogens**, substances with **estrogen-like** properties found in certain herbs, such as ginseng, black cohosh, dong quai, fenugreek, and licorice, and certain foods, especially carrots, yams, and soy products. Another menopause treatment option the practitioner should consider is nutritional supplements for a diet rich in **calcium** and **vitamins E, D, and B complex**. In addition, menopausal women should avoid foods such as **caffeine**, **alcohol**, and spicy foods that can trigger vasomotor symptoms (Olds et al, 2004). Alternative therapies for symptoms of menopause are presented in Table 48–3; herbal therapies are discussed in Chapter 10, and **HRT** is discussed in detail in Chapter 38.

Although managing menopausal symptoms is important, it is also vital at this time of life for a woman to achieve and/or maintain good health. Emphasis in the care of women in their 50s should be on health promotion and prevention of the diseases of older age. Classically, after menopause the lipid profile of women changes. The decline in endogenous **estrogen** removes a protective physiological mechanism that supports higher levels of high-density lipoprotein (HDL) and lowers low-density lipoproteins (LDL). Loss of **estrogen** places a woman at

Table 48–3 **Alternative Therapies for Menopause Symptoms**

Symptom	Alternative Therapy and Its Effects
Hot flashes	• **Suggest taking vitamin E 400 bid:** affects blood vessel walls; some women have blood pressure changes; monitor patients with hypertension. • **Suggest taking soy 2 oz:** contains 45 mg phytoestrogens (genistein); may protect from cancer. • **Suggest taking evening primrose 3 oz:** eliminate breast tenderness: stabilizes hormone fluctuations. • **Suggest taking remifemin (black cohosh) 1 tablet bid:** suppresses LH but not FSH; progesterone precursor; reduces hot flashes; used in Germany. • **Suggest taking dong quai:** estrogen precursor. • **Suggest taking bioidentical hormones:** contain equivalent hormones but from plant sources.
Reduced libido (or lack of sex drive)	• **Talk with the patient, sexual counseling/therapy:** ensure that spousal issues are not a hidden factor; if the intimate relationship is not good, menopause may not be the primary problem. • **Investigate sleep issues**: sleep disturbances can cause depression. • **Screen for depression**: depression often associated with altered libido. • **Suggest using alternative therapies listed for weight fluctuation:** improves self-image, which weight gain may hinder; increases energy after minimal weight loss (5 to 10 lb). • **Suggest using alternative therapies for vaginal dryness or soreness:** reduces vaginal dryness and pain; allows for anticipation of positive sensations.
Mood changes (irritability, depression)	• **Take vitamin B_6 (pyridoxine) 1.3 mg daily:** turns amino acids into serotonin, which affects mood. • **Practice meditation, yoga, or prayer:** calms nervous system; stimulates immunity; enhances personal control. • **Obtain adequate sleep:** aids relaxation. • **Improvise stress management techniques:** improves relaxation.
Sleep disturbances	• **Suggest taking valerian root, chamomile, melatonin:** aids relaxation. • **Exercise:** stimulates serotonin production after 40 min; affects mood. • **Decrease intake of or avoid stimulants (caffeine, nicotine, large protein-rich meals):** allows relaxation of nervous system. • **Avoid alcohol:** negatively affects all stages of sleep. • **Meditate, pray:** calms nervous system; stimulates immunity; enhances personal control.
Stress incontinence (urinary)	• **Decrease intake of caffeine beverages and diuretics:** reduces irritated detrusor muscle; results in less urgency. • **Perform Kegel exercises:** strengthens pelvic floor muscles. • **Treat/reduce constipation:** relieves pressure on urethra and bladder. • **Participate in bladder training programs:** reduces incidence of incontinence.
Vaginal dryness or soreness	• **Reduce or avoid use of medications such as antihistamines, decongestants, anticholinergics, and diuretics:** improves tissue moisture. • **Suggest using alternative therapies listed for hot flashes:** increases epithelial lining of vaginal tissues. • **Use water-soluble lubricants daily (e.g., Replens, Astroglide, Lubrin):** facilitates penetration; enhances foreplay (ensure that the patient knows areas to apply for maximum stimulation).
Weight fluctuations	• **Exercise 20 to 40 min, 3 to 4 times per week:** reduces weight gain; stabilizes mood; strengthens muscles; improves balance; stimulates good bone metabolism.

LH = luteinizing hormone; FSH = follicle-stimulating hormone.

increased risk for coronary artery disease, hypertension, and strokes (Olds et al, 2004). In fact, menopausal women "catch up" to men in relation to risks for these diseases and may experience "silent" coronary artery disease, which can become their greatest risk factor for death. Studies show that fewer women than men survive their first heart attack (Olds et al, 2004). Providers need to educate themselves and their female patients about the signs and symptoms of cardiac disease in women, and how the symptoms differ from those in men, with particular emphasis on the need to seek early treatment. Angina and ischemic heart disease are discussed in Chapter 28. Hypertension is discussed in Chapter 40, and hyperlipidemia in Chapter 39.

Genetics play a role in the diseases that afflict women at midlife, including heart disease, but preventive measures can be taught as well as prescribed. Primary prevention studies demonstrate that diets high in complex carbohydrates, fiber and protein, and low in animal fat are best. Balanced diets such as those recommended in *My Pyramid*

(U.S. Department of Agriculture [USDA], 2005) can lead to a lower body mass index (BMI). Normal BMI is considered between 19 and 24; 25 to 29 is considered overweight, and greater than 30 is obese (National Heart, Lung and Blood Institute, 2006).

Persons with BMI greater than 30 are associated with morbidity and shortened life expectancy.

Exercise is a nonpharmacological health promotion strategy. The exercise does not have to be strenuous, just consistent. Walking, yard work, bicycling, and swimming are all good forms of exercise. Brisk walking for 30 minutes three to five times a week is the activity recommended by most health-care providers.

Other postmenopausal physical changes seen in women are the results of normal human aging, and are shared by both sexes. These changes include thinning and graying of the hair, weight gain, drying skin, vision changes associated with presbyopia, and increased healing time for musculoskeletal injuries. Female genitourinary tract changes, affecting the vagina and urinary system, are the result of the cessation of ovarian function and decreased estrogen levels. Loss of the ureterovesicular angle and detrusor muscle instability result in urinary frequency and leakage, with increased residual bladder volume. Breast composition changes from dense glandular tissue to fatty replacement.

Older Age

In this millennium, many women are living as long after menopause as they did before it. If a woman reaches 50 years and is healthy, she has a good chance to live at least 80 years. Race is a major determinant of women's life spans. In the United States, white women have a life expectancy of 80.5 years, in contrast to African Americans, whose life expectancy is with 76.1 years (Hoyert, Matthews, Manacher, Strobino, & Guyler, 2006). Cardiovascular disease causes the greatest morbidity and mortality for the aging woman, followed by cancer and cerebrovascular disease (U.S. DHHS, Health Resources and Services Administration, 2005).

Aging women experience more frequent autoimmune disease, which manifests itself in joint and soft tissue pain and deformity. Although the risks for cancer increase with age and an estimated 250,000 new cases of breast cancer are diagnosed in the United States every year, many women never have mammograms because of lack of information, poor access to health care, or insufficient insurance coverage. Smoking by women has increased since the post–World War II years, which is hypothesized as the reason for their increased lung cancer rates. Geriatric patients are discussed in Chapter 51.

FACTORS THAT INFLUENCE POSITIVE OUTCOMES

Factors that produce positive outcomes are discussed in detail in Chapter 6. This section will discuss only those specific to women.

Number of Drugs Taken

Adult women receive more prescription drugs than men of the same age. Women are more apt to take medications for their skin, muscles, urinary tract, ophthalmological and otological problems, fatigue, extremity pain, weight, hypertension, and emotional complaints. Depression and connective tissue diseases are much more common in women. The risk for adverse reactions and drug interactions increases proportionately with the number of drugs being taken concurrently. The overall treatment regimen of each female patient should be regularly reviewed to eliminate any drugs that have "outlived" their usefulness or are duplicates.

Duration of Medication Therapy

Most patients can remember to take medications for a few days, especially if they are feeling ill, but drugs that must be taken daily and for many years are subject to poor adherence rates. Women may find themselves responsible for taking **oral contraceptive drugs (OCDs)** for 10 to 40 years, with other drugs added in from time to time. Adherence with OCD use varies over time, but generally averages below 60 percent. Providers who care for women of childbearing age need to be ever cognizant of the risk of pregnancy, even in women who using contraception.

Strategies to improve compliance, such as taking medications along with other routine activities of daily living, have been shown to work well. Women are frequently the primary caregivers of children and may also care for other family members (spouses, elderly parents, and relatives). The busyness of women's lives can complicate medication administration and decrease adherence.

Fear That Medications Cause Disease

Because social networking is frequently the way that women access health information, they hear about drugs (such as **hormones**) causing cancer or other disease from the media (e.g., television, newspapers) and from friends and relatives. This information is often sensational and can be inflammatory while being nonspecific. Concerns about exogenous hormones being carcinogenic can drive patient behavior, and it behooves providers to take time to explore them with patients. Education is needed to help women understand the results of studies done when much higher levels of potent **estrogen** were used in OCD and HRT formulations. Recent studies on the risk of gynecological cancers have shown a large hereditary component in breast cancer, especially when it occurs in women younger than 45 years. Genetic testing is now available for breast and ovarian cancers. Women may have a hard time deciding if they should use **hormonal therapies** because it is difficult to calculate their own absolute risk. What they hear in the media are relative risks, which refer to populations of women in certain age brackets. The results of the Women's Health Initiative (WHI) have further complicated decision making for both providers and patients. Providers need to read current research and be accurate in their knowledge in this area and share updated data with patients (Brucker & Youngkin, 2002).

Nutritional Status

Appropriate diet and good nutritional status are necessary for facilitating optimal growth in adolescents and for promoting health and wellness in women of all ages.

Obesity is a growing problem in all segments of the U.S. population. Women are at higher risk than men for eating disorders, which can lead to both overweight and underweight conditions. Obesity carries with it increased risks of cardiovascular and organ disease, hypertension, and diabetes. Anorexia nervosa and bulimia are complicated disorders with mental, emotional, and physical components that can lead to underweight as well as dental problems, osteopenia/osteoporosis, organ failure, and death. Of note, depression—more women than men suffer from this chronic mental illness—is the most common comorbidity with both obesity and anorexia (Ward & Hisley, 2009). Treatment for both overweight and underweight women can be challenging, with the best results involving an interdisciplinary team of providers. Polypharmacy can be a hazard in these patients, and prescriber vigilance in monitoring both drugs and changing doses, as weight and other body parameters change, is needed.

Safety of Medications While Breastfeeding

The benefits conferred to infants by breastfeeding, especially in the first year of life, are well described in the literature. Points to be considered in prescribing to lactating mothers are the acidity of breast milk in relation to the pH of plasma, the protein-binding effects of the drug prescribed, the liposolubility of the drug prescribed, and the molecular weight of the drug prescribed. (See Chap. 50 for specific information on drugs in breast milk.)

Ethnic, Cultural, and Religious Differences

Although women from diverse cultures commonly seek health care more often than do men (this is true in most cultures), many cultures are patriarchies. In patriarchal societies, men make the decisions about **birth control**, whether women work outside the home, and how much money women receive to run the household. Women may not have the choice to refuse sexual relations. The lack of power and control over their own bodies can generate many somatic complaints. These women patients often present on multiple occasions with what may appear to be nonspecific and unrelated symptoms. Pelvic pain and genital pain are frequent complaints, and unplanned pregnancies are not unusual. Adherence to prescribed **contraceptive** regimens is difficult, if not impossible, for women in many of these situations.

Religion can also raise issues related to the prescribing of medications. If a patient's belief system does not support a treatment that the provider is prescribing, adherence may become a problem. Cultural issues are discussed in detail in Chapter 7.

> **CLINICAL PEARL**
>
> **Prescribing During Breastfeeding**
>
> When prescribing for a breastfeeding woman, ask yourself: Is this drug safe for infants?

> **CLINICAL PEARL**
>
> **Mothers and Smoking**
>
> Mothers who smoke should be told that infants of mothers who smoked in the home had the same level of drug **(nicotine)** excreted in their urine as those infants with mothers who always smoked outside.

COMMON PROBLEMS THAT REQUIRE MEDICATIONS

In addition to the array of medical problems shared by both genders—hypertension, cardiovascular disease, diabetes, cancer, glaucoma, organ disease, arthritis, mental illnesses, autoimmune disorders, and pain management—specific problems in women that require medications include urinary tract infection and urinary incontinence, sexually transmitted infections and vaginitis, premenstrual disorders, endometriosis, polycystic ovarian syndrome (PCOS), contraception, infertility, menopause, gynecological cancers, osteoporosis, depression, and hypothyroidism. Many of these problems are discussed in the appropriate chapters in Unit III. Problems not discussed in Unit III chapters are

> **CLINICAL PEARL**
>
> **Prescribing in a Diverse Culture**
>
> Be aware of the common ethnic groups in your patient population. Get to know the cultures. Frequently, community programs that teach cultural awareness and some simple ethnic phrases are available for health-care personnel. Bookstores carry pocket-sized books to facilitate a simple medical interview in different languages.

included here: menopause, premenstrual syndrome and premenstrual dysphoric disorder, endometriosis, PCOS, AIDS in pregnancy, and infertility.

Menopause

Menopause is a normal physiological process in women, with the mean age of menopause in the United States at 51.3 years (Olds et al, 2004; Smith, 2005). Several years of gradual decline or erratic levels of endogenous **estrogen** precede cessation of ovarian function. All women experience changes in their secondary sexual characteristics. Some women barely notice vasomotor instability, whereas hot flashes and insomnia incapacitate others. **Estrogen** and **progesterone** may interact at more than 200 receptor sites in a woman's body, so exogenous treatment may affect women in many different ways. Alternative therapies for symptoms of menopause are presented in Table 48–3. When women are postmenopausal and choose to use drug therapy (HRT) absolute risks versus benefits for the individual should be assessed and discussed. Present recommendations are for the lowest amount of drug to be used for the shortest period of time to alleviate problematic symptoms (National Association of Nurse Practitioners in Women's Health, 2002).

Dysmenorrhea, Premenstrual Syndrome, and Premenstrual Dysphoric Disorder

Women typically have menstrual cycles for about 40 years. Cyclic perimenstrual pain and discomfort (CPPD) is the name of a concept developed by a team of American Women's Health, Obstetric and Neonatal Nurses (AWHONN) nurse-researchers (Collins-Sharp, Taylor, Thanas, Killeen, & Danwood, 2002). This concept includes dysmenorrhea, premenstrual syndrome (PMS), and premenstrual dysphoric disorder (PMDD). CPPD can have a significant impact on a woman's quality of life. Nurse practitioners play a vital role in identifying and diagnosing dysmenorrhea, PMS, and the more disabling PMDD and in managing the symptom of these disorders. Bhati and Bhati (2002) report that as many as 20 to 40 percent of menstruating women experience one of the disorders.

Dysmenorrhea

Dysmenorrhea, pain shortly before or during menstruation, is one of the most common gynecological complaints. Young adult women (ages 17 to 24) present most frequently with this complaint, but the condition affects women of all ages. Between 30 and 40 percent of women report some level of discomfort with menses, and 7 to 15 percent report severe pain (Parent-Stevens & Burns, 2000). Primary dysmenorrhea is due to increased myometrial activity, with contractions induced by prostaglandins in the second half of the menstrual cycle. **NSAIDS** are the first line of drug treatment for women not desiring contraception (American College of Obstetricians and Gynecologists [ACOG], 2004) and are particularly effective if begun 2 to 3 days before menses or at the first sign of bleeding. OTC **NSAIDs** have the same active ingredients (e.g., **ibuprofen, naproxen sodium**) as prescription drugs; however, the labeled recommended dose for general discomfort may be subtherapeutic for dysmenorrhea. Preparations containing **acetaminophen**, which is not an **NSAID**, are ineffective because of the absence of antiprostaglandin properties. For women who want contraception, oral contraceptive pills (**OCPs**) are a good therapeutic choice. Decreased prostaglandin synthesis results from an atrophic endometrium (ACOG, 2004; Speroff & Fritz, 2005). No single brand of **OCP** has been shown to be superior for this indication.

Many nonpharmacological measures can be used to relieve primary dysmenorrhea, and often the best treatment strategies involve using both medications and comfort measures along with lifestyle modifications. Heat (poultices or heating pads), massage/effleurage, guided imagery, progressive relaxation, yoga, exercise, and meditation have been successful in managing menstrual discomfort. Decreasing dietary intake of salt, sugar, and red meat in the luteal phase and increasing water intake may reduce edema (Lowdermilk & Perry, 2007).

If dysmenorrheal discomfort is not relieved by one of the **NSAIDS**, further investigation into the cause of symptoms is required. Secondary dysmenorrhea usually develops later in a woman's life (after age 25). Pelvic pathology—such as adenomyosis, endometriosis, pelvic inflammatory disease (PID), endometrial polyps, and myomas (fibroids)—is associated with secondary dysmenorrheal (Lowdermilk & Perry, 2007). Many of the relief measures for primary dysmenorrhea are also helpful for women with secondary dysmenorrhea, but treatment is aimed at removal of the underlying pathology.

Premenstrual Syndrome (PMS)

The diagnostic criteria for PMS were written by the American College of Obstetricians and Gynecologists (ACOG Practice Bulletin, 2006). Symptoms include irritability, depression, angry outbursts, anxiety, confusion, social withdrawal, and mood swings. Somatic symptoms include fatigue, insomnia, dizziness, headaches, breast tenderness, weight gain, abdominal bloating, edema secondary to water retention, and muscle and joint pain (Dickerson, Mazyck, & Hunter, 2003). Women often respond to exercising aerobically, decreasing **caffeine**, reducing salt intake, and taking **ibuprofen** 500 to 1,000 mg/day during the luteal phase: days 17 to 28 of the menstrual cycle (Frackiewicz & Shiovitz, 2001). Pritham (2002) recommends eating smaller, more frequent meals that are high in complex carbohydrates and fiber; reducing intake of salty foods, sugar, **caffeine**, chocolate, red meat, dairy products, and **alcohol**; and increasing the dose of **calcium** supplementation. She also recommends relaxation techniques, yoga, stress management, and good sleep hygiene.

Premenstrual Dysphoric Disorder

A small subgroup of CPPD patients (2% to 10%) has a more severe form of the disorder: premenstrual dysphoric disorder (PMDD) (Bhati & Bhati, 2002; Dickerson et al, 2003). Diagnosis of PMDD is based on criteria established by the American Psychiatric Association (APA) (2000). To meet diagnostic criteria, patients must exhibit five or more symptoms, including at least one "core" symptom. Severely affected women typically have symptoms for 6 to 7 days each cycle. Symptoms of PMDD include the core symptoms of markedly depressed moods, heightened anxiety/tension/edginess/nervousness, affective lability, persistent and marked anger and irritability; plus other symptoms, such as decreased interest in usual activities, marked lack of energy (fatigue, lethargy), hypersomnia or insomnia, difficulty concentrating, appetite changes or cravings, and a subjective sense of being overwhelmed or "out of control," *plus* any of the physical symptoms already described in the PMS section of this chapter (Minkin & Moore, 2006). Symptoms are cyclical, occurring during the luteal phase of the menstrual cycle and are significantly reduced or disappear completely during menstruation. The morbidity of this condition is staggering when one considers that an average woman might have more than 400 cycles between the ages of 14 and 51, depending on the number of pregnancies and how long she breastfeeds. Some women can experience approximately *8 cumulative years* of severe PMDD during their reproductive years!

Pathophysiology

The exact cause of PMS and PMDD is unknown, but clearly multifaceted interactions among the central nervous system, hormones, and other chemical modulators occur. Genetic influences mediated phenotypically through neurotransmitters and neuroreceptors seem to play a large role. Seventy percent of women whose mothers have PMS will have PMS themselves, and a 93 percent concordance rate occurs in monozygotic twins compared to 44 percent in dizygotic twins (Bhati & Bhati, 2002). Theories about the pathophysiological cause that are supported in research suggest that PMDD may be caused by altered sensitivity in the **serotonergic system** to phasic fluctuation in female **gonadal hormones.** Some of the nutritional interventions are based in studies of the effectiveness of **L-tryptophan,** a precursor of **serotonin,** and of **pyridoxine,** a cofactor in the conversion of **tryptophan** into **serotonin,** in relieving PMDD symptoms. The success of **SSRIs,** which are considered first-line therapy in this disorder (Bhati & Bhati, 2002; Frackiewicz & Shiovitz, 2001; Kaur, Gonsalves, & Thacker, 2004), also supports this hypothesis. **Spironolactone** has demonstrated benefits for symptoms in the premenstrual phase of the cycle (Ginsburg & Dinsay, 2000). **Prostaglandins** appear to play a role in some of the symptoms, and **NSAIDs** seem to be effective through their action on **prostaglandins.** In October 2009, the FDA approved an **oral contraceptive pill** (**OCP**) for the treatment of emotional and physical symptoms of PMDD in women who choose OCPs as their method of contraception. Each pill contains 3 mg **drospirenone** (which is derived from **spirolactone**) and 20 mcg ethinyl estradiol (Minkin & Moore, 2006).

Treatments

The same lifestyle modifications used with PMS are also useful with PMDD. The outcome most suited to pharmacological therapy in PMDD is symptom reduction. Nutritional, herbal, and drug therapies play a role in this complex disorder. The dosing of selected nutritional, herbal, and drug therapies is presented in Table 48–4.

Table 48–4 **Treatment Options for PMDD**

Therapy	Dosing	Symptom Improvement
	Nutritional Supplements	
Calcium carbonate	1,200–1,600 mg/d	Core symptoms.
Magnesium	Up to 500 mg/d	Bloating.
Tryptophan	Up to 6 g/d	Insomnia; affective symptoms.
Vitamin B_6	Up to 100 mg/d	Core symptoms; depression.
Vitamin E	200–400 mg/d	Stabilizes hormonal fluctuations.
	Herbals	
Evening primrose oil	500 mg daily to 1,000 mg tid	Anti-inflammatory; breast tenderness.
Chaste tree berry	30–40 mg/d	Breast engorgement.
	Drugs (SRIs)	
Citalopram (off-labeled)*	10–30 mg/d	All symptoms. Fewer side effects than other SRIs.
Fluoxetine (indication)	20 mg/d	All symptoms. Sexual side effects.
Paroxetine (off-labeled)	10–30 mg/d	All symptoms. GI and sexual side effects.
Sertraline (indication)	50–150 mg/d	All symptoms. GI and sexual side effects.

Continued

Table 48–4 **Treatment Options for PMDD—cont'd**

Therapy	Dosing	Symptom Improvement
	Drugs (Other)	
Alprazolam	0.375–1.5 mg/d	Anxiety and other affective symptoms.
Bromocriptine	Up to 2.5 mg tid	Breast engorgement.
Clomipramine	25–75 mg/d	All symptoms. Anticholinergic effects.
Ibuprofen	500–1000 mg/d	Pain; breast engorgement.
Spironolactone	100 mg/d	Water retention.

*This drug is best given during the luteal phase of the menstrual cycle.
PMDD = premenstrual dysphoric disorder.

Nutritional Supplements

Randomized, placebo-controlled trials have shown **vitamin B6** in dosages up to 100 mg per day to benefit patients with premenstrual symptoms and premenstrual depression. **Calcium carbonate** in dosages of 1,200 to 1,600 mg per day reduced core premenstrual symptoms by 48 percent for 466 patients in one study (Bhati & Bhati, 2002). **Vitamin E**, an antioxidant, reduces affective and physical symptoms in some patients. Finally, **magnesium** and **tryptophan** may also benefit PMS/PMDD patients. Nutritional supplements are generally considered second-line therapies, though they may be tried initially by women who are reticent to take pharmaceuticals.

Herbals

Data on the efficacy and safety of herbal supplements marketed for women with PMS/PMDD have been inconsistent for many products. In addition, manufacturing standards for herbal products are not uniform. Given these caveats, two products based on research are recommended by Bhati and Bhati (2002). The most studied is **evening primrose oil**, which may be a precursor for **prostaglandin synthesis** and so may benefit symptoms associated with **prostaglandins.** Doses are 500 mg daily to 1,000 mg tid. Chaste tree berry has also been studied, although less so. Doses of 30 to 40 mg per day may benefit breast symptoms because it inhibits **prolactin** production. Studies of **vitamin A** do not support its use: Other studies do not support the use of other herbals, such as black cohosh.

Drug Therapies

First-line therapy for PMDD is **SSRIs.** Three of them have been FDA approved for PMDD: **fluoxetine, paroxetine,** and **sertraline** (Bhati & Bhati, 2002; Dickerson et al, 2001; Freeman, Rickels, Sondheimer, Polansky, & Xiao, 2004; Halbreich & Kahn, 2003; Kaur et al, 2004; Luisi & Pawasaukas, 2003; Minkin & Moore, 2006). **Sertraline** is the most studied. Researchers disagree on whether it should be used only during the luteal phase (Halbreich & Kahn, 2003). Freeman and colleagues (2004) found no difference between continuous use and luteal phase only in reducing PMDD symptoms. Steiner and colleagues (2003) looked at **fluoxetine** efficacy related to affective and occupational functioning rather than physical symptoms. They found it reduced these symptoms relatively quickly at a low dose of 20 mg per day. Although they have been used for PMDD, the **anxiolytics, citalopram** and **alprazolam,** are off-labeled for this indication.

Second-line drug therapy includes **tricyclic clomipramine** and **benzodiazepine.** Although they are often helpful, **tricyclic clomipramine** has **anticholinergic** side effects and **benzodiazepine** is associated with tolerance if used long term.

Ibuprofen, spironolactone, and **bromocriptine** are focused on specific PMS/PMDD symptoms and are useful for patients with those symptoms. Table 48–4 gives doses for these drugs and the types of symptoms they are most effective in relieving.

Gonadotropin-releasing hormone (GnRH) agonists, and **danazol,** a weak **androgen,** have been used to treat PMDD (Bhati & Bhati, 2002; Dickerson et al, 2003; Minkin & Moore, 2006; Pritham, 2002). GnRH agonists inhibit follicle-stimulating hormone (FSH) and luteinizing hormone (LH), suppressing ovarian steroid hormone production and preventing ovulation. As the effect is equivalent to a medically induced oophorectomy, these drugs are best prescribed by a specialist.

Endometriosis

Endometriosis is primarily a disorder of young women. The incidence is hard to determine in asymptomatic adolescents and fertile women, but it has been estimated that 10 to 15 percent of reproductive-age women and 2 to 4 percent of menopausal women have endometriosis. As many as 50 percent of women evaluated for pelvic pain, infertility, or a pelvic mass are diagnosed with this disorder (McCance & Huether, 2006). The frequency and severity of symptoms do not correlate with the extent or site of the lesions, and as many as 31 percent of asymptomatic fertile women are found to have endometriosis when undergoing laparoscopy.

Pathophysiology

Endometriosis is the presence of functioning endometrial tissue (called implants) outside the uterus. The cause is unknown, but theories include retrograde menstruation, depressed cytotoxic T-cell response to endometrial cells in ectopic locations, and a genetic hypothesis that proposes abnormal development of epithelial cells of the reproductive organs (Georgia Reproductive Specialists, 2006; McCance & Huether, 2006). Endometriosis appears to have a genetic predisposition; the condition is six to seven times more prevalent in women who have a first-degree relative with endometriosis as compared to the general population (Speroff & Fritz, 2005). Women who have endometriosis may also have other conditions such as chronic fatigue syndrome, fibromyalgia, endocrine disorders, and autoimmune disorders ("Conversations with Colleagues," 2002–2003).

Endometrial implants can occur throughout the body, but are most often found on the ovaries, uterine ligaments, rectovaginal septum, and pelvic peritoneum. Other common sites include the surface of the intestines, the bladder, the vulva and vagina, and the pleural cavity and lungs (McCance & Huether, 2006). Cyclical changes in **gonadal hormones** results in proliferation of the ectopic endometrium with the subsequent breakdown and bleeding that is part of the normal menstrual cycle. The bleeding produces inflammation with the usual release of inflammatory mediators. Pain occurs in the surrounding tissues and the inflammatory process can lead to fibrosis, scarring, and adhesions, which are the lesions often held responsible for infertility in these women. Symptoms relate to the inflammatory process caused by the bleeding and include pelvic pain, dysmenorrhea, dyspareunia, and, less commonly, constipation and abnormal vaginal bleeding (McCance & Huether, 2006; Pick & Holmes, 2006).

Drug Therapies

The ACOG (1999) issued the following recommendations based on reliable scientific evidence:

- For pain relief, **GnRH agonists** for at least 3 months or **danazol** for at least 6 months. Treatment with **danazol** is about one-third less costly than **GnRH** agonist treatment.
- When **GnRH agonist** treatment must continue for some time, "add-back" regimens with **progestin, bisphosphonates, pulsatile parathyroid hormone**, or nasal **calcitonin** should be considered to reduce GnRH-induced bone mineral loss.

Pick and Holmes (2006) recommend less dramatic treatments first. They report a high rate of success with a combination of dietary changes, nutrient support, emotional healing, and alternative therapies such as acupuncture. Their dietary recommendations remove **xenoestrogen** exposure by eliminating nonorganic dairy products, beef and chicken; increase nutrient-rich food such as cruciferous vegetables, soy, cold water fish and fiber; and suggest a lower carbohydrate diet to support healthy insulin metabolism. Supplementation with **calcium** and **magnesium** (see PMDD) and **omega-3**, an essential fatty acid, reduces inflammation. When drugs are chosen, **ibuprofen, naprosyn**, and other **NSAIDs** are used to decrease pain and inflammation. **OCDs** that give synthetic **progestin** are also suggested to block the stimulation of the endometriosis implants. These researchers leave **GnRH** agonists and **danazol** to the more severe cases.

The Mayo Clinic (2006) supports this less dramatic approach to management. Its researchers do not discuss dietary and alternative therapies, but agree with the use of **ibuprofen** for pain management, and **oral contraceptives** including **Depo-Provera. GnRH agonists** and **antagonists** and **danazol** are also mentioned, but the latter are used only if the former is ineffective.

HIV/AIDS in Pregnancy

Women are now the fastest-growing population with HIV infection and AIDS; an estimated 27 percent of new infections occur in women (CDC, 2006a). "More than half of infections are among black and non-Hispanic women" and "the majority of HIV-positive women are of reproductive age (13 to 44 years)" (Kirshenbaum et al, 2004, p. 106). Pregnant women who are HIV positive face many challenges, such as unpredictable symptoms and prognosis, the potential for maternal to infant transmission and problematic life circumstances that have the potential to compromise parenting such as poverty, substance abuse, and the stigma associated with this disease. Despite these challenges, HIV-infected women are no less likely to become pregnant, nor are they more likely to terminate a pregnancy (Kirshenbaum et al, 2004).

Other viral infections, such as herpes and cytomegalovirus, seem to be more prevalent in women infected with HIV than in men (Williams, 2003). HIV-positive women also may have more severe pelvic inflammatory disease than other women and rates of cervical dysplasia and human papillomavirus (HPV) may be higher in HIV-positive women, with the clinical course accelerated and more frequent recurrence (Lowdermilk & Perry, 2007).

An infected woman can pass the HIV virus to her baby during pregnancy, delivery, or breastfeeding. **Antiretroviral** prophylaxis (e.g., **zidovudine** [ZDV, AZT, **Retrovir**]) during pregnancy greatly reduces the risk of passing the HIV virus to the fetus. Reported rates of mother-to-child transmission are 2 percent when women begin prophylactic medication treatment early in pregnancy (Stephenson, 2005). This rate increases to 12 to 13 percent if treatment is not initiated until labor, delivery, or after birth; and shoots up to 25 percent should women receive no preventive treatment.

The use of **zidovudine** or another **highly active antiretroviral therapy (HAART)** for infected pregnant women has contributed to the decline in the number of new pediatric AIDS cases. Therefore, the CDC recommends that all pregnant women be offered voluntary HIV testing as part of routine prenatal care so that those who carry the virus can obtain treatment (Kirshenbaum et al,

2004; March of Dimes Birth Defects Foundation, 2002; Olds et al, 2004). Further discussion of the management of HIV/AIDS is found in Chapter 37.

Infertility

Infertility, defined as the absence of conception despite unprotected sexual intercourse for at least one year, has a profound emotional, psychological, and economic impact on the affected couple and society. A serious medical concern, the condition affects the quality of life for 10 to 15 percent of reproductive age couples (American Society for Reproductive Medicine [ASRM], 2002). About 35 percent of infertility problems are due to a male factor, 45 percent to a female factor, and the remaining 20 percent are due to problems with both partners or are unexplained. Incidence of infertility increases with a woman's age, particularly in women older than age 40 (Stenchever, Droegremuller, Herbst, & Mishell, 2001). Determination of hormone levels, such as prolactin, FSH, LH, estradiol (E2), progesterone, and thyroid, may be necessary to diagnose the cause of absent or irregular menstrual cycles. The **clomiphene citrate** challenge test (CCCT) can be given to assess ovarian reserves. Couples should undergo an infertility evaluation by a specialist if after 1 year of trying they have been unable to conceive. A woman older than 35 years may be referred earlier, for example, after only 6 to 9 months of unprotected intercourse without achieving conception (Olds et al, 2004).

Polycystic Ovarian Syndrome

An endocrine imbalance that results in high levels of estrogen, testosterone, and LH with decreased levels of FSH, polycystic ovarian syndrome (PCOS) is associated with a number of problems in the hypothalamic-pituitary-ovarian axis. The ovaries can double in size with multiple follicular cysts, producing excess estrogen. Impaired glucose tolerance and hyperinsulinemia (metabolic syndrome) occur in about 45 percent of women with PCOS (Stenchever et al, 2001). Affected women are at high risk of developing type 2 diabetes and cardiovascular diseases (Sheehan, 2004).

Analgesics may be prescribed for pain management, and regular examination is needed to monitor the size of the ovaries. **OCPs** may be indicated for few months to suppress functional cysts, if pregnancy is not desired. **GnRH analogues** may be used to treat hirsutism if **OCPs** do not improve this distressing symptom (Lowdermilk & Perry, 2007). If pregnancy is desired, medications for **ovulation induction** are given (Sheehan, 2004). **Insulin** and **metformin** are prescribed to manage the type 2 diabetes, lowering blood glucose and testosterone, which, in turn, can reduce acne, hirsutism, abdominal obesity, and amenorrhea in women with PCOS (ACOG, 2002; Lord & Wilkin, 2004).

HEALTH PROMOTION, DISEASE PREVENTION, AND SCREENING

Preventive screening and testing save lives by identifying previously undiagnosed conditions and by allowing for early intervention and treatments so that health outcomes are improved. Many simple, preventive measures can be taken by women to reduce morbidity and mortality. These measures include **immunizations** for **pneumonia** and **influenza;** and screening for high blood pressure, cholesterol, and blood sugar. Screening tests to identify heart disease, cancers, and diabetes are recommended by the American Cancer Society, the American Diabetes Association, the American Heart Association, the American Academy of Family Physicians, and the U.S. Preventive Services Task Force.

Some preventive health-care screening recommendations for adult women without symptoms of disease should begin at age 18 years and include an eye examination, blood pressure check, Pap test and pelvic examination, and breast self-examination. **Tetanus (Td or Tdap) immunizations** should be updated every 10 years. Anyone in a risk category should complete immunization series for **hepatitis A** and **B.** In 2006, the CDC recommended routine vaccination of girls aged 12 to 24 years against HPV (CDC, 2006b). Other screening tests should be implemented beginning at age 40 years, such as a breast examination performed by a health-care provider and mammograms (American Cancer Society, 2006). There is no consensus on the frequency of mammograms for women between 40 and 49 years of age; recommendations vary from annually over age 40 (American Cancer Society, 2006) to annually over age 50 (U.S. Preventive Services Task Force [USPSTF], 2005). Providers are urged to individualize recommendations for their patients. Since lung and colon cancers have increased in the past century, patients need to begin screening procedures, such as sigmoidoscopy at age 50 years. Skin examination for cancer should be done every 3 years between ages 20 and 40, and at least annually afterward. Bone mineral density (BMD) testing is recommended for all women aged 65 and older and younger women at risk for osteoporosis. A complete list of preventive health-care screening tests can be found at http://www.4women.gov.

GAY AND LESBIAN HEALTH

Membership in a sexual minority group is not in and of itself hazardous; however, risk factors may be conferred through "homophobia," the socialization of heterosexuals against homosexuals. "Homophobia places a huge cost on society and has been linked to increased rates in smoking, **alcohol** use, depression, HIV/AIDS, physical violence, and attempted suicide rates among members of the lesbian, gay, bisexual, transgendered, and queer (LGBTQ) community" (Goldberg,

2006, p. 464). Heterosexist and homophobic attitudes permeate health-care environments and are manifested through avoidance, inappropriateness, and distance, which create an atmosphere of nondisclosure of important health-related information to health-care providers. The assumption by health-care providers that heterosexuality is the relationship norm and any other variation is deviant makes it difficult and embarrassing for individuals to open up about their sexuality. Ignorance resulting from heterosexist assumptions has resulted in practitioners erroneously advising lesbians they cannot contract a sexually transmitted infection (STI) from a female partner or that screening for cervical cancer is not required. Evidence has demonstrated that lesbians who have had no history of sexual intercourse with males can have abnormal Pap smears (Goldberg, 2006; Olds et al, 2004).

Lesbian health is not completely the same as women's health because "their lived experiences and ways of being in the world are different" (Goldberg, 2006). As a group lesbian and bisexual women are less likely to have health-care insurance or access to health-care services. Those with access to care are less likely than heterosexual women to adequately use preventive health-care services because of fear of discrimination. This avoidance behavior is of concern because lesbian and bisexual women smoke more cigarettes and are less likely to use oral contraceptives, which increase their risk for breast cancer (Olds et al, 2004).

Providers have a professional and moral responsibility to treat all people with respect and dignity, regardless of their sexual orientation or preference. Providers working with the gay and lesbian community can use several helpful strategies to address homophobia and promote a positive environment. First and foremost the provider must be aware of his or her own biases and be open, knowledgeable, and comfortable with sexual differences. This "gay positive" posture creates a safe atmosphere for disclosure of information so appropriate diagnosis, treatment, and information can be provided to the patient. The provider should also reconsider how health histories are obtained. For example, consider creating a space for the client to document nonheterosexual relationships on written documents and modifying questions used to obtain information regarding sexuality. One method for acknowledging a current relationship status is to ask questions such as, "Are you at present in a relationship?" or "Who is your partner in your relationship?" In addition, an accepting physical environment can be achieved by having pamphlets about lesbian and bisexual health readily available. Finally, providers and others should avoid using euphemisms such as "special friend" when asking about the patient's partner (Goldberg, 2006). Providers can obtain additional facts and information about gay and lesbian health-care issues from the National Coalition for Lesbian, Gay, Bisexual, and Transgender Health at http://www.lgbthealth.net or the Gay and Lesbian Medical Association at http://www.glma.org.

REFERENCES

Agency for Healthcare Research and Quality (AHRQ). (2002). *AHRQ focus on research: Healthcare for women.* Washington, DC: Author.

American Academy of Pediatrics. (2009). Interim vaccine statement: Human papillomavirus (HPV). Updated March 30, 2010. Retrieved from http://www.healthychildren.org

American Cancer Society. (2006). *Cancer facts and figures, 2006.* New York: Author.

American College of Obstetricians and Gynecologists (ACOG). (1999). Medical management of endometriosis (ACOG Practice Bulletin 11). Washington, DC: Author.

American College of Obstetricians and Gynecologists (ACOG). (2002). Polycystic ovarian syndrome: Diagnosis and management. *Clinics in Medical Research, 2*(1), 3–27.

American College of Obstetricians and Gynecologists (ACOG). (2004). Chronic pelvic pain (ACOG Practice Bulletin No. 51). *Obstetrics and Gynecology, 103*(3), 589–605.

American College of Obstetricians and Gynecologists (ACOG). (2006). Premenstrual syndrome (ACOG Practice Bulletin No. 15). Washington, DC: Author.

American Pregnancy Association. (2005). What's the real scoop on caffeine during pregnancy? Retrieved November 11, 2005, from http://www.americanpregancny.org/pregnancyhealth/caffeine.html

American Psychiatric Association (APA). (2000). *Diagnostic and statistical manual of mental disorders* (4th ed., text revision). Washington, DC: Author.

American Society for Reproductive Medicine (ASRM). (2002). Assisted reproductive technology in the U.S: 1999 results generated for the ASRM/Society for Assisted Reproductive Registry. *Fertility and Sterility, 78*(5), 918–931.

Anderson, G. (2005). Sex and racial differences in pharmacological response: Where is the evidence? Pharmacogenetics, pharmacokinetics and pharmacodynamics. *Journal of Women's Health, 14,* 19–29.

Bhati, S., & Bhati, S. (2002). Diagnosis and treatment of premenstrual dysphoric disorder. *American Family Physician, 66*(7). Retrieved January 13, 2006, from http://www.aafp.org/afp/20021001/1239.html

Blumenthal, M., Goldberg, A., & Brinckman, J. (Eds.). (2000). *Herbal medicine: Expanded Commission E monographs.* Newton, MA: Integrated Medicine Communications.

Bohn, D., Tibben, J., & Campbell, J. (2004). Influences of income, education, age and ethnicity on physical abuse before and during pregnancy. *Journal of Obstetrics, Gynecologic, & Neonatal Nursing, 33,* 561–571.

Brucker, M., & Youngkin, E. (2002, October/November). What's a woman to do? *AWHONN Lifelines,* 407–417.

Cauley, J., Lucas, F., Kuller, L., Stone, K., Browner, W., & Cummings, S. (1999). Elevated serum estradiol and testosterone concentrations are associated with a high risk for breast cancer. *Annals of Internal Medicine, 130*(4), 270–277.

Centers for Disease Control and Prevention (CDC). (2005a). *Intimate partner violence: Fact sheet.* Retrieved January 5, 2005, from http://www.cdc.gov/ncipc/factsheets/ipvoverview.htm

Centers for Disease Control and Prevention (CDC). (2005b). *Intimate partner violence: Overview.* Retrieved January 5, 2005, from http://www.cdc.gov/ncipc/factsheets/ipvoverview.htm

Centers for Disease Control and Prevention (CDC). (2006a). *HIV/AIDS update: A glance at the epidemic.* Washington, DC: Author. Retrieved from http://www.cdc.gov.hiv/pubs/facts/at-a-glance.html

Centers for Disease Control and Prevention (CDC). (2006b). Sexually transmitted disease treatment guidelines. *Morbidity and Mortality Weekly Report, 55*(RRII), 1–94.

Collins-Sharp, B., Taylor, D., Thanas, K., Killeen, M., & Danwood, M. (2002). Cyclic premenstrual pain and discomfort: The scientific basis for practice. *Journal of Obstetrical, Gynecologic and Neonatal Nursing, 31*(6), 637–649.

Conversations with colleagues. (2002–2003). Endometriosis sufferers risk other diseases. *AWHONN Lifelines, 6*(6), 502–504.

Davis, W. (1998). Impact of gender on drug responses. *Drug Topics,* October 5, 91–98.

Dickerson, L., Mazyck, P., & Hunter, M. (2003). Premenstrual syndrome. *American Family Physician, 67*(8). Retrieved January 13, 2006, from http://www.aafp.org/afp/200304151743.html

Disability Statistics Center. (2002). *How does the Disability Statistics Center define disability?* San Francisco: Author.

Drug facts and comparisons. (2009). St. Louis, MO: Wolters Kluwer Health.

Frackiewicz, E., & Shiovitz, T. (2001). Evaluation and management of premenstrual syndrome and premenstrual dysphoric disorder. *Journal of American Pharmacology Association, 41*(3), 437–447.

Freeman, E., Rickels, K., Sondheimer, S., Polansky, M., & Xiao, S. (2004). Continuous or intermittent dosing with sertraline for patients with severe premenstrual syndrome or premenstrual dysphoric disorder. *American Journal of Psychiatry, 161*(2), 343–351.

Gandhi, M., Aweeka, F., Greenblatt, R., & Blaschke, T. (2004). Sex differences in pharmacokinetics and pharmacodynamics. *Annual Review of Pharmacology and Toxicology, 44,* 499–523.

Georgia Reproductive Specialists. (2006). Endometriosis. Retrieved January 13, 2006, from http://ivf.comendoassn/html

Gibson, E., & Coupey, S. (2007). The female athlete triad. *The Female Patient, 32,* 34–41.

Ginn, J., Street, D., & Arber, S. (2001). *Women, work and pensions: Interracial issues and prospects.* Buckingham, England: Open University Press.

Ginsburg, K. A., & Dinsay, R. (2000). Premenstrual syndrome. In S. B. Ransom (Ed.), *Practical strategies in obstetrics and gynecology.* Philadelphia: Saunders.

Goldberg, L. (2006). Understanding lesbian experience. *AWHONN Lifelines, 9*(6), 463–467.

Gottlieb, B. (2000). *Alternative cures.* Emmaus, PA: Rodale.

Halbreich, U., & Kahn, L. (2003). Treatment of premenstrual dysphoric disorder with luteal phase dosing of sertraline. *Expert Opinion in Pharmacotherapy, 4*(11), 2065–2078.

Hardy, M. (2000). Herbs of special interest to women. *Journal of the American Pharmaceutical Association, 40*(2), 234–242.

Hoyert, D., Matthews, J. T., Menacher, F., Strobino, D., & Guyler, B. (2006). Annual summary of vital statistics: 2004. *Pediatrics, 117*(1), 168–183.

Kaur, G., Gonsalves, L., & Thacker, H. (2004). Premenstrual dysphoric disorder: A review for the treating practitioner. *Cleveland Clinic Journal of Medicine, 71*(4), 303–305, 312–313, 317–318.

Kirshenbaum, S. B., Hirky, A. E., Correale, J., Goldstein, R. B., Johnson, M. O., Rotheram-Borus, M. J., et al. (2004). "Throwing in the dice": Pregnancy decision-making among HIV-positive women in four U.S. cities. *Perspectives on Sexual and Reproductive Health, 36*(3), 106–113.

Kleist, P. (2005, December). Women and trials: When is gender a consideration? *Applied Clinical Trials.* Retrieved January 4, 2006, from http://www.actmagazine.com/appliedclinicaltrials/article

Kotler, D., Thea, D., Heo, M., Allison, D., Engelson, E., Wang, J., et al. (1999). Relative influences of sex, race, environment, and HIV infection on body composition in adults. *American Journal of Clinical Nutrition, 69*(9), 432–439.

Levine, S. (1998). The sexual consequences of perimenopause and menopause. *Women's Health in Primary Care, 1*(10), 509–514.

Lord, J., & Wilkin, T. (2004). Metformin in polycystic ovarian syndrome. *Current Opinions in Obstetrics and Gynecology, 76*(6), 481–486.

Lowdermilk, D., & Perry, S. (2007). *Maternity and women's health care.* St. Louis, MO: Mosby/Elsevier.

Luisi, A., & Pawasaukas, J. (2003). Treatment of premenstrual dysphoric disorder with selective serotonin reuptake inhibitors. *Pharmacotherapy, 23*(9), 1131–1140.

March of Dimes Birth Defects Foundation. (2002). Medical References: HIV and AIDS in pregnancy. Retrieved January 13, 2006, from http://www.marchofdimes.com/professionals/681_1223.asp

Mayo Clinic. (2006). Endometriosis. Retrieved January 6, 2006, from http://www.mayoclinic.com

McCance, K., & Huether, S. (2006). *Pathophysiology: The biological basis for disease in adults and children* (5th ed.). St. Louis, MO: Elsevier Mosby.

Minkin, M., & Moore, A. (2006). Identifying and managing premenstrual disorders: Putting strategies into practice. *Clinical Advisor* (supplement, November). Montvale, NJ: Haymarket Media.

Moore, A., Sabin, C., Johnson, M., & Phillips, A. (2002). Gender and clinical outcomes after starting highly active antiretroviral treatment: A cohort study. *Journal of Acquired Immune Deficiency Syndrome, 29,* 197–202.

Moos, M. (2005). Have your teenagers had their calcium today? *AWHONN Lifelines, 9*(9), 324–326.

Naftolin, F. (2002). Cognitive function and menopause. *The Female Patient, 27*(2), 46–47.

National Heart, Lung and Blood Institute. (2006). Body mass index (BMI) table. Washington, DC: Author. Retrieved from http://www.nhlbl.nih.gov/guidelines/obesity/bmi_table.html

National Institutes of Health. (1999). Agenda for Research in Women's Health for the 21st Century: A report of the Task Force for the NIH Women's Health Research. NIH Publs. 99-4385 to 4390.

Olds, S., London, M., Ladewig, P., & Davidson, M. (2004). *Maternal-newborn nursing and women's health care* (7th ed.). Upper Saddle River, NJ: Prentice Hall.

Parent-Stevens, L., & Burns, E. (2000). Menstrual disorders. In M. Smith & L. Sharp (Eds.), *20 common problems in women's health care.* New York: McGraw-Hill.

Pick, M., & Holmes, M. (2006). What you should know about endometriosis. Retrieved January 13, 2006, from http://www.womentowomen.com/hysterectomyandalternatives/endometriosis.asp

Pritham, U. (2002). Managing PMS and PMDD: Exploring new treatment options. *AWHONN Lifelines, 6*(5), 428–437.

Rademaker, M. (2001). Do women have more adverse drug reactions? *American Journal of Clinical Dermatology, 2,* 349–351.

Rajaram, S., & Rashidi, A. (1998). Minority women and breast cancer screening: The role of cultural explanatory models. *Preventive Medicine, 27,* 757–764.

Sarto, G. (1998). How race, ethnicity, and culture influence women's health. *Women's Health in Primary Care, 1*(10), 7–14.

Schoening, A., Greenwood, J., McNichols, J., Heermann, J., & Agrawal, S. (2004). Effect of an intimate partner violence educational program on the attitudes of nurses. *Journal of Obstetric, Gynecologic, & Neonatal Nursing, 33,* 572–578.

Sheehan, M. (2004). Polycystic ovarian syndrome: Diagnosis and management. *Clinics in Medical Research, 2*(1), 3–27.

Smith, P. E. (2005). Menopause: Assessment, treatment, and patient education. *Nurse Practitioner, 30*(2), 33–38.

Speroff, L., & Fritz, M. (2005). *Clinical gynecologic endocrinology and infertility* (7th ed.). Philadelphia: Lippincott, Williams & Wilkins.

Steiner, M., Brown, E., Trzepacz, P., Dillon, J., Berger, C., Carter, D., et al. (2003). Fluoxetine improves functional work capacity in women with premenstrual dysphoric disorder. *Archives of Women's Mental Health, 6*(1), 71–77.

Stenchever, M., Droegemuller, W., Herbst, A., & Mishell, D. (2001). *Comprehensive gynecology* (4th ed.). St. Louis, MO: Mosby.

Stephenson, J. (2005). Reducing HIV vertical transmission scrutinized. *Journal of the American Medical Association, 293*(17), 2079–2081.

Teegarden, D., Lyle, R., McCabe, G., McCabe, L., Proulx, W., Michon, K., et al. (1998). Dietary calcium, protein, and phosphorus are related to bone mineral density and content in young women. *American Journal of Clinical Nutrition, 68,* 749–754.

Tranin, A. (2005). Hereditary breast and ovarian cancer. *AWHONN Lifelines, 9*(5), 372–376.

Trussell, J., Vaughn, B., and Stanford, J. (1999). Are all contraceptive failures unintended pregnancies? Evidence from the 1995 National Survey of Family Growth. *Family Planning Perspectives, 31*(5), 246–260.

United National Population Fund. (2008). *1999 annual report.* New York: Author.

U.S. Census Bureau. (2007). Internet access usage and online service usage. Retrieved March 15, 2010, from http://www.census.gov/compendia/statab/tables

U.S. Department of Agriculture (USDA). (2005). *My Pyramid*. Washington, DC: Author. Retrieved from http://www.mypyramid.gov

U.S. Department of Health and Human Services, Office of the Assistant Secretary for Planning and Evaluation. (2005). *Overview of the uninsured in the United States: An analysis of the 2005 current population survey.* Rockville, MD: Author.

U.S. Department of Health and Human Services, Health Resources and Services Administration. (2005). *Women's health, 2005.* Rockville, MD: Author.

U.S. Preventive Services Task Force (USPSTF). (2005). *Guide to clinical preventive services.* U.S. Department of Health and Human Services, Agency for Healthcare Research and Quality (AHRQ) (AHRQ Publication No. 05-0570). Baltimore: Williams & Wilkins.

Ward, S., & Hisley, S. (2009). *Maternal-child nursing care.* Philadelphia: F.A. Davis.

Williams, A. (2003). Gynecologic care for women with HIV infection. *Journal of Obstetric, Gynecologic and Neonatal Nursing, 32*(1), 87–93.

Woosley, R. (1998). Why women are at greater risk for torsades de pointes drug toxicity. *Women's Health in Primary Care, 1*(10), 15–20.

Young, M. G. (2000). Recognizing the signs of elder abuse. *Patient Care, 34*(20), 56.

CHAPTER 49

MEN AS PATIENTS

James Raper

Chapter Outline

Gender-related health disparity across the life span is significant for men. The Men's Health Network (2008) reports a number of disparities between males and females across their life spans. The male fetus is at greater risk for miscarriage and stillbirth, and male newborns have a 25 percent greater risk of mortality than do female newborns. Three-fifths of sudden infant death syndrome (SIDS) victims are boys. Men are 100 percent less likely to receive annual examinations and disease prevention services than are women. Men die at higher rates from the top 10 causes of death than do women. Men are four times more likely to commit suicide than women are. A total of 33 percent of men do not have health-care insurance, compared to 28 percent of women. Men account for 92 percent of deaths in the workplace. Men have fewer infection-fighting T cells and are thought to have weaker immune systems than women. Testosterone is linked to elevations of low-density lipids (LDLs) and declines in high-density lipids (HDLs). Men suffer hearing loss at twice the rate of women. Life expectancy of men is 5 years less than that of women; women outnumber men 8 to 1 by age 100 years. Clearly, there is a need to address health specific to men.

Some government agencies, such as the Agency for Healthcare Research and Quality (AHRQ), address the need for greater dissemination of men's health issues. AHRQ's campaign Real Men Wear Gowns (http://www.ahrq.gov/realmen/) is an example of how to increase public awareness the importance of men's health issues. Men's health issues do not fare as well when compared to efforts to promote awareness of disease conditions affecting women. It is common to see diseases affecting women grouped under the identifier of women's health (http://www.qualityforum.org/Topics/Disparities.aspx). The paucity of literature pertaining to men's health, the glaring absence of health-care policies addressing men's health, and the lack of health-care options available for men underscore the need for a greater focus on men's health.

Even with age-adjusted mortality rates, men have higher death rates compared with women for the 15 leading causes of death in the United States, except for Alzheimer's disease (Williams, 2003). The leading causes of death in men are heart disease, cancer, and unintentional accidents; whereas, the leading causes of death in women are heart disease, breast cancer, and stroke

(Centers for Disease Control and Prevention [CDC], 2007). According to the U.S. Department of Health and Human Services, men are two and a half times less likely to have seen a doctor than are women (2007). The determinants of men's poorer health status arise from cultural and social beliefs about men, manhood, and masculinity. Although socioeconomic status (SES) is considered the strongest determinant of men's health (Williams, 2003), men from all SES groups are considered disadvantaged as compared with women. Other determinants of men's health are absence of work, marginality, poor emotional processing ability, cumulative adversity over a life span, and access to and use of health services. Little is known about men's perception of health and the influences of masculinity on health care–seeking behaviors by men (Liburd, Namageyo-Funa, & Jack, 2007).

The cultural concept of masculinity begins with socialization at a young age. Edley and Wetherell (1996) define masculinity as a "shared understanding of what it means to be a man: what one looks like, how one should behave and so forth" (p. 185). Masculinity directly affects health care and health-care choices. The socialization of men helps determine to what degree men respond to pain (Braithwaite, 2001), make health-care selections, engage in risk-taking behaviors, achieve effective self-care in the management of type 2 diabetes (Liburid et al, 2007), and adhere to medical plans of care (Brooks, 2001).

Although culture plays a significant role in masculinity, steroid hormones known as androgens affect the development of male-specific phenotype during embryogenesis; in the establishment of sexual maturation at puberty; and in the maintenance of the male reproductive function, spermatogenesis, and sexual behavior during adult life. These steroid hormones also affect a wide variety of functions in nonreproductive tissues, such as bone and skeletal muscle (Matsumoto, Shiina, Kawano, Sato, & Kato, 2008). Testosterone and its active metabolite dihydrotestosterone (DHT) exert most of their effects by binding to the androgen receptor (AR), a ligand-activated transcription factor that results in the control of gene transcription by the interaction of AR with coregulators and specific DNA sequences of androgen-responsive genes of the target cells. Because of the involvement of androgens in a large number of pathological processes, several synthetic steroidal and nonsteroidal AR ligands have been developed and are widely used in clinical applications, including the treatment of male hypogonadism (AR agonists), prostate diseases (AR antagonists), and others.

In this chapter, the basic effects of androgen deficiency on various organ systems; reported improvement of features of metabolic syndrome, bone mineral density, mood and sexual function; and the potential complications of testosterone treatment are presented. Symptoms related to androgen deficiency are presented as psychosomatic complaints, metabolic disorders, and sexual health problems. Patients suffering from one of these three constellations of symptoms may exhibit distinct features in terms of androgen levels, age, and body mass index. In addition to discussing testosterone-related health conditions of men as patients, the chapter discusses other common conditions requiring medication along with racial and cultural differences affecting men's health.

A number of health issues in men respond to pharmacological treatment. The natural decline in testosterone levels as men age or in adolescents with hypogonadism may respond to **testosterone** therapy. Erectile dysfunction may respond to **phosphodiesterase type 5 (PDE-5) inhibitors.** Benign prostatic hypertrophy, prostatitis, and male pattern hair loss may also respond to pharmacological intervention.

HYPOGONADISM

Hypogonadism, thought to be one of the main causes of male fertility problems, occurs in an estimated 13 million men in the United States. The exact prevalence is uncertain, because less than 10 percent of those affected by hypogonadism seek treatment. Hypogonadism refers to the failure of the testes to produce androgen, sperm, or both. Hypogonadism affects a man's fertility because the lack of testosterone makes it difficult for men to properly produce sperm. Furthermore, a low testosterone level can contribute to a low sex drive as well as erectile dysfunction.

Pathophysiology

Circulating testosterone is largely protein bound. The major protein is sex hormone–binding globulin (SHBG) with only 2 percent present as the biologically active or free fraction. The bioavailable fraction, representing testosterone loosely bound predominantly to serum albumin, is probably more meaningful. Hepatic SHBG production rises with aging and thyroid hormone excess and declines in hyperinsulinemic states (obesity and type 2 diabetes), so that free values may not always be concordant with total testosterone values. The biological effects of testosterone may be mediated directly by testosterone or by its metabolites 5a-dihydrotestosterone or estradiol. See Figure 49–1.

Classifications

Men with classical hypogonadism are routinely classified into two categories: (1) those with primary hypogonadism (testicular failure) characterized by low testosterone and elevated gonadotropins and (2) those with secondary hypogonadism (hypothalamic-pituitary failure) with low testosterone and low or normal gonadotropins. Interestingly, a third category represents a significant proportion of older men that do not fit into either of the classical categories. These men are typically older and have high gonadotropins and testosterone within the normal range (Harkonen et al, 2003; van den Beld et al, 1999; Wu et al, 2008). This may represent a state of compensated, or subclinical, hypogonadism that could eventually develop into

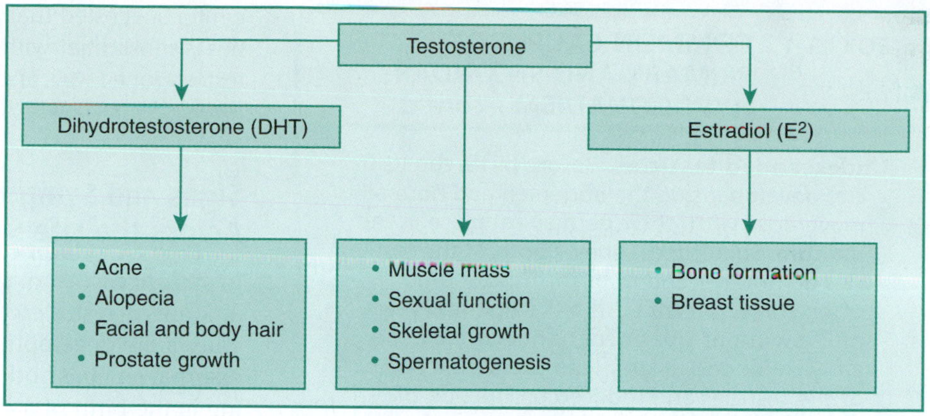

Figure 49–1. Effects of testosterone and its metabolites in men.

overt primary hypogonadism. A similar, well-recognized situation occurs in the pituitary-thyroid axis when high TSH is observed in the face of normal thyroid hormone levels, a hallmark of subclinical hypothyroidism.

Deficient testosterone production can happen at any point during a man's life. Common causes of hypogonadism are displayed in Box 49–1. In some men, hypogonadism is a congenital abnormality, as the deficiency has been present from birth. For other men, the deficiency does not present itself until the onset of puberty. In some cases, a man may not develop the testosterone disorder until well into adulthood.

Testosterone production declines with advancing age; 20 percent of men older than 60 years and 30 to 40 percent of men older than 80 years have serum testosterone levels that would be subnormal in their younger adult male counterparts. This physiological decline in circulating testosterone levels is compounded in frequency by permanent disorders of the hypothalamic-pituitary-gonadal axis, including transient deficiency states associated with acute stressful illnesses, such as surgery and myocardial infarction, and the more chronic deficiency states associated with wasting illnesses, such as cancer and AIDS.

The underlying etiologies and clinical management of secondary and primary hypogonadism are different. It may be informative to differentiate older men who are candidates for the diagnosis of late-onset hypogonadism (LOH) into different categories of hypogonadism by coupling testosterone with luteinizing hormone (LH) levels. Specific risk factors or clinical features can differentiate between secondary, primary, and the new subclinical form of compensated hypogonadism (Lee et al, 2009). Age-related symptoms of LOH, such as decreased bone density, energy, muscle mass and strength, erectile function, mood, and libido, are reminiscent of typical androgen deficiency in symptomatic hypogonadism due to pituitary or testicular disease in young men (Snyder, 2004). Other common terms used to describe LOH are andropause, male menopause, and androgen deficiency syndrome of the aging male (ADAM).

BOX 49–1 COMMON CAUSES OF PRIMARY AND SECONDARY HYPOGONADISM

Primary Hypogonadism

Cancer treatment. Chemotherapy or radiation therapy for the treatment of cancer can interfere with testosterone and sperm production. The effects of both treatments are often temporary, but permanent infertility may occur. Although many men regain their fertility within a few months after treatment ends, preserving sperm before starting cancer therapy is a consideration.

Hemochromatosis. Excess iron in the blood can cause testicular failure or pituitary gland dysfunction, affecting testosterone production.

Klinefelter syndrome. In this congenital abnormality of the sex chromosomes, X and Y, a male has two or more X chromosomes in addition to one Y chromosome. The Y chromosome contains the genetic material that determines the sex of a child and related development. In addition to other defects, the extra X chromosome causes abnormal development of the testicles, which in turn results in underproduction of testosterone.

Mumps orchitis. If a mumps infection involving the testicles (mumps orchitis) occurs during adolescence or adulthood, long-term testicular damage may occur. This may affect normal testicular function and testosterone production.

Normal aging. As men age, testosterone production slowly and continuously decreases. The rate of decline varies greatly among men. As many as 30 percent of men older than 75 years have a low testosterone level, according to the American Association of Clinical Endocrinologists. The value of treatment is controversial.

Trauma to the testicles. The testicles are prone to injury. Damage to normally developed testicles can cause hypogonadism. Damage to one testicle may not impair testosterone production.

Continued

BOX 49–1 **COMMON CAUSES OF PRIMARY AND SECONDARY HYPOGONADISM—cont'd**

Undescended testicles. Before birth, the testicles develop inside the abdomen and normally move down into their permanent place in the scrotum. Sometimes, one or both of the testicles do not descend at birth. This condition often corrects itself within the first few years of life without treatment. If not corrected in early childhood, it may lead to malfunction of the testicles and reduced production of testosterone.

Secondary Hypogonadism

HIV/AIDS. This virus can cause low levels of testosterone by affecting the hypothalamus, the pituitary and the testes.

Inflammatory disease. Certain inflammatory diseases, such as sarcoidosis, histiocytosis, and tuberculosis, involve the hypothalamus and pituitary gland and can decrease testosterone production.

Kallmann syndrome. Abnormal development of the hypothalamus can cause hypogonadism. This abnormality is also associated with impaired development of the ability to smell (anosmia).

Medications. Certain drugs and some hormones, can affect testosterone production.

Obesity. Being significantly overweight at any age may be linked to hypogonadism.

Opioid users. Commonly prescribed opioids in sustained-action dosage forms usually produce subnormal sex hormone levels, which may contribute to a diminished quality of life for many patients with painful chronic illness.

Pituitary disorders. An abnormality in the pituitary gland can impair the release of hormones from the pituitary gland to the testicles, affecting normal testosterone production. A pituitary tumor or other type of brain tumor located near the pituitary gland may cause testosterone or other hormone deficiencies. Surgery or radiation therapy for the treatment of brain tumor may impair pituitary function and cause hypogonadism.

Perhaps the minor contribution of adrenal androgens (or androgenic precursors) may substitute for testicular deficiency once the target tissues have been fully developed. Moreover, ingrained behavior patterns may be resistant to androgenic hormone deficiency. Certainly, prolactin excess, testosterone deficiency, or both in men may result in decreased libido and erectile dysfunction. The yield of finding hyperprolactinemia or testosterone deficiency, or both, in patients presenting with these symptoms is generally less than 5 percent. However, a large survey of patients with erectile dysfunction presenting to a Veterans Affairs center suggested that the prevalence of these abnormalities is substantial, with 18.7 percent of patients having low testosterone levels and 4.6 percent with elevated prolactin levels (Bodie, Lewis, Schow, & Monga, 2003).

Signs and Symptoms of Hypogonadism Across the Life Span

In instances of congenital hypogonadism, insufficient amounts of testosterone are produced by the gonads. This causes the developing fetus to have improperly formed external genitals and internal reproductive organs, resulting in the birth of a child whose sex is not entirely clear. Beginning at birth and through infancy the persistent failure of the testes to descend may be an early manifestation of testicular dysfunction. In addition, a normally formed but hypotrophic penis may provide a clue to an abnormality of the hypothalamic-pituitary-gonadal axis. Later, during puberty, delayed, arrested, or absent testicular growth and secondary sexual characteristic development are hallmarks of pubertal disorders. Males starting puberty with a testosterone deficiency suffer from a variety of symptoms affecting almost every part of their normal growth and development. Because the body does not produce enough testosterone, the voice does not deepen and little muscle mass increase occurs, although there may be some development of the breasts. The penis and testicles also do not develop and mature, the growth of facial hair is inhibited, and arms and legs grow out of proportion to the trunk of the body. Skeletal proportions may be abnormal (eunuchoid) with more than a 5-cm difference between span and height and between pubis-floor and pubis-vertex dimensions. During adulthood, manifestations are generally more subtle.

When hypogonadism presents itself in adulthood, the physical appearance of the man can be significantly altered. Normal reproductive functioning may cease, while emotionally a man can exhibit changes similar to those of menopausal women. Symptoms of this type of hypogonadism may include depression, development of male breasts, erectile dysfunction, failure of facial and body hair to grow, increase in body fat, loss of energy, inhibited sexual desire, loss of muscle mass; menopausal emotions including hot flashes, irritability and mood swings; onset of osteoporosis; and shrinking and softening of the testicles. Hypogonadism affects a man's fertility because the lack of testosterone makes it difficult for men to properly produce sperm. Male factor infertility is likely to be responsible for one-third of the 10 to 15 percent of couples who are unable to conceive within 1 year of unprotected intercourse. Most of these male-associated cases result from diminished, absent, or faulty spermatogenesis. In addition to abnormal sperm production, other associated conditions causing infertility include obstructive ductal disease, epididymal hostility, immunological disorders, and erectile or ejaculatory dysfunction. Furthermore, a low testosterone level can contribute to a low sex drive as well as erectile dysfunctions.

Older Men

The aging man represents a special case. There is a well-known decline in testosterone production with age in otherwise healthy men. This decline in mean testosterone values can be seen in free testosterone levels, beginning in the mid-40s (some clinicians suggest even earlier), as a consequence of increasing sex hormone–binding globulin levels. The physiological mechanism for this is unknown. Total testosterone levels decline on average beyond 70 years. The diurnal rhythm is lost beyond 60 years. Although testicular size also declines in this age group, spermatogenesis may be well maintained into the 80s or even beyond. Gonadotropin levels tend to rise after 70 years, indicating that the testosterone deficiency is usually primary. Using the criterion of a low testosterone value, and remembering that commercially available tests have considerable variability regarding normal young adult ranges, an estimated 7 percent of 40- to 60-year-olds, 22 percent of 60- to 80-year-olds, and 36 percent of 80- to 100-year-olds are hypogonadal (Vermeulen & Kaufman, 1995).

Increased longevity and population aging will increase the number of older men with LOH. The condition is common, but often underdiagnosed and undertreated. Although controversy remains regarding indications for testosterone supplementation in aging men because of lack of large-scale, long-term studies assessing the benefits and risks of testosterone replacement therapy (TRT), reports indicate that TRT may produce a wide range of benefits for men with hypogonadism that include improvement in body composition, bone density, cardiovascular (CV) disease, cognition, erythropoiesis, libido and sexual function, mood, muscle mass, and quality of life. The ultimate issue as to whether these changes are normal and physiological or should be considered pathological, thus demanding therapy, remains unresolved. Indeed, it is a situation analogous to the ongoing dilemma of hormone replacement therapy for postmenopausal women, although in women the hormonal deficiency state is usually more abrupt and symptomatic.

In the largest double-blind, placebo-controlled interventional study of testosterone replacement in elderly men to date, Srinivas-Shankar and colleagues (2010) report that for intermediate-frail and frail elderly community-dwelling hypogonadal men at least 65 years of age, TRT prevents deterioration in muscle strength and improves body composition and symptom-related quality of life. Furthermore, TRT was associated with improved physical function in older and frailer men, highlighting possible functional consequences of small changes in physical performance.

Diagnosis

Serum testosterone has a well-known diurnal rhythm that appears to be lost when a man reaches age 60 years. Because testosterone values are 30 percent or so higher near 8 a.m. versus the later day trough, a testosterone value should be determined first thing in the morning. Although normal testosterone ranges vary among reference laboratories, the usually quoted range for young men is 300 to 1,000 ng/dL. In general, values below 220 to 250 ng/dL are clearly low in most laboratories; values between 250 and 350 ng/dL should be considered borderline low. Because the acute effect of stressful illness may result in a transient lowering of testosterone levels, a confirmatory early morning specimen should be obtained. Measurement of free testosterone levels or bioavailable testosterone levels, determined adequately in some reference laboratories, may provide additional information. Free testosterone levels may be lower than expected from the total testosterone level as a result of aging and higher than expected in insulin-resistant individuals, such as in the case of obesity. In addition, serum follicle-stimulating hormone (FSH), luteinizing hormone (LH), and prolactin levels should be used to help determine the cause of hypogonadism.

If gonadotropin levels are not elevated, despite clearly subnormal testosterone values, anterior pituitary (thyroid-adrenal) function should be determined by measuring free thyroxine and thyroid-stimulating hormone levels, as well as an early morning cortisol level. A magnetic resonance imaging (MRI) scan of the brain and sella should be considered. An exception to this recommendation is the condition of morbid obesity, in which both total and free testosterone levels are typically low and gonadotropin values not elevated. Hyperprolactinemia, even of a small degree, may also warrant ordering an MRI, because interference of hypothalamic-pituitary vascular flow by space-occupying, stalk-compressing lesions will lead to disruption of the tonic inhibitory influence of hypothalamic dopamine, and result in modest hyperprolactinemia (20- to 50-ng/mL range). Semen analysis should be performed when fertility is in question.

TESTOSTERONE REPLACEMENT THERAPY

Pharmacodynamics

Restoring testosterone levels to within the normal range by using testosterone replacement therapy (TRT) can improve many of the effects of hypogonadism (see Table 49–1). Gooren (2010) presents a review of clinically based evidence from the past decade that denotes the benefits of TRT on multiple target organs of hypogonadal men. The review provides a comprehensive appraisal of the well-substantiated benefits of clinically indicated TRT and areas that need additional investigation.

Anemia

Endogenous androgens are known to stimulate erythropoiesis; increase reticulocyte count, blood hemoglobin levels and bone marrow erythropoietic activity in mammals, whereas castration has opposite effects. Hypogonadism results in a 10 percent to 20 percent decrease in the blood hemoglobin (Hgb) concentration that can

Table 49–1 **Postpubertal Hypogonadal-Related Problems and Effectiveness of Testosterone Replacement**

Postpubertal Problems Associated With Hypogonadism	Evidence of Improvement With Administration of Testosterone
Decreased bone mineral density	Increased bone mineral density
Decreased cognitive function	Increased cognitive function
Decreased energy, mood, and quality of life	Increased energy, mood, and quality of life
Erectile dysfunction	Increased sexual function
Decreased hematocrit and hemoglobin concentrations	Increased hematocrit and hemoglobin
Decreased muscle mass	Increased muscle mass
Decreased prostate glands	Increased prostate gland size—prostate symptom score, urine flow rate, and postvoiding residual urine in the bladder after voiding did not change significantly*
Decreased sexual desire	Increased libido

*Snyder, et al, 2000.

result in anemia. Young hypogonadal men usually have fewer red blood cells and lower Hgb levels than do age-matched controls

Bone Mineral Density

Osteopenia, osteoporosis, and fracture prevalence rates are higher in hypogonadal men because testosterone plays a major role in bone density (BMD). The prevalence of osteoporosis in hypogonadal males is twice that of those of eugonadal men. Bone density in hypogonadal men of all ages increases under appropriately dosed TRT, although normal adult bone mass is not achieved. Testosterone produces this effect by increasing osteoblastic activity and through aromatization to estrogen reducing osteoclastic activity. Part of testosterone's effect on bone is at least partially indirect, mediated via its aromatization product estradiol. Patients with prostate cancer treated with androgen deprivation therapy have an increased risk of osteoporotic fracture. The role of LOH in aging males in bone fracture rate is not known. The long-term benefit of TRT requires further investigation. Trials of the effects of TRT on BMD yield mixed results. The pooled results of a meta-analysis suggest a beneficial effect on lumbar spine bone density and equivocal findings on femoral neck BMD. Trials of intramuscular **testosterone** reported significantly larger effects on lumbar bone density than trials of transdermal **testosterone**, particularly among patients receiving chronic glucocorticoids. None of studies have been powered enough to show a fracture risk reduction with TRT.

Cognitive Function

Age-related decreases in testosterone predict age-related decline in visual and verbal memory. Evidence exists for a correlation between testosterone levels and cognitive performance, such as spatial abilities or mathematical reasoning. Higher free testosterone concentrations are associated with better performance in specific aspects of memory and cognitive function, optimally in men ranging from 35 to 90 years of age, even after adjustment for age, educational attainment, and CV morbidity. Total testosterone does not consistently have the same associations. Suppression of endogenous testosterone synthesis and blockade of the androgen receptor in men undergoing hormonal therapy for prostate cancer result in a beneficial effect on verbal memory but an adverse effect on spatial ability and slowed reaction time. There is no definitive proof of the beneficial effects of restoring testosterone levels to normal in elderly men. Trials of TRT in men to evaluate its effects on measures of cognitive function and memory are relatively small, are of a short duration and show mixed results (Beauchet, 2006; Hogervorst, Bandelow, Combrinck, & Smith, 2004). **Testosterone** treatment in men aged 34 to 70 years improved verbal memory, spatial memory, and constructional abilities in **nonhypogonadal** men with mild cognitive impairment and Alzheimer's disease (Cherrier, Craft, & Mastsumoto, 2003; Cherrier et al, 2005). In one study of healthy men aged 50 to 90 years, **testosterone** alone or in combination with the aromatase inhibitor **anastrozole** improved spatial memory, but verbal memory only improved in **testosterone**-treated men in the absence of **anastrozole** (Cherrier et al, 2005). This raises the possibility that part of the effect of exogenous **testosterone** is mediated by its aromatization to estradiol. Whereas the results from these observational studies are not uniform, it appears that lower free testosterone is associated with poorer outcomes on measures of cognitive function, particularly in older men and that **testosterone** therapy in hypogonadal men may have some benefit in cognitive performance.

Lower Urinary Tract Symptoms

In addition to improvement in sexual function, TRT may also improve lower urinary tract symptomatology and bladder functions by increasing bladder capacity and compliance and decreasing detrusor pressure at maximal flow in men with LOH.

Metabolic Syndrome and Type 2 Diabetes

Dyslipidemia-impaired glucose regulation, hypertension, insulin resistance, and obesity (all components of the metabolic syndrome) are also present in hypogonadal men. Lower testosterone levels are associated with surrogate markers for CV disease, including less favorable carotid intimal medial thickness, ankle/brachial index as a measure of peripheral arterial disease, and calcific aortic atheroma. There is a positive correlation between serum testosterone levels and insulin sensitivity in men across the full spectrum of glucose tolerance.

Improvement of insulin sensitivity is noted after TRT. The effects of TRT, diet, and exercise on glycemic control of men with diabetes mellitus indicate a favorable effect. By increasing lean body mass and reducing fat mass, **testosterone** therapy modulates insulin resistance and risk of metabolic syndrome. The mechanism of the fall in lipids may be related to the decrease in the visceral abdominal fat mass under the influence of testosterone, which inhibit lipoprotein lipase activity and increase lipolysis, with improvement of insulin sensitivity and mobilization of triglycerides from abdominal fat tissue. Hypogonadism is associated with an increased risk of CV disease in men (Muller et al, 2004). However, data are lacking as to whether higher testosterone levels predict reduced incidence of combined nonfatal and fatal major CV events. The inverse correlation between testosterone levels and the severity of coronary artery disease may be related to the fact that low testosterone levels are accompanied by an accumulation of abdominal visceral fat associated with increased CV risk factors, impaired glucose tolerance, and noninsulin-dependent diabetes mellitus (Caminiti et al, 2009).

Cardiovascular Disease

TRT does not increase the incidence of CV disease, myocardial infarction, stroke, or angina. The evidence supports no association between TRT and cardiac events. However, trials of TRT generally have not been designed or adequately powered to detect effects on clinically significant CV events. The outcome of most studies in men report either a favorable or neutral effect of normal testosterone levels on CV disease in men (Caminiti et al, 2009). TRT at physiological concentration increases coronary blood flow in patients with coronary heart disease. Beneficial effects on endothelial function and myocardial ischemia have been demonstrated, but not on CV mortality. Thus, although lower testosterone levels are associated with higher CV risk and mortality in aging men, adequately powered, randomized controlled clinical trials are needed to determine whether TRT will reduce morbidity and mortality from CV disease in hypogonadal or eugonadal men.

Mood and Energy and Quality of Life

Hypogonadal men older than 50 years report decreased quality of life, including common complaints of dysphoria, fatigue, loss of libido, and irritability (Wang, Cunningham, et al, 2004; Wang, Swerdloff, et al, 2000). These symptoms coincide with signs and symptoms of major depression. There is significant inverse correlation between free testosterone levels (but not with total testosterone) and a depression score in elderly men, regardless of age and weight. There are reduced libido and reduced feelings of well-being with hypogonadism; the depressive symptoms during the hypogonadal state are reversed by TRT. Men who received TRT report variable effects on mood, energy, and sense of well-being.

TRT at physiological doses to nondepressed eugonadal men does not result in significant effects on mood (Haren, Wittert, Chapman, Coates, & Morley, 2005; Tricker et al, 1996). In hypogonadal men, **testosterone** replacement was associated with improved mood and well-being, and reduced fatigue and irritability. Randomized controlled trials of TRT in men without or with underlying chronic illness report equivocal improvements in quality of life measures, including fatigue and general well-being (Gruenewald & Matsumoto, 2003; Livermann & Blazer, 2004). For patients with major depression and/or dysthymia, improvement was equal to that achieved with standard antidepressants with significant improvement in the depression inventory score. This effect may be a direct effect of **testosterone** or related to positive effects of **testosterone** on weight and/or other anthropometric measures. Additional research is needed to assess the effects of TRT on clinical depression in patients with human immunodeficiency virus. No relationship between testosterone level and depressive symptoms was found in the Massachusetts Male Aging Study (Harkonen et al, 2003; Seidman, Araujo, Roose, & McKinlay, 2001). Gooren (2010) postulates that the discrepancy in the results of the effects of TRT on mood is the result of a genetic polymorphism in the androgen receptor that defines a vulnerable group in whom depression is expressed when testosterone levels fall below a particular threshold.

Muscle Mass and Strength

Aging is accompanied by significant changes in body composition as evidenced by decreased fat free mass and increased and redistributed fat mass. These changes may impose functional limitations and increase morbidity. Maximal muscle strength correlates with muscle mass independently of age. In men, declining testosterone levels that occur with aging can contribute to these changes by direct effect on muscle cells or by stimulating IGF-1 expression directly and indirectly leading to increased muscle protein synthesis and growth. There is a correlation between free testosterone concentrations and fat-free mass; however, the correlation with grip strength is not clear. TRT may reverse age-dependent body composition changes and associated morbidity. TRT improves body composition: a decrease of fat mass, increase of lean body mass. In many studies, body weight change did not differ significantly (Morley et al, 1993; Page et al, 2005; Sih et al, 1997). TRT was associated with a greater improvement in grip strength than a placebo. Research supports the benefits of TRT on skeletal muscle performance in elderly men with chronic heart failure and its positive effects on the prevention of loss of muscle strength of the lower limbs (Caminiti et al, 2009; Srinivas-Shankar et al, 2010). Although TRT is promising for improving muscle mass in some patients, changes in lower extremity muscle strength and measures of physical function are inconsistent.

In aging men, positive correlations between testosterone and muscle strength parameters of upper and lower extremities also exist, as measured by leg extensor strength and isometric hand-grip strength (Srinivas-Shankar et al, 2010). **Testosterone** replacement is positively associated with functional parameters, including the doors test as well as the "get up and go" test and the 5-chair sit/stand test. Although increase in lean body mass has been observed, there is no proof of increase in physical function or in strength of knee extension or flexion. Although a potential role for TRT in the management of frailty exists, whether **testosterone** replacement improves physical function and other health-related outcomes, or reduces the risk of disability, falls, or fractures in older men with low testosterone levels is unknown.

Sexual Desire, Function, and Performance

The prevalence of erectile dysfunction (ED) increases with age. Free testosterone is correlated with erectile and orgasmic function. Compared with younger men, elderly men require higher levels of circulating testosterone for libido and erectile function. Decreased libido, with or without hypogonadism, might be related to other comorbidities or medications. Men with ED or decreased libido and documented hypogonadism may benefit from TRT. Adequate TRT can restore venous leakage in the corpus cavernosum, a condition that is a frequent factor in ED in elderly men. Research indicates some benefit of TRT on sexual health-related outcomes (Krause, Mueller, & Mazur, 2005). Long-term follow-up of TRT in hypogonadal males indicates that self-assessment of libido is higher with TRT (Bhasin et al, 2010). TRT also enhances libido and the frequency of sexual acts and sleep-related erections (Bhasin et al, 2010). Transdermal TRT is linked to positive effects on fatigue, mood, sexual function, and increases in sexual activity. In the presence of a clinical picture of hypogonadism and borderline testosterone levels, a short therapeutic trial may be reasonable. Evidence indicates that the combined use of **testosterone** and **PDE5 inhibitors** in hypogonadal or borderline eugonadal men have a synergetic effect (Shabsigh, Kaufman, Steidle, & Padma-Nathan, 2004). The combination treatment should be considered in hypogonadal patients with ED failing to respond to either single treatment. Testosterone produces this effect by enhancing the production of nitric oxide synthase.

Testosterone Clinical Use and Dosing

Testosterone replacement therapy (TRT) is relatively straightforward. See Table 49–2 for **testosterone** preparations available in the United States. Typically, the depot esters are administered by the deep IM route once every 2 weeks at a dose of 200 mg in adult men. A usual dosage for the transdermal or the buccal preparations results in the systemic absorption of 2.5 to 10 mg daily. If the parenteral route is chosen, patients should and can be taught to self-inject. The major disadvantage with the parenteral route is that testosterone levels exhibit a saw-toothed pattern, with high-normal or supranormal levels on days 2 to 4 and low-normal or borderline low trough values before the next injection. Mood, sense of well-being, and libido may vary accordingly in some individuals. Dosages may be adjusted by aiming for midnormal (400 to 600 ng/dL) testosterone levels after 1 week or at the low end (250 to 350 ng/dL) just before the next injection is due at 2 weeks. Testosterone values become stable within a few days or weeks after initiation of the buccal or skin gel or patch preparation. It should be ascertained whether the preparation was actually used on

Table 49–2 **Testosterone Preparations Available in the United States**

Drug	Dose
Buccal (Striant)	One buccal system (30 mg) to the gum region twice daily (q12h)
Depot esters—testosterone cypionate, enanthate, propionate, phenylpropionate, isocaproate, decanoate, acetate (Depo-T, Delatestryl)	For replacement in the hypogonadal male, 50–400 mg administered every 2 to 4 weeks
Topical Gel (AndroGel 1%, Testim)	5 g once a day to clean, dry intact skin of shoulders and/or upper arms or abdomen
Topical genital skin patch (Testoderm)	6 mg/d applied to scrotal area and worn for 22 to 24 h
Topical Non-genital skin patch (Androderm)	5 mg/d applied once daily to clean, dry, intact skin of the shoulders, upper arm or abdomen

the day that the sample was drawn. A testosterone value in the midnormal range (400 to 600 ng/dL) is the goal. Although comparable testosterone levels are reached via the patch and the gels, skin reactions at the application site are much more common with patch use. Because of the very high cost associated with transdermal preparations, many insurance plans do not include them on their formularies or require prior authorization. The buccal preparation is difficult for some patients to use because of gum irritation, pain, tenderness and/or swelling. Alkylated oral androgens should be viewed as potentially hepatotoxic and should not be used. Criteria for the selection of testosterone preparations are summarized in Table 49–3.

Risks and Contraindications

The most controversial issue related to TRT is associated risk (Bassil, Alkaade, & Morley, 2009; Bhasin et al, 2010). Erythrocytosis is a recognized risk of TRT; therefore, hemoglobin (Hgb) and hematocrit (Hct) levels should be checked periodically. Incremental increases are to be expected in the first 6 months of treatment, but an Hgb level higher than 17.5 g/dL, Hct higher than 54 percent, or both suggests overtreatment or occasionally abuse. Greater increments tend to occur more frequently with the IM preparations than with the transdermal. If the Hct is greater than 54 percent, therapy is stopped until the Hct decreases to a safe level. The patient should also be evaluated for hypoxia and sleep apnea (Bhasin et al, 2010). Restarting therapy at a reduced dose usually solves problems.

There is a risk of prostate cancer with the use of **testosterone** replacement. The Endocrine Society lists detection of subclinical prostate cancer and growth of metastatic prostate cancer as known risks of TRT (Bhasin et al, 2010). The Endocrine Society advises avoiding TRT in patients with metastatic prostate cancer or breast cancer (Bhasin et al, 2010). A digital rectal examination and PSA should be monitored throughout therapy. A urological consultation should be obtained if indicated by prostate symptom score, decreased urine flow rate, or postvoiding residual urine.

Additional risks of TRT have been identified. There is evidence of decreased sperm production and infertility reported among men receiving TRT by the Endocrine Society (Bhasin et al, 2010). Boys receiving TRT may experience acne and gynecomastia. The most serious risks of TRT in adolescents are aggressive behavior and premature closure of the epiphyses, leading to permanent short stature (Snyder, 2010).

Consideration of a number of clinical situations makes the risk of TRT an absolute or relative contraindication. Potential risks and contraindications are presented in Table 49–4. Clinical studies in large numbers of patients (either young or old) are limited, so potential risks and benefits should be individualized. Pierorazio and colleagues (2009) report that higher levels of serum-free testosterone are associated with an increased risk of aggressive prostate cancer among older men. Their data highlight the importance of prospective trials to ensure the safety of TRT in men older than age 65.

Drug–Drug Interactions

A total of 103 drugs (433 brand names and generics) are known to interact with **testosterone**. Of these, three medications have major interactions. The three high-risk medications are **anisindione**, **dicumarol**, and **warfarin**. Using **testosterone** with any of these medicines is usually not recommended, but may be required in some cases. Dose adjustment may be required for one or both of the interacting medicines. See Chapter 22 for further discussion of drug interactions with reproductive drugs, including **testosterone**.

Monitoring

The Endocrine Society recommends the monitoring the following in men receiving **testosterone** replacement therapy (Bhasin et al, 2010):

1. Evaluate the patient 3 to 6 months after treatment is started to determine efficacy in treating symptoms and if there are any adverse effects.
2. Evaluate the patient's testosterone level 3 to 6 months after starting therapy. The goal is the mid-normal range.
   a. Injectable **testosterone:** measure levels midway between injections
   b. Transdermal patches: measure levels 3 to 12 hours after applying patch

Table 49–3 **Comparison of Testosterone Replacement Therapies**

	Buccal	Intramuscular	Topical Gel	Topical Patch
Convenience	Yes	No	Yes	Yes
Cost	High	Low	Very high	High
Physiological	Yes	No (saw tooth)	Yes	Yes
Side effects	Local, moderate	Systemic & local	Local, minimal	Local, moderate
Stigma	No	No	No	Yes

Alkylated oral androgens should be viewed as potentially hepatotoxic and should not be used.

Table 49–4 **Contraindications and Associated Potential Risk for Testosterone Replacement Therapy**

Parameter	Contraindication vs. Potential Risk
Abnormal digital rectal examination	Contraindication
Breast carcinoma (history or presence)	Contraindication
Elevated levels of prostate-specific antigen	Contraindication
Erythrocytosis	Risk
Exacerbation of sleep apnea	Risk
Gynecomastia	Risk
Hypercoagulable states	Contraindication
Liver toxicity and liver tumor	Risk
Polycythemia (hematocrit >51%)	Contraindication
Prostate carcinoma (history or presence)	Contraindication
Psychopathology	Contraindication
Severe benign prostatic hyperplasia	Contraindication
Severe coronary heart failure (class III or IV)	Contraindication
Skin diseases	Risk
Stimulate growth of prostate cancer and breast cancer	Risk
Testicular atrophy and infertility	Risk
Untreated sleep apnea	Contraindication
Worsen symptoms of benign prostatic hypertrophy	Risk

c. Buccal **testosterone:** measure immediately after applying a new dose
d. **Testosterone** pellets: measure at the end of therapy
e. Oral **testosterone:** measure 3 to 5 hours after ingestion

3. Evaluate hematocrit at baseline, at 3 and 6 months, then annually.
4. Evaluate bone mineral density after 1 to 2 years of therapy.
5. Evaluate PSA levels and perform a digital rectal exam prior to beginning therapy, at 3 and 6 months, then per age-related guidelines for prostate cancer screening.

Obtain a urological consultation if there are concerns about response to therapy, an increase in PSA levels of greater than 1.4 ng/mL in a 12-month period, or if any prostatic abnormality is palpated on rectal exam (Bhasin et al, 2010).

COMMON PROBLEMS THAT REQUIRE MEDICATIONS

Erectile Dysfunction

Erectile dysfunction (ED) is a common sexual problem in men. The incidence increases with age and affects up to one-third of men at some time during their lives. ED causes a substantial negative impact on intimate relationships, quality of life, and self-esteem. Treatment includes **phosphodiesterase type 5 (PDE-5) inhibitors**, or **TRT** if appropriate. Penile self-injection and vacuum-assisted erection devices are not discussed in this chapter, as these are usually prescribed by urological specialists. Cognitive behavior therapy and therapy aimed at improving relationships may also help to improve ED (Heidelbaugh, 2010).

Pathophysiology

Normal erections require a complex interaction between hormonal, vascular, neurological, and psychological systems (Spark, 2011). Any disruption in any of these systems may cause ED. Risk factors for ED include chronic illnesses such as diabetes mellitus, hypertension, obesity, dyslipidemia, and cardiovascular disease (Spark, 2011). Smoking and medication use may also contribute to development of ED. Because there is no preferred first-line diagnostic test, in most cases history and physical examination are sufficient to make a diagnosis. Initial diagnostics are usually limited to a fasting serum glucose level and lipid panel, morning total testosterone level, and thyroid-stimulating hormone test. Screening for CV risk factors should be considered in men with ED because symptoms of ED present on average 3 years earlier than symptoms of coronary artery disease (Heidelbaugh, 2010).

Phosphodiesterase Type 5 (PDE-5) Inhibitors

Pharmacodynamics

First-line therapy for ED consists of lifestyle changes, modifying drug therapy that may cause ED, and pharmacotherapy with **PDE-5 inhibitors**. **PDE-5 inhibitors** are the most effective oral drugs for treatment of ED, including ED associated with antidepressants, diabetes mellitus, and spinal cord injury. There are three **PDE-5 inhibitors** available: **sildenafil (Viagra)**, **vardenafil (Levitra)**, and **tadalafil (Cialis)**. One aspect of a normal erection is the release of nitric oxide in the corpus cavernosum during sexual stimulation. Catabolism of cyclic GMP is responsible for detumescence. The **PDE-5 inhibitors** work by blocking the catabolism of cyclic GMP (guanosine monophosphate). Blocking cyclic GMP results in increased number and duration of erections in men with ED.

PDE-5 inhibitors are indicated for the treatment of ED. They vary in onset and duration of action (see Table 49–5 for dosing). **Sildenafil** and **vardenafil** have a 4-hour duration of effectiveness. **Tadalafil** may assist men with ED to have an erection in response to sexual stimulation for up to 36 hours after a single dose. **Sildenafil** and

Table 49–5 **Dosing Schedule of PDE-5 Inhibitors**

Drug Name	How Supplied	Dose
Sildenafil (Viagra)	25-mg, 50-mg, 100-mg tablets	Initial dose 50 mg. Take 1 dose as needed 1 to 4 hours before sexual activity, up to once daily. Decrease dose to 25 mg in patients with hepatic or renal impairment, or coadministration with CYP3A4 inhibitors.
Tadalafil (Cialis)	2.5-mg, 5-mg, 10-mg, 20-mg tablets	As needed dosing: Initial dose 10 mg. Take one dose as needed before sexual activity. May increase dose to 20 mg. May last up to 36 hours. Higher dose should not be used daily. Daily dosing: 2.5 mg taken at the same time each day. May increase dose to 5 mg daily.
Vardenafil (Levitra)	2.5-mg, 5-mg, 10-mg, 20-mg tablets	Initial dose 10 mg. Take 1 dose as needed 1 to 4 hours before sexual activity, up to once daily. Decrease dose to 5 mg in patients with hepatic or renal impairment, or coadministration with CYP3A4 inhibitors.

vardenafil should be taken on an empty stomach, as high fat meals or **alcohol** will delay absorption. **Tadalafil** absorption is not affected by food or **alcohol**. **Sildenafil** has the longest safety record of the three (Spark, 2010).

Risks and Contraindications

PDE-5 inhibitors are contraindicated in patients sensitive to any component of the medication.

There is a potential for fatal hypotension if **PDE-5 inhibitors** are taken concurrently with **nitrates (nitroglycerine)**.

Patients with cardiovascular disease, including acute myocardial infarction, stroke, or life-threatening arrhythmia within the past 6 months should not be prescribed **PDE-5 inhibitors**. Unstable angina, severe heart failure or prolonged QT, hypotension (systolic blood pressure less than 90 mg Hg) or hypertension (blood pressure greater than 170/110) requires caution in prescribing **PDE-5 inhibitors**.

Priapism is a rare occurrence. If the patient has an erection lasting longer than 4 hours, he should seek medical care.

Although **PDE-5 inhibitors** are specific for PDE-5, there have been reports of visual disturbances in some users of **PDE-5 inhibitors** most likely related to type 6 phosphodiesterase, which is required for the transformation of light into electrical signals.

PDE-5 inhibitors have been associated with rare reports of sudden hearing loss of unknown etiology. The hearing loss is temporary in one-third of patients and ongoing for the remaining patients (Spark, 2010). The U.S. Food and Drug Administration (FDA) is monitoring reports of hearing problems and any new hearing loss in patients who experience hearing problems while taking **PDE-5 inhibitors** should be reported to MedWatch (http://www.fda.gov/safety/medwatch).

Drug–Drug Interactions

The most concerning drug interactions with the **PDE-5 inhibitors** are the vasodilators, specifically the **nitrates** or **nitroprusside**.

Co-administration with **alpha blockers** may lead to additive hypotension. If considering co-administration the patient should be stable on his dose of **alpha blocker** before considering **PDE-5 inhibitors**. The lowest dose of a **PDE-5 inhibitor** should be used, and the patient monitored closely for hypotension.

PDE-5 inhibitors may interact with any of the **antihypertensives** and cause additive hypotension.

PDE-5 inhibitors should not be given concurrently with **class 1A** or **III antiarrhythmics** or drugs that cause prolonged QT interval.

Plasma levels of **PDE-5 inhibitors** may be increased by CYP3A4 inhibitors.

Monitoring

There is no specific laboratory monitoring for **PDE-5 inhibitors**. Patients should report symptoms of hypotension and any changes in self-monitored blood pressure readings.

Patient Education

Patients should be educated regarding the proper use of **PDE-5 inhibitors**. Drug interactions, specifically **nitrates** and other **antihypertensives**, should be discussed. Adverse drug reactions including priapism and visual and hearing disturbances should be explained and the patient advised to seek care if these occur.

Benign Prostatic Hyperplasia

Benign prostatic hyperplasia affects the prostate, a male sex gland beneath the urinary bladder. A donut-shaped gland, the prostate encircles the urinary outlet, or urethra. Contraction of the muscles in the prostate squeezes fluids into the urethral tract during ejaculation. An enlarged prostate is not cancerous but can cause disability and even serious illness if left untreated. When the prostate becomes too large, it presses against the urethral canal and interferes with normal urination. As a result, urine may back up in the kidneys, subsequently damaging them by excessive pressure and contaminated urine. Bladder infections such as cystitis commonly occur as well. These lower urinary tract symptoms (LUTS) are a common complaint among aging men: 8 percent of men aged 31 to 40 years, 50 percent in those aged 51 to 60 years, 70 percent in those aged 61 to 70 years, and 90 percent in those aged 81 to 90 years (Laborde & McVary, 2009). The symptoms are often caused by benign prostatic hyperplasia (BPH), and include nocturia, burning, decreased urine flow rates, difficulty in starting and stopping urination, hesitancy, incomplete bladder emptying, pain, progressive urinary frequency, urgency, and urinary frequency. A number of medical treatments for LUTS/BPH exist, such as **alpha blockers** (discussed in Chapter 14), **5-alpha-reductase inhibitors** (discussed in Chapter 22), **anticholinergics** (discussed in Chapter 14), **PDE-5 inhibitors**, and combination therapies.

Prostatitis and Male Pelvic Pain Syndrome

Prostatitis and male pelvic pain syndrome combine to form a multifactorial syndrome of largely unknown etiology. Prostatitis can partially or totally block the flow of urine from the bladder, resulting in urine retention. This causes the bladder to become distended, weak, tender, and susceptible to infection due to the increased amount of bacteria in the retained urine. Prostatitis is classified into a number of subtypes: acute bacterial prostatitis, chronic bacterial prostatitis, inflammatory and noninflammatory chronic pelvic pain syndrome, and asymptomatic prostatitis. Some symptoms of acute prostatitis include fever, chills, frequent urination accompanied by a burning sensation, pain between the scrotum and rectum, fatigue, blood or pus in the urine, lower back pain, and ED. It usually results from a bacterial infection and is common among males between the ages of 20 and 50. Pathogenic organisms can be cultured only in acute and chronic bacterial prostatitis. It is important for men who suffer from any of the symptoms associated with prostatitis to see a healthcare provider because the condition may progress to more severe complications, including kidney infection, orchitis (painful swelling of the testicles), and epididymitis (inflammation of the epididymis, a tube along the backside of the testicles). Acute prostatitis is treated with antibiotics, usually **fluoroquinolones**, for an adequate period of time. Treatment of prostatitis is covered in Chapter 44.

Premature ejaculation (PE) is a common sexual problem, and chronic prostatitis is an important cause of PE. **Antimicrobial** therapy is useful in the treatment of PE associated with inflammatory prostatitis (Zohdy, 2009).

Ninety percent of patients with prostatitis syndrome, however, suffer not from bacterial prostatitis but from chronic (abacterial) prostatitis / chronic pelvic pain syndrome (CP/CPPS). It remains unclear whether CP/CPPS is of infectious origin, and therefore the utility of a trial of antimicrobial treatment is debatable. (Wagenlehner, Naber, Schleipfer, Brähler & Weidner, 2009). Noninfective forms of prostatitis may be associated with autoimmune disorders. Bladder outlet obstruction and prostate stones may also occur if chronic prostatitis remains untreated.

Hair Loss

Rogers and Avram (2008) provide a comprehensive review discussing the current medications available to treat hair loss and medications currently under investigation. There has been extensive use of **minoxidil** (2% and 5%) topical solutions. **Minoxidil** maintains and thickens existing hair and, in some patients, it regrows hair follicles. **Minoxidil** is also available in a foam preparation. **Finasteride** is a **type II 5-alpha-reductase inhibitor** that is used to treat of BPH and androgenetic alopecia. **Finasteride** is an effective inhibitor of type II 5-alpha-reductase, the enzyme responsible for the reduction of testosterone to dihydrotestosterone (see Fig. 49–1). Its effects include increasing the hair growth rate, thickness, and hair count. Clinical use and dosing of **minoxidil** and **finasteride** are discussed in depth in Chapter 32.

Medications currently under investigation but not approved for the treatment of hair loss include **dutasteride**, **ketoconazole**, and **latanoprost**. **Dutasteride** is a potent type I and type II 5-alpha-reductase inhibitor that has shown superior hair count number and growth rate. **Ketoconazole** is an antifungal medication that has also been shown to promote hair growth. Its exact mechanism in hair loss treatment is poorly understood. In a clinical trial, Inui and Itami (2007) found that **ketoconazole** topical cream (2%) showed increased vertex hair growth in two of the five patients. **Latanoprost** is a prostaglandin analogue used for glaucoma and ocular hypertension that was found to encourage eyebrow and eyelash hair regrowth. Although no formal clinical studies exist using **latanoprost**, it appears to be a promising agent for further investigations.

In addition to the current medications and those under investigation, the field of hair transplantation has evolved considerably. The cosmetic results of contemporary hair transplantation are virtually undetectable. Large, pluggy "punch grafts" have been replaced with natural-appearing follicular unit grafts, which maintain their existing anatomy and with proper technique can match the orientation of surrounding hair follicles. Some of the important factors to consider include age of the patient, pattern of hair loss, and expected future hair loss (Lee & Minton, 2009).

HEALTH PROMOTION, DISEASE PREVENTION, AND SCREENING IN MEN

The top ten threats to the health of men in the United States include heart disease, cancer, injuries, stroke, chronic obstructive pulmonary disease (COPD), type 2 diabetes, influenza, suicide, kidney disease, and Alzheimer's disease (Mayo Clinic, 2010). Health promotion through preventive screening and testing is very important to preventing mortality and morbidity associated with these threats. Health promotion is about keeping healthy, living a healthy lifestyle, preventing illness, and preventing any existing illness from becoming worse. Immunizations also play an important role in health promotion. A schedule of recommended screening tests guidelines for men by age is presented in Table 49–6. Immunizations recommended for men of all ages are found in Chapter 19.

ETHNIC AND RACIAL ISSUES

Compared with African American (AF-AM) women and white men in the United States, AF-AM men have more health risks and a shorter life span. U.S. Department of Health and Human Services (2000) reported that AF-AM men live an average 6 years less than AF-AM women and 7 years less than white men. Reducing the life expectancy disparity between AF-AM men and other ethnic groups requires efforts to improve the overall health of AF-AM men with an emphasis on factors that

Table 49–6 **Screening Tests and Immunizations Guidelines for Men by Age**

Screening Tests	Ages 18–39	Ages 40–49	Ages 50–64	Ages 65 and Older
Blood pressure test	At least every 2 years	At least every 2 years	At least every 2 years	At least every 2 years
Cholesterol test	Start at age 20	Health-care provider to discuss with patient	Health-care provider to discuss with patient	Health-care provider to discuss with patient
Colorectal health (use 1 of these 3 methods): 1. Fecal occult blood test	Yearly			Yearly; older than age 75, discuss with patients
2. Flexible sigmoidoscopy (with fecal occult blood test)	Every 5 years			Every 5 years. Older than age 75, discuss with patient
3. Colonoscopy	Every 10 years			Every 10 years. Older than age 75, discuss with patients
Diabetes: blood sugar test	Health-care provider to discuss with patient	Start at age 45, then every 3 years	Every 3 years	Every 3 years
Eye and ear health: complete eye exam	At least once between the ages 20–29 and at least twice between the ages 30–39, or any time there is an eye problem	Get an exam at age 40, then every 2–4 years or as health-care provider advises	Every 2–4 years or as health-care provider advises	Every 1–2 years
Hearing test	Starting at age 18, then every 10 years	Every 10 years	Every 3 years	Every 3 years
General health: full checkup, including weight and height	Ages 18–39 Patient specific	Ages 40–49 Patient specific	Ages 50–64 Patient specific	Ages 65 and older Patient specific
HIV test	Test once for basic screening and then risk-based screening thereafter	Test once for basic screening and then risk-based screening thereafter	Test once for basic screening and then risk-based screening thereafter	Discuss with patient
Mental health screening	Patient specific	Patient specific	Patient specific	Patient specific
Oral health: dental exam	Routinely; discuss with dentist	Routinely; discuss with dentist	Routinely; discuss with dentist	Routinely; discuss with dentist
Prostate health: digital rectal exam (DRE)		Discuss with patient	Discuss with patient	Discuss with patient

Continued

Table 49–6 **Screening Tests and Immunizations Guidelines for Men by Age—cont'd**

Screening Tests	Ages 18–39	Ages 40–49	Ages 50–64	Ages 65 and Older
Prostate-specific antigen (PSA) test		Discuss with patient	Discuss with patient	Discuss with patient
Reproductive health: testicular exam	Discuss with patient	Discuss with patient	Discuss with patient	Discuss with patient
Sexually transmitted infection (STI) tests	Both partners should be tested for STIs, including HIV, before initiating sexual intercourse	Both partners should be tested for STIs, including HIV, before initiating sexual intercourse	Both partners should be tested for STIs, including HIV, before initiating sexual intercourse	Both partners should be tested for STIs, including HIV, before initiating sexual intercourse
Skin health: mole exam	Monthly mole self-exam; by a health-care provider as part of a routine full checkup starting at age 20	Monthly mole self-exam; by a health-care provider as part of routine full checkup	Monthly mole self-exam; by a provider as part of routine full checkup	Monthly mole self-exam; by a provider as part of routine full checkup

Source: Adapted from http://www.womenshealth.gov/prevention/men/men.pdf.

influence AF-AM men's health-related behaviors, the role of their health perceptions in perpetuating their behaviors, and strategies to overcome the disadvantages.

Factors such as socialization, structural barriers, and practitioner bias can adversely affect health behaviors and health outcomes in AF-AM men. Young African American males are socialized to accept masculine behavior through strength, dominance, autonomy, and physical aggression into adulthood. Difficulty expressing feelings leads to inner stress and adverse health consequences such as high rates of anxiety disorders and depression. Structural barriers such as poverty and lack of health insurance impede the delivery of health care to AF-AM men. AF-AM men hold a disproportional share of part-time, contract, or temporary jobs. Many of these jobs have no associated health-care benefits. Practitioner bias can have a negative impact on AF-AM men's health. Patronizing non-AF-AM providers heighten perceptions of mistrust. Some providers may inadvertently engage in negative racial stereotyping when caring for AF-AM men and thereby contribute to their patients' negative health perceptions and underuse or delayed use of health-care services.

HEALTH ISSUES FOR MEN WHO HAVE SEX WITH MEN

Health care for gay men and other men who have sex with men (MSM) is a complicated mix of physical, psychosocial, and cultural phenomena that requires provider awareness of the issues. Gay men's health issues are unique and need to be incorporated into clinical practice to provide comprehensive and culturally appropriate care.

HIV Infection and Sexually Transmitted Infections

Although HIV infection and sexually transmitted infections (STIs) are potential major health issues for all people, those issues remain of significant importance to gay men. The continued high rate of newly diagnosed HIV and STI cases signals that many gay men and other MSM are not taking the threat to their health seriously. Additionally, MSM are much more likely to become infected with HIV than their heterosexual counterparts. AF-AM and Latino-American MSM have twice the risk for acquiring HIV infection when compared to whites (CDC, 2006b).

Rates of three sexually transmitted infections (STIs)—chlamydia, gonorrhea, and syphilis—remain high in the United States (CDC, 2009). These infections can be cured, but can cause serious complications if untreated and can increase the risk of HIV acquisition and transmission. High STI rates among African Americans and teens are particularly alarming, and men who have sex with men account for the greatest prevalence of syphilis (CDC, 2009).

Additionally, recreational drug use with substances such as cocaine, ecstasy, inhalants, and methamphetamines influence unsafe sexual behavior in gay men and MSM (CDC, 2009). Many of these recreational drugs are used during "white" or "circuit" party activities in which gay men from various geographical locales gather in one large metropolitan gay community over an extended 2- or 3-day period for the purpose of intense recreation and sexual activity.

Anal Cancer

Anal cancer is increasing in MSM and particularly in HIV-infected MSM. From 1973 to 2000, the incidence of anal cancer (2.1 per 100,000) in the United States increased in the general population for both men (160%) and women (78%). The incidence is substantially higher in MSM, HIV-infected men and women, transplant recipients, and women with cervical squamous intraepithelial lesions. Data collected before the height of the HIV epidemic revealed the incidence of anal cancer in U.S. MSMs to be 35 per 100,000 (Daling, Weiss, & Hislop, 1987; Daling, Weiss, & Klopfenstein, 1982). Estimates now put the incidence among HIV-infected MSM at least twice as high; 70 to 100 per 100,000. The incidence of anal cancer is 17 times higher in gay and bisexual men than it is in heterosexual men (CDC, 2008b). In view of this increased incidence, there has been considerable discussion about whether regular anal screening using an anal PAP test should be implemented in the MSM population and specifically in the HIV-infected MSM population (CDC, 2008b). In 2010, a new recommendation has been suggested for all males to receive the HPV vaccine, which is discussed in Chapter 19.

Tobacco Abuse

Tobacco abuse continues to plague the gay community. Smoking among gay men occurs in nearly 33 percent of the population, whereas it remains at around 24 percent for the general public (CDC, 2006a). There is a paucity of interventions designed to target gay men with tobacco-abuse problems. Because HIV-infected individuals develop significant CV disease, a concerted effort must be taken to curtail smoking in this population. In addition, smokers who survive into later life may be at risk for significant cognitive decline. People who smoked 20 or more cigarettes daily have demonstrated faster declines in their verbal memory and slower visual search skills (Richards, Jarvis, Thompson, & Wadsworth, 2003). Smoking cessation programs designed to target gay men are being implemented slowly, but the need remains great. Smoking cessation is discussed in Chapter 43.

CONCLUSION

Most of the published studies addressing gender influence on health care focus on women's health or low income and minority groups (Galdas, Cheater, & Marshall, 2005). There is a gap in research pertaining to men's health and an absence of health-care policies addressing men's health. Although men are usually research subjects, they are rarely the subjects of research.

Limited health-care resources; inequitable options available to men in seeking health care; and the absence of policies addressing gender-specific issues such as learning styles, masculinity, influences of testosterone on health, and stereotypical male traits—such as risk taking behaviors—underscore the need for further studies and better understanding of men's health (Perls, Salzman, & Schaefer, 2006).

REFERENCES

Bassil, N., Alkaade, S., & Morley, J. E. (2009). The benefits and risks of testosterone replacement therapy: A review. *Therapeutics and Clinical Risk Management, 5,* 427–448.

Beauchet, O. (2006). Testosterone and cognitive function: Current clinical evidence of a relationship. *European Journal of Endocrinology, 155,* 773–781.

Bhasin, S., Cunningham, G. R., Hayes, F. J., Matsumoto, A. M., Snyder, P. J., Swerdloff, R. S., et al. (2010). Testosterone therapy in adult men with androgen deficiency syndromes: An Endocrine Society clinical practice guideline. *Journal of Clinical Endocrinology & Metabolism, 95*(6), 2536–2559.

Bodie, J., Lewis, J., Schow, D., & Monga, M. (2003). Laboratory evaluations of erectile dysfunction: An evidence-based approach. *Journal of Urology, 169,* 2262–2264.

Braithwaite, R. (2001). The health status of black men. In R. Braithwaite & S. Taylor (Eds.), *Health issues in the black community* (pp. 62–80). San Francisco, CA: Jossey-Bass.

Brooks, G. (2001). Masculinity and men's mental health. *Journal of American College of Health, 49*(6), 285–297.

Caminiti, G., Volterrani, M., Iellamo, F., Marazzi, G., Massaro, R., Miceli, M., et al. (2009). Effect of long-acting testosterone treatment on functional exercise capacity, skeletal muscle performance, insulin resistance, and baroreflex sensitivity in elderly patients with chronic heart failure: A double-blind, placebo-controlled, randomized study. *Journal of the American College of Cardiology, 54,* 919–927.

Centers for Disease Control and Prevention (CDC). (2006a). *Cigarette smoking among adults—United States. Mortality and Morbidity Weekly Report, 56,* 1157–1161.

Centers for Disease Control and Prevention (CDC). (2006b). *HIV and AIDS among gay and bisexual men.* Retrieved March 1, 2009, from http://www.cdc.gov/nchhstp/Newsroom/docs/FastFacts-MSM-FINAL508COMP.pdf

Centers for Disease Control and Prevention (CDC). (2007). *Top 20.* Retrieved April 20, 2008, from http://cdc.gov

Centers for Disease Control and Prevention (CDC). (2008a). *Sexually transmitted diseases surveillance.* Retrieved March 1, 2009, from http://www.cdc.gov/std/stats08/msm.htm

Centers for Disease Control and Prevention (CDC). (2008b). HPV and men—CDC fact sheet. Retrieved from http://www.cdc.gov/std/hpv/stdfact-hpv-and-men.htm

Centers for Disease Control and Prevention (CDC). (2009). NHBS: HIV risk taking and testing behaviors among young MSM. Retrieved from http://www.cdc.gov/hiv/topics/msm/ymsm.htm

Centers for Disease Control and Prevention (CDC). (2010). *Screening tests and immunizations guidelines for men.* Retrieved March 1, 2010, from http://www.womenshealth.gov/prevention/men/men.pdf

Cherrier, M. M., Craft, S., & Matsumoto, A. H. (2003). Cognitive changes associated with supplementation of testosterone or dihydrotestosterone in mildly hypogonadal men: A preliminary report. *Journal of Andrology, 24,* 568–576.

Cherrier, M. M., Matsumoto, A. M., Amory, J. K., Asthana, S., Bremner, W., Peskind, E.R., et al. (2005). Testosterone improves spatial memory in men with Alzheimer disease and mild cognitive impairment. *Neurology, 64,* 2063–2068.

Chin-Hong, P., & Palefsk, J. (2002). Natural history and clinical management of anal human papillomavirus disease in men and women infected with human immunodeficiency virus. *Clinical Infectious Diseases, 35,* 1127–1134.

Daling, J., Weiss, N., & Hislop, T. (1987). Sexual practices, sexually transmitted diseases, and the incidence of anal cancer. *New England Journal of Medicine, 317,* 973–977.

Daling, J., Weiss, N., & Klopfenstein, L. (1982). Correlates of homosexual behavior and the incidence of anal cancer. *Journal of the American Medical Association, 247,* 1988–1990.

Edley, N., & Wetherell, M. (1996). Masculinity, power and identity. In Mac an Ghaill, M. (Ed), *Understanding Masculinities* (pp. 185–201). Buckingham, England: Open University Press.

Galdas, P., Cheater, F., & Marshall, P. (2005). Men and health help-seeking behavior: Literature review. *Journal of Advanced Nursing, 49*(6), 616–623.

Goedert, J., Cote, T., & Virgo, P. (1998). Spectrum of AIDS-associated malignant disorders. *Lancet, 351,* 1833–1839.

Gooren, L. J. (2010). Androgens and male aging: Current evidence of safety and efficacy. *Asian Journal of Andrology, 12,* 136–151.

Gruenewald, D. A., & Matsumoto, A. M. (2003). Testosterone supplementation therapy for older men: Potential benefits and risks. *Journal of the American Geriatric Society, 51,* 101–115.

Haren, M. T., Wittert, G. A., Chapman, I. M., Coates, P., & Morley, J. E. (2005). Effect of oral testosterone undecanoate on visuospatial cognition, mood and quality of life in elderly men with low normal gonadal status. *Maturitas, 50* 124–133.

Harkonen, K., Huhtaniemi, I., Makinen, J., Hubler, D., Irjala, K., Koskenvuo, M., et al. (2003). The polymorphic androgen receptor gene CAG repeat, pituitary-testicular function and andropausal symptoms in ageing men. *International Journal of Andrology, 26,* 187–194.

Heidelbaugh, J. J. (2010). Management of erectile dysfunction. *American Family Physician, 81,* 305–312.

Hogervorst, E., Bandelow, S., Combrinck, M., & Smith, A. D. (2004). Low free testosterone is an independent risk factor for Alzheimer's disease. *Experimental Gerontology, 39,* 1633–1639.

Inui, S., & Itami, S. (2007). Reversal of androgenetic alopecia by topical ketoconazole: Relevance of antiandrogenic activity. *Journal of Dermatological Science, 45,* 66–68.

Krause, W., Mueller, U., & Mazur, A. (2005). Testosterone supplementation in the aging male: Which questions have been answered? *Aging Male, 8,* 31–38.

Laborde, E. E., & McVary, K. T. (2009). Medical management of lower urinary tract symptoms. *Reviews in Urology, 11,* S19–S25.

Lee, D. M., O'Neill, T. W., Pye, S. R., Silman, A. J., Finn, J. D., Pendleton, N., et al. (2009). The European Male Ageing Study (EMAS): Design, methods and recruitment. *International Journal of Andrology, 32,* 11–24

Lee, T. S., & Minton, T. J. (2009). An update on hair restoration therapy. *Current Opinion in Otolaryngology & Head and Neck Surgery, 17,* 287–294.

Liburd, L., Namageyo-Funa, A., & Jack, L. (2007). Understanding "masculinity" and the challenges of managing type-2 diabetes among African-American men. *Journal of the American Medical Association, 99*(5), 550–558.

Liverman, C. T., & Blazer, D. G. (Eds.). (2004). *Testosterone and aging: Clinical research directions.* Washington, DC: National Academies Press.

Matsumoto, T., Shiina, H., Kawano, H., Sato, T., & Kato, S. (2008). Androgen receptor functions in male and female physiology. *Journal of Steroid Biochemistry and Molecular Biology, 109*(3–5), 236–241.

Mayo Clinic. (2010). *Men's health: Preventing your top 10 threats.* Retrieved March 1, 2010, from http://www.mayoclinic.com/print/mens-health/MC00013

Men's Health Network. (2008). *Reports.* Retrieved April 20, 2008, from http://www.menshealthnetwork.org

Morley, J. E., Perry, H. M., III, Kaiser, F. E., Kraenzle, D., Jensen, J., Houston, K., et al. (1993). Effects of testosterone replacement therapy in old hypogonadal males: A preliminary study. *Journal of the American Geriatrics Society, 41,* 149–152.

Muller, M., van den Beld, A. W., Bots, M. L., Grobbee, D. E., Lamberts, S. W., & van der Schouw, Y. T. (2004). Endogenous sex hormones and progression of carotid atherosclerosis in elderly men. *Circulation, 109,* 2074–2079.

Page, S. T., Amory, J. K., Bowman, F. D., Anawalt, B. D., Matsumoto, A. M., Bremner, W. J., et al. (2005). Exogenous testosterone (T) alone or with finasteride increases physical performance, grip strength, and lean body mass in older men with low serum T. *Journal of Clinical Endocrinology and Metabolism, 90,* 1502–1510.

Perls, T., Salzman, B., & Schaefer, S. (2006, June). Why do men die at a younger age than women, and what can be done about it? *Patient Care,* 20–28.

Pierorazio, P. M., Ferrucci, L., Kettermann, A., Longo, D. L., Metter, E. J., & Carter, H. B. (2009). Serum testosterone is associated with aggressive prostate cancer in older men: Results from the Baltimore Longitudinal Study of Aging. *BJU International, 105*(6), 824–829.

Rhoden, E. L., & Morgentaler, A. (2004). Risk of testosterone-replacement therapy and recommendations for monitoring. *New England Journal of Medicine, 350*(5), 482–492.

Richards, M., Jarvis, M. J., Thompson, N., & Wadsworth, M. E. (2003). Cigarette smoking and cognitive decline in midlife: Evidence from a prospective birth cohort study. *American Journal of Public Health, 93,* 994–998.

Rogers, N., & Avram, M. (2008). Medical treatments for male and female pattern hair loss. *Journal of the American Academy of Dermatology, 59,* 547–566.

Seidman, S. N., Araujo, A. B., Roose, S. P., & McKinlay, J. B. (2001). Testosterone level, androgen receptor polymorphism, and depressive symptoms in middle-aged men. *Biological Psychiatry, 50,* 371–376.

Shabsigh R., Kaufman, J. M., Steidle, C., & Padma-Nathan, H. (2004). Randomized study of testosterone gel as adjunctive therapy to sildenafil in hypogonadal men with erectile dysfunction who do not respond to sildenafil alone. *Journal of Urology, 172,* 658–663.

Sih, R., Morley, J. E., Kaiser, F. E., Perry, H. M., III, Patrick, P., & Ross, C. (1997). Testosterone replacement in older hypogonadal men: A 12-month randomized controlled trial. *Journal of Clinical Endocrinology and Metabolism, 82,* 1661–1667.

Snyder, P. J. (2004). Hypogonadism in elderly men: What to do until the evidence comes. *New England Journal of Medicine, 350,* 440–442.

Snyder, P. J. (2010). Testosterone treatment in male hypogonadism. *Up ToDate Online.* Retrieved from http://www.uptodate.com

Snyder, P. J., Peachey, H., Berlin, J. A., Hannoush, P., Haddad, G., Dlewati, A., et al. (2000). Effects of testosterone replacement in hypogonadal men. *Journal of Clinical Endocrinology and Metabolism, 85,* 2670–2677.

Spark, R. F. (2011). Overview of male sexual dysfunction. UpToDate Online. Retrieved from http://www.uptodate.com/contents/overview-of-male-sexual-dysfunction?source=search_result&selectedTitle=3~150

Srinivas-Shankar, U., Roberts, S. A., Connolly, M. J., Adams, J. E., Oldham, J. A., & Wu, F. C. (2010). Effects of testosterone on muscle strength, physical function, body composition, and quality of life in intermediate-frail and frail elderly men: A randomized, double-blind, placebo-controlled study. *Journal of Clinical Endocrinology and Metabolism, 95*(2), 639–650.

Tricker, R., Casaburi, R., Storer, T. W., Clevenger, B., Berman, N., Shirazi, A., et al. (1996). The effects of supraphysiological doses of testosterone on angry behavior in healthy eugonadal men—a clinical research center study. *Journal of Clinical Endocrinology and Metabolism, 81*(10), 3754–3758.

U.S. Department of Health and Human Services. (2000). *National statistics reports.* Retrieved April 20, 2008, from http://www.hhs.gov

van den Beld, A., Huhtaniemi, I. T., Pettersson, K. S., Pols, H. A., Grobbee, D. E., de Jong, F. H., et al. (1999). Luteinizing hormone and different genetic variants, as indicators of frailty in healthy elderly men. *Journal of Clinical Endocrinology and Metabolism, 84,* 1334–1339.

Vermeulen, A., & Kaufman, J. M. (1995). Aging of the hypothalamic-pituitary-testicular axis in men. *Hormone Research, 43,* 25–28.

Wagenlehner, F. M. E., Naber, K. G., Schleipfer, T. Brähler, E., & Weidner, W. (2009). Prostatitis and male pelvic pain syndrome: Diagnosis and treatment. *Deutsches Ärzteblatt International, 106,* 175–183.

Wang, C., Cunningham, G., Dobs, A., Iranmanesh, A., Matsumoto, A. M., Snyder, P. J., et al. (2004). Long-term testosterone gel (AndroGel) treatment maintains beneficial effects on sexual function and mood, lean and fat mass, and bone mineral density in hypogonadal men. *Journal of Clinical Endocrinology and Metabolism, 89,* 2085–2098.

Wang, C., Swerdloff, R. S., Iranmanesh, A., Dobs, A., Snyder, P. J., Cunningham, G., et al. (2000). Transdermal testosterone gel improves sexual function, mood, muscle strength, and body composition parameters in hypogonadal men. *Journal of Clinical Endocrinology and Metabolism, 85,* 2839–2853.

Williams, D. (2003). The health of men: Structured inequalities and opportunities. *American Journal of Public Health, 93*(5), 724–731.

Wu, F. C., Tajar, A., Pye, S. R., Silman, A. J., Finn, J. D., O'Neill, T. W., et al. (2008). Hypothalamic-pituitary-testicular axis disruptions in older men are differentially linked to age and modifiable risk factors: The European Male Aging Study. *Journal of Clinical Endocrinology and Metabolism, 93,* 2737–2745.

Zohdy, W. (2009). Clinical parameters that predict successful outcome in men with premature ejaculation and inflammatory prostatitis. *Journal of Sexual Medicine, 6,* 3139–3146.

CHAPTER 50

PEDIATRIC PATIENTS

Teri Moser Woo

Chapter Outline

Pediatric patients present a special challenge to the primary care practitioner; they are constantly changing, both physiologically and developmentally. The practitioner who is making a treatment decision must consider the parent and the family situation, as well as the patient, in determining if the treatment will be appropriate. In addition, information on use of medications in children is limited, because many medications are labeled "not recommended in children." This chapter presents the factors that the prescriber will need to consider to safely prescribe to children.

HISTORICAL PERSPECTIVE ON PEDIATRIC PRESCRIBING

Federal Drug Regulation

Drug regulation in the United States has often been moved forward after tragedies have occurred that directly involved children. Regulation began with the passage of the Federal Food and Drug Act of 1906, which was enacted because children had died from ingesting tainted food products and soldiers had died from ingesting adulterated **quinine.** This law, known as the Wiley Act, prohibited the manufacture and interstate shipment of adulterated and misbranded foods and drugs. In 1938, the federal Food, Drug, and Cosmetic Act was the next major legislation enacted. It was passed as the result of continued adulteration of products, including **sulfanilamide,** which had caused more than 100 deaths in children because of the **diethylene glycol** used in the elixir. For the first time, documentation of drug safety was mandated. This act also mandated truthful labeling and established the new drug application process that required toxicology testing prior to drugs being promoted and distributed. In 1962 the Harris-Kefauver Amendment was passed, prompted by the births of thousands of deformed infants whose mothers had taken the sedative **thalidomide.** This amendment mandated preclinical animal trials before testing drugs in humans. It also established three phases of clinical testing: Phase I establishes safety and pharmacokinetics; phase II establishes initial effectiveness and dose range; phase III conducts comparative clinical trials. Although the Harris-Kefauver Amendment increased the safety of new drugs coming onto the market, it also slowed new drug development, increasing the time from investigational new drug to new drug approval to 8 or 9 years. In 1972 an over-the-counter (OTC) drug review process was begun to enhance the safety and labeling of nonprescription medications. In 1986 the Child Vaccine Act was passed requiring patients/parents be informed regarding the vaccines they are being given. In spite of all of these laws, as late as the 1990s the percentage of approved drugs that contained no labeling information for children was approximately 70 percent. The next major legislation that affected children was the U.S. Food and Drug Administration (FDA) Modernization Act of 1997. The act had two main components pertaining to pediatrics: (1) The FDA could require in writing that the manufacturer submit data on pediatric patients for drugs that appear to have a pediatric use. Previously, drugs were approved for use in adults and the pediatric prescribing information happened later. This law mandated that the FDA require the pediatric data up front. (2) Pharmaceutical companies were rewarded by a 6-month extension on any patent if they voluntarily test the medications for safety in children. The FDA Modernization Act was challenged by the drug companies and overturned in 2002, a setback for pediatric drug safety.

Best Pharmaceuticals for Children Act

Fortunately, the American Academy of Pediatrics and other groups concerned with pediatric drug safety went before Congress and the result was the passage in 2003 of the Best Pharmaceuticals for Children Act (BPCA). This reinstated the pediatric exclusivity rule, giving a 6-month extension on patents if a manufacturer studies a given drug in children. It also established a mandate for an annual list of requested drugs to be studied. Experts in pediatrics are consulted and a list is developed for priority testing. In addition, the Pediatric Research Equity Act (PREA) was signed into law in December 2003. It requires that all applications for new active ingredients, new indications, new dosage forms, new dosing regimens, and new routes of administration must contain a pediatric assessment unless the sponsor has obtained a waiver or deferral of pediatric studies. The BPCA was renewed in 2007. The outcome so far of these major moves toward pediatric drug safety has been 1,145 studies requested and 386 written requests for studies issued as of April 2010.

As of April 2010, 355 drugs have been relabeled or newly labeled for pediatric use (FDA, 2010). As more studies are completed, we will have a clearer picture of the safety and efficacy of the drug prescribed and pediatric providers will have to do less off-labeled prescribing of medications. When a relabeled drug contains the statement "Safety and effectiveness have not been established," it really means that the drug is either not safe or not effective in children as determined by pediatric studies. Providers can find current information regarding drug label changes at the FDA Pediatric Exclusivity Labeling Changes Web site: http://www.fda.gov/scienceresearch/specialtopics/pediatrictherapeuticsresearch/default.htm.

Another exciting development in pediatrics is an international movement toward improving pediatric drug safety. The World Health Organization (WHO) launched the "make medicines child size" campaign in December 2007, to raise awareness and encourage medication development for children younger than age 12 years (WHO, 2010). A global alliance in pediatric pharmacology has been formed and pediatric pharmacologists from more than 30 countries have met to share information from pharmacokinetic and pharmacodynamic studies and avoid unnecessary duplication of studies (Koren, Reider, & MacLeod, 2009).

PHARMACOKINETIC AND PHARMACODYNAMIC DIFFERENCES IN CHILDREN

Pharmacokinetics

Drug absorption, metabolism, and excretion can vary throughout infancy and early childhood. Even at puberty, there are differences in drug clearance between girls and boys as drug clearance rates reach adult levels. As more is learned about the metabolic pathways in the adult liver, more knowledge is gained about how to study the differences in children. Past disasters caused by lack of understanding about the physiology of newborn metabolism have led to caution regarding the use of medications in infants. Gray baby syndrome caused by inadequate glucuronidation of **chloramphenicol**, which led to dangerous drug accumulation, and **sulfonamide**-induced kernicterus (caused by displacement of bilirubin from plasma proteins by **sulfonamides**) are two such disasters that have been hard lessons in the use of medication in newborns. Well-designed pharmacokinetic studies in the newborn and careful therapeutic drug monitoring have improved our knowledge of neonatal pharmacology, yet care is essential when any new therapy is tried.

Drug Absorption

Drug absorption can be affected in children more than it is in adults by three factors: (1) the blood flow at the site of administration (intramuscular [IM] or subcutaneous [SC] administration), (2) gastrointestinal (GI) function, and (3) thin stratum corneum.

Neonates have more variability in the blood flow to the muscles, especially ill newborns, and poor blood flow can lead to delayed or variable absorption of medications. If perfusion suddenly improves, there can be a rapid absorption of the medication from the muscle, leading to possible toxic levels. Care should be taken when administering potentially toxic drugs such as **cardiac glycosides**, **aminoglycoside antibiotics**, and **anticonvulsants** IM to ill infants.

GI function is variable in neonates and young infants. Gastric acid function begins soon after birth and gradually increases over several hours. In premature infants, gastric acid secretion occurs more slowly and takes up to 4 days to reach normal levels. Gastric pH does not reach adult values until 20 to 30 months. Gastric emptying time is prolonged, reaching adult values by 6 to 8 months, meaning medications absorbed from the stomach may therefore have increased absorption. The neonate also has slow and irregular peristalsis, and medications absorbed primarily from the small intestine should be monitored for potential toxic levels. It is known that the neonate has decreased oral absorption of **acetaminophen, phenobarbital**, and **phenytoin**, whereas **ampicillin** and **penicillin G** have increased bioavailability when taken orally. Diarrhea, a common ailment in young children, lessens the extent of absorption from the intestine, causing decreased drug levels.

The developmental changes in gastric function alter drug absorption in a fairly predictable manner. The oral bioavailability of **acid labile compounds (beta-lactams)** is increased and the oral bioavailability of **weak organic acids (phenobarbital** and **phenytoin)** is decreased. Basic drugs, such as **diazepam** and **theophylline**, have increased absorption. Gastric motility greatly alters the absorption of drugs with limited water solubility (**phenytoin** and **carbamazepine**) (Kearns, 2000; Kearns et al, 2003; Rakhmanina & van den Anker, 2006).

It is well known that infants and young children have a thin stratum and larger body surface area in relation to size and this affects topical absorption of medication. Children absorb topical medications more readily than do adults, leading to systemic toxicity seen with topical medication use. This is seen with topical use of **lidocaine** or **diphenhydramine** in young children. Most providers are familiar with the concern for systemic absorption of topical **corticosteroids** in children, with systemic Cushingoid symptoms or hypothalamic-pituitary-adrenal (HPA)-axis suppression developing with topical use. Due to BPCA and pharmacokinetic studies that indicated HPA-axis suppression or adrenal suppression in children, a number of topical **corticosteroids** have been relabeled. **Diprolene (diprosone)** cream, ointment, and lotion are not recommended for use in children younger than 12 years due to HPA-axis suppression. In addition, **Diprolene AF** and **Elocon (mometasone)** lotion are not recommended, although **Elocon** cream and ointment may be used in children as young as 2 years. In an open-label study of **Lotrisone (clotrimazole** and **betamethasone dipropionate)** cream for the treatment of tinea pedis, 17 of 43 (39.5%) patients (12 to 16 years) demonstrated adrenal suppression as determined by cosyntropin testing. In an open-label study of **Lotrisone** cream for the treatment of tinea cruris, 8 of 17 (47.1%) patients (12 to 16 years) demonstrated adrenal suppression by cosyntropin testing. **Lotrisone** has been relabeled and is not recommended for children younger than 17 years and not recommended for diaper dermatitis; previously it was not recommended for children younger than 12 years. **Cutivate (fluticasone)** ointment has been similarly relabeled to be used only in adults (U.S. Food and Drug Administration, 2010b).

Distribution

There are clear changes in body composition in neonates, infants, children, and adolescents. Newborns have total body water (TBW) of 80 percent, which drops over the first few months to TBW of 60 percent at 6 months; therefore, infants require higher doses of **hydrophilic drugs**. Infants also have a decreased volume of distribution for **lipid-soluble drugs**. Infants younger than 6 months have decreased plasma proteins available for drug binding, which will cause elevated levels of unbound medication. Providers need to monitor for drug toxicity even if they have normal or low plasma concentration of total drug. **Phenytoin** is one drug that this is seen in, as it is only 80 to 85 percent bound in infants and 94 to 98 percent bound in adults (Kearns, 2000; Kearns et al, 2003).

The ratio of fat to lean muscle also shifts throughout childhood with a shift toward decreased total body fat in adolescence, a shift of approximately 50 percent in males between ages 10 and 20 years. Consequently, lean body mass increases more in males. The shift in females is less dramatic shifting from 28 to 25 percent from ages 10 to 20 years. (Kearns, 2000; Rakhmanina & van den Anker, 2006). Due to these changes it may be difficult to predict pharmacokinetics of some drugs during pubertal growth. Medications that the patient takes chronically, such as seizure medications, need to be monitored closely during pubertal growth.

Metabolism

Phase I Enzymes

The pathways of drug metabolism develop variably over the first year of life and may be influenced by medications that induce drug-metabolizing enzymes (e.g., **phenobarbital**). In adults, much has been learned about the cytochrome P450 (CYP450) enzymes, and much is still unknown. The exact developmental pattern is not known for most of the CYP450 isoenzymes although our knowledge is increasing rapidly. Recent studies recognize that the small intestine is a major site of drug metabolism because it contains enterocytes in the bowel mucosa, which have CYP450 drug metabolism enzymes. This information enhances our knowledge of drug metabolism, but there may be large interindividual variation in the capacity of the small bowel to metabolize drugs.

Studies of CYP450 1A2 using **caffeine** as the test substrate demonstrate limited metabolic clearance in the newborn, reaches adult levels at 4 months, and then exceeds adult levels at 1 to 2 years throughout childhood. At puberty (Tanner stage II), clearance begins to decline to adult levels, in girls sooner than in boys. Diseases such as cystic fibrosis (CF) can affect CYP1A2 activity and CF patients may need higher doses of medications metabolized via the CYP1A2 pathway.

There are many medications that are metabolized via the CYP1A2 enzymes including **theophylline, erythromycin, cimetadine, phenobarbitol, phenytoin, carbamazepine, clarithromycin**, and others. Foods that are affected by the CYP1A2 pathway are grapefruit juice, cruciferous vegetables, and charbroiled foods—foods not commonly eaten by children, but the provider should be aware of these food interactions. Cigarette smoking also affects CYP1A2 enzymes and providers should inquire if patients taking medications are smoking, as it may affect therapeutic levels of medication including a number of seizure medications. In practice this implies that drug dosages need to be adjusted as a child goes through phases of CYP1A2 maturation; higher dosages may be needed from 1 year until puberty and therapeutic drug levels will need to be monitored as a child goes through puberty.

The isoenzyme CYP3A4 is the most abundant CYP isoform, and undergoes a similar maturational process to CYP1A2. CYP3A4 has low activity at birth and reaches 30 to 40 percent of adult level by 1 month. By 6 months it is at full adult level and exceeds adult level at 1 to 4 years. At puberty it decreases to adult levels. The CYP3A4 enzymes are used to metabolize more than 20 commonly used pediatric medications including **carbamazepine, prednisone, oral contraceptives, macrolides, NSAIDS, antihistamines**, and others. The implications for pediatric practice include monitoring when prescribing more than one drug metabolized by CYP3A4 enzyme and monitoring during developmental changes.

Phase II Enzymes

Phase II enzymes are responsible for synthesis of water-soluble compounds. There is less information available on phase II activity in children. UDP glucuronosyltransferase (UGT) are responsible for the glucuronidation of hundreds of hydrophobic compounds. It is known that **morphine** is metabolized by UGT 2B7. It is known from **morphine** studies in neonates that premature infants (gestational age 24 to 37 weeks) have a much lower plasma clearance of **morphine** than children 1 to 16 years. It is thought that **morphine** clearance reaches adult levels at 2 to 6 months, although some children do not reach adult levels until 3 years (Blake, Castro, Leeder, & Kearns, 2005; Kearns, 2000; Rakhmanina & van den Anker, 2006). There appears to be ethnic variations in thiopurine methyltransferase (TPMT) activity, as Koreans do not reach adult activity levels until 7 to 9 years. Little is known about the phase II enzymes in children, but the knowledge base is growing. Commonly used medications such as **acetaminophen, morphine, propofol**, and **caffeine** are metabolized via the phase II enzymes and providers need to be aware of developmental as well as possible ethnic variations.

One essential consideration from our knowledge thus far is that, during times of great physiological change (the premature, the neonate, puberty), there are likely to be major changes in pharmacokinetics. More variability among individuals and within the individual is likely during these periods. Careful monitoring of therapeutic drug levels is critical to safe outcomes. In the neonatal period, frequent adjustments may be necessary because of the rapid changes the neonate is undergoing. A drug dosage that is at a therapeutic level in a 9-year-old girl has to be carefully monitored as she proceeds through puberty to ensure that she will not develop toxic levels as her drug clearance reaches adult levels.

Drug metabolism is an area in which the BPCA and Pediatric Research Equity Act (PREA) studies have expanded our knowledge. For example, females aged 8 to 11 years have higher therapeutic levels of **fluvoxamine (Luvox)** compared to boys the same age. The studies indicate that girls need lower doses of **fluvoxamine** (U.S. Food and Drug Administration, 2010b). Likewise, pharmacokinetic studies of **oxcarbazepine (Trileptal)** in children have determined clearance decreases with age, to the point that children aged 2 to younger than 4 years may require up to twice the dose per body weight compared to adults, and children aged 4 to 12 years may require a dose 50 percent higher per weight than adults (U.S. Food and Drug Administration, 2010b). Pharmacokinetic studies of **levetriacetam (Keppra)** found clearance increased with increased body weight; adults have 40 percent higher clearance than do children. Hence, prescribers need to be aware of nonlinear pharmacokinetics seen with some pediatric medications and prescribe and monitor accordingly.

Excretion

Drug excretion rates are affected by the lower glomerular filtration rate in newborns, which is only 30 to 40 percent of adult values. By age 6 to 12 months, the glomerular filtration rate reaches adult values (per unit surface area). Drugs that depend on renal excretion are cleared more slowly in neonates. Drug dosages and dosing intervals in newborns are adjusted accordingly for medications such as **ampicillin, aminoglycoside antibiotics**, and **digoxin.** Renal blood flow is also reduced in neonates and reaches adult levels at approximately 9 months.

Pharmacodynamics

There are pharmacodynamic differences between children and adults that need to be taken into consideration in prescribing for children. Like much medical knowledge, information on the differences between children and adults has been gained from an unexpected outcome in children in response to a medication that is safe for adults. The classic examples are **antihistamines** and **barbiturates**, which may cause hyperactivity rather than sedation when given to children. Another classic example is **tetracycline**, which deposits in developing teeth and causes permanent stains. **Systemic corticosteroids** stunt linear growth if taken for long periods, as well as producing all of the same adverse reactions found in adults. Some medications, such as **isoniazid**, are less toxic in children than they are in adults.

Another concern in children is the vehicle in which the medication is administered or the formulation of the vehicle. Children have sometimes had toxic or unexpected results, not from the medication, but from the additives or preservatives used. As recently as the 1980s, **benzyl alcohol**, a preservative used in drugs, was discovered to cause "gasping syndrome" when medications containing it were administered to newborns.

Topical ointments and creams are routinely prescribed to adults and children, yet there is a major difference between adults and children in the absorption rates from the skin. Infants and children have a thinner stratum corneum that allows medications to be more readily absorbed. Compared with older children and adults, infants have a larger skin surface area that is capable of greater weight-adjusted absorption of **hydrophilic drugs**. Occlusive dressings can increase the absorption of medications, which is of particular concern regarding **corticosteroids** in the diaper area. The plastic coating on the diaper can cause occlusion, thereby increasing absorption and producing systemic steroid effects.

DEVELOPMENTAL ASPECTS OF PEDIATRIC MEDICATION ADMINISTRATION

With adults, the provider can assume that, if reasonably clear instructions are given, the patient will take the medication as prescribed. With children, many added variables affect administration of the medication and compliance with the medication regimen. The first consideration is the developmental level of the child and the amount of parental control at each developmental level. This section addresses these differences and suggests strategies for improving compliance at each age level.

Breastfed infants

Breastfeeding an infant the first year of life is beneficial both physically and emotionally to the infant. Therefore, when prescribing medications to a lactating woman, the practitioner needs to be aware of which medications can be used safely and which are contraindicated (Box 50–1). The most up-to-date, peer-reviewed, and easily accessible resource is the LactMed database at the National Library of Medicine TOXNET Web site (http://toxnet.nlm.nih.gov/index.html). LactMed is searchable by drug name and gives recommendations for prescribers with updated safety information.

Drug Excretion in Breast Milk

The mammary gland can be viewed as an elimination organ in relation to maternal medication ingestion. Like other elimination organs, the properties of the medication determine how much of the medication will be in the breast milk. Because breast milk is more acidic than plasma, basic compounds **(beta blockers)** may be slightly more concentrated in the milk, and the concentration of acidic compounds **(penicillins** and **NSAIDs)** in the milk will be lower than plasma levels (Berlin & Briggs, 2005). Protein binding also affects the transfer of medications into breast milk. Highly plasma protein–bound drugs have a lower amount of drug available to transfer into milk because only the free drug is available for transfer. Liposolubility also affects the ability of drugs to cross the alveolar cells by diffusion and enter the milk. Another factor is the molecular weight of the drug: Drugs with high molecular weight are transferred less easily into milk than drugs with lower molecular weight.

Factors Influencing an Infant's Exposure to Drugs in Breast Milk

A number of factors must be accounted for in determining the infant's exposure to a drug (Table 50–1). The following variables encompass physiological processes in

(Text continues on page 9)

BOX 50–1 PRESCRIBING TO LACTATING WOMEN

Prescribing medications for lactating women should be undertaken with the same caution as prescribing for pregnant women. Assume that any drug prescribed will, in some amount, be found in the breast milk. Therefore, knowledge regarding safety of medications for lactating women is essential for all primary care practitioners. When prescribing, take the following steps:

1. Review the safety of the drug during lactation.
2. If the drug is relatively safe, discuss the risks with the mother and explain the symptoms of drug toxicity.
3. Explain that the drug should be taken just after nursing or before infant's sleep.
4. Measure drug concentrations in milk or infant's serum when toxicity is likely.
5. Monitor the infant for signs of pharmacological action or drug toxicity.
6. Report any symptoms or signs of drug toxicity to the American Academy of Pediatrics, Committee on Drugs.

A few medications are absolutely contraindicated in lactating women (Table 50–1). Contraindications include **antineoplastic drugs** because of immediate or delayed toxicity in the infant. Weekly use of **methotrexate** for rheumatic disease is acceptable during lactation, but the infant needs to be monitored closely, with routine laboratory

Continued

BOX 50–1 **PRESCRIBING TO LACTATING WOMEN—cont'd**

analysis of complete blood count with differential, liver enzymes, and renal function essential to infant safety. Another contraindication to breastfeeding is **iodine-containing radioactive medications** used in nuclear medicine studies. In this case, temporary cessation of breastfeeding ("pump and dump") is indicated. The length of time before resumption of breastfeeding is determined by the half-life of the **radiopharmaceutical agent.**

Drugs that should be avoided include **lithium** and **oral contraceptives,** yet both have been used in lactating women. **Lithium** is excreted in breast milk at about 40 percent of the concentration of maternal serum, and milk and infant serum levels are approximately equal. If, for maternal health reasons, **lithium** needs to be prescribed, the infant's serum **lithium** level needs to be monitored closely. The main contraindication to **oral contraceptives** containing **estrogen** is that they may decrease milk supply. An **oral contraceptive** with low **estrogen** levels can be prescribed once the milk supply is well established (more than 6 weeks postpartum), but the first choice should be a **progestin-only oral contraceptive.** Decreased milk supply should be discussed with the mother as an adverse effect of **estrogen-containing oral contraceptives** prior to prescribing.

All illicit drugs are contraindicated in lactating women, specifically **cocaine, heroin,** and **methamphetamine.** Infants exposed to **cocaine** via breast milk may show signs of toxicity (irritability, tremors, increased startle response). **Cocaine** metabolites can be found in breast milk for up 36 hours after the mother's last dose. **Heroin** enters breast milk and can cause neonatal depression. **Amphetamines** are excreted in breast milk and cause excitation in the infant. **Methamphetamine** poses an additional concern because some of the chemicals used to manufacture the illicit drug are toxic to both mother and infant, specifically lead, which is quite harmful to the infant. Any drug use during lactation should be explored and the mother encouraged to discontinue breastfeeding if illicit drug use is a concern.

Alcohol and **tobacco** are two commonly used legal drugs that can affect the breastfed infant. **Alcohol** passes freely into breast milk and reaches levels close to maternal serum levels. High levels of **alcohol** in the breast milk put the infant at risk for sedation and cause a reduction in the maternal milk-ejecting response. There is controversy regarding maternal **alcohol** use during lactation. It is probably safe for the mother to ingest small amounts of **alcohol** timed just after a feeding, when levels in the milk are the lowest possible. **Tobacco** is a concern because of both secondhand smoke exposure and the **nicotine** that passes into breast milk. **Nicotine** passes freely into breast milk, and therefore the breastfed infant is exposed to this toxin. If a **nicotine replacement patch** is used for maternal smoking cessation, then the **nicotine** blood levels and therefore breast milk levels are lower than with smoked **tobacco.**

Because drugs are almost never tested for use in lactating women prior to their release onto the market, questions regarding their safety during breastfeeding always exist. Understanding some basic principles regarding the transfer of drugs into breast milk and their pharmacokinetic actions helps the practitioner make decisions about safe prescribing. The practitioner should have ready reference to the most current information available about drugs during lactation, including, *Drug Facts and Comparisons; Drugs in Pregnancy and Lactation* by Biggs, Freeman, and Yaffe; and *Teratogen Information Services,* available from your local Poison Control Center.

The National Library of Medicine TOXNET (Toxicology Data Network) maintains a peer-reviewed, searchable online database of drugs in lactation: LactMed (http://toxnet.nlm.nih.gov/index.html)

Table 50–1 **Effects of Commonly Prescribed Medications on Infants During Lactation**

Drug	Effect on Infant	Comments
Acetaminophen	Minimal	Found in breast milk. No adverse reactions reported. Safer than aspirin when lactating.
Amoxicillin (all penicillins)	Minimal	Excreted in breast milk in low concentrations. May cause mild diarrhea in infant.
Amoxicillin-clavulanate (Augmentin)	Minimal	Excreted in breast milk. Infant may have diarrhea.
Amphetamine	Unknown	It is not known if levels prescribed for medical indications affects the neurological development of the infant.
Aripiprazole	Unknown	Found in breast milk. Avoid in nursing women until more information available.
Asenapine	Unknown	Avoid until more information is available.

Table 50–1 Effects of Commonly Prescribed Medications on Infants During Lactation—cont'd

Drug	Effect on Infant	Comments
Aspirin	Minimal, rare complication of bleeding	Occasional doses probably safe.
Atenolol	Moderate to significant	Excreted in breast milk in a milk to plasma (M:P) ratio of 1.5:6.8 (one patient had an estimated dose of 0.13 mg atenolol per feeding with a maternal dose of 100 mg/d). Cyanosis and bradycardia have been reported in breastfed infants with maternal intake of 100 mg/d. **Use with caution.**
Caffeine	Minimal	Excreted in breast milk. If mother has one cup of coffee, the infant probably ingests 1.5–3.1 mg of caffeine. Caffeine has a long half-life in young infants (82 h in term newborn, 14.4 h in 3- to 4.5/2-mo-old infants, and 2.6 h in 6-mo-old infants). Probably safe in small amounts, with variable reaction based on individual infant.
Bromocriptine	Minimal	Used to suppress lactation.
Carbamazepine	Moderate	Infants have measurable carbamazepine levels. Monitor the infant for jaundice, drowsiness, adequate weight gain, and developmental milestones, especially in younger, exclusively breastfed infants (LactMed).
Chloramphenicol	Significant	**Avoid while lactating.** Possible bone marrow suppression.
Cascara	Moderate	Excreted in breast milk. Causes colic and diarrhea in the infant. **Avoid.**
Cephalosporin antibiotics	Minimal	Excreted in small amounts in milk. Probably safe.
Chlorpromazine	Probably minimal	Excreted in breast milk. Monitor infant for drowsiness.
Citalopram	Minimal	Excreted in breast milk. Monitor infant for sedation or fussiness. OK if required by mother. Consider a trial of escitalopram, which appears safer.
Codeine	Minimal; infant may experience lethargy	Excreted in breast milk. Limit use to 4 d and keep dose low. Newborns particularly sensitive to effects of maternal codeine use (LactMed).
Diazepam (all benzodiazepines)	Significant; infant may experience lethargy; apnea reported	Infants metabolize benzodiazepines more slowly than adults; accumulation of toxic levels of drug is possible. **Avoid in nursing mothers** other than a single dose for procedures (LactMed).
Dicumarol	Minimal	Excreted in breast milk in **inactive** form. May want to monitor infant's prothrombin time.
Digoxin	Minimal	Small amounts excreted in breast milk. Probably safe.
Ergot	Significant; infant may experience vomiting, diarrhea, peripheral vasoconstriction	**Contraindicated** in lactation. May suppress lactation.
Escitalopram	Minimal	Maternal doses up to 20 mg/d produce low levels in breast milk. Safer than citalopram.
Fluoroquinolones	Unknown	Small amounts in breast milk. Little information available. Use an alternate drug for which safety information is available (LactMed).
Fluoxetine	Moderate	Colic, irritability, feeding and sleep disorders, slow weight gain. If mother requires fluoxetine, lactation is not a reason to stop. Monitor the infant.
Fluconazole	Minimal	Fluconazole is excreted in breast milk at concentrations similar to plasma. Safe.

Continued

Table 50–1 **Effects of Commonly Prescribed Medications on Infants During Lactation—cont'd**

Drug	Effect on Infant	Comments
Furosemide	Minimal or unknown	Excreted in breast milk. Use with close monitoring of the infant.
Gold salts	Significant hepatonephrotoxicity	**Contraindicated** in lactation. May be excreted in milk after therapy is discontinued.
Iodine (radioactive)	Significant; may cause thyroid suppression in the infant	**Contraindicated.** Maternal testing requiring radioactive iodine requires breast milk to be discarded according to the half-life of the drug.
Isoniazid (INH)	Minimal; possibility of pyridoxine deficiency developing in the infant	Milk levels same as maternal plasma levels. Observe infant for adverse effects. Probably safe. Nursing mothers who are taking isoniazid should take 25 mg of oral pyridoxine daily.
Lithium	Significant; infant may develop toxic lithium levels	Avoid breastfeeding if possible. If no other choice, lithium may be prescribed to the mother, but routine lithium levels need to be drawn on the infant and the infant observed for toxicity.
Macrolide antibiotics	Minimal	All macrolides are minimally excreted in breast milk. Monitor infant for diarrhea and *Candida* infection.
Methadone	Significant	May be used under close medical supervision. Infant may exhibit signs of withdrawal if methadone is discontinued abruptly or if breastfeeding is discontinued abruptly.
Metoprolol	Minimal	Excreted in very small amounts in breast milk. Infant consuming 1 L breast milk will get <1 mg metoprolol.
Metronidazole	Unknown	Milk levels similar to maternal plasma levels. Half-life in breast milk 8–10 h. **Contraindicated:** Nursing mothers should express and discard milk during and for 24–48 h after stopping drug therapy. Topical application is probably safe.
Olanzapine	Minimal	Doses up to 20 mg/d not detected in infant serum. Limited information available. Monitor the infant for drowsiness and developmental milestones, especially if other antipsychotics are used concurrently (LactMed).
Oral contraceptives	Minimal to moderate	Hormones are released into breast milk. May cause jaundice and breast enlargement in the infant. Estrogen compounds suppress lactation, decreasing the quantity and quality of breast milk. Use progestin-only preparations ("minipill") or wait until milk supply is well established (>6 wk postpartum) to use combined forms.
Paroxetine	Minimal	Minimal levels in breast milk. Preferred drug in lactating women (LactMed).
Phenobarbital	Moderate; lethargy in the infant	Excreted in breast milk. Monitor infant for lethargy and feeding problems.
Phenytoin	Minimal	Low levels in breast milk. Probably safe.
Prednisone	Moderate	Excreted in breast milk and may suppress growth and interfere with exogenous steroid production in the infant. Low maternal doses (<20 mg/d) probably safe. Larger doses for a short time may not harm the infant. It is best to time the medication dose just after a feeding and wait 3–4 h for next feeding.
Propranolol	Minimal	Excreted in breast milk in a amounts too small to have any effect.
Propoxyphene	Minimal; possible lethargy	Excreted in small amounts in breast milk.
Propylthiouracil	Significant; can suppress thyroid function in the infant	**Use with caution.** Avoid if possible.
Risperidone	Unknown	Little information available.

Table 50–1 **Effects of Commonly Prescribed Medications on Infants During Lactation—cont'd**

Drug	Effect on Infant	Comments
Radioactive material	Significant; carcinogenic	**Contraindicated**
Spironolactone	Minimal	Very small amounts (0.2%) of metabolite of mother's daily dose are excreted in breast milk. Safe for use with breastfeeding.
Tetracycline	Moderate; discolored teeth	Excreted in breast milk, M:P ratio of 0.6 to 0.8. **Avoid when lactating.** Use safer antibiotics.
Theophylline	Moderate	Excreted in breast milk. May cause irritability in the infant. Monitor for signs of toxicity.
Warfarin	Minimal	Excreted in breast milk in inactive form. Safe during breastfeeding.
Ziprasidone	Unknown	Avoid while breastfeeding until more information available.
Zolpidem	Minimal	Low levels excreted in breast milk. Short-acting. Essentially safe.

both the infant and the mother that influence the effects of a drug on the infant:

1. Maternal pharmacokinetics has a great impact on the level of drug found in breast milk; the higher the drug concentration in the maternal plasma, the higher the concentration of that drug in the milk. Pregnant women have altered pharmacokinetics in the last trimester of gestation. Failure to monitor doses and decrease medication dosages appropriately after delivery may lead to toxic effects in both the mother and the breastfed infant. Higher maternal drug dose or decreased clearance leads to increased amounts of a drug in breast milk.
2. The infant suckling pattern can determine the level of drug found in breast milk. The time of the feeding in relation to the maternal dosing determines how much of the drug is in the breast milk. A drug with a short half-life, given to the mother right after feeding, decreases the amount of drug the infant is exposed to. Likewise, drugs with a long half-life increase the infant's exposure to the drug. Infant suckling time and the number of feedings also have an impact on drug exposure. Some infants nurse for long periods or very frequently, which will increase the amount of drug that the infant ingests.
3. Infant pharmacokinetics also plays an important role in how maternal medication use affects the breastfed infant. As mentioned at the beginning of this chapter, gastric acid production and gastric emptying time are decreased and variable in neonates. The volume of distribution in infants is greater because of their greater total body water and their lower body fat. Infants also have significant differences in drug metabolism by the liver, as previously mentioned. Renal excretion, too, is altered in younger infants, which can affect their overall clearance rate of drugs. All of these factors need to be considered in prescribing to a lactating woman, especially if the breastfed infant is very young (less than 1 month old).
4. Susceptibility to a drug's effects can vary among infants. There is some dose-related predictability to a drug's effects that are related to the pharmacological properties of the drug. In some infants, however, there are unique effects that are not dose related and instead are idiosyncratic and therefore unpredictable. This reaction is fortunately uncommon, but must be considered if an infant is demonstrating some effects of maternal drug use.
5. The milk to plasma (M:P) drug ratio affects the infant's exposure to a medication because the infant's clearance of the drug affects the overall exposure. Even drugs with a low M:P ratio may produce a toxic level if the infant is unable to effectively excrete the drug.

Infants

Infants are totally dependent on their parents to administer their medication. Although the infant may balk at the taste of a medication, the parent is still in control of administering the medication. Intervention at this age is aimed at teaching parents or caregivers how to properly administer the medication. Parents need to be edified and encouraged as they take on the role of administering and monitoring a child's medication. Many parents are nervous the first time they give their child medication. Thorough education ensures better medication compliance. Discussing the reason for the medication, the dose, the length of treatment, medication administration tips, and expected and unexpected adverse effects (e.g., the mild diarrhea that is expected with some **antibiotics**) should increase a parent's comfort with administering medications. Written instructions are essential at all ages but especially for the infant, because the parent is more likely to be fatigued and less likely to retain instructions given orally. Dosing medications for parental convenience increases compliance. Ask parents if they are working outside their home and who else may be administering the medication. A medication with fewer daily doses may be indicated if the child is in a day-care setting or has multiple caregivers.

Toddlers and Preschoolers

Toddlers and preschoolers are beginning to exert their independence, and administering medications to this age group can be a challenge, even a battlefield. Even the most experienced parent can have difficulty administering oral medications to a toddler. The key to success with this age group is to discuss medication administration with the parent prior to prescribing and, if possible, choose a medication that poses the fewest problems with administration. Doses per day, palatability, and dosage forms should be taken into consideration. If the toddler is resistant to taking medication, prescribe a once- or twice-daily medication if possible. Using chewable formulations, if the child has molars, can increase compliance because the child can self-administer the medication. Using higher concentrations of medication, if possible, to decrease the volume administered can be helpful. By 2 or 3 years, children can often begin to self-administer oral medication by using a vertical medication spoon or medicine cup. Parents can help a child practice this skill with juice or another liquid before taking the medication. Discussing administration of the prescribed medication while the family is still in the clinic is essential. Ask the parent what has worked in the past to ease medication administration and what has not worked. Listen to parents; they know their child and can anticipate what will ease the medication administration.

CLINICAL PEARL

Infants

- Parents are often unsure how to administer medication to an infant. While the parents are in the clinic with the child, the practitioner should address this issue and demonstrate how to administer medication to an infant. For ease of administration, use a medication syringe and insert the syringe into the mouth along the inner cheek. To decrease choking, advise parents to squirt small amounts (1 mL) of medication at a time into the inner buccal space. Wait until the infant swallows, and then administer another small amount until all the medication is administered. Direct parents *not* to administer the medication directly over the tongue, which increases choking and allows the infant more easily to spit out the medication.
- Advise parents to check with the pharmacist before mixing any medication with formula or breast milk; some medications are bound with the calcium or other ingredients in the formula, causing them to be less effective.
- Breastfed infants often choke and sputter when medications are first administered because these infants are used to only the feel of the breast in their mouths. Warning parents of this response and teaching them proper technique will help them gain confidence in medication administration.
- Giving **acetaminophen** in suppository form is an option if administering oral medications to the infant is difficult. The practitioner can demonstrate this procedure, which works well in breastfed infants especially.

School-Age Children

Giving medication to school-age children is often easier than it is in other age groups. Developmentally, they are industrious and eager to learn. It is essential to include the child in the decision-making process, if possible. Let the child choose the formulation. Does he or she want liquid, chewable tablets, or pills to swallow? Some liquid medication doses become large in volume as the child gets to school age (e.g., **trimethoprim-sulfamethoxazole** and **prednisone**), so advise parents and the child who chooses a liquid formulation of this fact. Be sure the child can swallow pills before prescribing them. Some medications can be crushed and mixed with highly viscous fluid (e.g., chocolate syrup). Check with the pharmacist prior to suggesting this if you are not familiar with a medication. Teaching with this age group should be aimed at both the parent and the child. Children need to know the rationale for prescribing a particular medication. They are being taught in school to avoid "drugs," and they need clarification about helpful medication and illicit drugs. Schools have varying regulations regarding administration of medication at school. If possible, avoid school-hour dosing to simplify the medication regimen.

Adolescents

Adolescent patients often administer their own medications. The compliance rates vary with this age group. Some teenagers are excellent at medication self-administration, and others are poorly compliant. The adolescent is developmentally entering the period of formal operational thinking, characterized by propositional thinking and abstract reasoning. Younger adolescents may still be in the concrete-thinking stage, and their interactions with the health-care provider may reflect this stage, rather than the abstract thought process of older teenagers. Although adolescents may be able to self-administer medication and appear to be capable of the task, they may vary in their sophistication regarding medication use. The practitioner needs to form an alliance with teenagers and ask their perspective regarding their medications. Do they have an opinion regarding the medication? What schedule will work best with their lifestyle? Teenagers appreciate having their opinions taken into consideration as treatment is planned. When a medication history is taken with the parent present, the teenager may not be completely truthful. Practitioners need to be aware of the laws of the state in which they practice and, when treating teenagers, maintain confidentiality if necessary. Teenagers, too, must understand the confidentiality laws of their state and at what age they are able to receive confidential treatment. Parents often struggle with letting teenagers self-administer medications. The practitioner needs to be skilled at assisting family members as they move from parent-controlled to child- or teen-controlled medication administration. This transition varies by family.

FACTORS THAT INFLUENCE POSITIVE OUTCOMES

Compliance or adherence with the medication regimen is an issue for all patients. Pediatric patients pose a unique dilemma because the practitioner has to address both the child's compliance and the parent's, plus possibly that of other caregivers. The many factors that influence adherence include length of medication regimen, number of medications prescribed, medication interval, palatability, cost, and family issues. The practitioner needs to consider all of these issues when prescribing to ensure successful treatment.

There is little agreement in the definitions of *compliance* and *noncompliance.* Is anything less than full compliance considered noncompliance? If the therapeutic outcome is adequate, is less than full compliance with the treatment regimen acceptable? Often, compliance of a certain set percentage (e.g., less than or equal to 70%) is considered to be compliant with the regimen (Matsui, 1997). Dose omission and delay are the most common dosing errors, yet other forms of noncompliance may occur, including failure to fill the prescription, incorrect dosing or dosing intervals, and discontinuation of the medication prior to the recommended time. Compliance rates vary from 7 to 89 percent for short-term medications and from 11 to 83 percent for long-term medications when rates are studied in pediatric patients (Matsui, 1997). Few recent studies of medication compliance have been conducted in children, but older studies indicate that of patients treated for otitis media only 7.3 percent had complete compliance with the prescribed **antibiotics** and 53 percent took less than half of the prescribed medicine (Matter, Markello, & Yaffe, 1975). A systematic review and meta-analysis of 46 studies of antibiotic misuse found a mean compliance rate of 62.2 percent (95% confidence level, 56.4% to 68.0%), although this study was not specific to pediatric patients (Kardas, Devine, Golembesky, & Roberts, 2005). One older study of sexually active female teenagers found that only 44.6 percent were compliant with taking their **oral contraceptives** (Litt, Cuskey, & Rudd, 1980), whereas a more recent study of adolescent females (aged 14 to 17 years) taking **oral contraceptives pills (OCPs)** found only 45 percent of coital events were protected by **OCPs** (Woods et al, 2006). Even patients with life-threatening conditions, such as organ transplant or cancer, report compliance rates as low as 52 to 60 percent (Matsui, 1997).

Monitoring compliance can be a challenge in children. Direct methods of measuring compliance with the medication regimen, such as serum drug levels, are invasive and costly. Less invasive methods are being explored, such as urinalysis for drug metabolites, saliva analysis (for **theophylline, phenytoin, phenobarbital,** and **carbamazepine** levels), and hair analysis (used currently for **cocaine** and **nicotine** exposure in utero and can be expanded to other medications) (Bailey, Klein, & Koren, 1997). Indirect methods, such as patient and parental reports, are the most widely used and the most practical method of measuring medication compliance, but it is limited by the reliability of the person who is reporting. Pill counts and other methods of determining compliance have also been found to be unreliable (Matsui, 1997). A diary of medication doses taken may give a clearer picture of what doses the child has received, although this is also only as accurate as the recorder. In a review of the literature related to pediatric medication compliance, Winnock, Lucas, Hartman, and Toll (2005) found compliance ranged from 11 to 93 percent in the more than 250 articles they reviewed.

Specific Factors That Influence Compliance

Long-Term Versus Short-Term Medication Regimens

It is clear that compliance is poorer for long-term medications than it is for short-term medication regimens (Fotheringham & Sawyer, 1995). Compliance also decreases as soon as symptoms improve. For example, compliance with **antibiotics** is poor because the medication may be discontinued as soon as symptoms are relieved. Compliance in **penicillin** prescribed for streptococcal pharyngitis decreases sharply after symptoms improve. In a summary of eight randomized clinical trails, Paradise (1997) determined that a shortened course of **antibiotics** (5 d versus 10 d) for mild otitis media is often adequate treatment for children older than 6 years. This same analysis determined that in children younger than 6 years—in particular, children younger than 2 years—a shortened course of treatment is not adequate and that these younger children should be treated for 10 full days. Note that **azithromycin (Zithromax)**, which has a standard 5-day dosing schedule, was not included in this analysis. More studies are needed regarding a shortened length of treatment for other common childhood illnesses because briefer treatments could lead to increased compliance.

Chronic illness presents a number of problems for the family, often including a daily medication regimen. Compliance rates vary significantly for children with chronic illness (Matsui, 1997). Even patients for whom noncompliance can be life threatening are not taking their medications as prescribed. Self-reported compliance among children and adolescents with cancer was 60.5 percent in one study (Tebbi, Cummings, & Zevon, 1986). Children with sickle cell disease were found to have a refill rate for their daily medications of 58.4 percent (Patel, Lindsey, Strunk, & DeBaun, 2010).

Number of Medications Prescribed

The number of medications prescribed can have an impact on compliance with the regimen. The more medications that are prescribed, the lower the compliance rate is. Keeping medication schedules simple increases the likelihood of success for the treatment.

Medication Interval

Medication interval has a significant impact on the success of the treatment, especially given the number of families with both parents working and more children in day care. In a review of the literature (Greenberg, 1984), once-a-day and twice-a-day regimens were associated with significantly better compliance (73% and 70%, respectively). Three-times-a-day regimens had 52 percent compliance, and four-times-a-day medications were likely to be given as directed only 42 percent of the time. Children who are in school or have parents who are both working are probably not receiving their medications as often as recommended if they are taking any medication that needs to be administered more than twice a day.

CLINICAL PEARL

Electrolyte Solutions

- Pediatric **electrolyte solutions** are often not well accepted by children. One trick is to use **electrolyte Popsicles (Pedialyte)** or freeze the bottled solution into homemade Popsicles. The cold taste seems to be better accepted.
- Sugar-free Kool-Aid or another drink mix sweetened with Nutrasweet can be added to unflavored **electrolyte solutions** to make the taste of the **electrolyte solution** more acceptable to children.

Palatability

Palatability is often overlooked as a reason for noncompliance, yet in children it is a critical factor in medication compliance. Studies comparing the taste of a variety of **antibiotics** (Holas, Chiu, Notario, & Kapral, 2005; Matsui, Barron, & Rieder, 1996; Powers, Gooch, & Oddo, 2000; Ruff, Schotic, Bass, & Vincent, 1991) determined that some **antibiotics** were ranked better tasting than others, with the **cephalosporins (cefindir, cefixime, cephalexin,** and **cefaclor)** ranked as the best tasting overall. **Dicloxacillin** ranked the worst for taste. Although no published reports studied taste differences between brand-name and generic preparations, anecdotal reports from parents and patients suggest that brand-name preparations taste better. Of medications with the same efficacy profile, the best tasting is the easiest to administer to young children.

Cost

The cost of the medication needs to be addressed for patients who are not adequately insured for prescriptions. The cost of common **antibiotics** prescribed for otitis media range from $10 to more than $100 to treat a 15-kg child for 10 days. Prescribing an expensive **antibiotic** for a family who cannot afford to fill the prescription places the family in an uncomfortable position. Simply asking the family if they have insurance to cover the medication and then problem solving with them if they do not will increase the likelihood that the family will fill the prescription. For example if an antibiotic is indicated, the brand-name Zithromax costs $50.46 for a 15 ml 200 mg/5 ml bottle, the generic is $32.27 (http://www.drugstore.com), whereas amoxicillin suspension is on the Walmart Pharmacy's $4 list. If possible, give the family a few days of medication samples to defray the cost of the treatment if a less expensive medication is not available. Knowing which pharmacies in the local area are the least expensive or calling ahead for a price check before sending the family to the pharmacy is helpful. A family who knows the approximate amount that the medication will cost will not be surprised when the prescription is filled.

Family Issues

Family issues affect the family's ability to comply with the prescribed treatment regimen. Families in which both parents are working and therefore have limited time with their children have more problems with complex treatment regimens. Lack of social support can leave a parent isolated and make parenting more stressful. Parental fatigue is often overlooked as a factor in treatment outcomes. Parents who are fatigued can easily miss medication doses; even those who are usually well organized can miss medication doses when they are tired. Disruptive and dysfunctional families may have difficulty in following the plan of treatment because of the chaos present in the home. Another family situation that needs to be addressed when clinical improvement is less than satisfactory is parental use of the child's medications. For example, a child may be prescribed **stimulants** for attention deficit-hyperactivity disorder, and a parent or other family member may be abusing the child's medication. This is a situation no practitioner wants to encounter, yet there should always be some index of suspicion when the family history is not clear. All of these issues need to be accounted for when the practitioner is prescribing a medication and during follow-up on the patient's progress. They often present in an unclear fashion, and ferreting out the reason for noncompliance with the treatment regimen may take some time.

Improving Compliance in the Pediatric Patient

When poor compliance is identified, it is essential to address this issue and determine strategies with the patient and parent to improve the success of the treatment regimen. There are a variety of methods to improve the success of the treatment regimen, but first it is necessary to make sure that the diagnosis is accurate and that the drug therapy is beneficial.

Medication Concentration

Medication concentration can be adjusted in some of the liquid preparations. The practitioner can choose to prescribe a more concentrated form when a parent has difficulty administering medications to a patient. Many of the **antibiotics** come in different strengths, and giving one-half teaspoon is easier than administering a full teaspoon. **Prednisone** comes in two different strengths, as well as in tablets that can be crushed. By involving the parents in the decision to use a more concentrated form of a medication, you are allowing them some control over the treatment regimen, and they may therefore be more likely to administer the medication that is prescribed.

Written Versus Oral Instructions

Most practitioners should address the issue of written versus oral instructions in their own practice. Studies show that only 50 percent of instructions given by physicians are recalled immediately after the visit (Liptak, 1996). Therefore, giving written instructions along with the oral directions will improve compliance. This is especially important for over the counter medications such as **acetaminophen** and **ibuprofen**. Parents need to understand the different formulations and dosing by weight and every parent should have a weight based dosing chart (Box 50–2).

Self-Monitoring Calendars

Self-monitoring calendars should be a standard in the treatment of preschool and school-age children. Children can apply a sticker or color in a box as each dose is taken. Parents should be involved in the process and set a reward for completion of the medication regimen. In acute illness such as otitis media, in which the patient will be returning to the clinic, the practitioner may offer a reward for a full calendar. Children with chronic illness, who are often on long-term medication, need to have a set reward for a certain number of days of successfully taking their medication. Parents need to take an active role in medication calendar usage, and they, too, should be praised for their participation in the medication regimen.

Telephone Reminders

Telephone reminders are helpful in increasing compliance, especially if the parent is leaving the clinic with multiple prescriptions. A quick telephone call allows the parent to clarify the treatment regimen and reinforces teaching that took place in the clinic.

Contracts and Reinforcement Programs

Contracts or reinforcement programs may be necessary if compliance continues to be a problem. The practitioner,

---

BOX 50–2 PRESCRIBING OVER-THE-COUNTER PAIN MEDICATIONS FOR PEDIATRIC PATIENTS

Pain in children can range from teething pain to pain associated with otitis media. Parents often ask the practitioner about using **acetaminophen** or **ibuprofen** for the treatment of pain in children. For the safety of their children and the efficacy of the medication, parents should be taught how to administer over-the-counter (OTC) pain medications properly.

The two most commonly used **analgesics** in pediatric patients are **acetaminophen** and **ibuprofen. Aspirin** should never be given to children for acute pain management due to the risk of Reye syndrome, and the practitioner should teach parents this rule.

Acetaminophen can be administered orally or rectally (suppository), and it peaks in 30 to 60 minutes. Dosage for children is 10 to 15 mg/kg/dose q4–6h.

Continued

BOX 50–2 PRESCRIBING OVER-THE-COUNTER PAIN MEDICATIONS FOR PEDIATRIC PATIENTS—cont'd

Ibuprofen is effective for pain control and has on additive anti-inflammatory effect, which appears to provide better pain control in acute otitis media than **acetaminophen.** The correct dosage is 5 to 10 mg/kg/dose q6–8h.

Although **acetaminophen** and **ibuprofen** provide good pain relief for mild to moderate pain and both have antipyretic effects, **ibuprofen** may be the drug of choice for night pain associated with otitis media because of its longer duration. Both drugs are equally easy to administer, although **ibuprofen** is not available in suppository form. Combining acetaminophen and ibuprofen in an alternating schedule for fever or pain is not recommended in the outpatient setting. One or the other, properly dosed, should be used. The goal of antipyretic therapy is not to reduce temperature to normal, but to decrease discomfort associated with fever.

Give parents a dosing chart with their child's dose based on weight. The different strengths of **acetaminophen** must be dosed correctly. New parents may not be aware that drops and liquid or suspension are different strengths, which can lead to dosing errors. Different strengths of chewable tablets are also available.

CLINICAL PEARL

Improving Compliance with Ophthalmic Preparations

- Administration of ophthalmic preparations to toddlers and preschoolers is often difficult, and the incidence of noncompliance increases with each dose that is a battle to administer. Parents can safely restrain the child to administer eye medications as follows:
  1. Sit on the floor with the child sitting on the floor between the parent's legs.
  2. Place the child's feet near the parent's feet and the child's head between the parent's thighs.
  3. Slip the child's arms under the parent's thighs and, with the legs, hold the child's head and arms still.

  The parent then has both hands free to administer the eye medication. Although this procedure may sound drastic, it is a quick way for a parent to administer the medication when no other adult is around to assist with a squirming, resistant child.
- Older preschoolers and school-age children often cooperate with administration of eyedrops if they are told to lie back and close their eyes. Eyedrops can then be applied to the inner corner of the eyes (while the eyes are closed). Next, children are told to open their eyes, without any head movement. The medication rolls into the eye when the eye is opened. This is much easier than the bull's-eye approach of trying to get children to keep their eyes open for squeezing in drops.

the patient, and the family need to be in agreement about the goals of the treatment contract and the consequences of noncompliance. A case conference may be necessary to involve other disciplines in the treatment. A home visit may provide information that leads to an altered treatment program that will be better tolerated by the family. The role of the practitioner is to attempt to simplify the medication treatment and still have an adequate therapeutic outcome. This goal should be shared with the patient and family.

Childhood Obesity Influences Outcomes

Over the past 30 years pediatric overweight and obesity has steadily increased. In the 2007–2008 National Health and Nutrition Examination Survey (NHANES), 10.4 percent of 2- to 5-year-olds, 19.6 percent of 6- to 11-year-olds, and 18.1 percent of adolescents were considered obese (Centers for Disease Control and Prevention, 2010). Little is known about pharmacokinetic differences in obese children. A recent review of pharmacokinetics in obese adults indicated the obese patient may need a larger loading dose because of larger volume of distribution, but maintenance doses should not be increased because clearance of drugs is not altered (Hanley, Abernathy, & Greenblatt, 2010). Small studies on pediatric oncology patients indicate **doxorubicinol**, but not **doxorubicin** clearance is decreased in patients with body fat greater than 30 percent (Thompson et al, 2009).

For the obese patient, the prescriber needs to decide whether to calculate the dose based on actual body weight or ideal body weight. When young children weigh as much as an adult, dosing quickly becomes a challenge. Although body weight may be consistent in an adult, liver and kidney functions are still at the chronological age of the child. Currently, no guidelines are available for dosing obese children, other than not to exceed adult doses of most medications. Studies are in progress and until guidelines are published, the nurse practitioner prescriber will need to use clinical judgment and monitor the patient closely for adverse effects if dosed by weight and efficacy if dosed by age.

REFERENCES

Bailey, B., & Ito, S. (1997). Breast-feeding and maternal drug use. *Pediatric Clinics of North America, 44*(1), 41–54.

Bailey, B., Klein, J., & Koren, G. (1997). Noninvasive methods for drug measurement in pediatrics. *Pediatric Clinics of North America, 44*(1), 15–25.

Berlin, C. M. (1997). Advances in pediatric pharmacology and toxicology. *Advances in Pediatrics, 44,* 545.

Berlin, C. M., & Briggs, G. G. (2005). Drugs and chemicals in human milk. *Seminars in Fetal & Neonatal Medicine, 10,* 149–159.

Briggs, G. G., Freeman, R. K., & Yaffe, S. J. (1994). *Drugs in pregnancy and lactation.* Baltimore, MD: Williams & Wilkins.

Blake, M. J., Castro, L., Leeder, J. S., & Kearns, G. L. (2005). Ontogeny of drug metabolizing enzymes in the neonate. *Seminars in Fetal and Neonatal Medicine, 10,* 123–138.

Bolinger, A. M., & Chan, C. Y. J. (1996). Pediatric considerations. In L. Y. Young & M. A. Koda-Kimble (Eds.), *Applied therapeutics.* Vancouver, WA.

Centers for Disease Control and Prevention. (2010). Childhood overweight and obesity. Retrieved from http://www.cdc.gov/obesity/childhood/index.html

Conroy, S., & McIntyre, J. (2005). The use of unlicensed and off-label medicines in the neonate. *Seminars in Fetal & Neonatal Medicine, 10,* 115–122.

Fotheringham, M. J., & Sawyer, M. G. (1995). Adherence to recommended medical regimens in childhood and adolescence. *Journal of Pediatrics and Child Health, 31,* 72.

Giacoia, G. P., & Mattison, D. R. (2005). Newborns and drug studies: The NICHD/FDA drug development initiative. *Clinical Therapeutics, 27*(6), 796–813.

Goodman, J., & Gal, P. (1992). Pharmacokinetic and pharmacodynamic data collection in children and neonates. *Clinical Pharmacokinetics, 23*(1), 1–9.

Greenberg, R. N. (1984). Overview of patient compliance with medication dosing: A literature review. *Clinical Therapeutics, 6,* 592.

Gupta, A., & Waldhauer, L. K. (1997). Adverse drug reactions from birth to early childhood. *Pediatric Clinics of North America, 44*(1), 79–92.

Hanley, M. J., Abernathy, D. R., & Greenblatt, D. J. (2010). Effect of obesity on the pharmacokinetics of drugs in humans. *Clinical Pharmacokinetics, 49*(2), 71–87.

Holas, C., Chiu, Y. L., Notario, G., & Kapral, D. (2005). A pooled analysis of seven randomized crossover studies of the palatability of cefdinir oral suspension versus amoxicillin/clavulanate potassium, cefprozil, azithromycin, and amoxicillin in children aged 4 to 8 years. *Clinical Therapeutics, 27*(12), 1950–1960.

Kardas, P., Devine, S., Golembesky, A., & Roberts, C. (2005). A systematic review of misuse of antibiotic therapies in the community. *Journal of Antimicrobial Agents, 26*(2), 106–113.

Kearns, G. L. (2000). Impact of developmental pharmacology on pediatric study design: Overcoming the challenges. *Journal of Allergy and Clinical Immunology, 106,* S128–S138.

Kearns, G. L., Abdel-Rahman, S. M., Alander, S. W., Blowey, D. L., Leeder, S. L., & Kauffman R. E. (2003). Developmental pharmacology—drug disposition, action, and therapy in infants and children. *New England Journal of Medicine, 349*(12), 1157–1167.

Koren, G., Reider, M., & MacLeod, S. M. (2009). The global alliance for pediatric pharmacology: The future is here and now. *Paediatric Drugs, 11*(1), 4–5.

Liptak, G. S. (1996). Enhancing patient compliance in pediatrics. *Pediatrics in Review, 17,* 128.

Litt, I. F., Cuskey, W. R., & Rudd, S. (1980). Identifying adolescents at risk for noncompliance with contraceptive therapy. *Journal of Pediatrics, 96,* 742.

MacDonald, M. (1996). Eye problems. In C. E. Burns & A. Dunn (Eds.), *Pediatric primary care: A handbook for nurse practitioners.* Philadelphia: Saunders.

Mason, W. H. (1996). The management of common infections in ambulatory children. *Pediatric Annals, 25,* 621.

Matsui, D. M. (1997). Drug compliance in pediatrics. *Pediatric Clinics of North America, 44*(1), 1–13.

Matsui, D. M., Barron, A., & Rieder, M. J. (1996). Assessment of the palatability of antistaphylococcal antibiotics in pediatric volunteers. *Annals of Pharmacotherapy, 30,* 586–588.

Matter, M. E., Markello, J., & Yaffe, S. J. (1975). Inadequacies in the pharmacological management of ambulatory children. *Journal of Pediatrics, 87,* 137.

National Library of Medicine. (2010). Drugs and lactation data base (LactMed). Retrieved from http://toxnet.nlm.nih.gov/cgi-bin/sis/htmlgen?LACT

Niederhauser, V. P. (1997). Prescribing for children: Issues in pediatric pharmacology. *Nurse Practitioner, 22*(3), 16–30.

Nies, A. S., & Spielberg, S. P. (1996). Principles of therapeutics. In L. S. Goodman, L. E. Limbird, P. B. Milinoff, R. W. Russon, & A. G. Gilman (Eds.), *Goodman & Gilman's the pharmacological basis of therapeutics* (9th ed.). New York: McGraw-Hill.

O'Brien, K. L., Dowell, S. F., Schwartz, B., Marcy, S. M., Phillips, W. R., & Gerber, M. A. (1998). Acute sinusitis: Principles of judicious use of antimicrobial agents. *Pediatrics, 101*(Suppl.), 174.

Paradise, J. L. (1997). Short-course antimicrobial treatment for acute otitis media: Not best for infants and young children. *Journal of the American Medical Association, 278,* 1640.

Patel, N. G., Lindsey, T., Strunk, R. C., & DeBaun, M. R. (2010). Prevalence of daily medication adherence among children with sickle cell disease: A 1-year retrospective cohort analysis. *Pediatric Blood & Cancer, 55*(3), 554–556.

Powers, J. L., Gooch, W. M., III, & Oddo, L. P. (2000). Comparison of the palatability of the oral suspension of cefdinir vs. amoxicillin/clavulanate potassium, cefprozil and azithromycin in pediatric patients. *Pediatric Infectious Disease Journal, 19*(Suppl. 12), S174–S180.

Rakhmanina, N. Y., & van den Anker, J. N. (2006). Pharmacological research in pediatrics: From neonates to adolescents. *Advanced Drug Delivery Reviews, 58,* 4–14.

Ruff, M. E., Schotic, D. A., Bass, J. W., & Vincent, J. M. (1991). Antimicrobial drug suspensions: A blind comparison of taste of fourteen common pediatric drugs. *Pediatric Infectious Disease Journal, 10,* 30.

Stephenson, T. (2005). How children's responses to drugs differ from adults. *British Journal of Clinical Pharmacology, 59*(6), 670–673.

Tebbi, C. K., Cummings, M., & Zevon, M. A. (1986). Compliance of pediatric and adolescent cancer patients. *Cancer, 58,* 1179.

Tershakovec, A. M., & Stallings, V. A. (1998). Pediatric nutrition and nutritional disorders. In R. E. Behrman & R. M. Kliegman (Eds.), *Nelson essentials of pediatrics* (3rd ed., p. 56). Philadelphia: Saunders.

Thompson, P. A., Rosner, G. L., Matthay, K. K., Moore, T. B., Bomgaars, L. R., Ellis, K. J., et al. (2009). Impact of body composition of pharmacokinetics of doxorubicin in children: A Glaser Pediatric Research Network study. *Cancer Chemotherapy Pharmacology, 64,* 243–251.

Umetsu, D. T. (1998). Immunology and allergy. In R. E. Behrman & R. M. Kliegman (Eds.), *Nelson essentials of pediatrics* (3rd ed., p. 263). Philadelphia: Saunders.

U.S. Food and Drug Administration (FDA). (2009a). The story of the laws behind the labels: Part 1: 1906 Food and Drugs Act. Retrieved from http://www.fda.gov/AboutFDA/WhatWeDo/History/Overviews/ucm056044.htm

U.S. Food and Drug Administration. (2009b). The story of the laws behind the labels: Part 2: 1938 Federal Food, Drug and Cosmetic Act. Retrieved from http://www.fda.gov/AboutFDA/WhatWeDo/History/Overviews/ucm056044.htm

U.S. Food and Drug Administration. (2009c). The story of the laws behind the labels: Part 3: 1962 Drug Amendments. Retrieved from http://www.fda.gov/AboutFDA/WhatWeDo/History/Overviews/ucm056044.htm

U.S. Food and Drug Administration. (2010a). Milestones in food and drug law history. Retrieved from http://www.fda.gov/AboutFDA/WhatWeDo/History/Milestones/default.htm

U.S. Food and Drug Administration. (2010b). Pediatric labeling changes through April 12, 2010. Retrieved from http://www.fda.gov/downloads/ScienceResearch/SpecialTopics/PediatricTherapeuticsResearch/UCM163159.pdf

Winnock, S., Lucas, D. O., Hartman, A. L., & Toll, D. (2005). How do you improve compliance? *Pediatrics, 115,* e718–e724.

Woods, J. L., Shew, M. L., Tu, W., Ofner, S., Ott, M. A., & Fortenberry, J. D. (2006). Patterns of oral contraceptive pill-taking and condom use among adolescent contraceptive pill takers. *Journal of Adolescent Health, 39*(3), 381–387.

World Health Organization (WHO). (2010). Make medicines child size. Retrieved from http://www.who.int/childmedicines/en/

CHAPTER 51

GERIATRIC PATIENTS

Casey Shillam

Chapter Outline

The fastest growing segment of the population in the United States is people older than 65 years. Today, an estimated 37.9 million people aged 65 and older account for 12.6 percent of the total population (National Center for Health Statistics, 2009). This number is projected to grow to 71.5 million by 2030, and represents nearly 20 percent of the total U.S. population (Federal Interagency Forum on Aging Related Statistics, 2008). It is estimated that older adults consume about 30 percent of prescription drugs and about 40 percent of over-the-counter (OTC) drugs (Mahoney, Zhan, & Eckler, 1999). Increased chronic illness is associated with higher prescription drug costs. The older adult population takes four to six prescription drugs daily (Mahoney et al, 1999), and prescription drugs account for 15 percent of health-care costs among older adults (Federal Interagency Forum on Aging-Related Statistics, 2008).

Research indicates that as many as 84 percent of older adults over the age of 65 use prescription drugs on a regular basis (AARP, 2002; Kaufman, Kelly, Rosenberg, Anderson, & Mitchell, 2002), and approximately 33 percent of older adults use three or more prescription drugs in conjunction with three or more dietary **supplements** (Nahin et al, 2009). **Laxatives** are used by one-third of older adults, many of whom are not constipated (Mahoney et al, 1999). NSAIDs, sedating **antihistamines**, **sedatives**, and **histamine$_2$ blockers** are all available OTC and all may cause major adverse reactions and drug interactions with any prescription drugs being taken. With the high cost of prescribed drugs (rarely covered by insurance programs), complex medication schedules, inadequate teaching, poor vision, and loss of dexterity, it is not unusual for older adults to have unintended nonadherence with their drug regimens. Health-care providers contribute to the drug-related problems in the older adult with inadequate assessment of drugs being taken by these patients and the context within which the drugs are being taken, prescribing drugs that are inappropriate for older adults given their aging changes, and failing to provide effective patient education to foster adherence.

Bergman-Evans (2004) proposes three major outcomes to improve the management of drugs for older adults:

- Reduce inappropriate prescribing.
- Decrease polypharmacy.
- Avoid adverse events.

The focus of this chapter will be to provide information to assist in meeting those outcomes.

GENERAL PRINCIPLES FOR PRESCRIBING FOR OLDER ADULTS

Chapters 1 and 3 provide information about rational drug selection for the general population. All these recommendations also hold for older adults. For this population, however, some are especially important:

- Before prescribing, collect a complete drug history—including herbs, vitamins, and nonprescription drugs that the patient is taking. Ask specifically about the latter categories, because older adults may not consider these to be drugs.
- Evaluate if drug therapy is required. Determine if the problem can be treated with nonpharmacological interventions or if it can be resolved by removing unnecessary drugs from the patient's medication regimen. Discontinue drugs when possible if the benefit is unclear or the adverse effects of the drug result in nonadherence.
- Avoid a drug if the benefit is marginal or if a nonpharmacological alternative exists. This is especially true of high-cost newer drugs. Determine if the newer drug provides some unique benefit, and if the benefit of adding an additional drug to the medication regimen is sufficient to justify the cost, the increased complexity of the regimen, and the risk of adverse reactions. Keep the regimen as simple as possible.
- When therapy is deemed appropriate, start low and go slow. However, do not fail to prescribe appropriate therapy in doses that are sufficient to resolve or treat the problem.
- Evaluate if the drug and its formulation are appropriate for older adults based on the normal physiological changes associated with aging.
- Remember that older adults have a lifetime of experiences that make each of them unique. Consider the unique nature of individuals in terms of their diseases, comorbid conditions, and experiences with medications when prescribing.

PHARMACOKINETICS CHANGES

Absorption and Distribution

General absorption of drugs is not dramatically different in the older adult than it is in the younger population for the vast majority of prescribed and OTC medications. Oral drugs are absorbed by the gastrointestinal (GI) tract. With aging this tract produces less acid as fewer parietal cells are generated, but the change is too small to be clinically relevant. However, this small change does become clinically significant in the presence of drugs that compound this problem, such as proton pump inhibitors (Thjodleifsson, 2002). There is decreased active transport of some drugs, causing decreased bioavailability.

Older adults undergo normal age-related changes in the body that affect the action of bioactive substances. Aging results in a reduced lean muscle mass by about 20 percent and decreased total body water by 10 to 15 percent, implicating changes in the absorption of many drugs (Kyle et al, 2001). Pharmaceutical agents primarily distributed in lean body mass or body water may reach higher serum concentrations in older adults and their effects may be magnified when compared to similar doses in younger adults. These changes may affect drugs administered IM, which are often highly water soluble.

Water-soluble drugs, such as **lithium** and **digoxin**, can have a smaller volume of distribution, resulting in a higher peak plasma concentration at normal dosages (Zagaria, 2005). This is especially important for drugs with narrow therapeutic ranges. Changes are also suspected in the absorption of transdermal drugs, yet more studies are needed to understand how age-related changes in skin physiology are impacted (Zagaria, 2005).

Another normal, age-related change also occurs in body fat stores, increasing by 15 to 20 percent as a person ages (Kyle et al, 2001). Lipid-soluble drugs, such as **benzodiazepines**, have a higher tendency to accumulate in adipose tissue, resulting in lowered serum concentrations. This accumulation in the adipose tissue can result in a prolonged duration of action due to an increased half-life. The result is a less intense immediate medication effect as well as a prolonged or unpredictable effect in the older adult.

Normal aging also results in a decrease by as much as 20 percent in serum albumin levels, a main plasma drug-binding protein. The consequence of these lowered serum albumin levels is fewer molecules available for binding, and higher levels of unbound agent available for metabolism and tissue perfusion. This change becomes substantially worsened when combined with poor nutrition, age-related liver changes, or multiple medications competing for protein-binding sites, which are often concerns for many older adults. With decreased binding ability, more free drug is available, necessitating lower drug doses to prevent adverse drug interactions.

Metabolism and Excretion

Aging results in a decrease in both liver size and blood flow. The oxidative reactions of phase I metabolism decline secondary to a reduction in liver volume resulting in decreased drug clearance and an increase in half-life for such agents as **diazepam, theophylline, quinidine,** and **piroxicam** (Zagaria, 2005). The metabolic clearance is primarily reduced with drugs that display high hepatic extraction (blood-flow limited metabolism) (e.g., **morphine, propranolol, imipramine**) and not diminished for those drugs with low hepatic extraction (capacity-limited metabolism) (Turnheim, 2003). In contrast, phase II metabolism is relatively unaffected by age, so that **benzodiazepines (BDZs)** such as **lorazepam** and **oxazepam** are better tolerated than **diazepam.** Reduction in metabolism is more pronounced in malnourished or frail elders. Changes in first-pass metabolism due to a variable decline in hepatic blood flow are difficult to predict. In general, older adults have less first-pass effect than do younger people. This is especially important for drugs that have a large first-pass effect (e.g., **histamine$_2$ blockers**).

Acetylation and conjugation do not change appreciably with age. Oxidative metabolism through the cytochrome P450 (CYP450) system does decrease with aging, resulting in a decreased clearance of drugs. The CYP450 system is discussed in detail in Chapter 2 and included throughout the book for each drug class where metabolism by the system is important. Drugs that are potent inhibitors (e.g., **amiodarone, azole antifungals**, and **cimetidine**) or inducers (e.g., **barbiturates, phenytoin, rifampin**, and **tobacco**) should be avoided in older adults or used with caution.

There is a significant reduction in renal mass and blood flow associated with the aging process (Zagaria, 2005) but glomerular filtration rate (GFR) decline is extremely variable. About 30 percent of older adults have little change, 30 percent have a moderate decrease, and 30 percent have severe decreases. Tubular secretion of drugs is also decreased. Drugs that are eliminated by the renal system are potentially dangerous in the older adult; therefore, older adults should be treated as though they have renal impairment. This may mean dosage adjustments for some drugs. Examples of drugs for which there is evidence of age-related reduction in clearance include **acetazolamide, amantadine, atenolol, captopril, cimetidine, digoxin, lithium**, and **vancomycin.** Others are shown in the various chapters that discuss specific drug classes (Unit II). Disease processes may be more of a factor than normal aging. Diabetes, for example, and hypertension have been found to be powerful determinants of renal dysfunction in the very old (Wasen et al, 2004).

Determination of normal renal function is not easily established in the older adult. Although serum creatinine is the most reliable and easiest test to determine renal function in younger persons, it is an unreliable marker in older adults. Renal function tests are affected by poor nutrition and reduced lean muscle mass. Adequate protein ingestion is a requirement of evaluating accurate blood urea nitrogen levels, and adequate muscle mass is a requirement of determining accurate serum creatinine levels. Creatinine clearance (CCr) evaluated with the Cockcroft-Gault equation (discussed in Chapter 2) is the best method for this evaluation (Zagaria, 2005). Although it is the most accurate method of evaluation, this equation still has limitations, especially in frail elders, as it may overestimate CCr in older adults.

Table 51–1 presents common pharmacokinetic and pharmacodynamic age-related changes and the drug implications.

PHARMACODYNAMIC CHANGES

Aside from the pharmacokinetic changes, one of the characteristics of old age is a progressive decline in counterregulatory (homeostatic) mechanisms and altered receptor sensitivity.

The results of this decline include less mitigation of drug effects, more intense drug reactions than those experienced by younger patients, and a higher rate and intensity of adverse effects (Zagaria, 2005). Reflex tachycardia, commonly

Table 51–1 ▶ **Common Pharmacokinetic and Pharmacodynamic Changes in Older Adults**

Pharmacokinetic Process	Changes in Older Adults	Implications
Absorption	Change not clinically significant usually Oral drugs: Decreased acid production by parietal cells; delayed gastric emptying; reduced blood flow to GI tract. IM drugs: Decreased lean muscle mass	May decrease rate of absorption. Use of drugs that have same action as aging change may increase problem to level of clinical significance.
Distribution	Increased fat stores	Lipid-soluble drugs have greater Vd and longer half-lives.
	Decreased body water	Water-soluble drugs have smaller Vd and higher peak plasma levels.
	Decreased serum albumin levels	Decreased drug–protein binding; increased levels of free drug. Especially a problem for drugs with high protein-binding percentages. Changes onset and duration of action of highly tissue-bound drugs as well.

Continued

Table 51–1 ▶ **Common Pharmacokinetic and Pharmacodynamic Changes in Older Adults—cont'd**

Pharmacokinetic Process	Changes in Older Adults	Implications
Metabolism	Decreased hepatic blood flow	Less first-pass effect so increased amount of drugs that have high first-pass breakdown and decreased amount of prodrugs that require first-pass activation.
	Decreased CYP450 system function	Decreased metabolic clearance of drugs. Decreased metabolism of some drugs. Altered drug–drug interactions.
Excretion	Decreased renal mass and GFR Decreased tubular secretion	Decreased renal clearance of drugs. May require dosage adjustments. Treat older adults as if they had renal impairment.
Pharmacodynamic changes	Reduced thermoregulatory ability	Increased hypothermia risk. Direct effect on phenothiazines, BDZs, TCAs, and narcotics.
	Impaired baroreceptors function and altered fluid status	Postural hypotension with antihypertensives, TCAs, MAOIs, antihistamines.

BDZs = benzodiazepines; GI = gastrointestinal; MAOIs = monoamine oxidase inhibitors; TCAs = tricyclic antidepressants; Vd = volume of distribution.

seen with **vasodilator therapy**, is often blunted, possibly due to dampened baroreceptors response. **Anticholinergic agents** may cause urinary retention because the detrusor muscle tone of the bladder is decreased. **Tricyclic antidepressants** may cause confusion in the depressed patient, secondary to the **anticholinergic** adverse reactions. **Narcotic** and **psychoactive drugs** can cause oversedation, confusion, and respiratory depression and distort the patient's sense of balance. Drugs that lower blood pressure may exhibit more orthostatic hypotension. **Diabetic drugs** are more likely to produce hypoglycemia. **Diuretics** have increased risk for fluid and electrolyte adverse reactions. **NSAIDs** are more likely to produce GI bleeding. **Coumarin anticoagulants** have a greater effect on clotting factor synthesis. Some OTC cold remedies with **anticholinergic** adverse reactions may cause the patient with glaucoma to experience vision loss secondary to the increase of intraoptic pressure or urinary retention in the patient with benign prostatic hypertrophy. As a contrast, some older adults are less sensitive to certain other drugs, such as **beta blockers** and **beta agonists** (Mahoney et al, 1999). For example, when compared to younger patients' reactions, older adults may have a decreased response to a **beta blocker (propranolol)**, resulting in less of a slowed heart rate or only a mild increase in heart rate in response to a **beta agonist** (epinephrine).

PHARMACOTHERAPEUTICS

The best advice for evaluating pharmacological intervention in the older adult is to assess for drug–disease interactions, drug–drug interactions, and drug–metabolism interactions. The older adult often reacts to drugs in the same fashion as do individuals of all other ages, but the practitioner has to be aware of all compounding factors. Drugs may cause an adverse reaction in the older adult, but this reaction could occur later than it would in a younger person; for example, the half-life of the drug may take longer to clear the older adult's system because of slower metabolism.

Assessing Pharmacological Problems and Concerns of Older Adults

Older adults are at higher risk for drug interactions, not only because of physiological changes but also because of the medication practices of both health-care provider and patients. Nonadherence with drug therapy, either intentional or unintentional, is reported in up to 50 percent of older adults (Hughes, 2004). Health-care providers must be aware of the many compounding factors that make pharmacotherapeutics complex in the older adult population.

CLINICAL PEARL

Medication Review

Have the older adult bring all the drugs he or she is taking, including herbs, vitamins, and OTC drugs, in a brown bag to the annual visit. This will enable you to see all the drugs and to determine if there are overlapping drugs that could be eliminated, combinations that could reduce the total number of drugs, or drugs prescribed by other providers that the patient failed to mention. It also helps to evaluate the patient's knowledge of the drugs, including why the drug is being taken and if he or she understands the ADRs.

Using a thorough and quick checklist at each clinic visit with older adult patients provides an accurate evaluation of their understanding of the drugs and their ability to manage the regimen. Box 51–1 is a questionnaire that may be used for this assessment.

During the drug history assessment, providers need to inquire directly regarding the use of OTC drugs, herbs, and vitamins. Specific questions should be asked in the review of systems that relate to the common complaints that older adults experience (e.g., constipation). Providers should also instruct older adults to maintain a current list of all mediations being taken. This list should be kept accessible for use by emergency care providers.

COMMON PHARMACOLOGICAL ISSUES FOR OLDER ADULTS

Polypharmacy

Polypharmacy is the concurrent use of several differ drugs; this alone does not necessarily create a problem. The problem begins when more drugs are prescribed than is clinically indicated or warranted. Polypharmacy becomes an issue for older adults when the high number of drugs in a medication regimen includes overlapping drugs for the same therapeutic effect. Another serious concern is the prescription of optional drugs for an effect that could be managed by nonpharmacological approaches. Other situations contributing to polypharmacy include the use of inappropriate drugs whose adverse effects are facilitating nonadherence, drugs prescribed to treat the adverse effects of other drugs rather than to treat the underlying problem, and drugs whose benefit is marginal at best.

Polypharmacy contributes to adverse drug reactions (ADRs), drug–drug interactions, decreased adherence to drug regimens, unnecessary drug expenses, and poor quality of life for the patient (Andrejak et al, 2000; Barat, Andreasen, & Damsgaard, 2001; Gray, Mahoney, & Blough, 2001; Gurwitz et al, 2003; Patel, 2003).

Multiple factors contribute to polypharmacy in the older adult. Older adult patients will often underreport their symptoms, use multiple providers, and use other's medications. Providers also contribute to the problem by not communicating with one another when multiple providers are involved in the patient's care. Additionally, there is often limited time for assessment and discussion with each patient, limited knowledge of geriatric pharmacology, and a propensity to stick to old habits rather than to keep current in treatment options and try newer approaches. Both providers and patients need to work together to minimize polypharmacy.

Several steps can be taken to reduce polypharmacy (Bergman-Evans, 2004):

- Obtain a complete drug history and review current drugs (prescription and others) every 6 months. Look for drugs without indications and discontinue.
- Avoid prescribing when the benefit is questionable. Consider the age of the patient and the stage of the disease when evaluating the benefit of prescription drug use.
- Evaluate for duplications in drug therapy. Simplify the regimen by using drug combinations or by prescribing single drugs that will provide the appropriate therapeutic effect whenever possible. The use of combinations drugs improves adherence when compared to dual therapy.
- Review medication regimen for drugs prescribed for an ADR. If so, explore whether the original drug be withdrawn or changed to avoid this reaction. Avoid treating adverse reactions/side effects with more drugs. Treat the underlying condition, rather than the symptoms, if possible.
- Prescribe lifestyle changes and other nondrug therapies whenever possible. These may require support from family and other health-care providers.
- Clearly understand the difference between manifestations of the aging process and the disease state that must be treated.

BOX 51–1 QUESTIONNAIRE FOR ASSESSING MEDICATION MANAGEMENT

- Did you bring all of your medications with you?
- List your medications, and tell me how you take them.
- Do you have any new eyedrops, either over the counter or from your eye doctor?
- What over-the-counter medications are you taking, such as food supplements, vitamins, laxatives, pain relievers, and herbal or natural products?
- What medicine or herbs do you use for headaches, muscle aches or pains, nausea, or constipation?
- Do you have any problems opening the bottles?
- Do you sometimes skip some of the medicine? Why?
- What do you do when you run out of your pills?
- At what time of the day do you take your pills, and do you do this the same every day?
- How do you remember to take your pills?
- How do you tell the difference between your medications (size, color)?
- What questions do you have about your medications?

Adverse Drug Reactions

Because the prevalence of prescription medication use among older adults increases with advanced age, older adults are two to three times more at risk for ADRs.

Additionally, the risk of ADRs increases because of the following:

- Reduced renal and hepatic function (see the Pharmacokinetics section, above).
- Cumulative insults to the body by disease, diet, and drug use.
- Polypharmacy. (The most consistent risk factor for ADRs is the number of drugs being taken. Risk increases exponentially as the number of drugs increases.)
- Altered pharmacokinetics and pharmacodynamics (see above).
- Failure to follow the treatment regimen correctly.

Poor medication practices of older adults can also contribute to ADRs: using another's medications, changing the medication regimen without notifying the provider, and neglecting to inform the provider about all therapies being utilized. Of the ADRs that occur annually, up to 28 percent are considered preventable, with errors contributing to the ADR most often occurring at the stages of prescribing (58% of errors) and monitoring (61% of errors) (Gurwitz et al, 2003). **Aspirin (acetylsalicylic acid), NSAIDs, cardiovascular agents** (e.g., **diuretics, digoxin**), and **psychotropic agents** (e.g., **benzodiazepines, antidepressants, antipsychotics**) are most frequently implicated in ADRs (Atkin, Veitch, Veitch, & Ogle, 1999; Gurwitz et al, 2003).

Providers can avoid ADRs with consistent use of the "start low, go slow" axiom. Start with the lowest dose that will provide a therapeutic effect and titrate upward at a slower rate than is used with younger adults. Monitoring older adult patients closely for deterioration in function (including physiological) and cognition is also necessary.

Drug–Drug and Drug–Food Interactions

Empirical data about drug–drug interactions in community-living older adults are very likely underestimated. Pharmacological interventions contribute significantly to the treatment of diseases; however, ADRs also occur more frequently with the increased use of pharmacological treatments. Drug–drug interactions are implicated in 10 to 20 percent of acute geriatric hospital admissions (Atkin et al, 1999). Of the ADRs determined to be preventable, 58 percent are attributed to errors made in providers' writing of the prescription (Gurwtiz et al, 2003). For example, the prescription of a drug for which a known interaction with another drug exists is responsible for up to 13 percent of ADRs in older adults (Gurwtiz et al, 2003).

An older adult with multiple chronic illnesses may not recognize a new symptom as drug related. Rather, it may be attributed as a manifestation of the ongoing disease process and therefore may not be reported to the health-care provider. Drug-induced confusion, incontinence, depression, or fatigue may also be ascribed to the aging process instead of the effect of a drug interaction. Interactions can also occur between prescription drugs and OTC medications and herbal remedies. These nonprescription remedies should also be included on the comprehensive medication list maintained by the older adult.

Drug–food interactions are also important, so a dietary assessment should be done. The patient is the best source of information about any ADRs he or she might have experienced. Ask about allergies and adverse reactions to both medications and foods. Drug–drug and drug–food interactions are presented throughout this book in each drug class.

Drug–disease interactions may also occur. Patients with Parkinson's disease have increased risk for drug-induced confusion. **NSAIDs** can exacerbate heart failure and reduce the effect of other drugs used to treat hypertension. Urinary retention may occur in older adults with benign prostatic hyperplasia if they take **decongestants** or **anticholinergics.**

Constipation may be worsened by **calcium, anticholinergics,** or **calcium channel blockers. Neuroleptics** and **quinolones** lower seizure thresholds. Many drugs to be avoided in the older adult fall into this classification due to these interactions.

Self-Medication Practices

The older adult faces several factors that may result in self-medication practices. Self-medication is often the first or primary response to symptoms of illness but can also be a complicating factor. The current cohort of older adults grew up in a time when they went to the local druggist with their health/illness problems and together they decided on a drug/potion solution. They often also asked family members who were considered to be knowledgeable in the area of the problem or who had had similar symptoms. Health-care providers were considered "consultants" not "controllers" of their health/illness and its management.

In addition to use of prescribed drugs, older adults commonly use other products such as OTC drugs, herbal remedies, and dietary supplements. The widespread availability of potent drugs can further complicate an already complex drug regimen, which results in poor adherence, drug interactions, adverse effects, and high costs to patients and to society (Murray & Callahan, 2003). The semiannual review of the medication regimen, or the annual "brown bag" evaluation, is critical with the older adult population.

CLINICAL PEARL

Start Low, Go Slow

The Golden Rule of geriatrics: Start low, go slow, but go! Treat the problem, starting at lower dosages and titrate up slowly over a longer period of time than for a younger person. You will be able to evaluate for ADRs before they become serious and costly.

Older adults need an evaluation of their functional and cognitive capacity and the context (e.g., home environment and assistance available) in which they will be taking medications. The Gerontological Nursing Interventions Research Center at the University of Iowa (Bergman-Evans, 2004) has a Drug Regimen Unassisted Grading Scale (DRUGS) tool that can be administered at the initial visit where this evaluation is made and at least annually thereafter. This tool can help to identify older adults who may not be able to safely self-administer their medications. It can also identify specific problems that, if resolved, would maintain the older adult's independence to continue safely to self-administer medications.

Someone Else's Medication

Another area of concern is the older adult's practice of using someone else's prescribed drug. The symptoms may sound the same, and to save cost, the kindly neighbor or family member offers to help out by sharing a drug. Then, out of embarrassment or concern for the "helpful" friend, the patient may not tell the health-care provider about using someone else's drug. This results in problems for both the uninformed provider and the patient. Box 51–2 presents poor medication practices commonly seen in older adults. To address this issue, health-care providers need to be aware of its existence and inform their patients about the need to talk to their provider before taking any drugs to avoid untoward reactions and interactions.

Alternative Medicines

Utilization of alternative medicines is well worth investigating, and knowledge about this area is valuable. Several reputable drug information sources now provide data about these drugs and are discussed in Chapter 10. Diverse cultures, fads, and advertising have combined to make alternative medicines more prevalent now in the American culture. Use of complementary therapies is very common in older adults. Some common herbs and alternative therapies include the following:

- "Anti-aging" **DHEA** (dehydroepiandrosterone) and **growth hormone**.
- **Ginkgo biloba** to prevent or treat dementia.
- **Saw palmetto** to relieve the symptoms of benign prostatic hyperplasia. **Chondroitin sulfate** and **glucosamine sulfate** for osteoarthritis.
- **St. John's wort** and **SAMe** (S-Adenosyl-L-Methionine) to treat depression.

Many practitioners utilize herbal medications, but the practice is very diverse and complicated. If the practitioner has only a limited knowledge of herbal medications or cultural practices, opening the dialogue with the older adult to understand the patient's practices will help in avoiding the adverse reactions of polypharmacy. Contact with a local person who is knowledgeable concerning these topics will help the practitioner prescribe and recommend appropriate treatment. Chapter 7 deals with cultural influences on pharmacotherapeutics.

In addition to knowledge about how to use these products, it is important to recognize the risks of products that have limited to no control on their production, on the actual percentage of advertised drug in the product, or on the presence of adulterants. There have been multiple reports of adulterated products marketed to consumers, with a study by Ko finding 32 percent of the 250 products screened containing unlabeled medicines or substances (1998). While the FDA does not regulate dietary supplements, it maintains a webpage to notify consumers and providers of safety alerts related to supplements (www.fda.gov/Food/DietarySupplements/default.htm).

Inappropriate Prescribing: Drugs to Be Avoided in Older Adults

Medication toxic effects and drug-related problems can have profound medical and safety consequences for older adults and economically affect the health-care system. Beers, Ouslander, Rollingher, Reuben, and Beck (1991) first produced a list of explicit criteria for determining inappropriate medication use in the elderly. This list was updated in 1997 and again in 2003 (Beers, 1997; Fick et al, 2003). Commonly referred to as the Beers Criteria, authors have determined that medications found to be in conflict with these criteria should be discontinued, unless

BOX 51–2 POOR DRUG PRACTICES COMMONLY SEEN IN OLDER ADULTS

- Using another's medications or remedies.
- Changing the prescribed medication regimen without informing the provider.
- Utilizing self-care practices based on no or poor information.
- Neglecting to inform the health-care provider about all therapies being utilized.
- Hording medications.

CLINICAL PEARL

Resources

- Helpful Internet resources to evaluate the quality and content of herbs and supplements: http://www.consumerlab.com
- Helpful assessment tools: Try This:® and How to Try This:® Series—Resources for the care of older adults, including assessment tools and instructions for the proper use of those tools: http://consultgerirn.org/

compelling evidence exists for its use in the older adult (Bergman-Evans, 2004; Fick et al, 2003). The decision to put drugs on this list and to rate them as "high concern" or "low concern" was made by a group of experts using the Delphi method. Drugs rated "high concern" included those that should be generally avoided in persons 65 years or older because they are ineffective or they pose unnecessarily high risk for older persons and a safer alternative is available. Drugs rated "low concern" included those that should not be used in older persons known to have specific medical conditions. Table 52–5 in Chapter 52 contains the comprehensive Beers Criteria for potentially inappropriate medication use in older adults (Fick et al, 2003). It is imperative to seek out safer alternatives for those medications with a narrow therapeutic range, very slow elimination rates, or for which elimination is dependent on kidney function.

FACTORS INFLUENCING POSITIVE OUTCOMES OR ADHERENCE

Polypharmacy is only one of the possible influences that affects the outcome in the management of medications with older adults. Several other factors such as income, mobility, complicated medication dosages, and the patient's functional ability can also influence the older adult's ability to be adherent with a medication regimen. Refer to Chapter 6 for discussion of factors influencing positive outcomes.

Assessing functional ability may be one of the most important steps in evaluating appropriate pharmaceutical interventions. Older adults' abilities to manage their activities of daily living and their cognitive status and social systems are strong indicators of their ability to manage pharmaceutical interventions. Several assessment tools developed specifically for use with older adults include the Katz Index of Independence in Activities of Daily Living, the Lawton Instrumental Activities of Daily Living, the Folstein Mini Mental, and the Geriatric Depression Scale. These tools are short, quick, and provide evidence-based assessment data for the evaluation of an older adult's overall functional ability (see Clinical Pearl, "Resources").

In addition, assessing older adults' sensory functions (sight, hearing, taste, touch) is important because of the possible impairments that occur with aging that may affect the patient's ability to know what is expected in managing a medication regimen. An accurate functional assessment helps assess risk behaviors, prevent catastrophic events triggered by ADRs or inadvertent misuse of medications, and improve a patient's quality of life.

Cognitive function must also be assessed. The DRUGS tool evaluates cognitive function to determine if patients are able to self-administer medications. Patients with dementia are particularly prone to delirium from some medications. These further declines in their cognitive impairment are often reversible with the removal of the medication from the regimen. Medications known to potentially cause delirium in those with dementia include **anticholinergics**, **NSAIDs**, **cimetidine**, and **steroids**.

Adherence problems fall into two categories: intentional and unintentional. Intentional lack of adherence can occur because of doubt about the drug or its validity to treat their problem, lack of motivation, poor acceptability of the drug or the provider, poor tolerability of the drug and its effects or adverse effects, advice from others, dislike of the formulation, or financial concerns. Many older adults live on fixed incomes and have limited drug coverage on their health insurance. The Medicare Prescription Benefit is a good first step, but it does not cover all drugs or the full cost of a drug. Some older adults engage in "intelligent nonadherence." They believe they are making an informed or valid decision to stop the drug or change the dose, but they fail to discuss it with their provider.

Unintentional nonadherence can occur because instruction about the drug and its use was poor or lacking all together; the drug dosing regimen is complex and the older adult has some degree of cognitive, visual, or auditory impairment or dysphagia; the drug container is difficult to use; or the older adult has decreased mobility and may not be able to get to a pharmacy to fill the prescription. All of these are compounded if the person lives alone and has no family support.

Older adults often require small doses, but the dexterity needed to halve tablets may be a problem. Providers can help by prescribing the lower dose or by having the pharmacy halve the tablets for the patient and put them in blister packs. Pharmacies may change the company that supplies their generic drugs. The new generic may be a different color or shape. Whereas ordering generics can save the older adult money—sometimes a great deal of money—older adults often use color and shape to keep track of their medications. If a change is required, special attention needs to be taken to assure that they know about the new drug and that it is the same medication as they were previously taking. Taping one old tablet and one new tablet on a paper together with the instructions may be helpful.

A variety of other methods can be used to improve adherence. Calendars, charts, medication boxes, measured-dose systems, and other memory aids are helpful. Planning drug taking around daily activities or at the beginning of the day can serve as a memory aid and increase adherence. Home delivery of drugs can be

CLINICAL PEARL

Polypharmacy

The first step in avoiding ADRs is to establish risk predictions. Polypharmacy is only part of the picture. Take into account age, gender, multiple comorbidities, body weight, renal and hepatic failure, and previous drug reactions.

arranged. Regimens can be simplified. Caregivers and home health visits can be supplied if needed. Chapter 6 has other suggestions as well.

PHYSICAL CHANGES ASSOCIATED WITH AGING

Mental Changes

Mental changes in the healthy older adult are minimal. Although white brain matter does begin to deteriorate at about 60 years, an inability of the older adult to function independently is not a normal part of the aging process. Disease processes are the culprits that rob older adults of the ability to think clearly and maintain independence. Several diseases, such as Alzheimer's disease and cerebrovascular accidents, may impair a person's mental status. In addition, evaluation of a person's pharmaceutical practices may provide insight into the actual causes of a "dementia."

Dementia may present as mild confusion or as inability to perform even the simplest of tasks. Abrupt changes in an older adult's abilities are usually readily recognizable and often attributed to disease processes, whereas insidious, slow changes are attributed to "aging." However, both abrupt and slow changes could be the result of ADRs, a situation the practitioner should investigate. For example, "simple" cystitis, which may also bring complaints of dizziness, confusion, or ataxia, could be a result of a disease process, changes associated with aging, or an ADR.

Sensory Changes

Sight

The eye undergoes several changes (e.g., shape) with natural aging. Conditions associated with aging, such as cataracts, glaucoma, and macular degeneration, can present challenges to the practitioner who is prescribing and managing the patient's drug regimen. Fortunately, most of these changes can be either corrected or easily managed if identified, and most geriatric patients have insurance coverage, such as Medicare, that allows for at least one examination every 2 years for general eye health.

If the patient's vision is affected, it is crucial to adjust the medication regimen to accommodate these changes. Simplify the drug regimen to once or twice a day, and reduce the total number of drugs prescribed. For some patients with vision loss, having more than three drugs can create inadvertent devastating medication errors. Medisets or pill containers that can be set up for the week also greatly reduce the possibility of inadvertent medication mismanagement.

Hearing

Older adults should have their hearing evaluated. Inability to distinguish high-pitched sounds and muffling of the spoken word are two common occurrences of the aging process. The cerumen may become hardened near the tympanic membrane and form a plug that becomes almost impossible to hear through. Removal of this plug is simple and creates a remarkable hearing improvement.

Older adults may have lost their hearing gradually and be unaware that they are not fully hearing what is spoken. Missing one or two words in the instructions for a prescribed drug could have devastating consequences.

Smell and Taste

The senses of smell and taste are usually lost only through a disease process or in the very old (older than 90 years). Aging may reduce the perceived intensity of taste sensations, but the changes are usually small, so it very rarely causes any kind of drug mismanagement. However, it may create a situation of poorer nutrition secondary to the lack of stimulus in eating. Lack of dietary **iron** or the B vitamins can lead to atrophic changes of the oral mucosa, resulting in dry mouth and a change in taste.

Some older adults may complain of a burning mouth and tongue. Local trauma, poor nutrition, diabetes, or anemia can cause these symptoms. Thorough investigation and treatment of the cause, if possible, are the easy parts of managing this irritating problem.

Reassurance and empathy are the tools of management if no medical cause can be found.

Chapter 50 discusses the role of taste and texture in the willingness of children to take certain drugs. Older adults also respond to taste and texture in taking oral suspensions.

Musculoskeletal Changes

Musculoskeletal changes associated with aging range from impaired manual dexterity, which can prevent older adults from opening medication containers, to mobility problems, which can keep them from getting to the drugstore. These musculoskeletal changes can cause older adults to experience difficulty with drug administration and adherence.

Mobility problems, including disorders affecting gait, limb function, manual dexterity, and driving, can threaten the independence and functioning of older adults, specifically their adherence to drug therapy.

Neurological diseases, such as cerebrovascular disease, Parkinson's disease, and motor neuron disease, can lead to increased difficulties in the practical application of drug treatments. Such problems may range from the inability to visit the health-care provider's office to the inability to open the childproof containers.

Immobility from joint deformity, pain, and impaired manual dexterity may make activating **inhalers** or **nebulizers** or applying eyedrops impossible to perform. Some medications may dramatically improve patients' mobility (e.g., medications to treat Parkinson's disease), but others may dramatically exacerbate mobility problems (e.g., **antihypertensives**, **tricyclic antidepressants**).

CLINICAL PEARL

UTI in the Elderly

When ordering laboratory tests, always order at least a urine dip to rule out a urinary tract infection. A "simple" cystitis can cause dizziness, delirium, or ataxia, which may not be recognized as cystitis because the normal complaints of urinary burning, urgency, or frequency may not be present. Simple cystitis is much easier to manage pharmaceutically than the complications of ataxia.

Some practical guidelines that can be applied in most settings to facilitate drug therapy include the following:

1. While writing a prescription, assess potential problems that may create unintentional medication nonadherence. Can the patient open and remove the tablets from the childproof bottle or the prepackaged blister packs? Can the patient being asked to take half a tablet see the tablet well enough and have the manual dexterity to break or cut the tablet in half?
2. If an **inhaler** has been prescribed, does the older adult have the manual dexterity and inhalation volume to activate the **inhaler**? If a **metered-dose inhaler** (MDI) is more applicable to the situation, can the older adult actually utilize this device, which is difficult for about 40 percent of patients (Thwaites, 1999)? Many older adults require the use of a spacer (Aerochamber) in order to receive the fully inhaled dose from an **MDI. Breath-activated inhalers (BAIs)** have been developed to assist the patient with manual dexterity problems.
3. Home pharmacy assessments of frail older adults may reveal drug administration problems, including incorrect dosages, incorrect frequency, expired drug use, and drug omission. Home visits could lead to improved pharmaceutical interventions and adherence. Nurse practitioners are perfect for this type of assessment. With the recent changes in Medicare reimbursement, the nurse practitioner can be reimbursed for such a home visit.
4. Another study showed that, of patients who were asked whether they could manage the administration of drugs, 72 percent stated that this was the first time they had been asked and 69 percent said they would not tell their doctor about the problem even if asked (Thwaites, 1999). This area is obviously a concern for the practitioner and the patient. Developing good communication between provider and patient is critical to obtaining accurate information from this population.
5. Utilize a pharmacist, who certainly has information that can help the practitioner and the patient create a manageable, easy-to-follow pharmaceutical regimen. Have the older adult use the same pharmacy/pharmacist so that problems can be picked up and instructions will be more readily accepted from a familiar provider.

OTHER COMMON PROBLEMS AND CONCERNS

Nutrition

The economic position of the majority of geriatric patients has improved greatly over the past 15 years. However, the reality is that many older adults are still poor. Although many older adults are eligible for social welfare programs, many do not receive them. Explanations for this phenomenon include (1) older adults are unable to initiate and follow though the bureaucratic requirements to establish their eligibility, (2) older adults are unaware of the various benefits they are entitled to, and (3) many older adults have an ethical rejection of accepting "charity."

Malnutrition by itself is a major common health problem for older adults. Medication adherence is a strong component of malnutrition in that the older adult may forgo buying food in order to pay for drugs. Smell and taste changes discussed above can lead to anorexia. Anorexia is a major contributor to weight loss and undernutrition in adults 65 years and older. It can be a leading cause of morbidity and mortality in this population. The National Diet and Nutrition Survey revealed that 43 percent of independent older adults consume less than 1,500 calories per day and that 16 to 18 percent consume less than 1,000 calories per day (Endoy, 2005). The end result is decreased protein intake resulting in fewer protein-binding sites for drug distribution.

The older adult tends to have a gradual weight loss and a reduction in energy requirements as activity declines and body composition changes. It is possible to neglect gradually developing malnutrition and instead attribute the weight loss to a secondary effect of the aging process. Malnutrition can be the cause of many other disease problems and may have a role in the decline of the body's immune system.

Many older adults do not eat the recommended amounts of nutritional intake daily. Assessing nutrition in the older

CLINICAL PEARL

Medication Effect on Mobility

Remember that drugs present a double-edged sword of either a positive or negative effect on mobility. If the older adult has an increase in difficulty with dexterity or an increase in falls, closely scrutinize the medication regimen.

adult can be easily accomplished with the Mini-Nutritional Assessment® (Sheirlinkx, Nicholas, Nourhashemi, et al, 1998), or with using the DETERMINE mnemonic:

D: disease
E: eating poorly
T: toothless or mouth pain
E: economic hardship
R: reduced social contact
M: multiple medications
I: involuntary weight loss or gain
N: needs assistance in self-care
E: elder years above age 80

By reviewing each of these components, the nurse practitioner is better able to assess the older adult's nutritional status and determine if nutrition is playing a part in poor health. Consultation with a nutritionist or dietitian is also usually indicated. Chapter 9 discusses these and other issues related to nutrition.

Sleep Problems

Sleep problems are common complaints of about half of older adults (Dexter, 1999). Sleep-wake disturbances may be a result of physiological changes that appear to be part of the normal aging process, a primary sleep disorder, or a secondary sleep disorder resulting from numerous causes. Patients may complain, "I sleep all night, but I wake up so tired," indicating that they are not obtaining high-quality sleep.

Studies reveal that older adults have decreased rapid eye movement (REM) sleep and increased nighttime wakefulness as part of normal aging. As a result, the older adult often naps during the daytime. When sleep disorder becomes a problem for the person, such as missing meals or appointments or contributing to limited energy, the practitioner must identify the problem and treat accordingly. Box 51–3 lists common age-related factors that influence sleep problems.

Sleep problems affect more than half of older adults residing at home and about two-thirds of those residing in long-term care facilities (Beck-Little & Weinrich, 1998). Dyssomnias that affect older adults include obstructive sleep apnea, periodic limb movement, and restless legs syndrome. Pharmaceutical interventions may be used alone or in conjunction with environmental or surgical interventions. Surgery, weight loss, and use of continuous positive airway pressure may assist the patient with obstructive sleep apnea. Periodic limb movement disease, resulting in frequent waking, nocturnal restlessness, and daytime fatigue, may benefit from **clonazepam**, **trazodone**, or **benzodiazepines**. The parkinsonian symptoms of muscle ache, stiffness, and pain respond better to controlled-release **levodopa**. Patients with restless legs syndrome may respond to standard **levodopa** or to high doses of **vitamin E**. **Gabapentin (Neurontin)** in small doses may be used for managing restless legs syndrome.

BOX 51–3 AGE-RELATED FACTORS INFLUENCING SLEEP PROBLEMS

Biological Factors

- Increased micturition
- Apnea
- Restless legs syndrome
- Muscle cramps
- Arthritic pain
- Vascular changes
- Depression
- Dementia

Social/Psychological Factors

- Death of loved loves
- Loneliness
- Financial hardships
- Institutionalization

Medical-Psychiatric Disorders

Medical disorders that contribute to sleep problems in the older adult include cardiovascular disease, diabetes, GI reflux, and arthritis. Psychiatric disorders that affect sleep include anxiety disorder, depression, and cognitive deficits. Cardiovascular problems may cause nocturnal awakenings because of the increased heart rate that occurs during REM sleep (Asplund, 1999). Sustained-release **cardiac vasodilator agents** may resolve this problem. **Diuretics** and fluids should be avoided in late afternoon to prevent nocturnal enuresis. Hypoglycemia related to diabetes that occurs at night could be relieved with a bedtime snack. Evaluation of **insulin** doses or **oral hypoglycemics** may resolve this particular problem. Gastrointestinal reflux, which may result in prolonged sleep latency or awakenings, may be relieved by restricting intake after dinner, administering **antacids**, and elevating the head of the bed. The pain and muscle stiffness of arthritis often results in early morning awakenings. Prescribing a sustained-release **analgesic** to be taken at bedtime may help. Providing supportive care and **anti-anxiety medications** such as **anxiolytics** may assist the patient with an anxiety disorder. Depression may result in early morning awakenings with a decreased energy level. Providing counseling, encouraging socialization, and prescribing low-dose **tricyclic antidepressants** may help the patient overcome this sleep problem. Agitation at bedtime or nocturnal wandering, resulting in reduced sleep, may be a result of cognitive deficits. Providing a structured environment and prescribing **antipsychotic medications** may be indicated. **Psychotropic drugs** are discussed in Chapter 15.

Melatonin has been used with limited success to treat sleep disorders. It appears to have a greater effect in "resetting" the circadian rhythm than in treating insomnia. Resetting the circadian rhythm enables the patient to sleep at "normal" times of the night. This treatment is certainly more relevant for patients with age-related sleep problems than it is for those with sleep disorders.

Management of sleep disorders is second to incontinence in the diagnosis of admissions to long-term care facilities for the older adult. With improved sleep, the older adult has the potential for greater alertness and more social interaction. Recognition and proper treatment of sleep disorders improve quality of life.

Urinary Incontinence

Urinary incontinence affects approximately 12 to 13 million people in the United States. It is estimated that 50 to 74 percent of women in long-term care facilities and 20 percent of women aged 40 to 60 years have some degree of incontinence (Maloney, 1998). About 1.5 to 2.5 percent of men aged 15 to 64 years are affected by incontinence, with this percentage increasing to 15 to 25 percent after 60 years (Maloney, 1998).

There are several types of chronic urinary incontinence, each with a different etiology: stress incontinence, urge incontinence, overflow incontinence, and functional urinary incontinence. Stress and urge urinary incontinence usually occur because of a weakened pelvic floor, whereas overflow and functional urinary incontinence stem from a neurological impairment.

Drugs play a dominant role in the causes and cures of urinary incontinence. Nonneurological causes of urinary incontinence are predominantly related to drugs that directly affect smooth muscle (Gallo, Fallon, & Staskin, 1997). Commonly prescribed drugs for psychiatric, cardiac, and gastrointestinal disorders, as well as those prescribed for the treatment of colds and pain, have an **anticholinergic** effect that directly affects the smooth muscle of the bladder by relaxing the sphincter. This information again makes it important to obtain an accurate and complete list of the drugs the older adult is taking. Drugs also play an important part in "curing" stress and urge urinary incontinence by strengthening tissue.

Stress incontinence can usually be diagnosed through a basic health examination, including a history of duration and the situations of occurrence; a urinalysis; and a pelvic, rectal, and neurological examination (Gallo et al, 1997; Maloney, 1998). Treatments for stress incontinence include behavioral interventions, medications, and surgical repair. Drugs prescribed for stress urinary incontinence include the **alpha-adrenergic agonists**, which increase the bladder outlet resistance. However, in the older adult these drugs may be poorly tolerated. The **alpha-adrenergic agonists** also may increase blood pressure; create a dry mouth; and induce tachycardia, headache, or palpitations (see Chapter 14). Use this type of drug with caution in the older adult.

The older female patient with stress incontinence may benefit from the addition of **estrogen**, which may relieve many of the symptoms. However, some women are unwilling to tolerate symptoms of vaginal bleeding and breast tenderness secondary to the **hormone replacement**. Use of the lowest amount of **estrogen** appears to improve the urethral closure without causing the ADRs seen in many women. More recently, use of **estrogen** creams vaginally appears to be effective in treating this type of incontinence. Recommended effective dosage is application every night for 2 weeks, then two nights a week. **Vaginal estrogens** spare the patient the ADRs of the oral products. Inform the patient that it may take about 4 to 6 weeks before the beneficial effect is apparent.

Urge incontinence may have a functional or medication-related cause. **Diuretics** may cause urgency and frequency, which may create such emotional stress that patients may either not leave their room or not take the drug. If a patient has urge incontinence and must take **diuretics**, work with the patient about timing the drug so it does not interfere with his or her social life.

Functional urge incontinence can be caused by problems of the nervous system, bladder infection, thinning of the urethral tissue, fecal impaction, or enlarged prostate. Pharmacological interventions are **vaginal estrogen** as mentioned previously, **anticholinergics (oxybutynin, propantheline)**, or **tricyclic antidepressants (imipramine)**. The **anticholinergics** and **antidepressants** both have their particular ADRs, but the emotional relief of controlling the urine problem may outweigh them.

The Agency for Health Care Policy and Research has established basic criteria for a primary care provider for referral to a specialist for the incontinent patient (1996). This guideline is helpful in following treatment plans and well worth the practitioner's time to have the resource available.

Many practitioners use behavioral interventions first in treating urge and stress incontinence with relatively frequent success. Pharmacological interventions may become necessary, but keep in mind the possible ADRs.

Constipation

Of the possible GI problems, constipation is the most frequently encountered in the older adult population. There are several pathogenic reasons. Ignoring the urge to defecate; inadequate ingestion of food, fluid, and fiber; **diuretic therapy**; sedentary lifestyle; and the early, lifelong attitude that one must defecate every day (chronic **laxative** use) are common behaviors that are hard to treat. The various drug interactions, metabolic disorders, neurological diseases, and colonic disorders are more readily recognizable.

The complaint of constipation accounts for about 2.5 million health-care visits every year. Despite this high number of health-care visits, rarely does a significant abnormality exist. The abuse of OTC **laxatives** may contribute to the problem. Careful history taking and continued education are the keys to helping the older adult stop fearing constipation.

Constipation is a real problem with real consequences. Some patients have been told that no one has ever died from constipation. This attitude discredits patients' complaints and may cause them to use alternative therapies that are less than desirable. Some older adults have been taught that they should be "cleansed" at least weekly or daily, which means an enema. Others believe that they must have a daily bowel movement. To the younger population, many of these ideas are not consistent with their beliefs, and bias may create a barrier to open communication.

Nondrug therapies to treat constipation include increased fiber in the diet and increased fluid intake. Encourage the intake of up to 3,000 mL of "free" water every day, if there is no contradictory disease process (e.g., heart failure). Have the older adult fill a 2-quart (2,000 mL) container with water in the morning and drink it throughout the day until it is gone. The other 1,000 mL can be obtained by various other sources (e.g., juice or herbal teas). For better adherence, encourage the person to drink the water before 6 p.m., to avoid getting up more frequently at night to urinate.

Encourage exercise. If the older adult has the mobility, encourage abdominal and pelvic exercises in the morning. Walking is a terrific overall exercise but can be problematic if the older adult has physical limitations. Many who cannot tolerate the joint impact of walking can ride a stationary bike. Swimming is another overall exercise that can maintain the level of muscle activity needed without causing undue stress on joints. Exercise must be tailored to the individual and may not be an option.

Laxatives may be the only choice available if the constipation is not relieved through the preceding methods. The practitioner has the choice of **stool softeners, stimulant** or **saline laxatives**, and **bulk laxatives. Stool softeners** are used when the complaint is consistent with hard, dry stools. **Mineral oil** is a poorly tolerated **laxative** because of its interference with the absorption of the **fat-soluble vitamins, calcium, phosphate**, and other nutrients. Aspiration of **mineral oil** can cause lipid pneumonia and pulmonary fibrosis.

Bulk-forming laxatives include **bran, methylcellulose**, and **psyllium**. They act like **laxatives** because of their ability to hold water, which in turn softens the stool and promotes peristalsis. Do not recommend **bulk laxatives** to patients with bowel strictures, diabetics, and those on **salicylate** and **digoxin** therapy. **Stimulant laxatives** should be used only short term and only under specific conditions. They can be habit forming, in that the colon becomes dependent on the outside stimulation for peristalsis. There are appropriate times for this type of **laxative**, but proceed with caution in prescribing them. The **stimulant laxative** is normally utilized as the last choice when other **laxatives** have failed.

Each of these drug classes is discussed in Chapter 20.

Pain

Complaints of pain are reported by 25 to 50 percent of community-dwelling older adults and 45 to 80 percent of residents in long-term care facilities (Feldt, 2005). Untreated pain can have serious consequences including depression, decreased socialization, sleep disturbances, impaired ambulation, slow healing, and increased health-care costs.

Assessing pain in the older adult can present problems. Most older adults can accurately respond to questions about pain, but cognitively impaired older adults may have difficulty recognizing and describing their pain and may be unable to conceptualize the distressed feeling as pain. Feldt (2005) suggests that the key to optimal assessment of pain is use of pain assessment instruments that are simple, readily available, in large and bold print, and in language that patients understand. The Verbal Descriptor Scale was preferred in one study because it was most easily understood by older adults in the community. It was also understood by 73 percent of cognitively impaired hospitalized older adults (Feldt, 2005). The use of descriptive synonyms for pain (e.g., aching, stiff, dull, pressure, burning, shooting, cramping, sore, uncomfortable) is also recommended.

The American Medical Directors Association published a guideline for treating chronic pain in older adults in 1999, followed by the American Geriatric Society clinical practice guidelines for the management of persistent pain in older adults in 2002. They specifically recommend the following:

- Use the least invasive route (oral) to administer pain drugs whenever possible.
- Identify the underlying cause of the pain to select the best treatment.
- Avoid oversedation.
- Develop individually-tailored therapeutic regimens.
- Continue to monitor for side effects of opioid and adjuvant therapies.

Short-acting analgesics that have a rapid onset are best for acute flare-ups of pain. **Acetaminophen** is the drug of choice for mild to moderate pain, administered on a regular schedule. **NSAIDs** should be prescribed with caution, but are appropriate when the underlying problem is inflammation. Short-acting forms (e.g., **ibuprofen**) in lower doses (e.g., 400 mg) are best for this class. **Opioids** are appropriate for severe pain, but they should be titrated so that the lowest effective dose is used. Continuous pain can be treated with long-acting or sustained-release **analgesics**. Chapter 53 discusses the treatment of acute and chronic pain across the age groups.

In summary, when prescribing for older adults:

- Use single daily-dose regimens or the simplest effective regimen. Avoid polypharmacy wherever possible.
- Limit the use of prn drugs.
- Consider all new drugs as a therapeutic trial; stop the drug if it is ineffective.
- Do not prescribe drugs whose benefits are marginal or for which there is no clear indication.
- Discontinue drugs that have adverse reactions that produce nonadherence.
- Attempt to prescribe a drug that will treat more than one existing problem (e.g., an **ACE-inhibitor** to treat hypertension, heart failure, and/or as renal protection in diabetes).
- Provide legible written instructions and follow up on adherence to the treatment regimen.

REFERENCES

AARP. (2002). *Prescription drug use among persons age 45+: A chart book*. Washington, DC: AARP.

Agency for Health Care Policy and Research. (1996). *Urinary incontinence in adults: Acute and chronic management.* Clinical Practice Guideline Number 2. Public Health Service, Rockville, MD: US Department of Health and Human Services.

American Geriatrics Society. (2002). The management of persistent pain in older persons. *The Journal of the American Geriatrics Society, 50,* S205–S224.

American Medical Directors Association. (1999). *Chronic pain management in the long-term care setting.* Columbia, MD: Author.

Andrejak, M., Genes, N., Vaur, L., Poncelet, P., Clerson, P., & Carre, A. (2000). Electronic pill-boxes in the evaluation of antihypertensive treatment compliance: Comparison of once daily versus twice daily regimen. *American Journal of Hypertension, 13,* 184–190.

Asplund, R. (1999). Sleep disorders in the elderly. *Drugs and Aging, 14*(2), 91–104.

Atkin, P. A., Veitch, P. C., Veitch, E. M., & Ogle, S. J. (1999). The epidemiology of serious adverse drug reactions among the elderly. *Drugs and Aging, 14*(2), 141–152.

Barat, I., Andreasen, F., & Damsgaard, E. M. (2001). Drug therapy in the elderly: What doctors believe and patients actually do. *British Journal of Clinical Pharmacology, 51,* 615–622.

Beck-Little, R., & Weinrich, S. P. (1998). Assessment and management of sleep disorders in the elderly. *Journal of Gerontological Nursing, 24*(4), 21–29.

Beers, M. H. (1997). Explicit criteria for determining potentially inappropriate medication use by the elderly. *Archives of Internal Medicine, 157,* 1531–1536.

Beers, M. H., Ouslander, J. G., Rollingher, J., Reuben, D. B., & Beck, J. C. (1991). Explicit criteria for determining inappropriate medication use in nursing home residents. *Archives of Internal Medicine, 151,* 1825–1832.

Bergman-Evans, B. (2004). *Improving medication management for older adult clients*. Gerontological Nursing Interventions Research Center, Research Dissemination Care. Iowa City, IA: University of Iowa.

Bogunovic, O., & Greenfield, S. (2004). Use of benzodiazepines among elderly patients. *Psychiatric Services, 55*(3), 233–235.

Dexter, D. (1999). Sleep disorders in the elderly. *Annals of Long-Term Care, 7,* 33–36.

Endoy, M. (2005). Anorexia among older adults. *American Journal for Nurse Practitioners, 9*(5), 31–38.

Federal Interagency Forum on Aging-Related Statistics. (2008). *Older Americans 2008: Key indicators of well-being.* Washington, DC: U.S. Government Printing Office.

Feldt, K. (2005). Pain in the elderly. *Advance for Nurse Practitioners, 13*(6), 51–54.

Fick, D., Cooper, J., Wade, W., Waller, J., McClean, J., & Beers, M. (2003). Updating the Beers Criteria for potentially inappropriate medication use in older adults. *Archives of Internal Medicine, 163,* 2716–2724.

Gallo, M., Fallon, P. J., & Staskin, D. R. (1997). Urinary incontinence: Steps to evaluation, diagnosis and treatment. *Nurse Practitioner, 22*(2), 21–44.

Gray, S. L., Mahoney, F. E., & Blough, D. K. (2001). Medication adherence in the elderly patients receiving home health services following hospital discharge. *Annals of Pharmacotherapy, 35,* 539–545.

Gurwitz, J. H., Field, T. S., Harrold, L. R., Rothschild J., Debellis, K., Seger, A. C., Cadoret C., Fish, L. S., Garber, L., Kelleher, M., & Bates, D. W. (2003). Incidence and preventability of adverse drug events among older persons in the ambulatory setting. *Journal of the American Medical Association, 289,* 1107–1116.

Howard, M., Dolovich, I., Kaczorowski, J., Sellors, C., & Sellors, J. (2004). Prescribing of potentially inappropriate medications in elderly people. *Family Practice, 21,* 244–247.

Hsia Der, E., Rubenstein, L., & Choy, G. (1997). The benefits of in-home pharmacy evaluation for older persons. *Journal of the American Geriatric Society, 45,* 211–214.

Hughes, C. M. (2004). Medication non-adherence in the elderly: How big is the problem? *Drugs and Aging, 21*(12), 793–811.

Kaufman, D. W., Kelly, J. P., Rosenberg, L., Anderson, T. E., & Mitchell, A. A. (2002). Recent patterns of medication use in the ambulatory adult population of the United States: The Sloan survey. *Journal of the American Medical Association, 287*(3), 337–344.

Ko, R. (1998). Adulterants in Asian patent medicines. *New England Journal of Medicine, 339,* 847.

Kyle, U. G., Genton, L., Hans, D., Karsegard, V. L., Michel, J. P., Slosman, D. O., & Pichard, C. (2001). Total body mass, fat mass, fat-free mass, and skeletal muscle in older people: Cross-sectional differences . . . *Journal of the American Geriatrics Society, 49,* 1633–1640.

Leipzig, R. (2003). Update in geriatric medicine. *Annals of Internal Medicine, 139*(12), 1003–1008.

Masand, P., & Gupta, S. (2003). Long-acting injectable antipsychotics in the elderly. *Drugs and Aging, 20*(15), 1099–1110.

Mahoney, D., Zhan, L., & Eckler, M. (1999). Preventing drug-drug interactions among older adults: Guidelines and clinical application. *American Journal for Nurse Practitioners, 3*(1), 7–20.

Maloney, C. (1998). Urinary incontinence: A guide to the diagnosis of chronic and reversible causes in a primary care setting. *American Journal for Nurse Practitioners, 2*(3), 8–13.

Murray, M., & Callahan, C. (2003). Improving medication use for older adults: An integrated research agenda. *Annals of Internal Medicine, 139*(5), 425–429.

Nahin, R. L., Pecha, M., Welmerink, D. B., Sink, K., DeKosky, S. T., & Fitzpatrick, A. L. (2009). Concomitant use of prescription drugs and dietary supplements in ambulatory elderly people. *Journal of the American Geriatrics Society, 57*(7), 1197–1205.

National Center for Health Statistics. (2009). *Health, United States, 2009: With special feature on medical technology.* Hyattsville, MD: U.S. Government Printing Office.

Patel, R. (2003). Polypharmacy and the elderly. *Journal of Infusion Nursing, 26*(3), 166–169.

Sheirlinkx, K., Nicolas, A. S., Nourhashemi, F., Vellas, B., Albarèdem, J. L., & Garry, P. (1998). The MNA® score in successfully aging persons. In: B. Vellas, B. P. J. Garry, & Y. Guigoz (Eds.), *Mini Nutritional Assessment* (MNA®): *Research and practice in elderly* (pp. 61–66). Nestlé Clinical and Performance Nutrition Workshop Series, Vol 1. Philadelphia: Lippincott-Raven.

Thjodleifsson, B. (2002). Treatment of acid-related diseases in the elderly with emphasis on the use of proton pump inhibitors. *Drugs and Aging, 19*(12), 921–927.

Thwaites, J. H. (1999). Practical aspects of drug treatment in elderly patients with mobility problems. *Drugs and Aging, 2,* 105–114.

Turnheim, K. (2003). *When drug therapy gets old: Pharmacokinetics and pharmacodynamics in the elderly.* Vienna, Austria: Universitat Wien, Institut fur Pharmakologie.

Wasen, E., Isoaho, R., Mattila, K., Vahlberg, T., Kivela, S., & Irjala, K. (2004). Renal impairment associated with diabetes in the elderly. *Diabetes Care, 27*(11), 2648–2653.

Zagaria, M. (2005). The effects of aging on drug efficacy: Drug pharmacodynamics and pharmacokinetics. *U.S. Pharmacist, 30*(5), 54–57.

CHAPTER 52

CHRONIC ILLNESS AND LONG-TERM CARE

Casey Shillam

Chapter Outline

Health-care professionals face many major health and illness problems in the 21st century. Today, chronic diseases—such as cardiovascular disease (primarily heart disease and stroke), cancer, and diabetes—are among the most prevalent, costly, and preventable of all health problems (Centers for Disease Control and Prevention [CDC], 2010). Seven of every 10 deaths in Americans each year are due to a chronic disease: more than 1.7 million people annually. For millions of Americans, the prolonged course of illness and disability from chronic diseases such as diabetes and arthritis often result in extended pain, functional limitations, and changes in quality of life.

Almost one out of every two Americans, over 133 million people, has at least one chronic condition (CDC, 2010; Jack et al, 2006). Chronic diseases account for three-fourths of the nation's 1.4 trillion dollars in medical care costs and one-third of the years of potential life lost before age 65 (CDC, 2010). Individual, family, health system, community, and societal factors all contribute to the rise in chronic disease rates in the United States (American Association of Public Health, 2001). Many variables may explain the prevalence of chronic illness, such as increased individual risk factors, a lack of health-care resources for the poor and underserved, and environmental conditions that do not support the adoption and sustainability of healthy eating and physical activity (Litaker, Koroukian, & Love, 2005). Collectively, these factors may clinically express themselves differently from one person to another. As a result, the prescriber and members of a multidisciplinary health team must use various approaches to positively intervene for persons living with chronic illness. Moreover, the advanced practice nurse must attend to the emotional, intellectual, social, and spiritual needs of those living with chronic illness. So, the prescriber must be attuned to the ever-expanding knowledge base regarding chronic illness management and issues.

CHANGES IN THE ADVANCED PRACTICE PRESCRIBER'S ROLE IN CHRONIC ILLNESS

Chronic Illness

Chronic illness is a somewhat new idea that arose along with the 20th-century advancements in medical care. "Prior to the second half of the previous century, there were many children crippled with conditions such as polio and tuberculosis; many adults were handicapped or disabled from similar illnesses or farm and industrial accidents" (Kurz & Shepard, 2005, p. 416). Since the middle part of the 20th century, there have been many attempts to define chronic illness (Abram, 1972; Commission on Chronic Illness, 1957; Feldman, 1974). In the 21st century, the focus is now on operational definitions of chronic illness and diseases to guide health-care providers in the assessment, implementation, and evaluation of health for individuals, families, and populations. One of the most widely used definitions has been adopted by the Adherence Project of the World Health Organization (WHO) (2003): "Diseases which have one or more of the following characteristics: they are permanent, leave residual disability, are caused by nonreversible pathological alteration, require special training of the patient for rehabilitation, or may be expected to require a long period of supervision, observation, or care" (p. 4).

With multiple disciplines interested in chronic illness, nursing needed to describe and define its unique view of chronic illness so that the definition would be holistic and broad enough in scope to be useful and meaningful to nursing practice. Nurse-scholars Curtin and Lubkin (1995), in their classic definition, write about chronic illness as "the irreversible presence, accumulation, or latency of disease states or impairments that involve the total human environment for supportive care and self-care, maintenance of function, and prevention of further disability" (pp. 6–7). A chronic illness is further identified as existing for 3 months or longer, does not resolve spontaneously, and is rarely cured (Kurz & Shepard, 2005).

Advanced Practice Prescriber: Role Differences

The prescriber role of the advanced nurse practitioner focuses on health promotion and maintenance, increased knowledge about chronic conditions, and additional interpersonal communication and organizational skills (Jackson, 2000). All prescribers should focus on reducing the number of (1) acute illness exacerbations due to existing chronic illnesses, and (2) hospitalizations and/or admissions to skilled nursing units within long-term care centers through positive illness and disease management. "Client education and health promotion activities can accomplish this goal through timely, well-planned interventions and follow-up illness prevention care" (Meiner, 2002, p. 464).

The prescriber must be clear in how decisions are made regarding medication prescribing for persons living with a chronic illness. Most providers use a set of guidelines or theories to guide their interactions and actions to support: collaborating with others; listening to the client; educating the client, family, and interdisciplinary staff; initiating research; and consulting with others (Meiner, 2002). These foci utilize skills that benefit persons with chronic illness such as conducting health histories; physical examinations; diagnosing and treating common acute illnesses and injuries; and providing supportive, ongoing care of the person with a chronic illness. The prescribing aspect of advanced practice is deeply connected to the prescriber as nurse, consultant, educator, advocate, and practitioner.

Considerations Related to Adherence in the Chronically Ill

People are faced with managing increasingly complex health and illness situations as science and technology continue to advance. Treatment plans have become more complex and require the implementation of health-care regimens by people in their homes. Patients must be concerned with the self-management of short-term illnesses while learning to live their lives in new ways when a chronic illness becomes a part of daily life. Living with a chronic illness successfully centers on adhering to a recommended, yet personalized health-care regimen. Successful adherence to a complex treatment regimen, often consisting of multiple drugs from a variety of drug classes, requires a collaborative process designed to optimize practice outcomes. Adherence is discussed in Chapter 8. This chapter focuses on the additional considerations for the patient with a chronic illness.

Collaborative management is an important method of encouraging adherence to a complex health-care regimen. Collaborative management is care that "strengthens and supports self-care in chronic illness while assuring that effective medical, preventive, and health maintenance interventions can take place" (von Korff, 1997, p. 1097). The process of collaborative management is both dynamic and continuous. Collaborative management:

1. Begins with dialogue and mutual respect between the patient and the health-care team.
2. Is a starting point for care in chronic illness that includes choosing desirable and obtainable goals that provide direction for care management.
3. Is flexible in nature to enhance care and communication.
4. Does not end with regimen selection, but progresses through stages in the direction of improving adherence, optimal health, and survival. (Jani, Stewart, Nolen, & Tavel, 2002, p. 84)

Moreover, von Korff (1997, p. 1098) further outlines the essential elements of health care central to such collaborative management. These essential elements are the following:

1. Collaborative definition of problems.
2. Targeting, goal setting, and planning.
3. Creating a continuum of self-management training and support services.
4. Active and sustained follow-up.

These four elements provide a unique manner to address not only medication adherence issues but also chronic illness care in general. For example, patients and providers define problems differently. Patients may focus on functionality, subjective complaints, and lifestyle choices; providers may focus on disease prevention, medication therapy, nonadherence to recommendations, and risk factors related to prognosis. It is imperative that patients and providers have a mutual understanding of problems and understand one another's points of view (von Korff, 1997).

Nonadherence is centered on a person's lack of understanding of the prescribed medication regimen and the resulting behavior. Numerous factors contribute to nonadherence. Three basic forms of nonadherence are commonly seen in the chronically ill: erratic nonadherence, unwitting nonadherence, and intelligent nonadherence.

Erratic nonadherence is probably the most common form, composed of missed doses of medications and is the most acknowledged form of nonadherence by prescribers. Erratic nonadherence is often observed in individuals with forgetfulness, changing schedules, or busy lifestyles. People find it difficult to follow a prescribed regimen when the complexity of their lives interferes with adherence or when they have not prioritized the management of their chronic illness.

Unwitting nonadherence occurs when people fail to understand fully either the specifics of the regimen or the necessity for adherence. Often, people forget the instructions given to them by the health-care provider (Frank & Miramontes, 1998).

Intelligent nonadherence occurs when people purposely alter, discontinue, or fail to initiate a prescribed medication regimen (Rand, Bender, Boulet, Chaustre, & Weinstein, 2003). This form of lack of adherence reflects a person's reasoned choice to stop or alter what was prescribed. People who feel better may decide that they no longer need to take prescribed medications. Fear of apparent short- or long-term medication side effects may cause some people to decrease the dose or discontinue the medication. Also, people may stop a prescribed medication regimen because of the bad taste of the medication, the complexity of the regimen, or the interference with daily life, convincing them that the disadvantages of the prescribed regimen outweigh the benefits.

CHRONIC ILLNESS AND MEDICATION ADHERENCE: DISEASE-SPECIFIC EXAMPLES

People living with chronic illness face a variety of issues that affect medication adherence. These issues reflect each person's unique concerns and needs. For example, one person may have a priority to understand the health-care regimen focusing on exactly how and when to take medications. Another person may focus on fear of side effects and the ability to control them. Anticipatory fear or actual occurrence of side effects is a significant contributor to nonadherence. Prescribers must be skilled in providing information about possible side effects and approaches to dealing with them prior to the occurrence (Frank & Miramontes, 1998). Several of the major contributing factors in medication adherence with chronic illness are listed in Table 52–1.

Asthma

The use of medication in asthma patients is varied and best described by three illustrations of medication adherence patterns. The first adherence pattern is usually the most obvious: the chronic underuse of medication. Chronic undertreatment of asthma may lead to poor control of symptoms and greater reliance on "as needed" (prn) treatments for the relief of acute asthma symptoms (Rand et al, 2003).

A second adherence pattern is the erratic use of medication: alternating between fully adherent (usually when symptomatic) and underuse or total nonuse (most likely when asymptomatic). The person with erratic adherence may present for treatment of acute asthma, although the person appears to adhere completely to the prescribed regimen. Some people relying solely on inhaled **beta antagonists** for symptom relief may be prone to overuse during acute bronchospasm. This misuse may cause a delay in seeking care or lead to complications associated with excessive use of **beta antagonists** (Rand et al, 2003).

The third adherence pattern is a combination of the previous two: adhering differently to the various medications prescribed for asthma management. For instance, a person may underuse the prescribed prophylactic **anti-inflammatory** while remaining appropriately adherent to the **beta agonists** (Rand et al, 2003). Moreover, a person may or may not use a **metered-dose inhaler (MDI)** appropriately. Although MDI adherence is difficult to assess, poor technique is usually a significant contributor to nonadherence and most likely results from "inadequate

Table 52–1 Factors Contributing to Medication Adherence With Chronic Illness

Understanding treatment regimen	Beliefs in effectiveness
Fitting with current routine	Cultural relevancy (see Chapter 9)
Having the skills to carry out the regimen	The staging of disease and level of wellness
Fear of side effects	The ability to control side effects
Remembering to take the medications	Mental health
Family/caregiver support	Interaction with street drugs
Personal views of health	Trust in provider

Adapted from Frank, L., & Miramontes, H. (1998). *Health care provider adherence curriculum.* Pittsburgh, PA: AIDS Education and Training Centers Program.

instruction and a person's forgetfulness" (Rand et al, 2003, p. 48). Treatment of asthma and the appropriate techniques for use of **MDIs** is discussed in Chapter 30.

Depression

The efficacy of pharmacological therapy for depression depends on a person's adherence to the prescribed regimen and the appropriate diagnosis and treatment regimen by the advanced practice nurse prescriber. The focus here, however, is on medication adherence. The best predictors of adherence in persons living with depression are frequency of dosing, education, drug type, comedication, psychiatric comorbidity, and personality traits (Peveler & Tejada, 2003). Frequency of medication dosing is influential on a person's adherence to a medication regimen. Prescribers need to provide some personal control over the frequency of medication dosing as much as possible (Peveler & Tejada, 2003). For example, Claxton (2000) has suggested that prescribing a once-weekly dose of enteric-coated **fluoxetine** may lead to better adherence than a once-daily dose, whereas a person taking other medications daily may be more likely to adhere to a daily dose. The prescriber should assess what will work best in the patient's life.

Consideration may also be given to the link between the drug type and enhanced adherence, as different **antidepressants** may be associated with improved adherence. Tai-Seale, Groghan, and Obenchain (2000) propose that adherence may be compromised in people treated with **tricyclic antidepressants** because of the many adverse reactions. They suggest that psychotherapy improves medication adherence in persons with depression. Furthermore, the provider must consider psychiatric comorbidities and personality traits to improve adherence. For example, people with alcohol use disorders, psychotic disorders, and mood disorders have significantly lower levels of medication adherence than those with neurotic or somatoform disorders (Kim, Park, Park, & Kim, 2010). Anxiety and depression and medication management are discussed further in Chapter 29.

COLLABORATIVE PROCESS TO IMPROVE MEDICATION ADHERENCE

Medication adherence is important for the effective management of chronic conditions. A collaborative four-step process can be used by providers to approach a variety of people with chronic illness (Jani et al, 2002). The four steps to this process are the following:

1. Assess clinical factors that may influence adherence.
2. Create and maintain a therapeutic alliance between the patient and the provider.
3. Monitor the level of medication adherence.
4. Identify strategies to improve medication adherence (p. 85).

This process incorporates principles of learning theory, the daily living challenges of the person living with a chronic illness, and the complexity of medical and psychosocial factors specific to chronic illness diseases.

Assessing Clinical Factors

Many factors influence medication adherence. Treatment readiness and a person's self-efficacy are particularly central to adherence. Other factors assessed for medication adherence are described in Table 52–2.

Table 52–2 **Factors Influencing Adherence**

General Health Status	Medical History, Nutritional Assessment, and Comorbidities
Life goals	To understand deeper issues such as • what gives meaning to a patient's life • the context of illness and treatment on a patient's life • the patient's definition of quality of life • a patient's attitudes and motivations based on one's self-perception
Medication history	Past experience, current regimens, and side effects from all medications
Comorbidities	Psychiatric, substance use, and medical illnesses
Social stability	Housing status, food resources, transportation needs, financial status, and insurance status
Employment status	Type of job, constraints, and disclosure issues
Health beliefs & cultural background	Language and perceptions toward illness & chronic illness, diagnosis, prognosis, role of medications, understanding of consequences of medication nonadherence, and spiritual/religious orientation in reference to one's life and health goals
Family & social support	Identification of personalized medication facilitator and network of social support
Educational background	Educational level, literacy level, baseline knowledge regarding specific chronic illness, medications, and importance of adherence

Adapted from Jani, A. A., Stewart, A., Nolen, R. D., & Tavel, L. (2002). Medication adherence and patient education. Florida AIDS Education & Training Center. In *HIV/AIDS primary care guide* (p. 86). Gainesville, FL: University of Florida Press.

Assessment of these factors takes time and will likely occur over several visits. The provider should integrate as many of these factors into the treatment plan as possible.

Therapeutic Alliance

Creating and maintaining a therapeutic alliance between the patient and provider is critical to adherence in medication regimens. The prescriber must support and guide a person to take an active role in his or her own health care. The therapeutic alliance is further enhanced and created through trust and respect of the person as life and health decisions are made. It is important to understand and seek clarification about the person's values, health beliefs, and goals before attempting to prescribe a plan of care or medication regimen (Jani et al, 2002). In fact, "better adherence is likely to be achieved if and when the patient feels more *in control* of the illness, therapy choices, regimen efficacy, and clinical outcomes" (p. 86).

Furthermore, there are several other issues that must be addressed in order to create and maintain a therapeutic alliance (Table 52–3).

The process of creating and maintaining a therapeutic alliance involves many contributing and complex factors. The prescriber must be patient and open to each person's unique experience in living with a chronic illness. The therapeutic alliance is an important way to support and guide people in practice.

Medication Adherence Monitoring

Adhering to a medication regimen is ongoing and must continually be addressed and monitored by the patient and the advanced nurse practitioner prescriber. "Adherence must always be assessed and not assumed" (Jani et al, 2002, p. 87). There are various strategies to measure adherence: clinical and laboratory values and measurements, pill counts, and self-report measures such as the Morisky four-question self-reporting tool and scale (Morisky, Green, & Levine, 1986). An important use of this scale lies in the ability of the prescriber to uncover nonadherence and promote further dialogue with the person to better characterize the nonadherence in terms of its frequency and causation (Box 52–1).

Monitoring the level of medication adherence is another step in the process of collaborative care. The prescriber and the patient need to work together to create a dialogue about methods for taking medications.

BOX 52–1 MORISKY SIMPLIFIED SELF-REPORT MEASURE OF ADHERENCE

Scoring: 0 = High Adherence;
1–2 Medium Adherence; 3–4 Low Adherence

1. Do you ever forget to take your medicine?
2. Are you careless at times about taking your medicine?
3. When you feel better do you sometimes stop taking your medicine?
4. Sometimes if you feel worse when you take your medications, do you stop taking it?

Adapted from Jani, A. A., Stewart, A., Nolen, R. D., & Tavel, L. (2002). Medication adherence and patient education. Florida AIDS Education & Training Center. In *HIV/AIDS primary care guide* (p. 87). Gainesville, FL: University of Florida Press.

Table 52–3 **Therapeutic Alliance Issues**

Communication process & Informed consent	• Specific training and skills development for clinical interviewing is needed in order to establish a therapeutic alliance, keeping in mind the specific cultural and language background of the patient. • A contractual agreement based on informed consent can assist in galvanizing the patient–provider rapport and commitment to medication adherence.
Individualized profile of pertinent factors	This profile of pertinent factors that may influence issues regarding medication adherence should be created. These factors should be identified in the preliminary assessment.
Identified barriers to reaching health goals	Potential and actual barriers to reaching health goals of the patient should be identified, including medication adherence. Conversely, identifying special support systems that may be present and could be strengthened is key.
Assessment of patient readiness	Assess the patient's readiness for behavior change, including medication usage and adherence. This will assist the provider in the potential application of motivational interviewing to move the patient to positive and consistent adherence.
Determination of medication regimen and implementation	Establish definitions of success and failure that are tailored to the patient's daily lifestyle.

Adapted from Jani, A. A., Stewart, A., Nolen, R. D., & Tavel, L. (2002). Medication adherence and patient education. Florida AIDS Education & Training Center. In *HIV/AIDS primary care guide* (p. 86). Gainesville, FL: University of Florida Press.

Identifying Adherence Strategies

Identifying strategies to improve medication adherence aids the nurse practitioner in management of chronic illnesses. In this process, the prescriber defines the pattern(s) of nonadherence (as discussed previously in the chapter). The prescriber must also identify specific barriers that promote nonadherence and identify factors that can be modified that will enhance the person's ability to adhere to the regimen (Jani et al, 2002). Moreover, the prescriber must engage in ongoing dialogue with each patient regarding perceptions of the health goals, the disease process, the purpose of the medication, the role of adherence, and the consequences of nonadherence. This dialogue will facilitate individual and specific strategies to improve medication adherence. Above all, it is paramount to tailor the regimen to fit the lifestyle, job situation, and food habits of each person.

These four steps of the collaborative process to medication adherence serve as a framework for the prescriber to create and refine a systematic approach to working with people with chronic illness to improve medication adherence. This collaborative process strengthens and supports self-care in chronic illness while assuring that effective medical, preventative, and health maintenance interventions can take place (von Korff, 1997). The prescriber is best positioned to support and guide patients in a dialogue of mutual respect.

SPECIAL CONSIDERATIONS IN PRESCRIBING FOR PATIENTS IN LONG-TERM CARE FACILITIES

Today there are an estimated 37.9 million people are over the age of 65; this number is projected to grow to 71.5 million by 2030 (Federal Interagency Forum on Aging Related Statistics, 2008; National Center for Health Statistics, 2009). Additional projections estimate that 43 percent of these older adults will need to enter a long-term care facility (U.S. Census Bureau, 2006). These trends reflect the positive outcomes in "health practices, pharmaceutical advances, medical care, and nursing innovations" (Barnes, 2002, p. 533). These changes dictate that prescribers must be aware of the changing and increasing needs of persons residing in long-term care facilities. With the present and projected increase in this population, prescribers will be on the front lines of treating and managing the health-care needs of this unique population.

One of the primary considerations in prescribing for persons living in long-term care facilities is inappropriate medication use (Fick et al, 2003; Luggen, 2005; Molony, 2004). The prescriber must be aware of many of high-risk medications used to reduce medication-related risk.

The adapted Beers' Criteria identifies medications noted by an expert panel to have potential risks that outweigh potential benefits of the drug. The criteria are appropriate for persons older than 65 years of age, regardless of their level of frailty. The criteria provide a rating of severity for adverse outcomes (severe vs. less severe) as well as a descriptive summary of the prescribing concerns associated with the medication. (Molony, 2004)

Another consideration in prescribing for those in long-term care is the prevalence of medication errors. Medication errors occur in up to 70 percent of patients in long-term care settings and are most often attributed to inaccessibility of the prescriber, the prescriber not knowing the resident, wrong prescription dose, and administration of an inappropriate medication (Barber et al, 2009; Pepper & Towsley, 2007).

The adverse drug events in long-term care are preventable and fall into less-serious and serious categories (Fig. 52–1). The prescriber must be attuned to the changes he or she must make in their prescribing patterns to lower the risk of adverse drug events.

The prescriber must also be aware of the most common errors made in prescribing within long-term care facilities (Fig. 52–2).

The Beers Criteria for Potentially Inappropriate Medication Use in Older Adults (Fick et al, 2003) must be used by primary care prescribers not only to increase their awareness "of medications that may present increased risk for adverse drug reactions" (Molony, 2004), but should

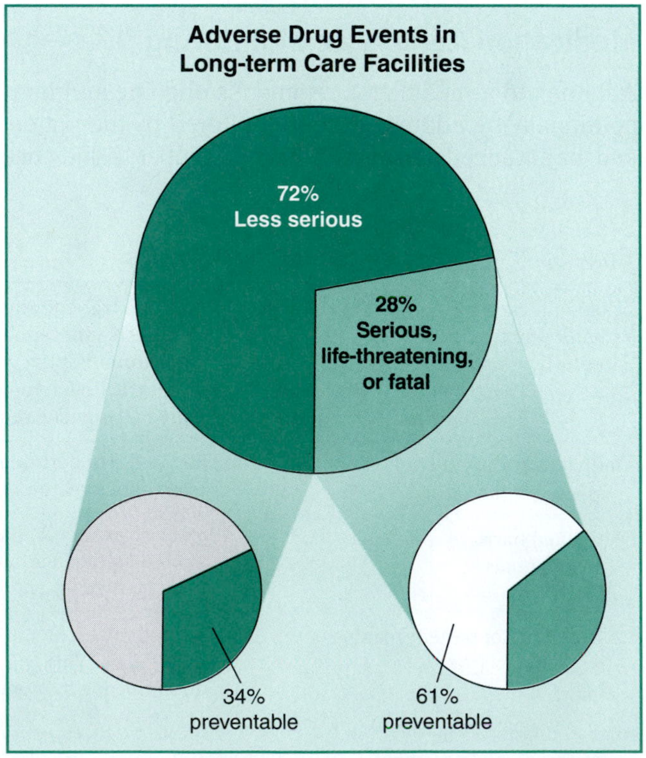

Figure 52–1. Adverse drug events in long-term care facilities.

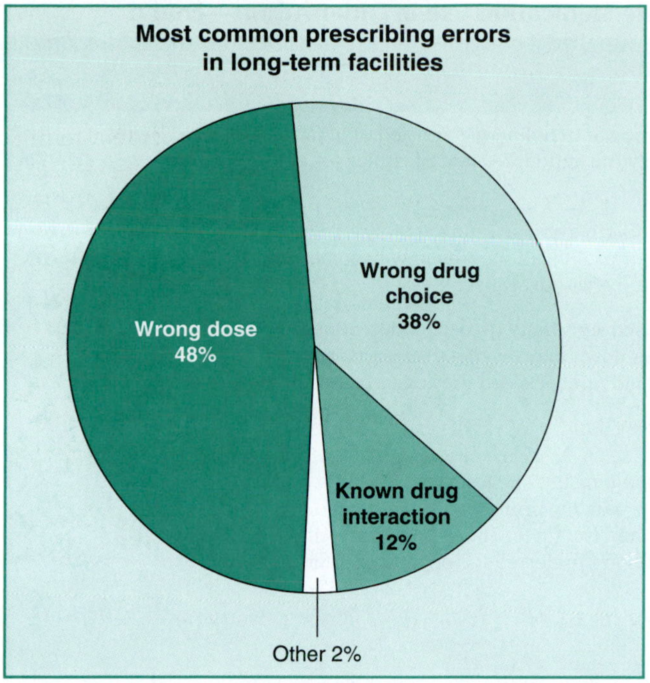

Figure 52–2. Most common prescribing errors in long-term care facilities.

use the updated criteria "to individualize medication regimes and provide appropriate clinical monitoring and education" as well (Molony, 2004). The final criteria are 48 individual medications or classes of medications to avoid in older adults and 20 diseases or conditions and medications to be avoided in older adults with these conditions. "Sixty-six of these potentially inappropriate drugs were considered by the panel to have adverse outcomes of high severity" (Fick et al, 2003, p. 2718).

Table 52–4 contains the Updated Beers Criteria for Potentially Inappropriate Medication Use in Older Adults (derived from Fick et al, 2003, p. 2722).

The Updated Beers Criteria for Potentially Inappropriate Medication Use in Older Adults (Fick et al, 2003) must be used as well-researched–based guidelines that "are not meant to regulate practice in a manner to which they supersede the clinical judgment and assessment of the physician or practitioner" (Fick et al, 2003, p. 2723). Therefore, the prescriber must use many professional learned skills and knowledge to carefully assess, evaluate, and prescribe any therapeutic regimen for persons living in long-term care settings.

Table 52–4 **Beers Criteria for Potentially Inappropriate Medication Use in Older Adults**

Drug	Concern	Severity Rating (High or Low)
Propoxyphene (Darvon) and combination products (Darvon with ASA, Darvon-N, and Darvon-N)	Offers few analgesic advantages ever acetaminophen, yet has the adverse effects of other narcotic drugs.	Low
Indomethacin (Indocin and Indocin SR)	Of all available nonsteroidal anti-inflammatory drugs, this drug produces the most CNS adverse effects.	High
Pentazocine (Talwin)	Narcotic analgesic that causes more CNS adverse effects, including confusion and hallucinations, more commonly than other narcotic drugs. Additionally, it is a mixed agonist and antagonist.	High
Trimethobenzamide (Tigan)	One of the least effective antiemetic drugs, yet it can cause extrapyramidal adverse effects.	
Muscle relaxants and antispasmodics: methocarbamol (Robaxin), carisoprodol (Soma), chlorzoxazone (Paraflex), metaxalone (Skelaxin), cyclobenzaprine (Flexeril), and oxybutynin (Ditropan). Do not consider the extended-release Ditropan XL.	Most muscle relaxants and antispasmodic drugs are poorly tolerated by elderly patients, since these cause anticholinergic adverse effects, sedation, and weakness. Additionally, their effectiveness at doses tolerated by elderly patients is questionable.	High
Flurazepam (Dalmane)	This benzodiazepine hypnotic has an extremely long half-life in elderly patients (often days), producing prolonged sedation and increasing the incidence of falls and fracture. Medium- or short-acting benzodiazepines are preferable.	High
Amitriptyline (Elavil), chlordiazepoxide-amitriptyline (Limbitrol), and perphenazine-amitriptyline (Triavil)	Because of its strong anticholinergic and sedation properties, amitriptyline is rarely the antidepressant of choice for elderly patients.	High

Continued

Table 52–4 **Beers Criteria for Potentially Inappropriate Medication Use in Older Adults—cont'd**

Drug	Concern	Severity Rating (High or Low)
Doxepin (Sinequan)	Because of its strong anticholinergic and sedating properties, doxepin is rarely the antidepressant of choice for elderly patients.	High
Meprobamate (Miltown and Equanil)	This is a highly addictive and sedating anxiolytic. Those using meprobamate for prolonged periods may become addicted and may need to be withdrawn slowly.	High
Doses of short-acting benzodiazepines: doses greater than lorazepam (Ativan), 3 mg; oxazepam (Serax), 60 mg; alprazolam (Xanax), 2 mg; temazepam (Restoril), 15 mg; and triazolam (Halcion), 0.25 mg	Because of increased sensitivity to benzoadiazepines in elderly patients, smaller doses may be effective as well as safer. Total daily doses should rarely exceed the suggested maximums.	High
Long-acting banzodiazepines: chlordiazepoxide (Librium), chlordiazepoxide-amitriptyline (Limbitrol) clidinium-chlordiazepoxide (Librax), diazapam (Valium), quazepam (Doral), halazepam (Paxipam), and chlorazepate (Tranxene)	These drugs have a long half-life in elderly patients (often several days), producing prolonged sedation and increasing the risk of falls and fractures. Short- and intermediate-acting benzodiazepines are preferred if a benzodiazepine is required.	High
Disopyramide (Norpace and Norpace CR)	Of all antiarrhythmic drugs, this is the most potent negative inotrope and therefore may induce heart failure in elderly patients. It is also strongly anticholinergic. Other antiarrhythmic drugs should be used.	High
Digoxin (Lanoxin) (should not exceed >0.125 mg/d except when treating atrial arrhythmias)	Decreased renal clearance may lead to increased risk of toxic effects.	Low
Short-acting dipyridamole (Persantine). Do not consider the long-acting dipyridamole (which has better properties than the short-acting in older adults) except with patients with artificial heart valves	May cause orthostatic hypotension.	Low
Methyldopa (Aldomet) and methyldopa-hydrochlorothiazide (Aldoril)	May cause bradycardia and exacerbate depression in elderly patients.	High
Reserpine at doses >0.25 mg	May induce depression, impotence, sedation, and orthostatic hypotension.	Low
Chlorpropamide (Diabinese)	It has a prolonged half-life in elderly patients and could cause prolonged hypoglycemia. Additionally, it is the only oral hypoglycemic agent that causes SIADH.	High
Gastrointestinal antispasmodic drugs: dicyclomine (Bentyl), hyoscyamine (Levsin and Levsinex), propantheline (Pro-Banthine), belladonna alkaloids (Donnatal and others), and clidinium-chlordiazepoxide (Librax)	GI antispasmodic drugs are highly anticholinergic and have uncertain effectiveness. These drugs should be avoided (especially for long-term use).	High
Anticholinergics and antihistamines: chlorpheniramine (Chlor-Trimeton), diphenhydramine (Benadryl), hydroxyzine (Vistaril and Atarax), cyproheptadine (Periactin), promethazine (Phenergan), tripelennamine, dexchlorpheniramine (Polaramine)	All nonprescription and many prescription antihistamines may have potent anticholinergic properties. Nonanticholinergic antihistamines are preferred in elderly patients when treating allergic reactions.	High
Diphenhydramine (Benadryl)	May cause confusion and sedation. Should not be used as a hypnotic, and when used to treat emergency allergic reactions, it should be used in the smallest possible dose.	High
Ergot mesyloids (Hydergine) and cyclandelate (Cyclospasmol)	Have not been shown to be effective in the doses studied.	Low

Table 52–4 **Beers Criteria for Potentially Inappropriate Medication Use in Older Adults—cont'd**

Drug	Concern	Severity Rating (High or Low)
Ferrous sulfate >325 mg/d	Doses >325 mg/d do not dramatically increase the amount absorbed but greatly increase the incidence of constipation.	Low
All barbiturates (except phenobarbital) except when used to control seizures	Are highly addictive and cause more adverse effects than most sedative or hypnotic drugs in elderly patients.	High
Meperidine (Demerol)	Not an effective oral analgesic in doses commonly used. May cause confusion and has many disadvantages to other narcotic drugs.	High
Ticlopidine (Ticlid)	Has been shown to be no better than aspirin in preventing clotting and may be considerably more toxic. Safer, more effective alternatives exist.	High
Ketorolac (Toradol)	Immediate and long-term use should be avoided in older persons since a significant number have asymptomatic GI pathologic conditions.	High
Amphetamines and anorexic agents	These drugs have potential for causing dependence, hypertension, angina, and myocardial infarction.	High
Long-term use of full-dosage, longer half-life, non—COX-selective NSAIDs: naproxen (Naprosyn, Avaprox, and Aleve), oxaprozin (Daypro), and piroxicam (Feldene)	Have the potential to produce GI bleeding, renal failure, high blood pressure, and heart failure.	High
Daily fluoxetine (Prozac)	Long half-life of drug and risk of producing excessive CNS stimulation, sleep disturbances, and increasing agitation. Safer alternatives exist.	High
Long-term use of stimulant laxatives: bisacodyl (Dulcolax), cascara sagrada, and Neoloid except in the presence of opiate analgesic use	May exacerbate bowel dysfunction.	High
Amiodarone (Cordarone)	Associated with QT interval problems and risk of provoking torsades de pointes. Lack of efficacy in older adults.	High
Orphenadrine (Norflex)	Causes more sedation and anticholinergic adverse effects than safer alternatives.	High
Guanethidine (Ismelin)	May cause orthostatic hypotension. Safer alternatives exist.	High
Guanedrel (Hylorel)	May cause orthostatic hypotension.	High
Cyclandelate (Cyclospasmol)	Lack of efficacy.	Low
Isoxsurpine (Vasodailan)	Lack of efficacy.	Low
Nitrofurantoin (Macrodantin)	Potential for renal impairment. Safer alternatives available.	High
Doxazosin (Cardura)	Potential for hypotension, dry mouth, and urinary problems.	Low
Methyltestosterone (Android, Virilon, and Testrad)	Potential for prostatic hypertrophy and cardiac problems.	High
Thioridazine (Mellaril)	Greater potential for CNS and extrapyramidal adverse effects.	High
Mesondazine (Serentil)	CNS and extrapyramidal adverse effects.	High
Short acting nifedipine (Procardia and Adalat)	Potential for hypotension and constipation.	High
Clonidine (Catapres)	Potential for orthostatic hypotension and CNS adverse effects.	Low
Mineral oil	Potential for aspiration and adverse effects. Safer alternatives available.	High

Continued

Table 52–4 **Beers Criteria for Potentially Inappropriate Medication Use in Older Adults—cont'd**

Drug	Concern	Severity Rating (High or Low)
Cimetidine (Tagamet)	CNS adverse effects including confusion.	Low
Ethacrynic acid (Edecrin)	Potential for hypertension and fluid imbalances. Safer alternatives available.	Low
Desiccated thyroid	Concerns about cardiac effects. Safer alternatives available.	High
Amphetamines (excluding methylphenidate hydrochloride and anorexics)	CNS stimulant adverse effects.	High
Estrogens only (oral)	Evidence of the carcinogenic (breast and endometrial cancer) potential of these agents and lack of cardioprotective effect in older woman.	Low

Medicines Modified Since 1997 Beers Criteria

1. Reserpine (Serpasil and Hydropres)*
2. Extended-release oxybutynin (Ditropan XL)[†]
3. Iron supplements >325 mg[†]
4. Short-acting dipyridamole (Persantine)‡

Medicines Dropped Since 1997 Beers Criteria

Independent of Diagnoses

1. Phenylbutazone (Butazolidin)

Considering Diagnoses

2. Recently started corticosteroid therapy with diabetes
3. β-Blockers with diabetes, COPD or asthma, peripheral vascular disease, and syncope or falls
4. Sedative hypnotics with COPD
5. Potassium supplements with gastric or duodenal ulcers
6. Metoclopramide (Reglan) with seizures or epilepsy
7. Narcotics with bladder outflow obstruction and narcotics with constipation
8. Desipramine (Norpramin) with insomnia
9. All SSRIs with insomnia
10. β-Agonists with insomnia
11. Bethanechol chloride with bladder outflow obstruction

Medicines Added Since 1997 Beers Criteria

Independent of Diagnoses

1. Ketorolac tromethamine (Toradol)
2. Orphenadrine (Norflex)
3. Guanethidine (Ismelin)
4. Guanadrel (Hylorel)
5. Cyclandelate (Cyclospasmol)
6. Isoxsuprine (Vasodilan)
7. Nitrofurantoin (Macrodantin)
8. Doxazosin (Cardura)
9. Methyltestosterone (Android, Virilon, and Testrad)
10. Mesoridazine (Serentil)
11. Clonidine (Catapres)
12. Mineral oil
13. Cimetidine (Tagamet)
14. Ethacrynic acid (Edecrin)
15. Desiccated thyroid
16. Ferrous sulfate >325 mg
17. Amphetamines (excluding methylpenidate and anorexics)
18. Thioridazine (Mellaril)
19. Short-acting nifedipine (Procardia and Adalat)
20. Daily fluoxetine (Prozac)
21. Stimulant laxatives may exacerbate bowel dysfunction (except in presence of chronic pain requiring opiate analgesics)
22. Amiodarone (Cordarone)
23. Non—COX-selective NSAIDs (naproxen [Naprosyn], oxaprozin, and piroxicam)
24. Reserpine doses >0.25 mg/d
25. Estrogens in older women

Considering Diagnoses

26. Long-acting benzodiazepines: chlordiazepoxide (Librium), chlordiazepoxide-amitriptyline (Limbitrol),clidinium-chlordiazepoxide (Librax), diazepam (Valium),quazepam (Doral), halazepam (Paxipam), and chlorazepate (Tranxene) with COPD, stress incontinence, depression, and falls
27. Propanolol with COPD/asthma
28. Anticholinergics with stress incontinence
29. Tricyclic antidepressants (imipramine hydrochloride, doxepine hydrochloride, and amitriptyline hydrochloride) with syncope or falls and stress incontinence
30. Short to intermediate and long-acting benzodiazepines with syncope or falls
31. Clopidogrel (Plavix) with blood-clotting disorders receiving anticoagulant therapy
32. Tolterodine (Detrol) with bladder outflow obstruction
33. Decongestants with bladder outflow obstruction
34. Calcium channel blockers with constipation
35. Phenylpropanolamine with hypertension
36. Bupropion (Wellbutrin) with seizure disorder
37. Olanzapine (Zyprexa) with obesity

Table 52–4 **Beers Criteria for Potentially Inappropriate Medication Use in Older Adults—cont'd**

Drug	Concern	Severity Rating (High or Low)
38. Metoclopramide (Reglan) with Parkinson disease 39. Conventional antipsychotics with Parkinson disease 40. Tacrine (Cognex) with Parkinson disease 41. Barbiturates with cognitive impairment	42. Antispasmodics with cognitive impairment 43. Muscle relaxants with cognitive impairment 44. CNS stimulants with anorexia, malnutrition, and cognitive impairment	

Abbreviations: CNS, central nervous system; COPD, chronic obstructive pulmonary disease; COX, cyclooxygenase; GI, gastrointestinal; NSAIDs, nonsteroidal anti-inflamnatory drugs; SIADH, syndrome of inappropriate antidiuretic hormone secretion. SSRIs, selective serotonin reuptake inhibitors.

*Reserpine in doses >0.25 mg was added to the list.

†Ditropan was modified to refer to the immediate-release formulation only and not Ditropan XL and iron supplements was modified to include only ferrous sulfate.

‡Do not consider the long-acting dipyridamole, which has better properties than the short-acting dipyridamole in older adults (except with patients with artificial heart valves).

REFERENCES

Abram, H. S. (1972). The psychology of chronic illness. *Journal of Chronic Disease, 25*(12), 659-64.

American Association of Public Health. (2001). Effective interventions for reducing racial and ethnic disparities in health. *American Journal of Public Health, 91*, 485–486.

Baena-Cagnani, C. E. (2001). The global burden of asthma and allergic diseases: The challenge for the new century. *Current Allergy & Asthma Reports, 1,* 297–298.

Barber, N. D., Alldred, D. P., Raynor, D. K., Dickinson, R., & Zermansky, A. G. (2009). Care homes' use of medicines study: Prevalence, causes and potential harm of medication errors in care homes for older people. *Quality & Safety in Health Care, 18*(5), 341–346.

Barnes, S. J. (2002). Long-term care. In I. M. Lubkin & P. D. Larsen (Eds.), *Chronic illness: Impact and interventions* (5th ed., pp. 533–554). Sudbury, MA: Jones & Bartlett.

Centers for Disease Control and Prevention (CDC). (2010). Chronic disease prevention and health promotion. Retrieved April 3, 2010, from http://www.cdc.gov/chronicdisease/overview/index.htm

Claxton, A. (2000). Patient compliance to a new enteric-coated weekly formulation of fluoxetine during continuation treatment of major depressive disorder. *Journal of Clinical Psychiatry, 6,* 928–932.

Commission on Chronic Illness. (1957). *Chronic illness in the United States, prevention of chronic illness.* Cambridge, MA: Harvard University Press.

Curtin, M, & Lubkin, I. (1995). What is chronicity? In Lubkin, I., Editor *Chronic Illness: Impact and Intervention, 3rd Ed.* Sudbury, MA: Jones & Bartlett.

Federal Interagency Forum on Aging-Related Statistics. (2008). *Older Americans 2008: Key indicators of well-being.* Washington, DC: U.S. Government Printing Office.

Feldman, D. (1974). Chronic disabling illness: A holistic view. *Journal of Chronic Diseases, 27,* 287–291.

Fick, D. M., Cooper, J. W., Wade, W. E., Waller, J. L., Maclean, J. R., & Beers, M. H. (2003). Updating the Beers Criteria for Potentially Inappropriate Medication Use in Older Adults: Results of a U.S. census panel of experts. *Archives of Internal Medicine, 163,* 2716–2724.

Frank, L., & Miramontes, H. (1998). *Health care provider adherence curriculum.* Pittsburgh, PA: AIDS Education and Training Centers Program.

Furukawa, T. A., Streiner, D. L., & Young, L. T. (2001). Is antidepressant benzodiazepine combination therapy clinically more useful? A meta-analytic study. *Journal of Affective Disorders, 65,* 173–177.

Jack, L., Jr., Mukhtar, Q., Martin, M., Rivera, M., Lavinghouze, S. R., Jernigan, J., et al. (2006). Program evaluation and chronic diseases: Methods, approaches, and implications for public health. In *Preventing chronic disease: Public health research, practice, and policy* [Serial online]. Retrieved February 21, 2006, from http://www.cdc.gov/pcd/issues/2006jan/05_0141.htm

Jackson, P. L. (2000). The primary care provider and children with chronic conditions. In P. L. Jackson & J. A. Vessey (Eds.), *Primary care of the child with a chronic condition* (3rd ed., pp. 3–19). St. Louis, MO: Mosby.

Jani, A. A., Stewart, A., Nolen, R. D., & Tavel, L. (2002). Medication adherence and patient education. Florida AIDS Education & Training Center. In *HIV/AIDS primary care guide* (pp. 83–92). Gainesville, FL: University of Florida Press.

Kim, H. K., Park, J. H., Park, J. H., & Kim, J. H. (2010). Differences in adherence to antihypertensive medication regimens according to psychiatric diagnosis: Results of a Korean population-based study. *Psychosomatic Medicine, 72*(1), 80-87.

Kurz, J. M., & Shepard, M. P. (2005). Families with chronic illness. In S. Harmon-Hanson, V. Gedaly-Duff, & J. Rowe Kaakinen (Eds.), *Family healthcare nursing: Theory, practice, and research* (3rd ed., pp. 413–435). Philadelphia: F.A. Davis.

Litaker, D., Koroukian, S. M., & Love, T. E. (2005). Context and healthcare access: Looking beyond the individual. *Medical Care, 43,* 531–540.

Lubkin, I., & Larsen, P. D. (2002). What is chronicity? In I. M. Lubkin & P. D. Larsen (Eds.), *Chronic illness: Impact and interventions* (5th ed., pp. 3–24). Sudbury, MA: Jones & Bartlett.

Luggen, A. S. (2005). Pharmacology update: Inappropriate prescribing in the long-term care setting. *Geriatric Nursing, 26*(4), 233.

Meiner, S. E. (2002). The advanced practice nurse in chronic illness. In I. M. Lubkin & P. D. Larson (Eds.), *Chronic illness: Impact and interventions* (5th ed., pp. 453–467). Sudbury, MA: Jones & Bartlett.

Mendis, S., & Salas, M. (2003). Hypertension. In *Adherence to long-term therapies: Evidence for action* (pp. 107–114). Geneva, Switzerland: World Health Organization.

Molony, S. (2004). Beers Criteria for Potentially Inappropriate Medication Use in the Elderly. *Dermatology Nursing, 16,* 547–548. Retrieved April 19, 2006, from www.medscape.com/viewarticle/496383

Morisky, D. E., Green, L. W., & Levine, D. M. (1986). Concurrent and predictive validity of a self-reported measure of medication adherence. *Medical Care, 24,* 67–74.

National Center for Health Statistics. (2009). *Health, United States, 2009: With special feature on medical technology.* Hyattsville, MD: U.S. Government Printing Office.

Pepper, G. A., & Towsley, G. L. (2007). Medication errors in nursing homes: Incidence and reduction strategies. *Journal of Pharmaceutical Finance, Economics & Policy, 16*(1), 5–133.

Peveler, R., & Tejada, M. L. (2003). Depression. In *Adherence to long-term therapies: Evidence for action* (pp. 65–70). Geneva, Switzerland: World Health Organization.

Rand, C., Bender, B., Boulet, L. P., Chaustre, I., & Weinstein, A. (2003). Asthma. In *Adherence to long-term therapies: Evidence for action* (pp. 47–58). Geneva, Switzerland: World Health Organization.

Tai-Seale, M., Groghan, T. W., & Obenchain, R. (2000). Determinants of antidepressant treatment compliance: Implications for policy. *Medical Care Research & Review, 57,* 491–512.

U.S. Census Bureau. (2006). S0103. Population 65 Years and Over in the United States: American FactFinder. Retrieved from http://factfinder.census.gov/servlet/STTable?_bm=y&-geo_id=01000US&-qr_name=ACS_2009_5YR_G00_S0103&-ds_name=ACS_2009_5YR_G00_&-_lang=en&-redoLog=false&-format=&-CONTEXT=st

von Korff, M. (1997). Collaborative management of chronic illness. *Annals of Internal Medicine, 172,* 1097–1102.

World Health Organization (2003). Adherence to Long Term Therapies – Evidence for Action. World Health Organization: Geneva. Retrieved from http://apps.who.int/medicinedocs/en/d/Js4883e/6.html

Wright, J. M. (2000). Choosing a first line drug in the management of elevated blood pressure. What is the evidence? *Canadian Medical Association Journal, 163,* 57–60.

Wright, J. M., Lee, C., & Chambers, G. K. (2000). Real-world effectiveness of antihypertensive drugs. *Canadian Medical Association Journal, 162,* 190–191.

CHAPTER 53

PAIN MANAGEMENT: ACUTE AND CHRONIC PAIN

Anita Lee Wynne and Victoria LaPorte

Chapter Outline

OVERVIEW OF PAIN CONCEPTS

The International Association for the Study of Pain (IASP) defines pain as "an unpleasant sensory and emotional experience associated with actual or potential tissue damage, or described in terms of such damage." Pain is always subjective and is, therefore, often undertreated by many providers when they look for objective signs of its existence. This undertreatment can lead to serious clinical consequences (Institute for Clinical Systems Improvement [ICSI], 2008a) The focus of this chapter is on the physiological aspects of pain and its management with drugs. Pain is far more complex that this simple explanation. The discussion of the pain experience that follows is based on material in McCance and Huether (2006).

The Experience of Pain

Pain involves the interactions of three major systems:

- **Sensory/discriminative system.** This system processes information about the strength, intensity, and temporal/spatial aspects of pain. Afferent nerve fibers, the spinal cord, the brainstem, and higher brain centers are all involved. The result is prompt withdrawal from the painful stimulus, when possible.
- **Motivational/affective system.** This system determines the conditioned or learned approach and avoidance behaviors related to experiencing pain. The reticular formation, limbic system, and brainstem are involved. The reticular system helps maintain an alert state; the limbic system regulates the emotional response.
- **Cognitive/evaluative system.** This system allows the person to interpret the pain experience and decide what behavior is appropriate in the circumstances in which the pain is occurring. Cultural input, male and female roles, and past experiences with pain contribute to this interpretation. Influences from this system may block, modulate, or enhance the perception of pain. Higher brain centers are mainly involved.

Pain Threshold and Pain Tolerance

There is no direct relationship between a nociceptive (pain) stimulus and the experience of or response to that stimulus. The pain threshold is the point at which that stimulus is experienced as pain. It varies significantly among people and within the same person over time. Sometimes, pain in one area may make pain in another area seem less or it may be ignored. This is especially true if the initial pain is perceived to represent a significant threat to the person (e.g., chest pain). This is referred to as *perceptual dominance.* Even if pain is occurring in several sites, only the most severe or the important in the perception of the person experiencing the pain may be reported. Patients need to be questioned about all pain sites; the one they perceive as most important may be less so in terms of what may be necessary to treat.

Pain tolerance is the duration of time or the intensity of pain that a person will endure before taking overt action to relieve the pain. The cognitive/evaluative system plays a large role in pain tolerance. Past experiences with pain are also a factor.

Pain tolerance generally decreases with repeated exposure to pain. Tolerance is also decreased by fatigue, anger, fear, and sleep deprivation. It may be increased by drugs, including **alcohol**; hypnosis; warmth; distracting activities; and strong beliefs or faith.

Neurological Basis of Pain

Anatomy

There are three integrated systems for the perception of pain. The *afferent pathways* bring pain signals to the spinal cord system, which consists of (1) A-delta fibers, which transmit rapid information and precise location of the stimulus; (2) C-fibers, which are slower and send poorly localized signals; and (3) the lamina in the dorsal horn of the cord where first-order neurons that received the initial stimulus synapse with second-order neurons that decussate and transmit the signal to the *brain (central nervous system [CNS])* via two divisions of the spinothalamic tract. The neospinothalamic tract carries sharp and intense acute pain signals to the midbrain, postcentral gyrus, and the cortex; the paleospinothalamic tract carries dull and burning (often visceral) pain signals to the reticular formation, pons, limbic system, and midbrain. Various portions of the CNS facilitate discrimination and localization of pain (ventroposterior and medial thalamic nuclei); arouse and alert the body; deal with motivational factors (limbic and reticular tracts, see previous discussion); and activate "fight or flight" responses through the release of cortisol (medulla and hypothalamus). *Efferent pathways* modulate the pain sensation through fibers that connect the reticular formation, midbrain, and substantia gelatinoza. Figure 53–1 depicts the anatomy of pain transmission.

Physiology

A wide range of neurotransmitters are involved in the neuromodulation of pain. Tissue injury results in the production of arachidonic acid, which cyclooxygenase (COX) catalyzes to produce prostaglandins (e.g., PGE_2, PGI_2, nitric oxide, bradykinins, and histamine). These inflammatory mediators depolarize adjacent nociceptors, causing acute pain. Lymphokines released from lymphocytes in chronic inflammatory states may contribute to some types of chronic pain. The role of anti-inflammatory agents can be explained by this mechanism.

Substance P, neurokinin A, and calcitonin gene–related peptide are released from peripheral pain receptors and promote the spread of pain locally. Norepinephrine (NE) and serotonin (5-hydroxytryptamine [5-HT]) modulate pain in the medulla and pons. They also inhibit pain sensations by traveling down the efferent fibers of the spinal cord. In pain management, the use of **tricyclic antidepressants (TCAs)** and **serotonin-norepinephrine reuptake inhibitors (SNRIs)**, both of which increase the levels of these neurotransmitters, can be partially explained by these mechanisms.

Endorphins (endogenous **morphines**) form three classifications of neuropeptides that inhibit pain transmission in the spinal cord and brain. *Beta-lipotropin* is a potent endorphin located in the hypothalamus and the pituitary gland. It is responsible for a general sensation of well-being. *Enkephalin* is a weaker analgesic but is longer lasting than morphine. *Dynorphin* is 50 times more potent than beta-lipotropin and originates in the neural lobe of the pituitary. All endorphins act by attaching to opiate receptors on the plasma membrane of the afferent neuron. When attached, they inhibit the release of excitatory neurotransmitters, such as substance P, to block the transmission of painful stimuli. *Narcotics are exogenous opiates*; this is their mode of action. Over 20 different opiate receptors have been identified in the hypothalamus. **Opiates** attach themselves to different receptors. Receptors that are sensitive to exogenous opiates vary among patients. Genetics and current and/or prior use of particular **opiates** affect one's unique response to **opiate** therapy.

Stress, excessive physical exertion, acupuncture, intercourse, and other nonpharmacological factors may increase the levels of circulating endogenous endorphins, NE, and 5-HT to raise the pain threshold. Some complementary and alternative therapies, including herbs, massage, and transdermal nerve stimulation, may be explained by these mechanisms.

Differences in Children and Older Adults

Pediatrics

There is a myth that children, especially infants, do not feel pain the way adults do, or if they do, there is no untoward consequence (Richeimer, 2009). Children, from preterm and newborn infants to older children, have functional pain pathways, centers for pain perception, and the neurotransmitters associated with pain transmission and modulation. In fact, the nociceptive system is functional in fetuses by 24 weeks of gestation. However, the enzyme systems involved in drug metabolism are

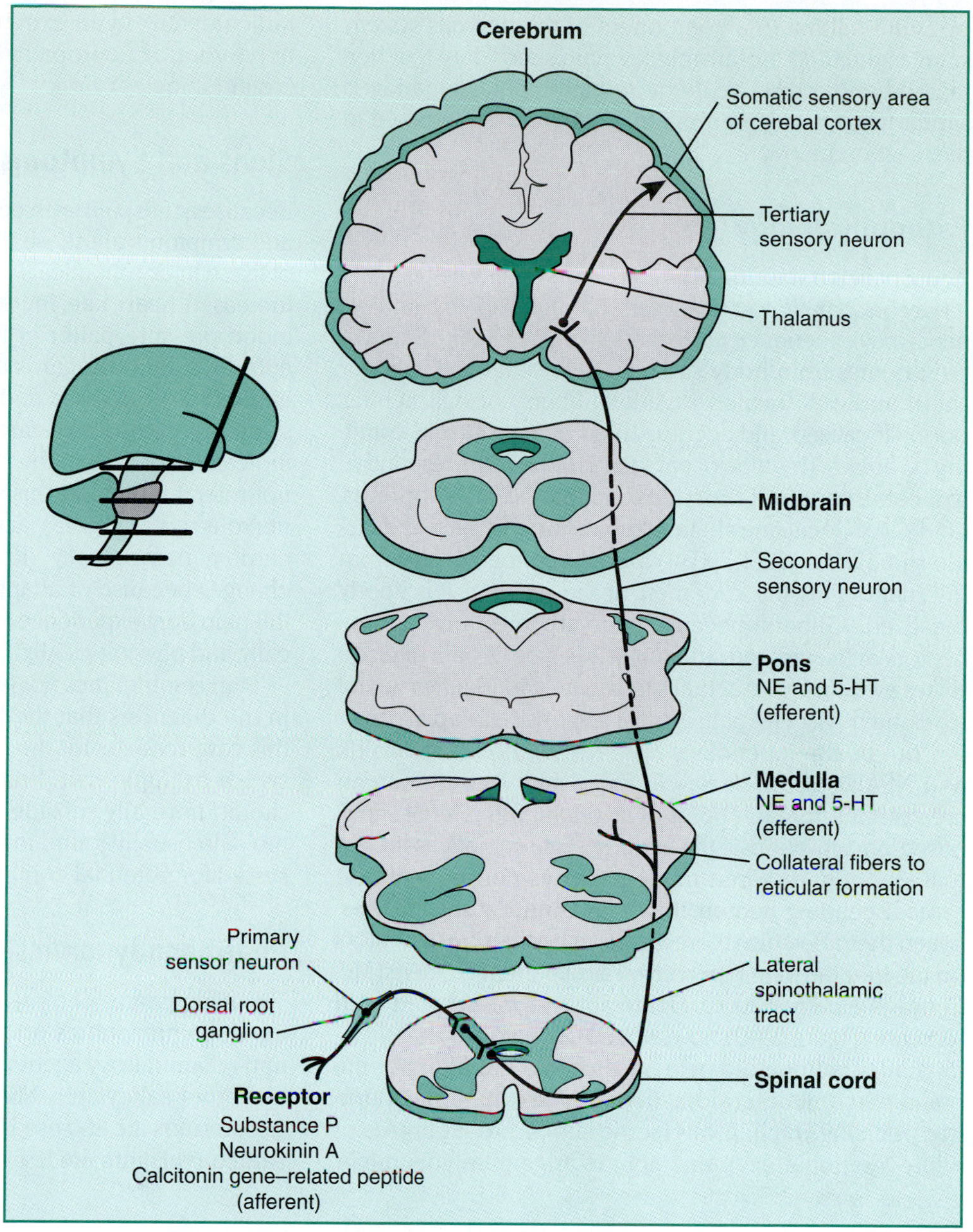

Figure 53–1. Anatomy of pain transmission.

immature in neonates and preterm infants (Richeimer, 2009). Prescribing drugs during pregnancy and the neonatal period should be done with the knowledge that repetitive, painful experiences and prolonged exposure to **analgesic drugs** during these periods may permanently alter synaptic and neuronal organization.

Children 5 to 18 years tend to have higher pain thresholds than do adults, but infants and children of all ages have the same highly individualized responses to pain as do adults.

Older Adults

Studies about pain in the older population have yielded conflicting results. Pain threshold is increased in some studies, but others show no change. It is possible that when increases in pain threshold occur, they are related to peripheral neuropathies and changes in the thickness of the skin rather than changes in pain pathways or neurotransmitters. A decrease in pain tolerance is evident in older adults, and women appear to be more sensitive to pain than men.

ACUTE PAIN

Acute pain is an event of recent onset, usually sudden and limited in duration. It can last from 1 second to less than 6 months. It characteristically has an identifiable source, suffering decreases over time; defining characteristics are more obvious; and there is a likelihood of eventual, complete relief. Acute pain is usually initiated by stimulation of nociceptive receptors on the body surfaces (somatic) or viscera. Acute pain may also be neuropathic, initiated by acute trauma to a component of the nervous system, such as the tingling, burning leg pain secondary to a herniated lumbar disc. Acute neuropathic pain is managed similarly to chronic neuropathic pain and is discussed in that section below.

Pathophysiology

Acute pain is a warning of actual or impending tissue injury. It may be somatic, visceral, referred, or neuropathic and patients may experience more than one type of pain. Somatic pain comes from body surfaces (e.g., skin) and is either sharp and well localized (A-delta fibers) or dull, aching, poorly localized, and accompanied by nausea and vomiting (C-fibers). This type of pain tends to be more responsive to **acetaminophen, corticosteroids, NSAIDs, opiates,** cold packs, local anesthetics (topical or infiltrate), and tactile stimulation (ICSI, 2008a) *Visceral pain* emanates from internal organs, the abdomen, or the skeleton. It is poorly localized (C-fibers) because there are fewer mechanoreceptors in the visceral structures. This type of pain often radiates away from the actual site of pain and requires skillful assessment. Visceral pain is most responsive to **opiate** therapy, but treatment choices also include **corticosteroids** and **NSAIDs** (ICSI, 2008a). *Referred pain* is present in an area distant from the point of its origin. The referral site is based on activation of the same spinal segment as the actual site of pain. When many impulses converge on the same ascending neuron, the brain cannot distinguish between them. Because there are more nociceptive receptors on the skin, the pain is perceived as experienced there (McCance & Huether, 2006). Figure 53–2 shows referred pain sites, and Figure 53–3 shows spinal dermatomes.

Acute neuropathic pain arises from central or peripheral nerve irritation (along dermatomes). It is often burning, prickling, tingling, or electric shock like. Examples of acute neuropathic pain include trigeminal neuralgia, radiculopathy in an extremity from pressure on a spinal nerve root, or neuropathy that accompanies the herpes zoster (shingles) virus.

Signs and Symptoms

Because acute pain is associated with tissue injury, the signs and symptoms are those that occur based on the release of tissue injury chemicals. Physiological responses include increased heart rate, increased respiratory rate, elevated blood pressure, pallor or flushing, dilated pupils, and diaphoresis. Blood sugar is elevated, gastric acid secretion and motility decrease, and blood flow to the viscera and skin decreases. Health-care providers often look for these indications of pain in their assessment of it. The body cannot tolerate being in this state of increased sympathetic nervous system (SNS) activation for long. Patients with chronic pain usually do not exhibit these acute SNS changes because of adaptation. This does not mean that the pain they experience is any less real, both psychologically and physiologically.

Pain is sometimes not proportional to what is expected in the diagnosis that the health-care provider makes. In this case, reassess for the possibility of a different diagnosis. For example, pain from a fracture that persists after it should normally subside and that is not proportional to the pain usually found in a healing fracture should be assessed for potential compartment syndrome.

Pharmacodynamics

Two main groups of drugs are used to treat acute pain: **exogenous morphines** and their derivatives (**opiates**) and **anti-inflammatory agents.** The latter group includes **aspirin** and **other salicylates, NSAIDs,** and **acetaminophen. Corticosteroids** are also used for their anti-inflammatory effects. **Anticonvulsants** are less commonly used in the treatment

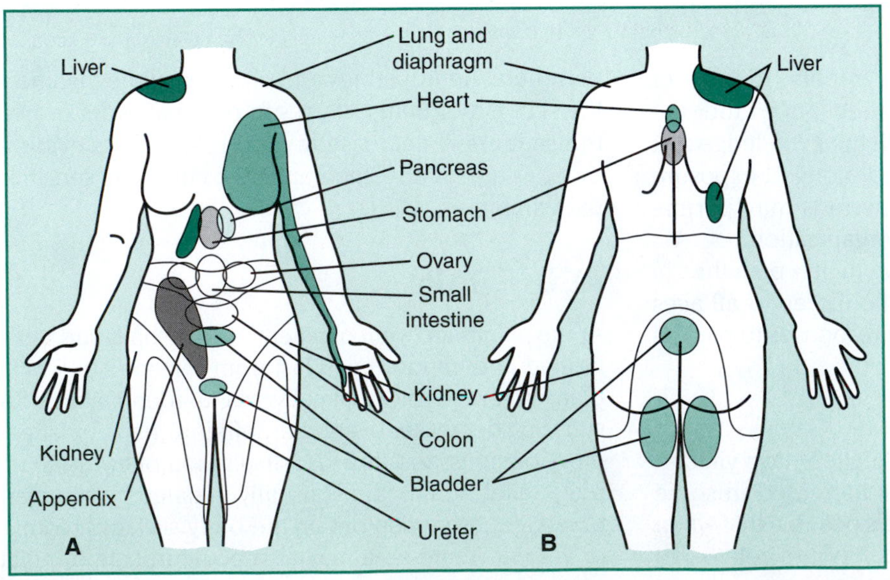

Figure 53–2. Referred pain sites.

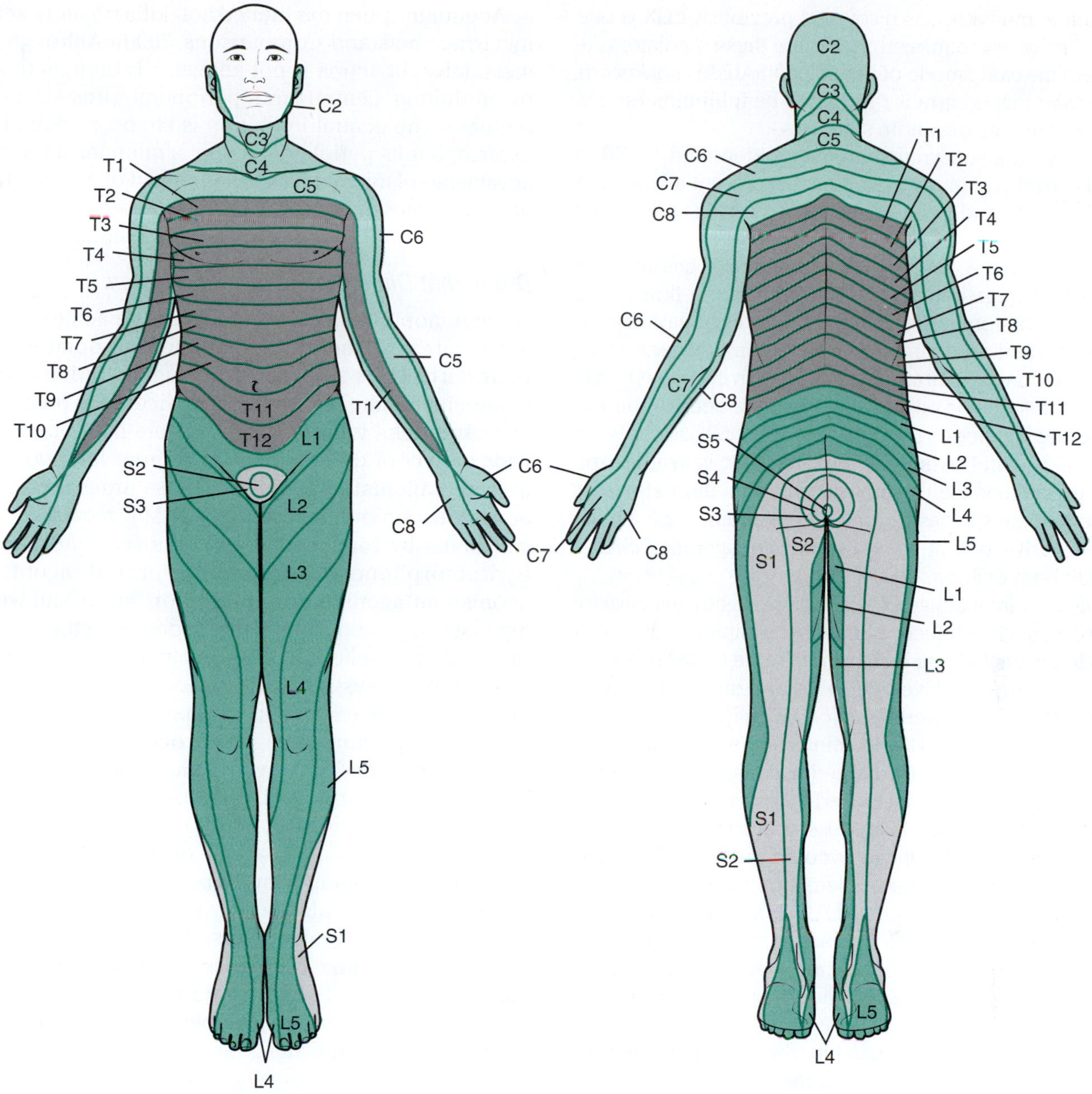

Levels of principal dermatomes

C5	Clavicles	**T10**	Level of umbilicus
C5, 6, 7	Lateral parts of upper limbs	**T12**	Inguinal or groin regions
C8, T1	Medial sides of upper limbs	**L1, 2, 3, 4**	Anterior and inner surfaces of lower limbs
C6	Thumb	**L4, 5, S1**	Foot
C6, 7, 8	Hand	**L4**	Medial side of great toe
C8	Ring and little fingers	**S1, S2, L5**	Posterior and outer surfaces of lower limbs
T4	Level of nipples	**S1**	Lateral margin of foot and little toe
		S2, 3, 4	Perineum

Figure 53–3. Spinal dermatomes.

of acute pain, and are indicated when acute pain has a neuropathic component, such as shingles.

Drugs That Reduce Inflammation

Inflammation is a common cause of pain and drugs that reduce inflammation and "turn off" the inflammatory mediators of pain are often the first drugs used in managing acute pain. **Salicylates** and **NSAIDs** reduce inflammation through their reduction of prostaglandins. Chapter 25 discusses these drugs. Their advantage in treating pain includes the fact that they reduce the need for **opioid** analgesics. Destruction of cell membranes results in release of chemical mediators, as discussed previously. COX is one of the enzymes required to produce these mediators. Although the exact mode of action of NSAIDs is not known, the major mechanism is thought to be inhibition of COX activity and prostaglandin synthesis.

Two COX isoenzymes have been identified. COX-1 is synthesized continuously so that it is present all the time in all tissues and cells, especially platelets; endothelial cells; the gastrointestinal (GI) tract; and renal microvasculature, glomeruli, and collecting ducts. It has roles in platelet aggregation, the regulation of blood flow to the kidney and stomach, and the regulation of gastric acid secretion and production of protective mucus, especially in the stomach. Inhibition of these activities by **NSAIDs** accounts for their adverse reactions, especially on the renal and GI tracts.

COX-2 is an "inducible" enzyme that is synthesized mainly in response to pain and inflammation. However, there is some synthesis in the kidney, brain, bone, female reproductive system, and GI tract. Nonspecific **NSAIDs** inhibit both COX-1 and COX-2.

NSAIDs are mainly COX-1 selective, slightly selective for COX-1, or slightly selective for COX-2. Chapter 25 discusses the drugs that fall into each group. Three COX-2–selective drugs have been developed that appear not to inhibit COX-1. These drugs were used for patients who had higher risks for GI bleeding. However, in 2004, research indicated that the overall risk for GI bleeding was not sufficient to compensate for the increased risk for cardiovascular events that occurred with these drugs (Drug Facts and Comparisons, 2009). Only **celocoxib (Celebrex)** remains on the market, and it has a black box warning related to this risk. All over-the-counter (OTC) **NSAIDs** also had their labeling revised in 2004 to include more specific information about potential GI and cardiovascular risks. In addition, a medication guide must now be provided with each prescription.

NSAIDs are primarily used for their anti-inflammatory activity, but they are effective for the relief of mild to moderate pain or, in the case of **ketorolac (Toradol)**, for moderate to severe pain (ICSI, 2008a). Their other actions and uses are discussed in Chapter 25. Before using **NSAIDS**, the hematological, gastrointestinal, and renal effects of these drugs should be taken into account.

All **salicylates** have analgesic properties, but **aspirin** is the prototype drug in this class. Their anti-inflammatory and analgesic activities are mediated through inhibition of prostaglandin synthesis in the same manner as **NSAIDs**. However, **aspirin** more potently inhibits prostaglandin synthesis and has greater anti-inflammatory activity than the **NSAIDs**. The acetyl group of the **aspirin** molecule is thought to be responsible for these differences. **Aspirin** acetylates the COX enzyme in the prostaglandin biosynthesis pathway. **Salicylates** are also effective for mild to moderate pain. Their other actions and uses are discussed in Chapter 25.

Acetaminophen has limited anti-inflammatory activity. (Drug Facts and Comparisons, 2009). Although its mechanism of action is not known, it is thought to act by inhibiting central and peripheral prostaglandin synthesis. The central inhibition is almost as potent as **aspirin**, but its peripheral action is minimal. It has the advantages of minimum GI irritation and of not affecting bleeding times or respiration. It is also useful for mild to moderate pain. It is also discussed in Chapter 25.

Drugs That Directly Affect Pain Receptors

When **nonopioid drugs** are ineffective for acute pain relief, **opiates** are the next logical step. All **opiates and their derivatives** are scheduled drugs requiring a Drug Enforcement Administration (DEA) license to prescribe. They are useful for moderate to severe pain. There is a wide variety of **opiates** that range from full **agonists** to mixed **agonist-antagonists**. These drugs are active at various opioid receptor sites. Mu receptors are stimulated by some strong **agonists** (e.g., **morphine, hydromorphone, levorphanol**), **partial agonists/ agonist- antagonists** (e.g., **buprenorphine**), and **weak agonists** (e.g., **meperidine, methadone**) for the control of pain. Adverse effects at this receptor include euphoria, respiratory depression, constipation, urinary retention, and drug dependence. Kappa receptors also have **strong agonists** (e.g., **morphine, pentazocaine, nalbuphine, butorphanol**) and some with little or no activity (e.g., **methadone, levorphanol, meperidine**). Kappa receptors produce sedation, but little to no euphoria, respiratory depression, constipation, or urinary retention. **Naloxone** is an **antagonist** for both receptors. Delta receptors produce analgesia only when stimulated simultaneously with mu receptors, and sigma receptors apparently have no clear analgesic role and are associated with dysphoria and confusion. Nociceptive impulses appear to stimulate multiple receptors at the same time, so that both the analgesic effects and the adverse effects of all receptors may occur simultaneously. **Tramadol** and **tapentadol** are weak mu receptor agonists that also inhibit reuptake of norepinephrine, thereby demonstrating a dual-action analgesic effect. These drugs are discussed in more detail in Chapter 15 In addition to producing analgesia, **opiates** may also alter the perception of and emotional response to pain because these receptors are widely distributed in the CNS, including the limbic system, thalamus, hypothalamus, and midbrain. Some **opiate derivatives**, such as **codeine**, also have antitussive effects.

Goals of Treatment

The goal for treatment of acute pain is reduction or elimination of the pain sensation with a minimum of adverse reactions. Because acute pain has a high probability of complete relief, this is a realistic goal.

Rational Drug Selection

Algorithm

Figure 53–4 depicts the algorithm for the management of acute pain. Because acute pain is a short-term phenomenon, lifestyle modifications are largely directed toward reduction of the source of the painful stimulus, rest or immobilization of the affected part, elevation when possible, ice, or compression. Several of these are largely intended to reduce the effects of inflammation.

Oral administration of any pain drug is the route of choice if the patient has a functioning GI system. This route is the safest, least expensive, and most convenient. Other routes (e.g., IM, IV) are available for many pain drugs, but these are more expensive and less convenient and may require that they be given only at the clinic site or require additional patient instruction in their administration. For older adults the issue also arises of decreased muscle mass and less fatty tissue so that absorption via the IM route is significantly affected. The transdermal route falls somewhere between these two in safety, expense, and convenience. Epidural and intrathecal routes are rarely used in primary care

Drug Therapy

Analgesic/Anti-Inflammatory Drugs

Chapter 25 discusses in some detail the choice among these drugs related to pain management. **Ibuprofen** is the

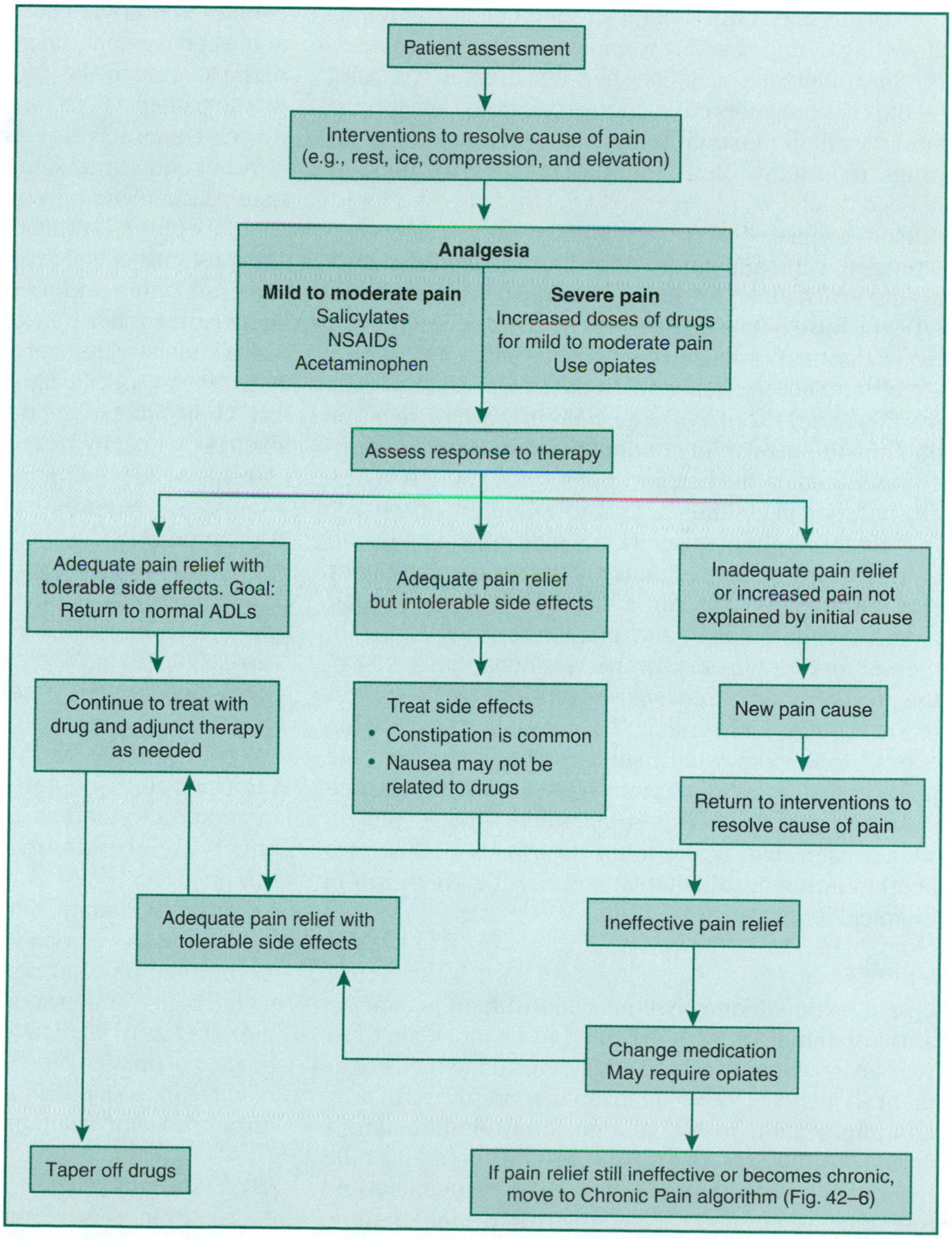

Figure 53–4. Acute pain management algorithm.

most commonly used NSAID because it is inexpensive, available OTC, and short acting, so that acute pain can be managed without long-term effects and adverse reactions. For women of childbearing age, it is Pregnancy Category B. For nursing women, it is not detected in breast milk, unlike many other NSAIDs. However, all NSAIDs are Pregnancy Category D during the third trimester. Ibuprofen has been approved for children 6 months of age or older (http://www.fda.gov). Naproxen sodium reaches its peak of action more rapidly; however, safety has not been established for children 2 years of age or younger. This drug is also Pregnancy Category B except during the last trimester. When an injectable NSAID is needed, only ketorolac has such a formulation. It is Pregnancy Category C, but found in breast milk in quantities that contradict its use in nursing mothers. It has no published doses for children of any age. NSAIDs come in short-acting, intermediate-acting, and long-acting formulations. Because there is no clear difference in efficacy between drugs in this class, health-care providers often choose one from each formulation for their personal formulary and prescribe these drugs repeatedly based on the duration of therapy needed.

Pain associated with inflammation is especially well managed with salicylates. Aspirin is the gold standard against which others are judged. It is inexpensive, available OTC, the most potent analgesic in the class, and short acting, so that acute pain can be managed without long-term effects and adverse reactions. It has limitations, however. It is Pregnancy Category D, especially in the third trimester, and contraindicated in children with influenza or chickenpox. Based on the risk for Reye's syndrome, it is generally not used in children.

Acetaminophen is useful in treating mild to moderate pain in which inflammation is not the major component. It is not intended for pain management for more than 5 days in children or 10 days in adults because of the increased risk for hepatic adverse reactions. Immaturity of the newborn hepatic enzymes severs a protective role in this age group (Richeimer, 2009). For adults, 325 to 650 mg every 4 to 6 hours usually suffices. Children's doses are published for ages from 3 months to 14 years; however, the dosing of this drug is more accurate when based on weight. After age 14, the adult dose is used. Doses for acetaminophen, salicylates, and NSAIDs are shown in Chapter 25.

Opiates

If pain is not adequately controlled with an analgesic/anti-inflammatory or is expected to be moderate to severe, an appropriate opiate should be added to the treatment. If patients have an absolute or strong relative contraindication to the analgesic/anti-inflammatory group of drugs, an opiate can be considered for mild to moderate pain. Opiates have high abuse potential and tolerance is common. Fixed-interval dosing is more effective in achieving pain relief than "as-needed" dosing. Morphine is considered to be the standard opiate, but selection among these drugs may be based on a variety of factors. Opiates are discussed in more detail in Chapter 15.

Severity of Pain

Codeine, oxycodone, and hydrocodone are drugs of choice for moderate pain. Although they are available as independent formulations, they often work better in combination with aspirin or acetaminophen. One advantage of these drugs is their oral formulation. Tramadol and tapentadol, alone or in combination with acetaminophen, may also be used. Keep in mind that these latter two opiates are also norepinephrine reuptake inhibitors, and have more drug interactions than pure opiates.

For severe pain, morphine, oxycodone, oxymorphone, hydromorphone, and fentanyl are better choices. Fentanyl is available in a transdermal formulation when the ability to swallow is a problem or there is a desire to avoid the IM route. This drug is generally reserved for the patient who is tolerant to opiates and rarely used for acute pain. It is also less likely to produce the adverse effects common to stimulation of the mu receptor, because it stimulates only one subset (mu-1) of these receptors. Morphine is available in many formulations and is the most cost effective. Hydromorphone is more potent than morphine and used when high doses are needed. Meperidine is less potent than morphine and has a neurotoxic metabolite (normeperidine) that affects its use. ICSI (2008b) specifically recommends that it not be a first-line choice due to the dosing limitations to prevent CNS excitatory toxicity from normeperidine accumulation. Patients with impaired renal function, including older adults, are at particularly high risk for CNS toxicity. Morphine (MS Contin), oxycodone (OxyContin), and fentanyl (Duragestic patches) come in long-acting formulations. These latter formulations are used less often in acute pain. Oral formulations of many of these drugs tend to be less effective than IM formulations and may require higher doses. Equianalgesic doses are found in Table 53–1.

Antitussive Effects

Choosing among opiates may also be based on factors in addition to their ability to relieve pain. If antitussive effects are also desired, codeine is probably best in this area.

Anticonvulsants, such as neurontin, are powerful modulators of neuropathic pathways, thereby decreasing the burning, prickling sensations that accompany neuropathic pain. Caution should be observed when introducing this class of medication, as they are sedating, and they potentiate opiates. Another side effect of anticonvulsant medication is suicidal ideation and abrupt withdrawal is associated with a withdrawal syndrome.

Route of Administration

Although most have multiple formulations, the route chosen may be influenced by the amount of skeletal

Table 53–1 **Equianalgesic Doses of Oral, Intramuscular, and Transdermal Opiates**

Drug/Dose	Ratio	Comparable Morphine	Comparable Analgesic
Codeine 30–60 mg (PO/IR)			Aspirin 650 mg
Codeine 90 mg (PO) or 60 mg IM	0.15:1	Morphine 10 mg (PO)	
Fentanyl (TD)† 25 mcg/h 50 mcg/h 75 mcg/h 100 mcg/h	1:3.5	Oral morphine/24 h 45–134 mg 135–224 mg 225–314 mg 315–404 mg Oral morphine 30 mg (SR) q8h	Oxycontin 10 mg q12h Oxycontin 20 mg q12h
Hydrocodone (PO) 5 mg	1:1	Morphine 10 mg (IM) Morphine 5 mg (PO)	
Hydromorphone 4 mg (PO) or 2 mg (IM)	1:4	Morphine 15 mg (PO) Morphine 10 mg (IM)	
Meperidine 50 mg (PO)§			Aspirin 650 mg
Meperidine 100 mg (PO)§	0.1:1	Morphine 10 mg (PO)	
Methadone 10 mg (PO)	‡	Morphine 10 mg (IM) Morphine 30–45 mg (PO)	
Morphine 15 mg (PO/IR) 30 mg (SR)		Morphine 10 mg (IM) Morphine 10 mg (IM)	
Oxycodone (PO) 5 mg 20 mg 10 mg q12h (CR)	1:1.5	Morphine 30 mg (IM) Morphine 15 mg q8h	Codeine 60 mg (PO)
Pentazocine 30 mg (PO) 60 mg (IM)	0.17:1	Morphine 10 mg (IM)	Aspirin 650 mg
Tramadol 50 (PO)			

CR = controlled release; IR = immediate release; SR = sustained release; TD = transdermal.
When converting from short-acting opiates to timed release, start with half to two-thirds of the equianalgesic dose.
† Maximum effect of fentanyl is achieved in 12–18 h. Allow 12–18 h for fentanyl to wash out before initiating oral timed-release opiates.
‡ The half-life of methadone varies from 15–40 h and, with chronic administration, methadone accumulates in body tissues. Ratio between methadone and other opiates may vary widely as a function of previous dose exposure.
§ These drugs should be avoided in adults over 65 years, or in those with renal insufficiency or chronic pain. Do not exceed 600 mg/24 h and total duration is not to exceed 48 h for meperidine. Toxic metabolites accumulate, which are not reversible by naloxone.

muscle tissue (IM) or fatty tissue (subcutaneous). Skeletal muscle and fatty tissue have fairly slow absorption and release and can act as storage reservoirs. IM administration should be avoided in older adults because of muscle wasting and less fatty tissue in this population compared to younger adults. In addition, IM absorption of **analgesics** is slower and may result in delayed/prolonged effect of the drug, altered **analgesic** serum levels and possible toxicity with repeated injections. This is more common with **meperidine** than it is with **morphine** (Herr, Bjoro, Steffensmeier, & Rakel, 2006). Rectal absorption is erratic.

Transdermal **opiate** formulations give a consistent, slow release of drug over 24 hours. When using the transdermal route, calculate 24-hour drug requirements in determining dose of patch to use.

Dermal **lidocaine** is an excellent choice for the acute neuropathic pain that accompanies the herpes zoster virus. Apply no more than three patches to the allodynic dermatome at one time, and make certain that the skin is intact. It is not appropriate to apply **lidocaine** cream or patches to blistered or crusted skin.

Patient Variables

Age

Issues related to infants and children are discussed previously for **anti-inflammatories/analgesics.** However, **opiate** metabolism in the neonate is different. Because hepatic enzymes take 3 to 6 months to mature, the half-life of **morphine** is twice as long in the neonate as in the adult (Richeimer, 2009). Older adults have reduced renal function, and **aspirin** and **NSAIDs** are heavily dependent on the renal system for excretion. Use of these drugs in older adults may require dosage adjustments. Use the lowest effective dose for the shortest possible time. Age also appears to increase the risk for adverse reactions to **NSAIDs**. The risk for serious ulcer disease is greater in adults over age 65. This risk appears to be dose dependent, and reduced dosages may be necessary. GI and renal function should be monitored closely in all older adults taking these drugs for more than a few days. **Ibuprofen** and **naproxen** are preferred nonselective **NSAIDs** for use with older adults due to the lower adverse effects profiles compared to other nonselective **NSAIDs** (Herr et al, 2006). **Piroxicam (Feldene)** should be avoided in the older adults because its long half-life results in drug accumulation and can lead to toxicity.

Indomethacin produces the most CNS adverse effects and should be avoided in the older adult (Howard, Dolovich, Kaczorowski, Sellors, & Sellors, 2004). **Ketorolac** is cleared more slowly in older adults. **Nabumetone** shows no difference in overall efficacy and safety between older adults and younger patients.

Acetaminophen is the preferred **nonopiate** for mild to moderate pain in children and older adults because it is cost effective, has no effect on platelets, and has fewer adverse effects than **NSAIDs** or **aspirin** (Herr et al, 2006). The dose must not exceed 4 gm/day in older adults with a maximum dose of 3 g/day in the frail older adult, with the trend being toward lower doses. **Opiates** are useful in the management of moderate to severe pain in older adults. The mu agonists (**morphine, oxycodone**) are the first-line drugs in this group (Herr et al, 2006). **Opiates** with short half-lives are the best choices (**hydrocodone, morphine, hydromorphone, oxycodone**). **Morphine** is the drug of choice because it has a short half-life formulation and can be easily administered and titrated, and its metabolites are usually not clinically significant when used short term. **Hydromorphone** is an acceptable alternative because it also has a short half-life and can be used in patients with renal impairment (Herr et al, 2006). Its metabolites are also not clinically significant when used short term. **Oxycodone** provides excellent pain relief with no clinically significant metabolites. It is available in both short-acting and long-acting formulations. Because these drugs also have increased risk for adverse reactions in older adults, it is best to initiate therapy at a 25 to 50 percent lower dose than used for younger adults and slowly titrate the dose up by 25 percent on a individual basis until there is either a 50 percent reduction in the pain rating or the patient reports satisfactory pain relief (Herr et al, 2006). Although there is no maximum dose for the mu agonists, **opiate** adverse effects are dose related. For breakthrough pain, a fast-acting mu agonist with a short half-life is preferred. Breakthrough doses are 10 to 15 percent of the total daily around-the-clock dose and may be made available every 3 to 4 hours when the patient is on oral therapy. The adverse reactions of constipation and urinary retention are commonly related to the normal physiological changes of aging. Decreased pulmonary function associated with aging may be accentuated by the respiratory depressant effects of **opiates**. Care should be used if older adults require these drugs for pain management, and the duration of therapy should be short.

Certain drugs should be used with extreme caution, if at all, in older adults. **Benzodiazepines** do not provide analgesia and can cause severe adverse effects in the older adult. They can be used to diminish muscle spasm and reduce anxiety. Short- and intermediate-acting agents (**alprazolam [Xanax], lorazepam [Ativan], oxazepam [Serax]**) are preferred. **Codeine** should be avoided because the dose required to effectively relieve pain is associated with an increased incidence of adverse effects. It is also ineffective in patients with impaired CYP2D6 activity (admittedly not a large number of patients) because it cannot covert to **morphine** in this population. **Meperidine** is contraindicated in older adults because its metabolite is toxic to the CNS. The incidence of CNS adverse effects is higher in older patients.

Opiate pharmacokinetics in the neonate are different even from other children. Because hepatic enzymes take time to mature (3 to 6 months), the half-life of **morphine** is twice as long in this population, requiring adjustments in dose and time between doses. **Opiates** generally should be avoided in children except for very short duration. Some specific **opiates** (e.g., **oxycodone, propoxyphene, methadone, oxymorphone, tramodol, tapendadol,** and **hydromorphone**) should not be used in children.

Dementia

Dementia is considered separately from age because not all older adults have dementia and dementia may occur prior to age 65. Older adults and others with cognitive impairment experience pain but are often unable to verbalize it effectively (Horgas & Yoon, 2008). Acute pain can occur in persons with dementia, but the lack of objective markers means it is underrecognized and undertreated. Poorly managed pain can result in behavioral symptoms and lead to unnecessary use of psychotropic drugs in this population. For this reason, careful observation of patients with dementia when they move may uncover problems that may not occur at rest

In addition, behavioral symptoms such as agitation and mood changes, physical indications of pain, and withdrawal from usual activities may indicate pain. Potential sources of pain that the cognitively impaired may be unable to report such as distended bladder, infection, inflammation, positioning, urinary tract infection, and constipation, should also be assessed (Herr et al, 2006). Assessment tools for determining pain in dementia patients may be found by contacting the Alzheimer's Disease Association at http://www.alz.org. Commonly used tools include the Mini Mental Status Examination and the Six-Item Mental Status Screener (Herr et al, 2006). The Checklist of Nonverbal Pain Indications (Feldt, 2000, reported in Herr et al, 2006) is an observational tool developed for use with nonverbal older adults and includes six pain behavioral items commonly observed in older adults in acute pain. Pain scales have been developed for noncommunicating children (Breau, McGrath, Camfield, & Finley, 2002) and one such pain scale has been adapted for use with adults with severe to profound mental retardation (Bodfish, Harper, Deacon, Deacon, & Symons, 2006). This pain scale (Pain and Discomfort Scale—PADS) is also appropriate for use with older adults who have dementia. It includes a standardized physical exam, pain exam procedure and requires no more than 10 minutes to complete. The scale can be downloaded from http://www.dads.tx.state.us/quality matters/qcp/pain/PADS.pdf. Another pain scale developed specifically for older adults with advanced dementia is the PAINAD scale, which was developed by Ladislav Volicer and others. It can be downloaded from the http://www.dads site. Dr. Volicer can be contacted for questions about the scale at lvolicer@cas.usf.edu.

Reduced mental capacity does not mean reduced ability to feel pain, and pain should be adequately managed in this population. When choosing a pain medication, consider all the adverse reactions to the drug chosen including effects on dementia and cognitive functioning (Alzheimer's Disease Association, 2005). In addition to affecting the ability to accurately assess pain in these older adults, cognitive-behavioral therapies that focus on changing pain perception (e.g., relaxation, education, and distraction) may not be appropriate for cognitively impaired persons (Horgas & Yoon, 2008)

Pregnancy

Pregnancy categories are discussed previously for **anti-inflammatories/analgesics**. Safe use of **opiates** during pregnancy and in nursing women has not been established, and they are Pregnancy Category C. Short-term use for acute pain, however, appears to be acceptable. Infants born to mothers addicted to these drugs suffer from sedation and respiratory depression and experience physiological withdrawal during the neonatal period.

Concomitant Diseases

Patients with a history of GI bleeding probably should not use **aspirin** or **NSAIDs**. Serious GI bleeding, ulceration, and perforation can occur at any time without warning symptoms. Studies have not identified any subset of patients not at risk for these problems. A history of serious GI events, alcoholism, and smoking are the only specific factors associated with increased risk. Based on these data, active or chronic inflammation or ulceration of the GI tract relatively contraindicates use of all NSAIDs, especially **indomethacin** and **sulindac**.

Concurrent liver disease means cautious use of NSAIDs and contraindicates the use of **acetaminophen**. Further discussion of specific diseases is found in Chapter 25.

Patients with adrenal insufficiency or hypothyroidism may have prolonged and exaggerated responses to **opiates**. Patients with impaired hepatic or renal function will have prolonged half-lives of **opiates** and **anticonvulsants**. Doses should be reduced for these patients. **Fentanyl** and **methadone** are the safest drugs to use with renal failure patients.

Monitoring

The best monitoring system for acute pain is simply asking patients about their pain, having them rate it on an appropriate scale, and adjusting drug dosages and schedules based on responses. Table 53–2 shows the history and physical examination data assessed for acute pain. Table 53–3 compares some pain assessment tools used in children including the appropriate age for the use of each one and the advantages and disadvantage of each.

Table 53–2 **Assessment of Acute Pain**

History Data
• Severity of pain on a numerical rating scale or other appropriate scale based on age and mental status (rating 1–6 mild to moderate pain; 7–10 severe pain) • Characteristics of pain: pain onset, quality, duration, and variability • Previous pain experiences and treatments • Alleviating and aggravating patterns • Parents can help assess pain in children by what the child says and does and how his or her body is reacting, based on what are normal responses for that child.
Physical Examination Data
• Location and source of pain with consideration of possible referred source • Indications of inflammation (redness, swelling, heat) • Objective signs of pain: grimacing, guarding, vital sign changes, etc. (vital signs may be normal based on physiological adaptation)

Table 53–3 **Self-Report Measures of Pain in Children**

Device	Description	Age Range	Advantages	Disadvantages
Faces Scale	Faces showing intensity of pain	6–8 yr	Test/retest reliability	No validity test completed
Visual Analog Scale	Vertical line with numerical anchors	5 yr +	Reliable, valid, and versatile. Can relate to dimensions	Must understand proportionality
Oucher Scale	6 photos of children showing pain	3–12 yr	Pictorial and numerical range; broader age proportionality	Must understand concept
Poker Chip Scale	Quantifies pain by the number of chips (0–4) child sees	5 yr +	Proportionality	Requires ability to understand concept
Body Outlines	Children color area that hurts	3 yr +	Can show exact area of pain. May indicate intensity.	Children tend to associate blue with cold and red with hot. What color is "pain"?
Pain Diary	Numerical rating along with time, activity, drugs, etc.	Adolescent	Useful to determine patterns of pain and self-taught management strategies	Requires commitment

Source: Adapted from Suresh, S. (2002). Chronic pain management in children and adolescents. *The Children's Doctor: Journal of Children's Memorial Hospital, Chicago*. Retrieved October 22, 2009, from http://www.childsdoc.org/spring2002/chronic pain.asp. Richeimer, S. (2009). Acute and post operative pain management for children. Retrieved October 22, 2009, from http://www.spineuniverse.com/displayarticle.php/article392.html

Outcome Evaluation

Figure 53–4 shows the treatment algorithm for acute pain. Outcome evaluation targets relief of symptoms. Patients who have adequate pain relief based on their own assessment of their pain and who remain symptom free require no specific follow-up.

Patients who do not respond to standard therapy should have their pain reassessed to determine if the diagnoses of the sources of the pain are correct, and different drugs or different combinations of drugs and nonpharmacological therapy should be tried. Questions to ask include the following:

- Are several pain-relief measures being used? Should additional measures be taken?
- Are the pain relief measures being used before the pain becomes severe? Studies have shown that fixed-interval dosing that provides anticipatory analgesia is more effective than "as-needed" dosing.
- Is what the patient believes to be effective included in the treatment? There is a placebo effect for all pain treatment, and if the patient does not believe the chosen treatment will be effective, it probably will not be.
- Is the patient willing and able to be an active participant in the pain management?
- How can this active participation be facilitated?

If the patient still does not respond to standard therapy or appropriate adjustments with adequate pain relief, or if he or she develops complications associated with the source of the pain, consultation with or referral to a pain specialist may be needed. Such consultation may also be helpful in the case of chemical dependency, even if adequate pain relief is gained.

Patient Education

Patient education should include a discussion of information related to the overall treatment plan as well as that specific to the drug therapy, reasons for the drug being taken, drugs as part of the total treatment regimen, and adherence issues.

ACUTE PAIN MANAGEMENT

PATIENT EDUCATION

Related to the Overall Treatment Plan and Disease Process

- Pathophysiology of pain and its cause (where appropriate), at a level the patient can understand, to explain how the drugs work.
- Importance of adherence to the treatment regimen.
- Indications for contacting the health-care provider when pain relief is ineffective.
- Need for follow-up visit(s) with the primary care provider.

ACUTE PAIN MANAGEMENT—CONT'D

PATIENT EDUCATION

Specific to the Drug Therapy

- Reasons for taking the drug(s) and the anticipated action of these drug(s) in pain relief.
- Doses and schedules for taking the drug(s), including early round-the-clock dosing of drugs.
- Possible adverse reactions and what to do if they occur.

Reasons for Taking the Drug(s)

- Patient education about specific drugs is provided in Chapters 15 and 25. The explanations should be clear about what pain drugs can and cannot do.

Drugs as Part of the Total Treatment Regimen

- Role of both pharmacological and nonpharmacological treatments for pain and their interconnection.

Adherence Issues

- The fact that most acute pain can be resolved should be stressed. The importance of that resolution to avoid the development of chronic pain should be addressed.
- Adherence to the drug regimen is important to resolving acute pain.

CHRONIC PAIN

Chronic pain, unlike acute pain, is less easily differentiated, and defining characteristics are less obvious. Its intensity is more difficult to evaluate; suffering usually increases over time; and there is little chance of complete relief. The source of the pain may have originally been determined, but it is no longer clear. Duration is often greater than 6 months. To clearly differentiate between untreated acute pain and ongoing chronic pain, ICSI (2008b) suggest that any pain that persists for 6 weeks (or longer than the anticipated healing time) requires a thorough evaluation to determine if it is chronic in nature. An effective tool for the assessment of changes in chronic pain severity over time is the Chronic Pain Grade (Elliott, Smith, Smith, & Chambers, 2000). Chronic pain includes cancer pain (malignant pain) and nonmalignant pain. Many medicolegal issues arise when managing chronic nonmalignant pain. The treatment areas of this section focus on nonmalignant pain, and this chapter deals with the multifaceted dynamics of managing the patient with this type of pain, including the relevant medicolegal issues.

Pathophysiology

Chronic pain may be persistent (e.g., back pain) or intermittent (migraines). It is physiologically different from acute pain. Differences include the following:

- Decreased levels of endorphins
- Predominance of C-neuron stimulation
- Lower threshold in sensitivity of neurons
- Spontaneous impulses from regenerating peripheral nerve
- Alterations in the dorsal root ganglion resulting in reorganization of nociceptive neurons
- Loss of pain inhibition in the spinal cord

Prolonged firing of peripheral C-fibers leads to *central sensitization* with an increase in excitability of medullary and spinal neurons. This stimulation causes the release of glutamate and aspartate, which act on *N*-methyl-D-aspartate (NMDA) receptors in the spinal cord to release nitric oxide (see prostaglandins in the Drugs That Reduce Inflammation section, earlier in this chapter). At this point, the spinal cord is more sensitive to all of its inputs, including ascending pain stimuli.

The four major forms of chronic pain are central pain, nonneuropathic pain, neuropathic pain, and psychogenic pain.

Central Pain

Central pain is caused by a lesion or dysfunction in the CNS. Possible lesions include infarction, hemorrhage, abscess, degeneration, tumors, or traumatic injury. Migraine and other headaches (see Chapter 35) also fall into this category. The pain may be experienced over a large or defined body area. This type of pain is usually irritating and constant and can cause considerable suffering. Treatment involves both correction and management of the central lesion and pain medication.

Nonneuropathic Pain

Nonneuropathic chronic pain is the result of any lesion that is noncancerous and not the result of nerve damage. The most common causes are inflammatory in nature, but the exact physiological basis may be unclear. A wide variety of general chronic pain syndromes is included in this classification. Myofascial pain syndromes are the second most common cause of chronic pain. These conditions include fibromyalgia (which is not inflammatory) and myositis, myalgia, and muscle strain (which have an inflammatory component). The pain is the result of muscle spasm, tenderness, and stiffness. These conditions lead to muscle guarding, resulting in limited muscle motion. Limited muscle motion leads to weakness and stiffness. The pain is described as dull and aching and may be mild to disabling. Early in the disease process, the pain tends to be localized, but later, it becomes generalized. When the pain has an inflammatory component, **anti-inflammatory/ analgesics** are appropriate. In other cases, TCAs and **serotonin reuptake inhibitors** may be used.

Fibromyalgia symptoms and myofascial pain syndromes are common chronic musculoskeletal disorders in which chronic pain is a major component. They deserve a brief specific discussion. Both syndromes have some degree of controversy associated with them because the cause of each is not clearly known. Although extensive literature exists about diagnosis and treatment, few randomized, controlled studies have been done (ICSI, 2008b).

Fibromyalgia and myofascial pain syndrome both result in sore, stiff, aching, painful muscles and soft tissues. Both also share symptoms including fatigue, poor sleep, depression, headaches, and irritable bowel syndrome. Most patients with these disorders function satisfactorily in their activities of daily living (ADLs) despite chronic pain, but some report pain-related disability.

The American College of Rheumatology Criteria for classification of fibromyalgia (one of the most common pain clinic diagnoses) includes the following:

- Widespread pain (trunk and upper/lower extremities)
- Pain in at least 11 of 18 specific tender spots
- Pain present for at least 3 months
- Other symptoms that are chronic but not diagnostic including insomnia, depression, stress, fatigue and irritable bowel syndrome (ICSI, 2008b)

Neuropathic Pain

Neuropathic pain is the result of trauma or disease of the peripheral nerves. The pain is often paroxysmal, tingling, burning, or shooting. It can be evoked by movement, and there may be hypersensitivity in the part of the body innervated by that peripheral nerve. The pathophysiology is complex. Injured nerves can become hyperexcitable and generate ectopic discharges, with spontaneous firing at low thresholds for stimuli. The source of the hyperexcitability may be increased sodium ion channels at the sites of nerve injury and demyelination. Alterations in the structure of the nerve, which is possible after injury, may produce changes in the brain and spinal cord in the pain pathways. A variety of conditions fall into this category.

Neuralgias are painful conditions that result from an infection or disease that damages a peripheral nerve. Postherpetic neuralgia ("shingles") is an example. Recently, the IASP has grouped the terms *causalgia* and *reflex sympathetic dystrophy* under the term *complex regional pain syndrome (CRPS)*, a chronic neurological disease affecting one or more extremities. Subclassifications include CRPS-I, previously called *reflex sympathetic dystrophy,* and CRPS-II, previously called *causalgia.* CRPS-II has the same clinical features as CRPS-I, except for the presence of clinical signs and history consistent with a nerve injury. The pathophysiology of CRPS is not entirely clear. Current theories involve both peripheral and central sites of involvement. Preclinical models of neuropathic and inflammatory pain show up-regulation of alpha-adrenergic receptors, adrenergic receptor super-sensitivity, and functional coupling between sympathetic efferent and sensory afferent fibers (Schurmann, Gradl, Andress, Furst, & Schildberg, 1999). Sympathetically maintained pain (SMP) and sympathetically independent pain (SIP) are components of CRPS-I and II. SMP is defined as that aspect of pain that is maintained by the SNS activity, including circulating catecholamines. Blockade of the efferent sympathetic nerve (sympathetic nerve block) for that extremity, which results in pain relief, is diagnostic of SMP. This is often seen in CRPS-I. Defining the SMP and SIP components of the overall pain in any given patient will affect the treatment plan. CRPS-I is usually preceded by trauma or surgery and is often associated with prolonged immobilization, such as a cast. The event may have occurred several weeks or months prior to onset of symptoms. The patient presents with a triad of sensory, autonomic, and motor signs and symptoms in an extremity. Telltale signs of CRPS-I are the following:

- Deep, aching, cold, burning pain
- Allodynia
- Hyperpathia—duration of pain response is prolonged
- Swelling of extremity without definable cause
- Abnormal hair or nail growth
- Shiny skin, intermittent rubor/blotching/cyanosis
- Abnormal skin temperature
- Abnormal sweating
- Weakness, dystonia, contractures

When suspecting CRPS, the provider should refer the patient promptly to an interventional pain specialist for definitive diagnostic evaluation and treatment. Early recognition and aggressive treatment with sympathetic nerve blocks can greatly improve outcomes.

Hyperesthesias are characterized by increased sensitivity and decreased pain threshold to tactile and painful stimuli. As with CRPS, normally nonnoxious stimuli may produce pain. The pain is usually diffuse and modified by fatigue and emotion.

Phantom limb pain is the result of stimulation of the neuronal pathway from the amputated limb at any point along its pathway. Action potentials are propagated toward the CNS, where integration results in the perception of pain from the receptors in the amputated limb. This type of pain may be influenced by emotions and sympathetic stimulation and may be associated with trigger points.

Psychogenic Pain

Psychogenic pain is related to a psychological disorder. Pain that is purely psychogenic, such as "conversion reaction" is rare. Psychogenic pain is often a component of the overall pain experience. For example, 76 percent of patients with major depressive disorder (MDD) report pain (Fava, 2002). The patient with MDD reports levels of pain and disability out of proportion to what most people with a similar disorder experience. For many years, the mind–body connection has been hypothesized. 5-HT and NE are involved in the pathophysiology of depression. These neurotransmitters also modulate pain sensitivity via the descending pain pathway.

Pharmacodynamics

In addition to **NSAIDs** and **opiates**, patients with chronic neuropathic pain may require **SNRIs**, **TCAs**, or **anticonvulsants** to effectively treat their pain. **NSAIDs** and **opiates** have been previously discussed. **Opiates** have a role in chronic pain, but high doses may be necessary because of receptor up-regulation and ineffective cellular membrane transport of these drugs in chronic pain.

NE from the rostral pons and 5-HT from the periaqueductal gray matter (PAG) inhibit pain transmission in the medulla and pons and activate the efferent pain pathways that modulate pain. **SNRIs** and **TCAs** increase both NE and 5-HT at these synapses.

Anticonvulsants are helpful because they prevent the "wind-up" phenomenon common to central sensitization found in chronic pain. Their action is to reduce the hyperexcitability of medullary and spinal neurons arising from persistent stimulation of injured peripheral nerves.

Goals of Treatment

The goal of treatment for all patients with pain is elimination of the pain. With chronic pain, this is often not possible. An acceptable goal for treatment in chronic pain is the reduction of pain to a level that the patient finds tolerable with a minimum of medication side effects. A patient-centered, multifactorial, and comprehensive approach to chronic pain that includes biopsychosocial factors is necessary. Spiritual and cultural factors should also be addressed. Goals should be (1) negotiated between the patient and the provider, (2) specific, and (3) measurable. Goals should be tied to physical and psychological function.

Model Guidelines for Treatment of the Patient With Chronic Nonmalignant Pain

Health-care providers must decide at what point to manage pain using an acute or a chronic model. Sometimes, the diagnosis is sufficient to justify medicating the patient using a chronic pain model. Often, it is not. Factors to consider when making the decision include the following: (1) duration—usually over 6 months, (2) whether the amount of short-acting medication required exceeds the provider's level of comfort, (3) whether the amount of **acetaminophen** in the short-acting medication exceeds the recommended daily dose, and (4) failure of current therapy to eradicate pain and disability. Some states require that the provider secure a second opinion before prescribing **opiates** for the management of chronic nonmalignant pain.

Review the Patient's History

Review of the patient's history related to chronic pain includes the medical aspects of the chief complaint, history of the present illness, and past and current treatments. A pain diagram may be helpful. Note the patient's affect during the history-taking process. Elicit the physical, psychological, social, vocational, and lifestyle changes that have occurred as the result of chronic and persistent pain. Baseline functional ability assessment can provide objectively verifiable data about quality of life and ability to participate in normal life activities. A preliminary sleep history should be gathered.

In addition to the data mentioned in Table 53–2 related to acute pain, it is also important to assess the progression of the problem (e.g., from localized pain to generalized pain) and the addition of related problems (e.g., depression, insomnia). Chronic pain frequently involves the musculoskeletal and nervous systems and these systems should be examined more carefully with attention to possible sources of pain relative to the patient history.

Chemical dependency assessment is integral to the initial assessment of the patient with chronic pain because the drugs used to treat chronic pain are mostly controlled substances. The DAST-20 and CAGE-AID questions discussed in the Chemical Dependency section later in this chapter are useful for this purpose. State medical and nursing boards, professional associations, and the federal government all currently recognize the need for assessment of risk of chemical dependency and substance abuse prior to prescribing **opiates**. A urine toxicology screen should also be gathered prior to writing the initial prescription. The NIDA-5 (National Institute on Drug Abuse) is the most commonly used basic urine drug test that screens for five common drug classes: **cannabinoids**, **cocaine**, **amphetamines**, **opioids**, and **phencyclidine**. This test does not screen many other drugs of abuse (**barbiturates**, **benzodiazepines**, **hydrocodone**, **methadone**, **oxycodone**, **propoxyphene**, and other synthetic drugs). If these latter drugs are suspected, an expanded drug screen can be ordered (Washington State Agency Medical Director's Group, 2007). Combined with risk assessment, drug screening helps to identify the patient at risk for abuse. Results can influence psychological evaluation and

CLINICAL PEARL

Three simple questions can clue you in to sleep apnea, a common problem among patients who experience chronic pain. (1) Do you experience excessive daytime sleepiness? (2) Do you snore? (3) Do you experience nonrestorative sleep (e.g., tired on awakening)? A "yes" response to any of these questions should trigger an evaluation for sleep apnea. Also, obesity is nearly always suggestive for sleep apnea. Treating sleep apnea often reduces pain levels.

treatment. Periodic urine toxicology screens reflect the provider's attention to adherence issues.

Develop a Treatment Plan

A written plan using the biopsychosocial model is essential for ensuring a comprehensive approach to treatment of the patient with chronic pain. The treatment plan, negotiated with the patient's active participation, is tailored to assist the patient in five major areas (ICSI, 2008b):

- Setting personal goals
- Improving sleep
- Increasing physical activity
- Managing stress
- Decreasing pain

This plan should include multidisciplinary therapies, made up of but not limited to physical therapy, psychological assessment and therapy, and drug therapy. ICSI (2008b) recommends that all patients with chronic pain participate in an exercise program to improve function and fitness. Integration of alternative therapies, chiropractic, and massage may also be appropriate. Interventional therapies are not discussed in this chapter, as they are in the realm of the specialty pain clinic.

Obtain Informed Consent

Informed consent should be obtained prior to the onset of **opiate** therapy (at the minimum) and should be documented in the medical record (ICSI, 2008b). The Materials Risk Sheet (Fig. 53–5) serves as informed consent to use controlled substances for the treatment of pain. The Pain Management Contract (Fig. 53–6), a separate document, lays out the ground rules regarding collection of urine

This will confirm that you (name of patient), have been diagnosed with (specify diagnosis), a condition causing you intractable pain. I have recommended treating your condition with the following controlled substances:

____

Your goals of therapy are:

1. ____

2. ____

Alternatives and adjuncts to this therapy are: (e.g., physical or psychological therapy)

1. ____

2. ____

NOTICE OF RISK: Use of controlled substances is associated with certain risks such as:

1. CNS: sleepiness, decreased mental ability, and confusion. Avoid alcohol while taking these medications and use care when driving and operating machinery.
   Your ability to make decisions may be impaired.
2. RESPIRATORY: Depression (slowing) of breathing and possible bronchospasm (wheezing), causing difficulty in catching your breath or shortness of breath.
3. GASTROINTESTINAL: Nausea, vomiting, and constipation that can be severe.
4. DERMATOLOGICAL: Itching and rash
5. URINARY: Urinary retention (difficulty urinating)
6. DRUG INTERACTIONS: Possible interaction with or altering the effect of drugs.
7. TOLERANCE: Increasing doses of the drug may be needed over time to achieve the same effect.
8. PHYSICAL DEPENDENCE AND WITHDRAWAL: Physical dependence develops within 3–4 weeks in most patients receiving daily doses of these drugs. If your medications are abruptly stopped, symptoms of withdrawal (nausea, vomiting, sweating, flu-like symptoms, abdominal cramps, abnormal heart beats, and increased blood pressure) may occur. All controlled substances need to be slowly tapered off under the direct supervision of your health-care provider.
9. ADDICTION: Addiction is abnormal behavior directed towards acquiring or using drugs in a non-medically supervised manner. Patients with a history of alcohol and/or drug abuse are at increased risk for developing addiction. Tolerance and physical dependence are normal for the medications that have been prescribed for you. These are not addiction.
10. POTENTIAL ALLERGIC REACTIONS: Allergic reactions are possible with any medication.

*Most side effects are transient and can be controlled by continued therapy or the use of other medications.
I have read and understand this document. This document represents my informed consent to use these controlled substances for the treatment and management of my intractable pain.

____

Patient Signature Date

____

Provider Signature Date

Figure 53–5. Material risk notification for controlled substances used to treat intractable pain.

I, (patient's name), agree to the following conditions. If I deviate from these conditions, I understand that I jeopardize my medical relationship with this clinic, and that future services at (clinic name) may be terminated.

1. I will obtain prescriptions for controlled substances ONLY from (provider name) ____________________
2. Refills are to be requested ONLY during normal business hours, allowing 48 hours completion.
3. I will not obtain controlled substance prescriptions from any other provider, without prior consent from this clinic.
4. I will fill prescriptions at only one pharmacy: Name of pharmacy: ____________________

   Phone of pharmacy: ____________________
5. I will take the medication for the treatment of intractable pain ONLY as prescribed. I will not increase the use of these medications without prior discussion of such changes with the above-named provider.
6. I agree to submit urine for screening to assess adherence at any time.
7. I will meet regularly, as requested, with the above-named provider. I understand that I will not receive refills of controlled substances unless I attend these regular appointments.
8. I will not make multiple telephone calls for non-urgent requests.
9. I will not exhibit hostile, aggressive behavior towards the provider and staff.
10. I will not ingest recreational drugs, including, but not restricted to, alcohol, marijuana, and other illegal substances, while under the care of the providers in this clinic.

GOALS OF THERAPY: (patient is to list functional goals, such as return to work, resume exercise, improved relationships with friends and family, manageable pain. A goal of ZERO pain is a red flag.)

____

____

____

Signed ____________________ Date ____________________

Witness ____________________

Figure 53–6. Pain management contract.

samples, refills, and other issues that frequently arise during the course of treatment. Goals of therapy are written in the contract. These goals are referred to periodically when evaluating response to treatment.

Periodic Evaluation of the Patient

Routine, often monthly, office visits provide for evaluation of pain levels as well as progress toward functional goals. Adverse effects and adherence to drug therapy are routinely evaluated in every patient. Systematic documentation of these four domains (pain relief, patient functioning, adverse effects, and aberrant behaviors and measures taken to correct them) provides a framework for managing these patients. The Pain Assessment and Documentation Tool (PADT), developed by Passik and colleagues (2004), is useful to guide evaluation of outcomes of therapy to manage chronic pain. This tool is a comprehensive, yet concise, framework for documenting the information that legal and regulatory bodies seek. Using this tool can reduce the provider's reluctance to manage chronic pain (Table 53–4).

The Visual Analog Scale (VAS) is considered the fifth vital sign. The pain domain of the PADT elaborates on this scale, providing additional insight into patterns of pain and function. Documentation of activity relates to goals of therapy, which are clear and measurable. The importance of asking about side effects, especially constipation and sedation, cannot be overstated, as many of the adverse events related to opiate therapy can be life threatening. Aberrant behavior includes overt addictive behaviors listed in the PADT, as well as missed appointments, frequent phone calls, refusal to submit urine for screening, urine containing illegal substances or controlled substances not prescribed, or an "empty" urine that does not contain the medication prescribed. Reports of injury, loss of employment, motor vehicle accidents, divorce, and otherwise chaotic events in the patient's life are not overtly aberrant behavior, but should serve as red flags, alerting the provider to real or potential problems with opiate therapy.

Refer for Additional Evaluation and Treatment as Needed

A multidisciplinary approach should be considered during ongoing therapy. Pain is not static. Drug therapy alone may fail to reduce pain levels and improve function. Failure of therapy can occur for many reasons, including the

Table 53–4 The Four A's of Documenting for Chronic Pain

ANALGESIA	Visual analogue scale (1–10)
ACTIVITY	Function related to goals of therapy
ADVERSE EFFECTS	Medication side effects
ABERRANT BEHAVIOR	Noncompliance, behavioral problems

Source: Printed with permission of Steve Passik, PhD.

following: (1) progression of disease, (2) new disease, and (3) the development of drug tolerance. Other valid reasons to refer the patient include the following: (1) nonadherence, (2) second opinion required by state law or other regulatory body, and (3) the provider's own comfort level in managing the patient. As mentioned in the Acute Pain section, when the pain is not proportional to the diagnosis or the progression of the disease, reevaluation for another possible cause of the pain is important.

Accurate and Complete Documentation

Keep accurate and complete records of all contacts with the patient. Although this is important for all patients, it is especially important should the patient's chart come under review by regulatory bodies. The review process may be initiated by many parties, including a dissatisfied patient, a family member, a concerned pharmacist, or an insurance company.

State and Federal Controlled Substance Laws and Regulations

The provider must be familiar with the laws and regulations in his or her treatment area. The treatment model outlined previously is the law in many states. Following is a brief comment related to medical marijuana, a situation in which conflicting state and federal laws have huge implications.

Realize that federal law trumps state law in terms of **medical marijuana.** Many states have laws that allow the prescribing of **marijuana** for well-defined medical conditions. The DEA currently does not support the concept of **medical marijuana.** Concurrent ingestion of **marijuana** with other controlled substances may be legal in some states for the treatment of malignant (cancer) pain, but not legal for the treatment of nonmalignant pain. The decision to treat a chronic pain condition with **marijuana** as monotherapy, or in combination with other controlled substances, is not discussed in this book. The provider must be familiar with the pharmacology of **marijuana,** as well as the laws and regulations in her or his treatment area when considering using this substance to manage chronic pain.

Rational Drug Selection

Algorithm

Figure 53–7 depicts the algorithm for management of chronic pain. Unlike acute pain, a multidisciplinary approach is often needed when treating chronic pain, and this approach is presented in the algorithm.

Lifestyle Modifications

Acute pain rarely requires lifestyle modifications, at least not for any length of time. Chronic pain frequently requires them. The following modifications should be addressed in the overall treatment plan:

- **Weight loss.** Achieving ideal body weight may not be realistic, but even small amounts of weight loss in patients who are overweight can be helpful—especially if the pain has a component that involves stress on joints and muscles.
- **Increased aerobic activity.** Chronic pain often results in limitations of activity. Being able to engage in even limited amounts of activity improves both the physical condition of the patient through decreasing the hazards of reduced mobility and the depression that commonly accompanies chronic pain. Increased activity also improves sleep. A graded, gradually progressive exercise program should focus on endurance activity such as walking, strengthening such as resistance training, balancing activities, and flexibility.

Cognitive-Behavioral Strategies

ICSI (2008b) recommends several cognitive-behavioral strategies that can be used by the primary care provider and do not require a specialist to implement. These are outlined below:

- Chronic pain is a complicated problem requiring a team approach. The patient should expect help from a variety of providers to deal with sleep, mood, levels of strength and fitness, ability to work, family relationships, and many other aspects of the person's life.
- The patient should understand that the provider believes the pain is *real* and not imagined.
- The patient should be encouraged to take an active role in the management of his or her pain.
- The provider should avoid telling patient to "let pain be your guide," whether it is stopping activity because of pain or taking drugs or rest in response to pain.
- The provider should prescribe time-contingent pain medications rather than prn, and dissociate the pain drug from the pain behavior. The powerfully reinforcing properties of pain-relieving drugs are not then contingent on high levels of pain.
- The provider should schedule return visits on a regular schedule and not allow the appointment to be driven by increasing levels of pain.
- The provider should reinforce wellness behaviors, especially exercise programs.
- The provider should enlist the help of family and other supports to reinforce gains made toward improved functioning.

Drug Therapy

Nonneuropathic chronic pain may be treated with **anti-inflammatory/analgesics** when there is an inflammatory component and the pain is mild to moderate. They are usually the first-line drug choice. GI bleeding risk and renal function should be assessed when choosing **aspirin** or **NSAIDs. Ketorolac** should *not* be used for longer than 5 days, and is, therefore, not appropriate in the treatment of chronic pain. It is important to remember the increased risk for bleeding and the reduced

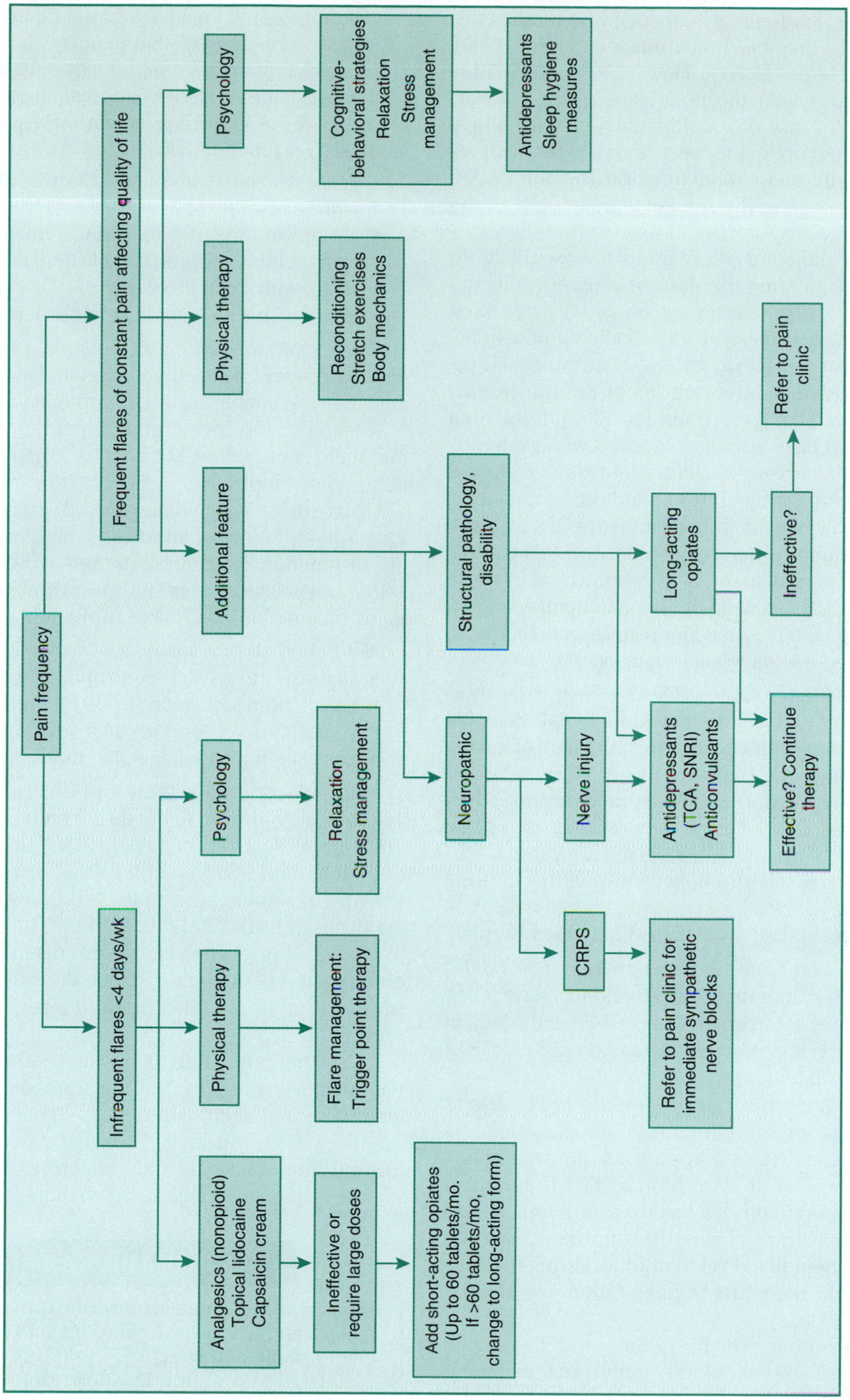

Figure 53–7. Chronic pain management algorithm.

renal function in older adults. **Indomethacin (Indocin)** and **piroxicam (Feldene)** are especially high risk in this population, and they also have unacceptable CNS adverse effects (Herr et al, 2006; Howard et al, 2004). They are rarely appropriate in this population. Chronic **NSAID** use increases the risk of renal insufficiency for all patients, but especially for those with diabetes. Patients should be monitored for renal function. The only **COX-2 inhibitor** currently on the market is **celecoxib (Celebrex)**. It is especially effective in treating musculoskeletal and skeletal pain and is very useful in doses of 200 to 400 mg/day for treating the pain of osteoarthritis and rheumatoid arthritis (Garner et al, 2002). **Naproxen sodium** 1 g/day also showed statistically significant improvements over placebo in a 12-week study of 1,061 patients with moderate osteoarthritis of the hip (Kaiser Permanente Medical Care Program, 2004). **Ibuprofen** and **ketoprofen** have also been studied, with similar results. **Celecoxib** carries a warning about cardiac disease and requires monitoring in this area. Studies of patients with chronic low back pain had similar results with **salicylates**. **Acetaminophen** may be used in this population, but it is important to monitor liver function because long-term use is associated with hepatic damage.

Opiates should be reserved for patients with moderate to severe pain in the following instances:

- Clinical evidence suggests they are likely to be effective in pain that is not relieved by initial therapies. They are rarely beneficial in the treatment of inflammatory pain.
- They have an equal or better therapeutic index than alternatives.
- The medical risk of their use is relatively low.
- The patient is likely to behave responsibly in using the drug.
- **Opiate** therapy is part of the overall treatment plan.

The Washington State Interagency guideline (2007) states that conservative measures should first have failed and **opiates** have not been tried and/or when the patient has demonstrated improvement in function and pain level in a previous **opiate** trial.

Opiates do not appear to be superior to **NSAIDs** as first-line drugs for mild to moderate chronic non-neuropathic pain. They are appropriate as second-line therapy (Caldwell et al, 2002; ICSI, 2008b). If the initial **opiate** tried is ineffective, a trial of a different **opiate** is appropriate. Failure of one drug in this class does not predict patient response to another owing to differences in **opioid** receptors (Quang-Cantagrel, Wallace, & Magnuson, 2000).

Adverse reactions will be common at the higher doses required. Doses should be titrated so that there is a balance between pain control and acceptable adverse reactions. Patients usually experience tachyphylaxis to most adverse responses over time owing to tolerance, but constipation usually persists. Patients should be treated prophylactically with a stimulant laxative and a stool softener. Bulk laxatives should be avoided.

Some evidence exists that indicates both long-acting and short-acting **opiates** are equally effective in chronic pain management. However, long-acting formulations are best for the following patients (Kaiser Permanente Medical Care Program, 2004):

- Those who need around-the-clock coverage because pain lasts at least 12 hours of each day
- Those with difficulty following a treatment regimen with multiple daily dosing of short-acting agents
- Those with sleep problems
- Those with a history of chemical dependency

For those on long-acting formulation, a short-acting formulation should be used until the analgesia is stabilized and made available for breakthrough pain. Dosing for older adults for breakthrough pain is discussed in the Acute Pain section. Long-acting formulations are not appropriate for prn use.

Opiate therapy should be tapered when the drug is no longer contributing to improved pain control, quality of life, or function. Tapering drug therapy helps to prevent withdrawal-related adverse responses. The following tapering is recommended (Kaiser Permanente Medical Care program, 2004):

- Decrease dose by 10 percent each week.
- Switch from long-acting to short-acting formulations.
- Give only a 7-day supply at any one time.
- Use scheduled dosing rather than prn.

Many drugs other than **opiates** also display a withdrawal syndrome. Acute discontinuation of **anticonvulsant medications** can result in seizure. SNRI discontinuation can include confusion and agitation, for example, serotonin syndrome. Withdrawal from moderate doses of **butalbital** formulations (often used in the treatment of migraine) can result in seizure. Acute discontinuation of moderate to high daily doses of **carisoprodol (Soma)** can also result in a severe withdrawal syndrome.

Of special note is the use is **methadone** in chronic pain management. This drug has unpredictable pharmacokinetics and accumulates with repeated doses, often requiring a decrease in dosage size and frequency. Consultation with a pain management specialist is recommended when initiating therapy with methadone.

CLINICAL PEARL

When tapering **opiates,** prescribe drugs to manage nausea and withdrawal symptoms. **Promethazine** is affordable and effective. **Clonidine** 0.1 mg 1 to 2 tablets bid prn, or a **low-dose clonidine** patch, will eliminate most of the agitation and sensations of "skin crawling" that often accompany opiate withdrawal.

Neuropathic chronic pain is often resistance to standard **opioid** therapy (ICSI, 2008b) and is best treated with a **secondary amine tricyclic antidepressant (nortriptyline, desipramine), a selective serotonin or norepinephrine reuptake inhibitor (SSNRI) (duloxetine, venlafaxine)**, or a **calcium channel alpha$_2$ delta ligand (anticonvulsants) (gabapentin or pregabalin)**. For patients with localized peripheral neuropathic pain, topical **lidocaine** can be used alone or in combination with one of the other first line therapies. (Dworkin et al, 2007). Their mechanisms of action are discussed previously.

TCAs are first-line therapy for neuropathic pain and have shown promise with central pain as well. They are typically inexpensive and usually administered once daily. **Secondary amines (nortriptyline [Aventyl, Pamelor], desipramine [Norpramin])** are preferred for diabetic neuropathy and postherpetic neuralgia. Alleviation of pain is usually accomplished at much lower doses than are required for depression. Starting doses should be low and titrated upward slowly until pain is adequately controlled or adverse effects limit continued titration (Dworkin et al, 2007). Pain reduction usually occurs within 2 weeks, but up to 6 weeks may be needed for full effects. Because these drugs affect different receptors in different ways, if the initial drug is ineffective or does not relieve pain sufficiently, trial with a different TCA is recommended. **Tertiary amines (amitriptyline [Elavil, Endep], doxepin [Sinequan, Zonalon], imipramine [Tofranil])** may also be used, but they are less well tolerated than are the **secondary amines. Amitriptyline** should be avoided in older adults because of its higher incidence of **anticholinergic** effects, including the risk for orthostatic hypotension. They have also been associated with exacerbation of cognitive impairment and gait disturbances in older adults, which may predispose them to falls. **TCAs** should also be avoided in patients who have ischemic heart disease or an increased risk of sudden cardiac death. A screening electrocardiogram (ECG) is recommended before beginning treatment with these drugs in patients over 40 years of age (Dworkin et al, 2007). Additional information on these drugs is found in Chapter 15.

Among the **SNRIs, duloxetine (Cymbalta)** is indicated for management of diabetic peripheral neuropathies. It has not been studied in other types of neuropathic pain (Dworkin et al, 2007). It has a generally favorable adverse effects profile and dosing is simple. Dosage for this indication is initiated at 30 mg given once daily and titrated up to 60 mg/day given once daily. There is no evidence that lower doses are effective or that higher doses confer any additional benefit. Pain relief usually occurs within 1 week.

Venlafaxine inhibits serotonin reuptake at lower doses and both serotonin and norepinephrine reuptake at higher doses. Randomized clinical trials in patients with painful diabetic peripheral neuropathies (DPN) and painful polyneuropathies of various types demonstrated efficacy at doses of 150 to 225 mg/day. Trials with other neuropathic pain entities did not show consistent results or showed negative results. Effectiveness for treatment of depression in pediatric patients has not been established (http://www.fda.gov) and it has not been studied in chronic pain in children. This drug is available in both short- and long-acting formulations. Pain relief usually occurs in 2 to 4 weeks because it takes this long to titrate an effective dose. Patients should be tapered gradually from **venlafaxine** due to a risk of discontinuation syndrome. Further discussion is found in Chapter 15.

Calcium channel alpha$_2$-delta ligands (anticonvulsants) have also been shown to be effective in treating neuropathic pain (Dworkin et al, 2007). **Gabapentin (Neurontin)** is generally safe, has no clinically important drug interactions, and is available in generic formulations. It is also first-line therapy. It has demonstrated efficacy in the treatment of neuropathies (Sindrup & Jensen, 2000; ICSI, 2008b). The ones most responsive to this drug are diabetic neuropathies and postherpetic neuralgia. Several weeks can be required to reach an effective dose, which is usually between 1,800 and 3,600 mg/day administered in three divided doses, with the nighttime dose being the largest of the three. Dosage reduction is required for renal insufficiency and exacerbation of cognitive, and gait impairment has been shown in the older adult (Dworkin et al, 2007). It is not the best choice in this population. Safety and effectiveness in the treatment of seizures have been demonstrated in children as young as 3 years of age. There are no trials on its use in chronic pain in children. **Gabapentin** has shown greater efficacy than **TCAs** in some studies of postherpetic neuralgia.

Pregabalin produces dose-dependent adverse effects similar to **gabapentin**. It has demonstrated anxiolytic effects in trial involving patients with generalized anxiety disorder, so it may provide an added benefit in patient with chronic pain. It also required dosage reduction in patients with renal impairment. Treatment is initiated at 150 mg/day in two or three divided doses, although some providers have used 75 mg/day at bedtime to reduce the chance of adverse effects, especially in older adults. Maximum benefit occurs in 1 to 2 weeks with dosages of 300 to 600 mg/day (Dworkin et al, 2007). In a randomized, double-blind placebo-controlled trial, **pregabalin** at 300-mg, 450-mg, and 600-mg doses showed significant improvement in pain, in the Fibromyalgia Impact Score and in sleep (Arnold et al, 2008).

Carbamazepine (Tegretol), another **anticonvulsant**, has also been shown to have clinical efficacy in treating some neuropathies (Sindrup & Jensen, 2000). It is best for trigeminal neuralgias and useful in diabetic neuropathy and postherpetic neuralgia. It is generally reserved for third-line therapy. Suresh (2002) recommends **carbamazepam** or **cloanazepam** over other **anticonvulsant** drug choices in treating chronic neuropathic pain in children.

Opiates have a role in the treatment of neuropathic pain; however, studies have shown that high doses are required to achieve adequate pain relief (Rowbotham et al, 2003). At these higher doses, more adverse effects are found. Another study compared **opiates** with **TCAs** (Raja et al, 2002) and found no significant difference between the efficacy of the two classes of drugs. **Opiates** do not have clear evidence to make them more than second-line therapy. They should be reserved for patient who have failed to respond to or cannot tolerate the first-line drugs or for short-term use (Dworkin et al, 2007).

Before initiating treatment with **opiates**, risk factors for abuse should be identified and addressed. These risk factors include active or prior history of drug abuse, major psychiatric pathology, and family history of substance abuse. Dworkin and colleagues (2007) recommend that providers who are without **opioid** experience obtain consultation from appropriate specialists in developing a treatment plan for challenging patients.

The effective **opioid** dose varies widely among patients. Two strategies for achieving the most appropriate dose are recommended by Dworkin and colleagues (2007). **Opioid**-naïve patients can be started on an oral immediate-release drug at a dose equivalent to 10 to 15 mg of **morphine** every 4 hours or on an as-needed basis with conversion to a long-acting drug in a few days when the approximate daily dose has been determined. Treatment can also be initiated with a long-acting **opioid** such as extended-release oral **morphine** or **oxycodone** or transdermal **fentanyl**. Fixed-schedule dosing is preferred for these drugs. Titration continues until pain relief is achieved. Short-acting formulations can also be used as "rescue" treatment for selected patients.

Patient Variables

Age

Neuropathies are not common in the pediatric population, and many of the drugs used to treat neuropathic pain do not have pediatric doses. Consultation with a pediatric specialist is recommended if chronic neuropathic pain occurs and requires treatment. Older adults are more likely to experience adverse reactions to any drug, but the administration of pain medications is safe and effective in this population and should not be omitted. **Opiates** are recommended for older adults only when they cannot tolerate **NSAIDs** or their pain is poorly controlled with **nonopioid analgesics**. Because this population usually has reduced hepatic and renal function, low initial doses and slow titration with frequent assessment of pain management should be the rule. See further discussion of this topic in the Acute Pain section.

Tertiary amines (amitriptyline [Elavil, Endep], doxepin [Sinequan, Zonalon], imipramine [Tofranil]) are generally not used for adults older than 65 years because of their strong sedative, anticholinergic, and orthostatic hypotensive effects in this population.

Caution and increased monitoring are recommended when using any **TCA** in patients with severe heart disease, symptomatic benign prostatic hyperplasia (BPH), neurogenic bladder, dementia, and narrow-angle glaucoma. These conditions are more common in older adults. Once again, the recommendation is "start low and go slow" in titration.

Gabapentin is a good choice for older adults and those taking medications for comorbid conditions because it has fewer drug–drug interactions than do **TCAs**. **Pregabalin** is expensive, but has fewer side effects.

Detailed discussion of **TCAs**, **SNRIs**, and **anticonvulsants** is found in Chapter 15. Specific considerations, besides age, in choosing and using these drugs are provided in that chapter.

Cultural Considerations in Chronic Pain

Culture plays a role in how pain is defined and what treatments will be accepted, whether the pain is acute or chronic. In chronic pain, however, culture takes on a larger role because of the length of time and the variety of treatments that must be applied. It is important that health-care providers interpret the patient's pain-related behaviors in the patient's cultural context instead of on solely non-Hispanic, white biomedical standards or the provider's own culturally specific values.

A shared decision-making process that involves questions about various cultural health-care beliefs and expectations is important in order to attain effective patient–provider communication and understand and create a mutually acceptable treatment plan. Chapter 7 discusses overall cultural influences on pharmacotherapeutics. Some specific suggestions related to pain include the following:

- Use cross-culturally validated assessment tools such as the Brief Pain Inventory.
- Use certified medical interpreters for non-English- and limited-English-speaking patients. Have family members translate only as a last resort. Patients may not wish to share specific information through a family member; family members may "color" the translation based on their own values; and family members may not be clear in their own understanding of the medically based questions.
- Ask patients about the following:
    1. Preferences for treatment that may include integrating complementary and alternative medicine or traditional healers.
    2. Beliefs about or explanations of their pain or the meaning of pain. If they have an external locus of control, they may require more support for self-management. If they have a strong belief in mind–body relationships, they may prefer to integrate physical and behavioral modalities with the drug therapy.
    3. Social context with family, work, and home environment to determine available supports.
- Factors affecting the pain experience that may differ between cultural groups may include the following:

1. Meaning of pain; cultural and religious beliefs regarding pain.
2. Locus of control style.
3. Ethnic group affiliation. Being genetically from a specific race does not always mean subscribing to that culture.
4. Generation. The closer the patient is to initial immigration to the United States, either familial or directly, the more likely there will be cultural differences between the patient and the larger society.
5. Cultural standards of pain expression and treatment modalities.
6. Language spoken. Having a surname of a specific ethnic group does not necessarily mean the patient speaks a specific language.

Chemical Dependency

Chemical dependency is not an absolute contraindication for pain management with either **anti-inflammatories/analgesics** or **opiates.** Although **opiates** carry a high risk for physical tolerance and dependence, as well as having "street value," they are still appropriate for the treatment of severe pain. The health-care provider needs to obtain a thorough history of current and past chemical dependency because of the dangers of cross-tolerance and additive CNS depression. It is also important to keep in mind that the risk exists for misinterpretation of requests for more **opiates** as addiction, when the cause is actually inadequate pain management, tolerance, or physical dependence.

Red flags for addiction or chemical dependency include the following:

- Concurrent abuse of **alcohol** or illicit drugs.
- Multiple dose escalations or other nonadherence to therapy, despite warnings.
- Multiples episodes of prescription loss.
- Repeatedly seeking prescriptions from other clinicians without informing the prescriber or after warnings to desist from such action.
- Evidence of deterioration in the ability to function at work, in the family, or socially that appears related to drug use.
- Repeated resistance to changes in therapy despite adverse physical or psychosocial effects from the drug.
- Selling prescription drugs.
- Stealing or "borrowing" drugs from others.
- Prescription forgery.
- Injecting oral formulations.
- Obtaining prescription drugs from nonmedical sources.

The CAGE-AID questionnaire is an addiction risk tool to determine whether a patient may be suffering from addiction. This tool asks if the patient has ever in the past:

- Felt that you want or need to Cut down on your drinking or drug use?
- Been Annoyed or Angered by others complaining about your drug use?
- Felt Guilty about the consequences of your drinking or drug use?
- Had a drink or taken a drink in the morning (Eye opener) to decrease hangover or withdrawal?
- Adapted your life to Include Drugs?

One positive response suggests caution in prescribing **opiates**; two or more positive responses suggest the need for increased vigilance by the health-care provider prescribing **opiates** (Gardner-Nix, 2003).

The DAST-20 uses a similar set of questions to assess for chemical dependency. They admittedly seem to assume drug abuse and are probably not as appropriate as the CAGE-AID questionnaire for patients in whom chemical dependency is more possible than probable. The following questions are included:

- Have you used drugs other than those required for medical reasons?
- Have you abused prescription drugs?
- Do you abuse more than one drug at a time?
- Can you get through the week without using drugs?
- Are you always able to stop using drugs when you want to?
- Have you had "blackouts" or "flashbacks" as a result of drug use?
- Do you ever feel bad or guilty about your drug use?
- Does your spouse (or parents) ever complain about your involvement with drugs?
- Has your drug abuse ever created problems between you and your spouse or parents?
- Have you ever lost friends because of your use of drugs?
- Have you neglected your family because of your use of drugs?
- Have you ever been in trouble at work because of drug abuse?
- Have you lost a job because of drug abuse?
- Have you gotten into fights when under the influence of drugs?
- Have you ever engaged in illegal activities in order to obtain drugs?
- Have you been arrested for possession of illegal drugs?
- Have you ever experienced withdrawal symptoms when you stopped taking drugs?
- Have you had medical problems as a result of your drug use (e.g., memory loss, hepatitis, convulsions, bleeding)?
- Have you gone to anyone for help for a drug problem?
- Have you been involved in a treatment program specifically related to drug abuse?

The DAST-20 is scored by summing the responses to the questions with each question receiving one point. "No" responses to the fourth and fifth questions indicate drug use problems. For all other questions, a "yes" response indicates drug use problems. A score of 1 to 5 indicates a low-level problem; 6 to 10, a moderate level; 11 to 15, a substantial level; and 16 to 20, a severe level of problems owing to drug abuse (Skinner, 1982).

When chemical dependency is suspected or known, a pain contract may be appropriate. These contracts are discussed in the Model Guidelines for Treatment of the Patient With Chronic Nonmalignant Pain section, earlier in this chapter, and the Monitoring section. **Opiates** have been implicated in suicide or accidental death, particularly in combination with **alcohol.**

Do not use **partial agonists** or **mixed agonist-antagonists** for patients who have a history of chemical dependency or who may be currently using **opiate derivatives.** Patients may undergo physical withdrawal symptoms. **Methadone** is a pure **opiate agonist** that is used to prevent withdrawal symptoms. Nurse practitioners may legally prescribe this drug in many states, but only for chronic pain management.

Monitoring

Monitoring for chronic pain includes the same variables as for acute pain with some additions that may relate to the specific cause of the pain, such as ongoing diagnostic tests for disease process changes. Monitoring requires regular in-office evaluation. Refilling **opiate** prescriptions is a strong motivator for the patient to attend monthly office visits. Ideally, refills are written ONLY at regularly scheduled office visits. Because schedule II **opiate** prescriptions must be handwritten each time, with duplicate or triplicate copies (depending on individual state law), an office visit should be required in order to obtain it. By law, a 30-day supply is the maximum amount of a schedule II **opiate** that can be written at one time. Multiple prescriptions for 30-day supplies of schedule II **opiates** cannot be written on the same date (federal law). Schedules III, IV, and V controlled substances may be refilled by telephone, or with refills written on the prescription, but this is not advisable.

Observation of mood, affect, gait, and speech are strong indicators of response to therapy. Documentation of pain level, side effects, function, and aberrant behavior (the FOUR A's shown in Table 53-4) can be accomplished with a short appointment. Keep track of referrals made to other specialists (e.g., physical therapy and psychological therapy). Patients who are interested in pills only should be considered higher risk.

Physical exams at "refill visits" may be brief if the patient is stable. Frequency of an in-depth physical examination is guided by the severity of disease, concurrent diseases, and changes in condition. If the patient presents with new problems at his or her brief "refill visit," have the patient return for full evaluation at a later appointment if it is safe to do so.

Acute pain can lead to chronic pain. The following acute pain patients are at high risk for developing chronic pain and should be monitored for it:

- Unrelieved severe pain intensity.
- Age over 60 years (moderate risk) or over 80 years (severe risk).
- Self-perceived risk of developing chronic pain.
- Previous history of low back pain.
- Psychological distress, stressful life event, and depression.
- Poor functional status or having a level of disability. Ask the patient to rate how much the pain interferes with daily activities.
- Low level of education.
- Lack of coping skills such as realistic goal setting, pacing, and realistic beliefs about the condition causing the pain.
- Involvement in litigation related to an accident that caused pain.

Pain Contracts

For patients who have a history of chemical dependency or for whom questions arise about possible inappropriate use of pain medications, a pain contract may be useful. Pain contracts are discussed previously, and a sample contract is found in Figure 42–5.

Outcome Evaluation

Outcome evaluation is tied to goals of therapy, balancing pain relief with adverse effects. The outcome of intervention in chronic pain may not be complete pain relief. When pain is at a level that the patient describes as tolerable and the patient has increased functional ability, the goal has been achieved. Use the baseline rating of pain, the negotiated level of pain that the patient states will be acceptable, and the baseline description of functional capacity to evaluate the outcome of treatment.

Chronic pain itself is rarely measurable by objective indicators. Relief must be tied to other measurable, observable outcomes. Physical measures may include being able to walk 30 min/day or getting a good night's sleep. Vocational measures may include the ability to return to work or enjoy a hobby. Social measures include improved relationships with friends and family. Psychological measures include improved coping skills and less depression.

Patient Education

Patients need definitions of terms commonly used in the treatment of pain. Providers also need to know and use these terms correctly. For instance, patients often feel reluctant to take **opiates** for fear of becoming what they perceive as addicted. *Addiction* is the nonmedical use of a drug, overwhelming and compulsive use of the drug, and continued use despite harm. *Physical dependence* is a state characterized by the onset of physical withdrawal symptoms when the drug is precipitously stopped or a specific antagonist is administered. *Tolerance* is the need for increasing dosages over time to achieve the desired effect. It usually develops as a cellular adaptation to continued blockade of nociceptive receptors resulting in up-regulation. *Pseudoaddiction* is defined as a behavioral pattern similar to addiction, but the reason for drug-seeking behavior often arises owing to undertreatment of pain.

Some key messages to give to chronic pain patients include the following:

- I understand you are in pain. It is not all in your head. It is a real condition.
- Your active role in the management of your pain will help improve your quality of life.
- It is important to set realistic treatment goals. We can decrease your pain to improve your everyday functioning.
- There will be better and worse days, but we can work together to help you feel better.
- Chronic pain can affect one's mood, disrupt sleep, interfere with work and relationships, and have a profound effect on other family members. Treatment for chronic pain involves a team approach with a variety of specialists and therapies—not just pain medications.

CHRONIC PAIN MANAGEMENT

PATIENT EDUCATION

Related to the Overall Treatment Plan and Disease Process

- Pathophysiology of pain and its cause (where appropriate), at a level the patient can understand, to explain how the drugs work.
- Role of lifestyle modification in improving prognosis and keeping the number and cost of required drugs and other treatments down.
- Indications for contacting the health-care provider when pain relief is ineffective.
- Need for follow-up visit(s) with the primary care provider.

Specific to the Drug Therapy

- Reasons for taking the drug(s) and the anticipated action of these drug(s) in pain relief.
- Doses and schedules for taking the drug(s), including round-the-clock dosing of drugs.
- Possible adverse reactions and what to do if they occur.
- Coping mechanisms to deal with the complex and costly treatment regimens.

Reasons for Taking the Drug(s)

- Patient education about specific drugs is provided in Chapters 15 and 25. The explanations should be clear about what pain drugs can and cannot do.
- Patients should be made aware that the drug(s) may need to be taken over a long period of time, so interventions to reduce adverse reactions and reporting them when they occur are important.

Drugs as Part of the Total Treatment Regimen

- Role of both pharmacological and nonpharmacological treatments for pain and their interconnection.

Adherence Issues

- The fact that most chronic pain cannot be completely relieved should be addressed.
- Adherence to the drug regimen is important to improving chronic pain.
- Adherence to lifestyle issues is equally important.
- Discussion of ways to remove barriers to adherence should occur.

REFERENCES

Alzheimer's Disease Association. (2005). *Dementia care practice recommendations for assisted living residences and nursing homes.* Retrieved September 12, 2005, from http://www.alz.org

Arnold, L., Russell, J., Diri, E., Duan, W., Young, J., Sharma, U., et al. (2008). A 14-week, randomized, double-blinded, placebo-controlled monotherapy trial of pregabalin in patients with fibromyalgia. *Journal of Pain, 9*(9), 792–805.

Bodfish, J., Harper, V., Deacon, J. M., Deacon, J. R., & Symons, F. (2006). Issues in pain assessment for adults with severe to profound mental retardation. In F. Oberland & F. Symons (Eds.), *Pain in children and adults with developmental disabilities* (pp. 149–172). Baltimore: Brookes.

Breau, L., McGrath, P., Camfield, A., & Finley, G. (2002). Psychometric properties of the Con-communicating Children's Pain Checklist—Revised. *Pain, 99,* 349–357.

Caldwell, J., Rapoport, R., Davis, J., Offenberg, H., Marker, H., & Roth, S. (2002). Efficacy and safety of a once-daily morphine formulation in chronic, moderate-to-severe osteoarthritis pain: Results from a randomized, placebo-controlled, double-blind trial and an open-label extension trial. *Journal of Pain Symptom Management, 23*(4), 278–291.

Dworkin, R., O'Conner, A., Backonja, M., Farrar, J., Finnerup, N., Jensen, T., et al. (2007). Pharmacologic management of neuropathic pain: Evidence-based recommendations. *Pain, 132*(3), 237–251.

Elliott, A., Smith, B., Smith, W., & Chambers, W. (2000). Changes in chronic pain severity over time: The Chronic Pain Grade as a valid measure. *Pain, 88*(3), 303–308.

Fava, M. (2002). Somatic symptoms, depression, and antidepressant treatment. *Journal of Clinical Psychiatry, 63,* 305–307.

Federation of State Medical Boards of the United States. (1998). *Model guidelines for the use of controlled substances for the treatment of pain.* Euless, TX: Federation of State Medical Boards of the United States. Retrieved September 30, 2005, from http://www.fsmb.org "Policy Documents."

Gardner-Nix, J. (2003). Principles of opioid use in chronic noncancer pain. *Canadian Medical Journal, 169*(1), 38–43.

Garner, S., Fidan, D., Frankish, R., Judd, M., Shea, B., & Towheed, T. (2002). Celecoxib for rheumatoid arthritis. *Cochrane Database Systematic Reviews, 2002*(4), CD003831.

Herr, K., Bjoro, K., Steffensmeier, J., & Rakel, B. (2006). Acute pain management in older adults. Iowa City, IA: University of Iowa Gerontological Nursing Interventions Research Center, Research Translation and Dissemination Core. 113 pp. Retrieved October 11, 2009, from http://www/guideline/gov/summary/summary.aspx

Horgas, A., & Yoon, S. (2008). Pain management. In E. Capezuti, D. Zwicker, M. Mezey, & T. Fulmer (Eds.), *Evidence-based geriatric nursing protocols for best practice* (3rd ed., pp. 199–222). New York: Springer.

Howard, M., Dolovich, I., Kaczorowski, J., Sellors, C., & Sellors, J. (2004). Prescribing of potentially inappropriate medications in elderly people. *Family Practice, 21,* 244–247.

Institute for Clinical Systems Improvement (ICSI). (2008a). Assessment and management of acute pain. Bloomington, MN: Institute for Clinical Systems Improvement. 58 pp. Retrieved October 11, 2009, from http://www.guideline/gov/summary/summary.aspx

Institute for Clinical Systems Improvement (ICSI). (2008b). Assessment and management of chronic pain. Bloomington, MN: Institute for Clinical Systems Improvement. 84 pp. Retrieved October 11, 2009, from http://www.guideline/gov/summary/summary.aspx

Kaiser Permanente Medical Care Program. (2004). *Evidence-based guidelines and technical review from chronic pain management in primary care.* Revised May 2004. Portland, OR: Kaiser Permanente's Care Management Institute Chronic Pain Guidelines Group.

McCance, K., & Huether, S. (2006). *Pathophysiology: The biological basis for disease in adults and children* (5th ed.). St. Louis, MO: Mosby.

Passik, S., Kirsh, K., Whitcomb, L., Portenoy, R., Katz, N., Kleinman, L., et al. (2004). A new tool to assess and document pain outcomes in chronic pain patients receiving opioid therapy. *Clinical Therapeutics, 26*(4), 552–561.

Quang-Cantagrel, N., Wallace, M., & Magnuson, S. (2000). Opioid substitution to improve the effectiveness of chronic noncancer pain control: A chart review. *Anesthesia Analogues, 90*(4), 933–937.

Raja, S., Haythornthwaite, J., Pappagallo, M., Clark, M., Travison, T., & Sabeen, A. (2002). Opioids versus antidepressants in postherpetic neuralgia: A randomized, placebo-controlled trial. *Neurology, 59*(7), 1015–1021.

Richeimer, S. (2009). Acute and post operative pain management for children. Retrieved October 22, 2009, from http://www.spineuniverse.com/displayarticle.php/article392.html

Rowbotham, M., Twilling, L., Davies, P., Reisner, L., Taylor, K., & Mohr, D. (2003). Oral opioid therapy for chronic peripheral and central neuropathic pain. *New England Journal of Medicine, 348*(13), 1223–1232.

Schurmann M., Gradl, G., Andress, J., II, Furst, I., & Schildberg, F. (1999). Assessment of peripheral sympathetic nervous system function in diagnosing early post-traumatic complex regional pain syndrome type I. *Pain, 80,* 149–159.

Sindrup, S., & Jensen, T. (2000). Pharmacologic treatment of pain in polyneuropathy. *Neurology, 55*(7), 915–920.

Skinner, H. (1982). The drug abuse screening text. *Addictive Behavior, 7*(4), 363–371.

Suresh, S. (2002). Chronic pain management in children and adolescents. *The Children's Doctor: Journal of Children's Memorial Hospital, Chicago.* Retrieved October 22, 2009, from http://www.childsdoc.org/spring2002/chronic pain.asp

Washington State Agency Medical Director's Group. (2007). Interagency guideline on opioid dosing for chronic non-cancer pain: An educational pilot to improve care and safety with opioid treatment. Olympia, WA: Washington State Department of Labor and Industries. 14 pp. Retrieved October 11, 2009, from http://www.guideline.gov/summary/summary.aspx

Wolters Kluwer Health. (2009). *Drug facts and comparisons.* St. Louis, MO: Wolters Kluwer Health.

INDEX

Page numbers followed by "b" indicate boxes; by "f" indicate figures; and by "t" indicate tables.

A

B

C

D

E

H

I

J

K

L

M

N

O

P

Q

R

S

T

Z